SIXTH EDITION

UNDERSTANDING PATHOPHYSIOLOGY

Sue E. Huether, MS, PhD
Professor Emeritus
College of Nursing
University of Utah
Salt Lake City, Utah

Kathryn L. McCance, MS, PhD
Professor Emeritus
College of Nursing
University of Utah
Salt Lake City, Utah

SECTION EDITORS

Valentina L. Brashers, MD
Professor of Nursing and Woodard Clinical Scholar
Attending Physician in Internal Medicine
University of Virginia Health System
Charlottesville, Virginia

Neal S. Rote, PhD
Academic Vice-Chair and Director of Research
Department of Obstetrics and Gynecology
University Hospitals Case Medical Center
William H. Weir, MD, Professor of Reproductive Biology
    and Pathology
Case Western Reserve University School of Medicine
Cleveland, Ohio

ELSEVIER

With more than 1000 illustrations

ELSEVIER

3251 Riverport Lane
St. Louis, Missouri 63043

Library of Congress Cataloging-in-Publication Data
Names: Huether, Sue E., editor. | McCance, Kathryn L., editor.
Title: Understanding pathophysiology / [edited by] Sue E. Huether,
　　Kathryn L. McCance ; section editors, Valentina L. Brashers,
　　Neal S. Rote.
Description: Sixth edition. | St. Louis, Missouri : Elsevier, [2017] |
　　Includes bibliographical references and index.
Identifiers: LCCN 2015037586 | ISBN 9780323354097 (pbk. : alk.
　　paper)
Subjects: | MESH: Pathology—Nurses' Instruction. | Disease—
　　Nurses' Instruction. | Physiology—Nurses' Instruction.
Classification: LCC RB113 | NLM QZ 4 | DDC 616.07—dc23 LC
　　record available at http://lccn.loc.gov/2015037586

Executive Content Strategist: Kellie White
Content Development Manager: Laurie Gower
Senior Content Development Specialist: Karen C. Turner
Publishing Services Manager: Jeffrey Patterson
Senior Project Managers: Jeanne Genz and Tracey Schriefer
Designer: Margaret Reid

**ABOUT
THE COVER**

Microbiome. This colored scanning electron micrograph of *Escherichia coli* bacteria (red rods) was taken from the small intestine of a child. *E. coli* are part of the normal flora or microbiota of the human gut and many normal flora are essential for health. The terms microbiota or microbiome refer to the community of microbes that normally reside on and within the human body. The microbiome also means the full collection of genes of all the microbes in the community. DNA-sequencing tools have helped define the microbiome and they outnumber our own cells by about 10 to 1. These resident microbes are highly skilled and provide crucial functions—they sense what food is present, if pathogens are lurking, and the inflammatory state of the gut. Shifts in the bacterial composition of the gut microbiota have been correlated with intestinal dysfunctions such as inflammatory bowel disease, antibiotic-associated diarrhea and metabolic dysfunction including obesity. Gut microflora have protective, metabolic, growth, and immunologic functions because the microbiota interact with both innate and adaptive immune systems. If the overall interaction is flawed autoimmune or inflammatory diseases may occur. We acquire our microbiomes from the environment at birth. Our microbial profiles change with aging because microbial populations shift with changes in the environment. Credit: STEPHANIE SCHULLER/SCIENCE PHOTO LIBRARY

CONTRIBUTORS

Barbara J. Boss, RN, PHD, CFNP, CANP
Retired Professor of Nursing
University of Mississippi Medical Center
Jackson, Mississippi

Kristen Lee Carroll, MD
Chief of Staff
Medical Staff/Orthopedics
Shriners Hospital for Children
Professor of Orthopedics
University of Utah
Salt Lake City, Utah

Margaret F. Clayton, PhD, APRN
Associate Professor and Assistant Dean for
    the PhD Program
College of Nursing
University of Utah
Salt Lake City, Utah

**Christy L. Crowther-Radulewicz, RN, MS,
CRNP**
Nurse Practitioner
Orthopedic Surgery
Anne Arundel Orthopedic Surgeons
Annapolis, Maryland

**Susanna G. Cunningham, BSN, MA, PhD,
RN, FAHA, FAAN**
Professor Emeritus
Department of Biobehavioral Nursing
School of Nursing
University of Washington
Seattle, Washington

**Sara J. Fidanza, MS, RN, CNS-BC,
CPNP-BC**
Digestive Health Institute
Children's Hospital Colorado
Clinical Faculty
University of Colorado College of Nursing
Aurora, Colorado

Diane P. Genereux, PhD
Assistant Professor
Department of Biology
Westfield State
Westfield, Massachusetts

Todd Cameron Grey, MD
Chief Medical Examiner
Office of the Medical Examiner
State of Utah
Salt Lake City, Utah

Robert E. Jones, MD, FACP, FACE
Professor of Medicine
Endocrinology Division
University of Utah School of Medicine
Salt Lake City, Utah

Lynn B. Jorde, PhD
H.A. and Edna Benning Presidential
    Professor and Chair
Department of Human Genetics
University of Utah School of Medicine
Salt Lake City, Utah

Lynne M. Kerr, MD, PhD
Associate Professor
Department of Pediatrics, Division of
    Pediatric Neurology
University of Utah Medical Center
Salt Lake City, Utah

Nancy E. Kline[†], PhD, RN, CPNP, FAAN
Director, Nursing Research, Medicine
Patient Services/Emergency Department
Boston Children's Hospital
Boston, Massachusetts

Lauri A. Linder, PhD, APRN, CPON
Assistant Professor
College of Nursing
University of Utah
Clinical Nurse Specialist
Cancer Transplant Center
Primary Children's Hospital
Salt Lake City, Utah

Sue Ann McCann, MSN, RN, DNC
Programmatic Nurse Specialist
Nursing
Clinical Research Coordinator
Dermatology
University of Pittsburgh Medical Center
Pittsburgh, Pennsylvania

Nancy L. McDaniel, MD
Associate Professor of Pediatrics
University of Virginia
Charlottesville, Virginia

Afsoon Moktar, PhD, EMBA, CT (ASCP)
Associate Professor
School of Physician Assistant Studies
Massachusetts College of Pharmacy and
    Health Sciences University
Boston, Massachusetts

**Noreen Heer Nicol, PhD, RN, FNP,
NEA-BC**
Associate Professor
College of Nursing
University of Colorado
Denver, Colorado

Nancy Pike, PhD, RN, CPNP-AC, FAAN
Assistant Professor
UCLA School of Nursing
Pediatric Nurse Practitioner
Cardiothoracic Surgery
Children's Hospital Los Angeles
Los Angeles, California

Patricia Ring, RN, MSN, PNP, BC
Pediatric Nephrology
Children's Hospital of Wisconsin
Wauwatosa, Wisconsin

Anna E. Roche, MSN, RN, CPNP, CPON
Pediatric Nurse Practitioner
Dana Farber/Boston Children's Cancer and
    Blood Disorders Center
Boston, Massachusetts

George W. Rodway, PhD, APRN
Associate Clinical Professor
Betty Irene Moore School of Nursing
    at UC Davis
Sacramento, California

**Sharon Sables-Baus, PhD, MPA, RN,
PCNS-BC**
Associate Professor
University of Colorado
College of Nursing and School of Medicine
Department of Pediatrics
Pediatric Nurse Scientist
Children's Hospital Colorado
Aurora, Colorado

Anna Schwartz, PhD, FNP-C, FAAN
Associate Professor
School of Nursing
Northern Arizona University
Flagstaff, Arizona;
Affiliate Associate Professor
Biobehavioral Nursing and Health Systems
University of Washington
Seattle, Washington

---

†Deceased.

Joan Shea, MSN, RN, CPON
Staff Nurse III
Hematology/Oncology/Clinical Research
Boston Children's Hospital
Boston, Massachusetts

Lorey K. Takahashi, PhD
Professor of Psychology
Department of Psychology
University of Hawaii at Manoa
Honolulu, Hawaii

David M. Virshup, MD
Professor and Director
Program in Cancer and Stem Cell Biology
Duke-NUS Graduate Medical School
Singapore;
Professor of Pediatrics
Duke University School of Medicine
Durham, North Carolina

Deborah Cipale, RN, MSN
Nursing Resource Lab Coordinator
Des Moines Area Community College
Ankeny, Iowa

David J. Derrico, RN, MSN
Clinical Assistant Professor
Department of Adult and Elderly Nursing
University of Florida College of Nursing
Gainesville, Florida

Sandra L. Kaminski, MS, PA-C
Adjunct Professor
Physician Assistant Program
Pace University
New York, New York

Stephen D. Krau, PhD, RN, CNE
Associate Professor
Vanderbilt University School of Nursing
Nashville, Tennessee

Lindsay McCrea, PhD, RN, FNP-BC, CWOCN
Professor
Nursing Program Assistant Director
California State University, East Bay
Hayward, California

Afsoon Moktar, PhD, EMBA, CT (ASCP)
Associate Professor
School of Physician Assistant Studies
Massachusetts College of Pharmacy and Health Sciences University
Boston, Massachusetts

Kathleen S. Murtaugh, RN, MSN, CAN
Assistant Professor of Nursing
Saint Joseph College—St. Elizabeth School of Nursing Cooperative
    Program
Rensselaer, Indiana

Judith L. Myers, MSN, RN
Assistant Professor of Nursing
Grand View University
Nursing Department
Des Moines, Iowa

Holldrid Odreman, MScN-Ed, BScN, RN
Professor
Program Coordinator of Nursing
Niagara College Canada
Certified Simulationist
SIMone Ontario Simulation Network
Welland, Ontario, Canada

Jay Schulkin, PhD
Director of Research
The American Congress of Obstetricians and Gynecologists
Washington, DC;
Acting Professor
Obstetrics & Gynecology
University of Washington School of Medicine
Seattle, Washington

Crystal R. Sherman, DNP, RN, APHN-BC
Associate Professor of Nursing
Shawnee State University
Portsmouth, Ohio

Lorey K. Takahashi, PhD
Professor of Psychology
Department of Psychology
University of Hawaii at Manoa
Honolulu, Hawaii

Cheryl A. Tucker, MSN, RN, CNE
Senior Lecturer and Undergraduate Theory Coordinator
Baylor University
Louise Herrington School of Nursing
Dallas, Texas

Linda Turchin, MSN, CNE
Associate Professor of Nursing
Fairmont State University
Fairmont, West Virginia

Jo A. Voss, PhD, RN, CNS
Associate Professor
South Dakota State University
West River Department of Nursing
Rapid City, South Dakota

Kim Webb, MN, RN
Part-time Nursing Instructor
Pioneer Technology Center
Ponca City, Oklahoma

The sixth edition of *Understanding Pathophysiology,* like other editions, has been rigorously updated and revised with consideration of the rapid advances in molecular and cell biology. Many sections have been rewritten or reorganized to provide a foundation for better understanding of the mechanisms of disease. Integrated throughout the text are concepts from the basic sciences, including genetics, epigenetics, gene–environment interaction, immunity, and inflammation. The text has been written to assist students with the translation of the concepts and processes of pathophysiology into clinical practice and to promote lifelong learning.

Although the primary focus of the text is pathophysiology, we continue to include discussions of the following interconnected topics to highlight their importance for clinical practice:

- A life-span approach that includes special sections on aging and separate chapters on children
- Epidemiology and incidence rates showing regional and worldwide differences that reflect the importance of environmental and lifestyle factors on disease initiation and progression
- Sex differences that affect epidemiology and pathophysiology
- Molecular biology—mechanisms of normal cell function and how their alteration leads to disease
- Clinical manifestations, summaries of treatment, and health promotion/risk reduction

ORGANIZATION AND CONTENT: WHAT'S NEW IN THE SIXTH EDITION

The book is organized into two parts: Part One, Basic Concepts of Pathophysiology, and Part Two, Body Systems and Diseases. Two new chapters have been added.

Part One: Basic Concepts of Pathophysiology

Part One introduces basic principles and processes that are important for a contemporary understanding of the pathophysiology of common diseases. The concepts include descriptions of cellular communication; forms of cell injury; genes and genetic disease; epigenetics; fluid and electrolytes and acid and base balance; immunity and inflammation; mechanisms of infection; stress, coping, and illness; and tumor biology. A new chapter, *Epigenetics and Disease* (Chapter 3), has been added since significant progress is emerging that explains the way heritable changes in gene expression—*phenotype* without a change in *genotype*—are influenced by several factors, including age, environment/lifestyle, and disease state.

Significant revisions to Part One also include new or updated information on the following topics:

- Updated content on cell membranes, cell junctions, intercellular communication, transport by vesicles, and stem cells (Chapter 1)
- New chapter on epigenetics and disease (Chapter 3)
- Updated content on cellular adaptations, oxidative stress, chemical injury, types of cell death, and aging (Chapter 4)
- Updates regarding mechanisms of human defense—characteristics of innate and adaptive immunity (Chapters 6 and 7)
- Updated content on mechanisms of infection, antibiotic-resistant disease, and alterations in immune defense (Chapter 8)
- Updated content on stress, inflammation, hormones, and disease (Chapter 9)

- Extensive entire chapter revisions and reorganization of tumor biology (Chapter 10)
- Extensive entire chapter revisions and updated epidemiology of cancer (Chapter 11)

Part Two: Body Systems and Diseases

Part Two presents the pathophysiology of the most common alterations according to body system. To promote readability and comprehension, we have used a logical sequence and uniform approach in presenting the content of the units and chapters. Each unit focuses on a specific organ system and contains chapters related to anatomy and physiology, the pathophysiology of the most common diseases, and common alterations in children. The anatomy and physiology content is presented as a review to enhance the learner's understanding of the structural and functional changes inherent in pathophysiology. A brief summary of normal aging effects is included at the end of these review chapters. The general organization of each disease/disorder discussion includes an introductory paragraph on relevant risk factors and epidemiology, a significant focus on pathophysiology and clinical manifestations, and then a brief review of evaluation and treatment.

The information on reproductive pathophysiology is now presented in two chapters, with a new chapter, *Alterations of the Male Reproductive System.* Other significant revisions to Part Two include new and/or updated information on the following topics:

- Mechanisms of pain transmission, pain syndromes, and categories of sleep disorders (Chapter 14)
- Alterations in levels of consciousness, seizure disorders, and delirium. Pathogenesis of degenerative brain diseases, the dementias, movement disorders, traumatic brain and spinal cord injury, stroke syndromes, headache, and infections and structural malformations of the CNS (Chapters 15, 16, 17)
- The pathogenesis of type 2 diabetes mellitus (Chapter 19)
- Platelet function and coagulation; anemias, alterations of leukocyte function and myeloid and lymphoid tumors (Chapters 20 and 21)
- Extensive chapter revisions of alterations of hematologic function in children (Chapter 22)
- Extensive chapter revisions on structure and function of the cardiovascular and lymphatic systems (Chapter 23)
- Mechanisms of atherosclerosis, hypertension, coronary artery disease, heart failure, and shock (Chapter 24)
- Pediatric valvular disorders, heart failure, hypertension, obesity, and heart disease (Chapter 25)
- Pathophysiology of acute lung injury, asthma, pneumonia, lung cancer, respiratory distress in the newborn, and cystic fibrosis (Chapters 27 and 28)
- Mechanisms of kidney stone formation, immune processes of glomerulonephritis, and acute and chronic kidney injury (Chapters 30 and 31)
- Female and male reproductive disorders, female and male reproductive cancers, breast diseases and mechanisms of breast cancer, prostate cancer, male breast cancer, and sexually transmitted infections (Chapters 33 and 34)
- Gastroesophageal reflux, nonalcoholic liver disease, inflammatory bowel disease, viral hepatitis, obesity, gluten-sensitive enteropathy, and necrotizing enterocolitis (Chapters 36 and 37)
- Bone cells, bone remodeling, joint and tendon diseases, osteoporosis, rheumatoid arthritis, and osteoarthritis (Chapters 38 and 39)

- Congenital and acquired musculoskeletal disorders, and muscular dystrophies in children (Chapter 40)
- Psoriasis, discoid lupus erythematosus, and atopic dermatitis (Chapters 41 and 42)

Cancer of the various organ systems was updated for all of the chapters.

FEATURES TO PROMOTE LEARNING

A number of features are incorporated into this text that guide and support learning and understanding, including:

- *Chapter Outlines* including page numbers for easy reference
- *Quick Check* questions strategically placed throughout each chapter to help readers confirm their understanding of the material; answers are included on the textbook's Evolve website
- *Health Alerts* with concise discussions of the latest research
- *Risk Factors* boxes for selected diseases
- End-of-chapter *Did You Understand?* summaries that condense the major concepts of each chapter into an easy-to-review list format; printable versions of these are available on the textbook's Evolve website
- *Key Terms* set in blue boldface in text and listed, with page numbers, at the end of each chapter
- Special boxes for *Aging* and *Pediatrics* content that highlight discussions of life-span alterations

ART PROGRAM

All of the figures and photographs have been carefully reviewed, revised, or updated. This edition features approximately 100 new or heavily revised illustrations and photographs with a total of approximately 1000 images. The figures are designed to help students visually understand sometimes difficult and complex material. Hundreds of high-quality photographs show clinical manifestations, pathologic specimens, and clinical imaging techniques. Micrographs show normal and abnormal cellular structure. The combination of illustrations, algorithms, photographs, and use of color for tables and boxes allows a more precise understanding of essential information.

TEACHING/LEARNING PACKAGE

For Students

The free electronic **Student Resources** on Evolve include review questions and answers, numerous animations, answers to the Quick Check questions in the book, printable key points, and bonus case studies with questions and answers. A comprehensive *Glossary* for the textbook of more than 600 terms helps students with the often difficult terminology related to pathophysiology; this is available both on Evolve and in the electronic version of the textbook. These electronic resources enhance learning options for students. Go to http://evolve.elsevier.com/Huether.

The newly rewritten **Study Guide** includes many different question types, aiming to help the broad spectrum of student learners. Question types include the following:

- Choose the Correct Words
- Complete These Sentences
- Categorize These Clinical Examples
- Explain the Pictures
- Teach These People about Pathophysiology
- Plus many more…

Answers are found in the back of the **Study Guide** for easy reference for students.

For Instructors

The electronic **Instructor Resources** on Evolve are available free to instructors with qualified adoptions of the textbook and include the following: TEACH Lesson Plans with case studies to assist with clinical application; a Test Bank of more than 1200 items; PowerPoint Presentations for each chapter, with integrated images, audience response questions, and case studies; and an Image Collection of approximately 1000 key figures from the text. All of these teaching resources are also available to instructors on the book's Evolve site. Plus the *Evolve Learning System* provides a comprehensive suite of course communication and organization tools that allow you to upload your class calendar and syllabus, post scores and announcements, and more. Go to http://evolve.elsevier.com/Huether.

The most exciting part of the learning support package is **Pathophysiology Online,** a complete set of online modules that provide thoroughly developed lessons on the most important and difficult topics in pathophysiology supplemented with illustrations, animations, interactive activities, interactive algorithms, self-assessment reviews, and exams. Instructors can use it to enhance traditional classroom lecture courses or for distance and online-only courses. Students can use it as a self-guided study tool.

ACKNOWLEDGMENTS

This book would not be possible without the knowledge and expertise of our contributors, both those who have worked with us through previous editions and the new members of our team. Their reviews and synthesis of the evidence and clear concise presentation of information is a strength of the text. We thank them.

Nancy Kline, PhD, RN was a highly respected colleague, researcher, nurse, and contributor to our textbooks. We dedicate this edition to her memory and the many contributions she made to nursing research, medicine, patient services, and children's health. We will miss her.

The reviewers for this edition provided excellent recommendations for focus of content and revisions. We appreciate their insightful work.

For more than 30 years Sue Meeks has been the rock of our manuscript preparation. She is masterful at managing details of the numerous revisions, maintains the correct formatting, provides helpful recommendations, and manages the complexity and chaos—all with a wonderful sense of humor. We cannot thank her enough.

Tina Brashers, MD, and Neal Rote, PhD, continued to serve as section editors and contributing authors. Tina is a distinguished teacher and has received numerous awards for her teaching and work with nursing and medical students and faculty. She is nationally known for her leadership and development in promoting and teaching interprofessional collaboration. Tina brings innovation and clarity to the subject of pathophysiology. Her contributions to the online course continue to be intensive and creative, and a significant learning enhancement for students. Thank you, Tina, for the outstanding quality of your work. Neal has major expertise, passion, and hard-to-find precision in the topics of immunity, reproductive biology, and human defenses. His expertise was well placed to rewrite and update the challenging tumor biology chapter. Neal has held many appointments, including department chair, associate dean, and professor in both reproductive biology and pathology. He is a top-notch researcher and reviewer of grants and has received numerous awards and recognition for his teaching. Neal has a gift for creating images that bring clarity to the complex content of immunology. He also completely updated the glossary. Thank you, Neal, for your persistence in promoting understanding and for your continuing devotion to students.

Karen Turner was our excellent Senior Content Development Specialist. Always gracious and efficient, Karen guided us through the hardest times and even the redo times. Thank you, Karen, especially for another set of "eagle eyes." Jeanne Genz retired as the Project Manager during the preparation of this edition and we will miss her expertise. Always dedicated and an amazing "can do" attitude, we thank you, Jeanne. Tracey Schriefer picked up the reins without missing a step. Thank you, Tracey, for such diligence—finding and correcting obscure errors. We also thank Beth Welch, who has copyedited our last four editions. Kellie White was our Executive Content Strategist and was responsible for overseeing the entire project. Very organized and a delightful sense of humor, we thank you Kellie. The internal layout, selection of colors, and design of the cover highlight the pedagogy and were done by our Designer, Margaret Reid. Thanks to the team from Graphic World, who created many new images and managed the cleanup and scanning of artwork obtained from many resources.

We thank the Department of Dermatology at the University of Utah School of Medicine, which provided numerous photos of skin lesions. Thank you to our many colleagues and friends at the University of Utah College of Nursing, School of Medicine, Eccles Medical Library, and College of Pharmacy for their helpfulness, suggestions, and critiques.

We extend gratitude to those who contributed to the book supplements. Linda Felver has created an all new inventive and resourceful Study Guide. Thank you, Linda, for your very astute edits. Additional thanks to the reviewers of the Study Guide, Janie Corbitt, Kathleen Murtaugh, and Linda Turchin. A special thanks to Linda Turchin, Joanna Cain, Stephen Krau, and Melanie Cole for their thorough approach in preparing the materials for the Evolve website, and to Linda Turchin, Kim Webb, and Lauren Mussig for the valuable reviews of these resources. Tina Brashers, Nancy Burruss, Mandi Counters, Joe Gordon, Melissa Geist, Kay Gaehle, Stephen Krau, Jason Mott, and Kim Webb also updated the interactive online lessons and activities for *Pathophysiology Online*.

Special thanks to faculty and nursing students and other health science students for your questions and suggestions. It is because of you, the future clinicians, that we are so motivated to put our best efforts into this work.

Sincerely and with great affection we thank our families, especially Mae and John. Always supportive, you make the work possible!

Sue E. Huether
Kathryn L. McCance

INTRODUCTION TO PATHOPHYSIOLOGY

The word root *"patho"* is derived from the Greek word *pathos,* which means suffering. The Greek word root *"logos"* means discourse or, more simply, system of formal study, and *"physio"* refers to functions of an organism. Altogether, pathophysiology is the study of the underlying changes in body physiology (molecular, cellular, and organ systems) that result from disease or injury. Important, however, is the inextricable component of suffering and the psychological, spiritual, social, cultural, and economic implications of disease.

The science of pathophysiology seeks to provide an understanding of the mechanisms of disease and to explain how and why alterations in body structure and function lead to the signs and symptoms of disease. Understanding pathophysiology guides healthcare professionals in the planning, selection, and evaluation of therapies and treatments.

Knowledge of human anatomy and physiology and the interrelationship among the various cells and organ systems of the body is an essential foundation for the study of pathophysiology. Review of this subject matter enhances comprehension of pathophysiologic events and processes. Understanding pathophysiology also entails the utilization of principles, concepts, and basic knowledge from other fields of study including pathology, genetics, epigenetics, immunology, and epidemiology. A number of terms are used to focus the discussion of pathophysiology; they may be used interchangeably at times, but that does not necessarily indicate that they have the same meaning. Those terms are reviewed here for the purpose of clarification.

Pathology is the investigation of structural alterations in cells, tissues, and organs, which can help identify the cause of a particular disease. Pathology differs from pathogenesis, which is the pattern of tissue changes associated with the *development* of disease. Etiology refers to the study of the *cause* of disease. Diseases may be caused by infection, heredity, gene–environment interactions, alterations in immunity, malignancy, malnutrition, degeneration, or trauma. Diseases that have no identifiable cause are termed idiopathic. Diseases that occur as a result of medical treatment are termed iatrogenic (for example, some antibiotics can injure the kidney and cause renal failure). Diseases that are acquired as a consequence of being in a hospital environment are called nosocomial. An infection that develops as a result of a person's immune system being depressed after receiving cancer treatment during a hospital stay would be defined as a nosocomial infection.

Diagnosis is the naming or identification of a disease. A diagnosis is made from an evaluation of the evidence accumulated from the presenting signs and symptoms, health and medical history, physical examination, laboratory tests, and imaging. A prognosis is the expected outcome of a disease. Acute disease is the sudden appearance of signs and symptoms that last only a short time. Chronic disease develops more slowly and the signs and symptoms last for a long time, perhaps for a lifetime. Chronic diseases may have a pattern of remission and exacerbation. Remissions are periods when symptoms disappear or diminish significantly. Exacerbations are periods when the symptoms become worse or more severe. A complication is the onset of a disease in a person who is already coping with another existing disease (for example, a person who has undergone surgery to remove a diseased appendix may develop the complication of a wound infection or pneumonia). Sequelae are unwanted outcomes of having a disease or are the result of trauma, such as paralysis resulting from a stroke or severe scarring resulting from a burn.

Clinical manifestations are the signs and symptoms or *evidence* of disease. Signs are objective alterations that can be observed or measured by another person, measures of bodily functions such as pulse rate, blood pressure, body temperature, or white blood cell count. Some signs are local, such as redness or swelling, and other signs are systemic, such as fever. Symptoms are subjective experiences reported by the person with disease, such as pain, nausea, or shortness of breath; and they vary from person to person. The prodromal period of a disease is the time during which a person experiences vague symptoms such as fatigue or loss of appetite before the onset of specific signs and symptoms. The term insidious symptoms describes vague or nonspecific feelings and an awareness that there is a change within the body. Some diseases have a latent period, a time during which no symptoms are readily apparent in the affected person, but the disease is nevertheless present in the body; an example is the incubation phase of an infection or the early growth phase of a tumor. A syndrome is a group of symptoms that occur together and may be caused by several interrelated problems or a specific disease; severe acute respiratory syndrome (SARS), for example, presents with a set of symptoms that include headache, fever, body aches, an overall feeling of discomfort, and sometimes dry cough and difficulty breathing. A disorder is an abnormality of function; this term also can refer to an illness or a particular problem such as a bleeding disorder.

Epidemiology is the study of tracking patterns or disease occurrence and transmission among populations and by geographic areas. Incidence of a disease is the number of new cases occurring in a specific time period. Prevalence of a disease is the number of existing cases within a population during a specific time period.

Risk factors, also known as predisposing factors, increase the probability that disease will occur, but these factors are not the *cause* of disease. Risk factors include heredity, age, gender, race, environment, and lifestyle. A precipitating factor is a condition or event that *does* cause a pathologic event or disorder. For example, asthma is precipitated by exposure to an allergen, or angina (pain) is precipitated by exertion.

Pathophysiology is an exciting field of study that is ever-changing as new discoveries are made. Understanding pathophysiology empowers healthcare professionals with the knowledge of how and why disease develops and informs their decision making to ensure optimal healthcare outcomes. Embedded in the study of pathophysiology is understanding that suffering is a personal, individual experience and a major component of disease.

CONTENTS

PART TWO Body Systems and Diseases

Unit 4 The Neurologic System

Cellular Biology

Kathryn L. McCance

ⓔ EVOLVE WEBSITE

http://evolve.elsevier.com/Huether/
Student Review Questions
Audio Key Points

Case Studies
Animations
Quick Check Answers

CHAPTER OUTLINE

All body functions depend on the integrity of cells. Therefore an understanding of cellular biology is increasingly necessary to comprehend disease processes. An overwhelming amount of information reveals how cells behave as a multicellular "social" organism. At the heart of it all is cellular communication (cellular "crosstalk")—how messages originate and are transmitted, received, interpreted, and used by the cell. Streamlined conversation between, among, and within cells maintains cellular function and specialization. Cells must demonstrate a "chemical fondness" for other cells to maintain the integrity of the entire organism. When they no longer tolerate this fondness, the conversation breaks down, and cells either adapt (sometimes altering function) or become vulnerable to isolation, injury, or disease.

PROKARYOTES AND EUKARYOTES

Living cells generally are divided into eukaryotes and prokaryotes. The cells of higher animals and plants are eukaryotes, as are the single-celled organisms, fungi, protozoa, and most algae. Prokaryotes include cyanobacteria (blue-green algae), bacteria, and rickettsiae. Prokaryotes traditionally were studied as core subjects of molecular biology. Today, emphasis is on the eukaryotic cell; much of its structure and function have no counterpart in bacterial cells.

Eukaryotes (*eu* = good; *karyon* = nucleus; also spelled eucaryotes) are larger and have more extensive intracellular anatomy and organization than prokaryotes. Eukaryotic cells have a characteristic set of membrane-bound intracellular compartments, called *organelles,* that includes a well-defined nucleus. The prokaryotes contain no organelles, and their nuclear material is not encased by a nuclear membrane. Prokaryotic cells are characterized by lack of a distinct nucleus.

Besides having structural differences, prokaryotic and eukaryotic cells differ in chemical composition and biochemical activity. The *nuclei* of prokaryotic cells carry genetic information in a single circular chromosome, and they lack a class of proteins called *histones,* which in eukaryotic cells bind with deoxyribonucleic acid (DNA) and are involved in the supercoiling of DNA. Eukaryotic cells have several or many chromosomes. Protein production, or synthesis, in the two classes of cells also differs because of major structural differences in ribonucleic acid (RNA)–protein complexes. Other distinctions include differences in mechanisms of transport across the outer cellular membrane and in enzyme content.

CELLULAR FUNCTIONS

Cells become specialized through the process of differentiation, or maturation, so that some cells eventually perform one kind of function and other cells perform other functions. Cells with a highly developed function, such as movement, often lack some other property, such as hormone production, which is more highly developed in other cells.

The eight chief cellular functions are as follows:

1. *Movement.* Muscle cells can generate forces that produce motion. Muscles that are attached to bones produce limb movements, whereas those muscles that enclose hollow tubes or cavities move or empty contents when they contract (e.g., the colon).
2. *Conductivity.* Conduction as a response to a stimulus is manifested by a wave of excitation, an electrical potential that passes along the surface of the cell to reach its other parts. Conductivity is the chief function of nerve cells.
3. *Metabolic absorption.* All cells can take in and use nutrients and other substances from their surroundings.
4. *Secretion.* Certain cells, such as mucous gland cells, can synthesize new substances from substances they absorb and then secrete the new substances to serve as needed elsewhere.
5. *Excretion.* All cells can rid themselves of waste products resulting from the metabolic breakdown of nutrients. Membrane-bound sacs (lysosomes) within cells contain enzymes that break down, or digest, large molecules, turning them into waste products that are released from the cell.
6. *Respiration.* Cells absorb oxygen, which is used to transform nutrients into energy in the form of adenosine triphosphate (ATP). Cellular respiration, or oxidation, occurs in organelles called mitochondria.
7. *Reproduction.* Tissue growth occurs as cells enlarge and reproduce themselves. Even without growth, tissue maintenance requires that new cells be produced to replace cells that are lost normally through cellular death. Not all cells are capable of continuous division (see Chapter 4).
8. *Communication.* Communication is vital for cells to survive as a society of cells. Appropriate communication allows the maintenance of a dynamic steady state.

STRUCTURE AND FUNCTION OF CELLULAR COMPONENTS

Figure 1-1, *A*, shows a "typical" eukaryotic cell, which consists of three components: an outer membrane called the plasma membrane, or plasmalemma; a fluid "filling" called cytoplasm (Figure 1-1, *B*); and the "organs" of the cell—the membrane-bound intracellular organelles, among them the nucleus.

Nucleus

The nucleus, which is surrounded by the cytoplasm and generally is located in the center of the cell, is the largest membrane-bound organelle. Two pliable membranes compose the nuclear envelope (Figure 1-2, *A*). The nuclear envelope is pockmarked with pits, called nuclear pores, which allow chemical messages to exit and enter the nucleus (see Figure 1-2). The outer membrane is continuous with membranes of the endoplasmic reticulum (see Figure 1-1). The nucleus contains the nucleolus (a small dense structure composed largely of ribonucleic acid), most of the cellular DNA, and the DNA-binding proteins (i.e., the histones) that regulate its activity. The DNA "chain" in eukaryotic cells is so long that it is easily broken. Therefore the histones that bind to DNA cause DNA to fold into chromosomes (Figure 1-2, *C*), which decreases the risk of breakage and is essential for cell division in eukaryotes.

The primary functions of the nucleus are cell division and control of genetic information. Other functions include the replication and repair of DNA and the transcription of the information stored in DNA.

Genetic information is transcribed into ribonucleic acid (RNA), which can be processed into messenger, transport, and ribosomal RNAs and introduced into the cytoplasm, where it directs cellular activities. Most of the processing of RNA occurs in the nucleolus. (The roles of DNA and RNA in protein synthesis are discussed in Chapter 2.)

Cytoplasmic Organelles

Cytoplasm is an aqueous solution (cytosol) that fills the cytoplasmic matrix—the space between the nuclear envelope and the plasma membrane. The cytosol represents about half the volume of a eukaryotic cell. It contains thousands of enzymes involved in intermediate metabolism and is *crowded* with ribosomes making proteins (see Figure 1-1, *B*). Newly synthesized proteins remain in the cytosol if they lack a signal for transport to a cell organelle.[1] The organelles suspended in the cytoplasm are enclosed in biologic membranes, so they can simultaneously carry out functions requiring different biochemical environments. Many of these functions are directed by coded messages carried from the nucleus by RNA. The functions include synthesis of proteins and hormones and their transport out of the cell, isolation and elimination of waste products from the cell, performance of metabolic processes, breakdown and disposal of cellular debris and foreign proteins (antigens), and maintenance of cellular structure and motility. The cytosol is a storage unit for fat, carbohydrates, and secretory vesicles. Table 1-1 lists the principal cytoplasmic organelles.

 QUICK CHECK 1-1
1. Why is the process of differentiation essential to specialization? Give an example.
2. Describe at least two cellular functions.

Plasma Membranes

Every cell is contained within a membrane with gates, channels, and pumps. Membranes surround the cell or enclose an intracellular organelle and are exceedingly important to normal physiologic function because they control the composition of the space, or compartment, they enclose. Membranes can allow or exclude various molecules and, because of selective transport systems, they can move molecules in or out of the space (Figure 1-3). By controlling the movement of substances from one compartment to another, membranes exert a powerful influence on metabolic pathways. Directional transport is facilitated by polarized domains, distinct apical and basolateral domains. Cell polarity, the direction of cellular transport, maintains normal cell and tissue structure for numerous functions (for example, movement of nutrients in and out of the cell) and becomes altered with diseases (Figure 1-4). The plasma membrane also has an important role in cell-to-cell recognition. Other functions of the plasma membrane include cellular mobility and the maintenance of cellular shape (Table 1-2).

Membrane Composition

The basic structure of cell membranes is the lipid bilayer, composed of two apposing leaflets and proteins that span the bilayer or interact with the lipids on either side of the two leaflets (Figure 1-5). Lipid research is growing and principles of membrane organization are being overhauled.[2] In short, the main constituents of cell membranes are lipids and proteins. Historically, the plasma membrane was described as a fluid lipid bilayer (fluid mosaic model) composed of a *uniform*

FIGURE 1-1 Typical Components of a Eukaryotic Cell and Structure of the Cytoplasm. A, Artist's interpretation of cell structure. Note the many mitochondria known as the "power plants of the cell." **B,** Color-enhanced electron micrograph of a cell. The cell is crowded. Note, too, the innumerable dots bordering the endoplasmic reticulum. These are ribosomes, the cell's "protein factories." (**B,** from Patton KT, Thibodeau GA: *Anatomy & physiology,* ed 8, St Louis, 2013, Mosby.)

lipid distribution with inserted moving proteins. It now appears that the lipid bilayer is a much more complex structure where lipids and proteins are not uniformly distributed but can separate into discrete units called *microdomains,* differing in their protein and lipid compositions.[3] Different membranes have varying percentages of lipids and proteins. Intracellular membranes may have a higher percentage of proteins than do plasma membranes, presumably because most enzymatic activity occurs within organelles. The membrane organization is achieved through noncovalent bonds that allow different physical states called phases. The lipid bilayer can be structured in three main phases: solid gel phase, fluid liquid-crystalline phase, and liquid-ordered phase (Figure 1-5, *B*). These phases can change under physiologic factors such as temperature and pressure fluctuations. Carbohydrates are mainly associated with plasma membranes, in which they are chemically combined with lipids, forming **glycolipids,** and with proteins, forming **glycoproteins** (see Figure 1-5).

The outer surface of the plasma membrane in many types of cells, especially endothelial cells and adipocytes, is not smooth but dimpled with flask-shaped invaginations known as caveolae ("tiny caves"). Caveolae serve as a storage site for many receptors, provide a route for transport into the cell, and act as the initiator for relaying signals from several extracellular chemical messengers into the cell's interior (see p. 24).

Lipids. Each lipid molecule is said to be polar, or **amphipathic,** which means that one part is hydrophobic (uncharged, or "water hating") and another part is hydrophilic (charged, or "water loving") (Figure 1-6). The membrane spontaneously organizes itself into two layers because of these two incompatible solubilities. The hydrophobic region (hydrophobic tail) of each lipid molecule is protected from water, whereas the hydrophilic region (hydrophilic head) is immersed in it. The bilayer serves as a barrier to the diffusion of water and hydrophilic substances, while allowing lipid-soluble molecules, such as

FIGURE 1-2 The Nucleus. The nucleus is composed of a double membrane, called a nuclear envelope, that encloses the fluid-filled interior, called nucleoplasm. The chromosomes are suspended in the nucleoplasm (illustrated here much larger than actual size to show the tightly packed DNA strands). Swelling at one or more points of the chromosome, shown in **A**, occurs at a nucleolus where genes are being copied into RNA. The nuclear envelope is studded with pores. **B,** The pores are visible as dimples in this freeze-etch of a nuclear envelope. **C,** Histone-folding DNA in chromosomes. (**B,** from Raven PH, Johnson GB: *Biology*, St Louis, 1992, Mosby.)

TABLE 1-1	Principal Cytoplasmic Organelles
Organelle	**Characteristics and Description**
Ribosomes	RNA-protein complexes (nucleoproteins) synthesized in nucleolus and secreted into cytoplasm. Provide sites for cellular protein synthesis.
Endoplasmic reticulum	Network of tubular channels (cisternae) that extend throughout outer nuclear membrane. Specializes in synthesis and transport of protein and lipid components of most organelles.
Golgi complex	Network of smooth membranes and vesicles located near nucleus. Responsible for processing and packaging proteins onto secretory vesicles that break away from the complex and migrate to various intracellular and extracellular destinations, including plasma membrane. Best-known vesicles are those that have coats largely made of the protein *clathrin*. Proteins in the complex bind to the cytoskeleton, generating tension that helps organelle function and keep its stretched shape intact.
Lysosomes	Saclike structures that originate from Golgi complex and contain enzymes for digesting most cellular substances to their basic form, such as amino acids, fatty acids, and carbohydrates (sugars). Cellular injury leads to release of lysosomal enzymes that cause cellular self-destruction.
Peroxisomes	Similar to lysosomes but contain several oxidative enzymes (e.g., catalase, urate oxidase) that produce hydrogen peroxide; reactions detoxify various wastes.
Mitochondria	Contain metabolic machinery needed for cellular energy metabolism. Enzymes of respiratory chain (electron-transport chain), found in inner membrane of mitochondria, generate most of cell's ATP (oxidative phosphorylation). Have a role in osmotic regulation, pH control, calcium homeostasis, and cell signaling.
Cytoskeleton	"Bone and muscle" of cell. Composed of a network of protein filaments, including microtubules and actin filaments (microfilaments); forms cell extensions (microvilli, cilia, flagella).
Caveolae	Tiny indentations (caves) that can capture extracellular material and shuttle it inside the cell or across the cell.
Vaults	Cytoplasmic ribonucleoproteins shaped like octagonal barrels. Thought to act as "trucks," shuttling molecules from nucleus to elsewhere in cell.

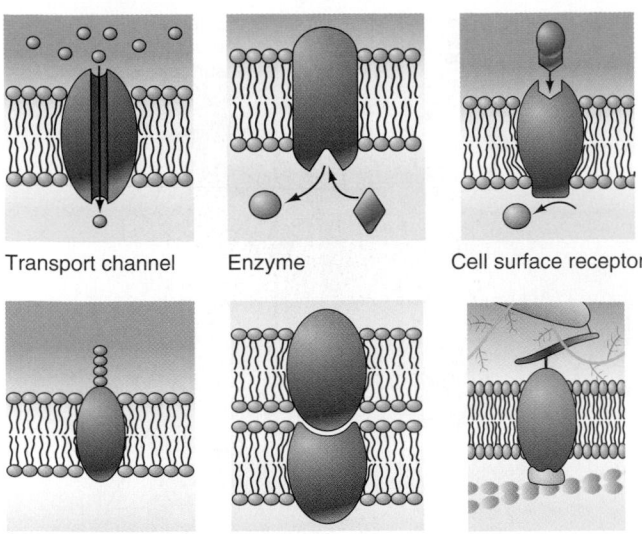

Transport channel   Enzyme   Cell surface receptor

Cell surface markers   Cell adhesion   Attachment of cytoskeleton

FIGURE 1-3 Functions of Plasma Membrane Proteins. The plasma membrane proteins illustrated here show a variety of functions performed by the different types of plasma membranes. (From Raven PH, Johnson GB: *Understanding biology,* ed 3, Dubuque, Iowa, 1995, Brown.)

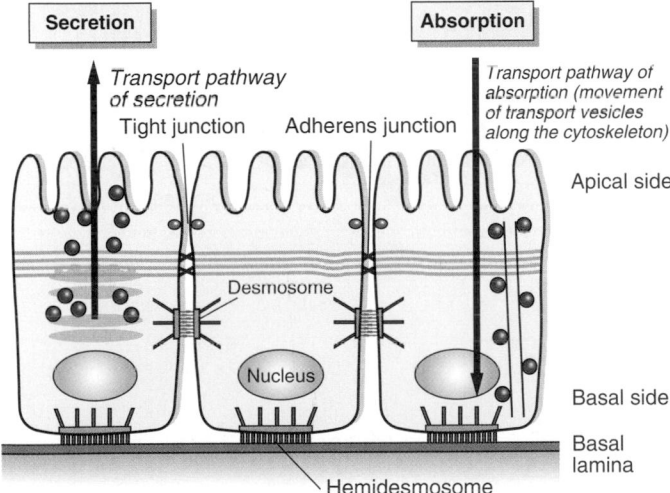

FIGURE 1-4 Cell Polarity of Epithelial Cells. Schematic of cell polarity (cell direction) of epithelial cells. Shown are the directions of the basal side and the apical side. Organelles and cytoskeleton are also arranged directionally to enable, for example, intestinal cell secretion and absorption. (Adapted from *Life science web textbook,* The University of Tokyo.)

oxygen (O_2) and carbon dioxide (CO_2), to diffuse through the membrane readily.

A major component of the plasma membrane is a bilayer of lipid molecules—glycerophospholipids, sphingolipids, and sterols (for example, cholesterol). The most abundant lipids are phospholipids. **Phospholipids** have a phosphate-containing hydrophilic head connected to a hydrophobic tail. Phospholipids and glycolipids form self-sealing lipid bilayers. Lipids along with protein assemblies act as "molecular glue" for the structural integrity of the membrane. Investigators are studying the concept of lipid rafts. **Membrane lipid rafts**

TABLE 1-2	**Plasma Membrane Functions**
Cellular Mechanism	**Membrane Functions**
Structure	Usually thicker than membranes of intracellular organelles
	Containment of cellular organelles
	Maintenance of relationship with cytoskeleton, endoplasmic reticulum, and other organelles
	Maintenance of fluid and electrolyte balance
	Outer surfaces of plasma membranes in many cells are not smooth but are dimpled with cavelike indentations called *caveolae;* they are also studded with cilia or even smaller cylindrical projections called *microvilli;* both are capable of movement
Protection	Barrier to toxic molecules and macromolecules (proteins, nucleic acids, polysaccharides)
	Barrier to foreign organisms and cells
Activation of cell	Hormones (regulation of cellular activity)
	Mitogens (cellular division; see Chapter 2)
	Antigens (antibody synthesis; see Chapter 6)
	Growth factors (proliferation and differentiation; see Chapter 10)
Storage	Storage site for many receptors
	Transport
	Diffusion and exchange diffusion
	Endocytosis (pinocytosis, phagocytosis)
	Exocytosis (secretion)
	Active transport
Cell-to-cell interaction	Communication and attachment at junctional complexes
	Symbiotic nutritive relationships
	Release of enzymes and antibodies to extracellular environment
	Relationships with extracellular matrix

Modified from King DW, Fenoglio CM, Lefkowitch JH: *General pathology: principles and dynamics,* Philadelphia, 1983, Lea & Febiger.

(MLRs) appear to be structurally and functionally distinct regions of the plasma membrane[4,5] and consist of cholesterol and sphingolipid-dependent microdomains that form a network of lipid-lipid, protein-protein, and protein-lipid interactions (Figures 1-5, *B,* and 1-7) Although discrepancies between experimental results exist, two main types of MLRs are hypothesized: those that contain the cholesterol-binding protein caveolin (see p. 24) and those that do not.[4] Researchers hypothesized there are lipid rafts that have several functions, including (1) providing cellular polarity and organization of signaling trafficking; (2) acting as platforms for extracellular matrix (ECM) adhesion and intracellular cytoskeletal tethering to the plasma membrane through cellular adhesion molecules (CAMs, see p. 8); (3) enabling signaling across the membrane, which can rearrange cytoskeletal architecture and regulate cell growth, migration, and other functions; and (4) allowing entry of viruses, bacteria, toxins, and nanoparticles.[4]

Proteins. A **protein** is made from a chain of amino acids known as **polypeptides.** There are 20 types of amino acids in proteins and each type of protein has a unique sequence of amino acids. Proteins are the major workhorses of the cell. After translation (the synthesis of protein from RNA, see Chapter 2) of a protein, **posttranslational modifications (PTMs)** are the methods used to diversify the limited numbers of proteins generated. These modifications alter the activity and functions of proteins and have become very important in understanding diseases. Researchers have known for decades that pathogens

A

B

C

FIGURE 1-5 Lipid Bilayer Membranes. A, Concepts of biologic membranes have markedly changed in the last two decades, from the classic fluid mosaic model to the current model that lipids and proteins are not evenly distributed but can isolate into microdomains, differing in their protein and lipid composition. **B,** An example of a microdomain is lipid rafts *(yellow)*. Rafts are dynamic domain structures composed of cholesterol, sphingolipids, and membrane proteins important in different cellular processes. Various models exist to clarify the functions of domains. The three major phases of lipid bilayer organization include a solid gel phase (e.g., with low temperatures), a liquid-ordered phase (high temperatures), and a fluid liquid-crystalline (or liquid-disordered) phase. Some membrane-associated proteins are integrated into the lipid bilayer; other proteins are loosely attached to the outer and inner surfaces of the membrane. Transmembrane proteins protrude through the entire outer and inner surfaces of the membrane, and they can be attracted to microdomains through specific interactions with lipids. Interaction of the membrane proteins with distinct lipids depends on the hydrophobic thickness of the membrane, the lateral pressures of the membrane (mechanical force may shift protein channels from an open to closed state), the polarity or electrical charges at the lipid-protein interface, and the presence on the protein side of amino acid side chains. Important for pathophysiology is the proposal that protein-lipid interactions can be critical for correct insertion, folding, and orientation of membrane proteins. For example, diseases related to lipids that interfere with protein folding are becoming more prevalent. **C,** The cell membrane is not static but is always moving. Observed for the first time from measurements taken at the National Institute of Standards and Technology (NIST) and France's Institut Laue-Langevin (ILL). (Adapted from Bagatolli LA et al: *Prog Lipid Res* 49[4]:378-389, 2010; Contreras FX et al: *Cold Spring Harb Perspect Biol* 3[6]:pii a004705, 2011; Cooper GM: *The cell—a molecular approach,* ed 2, Sunderland (MA): Sinauer Associates, 2000; Defamie N, Mesnil M: *Biochim Biophys Acta* 1818(8):1866-1869, 2012; Woodka AC et al: *Phys Rev Lett* 9(5):058102, 2012.)

FIGURE 1-6 Structure of a Phospholipid Molecule. A, Each phospholipid molecule consists of a phosphate functional group and two fatty acid chains attached to a glycerol molecule. **B,** The fatty acid chains and glycerol form nonpolar, hydrophobic "tails," and the phosphate functional group forms the polar, hydrophilic "head" of the phospholipid molecule. When placed in water, the hydrophobic tails of the molecule face inward, away from the water, and the hydrophilic head faces outward, toward the water. (From Raven PH, Johnson GB: *Understanding biology,* ed 3, Dubuque, Iowa, 1995, Brown.)

FIGURE 1-7 Lipid Rafts. The plasma membrane is composed of many lipids, including sphingomyelin *(SM)* and cholesterol, shown here as a small raft in the external leaflet. *GS,* Glycosphingolipid; *PC,* phosphatidyl-choline; *PE,* phosphatidylethanolamine; *PS,* phosphatidylserine. (From Pollard TD, Ernshaw WC: *Cell biology,* St Louis, 2004, Saunders Elsevier.)

interfere with the host's PTMs.[6] New approaches are being used to understand changes in proteins—a field called **proteomics** is the study of the **proteome,** or entire set of proteins expressed by a genome from synthesis, translocation, and modification (e.g., folding), and the analysis of the roles of proteomes in a staggering number of diseases.

Membrane proteins associate with the lipid bilayer in different ways (Figure 1-8), including (1) **transmembrane proteins** that extend across the bilayer and exposed to an aqueous environment on both sides of the membrane (see Figure 1-8, *A*); (2) proteins located almost entirely in the cytosol and associated with the cytosolic half of the lipid bilayer by an α helix exposed on the surface of the protein (see Figure 1-8, *B*); (3) proteins that exist outside the bilayer, on one side or the other, and attached to the membrane by one or more covalently attached lipid groups (see Figure 1-8, *C*); and (4) proteins bound indirectly to one or the other bilayer membrane face and held in place by their interactions with other proteins (see Figure 1-8, *D*).[1]

Proteins directly attached to the membrane bilayer can be removed by dissolving the bilayer with detergents called **integral membrane proteins.** The remaining proteins that can be removed by gentler procedures that interfere with protein-protein interactions but do not dissolve the bilayer are known as **peripheral membrane proteins.**

Proteins exist in densely folded molecular configurations rather than straight chains; so most hydrophilic units are at the surface of the molecule and most hydrophobic units are inside. Membrane proteins, like other proteins, are synthesized by the ribosome and then make their way, called *trafficking,* to different membrane locations of a cell.[7] Trafficking places unique demands on membrane proteins for folding, translocation, and stability.[7] Thus, much research is now being done to understand misfolded proteins (for example, as a cause of disease; Box 1-1).

Although membrane structure is determined by the lipid bilayer, membrane functions are determined largely by proteins. Proteins act as (1) recognition and binding units (receptors) for substances moving into and out of the cell; (2) pores or transport channels for various electrically charged particles, called **ions** or *electrolytes,* and specific carriers for amino acids and monosaccharides; (3) specific enzymes that drive active pumps to promote concentration of certain ions, particularly potassium (K^+), within the cell while keeping

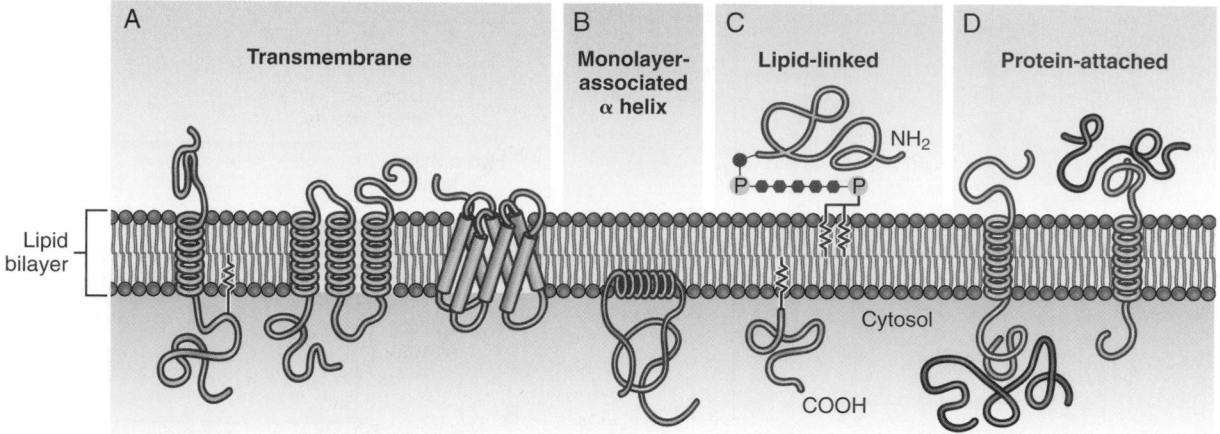

FIGURE 1-8 Proteins Attach to the Plasma Membrane in Different Ways. A, Transmembrane proteins extend through the membrane as a single α helix, as multiple α helices, or as a rolled up barrel-like sheet called a β barrel. **B,** Some membrane proteins are anchored to the cytosolic side of the lipid bilayer by an amphipathic α helix. **C,** Some proteins are linked on either side of the membrane by a covalently attached lipid molecule. **D,** Proteins are attached by weak noncovalent interactions with other membrane proteins. All are integral membrane proteins except. (D, adapted from Alberts B: *Essential cell biology,* ed 4, New York, 2014, Garland.)

BOX 1-1   Endoplasmic Reticulum, Protein Folding, and ER Stress

Protein folding in the endoplasmic reticulum (ER) is critical for us. As the biologic workhorses, proteins perform vital functions in every cell. To do these tasks proteins must fold into complex three-dimensional structures (see figure). Most secreted proteins *fold* and are modified in an error-free manner, but ER or cell stress, mutations, or random (stochastic) errors during protein synthesis can decrease the folding amount or the rate of folding. Pathophysiologic processes, such as viral infections, environmental toxins, and mutant protein expression, can perturb the sensitive ER environment. Natural processes also can perturb the environment, such as the large protein-synthesizing load placed on the ER. These perturbations cause the accumulation of immature and abnormal proteins in cells, leading to **ER stress**. Fortunately, the ER is loaded with protective ways to help folding; for example, protein *chaperones* facilitate folding and prevent the formation of off-pathway types. Because specialized cells produce large amounts of secreted proteins, the movement or flux through the ER is tremendous. Therefore misfolded proteins not repaired in the ER are observed in some diseases and can initiate apoptosis or cell death. It has recently been shown that the endoplasmic reticulum mediates intracellular signaling pathways in response to the accumulation of unfolded or misfolded proteins; collectively, the pathways are known as the **unfolded-protein response (UPR)**. Investigators are studying UPR-associated inflammation and how the UPR is coupled to

inflammation in health and disease. Specific diseases include Alzheimer disease, Parkinson disease, prion disease, amyotrophic lateral sclerosis, and diabetes mellitus. Additionally being studied is ER stress and how it may accelerate age-related dysfunction.

Protein Folding. Each protein exists as an unfolded polypeptide *(left)* or a random coil after the process of translation from a sequence of mRNA to a linear string of amino acids. From amino acids interacting with each other they produce a three-dimensional structure called the folded protein *(right)* that is its native state.

Data from Brodsky J, Skach WR: *Curr Opin Cell Biol* 23:464-475, 2011; Jäger R et al: *Biol Cell* 104(5):259-270,2012; Ron D, Walter P: *Nat Rev Mol Cell Biol* 8:519-529, 2007.

---

concentrations of other ions (for example, sodium, Na^+), less than concentrations found in the extracellular environment; (4) cell surface markers, such as **glycoproteins** (proteins attached to carbohydrates), that identify a cell to its neighbor; (5) cell adhesion molecules (CAMs), or proteins that allow cells to hook together and form attachments of the cytoskeleton for maintaining cellular shape; and (6) catalysts of chemical reactions (for example, conversion of lactose to glucose; see Figure 1-3). Membrane proteins are key components of energy transduction, converting chemical energy into electrical energy, or electrical energy into either mechanical energy or synthesis of ATP.[7] Investigators

are studying ATP enzymes and the changes in shape of biologic membranes, particularly mitochondrial membranes, and their relationship to aging and disease.[8-10]

In animal cells, the plasma membrane is stabilized by a meshwork of proteins attached to the underside of the membrane called the cell cortex. Human red blood cells have a cell cortex that maintains their flattened biconcave shape.[1]

Protein regulation in a cell: protein homeostasis. The cellular protein pool is in constant change or flux. The number of copies of a protein in a cell depends on how quickly it is made and how long it

FIGURE 1-9 Protein Homeostasis System and Outcomes. A main role of the protein homeostasis network *(proteostasis)* is to minimize protein misfolding and protein aggregation. The network includes ribosome-mediated protein synthesis, chaperone (folding helpers in the ER) and enzyme mediated folding, breakdown systems of lysosome and proteasome-mediated protein degradation, and vesicular trafficking. The network integrates biologic pathways that balance folding, trafficking, and protein degradation depicted by arrows *b, d, e, f, g, h,* and *i. ER,* Endoplasmic reticulum. (Adapted from Lindquist SL, Kelly JW: *Cold Spring Harb Perspect Biol* 3[12]:pii: a004507, 2011.)

survives or is broken down. This adaptable system of protein homeostasis is defined by the "proteostasis" network comprised of ribosomes (makers); chaperones (helpers); and two protein breakdown systems or proteolytic systems—lysosomes and the ubiquitin-proteasome system (UPS). These systems regulate protein homeostasis under a large variety of conditions, including variations in nutrient supply, the existence of oxidative stress or cellular differentiation, changes in temperature, and the presence of heavy metal ions and other sources of stress.[11] Malfunction or failure of the proteostasis network is associated with human disease[12] (Figure 1-9).

Carbohydrates. The short chains of sugars or carbohydrates *(oligosaccharides)* contained within the plasma membrane are generally bound to membrane proteins (glycoproteins) and lipids (glycolipids). Long polysaccharide chains attached to membrane proteins are called *proteoglycans.* All of the carbohydrate on the glycoproteins, proteoglycans, and glycolipids is located on the outside of the plasma membrane and the carbohydrate coating is called the glycocalyx. The glycocalyx helps protect the cell from mechanical damage.[1] Additionally, the layer of carbohydrate gives the cell a slimy surface that assists the mobility of other cells, like leukocytes, to squeeze through the narrow spaces.[1] The functions of carbohydrates are more than protection and lubrication and include specific cell-cell recognition and adhesion. Intercellular recognition is an important function of membrane oligosaccharides; for example, the transmembrane proteins called *lectins,* which bind to a particular oligosaccharide, recognize neutrophils at the site of bacterial infection. This recognition allows the neutrophil to adhere to the blood vessel wall and migrate from the blood into the infected tissue to help eliminate the invading bacteria.[1]

Cellular Receptors

Cellular receptors are protein molecules on the plasma membrane, in the cytoplasm, or in the nucleus that can recognize and bind with specific smaller molecules called ligands (from the Latin *ligare,* "to bind") (Figure 1-10). The region of a protein that associates with a ligand is called its binding site. Hormones, for example, are ligands. Recognition and binding depend on the chemical configuration of the receptor and its smaller ligand, which must fit together somewhat like pieces of a jigsaw puzzle (see Chapter 18). Binding selectively to a protein receptor with high affinity to a ligand depends on formation of weak, noncovalent interactions—hydrogen bonds, electrostatic attractions, and van der Waals attractions—and favorable hydrophobic forces.[1] Numerous receptors are found in most cells, and ligand binding to receptors activates or inhibits the receptor's associated signaling or biochemical pathway (see p. 12).

Plasma membrane receptors protrude from or are exposed at the external surface of the membrane and are important for cellular uptake of ligands (see Figure 1-10). The ligands that bind with membrane receptors include hormones, neurotransmitters, antigens, complement components, lipoproteins, infectious agents, drugs, and metabolites. Many new discoveries concerning the specific interactions of cellular receptors with their respective ligands have provided a basis for understanding disease.

Although the chemical nature of ligands and their receptors differs, receptors are classified based on their location and function. Cellular type determines overall cellular function, but plasma membrane receptors determine which ligands a cell will bind with and how the cell will respond to the binding. Specific processes also control intracellular mechanisms.

Receptors for different drugs are found on the plasma membrane, in the cytoplasm, and in the nucleus. Membrane receptors have been found for certain anesthetics, opiates, endorphins, enkephalins, antibiotics, cancer chemotherapeutic agents, digitalis, and other drugs. Membrane receptors for endorphins, which are opiate-like peptides isolated from the pituitary gland, are found in large quantities in pain pathways of the nervous system (see Chapters 13 and 14). With binding to the receptor, the endorphins (or drugs such as morphine) change the cell's permeability to ions, increase the concentration of molecules that regulate intracellular protein synthesis, and initiate molecular events that modulate pain perception.

Receptors for infectious microorganisms, or antigen receptors, bind bacteria, viruses, and parasites to the cell membrane. Antigen receptors on white blood cells (lymphocytes, monocytes, macrophages,

FIGURE 1-10 Cellular Receptors. (A) 1, Plasma membrane receptor for a ligand (here, a hormone molecule) on the surface of an integral protein. A neurotransmitter can exert its effect on a postsynaptic cell by means of two fundamentally different types of receptor proteins: **2,** channel-linked receptors, and **3,** non–channel-linked receptors. Channel-linked receptors are also known as *ligand-gated channels.* **(B)** Example of ligand-receptor interaction. Insulin-like growth factor 1 (IGF-1) is a ligand and binds to the insulin-like growth factor 1 receptor (IGF-1R). With binding at the cell membrane the intracellular signaling pathway is activated, causing translation of new proteins to act as intracellular communicators. This pathway is important for cancer growth. Researchers are developing pharmacologic strategies to reduce signaling at and downstream of the insulin-like growth factor 1 receptor (IGF-1R), hoping this will lead to compounds useful in cancer treatment.

granulocytes) recognize and bind with antigenic microorganisms and activate the immune and inflammatory responses (see Chapter 6).

CELL-TO-CELL ADHESIONS

Cells are small and squishy, *not* like bricks. They are enclosed only by a flimsy membrane, yet the cell depends on the integrity of this membrane for its survival. How can cells be connected strongly, with their membranes intact, to form a muscle that can lift this textbook? Plasma membranes not only serve as the outer boundaries of all cells but also allow groups of cells to be held together robustly, in cell-to-cell adhesions, to form tissues and organs. Once arranged, cells are linked by three different means: (1) cell adhesion molecules in the cell's plasma membrane (see p. 8), (2) the extracellular matrix, and (3) specialized cell junctions.

Extracellular Matrix

Cells can be united by attachment to one another or through the extracellular matrix (including the basement membrane), which the cells secrete around themselves. The extracellular matrix is an intricate meshwork of fibrous proteins embedded in a watery, gel-like substance composed of complex carbohydrates (Figure 1-11). The matrix is similar to glue; however, it provides a pathway for diffusion of nutrients, wastes, and other water-soluble substances between the blood and

tissue cells. Interwoven within the matrix are three groups of macro-molecules: (1) fibrous structural proteins, including collagen and elastin; (2) adhesive glycoproteins, such as fibronectin; and (3) proteoglycans and hyaluronic acid.

1. Collagen forms cablelike fibers or sheets that provide tensile strength or resistance to longitudinal stress. Collagen breakdown, such as occurs in osteoarthritis, destroys the fibrils that give cartilage its tensile strength.
2. Elastin is a rubber-like protein fiber most abundant in tissues that must be capable of stretching and recoiling, such as found in the lungs.
3. Fibronectin, a large glycoprotein, promotes cell adhesion and cell anchorage. Reduced amounts have been found in certain types of cancerous cells; this allows cancer cells to travel, or metastasize, to other parts of the body. All of these macromolecules occur in intercellular junctions and cell surfaces and may assemble into two different components: interstitial matrix and basement membrane (BM) (see Figure 1-11).

The **basement membrane** is a thin, tough layer of extracellular matrix (connective tissue) underlying the epithelium of many organs and is also called the basal lamina (see Figure 1-11, *B*).

The extracellular matrix is secreted by fibroblasts ("fiber formers") (Figure 1-12), local cells that are present in the matrix. The matrix and the cells within it are known collectively as connective tissue because

Epithelium

Integrins

Basement membrane

Integrins

Endothelial cells

Capillary

Fibroblasts

Integrins

Cross-linked collagen triple helices

Type IV collagen

Basement membrane
- Type IV collagen
- Laminin
- Proteoglycan

Laminin

Proteoglycans

Interstitial matrix
- Fibrillar collagens
- Elastin
- Proteoglycan and hyaluronan

Adhesive glycoproteins

A

B

FIGURE 1-11 Extracellular Matrix. A, Tissues are not just cells but also extracellular space. The extracellular space is an intricate network of macromolecules called the *extracellular matrix (ECM)*. The macromolecules that constitute the ECM are secreted locally (by mostly fibroblasts) and assembled into a meshwork in close association with the surface of the cell that produced them. Two main classes of macromolecules include proteoglycans, which are bound to polysaccharide chains called *glycosaminoglycans,* and fibrous proteins (e.g., collagen, elastin, fibronectin, and laminin), which have structural and adhesive properties. Together the proteoglycan molecules form a gel-like ground substance in which the fibrous proteins are embedded. The gel permits rapid diffusion of nutrients, metabolites, and hormones between the blood and the tissue cells. Matrix proteins modulate cell-matrix interactions, including normal tissue remodeling (which can become abnormal, for example, with chronic inflammation). Disruptions of this balance result in serious diseases such as arthritis, tumor growth, and other pathologic conditions. **B,** Scanning electron micrograph of a chick embryo where a portion of the epithelium has been removed, exposing the curtain-like extracellular matrix. (**A,** adapted from Kumar V et al: *Robbins and Cotran pathologic basis of disease,* ed 9, Philadelphia, 2015, Saunders; **B,** © Robert L Trelstad; from Gartner LP, Hiatt JL: *Color textbook of histology,* ed 3, St Louis, 2006, Saunders/Elsevier.)

they interconnect cells to form tissues and organs. Human connective tissues are enormously varied. They can be hard and dense, like bone; flexible, like tendons or the dermis of the skin; resilient and shock absorbing, like cartilage; or soft and transparent, similar to the jelly-like substance that fills the eye. In all these examples, the majority of the tissue is composed of extracellular matrix, and the cells that produce the matrix are scattered within it like raisins in a pudding (see Figure 1-12).

The matrix is not just passive scaffolding for cellular attachment but also helps regulate the function of the cells with which it interacts. The matrix helps regulate such important functions as cell growth and differentiation.

Specialized Cell Junctions

Cells in direct physical contact with neighboring cells are often interconnected at specialized plasma membrane regions called **cell junctions.** Cell junctions are classified by their function: (1) some hold cells together and form a tight seal (tight junctions); (2) some provide strong mechanical attachments (adherens junctions, desmosomes, hemidesmosomes); (3) some provide a special type of chemical communication (for example, inorganic ions and small water-soluble molecules to move from the cytosol of one cell to the cytosol of another cell), such as those causing an electrical wave (gap junctions); and (4) some maintain apico-basal polarity of individual epithelial cells (tight junctions) (Figure 1-13). Overall, cell junctions make the epithelium leak-proof and mediate mechanical attachment of one cell to another, allow communicating tunnels and maintaining cell polarity.

Cell junctions can be classified as symmetric and asymmetric. Symmetric junctions include tight junctions, the belt desmosome (zonula adherens), desmosomes (macula adherens), and gap junctions (also called intercellular channel or communicating junctions).[13] An asymmetric junction is the hemidesmosome (see Figure 1-13). Together they

FIGURE 1-12 Fibroblasts in Connective Tissue. This micrograph shows tissue from the cornea of a rat. The extracellular matrix surrounds the fibroblasts *(F)*. (From Nishida T et al: The extracellular matrix of animal connective tissues, *Invest Ophthalmol Vis Sci* 29:1887-1880, 1998.)

0.1 μm

form the **junctional complex**. **Desmosomes** unite cells either by forming continuous bands or belts of epithelial sheets or by developing button-like points of contact. Desmosomes also act as a system of braces to maintain structural stability. **Tight junctions** are barriers to diffusion, prevent the movement of substances through transport proteins in the plasma membrane, and prevent the leakage of small molecules between the plasma membranes of adjacent cells. **Gap junctions** are clusters of communicating tunnels or connexons that allow small ions and molecules to pass directly from the inside of one cell to the inside of another. **Connexons** are hemichannels that extend outward from each of the adjacent plasma membranes (Figure 1-13, *C*).

Multiple factors regulate gap junction intercellular communication, including voltage across the junction, intracellular pH, intracellular Ca^{++} concentration, and protein phosphorylation. The most abundant human connexin is connexin 43 (Cx43).[14] Investigators recently showed that loss of Cx43 expression in colorectal tumors is correlated with a shorter cancer-free survival rate.[15] This study is the first evidence that Cx43 acts as a tumor suppressor for colorectal cancer (enhances apoptosis) and therefore may be an important prognostic marker and target for therapy.[15] Investigators also recently reported that glycyrrhizic acid (GA), a glycoside of licorice root extracts, may be a strong chemopreventive agent against carcinogens; induced colon cancer in rats and Cx43 is one target.[16] Too much GA often in humans may lead to hypokalemia and hypertension.[17]

The junctional complex is a highly permeable part of the plasma membrane. Its permeability is controlled by a process called **gating**. Increased levels of cytoplasmic calcium cause decreased permeability at the junctional complex. Gating enables uninjured cells to protect themselves from injured neighbors. Calcium is released from injured cells.

CELLULAR COMMUNICATION AND SIGNAL TRANSDUCTION

Cells need to communicate with each other to maintain a stable internal environment, or **homeostasis**; to regulate their growth and division; to oversee their development and organization into tissues; and to coordinate their functions. Cells communicate by using hundreds of kinds of signal molecules, for example, insulin (see Figure 1-10, *B*). Cells communicate in three main ways: (1) they display plasma membrane–bound signaling molecules (receptors) that affect the cell itself and other cells in direct physical contact (Figure 1-14, *A*); (2) they affect receptor proteins *inside* the target cell and the signal molecule has to enter the cell to bind to them (Figure 1-14, *B*); and (3) they form protein channels (gap junctions) that directly coordinate the activities of adjacent cells (Figure 1-14, *C*). Alterations in cellular communication affect disease onset and progression. In fact, if a cell cannot perform gap junctional intercellular communication, normal growth control and cell differentiation is compromised, thereby favoring cancerous tumor development (see Chapter 10). (Communication through gap junctions was discussed earlier, and contact signaling by plasma membrane–bound molecules is discussed on this page and on p. 15.) Secreted chemical signals involve communication locally and at a distance. Primary modes of intercellular signaling are contact-dependent, paracrine, hormonal, neurohormonal, and neurotransmitter. Autocrine stimulation occurs when the secreting cell targets itself (Figure 1-15).

Contact-dependent signaling requires cells to be in close membrane-membrane contact. In **paracrine signaling**, cells secrete local chemical mediators that are quickly taken up, destroyed, or immobilized. Paracrine signaling usually involves different cell types; however, cells also can produce signals to which they alone respond, called **autocrine signaling** (see Figure 1-15). For example, cancer cells use this form of signaling to stimulate their survival and proliferation. The mediators act only on nearby cells. **Hormonal signaling** involves specialized endocrine cells that secrete chemicals called hormones; hormones are released by one set of cells and travel through the bloodstream to produce a response in other sets of cells (see Chapter 18). In **neurohormonal signaling** hormones are released into the blood by neurosecretory neurons. Like endocrine cells, neurosecretory neurons release blood-borne chemical messengers, whereas ordinary neurons secrete short-range neurotransmitters into a small discrete space (i.e., synapse). Neurons communicate directly with the cells they innervate by releasing chemicals or **neurotransmitters** at specialized junctions called **chemical synapses**; the neurotransmitter diffuses across the synaptic cleft and acts on the postsynaptic target cell (see Figure 1-15). Many of these same signaling molecules are receptors used in hormonal, neurohormonal, and paracrine signaling. Important differences lie in the speed and selectivity with which the signals are delivered to their targets.[1]

Plasma membrane receptors belong to one of three classes that are defined by the signaling (transduction) mechanism used. Table 1-3 summarizes these classes of receptors. Cells respond to external stimuli by activating a variety of **signal transduction pathways**, which are communication pathways, or signaling cascades (Figure 1-16, *C*). Signals are passed between cells when a particular type of molecule is produced by one cell—the **signaling cell**—and received by another—the **target cell**—by means of a **receptor protein** that recognizes and responds specifically to the signal molecule (Figure 1-16, *A* and *B*). In turn, the signaling molecules activate a pathway of intracellular protein kinases that results in various responses, such as grow and reproduce, die, survive, or differentiate (Figure 1-16, *D*). If deprived of appropriate

A

Junctional complex

Tight junction
(zonula occludens)

Belt desmosome
(zonula adherens)

Filamentous
material in
intercellular
space

Spot desmosome
(macula adherens)

Intercellular filaments

Intercellular channel

Gap
junction

Intercellular units
forming channels for
extracellular transport

Epithelial cells

Belt
desmosome

Spot
desmosomes

Hemidesmosomes

B

Cell 1 cytosol

Diameter of
channel = 1.5 nm

Connexon

Gap junction
Longitudinal section
of connexon

Passage of ions
and small molecules

No passage of
large molecules

2.4 nm

Cell 2 cytosol

Interacting plasma membranes

C

FIGURE 1-13 Junctional Complex. A, Schematic drawing of a belt desmosome between epithelial cells. This junction, also called the *zonula adherens,* encircles each of the interacting cells. The spot desmosomes and hemidesmosomes, like the belt desmosomes, are adhering junctions. This tight junction is an impermeable junction that holds cells together but seals them in such a way that molecules cannot leak between them. The gap junction, as a communicating junction, mediates the passage of small molecules from one interacting cell to the other. **B,** Connexons. The connexin gap junction proteins have four transmembrane domains and they play a vital role in maintaining cell and tissue function and homeostasis. Cells connected by gap junctions are considered ionically (electrically) and metabolically coupled. Gap junctions coordinate the activities of adjacent cells; for example, they are important for synchronizing contractions of heart muscle cells through ionic coupling and for permitting action potentials to spread rapidly from cell to cell in neural tissues. The reason gap junctions occur in tissues that are not electrically active is unknown. Although most gap junctions are associated with junctional complexes, they sometimes exist as independent structures. **C,** Electron micrograph of desmosomes. (**A** and **C** from Raven PH, Johnson GB: *Biology,* St Louis, 1992, Mosby; **B,** adapted from Gartner LP, Hiatt JL: *Color textbook of histology,* ed 3, St Louis, 2006, Saunders Elsevier; Sherwood L: *Learning,* ed 8, Belmont, Calif, 2013, Brooks/Cole CENGAGE.)

FIGURE 1-14 Cellular Communication. Three primary ways cells communicate with one another. (**B** adapted from Alberts B et al: *Molecular biology of the cell,* ed 5, New York, 2008, Garland.)

FIGURE 1-15 Primary Modes of Chemical Signaling. Five forms of signaling mediated by secreted molecules. Hormones, paracrines, neurotransmitters, and neurohormones are all intercellular messengers that accomplish communication between cells. Autocrines bind to receptors on the same cell. Not all neurotransmitters act in the strictly synaptic mode shown; some act in a contact-dependent mode as local chemical mediators that influence multiple target cells in the area.

signals, most cells undergo a form of cell suicide known as *programmed cell death,* or *apoptosis* (see p. 104).

CELLULAR METABOLISM

All of the chemical tasks of maintaining essential cellular functions are referred to as cellular metabolism. The energy-using process of metabolism is called anabolism (*ana* = upward), and the energy-

releasing process is known as catabolism (*kata* = downward). Metabolism provides the cell with the energy it needs to produce cellular structures.

Dietary proteins, fats, and starches (i.e., carbohydrates) are hydrolyzed in the intestinal tract into amino acids, fatty acids, and glucose, respectively. These constituents are then absorbed, circulated, and incorporated into the cell, where they may be used for various vital cellular processes, including the production of ATP. The process by

TABLE 1-3   Classes of Plasma Membrane Receptors

Type of Receptor	Description
Ion channel coupled	Also called *transmitter-gated* ion channels; involve rapid synaptic signaling between electrically excitable cells. Channels open and close briefly in response to neurotransmitters, changing ion permeability of plasma membrane of postsynaptic cell.
Enzyme coupled	Once activated by ligands, function directly as enzymes or associate with enzymes.
G-protein coupled	Indirectly activate or inactivate plasma membrane enzyme or ion channel; interaction mediated by *GTP-binding regulatory protein (G-protein)*. May also interact with inositol phospholipids, which are significant in cell signaling, and with molecules involved in *inositol-phospholipid transduction pathway*.

FIGURE 1-16 Schematic of a Signal Transduction Pathway. Like a telephone receiver that converts an electrical signal into a sound signal, a cell converts an extracellular signal, A, into an intracellular signal, B. C, An extracellular signal molecule (ligand) bonds to a receptor protein located on the plasma membrane, where it is transduced into an intracellular signal. This process initiates a signaling cascade that relays the signal into the cell interior, amplifying and distributing it during transit. Amplification is often achieved by stimulating enzymes. Steps in the cascade can be modulated by other events in the cell. D, Different cell behaviors rely on multiple extracellular signals.

which ATP is produced is one example of a series of reactions called a **metabolic pathway**. A metabolic pathway involves several steps whose end products are not always detectable. A key feature of cellular metabolism is the directing of biochemical reactions by protein catalysts or enzymes. Each enzyme has a high affinity for a **substrate**, a specific substance converted to a product of the reaction.

Role of Adenosine Triphosphate

Best known about ATP is its role as a universal "fuel" *inside* living cells. This fuel or energy drives biologic reactions necessary for cells to function. For a cell to function, it must be able to extract and use the chemical energy in organic molecules. When 1 mole (mol) of glucose metabolically breaks down in the presence of oxygen into carbon dioxide and water, 686 kilocalories (kcal) of chemical energy are released. The chemical energy lost by one molecule is transferred to the chemical structure of another molecule by an energy-carrying or energy-transferring molecule, such as ATP. The energy stored in ATP can be used in various energy-requiring reactions and in the process is generally converted to adenosine diphosphate (ADP) and inorganic phosphate (Pi). The energy available as a result of this reaction is about 7 kcal/mol of ATP. The cell uses ATP for muscle contraction and active transport of molecules across cellular membranes. ATP not only stores energy but also *transfers* it from one molecule to another. Energy stored by carbohydrate, lipid, and protein is catabolized and transferred to ATP.

Emerging understandings are the role of ATP *outside* cells—as a messenger. In animal studies, using the newly developed ATP probe, ATP has been measured in pericellular spaces. New research is clarifying the role of ATP as an extracellular messenger and its role in many physiologic processes, including inflammation.[18-20]

Food and Production of Cellular Energy

Catabolism of the proteins, lipids, and polysaccharides found in food can be divided into the following three phases (Figure 1-17):

Phase 1: Digestion. Large molecules are broken down into smaller subunits: proteins into amino acids, polysaccharides into simple sugars (i.e., monosaccharides), and fats into fatty acids and glycerol. These processes occur outside the cell and are activated by secreted enzymes.

Phase 2: Glycolysis and oxidation. The most important part of phase 2 is glycolysis, the splitting of glucose. Glycolysis produces two molecules of ATP per glucose molecule through oxidation, or the removal and transfer of a pair of electrons. The total process is called *oxidative cellular metabolism* and involves ten biochemical reactions (Figure 1-18).

Phase 3: Citric acid cycle (Krebs cycle, tricarboxylic acid cycle). Most of the ATP is generated during this final phase, which begins with the citric acid cycle and ends with oxidative phosphorylation. About two thirds of the total oxidation of carbon compounds in most cells is accomplished during this phase. The major end products are carbon dioxide (CO_2) and two dinucleotides—reduced nicotinamide adenine dinucleotide (NADH) and the reduced form of flavin adenine dinucleotide ($FADH_2$)—both of which transfer their electrons into the electron-transport chain.

Oxidative Phosphorylation

Oxidative phosphorylation occurs in the mitochondria and is the mechanism by which the energy produced from carbohydrates, fats, and proteins is transferred to ATP. During the breakdown (catabolism) of foods, many reactions involve the removal of electrons from various intermediates. These reactions generally require a coenzyme (a nonprotein carrier molecule), such as nicotinamide adenine dinucleotide

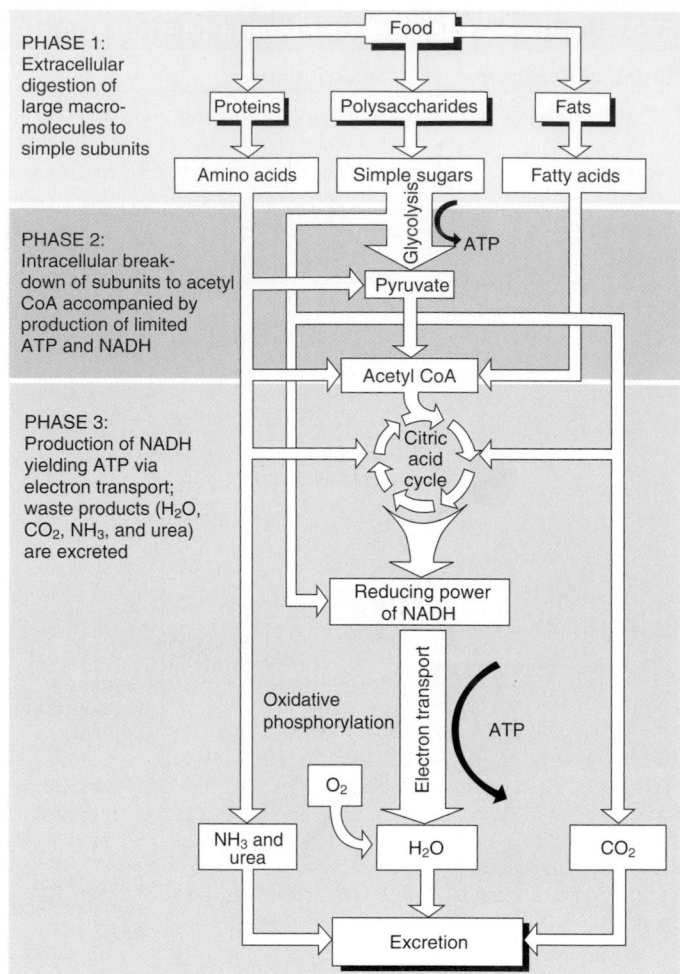

FIGURE 1-17 Three Phases of Catabolism, Which Lead from Food to Waste Products. These reactions produce adenosine triphosphate (ATP), which is used to power other processes in the cell.

(NAD), to transfer the electrons and thus are called **transfer reactions**.

Molecules of NAD and flavin adenine dinucleotide (FAD) transfer electrons they have gained from the oxidation of substrates to molecular oxygen, O_2. The electrons from reduced NAD and FAD, NADH and $FADH_2$, respectively, are transferred to the **electron-transport chain** on the inner surfaces of the mitochondria with the release of hydrogen ions. Some carrier molecules are brightly colored, iron-containing proteins known as cytochromes that accept a pair of electrons. These electrons eventually combine with molecular oxygen.

If oxygen is not available to the electron-transport chain, ATP will not be formed by the mitochondria. Instead, an anaerobic (without oxygen) metabolic pathway synthesizes ATP. This process, called **substrate phosphorylation** or **anaerobic glycolysis**, is linked to the breakdown (glycolysis) of carbohydrate (see Figure 1-18). Because glycolysis occurs in the cytoplasm of the cell, it provides energy for cells that lack mitochondria. The reactions in anaerobic glycolysis involve the conversion of glucose to pyruvic acid (pyruvate) with the simultaneous production of ATP. With the glycolysis of one molecule of glucose, two ATP molecules and two molecules of pyruvate are liberated. If oxygen is present, the two molecules of pyruvate move into the mitochondria, where they enter the citric acid cycle (Figure 1-19).

FIGURE 1-18 Glycolysis. Sugars are important for fuel or energy and they are oxidized in small steps to carbon dioxide (CO_2) and water. Glycolysis is the process for oxidizing sugars or glucose. Breakdown of glucose. **A,** Anaerobic catabolism, to lactic acid and little ATP. **B,** Aerobic catabolism, to carbon dioxide, water, and lots of ATP. (From Herlihy B: *The human body in health and illness,* ed 5, St Louis, 2015, Saunders.)

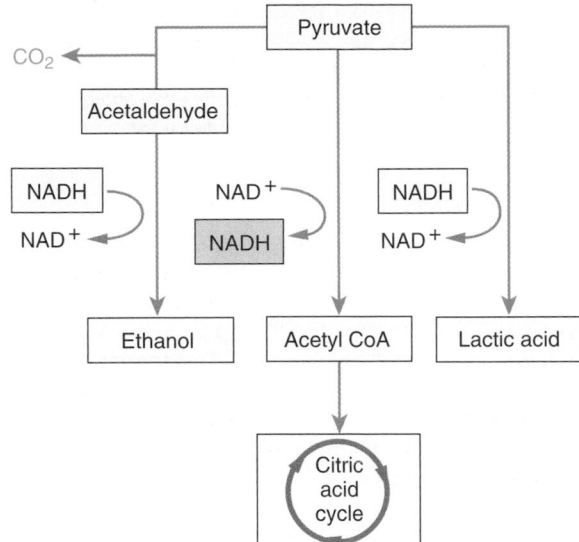

FIGURE 1-19 What Happens to Pyruvate, the Product of Glycolysis? In the presence of oxygen, pyruvate is oxidized to acetyl coenzyme A *(Acetyl CoA)* and enters the citric acid cycle. In the absence of oxygen, pyruvate instead is reduced, accepting the electrons extracted during glycolysis and carried by reduced nicotinamide adenine dinucleotide *(NADH).* When pyruvate is reduced directly, as it is in muscles, the product is lactic acid. When CO_2 is first removed from pyruvate and the remainder is reduced, as it is in yeasts, the resulting product is ethanol.

If oxygen is absent, pyruvate is converted to lactic acid, which is released into the extracellular fluid. The conversion of pyruvic acid to lactic acid is reversible; therefore once oxygen is restored, lactic acid is quickly converted back to either pyruvic acid or glucose. The anaerobic generation of ATP from glucose through glycolysis is not as efficient as the aerobic generation process. Adding an oxygen-requiring stage to the catabolic process (phase 3; see Figure 1-17) provides cells with a much more powerful method for extracting energy from food molecules.

MEMBRANE TRANSPORT: CELLULAR INTAKE AND OUTPUT

Cell survival and growth depend on the constant exchange of molecules with their environment. Cells continually import nutrients, fluids, and chemical messengers from the extracellular environment and expel metabolites, or the products of metabolism, and end products of lysosomal digestion. Cells also must regulate ions in their cytosol and organelles. Simple diffusion across the lipid bilayer of the plasma membrane occurs for such important molecules as O_2 and CO_2. However, the majority of molecular transfer depends on specialized membrane transport proteins that span the lipid bilayer and provide private conduits for select molecules.[1] Membrane transport proteins occur in many forms and are present in all cell membranes.[1] Transport by membrane transport proteins is sometimes called mediated transport. Most of these transport proteins allow selective passage (for example, Na^+ but not K^+ or K^+ but not Na^+). Each type of cell

membrane has its own transport proteins that determine which solute can pass into and out of the cell or organelle.[1] The two main classes of membrane transport proteins are *transporters* and *channels.* These transport proteins differ in the type of solute—small particles of dissolved substances—they transport. A transporter is specific, allowing only those ions that fit the unique binding sites on the protein (Figure 1-20, *A*). A transporter undergoes conformational changes to enable membrane transport. A channel, when open, forms a pore across the lipid bilayer that allows ions and selective polar organic molecules to diffuse across the membrane (see Figure 1-20, *B*). Transport by a channel depends on the size and electrical charge of the molecule. Some channels are controlled by a gate mechanism that determines which solute can move into it. Ion channels are responsible for the electrical excitability of nerve and muscle cells and play a critical role in the membrane potential.

The mechanisms of membrane transport depend on the characteristics of the substance to be transported. In passive transport, water and small, electrically uncharged molecules move easily through pores in the plasma membrane's lipid bilayer (see Figure 1-20). This process occurs naturally through any semipermeable barrier. Molecules will easily flow "downhill" from a region of high concentration to a region of low concentration; this movement is called *passive* because it does not require expenditure of energy or a driving force. It is driven by osmosis, hydrostatic pressure, and diffusion, all of which depend on the laws of physics and do not require life.

Other molecules are too large to pass through pores or are ligands bound to receptors on the cell's plasma membrane. Some of these molecules are moved into and out of the cell by active transport, which requires life, biologic activity, and the cell's expenditure of metabolic energy (see Figure 1-20). Unlike passive transport, active transport occurs across only living membranes that have to drive the flow

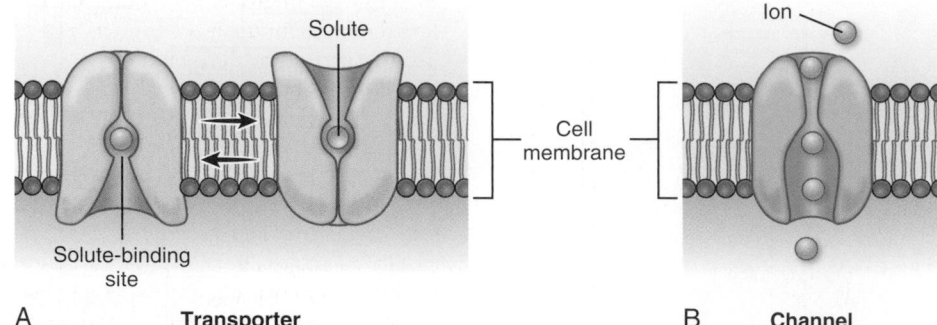

FIGURE 1-20 Inorganic Ions and Small, Polar Organic Molecules Can Cross a Cell Membrane Through Either a Transporter or a Channel. (Adapted from Alberts B: *Essential cell biology,* ed 4, New York, 2014, Garland.)

FIGURE 1-21 Pumps Carry Out Active Transport in Three Ways. 1, *Coupled pumps* link the uphill transport of one solute to the downhill transport of another solute. **2,** *ATP-driven pumps* drive uphill transport from hydrolysis of ATP. **3,** *Light-driven pumps* are mostly found in bacteria and use energy from sunlight to drive uphill transport. (Adapted from Alberts B: *Essential cell biology,* ed 4, New York, 2014, Garland.)

"uphill" by coupling it to an energy source (see p. 21). Movement of a solute against its concentration gradient occurs by special types of transporters called *pumps* (see Figure 1-20). These transporter pumps must harness an energy source to power the transport process. Energy can come from ATP hydrolysis, a transmembrane ion gradient, or sunlight (Figure 1-21). The best-known energy source is the Na$^+$-K$^+$–dependent adenosine triphosphatase (ATPase) pump (see Figure 1-26). It continuously regulates the cell's volume by controlling leaks through pores or protein channels and maintaining the ionic concentration gradients needed for cellular excitation and membrane conductivity (see p. 24). The maintenance of intracellular K$^+$ concentrations is required also for enzyme activity, including enzymes involved in protein synthesis (see Figure 1-21). Large molecules (macromolecules), along with fluids, are transported by endocytosis (taking

in) and exocytosis (expelling) (see p. 21). Receptor-macromolecule complexes enter the cell by means of receptor-mediated endocytosis (see p. 24).

Mediated transport systems can move solute molecules singly or two at a time. Two molecules can be moved simultaneously in one direction (a process called **symport**; for example, sodium-glucose in the digestive tract) or in opposite directions (called **antiport**; for example, the sodium-potassium pump in all cells), or a single molecule can be moved in one direction (called **uniport**; for example, glucose) (Figure 1-22).

Electrolytes as Solutes

Body fluids are composed of **electrolytes**, which are electrically charged and dissociate into constituent **ions** when placed in solution, and

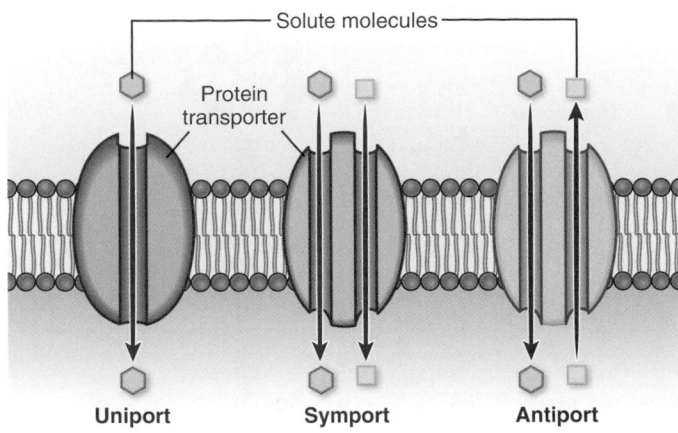

FIGURE 1-22 Mediated Transport. Illustration shows simultaneous movement of a single solute molecule in one direction *(Uniport),* of two different solute molecules in one direction *(Symport),* and of two different solute molecules in opposite directions *(Antiport).*

nonelectrolytes, such as glucose, urea, and creatinine, which do not dissociate. Electrolytes account for approximately 95% of the solute molecules in body water. Electrolytes exhibit **polarity** by orienting themselves toward the positive or negative pole. Ions with a positive charge are known as **cations** and migrate toward the negative pole, or cathode, if an electrical current is passed through the electrolyte solution. **Anions** carry a negative charge and migrate toward the positive pole, or anode, in the presence of electrical current. Anions and cations are located in both the intracellular fluid (ICF) and the extracellular fluid (ECF) compartments, although their concentration depends on their location. (Fluid and electrolyte balance between body compartments is discussed in Chapter 5.) For example, sodium (Na^+) is the predominant extracellular cation, and potassium (K^+) is the principal intracellular cation. The difference in ICF and ECF concentrations of these ions is important to the transmission of electrical impulses across the plasma membranes of nerve and muscle cells.

Electrolytes are measured in milliequivalents per liter (mEq/L) or milligrams per deciliter (mg/dl). The term *milliequivalent* indicates the chemical-combining activity of an ion, which depends on the electrical charge, or **valence**, of its ions. In abbreviations, valence is indicated by the number of plus or minus signs. One milliequivalent of any cation can combine chemically with 1 mEq of any anion: one monovalent anion will combine with one monovalent cation. Divalent ions combine more strongly than monovalent ions. To maintain electrochemical balance, one divalent ion will combine with two monovalent ions (e.g., $Ca^{++} + 2Cl^- \rightleftharpoons CaCl_2$).

Passive Transport: Diffusion, Filtration, and Osmosis

Diffusion. **Diffusion** is the movement of a solute molecule from an area of greater solute concentration to an area of lesser solute concentration. This difference in concentration is known as a **concentration gradient**. Although particles in a solution move randomly in any direction, if the concentration of particles in one part of the solution is greater than that in another part, the particles distribute themselves evenly throughout the solution. According to the same principle, if the concentration of particles is greater on one side of a *permeable*

membrane than on the other side, the particles diffuse spontaneously from the area of greater concentration to the area of lesser concentration until equilibrium is reached. The higher the concentration on one side, the greater the diffusion rate.

The diffusion rate is influenced by differences of electrical potential across the membrane (see p. 24). Because the pores in the lipid bilayer are often lined with Ca^{++}, other cations (e.g., Na^+ and K^+) diffuse slowly because they are repelled by positive charges in the pores.

The rate of diffusion of a substance depends also on its size (diffusion coefficient) and its lipid solubility (Figure 1-23). Usually, the smaller the molecule and the more soluble it is in oil, the more hydrophobic or nonpolar it is and the more rapidly it will diffuse across the bilayer. Oxygen, carbon dioxide, and steroid hormones (for example, androgens and estrogens) are all nonpolar molecules. Water-soluble substances, such as glucose and inorganic ions, diffuse very slowly, whereas uncharged lipophilic ("lipid-loving") molecules, such as fatty acids and steroids, diffuse rapidly. Ions and other polar molecules generally diffuse across cellular membranes more slowly than lipid-soluble substances.

Water readily diffuses through biologic membranes because water molecules are small and uncharged. The dipolar structure of water allows it to rapidly cross the regions of the bilayer containing the lipid head groups. The lipid head groups constitute the two outer regions of the lipid bilayer.

Filtration: hydrostatic pressure. **Filtration** is the movement of water and solutes through a membrane because of a greater pushing pressure (force) on one side of the membrane than on the other side. **Hydrostatic pressure** is the mechanical force of water pushing against cellular membranes (Figure 1-24, *A*). In the vascular system, hydrostatic pressure is the *blood pressure* generated in vessels when the heart contracts. Blood reaching the capillary bed has a hydrostatic pressure of 25 to 30 mm Hg, which is sufficient force to push water across the thin capillary membranes into the interstitial space. Hydrostatic pressure is partially balanced by osmotic pressure, whereby water moving *out* of the capillaries is partially balanced by osmotic forces that tend to *pull* water *into* the capillaries (Figure 1-24, *B*). Water that is not osmotically attracted back into the capillaries moves into the lymph system (see the discussion of Starling forces in Chapter 5).

Osmosis. **Osmosis** is the movement of water "down" a concentration gradient—that is, across a semipermeable membrane from a region of higher water concentration to one of lower concentration. For osmosis to occur, (1) the membrane must be more permeable to water than to solutes and (2) the concentration of solutes on one side of the membrane must be greater than that on the other side so that water moves more easily. Osmosis is directly related to both hydrostatic pressure and solute concentration but *not* to particle size or weight. For example, particles of the plasma protein albumin are small but are more concentrated in body fluids than the larger and heavier particles of globulin. Therefore albumin exerts a greater osmotic force than does globulin.

Osmolality controls the distribution and movement of water between body compartments. The terms *osmolality* and *osmolarity* often are used interchangeably in reference to osmotic activity, but they define different measurements. **Osmolality** measures the number of milliosmoles per kilogram (mOsm/kg) of water, or the concentration of molecules per *weight* of water. **Osmolarity** measures the number of milliosmoles per liter of solution, or the concentration of molecules per *volume* of solution.

In solutions that contain only dissociable substances, such as sodium and chloride, the difference between the two measurements is

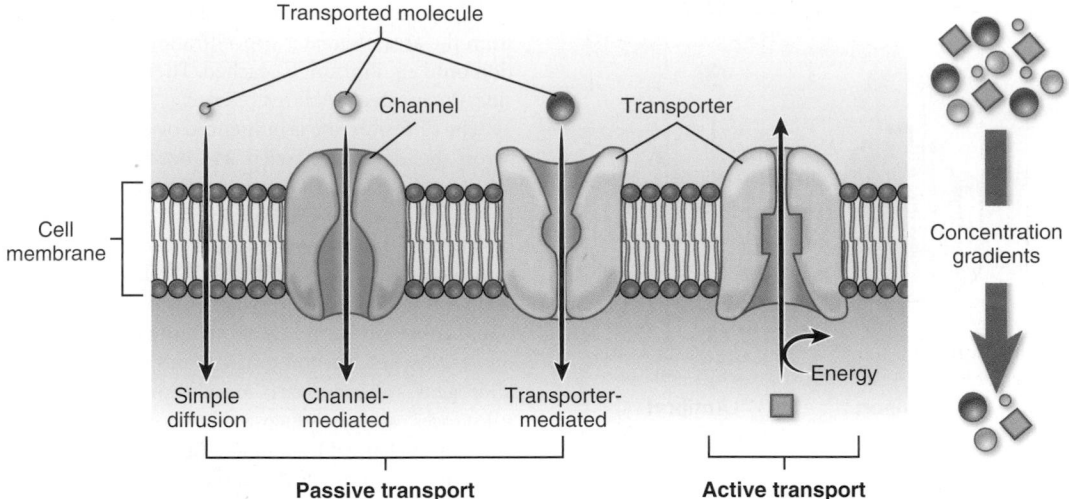

FIGURE 1-23 Passive Diffusion of Solute Molecules Across the Plasma Membrane. Oxygen, nitrogen, water, urea, glycerol, and carbon dioxide can diffuse readily down the concentration gradient. Macromolecules are too large to diffuse through pores in the plasma membrane. Ions may be repelled if the pores contain substances with identical charges. If the pores are lined with cations, for example, other cations will have difficulty diffusing because the positive charges will repel one another. Diffusion can still occur, but it occurs more slowly.

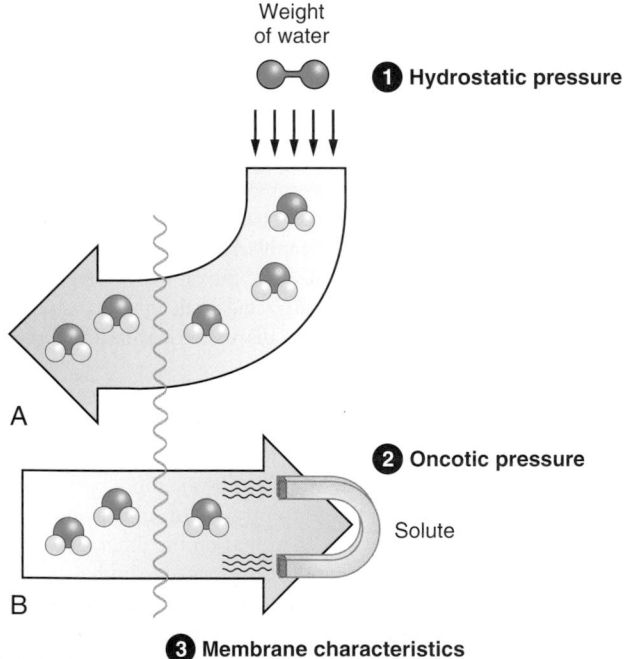

FIGURE 1-24 Hydrostatic Pressure and Oncotic Pressure in Plasma. 1, Hydrostatic pressure in plasma. **2,** Oncotic pressure exerted by proteins in the plasma usually tends to *pull* water into the circulatory system. **3,** Individuals with low protein levels (e.g., starvation) are unable to maintain a normal oncotic pressure; therefore water is not reabsorbed into the circulation and, instead, causes body edema.

negligible. When considering all the different solutes in plasma (e.g., proteins, glucose, lipids), however, the difference between osmolality and osmolarity becomes more significant. Less of plasma's weight is water, and the overall concentration of particles is therefore greater. The osmolality will be greater than the osmolarity because of the smaller proportion of water. Osmolality is thus preferred in human clinical assessment.

The normal osmolality of body fluids is 280 to 294 mOsm/kg. The osmolalities of intracellular and extracellular fluids tend to equalize, providing a measure of body fluid concentration and thus the body's hydration status. Hydration is affected also by hydrostatic pressure because the movement of water by osmosis can be opposed by an equal amount of hydrostatic pressure. The amount of hydrostatic pressure required to oppose the osmotic movement of water is called the osmotic pressure of the solution. Factors that determine osmotic pressure are the type and thickness of the plasma membrane, the size of the molecules, the concentration of molecules or the concentration gradient, and the solubility of molecules within the membrane.

Effective osmolality is sustained osmotic activity and depends on the concentration of solutes remaining on one side of a permeable membrane. If the solutes penetrate the membrane and equilibrate with the solution on the other side of the membrane, the osmotic effect will be diminished or lost.

Plasma proteins influence osmolality because they have a negative charge (see Figure 1-24, *B*). The principle involved is known as *Gibbs-Donnan equilibrium;* it occurs when the fluid in one compartment contains small, diffusible ions, such as Na^+ and chloride (Cl^-), together with large, nondiffusible, charged particles, such as plasma proteins. Because the body tends to maintain an electrical equilibrium, the nondiffusible protein molecules cause asymmetry in the distribution of small ions. Anions such as Cl^- are thus driven out of the cell or plasma, and cations such as Na^+ are attracted to the cell. The protein-containing compartment maintains a state of electroneutrality, but the osmolality is higher. The overall osmotic effect of colloids, such as plasma proteins, is called the oncotic pressure, or colloid osmotic pressure.

Tonicity describes the effective osmolality of a solution. (The terms osmolality and tonicity may be used interchangeably.) Solutions have relative degrees of tonicity. An isotonic solution (or isosmotic solution) has the same osmolality or concentration of particles (285 mOsm) as

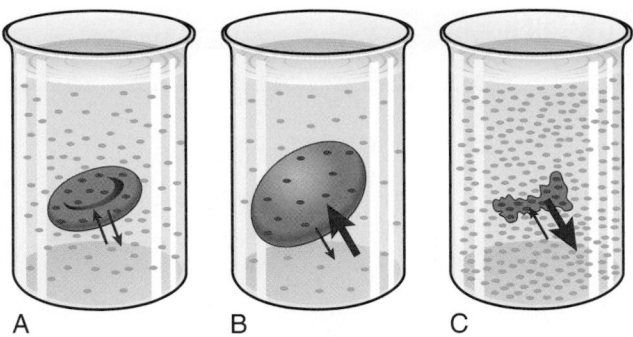

FIGURE 1-25 Tonicity. Tonicity is important, especially for red blood cell function. **A**, Isotonic solution. **B**, Hypotonic solution. **C**, Hypertonic solution. (From Waugh A, Grant A: *Ross and Wilson anatomy and physiology in health and illness*, ed 12, London, 2012, Churchill Livingstone.)

the ICF or ECF. A hypotonic solution has a lower concentration and is thus more dilute than body fluids (Figure 1-25). A hypertonic solution has a concentration of more than 285 to 294 mOsm/kg. The concept of tonicity is important when correcting water and solute imbalances by administering different types of replacement solutions (see Figure 1-25) (see Chapter 5).

✔ QUICK CHECK 1-2

1. What does glycolysis produce?
2. Define membrane transport proteins.
3. What are the differences between passive and active transport?
4. Why do water and small, electrically charged molecules move easily through pores in the plasma membrane?

Active Transport of Na⁺ and K⁺

The active transport system for Na^+ and K^+ is found in virtually all mammalian cells. The Na^+-K^+–antiport system (i.e., Na^+ moving out of the cell and K^+ moving into the cell) uses the direct energy of ATP to transport these cations. The transporter protein is ATPase, which requires Na^+, K^+, and magnesium (Mg^{++}) ions. The concentration of ATPase in plasma membranes is directly related to Na^+-K^+–transport activity. Approximately 60% to 70% of the ATP synthesized by cells, especially muscle and nerve cells, is used to maintain the Na^+-K^+–transport system. Excitable tissues have a high concentration of Na^+-K^+ ATPase, as do other tissues that transport significant amounts of Na^+. For every ATP molecule hydrolyzed, three molecules of Na^+ are transported out of the cell, whereas only two molecules of K^+ move into the cell. The process leads to an electrical potential and is called *electrogenic*, with the inside of the cell more negative than the outside. Although the exact mechanism for this transport is uncertain, it is possible that ATPase induces the transporter protein to undergo several conformational changes, causing Na^+ and K^+ to move short distances (Figure 1-26). The conformational change lowers the affinity for Na^+ and K^+ to the ATPase transporter, resulting in the release of the cations after transport.

Table 1-4 summarizes the major mechanisms of transport through pores and protein transporters in the plasma membranes. Many disease

FIGURE 1-26 Active Transport and the Sodium-Potassium Pump. 1, Three Na^+ ions bind to sodium-binding sites on the carrier's inner face. 2, At the same time, an energy-containing adenosine triphosphate *(ATP)* molecule produced by the cell's mitochondria binds to the carrier. The ATP dissociates, transferring its stored energy to the carrier. 3 and 4, The carrier then changes shape, releases the three Na^+ ions to the outside of the cell, and attracts two potassium *(K⁺)* ions to its potassium-binding sites. 5, The carrier then returns to its original shape, releasing the two K^+ ions and the remnant of the ATP molecule to the inside of the cell. The carrier is now ready for another pumping cycle.

states are caused or manifested by loss of these membrane transport systems.

Transport by Vesicle Formation
Endocytosis and Exocytosis

The active transport mechanisms by which the cells move large proteins, polynucleotides, or polysaccharides (macromolecules) across the plasma membrane are very different from those that mediate small solute and ion transport. Transport of macromolecules involves the sequential formation and fusion of membrane-bound vesicles.

TABLE 1-4   Major Transport Systems in Mammalian Cells

Substance Transported	Mechanism of Transport*	Tissues
Carbohydrates		
Glucose	Passive: protein channel	Most tissues
	Active: symport with Na^+	
Fructose	Active: symport with Na^+	Small intestines and renal tubular cells
	Passive	Intestines and liver
Amino Acids		
Amino acid specific transporters	Coupled channels	Intestines, kidney, and liver
All amino acids except proline	Active: symport with Na^+	Liver
Specific amino acids	Active: group translocation	Small intestine
	Passive	
Other Organic Molecules		
Cholic acid, deoxycholic acid, and taurocholic acid	Active: symport with Na^+	Intestines
Organic anions (e.g., malate, α-ketoglutarate, glutamate)	Antiport with counter–organic anion	Mitochondria of liver cells
ATP-ADP	Antiport transport of nucleotides; can be active	Mitochondria of liver cells
Inorganic Ions		
Na^+	Passive	Distal renal tubular cells
Na^+/H^+	Active antiport, proton pump	Proximal renal tubular cells and small intestines
Na^+/K^+	Active: ATP driven, protein channel	Plasma membrane of most cells
Ca^{++}	Active: ATP driven, antiport with Na^+	All cells, antiporter in red cells
H^+/K^+	Active	Parietal cells of gastric cells secreting H^+
Cl^-/HCO_3^- (perhaps other anions)	Mediated: antiport (anion transporter–band 3 protein)	Erythrocytes and many other cells
Water	Osmosis passive	All tissues

Data from Alberts B et al: *Molecular biology of the cell,* ed 4, New York, 2001, Wiley; Alberts B et al: *Essential cell biology,* ed 4, New York, 2014, Garland, Devlin TM, editor: *Textbook of biochemistry: with clinical correlations,* ed 3, New York, 1992, Wiley; Raven PH, Johnson GB: *Understanding biology,* ed 3, Dubuque, IA, 1995, Brown.
*NOTE: The known transport systems are listed here; others have been proposed. Most transport systems have been studied in only a few tissues and their sites of activity may be more limited than indicated.
ADP, Adenosine diphosphate; *ATP,* adenosine triphosphate.

In endocytosis, a section of the plasma membrane enfolds substances from outside the cell, invaginates (folds inward), and separates from the plasma membrane, forming a vesicle that moves into the cell (Figure 1-27, *A*). Two types of endocytosis are designated based on the size of the vesicle formed. Pinocytosis (cell drinking) involves the ingestion of fluids, bits of the plasma membrane, and solute molecules through formation of small vesicles; and phagocytosis (cell eating) involves the ingestion of large particles, such as bacteria, through formation of large vesicles (vacuoles).

Because most cells continually ingest fluid and solutes by pinocytosis, the terms *pinocytosis* and *endocytosis* often are used interchangeably. In pinocytosis, the vesicle containing fluids, solutes, or both fuses with a lysosome, and lysosomal enzymes digest the vesicle's contents for use by the cell. Vesicles that bud from membranes have a particular protein coat on their cytosolic surface and are called coated vesicles. The best studied are those that have an outer coat of bristlelike structures—the protein clathrin. Pinocytosis occurs mainly by the clathrin-coated pits and vesicles (Figure 1-28). After the coated pits pinch off from the plasma membrane, they quickly shed their coats and fuse with an endosome. An endosome is a vesicle pinched off from the plasma membrane from which its contents can be recycled to the plasma membrane or sent to lysosomes for digestion. In phagocytosis, the large molecular substances are engulfed by the plasma membrane and enter the cell so that they can be isolated and destroyed by lysosomal enzymes (see Chapter 6). Substances that are not degraded by lysosomes are isolated in residual bodies and released by exocytosis.

BOX 1-2   The New Endocytic Matrix

An explosion of new data is disclosing a much more involved role for endocytosis than just a simple way to internalize nutrients and membrane-associated molecules. These new data show that endocytosis not only is a master organizer of signaling pathways but also has a major role in managing signals in time and space. Endocytosis appears to control signaling; therefore it determines the net output of biochemical pathways. This occurs because endocytosis modulates the presence of receptors and their ligands as well as effectors at the plasma membrane or at intermediate stations of the endocytic route. The overall processes and anatomy of these new functions are sometimes called the "endocytic matrix." All of these functions ultimately have a large impact on almost every cellular process, including the nucleus.

Both pinocytosis and phagocytosis require metabolic energy and often involve binding of the substance with plasma membrane receptors before membrane invagination and fusion with lysosomes in the cell. New data are revealing that endocytosis has an even larger and more important role than previously known (Box 1-2).

In eukaryotic cells, secretion of macromolecules almost always occurs by exocytosis (see Figure 1-27). Exocytosis has two main functions: (1) replacement of portions of the plasma membrane that have been removed by endocytosis and (2) release of molecules synthesized by the cells into the extracellular matrix.

FIGURE 1-27 Endocytosis and Exocytosis. A, Endocytosis and fusion with lysosome and exocytosis. **B,** Electron micrograph of exocytosis. (**B** from Raven PH, Johnson GB: *Biology*, ed 5, New York, 1999, McGraw-Hill.)

FIGURE 1-28 Ligand Internalization by Means of Receptor-Mediated Endocytosis. A, The ligand attaches to its surface receptor (through the bristle coat or clathrin coat) and, through receptor-mediated endocytosis, enters the cell. The ingested material fuses with a lysosome and is processed by hydrolytic lysosomal enzymes. Processed molecules can then be transferred to other cellular components. **B,** Electron micrograph of a coated pit showing different sizes of filaments of the cytoskeleton (×82,000). (**B** from Erlandsen SL, Magney JE: *Color atlas of histology*, St Louis, 1992, Mosby.)

Receptor-Mediated Endocytosis

The internalization process, called receptor-mediated endocytosis (ligand internalization), is rapid and enables the cell to ingest large amounts of receptor-macromolecule complexes in clathrin-coated vesicles without ingesting large volumes of extracellular fluid (see Figure 1-28). The cellular uptake of cholesterol, for example, depends on receptor-mediated endocytosis. Additionally, many essential metabolites (for example, vitamin B_{12} and iron) depend on receptor-mediated endocytosis and, unfortunately, the influenza flu virus.

Caveolae

The outer surface of the plasma membrane is dimpled with tiny flask-shaped pits (cavelike) called caveolae. Caveolae are thought to form from membrane microdomains or lipid rafts. Caveolae are cholesterol- and glycosphingolipid-rich microdomains where the protein *caveolin* is thought to be involved in several processes, including clathrin-independent endocytosis, cellular cholesterol regulation and transport, and cellular communication. Many proteins, including a variety of receptors, cluster in these tiny chambers.

Caveolae are not only uptake vehicles but also important sites for signal transduction, a tedious process in which extracellular chemical messages or *signals* are communicated to the cell's interior for execution. For example, in vitro evidence now exists that plasma membrane estrogen receptors can localize in caveolae, and crosstalk with estradiol facilitates several intracellular biologic actions.[21]

Movement of Electrical Impulses: Membrane Potentials

All body cells are electrically polarized, with the inside of the cell more negatively charged than the outside. The difference in electrical charge, or voltage, is known as the resting membrane potential and is about −70 to −85 millivolts (mV). The difference in voltage across the plasma membrane results from the differences in ionic composition of ICF and ECF. Sodium ions are more concentrated in the ECF, and potassium ions are in greater concentration in the ICF. The concentration difference is maintained by the active transport of Na^+ and K^+ (the sodium-potassium pump), which transports sodium outward and potassium inward (Figure 1-29). Because the resting plasma membrane is more permeable to K^+ than to Na^+, K^+ diffuses easily from the ICF to the ECF. Because both sodium and potassium are cations, the net result is an excess of anions inside the cell, resulting in the resting membrane potential.

Nerve and muscle cells are excitable and can change their resting membrane potential in response to electrochemical stimuli. Changes in resting membrane potential convey messages from cell to cell. When a nerve or muscle cell receives a stimulus that exceeds the membrane threshold value, a rapid change occurs in the resting membrane potential, known as the action potential. The action potential carries signals along the nerve or muscle cell and conveys information from one cell to another in a domino-like fashion. Nerve impulses are described in Chapter 13. When a resting cell is stimulated through voltage-regulated channels, the cell membranes become more permeable to sodium, so a net movement of sodium into the cell occurs and the membrane potential decreases, or moves forward, from a negative value (in millivolts) to zero. This decrease is known as depolarization. The depolarized cell is more positively charged, and its polarity is neutralized.

To generate an action potential and the resulting depolarization, the threshold potential must be reached. Generally this occurs when the cell has depolarized by 15 to 20 millivolts. When the threshold is

FIGURE 1-29 Sodium-Potassium Pump and Propagation of an Action Potential. A, Concentration difference of sodium *(Na⁺)* and potassium *(K⁺)* intracellularly and extracellularly. The direction of active transport by the sodium-potassium pump is also shown. **B,** The left diagram represents the polarized state of a neuronal membrane when at rest. The middle and right diagrams represent changes in sodium and potassium membrane permeabilities with depolarization and repolarization.

reached, the cell will continue to depolarize with no further stimulation. The sodium gates open, and sodium rushes into the cell, causing the membrane potential to drop to zero and then become positive (depolarization). The rapid reversal in polarity results in the action potential.

During repolarization, the negative polarity of the resting membrane potential is reestablished. As the voltage-gated sodium channels begin to close, voltage-gated potassium channels open. Membrane permeability to sodium decreases and potassium permeability increases, so potassium ions leave the cell. The sodium gates close, and with the loss of potassium the membrane potential becomes more negative. The Na^+, K^+ pump then returns the membrane to the resting potential by pumping potassium back into the cell and sodium out of the cell.

During most of the action potential, the plasma membrane cannot respond to an additional stimulus. This time is known as the absolute refractory period and is related to changes in permeability to sodium. During the latter phase of the action potential, when permeability to potassium increases, a stronger-than-normal stimulus can evoke an action potential; this time is known as the relative refractory period.

When the membrane potential is more negative than normal, the cell is in a hyperpolarized state (less excitable: decreased K^+ levels within the cell). A stronger-than-normal stimulus is then required to reach the threshold potential and generate an action potential. When the membrane potential is more positive than normal, the cell is in a hypopolarized state (more excitable than normal: increased K^+ levels within the cell) and a weaker-than-normal stimulus is required to reach the threshold potential. Changes in the intracellular and extracellular concentrations of ions or a change in membrane permeability can cause these alterations in membrane excitability.

CELLULAR REPRODUCTION: THE CELL CYCLE

Human cells are subject to wear and tear, and most do not last for the lifetime of the individual. In most tissues, new cells are created as fast as old cells die. Cellular reproduction is therefore necessary for the maintenance of life. Reproduction of gametes (sperm and egg cells) occurs through a process called *meiosis*, described in Chapter 2. The reproduction, or division, of other body cells (somatic cells) involves two sequential phases—mitosis, or nuclear division, and cytokinesis, or cytoplasmic division. Before a cell can divide, however, it must double its mass and duplicate all its contents. Separation for division occurs during the growth phase, called interphase. The alternation between mitosis and interphase in all tissues with cellular turnover is known as the cell cycle.

The four designated phases of the cell cycle (Figure 1-30) are (1) the S phase (S = synthesis), in which DNA is synthesized in the cell nucleus; (2) the G_2 phase (G = gap), in which RNA and protein synthesis occurs, namely, the period between the completion of DNA synthesis and the next phase (M); (3) the M phase (M = mitosis),

FIGURE 1-30 Interphase and the Phases of Mitosis. A, The G_1/S checkpoint is to "check" for cell size, nutrients, growth factors, and DNA damage. See text for resting phases. The G_2/M checkpoint checks for cell size and DNA replication. **B,** The orderly progression through the phases of the cell cycle is regulated by *cyclins* (so called because levels rise and fall) and *cyclin-dependent protein kinases* (CDKs) and their inhibitors. When cyclins are complexed with CDKs, cell cycle events are triggered.

TABLE 1-5　Examples of Growth Factors and Their Actions

Growth Factor	Physiologic Actions
Platelet-derived growth factor (PDGF)	Stimulates proliferation of connective tissue cells and neuroglial cells
Epidermal growth factor (EGF)	Stimulates proliferation of epidermal cells and other cell types
Insulin-like growth factor 1 (IGF-1)	Collaborates with PDGF and EGF; stimulates proliferation of fat cells and connective tissue cells
Vascular endothelial growth factor (VEGF)	Mediates functions of endothelial cells; proliferation, migration, invasion, survival, and permeability
Insulin-like growth factor 2 (IGF-2)	Collaborates with PDGF and EGF; stimulates or inhibits response of most cells to other growth factors; regulates differentiation of some cell types (e.g., cartilage)
Transforming growth factor-beta (TGF-β; multiple subtypes)	Stimulates or inhibits response of most cells to other growth factors; regulates differentiation of some cell types (e.g., cartilage)
Fibroblast growth factor (FGF; multiple subtypes)	Stimulates proliferation of fibroblasts, endothelial cells, myoblasts, and other multiple subtypes
Interleukin-2 (IL-2)	Stimulates proliferation of T lymphocytes
Nerve growth factor (NGF)	Promotes axon growth and survival of sympathetic and some sensory and central nervous system (CNS) neurons
Hematopoietic cell growth factors (IL-3, GM-CSF, G-CSF, erythropoietin)	Promote proliferation of blood cells

G-CSF, Granulocyte colony-stimulating factor; *GM-CSF,* granulocyte-macrophage colony-stimulating factor.

which includes both nuclear and cytoplasmic division; and (4) the G₁ phase, which is the period between the M phase and the start of DNA synthesis.

Phases of Mitosis and Cytokinesis

Interphase (the G₁, S, and G₂ phases) is the longest phase of the cell cycle. During interphase, the chromatin consists of very long, slender rods jumbled together in the nucleus. Late in interphase, strands of chromatin (the substance that gives the nucleus its granular appearance) begin to coil, causing shortening and thickening.

The M phase of the cell cycle, mitosis and cytokinesis, begins with prophase, the first appearance of chromosomes. As the phase proceeds, each chromosome is seen as two identical halves called chromatids, which lie together and are attached by a spindle site called a centromere. (The two chromatids of each chromosome, which are genetically identical, are sometimes called sister chromatids.) The nuclear membrane, which surrounds the nucleus, disappears. Spindle fibers are microtubules formed in the cytoplasm. They radiate from two centrioles located at opposite poles of the cell and pull the chromosomes to opposite sides of the cell, beginning metaphase. Next, the centromeres become aligned in the middle of the spindle, which is called the equatorial plate (or metaphase plate) of the cell. In this stage, chromosomes are easiest to observe microscopically because they are highly condensed and arranged in a relatively organized fashion.

Anaphase begins when the centromeres split and the sister chromatids are pulled apart. The spindle fibers shorten, causing the sister chromatids to be pulled, centromere first, toward opposite sides of the cell. When the sister chromatids are separated, each is considered to be a chromosome. Thus the cell has 92 chromosomes during this stage. By the end of anaphase, there are 46 chromosomes lying at each side of the cell. Barring mitotic errors, each of the 2 groups of 46 chromosomes is identical to the original 46 chromosomes present at the start of the cell cycle.

During telophase, the final stage, a new nuclear membrane is formed around each group of 46 chromosomes, the spindle fibers disappear, and the chromosomes begin to uncoil. Cytokinesis causes the cytoplasm to divide into almost equal parts during this phase. At the end of telophase, two identical diploid cells, called daughter cells, have been formed from the original cell.

Rates of Cellular Division

Although the complete cell cycle lasts 12 to 24 hours, about 1 hour is required for the four stages of mitosis and cytokinesis. All types of cells undergo mitosis during formation of the embryo, but many adult cells—such as nerve cells, lens cells of the eye, and muscle cells—lose their ability to replicate and divide. The cells of other tissues, particularly epithelial cells (e.g., cells of the intestine, lung, or skin), divide continuously and rapidly, completing the entire cell cycle in less than 10 hours.

The difference between cells that divide slowly and cells that divide rapidly is the length of time spent in the G₁ phase of the cell cycle. Once the S phase begins, however, progression through mitosis takes a relatively constant amount of time.

The mechanisms that control cell division depend on the integrity of genetic, epigenetic (heritable changes in genome function that occur without alterations in the DNA sequence; see Chapter 3), and protein growth factors. Protein growth factors govern the proliferation of different cell types. Individual cells are members of a complex cellular society in which survival of the entire organism is key—not survival or proliferation of just the individual cells. When a need arises for new cells, as in repair of injured cells, previously nondividing cells must be triggered rapidly to reenter the cell cycle. With continual wear and tear, the cell birth rate and the cell death rate must be kept in balance.

Growth Factors

Growth factors, also called cytokines, are peptides (protein fractions) that transmit signals within and between cells. They have a major role in the regulation of tissue growth and development (Table 1-5). Having nutrients is not enough for a cell to proliferate; it must also receive stimulatory chemical signals (growth factors) from other cells, usually its neighbors or the surrounding supporting tissue called stroma. These signals act to overcome intracellular braking mechanisms that tend to restrain cell growth and block progress through the cell cycle (Figure 1-31).

An example of a brake that regulates cell proliferation is the retinoblastoma (Rb) protein, first identified through studies of a rare childhood eye tumor called *retinoblastoma*, in which the Rb protein is missing or defective. The Rb protein is abundant in the nucleus of all

FIGURE 1-31 How Growth Factors Stimulate Cell Proliferation. **A,** Resting cell. With the absence of growth factors, the retinoblastoma *(Rb)* protein is not phosphorylated; thus it holds the gene regulatory proteins in an inactive state. The gene regulatory proteins are required to stimulate the transcription of genes needed for cell proliferation. **B,** Proliferating cell. Growth factors bind to the cell surface receptors and activate intracellular signaling pathways, leading to activation of intracellular proteins. These intracellular proteins phosphorylate and thereby inactivate the Rb protein. The gene regulatory proteins are now free to activate the transcription of genes, leading to cell proliferation.

vertebrate cells. It binds to gene regulatory proteins, preventing them from stimulating the transcription of genes required for cell proliferation (see Figure 1-31). Extracellular signals, such as growth factors, activate intracellular signaling pathways that inactivate the Rb protein, leading to cell proliferation.

Different types of cells require different growth factors; for example, **platelet-derived growth factor (PDGF)** stimulates the production of connective tissue cells. Table 1-5 summarizes the most significant growth factors. Evidence shows that some growth factors also regulate other cellular processes, such as cellular differentiation. In addition to growth factors that stimulate cellular processes, there are factors that inhibit these processes; these factors are not well understood. Cells that are starved of growth factors come to a halt after mitosis and enter the **arrested (resting) (G₀) state** of the cell cycle (see p. 25 for cell cycle).[1]

TISSUES

Cells of one or more types are organized into tissues, and different types of tissues compose organs. Finally, organs are integrated to perform complex functions as tracts or systems.

All cells are in contact with a network of extracellular macromolecules known as the extracellular matrix (see p. 10). This matrix not only holds cells and tissues together but also provides an organized latticework within which cells can migrate and interact with one another.

Tissue Formation

To form tissues, cells must exhibit intercellular recognition and communication, adhesion, and memory. Specialized cells sense their environment through signals, such as growth factors, from other cells. This type of communication ensures that new cells are produced only when and where they are required. Different cell types have different adhesion molecules in their plasma membranes, sticking selectively to other cells of the same type. They can also adhere to extracellular matrix components. Because cells are tiny and squishy and enclosed by a flimsy membrane, it is remarkable that they form a strong human being. Strength can occur because of the extracellular matrix and the strength of the cytoskeleton with cell-cell adhesions to neighboring cells. Cells have memory because of specialized patterns of gene expression evoked by signals that acted during embryonic development. Memory allows cells to autonomously preserve their distinctive character and pass it on to their progeny.[1]

Fully specialized or **terminally differentiated** cells that are lost are regenerated from proliferating *precursor cells.* These precursor cells have been derived from a smaller number of stem cells.[1] **Stem cells** are cells with the potential to develop into many different cell types during early development and growth. In many tissues, stem cells serve as an internal repair and maintenance system, dividing indefinitely. These cells can maintain themselves over very long periods of time, called **self-renewal,** and can generate all the differentiated cell types of the tissue or **multipotency.** This stem cell–driven tissue renewal is very evident in the epithelial lining of the intestine, stomach, blood cells, and skin, which is continuously exposed to environmental factors. A class of extracellular signaling proteins, known as **Wnt signals,** sustain tissue renewal and enable tissue to be continuously replenished and maintained over a lifetime.[22] When a stem cell divides, each daughter cell has a choice: it can remain as a stem cell or it can follow a pathway that results in terminal differentiation (Figure 1-32).

Types of Tissues

The four basic types of tissues are nerve, epithelial, connective, and muscle. The structure and function of these four types underlie the structure and function of each organ system. Neural tissue is composed of highly specialized cells called *neurons,* which receive and transmit electrical impulses rapidly across junctions called *synapses* (see Figure 13-1). Different types of neurons have special characteristics that depend on their distribution and function within the nervous system. Epithelial, connective, and muscle tissues are summarized in Tables 1-6, 1-7, and 1-8, respectively.

✓ QUICK CHECK 1-4
1. What is the cell cycle?
2. Discuss the five types of intracellular communication.
3. Why is the extracellular matrix important for tissue cells?

Text continued on p. 34

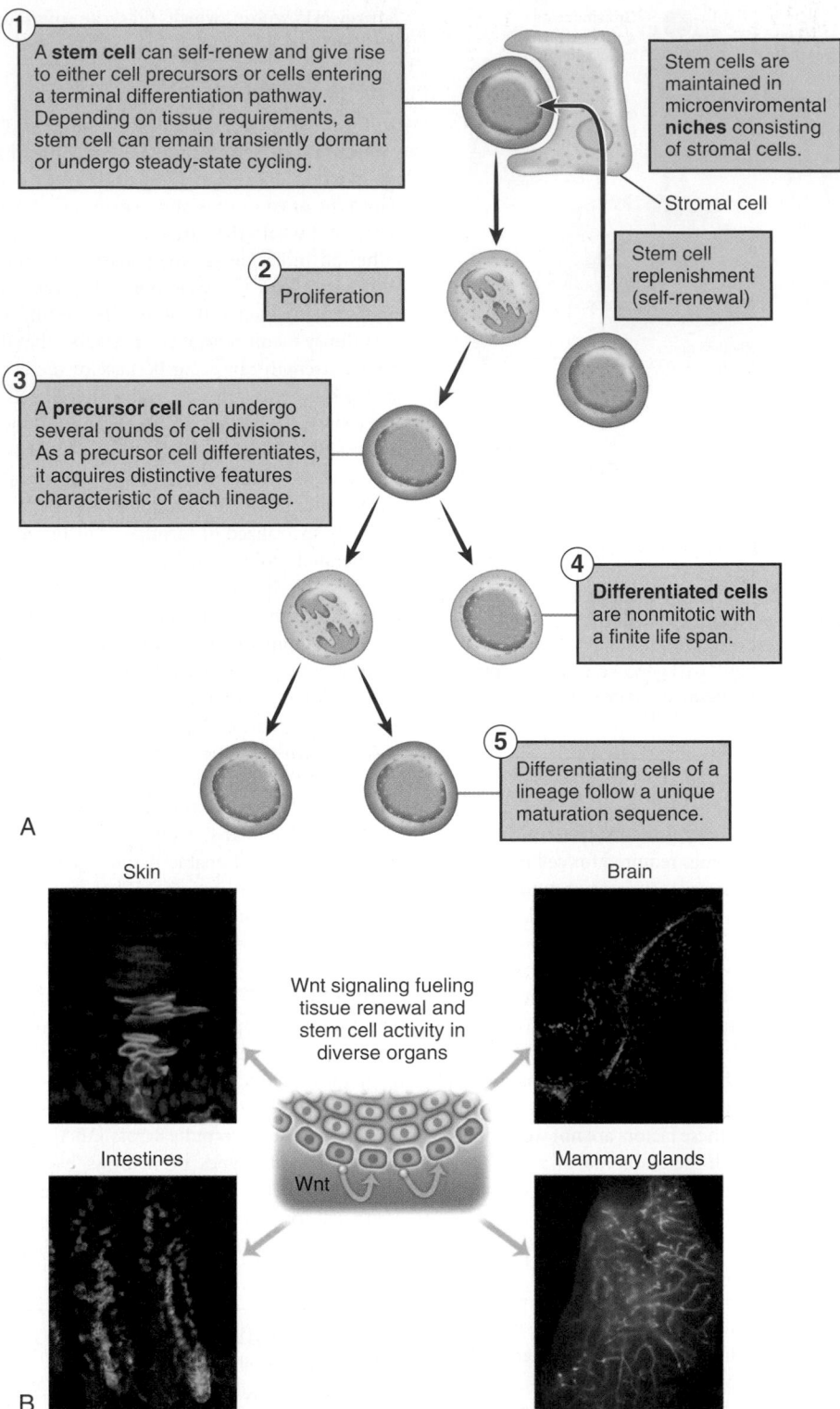

1 A **stem cell** can self-renew and give rise to either cell precursors or cells entering a terminal differentiation pathway. Depending on tissue requirements, a stem cell can remain transiently dormant or undergo steady-state cycling.

Stem cells are maintained in microenviromental **niches** consisting of stromal cells.

Stromal cell

Stem cell replenishment (self-renewal)

2 Proliferation

3 A **precursor cell** can undergo several rounds of cell divisions. As a precursor cell differentiates, it acquires distinctive features characteristic of each lineage.

4 **Differentiated cells** are nonmitotic with a finite life span.

5 Differentiating cells of a lineage follow a unique maturation sequence.

A

Skin

Brain

Wnt signaling fueling tissue renewal and stem cell activity in diverse organs

Intestines

Mammary glands

Wnt

B

FIGURE 1-32 Properties of Stem Cell Systems. A, Stem cells have three characteristics: *self-renewal, proliferation,* and *differentiation* into mature cells. Stem cells are housed in *niches* consisting of *stromal cells* that provide factors for their maintenance. Stem cells of the embryo can give rise to cell precursors that generate all the tissues of the body. This property defines stem cells as *multipotent.* Stem cells are difficult to identify anatomically. Their identification is based on specific *cell surface markers* (cell surface antigens recognized by specific monoclonal antibodies) and on the lineage they generate following *transplantation.* **B,** Wnt signaling fuels tissue renewal. (**A,** from Kierszenbaum A: *Histology and cell biology: an introduction to pathology,* ed 3, St Louis, 2012, Elsevier. **B,** from Clevers H, et al: *Science* 346(3), 2014.)

TABLE 1-6 Characteristics of Epithelial Tissues

Simple Squamous Epithelium
Structure
Single layer of cells

Location and Function
Lining of blood vessels leads to diffusion and filtration
Lining of pulmonary alveoli (air sacs) leads to separation of blood from fluids in tissues
Bowman's capsule (kidney), where it filters substances from blood, forming urine

Simple Squamous Epithelial Cell. Photomicrograph of simple squamous epithelial cell in parietal wall of Bowman's capsule in kidney. (From Erlandsen SL, Magney JE: *Color atlas of histology*, St Louis, 1992, Mosby.)

Stratified Squamous Epithelium
Structure
Two or more layers, depending on location, with cells closest to basement membrane tending to be cuboidal

Location and Function
Epidermis of skin and linings of mouth, pharynx, esophagus, and anus provide protection and secretion

Cornified layer

Basement membrane   Basal cells   Dermis

Cornified Stratified Squamous Epithelium. Diagram of stratified squamous epithelium of skin. (Copyright Ed Reschke. Used with permission.)

Transitional Epithelium
Structure
Vary in shape from cuboidal to squamous depending on whether basal cells of bladder are columnar or are composed of many layers; when bladder is full and stretched, the cells flatten and stretch like squamous cells

Location and Function
Linings of urinary bladder and other hollow structures stretch, allowing expansion of the hollow organs

Stratified transitional epithelial cells

Binucleate cell

Basement membrane   Connective tissue

Stratified Squamous Transitional Epithelium. Photomicrograph of stratified squamous transitional epithelium of urinary bladder. (Copyright Ed Reschke. Used with permission.)

Simple Cuboidal Epithelium
Structure
Simple cuboidal cells; rarely stratified (layered)

Location and Function
Glands (e.g., thyroid, sweat, salivary) and parts of the kidney tubules and outer covering of ovary secrete fluids

Simple Cuboidal Epithelium. Photomicrograph of simple cuboidal epithelium of pancreatic duct. (From Erlandsen SL, Magney JE: *Color atlas of histology*, St Louis, 1992, Mosby.)

Continued

TABLE 1-6   Characteristics of Epithelial Tissues—cont'd

Simple Columnar Epithelium
Structure
Large amounts of cytoplasm and cellular organelles

Location and Function
Ducts of many glands and lining of digestive tract allow secretion and absorption from stomach to anus

Goblet cells

Columnar epithelial cell

Simple Columnar Epithelium. Photomicrograph of simple columnar epithelium. (Copyright Ed Reschke. Used with permission.)

Ciliated Simple Columnar Epithelium
Structure
Same as simple columnar epithelium but ciliated

Location and Function
Linings of bronchi of lungs, nasal cavity, and oviducts allow secretion, absorption, and propulsion of fluids and particles

Stratified Columnar Epithelium
Structure
Small and rounded basement membrane (columnar cells do not touch basement membrane)

Location and Function
Linings of epiglottis, part of pharynx, anus, and male urethra provide protection

Pseudostratified Ciliated Columnar Epithelium
Structure
All cells in contact with basement membrane
Nuclei found at different levels within cell, giving stratified appearance
Free surface often ciliated

Location and Function
Linings of large ducts of some glands (parotid, salivary), male urethra, respiratory passages, and eustachian tubes of ears transport substances

Cilia   Columnar cell   Goblet cell   Basement membrane

Mucous glands

Pseudostratified Ciliated Columnar Epithelium. Photomicrograph of pseudostratified ciliated columnar epithelium of trachea. (Copyright Robert L. Calentine. Used with permission.)

TABLE 1-7 Connective Tissues

Loose or Areolar Tissue

Structure

Unorganized; spaces between fibers

Most fibers collagenous, some elastic and reticular

Includes many types of cells (fibroblasts and macrophages most common) and large amount of intercellular fluid

Location and Function

Attaches skin to underlying tissue; holds organs in place by filling spaces between them; supports blood vessels

Intercellular fluid transports nutrients and waste products

Fluid accumulation causes swelling (edema)

Bundle of collagenous fibers

Elastic fibers

Loose Areolar Connective Tissue. (Copyright Ed Reschke. Used with permission.)

Dense Irregular Tissue

Structure

Dense, compact, and areolar tissue, with fewer cells and greater number of closely woven collagenous fibers than in loose tissue

Location and Function

Dermis layer of skin; acts as protective barrier

Fibroblast   Collagenous fibers

Dense, Irregular Connective Tissue. (Copyright Ed Reschke. Used with permission.)

Dense, Regular (White Fibrous) Tissue

Structure

Collagenous fibers and some elastic fibers, tightly packed into parallel bundles, with only fibroblast cells

Location and Function

Forms strong tendons of muscle, ligaments of joints, some fibrous membranes, and fascia that surrounds organs and muscles

Fibroblast   Collagenous fibers

Dense, Regular (White Fibrous) Connective Tissue. (Copyright Phototake. Used with permission.)

Elastic Tissue

Structure

Elastic fibers, some collagenous fibers, fibroblasts

Location and Function

Lends strength and elasticity to walls of arteries, trachea, vocal cords, and other structures

Elastic Connective Tissue. (From Erlandsen SL, Magney JE: *Color atlas of histology*, St Louis, 1992, Mosby.)

Continued

TABLE 1-7 Connective Tissues—cont'd

Adipose Tissue
Structure
Fat cells dispersed in loose tissues; each cell containing a large droplet of fat flattens nucleus and forces cytoplasm into a ring around cell's periphery

Location and Function
Stores fat, which provides padding and protection

Storage area for fat   Plasma membrane

Nucleus of adipose cell

Adipose Tissue. A, Fat storage areas—distribution of fat in male and female bodies. **B,** Photomicrograph of adipose tissue. (**A** from Thibodeau GA, Patton KT: *Anatomy & physiology*, ed 6, St Louis, 2007, Mosby; **B** copyright Ed Reschke. Used with permission.)

Cartilage (Hyaline, Elastic, Fibrous)
Structure
Collagenous fibers embedded in a firm matrix (chondrin); no blood supply

Location and Function
Gives form, support, and flexibility to joints, trachea, nose, ear, vertebral disks, embryonic skeleton, and many internal structures

Matrix   Chondrocyte in lacuna   Perichondrium layer

Lacuna   Chondrocyte (within lacuna)   Elastic fibers

Matrix   Collagenous fibers   Cartilage cell in lacuna

Cartilage. A, Hyaline cartilage. **B,** Elastic cartilage. **C,** Fibrous cartilage. (**A** and **C** copyright Robert L. Calentine; **B** copyright Ed Reshke. Used with permission.)

TABLE 1-7 Connective Tissues—cont'd

Bone
Structure
Rigid connective tissue consisting of cells, fibers, ground substances, and minerals

Location and Function
Lends skeleton rigidity and strength

Osteon (haversian system)

Bone. (Copyright Phototake. Used with permission.)

Special Connective Tissues
Plasma
Structure
Fluid

Location and Function
Serves as matrix for blood cells

Macrophages in Tissue, Reticuloendothelial, or Macrophage System
Structure
Scattered macrophages (phagocytes) called Kupffer cells (in liver), alveolar macrophages (in lungs), microglia (in central nervous system)

Location and Function
Facilitate inflammatory response and carry out phagocytosis in loose connective, lymphatic, digestive, medullary (bone marrow), splenic, adrenal, and pituitary tissues

TABLE 1-8 Muscle Tissues

Skeletal (Striated) Muscle
Structure Characteristics of Cells
Long, cylindrical cells that extend throughout length of muscles
Striated myofibrils (proteins)
Many nuclei on periphery

Location and Function
Attached to bones directly or by tendons and provide voluntary movement of skeleton and maintenance of posture

Cross striations of muscle cell

Nuclei of muscle cell   Muscle fiber

Skeletal (Striated) Muscle. (From Thibodeau GA, Patton KT: *Anatomy & physiology*, ed 6, St Louis, 2007, Mosby.)

Cardiac Muscle
Structure Characteristics of Cells
Branching networks throughout muscle tissue
Striated myofibrils

Location and Function
Cells attached end-to-end at intercalated disks with tissue forming walls of heart (myocardium) to provide involuntary pumping action of heart

Nucleus

Intercalated disks

Cardiac Muscle. (Copyright Ed Reschke. Used with permission.)

Continued

TABLE 1-8   Muscle Tissues—cont'd

Smooth (Visceral) Muscle
Structure Characteristics of Cells
Long spindles that taper to a point
Absence of striated myofibrils

Location and Function
Walls of hollow internal structures, such as digestive tract and blood vessels
(viscera), provide voluntary and involuntary contractions that move
substances through hollow structures

Smooth muscle cells

Smooth (Visceral) Muscle. (Copyright Phototake. Used with permission.)

DID YOU UNDERSTAND?

Cellular Functions

1. Cells become specialized through the process of differentiation or maturation.
2. The eight specialized cellular functions are movement, conductivity, metabolic absorption, secretion, excretion, respiration, reproduction, and communication.

Structure and Function of Cellular Components

1. The eukaryotic cell consists of three general components: the plasma membrane, the cytoplasm, and the intracellular organelles.
2. The nucleus is the largest membrane-bound organelle and is found usually in the cell's center. The chief functions of the nucleus are cell division and control of genetic information.
3. Cytoplasm, or the cytoplasmic matrix, is an aqueous solution (cytosol) that fills the space between the nucleus and the plasma membrane.
4. The organelles are suspended in the cytoplasm and are enclosed in biologic membranes.
5. The endoplasmic reticulum is a network of tubular channels (cisternae) that extend throughout the outer nuclear membrane. It specializes in the synthesis and transport of protein and lipid components of most of the organelles.
6. The Golgi complex is a network of smooth membranes and vesicles located near the nucleus. The Golgi complex is responsible for processing and packaging proteins into secretory vesicles that break away from the Golgi complex and migrate to a variety of intracellular and extracellular destinations, including the plasma membrane.
7. Lysosomes are saclike structures that originate from the Golgi complex and contain digestive enzymes. These enzymes are responsible for digesting most cellular substances to their basic form, such as amino acids, fatty acids, and carbohydrates (sugars).
8. Cellular injury leads to a release of the lysosomal enzymes, causing cellular self-digestion.
9. Peroxisomes are similar to lysosomes but contain several enzymes that either produce or use hydrogen peroxide.
10. Mitochondria contain the metabolic machinery necessary for cellular energy metabolism. The enzymes of the respiratory chain (electron-transport chain), found in the inner membrane of the mitochondria, generate most of the cell's ATP.
11. The cytoskeleton is the "bone and muscle" of the cell. The internal skeleton is composed of a network of protein filaments, including microtubules and actin filaments (microfilaments).
12. The plasma membrane encloses the cell and, by controlling the movement of substances across it, exerts a powerful influence on metabolic pathways. Principles of membrane structure are being overhauled.
13. Proteins are the major workhorses of the cell. Membrane proteins, like other proteins, are synthesized by the ribosome and then make their way, called trafficking, to different locations in the cell. Trafficking places unique demands on membrane proteins for folding, translocation, and stability. Misfolded proteins are emerging as an important cause of disease.
14. Protein regulation in a cell is called protein homeostasis and is defined by the proteostasis network. This network is composed of ribosomes (makers), chaperones (helpers), and protein breakdown or proteolytic systems. Malfunction of these systems is associated with disease.
15. Carbohydrates contained within the plasma membrane are generally bound to membrane proteins (glycoproteins) and lipids (glycolipids).
16. Protein receptors (recognition units) on the plasma membrane enable the cell to interact with other cells and with extracellular substances.
17. Membrane functions are determined largely by proteins. These functions include recognition by protein receptors and transport of substances into and out of the cell.

Cell-to-Cell Adhesions

1. Cell-to-cell adhesions are formed on plasma membranes, thereby allowing the formation of tissues and organs. Cells are held together by three different means: (1) the extracellular membrane, (2) cell adhesion molecules in the cell's plasma membrane, and (3) specialized cell junctions.
2. The extracellular matrix includes three groups of macromolecules: (1) fibrous structural proteins (collagen and elastin), (2) adhesive

glycoproteins, and (3) proteoglycans and hyaluronic acid. The matrix helps regulate cell growth, movement, and differentiation.
3. The basement membrane is a tough layer of extracellular matrix underlying the epithelium of many organs; it is also called the basal lamina.
4. Cell junctions can be classified as symmetric and asymmetric. Symmetric junctions include tight junctions, the belt desmosome, desmosomes, and gap junctions. An asymmetric junction is the hemidesmosome.

Cellular Communication and Signal Transduction
1. Cells communicate in three main ways: (1) they form protein channels (gap junctions); (2) they display receptors that affect intracellular processes or other cells in direct physical contact; and (3) they use receptor proteins *inside* the target cell.
2. Primary modes of intercellular signaling include contact-dependent, paracrine, hormonal, neurohormonal, and neurotransmitter.
3. Signal transduction involves signals or instructions from extracellular chemical messengers that are conveyed to the cell's interior for execution. If deprived of appropriate signals, cells undergo a form of cell suicide known as programmed cell death or apoptosis.

Cellular Metabolism
1. The chemical tasks of maintaining essential cellular functions are referred to as *cellular metabolism*. Anabolism is the energy-using process of metabolism, whereas catabolism is the energy-releasing process.
2. Adenosine triphosphate (ATP) functions as an energy-transferring molecule. It is fuel for cell survival. Energy is stored by molecules of carbohydrate, lipid, and protein, which, when catabolized, transfers energy to ATP.
3. Oxidative phosphorylation occurs in the mitochondria and is the mechanism by which the energy produced from carbohydrates, fats, and proteins is transferred to ATP.

Membrane Transport: Cellular Intake and Output
1. Cell survival and growth depends on the constant exchange of molecules with their environment. The two main classes of membrane transport proteins are transporters and channels. The majority of molecular transfer depends on specialized membrane transport proteins.
2. Water and small, electrically uncharged molecules move through pores in the plasma membrane's lipid bilayer in the process called *passive transport*.
3. Passive transport does not require the expenditure of energy; rather, it is driven by the physical effect of osmosis, hydrostatic pressure, and diffusion.
4. Larger molecules and molecular complexes are moved into the cell by active transport, which requires the cell to expend energy (by means of ATP).
5. The largest molecules (macromolecules) and fluids are transported by the processes of endocytosis (ingestion) and exocytosis (expulsion). Endocytosis, or vesicle formation, is when the substance to be transported is engulfed by a segment of the plasma membrane, forming a vesicle that moves into the cell.
6. Pinocytosis is a type of endocytosis in which fluids and solute molecules are ingested through formation of small vesicles.
7. Phagocytosis is a type of endocytosis in which large particles, such as bacteria, are ingested through formation of large vesicles, called *vacuoles*.

8. In receptor-mediated endocytosis, the plasma membrane receptors are clustered, along with bristlelike structures, in specialized areas called *coated pits*.
9. Endocytosis occurs when coated pits invaginate, internalizing ligand-receptor complexes in coated vesicles.
10. Inside the cell, lysosomal enzymes process and digest material ingested by endocytosis.
11. Two types of solutes exist in body fluids: electrolytes and nonelectrolytes. Electrolytes are electrically charged and dissociate into constituent ions when placed in solution. Nonelectrolytes do not dissociate when placed in solution.
12. Diffusion is the passive movement of a solute from an area of higher solute concentration to an area of lower solute concentration.
13. Filtration is the measurement of water and solutes through a membrane because of a greater pushing pressure.
14. Hydrostatic pressure is the mechanical force of water pushing against cellular membranes.
15. Osmosis is the movement of water across a semipermeable membrane from a region of lower solute concentration to a region of higher solute concentration.
16. The amount of hydrostatic pressure required to oppose the osmotic movement of water is called the *osmotic pressure of solution*.
17. The overall osmotic effect of colloids, such as plasma proteins, is called the *oncotic pressure* or *colloid osmotic pressure*.
18. All body cells are electrically polarized, with the inside of the cell more negatively charged than the outside. The difference in voltage across the plasma membrane is the resting membrane potential.
19. When an excitable (nerve or muscle) cell receives an electrochemical stimulus, cations enter the cell and cause a rapid change in the resting membrane potential known as the *action potential*. The action potential "moves" along the cell's plasma membrane and is transmitted to an adjacent cell. This is how electrochemical signals convey information from cell to cell.

Cellular Reproduction: The Cell Cycle
1. Cellular reproduction in body tissues involves mitosis (nuclear division) and cytokinesis (cytoplasmic division).
2. Only mature cells are capable of division. Maturation occurs during a stage of cellular life called *interphase (growth phase)*.
3. The cell cycle is the reproductive process that begins after interphase in all tissues with cellular turnover. There are four phases of the cell cycle: (1) the S phase, during which DNA synthesis takes place in the cell nucleus; (2) the G_2 phase, the period between the completion of DNA synthesis and the next phase (M); (3) the M phase, which involves both nuclear (mitotic) and cytoplasmic (cytokinetic) division; and (4) the G_1 phase (growth phase), after which the cycle begins again.
4. The M phase (mitosis) involves four stages: prophase, metaphase, anaphase, and telophase.
5. The mechanisms that control cellular division depend on the integrity of genetic, epigenetic, and protein growth factors.

Tissues
1. Cells of one or more types are organized into tissues, and different types of tissues compose organs. Organs are organized to function as tracts or systems.
2. Three key factors that maintain the cellular organization of tissues are (1) recognition and cell communication, (2) selective cell-to-cell adhesion, and (3) memory.

3. Fully specialized or terminally differentiated cells that are lost are generated from proliferating *precursor cells* and they, in turn, have been derived from a smaller number of stem cells. Stem cells are cells with the potential to develop into many different cell types during early development and growth. In many tissues, stem cells serve as an internal repair and maintenance system dividing indefinitely. These cells can maintain themselves over very long periods of time, called self-renewal, and can generate all the differentiated cell types of the tissue or multipotency.

4. Tissue cells are linked at cell junctions, which are specialized regions on their plasma membranes. Cell junctions attach adjacent cells and allow small molecules to pass between them.

5. The four basic types of tissues are epithelial, muscle, nerve, and connective tissues.

6. Neural tissue is composed of highly specialized cells called neurons that receive and transmit electrical impulses rapidly across junctions called *synapses*.

7. Epithelial tissue covers most internal and external surfaces of the body. The functions of epithelial tissue include protection, absorption, secretion, and excretion.

8. Connective tissue binds various tissues and organs together, supporting them in their locations and serving as storage sites for excess nutrients.

9. Muscle tissue is composed of long, thin, highly contractile cells or fibers called *myocytes*. Muscle tissue that is attached to bones enables voluntary movement. Muscle tissue in internal organs enables involuntary movement, such as the heartbeat.

KEY TERMS

Absolute refractory period, 25
Action potential, 24
Active transport, 17
Amphipathic, 3
Anabolism, 14
Anaphase, 26
Anion, 19
Antiport, 18
Arrested (resting) (G_0) state, 27
Autocrine signaling, 12
Basal lamina, 10
Basement membrane, 10
Binding site, 9
Catabolism, 14
Cation, 19
Caveolae, 24
Cell adhesion molecule (CAM), 8
Cell cortex, 8
Cell cycle, 25
Cell junction, 11
Cell polarity, 2
Cell-to-cell adhesion, 10
Cellular metabolism, 14
Cellular receptor, 9
Centromere, 26
Channel, 17
Chemical synapse, 12
Chromatid, 26
Chromatin, 26
Citric acid cycle (Krebs cycle, tricarboxylic acid cycle), 16
Clathrin, 22
Coated vesicle, 22
Collagen, 10
Concentration gradient, 19
Connective tissue, 10
Connexon, 12
Contact-dependent signaling, 12
Cytokinesis, 25
Cytoplasm, 2

Cytoplasmic matrix, 2
Cytosol, 2
Daughter cell, 26
Depolarization, 24
Desmosome, 12
Differentiation, 1
Diffusion, 19
Digestion, 16
Effective osmolality, 20
Elastin, 10
Electrolyte, 18
Electron-transport chain, 16
Endocytosis, 22
Endosome, 22
Equatorial plate (metaphase plate), 26
ER stress, 8
Eukaryote, 1
Exocytosis, 22
Extracellular matrix, 10
Fibroblast, 10
Fibronectin, 10
Filtration, 19
G_1 phase, 26
G_2 phase, 25
Gap junction, 12
Gating, 12
Glycocalyx, 9
Glycolipid, 3
Glycolysis, 16
Glycoprotein, 3
Growth factor (cytokine), 26
Homeostasis, 12
Hormonal signaling, 12
Hydrostatic pressure, 19
Hyperpolarized state, 25
Hypopolarized state, 25
Integral membrane protein, 7
Interphase, 25
Ions, 7
Junctional complex, 12

Ligand, 9
Lipid bilayer, 2
M phase, 25
Macromolecule, 10
Mediated transport, 17
Membrane lipid raft (MLR), 5
Membrane transport protein, 17
Metabolic pathway, 16
Metaphase, 26
Mitosis, 25
Multipotency, 27
Neurohormonal signaling, 12
Neurotransmitter, 12
Nuclear envelope, 2
Nuclear pores, 2
Nucleolus, 2
Nucleus, 2
Oncotic pressure (colloid osmotic pressure), 20
Organelle, 2
Osmolality, 19
Osmolarity, 19
Osmosis, 19
Osmotic pressure, 20
Oxidation, 16
Oxidative phosphorylation, 16
Paracrine signaling, 12
Passive transport, 17
Peripheral membrane protein, 7
Phagocytosis, 22
Phospholipid, 5
Pinocytosis, 22
Plasma membrane (plasmalemma), 2
Plasma membrane receptor, 9
Platelet-derived growth factor (PDGF), 27
Polarity, 19
Polypeptide, 5
Posttranslational modification (PTM), 5

Prokaryote, 1
Prophase, 26
Protein, 5
Proteolytic, 9
Proteome, 7
Proteomic, 7
Receptor protein, 12
Receptor-mediated endocytosis (ligand internalization), 24
Relative refractory period, 25
Repolarization, 25
Resting membrane potential, 24
Retinoblastoma (Rb) protein, 26
Self-renewal, 27
S phase, 25
Signal transduction pathway, 12
Signaling cell, 12
Solute, 17
Spindle fiber, 26
Stem cell, 27
Stroma, 26
Substrate, 16
Substrate phosphorylation (anaerobic glycolysis), 16
Symport, 18
Target cell, 12
Telophase, 26
Terminally differentiated, 27
Threshold potential, 24
Tight junction, 12
Tonicity, 20
Transfer reaction, 16
Transmembrane protein, 7
Transporter, 17
Unfolded-protein response, 8
Uniport, 18
Valence, 19
Wnt signals, 27

REFERENCES

1. Alberts B: *Essential cell biology,* ed 4, New York, 2014, Garland.
2. Simons K, Sampaio JL: Membrane organization and lipid rafts, *Cold Spring Harb Perspect Biol* 3(10):a004697, 2011.
3. Contreras FX et al: Specificity of intramembrane protein-lipid interactions, *Cold Spring Harb Perspec Biol* 3(6):pii a004705, 2011.
4. Head BP et al: Interaction of membrane/lipid rafts with the cytoskeleton: impact on signaling and function: membrane/lipid rafts, mediators of cytoskeletal arrangement and cell signaling, *Biochim Biophys Acta* 1838(2):532-545, 2014.
5. Karnovsky MJ et al: The concept of lipid domains in membranes, *J Cell Biol* 94:1-6, 1982.
6. Ribert D, Cossart P: Pathogen-mediated postranslational modification: a re-emerging field, *Cell* 143:694-702, 2010.
7. Vinothkumar KR, Henderson R: Structure of membrane proteins, *Q Rev Biophysics* 43(1):65-158, 2010.
8. Cogliati S et al: Mitochondrial cristae shape determines respiratory chain supercomplexes assembly and respiratory efficiency, *Cell* 155(1):160-171, 2013.
9. Daum B et al: Age-dependent dissociation of ATP synthase dimers and loss of inner-membrane cristae in mitochondria, *Proc Natl Acad Sci U S A* 110(38):15301-15306, 2013.
10. Friedman JR, Nunnari J: Mitochondrial form and function, *Nature* 505:335-343, 2014.
11. Amm I et al: Protein quality control and elimination of protein waste: the role of the ubiquitin-proteosome system, *Biochim Biophys Acta* 1843:182-196, 2014.
12. Lindquist SL, Kelly JW: Chemical and biological approaches for adapting proteostasis to ameliorate protein misfolding and aggregation diseases: progress and prognosis, *Cold Spring Harb Perspect Biol* 3(12), 2011.
13. Kierszenbaum AL, Tres LT: *Histology and cell biology: an introduction to pathology,* ed 3, St Louis, 2011, Elsevier.
14. Xu Q et al: Gating of connexin 43 gap junctions by a cytoplasmic loop calmodulin binding domain, *Am J Physiol Cell Physiol* 302(10):C1548-C1556, 2012.
15. Sirnes S et al: Connexin43 acts as a colorectal tumor suppressor and predicts disease outcome, *Int J Cancer* 131(3):570-581, 2012.
16. Khan R et al: Glycyrrhizic acid suppresses the development of precancerous lesions via regulating the hyperproliferation, inflammation, angiogenesis ad apoptosis in the colon of Wistar rats, *PLoS One* 8(2), e56020, 2013.
17. Zhang MZ et al: Inhibition of 11β hydroxysteroid dehydrogenase type II selectively blocks the tumor COX-2 pathway and suppresses colon carcinogenesis in mice and humans, *J Clin Invest* 119:876-885, 2009.
18. Burnstock G: Physiology and pathophysiology in purinergic neurotransmission, *Physiol Rev* 87(2):659-797, 2007.
19. Falzoni S et al: Detecting adenosine triphosphate in the pericellular space, *Interface Focus* 3(3): 20120101, 2013.
20. Nurse CA, Piskuric NA: Signal processing at mammalian carotid body chemoreceptors, *Semin Cell Dev Biol* 24(1):22-30, 2012.
21. Chaudhri RA et al: Role of ERα36 in membrane-associated signaling by estrogen, *Steroids* 81:74-80, 2014.
22. Clevers H et al: Stem cell signaling. An integral program for tissue renewal and regeneration: Wnt signaling and stem cell control, *Science* 346(6205): 1248012, 2014.

2

Genes and Genetic Diseases

Lynn B. Jorde

CHAPTER OUTLINE

Genetics occupies a central position in the entire study of biology. An understanding of genetics is essential to study human, animal, plant, or microbial life. Genetics is the study of biologic inheritance. In the nineteenth century, microscopic studies of cells led scientists to suspect the nucleus of the cell contained the important mechanisms of inheritance. Scientists found chromatin, the substance giving the nucleus a granular appearance, is observable in nondividing cells. Just before the cell divides, the chromatin condenses to form discrete, dark-staining organelles, which are called **chromosomes**. (Cell division is discussed in Chapter 1.) With the rediscovery of Mendel's important breeding experiments at the turn of the twentieth century, it soon became apparent the chromosomes contained **genes**, the basic units of inheritance (Figure 2-1).

The primary constituent of chromatin is **deoxyribonucleic acid (DNA)**. Genes are composed of sequences of DNA. By serving as the blueprints of proteins in the body, genes ultimately influence all aspects of body structure and function. Humans have approximately 20,000 protein-coding genes and an additional 9000 to 10,000 genes that encode various types of RNA (see below) that are not translated into proteins. An error in one of these genes often leads to a recognizable genetic disease.

To date, more than 20,000 genetic traits and diseases have been identified and cataloged. As infectious diseases continue to be more effectively controlled, the proportion of beds in pediatric hospitals occupied by children with genetic diseases has risen. In addition to children, many common diseases primarily affecting adults, such as hypertension, coronary heart disease, diabetes, and cancer, are now known to have important genetic components.

Great progress is being made in the diagnosis of genetic diseases and in the understanding of genetic mechanisms underlying them. With the huge strides being made in molecular genetics, "gene therapy"—the utilization of normal genes to correct genetic disease—has begun.

DNA, RNA, AND PROTEINS: HEREDITY AT THE MOLECULAR LEVEL

Definitions

Composition and Structure of DNA

Genes are composed of DNA, which has three basic components: the five-carbon monosaccharide deoxyribose; a phosphate molecule; and four types of nitrogenous bases. Two of the bases, **cytosine** and **thymine**, are single carbon-nitrogen rings called **pyrimidines**. The other two bases, **adenine** and **guanine**, are double carbon-nitrogen rings called **purines**. The four bases are commonly represented by their first letters: A (adenine), C (cytosine), T (thymine), and G (guanine).

Watson and Crick demonstrated how these molecules are physically assembled as DNA, proposing the **double-helix model**, in which DNA appears like a twisted ladder with chemical bonds as its rungs (Figure 2-2). The two sides of the ladder consist of deoxyribose and phosphate molecules, united by strong phosphodiester bonds. Projecting from each side of the ladder, at regular intervals, are the nitrogenous bases. The base projecting from one side is bound to the base projecting from the other by a weak hydrogen bond. Therefore the nitrogenous bases form the rungs of the ladder; adenine pairs with thymine, and guanine pairs with cytosine. Each DNA subunit—consisting of one

FIGURE 2-1 Successive Enlargements from a Human to the Genetic Material.

deoxyribose molecule, one phosphate group, and one base—is called a nucleotide.

DNA as the Genetic Code

DNA directs the synthesis of all the body's proteins. Proteins are composed of one or more polypeptides (intermediate protein compounds), which in turn consist of sequences of amino acids. The body contains 20 different types of amino acids; they are specified by the 4 nitrogenous bases. To specify (code for) 20 different amino acids with only 4 bases, different combinations of bases, occurring in groups of 3 (triplets), are used. These triplets of bases are known as codons. Each codon specifies a single amino acid in a corresponding protein. Because there are 64 ($4 \times 4 \times 4$) possible codons but only 20 amino acids, there are many cases in which several codons correspond to the same amino acid.

The genetic code is universal: *all* living organisms use precisely the same DNA codes to specify proteins except for mitochondria, the cytoplasmic organelles in which cellular respiration takes place (see Chapter 1)—they have their own extranuclear DNA. Several codons of mitochondrial DNA encode different amino acids, as compared to the same nuclear DNA codons.

Replication of DNA

DNA replication consists of breaking the weak hydrogen bonds between the bases, leaving a single strand with each base unpaired (Figure 2-3). The consistent pairing of adenine with thymine and of guanine with cytosine, known as complementary base pairing, is the key to accurate replication. The unpaired base attracts a free nucleotide only if the nucleotide has the proper complementary base. When replication is complete, a new double-stranded molecule identical to the original is formed. The single strand is said to be a template, or molecule on which a complementary molecule is built, and is the basis for synthesizing the new double strand.

Several different proteins are involved in DNA replication. The most important of these proteins is an enzyme known as DNA polymerase. This enzyme travels along the single DNA strand, adding the correct nucleotides to the free end of the new strand and checking to ensure that its base is actually complementary to the template base. This mechanism of DNA proofreading substantially enhances the accuracy of DNA replication.

Mutation

A mutation is any inherited alteration of genetic material. One type of mutation is the base pair substitution, in which one base pair replaces another. This replacement *can* result in a change in the amino acid sequence. However, because of the redundancy of the genetic code, many of these mutations do not change the amino acid sequence and thus have no consequence. Such mutations are called silent mutations. Base pair substitutions altering amino acids consist of two basic types: missense mutations, which produce a change (i.e., the "sense") in a single amino acid; and nonsense mutations, which produce one of the three stop codons (UAA, UAG, or UGA) in the messenger RNA (mRNA) (Figure 2-4). Missense mutations (see Figure 2-4, *A*) produce a single amino acid change, whereas nonsense mutations (see Figure 2-4, *B*) produce a premature stop codon in the mRNA. Stop codons terminate translation of the polypeptide.

The frameshift mutation involves the insertion or deletion of one or more base pairs of the DNA molecule. As Figure 2-5 shows, these mutations change the entire "reading frame" of the DNA sequence because the deletion or insertion is not a multiple of three base pairs (the number of base pairs in a codon). Frameshift mutations can thus greatly alter the amino acid sequence. (*In-frame* insertions or deletions, in which a multiple of three bases is inserted or lost, tend to have less severe disease consequences than do frameshift mutations.)

Agents known as mutagens increase the frequency of mutations. Examples include radiation and chemicals such as nitrogen mustard, vinyl chloride, alkylating agents, formaldehyde, and sodium nitrite.

Mutations are rare events. The rate of spontaneous mutations (those occurring in the absence of exposure to known mutagens) in humans is about 10^{-4} to 10^{-7} per gene per generation. This rate varies from one gene to another. Some DNA sequences have particularly high mutation rates and are known as mutational hot spots.

From Genes to Proteins

DNA is formed and replicated in the cell nucleus, but protein synthesis takes place in the cytoplasm. The DNA code is transported from nucleus to cytoplasm, and subsequent protein is formed through two basic processes: transcription and translation. These processes are mediated by ribonucleic acid (RNA), which is chemically similar to DNA except the sugar molecule is ribose rather than deoxyribose, and uracil rather than thymine is one of the four bases. The other bases of RNA, as in DNA, are adenine, cytosine, and guanine. Uracil is structurally similar to thymine, so it also can pair with adenine. Whereas DNA usually occurs as a double strand, RNA usually occurs as a single strand.

Transcription

In transcription, RNA is synthesized from a DNA template, forming messenger RNA (mRNA). RNA polymerase binds to a promoter site, a sequence of DNA that specifies the beginning of a gene. RNA polymerase then separates a portion of the DNA, exposing unattached DNA bases. One DNA strand then provides the template for the sequence of mRNA nucleotides.

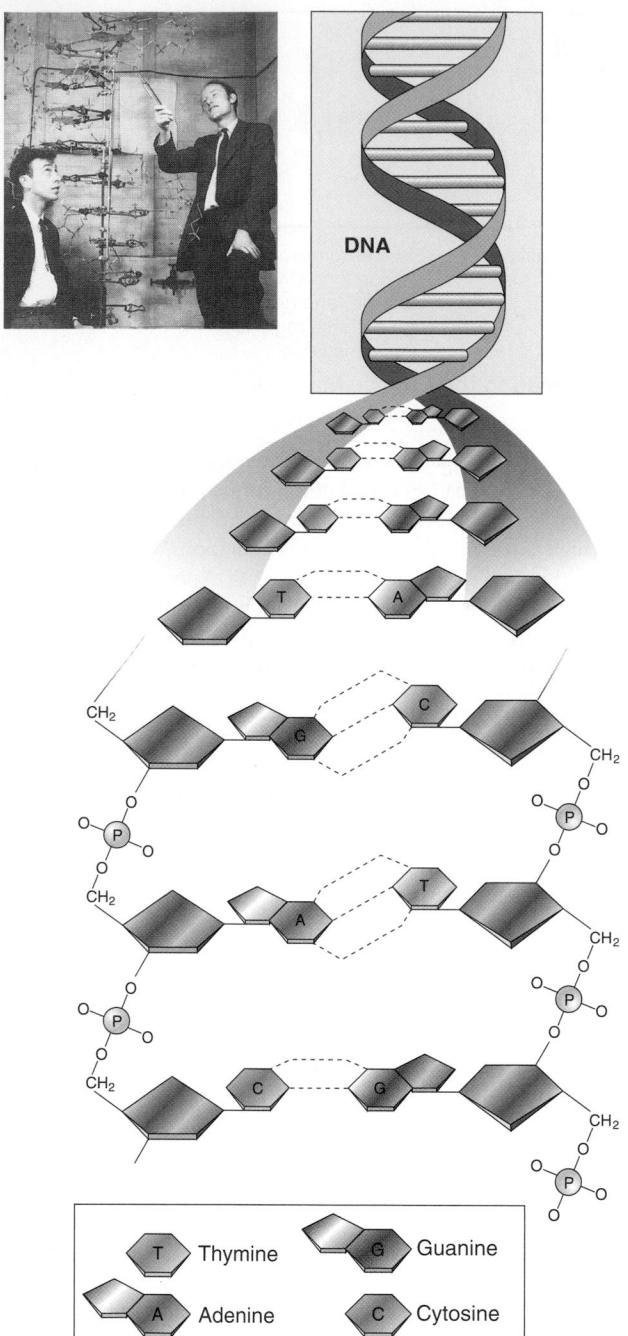

FIGURE 2-2 Watson-Crick Model of the DNA Molecule. The DNA structure illustrated here is based on that published by James Watson *(photograph, left)* and Francis Crick *(photograph, right)* in 1953. Note that each side of the DNA molecule consists of alternating sugar and phosphate groups. Each sugar group is bonded to the opposing sugar group by a pair of nitrogenous bases (adenine-thymine or cytosine-guanine). The sequence of these pairs constitutes a genetic code that determines the structure and function of a cell. (Illustration from Herlihy B: *The human body in health and illness,* ed 5, St Louis, 2015, Saunders.)

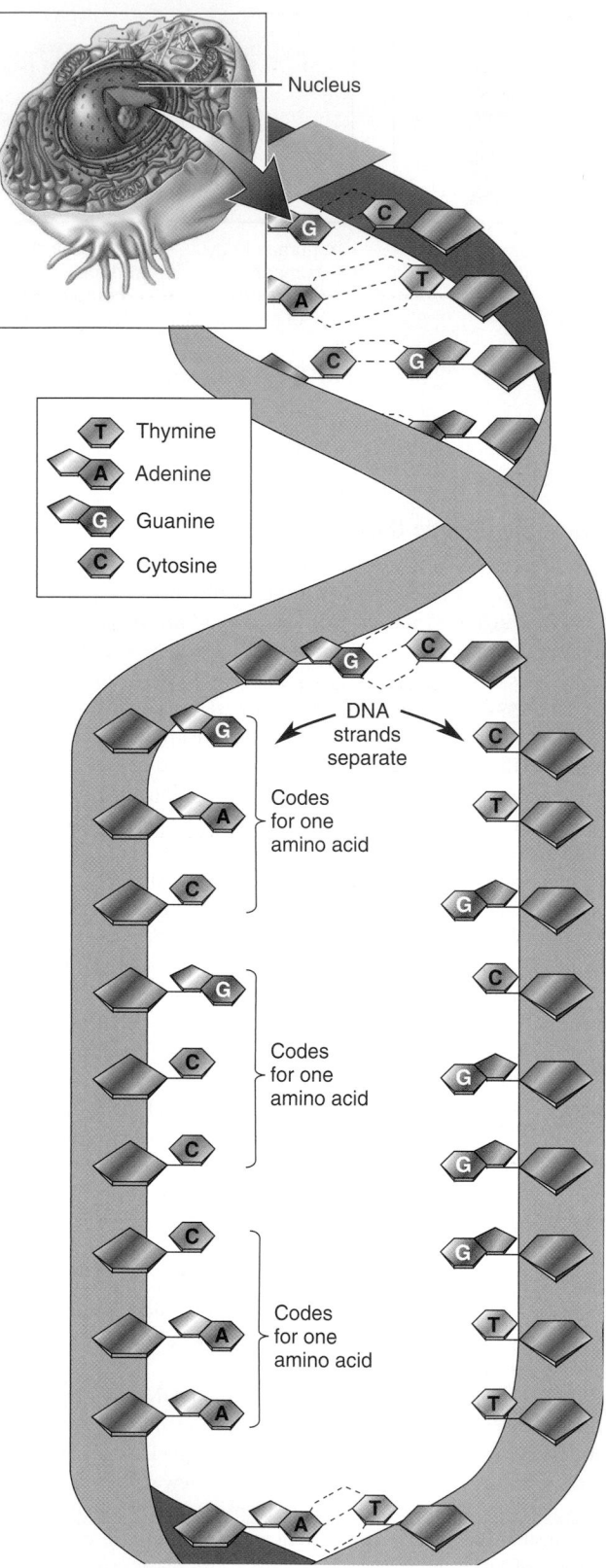

FIGURE 2-3 Replication of DNA. The two chains of the double helix separate and each chain serves as the template for a new complementary chain. (From Herlihy B: *The human body in health and illness,* ed 5, St Louis, 2015, Saunders.)

FIGURE 2-4 Base Pair Substitution. Missense mutations (A) produce a single amino acid change, whereas nonsense mutations (B) produce a stop codon in the mRNA. Stop codons terminate translation of the polypeptide. (From Jorde L et al: *Medical genetics,* ed 4, St Louis, 2010, Mosby.)

FIGURE 2-5 Frameshift Mutations. Frameshift mutations result from the addition or deletion of a number of bases that is not a multiple of 3. This mutation alters all of the codons downstream from the site of insertion or deletion. (From Jorde L et al: *Medical genetics,* ed 4, St Louis, 2010, Mosby.)

The sequence of bases in the mRNA is thus complementary to the template strand, and except for the presence of uracil instead of thymine, the mRNA sequence is identical to that of the other DNA strand. Transcription continues until a **termination sequence**, codons that act as signals for the termination of protein synthesis, is reached. Then the RNA polymerase detaches from the DNA, and the transcribed mRNA is freed to move out of the nucleus and into the cytoplasm (Figures 2-6 and 2-7).

Gene Splicing

When the mRNA is first transcribed from the DNA template, it reflects exactly the base sequence of the DNA. In eukaryotes, many RNA sequences are removed by nuclear enzymes, and the remaining sequences are spliced together to form the functional mRNA that migrates to the cytoplasm. The excised sequences are called **introns** (intervening sequences), and the sequences that are left to code for proteins are called **exons**.

Translation

In **translation**, RNA directs the synthesis of a polypeptide (see Figure 2-7), interacting with **transfer RNA (tRNA)**, a cloverleaf-shaped strand of about 80 nucleotides. The tRNA molecule has a site where an amino acid attaches. The three-nucleotide sequence at the opposite side of the cloverleaf is called the **anticodon**. It undergoes complementary base pairing with an appropriate codon in the mRNA, which specifies the sequence of amino acids through tRNA.

The site of actual protein synthesis is in the **ribosome**, which consists of approximately equal parts of protein and **ribosomal RNA (rRNA)**. During translation, the ribosome first binds to an initiation site on the mRNA sequence and then binds to its surface, so that base

FIGURE 2-6 General Scheme of Ribonucleic Acid (RNA) Transcription. In transcription of messenger RNA (mRNA), a DNA molecule "unzips" in the region of the gene to be transcribed. RNA nucleotides already present in the nucleus temporarily attach themselves to exposed DNA bases along one strand of the unzipped DNA molecule according to the principle of complementary pairing. As the RNA nucleotides attach to the exposed DNA, they bind to each other and form a chainlike RNA strand called a messenger RNA (mRNA) molecule. Notice that the new mRNA strand is an exact copy of the base sequence on the opposite side of the DNA molecule. As in all metabolic processes, the formation of mRNA is controlled by an enzyme—in this case, the enzyme is called RNA polymerase. (From Ignatavicius DD, Workman LD: *Medical-surgical nursing,* ed 6, St Louis, 2010, Saunders.)

pairing can occur between tRNA and mRNA. The ribosome then moves along the mRNA sequence, processing each codon and translating an amino acid by way of the interaction of mRNA and tRNA.

The ribosome provides an enzyme that catalyzes the formation of covalent peptide bonds between the adjacent amino acids, resulting in a growing polypeptide. When the ribosome arrives at a termination signal on the mRNA sequence, translation and polypeptide formation cease; the mRNA, ribosome, and polypeptide separate from one another; and the polypeptide is released into the cytoplasm to perform its required function.

CHROMOSOMES

Human cells can be categorized into **gametes** (sperm and egg cells) and **somatic cells,** which include all cells other than gametes. Each somatic cell nucleus has 46 chromosomes in 23 pairs (Figure 2-8). These are **diploid cells,** and the individual's father and mother each donate one chromosome per pair. New somatic cells are formed through **mitosis** and **cytokinesis.** Gametes are **haploid cells:** they have only 1 member of each chromosome pair, for a total of 23 chromosomes. Haploid cells are formed from diploid cells by **meiosis** (Figure 2-9).

In 22 of the 23 chromosome pairs, the 2 members of each pair are virtually identical in microscopic appearance: thus they are **homologous** (Figure 2-10, *B*). These 22 chromosome pairs are homologous in both males and females and are termed **autosomes.** The remaining pair of chromosomes, the sex chromosomes, consists of two homologous X chromosomes in females and a nonhomologous pair, X and Y, in males.

Figure 2-10, *A,* illustrates a **metaphase spread,** which is a photograph of the chromosomes as they appear in the nucleus of a somatic cell during metaphase. (Chromosomes are easiest to visualize during this stage of mitosis.) In Figure 2-10, *A,* the chromosomes are arranged according to size, with the homologous chromosomes paired. The 22 autosomes are numbered according to length, with chromosome 1 being the longest and chromosome 22 the shortest. A **karyotype,** or **karyogram,** is an ordered display of chromosomes. Some natural variation in relative chromosome length can be expected from person to person, so it is not always possible to distinguish each chromosome by its length. Therefore the position of the centromere (region of DNA responsible for movement of the replicated chromosomes into the two daughter cells during mitosis and meiosis) also is used to classify chromosomes (Figures 2-10, *B* and 2-11).

The chromosomes in Figure 2-10 were stained with Giemsa stain, resulting in distinctive **chromosome bands.** These form various patterns in the different chromosomes so that each chromosome can be distinguished easily. Using banding techniques, researchers can number chromosomes and study individual variations. Missing or duplicated portions of chromosomes, which often result in serious diseases, also are readily identified. More recently, techniques have been devised permitting each chromosome to be visualized with a different color.

Chromosome Aberrations and Associated Diseases

Chromosome abnormalities are the leading known cause of intellectual disability and miscarriage. Estimates indicate that a major chromosome aberration occurs in at least 1 in 12 conceptions. Most of these fetuses do not survive to term; about 50% of all recovered first-trimester spontaneous abortuses have major chromosome aberrations.[1] The number of live births affected by these abnormalities is, however, significant; approximately 1 in 150 has a major diagnosable chromosome abnormality.[1]

Polyploidy

Cells with a multiple of the normal number of chromosomes are **euploid cells** (Greek *eu* = good or true). Because normal gametes are haploid and most normal somatic cells are diploid, they are both euploid forms. When a euploid cell has more than the diploid number of chromosomes, it is said to be a **polyploid cell.** Several types of body tissues, including some liver, bronchial, and epithelial tissues, are normally polyploid. A zygote that has three copies of each chromosome, rather than the usual two, has a form of polyploidy called **triploidy.** Nearly all triploid fetuses are spontaneously aborted or stillborn. The prevalence of triploidy among live births is approximately 1 in 10,000. **Tetraploidy,** a condition in which euploid cells have 92 chromosomes, has been found primarily in early abortuses, although occasionally affected infants have been born alive. Like triploid infants, however, they do not survive. Triploidy and tetraploidy are relatively common conditions, accounting for approximately 10% of all known miscarriages.[2]

Aneuploidy

A cell that does not contain a multiple of 23 chromosomes is an **aneuploid cell.** A cell containing three copies of one chromosome is said to be trisomic (a condition termed **trisomy**) and is aneuploid.

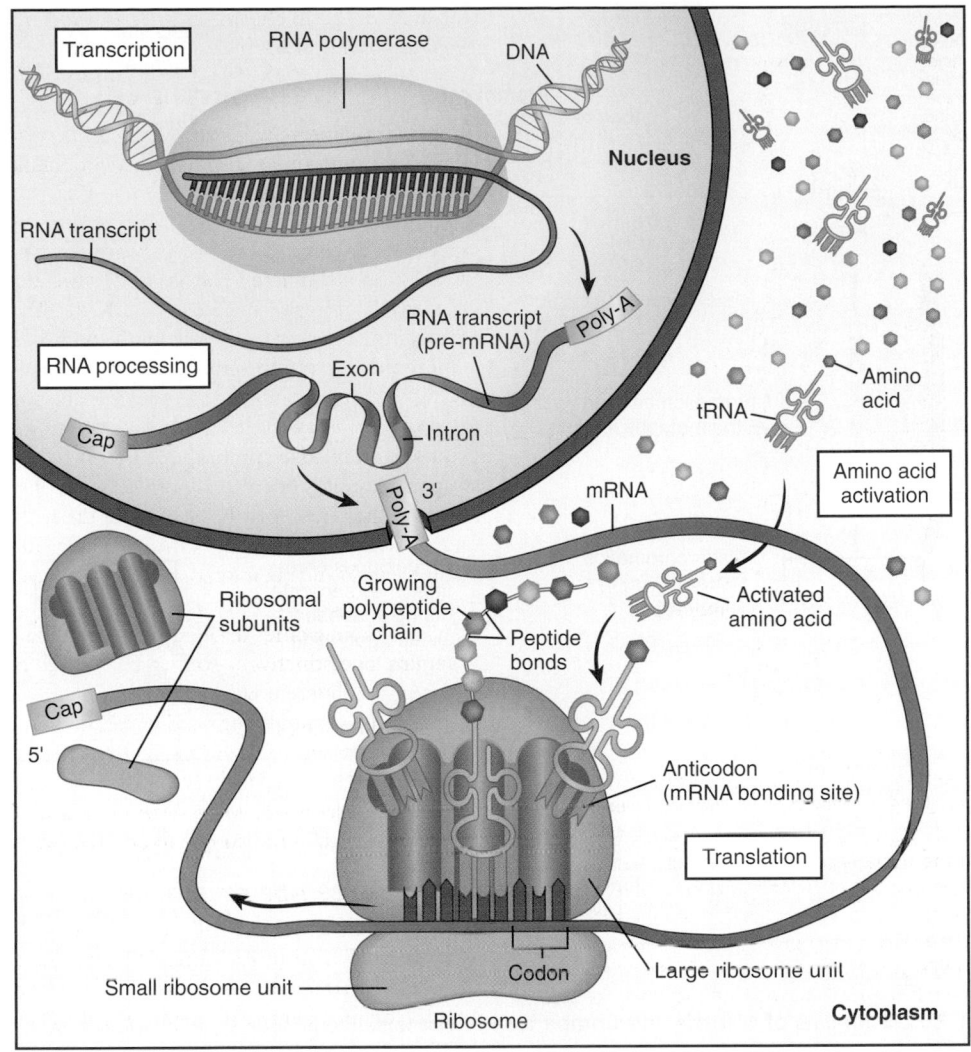

FIGURE 2-7 Protein Synthesis. The site of transcription is the nucleus and the site of translation is the cytoplasm. See the text for details.

DNA
The structure of DNA is similar to a twisted ladder, with base pairs forming the rungs. **Genes** are composed of DNA segments.

COILED DNA
The DNA in each cell would be about 6 feet long if stretched out. To fit inside the cell, the DNA is tightly coiled.

CHROMOSOMES
One chromosome of every pair is from each parent.

NUCLEUS
Each nucleus of a somatic cell contains 46 chromosomes arranged in 23 pairs.

CELLS
A nucleus resides in most human cells.

FIGURE 2-8 From Molecular Parts to the Whole Somatic Cell.

Monosomy, the presence of only one copy of a given chromosome in a diploid cell, is the other common form of aneuploidy. Among the autosomes, monosomy of any chromosome is lethal, but newborns with trisomy of chromosomes 13, 18, 21, or X can survive. This difference illustrates an important principle: *in general, loss of chromosome*

material has more serious consequences than duplication of chromosome material.

Aneuploidy of the sex chromosomes is less serious than that of the autosomes. Very little genetic material—only about 40 genes—is located on the Y chromosome. For the X chromosome, inactivation of

MITOSIS	MEIOSIS

MITOSIS

Prophase

Duplicated chromosome (two sister chromatids)

Parent cell (before chromosome replication)

Chromosome replication

$2n = 4$

Chromosome replication

Chiasma (site of crossing over)

Tetrad formed by synapsis of homologous chromosomes

MEIOSIS I Prophase I

Metaphase

Chromosomes align at the metaphase plate

Tetrads align at the metaphase plate

Metaphase I

Anaphase Telophase

Sister chromatids separate during anaphase

$2n$ $2n$

Daughter cells of mitosis

Homologous chromosomes separate during anaphase 1; sister chromatids remain together

Haploid $n = 2$

Anaphase I Telophase I

Daughter cells of mitosis I

n n n n

MEIOSIS II

Daughter cells of mitosis II
No further chromosomal replication; sister chromatids separate during anaphase II

FIGURE 2-9 Phases of Meiosis and Comparison to Mitosis. (From Jorde LB et al: *Medical genetics,* ed 4, St Louis, 2010, Mosby.)

1   2   3   4   5
6   7   8   9   10
11   12   13   14   15
16   17   18   Y
19   20   21   22   X

9.2 µm

A

Homologous chromosomes   Homologous chromosomes

Kinetochore

Replication

Centromere

Cohesin proteins

Kinetochores

Sister chromatids

Sister chromatids

B

FIGURE 2-10 Karyotype of Chromosomes. A, Human karyotype. **B,** Homologous chromosomes and sister chromatids. (From Raven PH et al: *Biology,* ed 8, New York, 2008, McGraw-Hill.)

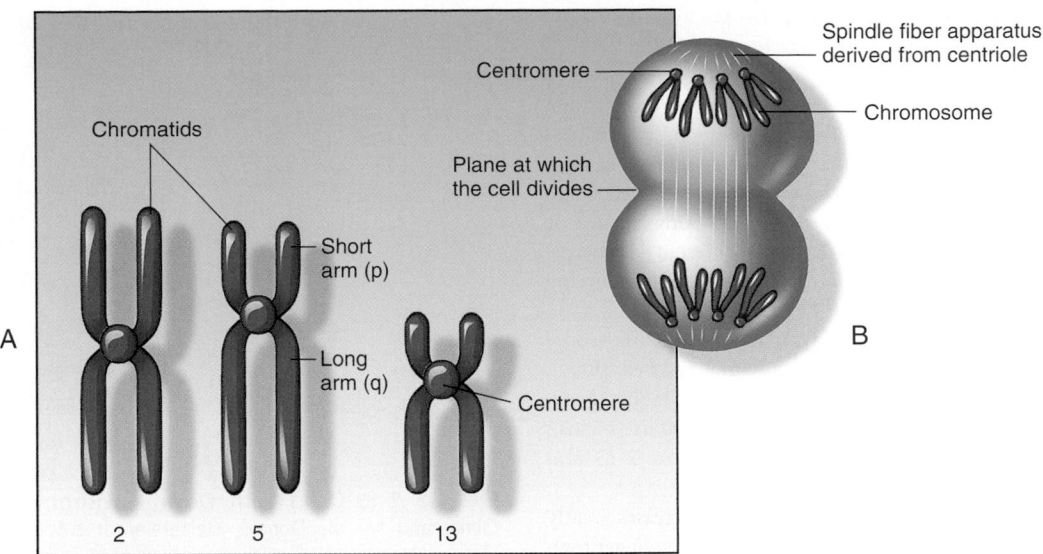

FIGURE 2-11 Structure of Chromosomes. A, Human chromosomes 2, 5, and 13. Each is replicated and consists of two chromatids. Chromosome 2 is a metacentric chromosome because the centromere is close to the middle; chromosome 5 is submetacentric because the centromere is set off from the middle; chromosome 13 is acrocentric because the centromere is at or very near the end. **B,** During mitosis, the centromere divides and the chromosomes move to opposite poles of the cell. At the time of centromere division, the chromatids are designated as chromosomes.

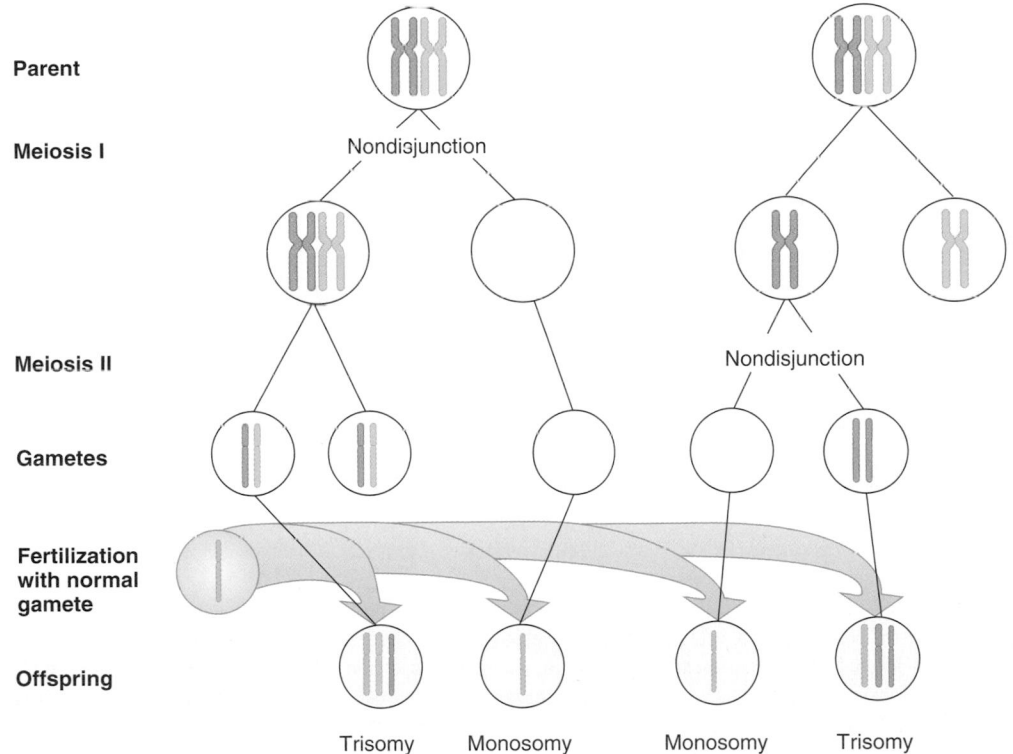

FIGURE 2-12 Nondisjunction. Nondisjunction causes aneuploidy when chromosomes or sister chromatids fail to divide properly. (From Jorde LB et al: *Medical genetics,* ed 4, St Louis, 2010, Mosby.)

extra chromosomes (see p. 54) largely diminishes their effect. A zygote bearing *no* X chromosome, however, will not survive.

Aneuploidy is usually the result of **nondisjunction,** an error in which homologous chromosomes or sister chromatids fail to separate normally during meiosis or mitosis (Figure 2-12). Nondisjunction produces some gametes that have two copies of a given chromosome and others that have no copies of the chromosome. When such gametes unite with normal haploid gametes, the resulting zygote is monosomic or trisomic for that chromosome. Occasionally, a cell can be monosomic or trisomic for more than one chromosome.

Autosomal aneuploidy. Trisomy can occur for any chromosome, but fetuses with other trisomies of chromosomes (other than 13, 18,

21, or X) do not survive to term. Trisomy 16, for example, is the most common trisomy among abortuses, but it is not seen in live births.[3]

Partial trisomy, in which only an extra portion of a chromosome is present in each cell, can occur also. The consequences of partial trisomies are not as severe as those of complete trisomies. Trisomies may occur in only some cells of the body. Individuals thus affected are said to be chromosomal mosaics, meaning that the body has two or more different cell lines, each of which has a different karyotype. Mosaics are often formed by early mitotic nondisjunction occurring in one embryonic cell but not in others.

The best-known example of aneuploidy in an autosome is trisomy of chromosome 21, which causes Down syndrome (named after J. Langdon Down, who first described the syndrome in 1866). Down syndrome is seen in approximately 1 in 800 to 1 in 1000 live births;[4] its principal features are shown and outlined in Figure 2-13 and Table 2-1.

The risk of having a child with Down syndrome increases greatly with maternal age. As Figure 2-14 demonstrates, women younger than 30 years have a risk ranging from about 1 in 1000 births to 1 in 2000

FIGURE 2-13 Child with Down Syndrome. (Courtesy Drs. A. Olney and M. MacDonald, University of Nebraska Medical Center, Omaha, Neb.)

TABLE 2-1   Characteristics of Various Chromosome Disorders

Disease/Disorder	Features
Down Syndrome	
Trisomy of Chromosome 21	
IQ	Usually ranges from 20 to 70 (intellectual disability)
Male/female findings	Virtually all males are sterile; some females can reproduce
Face	Distinctive: low nasal bridge, epicanthal folds, protruding tongue, low-set ears
Musculoskeletal system	Poor muscle tone (hypotonia), short stature
Systemic disorders	Congenital heart disease (one third to half of cases), reduced ability to fight respiratory tract infections, increased susceptibility to leukemia—overall reduced survival rate; by age 40 years usually develop symptoms similar to those of Alzheimer disease
Mortality	About 75% of fetuses with Down syndrome abort spontaneously or are stillborn; 20% of infants die before age 10 years; those who live beyond 10 years have life expectancy of about 60 years
Causative factors	97% caused by nondisjunction during formation of one of parent's gametes or during early embryonic development; 3% result from translocations; in 95% of cases, nondisjunction occurs when mother's egg cell is formed; remainder involve paternal nondisjunction; 1% are mosaics—these have a large number of normal cells, and effects of trisomic cells are attenuated and symptoms are generally less severe
Turner Syndrome	
(45,X) Monosomy of X Chromosome	
IQ	Not considered to be intellectually disabled, although some impairment of spatial and mathematical reasoning ability is found
Male/female findings	Found only in females
Musculoskeletal system	Short stature common, characteristic webbing of neck, widely spaced nipples, reduced carrying angle at elbow
Systemic disorders	Coarctation (narrowing) of aorta, edema of feet in newborns, usually sterile and have gonadal streaks rather than ovaries; streaks are sometimes susceptible to cancer
Mortality	About 15-20% of spontaneous abortions with chromosome abnormalities have this karyotype, most common single-chromosome aberration; highly lethal during gestation, only about 0.5% of these conceptions survive to term
Causative factors	75% inherit X chromosome from mother, thus caused by meiotic error in father; frequency low compared with other sex chromosome aneuploidies (1:5000 newborn females); 50% have simple monosomy of X chromosome; remainder have more complex abnormalities; combinations of 45, X cells with XX or XY cells common
Klinefelter Syndrome	
(47,XXY) XXY Condition	
IQ	Moderate degree of mental impairment may be present
Male/female findings	Have a male appearance but usually sterile; 50% develop female-like breasts (gynecomastia); occurs in 1:1000 male births
Face	Voice somewhat high pitched
Systemic disorders	Sparse body hair, sterile, small testicles
Causative factors	50% of cases the result of nondisjunction of X chromosomes in mother, frequency rises with increasing maternal age; also involves XXY and XXXY karyotypes with degree of physical and mental impairment increasing with each added X chromosome; mosaicism fairly common with most prevalent combination of XXY and XY cells

FIGURE 2-14 Down Syndrome Increases with Maternal Age.
Rate is per 1000 live births related to maternal age.

B

FIGURE 2-15 Turner Syndrome. A, A sex chromosome is missing, and the person's chromosomes are 45,X. Characteristic signs are short stature, female genitalia, webbed neck, shieldlike chest with underdeveloped breasts and widely spaced nipples, and imperfectly developed ovaries. **B,** As this karyotype shows, Turner syndrome results from monosomy of sex chromosomes (genotype XO). (From Patton KT, Thibodeau GA: *Anatomy & physiology,* ed 8, St Louis, 2013, Mosby. Courtesy Nancy S. Wexler, PhD, Columbia University.)

births. The risk begins to rise substantially after 35 years of age, and reaches 3% to 5% for women older than 45 years. This dramatic increase in risk is caused by the age of maternal egg cells, which are held in an arrested state of prophase I from the time they are formed in the female embryo until they are shed in ovulation. Thus an egg cell formed by a 45-year-old woman is itself 45 years old. This long suspended state may allow defects to accumulate in the cellular proteins responsible for meiosis, leading to nondisjunction. The risk of Down syndrome, as well as other trisomies, does not increase with paternal age.[4]

Sex chromosome aneuploidy. The incidence of sex chromosome aneuploidies is fairly high. Among live births, about 1 in 500 males and 1 in 900 females have a form of sex chromosome aneuploidy.[5] Because these conditions are generally less severe than autosomal aneuploidies, all forms except complete absence of any X chromosome material allow at least some individuals to survive.

One of the most common sex chromosome aneuploidies, affecting about 1 in 1000 newborn females, is trisomy X. Instead of two X chromosomes, these females have three X chromosomes in each cell. Most of these females have no overt physical abnormalities, although sterility, menstrual irregularity, or intellectual disability is sometimes seen. Some females have four X chromosomes, and they are more often intellectually disabled. Those with five or more X chromosomes generally have more severe intellectual disability and various physical defects.

A condition that leads to somewhat more serious problems is the presence of a single X chromosome and no homologous X or Y chromosome, so that the individual has a total of 45 chromosomes. The karyotype is usually designated 45,X, and it causes a set of symptoms known as Turner syndrome (Figure 2-15; see Table 2-1). Individuals with at least two X chromosomes and one Y chromosome in each cell (47,XXY karyotype) have a disorder known as Klinefelter syndrome (Figure 2-16; see Table 2-1).

Abnormalities of Chromosome Structure

In addition to the loss or gain of whole chromosomes, parts of chromosomes can be lost or duplicated as gametes are formed, and the arrangement of genes on chromosomes can be altered. Unlike aneuploidy and polyploidy, these changes sometimes have no serious consequences for an individual's health. Some of them can even remain entirely unnoticed, especially when very small pieces of chromosomes

are involved. Nevertheless, abnormalities of chromosome structure can also produce serious disease in individuals or their offspring.

During meiosis and mitosis, chromosomes usually maintain their structural integrity, but chromosome breakage occasionally occurs. Mechanisms exist to "heal" these breaks and usually repair them perfectly with no damage to the daughter cell. However, some breaks remain or heal in a way that alters the chromosome's structure. The risk of chromosome breakage increases with exposure to harmful agents called clastogens (e.g., ionizing radiation, viral infections, or some types of chemicals).

FIGURE 2-16 Klinefelter Syndrome. This young man exhibits many characteristics of Klinefelter syndrome: small testes, some development of the breasts, sparse body hair, and long limbs. This syndrome results from the presence of two or more X chromosomes with one Y chromosome (genotypes XXY or XXXY, for example). (From Patton KT, Thibodeau GA: *Anatomy & physiology,* ed 9, St Louis, 2016, Mosby. Courtesy Nancy S. Wexler, PhD, Columbia University.)

Deletions. Broken chromosomes and lost DNA cause **deletions** (Figure 2-17). Usually, a gamete with a deletion unites with a normal gamete to form a zygote. The zygote thus has one chromosome with the normal complement of genes and one with some missing genes. Because many genes can be lost in a deletion, serious consequences result even though one normal chromosome is present. The most often cited example of a disease caused by a chromosomal deletion is the **cri du chat syndrome.** The term literally means "cry of the cat" and describes the characteristic cry of the affected child. Other symptoms include low birth weight, severe intellectual disability, microcephaly (smaller than normal head size), and heart defects. The disease is caused by a deletion of part of the short arm of chromosome 5.

Duplications. A deficiency of genetic material is more harmful than an excess, so **duplications** usually have less serious consequences than deletions. For example, a deletion of a region of chromosome 5 causes cri du chat syndrome, but a duplication of the same region causes mental retardation but less serious physical defects.

Inversions. An **inversion** occurs when two breaks take place on a chromosome, followed by the reinsertion of the missing fragment at its original site but in inverted order. Therefore a chromosome symbolized as ABCDEFG might become ABEDCFG after an inversion.

Unlike deletions and duplications, no loss or gain of genetic material occurs, so inversions are "balanced" alterations of chromosome structure, and they often have no apparent physical effect. Some genes are influenced by neighboring genes, however, and this **position effect,** a change in a gene's expression caused by its position, sometimes results in physical defects in these persons. Inversions can cause serious

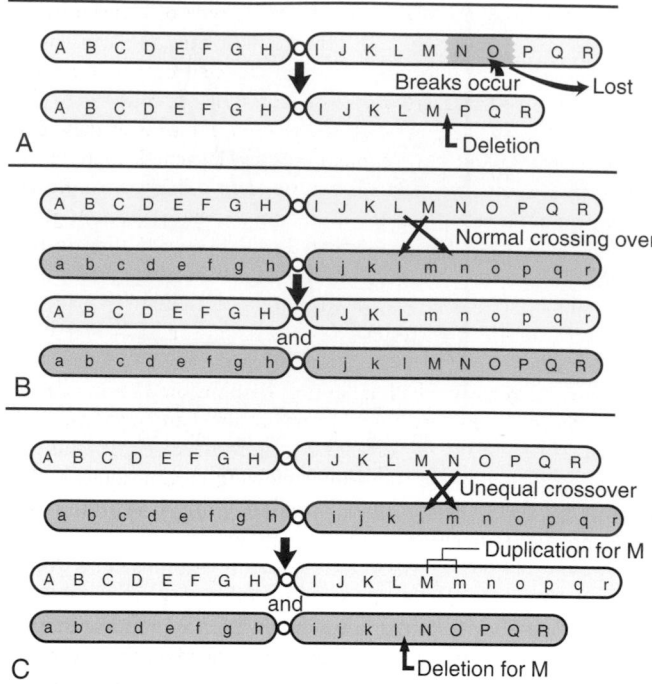

FIGURE 2-17 Abnormalities of Chromosome Structure. A, Deletion occurs when a chromosome segment is lost. **B,** Normal crossing over. **C,** The generation of duplication and deletion through unequal crossing over.

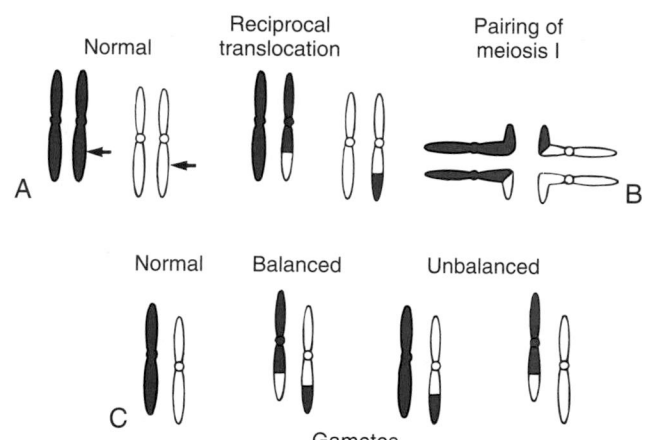

FIGURE 2-18 Normal and Abnormal Chromosome Translocation. A, Normal chromosomes and reciprocal translocation. **B,** Pairing at meiosis. **C,** Consequences of translocation in gametes; unbalanced gametes result in zygotes that are partially trisomic and partially monosomic and consequently develop abnormally.

problems in the offspring of individuals carrying the inversion because the inversion can lead to duplications and deletions in the chromosomes transmitted to the offspring.

Translocations. The interchange of genetic material between nonhomologous chromosomes is called **translocation.** A **reciprocal translocation** occurs when breaks take place in two different chromosomes and the material is exchanged (Figure 2-18, *A*). As with inversions, the carrier of a reciprocal translocation is usually normal, but his or her offspring can have duplications and deletions.

A second and clinically more important type of translocation is **Robertsonian translocation**. In this disorder, the long arms of two nonhomologous chromosomes fuse at the centromere, forming a single chromosome. Robertsonian translocations are confined to chromosomes 13, 14, 15, 21, and 22 because the short arms of these chromosomes are very small and contain no essential genetic material. The short arms are usually lost during subsequent cell divisions. Because the carriers of Robertsonian translocations lose no important genetic material, they are unaffected although they have only 45 chromosomes in each cell. Their offspring, however, may have serious monosomies or trisomies. For example, a common Robertsonian translocation involves the fusion of the long arms of chromosomes 21 and 14. An offspring who inherits a gamete carrying the fused chromosome can receive an extra copy of the long arm of chromosome 21 and develop Down syndrome. Robertsonian translocations are responsible for approximately 3% to 5% of Down syndrome cases. Parents who carry a Robertsonian translocation involving chromosome 21 have an increased risk for producing multiple offspring with Down syndrome.

Fragile sites. A number of areas on chromosomes develop distinctive breaks and gaps (observable microscopically) when the cells are cultured. Most of these fragile sites do not appear to be related to disease. However, one fragile site, located on the long arm of the X chromosome, is associated with *fragile X syndrome.* The most important feature of this syndrome is intellectual disability. With a relatively high population prevalence (affecting approximately 1 in 4000 males and 1 in 8000 females), fragile X syndrome is the second most common genetic cause of intellectual disability (after Down syndrome).

In fragile X syndrome, females who inherit the mutation do not necessarily express the disease condition, but they can pass it on to descendants who do express it. Ordinarily, a male who inherits a disease gene on the X chromosome expresses the condition, because he has only one X chromosome. An uncommon feature of this disease is that about one third of carrier females are affected, although less severely than males. Unaffected transmitting males have been shown to have more than about 50 repeated DNA sequences near the beginning of the fragile X gene. These trinucleotide sequences, which consist of CGG sequences duplicated many times, cause fragile X syndrome when the number of copies exceeds 200.[6] The number of these repeats can increase from generation to generation. More than 20 other genetic diseases, including Huntington disease and myotonic dystrophy, also are caused by this mechanism.[7]

✔ QUICK CHECK 2-1
1. What is the major composition of DNA?
2. Define the terms mutation, autosomes, and sex chromosomes.
3. What is the significance of mRNA?
4. What is the significance of chromosomal translocation?

ELEMENTS OF FORMAL GENETICS

The mechanisms by which an individual's set of paired chromosomes produces traits are the principles of genetic inheritance. Mendel's work with garden peas first defined these principles. Later geneticists have refined Mendel's work to explain patterns of inheritance for traits and diseases that appear in families.

Analysis of traits that occur with defined, predictable patterns has helped geneticists to assemble the pieces of the human gene map. Current research focuses on determining the RNA or protein products of each gene and understanding the way they contribute to disease. Eventually, diseases and defects caused by single genes can be traced and therapies to prevent and treat such diseases can be developed.

Traits caused by single genes are called mendelian traits (after Gregor Mendel). Each gene occupies a position along a chromosome known as a locus. The genes at a particular locus can have different forms (i.e., they can be composed of different nucleotide sequences) called alleles. A locus that has two or more alleles that each occur with an appreciable frequency in a population is said to be polymorphic (or a polymorphism).

Because humans are diploid organisms, each chromosome is represented twice, with one member of the chromosome pair contributed by the father and one by the mother. At a given locus, an individual has one allele whose origin is paternal and one whose origin is maternal. When the two alleles are identical, the individual is homozygous at that locus. When the alleles are not identical, the individual is heterozygous at that locus.

Phenotype and Genotype

The composition of genes at a given locus is known as the genotype. The outward appearance of an individual, which is the result of both genotype and environment, is the phenotype. For example, an infant who is born with an inability to metabolize the amino acid phenylalanine has the single-gene disorder known as phenylketonuria (PKU) and thus has the PKU genotype. If the condition is left untreated, abnormal metabolites of phenylalanine will begin to accumulate in the infant's brain and irreversible intellectual disability will occur. Intellectual disability is thus one aspect of the PKU phenotype. By imposing dietary restrictions to exclude food that contains phenylalanine, however, intellectual disability can be prevented. Foods high in phenylalanine include proteins found in milk, dairy products, meat, fish, chicken, eggs, beans, and nuts. Although the child still has the PKU genotype, a modification of the environment (in this case, the child's diet) produces an outwardly normal phenotype.

Dominance and Recessiveness

In many loci, the effects of one allele mask those of another when the two are found together in a heterozygote. The allele whose effects are observable is said to be dominant. The allele whose effects are hidden is said to be recessive (from the Latin root for "hiding"). Traditionally, for loci having two alleles, the dominant allele is denoted by an uppercase letter and the recessive allele is denoted by a lowercase letter. When one allele is dominant over another, the heterozygote genotype *Aa* has the same phenotype as the dominant homozygote *AA.* For the recessive allele to be expressed, it must exist in the homozygote form, *aa.* When the heterozygote is distinguishable from both homozygotes, the locus is said to exhibit codominance.

A carrier is an individual who has a disease gene but is phenotypically normal. Many genes for a recessive disease occur in heterozygotes who carry one copy of the gene but do not express the disease. When recessive genes are lethal in the homozygous state, they are eliminated from the population when they occur in homozygotes. By "hiding" in carriers, however, recessive genes for diseases are passed on to the next generation.

TRANSMISSION OF GENETIC DISEASES

The pattern in which a genetic disease is inherited through generations is termed the mode of inheritance. Knowing the mode of inheritance can reveal much about the disease-causing gene itself, and members of families with the disease can be given reliable genetic counseling.

Gregor Mendel systematically studied modes of inheritance and formulated two basic laws of inheritance. His **principle of segregation** states that homologous genes separate from one another during reproduction and that each reproductive cell carries only one copy of a homologous gene. Mendel's second law, the **principle of independent assortment**, states that the hereditary transmission of one gene does not affect the transmission of another. Mendel discovered these laws in the mid-nineteenth century by performing breeding experiments with garden peas, even though he had no knowledge of chromosomes. Early twentieth century geneticists found that chromosomal behavior essentially corresponds to Mendel's laws, which now form the basis for the **chromosome theory of inheritance**.

The known single-gene diseases can be classified into four major modes of inheritance: autosomal dominant, autosomal recessive, X-linked dominant, and X-linked recessive. The first two types involve genes known to occur on the 22 pairs of autosomes. The last two types occur on the X chromosome; very few disease-causing genes occur on the Y chromosome.

The **pedigree** chart summarizes family relationships and shows which members of a family are affected by a genetic disease (Figure 2-19). Generally, the pedigree begins with one individual in the family, the **proband**. This individual is usually the first person in the family diagnosed or seen in a clinic.

Autosomal Dominant Inheritance
Characteristics of Pedigrees

Diseases caused by autosomal dominant genes are rare, with the most common occurring in fewer than 1 in 500 individuals. Therefore it is uncommon for two individuals who are both affected by the same autosomal dominant disease to produce offspring together. Figure 2-20, *A*, illustrates this unusual pattern. Affected offspring are usually produced by the union of a normal parent with an affected heterozygous parent. The Punnett square in Figure 2-20, *B*, illustrates this mating. The affected parent can pass either a disease-causing allele or a normal allele to the next generation. On average, half the children will be heterozygous and will express the disease, and half will be normal.

The pedigree in Figure 2-21 shows the transmission of an autosomal dominant allele. Several important characteristics of this pedigree support the conclusion that the trait is caused by an autosomal dominant gene:

1. The two sexes exhibit the trait in approximately equal proportions; males and females are equally likely to transmit the trait to their offspring.
2. No generations are skipped. If an individual has the trait, one parent must also have it. If neither parent has the trait, none of the children have it (with the exception of new mutations, as discussed later).
3. Affected heterozygous individuals transmit the trait to approximately half their children, and because gamete transmission is subject to chance fluctuations, all or none of the children of an affected parent may have the trait. When large numbers of matings of this type are studied, however, the proportion of affected children closely approaches one half.

Recurrence Risks

Parents at risk for producing children with a genetic disease nearly always ask the question, "What is the *chance* that our child will have this disease?" The probability that an individual will develop a genetic

FIGURE 2-19 Symbols Commonly Used in Pedigrees. (From Jorde LB et al: *Medical genetics,* ed 4, St Louis, 2010, Mosby.)

disease is termed the **recurrence risk**. When one parent is affected by an autosomal dominant disease (and is a heterozygote) and the other is unaffected, the recurrence risk for each child is one half.

An important principle is that each birth is an independent event, much like a coin toss. Thus, even though parents may have already had a child with the disease, their recurrence risk remains one half. Even if they have produced several children, all affected (or all unaffected) by the disease, the law of independence dictates the probability their next child will have the disease is still one half. Parents' misunderstanding of this principle is a common problem encountered in genetic counseling.

FIGURE 2-20 Punnett Square and Autosomal Dominant Traits. A, Punnett square for the mating of two individuals with an autosomal dominant gene. Here both parents are affected by the trait. B, Punnett square for the mating of a normal individual with a carrier for an autosomal dominant gene.

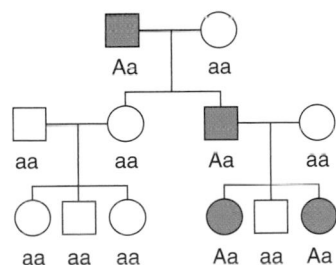

FIGURE 2-21 Pedigree Illustrating the Inheritance Pattern of Postaxial Polydactyly, an Autosomal Dominant Disorder. Affected individuals are represented by shading. (From Jorde LB et al: *Medical genetics*, ed 4, St Louis, 2010, Mosby.)

If a child is born with an autosomal dominant disease and there is no history of the disease in the family, the child is probably the product of a new mutation. The gene transmitted by one of the parents has thus undergone a mutation from a normal to a disease-causing allele. The alleles at this locus in most of the parent's other germ cells are still normal. In this situation the recurrence risk for the parent's subsequent offspring is not greater than that of the general population. The offspring of the affected child, however, will have a recurrence risk of one half. Because these diseases often reduce the potential for reproduction, many autosomal dominant diseases result from new mutations.

Occasionally, two or more offspring have symptoms of an autosomal dominant disease when there is no family history of the disease. Because mutation is a rare event, it is unlikely that this disease would be a result of multiple mutations in the same family. The mechanism most likely responsible is termed germline mosaicism. During the embryonic development of one of the parents, a mutation occurred that affected all or part of the germline. Few or none of the somatic cells of the embryo were affected. Thus the parent carries the mutation

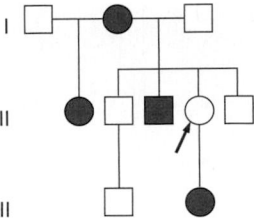

FIGURE 2-22 Pedigree for Retinoblastoma Showing Incomplete Penetrance. Female with marked arrow in line II must be heterozygous, but she does not express the trait.

in his or her germline but does not actually express the disease. As a result, the unaffected parent can transmit the mutation to multiple offspring. This phenomenon, although relatively rare, can have significant effects on recurrence risks.[8]

Delayed Age of Onset

One of the best-known autosomal dominant diseases is Huntington disease, a neurologic disorder whose main features are progressive dementia and increasingly uncontrollable limb movements (chorea; discussed further in Chapter 15). A key feature of this disease is its delayed age of onset: symptoms usually are not seen until 40 years of age or later. Thus those who develop the disease often have borne children before they are aware they have the disease-causing mutation. If the disease was present at birth, nearly all affected persons would die before reaching reproductive age and the occurrence of the disease-causing allele in the population would be much lower. An individual whose parent has the disease has a 50% chance of developing it during middle age. He or she is thus confronted with a torturous question: Should I have children, knowing that there is a 50:50 chance that I may have this disease-causing gene and will pass it to half of my children? A DNA test can now be used to determine whether an individual has inherited the trinucleotide repeat mutation that causes Huntington disease.

Penetrance and Expressivity

The penetrance of a trait is the percentage of individuals with a specific genotype who also exhibit the expected phenotype. Incomplete penetrance means individuals who have the disease-causing genotype may not exhibit the disease phenotype at all, even though the genotype and the associated disease may be transmitted to the next generation. A pedigree illustrating the transmission of an autosomal dominant mutation with incomplete penetrance is provided in Figure 2-22. Retinoblastoma, the most common malignant eye tumor affecting children, typically exhibits incomplete penetrance. About 10% of the individuals who are obligate carriers of the disease-causing mutation (i.e., those who have an affected parent and affected children and therefore must themselves carry the mutation) do not have the disease. The penetrance of the disease-causing genotype is then said to be 90%.

The gene responsible for retinoblastoma is a tumor-suppressor gene: the normal function of its protein product is to regulate the cell cycle so cells do not divide uncontrollably. When the protein is altered because of a genetic mutation, its tumor-suppressing capacity is lost and a tumor can form[9] (see Chapters 10 and 17).

Expressivity is the extent of variation in phenotype associated with a particular genotype. If the expressivity of a disease is variable, penetrance may be complete but the severity of the disease can vary greatly. A good example of variable expressivity in an autosomal dominant disease is neurofibromatosis type 1, or von Recklinghausen disease. As in retinoblastoma, the mutations that cause neurofibromatosis type 1

FIGURE 2-23 Neurofibromatosis. Tumors. The most common is sessile or pedunculated. Early tumors are soft, dome-shaped papules or nodules that have a distinctive violaceous hue. Most are benign. (From Habif et al: *Skin disease: diagnosis and treatment,* ed 2, St Louis, 2005, Mosby.)

occur in a tumor-suppressor gene.[10] The expression of this disease varies from a few harmless café-au-lait (light brown) spots on the skin to numerous neurofibromas, scoliosis, seizures, gliomas, neuromas, malignant peripheral nerve sheath tumors, hypertension, and learning disorders (Figure 2-23).

Several factors cause variable expressivity. Genes at other loci sometimes modify the expression of a disease-causing gene. Environmental factors also can influence expression of a disease-causing gene. Finally, different mutations at a locus can cause variation in severity. For example, a mutation that alters only one amino acid of the factor VIII gene usually produces a mild form of hemophilia A, whereas a "stop" codon (premature termination of translation) usually produces a more severe form of this blood coagulation disorder.

Epigenetics and Genomic Imprinting

Although this chapter focuses on DNA sequence variation and its consequence for disease, there is increasing evidence that the same DNA sequence can produce dramatically different phenotypes because of chemical modifications altering the *expression* of genes (these modifications are collectively termed epigenetic, Chapter 3). An important example of such a modification is DNA methylation, the attachment of a methyl group to a cytosine base followed by a guanine base in the DNA sequence (Figure 2-24). These sequences, which are common near many genes, are termed CpG islands. When the CpG islands located near a gene become heavily methylated, the gene is less likely to be transcribed into mRNA. In other words, the gene becomes transcriptionally inactive. One study showed that identical (monozygotic) twins accumulate different methylation patterns in the DNA sequences of their somatic cells as they age, causing increasing numbers of phenotypic differences.[11] Intriguingly, twins with more differences in their lifestyles (e.g., smoking versus nonsmoking) accumulated larger

numbers of differences in their methylation patterns. The twins, despite having identical DNA sequences, become more and more different as a result of epigenetic changes, which in turn affect the expression of genes (see Figure 3-5).

Epigenetic alteration of gene activity can have important disease consequences. For example, a major cause of one form of inherited colon cancer (termed hereditary nonpolyposis colorectal cancer [HNPCC]) is the methylation of a gene whose protein product repairs damaged DNA. When this gene becomes inactive, damaged DNA accumulates, eventually resulting in colon tumors. Epigenetic changes are also discussed in Chapters 3, 10 and 11.

Approximately 100 human genes are thought to be methylated differently, depending on which parent transmits the gene. This epigenetic modification, characterized by methylation and other changes, is termed genomic imprinting. For each of these genes, one of the parents *imprints* the gene (inactivates it) when it is transmitted to the offspring. An example is the insulin-like growth factor 2 gene *(IGF2)* on chromosome 11, which is transmitted by both parents, but the copy inherited from the mother is normally methylated and inactivated (imprinted). Thus only one copy of *IGF2* is active in normal individuals. However, the maternal imprint is occasionally lost, resulting in two active copies of *IGF2*. This causes excess fetal growth and contributes to a condition known as *Beckwith-Weidemann syndrome* (see p. 65).

A second example of genomic imprinting is a deletion of part of the long arm of chromosome 15 (15q11-q13), which, when inherited from the father, causes the offspring to manifest a disease known as *Prader-Willi syndrome* (short stature, obesity, hypogonadism). When the same deletion is inherited from the mother, the offspring develop *Angelman syndrome* (intellectual disability, seizures, ataxic gait). The two different phenotypes reflect the fact that different genes are normally active in the maternally and paternally transmitted copies of this region of chromosome 15 (see p. 65).

Autosomal Recessive Inheritance
Characteristics of Pedigrees

Like autosomal dominant diseases, diseases caused by autosomal recessive genes are rare in populations, although there can be numerous carriers. The most common lethal recessive disease in white children, cystic fibrosis, occurs in about 1 in 2500 births. Approximately 1 in 25 whites carries a copy of a mutation that causes cystic fibrosis (see Chapter 28). Carriers are phenotypically unaffected. Some autosomal recessive diseases are characterized by delayed age of onset, incomplete penetrance, and variable expressivity.

Figure 2-25 shows a pedigree for cystic fibrosis. The gene responsible for cystic fibrosis encodes a chloride ion channel in some epithelial cells. Defective transport of chloride ions leads to a salt imbalance that results in secretions of abnormally thick, dehydrated mucus. Some digestive organs, particularly the pancreas, become obstructed, causing malnutrition, and the lungs become clogged with mucus, making them highly susceptible to bacterial infections. Death from lung disease or heart failure occurs before 40 years of age in about half of persons with cystic fibrosis.

The important criteria for discerning autosomal recessive inheritance include the following:
1. Males and females are affected in equal proportions.
2. Consanguinity (marriage between related individuals) is sometimes present, especially for rare recessive diseases.
3. The disease may be seen in siblings of affected individuals but usually not in their parents.
4. On average, one fourth of the offspring of carrier parents will be affected.

FIGURE 2-24 Epigenetic Modifications. Because DNA is a long molecule, it needs packaging to fit in the tiny nucleus. Packaging involves *coiling* of the DNA in a "left-handed" spiral around spools, made of four pairs of proteins individually known as histones and collectively termed the histone octamer. The entire spool is called a nucleosome (also see Figure 1-2). Nucleosomes are organized into chromatin, the repeating building blocks of a chromosome. Histone modifications are correlated with methylation, are reversible, and occur at multiple sites. Methylation occurs at the 5 position of cytosine and provides a "footprint" or signature as a unique epigenetic alteration *(red)*. When genes are expressed, chromatin is open or active; however, when chromatin is condensed because of methylation and histone modification, genes are inactivated.

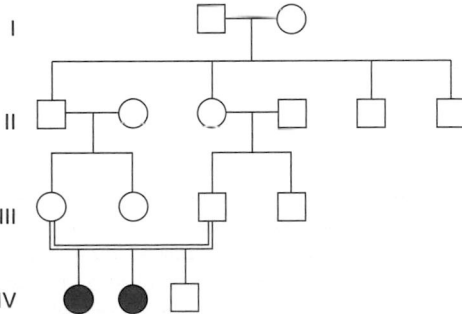

FIGURE 2-25 Pedigree for Cystic Fibrosis. Cystic fibrosis is an autosomal recessive disorder. The double bar denotes a consanguineous mating. Because cystic fibrosis is relatively common in European populations, most cases do not involve consanguinity.

	D	d
D	DD Homozygous normal	Dd Heterozygous carrier
d	Dd Heterozygous carrier	dd Homozygous affected

FIGURE 2-26 Punnett Square for the Mating of Heterozygous Carriers Typical of Most Cases of Recessive Disease.

Recurrence Risks

In most cases of recessive disease, both of the parents of affected individuals are heterozygous carriers. On average, one fourth of their offspring will be normal homozygotes, half will be phenotypically normal carrier heterozygotes, and one fourth will be homozygotes with the disease (Figure 2-26). Thus the recurrence risk for the offspring of carrier parents is 25%. However, in any given family, there are chance fluctuations.

If two parents have a recessive disease, they each must be homozygous for the disease. Therefore all their children also must be affected. This distinguishes recessive from dominant inheritance because two parents both affected by a dominant gene are nearly always both heterozygotes and thus one fourth of their children will be unaffected.

Because carrier parents usually are unaware that they both carry the same recessive allele, they often produce an affected child before becoming aware of their condition. Carrier detection tests can identify heterozygotes by analyzing the DNA sequence to reveal a mutation. Some recessive diseases for which carrier detection tests are routinely used include phenylketonuria (PKU), sickle cell disease, cystic fibrosis, Tay-Sachs disease, hemochromatosis, and galactosemia.

Consanguinity

Consanguinity and inbreeding are related concepts. Consanguinity refers to the mating of two related individuals, and the offspring of such matings are said to be *inbred*. Consanguinity is sometimes an important characteristic of pedigrees for recessive diseases because relatives share a certain proportion of genes received from a common ancestor. The proportion of shared genes depends on the closeness of their biologic relationship. Consanguineous matings produce a significant increase in recessive disorders and are seen most often in pedigrees for rare recessive disorders.

X-Linked Inheritance

Some genetic conditions are caused by mutations in genes located on the sex chromosomes, and this mode of inheritance is termed sex linked. Only a few diseases are known to be inherited as X-linked dominant or Y chromosome traits, so only the more common X-linked recessive diseases are discussed here.

Because females receive two X chromosomes, one from the father and one from the mother, they can be homozygous for a disease allele at a given locus, homozygous for the normal allele at the locus, or heterozygous. Males, having only one X chromosome, are hemizygous for genes on this chromosome. If a male inherits a recessive disease gene on the X chromosome, he will be affected by the disease because the Y chromosome does not carry a normal allele to counteract the effects of the disease gene. Because a single copy of an X-linked recessive gene will cause disease in a male, whereas two copies are required for disease expression in females, more males are affected by X-linked recessive diseases than are females.

X Inactivation

In the late 1950s Mary Lyon proposed that one X chromosome in the somatic cells of females is permanently inactivated, a process termed X inactivation.[12,13] This proposal, the Lyon hypothesis, explains why most gene products coded by the X chromosome are present in equal amounts in males and females, even though males have only one X chromosome and females have two X chromosomes. This phenomenon is called dosage compensation. The inactivated X chromosomes are observable in many interphase cells as highly condensed intranuclear chromatin bodies, termed Barr bodies (after Barr and Bertram, who discovered them in the late 1940s). Normal females have one Barr body in each somatic cell, whereas normal males have no Barr bodies.

X inactivation occurs very early in embryonic development—approximately 7 to 14 days after fertilization. In each somatic cell, one of the two X chromosomes is inactivated. In some cells, the inactivated X chromosome is the one contributed by the father; in other cells it is the one contributed by the mother. Once the X chromosome has been inactivated in a cell, all the descendants of that cell have the same chromosome inactivated (Figure 2-27). Thus inactivation is said to be random but *fixed*.

Some individuals do not have the normal number of X chromosomes in their somatic cells. For example, males with Klinefelter syndrome typically have two X chromosomes and one Y chromosome. These males do have one Barr body in each cell. Females whose cell nuclei have three X chromosomes have two Barr bodies in each cell,

FIGURE 2-27 The X Inactivation Process. The maternal *(m)* and paternal *(p)* X chromosomes are both active in the zygote and in early embryonic cells. X inactivation then takes place, resulting in cells having either an active paternal X or an active maternal X. Females are thus X chromosome mosaics, as shown in the tissue sample at the bottom of the page. (From Jorde LB et al: *Medical genetics*, ed 4, St Louis, 2010, Mosby.)

and females whose cell nuclei have four X chromosomes have three Barr bodies in each cell. Females with Turner syndrome have only one X chromosome and no Barr bodies. Thus the number of Barr bodies is always one less than the number of X chromosomes in the cell. All but one X chromosome are always inactivated.

Persons with abnormal numbers of X chromosomes, such as those with Turner syndrome or Klinefelter syndrome, are not physically normal. This situation presents a puzzle because they presumably have only one active X chromosome, the same as individuals with normal numbers of chromosomes. This is probably because the distal tips of the short and long arms of the X chromosome, as well as several other regions on the chromosome arm, are not inactivated. Thus X inactivation is also known to be *incomplete*.

The inactivated X chromosome DNA is heavily methylated. Inactive X chromosomes can be at least partially reactivated in vitro by administering 5-azacytidine, a demethylating agent.

Sex Determination

The process of sexual differentiation, in which the embryonic gonads become either testes or ovaries, begins during the sixth week of gestation. A key principle of mammalian sex determination is that one copy of the Y chromosome is sufficient to initiate the process of gonadal differentiation that produces a male fetus. The number of X chromosomes does not alter this process. For example, an individual with two X chromosomes and one Y chromosome in each cell is still phenotypically a male. Thus the Y chromosome contains a gene that begins the process of male gonadal development.

This gene, termed *SRY* (for "sex-determining region on the Y"), has been located on the short arm of the Y chromosome.[14] The *SRY* gene lies just outside the pseudoautosomal region (Figure 2-28), which pairs with the distal tip of the short arm of the X chromosome during meiosis and exchanges genetic material with it (crossover), just as autosomes do. The DNA sequences of these regions on the X and Y chromosomes are highly similar. The rest of the X and Y chromosomes,

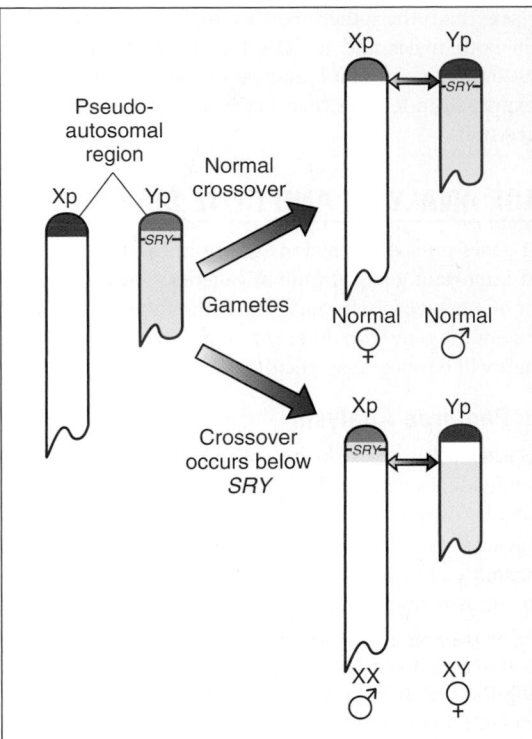

FIGURE 2-28 Distal Short Arms of the X and Y Chromosomes Exchange Material During Meiosis in the Male. The region of the Y chromosome in which this crossover occurs is called the *pseudoautosomal region*. The *SRY* gene, which triggers the process leading to male gonadal differentiation, is located just outside the pseudoautosomal region. Occasionally, the crossover occurs on the centromeric side of the *SRY* gene, causing it to lie on an X chromosome instead of a Y chromosome. An offspring receiving this X chromosome will be an XX male, and an offspring receiving the Y chromosome will be an XY female.

however, do not exchange material and are not similar in DNA sequence.

Other genes that contribute to male differentiation are located on other chromosomes. Thus *SRY* triggers the action of genes on other chromosomes. This concept is supported by the fact that the *SRY* protein product is similar to other proteins known to regulate gene expression.

Occasionally, the crossover between X and Y occurs closer to the centromere than it should, placing the *SRY* gene on the X chromosome after crossover. This variation can result in offspring with an apparently normal XX karyotype but a male phenotype. Such XX males are seen in about 1 in 20,000 live births and resemble males with Klinefelter syndrome. Conversely, it is possible to inherit a Y chromosome that has lost the *SRY* gene (the result of either a crossover error or a deletion of the gene). This situation produces an XY female. Such females have gonadal streaks rather than ovaries and have poorly developed secondary sex characteristics.

✔**QUICK CHECK 2-2**
1. Why is the influence of environment significant to phenotype?
2. Discuss the differences between a dominant and a recessive allele.
3. Why are the concepts of variable expressivity, incomplete penetrance, and delayed age of onset so important in relation to genetic diseases?
4. What is the recurrence risk for autosomal dominant inheritance and recessive inheritance?

Characteristics of Pedigrees

X-linked pedigrees show distinctive modes of inheritance. The most striking characteristic is that females seldom are affected. To express an X-linked recessive trait fully, a female must be homozygous: either both her parents are affected, or her father is affected and her mother is a carrier. Such matings are rare.

The following are important principles of X-linked recessive inheritance:
1. The trait is seen much more often in males than in females.
2. Because a father can give a son only a Y chromosome, the trait is never transmitted from father to son.
3. The gene can be transmitted through a series of carrier females, causing the appearance of one or more "skipped generations."
4. The gene is passed from an affected father to all his daughters, who, as phenotypically normal carriers, transmit it to approximately half their sons, who are affected.

A relatively common X-linked recessive disorder is Duchenne muscular dystrophy (DMD), which affects approximately 1 in 3500 males. As its name suggests, this disorder is characterized by progressive muscle degeneration. Affected individuals usually are unable to walk by age 10 or 12 years. The disease affects the heart and respiratory muscles, and death caused by respiratory or cardiac failure usually occurs before 20 years of age. Identification of the disease-causing gene (on the short arm of the X chromosome) has greatly increased our understanding of the disorder.[15] The *DMD* gene is the largest gene ever found in humans, spanning more than 2 million DNA bases. It encodes a previously undiscovered muscle protein, termed **dystrophin**. Extensive study of dystrophin indicates that it plays an essential role in maintaining the structural integrity of muscle cells; it may also help to regulate the activity of membrane proteins. When dystrophin is absent, as in DMD, the cell cannot survive, and muscle deterioration ensues. Most cases of DMD are caused by frameshift deletions of portions of the *DMD* gene and thus involve alterations of the amino acids encoded by the DNA following the deletion.

Recurrence Risks

The most common mating type involving X-linked recessive genes is the combination of a carrier female and a normal male (Figure 2-29, *A*). On average, the carrier mother will transmit the disease-causing allele to half her sons (who are affected) and half her daughters (who are carriers).

The other common mating type is an affected father and a normal mother (see Figure 2-29, *B*). In this situation, all the sons will be normal because the father can transmit only his Y chromosome to them. Because all the daughters must receive the father's X chromosome, they will all be heterozygous carriers. Because the sons *must* receive the Y chromosome and the daughters *must* receive the X chromosome with the disease gene, these are precise outcomes and not probabilities. None of the children will be affected.

The final mating pattern, less common than the other two, involves an affected father and a carrier mother (see Figure 2-29, *C*). With this pattern, on average, half the daughters will be heterozygous carriers, and half will be homozygous for the disease allele and thus affected. Half the sons will be normal, and half will be affected. Some X-linked recessive diseases, such as DMD, are fatal or incapacitating before the affected individual reaches reproductive age, and therefore affected fathers are rare.

Sex-Limited and Sex-Influenced Traits

A **sex-limited trait** can occur in only one sex, often because of anatomic differences. Inherited uterine and testicular defects are two obvious examples. A **sex-influenced trait** occurs much more often

FIGURE 2-29 Punnett Square and X-Linked Recessive Traits.
A, Punnett square for the mating of a normal male ($X_H Y$) and a female carrier of an X-linked recessive gene ($X_H X_h$). **B,** Punnett square for the mating of a normal female ($X_H X_H$) with a male affected by an X-linked recessive disease ($X_h Y$). **C,** Punnett square for the mating of a female who carries an X-linked recessive gene ($X_H X_h$) with a male who is affected with the disease caused by the gene ($X_h Y$).

in one sex than the other. For example, male-pattern baldness occurs in both males and females but is much more common in males. Autosomal dominant breast cancer, which is much more commonly expressed in females than males, is another example of a sex-influenced trait.

LINKAGE ANALYSIS AND GENE MAPPING

Locating genes on specific regions of chromosomes has been one of the most important goals of human genetics. The location and identification of a gene can tell much about the function of the gene, the interaction of the gene with other genes, and the likelihood that certain individuals will develop a genetic disease.

Classic Pedigree Analysis

Mendel's second law, the principle of independent assortment, states that an individual's genes will be transmitted to the next generation independently of one another. This law is only partly true, however, because genes located close together on the same chromosome do tend to be transmitted together to the offspring. Thus Mendel's principle of independent assortment holds true for most pairs of genes but not those that occupy the same region of a chromosome. Such loci demonstrate linkage and are said to be linked.

During the first meiotic stage, the arms of homologous chromosome pairs intertwine and sometimes exchange portions of their DNA (Figure 2-30) in a process known as crossover. During crossover, new combinations of alleles can be formed. For example, two loci on a chromosome have alleles *A* and *a* and alleles *B* and *b*. Alleles *A* and *B* are located together on one member of a chromosome pair, and alleles *a* and *b* are located on the other member. The genotype of this individual is denoted as *AB/ab*.

As Figure 2-30, *A*, shows, the allele pairs *AB* and *ab* would be transmitted together when no crossover occurs. However, when crossover occurs (see Figure 2-30, *B*), all four possible pairs of alleles can be transmitted to the offspring: *AB*, *aB*, *Ab*, and *ab*. The process of forming such new arrangements of alleles is called recombination. Crossover does not necessarily lead to recombination, however, because double

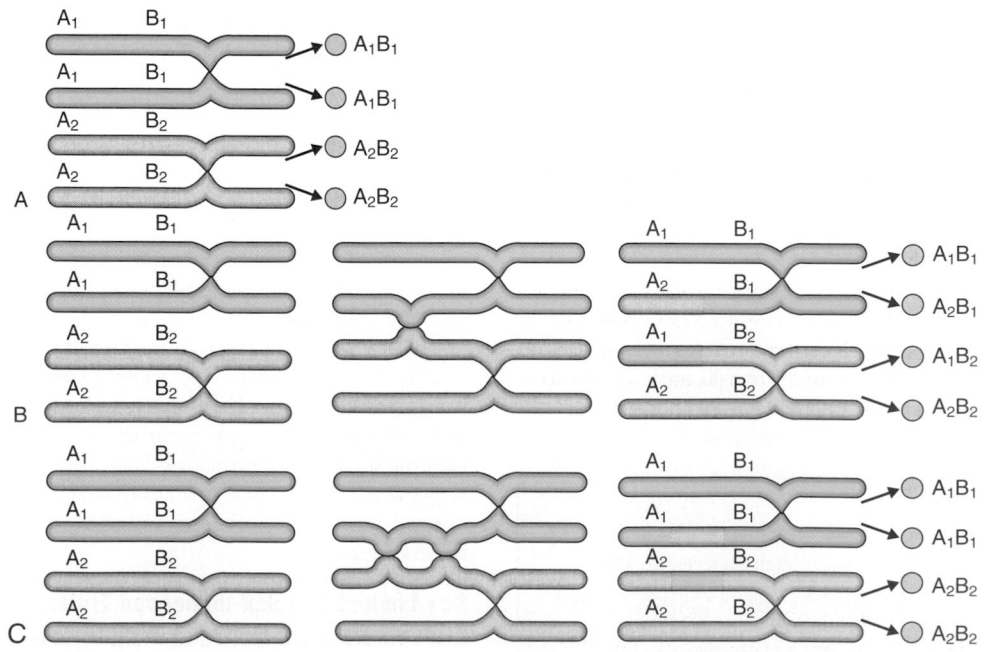

FIGURE 2-30 Genetic Results of Crossing Over. A, No crossing over. **B,** Crossing over with recombination. **C,** Double crossing over, resulting in no recombination.

FIGURE 2-31 Example of Diseases: A Gene Map. *ADA,* Adenosine deaminase; *ALD,* adrenoleukodystrophy; *PKU,* phenylketonuria.

crossover between two loci can result in no actual recombination of the alleles at the loci (see Figure 2-30, *C*).

Once a close linkage has been established between a disease locus and a "marker" locus (a DNA sequence that varies among individuals) and once the alleles of the two loci that are inherited together within a family have been determined, reliable predictions can be made as to whether a member of a family will develop the disease. Linkage has been established between several DNA polymorphisms and each of the two major genes that can cause autosomal dominant breast cancer (about 5% of breast cancer cases are caused by these autosomal dominant genes). Determining this kind of linkage means that it is possible for offspring of an individual with autosomal dominant breast cancer to know whether they also carry the gene and thus could pass it on to their own children. In most cases, specific disease-causing mutations can be identified, allowing direct detection and diagnosis. For some genetic diseases, prophylactic treatment is available if the condition can be diagnosed in time. An example of this is hemochromatosis, a recessive genetic disease in which excess iron is absorbed, causing degeneration of the heart, liver, brain, and other vital organs. Individuals at risk for developing the disease can be determined by testing for a mutation in the hemochromatosis gene and through clinical tests, and preventive therapy (periodic phlebotomy) can be initiated to deplete iron stores and ensure a normal life span.

Complete Human Gene Map: Prospects and Benefits

The major goals of the Human Genome Project were to find the locations of all human genes (the "gene map") and to determine the entire human DNA sequence. These goals have now been accomplished and the genes responsible for more than 4000 mendelian conditions have been identified (Figure 2-31).[1,16,17] This has greatly increased our understanding of the mechanisms that underlie many diseases, such as retinoblastoma, cystic fibrosis, neurofibromatosis, and Huntington disease. The project also has led to more accurate diagnosis of these conditions, and in some cases more effective treatment.

DNA sequencing has become much less expensive and more efficient in recent years. Consequently, many thousands of individuals have now been completely sequenced, leading in some cases to the identification of disease-causing genes (see *Health Alert:* Gene Therapy).[18]

HEALTH ALERT

Gene Therapy

Thousands of subjects are currently enrolled in more than 1000 gene therapy protocols. Most of these protocols involve the genetic alteration of cells to combat various types of cancer. Others involve the treatment of inherited diseases, such as β-thalassemia, hemophilia B, severe combined immunodeficiency, and retinitis pigmentosa.

MULTIFACTORIAL INHERITANCE

Not all traits are produced by single genes; some traits result from several genes acting together. These are called **polygenic traits.** When environmental factors influence the expression of the trait (as is usually

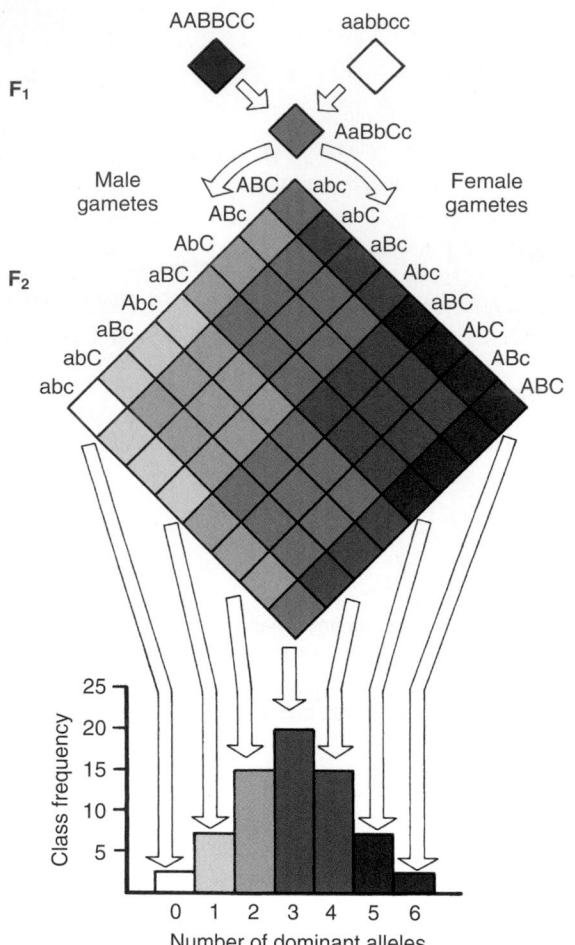

FIGURE 2-32 **Multifactorial Inheritance.** Analysis of mode of inheritance for grain color in wheat. The trait is controlled by three independently assorted gene loci.

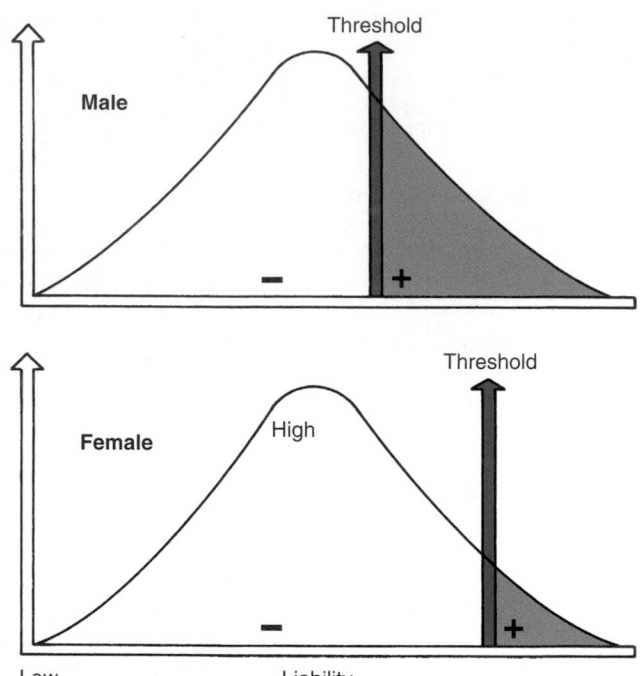

FIGURE 2-33 Threshold of Liability for Pyloric Stenosis in Males and Females.

the case), the term **multifactorial inheritance** is used. Many multifactorial and polygenic traits tend to follow a normal distribution in populations (the familiar bell-shaped curve). Figure 2-32 shows how three loci acting together can cause grain color in wheat to vary in a gradual way from white to red, exemplifying multifactorial inheritance. If both alleles at each of the three loci are white alleles, the color is pure white. If most alleles are white but a few are red, the color is somewhat darker; if all are red, the color is dark red.

Other examples of multifactorial traits include height and IQ. Although both height and IQ are determined in part by genes, they are influenced also by environment. For example, the average height of many human populations has increased by 5 to 10 cm in the past 100 years because of improvements in nutrition and health care. Also, IQ scores can be improved by exposing individuals (especially children) to enriched learning environments. Thus both genes and environment contribute to variation in these traits.

A number of diseases do not follow the bell-shaped distribution. Instead they appear to be either present in or absent from an individual. Yet they do not follow the patterns expected of single-gene diseases. Many of these are probably polygenic or multifactorial, but a certain **threshold of liability** must be crossed before the disease is expressed. Below the threshold the individual appears normal; above it, the individual is affected by the disease (Figure 2-33).

A good example of such a threshold trait is pyloric stenosis, a disorder characterized by a narrowing or obstruction of the pylorus, the area between the stomach and small intestine. Chronic vomiting, constipation, weight loss, and electrolyte imbalance can result from the condition, but it is easily corrected by surgery. The prevalence of pyloric stenosis is about 3 in 1000 live births in whites. This disorder is much more common in males than females, affecting 1 in 200 males and 1 in 1000 females. The apparent reason for this difference is the threshold of liability is much lower in males than females, as shown in Figure 2-33. Thus fewer defective alleles are required to generate the disorder in males. This situation also means the offspring of affected females are more likely to have pyloric stenosis because affected females necessarily carry more disease-causing alleles than do most affected males.

A number of other common diseases are thought to correspond to a threshold model. They include cleft lip and cleft palate, neural tube defects (anencephaly, spina bifida), clubfoot (talipes), and some forms of congenital heart disease.

Although recurrence risks can be given with confidence for single-gene diseases (e.g., 50% for autosomal dominants, 25% for autosomal recessives), it is considerably more difficult to do so for multifactorial diseases. The number of genes contributing to the disease is not known, the precise allelic constitution of the biologic parents is not known, and the extent of environmental effects can vary from one population to another. For most multifactorial diseases, **empirical risks** (i.e., those based on direct observation) have been derived. To determine empirical risks, a large sample of biologic families in which one child has developed the disease is examined. The siblings of each child are then surveyed to calculate the percentage who also develop the disease.

Another difficulty is distinguishing polygenic or multifactorial diseases from single-gene diseases having incomplete penetrance or variable expressivity. Large data sets and good epidemiologic data often are necessary to make the distinction. Box 2-1 lists criteria commonly used to define multifactorial diseases.

BOX 2-1 Criteria Used to Define Multifactorial Diseases

1. The recurrence risk becomes higher if more than one family member is affected. For example, the recurrence risk for neural tube defects in a British family increases to 10% if two siblings have been born with the disease. By contrast, the recurrence risk for single-gene diseases remains the same regardless of the number of siblings affected.

2. If the expression of the disease is more severe, the recurrence risk is higher. This is consistent with the liability model; a more severe expression indicates that the individual is at the extreme end of the liability distribution. Relatives of the affected individual are thus at a higher risk for inheriting disease genes. Cleft lip or cleft palate is a condition in which this has been shown to be true.

3. Relatives of probands of the less commonly affected are more likely to develop the disease. As with pyloric stenosis, this occurs because an affected individual of the less susceptible sex is usually at a more extreme position on the liability distribution.

4. Generally, if the population frequency of the disease is f, the risk for offspring and siblings of probands is approximately $\sqrt{f}$. This does not usually hold true for single-gene traits.

5. The recurrence risk for the disease decreases rapidly in more remotely related relatives. Although the recurrence risk for single-gene diseases decreases by 50% with each degree of relationship (e.g., an autosomal dominant disease has a 50% recurrence risk for siblings, 25% for uncle-nephew relationship, 12.5% for first cousins), the risk for multifactorial inheritance decreases much more quickly.

The genetics of common disorders such as hypertension, heart disease, and diabetes is complex and often confusing. Nevertheless, the public health impact of these diseases, together with the evidence for hereditary factors in their etiology, demands that genetic studies be pursued. Hundreds of genes contributing to susceptibility for these diseases have been discovered, and the next decade will undoubtedly witness substantial advancements in our understanding of these disorders.

QUICK CHECK 2-3

1. Define linkage analysis; cite an example.
2. Why is "threshold of liability" an important consideration in multifactorial inheritance?
3. Discuss the concept of multifactorial inheritance, and include two examples.

DID YOU UNDERSTAND?

DNA, RNA, and Proteins: Heredity at the Molecular Level

1. Genes, the basic units of inheritance, are composed of deoxyribonucleic acid (DNA) and are located on chromosomes.
2. DNA is composed of deoxyribose, a phosphate molecule, and four types of nitrogenous bases. The physical structure of DNA is a double helix.
3. The DNA bases code for amino acids, which in turn make up proteins. The amino acids are specified by triplet codons of nitrogenous bases.
4. DNA replication is based on complementary base pairing, in which a single strand of DNA serves as the template for attracting bases that form a new strand of DNA.
5. DNA polymerase is the primary enzyme involved in replication. It adds bases to the new DNA strand and performs "proofreading" functions.
6. A mutation is an inherited alteration of genetic material (i.e., DNA).
7. Substances that cause mutations are called mutagens.
8. The mutation rate in humans varies from locus to locus and ranges from 10^{-4} to 10^{-7} per gene per generation.
9. Transcription and translation, the two basic processes in which proteins are specified by DNA, both involve ribonucleic acid (RNA). RNA is chemically similar to DNA, but it is single stranded, has a ribose sugar molecule, and has uracil rather than thymine as one of its four nitrogenous bases.
10. Transcription is the process by which DNA specifies a sequence of messenger RNA (mRNA).
11. Much of the RNA sequence is spliced from the mRNA before the mRNA leaves the nucleus. The excised sequences are called introns, and those that remain to code for proteins are called exons.
12. Translation is the process by which RNA directs the synthesis of polypeptides. This process takes place in the ribosomes, which consist of proteins and ribosomal RNA (rRNA).
13. During translation, mRNA interacts with transfer RNA (tRNA), a molecule that has an attachment site for a specific amino acid.

Chromosomes

1. Human cells consist of diploid somatic cells (body cells) and haploid gametes (sperm and egg cells).
2. Humans have 23 pairs of chromosomes. Twenty-two of these pairs are autosomes. The remaining pair consists of the sex chromosomes. Females have two homologous X chromosomes as their sex chromosomes; males have an X and a Y chromosome.
3. A karyotype is an ordered display of chromosomes arranged according to length and the location of the centromere.
4. Various types of stains can be used to make chromosome bands more visible.
5. About 1 in 150 live births has a major diagnosable chromosome abnormality. Chromosome abnormalities are the leading known cause of mental retardation and miscarriage.
6. Polyploidy is a condition in which a euploid cell has some multiple of the normal number of chromosomes. Humans have been observed to have triploidy (three copies of each chromosome) and tetraploidy (four copies of each chromosome); both conditions are lethal.
7. Somatic cells that do not have a multiple of 23 chromosomes are aneuploid. Aneuploidy is usually the result of nondisjunction.
8. Trisomy is a type of aneuploidy in which one chromosome is present in three copies in somatic cells. A partial trisomy is one in which only part of a chromosome is present in three copies.

9. Monosomy is a type of aneuploidy in which one chromosome is present in only one copy in somatic cells.

10. In general, monosomies cause more severe physical defects than do trisomies, illustrating the principle that the loss of chromosome material has more severe consequences than the duplication of chromosome material.

11. Down syndrome, a trisomy of chromosome 21, is the best-known disease caused by a chromosome aberration. It affects 1 in 800 live births and is much more likely to occur in the offspring of women older than 35 years.

12. Most aneuploidies of the sex chromosomes have less severe consequences than those of the autosomes.

13. The most commonly observed sex chromosome aneuploidies are the 47,XXX karyotype, 45,X karyotype (Turner syndrome), 47,XXY karyotype (Klinefelter syndrome), and 47,XYY karyotype.

14. Abnormalities of chromosome structure include deletions, duplications, inversions, and translocations.

Elements of Formal Genetics

1. Mendelian traits are caused by single genes, each of which occupies a position, or locus, on a chromosome.

2. Alleles are different forms of genes located at the same locus on a chromosome.

3. At any given locus in a somatic cell, an individual has two genes, one from each parent. An individual may be homozygous or heterozygous for a locus.

4. An individual's genotype is his or her genetic makeup, and the phenotype reflects the interaction of genotype and environment.

5. In a heterozygote, a dominant gene's effects mask those of a recessive gene. The recessive gene is expressed only when it is present in two copies.

Transmission of Genetic Diseases

1. Genetic diseases caused by single genes usually follow autosomal dominant, autosomal recessive, or X-linked recessive modes of inheritance.

2. Pedigree charts are important tools in the analysis of modes of inheritance.

3. Recurrence risks specify the probability that future offspring will inherit a genetic disease. For single-gene diseases, recurrence risks remain the same for each offspring, regardless of the number of affected or unaffected offspring.

4. The recurrence risk for autosomal dominant diseases is usually 50%.

5. Germline mosaicism can alter recurrence risks for genetic diseases because unaffected parents can produce multiple affected offspring. This situation occurs because the germline of one parent is affected by a mutation but the parent's somatic cells are unaffected.

6. Skipped generations are not seen in classic autosomal dominant pedigrees.

7. Males and females are equally likely to exhibit autosomal dominant diseases and to pass them on to their offspring.

8. Many genetic diseases have a delayed age of onset.

9. A gene that is not always expressed phenotypically is said to have incomplete penetrance.

10. Variable expressivity is a characteristic of many genetic diseases.

11. Genomic imprinting, which is associated with methylation, results in differing expression of a disease gene, depending on which parent transmitted the gene.

12. Epigenetics involves changes, such as the methylation of DNA bases, that do not alter the DNA sequence but can alter the expression of genes.

13. Most commonly, biologic parents of children with autosomal recessive diseases are both heterozygous carriers of the disease gene.

14. The recurrence risk for autosomal recessive diseases is 25%.

15. Males and females are equally likely to be affected by autosomal recessive diseases.

16. Consanguinity is sometimes present in families with autosomal recessive diseases, and it becomes more prevalent with rarer recessive diseases.

17. Carrier detection tests for an increasing number of autosomal recessive diseases are available.

18. The frequency of genetic diseases approximately doubles in the offspring of first-cousin matings.

19. In each normal female somatic cell, one of the two X chromosomes is inactivated early in embryogenesis.

20. X inactivation is random, fixed, and incomplete (i.e., only part of the chromosome is actually inactivated). It may involve methylation.

21. Gender is determined embryonically by the presence of the *SRY* gene on the Y chromosome. Embryos that have a Y chromosome (and thus the *SRY* gene) become males, whereas those lacking the Y chromosome become females. When the Y chromosome lacks the *SRY* gene, an XY female can be produced. Similarly, an X chromosome that contains the *SRY* gene can produce an XX male.

22. X-linked genes are those that are located on the X chromosome. Nearly all known X-linked diseases are caused by X-linked recessive genes.

23. Males are hemizygous for genes on the X chromosome.

24. X-linked recessive diseases are seen much more often in males than in females because males need only one copy of the gene to express the disease.

25. Biologic fathers cannot pass X-linked genes to their sons.

26. Skipped generations often are seen in X-linked recessive disease pedigrees because the gene can be transmitted through carrier females.

27. Recurrence risks for X-linked recessive diseases depend on the carrier and affected status of the mother and father.

28. A sex-limited trait is one that occurs only in one sex (gender).

29. A sex-influenced trait is one that occurs more often in one sex than in the other.

Linkage Analysis and Gene Mapping

1. During meiosis I, crossover occurs and can cause recombinations of alleles located on the same chromosome.

2. The frequency of recombinations can be used to infer the map distance between loci on the same chromosome.

3. A marker locus, when closely linked to a disease-gene locus, can be used to predict whether an individual will develop a genetic disease.

4. The major goals of the Human Genome Project were to find the locations of all human genes (the "gene map") and to determine the entire human DNA sequence. These goals have now been accomplished and the genes responsible for more than 4000 mendelian conditions have been identified.

Multifactorial Inheritance

1. Traits that result from the combined effects of several loci are polygenic. When environmental factors also influence the trait, it is multifactorial.

2. Many multifactorial traits have a threshold of liability. Once the threshold of liability has been crossed, the disease may be expressed.

3. Empirical risks, based on direct observation of large numbers of families, are used to estimate recurrence risks for multifactorial diseases.

4. Recurrence risks for multifactorial diseases become higher if more than one biologic family member is affected or if the expression of the disease in the proband is more severe.

5. Recurrence risks for multifactorial diseases decrease rapidly for more remote relatives.

KEY TERMS

Adenine, 38
Allele, 49
Amino acid, 39
Aneuploid cell, 42
Anticodon, 41
Autosome, 42
Barr body, 54
Base pair substitution, 39
Carrier, 49
Carrier detection test, 54
Chromosomal mosaic, 46
Chromosome, 38
Chromosome band, 42
Chromosome breakage, 47
Chromosome theory of
    inheritance, 50
Clastogen, 47
Codominance, 49
Codon, 39
Complementary base pairing, 39
Consanguinity, 54
CpG islands, 52
Cri du chat syndrome, 48
Crossover, 56
Cytokinesis, 42
Cytosine, 38
Delayed age of onset, 51
Deletion, 48
Deoxyribonucleic acid
    (DNA), 38
Diploid cell, 42
DNA methylation, 52

DNA polymerase, 39
Dominant, 49
Dosage compensation, 54
Double-helix model, 38
Down syndrome, 46
Duplication, 48
Dystrophin, 55
Empirical risk, 58
Epigenetic, 52
Euploid cell, 42
Exon, 41
Expressivity, 51
Fragile site, 49
Frameshift mutation, 39
Gamete, 42
Gene, 38
Genomic imprinting, 52
Genotype, 49
Germline mosaicism, 51
Guanine, 38
Haploid cell, 42
Hemizygous, 54
Heterozygote, 49
Heterozygous, 49
Homologous, 42
Homozygote, 49
Homozygous, 49
Inbreeding, 54
Intron, 41
Inversion, 48
Karyotype (karyogram), 42
Klinefelter syndrome, 47

Linkage, 56
Locus, 49
Meiosis, 42
Messenger RNA (mRNA), 39
Metaphase spread, 42
Methylation, 52
Missense, 39
Mitosis, 42
Mode of inheritance, 49
Multifactorial inheritance, 58
Mutagen, 39
Mutation, 39
Mutational hot spot, 39
Nondisjunction, 45
Nonsense, 39
Nucleotide, 39
Obligate carrier, 51
Partial trisomy, 46
Pedigree, 50
Penetrance, 51
Phenotype, 49
Polygenic trait, 57
Polymorphic
    (polymorphism), 49
Polypeptide, 39
Polyploid cell, 42
Position effect, 48
Principle of independent
    assortment, 50
Principle of segregation, 50
Proband, 50
Promoter site, 39

Pseudoautosomal, 54
Purine, 38
Pyrimidine, 38
Recessive, 49
Reciprocal translocation, 48
Recombination, 56
Recurrence risk, 50
Ribonucleic acid (RNA), 39
Ribosomal RNA (rRNA), 41
Ribosome, 41
RNA polymerase, 39
Robertsonian translocation, 49
Sex-influenced trait, 55
Sex-limited trait, 55
Sex linked (inheritance), 54
Silent mutation, 39
Somatic cell, 42
Spontaneous mutation, 39
Template, 39
Termination sequence, 41
Tetraploidy, 42
Threshold of liability, 58
Thymine, 38
Transcription, 39
Transfer RNA (tRNA), 41
Translation, 41
Translocation, 48
Triploidy, 42
Trisomy, 42
Tumor-suppressor gene, 51
Turner syndrome, 47
X inactivation, 54

REFERENCES

1. Jorde LB et al: *Medical genetics*, ed 4, St Louis, 2010, Mosby-Elsevier.
2. Gardner RJM et al: *Chromosome abnormalities and genetic counseling*, Oxford, 2012, Oxford University Press.
3. Nagaoka SI et al: Human aneuploidy: mechanisms and new insights into an age-old problem, *Nat Rev Genet* 13(7):493-504, 2012.
4. Antonarakis SE, Epstein CJ: The challenge of Down syndrome, *Trends Mol Med* 12(10):473-479, 2006.
5. Gravholt CH: Sex chromosome abnormalities. In Rimoin DL, Pyeritz RE, Korf BR, editors: *Emery and Rimoin's principles and practice of medical genetics*, ed 6, Philadelphia, 2013, Elsevier.
6. Rooms L, Kooy RF: Advances in understanding fragile X syndrome and related disorders, *Curr Opin Pediatr* 23(6):601-606, 2011.

7. Nelson DL et al: The unstable repeats—three evolving faces of neurological disease, *Neuron* 77(5):825-843, 2013.
8. Biesecker LG, Spinner NB: A genomic view of mosaicism and human disease, *Nat Rev Genet* 14(5):307-320, 2013.
9. Foulkes WD: Inherited susceptibility to common cancers, *N Engl J Med* 359(20):2143-2153, 2008.
10. Pasmant E et al: Neurofibromatosis type 1: from genotype to phenotype, *J Med Genet* 49(8):483-489, 2012.
11. Fraga MF et al: Epigenetic differences arise during the lifetime of monozygotic twins, *Proc Natl Acad Sci U S A* 102(30):10604-10609, 2005.
12. Lyon MF: X-chromosome inactivation, *Curr Biol* 9(7):R235-R237, 1999.

13. Lee JT, Bartolomei MS: X-inactivation, imprinting, and long noncoding RNAs in health and disease, *Cell* 152(6):1308-1323, 2013.
14. Larney C et al: Switching on sex: transcriptional regulation of the testis-determining gene *Sry*, *Development* 141(11):2195-2205, 2014.
15. Flanigan KM: The muscular dystrophies, *Semin Neurol* 32(3):255-263, 2012.
16. Lander ES: Initial impact of the sequencing of the human genome, *Nature* 470(7333):187-197, 2011.
17. Yang Y et al: Clinical whole-exome sequencing for the diagnosis of mendelian disorders, *N Engl J Med* 369(16):1502-1511, 2013.
18. Koboldt DC et al: The next-generation sequencing revolution and its impact on genomics, *Cell* 155(1):27-38, 2013.

3

Epigenetics and Disease

Diane P. Genereux and Lynn B. Jorde

EVOLVE WEBSITE

CHAPTER OUTLINE

Human beings exhibit an impressive diversity of physical and behavioral features. Some of this diversity is attributable to genetic variation. Another contributor to human diversity is epigenetic ("upon genetic") modification (a change in phenotype or gene expression that does not involve DNA mutation or changes in nucleotide sequence). Basically, epigenetics is the study of mechanisms that will switch genes "on," such that they are *expressed*, and "off," such that they are *silenced*. Epigenetic mechanisms include chemical modifications to DNA and associated histones, and the production of small RNA molecules. Gene regulation by epigenetic processes can occur at the level of either transcription or translation. Epigenetic modification is critical for fundamental processes of human development, including the differentiation of embryonic stem cells into specific cell types, and the inactivation of one of the two X chromosomes in each cell of a genetic female. Some genes are noted to be *imprinted*, a form of epigenetic regulation where the expression of a gene depends on whether it is inherited from the mother or the father.

EPIGENETIC MECHANISMS

A variety of diseases can result from abnormal epigenetic states. Metabolic disease can occur when there is aberrant expression of both copies of a locus that is typically imprinted. Environmental stressors can markedly increase the risk of aberrant epigenetic modification and

are strongly associated with some cancers. It is because of their increasing clear role in a wide range of pathologies that abnormal epigenetic states are currently a focus of both preventative efforts and pharmaceutical intervention. Currently known epigenetic mechanisms include DNA methylation, histone modifications, and RNA-based mechanisms (Figure 3-1).

DNA Methylation

DNA methylation (see Figure 3-1) occurs through the attachment of a methyl group (CH_3) to a cytosine. Dense DNA methylation can be thought of as "insulation" that renders genes silent by blocking access by transcription factors. Dense methylation is typically coincident with hypoacetylation (decrease of the functional group acetyl) of the histone proteins around which the DNA is wound (see Histone Modifications). Together, DNA methylation and histone hypoacetylation can render a gene transcriptionally silent, preventing production of the encoded protein. Methylated cytosines have been found to occur principally at cytosines that are followed by a guanine base (sometimes known as cytosines in "CpG dinucleotides"). In human embryonic stem cells, methylation also can occur at cytosines outside of the CpG context (see Figure 2-24).

DNA methylation plays a prominent role in both human health and disease. For example, in each cell of a normal human female, one of the two X chromosomes is silenced by dense methylation and

FIGURE 3-1 Three Types of Epigenetic Processes. Investigators are studying three epigenetic mechanisms: **(1)** DNA methylation, **(2)** histone modifications, and **(3)** RNA based-mechanisms. See text for discussion.

associated molecular marks, whereas the other X chromosome is transcriptionally active and largely devoid of methylation. During early embryonic development, there is epigenetic inactivation of one of the two X chromosomes in each cell of a human female—either the X chromosome inherited from her mother or the X chromosome inherited from her father. The determination of which chromosome is to be silenced occurs at random and independently in each of the cells present at this stage of development; the silent state of that chromosome is inherited by all subsequent copies. If a woman's two X chromosomes carry different alleles at a given locus, random X inactivation can lead to somatic mosaicism, wherein the alleles active in two different cells can confer two very different traits. Striking examples include the patchy coloration of calico cats and *anhidrotic ectodermal dysplasia,* a condition characterized by patchy presence and absence of sweat glands in the skin of human females who have one X chromosome bearing a normal allele and one X chromosome bearing a mutant allele at the X-encoded locus. Because of the somatic mosaicism that arises through random inactivation of the X chromosome, females tend to have less severe phenotypes than do males for a variety of X-linked disorders, including color blindness and fragile X syndrome.

Aberrant DNA methylation, either the presence of dense methylation where it is typically absent or the absence of methylation where it is typically present, can lead to misregulation of tumor-suppressor genes and oncogenes. Abnormal DNA methylation states are a common feature of several human cancers, including those of the colon[1-3] (see Figures 3-1 and 3-6 [p. 69]; also see Chapter 10).

Histone Modifications

Histone modifications (see Figure 3-1) include histone acetylation (adding an acetyl group) and deacetylation (deletion of an acetyl group) to the end of a histone protein. Like DNA methylation, these changes can alter the expression state of chromatin. **Histones** are proteins that facilitate compaction of genomic DNA into the nucleus of a cell, much as a spool helps to organize a long piece of thread for storage in a small space. When the DNA of the human genome is wound around histones, it is only $\approx 1/40,000$ as long as it would be in its uncondensed state. Chemical modification of histones in a region of DNA can either up-regulate or down-regulate nearby gene expression by increasing or decreasing the tightness of the interaction between DNA and histones, thus modulating the extent to which DNA is accessible to transcription factors. DNA in association with histones is referred to as "chromatin." At any given time, various regions of chromatin are typically in one of two forms: *euchromatin,* an open state in which most or all nearby genes are transcriptionally active; or *heterochromatin,* a closed state in which most or all nearby genes are transcriptionally inactive.

Chromatin structure plays a critical role in determining the developmental potential of a given cell lineage, and can undergo dramatic changes during organismal development. For example, chromatin states differ substantially between embryonic stem cells, which are poised to give rise to all of the different cell types that make up an individual, and terminally differentiated cells, which are committed to a specific developmental path. The fraction of DNA that is in the heterochromatic state increases as cells differentiate, consistent with the reduction in the number of genes that are active as a cell lineage transitions from pluripotency to terminal differentiation.[4] Mutations in genes that encode histone-modifying proteins have been implicated in congenital heart disease,[5] for example, highlighting histone modification states as critical for normal development.

In contrast to the vast majority of other cell types, including oocytes, sperm cells express not histones but *protamines,* which are evolutionarily derived from histones.[6] Protamines enable sperm DNA to wind into an even more compact state than does the histone-bound DNA in somatic cells. This tight compaction improves the hydrodynamic features of the sperm head, facilitating its movement toward the egg.

RNA-Based Mechanisms

Noncoding RNAs (ncRNAs) and other RNA-based mechanisms (see Figure 3-1) play an important role in regulating a wide variety of cellular processes, including RNA splicing and DNA replication. These ncRNAs have been likened to "sponges" in so far as they can "sop up" complementary RNAs, thus inhibiting their function (see, for example, www.ncbi.nlm.nih.gov/pmc/articles/PMC2957044/). Of particular relevance to gene regulation are the hairpin-shaped microRNAs (miRNAs), which are encoded by DNA sequences of approximately 22 nucleotides, typically within the introns (a segment of a DNA molecule that does not code for proteins) of genes or in noncoding DNA located between genes (see Chapter 2). In contrast to DNA methylation and histone modification, both of which principally affect gene expression at the level of transcription, miRNAs typically modulate the stability and translational efficiency of existing messenger RNAs (mRNAs) encoded at other loci. Interaction between miRNAs and mRNAs target for degradation is typically mediated by regions of partial sequence complementarity. As a result, miRNAs can at once be specific enough so that they do not bind to *all* of the mRNAs in a cell and general enough to regulate a large number of different mRNA sequences. miRNAs also directly modulate translation by impairing ribosomal function. miRNAs regulate diverse signaling pathways; those that stimulate cancer development and progression are called oncomirs. For example, miRNAs have been linked to carcinogenesis because they alter the activity of oncogenes and tumor-suppressor genes (see Chapter 10).

EPIGENETICS AND HUMAN DEVELOPMENT

Each of the cells in the very early embryo has the potential to give rise to a somatic cell of any type. These embryonic stem cells are therefore said to be totipotent ("possessing all powers"). A key process in early development then is the differential epigenetic modification of specific DNA nucleotide sequences in these embryonic stem cells, ultimately leading to the differential gene-expression profiles that characterize the various differentiated somatic cell types. These early modifications ensure that specific genes are expressed only in the cells and tissue types in which their gene products typically function (e.g., factor VIII expression primarily in hepatocytes, or dopamine receptor expression in neurons).

Epigenetic modifications early in development also highlight a fundamental feature of genetics as compared to epigenetic information:

all of the cells in a given individual contain almost exactly the same genetic information. It is the epigenetic information eventually placed on top of these sequences that enables them to achieve the diverse functions of differentiated somatic cells. A small percentage of genes, termed housekeeping genes, are necessary for the function and maintenance of all cells. These genes escape epigenetic silencing and remain transcriptionally active in all or nearly all cells. Housekeeping genes include encoding histones, DNA and RNA polymerases, and ribosomal RNA genes.

How do embryonic stem cells achieve epigenetic states typical of totipotency, whereby they can give rise to all of the diverse cell types that make up a fully developed organism? One explanation is that early embryogenesis (approximately the 10 days just after fertilization) is characterized by rapid fluctuation in genome-wide DNA methylation densities. Fertilization triggers a global loss of DNA methylation at most loci in both the oocyte-contributed and the sperm-contributed genomes. This loss of methylation is accomplished in part by suppression of the DNA methyltransferases, the enzymes that add methyl groups to DNA. Methylation is not directly copied by the DNA replication process. Instead, immediately following replication, the methyltransferases read the pattern of methylation on the parent DNA strand and use that information to determine which daughter-strand cytosines should be methylated. As embryonic cell division proceeds in the absence of DNA methyltransferases, cell division continues, eventually yielding cells that have nearly all of their loci in unmethylated, transcriptionally active states. Around the time of implantation in the uterus, the DNA methyltransferases become active again, permitting establishment of the cell-lineage–specific marks required for the establishment of organ systems.

GENOMIC IMPRINTING

A baby inherits two copies of each autosomal gene: one from its mother and one from its father. For a large subset of these genes, expression is biallelic, meaning that both the maternally and the paternally inherited copies contribute to offspring phenotype. For another, smaller subset of these genes, expression is stochastically monoallelic,[7] meaning that the maternal copy is randomly chosen for inactivation in some somatic cells and the paternal copy is randomly chosen for inactivation in other somatic cells. For a third and smaller subset of autosomes (about 1%) either the maternal copy or the paternal copy is imprinted, meaning that either the copy inherited through the sperm or the copy inherited through the egg is inactivated and remains in this inactive state in all of the somatic cells of the individual.

The subset of genes that are subject to imprinting is highly enriched for loci relevant to organismal growth. The *genetic conflict hypothesis*[7] was developed as a potential explanation for this pattern. Although both the mother and the father benefit genetically from the birth and survival of offspring, their interests are not entirely aligned. Because a mother makes a large physiologic investment in each child, it is in her evolutionary best interest to limit the flow of energetic resources to any given offspring so as to maintain her physiologic capacity to bear subsequent children. By contrast, except in cases of certain permanent, certain monogamy, it is in the best interest of the father for his child to extract maximal resources from its mother, as his own future fecundity, or fertility, is not contingent on the sustained fecundity of the mother. In general, imprinting of maternally inherited genes tends to reduce offspring size; imprinting of paternally inherited genes tends to increase offspring size. One hallmark of imprinting-associated disease is that the phenotype of affected individuals is critically dependent on whether the mutation is inherited from the mother or from the father. Some examples are included in the following syndromes.

FIGURE 3-2 Prader-Willi and Angelman Syndromes. **A,** A child with Prader-Willi syndrome (truncal obesity, small hands and feet, inverted V-shaped upper lip). **B,** A child with Angelman syndrome (characteristic posture, ataxic gait, bouts of uncontrolled laughter). (From Jorde LB, Carey JC, Bamshad MJ: *Medical genetics,* ed 4, Philadelphia, 2010, Mosby.)

Prader-Willi and Angelman Syndromes

A well-known disease example of imprinting is associated with a deletion of about 4 million base (Mb) pairs of the long arm of chromosome 15. When this deletion is inherited from the father, the child manifests Prader-Willi syndrome, with features including short stature, hypotonia, small hands and feet, obesity, mild to moderate intellectual disability, and hypogonadism[8] (Figure 3-2, *A*). The same 4-Mb deletion, when inherited from the mother, causes Angelman syndrome, which is characterized by severe intellectual disability, seizures, and an ataxic gait (Figure 3-2, *B*).[9] These diseases are each observed in about 1 of every 15,000 live births; chromosome deletions are responsible for about 70% of cases of both diseases. The deletions that cause Prader-Willi and Angelman syndromes are indistinguishable at the DNA sequence level and affect the same group of genes.

For several decades, it was unclear how the same deletion could produce such disparate results in different individuals. Further analysis showed that the 4-Mb deletion (the *critical region*) contains several genes that are normally transcribed only on the copy of chromosome 15 that is inherited from the father.[10] These genes are transcriptionally inactive (imprinted) on the copy of chromosome 15 inherited from the mother. Similarly, other genes in the critical region are transcriptionally active only on the chromosome copy inherited from the mother and are inactive on the chromosome inherited from the father. Thus, several genes in this region are normally active on only one chromosome copy (Figure 3-3). If the single active copy of one of these genes is lost because of a chromosome deletion, then no gene product is produced, resulting in disease.

Molecular analysis has revealed much about genes in this critical region of chromosome 15.[10] The gene responsible for Angelman syndrome encodes a ligase involved in protein degradation during brain development (consistent with the mental retardation and ataxia observed in this disorder). In brain tissue, this gene is active only on the chromosome copy inherited from the mother. Consequently, a maternally transmitted deletion removes the single active copy of this gene. Several genes in the critical region are associated with Prader-Willi syndrome and they are transcribed only on the chromosome transmitted by the father. A paternally transmitted deletion removes the only active copies of these genes producing the features of Prader-Willi syndrome.

Beckwith-Wiedemann Syndrome

Another well-known example of imprinting is Beckwith-Wiedemann syndrome, an overgrowth condition accompanied by an increased predisposition to cancer. Beckwith-Wiedemann syndrome is usually identifiable at birth because of the presence of large size for gestational age, neonatal hypoglycemia, a large tongue, creases on the earlobe, and omphalocele (birth defect of infant intestines).[11] Children with Beckwith-Wiedemann syndrome have an increased risk of developing Wilms tumor or hepatoblastoma. Both of these tumors can be treated effectively if they are detected early; thus screening at regular intervals is an important part of management. Some children with Beckwith-Wiedemann syndrome also develop asymmetric overgrowth of a limb or one side of the face or trunk (hemihyperplasia).

As with Angelman syndrome, a minority of Beckwith-Wiedemann syndrome cases (about 20% to 30%) are caused by the inheritance of two copies of a chromosome from the father and no copy of the chromosome from the mother (*uniparental disomy,* in this case affecting chromosome 11). Several genes on the short arm of chromosome 11 are imprinted on either the paternally or the maternally transmitted chromosome. These genes are found in two separate, differentially

FIGURE 3-3 Prader-Willi Syndrome Pedigrees. These pedigrees illustrate the inheritance patterns of Prader-Willi syndrome, which can be caused by a 4-Mb deletion of chromosome 15q when inherited from the father. In contrast, Angelman syndrome can be caused by the same deletion but only when it is inherited from the mother. The reason for this difference is that different genes in this region are normally imprinted (inactivated) in the copies of 15q transmitted by the mother and the father. (From Jorde LB, Carey JC, Bamshad MJ: *Medical genetics,* ed 4, Philadelphia, 2010, Mosby.)

methylated regions (DMRs). In DMR1, the gene that encodes insulin-like growth factor 2 *(IGF2)* is inactive on the maternally transmitted chromosome but active on the paternally transmitted chromosome. Thus, a normal individual has only one active copy of *IGF2.* When two copies of the paternal chromosome are inherited (i.e., paternal uniparental disomy) or there is loss of imprinting on the maternal copy of *IGF2,* an active *IGF2* gene is present in double dose. These changes produce increased levels of insulin-like growth factor 2 during fetal development, contributing to the overgrowth features of Beckwith-Wiedemann syndrome. Note that, in contrast to Prader-Willi and Angelman syndromes, which are produced by a missing gene product, Beckwith-Wiedemann syndrome is caused, in part, by overexpression of a gene product.

Russell-Silver Syndrome

Russell-Silver syndrome is characterized by growth retardation, proportionate short stature, leg length discrepancy, and a small, triangular face. About one third of Russell-Silver syndrome cases are caused by imprinting abnormalities of chromosome 11p15.5 that lead to down-regulation of *IGF2* and therefore diminished growth. Another 10% of cases of Russell-Silver syndrome are caused by maternal uniparental disomy. Thus, whereas up-regulation, or extra copies, of active *IGF2* causes overgrowth in Beckwith-Wiedemann syndrome, down-regulation of *IGF2* causes the diminished growth seen in Russell-Silver syndrome.

> ✔ **QUICK CHECK 3-1**
> 1. Define epigenetics.
> 2. What are the three kinds of epigenetic mechanisms?
> 3. What is meant by the genetic conflict hypothesis?
> 4. Compare and contrast the molecular and phenotypic features of Prader-Willi and Angelman syndromes.

LONG-TERM AND MULTIGENERATIONAL PERSISTENCE OF EPIGENETIC STATES INDUCED BY STOCHASTIC AND ENVIRONMENTAL FACTORS

It is increasingly clear that imprinted genes are not the only loci for which epigenetic modifications persist over time. Conditions encountered in utero, during childhood, and even during adolescence or later can have long-term impacts on epigenetic states, sometimes with impacts that can be transmitted across generations. A few such examples are listed below.

Epigenetics and Nutrition

During the winter of 1943, millions of people in urban areas of the Netherlands suffered starvation conditions as a result of a Nazi blockage that prevented shipments of food from agricultural areas. When researchers sought to investigate how exposure to famine in utero had affected individuals born in a historically prosperous country, they found individuals who suffered nutritional deprivation in utero were more likely to suffer from obesity and diabetes as adults than individuals in the Netherlands who had not experienced nutritional deprivation during gestation. There also seemed to be a transgenerational impact, in that the children of individuals who were in utero during the Dutch Hunger Winter were found to be significantly smaller than the children of those not affected by the blockade. Other data sets reveal elevated risk of cardiovascular and metabolic disease for offspring of individuals exposed during early development to fluctuations in agricultural yields.[12]

The specific molecular mechanisms that may mediate these apparent relationships between nutritional deprivation and disease risk on one or more generations are largely unknown. From some animal models, it seems that the insulin-like growth factor 2 gene *(IGF2)* is a possible target of epigenetic modifications arising through nutritional deprivation. Exposure in utero and through lactation to some chemicals (including bisphenol A, a constituent of plastics sometimes used in food preparation and storage) seems to lead to epigenetic modifications similar to those that arise through nutritional deprivation in early life.[13]

Epigenetics and Maternal Care

It is increasingly clear that parenting style can affect epigenetic states, and that this information can be transmitted from one generation to the next. Mice and other rodents can exhibit two alternate styles of nursing behavior: frequent arched-back nursing with a high level of licking and grooming behavior, and an alternate style with infrequent arched-back nursing and much reduced licking and grooming behavior. In one especially compelling study,[14] pups of mothers that engaged in frequent arched-backed nursing were found to have significantly lower methylation levels and higher transcription activity of a glucocorticoid receptor–encoding locus. Because the glucocorticoid receptor is involved in a pathway that intensifies fearfulness and response to stress, these findings suggest that alteration to methylation states could help explain the finding that exposure to stress early in life can modulate behavior in adulthood. These findings also highlight the concept that epigenetic processes can help store information about the environment, and that the relevant epigenetic modifications can modulate behavior later in life.

Epigenetics and Mental Illness
Epigenetics and Ethanol Exposure During Gestation

The impact of ethanol exposure in utero on skeletal and neural development was first reported in 1973[15] and led to broad awareness of fetal alcohol syndrome. It was not until recently, however, that population-based and molecular-level studies began to clarify the epigenetic signals that mediate these impacts. At first, researchers found alcohol exposure in utero can affect the DNA methylation states of various genomic elements but without specific emphasis on loci directly relevant to skeletal and neural development.[11] More recently, it has been found that treating cultured neural stem cells with ethanol impairs their ability to differentiate to functional neurons; this impairment seems to be correlated with aberrant, dense methylation at loci that are active in normal neuronal tissue.[16] One possible explanation for these effects is that ethanol exposure in utero modulates fetal expression of the DNA methyltransfereases.[17]

Epigenetic Disease in the Context of Genetic Abnormalities

In some diseases, both genetic and epigenetic factors contribute to the origin of abnormal phenotypes. For example, several abnormal phenotypes can arise in individuals with mutations at the fragile X locus *FMR1* (Figure 3-4, *A*). Some of these phenotypes arise in individuals for whom epigenetic changes are coincident with genetic changes. The most common genetic abnormality at *FMR1* involves expansion in the number of cytosine-guanine (CG) dinucleotide repeats in the gene promoter. Females who have CG repeats in excess of the approximately 35 that are typical at this locus are at risk for fragile X–associated primary ovarian insufficiency, characterized by an elevated risk of early menopause.[18] Males with moderate expansions are at risk of fragile X

FIGURE 3-4 Comparing the Molecular Mechanisms of Fragile X and FSHD. **A**, *FMR1* in normal, expanded permutation, and full-mutation states. **B**, *DUX4* in normal and contracted states.

tremor ataxia syndrome (FXTAS), characterized by a late-onset intention tremor.[19] Both of these conditions seem to arise through accumulation of excess levels of *FMR1* mRNAs in nuclear inclusion bodies.[18,20] Individuals with 200 repeats are at risk of fragile X syndrome, characterized by reduced IQ and a set of behavioral abnormalities. Remarkably, although possession of a large CG repeat in the *FMR1* promoter dramatically increases the probability that an individual will have fragile X syndrome, the disease can be present in males who have the large repeat but be absent in their brothers who have inherited an allele of very similar size.[21] This can be explained, at least in part, by the observation that acquisition of methylation-based silencing at *FMR1* is stochastic, meaning that the presence of a large repeat increases the probability of the dense promoter methylation that could lead to gene silencing, but does not guarantee it. It remains to be seen whether dietary or environmental features can modulate the probability that dense methylation at *FMR1* will accrue in individuals with the full-mutation allele.

In another genetic-epigenetic disease, **fascioscapulohumeral muscular dystrophy (FSHMD)** (see Figure 3-4, *B*), the disease phenotype arises through loss of normal methylation rather than gain of abnormal methylation. Symptoms of the disease include adverse impacts on skeletal musculature. Though lifespan is not typically reduced by the disease, wheelchair use becomes necessary late in life for a subset of individuals. The primary genetic event in FSHMD is deletion of a nucleotide repeat in the *DUX4* gene (see Figure 3-4, *A*). In normal individuals, the *D4Z4* gene promoter has between 11 and 150 copies. This number is typically found to have been reduced by mutation in individuals with FSHMD, who usually have only 1 to 10 such repeats. In healthy individuals with a normal-sized allele, the *D4Z4* promoter typically has dense methylation. In individuals with reduced copy-counts, the normally dense methylation is lost (see Figure 3-4, *A*).[22] The disease allele typically also has fewer repressive histone marks than does the normal allele.[23] Together, fragile X syndrome and FSHMD highlight that both abnormal gain and abnormal loss of epigenetic modifications can result in disease.

Twin Studies Provide Insights on Epigenetic Modification

Identical (monozygotic) twin pairs, whose DNA sequences are essentially the same, offer a unique opportunity to isolate and examine the impacts of epigenetic modifications. A recent study found that as twins age, they exhibit increasingly substantial differences in methylation patterns of the DNA sequences of their somatic cells; these changes are often reflected in increasing numbers of phenotypic differences. Twins with significant lifestyle differences (e.g., smoking versus nonsmoking) tend to accumulate larger numbers of differences in their methylation patterns. These results, along with findings generated in animal studies, suggest that changes in epigenetic patterns may be an important part of the aging process[24] (Figure 3-5).

Molecular Approaches to Understand Epigenetic Disease

Because epigenetic information is not encoded by DNA molecules but instead by chemical modifications to those molecules, conventional sequencing approaches are not sufficient to reveal epigenetic differences between normal individuals and those who have epigenetic modifications associated with disease. To collect information on DNA methylation states of individual nucleotides, DNA is typically subjected to bisulfite conversion before sequencing. Bisulfite treatment does not alter most nucleotides, including methylated cytosines, but deaminates unmethylated cytosines to uracil.[25] Because uracil complements adenine, not guanine, methylated and unmethylated

FIGURE 3-5 Twins and Aging. A, Twins as babies look very much alike but, **B,** as adults, have slight differences in appearance, possibly because of epigenetics. (**A,** vgm/Shutterstock. **B,** Stacey Bates/Shutterstock.)

cytosines can be distinguished in resulting sequence data, so long as the genetic sequence is known. Histone modification states can be assayed through the use of antibodies specific for histones with various modifications.[26]

✔ QUICK CHECK 3-2

1. Evaluate the statement: "Epigenetic information is highly dynamic in early development."
2. How does the epigenetic regulation of imprinted genes compare with that of the rest of the genome?
3. Compare and contrast the molecular mechanisms leading to FX syndrome and to FSHMD.

EPIGENETICS AND CANCER

DNA Methylation and Cancer

Some of the most extensive evidence for the role of epigenetic modification in human disease comes from studies of cancer (Figure 3-6).[27,28] Tumor cells typically exhibit genome-wide hypomethylation (decreased methylation), which can increase the activity of oncogenes (see Chapter 10). Hypomethylation increases as tumors progress from

FIGURE 3-6 Global Epigenomic Alterations and Cancer. Oncogenesis often occurs through a combination of genetic mutations and epigenetic change. In cancer cells, the promoters of tumor-suppressor genes typically become hypermethylated, leading, in combination with histone modifications, to abnormal gene silencing. Because tumor-suppressor genes typically help to control cell division, their silencing can result in tumor progression. Global hypomethylation leads to chromosomal instability and fragility, and increases the risk of additional genetic mutations. Additionally, these modifications create abnormal mRNA and miRNA expression, which leads to activation of oncogenes and silencing of tumor-suppressor genes. (Adapted from Sandoval J, Esteller M. Cancer epigenomics: beyond genomics, *Curr Opin Genet Dev* 22:50-55, 2012.)

benign neoplasms to malignancy. In addition, the promoter regions of tumor-suppressor genes are often hypermethylated, which decreases their rate of transcription and their ability to inhibit tumor formation. Hypermethylation of the promoter region of the *RB1* gene is often seen in retinoblastoma[29]; hypermethylation of the *BRCA1* gene is seen in some cases of inherited breast cancer (Chapter 33).[30]

A major cause of one form of inherited colon cancer (hereditary nonpolyposis colorectal cancer [HNPCC]) is the methylation of the promoter region of a gene, *MLH1*, whose protein product repairs damaged DNA. When *MLH1* becomes inactive, DNA damage accumulates, eventually resulting in colon tumors[31,32]. Abnormal methylation of tumor-suppressor genes also is common in the progression of Barrett esophagus, a condition in which the lining of the esophagus is replaced by cells that have features associated with the lower intestinal tract, and to adenocarcinoma possibly through up-regulation of one of the enzymes that adds methyl groups to DNA.[33]

miRNAs and Cancer

Hypermethylation also is seen in microRNA genes, which encode small (22 base pair) RNA molecules that bind to the ends of mRNAs, degrading them and preventing their translation. More than 1000 microRNA sequences have been identified in humans, and hypermethylation of specific subgroups of microRNAs is associated with tumorigenesis.

When microRNA genes are methylated, their mRNA targets are overexpressed, and this overexpression has been associated with metastasis.[27]

Epigenetic Screening for Cancer

The common finding of epigenetic alteration in cancerous tissue raises the possibility that epigenetic screening approaches could complement or even replace existing early-detection methods. In some cases, epigenetic screening could be done using bodily fluids, such as urine or sputum, eliminating the need for the more invasive, costly, and risky strategies currently in place. Monitoring for misregulation of miRNAs has shown promise as a tool for early diagnosis of cancers of the colon,[34] breast,[35] and prostate.[36] Other epigenetics-based screening approaches have shown promise for detection of cancers of the bladder,[37] lung,[38] and prostate.[39]

Emerging Strategies for the Treatment of Epigenetic Disease

Epigenetic modifications are potentially reversible: DNA can be demethylated, histones can be modified to change the transcriptional state of nearby DNA, and miRNA-encoding loci can be up-regulated or down-regulated. This raises the prospect for treating epigenetic disease with pharmaceutical agents that directly reverse the changes

FIGURE 3-7 5-Azacytosine as Demethylating Agent. A, Unmethylated cytosines in DNA are typically subject to the addition of methyl groups by DNMT1, a DNA methyltransferase, using methyl groups supplied by the methyl donor S-adenosylmethionine. **B,** In 5-Azacytosine, the 5′ carbon of cytosine is replaced with a nitrogen. This chemical difference is sufficient both to block the addition of a methyl group and to confer irreversible binding to DNMT1. Incorporation of 5-Azacytosine into DNA is therefore sufficient to drive passive loss of methylation from replicating DNA, and thus to reactivate hypermethylated loci. 5-Azacytosine, bound to a sugar, can be integrated into DNA, and has been administered with some success in treating epigenetic diseases that arise through hypermethylation of individual loci.

associated with the disease phenotype. In recent years, interventions involving all three types of epigenetic modulators (DNA methylation, histone modification, and miRNAs) have shown considerable promise for the treatment of disease.

DNA Demethylating Agents

5-Azacytidine (Figure 3-7) has been used as a therapeutic drug in the treatment of leukemia and myelodysplastic syndrome.[40] A cytosine analog, 5-azacytidine, is incorporated into DNA opposite its complementary nucleotide, guanine. 5-Azacytidine differs from cytosine in that it has a nitrogen, rather than a carbon, in the 5th position of its cytidine ring. As result, the DNMTs cannot add methyl groups to 5-azacytidine, and DNAs that contain 5-azacytidine decline in their methylation density over successive rounds of DNA replication.[41] Administration of 5-azacytidine is associated with various side effects, including digestive disturbance, but has shown promise in the treatment of diseases, including pancreatic cancer[42] and myelodysplastic syndromes.[43,44]

Histone Deacetylase Inhibitors

The activity of the histone deacetylases (HDACs) increases chromatin compaction, decreasing transcriptional activity (see Figure 3-7). In many cases, excessive activity of HDACs results in transcriptional inactivation of tumor-suppressor genes, leading ultimately to the development of tumors. Treatment with HDAC inhibitors, either alone or in combination with other drugs, has shown promise in the treatment of cancers of the breast[45] and prostate,[46] but only very limited success in the treatment of pancreatic cancer.[47]

miRNA Coding

A major challenge in developing drugs that modify epigenetic alterations is to target only the genes responsible for a specific cancer. Therapeutic approaches that use microRNA offer a potential solution to this problem as treatment can be targeted to individual loci using sequence characteristics of relevant RNA molecules.

✔ QUICK CHECK 3-3

1. Assess the statement that cancer is, in many cases, an epigenetic disease.
2. Discuss the role of miRNAs in cancer.
3. Describe a potential strategy for the treatment of epigenetic disease.

FUTURE DIRECTIONS

Robust experimental observations are clarifying the roles of epigenetic states in determining cell fates and disease phenotypes. The well-documented involvement of epigenetic abnormalities in carcinogenesis and the mounting evidence for these epigenetic changes in other common diseases (discussed in other chapters) will likely elucidate possibilities for reversing the epigenetic abnormalities and possibly preventing their establishment in utero.

■ DID YOU UNDERSTAND?

Overview

1. Why are pairs of identical twins especially useful in the study of epigenetic phenomena?
2. Describe some of the challenges of developing pharmaceutical approaches to remedy abnormal epigenetic states.

Epigenetics and Human Development

1. Epigenetics modification alters gene expression without changes to DNA sequence.
2. Investigators are studying three major types of epigenetic processes: (1) DNA methylation, which results from attachment of a methyl group to a cytosine; in the somatic cells, all or nearly all methylation occurs at cytosines that are followed by guanines ("CpG dinucleotides"); (2) histone modification, through the addition of various chemical groups, including methyl and acetyl; and (3) noncoding RNAs (ncRNAs or miRNAs), short nucleotides derived from introns of protein coding genes or transcribed as independent genes from regions of the genome whose functions, if any, remain poorly understood. MicroRNAs regulate diverse signaling pathways.
3. DNA methylation is, at present, the best-studied epigenetic process. When a gene becomes heavily methylated the DNA is less likely to be transcribed into mRNA.
4. Methylation, along with histone hypoacetylation and condensation of chromatin, inhibits the binding of proteins that promote transcription, such that the gene becomes transcriptionally inactive.
5. Environmental factors, such as diet and exposure to certain chemicals, may cause epigenetic modifications.

6. The heritable transmission to future generations of epigenetic modifications is called transgenerational inheritance.

7. As twins age, they demonstrate increasing differences in methylation patterns of their DNA sequences, causing increasing numbers of phenotypic differences.

8. In studies of twins with significant lifestyle differences (e.g., smoking versus nonsmoking) large numbers of differences in their methylation patterns are observed to accrue over time.

Genomic Imprinting

1. Gregor Mendel's experiments with garden peas demonstrated that the phenotype is the same whether a given allele is inherited from the mother or the father. This principle, which has long been part of the central dogma of genetics, does not always hold. For some human genes, a given gene is transcriptionally active on only one copy of a chromosome (e.g., the copy inherited from the father). On the other copy of the chromosome (the one inherited from the mother) the gene is transcriptionally inactive. This process of gene silencing, in which genes are silenced depending on which parent transmits them, is known as *imprinting;* the transcriptionally silenced genes are said to be "imprinted."

2. When an allele is imprinted, it typically has heavy methylation. By contrast, the nonimprinted allele is typically not methylated.

3. A well-known disease example of imprinting is associated with a deletion of about 4 million base pairs (Mb) of the long arm of chromosome 15. When this deletion is inherited from the father, the child manifests Prader-Willi syndrome.

4. The same 4 Mb deletion, when inherited from the mother, causes Angelman syndrome.

5. Another well-known example of imprinting is Beckwith-Wiedemann syndrome, an overgrowth condition accompanied by an increased predisposition to cancer.

6. Whereas up-regulation, or extra copies, of active *IGF2* causes overgrowth in Beckwith Wiedemann syndrome, down-regulation of *IGF2* causes the diminished growth seen in Russell-Silver syndrome.

Long-Term and Multigenerational Persistence of Epigenetic States Induced by Stochastic and Environmental Factors

1. Events encountered in utero, in childhood, and in adolescence can result in specific epigenetic changes that yield a wide range of phenotypic abnormalities, including metabolic syndromes.

2. Fetal alcohol syndrome, which results from ethanol exposure in utero, may be mediated by the repressive impact of ethanol on the DNA methyltransferases.

3. Both abnormal gain of methylation, as in the case of fragile X syndrome, and abnormal loss of methylation, as in the case of FSHMD, can produce disease phenotypes.

Epigenetics and Cancer

1. The best evidence for epigenetic effects on disease risk comes from studies of human cancer.

2. Methylation densities decline as tumors progress, which can increase the activity of oncogenes, causing tumors to progress from benign neoplasms to malignancy. Additionally, the promoter regions of tumor-suppressor genes are often hypermethylated. These elevated methylation levels decreases their rate of transcription at these critical genes, thus reducing the ability to inhibit tumor formation.

3. Hypermethylation also is seen in microRNA genes and is associated with tumorigenesis.

4. Unlike DNA sequence mutations, epigenetic modifications can be reversed through pharmaceutical intervention. For example, 5-azacytidine, a demethylating agent, has been used as a therapeutic drug in the treatment of leukemia and myelodysplastic syndrome.

Future Directions

1. Robust experimental observations are defining the roles of epigenetic states in shaping cell fates.

2. The well-documented involvement of epigenetic abnormalities in carcinogenesis and the mounting evidence for these epigenetic changes in other common diseases (discussed throughout the text) will likely elucidate new therapies with the possibilities of reversing the epigenetic abnormalities.

▮ KEY TERMS

5-Azacytidine, 70
Angelman syndrome, 65
Beckwith-Wiedemann syndrome, 65
Biallelic, 64
DNA methylation, 62
Embryonic stem cell, 64
Epigenetics, 62
Fascioscapulohumeral muscular dystrophy (FSHMD), 68
Fragile X, 67
Histone, 63
Histone modification, 63
Housekeeping genes, 64
Imprinted, 64
MicroRNA (miRNA), 64
Monoallelic, 64
Noncoding RNA (ncRNA), 64
Prader-Willi syndrome, 65
Russell-Silver syndrome, 66

REFERENCES

1. King WD et al: A cross-sectional study of global DNA methylation and risk of colorectal adenoma, *BMC Cancer* 14(1):488, 2014.
2. Dhimolea E et al: Prenatal exposure to BPA alters the epigenome of the rat mammary gland and increases the propensity to neoplastic development, *PLoS One* 9(7):e99800, 2014.
3. Ashour N et al: A DNA hypermethylation profile reveals new potential biomarkers for prostate cancer diagnosis and prognosis, *Prostate* 74(12):1171-1182, 2014.
4. Meshorer E, Misteli T: Chromatin in pluripotent embryonic stem cells and differentiation, *Nat Rev Mol Cell Biol* 7(7):540-546, 2006.
5. Zaidi S et al: De novo mutations in histone-modifying genes in congenital heart disease, *Nature* 498(7453):220-223, 2013.
6. Balhorn R: The protamine family of sperm nuclear proteins, *Genome Biol* 8(9):227, 2007.
7. Deng Q et al: Single-cell RNA-seq reveals dynamic, random monoallelic gene expression in mammalian cells, *Science* 343(6167):193-196, 2014.
8. Cassidy SB et al: Prader-Willi syndrome, *Genet Med* 14:10-26, 2012.
9. Williams CA et al: Angelman syndrome 2005: updated consensus for diagnostic criteria, *Am J Med Genet A* 140:413-418, 2006.
10. Horsthemke B, Wagstaff J: Mechanisms of imprinting of the Prader-Willi/Angelman region, *Am J Med Genet A* 146A:2041-2052, 2008.
11. Kaminen-Ahola N et al: Maternal ethanol consumption alters the epigenotype and the phenotype of offspring in a mouse model, *PLoS Genet* 6(1):e1000811, 2010.
12. Bygren LO et al: Change in paternal grandmothers' early food supply influenced cardiovascular mortality of the female grandchildren, *BMC Genet* 15:12, 2014.
13. van Esterik JC et al: Programming of metabolic effects in C57BL/6JxFVB mice by exposure to bisphenol A during gestation and lactation, *Toxicology* 321:40-52, 2014.
14. Weaver IC et al: Epigenetic programming by maternal behavior, *Nat Neurosci* 7(8):847-854, 2004.
15. Jones KL et al: Pattern of malformation in offspring of chronic alcoholic mothers, *Lancet* 1(7815):1267-1271, 1973.
16. Zhou FC et al: Alcohol alters DNA methylation patterns and inhibits neural stem cell differentiation, *Alcohol Clin Exp Res* 35(4):735-746, 2011.

17. Mukhopadhyay P et al: Alcohol modulates expression of DNA methyltransferases and methyl CpG-/CpG domain-binding proteins in murine embryonic fibroblasts, *Reprod Toxicol* 37:40-48, 2013.

18. Lu C et al: Fragile X premutation RNA is sufficient to cause primary ovarian insufficiency in mice, *Hum Mol Genet* 21(23):5039-5047, 2012.

19. Jacquemot S: Penetrance of the fragile X–associated tremor/ataxia syndrome in a premutation carrier population, *J Am Med Assoc* 291(4):460-469, 2004.

20. Tassone F et al: Intranuclear inclusions in neural cells with premutation alleles in fragile X associated tremor/ataxia syndrome, *J Med Genet* 41(4):e43, 2004.

21. Stöger R et al: Epigenetic variation illustrated by DNA methylation patterns of the fragile-X gene FMR1, *Hum Mol Genet* 6(11):1791-1801, 1997.

22. Cabianca DS, Gabellini D: The cell biology of disease: FSHD: copy number variations on the theme of muscular dystrophy, *J Cell Biol* 191(6): 1049-1060, 2010.

23. Bodega B et al: Remodeling of the chromatin structure of the facioscapulohumeral muscular dystrophy (FSHD) locus and upregulation of FSHD-related gene 1 (FRG1) expression during human myogenic differentiation, *BMC Biol* 7:41, 2009.

24. Fraga MF et al: Epigenetic differences arise during the lifetime of monozygotic twins, *Proc Natl Acad Sci U S A* 102:10604-10609, 2005.

25. Frommer M et al: A genomic sequencing protocol that yields a positive display of 5-methylcytosine residues in individual DNA strands, *Proc Natl Acad Sci U S A* 89(5):1827-1831, 1992.

26. Peters AH et al: Partitioning and plasticity of repressive histone methylation states in mammalian chromatin, *Mol Cell* 12(6):1577-1589, 2003.

27. Esteller M: Epigenetics in cancer, *N Engl J Med* 358:1148-1159, 2008.

28. Sandoval J, Esteller M: Cancer epigenomics: beyond genomics, *Curr Opin Genet Dev* 22:50-55, 2012.

29. Giacinti C, Giordano A: RB and cell cycle progression, *Oncogene* 25(38):5220-5227, 2006.

30. Hansmann T et al: Constitutive promoter methylation of BRCA1 and RAD51C in patients with familial ovarian cancer and early-onset sporadic breast cancer, *Hum Mol Genet* 21(21): 4669-4679, 2012.

31. Lynch HT, de la Chapelle A: Hereditary colorectal cancer, *N Engl J Med* 348:919-932, 2003.

32. Pino MS, Chung DC: Microsatellite instability in the management of colorectal cancer, *Expert Rev Gastroenterol Hepatol* 5(3):385-399, 2011.

33. Hong J et al: Role of NADPH oxidase NOX5-S, NF-κB, and DNMT1 in acid-induced p16 hypermethylation in Barrett's cells, *Am J Physiol Cell Physiol* 305(10):C1069-C1079, 2013.

34. Tao K et al: Prognostic value of miR-221-3p, miR-342-3p and miR-491-5p expression in colon cancer, *Am J Transl Res* 6(4):391-401, 2014.

35. Ahmad A et al: Up-regulation of microRNA-10b is associated with the development of breast cancer brain metastasis, *Am J Transl Res* 6(4):384-390, 2014.

36. Ren Q et al: Epithelial and stromal expression of miRNAs during prostate cancer progression, *Am J Transl Res* 6(4):329-339, 2014.

37. Dulaimi E et al: Detection of bladder cancer in urine by a tumor suppressor gene hypermethylation panel, *Clin Cancer Res* 10(6):1887-1893, 2004.

38. Guzmán L et al: Analysis of aberrant methylation on promoter sequences of tumor suppressor genes and total DNA in sputum samples: a promising tool for early detection of COPD and lung cancer in smokers, *Diagn Pathol* 7:87, 2012.

39. Henrique R, Jerónimo C: Molecular detection of prostate cancer: a role for GSTP1 hypermethylation, *Eur Urol* 46(5):660-669, discussion 669, 2004.

40. Di Costanzo A et al: Epigenetic drugs against cancer: an evolving landscape, *Toxicology* 88(9): 1651-1668, 2014.

41. Christman JK: 5-Azacytidine and 5-aza-2′-deoxycytidine as inhibitors of DNA methylation: mechanistic studies and their implications for cancer therapy, *Oncogene* 21(35):5483-5495, 2002.

42. Zhang H et al: 5-Azacytidine suppresses the proliferation of pancreatic cancer cells by inhibiting the Wnt/β-catenin signaling pathway, *Genet Mol Res* 13(3):5064-5072, 2014.

43. Jabbour E, Garcia-Manero G: Deacetylase inhibitors for the treatment of myelodysplastic syndromes, *Leuk Lymphoma* 2015 Feb 24:1-8. [Epub ahead of print.]

44. Müller-Thomas C et al: Response to azacitidine is independent of p53 expression in higher-risk myelodysplastic syndromes and secondary acute myeloid leukemia, *Haematologica* 99(10): e179-e181, 2014.

45. Tate CR et al: Targeting triple-negative breast cancer cells with the histone deacetylase inhibitor panobinostat, *Breast Cancer Res* 14(3):R79, 2012.

46. Chen CS et al: Histone deacetylase inhibitors sensitize prostate cancer cells to agents that produce DNA double-strand breaks by targeting Ku70 acetylation, *Cancer Res* 67(11):5318-5327, 2007.

47. Koutsounas I et al: Histone deacetylase inhibitors and pancreatic cancer: are there any promising clinical trials? *World J Gastroenterol* 19(8): 1173-1181, 2013.

4

Altered Cellular and Tissue Biology

Kathryn L. McCance and Todd Cameron Grey

ⓔ EVOLVE WEBSITE

http://evolve.elsevier.com/Huether/
Student Review Questions
Audio Key Points

Case Studies
Animations
Quick Check Answers

CHAPTER OUTLINE

The majority of diseases are caused by many factors acting together (i.e., *multifactorial*) or interacting with a genetically susceptible person. Injury to cells and their surrounding environment, called the extracellular matrix, leads to tissue and organ injury. Although the normal cell is restricted by a narrow range of structure and functions, including metabolism and specialization, it can *adapt* to physiologic demands or stress to maintain a steady state called *homeostasis*. Adaptation is a reversible, structural, or functional response both to normal or physiologic conditions and to adverse or pathologic conditions. For example, the uterus adapts to pregnancy—a normal physiologic state—by enlarging. Enlargement occurs because of an increase in the size and number of uterine cells. In an adverse condition, such as high blood pressure, myocardial cells are stimulated to enlarge by the increased work of pumping. Like most of the body's adaptive mechanisms, however, cellular adaptations to adverse conditions are usually only temporarily successful. Severe or long-term stressors overwhelm adaptive processes and cellular injury or death ensues. Altered cellular and tissue biology can result from adaptation, injury, neoplasia, accumulations, aging, or death. (Neoplasia is discussed in Chapters 10 and 11.)

Knowledge of the structural and functional reactions of cells and tissues to injurious agents, including genetic defects, is vital to understanding disease processes. Cellular injury can be caused by any factor that disrupts cellular structures or deprives the cell of oxygen and nutrients required for survival. Injury may be reversible *(sublethal)* or irreversible *(lethal)* and is classified broadly as chemical, hypoxic (lack of sufficient oxygen), free radical, intentional, unintentional, immunologic, infection, and inflammatory. Cellular injuries from various causes have different clinical and pathophysiologic manifestations. Stresses from metabolic derangements may be associated with intracellular *accumulations* and include carbohydrates, proteins, and lipids. Sites of cellular death can cause accumulations of calcium resulting in *pathologic calcification*. Cellular death is confirmed by structural changes seen when cells are stained and examined under a microscope. The two main types of cell death include *necrosis* and *apoptosis* and nutrient deprivation can initiate *autophagy* that results in cell death. All of these pathways of cellular death are discussed later in this chapter.

Cellular aging causes structural and functional changes that eventually may lead to cellular death or a decreased capacity to recover from injury. Mechanisms explaining how and why cells age are not known, and distinguishing between pathologic changes and physiologic changes that occur with aging is often difficult. Aging clearly causes alterations in cellular structure and function, yet *senescence*, growing old, is both inevitable and normal.

CELLULAR ADAPTATION

Cells adapt to their environment to escape and protect themselves from injury. An adapted cell is neither normal nor injured—its condition lies somewhere between these two states. Adaptations are reversible changes in cell size, number, phenotype, metabolic activity, or functions of cells.[1] Adaptive responses have limits, however, and additional cell stresses can affect essential cell function leading to *cell injury*. Cellular adaptations also can be a common and central part of many disease states. In the early stages of a successful adaptive response, cells may have enhanced function; thus, it is hard to distinguish a pathologic response from an extreme adaptation to an excessive functional demand. The most significant adaptive changes in cells include atrophy (decrease in cell size), hypertrophy (increase in cell size), hyperplasia (increase in cell number), and metaplasia (reversible replacement of one mature cell type by another less mature cell type or a change in the phenotype). Dysplasia (deranged cellular growth) is not considered a true cellular adaptation but rather an atypical hyperplasia. These changes are shown in Figure 4-1.

Atrophy

Atrophy is a decrease or shrinkage in cellular size. If atrophy occurs in a sufficient number of an organ's cells, the entire organ shrinks or

FIGURE 4-1 Adaptive and Dysplastic Alterations in Simple Cuboidal Epithelial Cells.

becomes atrophic. Atrophy can affect any organ, but it is most common in skeletal muscle, the heart, secondary sex organs, and the brain. Atrophy can be classified as *physiologic* or *pathologic*. **Physiologic atrophy** occurs with early development. For example, the thymus gland undergoes physiologic atrophy during childhood. **Pathologic atrophy** occurs as a result of decreases in workload, pressure, use, blood supply, nutrition, hormonal stimulation, and nervous system stimulation (Figure 4-2). Individuals immobilized in bed for a prolonged time exhibit a type of skeletal muscle atrophy called **disuse atrophy**. Aging causes brain cells to become atrophic and endocrine-dependent organs, such as the gonads, to shrink as hormonal stimulation decreases. Whether atrophy is caused by normal physiologic conditions or by pathologic conditions, atrophic cells exhibit the same basic changes.

The atrophic muscle cell contains less endoplasmic reticulum (ER) and fewer mitochondria and myofilaments (part of the muscle fiber that controls contraction) than found in the normal cell. In muscular atrophy caused by nerve loss, oxygen consumption and amino acid uptake are immediately reduced. The mechanisms of atrophy include decreased protein synthesis, increased protein catabolism, or both. A new hypothesis includes ribosome function and its role as translation machinery or the conversion of mRNA into protein called ribosome biogenesis. Ribosome biogenesis has an important role in the regulation of skeletal muscle mass.[2] The primary pathway of protein catabolism is the **ubiquitin-proteasome pathway** and catabolism involves **proteasomes** (protein-degrading complexes. Proteins degraded in this pathway are first conjugated to **ubiquitin** (another small protein) and then degraded by proteasomes. An increase in proteasome activity is characteristic of atrophic muscle changes. Deregulation of this pathway often leads to abnormal cell growth and is associated with cancer and other diseases.

Atrophy as a result of chronic malnutrition is often accompanied by a "self-eating" process called *autophagy* that creates **autophagic vacuoles** (see p. 105). These vacuoles are membrane-bound vesicles within the cell that contain cellular debris and hydrolytic enzymes, which function to break down substances to the simplest units of fat, carbohydrate, or protein. The levels of hydrolytic enzymes rise rapidly in atrophy. The enzymes are isolated in autophagic vacuoles to prevent

FIGURE 4-2 Atrophy. A, Normal brain of a young adult. **B,** Atrophy of the brain in an 82-year-old male with atherosclerotic cerebrovascular disease, resulting in reduced blood supply. Note that loss of brain substance narrows the gyri and widens the sulci. The meninges have been stripped from the right half of each specimen to reveal the surface of the brain. (From Kumar V et al, editors: *Robbins and Cotran pathologic basis of disease,* ed 9, Philadelphia, 2015, Elsevier.)

uncontrolled cellular destruction. Thus the vacuoles form as needed to protect uninjured organelles from the injured organelles and are eventually engulfed and destroyed by lysosomes. Certain contents of the autophagic vacuole may resist destruction by lysosomal enzymes and persist in membrane-bound residual bodies. An example of this is granules that contain lipofuscin, the yellow-brown age pigment. Lipofuscin accumulates primarily in liver cells, myocardial cells, and atrophic cells.

Hypertrophy

Hypertrophy is a compensatory increase in the size of cells in response to mechanical stimuli (also called mechanical load or stress, such as from repetitive stretching, chronic pressure, or volume overload) and consequently increases the size of the affected organ (Figures 4-3 and 4-4). The cells of the heart and kidneys are particularly prone to enlargement. Hypertrophy, as an adaptive response (muscular enlargement), occurs in the striated muscle cells of both the heart and skeletal

FIGURE 4-3 Hypertrophy of Cardiac Muscle in Response to Valve Disease. A, Transverse slices of a normal heart and a heart with hypertrophy of the left ventricle (*L,* normal thickness of left ventricular wall; *T,* thickened wall from heart in which severe narrowing of aortic valve caused resistance to systolic ventricular emptying). **B,** Histology of cardiac muscle from the normal heart. **C,** Histology of cardiac muscle from a hypertrophied heart. (From Stevens A, Lowe J: *Pathology: illustrated review in color,* ed 2, Edinburgh, 2000, Mosby.)

FIGURE 4-4 Mechanisms of Myocardial Hypertrophy. Mechanical sensors appear to be the main stimulators for physiologic hypertrophy. Other stimuli possibly more important for pathologic hypertrophy include agonists (initiators) and growth factors. These factors then signal transcription pathways whereby transcription factors then bind to DNA sequences, activating muscle proteins that are responsible for hypertrophy. These pathways include induction of embryonic/fetal genes, increased synthesis of contractile proteins, and production of growth factors. (Adapted from Kumar V et al, editors: *Robbins and Cotran pathologic basis of disease,* ed 9, Philadelphia, 2015, Elsevier.)

muscles. Initial cardiac enlargement is caused by dilation of the cardiac chambers, is short lived, and is followed by increased synthesis of cardiac muscle proteins, allowing muscle fibers to do more work. The increase in cellular size is associated with an increased accumulation of protein in the cellular components (plasma membrane, ER, myofilaments, mitochondria) and *not* with an increase in cellular fluid. Yet, individual protein pools may expand or shrink.[3] Cardiac hypertrophy involves changes in signaling and transcription factor pathways resulting in increased protein synthesis leading to left ventricular hypertrophy (LVH). Emerging evidence suggests that the ubiquitin-proteasome system (UPS) not only attends to damaged, misfolded, or mutant proteins by protein breakdown but also may attend to cell growth eventually leading to LVH.[4] With time, cardiac hypertrophy is characterized by extracellular matrix remodeling and increased growth of adult myocytes. The myocytes progressively increase in size and reach a limit beyond which no further hypertrophy can occur.[5,6]

Although hypertrophy can be classified as *physiologic* or *pathologic,* time may be the critical factor or determinant of the transition from physiologic to pathologic cardiac hypertrophy. With *physiologic hypertrophy,* preservation of myocardial structure characterizes postnatal development, moderate endurance exercise training, pregnancy, and the early phases of increased pressure and volume loading on the adult human heart. This physiologic response is temporary; however, aging, strenuous exercise, and sustained workload or stress lead to pathologic hypertrophy with structural and functional manifestations. *Pathologic hypertrophy* in the heart is secondary to hypertension, coronary heart disease, or problem valves and is presumably a key risk factor for heart failure. Additionally, it is associated with increased interstitial fibrosis, cell death, and abnormal cardiac function (see Figure 4-3). Historically, the progression of pathologic cardiac hypertrophy has been considered irreversible. Emerging data, however, from experimental studies and clinical observations show in certain cases reversal of pathologic cardiac hypertrophy. Cardiac hypertrophy can be reversed when the increased wall stress is normalized, a process termed *regression.*[7] For example, unloading of hemodynamic stress by a left ventricular assist device (used in individuals with heart failure for bridging to heart transplantation) induces regression of cardiac hypertrophy and improvement of left ventricular (LV) function in those with end-stage heart failure.[8] Regression of cardiac hypertrophy is accompanied by activation of unique sets of genes, including fetal-type genes and those involved in protein degradation.[9,10] However, the signaling mechanisms mediating regression of cardiac hypertrophy have been poorly understood. Improvement in new blood vessel development (angiogenesis) in the hypertrophic heart can lead to regression of the hypertrophy and prevention of heart failure.[11,12] In mice, dietary supplementation of physiologically relevant levels of copper can reverse pathologic cardiac hypertrophy.[12,13]

When a diseased kidney is removed, the remaining kidney adapts to the increased workload with an increase in both the size and the number of cells. The major contributing factor to this renal enlargement is hypertrophy. Another example of normal or physiologic hypertrophy is the increased growth of the uterus and mammary glands in response to pregnancy.

Hyperplasia

Hyperplasia is an increase in the number of cells, resulting from an increased rate of cellular division. Hyperplasia, as a response to injury, occurs when the injury has been severe and prolonged enough to have caused cell death. Loss of epithelial cells and cells of the liver and kidney triggers deoxyribonucleic acid (DNA) synthesis and mitotic division. Increased cell growth is a multistep process involving the production of growth factors, which stimulate the remaining cells to

synthesize new cell components and, ultimately, to divide. Hyperplasia and hypertrophy often occur together, and both take place if the cells can synthesize DNA.

Two types of normal, or physiologic, hyperplasia are compensatory hyperplasia and hormonal hyperplasia. Compensatory hyperplasia is an adaptive mechanism that enables certain organs to regenerate. For example, removal of part of the liver leads to hyperplasia of the remaining liver cells (hepatocytes) to compensate for the loss. Even with removal of 70% of the liver, regeneration is complete in about 2 weeks. Several growth factors and cytokines (chemical messengers) are induced and play critical roles in liver regeneration.

Not all types of mature cells have the same capacity for compensatory hyperplastic growth. Nondividing tissues contain cells that can no longer (i.e., postnatally) go through the cell cycle and undergo mitotic division. These highly specialized cells, for example, neurons and skeletal muscle cells, never divide again once they have differentiated—that is, they are *terminally differentiated.*[14] In human cells, cell growth and cell division depend on signals from other cells; but cell growth, unlike cell division, does not depend on the cell-cycle control system.[14] Nerve cells and most muscle cells do most of their growing after they have terminally differentiated and permanently ceased dividing.[14] Significant compensatory hyperplasia occurs in epidermal and intestinal epithelia, hepatocytes, bone marrow cells, and fibroblasts; and some hyperplasia is noted in bone, cartilage, and smooth muscle cells. Another example of compensatory hyperplasia is the callus, or thickening, of the skin as a result of hyperplasia of epidermal cells in response to a mechanical stimulus.

Hormonal hyperplasia occurs chiefly in estrogen-dependent organs, such as the uterus and breast. After ovulation, for example, estrogen stimulates the endometrium to grow and thicken in preparation for receiving the fertilized ovum. If pregnancy occurs, hormonal hyperplasia, as well as hypertrophy, enables the uterus to enlarge. (Hormone function is described in Chapters 19 and 33.)

Pathologic hyperplasia is the abnormal proliferation of normal cells, usually in response to excessive hormonal stimulation or growth factors on target cells (Figure 4-5). The most common example is pathologic hyperplasia of the endometrium (caused by an imbalance

Lumen

Enlarged prostate

FIGURE 4-5 Hyperplasia of the Prostate with Secondary Thickening of the Obstructed Urinary Bladder (Bladder Cross Section). The enlarged prostate is seen protruding into the lumen of the bladder, which appears trabeculated. These "trabeculae" result from hypertrophy and hyperplasia of smooth muscle cells that occur in response to increased intravesical pressure caused by urinary obstruction. (From Damjanov I: *Pathology for the health professions,* ed 4, St Louis, 2012, Saunders.)

between estrogen and progesterone secretion, with oversecretion of estrogen) (see Chapter 33). Pathologic endometrial hyperplasia, which causes excessive menstrual bleeding, is under the influence of regular growth-inhibition controls. If these controls fail, hyperplastic endometrial cells can undergo malignant transformation. Benign prostatic hyperplasia is another example of pathologic hyperplasia and results from changes in hormone balance. In both of these examples, if the hormonal imbalance is corrected, hyperplasia regresses.[1]

Dysplasia: Not a True Adaptive Change

Dysplasia refers to abnormal changes in the size, shape, and organization of mature cells (Figure 4-6). Dysplasia is not considered a true adaptive process but is related to hyperplasia and is often called atypical hyperplasia. Dysplastic changes often are encountered in epithelial tissue of the cervix and respiratory tract, where they are strongly associated with common neoplastic growths and often are found adjacent to cancerous cells. Importantly, however, the term *dysplasia* does *not* indicate cancer and may not progress to cancer. Dysplasia is often classified as mild, moderate, or severe; yet, because this classification scheme is somewhat subjective, it has prompted some to recommend the use of either "low grade" or "high grade" instead. If the inciting stimulus is removed, dysplastic changes often are reversible. (Dysplasia is discussed further in Chapter 10.)

Metaplasia

Metaplasia is the reversible replacement of one mature cell type (epithelial or mesenchymal) by another, sometimes less differentiated, cell type. It is thought to develop, as an adaptive response better suited to withstand the adverse environment, from a reprogramming of stem cells that exist on most epithelia or of undifferentiated mesenchymal (tissue from embryonic mesoderm) cells present in connective tissue. These precursor cells mature along a new pathway because of signals generated by growth factors in the cell's environment. The best example of metaplasia is replacement of normal columnar ciliated epithelial cells of the bronchial (airway) lining by stratified squamous epithelial cells (Figure 4-7). The newly formed cells do not secrete mucus or have cilia, causing loss of a vital protective mechanism. Bronchial metaplasia can be reversed if the inducing stimulus, usually cigarette smoking, is removed. With prolonged exposure to the inducing stimulus, however, dysplasia and cancerous transformation can occur.

CELLULAR INJURY

Injury to cells and to the extracellular matrix (ECM) leads to injury of tissues and organs, ultimately determining the structural patterns of disease. Loss of function is derived from cell and ECM injury and cell death. Cellular injury occurs if the cell is unable to maintain

FIGURE 4-6 Dysplasia of the Uterine Cervix. A, Mild dysplasia. **B,** Severe dysplasia. (From Damjanov I, Linder J: *Anderson's pathology,* ed 10, St Louis, 1996, Mosby.)

Normal ciliated epithelium

Metaplasia
Chronic injury or irritation

Dysplasia
Persistent severe injury or irritation

FIGURE 4-7 Reversible Changes in Cells Lining the Bronchi.

homeostasis—a normal or adaptive steady state—in the face of injurious stimuli or stress. Injured cells may recover (**reversible injury**) or die (**irreversible injury**). Injurious stimuli include chemical agents, lack of sufficient oxygen (hypoxia), free radicals, infectious agents, physical and mechanical factors, immunologic reactions, genetic factors, and nutritional imbalances. Types of injuries and their responses are summarized in Table 4-1 and Figure 4-8.

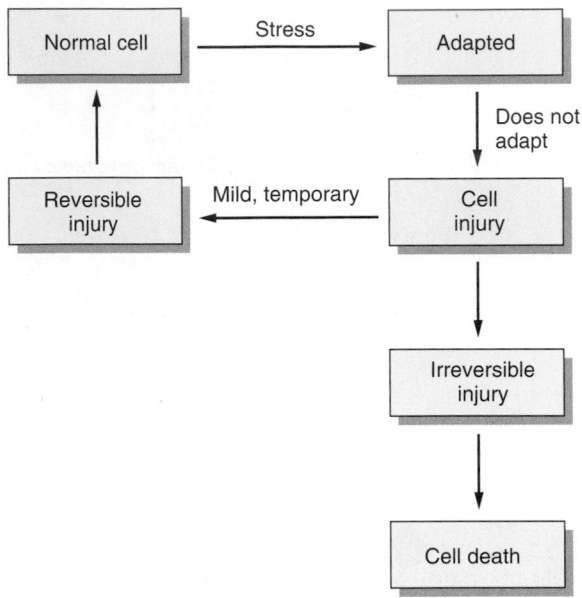

FIGURE 4-8 Stages of Cellular Adaptation, Injury, and Death. The normal cell responds to physiologic and pathologic stresses by adapting (atrophy, hypertrophy, hyperplasia, metaplasia). Cell injury occurs if the adaptive responses are exceeded or compromised by injurious agents, stress, and mutations. The injury is reversible if it is mild or transient, but if the stimulus persists the cell suffers irreversible injury and eventually death.

The extent of cellular injury depends on the type, state (including level of cell differentiation and increased susceptibility to fully differentiated cells), and adaptive processes of the cell, as well as the type, severity, and duration of the injurious stimulus. Two individuals exposed to an identical stimulus may incur varying degrees of cellular injury. Modifying factors, such as nutritional status, can profoundly influence the extent of injury. The precise "point of no return" that leads to cellular death is a biochemical puzzle, but once changes to the nucleus occur and cell membranes are disrupted, the cell moves to irreversible injury and death.

General Mechanisms of Cell Injury

Common biochemical themes are important to understanding cell injury and cell death regardless of the injuring agent. These include adenosine triphosphate (ATP) depletion, mitochondrial damage, oxygen and oxygen-derived free radical membrane damage (depletion of ATP), protein folding defects, DNA damage defects, and calcium level alterations (Table 4-2). Examples of common forms of cell injury are (1) hypoxic injury, (2) free radicals and reactive oxygen species injury, and (3) chemical injury.

Hypoxic Injury

Hypoxia, or lack of sufficient oxygen within cells, is the single most common cause of cellular injury (Figure 4-9). Hypoxia can result from

TABLE 4-1 Types of Progressive Cell Injury and Responses	
Type	**Responses**
Adaptation	Atrophy, hypertrophy, hyperplasia, metaplasia
Active cell injury	Immediate response of "entire" cell
Reversible	Loss of ATP, cellular swelling, detachment of ribosomes, autophagy of lysosomes
Irreversible	"Point of no return" structurally when severe vacuolization of mitochondria occurs and Ca++ moves into cell
Necrosis	Common type of cell death with severe cell swelling and breakdown of organelles
Apoptosis, or programmed cell death	Cellular self-destruction for elimination of unwanted cell populations
Autophagy	Eating of self, cytoplasmic vesicles engulf cytoplasm and organelles, recycling factory
Chronic cell injury (subcellular alterations)	Persistent stimuli response may involve only specific organelles or cytoskeleton (e.g., phagocytosis of bacteria)
Accumulations or infiltrations	Water, pigments, lipids, glycogen, proteins
Pathologic calcification	Dystrophic and metastatic calcification

ATP, Adenosine triphosphate; *Ca++*, calcium.

TABLE 4-2 Common Themes in Cell Injury and Cell Death	
Theme	**Comments**
ATP depletion	Loss of mitochondrial ATP and decreased ATP synthesis; results include cellular swelling, decreased protein synthesis, decreased membrane transport, and lipogenesis, all changes that contribute to loss of integrity of plasma membrane
Reactive oxygen species (↑ROS)	Lack of oxygen is key in progression of cell injury in ischemia (reduced blood supply); activated oxygen species (ROS, O$_2^-$, H$_2$O$_2$, OH•) cause destruction of cell membranes and cell structure
Ca++ entry	Normally intracellular cytosolic calcium concentrations are very low; ischemia and certain chemicals cause an increase in cytosolic Ca++ concentrations; sustained levels of Ca++ continue to increase with damage to plasma membrane; Ca++ causes intracellular damage by activating a number of enzymes
Mitochondrial damage	Can be damaged by increases in cytosolic Ca++, ROS; two outcomes of mitochondrial damage are loss of membrane potential, which causes depletion of ATP and eventual death or necrosis of cell, and activation of another type of cell death (apoptosis) (see p. 104)
Membrane damage	Early loss of selective membrane permeability found in all forms of cell injury, lysosomal membrane damage with release of enzymes causing cellular digestion
Protein misfolding, DNA damage	Proteins may misfold, triggering *unfolded protein response* that activates corrective responses; if overwhelmed, response activates cell suicide program or apoptosis; DNA damage (genotoxic stress) also can activate apoptosis (see p. 104)

ATP, Adenosine triphosphate; *Ca++*, calcium.

FIGURE 4-9 Hypoxic Injury Induced by Ischemia. **A,** Consequences of decreased oxygen delivery or ischemia with decreased ATP. The structural and physiologic changes are reversible if oxygen is delivered quickly. Significant decreases in ATP result in cell death, mostly by necrosis. **B,** Mitochondrial damage can result in changes in membrane permeability, loss of membrane potential, and decrease in ATP concentration. Between the outer and inner membranes of the mitochondria are proteins that can activate the cell's suicide pathways, called apoptosis. **C,** Calcium ions are critical mediators of cell injury. Calcium ions are usually maintained at low concentrations in the cell's cytoplasm; thus ischemia and certain toxins can initially cause an increase in the release of Ca^{++} from intracellular stores and later an increased movement (influx) across the plasma membrane. (Adapted from Kumar V et al, editors: *Pathology,* St Louis, 2014, Elsevier.)

a reduced amount of oxygen in the air, loss of hemoglobin or decreased efficacy of hemoglobin, decreased production of red blood cells, diseases of the respiratory and cardiovascular systems, and poisoning of the oxidative enzymes (cytochromes) within the cells. Hypoxia plays a role in physiologic processes including cell differentiation, angiogenesis, proliferation, erythropoiesis, and overall cell viability.[15] The main consumers of oxygen are mitochondria and the cellular responses to hypoxia are reported to be mediated by the production of reactive oxygen species (ROS) at the mitochondrial complex III.[15] Investigators are studying the role of ROS as hypoxia signaling molecules. More commonly, hypoxia is associated with the pathophysiologic conditions such as inflammation, ischemia, and cancer. Hypoxia can induce inflammation and inflamed lesions can become hypoxic (Figure 4-10).[16] The cellular mechanisms involved in hypoxia and inflammation are emerging and include activation of immune responses and oxygen-sensing compounds called *prolyl hydroxylases (PHDs)* and *hypoxia-inducible transcription factor (HIF).* The **hypoxia-inducible factor (HIF)** is a family of transcription regulators that coordinate the expression of many genes in response to oxygen deprivation. Mammalian development occurs in a hypoxic environment.[17] Hypoxia-induced signaling involves complicated crosstalk between hypoxia and inflammation, linking hypoxia and inflammation to inflammatory bowel disease, certain cancers, and infections.[16] Research is ongoing to understand the mechanisms of how tumors adapt to low oxygen levels by inducing angiogenesis, increasing glucose consumption, and promoting the metabolic state of glycolysis.[18]

The most common cause of hypoxia is **ischemia** (reduced blood supply). Ischemic injury often is caused by the gradual narrowing of

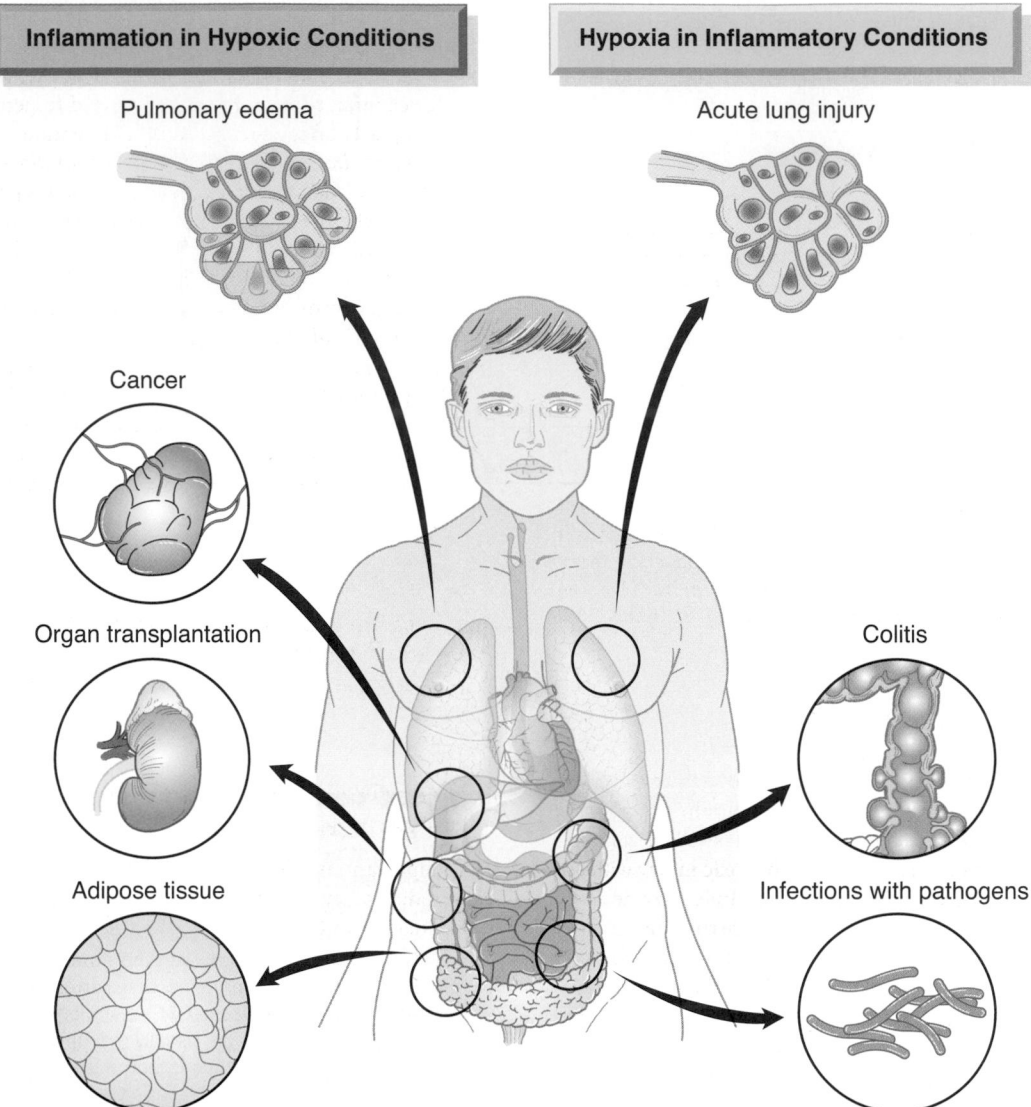

Inflammation in Hypoxic Conditions

Hypoxia in Inflammatory Conditions

Pulmonary edema

Acute lung injury

Cancer

Organ transplantation

Adipose tissue

Colitis

Infections with pathogens

FIGURE 4-10 Hypoxia and Inflammation. Shown is a simplified drawing of clinical conditions characterized by tissue hypoxia that causes inflammatory changes *(left)* and inflammatory diseases that ultimately lead to hypoxia *(right)*. These diseases and conditions are discussed in more detail in their respective chapters. (Adapted from Eltzschig HK, Carmeliet P: Hypoxia and inflammation, *N Engl J Med* 364:656-665, 2011.)

arteries (arteriosclerosis) or complete blockage by blood clots (thrombosis), or both. Progressive hypoxia caused by gradual arterial obstruction is better tolerated than the acute anoxia (total lack of oxygen) caused by a sudden obstruction, as with an embolus (a blood clot or other blockage in the circulation). An acute obstruction in a coronary artery can cause myocardial cell death (infarction) within minutes if the blood supply is not restored, whereas the gradual onset of ischemia usually results in myocardial adaptation. Myocardial infarction and stroke, which are common causes of death in the United States, generally result from atherosclerosis (a type of arteriosclerosis) and consequent ischemic injury. (Vascular obstruction is discussed in Chapter 24.)

Cellular responses to hypoxic injury caused by ischemia have been demonstrated in studies of the heart muscle. Within 1 minute after blood supply to the myocardium is interrupted, the heart becomes pale and has difficulty contracting normally. Within 3 to 5 minutes, the ischemic portion of the myocardium ceases to contract because of a rapid decrease in mitochondrial phosphorylation, causing insufficient ATP production. Lack of ATP leads to increased anaerobic metabolism, which generates ATP from glycogen when there is insufficient oxygen. When glycogen stores are depleted, even anaerobic metabolism ceases.

A reduction in ATP levels causes the plasma membrane's sodium-potassium (Na^+-K^+) pump and sodium-calcium exchange mechanism to fail, which leads to an intracellular accumulation of sodium and calcium and diffusion of potassium out of the cell. Sodium and water then can enter the cell freely, and cellular swelling, as well as early dilation of the endoplasmic reticulum (ER), results. Dilation causes the ribosomes to detach from the rough ER, reducing protein synthesis. With continued hypoxia, the entire cell becomes markedly swollen, with increased concentrations of sodium, water, and chloride and decreased concentrations of potassium. These disruptions are

FIGURE 4-11 Reperfusion Injury. Without oxygen, or anoxia, the cells display hypoxic injury and become swollen. With reoxygenation, reperfusion injury increases because of the formation of reactive oxygen radicals that can cause cell necrosis. (Redrawn from Damjanov I: *Pathology for the health professions,* ed 3, St Louis, 2006, Saunders.)

injury.[19] The PREVEC Trial (Prevention of reperfusion damage associated with percutaneous coronary angioplasty following acute myocardial infarction) seeks to evaluate whether vitamins C and E reduce infarct size in patients subjected to percutaneous coronary angioplasty after acute myocardial infarction.[20]

- *Increased intracellular calcium concentration*—Intracellular and mitochondrial calcium overload the cell; this process begins during acute ischemia. Reperfusion causes even more calcium influx because of cell membrane damage and ROS-induced injury to the sarcoplasmic reticulum. The increased calcium increases mitochondrial permeability, eventually leading to depletion of ATP and further cell injury.
- *Inflammation*—Ischemic injury increases inflammation because danger signals (from cytokines) are released by resident immune cells when cells die and this signaling initiates inflammation.
- *Complement activation*—The activation of complement may increase the tissue damage from reperfusion-ischemia injury.[1]

✔ **QUICK CHECK 4-1**
1. When does a cell become irreversibly injured?
2. Discuss the pathogenesis of hypoxic injury?
3. What are the mechanisms of ischemia-reperfusion injury?

---

reversible if oxygen is restored. If oxygen is not restored, however, vacuolation (formation of vacuoles) occurs within the cytoplasm and swelling of lysosomes and marked mitochondrial swelling result from damage to the outer membrane. Continued hypoxic injury with accumulation of calcium subsequently activates multiple enzyme systems resulting in membrane damage, cytoskeleton disruption, DNA and chromatin degradation, ATP depletion, and eventual cell death (see Figures 4-9, *C*, and 4-27). Structurally, with plasma membrane damage, extracellular calcium readily moves into the cell and intracellular calcium stores are released. Increased intracellular calcium levels activate cell enzymes (caspases) that promote cell death by apoptosis (see Figures 4-29 and 4-33). Persistent ischemia is associated with irreversible injury and necrosis. Irreversible injury is associated structurally with severe swelling of the mitochondria, severe damage to plasma membranes, and swelling of lysosomes. Overall, death is mainly by necrosis but apoptosis also contributes.[1]

Restoration of blood flow and oxygen, however, can cause additional injury called ischemia-reperfusion injury (Figure 4-11). Ischemia-reperfusion injury is very important clinically because it is associated with tissue damage during myocardial and cerebral infarction. Several mechanisms are now proposed for ischemia-reperfusion injury and include:

- *Oxidative stress*—Reoxygenation causes the increased generation of reactive oxygen species (ROS) and nitrogen species.[1] Highly reactive oxygen intermediates (oxidative stress) generated include hydroxyl radical (OH^-), superoxide radical (O_2^-), and hydrogen peroxide (H_2O_2) (see pp. 82-83). The nitrogen species include nitric oxide (NO) generated by endothelial cells, macrophages, neurons, and other cells. These radicals can all cause further membrane damage and mitochondrial calcium overload. The white blood cells (neutrophils) are especially affected with reperfusion injury, including neutrophil adhesion to the endothelium. Antioxidant treatment not only reverses neutrophil adhesion but also can reverse neutrophil-mediated heart injury. In one study of individuals undergoing elective percutaneous coronary intervention (PCI), pretreatment with vitamin C was associated with less myocardial

Free Radicals and Reactive Oxygen Species—Oxidative Stress

An important mechanism of cellular injury is injury induced by free radicals, especially by reactive oxygen species (ROS); this form of injury is called oxidative stress. Oxidative stress occurs when *excess* ROS overwhelm endogenous antioxidant systems. A free radical is an electrically uncharged atom or group of atoms that has an unpaired electron. Having one unpaired electron makes the molecule unstable; the molecule becomes stabilized either by donating or by accepting an electron from another molecule. When the attacked molecule loses its electron, it becomes a free radical. Therefore it is capable of injurious chemical bond formation with proteins, lipids, and carbohydrates—key molecules in membranes and nucleic acids. Free radicals are difficult to control and initiate chain reactions. They are *highly* reactive because they have low chemical specificity, meaning they can react with most molecules in their proximity. Oxidative stress can activate several intracellular signaling pathways because ROS can modulate enzymes and transcription factors. This is an important mechanism of cell damage in many conditions including chemical and radiation injury, ischemia-reperfusion injury, cellular aging, and microbial killing by phagocytes, particularly neutrophils and macrophages.[1]

Free radicals may be generated within cells, first by the reduction-oxidation reactions (redox reactions) in normal metabolic processes such as respiration. Under normal physiologic conditions ROS serve as "redox messengers" in the regulation of intracellular signaling; however, excess ROS may produce irreversible damage to cellular components. All biologic membranes contain redox systems, which also are important for cell defense (e.g., inflammation, iron uptake, growth and proliferation, and signal transduction) (Figure 4-12). Second, absorption of extreme energy sources (e.g., ultraviolet light, radiation) produces free radicals. Third, enzymatic metabolism of exogenous chemicals or drugs (e.g., CCl_3, a product of carbon tetrachloride [CCl_4]) results in the formation of free radicals. Fourth, transition metals (i.e., iron and copper) donate or accept free electrons during

FIGURE 4-12 Generation of Reactive Oxygen Species and Antioxidant Mechanisms in Biologic Systems. Free radicals are generated within cells in several ways, including from normal respiration; absorption of radiant energy; activation of leukocytes during inflammation; metabolism of chemicals or drugs; transition metals, such as iron (Fe^{+++}) or copper (Cu^+), where the metals donate or accept electrons as in the Fenton reaction; nitric oxide (NO) generated by endothelial cells (not shown); and reperfusion injury. Ubiquinone (coenzyme Q), a lipophilic molecule, transfers electrons in the inner membrane of mitochondria, ultimately enabling their interaction with oxygen (O_2) and hydrogen (H_2) to yield water (H_2O). In so doing, the transport allows free energy change and the synthesis of 1 mole of adenosine triphosphate (ATP). With the transport of electrons, free radicals are generated within the mitochondria. Reactive oxygen species (O_2^-, H_2O_2, OH•) act as physiologic modulators of some mitochondrial functions but may also cause cell damage. O_2 is converted to superoxide (O_2^-) by oxidative enzymes in the mitochondria, endoplasmic reticulum *(ER)*, plasma membrane, peroxisomes, and cytosol. O_2 is converted to H_2O_2 by superoxide dismutase *(SOD)* and further to OH• by the Cu/Fe Fenton reaction. Superoxide catalyzes the reduction of Fe^{++} to Fe^{+++}, thus increasing OH• formation by the Fenton reaction. H_2O_2 is also derived from oxidases in peroxisomes. The three reactive oxygen species (H_2O_2, OH•, and O_2^-) cause free radical damage to lipids (peroxidation of the membrane), proteins (ion pump damage), and DNA (impaired protein synthesis). The major antioxidant enzymes include SOD, catalase, and glutathione peroxidase.

intracellular reactions and activate the formation of free radicals such as in the Fenton reaction (see Figure 4-12). Finally, nitric oxide (NO) is an important colorless gas that is an intermediate in many reactions generated by endothelial cells, neurons, macrophages, and other cell types. NO can act as a free radical and can be converted to highly reactive peroxynitrite anion ($ONOO^-$), NO_2, and NO_3^-. Table 4-3 describes the most significant free radicals.

Free radicals cause several damaging effects by (1) **lipid peroxidation**, which is the destruction of polyunsaturated lipids (the same process by which fats become rancid), leading to membrane damage and increased permeability; (2) protein alterations, causing fragmentation of polypeptide chains that can lead to loss and protein misfolding; and (3) DNA damage, causing mutations (Figure 4-13; also see p. 39). Because of the increased understanding of free radicals, a growing number of diseases and disorders have been linked either directly or indirectly to these reactive species (Box 4-1).

The body can eliminate free radicals. The oxygen free radical superoxide may spontaneously decay into oxygen and hydrogen peroxide.

Table 4-4 summarizes other methods that contribute to inactivation or termination of free radicals. The toxicity of certain drugs and chemicals can be attributed either to conversion of these chemicals to free radicals or to the formation of oxygen-derived metabolites (see the following discussion).

Mitochondrial Effects

Mitochondria are key players in cell injury and cell death because they produce ATP or life-sustaining energy. Mitochondria can be damaged by ROS and by increases of cytosolic Ca^{++} concentration (see Figure 4-9). Box 4-2 summarizes the three major types and consequences of mitochondrial damage. Currently, investigators are trying to identify the polypeptides (i.e., proteomes) directly involved in diseases associated with mitochondrial dysfunction. ROS not only damage proteins and mitochondria but also can promote damage in neighboring cells. An important area of research emphasis is that protein aggregates can increase mitochondrial damage and damaged mitochondria can further induce protein damage, thus resulting in neurodegeneration.

TABLE 4-3 Biologically Relevant Free Radicals

Reactive oxygen species (ROS) Superoxide O_2^- $$O_2 \xrightarrow{\text{Oxidase}} O_2^-$$	Generated either (1) directly during autoxidation in mitochondria or (2) enzymatically by enzymes in cytoplasm, such as xanthine oxidase or cytochrome P-450; once produced, it can be inactivated spontaneously or more rapidly by enzyme superoxide dismutase (SOD): $$O_2^- + O_2^- + -H_2^- \xrightarrow{\text{SOD}} H_2O_2 + O_2$$
Hydrogen peroxide (H_2O_2) $$O_2^- + O_2^- + -H \xrightarrow{\text{SOD}} H_2O_2 + O_2$$ *Or* Oxidases present in peroxisomes $$O_2 \text{ peroxisome } O_2^- \xrightarrow{\text{SOD}} H_2O_2$$	Generated by SOD or directly by oxidases in intracellular peroxisomes; NOTE: SOD is considered an antioxidant because it converts superoxide to H_2O_2; catalase (another antioxidant) can then decompose H_2O_2 to $O_2 + H_2O$.)
Hydroxyl radicals (OH^-) $$H_2O \rightarrow H \cdot + OH \cdot$$ *Or* $$Fe^{++} + H_2O_2 \rightarrow Fe^{++} + OH \cdot + OH^-$$ *Or* $$H_2O_2 + O_2^- \rightarrow OH \cdot + OH^- + O_2$$ Nitric oxide (NO) $$NO \cdot + O_2^- \rightarrow ONOO^- + H^+$$	Generated by hydrolysis of water caused by ionizing radiation or by interaction with metals—especially iron (Fe) and copper (Cu); iron is important in toxic oxygen injury because it is required for maximal oxidative cell damage NO by itself is an important mediator that can act as a free radical; it can be converted to another radical—peroxynitrite anion ($ONOO^-$), as well as NO_2 and CO_3^-

Data from Cotran RS et al: *Robbins pathologic basis of disease*, ed 6, Philadelphia, 1999, Saunders.

TABLE 4-4 Methods Contributing to Inactivation or Termination of Free Radicals

Method	Process
Antioxidants	Endogenous or exogenous; either blocks synthesis or inactivates (e.g., scavenges) free radicals; includes vitamin E, vitamin C, cysteine, glutathione, albumin, ceruloplasmin, transferrin, γ-lipoacid, others
Enzymes	Superoxide dismutase,* which converts superoxide to H_2O_2; catalase* (in peroxisomes) decomposes H_2O_2; glutathione peroxidase* decomposes OH• and H_2O_2

*These enzymes are important in modulating the cellular destructive effects of free radicals, also released in inflammation.

BOX 4-1 Diseases and Disorders Linked to Oxygen-Derived Free Radicals

Deterioration noted in aging
  Atherosclerosis
  Ischemic brain injury
  Alzheimer disease
Neurotoxins
Cancer
Cardiac myopathy
Chronic granulomatous disease
Diabetes mellitus
Eye disorders
  Macular degeneration
  Cataracts
Inflammatory disorders
Iron overload

Lung disorders
  Asbestosis
  Oxygen toxicity
  Emphysema
Nutritional deficiencies
Radiation injury
Reperfusion injury
Rheumatoid arthritis
Skin disorders
Toxic states
  Xenobiotics (CCl_4, paraquat, cigarette smoke, etc.)
  Metal irons (Ni, Cu, Fe, etc.)

FIGURE 4-13 The Role of Reactive Oxygen Species (ROS) in Cell Injury. The production of ROS can be initiated by many cell stressors, such as radiation, toxins, and reperfusion of oxygen. Free radicals are removed by normal decay and enzymatic systems. ROS accumulates in cells because of insufficient removal or excess production leading to cell injury, including lipid peroxidation, protein modifications, and DNA damage or mutations. (Adapted from Kumar V et al, editors: *Robbins and Cotran pathologic basis of disease*, ed 9, Philadelphia, 2015, Elsevier.)

BOX 4-2   Three Major Types and Consequences of Mitochondrial Damage

1. Damage to the mitochondria results in the formation of the *mitochondrial permeability transition pore,* a high-conductance channel or pore. The opening of this channel results in the loss of mitochondrial membrane potential, causing failure of oxidative phosphorylation, depletion of ATP, and damage to **mitochondrial DNA (mtDNA),** leading to necrosis of the cell.
2. Altered oxidative phosphorylation leads to the formation of ROS that can damage cellular components.
3. Because mitochondria store several proteins between their membranes, increased permeability of the outer membrane may result in leakage of pro-apoptotic proteins and cause cell death by apoptosis.

Data from Kumar V et al, editors: *Robbins and Cotran pathologic basis of disease,* ed 9, Philadelphia, 2015, Elsevier.

An emerging area of research concerns mitochondrial DNA that escapes from autophagy, which may be a mechanism of tissue inflammation.[21]

Chemical or Toxic Injury
Mechanisms

Humans are exposed to thousands of chemicals that have inadequate toxicologic data.[22] The given societal considerations of time, cost, and reduced animal use have increased the need to develop new methods for toxicity testing. To meet this public health need, many agencies have partnered to investigate how chemicals interact with biologic systems. Advances in molecular and systems biology, computational toxicology, and bioinformatics have increased the development of powerful new tools.

The systems biology approach includes delineation of toxicity pathways that may be defined as cellular response pathways, which when disturbed are expected to result in adverse health effects. Using this model of testing, investigators proposed screening and classifying compounds using a "cellular stress response pathway." Components or mechanisms of these pathways include oxidative stress, heat shock response, DNA damage response, hypoxia, ER stress (see Chapter 1), mental stress, inflammation, and osmotic stress. Many chemicals have already been classified under these mechanisms.

Humans are constantly exposed to a variety of compounds termed xenobiotics (Greek *xenos,* "foreign"; *bios,* "life") that include toxic, mutagenic, and carcinogenic chemicals (Figure 4-14). Some of these chemicals are found in the human diet, for example, fungal mycotoxins such as aflatoxin B_1. Many xenobiotics are toxic to the liver (hepatotoxic). The liver is the initial site of contact for many ingested xenobiotics, drugs, and alcohol, making this organ most susceptible to chemically induced injury. The toxicity of many chemicals results from absorption through the gastrointestinal tract after oral ingestion. A main cause for withdrawing medications from the market is hepatotoxicity. Dietary supplements, for example, chaparral and ma huang, are potent hepatotoxins.[23] Other common routes of exposure for xenobiotics are absorption through the skin and inhalation. The severity of chemically induced liver injury varies from minor liver injury to acute liver failure, cirrhosis, and liver cancer.[24]

The liver as the principal site for xenobiotic metabolism, called *biotransformation,* converts the lipophilic xenobiotics to more hydrophilic forms for efficient excretion. Biotransformation, however, also can produce short-lived unstable highly reactive chemical intermediates that can lead to adverse effects.[25] These harmful intermediates,

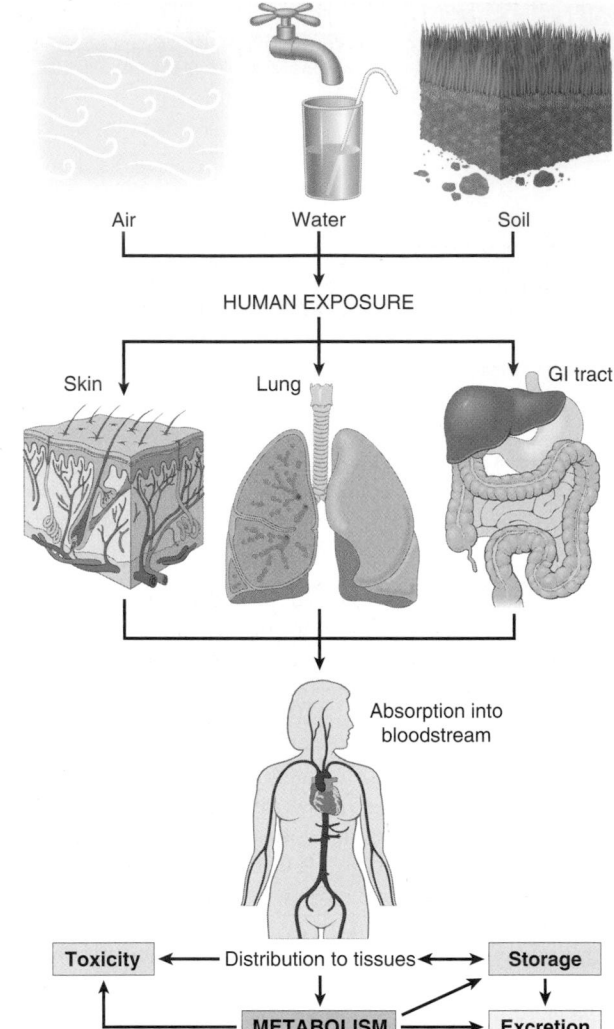

FIGURE 4-14 Human Exposure to Pollutants. Pollutants contained in air, water, and soil are absorbed through the lungs, gastrointestinal tract, and skin. In the body, the pollutants may act at the site of absorption but are generally transported through the bloodstream to various organs where they can be stored or metabolized. Metabolism of xenobiotics may result in the formation of water-soluble compounds that are excreted, or a toxic metabolite may be created by activation of the agent. (From Kumar V et al, editors: *Robbins and Cotran pathologic basis of disease,* ed 9, Philadelphia, 2015, Elsevier.)

classified and cataloged, are called toxicophores. The intermediates include electrophiles, nucleophiles, free radicals, and redox-active reactants. Electrophiles (electron lovers) are an atom or molecule attracted to electrons and accepts a pair of electrons to make a covalent bond. This process creates a partially or fully charged center in electrophilic molecules.[25] A nucleophile is an atom or molecule that donates an electron pair to an electrophile to make a chemical bond. All chemical species with a free pair of electrons can act as nucleophiles. Nucleophiles are strongly attracted to positively charged regions in other chemicals and can be oxidized to free radicals and electrophiles.[25] In general, the majority of all *reactive* chemical species are electrophilic because the formation of nucleophiles is rare[25] (for a discussion on free radicals, see p. 81). The generation of these excess reactive chemical species leads to molecular damage in liver cells (Figure 4-15). These reactive intermediates can interact with cellular macromolecules (such

FIGURE 4-15 Liver Toxicants: Chemical Injury.

The Percentage of Child Medication–Related Poisoning Deaths Is Increasing

Today, the leading cause of child poisoning is medications. Each year, more than 500,000 children, ages 5 and younger, experience a potential poisoning related to medications. More than 60,000 children are treated in emergency departments because of accidental medication exposure or overdose. Of every 150 2-year-old children, one is being sent to the emergency department for an unintentional medication overdose. Among children younger than age 5, 95% of emergency department visits are caused by unsupervised accidental ingestions and about 5% from dosing errors made by clinicians.

Importantly, investigators analyzed records from the American Association of Poison Control Centers' National Poison Data System (NPDS), an electronic database of all calls to the 61 poison control centers across the United States. Their analysis included all calls for children age 5 years or younger who were seen in a hospital emergency department between 2001 and 2008 for either unintentional self-exposure to a single drug (prescription or over-the-counter [OTC]) or unintentional therapeutic error for a single drug (prescription or OTC). The number of such calls during this 8-year period totaled 453,559. Medication-related poisoning deaths among children 5 years and younger now most frequently involve exposures to opioid analgesics and cardiovascular medications. About half of all poisoning-related deaths involve analgesics, antihistamines, and sedatives.

Development of new medications also has led to more of them being available in American homes. With aging, more adults are taking OTC and prescription medications as well as multiple medications. Oxycodone, morphine, and methadone prescriptions have increased between 159% and 559% between 2000 and 2009, depending on the drug; the number of prescribed cardiovascular drugs (e.g., metoprolol) has increased about fivefold. Additionally, more medications, such as those utilized for attention-deficit disorder and diabetes, are being prescribed to younger adults and children. Prescription pain killer overdose is a growing epidemic, especially among women.

How can we increase the safety of children exposed to so many medications? Safe storage is the *most* important solution and safe dosing from clinicians will reduce dosing errors. Additionally, improvements are continuing through improved packaging and labeling of medications as well as education of parents and consumers on dosing information.

Data from Bond GR et al: *J Pediatr* 160(2):265-270, 2011; Bronstein AC et al: *Clin Toxicol* 49:910-941, 2011; Budnitz DS, Lovegrove MC: *J Pediatr* 160(2):190-192, 2012; Bunitz DS, Salis S: *Pediatrics* 127(6):e1597-e1599, 2011; Centers for Disease Control and Prevention: Available at www.cdc/gov/features/medicationstorage/. Accessed February 9, 2010.

as proteins and DNA), can covalently bind to proteins and form **protein adducts** (chemical bound to protein) and DNA adducts, or can react directly with cell structures to cause cell damage.[26] Adduct formation can lead to adverse conditions including disruption in protein function, excess formation of fibrous connective tissue (fibrogenesis), and activation of immune responses.[25] The identity of proteins modified by xenobiotics can be found in the resource known as the reactive metabolite target protein database.[27] The body has two major defense systems for counteracting these effects: (1) detoxification enzymes and their cofactors and (2) antioxidant systems (see p. 82). Phases of detoxification include phase I enzymes, such as cytochrome P-450 (CYP) oxidases, which are the most important oxidative reactions. Other phase I detoxification enzymes include those for reduction and hydrolysis. In phase II detoxification, conjugation enzymes, such as glutathione (GSH), detoxify reactive electrophiles and produce polar metabolites that cannot diffuse across membranes. Most conjugation enzymes are located in the cytosol. Phase III detoxification is often called the efflux transporter system because enzymes remove the parent drugs, metabolites, and xenobiotics from cells. The liver has the highest supply of biotransformation enzymes of all organs and, therefore, has the key role in protection from chemical toxicity.[25] Figure 4-16 is a summary of chemically induced liver injury.

The consequence of self-propagating chain reactions of free radicals is lipid peroxidation (also see p. 82). Free radicals react mainly with polyunsaturated fatty acids in membranes and can initiate lipid peroxidation. The breakdown of membrane lipids results in altered function of the mitochondria, ER, plasma membranes, and Golgi apparatus, and therefore has a role in acute liver cell death (necrosis) and progression of liver injury (Figure 4-17).[25]

Chemical Agents Including Drugs

Numerous chemical agents cause cellular injury. Because chemical injury remains a constant problem in clinical settings, it is a major limitation to drug therapy. Over-the-counter and prescribed drugs can cause cellular injury, sometimes leading to death. The leading cause of child poisoning is medications (see *Health Alert:* The Percentage of Child Medication–Related Poisoning Deaths Is Increasing). The site of injury is frequently the liver, where many chemicals and drugs are metabolized (see Figure 4-17). Long-term exposure to air pollutants, insecticides, and herbicides can cause cellular injury (see *Health Alert:* Air Pollution Reported as Largest Single Environmental Health Risk).

Another way to classify mechanisms by which drug actions, chemicals, and toxins produce injury includes (1) direct damage, also called on-target toxicity; (2) exaggerated response at the target, including overdose; (3) biologic activation to toxic metabolites, including free radicals; (4) hypersensitivity and related immunologic reactions; and (5) rare toxicities.[28] These mechanisms are not mutually exclusive; thus several may be operating concurrently.

Direct damage is when chemicals and drugs injure cells by combining *directly* with critical molecular substances. For example, cyanide is highly toxic (e.g., poisonous) because it inhibits mitochondrial cytochrome oxidase and hence blocks electron transport. Many chemotherapeutic drugs, known as antineoplastic agents, induce cell damage by direct cytotoxic effects. Exaggerated pharmacologic responses at the target include tumors caused by industrial chemicals and the birth defects attributed to thalidomide.[28] Importantly, another example includes common drugs of abuse (Table 4-5). Drug abuse can involve

FIGURE 4-16 Chemical Liver Injury. Liver injury is a result of genetic, environmental, biologic, and dietary factors. Certain chemicals can form toxic or chemically reactive metabolites. The risk of liver injury also can increase with increasing doses of a toxicant. Xenobiotic enzyme induction can lead to altered metabolism of chemicals, and drugs can either inhibit or induce drug-metabolizing enzymes. These changes can lead to greater toxicity. The dose at the site of action is controlled by the Phase I to III xenobiotic metabolites and metabolizing enzymes are encoded by numerous different genes. Therefore, the metabolism and toxicity outcomes can vary greatly among individuals. Additionally, all aspects of xenobiotic metabolism are regulated by certain transcription factors (cellular mediators of gene regulation). Overall, the extent of cell damage depends on the balance between reactive chemical species and protective responses aimed at decreasing oxidative stress, repairing macromolecular damage, or preserving cell health by inducing apoptosis or cell death. Significant clinical outcomes of chemical-induced liver injury occur with necrosis and the immune response. Covalent binding of reactive metabolites to cellular proteins can produce new antigens (haptens) that initiate autoantibody production and cytotoxic T-cell responses. Necrosis, a form of cell death (see p. 102), can result from extensive damage to the plasma membrane with altered ion transport, changes of membrane potential, cell swelling, and eventual dissolution. Altogether the pathogenesis of chemically induced liver injury is determined by genetics, environmental factors, and other underlying pathologic conditions. Green arrows are pathways leading to cell recovery; red arrows indicate pathways to cell damage or death; black arrows are pathways leading to chemically induced liver injury. (Adapted from Gu X, Manautou JE: Molecular mechanisms underlying chemical liver injury, *Exp Rev Mol Med* 14:e4, 2013.)

Air Pollution Reported as Largest Single Environmental Health Risk

The World Health Organization (WHO) reports that about 7 million people died in 2012 as a result of air pollution exposure. Improved measurements and better technology have enabled scientists to make more detailed analyses of health risks. These findings confirm that air pollution is now the world's largest single environmental health risk and reducing air pollution could save millions of lives. New data show a stronger link between indoor and outdoor air pollution exposure and cardiovascular diseases, for example, strokes and ischemic heart disease, as well as the link between air pollution and cancer. These data are in addition to the role of air pollution and the development of respiratory diseases including infections and chronic obstructive pulmonary diseases. Using these 2012 data for low- and middle-income countries, Southeast Asia and Western Pacific regions had the largest air pollution burden. Included in the analysis is a breakdown of deaths for adults and children attributed to specific diseases:

Outdoor Air Pollution–Caused Deaths—Breakdown by Disease:

- 40% ischemic heart disease
- 40% stroke
- 11% chronic obstructive pulmonary disease (COPD)
- 6% lung cancer
- 3% acute lower respiratory tract infections in children

Indoor Air Pollution–Caused Deaths—Breakdown by Disease:

- 34% stroke
- 26% ischemic heart disease
- 22% COPD
- 12% acute lower respiratory tract infections in children
- 6% lung cancer

The WHO estimates that indoor air pollution was linked to 4.3 million deaths in 2012 from cooking over coal, wood, dung, and biomass stoves. Outdoor air pollution estimates were 3.7 million deaths in 2012 from urban and rural sources.

Data from World Health Organization (WHO): *7 million premature deaths annually linked to air pollution.* Available from www.who.int/mediacentre/news/releases/2014/air-pollution/en/#.

FIGURE 4-17 Chemical Injury of Liver Cells Induced by Carbon Tetrachloride (CCl₄) Poisoning. Light blue boxes are mechanisms unique to chemical injury, purple boxes involve hypoxic injury, and green boxes are clinical manifestations.

mind-altering substances beyond therapeutic or social norms (Table 4-6). Drug addiction and overdose are serious public health issues.

Most toxic chemicals are not biologically active in their parent (native) form but must be converted to reactive metabolites, which then act on target molecules. This conversion is usually performed by the cytochrome P-450 oxidase enzymes in the smooth ER of the liver and other organs. These toxic metabolites cause membrane damage and cell injury mostly from formation of *free radicals* and subsequent membrane damage from lipid peroxidation (see Figure 4-17). For example, acetaminophen (paracetamol) is converted to a toxic metabolite in the liver, causing cell injury (Figure 4-18). Acetaminophen is one of the most common causes of poisoning worldwide.[29] Many investigators are studying hepatoprotective strategies.[30]

Hypersensitivity reactions are a common drug toxicity and range from mild skin rashes to immune-mediated organ failure.[28] One type of hypersensitivity reaction is the delayed-onset reaction, which occurs after multiple doses of a drug are administered. Some protein drugs and large polypeptide drugs (e.g., insulin) can directly stimulate

antibody production (see Chapter 8). Most drugs, however, act as haptens and bind covalently to serum or cell-bound proteins. The binding makes the protein immunogenic, stimulating antidrug antibody production, T-cell responses against the drug, or both. For example, penicillin itself is not antigenic but its metabolic degradation products can become antigenic and cause an allergic reaction. Rare toxicities simply mean infrequent occurrences as described previously by the other four mechanisms. These toxicities reflect individual genetic predispositions that affect drug or chemical metabolism, disposition, and immune responses.

Carbon monoxide, carbon tetrachloride, and social drugs, such as alcohol, can significantly alter cellular function and injure cellular structures. Accidental or suicidal poisonings by chemical agents cause numerous deaths. The injurious effects of some agents—lead, carbon monoxide, ethyl alcohol, mercury—are common cellular injuries.

Lead. Lead (Pb) is a heavy toxic metal that persists in older homes, the environment, and the workplace. Lead may be found in hazardous concentrations in food, water, and air and it is one of the most common overexposures found in industry.[31] Despite efforts to reduce exposure through government regulation, exposure still persists for many people and toxicity is still a primary hazard for children[32] (see *Health Alert:*

TABLE 4-5 Common Drugs of Abuse

Class	Molecular Target	Example
Opioid narcotics	Mu opioid receptor (agonist)	Heroin, hydromorphone (Dilaudid) Oxycodone (Percodan, Percocet, OxyContin) Methadone (Dolophine) Meperidine (Demerol)
Sedative-hypnotics	GABA$_A$ receptor (agonist)	Barbiturates Ethanol Methaqualone (Quaalude) Glutethimide (Doriden) Ethchlorvynol (Placidyl)
Psychomotor stimulants	Dopamine transporter (antagonist) Serotonin receptors (toxicity)	Cocaine Amphetamines 3,4-Methylenedioxymethamphetamine (MDMA, ecstasy)
Phencyclidine-like drugs	NMDA glutamate receptor channel (antagonist)	Phencyclidine (PCP, angel dust) Ketamine
Cannabinoids	CB$_1$ cannabinoid receptors (agonist)	Marijuana Hashish
Hallucinogens	Serotonin 5-HT$_2$ receptors (agonist)	Lysergic acid diethylamide (LSD) Mescaline Psilocybin

From Kumar V et al: Cellular responses to stress and toxic insults: adaptation, injury, and death. In Kumar V et al, editors: *Robbins and Cotran pathologic basis of disease*, ed 9, St Louis, 2014, Saunders; Hyman SE: *JAMA* 286:2586, 2001.

CB$_1$, Cannabinoid receptor type 1; *GABA*, γ-aminobutyric acid; *5-HT$_2$*, 5-hydroxytryptamine; *NMDA*, N-methyl-D-aspartate.

TABLE 4-6 Social or Street Drugs and Their Effects

Type of Drug	Description and Effects
Marijuana (pot)	*Active substance:* Δ9-Tetrahydrocannabinol (THC), found in resin of *Cannabis sativa* plant With smoking (e.g., "joints"), about 5% to 10% is absorbed through lungs; with heavy use the following adverse effects have been reported: alterations of sensory perception; cognitive and psychomotor impairment (e.g., inability to judge time, speed, distance); it increases heart rate and blood pressure; increases susceptibility to laryngitis, pharyngitis, bronchitis; causes cough and hoarseness; may contribute to lung cancer (different dosages need study; contains large number of carcinogens); data from animal studies only indicate reproductive changes include reduced fertility, decreased sperm motility, and decreased levels of circulatory testosterone; fetal abnormalities include low birth weight; increased frequency of infectious illness is thought to be result of depressed cell-mediated and humoral immunity; beneficial effects include decreased nausea secondary to cancer chemotherapy and decreased pain in certain chronic conditions

Methamphetamine (meth)	An amine derivation of amphetamine (C$_{10}$H$_{15}$N) used as crystalline hydrochloride
	CNS stimulant; in large doses causes irritability, aggressive (violent) behavior, anxiety, excitement, auditory hallucinations, and paranoia (delusions and psychosis); mood changes are common and abuser can swiftly change from friendly to hostile; paranoiac swings can result in suspiciousness, hyperactive behavior, and dramatic mood swings
	Appeals to abusers because body's metabolism is increased and produces euphoria, alertness, and perception of increased energy
	Stages:
	    Low intensity: User is not psychologically addicted and uses methamphetamine by swallowing or snorting
	    Binge and high intensity: User has psychologic addiction and smokes or injects to achieve a faster, stronger high
	    Tweaking: Most dangerous stage; user is continually under the influence, not sleeping for 3-15 days, extremely irritated, and paranoid

Cocaine and crack	Extracted from leaves of cocoa plant and sold as a water-soluble powder (cocaine hydrochloride) liberally diluted with talcum powder or other white powders; extraction of pure alkaloid from cocaine hydrochloride is "free-base" called *crack* because it "cracks" when heated Crack is more potent than cocaine; cocaine is widely used as an anesthetic, usually in procedures involving oral cavity; it is a potent CNS stimulant, blocking reuptake of neurotransmitters norepinephrine, dopamine, and serotonin; also increases synthesis of norepinephrine and dopamine; dopamine induces sense of euphoria, and norepinephrine causes adrenergic potentiation, including hypertension, tachycardia, and vasoconstriction; cocaine can therefore cause severe coronary artery narrowing and ischemia; reason cocaine increases thrombus formation is unclear; other cardiovascular effects include dysrhythmias, sudden death, dilated cardiomyopathy, rupture of descending aorta (i.e., secondary to hypertension); effects on fetus include premature labor, retarded fetal development, stillbirth, hyperirritability
Heroin	Opiate closely related to morphine, methadone, and codeine Highly addictive, and withdrawal causes intense fear ("I'll die without it"); sold "cut" with similar-looking white powder; dissolved in water it is often highly contaminated; feeling of tranquility and sedation lasts only a few hours and thus encourages repeated intravenous or subcutaneous injections; acts on the receptors enkephalins, endorphins, and dynorphins, which are widely distributed throughout body with high affinity to CNS; effects can include infectious complications, especially *Staphylococcus aureus*, granulomas of lung, septic embolism, and pulmonary edema—in addition, viral infections from casual exchange of needles and HIV; sudden death is related to overdosage secondary to respiratory depression, decreased cardiac output, and severe pulmonary edema

Data from Kumar V et al, editors: *Robbins and Cotran pathologic basis of disease*, ed 9, Philadelphia, 2015, Elsevier; Nahas G et al: *N Engl J Med* 343(7):514, 2000.

CNS, Central nervous system; *HIV*, human immunodeficiency virus.

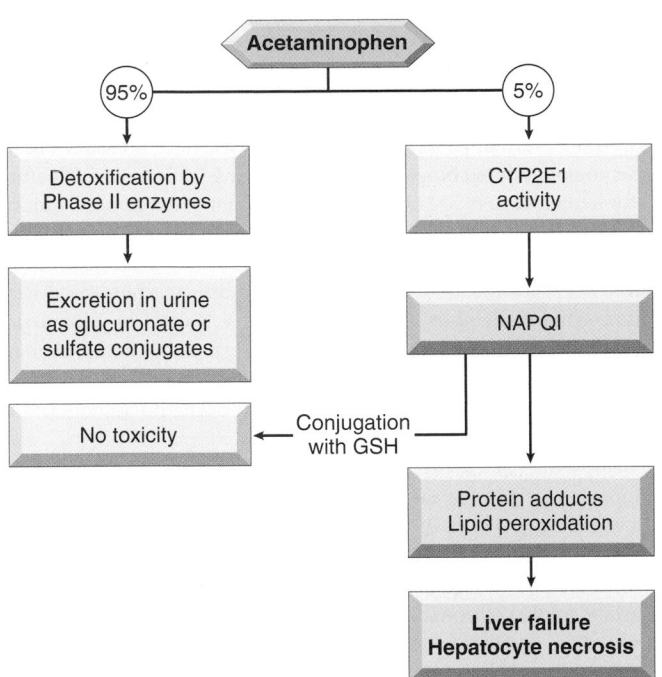

FIGURE 4-18 Acetaminophen Metabolism and Toxicity. *CYP2E1,* A cytochrome; *GSH,* glutathione; *NAPQI,* toxic byproduct.

TABLE 4-7	Common Sources of Lead Exposure
Exposure	**Source**
Environmental	Lead paint, soil, or dust near roadways or lead-painted homes; plastic window blinds; plumbing materials (from pipes or solder); pottery glazes and ceramic ware; lead-core candle wicks; leaded gasoline; water (pipes)
Occupational	Lead mining and refining, plumbing and pipe fitting, auto repair, glass manufacturing, battery manufacturing and recycling, printing shop, construction work, plastic manufacturing, gas station attendant, firing-range attendant
Hobbies	Glazed pottery making, target shooting at firing ranges, lead soldering, preparing fishing sinkers, stained-glass making, painting, car or boat repair
Other	Gasoline sniffing, costume jewelry, cosmetics, contaminated herbal products

Data from Sanborn MD et al: *CMAJ* 166(10):1287-1292, 2002.

HEALTH ALERT

Low-Level Lead Exposure Harms Children: A Renewed Call for Primary Prevention

An advisory committee of the CDC recently suggested that the current threshold for harmful lead exposure in children should be cut in half because even lower levels cause irreversible harm. The report noted that studies have found reduced intelligence quotients (IQs) and behavioral problems in children with exposure levels less than 10 mcg/dl and that such low levels have effects on cardiovascular, endocrine, and immunologic systems. Based on these data, the panel recommended reducing the threshold for harmful levels of lead in the blood to 5 mcg/dl. Despite progress in reducing blood lead levels (BLLs), racial and income disparities persist. An internal review process from both the Centers for Disease Control and Prevention and the U.S. Department of Health and Human Services will determine how to implement any accepted recommendations. This is a very important process because BLLs appear to be irreversible, underscoring the need for primary prevention.

Data from Advisory Committee for Childhood Lead Poisoning Prevention of the Centers for Disease Control and Prevention: *Low level lead exposure harms children: a renewed call for primary prevention,* 2012. Available at www.cdc.gov/nceh/lead/ACCLPP/FinalDocument030712.pdf. Accessed September 24, 2012.

Low-Level Lead Exposure Harms Children: A Renewed Call for Primary Prevention). Although Pb was removed from paint in Europe in 1922 and removed in the United States in 1978, many homes in the United States still contain leaded paint and chipped and peeling leaded paint constitutes a major source of current childhood exposure.[33-36] The chipped paint can disintegrate at friction surfaces to form Pb dust.[36] Another source of contamination is Pb dust dispersed along roadways from previous leaded gasoline emissions.[36] When Pb was removed from gasoline, blood lead levels (BLLs) dropped significantly.[37-39] Previous emissions of leaded fuel created large dispersions of lead dust in the environment. Particulate lead (2 to 10 μm) does not degrade and persists in the environment, making it a notable source of human exposure.[40] Other airborne sources include smelters and piston-engine airplanes.[41] Drinking water exposed to Pb occurs from outdated fixtures, plumbing without corrosion control, and solders.[36] Because well water is not subject to EPA regulation it may not be tested for Pb.[36] Although the average blood levels of Pb in children in the United States have dropped since the 1970s, there are at-risk populations with higher than average BLLs.[36] Children of lower social economic status or racial minority status are still at higher risk of Pb poisoning and some regions in the United States have an increased prevalence of higher BLLs in children.[36] Importantly, the CDC reports "no safe blood lead level in children has been identified."[42] Common sources of Pb are included in Table 4-7.

Children are more susceptible to the effects of Pb than adults for several reasons, including (1) children have increased hand-to-mouth behavior and exposure from the ingestion of Pb dust; (2) the blood-brain barrier in children is immature during fetal development, contributing to greater accumulation in the developing brain; and (3) infant absorption of Pb is greater than that in adults and bone turnover (in adults the body burden of lead is found in bone) in children from skeletal growth results in continuous leaching of Pb into blood, causing constant body exposure.[36,42] If nutrition is compromised, especially if dietary intake of iron and calcium is insufficient, children are more likely to have elevated BLLs.[36] Particularly worrisome is lead

exposure during pregnancy because the developing fetal nervous system is especially vulnerable; lead exposure can result in lower IQs, learning disorders, hyperactivity, and attention problems.[32]

The organ systems primarily affected by lead ingestion include the nervous system, the hematopoietic system (tissues that produce blood cells), and the kidneys of the urologic system. The neurologic effect of Pb in exposed children is the driving factor for reducing Pb levels in the environment.[36] Elevated BLLs not only are linked to cognitive deficits but also are associated with behavioral changes including antisocial behavior, acting out in school, and difficulty paying attention.[36] The cognitive and behavioral changes of Pb-exposed children persist after complete cessation of Pb exposure.[36] In 1991 the CDC lowered the definition of Pb intoxication to 10 μm/dl BLL because several studies reported that children with BLLs of at least 10 μm/dl had impaired intellectual functioning[36] (Figure 4-19). Studies in animals have led to the hypothesis that Pb targets the learning and memory processes by

μg/mL

150 ← Death

100 ← Encephalopathy
← Nephropathy
← Frank anemia

← Colic

50

40 ← Decreased hemoglobin synthesis

30

20 ← Decreased nerve conduction velocity
← Increased level of erythrocyte protoporphyrin
← Altered vitamin D metabolism
← Altered calcium homeostasis

10 ← Developmental toxicity
Decreased IQ level
Decreased hearing
Decreased growth
Impaired peripheral nerve function
Fetal effects by transplacental transfer

0

FIGURE 4-19 Lead Poisoning in Children Related to Blood Levels. (From Kumar V et al, editors: *Robbins and Cotran pathologic basis of disease,* ed 9, Philadelphia, 2015, Elsevier.)

inhibiting the *N*-methyl-D-aspartate receptor (NMDAR), which is necessary for hippocampus-mediated learning and memory.[36,43] Similar changes also have been found in cultured neuron systems.[36] Inhibition of either voltage-gated calcium channels or NMDARs by Pb results in reduction of Ca^{++} entry into the cell, thereby disrupting the necessary Ca^{++} signaling for neurotransmission.[44,45] Lead induces cellular damage by increasing oxidative stress.[46] Lead toxicity involves the direct formation of ROS (singlet oxygen, hydrogen peroxides, hydroperoxides) and depletion of antioxidants.[46] Pb exposure leads to lowered levels of glutathione; and because glutathione is important for the metabolism of specific drugs and other toxins, low Pb levels can increase their toxicity, as well as the levels of other metals.[46] From animal studies and human population studies, low-level lead exposure may cause hypertension.[47] Lead interferes with the normal remodeling of cartilage and bone in children. From radiologic studies of bone, "lead lines" are detectable and lead also can be found in the gums as a result of hyperpigmentation. Lead inhibits several enzymes involved in hemoglobin synthesis and causes anemia (most obvious is a microcytic hypochromic anemia). Renal lesions can cause tubular dysfunction resulting in glycosuria (glucose in the urine), aminoaciduria (amino acids in the urine), and hyperphosphaturia (excess phosphate in the urine). Gastrointestinal symptoms are less severe and include nausea, loss of appetite, weight loss, and abdominal cramping.

Carbon monoxide. Gaseous substances can be classified according to their ability to asphyxiate (interrupt respiration) or irritate. Toxic asphyxiants, such as carbon monoxide, hydrogen cyanide, and hydrogen sulfide, directly interfere with cellular respiration.

Carbon monoxide (CO) is an odorless, colorless, nonirritating, and undetectable gas unless it is mixed with a visible or odorous pollutant.

CO is produced by the incomplete combustion of fuels such as gasoline. Although CO is a chemical agent, the ultimate injury it produces is a hypoxic injury—namely, oxygen deprivation. As a systemic asphyxiant, CO causes death by inducing central nervous system (CNS) depression. Normally, oxygen molecules are carried to tissues bound to hemoglobin in red blood cells (see Chapter 27). Because CO's affinity for hemoglobin is 300 times greater than that of oxygen, CO quickly binds with the hemoglobin, preventing the oxygen molecules' ability to bind to the hemoglobin. Minute amounts of CO can produce a significant percentage of carboxyhemoglobin (carbon monoxide bound with hemoglobin). With increasing levels of carboxyhemoglobin, hypoxia occurs insidiously, evoking widespread ischemic changes in the CNS, and individuals are often unaware of their plight. The diagnosis is made from measurement of carboxyhemoglobin levels in the blood.

Symptoms related to CO poisoning include headache, giddiness, tinnitus (ringing in the ears), chest pain, confusion, nausea, weakness, and vomiting. CO is an *air pollutant* found in combustion fumes produced by cars and trucks, small gasoline engines, stoves, gas ranges, gas refrigerators, heating systems, lanterns, burning charcoal or wood, and cigarette smoke. Chronic exposure can occur in people working in confined spaces, such as underground garages and tunnels. Fumes can accumulate in enclosed or semi-enclosed spaces, and poisoning from breathing CO can occur in humans and animals. High levels of CO can cause loss of consciousness and death. Death can occur in individuals sleeping or intoxicated before experiencing any symptoms. Although all people and animals are at risk, those most susceptible to poisoning include unborn babies, infants, and people with chronic heart disease, respiratory problems, and anemia. For information on preventing CO poisoning from home appliances and proper venting, see the Centers for Disease Control and Prevention (CDC) website at www.cdc.gov/co/faqs.htm.

Ethanol. Alcohol (ethanol) is the primary choice among mood-altering drugs available in the United States. It is estimated there are more than 10 million chronic alcoholics in the United States. Alcohol contributes to more than 100,000 deaths annually with 50% of these deaths from drunk driving accidents, alcohol-related homicides, and suicides.[48] A blood concentration of 80 mg/dl is the legal definition for drunk driving in the United States. This level of alcohol in an average person may be reached after consumption of three drinks (three 12-ounce bottles of beer, 15 ounces of wine, and 4 to 5 ounces of distilled liquor). The effects of alcohol vary by age, gender, and percent body fat; the rate of metabolism affects the blood alcohol level. Because alcohol is not only a psychoactive drug but also a food, it is considered part of the basic food supply in many societies.

A large intake of alcohol has enormous effects on nutritional status. Liver and nutritional disorders are the most serious consequences of alcohol abuse. Major nutritional deficiencies include magnesium, vitamin B_6, thiamine, and phosphorus. Folic acid deficiency is a common problem in chronic alcoholic populations. Ethanol alters folic acid (folate) homeostasis by decreasing intestinal absorption of folate, increasing liver retention of folate, and increasing the loss of folate through urinary and fecal excretion.[49] Folic acid deficiency becomes especially serious in pregnant women who consume alcohol and may contribute to fetal alcohol syndrome (see p. 92).

Most of the alcohol in blood is metabolized to *acetaldehyde* in the liver by three enzyme systems: alcohol dehydrogenase (ADH), the microsomal ethanol-oxidizing system (MEOS; CYP2E1), and catalase (Figure 4-20). The major pathway involves ADH, an enzyme located in the cytosol of hepatocytes. The microsomal ethanol oxidizing system (MEOS) depends on cytochrome P-450 (CYP2E1), an enzyme needed for cellular oxidation. Activation of CYP2E1 requires a high ethanol

FIGURE 4-20 Ethanol Metabolism Pathway. Ethanol is metabolized into acetaldehyde through the cytosolic enzyme alcohol dehydrogenase *(ADH)*, the microsomal enzyme cytochrome P-450 2E1 *(CYP2E1)*, and the peroxisomal enzyme catalase. The ADH enzyme reaction is the main ethanol metabolic pathway involving an intermediate carrier of electrons, namely, nicotinamide adenine dinucleotide *(NAD+)*, which is reduced by two electrons to form NADH. Acetaldehyde is metabolized mainly by aldehyde dehydrogenase 2 *(ALDH2)* in the mitochondria to acetate and NADH before being cleared into the systemic circulation. (Adapted from Zhang Y, Ren J: *Pharmacol Ther* 132[1]:86-92, 2011.)

concentration and thus is thought to be important in the accelerated ethanol metabolism (i.e., tolerance) noted in persons with chronic alcoholism. Acetaldehyde has many toxic tissue effects and is responsible for some of the acute effects of alcohol and for development of head and neck cancer (HNC).[48] A recent and first study showed that head and neck cancer risk may be influenced by alcohol-metabolizing genes (*ADH1B* and *ALDH2*) and oral hygiene.[50]

The major effects of acute alcoholism involve the central nervous system (CNS). After alcohol is ingested, it is absorbed, unaltered, in the stomach and small intestine. Fatty foods and milk slow absorption. Alcohol then is distributed to all tissues and fluids of the body in direct proportion to the blood concentration. Individuals differ in their capability to metabolize alcohol. Genetic differences in the metabolism of liver alcohol, including levels of aldehyde dehydrogenases, have been identified.[51] These genetic polymorphisms may account for ethnic and gender differences in ethanol metabolism. Persons with chronic alcoholism develop tolerance because of production of enzymes, leading to an increased rate of metabolism (e.g., P-450).

Numerous studies have validated the so-called *J-* or *U-shaped* inverse association between alcohol and overall or cardiovascular mortality, such as from myocardial infarction and ischemic stroke. These studies have found that light to moderate (nonbinge) drinkers tend to have lower mortality than nondrinkers and heavy drinkers have higher mortality.[52] For both men and women, former drinkers and regular heavy drinkers had higher mortality.[52] Light to moderate drinkers in the United States may have reduced mortality but this may be confounded by medical care and social relationships, especially among women.[52,53] These relationships need further study. The suggested mechanisms for cardioprotection for light to moderate drinkers include increase in levels of high-density lipoprotein–cholesterol (HDL-C), decrease in levels of low-density lipoprotein (LDL), prevention of clot formation, reduction in platelet aggregation, decrease

in blood pressure, increase in coronary vessel vasodilation, increase in coronary blood flow, decrease in coronary inflammation, decrease in atherosclerosis, limited ischemia-reperfusion injury (I/R injury), and a decrease in diabetic vessel pathology.[54] The American Heart Association recommends no more than two drinks per day for men and one drink per day for women (one 12-oz beer, 4 oz of wine, 1.5 oz of 80-proof spirits, or 1 oz of 100-proof spirits). Drinking more alcohol can increase the risks of alcoholism, high blood pressure, obesity, stroke, breast cancer, suicide, and accidents.[55] Individuals who do not consume alcohol should not be encouraged to start drinking.[56]

Acute alcoholism (drunkenness) affects the CNS (see *Health Alert:* Alcohol: Global Burden, Adolescent Onset, Chronic or Binge Drinking). Alcohol intoxication causes CNS depression. Depending on the amount consumed, CNS depression is associated with sedation, drowsiness, loss of motor coordination, delirium, altered behavior, and loss of consciousness. Toxic amounts (300 to 400 mg/dl) result in a lethal coma or respiratory arrest because of medullary center depression. Investigators studied the effects of snoring and multiple variables including alcohol. They found that a low level of self-reported physical activity is a risk factor for future habitual snoring complaints in women independent of alcohol dependence, smoking, current weight, and weight gain. Furthermore, increased physical activity can modify the risk.[57] Acute alcoholism may induce reversible hepatic and gastric changes.[48] Acute alcoholism contributes significantly to motor vehicle fatalities.

Chronic alcoholism causes structural alterations in practically all organs and tissues in the body because most tissues contain enzymes capable of ethanol oxidation or nonoxidative metabolism. The most significant activity, however, occurs in the liver. Alcohol is the leading cause of liver-related morbidity and mortality.[58] In general, hepatic changes, initiated by acetaldehyde, include inflammation, deposition of fat, enlargement of the liver, interruption of microtubular transport

Alcohol: Global Burden, Adolescent Onset, Chronic or Binge Drinking

Alcohol is widely consumed worldwide, and in the United States 50% of the adult population (18 years and older) consumes alcohol regularly. Alcohol continues to be the drug of choice among teens and young adults with one third of twelfth graders and 40% of college students reporting "binge drinking" (four standard alcohol drinks on one occasion in females and five in males). Alcohol abuse is the leading cause of liver-related morbidity and mortality. Chronic and binge drinking causes alcoholic liver disease (ALD) with a spectrum from hepatic steatosis (fatty change) to steatohepatitis (fatty change and inflammation) and cirrhosis (see Chapter 36). These alterations can eventually lead to hepatocellular carcinoma. The pathogenesis of ALD is not fully characterized and recent studies reveal a major role of mitochondria. Animal studies have shown that alcohol causes mitochondrial DNA damage, lipid accumulation, and oxidative stress. Understanding the role of the mitochondria may help identify therapeutic targets.

Investigations of adolescent drinking behaviors, especially binge drinking, is providing evidence of neurocognitive changes, including changes in both gray and white matter. These studies are examining risk-taking behaviors that begin in adolescence and coincide with vulnerable and significant neurodevelopmental changes.

Data from Adams PF et al: *Vital Health Stat* 10(255), 2012; available from www.cdc.gov/nchs/data/series/sr_10/sr10_255.pdf; Hicks BM et al: *Addiction* 107:540-548, 2012; Johnston LD et al: *Monitoring the future national results on adolescent drug use: overview of key findings*, Bethesda, Md, 2009, National Institute on Drug Abuse; Lisdahl KM et al: *Front Psychiatry* 4:53, 2013; Mathews S et al: *Am J Physiol Gastrointest Liver Physiol* 2014 Apr 3 [Epub ahead of print]; Nassir F, Ibdah JA: *World J Gastroenterol* 20(9):2136-2142, 2014; White HR et al: *Alcohol Clin Exp Res* 35:295-303, 2010.

FIGURE 4-21 Alcoholic Hepatitis. Chicken-wire fibrosis extending between hepatocytes (Mallory trichrome stain). (From Damjanov I, Linder J, editors: *Anderson's pathology*, ed 10, St Louis, 1996, Mosby.)

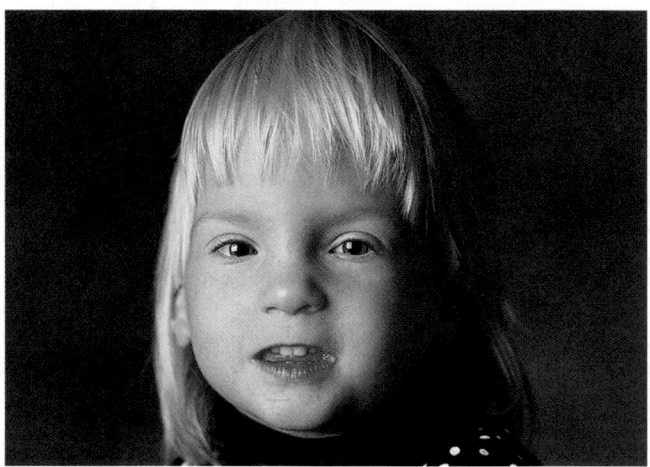

FIGURE 4-22 Fetal Alcohol Syndrome. When alcohol enters the fetal blood, the potential result can cause tragic congenital abnormalities, such as microcephaly ("small head"), low birth weight, and cardiovascular defects, as well as developmental disabilities, such as physical and intellectual disability, and even death. Note the small head, thinned upper lip, small eye openings (palpebral fissures), epicanthal folds, and receded upper jaw (retrognathia) typical of fetal alcohol syndrome. (From Fortinash KM, Holoday Worret PA: *Psychiatric mental health nursing*, ed 5, St Louis, 2012, Mosby.)

of proteins and their secretion, increase in intracellular water, depression of fatty acid oxidation in the mitochondria, increase in membrane rigidity, and acute liver cell necrosis (see Chapter 36). Specifically, chronic or binge alcohol consumption causes alcoholic liver disease (ALD) with a spectrum ranging from simple fatty liver (steatosis), to steatohepatitis (fatty with inflammation), to cirrhosis (Figure 4-21) (see Chapter 36). Cirrhosis is associated with portal hypertension and an increased risk for hepatocellular carcinoma. Cellular damage is increased by reactive oxygen species (ROS) and oxidative stress (see p. 81). Activation of proinflammatory cytokines from neutrophils and lymphocytes mediates liver damage.[59] Oxidative stress is associated with cell membrane phospholipid depletion, which alters the fluidity and function of cell membranes as well as intercellular transport. Chronic alcoholism is related to several disorders, including injury to the myocardium (alcoholic cardiomyopathy); increased tendency to hypertension, acute gastritis, and acute and chronic pancreatitis; and regressive changes in skeletal muscle. Chronic alcohol consumption is associated with an increased incidence of cancer of the oral cavity, liver, esophagus, and breast (see *Health Alert:* Alcohol: Global Burden, Adolescent Onset, Chronic or Binge Drinking).

Ethanol is implicated in the onset of a variety of immune defects, including effects on the production of cytokines involved in inflammatory responses. Alcohol can induce epigenetic variations in the developmental pathways of many types of immune cells (e.g., granulocytes, macrophages, and T-lymphocytes) that promote increased inflammation.[60] Alcohol increases the development of serious medical conditions related to immune system dysfunction, including acute respiratory distress syndrome (ARDS) as well as liver cancer and

alcoholic liver disease (ALD).[60] Binge and chronic drinking increases susceptibility to many infectious microorganisms and can enhance the progression of human immunodeficiency virus (HIV) by affecting innate and adaptive immunity.[60]

The deleterious effects of prenatal alcohol exposure can cause mental deficiency and neurobehavioral disorders, as well as fetal alcohol syndrome. Fetal alcohol syndrome includes growth retardation, facial anomalies, cognitive impairment, and ocular malformations (Figure 4-22). It is among the common causes of mental deficiency.[61] Evidence of epigenetic alterations has led to the hypothesis that alcohol effects on fetal development may be caused not only by maternal alcohol consumption but also by the father's exposure as well.[61] Epigenetic alterations may be carried through the male germline for generations.[62] Alcohol crosses the placenta, reaching the fetus, and blood levels of the fetus may reach equivalent levels to maternal levels in 1 to 2 hours.[63] Research has demonstrated an unimpeded bidirectional movement of alcohol between the fetus and the mother. The fetus may completely depend on maternal hepatic detoxification because the activity of alcohol dehydrogenase (ADH) in fetal liver is less than 10% of that in the adult liver.[63] Additionally, the amniotic fluid acts as a reservoir for alcohol, prolonging fetal exposure.[63] The specific mechanisms of injury are unknown; however, acetaldehyde can alter fetal development by disrupting differentiation and growth; DNA and protein synthesis; modification of carbohydrates, proteins, and fats; flow of nutrients across the placenta; and neuro-circuitry dysfunction that may be long-lasting.[61,63]

Mercury. Mercury is a global threat to human and environmental health. A recent report presents an overview of the *Global Mercury Assessment 2013.*[64] This report provides the most recent information on worldwide atmospheric mercury emissions, releases to the aquatic environment, and the fate of mercury in the global environment. Causes from human activity, called anthropogenic, are responsible for about 30% of annual emissions of mercury to air, another 10% arise from natural geologic sources, and the remainder (60%) occurs from re-emissions or earlier released mercury that has increased over decades and centuries in surface soil and water.[64] The major sources of anthropogenic mercury emissions to air are artisanal and small-scale gold mining (ASGM) and coal burning. The next major sources are the production of ferrous and nonferrous metals, and cement production. Importantly, investigators report that emissions from industrial sectors have increased since 2005.[64] Types of aquatic releases of mercury include industrial sites (power plants, factories), old mines, landfills, and waste disposal locations. Artisanal and small-scale gold mining are significant producers of aquatic mercury release. It is estimated that more than 90% of mercury in marine animals is from anthropogenic emissions.[64] Large amounts of inorganic mercury have accumulated in surface soils and in the oceans. Climate change, with thawing of enormous areas of frozen lands, may release even more long-stored mercury and organic matter into lakes, rivers, and oceans.[64]

Dental amalgams, or "silver fillings," are made of two almost equal parts of liquid mercury and a powder containing silver, tin, copper, zinc, and other metals.[41] When amalgams are placed or removed they can release a small amount of mercury vapor. Chewing can release a small amount of vapor and people absorb the vapor by inhalation or ingestion.[41] Researchers are studying the effects of exposure to magnetic fields, such as from mobile phone use, and the release of mercury from amalgams.[65] Susceptibility to mercury toxicity varies in a dose-dependent fashion, and among individuals based on multiple genes, not all have been identified.[66,67] Worldwide efforts are under way to phase down or eliminate the use of mercury dental amalgam.[67] Thimerosal, a mercury-containing preservative, was removed from all vaccines in 2001, with the exception of inactivated influenza vaccines.[68]

✔ QUICK CHECK 4-2
1. Why are children more susceptible to the toxic effects of lead exposure?
2. Discuss the sources of lead exposure?
3. Discuss the mechanisms of cell injury related to chronic alcoholism?
4. What are the sources of mercury exposure?

Unintentional and Intentional Injuries

Unintentional and intentional injuries are an important health problem in the United States. In 2012 there were 192,945 deaths, an injury death rate of 60.2/100,000.[69] The number of deaths because of poisoning was 48,545 with 15.4 deaths per 100,000. Motor vehicle traffic deaths were 33,804 with a rate of 10.7 deaths per 100,000. Deaths from all firearms were 33,636 with a rate of 10.6 deaths per 100,000. From data reporting in 2010, drug poisoning deaths were 12.4 per 100,000.[69] Death from injury is significantly more common for men than for women; the overall rate for men is 83.46/100,000 versus 39.28/100,000 for women. Significant racial differences are noted in the death rate, with whites at 64.85/100,000, blacks at 56.20/100,000, and other racial groups at a combined rate of 28.96/100,000. There also is a bimodal age distribution for injury-related deaths, with peaks in the young adult and elderly groups. Unintentional injury is the leading cause of death for people between the ages of 1 and 34 years; intentional injury (suicide, homicide) ranks between the second and fourth leading cause of death in this age group. The 1999 report published by the Institute of Medicine (IOM) indicated that between 44,000 and 98,000 unnecessary deaths per year occurred in hospitals alone as a result of errors by healthcare professionals (see *Health Alert:* Unintentional Injury Errors in Health Care and Patient Safety). Statistics on nonfatal injuries are harder to document accurately, but they are known to be a significant cause of morbidity and disability and to cost society billions of dollars annually. The more common terms used to describe and classify unintentional and intentional injuries and brief descriptions of important features of these injuries are discussed in Table 4-8.

HEALTH ALERT

Unintentional Injury Errors in Health Care and Patient Safety

According to a US Senate subcommittee hearing (July 17, 2014), despite more than a decade of national efforts to improve patient safety, hospitals and ambulatory care centers remain problematic for patients. This assessment follows the 15-year anniversary of the release of the IOM report on patient safety. Testimony from the senate hearings challenged the IOM report that patient harms were likely underestimated. A more recent estimate suggests the number of U.S. deaths as a result of medical error may be greater than 400,000 per year with more than 1000 each day.

Progress has been made in certain areas including the reduction of bloodstream infections from central lines. Success with this program has been expanded nationwide. Checklists are a very useful tool for improving patient safety. They have become more widely implemented and their success depends on appropriately targeting the intervention and utilizing a careful implementation strategy. Besides checklists, other examples of patient safety primers include adverse events after hospital discharge, computerized provider order entry, detection of safety hazards, diagnostic errors, disruptive and unprofessional behavior, error disclosure, handoffs and signouts, health care–associated infections, nursing and patient safety, and medication errors. In a testimony at the hearings it was stated "that one of the biggest barriers to improved patient safety is the lack of a robust national system for tracking patient safety data." Additionally, speakers testified that better systems of care are needed in understanding that a complex set of factors—complexity of hospital systems, time pressures, growing use of technology, financial incentives that reward hospitals by paying them to care for patients' complications, CEO compensation not tied to quality of care—all contribute to poor patient outcomes. The entrenched challenges of the U.S. health care system demand a transformed approach. Left unchanged, health care will continue to underperform; cause unnecessary harm; and strain national, state, and family budgets. The actions required to reverse this trend will be notable, substantial, sometimes disruptive—and absolutely necessary." (IOM Best Care at Lower Cost, The Path to Continuously Learning Health Care in America Institute of Medicine Report Brief Washington DC, 2012)

Data from Agency for Healthcare Research and Quality: *Patient safety primers*, Rockville, MD, 2014, U.S. Department of Health and Human Services; James JT: *J Patient Saf* 9(3):122-128, 2013; Kohn LT et al, editors: *To err is human: building a safer health system*, Washington DC, 1999, National Academy Press; Kuehn BM: *J Am Med Assoc* 312(9):879-880, 2014.

Asphyxial Injuries

Asphyxial injuries are caused by a failure of cells to receive or use oxygen. Deprivation of oxygen may be partial *(hypoxia)* or total *(anoxia)*. Asphyxial injuries can be grouped into four general categories: suffocation, strangulation, chemical asphyxiants, and drowning.

Suffocation. Suffocation, or oxygen failing to reach the blood, can result from a lack of oxygen in the environment (entrapment in an enclosed space or filling of the environment with a suffocating gas) or blockage of the external airways. Classic examples of these types of asphyxial injuries are a child who is trapped in an abandoned refrigerator or a person who commits suicide by putting a plastic bag over his or her head. A reduction in the ambient oxygen level to 16% (normal is 21%) is immediately dangerous. If the level is below 5%, death can ensue within a matter of minutes. The diagnosis of these types of asphyxial injuries depends on obtaining an accurate and thorough history because there will be no specific physical findings.

Diagnosis and treatment in choking asphyxiation (obstruction of the internal airways) depend on locating and removing the obstructing material. Injury or disease also may cause swelling of the soft tissues of the airway, leading to partial or complete obstruction and subsequent asphyxiation. Suffocation also may result from compression of the chest or abdomen (mechanical or compressional asphyxia),

---

TABLE 4-8 Unintentional and Intentional Injuries

Type of Injury	Description
BLUNT-FORCE INJURIES 	Mechanical injury to body resulting in tearing, shearing, or crushing; most common type of injury seen in healthcare settings; caused by blows or impacts; motor vehicle accidents and falls most common cause (see photo, A) *Contusion (bruise):* Bleeding into skin or underlying tissues; initial color will be red-purple, then blue-black, then yellow-brown or green (see Figure 4-26); duration of bruise depends on extent, location, and degree of vascularization; bruising of soft tissue may be confined to deeper structures; *hematoma* is collection of blood in soft tissue; *subdural hematoma* is blood between inner surface of dura mater and surface of brain; can result from blows, falls, or sudden acceleration/deceleration of head as occurs in *shaken baby syndrome;* *epidural hematoma* is collection of blood between inner surface of skull and dura; is most often associated with a skull fracture *Laceration:* Tear or rip resulting when tensile strength of skin or tissue is exceeded; is ragged and irregular with abraded edges; an extreme example is *avulsion,* where a wide area of tissue is pulled away; lacerations of internal organs are common in blunt-force injuries; lacerations of liver, spleen, kidneys, and bowel occur from blows to abdomen; thoracic aorta may be lacerated in sudden deceleration accidents; severe blows or impacts to chest may rupture heart with lacerations of atria or ventricles *Fracture:* Blunt-force blows or impacts can cause bone to break or shatter (see Chapter 39)
SHARP-FORCE INJURIES 	Cutting and piercing injuries accounted for 2734 deaths in 2007; men have a higher rate (1.37/100,000) than women (0.44/100,000); differences by race are whites 0.71/100,000, blacks 2.12/100,000, and other groups 0.80/100,000 *Incised wound:* A wound that is *longer* than it is *deep;* wound can be straight or jagged with sharp, distinct edges without abrasion; usually produces significant external bleeding with little internal hemorrhage; these wounds are noted in sharp-force injury suicides; in addition to a deep, lethal cut, there will be superficial incisions in same area called *hesitation marks* (see photo, B) *Stab wound:* A penetrating sharp-force injury that is *deeper* than it is *long;* if a sharp instrument is used, depths of wound are clean and distinct but can be abraded if object is inserted deeply and wider portion (e.g., hilt of a knife) impacts skin; depending on size and location of wound, external bleeding may be surprisingly small; after an initial spurt of blood, even if a major vessel or heart is struck, wound may be almost completely closed by tissue pressure, thus allowing only a trickle of visible blood despite copious internal bleeding *Puncture wound:* Instruments or objects with sharp points but without sharp edges produce puncture wounds; classic example is wound of foot after stepping on a nail; wounds are prone to infection, have abrasion of edges, and can be very deep *Chopping wound:* Heavy, edged instruments (axes, hatchets, propeller blades) produce wounds with a combination of sharp- and blunt-force characteristics

TABLE 4-8 Unintentional and Intentional Injuries—cont'd

Type of Injury	Description
GUNSHOT WOUNDS 	Accounted for more than 33,636 deaths in the United States in 2015; men more likely to die than women (18.16 vs. 2.73/100,000); black men between ages of 15 and 24 have greatest death rate (86.95/100,000); gunshot wounds are either penetrating (bullet remains in body) or perforating (bullet exits body); bullet also can fragment; most important factors or appearances are whether it is an entrance or exit wound and range of fire *Entrance wound:* All wounds share some common features; overall appearance is most affected by range of fire *Contact range entrance wound:* Distinctive type of wound when gun is held so muzzle rests on or presses into skin surface; there is searing of edges of wound from flame and soot or smoke on edges of wound in addition to hole; hard contact wounds of head cause severe tearing and disruption of tissue (because of thin layer of skin and muscle overlying bone); wound is gaping and jagged, known as *blow back;* can produce a patterned abrasion that mirrors weapon used (see photo, C) *Intermediate (distance) range entrance wound:* Surrounded by gunpowder tattooing or stippling; *tattooing* results from fragments of burning or unburned pieces of gunpowder exiting barrel and forcefully striking skin; *stippling* results when gunpowder abrades but does not penetrate skin (see photo, D) *Indeterminate range entrance wound:* Occurs when flame, soot, or gunpowder does not reach skin surface but bullet does; *indeterminate* is used rather than *distant* because appearance may be same regardless of distance; for example, if an individual is shot at close range through multiple layers of clothing the wound may look the same as if the shooting occurred at a distance *Exit wound:* Has the same appearance regardless of range of fire; most important factors are speed of projectile and degree of deformation; size cannot be used to determine if hole is an exit or entrance wound; usually has clean edges that can often be reapproximated to cover defect; skin is one of toughest structures for a bullet to penetrate; thus it is not uncommon for a bullet to pass entirely through body but stopped just beneath skin on "exit" side *Wounding potential of bullets:* Most damage done by a bullet is a result of amount of energy transferred to tissue impacted; speed of bullet has much greater effect than increased size; some bullets are designed to expand or fragment when striking an object, for example, *hollow-point* ammunition; lethality of a wound depends on what structures are damaged; wounds of brain may not be lethal; however, they are usually immediately incapacitating and lead to significant long-term disability; a person with a "lethal" injury (wound of heart or aorta) also may not be immediately incapacitated

preventing normal respiratory movements. Usual signs and symptoms include florid facial congestion and petechiae (pinpoint hemorrhages) of the eyes and face.

Strangulation. Strangulation is caused by compression and closure of the blood vessels and air passages resulting from external pressure on the neck. This causes cerebral hypoxia or anoxia secondary to the alteration or cessation of blood flow to and from the brain. It is important to remember that the amount of force needed to close the jugular veins (2 kg [4.5 lb]) or carotid arteries (5 kg [11 lb]) is significantly less than that required to crush the trachea (15 kg [33 lb]). It is the alteration of cerebral blood flow in most types of strangulation that causes injury or death—not the lack of airflow. With complete blockage of the carotid arteries, unconsciousness can occur within 10 to 15 seconds.

A noose is placed around the neck, and the weight of the body is used to cause constriction of the noose and compression of the neck in **hanging strangulations**. The body does not need to be completely suspended to produce severe injury or death. Depending on the type of ligature used, there usually is a distinct mark on the neck—an inverted V with the base of the V pointing toward the point of suspension. Internal injuries of the neck are actually quite rare in hangings, and only in judicial hangings, in which the body is weighted and dropped, is significant soft tissue or cervical spinal trauma seen. Petechiae of the eyes or face may be seen, but they are rare.

In ligature strangulation, the mark on the neck is horizontal without the inverted V pattern seen in hangings. Petechiae may be more common because intermittent opening and closure of the blood vessels may occur as a result of the victim's struggles. Internal injuries of the neck are rare.

Variable amounts of external trauma on the neck are found with contusions and abrasions in manual strangulation caused either by the assailant or by the victim clawing at his or her own neck in an attempt to remove the assailant's hands. Internal damage can be quite severe, with bruising of deep structures and even fractures of the hyoid bone and tracheal and cricoid cartilages. Petechiae are common.

Chemical asphyxiants. Chemical asphyxiants either prevent the delivery of oxygen to the tissues or block its utilization. Carbon monoxide is the most common chemical asphyxiant (see p. 90). Cyanide acts as an asphyxiant by combining with the ferric iron atom in cytochrome oxidase, thereby blocking the intracellular use of oxygen. A victim of cyanide poisoning will have the same cherry-red appearance as a carbon monoxide intoxication victim because cyanide blocks the use of circulating oxyhemoglobin. An odor of bitter almonds also may be detected. (The ability to smell cyanide is a genetic trait that is absent in a significant portion of the general population.) Hydrogen sulfide (sewer gas) is a chemical asphyxiant in which victims of hydrogen cyanide poisoning may have brown-tinged blood in addition to the nonspecific signs of asphyxiation.

Drowning. Drowning is an alteration of oxygen delivery to tissues resulting from the inhalation of fluid, usually water. In 2012 there were 3391 drowning deaths in the United States. Although research in the 1940s and 1950s indicated that changes in blood electrolyte levels and volume as a result of absorption of fluid from the lungs may be an important factor in some drownings, the major mechanism of injury is hypoxemia (low blood oxygen levels). Even in freshwater drownings, where large amounts of water can pass through the alveolar-capillary interface, there is no evidence that increases in blood volume cause significant electrolyte disturbances or hemolysis, or that the amount of fluid loading is beyond the compensatory capabilities of the kidneys and heart. Airway obstruction is the more important pathologic abnormality, underscored by the fact that in as many as 15% of drownings little or no water enters the lungs because of vagal nerve–mediated laryngospasms. This phenomenon is called dry-lung drowning.

No matter what mechanism is involved, cerebral hypoxia leads to unconsciousness in a matter of minutes. Whether this progresses to death depends on a number of factors, including the age and the health of the individual. One of the most important factors is the temperature of the water. Irreversible injury develops much more rapidly in warm water than it does in cold water. Submersion times of up to 1 hour with subsequent survival have been reported in children who were submerged in very cold water. Complete submersion is not necessary for a person to drown. An incapacitated or helpless individual (epileptic, alcoholic, infant) may drown in water that is only a few inches deep.

It is important to remember that no specific or diagnostic findings *prove* that a person recovered from the water is actually a drowning victim. In cases where water has entered the lung, there may be large amounts of foam exiting the nose and mouth, although this also can be seen in certain types of drug overdoses. A body recovered from water with signs of prolonged immersion could just as easily be a victim of some other type of injury with the immersion acting to obscure the actual cause of death. When working with a living victim recovered from water, it is essential to keep in mind that an underlying condition may have led to the person's becoming incapacitated and submerged—a condition that also may need to be treated or corrected while correcting hypoxemia and dealing with its sequelae.

Carbon monoxide is the most common chemical asphyxiant (see p. 90).

> ✔ **QUICK CHECK 4-3**
> 1. Give examples of intentional and unintentional injury in the United States..
> 2. Discuss unintentional injury as a form of injury with health care delivery in the United States.
> 3. What is the major mechanism of injury with drowning?

Infectious Injury

The pathogenicity (virulence) of microorganisms lies in their ability to survive and proliferate in the human body, where they injure cells and tissues. The disease-producing potential of a microorganism depends on its ability to (1) invade and destroy cells, (2) produce toxins, and (3) produce damaging hypersensitivity reactions. (See Chapter 8 for a description of infection and infectious organisms.)

Immunologic and Inflammatory Injury

Cellular membranes are injured by direct contact with cellular and chemical components of the immune and inflammatory responses, such as phagocytic cells (lymphocytes, macrophages) and substances such as histamine, antibodies, lymphokines, complement, and proteases (see Chapter 6). Complement is responsible for many of the membrane alterations that occur during immunologic injury.

Membrane alterations are associated with a rapid leakage of potassium (K^+) out of the cell and a rapid influx of water. Antibodies can interfere with membrane function by binding with and occupying receptor molecules on the plasma membrane. Antibodies also can block or destroy cellular junctions, interfering with intercellular communication. Other mechanisms of cellular injury are genetic and epigenetic factors, nutritional imbalances, and physical agents. These are summarized in Table 4-9.

MANIFESTATIONS OF CELLULAR INJURY: ACCUMULATIONS

An important manifestation of cell injury is the intracellular accumulation of abnormal amounts of various substances and the resultant metabolic disturbances. Cellular accumulations, also known as infiltrations, not only result from sublethal, sustained injury by cells, but also result from normal (but inefficient) cell function. Two categories of substances can produce accumulations: (1) a *normal cellular substance* (such as excess water, proteins, lipids, and carbohydrates) or (2) an *abnormal substance*, either endogenous (such as a product of abnormal metabolism or synthesis) or exogenous (such as infectious agents or a mineral). These products can accumulate transiently or permanently and can be toxic or harmless. Most accumulations are attributed to four types of mechanisms, all abnormal (Figure 4-23). Abnormal accumulations of these substances can occur in the cytoplasm (often in the lysosomes) or in the nucleus if (1) there is insufficient removal of the normal substance because of altered packaging and transport, for example, fatty change in the liver called *steatosis;* (2) an abnormal substance, often the result of a mutated gene, accumulates because of defects in protein folding, transport, or abnormal degradation; (3) an endogenous substance (normal or abnormal) is not effectively catabolized, usually because of lack of a vital lysosomal enzyme, called *storage diseases;* or (4) harmful exogenous materials, such as heavy metals,

TABLE 4-9   Mechanisms of Cellular Injury

Mechanism	Characteristics	Examples
Genetic Factors	Alter cell's nucleus and plasma membrane's structure, shape, receptors, or transport mechanisms	Sickle cell anemia, Huntington disease, muscular dystrophy, abetalipoproteinemia, familial hypercholesterolemia
Epigenetic Factors	Induction of mitotically heritable alterations in gene expression without changing DNA	Gene silencing in cancer
Nutritional Imbalances	Pathophysiologic cellular effects develop when nutrients are not consumed in diet and transported to body's cells *or* when excessive amounts of nutrients are consumed and transported	Protein deficiency, protein-calorie malnutrition, glucose deficiency, lipid deficiency (hypolipidemia), hyperlipidemia (increased lipoproteins in blood causing deposits of fat in heart, liver, and muscle), vitamin deficiencies
Physical Agents		
Temperature extremes	*Hypothermic injury* results from chilling or freezing of cells, creating high intracellular sodium concentrations; abrupt drops in temperature lead to vasoconstriction and increased viscosity of blood, causing ischemic injury, infarction, and necrosis; reactive oxygen species (ROS) are important in this process	Frostbite
	Hyperthermic injury is caused by excessive heat and varies in severity according to nature, intensity, and extent of heat	Burns, burn blisters, heat cramps usually from vigorous exercise with water and salt loss; heat exhaustion with salt and water loss causes heme contraction; heat stroke is life-threatening with a clinical rectal temperature of 106° F
	Tissue injury caused by compressive waves of air or fluid impinging on body, followed by sudden wave of decreased pressure; changes may collapse thorax, rupture internal solid organs, and cause widespread hemorrhage: carbon dioxide and nitrogen that are normally dissolved in blood precipitate from solution and form small bubbles (gas emboli), causing hypoxic injury and pain	Blast injury (air or immersion), decompression sickness (caisson disease or "the bends"); recently reported in a few individuals with subdural hematomas after riding high-speed roller coasters
Ionizing radiation	Refers to any form of radiation that can remove orbital electrons from atoms; source is usually environment and medical use; damage is to DNA molecule, causing chromosomal aberrations, chromosomal instability, and damage to membranes and enzymes; also induces growth factors and extracellular matrix remodeling; uncertainty exists regarding effects of low levels of radiation	X-rays, γ-rays, and α- and β-particles cause skin redness, skin damage, chromosomal damage, cancer
Illumination	Fluorescent lighting and halogen lamps create harmful oxidative stresses; ultraviolet light has been linked to skin cancer	Eyestrain, obscured vision, cataracts, headaches, melanoma
Mechanical stresses	Injury is caused by physical impact or irritation; they may be overt or cumulative	Faulty occupational biomechanics, leading to overexertion disorders
Noise	Can be caused by acute loud noise or cumulative effects of various intensities, frequencies, and duration of noise; considered a public health threat	Hearing impairment or loss; tinnitus, temporary threshold shift (TTS), or loss can occur as a complication of critical illness, from mechanical trauma, ototoxic medications, infections, vascular disorders, and noise

mineral dusts, or microorganisms, accumulate because of inhalation, ingestion, or infection.

In all storage diseases, the cells attempt to digest, or catabolize, the "stored" substances. As a result, excessive amounts of metabolites (products of catabolism) accumulate in the cells and are expelled into the extracellular matrix, where they are consumed by phagocytic cells called *macrophages* (see Chapter 6). Some of these scavenger cells circulate throughout the body, whereas others remain fixed in certain tissues, such as the liver or spleen. As more and more macrophages and other phagocytes migrate to tissues that are producing excessive metabolites, the affected tissues begin to swell. This is the mechanism that causes enlargement of the liver (hepatomegaly) or the spleen (splenomegaly) as a clinical manifestation of many storage diseases.

Water

Cellular swelling, the most common degenerative change, is caused by the shift of extracellular water into the cells. In hypoxic injury, movement of fluid and ions into the cell is associated with acute failure of metabolism and loss of ATP production. Normally, the pump that transports sodium ions (Na^+) out of the cell is maintained by the presence of ATP and adenosinetriphosphatase (ATPase), the active transport enzyme. In metabolic failure caused by hypoxia, reduced levels of ATP and ATPase permit sodium to accumulate in the cell while potassium (K^+) diffuses outward. The increased intracellular sodium concentration increases osmotic pressure, drawing more water into the cell. The cisternae of the ER become distended, rupture, and then unite to form large vacuoles that isolate the water from the cytoplasm, a process called *vacuolation*. Progressive vacuolation results in cytoplasmic swelling called oncosis (which has replaced the old term *hydropic [water] degeneration*) or vacuolar degeneration (Figure 4-24). If cellular swelling affects all the cells in an organ, the organ increases in weight and becomes distended and pale.

Cellular swelling is reversible and is considered sublethal. It is, in fact, an early manifestation of almost all types of cellular injury,

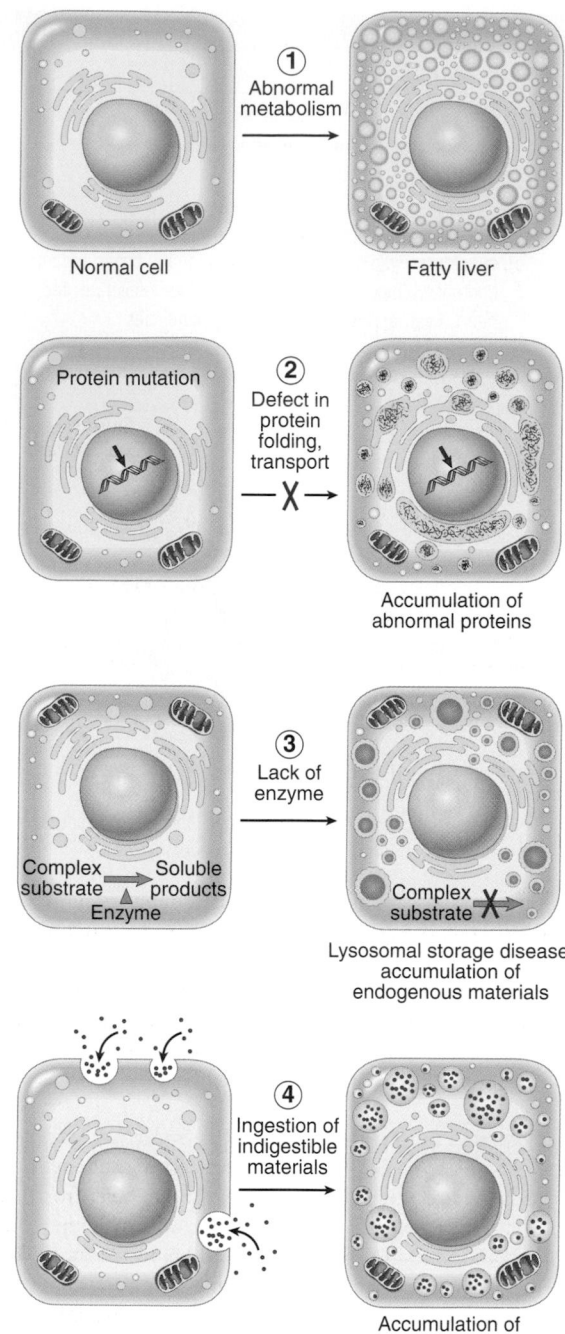

FIGURE 4-23 Mechanisms of Intracellular Accumulations. (From Kumar V et al, editors: *Robbins and Cotran pathologic basis of disease,* ed 9, Philadelphia, 2015, Elsevier.)

including severe or lethal cell injury. It is also associated with high fever, hypokalemia (abnormally low concentrations of potassium in the blood; see Chapter 5), and certain infections.

Lipids and Carbohydrates

Certain metabolic disorders result in the abnormal intracellular accumulation of carbohydrates and lipids. These substances may accumulate throughout the body but are found primarily in the spleen, liver, and CNS. Accumulations in cells of the CNS can cause neurologic dysfunction and severe intellectual disability. Lipids accumulate in Tay-Sachs disease, Niemann-Pick disease, and Gaucher disease; whereas in

the diseases known as mucopolysaccharidoses, carbohydrates are in excess. The mucopolysaccharidoses are progressive disorders that usually involve multiple organs, including liver, spleen, heart, and blood vessels. The accumulated mucopolysaccharides are found in reticuloendothelial cells, endothelial cells, intimal smooth muscle cells, and fibroblasts throughout the body. These carbohydrate accumulations can cause clouding of the cornea, joint stiffness, and intellectual disability.

Although lipids sometimes accumulate in heart, muscle, and kidney cells, the most common site of intracellular lipid accumulation, or **fatty change (steatosis)**, is liver cells (Figure 4-25). Because hepatic metabolism and secretion of lipids are crucial to proper body function, imbalances and deficiencies in these processes lead to major pathologic changes. In developed countries the most common cause of fatty change in the liver is alcohol abuse. Other causes of fatty change include diabetes mellitus, protein malnutrition, toxins, anoxia, and obesity. As lipids fill the cells, vacuolation pushes the nucleus and other organelles aside. The liver's outward appearance is yellow and greasy. Alcohol abuse is one of the most common causes of fatty liver (see Chapter 36).

Lipid accumulation in liver cells occurs after cellular injury instigates one or more of the following mechanisms:

1. Increased movement of free fatty acids into the liver (starvation, for example, increases the metabolism of triglycerides in adipose tissue, releasing fatty acids that subsequently enter liver cells)
2. Failure of the metabolic process that converts fatty acids to phospholipids, resulting in the preferential conversion of fatty acids to triglycerides
3. Increased synthesis of triglycerides from fatty acids (increased levels of the enzyme α-glycerophosphatase can accelerate triglyceride synthesis)
4. Decreased synthesis of apoproteins (lipid-acceptor proteins)
5. Failure of lipids to bind with apoproteins and form lipoproteins
6. Failure of mechanisms that transport lipoproteins out of the cell
7. Direct damage to the ER by free radicals released by alcohol's toxic effects

Many pathologic states show accumulation of cholesterol and cholesterol esters. These states include atherosclerosis, in which atherosclerotic plaques, smooth muscle cells, and macrophages within the intimal layer of the aorta and large arteries are filled with lipid-rich vacuoles of cholesterol and cholesterol esters. Other states include cholesterol-rich deposits in the gallbladder and Niemann-Pick disease (type C), which involve genetic mutations of an enzyme affecting cholesterol transport.

Glycogen

Glycogen storage is important as a readily available energy source in the cytoplasm of normal cells. Intracellular accumulations of glycogen are seen in genetic disorders called *glycogen storage diseases* and in disorders of glucose and glycogen metabolism. As with water and lipid accumulation, glycogen accumulation results in excessive vacuolation of the cytoplasm. The most common cause of glycogen accumulation is the disorder of glucose metabolism (i.e., diabetes mellitus) (see Chapter 19).

Proteins

Proteins provide cellular structure and constitute most of the cell's dry weight. The proteins are synthesized on ribosomes in the cytoplasm from the essential amino acids lysine, threonine, leucine, isoleucine, methionine, tryptophan, valine, phenylalanine, and histidine. The accumulation of protein probably damages cells in two ways. First, metabolites, produced when the cell attempts to digest some proteins,

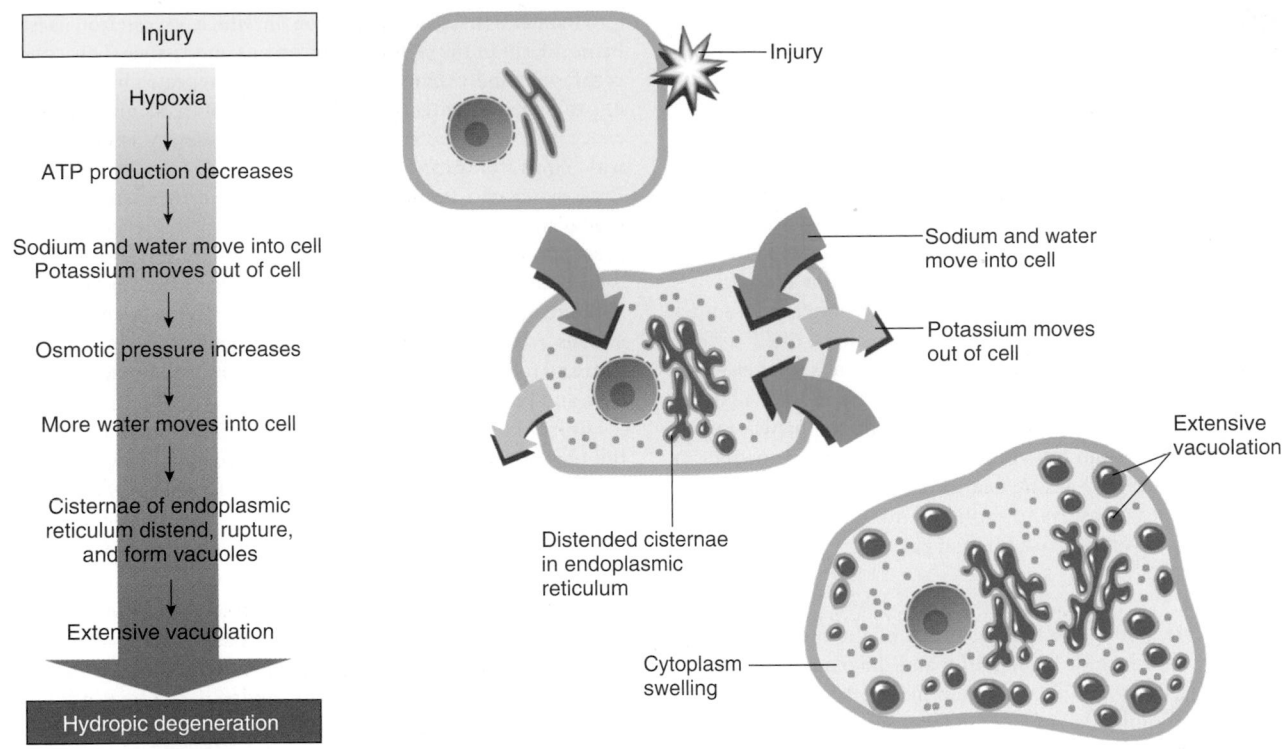

FIGURE 4-24 The Process of Oncosis (Formerly Referred to as "Hydropic Degeneration"). *ATP,* Adenosine triphosphate.

FIGURE 4-25 Fatty Liver. The liver appears yellow. (From Damjanov I, Linder J: *Pathology: a color atlas,* St Louis, 2000, Mosby.)

are enzymes that when released from lysosomes can damage cellular organelles. Second, excessive amounts of protein in the cytoplasm push against cellular organelles, disrupting organelle function and intracellular communication.

Protein excess accumulates primarily in the epithelial cells of the renal convoluted tubules of the nephron unit and in the antibody-forming plasma cells (B lymphocytes) of the immune system. Several types of renal disorders cause excessive excretion of protein molecules in the urine (proteinuria). Normally, little or no protein is present in the urine, and its presence in significant amounts indicates cellular injury and altered cellular function.

Accumulations of protein in B lymphocytes can occur during active synthesis of antibodies during the immune response. The excess aggregates of protein are called *Russell bodies* (see Chapter 6). Russell bodies have been identified in multiple myeloma (plasma cell tumor) (see Chapter 21).

Mutations in protein can slow protein folding, resulting in the accumulation of partially folded intermediates. An example is α_1-antitrypsin deficiency, which can cause emphysema. Certain types of cell injury are associated with the accumulation of cytoskeleton proteins. For example, the *neurofibrillary tangle* found in the brain in Alzheimer disease contains these types of proteins.

Pigments

Pigment accumulations may be normal or abnormal, endogenous (produced within the body) or exogenous (produced outside the body). Endogenous pigments are derived, for example, from amino acids (e.g., tyrosine, tryptophan). They include melanin and the blood proteins porphyrins, hemoglobin, and hemosiderin. Lipid-rich pigments, such as lipofuscin (the aging pigment), give a yellow-brown color to cells undergoing slow, regressive, and often atrophic changes. The most common exogenous pigment is carbon (coal dust), a pervasive air pollutant in urban areas. Inhaled carbon interacts with lung macrophages and is transported by lymphatic vessels to regional lymph nodes. This accumulation blackens lung tissues and involved lymph nodes. Other exogenous pigments include mineral dusts containing silica and iron particles, lead, silver salts, and dyes for tattoos.

Melanin

Melanin accumulates in epithelial cells (keratinocytes) of the skin and retina. It is an extremely important pigment because it protects the skin against long exposure to sunlight and is considered an essential factor in the prevention of skin cancer (see Chapters 11 and 41). Ultraviolet light (e.g., sunlight) stimulates the synthesis of melanin, which probably absorbs ultraviolet rays during subsequent exposure. Melanin also may protect the skin by trapping the injurious free radicals produced by the action of ultraviolet light on skin.

Melanin is a brown-black pigment derived from the amino acid *tyrosine*. It is synthesized by epidermal cells called *melanocytes* and is stored in membrane-bound cytoplasmic vesicles called *melanosomes.*

Melanin also can accumulate in melanophores (melanin-containing pigment cells), macrophages, or other phagocytic cells in the dermis. Presumably these cells acquire the melanin from nearby melanocytes or from pigment that has been extruded from dying epidermal cells. This is the mechanism that causes freckles. Melanin also occurs in the benign form of pigmented moles called *nevi* (see Chapter 41). Malignant melanoma is a cancerous skin tumor that contains melanin.

A decrease in melanin production occurs in the inherited disorder of melanin metabolism called *albinism*. Albinism is often diffuse, involving all the skin, the eyes, and the hair. Albinism is also related to phenylalanine metabolism. In classic types, the person with albinism is unable to convert tyrosine to DOPA (3,4-dihydroxyphenylalanine), an intermediate in melanin biosynthesis. Melanocytes are present in normal numbers, but they are unable to make melanin. Individuals with albinism are very sensitive to sunlight and quickly become sunburned. They are also at high risk for skin cancer.

Hemoproteins

Hemoproteins are among the most essential of the normal endogenous pigments. They include hemoglobin and the oxidative enzymes, the cytochromes. Central to an understanding of disorders involving these pigments is knowledge of iron uptake, metabolism, excretion, and storage (see Chapter 20). Hemoprotein accumulations in cells are caused by excessive storage of iron, which is transferred to the cells from the bloodstream. Iron enters the blood from three primary sources: (1) tissue stores, (2) the intestinal mucosa, and (3) macrophages that remove and destroy dead or defective red blood cells. The amount of iron in blood plasma depends also on the metabolism of the major iron transport protein, *transferrin.*

Iron is stored in tissue cells in two forms: as ferritin and, when increased levels of iron are present, as hemosiderin. Hemosiderin is a yellow-brown pigment derived from hemoglobin. With pathologic states, excesses of iron cause hemosiderin to accumulate within cells, often in areas of bruising and hemorrhage and in the lungs and spleen after congestion caused by heart failure. With local hemorrhage, the skin first appears red-blue and then lysis of the escaped red blood cells occurs, causing the hemoglobin to be transformed to hemosiderin. The color changes noted in bruising reflect this transformation (Figure 4-26).

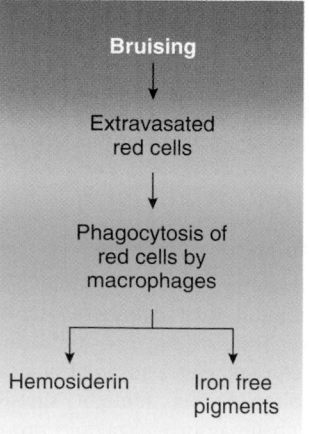

FIGURE 4-26 Hemosiderin Accumulation Is Noted as the Color Changes in a "Black Eye."

Hemosiderosis is a condition in which excess iron is stored as hemosiderin in the cells of many organs and tissues. This condition is common in individuals who have received repeated blood transfusions or prolonged parenteral administration of iron. Hemosiderosis is associated also with increased absorption of dietary iron, conditions in which iron storage and transport are impaired, and hemolytic anemia. Excessive alcohol (wine) ingestion also can lead to hemosiderosis. Normally, absorption of excessive dietary iron is prevented by an iron absorption process in the intestines. Failure of this process can lead to total body iron accumulations in the range of 60 to 80 g, compared with normal iron stores of 4.5 to 5 g. Excessive accumulations of iron, such as occur in hemochromatosis (a genetic disorder of iron metabolism and the most severe example of iron overload), are associated with liver and pancreatic cell damage.

Bilirubin is a normal, yellow-to-green pigment of bile derived from the porphyrin structure of hemoglobin. Excess bilirubin within cells and tissues causes jaundice (icterus), or yellowing of the skin. Jaundice occurs when the bilirubin level exceeds 1.5 to 2 mg/dl of plasma, compared with the normal values of 0.4 to 1 mg/dl. Hyperbilirubinemia occurs with (1) destruction of red blood cells (erythrocytes), such as in hemolytic jaundice; (2) diseases affecting the metabolism and excretion of bilirubin in the liver; and (3) diseases that cause obstruction of the common bile duct, such as gallstones or pancreatic tumors. Certain drugs (specifically chlorpromazine and other phenothiazine derivatives), estrogenic hormones, and halothane (an anesthetic) can cause the obstruction of normal bile flow through the liver.

Because unconjugated bilirubin is lipid soluble, it can injure the lipid components of the plasma membrane. Albumin, a plasma protein, provides significant protection by binding unconjugated bilirubin in plasma. Unconjugated bilirubin causes two cellular outcomes: uncoupling of oxidative phosphorylation and a loss of cellular proteins. These two changes could cause structural injury to the various membranes of the cell.

Calcium

Calcium salts accumulate in both injured and dead tissues (Figure 4-27). An important mechanism of cellular calcification is the influx of extracellular calcium in injured mitochondria. Another mechanism that causes calcium accumulation in alveoli (gas-exchange airways of the lungs), gastric epithelium, and renal tubules is the excretion of acid at these sites, leading to the local production of hydroxyl ions. Hydroxyl ions result in precipitation of calcium hydroxide, $Ca(OH)_2$, and hydroxyapatite, $(Ca_3[PO_4]_2)_3 \cdot Ca(OH)_2$, a mixed salt. Damage occurs when calcium salts cluster and harden, interfering with normal cellular structure and function.

Pathologic calcification can be dystrophic or metastatic. Dystrophic calcification occurs in dying and dead tissues in areas of necrosis (see also the types of necrosis: coagulative, liquefactive, caseous, and fatty). It is present in chronic tuberculosis of the lungs and lymph nodes, advanced atherosclerosis (narrowing of the arteries as a result of plaque accumulation), and heart valve injury (Figure 4-28). Calcification of the heart valves interferes with their opening and closing, causing heart murmurs (see Chapter 24). Calcification of the coronary arteries predisposes them to severe narrowing and thrombosis, which can lead to myocardial infarction. Another site of dystrophic calcification is the center of tumors. Over time, the center is deprived of its oxygen supply, dies, and becomes calcified. The calcium salts appear as gritty, clumped granules that can become hard as stone. When several layers clump together, they resemble grains of sand and are called psammoma bodies.

Metastatic calcification consists of mineral deposits that occur in undamaged normal tissues as the result of hypercalcemia (excess

FIGURE 4-27 Free Cytosolic Calcium: A Destructive Agent. Normally, calcium is removed from the cytosol by adenosine triphosphate (ATP)–dependent calcium pumps. In normal cells, calcium is bound to buffering proteins, such as calbindin or parvalbumin, and is contained in the endoplasmic reticulum and the mitochondria. If there is abnormal permeability of calcium-ion channels, direct damage to membranes, or depletion of ATP (i.e., hypoxic injury), calcium increases in the cytosol. If the free calcium cannot be buffered or pumped out of cells, uncontrolled enzyme activation takes place, causing further damage. Uncontrolled entry of calcium into the cytosol is an important final common pathway in many causes of cell death.

calcium in the blood; see Chapter 5). Conditions that cause hypercalcemia include hyperparathyroidism, toxic levels of vitamin D, hyperthyroidism, idiopathic hypercalcemia of infancy, Addison disease (adrenocortical insufficiency), systemic sarcoidosis, milk-alkali syndrome, and the increased bone demineralization that results from bone tumors, leukemia, and disseminated cancers. Hypercalcemia also may occur in advanced renal failure with phosphate retention. As phosphate levels increase, the activity of the parathyroid gland increases, causing higher levels of circulating calcium.

Urate

In humans, uric acid (**urate**) is the major end product of purine catabolism because of the absence of the enzyme urate oxidase. Serum urate concentration is, in general, stable: approximately 5 mg/dl in postpubertal males and 4.1 mg/dl in postpubertal females. Disturbances in maintaining serum urate levels result in hyperuricemia and the deposition of sodium urate crystals in the tissues, leading to painful disorders collectively called *gout*. These disorders include acute arthritis, chronic gouty arthritis, tophi (firm, nodular, subcutaneous deposits of urate crystals surrounded by fibrosis), and nephritis (inflammation of the nephron). Chronic hyperuricemia results in the deposition of urate in tissues, cell injury, and inflammation. Because urate crystals are not degraded by lysosomal enzymes, they persist in dead cells.

Systemic Manifestations

Systemic manifestations of cellular injury include a general sense of fatigue and malaise, a loss of well-being, and altered appetite. Fever is often present because of biochemicals produced during the inflammatory response. Table 4-10 summarizes the most significant systemic manifestations of cellular injury.

CELLULAR DEATH

In response to significant external stimuli, cell injury becomes irreversible and cells are forced to die. Cell death has historically been classified as necrosis and apoptosis. Necrosis is characterized by rapid loss of the plasma membrane structure, swelling of organelles, dysfunction of the mitochondria, and lack of typical features of apoptosis.[70] Apoptosis is known as a regulated or programmed cell process characterized by the "dropping off" of cellular fragments called apoptotic bodies. Too little or too much apoptosis is linked to many disorders, including neurodegenerative diseases, ischemic damage, autoimmune disorders, and cancers. Yet, apoptosis can have normal functions, and unlike necrosis it is not always linked with a pathologic process. Until recently, necrosis was only considered passive or accidental cell death occurring after severe and sudden injury. It is the main outcome in several common injuries including ischemia, toxin exposure, certain infections, and trauma. It has now been proposed that under certain conditions, such as activation of death proteases, necrosis may be *regulated* or *programmed* in a well-orchestrated way as a back-up for apoptosis (apoptosis may progress to necrosis)[71]—hence the new term **programmed necrosis**, or **necroptosis**. Necroptosis shares traits with both necrosis and apoptosis.[72] Although the identification of the signaling mechanisms for necroptosis is incomplete, necroptosis is recognized in both

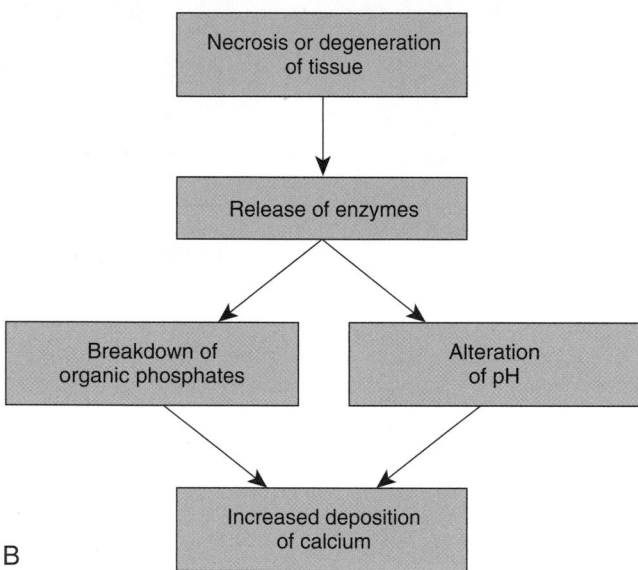

B

FIGURE 4-28 Aortic Valve Calcification. **A,** This calcified aortic valve is an example of dystrophic calcification. **B,** This algorithm shows the dystrophic mechanism of calcification. (**A** from Damjanov I: *Pathology for the health professions,* ed 4, St Louis, 2012, Saunders.)

TABLE 4-10	Systemic Manifestations of Cellular Injury
Manifestation	**Cause**
Fever	Release of endogenous pyrogens (interleukin-1, tumor necrosis factor-alpha, prostaglandins) from bacteria or macrophages; acute inflammatory response
Increased heart rate	Increase in oxidative metabolic processes resulting from fever
Increase in leukocytes (leukocytosis)	Increase in total number of white blood cells because of infection; normal is 5000-9000/mm³ (increase is directly related to severity of infection)
Pain	Various mechanisms, such as release of bradykinins, obstruction, pressure
Presence of cellular enzymes	Release of enzymes from cells of tissue* in extracellular fluid
Lactate dehydrogenase (LDH) (LDH isoenzymes)	Release from red blood cells, liver, kidney, skeletal muscle
Creatine kinase (CK) (CK isoenzymes)	Release from skeletal muscle, brain, heart
Aspartate aminotransferase (AST/SGOT)	Release from heart, liver, skeletal muscle, kidney, pancreas
Alanine aminotransferase (ALT/SGPT)	Release from liver, kidney, heart
Alkaline phosphatase (ALP)	Release from liver, bone
Amylase	Release from pancreas
Aldolase	Release from skeletal muscle, heart

*The rapidity of enzyme transfer is a function of the weight of the enzyme and the concentration gradient across the cellular membrane. The specific metabolic and excretory rates of the enzymes determine how long levels of enzymes remain elevated.

normal physiologic conditions and pathologic conditions, including bone growth plate disorders, cell death in fatty liver disease, acute pancreatitis, reperfusion injury, and certain neurodegenerative disorders, such as Parkinson disease.[1]

Historically, programmed cell death only referred to apoptosis. Figure 4-29 illustrates the structural changes in cell injury resulting in necrosis or apoptosis. Table 4-11 compares the unique features of necrosis and apoptosis. Other forms of cell loss include autophagy (self-eating) (see p. 105).

Necrosis

Cellular death eventually leads to cellular dissolution, or necrosis. Necrosis is the sum of cellular changes after local cell death and the process of cellular self-digestion, known as autodigestion or autolysis (see Figure 4-29). Cells die long before any necrotic changes are noted by light microscopy.[71] The structural signs that indicate irreversible injury and progression to necrosis are dense clumping and progressive disruption both of genetic material and of plasma cand organelle membranes. Because membrane integrity is lost, necrotic cell contents leak out and may cause the signaling of inflammation in surrounding

tissue. In later stages of necrosis, most organelles are disrupted, and **karyolysis** (nuclear dissolution and lysis of chromatin from the action of hydrolytic enzymes) is under way. In some cells the nucleus shrinks and becomes a small, dense mass of genetic material (**pyknosis**). The pyknotic nucleus eventually dissolves (by karyolysis) as a result of the action of hydrolytic lysosomal enzymes on DNA. **Karyorrhexis** means fragmentation of the nucleus into smaller particles or "nuclear dust."

Although necrosis still refers to death induced by nonspecific trauma or injury (e.g., cell stress or the heat shock response), with the very recent identification of molecular mechanisms regulating the process of necrosis, the study of necrosis has experienced a new twist. Unlike apoptosis, necrosis has been viewed as passive with cell death occurring in a disorganized and unregulated manner. Some molecular regulators governing programmed necrosis have been identified and demonstrated to be interconnected by a large network of signaling pathways.[71,73] Emerging evidence shows that programmed necrosis is associated with pathologic diseases and provides innate immune response to viral infection.[71,73]

Different types of necrosis tend to occur in different organs or tissues and sometimes can indicate the mechanism or cause of cellular injury. The four major types of necrosis are coagulative, liquefactive, caseous, and fatty. Another type, gangrenous necrosis, is *not* a distinctive type of cell death but refers instead to larger areas of tissue death. These necroses are summarized as follows:

1. **Coagulative necrosis.** Occurs primarily in the kidneys, heart, and adrenal glands; commonly results from hypoxia caused by severe

FIGURE 4-29 Schematic Illustration of the Morphologic Changes in Cell Injury Culminating in Necrosis or Apoptosis. Myelin figures come from degenerating cellular membranes and are noted within the cytoplasm or extracellularly. (From Kumar V et al, editors: *Robbins and Cotran pathologic basis of disease,* ed 9, Philadelphia, 2015, Elsevier.)

TABLE 4-11   Features of Necrosis and Apoptosis

Feature	Necrosis	Apoptosis
Cell size	Enlarged (swelling)	Reduced (shrinkage)
Nucleus	Pyknosis → karyorrhexis → karyolysis	Fragmentation into nucleosome-size fragments
Plasma membrane	Disrupted	Intact; altered structure, especially orientation of lipids
Cellular contents	Enzymatic digestion; may leak out of cell	Intact; may be released in apoptotic bodies
Adjacent inflammation	Frequent	No
Physiologic or pathologic role	Invariably pathologic (culmination of irreversible cell injury)	Often physiologic, means of eliminating unwanted cells; may be pathologic after some forms of cell injury, especially DNA damage

From Kumar V et al: Cellular responses to stress and toxic insults: adaptation, injury, and death. In Kumar V et al, editors: *Robbins and Cotran pathologic basis of disease*, ed 9, Philadelphia, 2015, Elsevier.

ischemia or hypoxia caused by chemical injury, especially ingestion of mercuric chloride. Coagulation is a result of protein denaturation, which causes the protein albumin to change from a gelatinous, transparent state to a firm, opaque state (Figure 4-30, *A*). The area of coagulative necrosis is called an **infarct.**

2. **Liquefactive necrosis.** Commonly results from ischemic injury to neurons and glial cells in the brain (Figure 4-30, *B*). Dead brain tissue is readily affected by liquefactive necrosis because brain cells are rich in digestive hydrolytic enzymes and lipids and the brain contains little connective tissue. Cells are digested by their own hydrolases, so the tissue becomes soft, liquefies, and segregates from healthy tissue, forming cysts. This can be caused by bacterial infection, especially *Staphylococci, Streptococci,* and *Escherichia coli.*

3. **Caseous necrosis.** Usually results from tuberculous pulmonary infection, especially by *Mycobacterium tuberculosis* (Figure 4-30, *C*). It is a combination of coagulative and liquefactive necroses. The dead cells disintegrate, but the debris is not completely digested by the hydrolases. Tissues resemble clumped cheese in that they are soft and granular. A granulomatous inflammatory wall encloses areas of caseous necrosis.

4. **Fatty necrosis.** Fat necrosis is cellular dissolution caused by powerful enzymes, called lipases, that occur in the breast, pancreas, and other abdominal structures (Figure 4-30, *D*). Lipases break down

FIGURE 4-30 Types of Necrosis. A, Coagulative necrosis. A wedge-shaped kidney infarct *(yellow).* **B,** Liquefactive necrosis of the brain. The area of infarction is softened as a result of liquefaction necrosis. **C,** Caseous necrosis. Tuberculosis of the lung, with a large area of caseous necrosis containing yellow-white and cheesy debris. **D,** Fat necrosis of pancreas. Interlobular adipocytes are necrotic; acute inflammatory cells surround these. (**A** and **C** from Kumar V et al, editors: *Robbins and Cotran pathologic basis of disease,* ed 9, Philadelphia, 2015, Elsevier. **B** from Damjanov I: *Pathology for the health professions,* ed 4, St Louis, 2012, Saunders. **D** from Damjanov I, Linder J, editors: *Anderson's pathology,* ed 10, St Louis, 1996, Mosby.)

triglycerides, releasing free fatty acids that then combine with calcium, magnesium, and sodium ions, creating soaps (saponification). The necrotic tissue appears opaque and chalk-white.

5. Gangrenous necrosis. Refers to death of tissue but is not a specific pattern of cell death and results from severe hypoxic injury, commonly occurring because of arteriosclerosis, or blockage, of major arteries, particularly those in the lower leg (Figure 4-31). With hypoxia and subsequent bacterial invasion, the tissues can undergo necrosis. *Dry gangrene* is usually the result of coagulative necrosis. The skin becomes very dry and shrinks, resulting in wrinkles, and its color changes to dark brown or black. *Wet gangrene* develops when neutrophils invade the site, causing liquefactive necrosis. This usually occurs in internal organs, causing the site to become cold, swollen, and black. A foul odor is present, and if systemic symptoms become severe, death can ensue.

6. Gas gangrene. Refers to a special type of gangrene caused by infection of injured tissue by one of many species of *Clostridium*. These anaerobic bacteria produce hydrolytic enzymes and toxins that destroy connective tissue and cellular membranes and cause bubbles of gas to form in muscle cells. This can be fatal if enzymes lyse the membranes of red blood cells, destroying their oxygen-carrying capacity. Death is caused by shock.

Apoptosis

Apoptosis ("dropping off") is an important distinct type of cell death that differs from necrosis in several ways (see Figure 4-29 and Table 4-11). Apoptosis is an active process of cellular self-destruction called *programmed cell death* and is implicated in both normal and pathologic tissue changes. Cells need to die; otherwise, endless proliferation would

lead to gigantic bodies. The average adult may create 10 billion new cells every day—and destroy the same number.[74] Death by apoptosis causes loss of cells in many pathologic states including the following:

- *Severe cell injury.* When cell injury exceeds repair mechanisms, the cell triggers apoptosis. *DNA damage* can result either directly or indirectly from production of free radicals.
- *Accumulation of misfolded proteins.* This may result from genetic mutations or free radicals. Excessive accumulation of misfolded proteins in the ER leads to a condition known as endoplasmic reticulum stress (ER stress) (see Chapter 1). ER stress results in apoptotic cell death. This mechanism has been linked to several degenerative diseases of the CNS and other organs (Figure 4-32).
- *Infections (particularly viral).* Apoptosis may be the result of the virus directly or indirectly by the host immune response. Cytotoxic T lymphocytes respond to viral infections by inducing apoptosis and, therefore, eliminating the infectious cells. This process can cause tissue damage and it is the same for cell death in tumors and rejection of tissue transplants.
- *Obstruction in tissue ducts.* In organs with duct obstruction, including the pancreas, kidney, and parotid gland, apoptosis causes pathologic atrophy.

Excessive or insufficient apoptosis is known as *dysregulated apoptosis.* A low rate of apoptosis can permit the survival of abnormal cells, for example, mutated cells that can increase cancer risk. Defective apoptosis may not eliminate lymphocytes that react against host tissue (self-antigens), leading to autoimmune disorders. Excessive apoptosis is known to occur in several neurodegenerative diseases, from ischemic injury (such as myocardial infarction and stroke), and from death of virus-infected cells (such as seen in many viral infections).

Thrombosis or embolism   Strangulated hernia   Volvulus   Intussusception   Gangrene

FIGURE 4-31 Gangrene, a Complication of Necrosis. In certain circumstances, necrotic tissue will be invaded by putrefactive organisms that are both saccharolytic and proteolytic. Foul-smelling gases are produced, and the tissue becomes green or black as a result of breakdown of hemoglobin. Obstruction of the blood supply to the bowel almost inevitably is followed by gangrene.

FIGURE 4-32 The Unfolded Protein Response, Endoplasmic Stress, and Apoptosis. A, In normal or healthy cells the newly made proteins are folded with help from chaperones and then incorporated into the cell or secreted. **B,** Various stressors can cause ER stress whereby the cell is challenged to cope with the increased load of misfolded proteins. The accumulation of the protein load initiates the *unfolded protein response* in the ER; if restoration of the protein fails, the cell dies by apoptosis. An example of a disease caused by misfolding of proteins is Alzheimer disease. (From Kumar V et al, editors: *Robbins and Cotran pathologic basis of disease,* ed 9, Philadelphia, 2015, Elsevier.)

Apoptosis depends on a tightly regulated cellular program for its initiation and execution.[74] This death program involves enzymes that divide other proteins—proteases, which are activated by proteolytic activity in response to signals that induce apoptosis. These proteases are called caspases, a family of aspartic acid–specific proteases. The activated suicide caspases cleave and, thereby, activate other members of the family, resulting in an amplifying "suicide" cascade. The activated caspases then cleave other key proteins in the cell, killing the cell quickly and neatly. The two different pathways that converge on caspase activation are called the *mitochondrial (intrinsic) pathway* and the *death receptor (extrinsic) pathway* (Figure 4-33). Cells that die by apoptosis release chemical factors that recruit phagocytes that quickly engulf the remains of the dead cell, thus reducing chances of

inflammation. With necrosis, cell death is not tidy because cells that die as a result of acute injury swell, burst, and spill their contents all over their neighbors, causing a likely damaging inflammatory response.

Autophagy

The Greek term autophagy means "eating of self." Autophagy, as a "recycling factory," is a self-destructive process and a survival mechanism. Basically, autophagy involves the delivery of cytoplasmic contents to the lysosome for degradation. Box 4-3 contains the terms used to describe autophagy.

When cells are starved or nutrient deprived, the autophagic process institutes cannibalization and recycles the digested contents.[48,75] Autophagy can maintain cellular metabolism under starvation

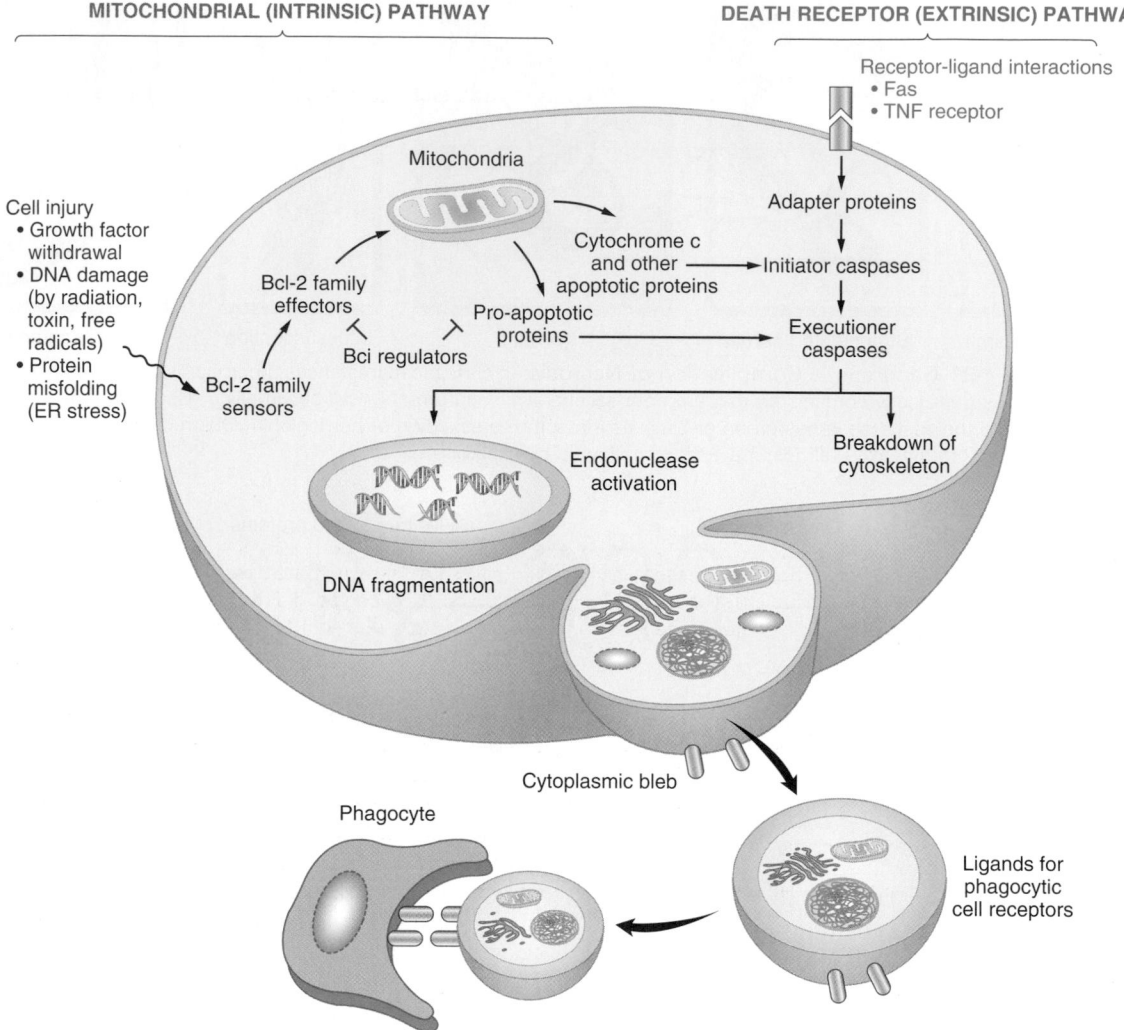

MITOCHONDRIAL (INTRINSIC) PATHWAY

DEATH RECEPTOR (EXTRINSIC) PATHWAY

FIGURE 4-33 Mechanisms of Apoptosis. The two pathways of apoptosis differ in their induction and regulation, and both culminate in the activation of "executioner" caspases. The induction of apoptosis by the mitochondrial pathway involves the Bcl-2 family, which causes leakage of mitochondrial proteins. The regulators of the death receptor pathway involve the proteases, called caspases. (Adapted from Kumar V et al, editors: *Robbins and Cotran pathologic basis of disease*, ed 9, Philadelphia, 2015, Elsevier.)

BOX 4-3 The Major Forms of Autophagy

Macroautophagy, the most common term to refer to autophagy, involves the sequestration and transportation of parts (cargo) of the cytosol in an autophagic vacuole (autophagosome).

Microautophagy is the inward invagination of the lysosomal membrane for cargo delivery.

Chaperone-mediated autophagy is the chaperone-dependent proteins that direct cargo across the lysosomal membrane.

---

conditions and remove damaged organelles under stress conditions, improving the survival of cells. With the central role of autophagy in cell homeostasis, autophagy has been implicated in cancer, heart disease, neurodegeneration diseases, inflammation, and infection.[76] Autophagy begins with a membrane, also known as a *phagophore* (although controversial) (Figure 4-34).[75] This cup-shaped, curved phagophore expands and engulfs intracellular cargo—organelles, ribosomes, proteins—forming a double membrane *autophagosome*. The cargo-laden autophagosome fuses with the lysosome, now called an

autophagolysosome, which promotes the degradation of the autophagosome by lysosomal acid proteases. The phagophore membrane is highly curved along the rim of the open cup, suggesting that mechanisms responsible for its formation and growth may depend on membrane curvature-dependent events.[77] Lysosomal transporters export amino acids and other byproducts of degradation out of the cytoplasm where they can be reused for the synthesis of macromolecules and for metabolism.[78,79] ATP is generated and cellular damage is reduced during autophagy that removes nonfunctional proteins and organelles.[75]

Investigators are excited about the utilization of autophagy for therapeutic strategies. Autophagy is a critical garbage collecting and recycling process in healthy cells, and this process becomes less efficient and less discriminating as the cell ages. Consequently, harmful agents accumulate in cells, damaging cells and leading to aging: for example, failure to clear protein products in neurons of the CNS can cause dementia; failure to clear ROS-producing mitochondria can lead to nuclear DNA mutations and cancer. Thus these processes may even partially define aging. Therefore normal autophagy may potentially rejuvenate an organism and prevent cancer development as well as

FIGURE 4-34 Autophagy. Cellular stresses, such as nutrient deprivation, activate autophagy genes that create vacuoles in which cellular organelles are sequestered and then degraded following fusion of the vesicles with lysosomes. The digested materials are recycled to provide nutrients for the cell.

other degenerative diseases.[80] In addition, autophagy may be the last immune defense against infectious microorganisms that penetrate intracellularly.[81]

AGING AND ALTERED CELLULAR AND TISSUE BIOLOGY

The terms *aging* and *life span* tend to be used synonymously; however, they are not equivalent. Aging is usually defined as a normal physiologic process that is universal and inevitable, whereas life span is the time from birth to death and has been used to study the aging process.[82] Aging is associated with a gradual loss of homeostatic mechanisms whose underlying cause is perplexing,[83] and is a complex process because of a multiplicity of factors. Investigators are focused on genetic, epigenetic, inflammatory, oxidative stress, and metabolic origins of aging, including the study of genetic signatures in humans with exceptional longevity; the identification and recent discovery of epigenetic mechanisms that modulate gene expression; the role of intrauterine environment and lifelong patterns of health; the effects of personality, behavior, and social support; the influence of insulin/insulin-like growth factor 1 (IGF-1) signaling; and the contributions of cellular dysfunction and senescence to an inflammatory microenvironment that leads to chronic disease, frailty, and decreased life span. To focus more simply, the factors that may be most important for aging include increased damage to the cell, reduced capacity to divide (replicative senescence), reduced ability to repair damaged DNA, and increased likelihood of defective protein balance or homeostasis.[1] A major challenge of aging research has been to separate the causes of cell and tissue aging from the vast changes that accompany it.[83] Public health issues

related to healthy aging require understanding of the nature of aging and the factors that predict healthy aging and delayed transition to increasing vulnerability and frailty.

Aging traditionally has not been considered a disease because it is "normal"; disease is usually considered "abnormal." Conceptually, this distinction seems clear until the concept of "injury" or "damage" is introduced; disease has been defined by some pathologists as the result of injury. *Chronologic aging* has been defined as the time-dependent loss of structure and function that proceeds very slowly and in such small increments that it appears to be the result of the accumulation of small, imperceptible injuries—a gradual result of wear and tear. One of the hallmarks of aging is the accumulation of damaged macromolecules. DNA damage can lead to cellular dysfunction both directly and indirectly as a consequence of cellular responses to damage that can lead to altered gene expression.[84,85] Age-related changes to macromolecules for long-lived cells, such as neurons and myofibers, lead to gradual loss of structure and function.

Replicative aging or *senescence* is the accumulation of cellular damage in continuously dividing cells, for example, epithelia of the skin or gastrointestinal tract. One mechanism of replicative senescence is the progressive shortening of telomeres—the repeated sequences of DNA at the ends of chromosomes. Replicative aging and chronologic aging are particularly important for adult stem cells because they divide throughout life.[86] As mutations increase with age, cell fates include apoptosis, malignant transformation, cell cycle arrest, or senescence.[87]

Despite the fact that aging and death are inevitable, life span, on the other hand, can be experimentally changed.[83] Genetic and environmental interventions have extended the life span of model organisms, such as the nematode worm *Caenorhabditis elegans (C. elegans)*, the fruit fly *Drosophilia melanogaster*, and mice.[88,89] Extending life span, however, is not equivalent to delaying aging![83] For example, treatment of an acute infection can prevent death but the fundamental *rate* of aging continues. Yet, investigators will study and try to isolate, manipulate, and reset so-called longevity genes to slow the rate of aging.

Recent advances in stem cell biology have begun to reveal the molecular mechanisms behind reprogramming events that occur during fertilization and when the nucleus of a mature somatic cell is transferred to an enucleated oocyte. Called somatic cell nuclear transfer (SCNT), this process gave rise to the first cloned mammal, Dolly the sheep, and lead to the explosion of research in cloning.[83] SCNT is important in terms of demonstrating the ability of the oocyte cytoplasm to reprogram the donor nucleus. These reprogramming events have led to the process to create induced pluripotent stem cells (iPSCs).[90] The major emphasis of reprogramming research is the reversal of the differentiated program and attainment of a pluripotent state (differentiated cells in all three germ layers of the embryo) and not the reversal of aging.[83,91] Nevertheless, each of these processes is discussed in the context of resetting the aging clock.

Restoration of youthfulness to aged cells and tissues has created so-called rejuvenating interventions. Experiments to test whether cells and tissues from an old animal can be restored to a younger self include the approach called *heterochronic* (i.e., young-to-old or old-to-young) transplantations and *heterochronic parabiosis,* when the systemic circulations of two animals are joined. The systemic environment may become more youthful with restoration of protein components in the blood and tissues, especially chemokines and cytokines.[92] For example, investigators found a protein, GDF-11, may reverse age-associated cardiac hypertrophy when injected into old animals.[93]

Administration of the drug rapamycin, an mTOR inhibitor, can extend the life span of mice.[94] These and future studies may not just change differentiation programs of cells and tissue, but also possibly alter the aging clock. Observations in *C. elegans* suggest strongly that the causes of aging may be largely epigenetic.[83,95,96]

Normal Life Span, Life Expectancy, and Quality-Adjusted Life Year

The maximal life span of humans is between 80 and 100 years and does not vary significantly among populations. Life expectancy is the *average* number of years of life remaining at a given age, however, it does not include quality of life. The **quality-adjusted life year (QALY)** is a measure of disease burden including quality and not just quantity of live lived. The Centers for Disease Control and Prevention reported in 2009 that the overall life expectancy at birth was 78.5 years. Between 2008 and 2009, life expectancy at birth increased for all groups reviewed. It increased for males, from 75.6 to 76.0 years, and females, 80.6 to 80.9 years; for the white population, 78.5 to 78.8 years; the black population, 74.0 to 74.5 years; the Hispanic population, 81.0 to 81.2 years; the non-Hispanic white population, 78.4 to 78.7 years; and the non-Hispanic black population, 73.7 to 74.0 years.[97]

Degenerative Extracellular Changes

Extracellular factors that affect the aging process include the binding of collagen; the increase in the effects of free radicals on cells; the structural alterations of fascia, tendons, ligaments, bones, and joints; and the development of peripheral vascular disease, particularly arteriosclerosis (see Chapter 24).

Aging affects the extracellular matrix with increased cross-linking (e.g., aging collagen becomes more insoluble, chemically stable but rigid, resulting in decreased cell permeability), decreased synthesis, and increased degradation of collagen. The extracellular matrix determines the tissue's physical properties.[98] These changes, together with the disappearance of elastin and changes in proteoglycans and plasma proteins, cause disorders of the ground substance that result in dehydration and wrinkling of the skin (see Chapter 41). Other age-related defects in the extracellular matrix include skeletal muscle alterations (e.g., atrophy, decreased tone, loss of contractility), cataracts, diverticula, hernias, and rupture of intervertebral disks.

Free radicals of oxygen that result from oxidative cellular metabolism, *oxidative stress* (e.g., respiratory chain, phagocytosis, prostaglan-

din synthesis), damage tissues during the aging process. The oxygen radicals produced include superoxide radical, hydroxyl radical, and hydrogen peroxide (see p. 81). These oxygen products are extremely reactive and can damage nucleic acids, destroy polysaccharides, oxidize proteins, peroxidize unsaturated fatty acids, and kill and lyse cells. Oxidant effects on target cells can lead to malignant transformation, presumably through DNA damage. That progressive and cumulative damage from oxygen radicals may lead to harmful alterations in cellular function is consistent with those alterations of aging. This hypothesis is founded on the wear-and-tear theory of aging, which states that damages accumulate with time, decreasing the organism's ability to maintain a steady state. Because these oxygen-reactive species not only can permanently damage cells but also may lead to cell death, there is new support for their role in the aging process.

Of much interest is the relationship between aging and the disappearance or alteration of extracellular substances important for vessel integrity. With aging, lipid, calcium, and plasma proteins are deposited in vessel walls. These depositions cause serious basement membrane thickening and alterations in smooth muscle functioning, resulting in arteriosclerosis (a progressive disease that causes such problems as stroke, myocardial infarction, renal disease, and peripheral vascular disease).

Cellular Aging

Cellular changes characteristic of aging include atrophy, decreased function, and loss of cells, possibly caused by apoptosis (Figure 4-35). Loss of cellular function from any of these causes initiates the compensatory mechanisms of hypertrophy and hyperplasia of the remaining cells, which can lead to metaplasia, dysplasia, and neoplasia. All of these changes can alter receptor placement and function, nutrient pathways, secretion of cellular products, and neuroendocrine control mechanisms. In the aged cell, DNA, RNA, cellular proteins, and

FIGURE 4-35 Some Biologic Changes Associated with Aging. Insets show the proportion of remaining functions in the organs of a person in late adulthood compared with those of a 20-year-old.

membranes are most susceptible to injurious stimuli. DNA is particularly vulnerable to such injuries as breaks, deletions, and additions. Lack of DNA repair increases the cell's susceptibility to mutations that may be lethal or may promote the development of neoplasia (see Chapter 10).

Mitochondria are the organelles responsible for the generation of most of the energy used by eukaryotic cells. **Mitochondrial DNA (mtDNA)** encodes some of the proteins of the electron-transfer chain, the system necessary for the conversion of adenosine diphosphate (ADP) to ATP. Mutations in mtDNA can deprive the cell of ATP, and mutations are correlated with the aging process. The accumulation of mutations could be caused by errors in replication or by unrepaired damage.[99,100]

The most common age-related mtDNA mutation in humans is a large rearrangement called the *4977 deletion,* or *common deletion,* and is found in humans older than 40 years. It is a deletion that removes all or part of 7 of the 13 protein-encoding mtDNA genes and 5 of the 22 tRNA genes. Individual cells containing this deletion have a condition known as *heteroplasmy.* Heteroplasmy levels rise with aging. Cumulative damage of mtDNA is implicated in the progression of such common diseases as diabetes, cancer, heart failure, and neurodegenerative disorders.

Tissue and Systemic Aging

It is probably safe to say that every physiologic process functions less efficiently with increasing age. The most characteristic tissue change with age is a progressive stiffness or rigidity that affects many systems, including the arterial, pulmonary, and musculoskeletal systems. A consequence of blood vessel and organ stiffness is a progressive increase in peripheral resistance to blood flow. The movement of intracellular and extracellular substances also decreases with age, as does the diffusion capacity of the lung. Blood flow through organs also decreases.

Changes in the endocrine and immune systems include thymus atrophy. Although this occurs at puberty, causing a decreased immune response to T-dependent antigens (foreign proteins), increased formation of autoantibodies and immune complexes (antibodies that are bound to antigens) and an overall decrease in the immunologic tolerance for the host's own cells further diminish the effectiveness of the immune system later in life. In women the reproductive system loses ova, and in men spermatogenesis decreases. Responsiveness to hormones decreases in the breast and endometrium.

The stomach experiences decreases in the rate of emptying and secretion of hormones and hydrochloric acid. Muscular atrophy diminishes mobility by decreasing motor tone and contractility. **Sarcopenia**, loss of muscle mass and strength, can occur into old age. The skin of the aged individual is affected by atrophy and wrinkling of the epidermis and by alterations in the underlying dermis, fat, and muscle.

Total body changes include a decrease in height; a reduction in circumference of the neck, thighs, and arms; widening of the pelvis; and lengthening of the nose and ears. Several of these changes are the result of tissue atrophy and of decreased bone mass caused by osteoporosis and osteoarthritis. Some body composition changes include an increase in body weight, which begins in middle age (men gain until 50 years of age and women until 70 years), and an increase fat mass followed by a decrease in stature, weight, fat-free mass, and body cell mass at older ages. **Fat-free mass (FFM)** includes all minerals, proteins, and water plus all other constituents except lipids. As the amount of fat increases, the percentage of total body water decreases. Increased body fat and centralized fat distribution (abdominal area) are associated with non–insulin-dependent diabetes and heart disease. Total body potassium concentration also decreases because of decreased cellular mass. An increased sodium/potassium ratio suggests that the decreased cellular mass is accompanied by an increased extracellular compartment.

Although some of these alterations are probably inherent in aging, others represent consequences of the process. Advanced age increases susceptibility to disease, and death occurs after an injury or insult because of diminished cellular, tissue, and organ function.

Frailty

Frailty is a common clinical syndrome in older adults, leaving a person vulnerable to falls, functional decline, disability, disease, and death. With an increasing aged population worldwide efforts to promote independence and decrease frailty are challenging and needed. Sarcopenia and cachexia are common as a consequence of aging and many acute and chronic illnesses.[101] Investigators are grappling with a common nomenclature to develop consensus for definitions of sarcopenia and cachexia. One proposal has been to define it simply as "muscle wasting disease," which can be applied in both acute and chronic settings.[101] An acceptable vocabulary and classification system is yet to be developed.

The determinants of sarcopenia include environmental and genetic factors, which presently are poorly understood.[102] Common themes of mechanisms for sarcopenia include the following: (1) decrease in the number of skeletal muscle fibers, mainly type II fibers; (2) decline in muscle protein synthesis with age; (3) decline in muscle fractions, such as myofibrillar and mitochondrial, with age; (4) reduction in protein turnover adversely affecting muscle function by inducing protein loss and protein accumulation; (5) loss of alpha motor neurons in the spinal column; (6) dysregulation of anabolic hormones; (7) cytokine productions and inflammation; (8) inadequate nutrition; and (9) sedentary history.[102,103] For research and clinical purposes, the criteria indicating compromised energetics include low grip strength, slowed walking speed, low physical activity, and unintentional weight loss.[104] The syndrome is complex and involves other alterations such as osteopenia, cognitive impairment, anemia, and gender differences.

SOMATIC DEATH

Somatic death is death of the entire person. Unlike the changes that follow cellular death in a live body, **postmortem change** is diffuse and does not involve components of the inflammatory response. Within minutes after death, postmortem changes appear, eliminating any difficulty in determining that death has occurred. The most notable manifestations are complete cessation of respiration and circulation. The surface of the skin usually becomes pale and yellowish; however, the lifelike color of the cheeks and lips may persist after death that is caused by carbon monoxide poisoning, drowning, or chloroform poisoning.[105]

Body temperature falls gradually immediately after death and then more rapidly (approximately 1.0° to 1.5° F/hour) until, after 24 hours, body temperature equals that of the environment.[106] After death caused by certain infective diseases, body temperature may continue to rise for a short time. Postmortem reduction of body temperature is called **algor mortis**.

Blood pressure within the retinal vessels decreases, causing muscle tension to decrease and the pupils to dilate. The face, nose, and chin become sharp or peaked-looking as blood and fluids drain from these areas.[105] Gravity causes blood to settle in the most dependent, or lowest, tissues, which develop a purple discoloration called **livor mortis**. Incisions made at this time usually fail to cause bleeding. The skin loses its elasticity and transparency.

Within 6 hours after death, acidic compounds accumulate within the muscles because of the breakdown of carbohydrates and the depletion of ATP. This interferes with ATP-dependent detachment of myosin from actin (contractile proteins), and muscle stiffening, or rigor mortis, develops. The smaller muscles are usually affected first, particularly the muscles of the jaw. Within 12 to 14 hours, rigor mortis usually affects the entire body.

Signs of putrefaction are generally obvious about 24 to 48 hours after death. Rigor mortis gradually diminishes, and the body becomes flaccid at 36 to 62 hours. Putrefactive changes vary depending on the temperature of the environment. The most visible is greenish discoloration of the skin, particularly on the abdomen. The discoloration is thought to be related to the diffusion of hemolyzed blood into the tissues and the production of sulfhemoglobin, choleglobin, and other denatured hemoglobin derivatives.[106,107] Slippage or loosening of the skin from underlying tissues occurs at the same time. After this, swelling or bloating of the body and liquefactive changes occur, sometimes causing opening of the body cavities. At a microscopic level, putrefactive changes are associated with the release of enzymes and lytic dissolution called postmortem autolysis.

✔ **QUICK CHECK 4-5**

1. Aging is a complex process, discuss the multitude of mechanisms of aging.
2. What are the body composition changes that occur with aging?
3. Define frailty and possible endocrine-immune system involvement.

DID YOU UNDERSTAND?

Cellular Adaptation

1. Cellular adaptation is a reversible, structural, or functional response both to normal or physiologic conditions and to adverse or pathologic conditions. Cells can adapt to physiologic demands or stress to maintain a steady state called homeostasis.
2. The most significant adaptive changes include atrophy, hypertrophy, hyperplasia, and metaplasia.
3. Atrophy is a decrease in cellular size caused by aging, disuse, or reduced/absent blood supply, hormonal stimulation, or neural stimulation. The amounts of ER, mitochondria, and microfilaments decrease. The mechanisms of atrophy probably include decreased protein synthesis, increased protein catabolism, or both. A new hypothesis called ribosome biogenesis involves the role of mRNA and protein translation.
4. Hypertrophy is an increase in the size of cells in response to mechanical stimuli and consequently increases the size of the affected organ. The amounts of protein in the plasma membrane, ER, microfilaments, and mitochondria increase. Hypertrophy can be classified as physiologic or pathologic.
5. Hyperplasia is an increase in the number of cells caused by an increased rate of cellular division. Hyperplasia is classified as physiologic (compensatory and hormonal) and pathologic.
6. Metaplasia is the reversible replacement of one mature cell type by another less mature cell type.
7. Dysplasia, or atypical hyperplasia, is an abnormal change in the size, shape, and organization of mature tissue cells. It is considered atypical rather than a true adaptational change.

Cellular Injury

1. Injury to cells and to the extracellular matrix (ECM) leads to injury of tissues and organs and ultimately determining the structural patterns of disease. Cellular injury occurs if the cell is unable to maintain homeostasis—a normal or adaptive steady state—in the face of injurious stimuli or stress. Injured cells may recover (reversible injury) or die (irreversible injury).
2. Injury is caused by lack of oxygen (hypoxia), free radicals, caustic or toxic chemicals, infectious agents, inflammatory and immune responses, genetic factors, insufficient nutrients, or physical and mechanical trauma from many causes.
3. Four biochemical themes are important to cell injury: (1) ATP depletion, resulting in mitochondrial damage; (2) accumulation of oxygen and oxygen-derived free radicals, causing membrane damage; (3) protein folding defects; and (4) increased intracellular calcium concentration and loss of calcium steady state.
4. The sequence of events leading to cell death is commonly decreased ATP production, failure of active transport mechanisms (the sodium-potassium pump), cellular swelling, detachment of ribosomes from the ER, cessation of protein synthesis, mitochondrial swelling as a result of calcium accumulation, vacuolation, leakage of digestive enzymes from lysosomes, autodigestion of intracellular structures, lysis of the plasma membrane, and death.
5. The initial insult in hypoxic injury is usually ischemia (the cessation of blood flow into vessels that supply the cell with oxygen and nutrients).
6. Free radicals cause cellular injury because they have an unpaired electron that makes the molecule unstable. To stabilize itself, the molecule either donates or accepts an electron from another molecule. Therefore it forms injurious chemical bonds with proteins, lipids, and carbohydrates—key molecules in membranes and nucleic acids.
7. The damaging effects of free radicals, especially activated oxygen species such as O_2^-, OH•, and H_2O_2, called oxidative stress, include (1) peroxidation of lipids, (2) alteration of ion pumps and transport mechanisms, (3) fragmentation of DNA, and (4) damage to mitochondria, releasing calcium into the cytosol.
8. Restoration of oxygen, however, can cause additional injury, called reperfusion injury. The mechanisms discussed for reperfusion-injury include oxidative stress, increased intracellular calcium concentration, inflammation, and complement activation.
9. Humans are exposed to thousands of chemicals that have inadequate toxicologic data. A systems biology approach is now being used to investigate toxicity pathways that include oxidative stress, heat shock proteins, DNA damage response, hypoxia, ER stress, mental stress, inflammation, and osmotic stress.
10. Unintentional and intentional injuries are an important health problem in the United States. Death as a result of these injuries is more common for men than women and higher among blacks than whites and other racial groups.
11. Injuries by blunt force are the result of the application of mechanical energy to the body, resulting in tearing, shearing, or crushing of tissues. The most common types of blunt-force injuries include motor vehicle accidents and falls.
12. A contusion is bleeding into the skin or underlying tissues as a consequence of a blow. A collection of blood in soft tissues or an enclosed space may be referred to as a hematoma.
13. An abrasion (scrape) results from removal of the superficial layers of the skin caused by friction between the skin and injuring object. Abrasions and contusions may have a patterned appearance that mirrors the shape and features of the injuring object.

14. A laceration is a tear or rip resulting when the tensile strength of the skin or tissue is exceeded.

15. An incised wound is a cut that is longer than it is deep. A stab wound is a penetrating sharp-force injury that is deeper than it is long.

16. Gunshot wounds may be either penetrating (bullet retained in the body) or perforating (bullet exits the body). The most important factors determining the appearance of a gunshot injury are whether it is an entrance or an exit wound and the range of fire.

17. Asphyxial injuries are caused by a failure of cells to receive or utilize oxygen. These injuries can be grouped into four general categories: suffocation, strangulation, chemical, and drowning.

18. Activation of inflammation and immunity, which occurs after cellular injury or infection, involves powerful biochemicals and proteins capable of damaging normal (uninjured and uninfected) cells.

19. Genetic disorders injure cells by altering the nucleus and the plasma membrane's structure, shape, receptors, or transport mechanisms.

20. Deprivation of essential nutrients (proteins, carbohydrates, lipids, vitamins) can cause cellular injury by altering cellular structure and function, particularly of transport mechanisms, chromosomes, the nucleus, and DNA.

21. Injurious physical agents include temperature extremes, changes in atmospheric pressure, ionizing radiation, illumination, mechanical stresses, and noise.

22. Errors in health care are a leading cause of injury or death in the United States. Errors involve medicines, surgery, diagnosis, equipment, and laboratory reports. They can occur anywhere in the healthcare system including hospitals, clinics, outpatient surgery centers, physicians' and nurse practitioners' offices, pharmacies, and the individual's home.

Manifestations of Cellular Injury

1. An important manifestation of cell injury is the resultant metabolic disturbances of intracellular accumulation (infiltration) of abnormal amounts of various substances. Two categories of accumulations are (1) normal cellular substances, such as water, proteins, lipids, and carbohydrate excesses; and (2) abnormal substances, either endogenous (e.g., from abnormal metabolism) or exogenous (e.g., a virus).

2. Most accumulations are attributed to four types of mechanisms, all abnormal: (1) An endogenous substance is produced in excess or at an increased rate; (2) an abnormal substance, often the result of a mutated gene, accumulates; (3) an endogenous substance is not effectively catabolized; and (4) a harmful exogenous substance accumulates because of inhalation, ingestion, or infection.

3. Accumulations harm cells by "crowding" the organelles and by causing excessive (and sometimes harmful) metabolites to be produced during their catabolism. The metabolites are released into the cytoplasm or expelled into the extracellular matrix.

4. Cellular swelling, the accumulation of excessive water in the cell, is caused by the failure of transport mechanisms and is a sign of many types of cellular injury. Oncosis is a type of cellular death resulting from cellular swelling.

5. Accumulations of organic substances—lipids, carbohydrates, glycogen, proteins, pigments—are caused by disorders in which (1) cellular uptake of the substance exceeds the cell's capacity to catabolize (digest) or use it or (2) cellular anabolism (synthesis) of the substance exceeds the cell's capacity to use or secrete it.

6. Dystrophic calcification (accumulation of calcium salts) is always a sign of pathologic change because it occurs only in injured or dead cells. Metastatic calcification, however, can occur in uninjured cells in individuals with hypercalcemia.

7. Disturbances in urate metabolism can result in hyperuricemia and deposition of sodium urate crystals in tissue—leading to a painful disorder called gout.

8. Systemic manifestations of cellular injury include fever, leukocytosis, increased heart rate, pain, and serum elevations of enzymes in the plasma.

Cellular Death

1. Cellular death has historically been classified as necrosis and apoptosis. Necrosis is characterized by rapid loss of the plasma membrane structure, organelle swelling, mitochondrial dysfunction, and the lack of features of apoptosis. Apoptosis is known as regulated or programmed cell death and is characterized by "dropping off" of cellular fragments, called apoptotic bodies. It is now understood that under certain conditions necrosis is regulated or programmed, hence the new term *programmed necrosis*, or necroptosis.

2. There are four major types of necrosis: coagulative, liquefactive, caseous, and fatty. Different types of necrosis occur in different tissues.

3. Structural signs that indicate irreversible injury and progression to necrosis are the dense clumping and disruption of genetic material and the disruption of the plasma and organelle membranes.

4. Apoptosis, a distinct type of sublethal injury, is a process of selective cellular self-destruction that occurs in both normal and pathologic tissue changes.

5. Death by apoptosis causes loss of cells in many pathologic states including (1) severe cell injury, (2) accumulation of misfolded proteins, (3) infections, and (4) obstruction in tissue ducts.

6. Excessive accumulation of misfolded proteins in the ER leads to a condition known as endoplasmic reticulum stress. ER stress results in apoptotic cell death and this mechanism has been linked to several degenerative diseases of the CNS and other organs.

7. Excessive or insufficient apoptosis is known as dysregulated apoptosis.

8. Autophagy means "eating of self," and as a recycling factory it is a self-destructive process and a survival mechanism. When cells are starved or nutrient deprived, the autophagic process institutes cannibalization and recycles the digested contents. Autophagy can maintain cellular metabolism under starvation conditions and remove damaged organelles under stress conditions, improving the survival of cells. Autophagy declines and becomes less efficient as the cell ages, thus contributing to the aging process.

9. Gangrenous necrosis, or gangrene, is tissue necrosis caused by hypoxia and the subsequent bacterial invasion.

Aging and Altered Cellular and Tissue Biology

1. It is difficult to determine the physiologic (normal) from the pathologic changes of aging. Investigators are focused on genetic, epigenetic, inflammatory, oxidative stress, and metabolic origins of aging.

2. Important factors in aging include increased damage to the cell, reduced capacity to divide, reduced ability to repair damaged DNA, and increased likelihood of defective protein balance or homeostasis.

3. Frailty is a common clinical syndrome in older adults, leaving a person vulnerable to falls, functional decline, disability, disease, and death. Sarcopenia and cachexia are common as a consequence of aging.

Somatic Death

1. Somatic death is death of the entire organism. Postmortem change is diffuse and does not involve the inflammatory response.
2. Manifestations of somatic death include cessation of respiration and circulation, gradual lowering of body temperature, dilation of the pupils, loss of elasticity and transparency in the skin, stiffening of the muscles (rigor mortis), and discoloration of the skin (livor mortis). Signs of putrefaction are obvious about 24 to 48 hours after death.

KEY TERMS

Adaptation, 73
Aging, 107
Algor mortis, 109
Anoxia, 80
Anthropogenic, 93
Apoptosis, 104
Asphyxial injury, 94
Atrophy, 74
Autolysis, 102
Autophagic vacuole, 74
Autophagy, 105
Bilirubin, 100
Carbon monoxide (CO), 90
Carboxyhemoglobin, 90
Caseous necrosis, 103
Caspase, 105
Cellular accumulations (infiltrations), 96
Cellular swelling, 97
Chemical asphyxiant, 96
Choking asphyxiation, 94
Coagulative necrosis, 102
Compensatory hyperplasia, 76
Cyanide, 96
Cytochrome, 100
Disuse atrophy, 74
Drowning, 96

Dry-lung drowning, 96
Dysplasia (atypical hyperplasia), 77
Dystrophic calcification, 100
Electrophile, 84
Endoplasmic reticulum stress (ER stress), 104
Ethanol, 90
Fat-free mass (FFM), 109
Fatty change (steatosis), 98
Fatty necrosis, 103
Fetal alcohol syndrome, 92
Frailty, 109
Free radical, 81
Gangrenous necrosis, 104
Gas gangrene, 104
Hanging strangulation, 95
Hemoprotein, 100
Hemosiderin, 100
Hemosiderosis, 100
Hormonal hyperplasia, 76
Hydrogen sulfide, 96
Hyperplasia, 76
Hypertrophy, 75
Hypoxia, 78
Hypoxia-inducible factor (HIF), 79

Infarct, 103
Irreversible injury, 78
Ischemia, 79
Ischemia-reperfusion injury, 81
Karyolysis, 102
Karyorrhexis, 102
Lead, 87
Life expectancy, 108
Life span, 107
Ligature strangulation, 96
Lipid peroxidation, 82
Lipofuscin, 75
Liquefactive necrosis, 103
Livor mortis, 109
Manual strangulation, 96
Maximal life span, 108
Melanin, 99
Mesenchymal (tissue from embryonic mesoderm) cell, 77
Metaplasia, 77
Metastatic calcification, 100
Mitochondrial DNA (mtDNA), 109
Necrosis, 102
Nucleophile, 84
Oncosis (vacuolar degeneration), 97

Oxidative stress, 81
Pathologic atrophy, 74
Pathologic hyperplasia, 76
Physiologic atrophy, 74
Postmortem autolysis, 110
Postmortem change, 109
Programmed necrosis (necroptosis), 101
Protein adduct, 85
Proteasome, 74
Psammoma body, 100
Pyknosis, 102
Reperfusion injury, 81
Reversible injury, 78
Rigor mortis, 110
Sarcopenia, 109
Somatic death, 109
Strangulation, 95
Suffocation, 94
Toxicophore, 84
Ubiquitin, 74
Ubiquitin-proteasome pathway, 74
Urate, 101
Vacuolation, 81
Xenobiotic, 84

REFERENCES

1. Kumar V et al, editors: *Pathology*, St Louis, 2014, Elsevier.
2. Chaillou T et al: Ribosome biogenesis: emerging evidence for a central role in the regulation of skeletal muscle mass, *J Cell Physiol* 2014 Mar 7. [Epub ahead of print.]
3. Lam MPY et al: Protein kinetic signatures of the remodeling heart following isoproterenol stimulation, *J Clin Invest* 124(4):1734-1744, 2014.
4. Cacciapuoti F: Role of ubiquitin-proteasome system (UPS) in left ventricular hypertrophy (LVH), *Am J Cardiovasc Dis* 4(1):1-5, 2014.
5. Hill JA, Olson EN: Cardiac plasticity, *N Engl J Med* 358(13):1370-1380, 2008.
6. Leri A et al: Role of cardiac stem cells in cardiac pathophysiology: a paradigm shift in human myocardial biology, *Circ Res* 109:941-961, 2011.
7. Hariharan N et al: Autophagy plays an essential role in mediating regression of hypertrophy during unloading of the heart, *PLos One* 8(1):e51632, 2013.
8. Zafeiridis A et al: Regression of cellular hypertrophy after left ventricular assist device support, *Circulation* 98:656d-662d, 1998.
9. Depre C et al: Unloaded heart in vivo replicates fetal gene expression of cardiac hypertrophy, *Nat Med* 4:1269-1275, 1998.
10. Friddle CJ et al: Expression profiling reveals distinct sets of genes altered during induction and regression of cardiac hypertrophy, *Proc Natl Acad Sci U S A* 97:6745-6750, 2000.
11. Jiang Y et al: Dietary copper supplementation reverses hypertrophic cardiomyopathy induced by chronic pressure overload in mice, *J Exp Med* 204:657-666, 2007.
12. Zhou Y et al: Copper reverses cardiomyocyte hypertrophy through vascular endothelial growth factor-mediated reduction in the cell size, *J Mol Cell Cardiol* 45:106-117, 2008.
13. Zhou Y et al: Copper-induced regression of cardiomyocyte hypertrophy is associated with enhanced vascular endothelial growth factor receptor-1 signalling pathway, *Cardiovasc Res* 84:54-63, 2009.
14. Alberts B et al: *Essential cell biology*, ed 4, New York, 2014, Garland Press.
15. Hamanaka RB, Chandel NS: Mitochondrial reactive oxygen species regulate hypoxic signaling, *Curr Opin Cell Biol* 21(6):894-899, 2009.
16. Eltzschig HK, Carmeliet P: Hypoxia and inflammation, *N Engl J Med* 364(7):656-665, 2011.
17. Choi HJ et al: ECM-dependent HIF induction directs trophoblast stem cell fate via LIMK1-mediated cytoskeletal rearrangement, *PLoS One* 8(2):e56949, 2013.
18. Choksi S et al: A HIF-1, ATIA, protects cells from apoptosis by modulating the mitochondrial thioredoxin, TRX2, *Mol Cell* 42(5):597-609, 2011.
19. Wang ZJ et al: The effect of intravenous vitamin C infusion on periprocedural myocardial injury for patients undergoing elective percutaneous coronary intervention, *Can J Cardiol* 30(1):96-101, 2014.
20. Rodrigo R et al: The effectiveness of antioxidant vitamins C and E in reducing myocardial infarct size in patients subjected to percutaneous coronary angioplasty (PREVEC Trial): study protocol for a pilot randomized double-blind controlled trial, *Trials* 15:192, 2014.
21. Oka T et al: Mitochondrial DNA that escapes from autophagy causes inflammation and heart failure, *Nature* 485(7397):251-255, 2012.
22. Tice RR et al: Improving the human hazard characterization of chemicals: a TOX21 update, *Environ Health Perspect* 121:756-765, 2013.
23. Seeff LB: Herbal hepatotoxicity, *Clin Liver Dis* 11:577-596, 2007.
24. Carithers RL Jr, McClain CJ: Alcoholic liver disease. In Sleisenger MH et al, editors: *Sleisenger and Fordtran's gastrointestinal and liver disease: pathophysiology, diagnosis, management*, ed 9, pp 1383-1400, Philadelphia, 2010, Saunders/Elsevier.
25. Gu X, Manautou JE: Molecular mechanisms underlying chemical liver injury, *Exp Rev Mol Med* 14:e4, 2013.
26. Jones DP, Delong MJ: Detoxification and protective functions of nutrients. In Stipanuk M, editor: *Biochemical and physiological aspects of nutrition*, Philadelphia, 2000, Saunders.
27. Hanzlik RP et al: The reactive metabolite target protein database (TPDB)—a web-accessible resource, *BMC Bioinformatics* 8:95, 2007.
28. Liebler DC, Guengerich FP: Elucidating mechanisms of drug-induced toxicity, *Nature* 4:410-420, 2005.
29. Gunnell D et al: Use of paracetamol (acetaminophen) for suicide and nonfatal

poisoning: worldwide patterns of use and misuse, *Suicide Life Threat Behav* 30:313-326, 2000.

30. Grespan R et al: Hepatoprotective effect of pretreatment with thymus vulgaris essential oil in experimental model of acetaminophen-induced injury, *Evid Based Complement Alternat Med* 2014:954136, 2014.

31. Occupational Safety and Health Administration: *Lead*, Washington, DC, 2012, U.S. Department of Labor.

32. Murata K et al: Lead toxicity: does the critical level of lead resulting in adverse effects differ between adults and children? *J Occup Health* 51(1):1-12, 2009.

33. Gibson JL: A plea for painted railings and painted walls of rooms as the source of lead poisoning amongst Queensland children, 1904, *Public Health Rep* 120:301, 2005.

34. Gilbert SG, Weiss B: A rationale for lowering the blood lead action level from 10 to 2 microg/dL, *Neurotoxicol* 27:693, 2006.

35. Jacobs DE et al: The prevalence of lead-based paint hazards in U.S. housing, *Environ Health Perspect* 110:599, 2002.

36. Neal AP, Guilarte TR: Mechanisms of lead and manganese neurotoxicity, *Toxicol Res* 2:99-114, 2013.

37. Nichani WI et al: Blood lead levels in children after phase-out of leaded gasoline in Bombay, India, *Sci Total Environ* 363:95, 2006.

38. Pirkle L et al: Exposure of the U.S. population to lead, 1991-1994, *Environ Health Perspect* 106:745, 1998.

39. Stromberg U et al: Yearly measurements of blood lead in Swedish children since 1978: the declining trend continues in the petrol-lead-free period 1995-2007, *Environ Res* 107:332, 2008.

40. Luo XS et al: Distribution, availability, and sources of trace metals in different particle size fractions of urban soils in Hong Kong: implications for assessing the risk to human health, *Environ Pollut* 159:1317, 2011.

41. United States Environmental Protection Agency: *Final Revisions to the National Quality Air Standards for Lead*, Lead fact sheet, Washington, DC, 2008, Author. Available at http://www.epa.gov/air/lead/pdfs/20081015pbfactsheet.pdf.

42. Centers for Disease Control and Prevention (CDC): *Blood lead levels in children aged 1-5 years—United States, 1999-2010*, Atlanta, GA, 2013, CDC.

43. Morris RG et al: Selective impairment of learning and blockade of long-term potentiation by an N-methyl-D-aspartate receptor antagonist, AP5, *Nature* 319(6056):774-776, 1986.

44. Konur S, Ghosh A: Calcium signaling and the control of dendritic development, *Neuron* 46:401-405, 2005.

45. Waites CL, Garner CC: Presynaptic function in health and disease, *Trends Neurosci* 34:326-337, 2011.

46. Jomova K, Valko M: Advances in metal-induced oxidative stress and human disease, *Toxicology* 283:65-87, 2011.

47. Abadin H et al: *Toxicological profile for lead*. Atlanta, GA, 2007, Agency for Toxic Substances and Disease Registry (US).

48. Kumar V et al, editors: *Robbins and Cotran pathologic basis of disease*, ed 9, St Louis, 2015, Saunders/Elsevier.

49. Romanoff R et al: Acute ethanol exposure inhibits renal folate transport, but repeated exposure upregulates folate transport proteins in rats and human cells, *J Nutr* 137:1260-1265, 2007.

50. Tsai ST et al: The interplay between alcohol consumption, oral hygiene, ALDH2, and ADH1B in the risk of head and neck cancer, *Int J Cancer* 2014 Apr10. [Epub ahead of print.]

51. Hines LM et al: Alcoholism: the dissection for endophenotypes, *Dialogues Clin Neurosci* 7(2):153-163, 2005.

52. Rostron B: Epidemiology alcohol consumption and mortality risks in the USA, *Alcohol Alcohol* 47(3):334-339, 2012.

53. Connor J: The life and times of the j-shaped curve, *Alcohol Alcohol* 41:583-584, 2006.

54. Krenz M, Korthuis RJ: Moderate ethanol ingestion and cardiovascular protection: from epidemiologic associations to cellular mechanisms, *J Mol Cell Cardiol* 52(1):93-104, 2013.

55. American Heart Association: *Alcohol and heart disease*, Dallas, TX, 2014, Author.

56. Costanzo S et al: Cardiovascular and overall mortality risk in relation to alcohol consumption in patients with cardiovascular disease, *Circulation* 121:1951-1959, 2010.

57. Spörndly-Nees S et al: Leisure-time physical activity predicts complaints of snoring in women: a prospective cohort study over 10 years, *Sleep Med* 15:415-421, 2014.

58. Nassir F, Ibdah JA: Role of mitochondria in alcoholic liver disease, *World J Gastroenterol* 20(9):2136-2142, 2014.

59. Leiber CS: Metabolism of alcohol, *Clin Liver Dis* 9(1):1-35, 2005.

60. Curtis BJ et al: Epigenetic targets for reversing immune defects caused by alcohol exposure, *Alcohol Res* 35(1):97-113, 2013.

61. Sadrian B et al: Long-lasting circuit dysfunction following developmental ethanol exposure, *Brain Sci* 3(2):704-727, 2013.

62. Govorko D et al: Male germline transmits fetal alcohol adverse effect on hypothalamic proopiomelanocortin gene across generations, *Biol Psychiatry* 72:378-388, 2012.

63. Burd L et al: Prenatal alcohol exposure, blood alcohol concentrations and alcohol elimination rates for the mother, fetus and newborn, *J Perinatol* 32(9):652-659, 2012.

64. UNEP: *Global mercury assessment 2013: sources, emissions, releases and environmental transport*, Geneva, Switzerland, 2013, UNEP Chemicals Branch.

65. Mortazavi SM et al: High-field MRI and mercury release from dental amalgam fillings, *Int J Occup Med* 5(2):101-105, 2014.

66. Geier DA et al: A dose-dependent relationship between mercury exposure from dental amalgams and urinary mercury levels: a further assessment of the Casa Pia Children's Dental Amalgam Trial, *Hum Exp Toxicol* 31(1):11-17, 2012.

67. Homme KG et al: New science challenges old notion that mercury dental amalgam is safe, *Biometals* 27(1):19-24, 2014.

68. Schecter R, Grether JK: Continuing increases in autism reported to California's developmental services system: mercury in retrograde, *Arch Gen Psychiatry* 65(1):19-24, 2008.

69. Centers for Disease Control and Prevention: CDC 24/7: Saving lives, protecting people. In: *All injuries. Health, United States*, 2013.

70. Hitomi J et al: Identification of a molecular signaling network that regulates a cellular necrotic cell death pathway by a genome wide siRNA screen, *Cell* 135(7):1311-1323, 2008.

71. Moquin D, Chan F: The molecular regulation of programmed necrotic cell injury, *Trends Biochem Sci* 35(8):434-441, 2010.

72. Smith CC, Yellon DM: Necroptosis, necrostatins and tissue injury, *J Cell Mol Med* 15(9):1797-1806, 2011.

73. Wang Z et al: The mitochondrial phosphatase PGAM5 functions at the convergence point of multiple necrotic death pathways, *Cell* 148:228-243, 2012.

74. Raloff J: Coming to terms with death: accurate descriptions of a cell's demise may offer clues to diseases and treatments, *Sci News* 159:378-380, 2001.

75. Glick D et al: Autophagy: cellular and molecular mechanisms, *J Pathol* 221(1):3-12, 2010.

76. Ge L et al: The protein-vesicle network of autophagy, *Curr Opin Cell Biol* 29:18-24, 2014.

77. Dancourt J, Melia TJ: Lipidation of the autophagy proteins LC3 and GABARAP is a membrane-curvature dependent process, *Autophagy* 10(8):2014 June 12. [Epub ahead of print.]

78. Mizushima N: Autophagy: process and function, *Genes Dev* 21(22):2861-2873, 2007, review.

79. Shen HM, Mizushima N: At the end of the autophagic road: an emerging understanding of lysosomal functions in autophagy, *Trends Biochem Sci* 39(2):61-71, 2014.

80. Butow RA, Avadhani NG: Mitochondrial signaling: the retrograde response, *Mol Cell* 14(1):1-15, 2004.

81. Levine B et al: Autophagy in immunity and inflammation, *Nature* 469:323-335, 2011.

82. Tissenbaum HA: Genetics, life span, health span, and the aging process in *Caenorhabditis elegans*, *J Gerontol A Biol Sci Med Sci* 67A(5):503-510, 2012.

83. Rando TA, Chang HY: Aging rejuvenation, and epigenetic reprogramming: resetting the aging clock, *Cell* 148:46-57, 2012.

84. Campisi J, Vijg J: Does damage to DNA and other macromolecules play a role in aging? If so, how? *J Gerontol A Biol Sci Med Sci* 64:175-178, 2009.

85. Seviour EG, Lin SY: The DNA damage response: balancing the scale between cancer and ageing, *Aging (Albany, NY)* 2:900-907, 2010.

86. Charville GW, Rando TA: Stem cell ageing and non-random chromosome segregation, *Philos Trans R Soc Lond B Biol Sci* 366:85-93, 2011.

87. Kuilman T et al: The essence of senescence, *Genes Dev* 24:2463-2479, 2010.

88. Fontana L et al: Extending healthy life span—from yeast to humans, *Science* 328:321-326, 2010.

89. Kenyon CJ: The genetics of ageing, *Nature* 464:504-512, 2010.

90. Takahashi K, Yamanaka S: Induction of pluripotent stem cells from mouse embryonic and adult fibroblast cultures by defined factors, *Cell* 126:663-676, 2006.

91. Hanna JH et al: Pluripotency and cellular reprogramming: facts, hypotheses, unresolved issues, *Cell* 143:508-525, 2010.

92. Villeda SA et al: Age-related changes in the systemic milieu regulate adult neurogenesis, *Nature* 477:90-94, 2011.

93. Loffredo FS et al: Growth differentiation factor 11 is a circulating factor that reverses age-related cardiac hypertrophy, *Cell* 153:828-839, 2013.

94. Harrison DE et al: Rapamycin fed late in life extends lifespan in genetically heterogeneous mice, *Nature* 460:392-395, 2009.

95. Armstrong L et al: The epigenetic contribution to stem cell ageing—can we rejuvenate our older cells? *Stem Cells* 2014 Apr 16. [Epub ahead of print.]

96. Greer EL et al: Transgenerational epigenetic inheritance of longevity in *Caenorhabditis elegans*, *Nature* 479:365-371, 2011.

97. Centers for Disease Control and Prevention (CDC): *National Vital Statist Rep* 62(7), 2009, United States Life Tables, Washington, DC, 2014, U.S. Department of Health and Human Services.

98. Fausto A et al: Liver regeneration, *Hepatology* 43:S45-S53, 2006.

99. Itsara LS et al: Oxidative stress is not a major contributor to somatic mitochondrial DNA mutations, *PLoS Genet* 10(2):e1003974, 2014.

100. Sevini F et al: mtDNA mutations in human aging and longevity: controversies and new perspectives opened by high-throughput technologies, *Exp Gerontol* 2014 Apr 5. [Epub ahead of print.] Available at http://dx.doi.org/10.1016/j.exger.2014.03.022.

101. Anker SD et al: Muscle wasting disease: a proposal for a new disease classification, *J Cachexia Sarcopenia Muscle* 5(1):1-3, 2014.

102. Walrand S et al: Physiopathological mechanism of sarcopenia, *Clin Geriatr Med* 27:365-385, 2011.

103. Ali S, Garcia JM: Sarcopenia, cachexia and aging: diagnosis, mechanism and therapeutic options—a mini-review, *Gerontology* 2014 Apr 8. [Epub ahead of print.]

104. Walston JD: *Clin Geriatr Med* 27(1), 2011.

105. Shennan T: *Postmortems and morbid anatomy*, ed 3, Baltimore, 1935, William Wood.

106. Riley MW: Foreword: the gender paradox. In Ory MG, Warner HR, editors: *Gender, health, and longevity: multidisciplinary perspectives*, New York, 1990, Springer.

107. Katsumata Y et al: Green pigments in epidermal blisters of decomposed cadavers, *Forensic Sci Int* 28(3-4):167-174, 1985.

5

Fluids and Electrolytes, Acids and Bases

Sue E. Huether

ⓔ EVOLVE WEBSITE

http://evolve.elsevier.com/Huether/
Student Review Questions
Audio Key Points

Case Studies
Animations
Quick Check Answers

The cells of the body live in a fluid environment with electrolyte and acid-base concentrations maintained within a narrow range. Changes in electrolyte concentration affect the electrical activity of nerve and muscle cells and cause shifts of fluid from one compartment to another. Alterations in acid-base balance disrupt cellular functions. Fluid fluctuations also affect blood volume and cellular function. Disturbances in these functions are common and can be life-threatening. Understanding how alterations occur and how the body compensates or corrects the disturbance is important for comprehending many pathophysiologic conditions.

DISTRIBUTION OF BODY FLUIDS AND ELECTROLYTES

The sum of fluids within all body compartments constitutes total body water (TBW)—about 60% of body weight in adults (Table 5-1). The volume of TBW is usually expressed as a percentage of body weight in kilograms. One liter of water weighs 2.2 lb (1 kg). The rest of the body weight is composed of fat and fat-free solids, particularly bone.

Body fluids are distributed among functional compartments, or spaces, and provide a transport medium for cellular and tissue function. Intracellular fluid (ICF) comprises all the fluid within cells, about two thirds of TBW. Extracellular fluid (ECF) is all the fluid outside the cells (about one third of TBW) and includes the interstitial fluid (the space between cells and outside the blood vessels) and the intravascular fluid (blood plasma) (Table 5-2). The total volume of body water for a 70-kg person is about 42 liters. Other ECF

compartments include lymph and transcellular fluids, such as synovial, intestinal, and cerebrospinal fluid; sweat; urine; and pleural, peritoneal, pericardial, and intraocular fluids.

Electrolytes and other solutes are distributed throughout the intracellular and extracellular fluid (Table 5-3). Note that the extracellular fluid contains a large amount of *sodium* and *chloride* and a small amount of *potassium*, whereas the opposite is true of the intracellular fluid. The concentrations of *phosphates* and *magnesium* are greater in the intracellular fluid and the concentration of *calcium* is greater in the extracellular fluid. These differences are important for the maintenance of electroneutrality between the extracellular and intracellular compartments, the transmission of electrical impulses, and the movement of water among body compartments (see Chapter 1).

Although the amount of fluid within the various compartments is relatively constant, solutes (e.g., salts) and water are exchanged between compartments to maintain their unique compositions. The percentage of TBW varies with the amount of body fat and age. Because fat is water repelling (hydrophobic), very little water is contained in adipose (fat) cells. Individuals with more body fat have proportionately less TBW and tend to be more susceptible to dehydration.

The distribution and the amount of TBW change with age (see the *Pediatric Considerations* and *Geriatric Considerations* boxes), and although daily fluid intake may fluctuate widely, the body regulates water volume within a relatively narrow range. Water obtained by drinking, water ingested in food, and water derived from oxidative metabolism are the primary sources of body water. Normally, the largest amounts of water are lost through renal excretion, with lesser

TABLE 5-1   Total Body Water (%) in Relation to Body Weight*

Body Build	Adult Male	Adult Female	Child (1-10 yr)	Infant (1 mo to 1 yr)	Newborn (Up to 1 mo)
Normal	60	50	65	70	70-80
Lean	70	60	50-60	80	
Obese	50	42	50	60	

*NOTE: Total body water is a percentage of body weight.

TABLE 5-2   Distribution of Body Water (70-kg Man)

Fluid Compartment	% of Body Weight	Volume (L)
Intracellular fluid (ICF)	40	28
Extracellular fluid (ECF)	20	14
Interstitial	15	11
Intravascular	5	3
Total body water (TBW)	60	42

TABLE 5-3   Representative Distribution of Electrolytes in Body Compartments

Electrolytes	ECF (mEq/L)	ICF (mEq/L)
Cations		
Sodium	142	12
Potassium	4.2	150
Calcium	5	0
Magnesium	2	24
TOTAL	153.2	186
Anions		
Bicarbonate	24	12
Chloride	103	4
Phosphate	2	100
Proteins	16	65
Other anions	8	6
TOTAL	153	187

ECF, Extracellular fluid; *ICF*, intracellular fluid.

TABLE 5-4   Normal Water Gains and Losses (70-kg Man)

	Daily Intake (mL)		Daily Output (mL)
Drinking	1400-1800	Urine	1400-1800
Water in food	700-1000	Stool	100
Water of oxidation	300-400	Skin	300-500
		Lungs	600-800
TOTAL	2400-3200	**TOTAL**	2400-3200

amounts lost through the stool and vaporization from the skin and lungs (insensible water loss) (Table 5-4).

Water Movement Between Plasma and Interstitial Fluid

The distribution of water and the movement of nutrients and waste products between the capillary and interstitial spaces occur as a result of changes in hydrostatic pressure (pushes water) and osmotic/oncotic pressure (pulls water) at the arterial and venous ends of the capillary (see Figure 1-24). Water, sodium, and glucose readily move across the capillary membrane. The plasma proteins normally do not cross the capillary membrane and maintain effective osmolality by generating plasma oncotic pressure (particularly albumin).

As plasma flows from the arterial to the venous end of the capillary, four forces determine if fluid moves out of the capillary and into the interstitial space (filtration) or if fluid moves back into the capillary from the interstitial space (reabsorption). These forces acting together are described as net filtration or Starling forces:

1. Capillary hydrostatic pressure (blood pressure) facilitates the outward movement of water from the capillary to the interstitial space.
2. Capillary (plasma) oncotic pressure osmotically attracts water from the interstitial space back into the capillary.
3. Interstitial hydrostatic pressure facilitates the inward movement of water from the interstitial space into the capillary.
4. Interstitial oncotic pressure osmotically attracts water from the capillary into the interstitial space.

The forces moving fluid back and forth across the capillary wall are summarized below:

Net filtration = (Forces favoring filtration) − (Forces opposing filtration)

Forces favoring filtration = Capillary hydrostatic pressure and interstitial oncotic pressure

Forces opposing filtration = Capillary oncotic pressure and interstitial hydrostatic pressure

At the arterial end of the capillary, hydrostatic pressure exceeds capillary oncotic pressure and fluid moves into the interstitial space (filtration). At the venous end of the capillary, capillary oncotic pressure exceeds capillary hydrostatic pressure and fluids are attracted back into the circulation (reabsorption). Interstitial hydrostatic pressure promotes the movement of about 10% of the interstitial fluid along with small amounts of protein into the lymphatics, which then returns to the circulation. Because albumin does not normally cross the capillary membrane, interstitial oncotic pressure is normally minimal. Figure 5-1 illustrates net filtration.

Water Movement Between ICF and ECF

Water moves between ICF and ECF compartments primarily as a function of osmotic forces (see Chapter 1 for definitions). Water moves freely by diffusion through the lipid bilayer cell membrane and through aquaporins, a family of water channel proteins that provide permeability to water.[1] Sodium is responsible for the ECF osmotic balance, and potassium maintains the ICF osmotic balance. The osmotic force of ICF proteins and other nondiffusible substances is balanced by the active transport of ions out of the cell. Water crosses cell membranes freely, so the osmolality of TBW is normally at equilibrium. Normally the ICF is not subject to rapid changes in osmolality, but when ECF osmolality changes, water moves from one compartment to another until osmotic equilibrium is reestablished (see Figure 5-7, p. 120).

ALTERATIONS IN WATER MOVEMENT

Edema

Edema is excessive accumulation of fluid within the interstitial spaces. The forces favoring fluid movement from the capillaries or lymphatic channels into the tissues are increased capillary hydrostatic pressure,

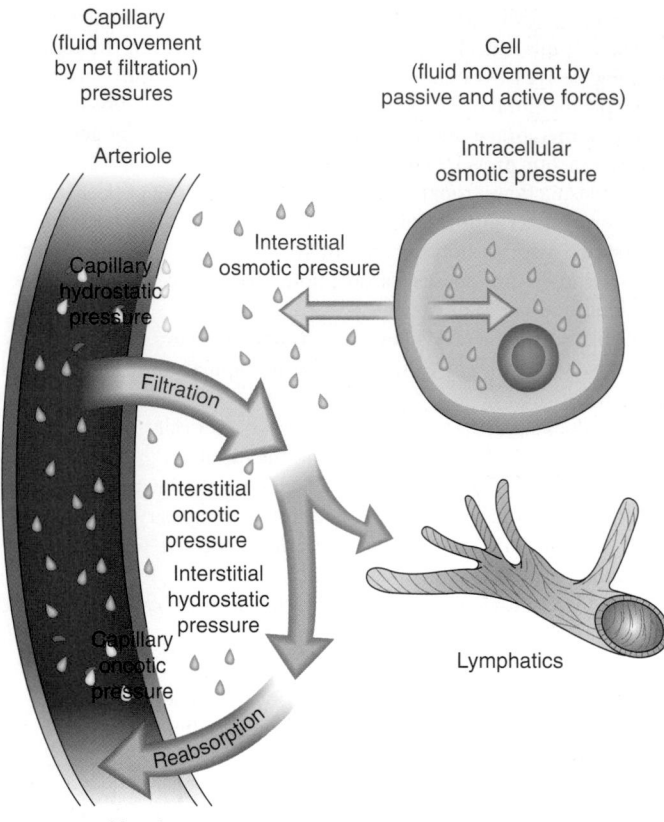

FIGURE 5-1 Net Filtration—Fluid Movement between Plasma and Interstitial Space. The movement of fluid between the vascular, interstitial spaces and the lymphatics is the result of net filtration of fluid across the semipermeable capillary membrane. Capillary hydrostatic pressure is the primary force for fluid movement out of the arteriolar end of the capillary and into the interstitial space. At the venous end, capillary oncotic pressure (from plasma proteins) attracts water back into the vascular space. Interstitial hydrostatic pressure promotes the movement of fluid and proteins into the lymphatics. Osmotic pressure accounts for the movement of fluid between the interstitial space and the intracellular space. Normally, intracellular and extracellular fluid osmotic pressures are equal (280 to 294 mOsm) and water is equally distributed between the interstitial and intracellular compartments.

decreased plasma oncotic pressure, increased capillary membrane permeability, and lymphatic channel obstruction[2] (Figure 5-2).

PATHOPHYSIOLOGY   Capillary hydrostatic pressure increases as a result of venous obstruction or salt and water retention. Venous obstruction causes hydrostatic pressure to increase behind the obstruction, pushing fluid from the capillaries into the interstitial spaces. Thrombophlebitis (inflammation of veins), hepatic obstruction, tight clothing around the extremities, and prolonged standing are common causes of venous obstruction. Congestive heart failure, renal failure, and cirrhosis of the liver are associated with excessive salt and water retention, which cause plasma volume overload, increased capillary hydrostatic pressure, and edema.

Since plasma albumin acts like a magnet to attract water, the loss or diminished production (e.g., from liver disease or protein malnutrition) contributes to decreased plasma oncotic pressure. Plasma proteins are lost in glomerular diseases of the kidney, serous drainage from open wounds, hemorrhage, burns, and cirrhosis of the liver. The

decreased oncotic attraction of fluid within the capillary causes filtered capillary fluid to remain in the interstitial space, resulting in edema.

Capillaries become more permeable with inflammation and immune responses, especially with trauma such as burns or crushing injuries, neoplastic disease, and allergic reactions. Proteins escape from the vascular space and produce edema through decreased capillary oncotic pressure and interstitial fluid protein accumulation.

The lymphatic system normally absorbs interstitial fluid and a small amount of proteins. When lymphatic channels are blocked or surgically removed, proteins and fluid accumulate in the interstitial space, causing **lymphedema**.[3] For example, lymphedema of the arm or leg occurs after surgical removal of axillary or femoral lymph nodes, respectively, for treatment of carcinoma. Inflammation or tumors may cause lymphatic obstruction, leading to edema of the involved tissues.

CLINICAL MANIFESTATIONS   Edema may be localized or generalized. *Localized edema* is usually limited to a site of trauma, as in a sprained finger. Another kind of localized edema occurs within particular organ systems and includes cerebral, pulmonary, and laryngeal edema; pleural effusion (fluid accumulation in the pleural space); pericardial effusion (fluid accumulation within the membrane around the heart); and ascites (accumulation of fluid in the peritoneal space). Edema of specific organs, such as the brain, lung, or larynx, can be life-threatening. *Generalized edema* is manifested by a more uniform distribution of fluid in interstitial spaces. Dependent edema, in which fluid accumulates in gravity-dependent areas of the body, might signal more generalized edema. Dependent edema appears in the feet and legs when standing and in the sacral area and buttocks when supine (lying on back). It can be identified by pressing on tissues overlying bony prominences. A pit left in the skin indicates edema (hence the term *pitting edema*) (Figure 5-3).

Edema usually is associated with weight gain, swelling and puffiness, tight-fitting clothes and shoes, limited movement of affected joints, and symptoms associated with the underlying pathologic condition. Fluid accumulations increase the distance required for nutrients and waste products to move between capillaries and tissues. Blood flow may be impaired also. Therefore wounds heal more slowly, and with prolonged edema the risks of infection and pressure sores over bony prominences increase. As edematous fluid accumulates, it is trapped in a "third space" (i.e., the interstitial space, pleural space, pericardial space) and is unavailable for metabolic processes or perfusion. Dehydration can develop as a result of this sequestering. Such sequestration occurs with severe burns, where large amounts of vascular fluid are lost to the interstitial spaces, reducing plasma volume and causing shock (see Chapter 24).

EVALUATION AND TREATMENT   Specific conditions causing edema require diagnosis. Edema may be treated symptomatically until the underlying disorder is corrected. Supportive measures include elevating edematous limbs, using compression stockings, avoiding prolonged standing, restricting salt intake, and taking diuretics. Administration of IV albumin can be required in severe cases.

QUICK CHECK 5-1
1. How does an increase in capillary hydrostatic pressure cause edema?
2. How does a decrease in capillary oncotic pressure cause edema?

SODIUM, CHLORIDE, AND WATER BALANCE

The kidneys and hormones have a central role in maintaining sodium and water balance. Because water follows the osmotic gradients

FIGURE 5-2 Mechanisms of Edema Formation.

FIGURE 5-3 Pitting Edema. (From Bloom A, Ireland J: *Color atlas of diabetes,* ed 2, St Louis, 1992, Mosby.)

established by changes in salt concentration, sodium concentration and water balance are intimately related. Sodium concentration is regulated by renal effects of aldosterone (see Figure 18-18). Water balance is regulated primarily by **antidiuretic hormone (ADH**; also known as *vasopressin*).

Sodium (Na$^+$) accounts for 90% of the ECF cations (positively charged ions) (see Table 5-3). Along with its constituent anions (negatively charged ions) chloride and bicarbonate, sodium regulates extracellular osmotic forces and therefore regulates water balance. Sodium is important in other functions, including maintenance of neuromuscular irritability for conduction of nerve impulses (in conjunction with potassium and calcium; see Figure 1-29), regulation of acid-base balance (using sodium bicarbonate and sodium phosphate),

participation in cellular chemical reactions, and transport of substances across the cellular membrane.

The kidney, in conjunction with neural and hormonal mediators, maintains normal serum sodium concentration within a narrow range (135 to 145 mEq/L) primarily through renal tubular reabsorption. Hormonal regulation of sodium (and potassium) balance is mediated by **aldosterone**, a mineralocorticoid synthesized and secreted from the adrenal cortex as a component of the **renin-angiotensin-aldosterone system.** Aldosterone secretion is influenced by circulating blood volume, by blood pressure, and by plasma concentrations of sodium and potassium. When circulating blood volume or blood pressure is reduced, or sodium levels are depressed or potassium levels are increased, **renin**, an enzyme secreted by the juxtaglomerular cells of the kidney, is released. Renin stimulates the formation of **angiotensin I**, an inactive polypeptide. Angiotensin-converting enzyme (ACE) in pulmonary vessels converts angiotensin I to **angiotensin II**, which stimulates the secretion of aldosterone and antidiuretic hormone (see below) and also causes vasoconstriction. The aldosterone promotes renal sodium and water reabsorption and excretion of potassium, increasing blood volume (Figure 5-4; also see Figure 29-9). Vasoconstriction elevates the systemic blood pressure and restores renal perfusion (blood flow). This restoration inhibits the further release of renin.

Natriuretic peptides are hormones primarily produced by the myocardium. Atrial natriuretic hormone (ANH) is produced by the atria. B-type natriuretic peptide (BNP) is produced by the ventricles. Urodilatin (an ANP analog) is synthesized within the kidney. Natriuretic peptides are released when there is an increase in transmural atrial pressure (increased volume), which may occur with congestive heart failure or when there is an increase in mean arterial pressure[4] (Figure 5-5). They are natural antagonists to the renin-angiotensin-aldosterone system. Natriuretic peptides cause vasodilation and increase sodium and water excretion, decreasing blood pressure. Natriuretic peptides are sometimes called a "third factor" in sodium regulation. (Increased glomerular filtration rate is thus the first factor and aldosterone the second factor.)

Chloride (Cl$^-$) is the major anion in the ECF and provides electroneutrality, particularly in relation to sodium. Chloride transport is generally passive and follows the active transport of sodium so that

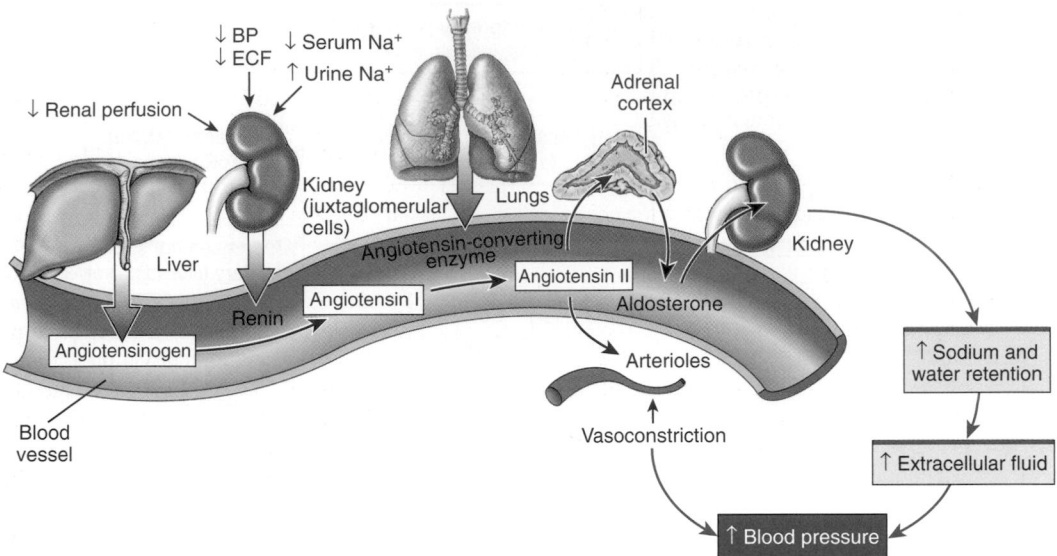

FIGURE 5-4 The Renin-Angiotensin-Aldosterone System. *ADH,* Antidiuretic hormone; *BP,* blood pressure; *ECF,* extracellular fluid; *Na,* sodium. (Modified from Herlihy B, Maebius N: *The human body in health and disease,* ed 4, Philadelphia, 2011, Saunders. Borrowed from Lewis et al: *Medical-surgical nursing: and management of clinical problems,* ed 9, St Louis, 2014, Mosby.)

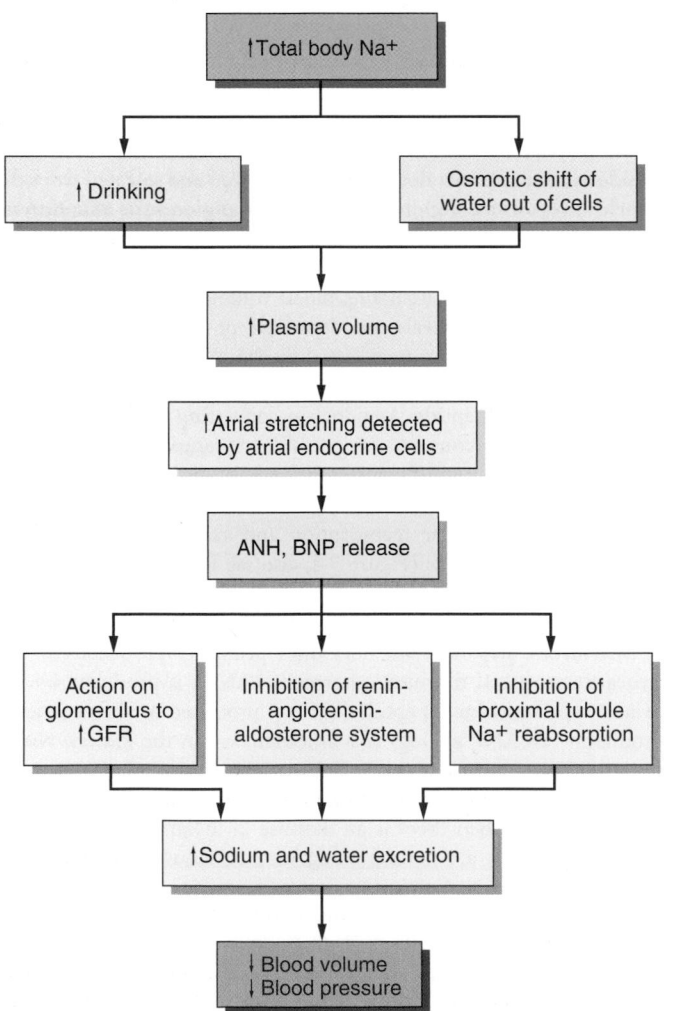

FIGURE 5-5 The Natriuretic Peptide System. *ANH,* Atrial natriuretic hormone; *BNP,* brain natriuretic peptide; *GFR,* glomerular filtration rate; *Na+,* sodium ion.

FIGURE 5-6 The Antidiuretic Hormone (ADH) System.

increases or decreases in chloride concentration are proportional to changes in sodium concentration. Chloride concentration tends to vary inversely with changes in the concentration of bicarbonate (HCO_3^-), the other major anion.

Water balance is regulated by the secretion of ADH (also known as vasopressin). ADH is secreted when plasma osmolality increases or circulating blood volume decreases and blood pressure drops (Figure 5-6). Increased plasma osmolality occurs with water deficit or sodium excess in relation to total body water. The increased osmolality stimulates hypothalamic **osmoreceptors**. In addition to causing thirst, these osmoreceptors signal the posterior pituitary gland to release ADH. Thirst stimulates water drinking and ADH increases water reabsorption into the plasma from the distal tubules and collecting ducts of the kidney (see Chapter 29). The reabsorbed water decreases plasma osmolality, returning it toward normal, and urine concentration increases.

With fluid loss (dehydration) from vomiting, diarrhea, or excessive sweating, a decrease in blood volume and blood pressure often occurs. Volume-sensitive receptors and baroreceptors (nerve endings that are sensitive to changes in volume and pressure) also stimulate the release of ADH from the pituitary gland and stimulate thirst. The volume receptors are located in the right and left atria and thoracic vessels; baroreceptors are found in the aorta, pulmonary arteries, and carotid sinus. ADH secretion also occurs when atrial pressure drops, as occurs with decreased blood volume and with the release of angiotensin II (see Figure 29-9). The reabsorption of water mediated by ADH then promotes the restoration of plasma volume and blood pressure (see Figure 5-6).

✔ **QUICK CHECK 5-2**
1. What forces promote net filtration?
2. How do hormones regulate salt and water balance?
3. What are aquaporins?

ALTERATIONS IN SODIUM, CHLORIDE, AND WATER BALANCE

Alterations in sodium and water balance are closely related. Sodium imbalances occur with gains or losses of body water. Water imbalances develop with gains or losses of salt. In general, these alterations can be classified as changes in tonicity, the change in the concentration of solutes in relation to water: isotonic, hypertonic, or hypotonic (Table 5-5 and Figure 5-7; also see Figure 1-25). Changes in tonicity also alter the volume of water in the intracellular and extracellular compartments, resulting in isovolemia, hypervolemia, or hypovolemia.

TABLE 5-5	**Water and Solute Imbalances**
Tonicity	**Mechanism**
Isotonic (isoosmolar) imbalance Serum osmolality = 280-294 mOsm/kg	Gain or loss of ECF resulting in concentration equivalent to 0.9% sodium chloride solution (normal saline); no shrinking or swelling of cells
Hypertonic (hyperosmolar) imbalance Serum osmolality >294 mOsm/kg	Imbalances that result in ECF concentration >0.9% salt solution (i.e., water loss or solute gain); cells shrink in hypertonic fluid
Hypotonic (hypoosmolar) imbalance Serum osmolality <280 mOsm/kg	Imbalance that results in ECF <0.9% salt solution (i.e., water gain or solute loss); cells swell in hypotonic fluid
Formula for calculating serum osmolarity	(2 × [Na] + [Glu])/18 + BUN/2.8

BUN, Blood serum urea nitrogen level (mg/dl); *ECF*, extracellular fluid; *[Glu]*, serum glucose concentration (mg/dl); *[Na]*, serum sodium concentration (mEq/dl).

Isotonic Alterations

Isotonic alterations are the most common and occur when TBW changes are accompanied by proportional changes in the concentrations of electrolytes (see Figure 5-7). Isotonic fluid loss causes dehydration and hypovolemia. For example, if an individual loses pure plasma or ECF, fluid volume is depleted but the concentration and type of electrolytes and the osmolality remain in the normal range (280 to 294 milliosmoles [mOsm]). Causes include hemorrhage, severe wound drainage, excessive diaphoresis (sweating), and inadequate fluid intake. There is loss of extracellular fluid volume with weight loss, dryness of skin and mucous membranes, decreased urine output, and symptoms of hypovolemia. Indicators of hypovolemia include a rapid heart rate, flattened neck veins, and normal or decreased blood pressure. In severe states, hypovolemic shock can occur (see Chapter 24). Isotonic fluids containing electrolytes and glucose are given orally, intravenously (i.e., 0.9% saline solution or 5% dextrose in 0.225% saline solution), or, in some cases, subcutaneously (hypodermoclysis).

Isotonic fluid excess causes hypervolemia. Common causes include excessive administration of intravenous fluids, hypersecretion of aldosterone, or the effects of drugs such as cortisone (which causes renal reabsorption of sodium and water). As plasma volume expands, hypervolemia develops with weight gain. The diluting effect of excess plasma volume leads to decreased hematocrit and decreased plasma protein concentration. The neck veins may distend, and the blood pressure increases. Increased capillary hydrostatic pressure leads to edema formation. Ultimately, pulmonary edema and heart failure may develop. Diuretics are commonly used for treatment.

Hypertonic Alterations

Hypertonic fluid alterations develop when the osmolality of the ECF is elevated above normal (greater than 294 mOsm). The most common causes are increased concentration of ECF sodium (hypernatremia) or deficit of ECF water, or both. In both instances, ECF hypertonicity attracts water from the intracellular space, causing ICF dehydration (see Figure 5-7).

Hypernatremia

PATHOPHYSIOLOGY Hypernatremia occurs when serum sodium levels exceed 145 mEq/L. Increased levels of serum sodium cause hypertonicity. Hypernatremia can be isovolemic, hypovolemic, or hypervolemic depending on the accompanying ECF water volume.

Isovolemic hypernatremia is the most common and occurs when there is a *loss of free water* with a near normal body sodium concentration. Causes include inadequate water intake; excessive sweating (sweat is hypotonic), fever, or respiratory tract infections, which increase the respiratory rate and enhance water loss from the lungs; burns; vomiting; diarrhea; and central or nephrogenic diabetes insipidus (lack of ADH or inadequate renal response to ADH). Infants with severe diarrhea are vulnerable and have increased risk because they cannot communicate thirst. Insufficient water intake occurs particularly in individuals who are comatose, confused, or immobilized or are receiving gastric feedings. Dehydration refers to water deficit but also is commonly used to indicate both sodium and water loss (isotonic or isoosmolar dehydration).[5]

Hypovolemic hypernatremia occurs where there is loss of sodium accompanied by a relatively greater loss of body water. Causes include use of loop diuretics, osmotic diuresis (i.e., from hyperglycemia related to uncontrolled diabetes mellitus or use of mannitol), or failure of the kidneys to concentrate urine.

Hypervolemic hypernatremia is rare and occurs when there is increased total body water and a greater increase in total body sodium

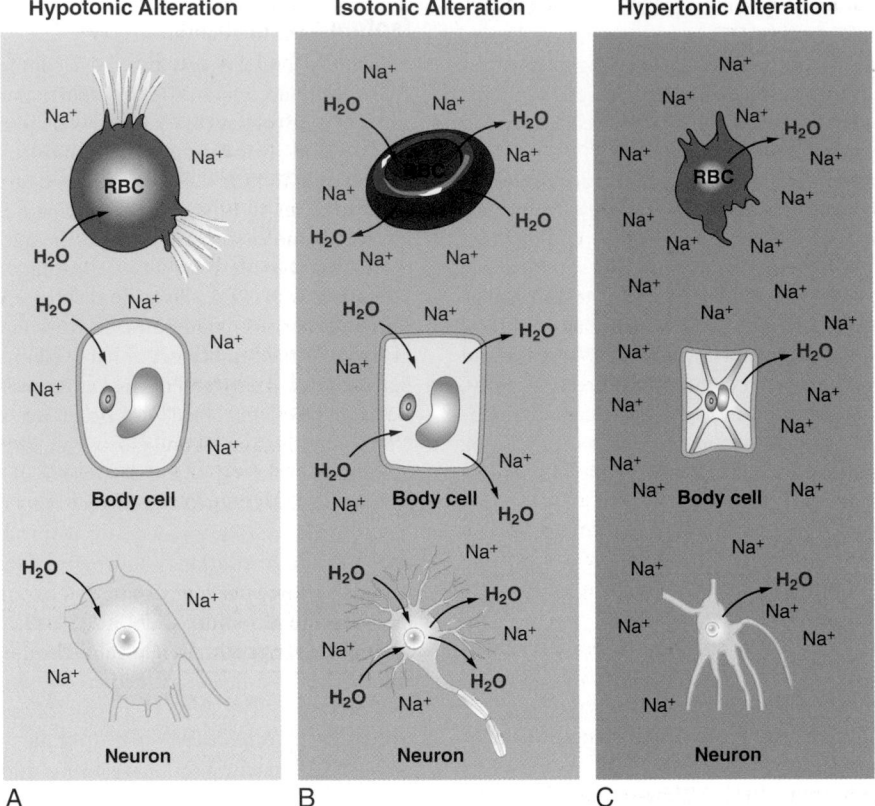

Hypotonic Alteration   **Isotonic Alteration**   **Hypertonic Alteration**

A   B   C

FIGURE 5-7 Effects of Alterations in Extracellular Sodium Concentration in RBC, Body Cell, and Neuron. **A,** Hypotonic alteration: Decrease in ECF sodium (Na⁺) concentration (hyponatremia) results in ICF osmotic attraction of water with swelling and potential bursting of cells. **B,** Isotonic alteration: Normal concentration of sodium in the ECF and no change in shifts of fluid in or out of cells. **C,** Hypertonic alteration: An increase in ECF sodium concentration (hypernatremia) results in osmotic attraction of water out of cells with cell shrinkage. *RBC,* Red blood cell.

level, resulting in hypervolemia. Causes include infusion of hypertonic saline solutions (e.g., as sodium replacement for treatment of salt depletion, which can occur with renal impairment, heart failure, or gastrointestinal [GI] losses); oversecretion of adrenocorticotropic hormone (ACTH) or aldosterone (e.g., Cushing syndrome, adrenal hyperplasia); and near salt water drowning.[6] High amounts of dietary sodium rarely cause hypernatremia in a healthy individual because the sodium is eliminated by the kidneys.

Because chloride follows sodium, **hyperchloremia** (elevation of serum chloride concentration greater than 105 mEq/L) often accompanies hypernatremia, as well as plasma bicarbonate deficits (such as in metabolic acidosis)[7] (see p. 127). There are no specific symptoms or treatment for chloride excess.

CLINICAL MANIFESTATIONS When there is excessive sodium intake or decreased sodium loss in relation to water, water is osmotically redistributed to the hypertonic extracellular space, resulting in hypervolemia, and intracellular dehydration ensues. Clinical manifestations include thirst, weight gain, bounding pulse, and increased blood pressure. Central nervous system signs are the most serious and are related to alterations in membrane potentials and shrinking of brain cells (sodium cannot cross brain capillaries because of their tight endothelial junctions). Signs include muscle twitching and hyperreflexia (hyperactive reflexes), confusion, coma, convulsions, and cerebral hemorrhage from stretching of veins. Hypernatremia with marked water deficit is manifested by signs and symptoms of

BOX 5-1 **Signs and Symptoms of Dehydration**

Increased serum sodium concentration	Soft eyeballs
	Sunken fontanels in infants
Thirst	Prolonged capillary refill time
Headache	Tachycardia
Weight loss	Weak pulses
Oliguria and concentrated urine	Low blood pressure
Hard stools	Postural hypotension
Decreased skin turgor	Hypovolemic shock
Dry mucous membranes	Confusion
Decreased sweating and tears	Coma
Elevated temperature	

intracellular and extracellular dehydration with volume depletion (Box 5-1).

EVALUATION AND TREATMENT Serum sodium levels are greater than 147 mEq/L and urine specific gravity will be greater than 1.030. The history and physical examination provide information about underlying disorders and events. The treatment of hypernatremia and water deficit is to give oral fluids or isotonic salt-free fluid (5% dextrose in water) until the serum sodium level returns to normal. Fluid replacement must be given slowly to prevent cerebral edema. Serum sodium levels need to be monitored. Hypervolemia or hypovolemia requires treatment of the underlying clinical condition.

Hypotonic Alterations

Hypotonic fluid imbalances occur when the osmolality of the ECF is less than 280 mOsm (see Figure 5-7). The most common causes are sodium deficit or water excess. Either leads to *intracellular overhydration* (cellular edema) and cell swelling. When there is a sodium deficit, the osmotic pressure of the ECF decreases and water moves into the cell where the osmotic pressure is greater. The plasma volume then decreases, leading to symptoms of hypovolemia. With water excess, increases in both the ICF and ECF volume occur, causing symptoms of hypervolemia and water intoxication with cerebral and pulmonary edema.

Hyponatremia

PATHOPHYSIOLOGY   Hyponatremia develops when the serum sodium concentration falls below 135 mEq/L. Hyponatremia occurs when there is loss of sodium, inadequate intake of sodium, or dilution of sodium by water excess.[8] Sodium depletion usually causes hypoosmolality with movement of water into cells with rupture of cell membranes.

Isovolemic hyponatremia occurs when there is loss of sodium without a significant loss of water (pure sodium deficit). Causes can include syndrome of inappropriate antidiuretic hormone[9] (SIADH [see Chapter 19], which enhances water retention), hypothyroidism, pneumonia, and glucocorticoid deficiency. Inadequate intake of dietary sodium is rare but possible in individuals on low-sodium diets, particularly with use of diuretics.

Hypervolemic hyponatremia occurs when total body sodium level increases. The increased sodium leads to an increase in total body water and dilution of sodium in the extracellular space. Causes include congestive heart failure, cirrhosis of the liver, and nephrotic syndrome. Edema is present.

Hypovolemic hyponatremia occurs with a loss of total body water, but there is a greater loss of body sodium. The extracelluar volume is decreased. Causes include prolonged vomiting, severe diarrhea, inadequate secretion of aldosterone (e.g., adrenal insufficiency), and renal losses from diuretics.

Dilutional hyponatremia (water intoxication) occurs when there is intake of large amounts of free water or replacement of fluid loss with intravenous 5% dextrose in water, which dilutes sodium. The glucose is metabolized to carbon dioxide and water, leaving a hypotonic solution with a diluting effect. Excessive sweating stimulates thirst and intake of large amounts of free water (as can occur in endurance athletes), which dilutes sodium. Some individuals with psychogenic disorders develop water intoxication from compulsive water drinking. Other causes can include tap water enemas, near fresh water drowning, and use of selective serotonin reuptake inhibitors (SSRIs). When the body is functioning normally, it is almost impossible to produce an excess of TBW because water balance is regulated by the kidneys.

Hypochloremia, a low level of serum chloride (less than 97 mEq/L), usually occurs with hyponatremia or an elevated bicarbonate concentration, as in metabolic alkalosis (see p. 127). Sodium deficit related to restricted intake, use of diuretics, vomiting, or nasogastric suction is accompanied by chloride deficiency. Cystic fibrosis is characterized by hypochloremia (see Chapter 28). Treatment of the underlying cause is required.

CLINICAL MANIFESTATIONS   The serum sodium concentration will be less than 135 mEq/L. Sodium depletion usually causes

hypoosmolality with movement of water into cells. The hematocrit is reduced from the dilutional effect of water excess in dilutional hyponatremia. The high amount of intracellular solutes compared to the low amount of extracellular solutes as a result of the hyponatremia causes an intracellular osmotic shift of water, resulting in cell swelling. The most life-threatening consequence is cerebral edema and increased intracranial pressure. Neurologic changes include lethargy, confusion, apprehension, seizures, and coma. A decrease in sodium concentration changes the cell's ability to depolarize and repolarize normally, altering the action potential in neurons and muscle (see Chapter 1). Muscle twitching, depressed reflexes, and weakness are common. Nausea and vomiting are more common with less severe hyponatremia (i.e., decreases between 120 and 130 mEq/L). Hypovolemic hyponatremia has signs of hypotension, tachycardia, and decreased urine output. Hypervolemic hyponatremia is accompanied by weight gain, edema, ascites, and jugular vein distension. Hyponatremia is a major cause of morbidity and mortality in intensive care units and in the elderly (see Health Alert: Hyponatremia and the Elderly).

HEALTH ALERT

Hyponatremia and the Elderly

Hyponatremia is the most common of the electrolyte disorders and prevalence is highest among elderly hospitalized individuals. Isovolemic hyponatremia caused by SIADH is thought to be the most common cause and can occur with central nervous system injury, pulmonary disease, malignancies, nausea, pain, and aging changes. Other contributing factors include use of thiazide diuretics, proton pump inhibitors, age-related decrease in thirst with dehydration, and diminished urine concentrating ability. Hyponatremia contributes to cognitive deficits, gait disturbances, falls, fractures, long-term hospitalization, the need for long-term care, and death. The elderly need to be assessed for risk, implementation of preventive strategies, and early intervention.

From Ayus JC et al: *Nephrol Dial Transplant* 27(10):3725-3731, 2012; Berl T. *Clin J Am Soc Nephrol* 8(3):469-475; Cowen LE et al: *Endocrinol Metab Clin North Am* 42(2):349-370, 2013; Cumming K et al: *PLoS One* 9(2):e88272, 2014; Mannesse CK et al. *Ageing Res Rev* 12(1):165-173, 2013; Schrier RW et al: *Nat Rev Nephrol* 9(1):37-50, 2013 (Erratum in: *Nat Rev Nephrol* 9(3):124, 2013). *SIADH*, Syndrome of inappropriate antidiuretic hormone.

EVALUATION AND TREATMENT   The cause of hyponatremia must be determined and treatment planned accordingly. Small amounts of intravenous hypertonic sodium chloride (i.e., 3% sodium chloride) can be given when neurologic manifestations are severe but must be given slowly to prevent osmotic demyelination syndrome in the brain.[9] Restriction of water intake is required in most cases of dilutional hyponatremia because body sodium levels may be normal or increased even though serum sodium levels are low. Arginine vasopressin (ADH) receptor antagonists (vaptans) are a class of drugs used for the treatment of hypervolemic and euvolemic hyponatremia.[10] Serum sodium concentration must be monitored.[8]

✓ QUICK CHECK 5-3
1. What causes isotonic imbalance?
2. What are some causes of hypernatremia?
3. What is the most severe complication of hyponatremia?

ALTERATIONS IN POTASSIUM AND OTHER ELECTROLYTES

Potassium

Potassium (K⁺) is the major intracellular electrolyte and is essential for normal cellular functions. Total body potassium content is about 4000 mEq, with most of it (98%) located in the cells. The ICF concentration of potassium is 150 to 160 mEq/L; the ECF potassium concentration is 3.5 to 5.0 mEq/L. The difference in concentration is maintained by a sodium-potassium adenosinetriphosphatase active transport system (Na^+-K^+ ATPase pump) (see Figure 1-26).

As the predominant ICF ion, potassium exerts a major influence on the regulation of ICF osmolality and fluid balance as well as on intracellular electrical neutrality in relation to hydrogen (H^+) and sodium. Potassium is required for glycogen and glucose deposition in liver and skeletal muscle cells. It also maintains the resting membrane potential, as reflected in the transmission and conduction of nerve impulses (see Figure 1-29), the maintenance of normal cardiac rhythms, and the contraction of skeletal muscle and smooth muscle.

Dietary potassium moves rapidly into cells after ingestion. However, the distribution of potassium between intracellular and extracellular fluids is influenced by several factors. Insulin, aldosterone, epinephrine, and alkalosis facilitate the shift of potassium into cells. Insulin deficiency, aldosterone deficiency, acidosis, cell lysis, and strenuous exercise facilitate the shift of potassium out of cells. Glucagon blocks entry of potassium into cells, and glucocorticoids promote potassium excretion. Potassium also will move out of cells along with water when there is increased ECF osmolarity.

Although potassium is found in most body fluids, the kidney is the most efficient regulator of potassium balance. Potassium is freely filtered by the renal glomerulus, and 90% is reabsorbed by the proximal tubule and loop of Henle. In the distal tubules, principal cells secrete potassium and intercalated cells reabsorb potassium. These cells determine the amount of potassium excreted from the body. The gut may also sense the amount of K⁺ ingested and stimulate renal K⁺ excretion independent of aldosterone.[11]

The potassium concentration in the distal tubular cells is determined primarily by the plasma concentration in the peritubular capillaries. When plasma potassium concentration increases from increased dietary intake or shifts of potassium from the ICF to the ECF occur, potassium is secreted into the urine by the distal tubules. Decreased levels of plasma potassium result in decreased distal tubular secretion, although approximately 5 to 15 mEq per day will continue to be lost. Changes in the rate of filtrate (urine) flow through the distal tubule also influence the concentration gradient for potassium secretion. When the urine flow rate is high, as with the use of diuretics, potassium concentration in the distal tubular urine is lower, leading to the secretion of potassium into the urine.

Changes in pH and thus in hydrogen ion concentration also affect potassium balance. During acute acidosis, hydrogen ions accumulate in the ICF and potassium shifts out of the cell to the ECF to maintain a balance of cations across the cell membrane. This occurs in part because of a decrease in sodium-potassium ATPase pump activity. Decreased ICF potassium results in decreased secretion of potassium by the distal tubular cells, contributing to hyperkalemia. In acute alkalosis, intracellular fluid levels of hydrogen diminish and potassium shifts into the cell; in addition, the distal tubular cells increase their secretion of potassium, further contributing to hypokalemia.[12]

Besides conserving sodium, *aldosterone* also regulates potassium concentration. Elevated plasma potassium concentration causes the release of renin by renal juxtaglomerular cells and the adrenal secretion of aldosterone through the renin-angiotensin-aldosterone system. Aldosterone then stimulates the release of potassium into the urine by the distal renal tubules. Aldosterone also increases the secretion of potassium from sweat glands.

Insulin helps regulate plasma potassium levels by stimulating the sodium-potassium ATPase pump, thus promoting the movement of potassium into liver and muscle cells, particularly after eating. Insulin can also be used to treat hyperkalemia. Dangerously low levels of plasma potassium can result when insulin is given while potassium levels are depressed. Potassium balance is especially significant in the treatment of conditions requiring insulin administration, such as insulin-dependent diabetes mellitus.

Potassium adaptation is the ability of the body to adapt to increased levels of potassium intake over time. A sudden increase in potassium may be fatal, but if the intake of potassium is slowly increased by amounts of more than 120 mEq per day, the kidney can increase the urinary excretion of potassium and maintain potassium balance.

Hypokalemia

PATHOPHYSIOLOGY Potassium deficiency, or hypokalemia, develops when the serum potassium concentration falls to less than 3.5 mEq/L. Because cellular and total body stores of potassium are difficult to measure, changes in potassium balance are described, although not always accurately, by the plasma concentration. Generally, lowered serum potassium level indicates loss of total body potassium. With potassium loss from the ECF, the concentration gradient change favors movement of potassium from the cell to the ECF. The ICF/ECF concentration ratio is maintained, but the amount of total body potassium is depleted.

Factors contributing to the development of hypokalemia include reduced intake of potassium, increased entry of potassium into cells, and increased losses of body potassium. Dietary deficiency of potassium is more common in elderly individuals with both low protein intake and inadequate intake of fruits and vegetables and in individuals with alcoholism or anorexia nervosa (see *Health Alert:* Potassium Intake: Hypertension and Stroke). Reduced potassium intake generally becomes a problem when combined with other causes of potassium depletion.

HEALTH ALERT

Potassium Intake: Hypertension and Stroke

Enriched dietary intake of potassium is associated with lower risk of hypertension and stroke. The American diet often exceeds recommendations for sodium intake and a deficiency in potassium intake. There is increased risk of high blood pressure, cardiovascular disease, and mortality when the plasma ratio of sodium concentration to potassium concentration is high. Potassium attenuates the effects of high dietary salt with reduction in blood pressure, stroke rates, and cardiovascular disease risk. The exact mechanism of how potassium affects blood pressure is unknown but is thought to be related to renal handling of sodium, endothelial cell function, decreased vascular resistance, and reduced oxidative stress. A large prospective study of older women showed they were found to have lower risk of ischemic but not hemorrhagic stroke associated with higher intakes of potassium, especially in women without hypertension. Lower risk of mortality was found in all women with higher intakes of potassium. Increased dietary intake of potassium is recommended for most individuals without impaired renal handling of potassium.

Data from Aaron KJ, Sanders PW: *Mayo Clin Proc* 88(9):987-995, 2013; Arjun S et al: *Stroke* September 4, 2014 [Epub ahead of print]; Castro H, Raij L: *Semin Nephrol* 33(3):277-289, 2013; Whelton PK, He J: *Curr Opin Lipidol* 25(1):75-79, 2014.

ECF hypokalemia can develop without losses of total body potassium. For example, potassium shifts from the ECF to the ICF in exchange for hydrogen to maintain plasma acid-base balance during respiratory or metabolic alkalosis. Insulin promotes cellular uptake of potassium and insulin administration may cause an ECF potassium deficit.

Potassium shifts from the ICF to the ECF in conditions such as diabetic ketoacidosis, in which the increased hydrogen ion concentration in the ECF causes H^+ to shift into the cell in exchange for potassium. A normal level of potassium is maintained in the plasma, but potassium continues to be lost in the urine, causing a deficit in the amount of total body potassium. Severe, even fatal, hypokalemia may occur if insulin is administered without also providing potassium supplements. Thus total body potassium depletion becomes evident when insulin treatment and rehydration therapy are initiated. Potassium replacement is instituted cautiously to prevent hyperkalemia.

Losses of potassium from body stores are usually caused by gastrointestinal and renal disorders. Diarrhea, intestinal drainage tubes or fistulae, and laxative abuse also result in hypokalemia. Normally, only 5 to 10 mEq of potassium and 100 to 150 ml of water are excreted in the stool each day. With diarrhea, fluid and electrolyte losses can be voluminous, with several liters of fluid and 100 to 200 mEq of potassium lost per day. Vomiting or continuous nasogastric suctioning often is associated with potassium depletion, partly because of the potassium lost from the gastric fluid but principally because of renal compensation for volume depletion and the metabolic alkalosis (elevated bicarbonate levels) that occurs from sodium, chloride, and hydrogen ion losses. The loss of fluid and sodium stimulates the secretion of aldosterone, which in turn causes renal losses of potassium.

Renal potassium losses occur with increased secretion of potassium by the distal tubule. Use of potassium-wasting diuretics, excessive aldosterone secretion, increased distal tubular flow rate, and low plasma magnesium concentration all may contribute to urinary losses of potassium. The elevated flow of bicarbonate at the distal tubule during alkalosis also contributes to renal excretion of potassium because the increased tubular lumen electronegativity attracts potassium. Many diuretics inhibit the reabsorption of sodium chloride, causing the diuretic effect. The distal tubular flow rate then increases, promoting potassium excretion. If sodium loss is severe, the compensating aldosterone secretion may further deplete potassium stores. Primary hyperaldosteronism with excessive secretion of aldosterone from an adrenal adenoma (tumor) also causes potassium wasting. Many kidney diseases reduce the ability to conserve sodium. The disordered sodium reabsorption produces a diuretic effect, and the increased distal tubule flow rate favors the secretion of potassium. Magnesium deficits increase renal potassium secretion and promote hypokalemia. Certain antibiotics (i.e., carbenicillin disodium and amphotericin B) are known to cause hypokalemia by increasing the rate of potassium excretion. Rare hereditary defects in renal potassium transport (e.g., Bartter and Gitelman syndromes) also can cause hypokalemia.

CLINICAL MANIFESTATIONS Mild losses of potassium are usually asymptomatic. Severe loss of potassium results in neuromuscular and cardiac manifestations. Neuromuscular excitability decreases, causing skeletal muscle weakness, smooth muscle atony, cardiac dysrhythmias, glucose intolerance, and impaired urinary concentrating ability.[13]

Symptoms occur in relation to the rate of potassium depletion. Because the body can accommodate slow losses of potassium, the decrease in ECF concentration may allow potassium to shift from the intracellular space, restoring the potassium concentration gradient toward normal, with less severe neuromuscular changes. With acute and severe losses of potassium, changes in neuromuscular excitability

are more profound. Skeletal muscle weakness occurs initially in the larger muscles of the legs and arms and ultimately affects the diaphragm and depresses ventilation. Paralysis and respiratory arrest can occur with severe losses. Loss of smooth muscle tone is manifested by constipation, intestinal distention, anorexia, nausea, vomiting, and paralytic ileus (paralysis of the intestinal muscles).

The cardiac effects of hypokalemia are related also to changes in membrane excitability. As ECF potassium concentration decreases, the resting membrane potential becomes more negative (i.e., from −90 millivolts to −100 millivolts [hypopolarization]). Because potassium contributes to the repolarization phase of the action potential, hypokalemia delays ventricular repolarization. Various dysrhythmias may occur, including sinus bradycardia, atrioventricular block, and paroxysmal atrial tachycardia. The characteristic changes in the electrocardiogram (ECG) reflect *delayed repolarization*. For instance, the amplitude of the T wave decreases, the amplitude of the U wave increases, and the ST segment is depressed (Figure 5-8). In severe states of hypokalemia, P waves peak, the QT interval is prolonged, and T wave inversions may be seen. Hypokalemia enhances the therapeutic effect of digitalis and increases the risk of digitalis toxicity.

A wide range of metabolic dysfunctions may result from potassium deficiency (Table 5-6). Carbohydrate metabolism is affected because hypokalemia depresses insulin secretion and alters hepatic and skeletal

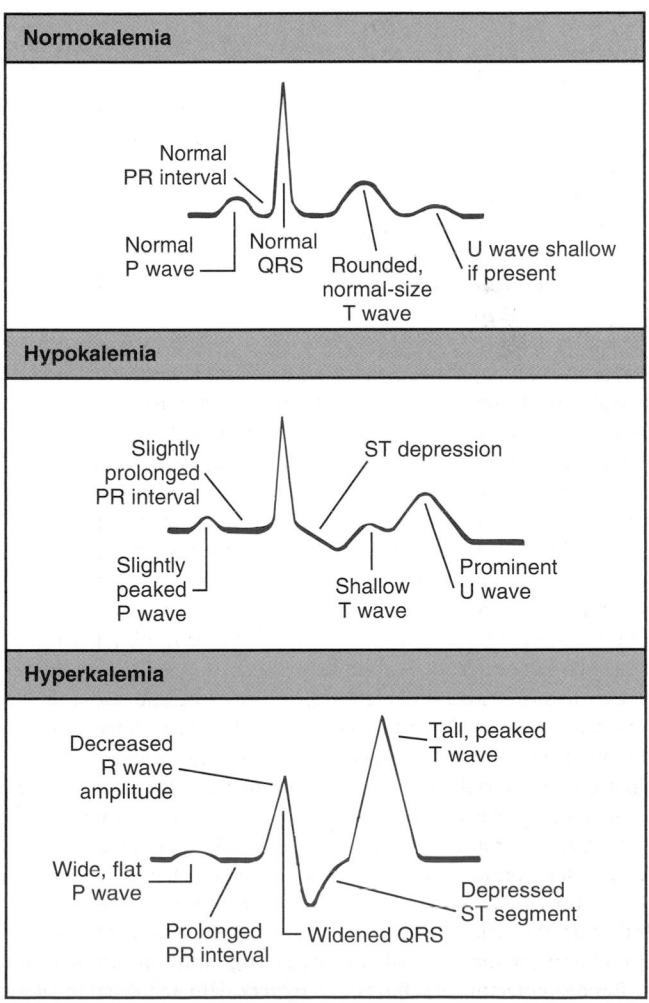

FIGURE 5-8 Electrocardiogram Changes with Potassium Imbalance.

TABLE 5-6   Clinical Manifestations of Potassium Level Alterations

Organ System	Hypokalemia	Hyperkalemia
Cardiovascular	Dysrhythmias	Dysrhythmias
	ECG changes (flattened T waves, U waves, ST depression, peaked P wave, prolonged QT interval)	ECG changes (peaked T waves, prolonged PR interval, absent P wave with widened QRS complex)
	Cardiac arrest	Bradycardia
	Weak, irregular pulse rate	Heart block
	Postural hypotension	Cardiac arrest
Nervous	Lethargy	Anxiety
	Fatigue	Tingling
	Confusion	Numbness
	Paresthesias	
Gastrointestinal	Nausea and vomiting	Nausea and vomiting
	Decreased motility	Diarrhea
	Distention	Colicky pain
	Decreased bowel sounds	
	Ileus	
Kidney	Water loss	Oliguria
	Thirst	Kidney damage
	Inability to concentrate urine	
	Increased tubular production of ammonia and ammonium	
	Kidney damage	
Skeletal and smooth muscle	Weakness	Early: hyperactive muscles
	Flaccid paralysis	Late: weakness and flaccid paralysis
	Respiratory arrest	
	Constipation	
	Bladder dysfunction	

muscle glycogen synthesis. Renal function is impaired, with a decreased ability to concentrate urine. Polyuria (increased urine) and polydipsia (increased thirst) are associated with decreased responsiveness to ADH. Long-term potassium deficits lasting more than 1 month may damage renal tissue, with interstitial fibrosis and tubular atrophy.

EVALUATION AND TREATMENT   The diagnosis of hypokalemia is significantly related to the medical history and the identification of disorders associated with potassium loss or shifts of extracellular potassium to the intracellular space. Treatment involves an estimation of total body potassium losses and correction of acid-base imbalances. Further losses of potassium should be prevented and the individual should be encouraged to eat foods rich in potassium. The maximal rate of oral replacement is 40 to 80 mEq/day if renal function is normal. A maximal safe rate of intravenous replacement is 20 mEq/hr. Because potassium is irritating to blood vessels, a maximal concentration of 40 mEq/L should be used. Serum potassium values are monitored until normokalemia is achieved.

Hyperkalemia

PATHOPHYSIOLOGY   Elevation of ECF potassium concentration greater than 5.5 mEq/L constitutes hyperkalemia.[14] Because of efficient renal excretion, increases in total body potassium level are relatively rare. Acute increases in serum potassium level are handled quickly through increased cellular uptake and renal excretion of body potassium excesses.

Hyperkalemia may be caused by increased intake, a shift of potassium from cells to the ECF, decreased renal excretion, or drugs that decrease renal potassium excretion (i.e., ACE inhibitors, angiotensin receptor blockers, and aldosterone antagonists). If renal function is normal, slow, long-term increases in potassium intake are usually well tolerated through potassium adaptation, although short-term potassium loading can exceed renal excretion rates. Dietary excesses of potassium are uncommon but accidental ingestion of potassium salt substitutes can cause toxicity. Use of stored whole blood and intravenous boluses of potassium penicillin G or replacement potassium can precipitate hyperkalemia, particularly with impaired renal function. Potassium moves from the ICF to the ECF with cell trauma or a change in cell membrane permeability, acidosis, insulin deficiency, or cell hypoxia. Burns, massive crushing injuries, and extensive surgeries can cause release of potassium to the ECF as a result of cell trauma. If renal function is sustained, potassium is excreted. As cell repair begins, hypokalemia develops without an adequate replacement of potassium.

In acidosis, ECF hydrogen ions shift into cells in exchange for ICF potassium and sodium; hyperkalemia and acidosis therefore often occur simultaneously. Because insulin promotes cellular entry of potassium, insulin deficits, which occur with such conditions as diabetic ketoacidosis, are accompanied by hyperkalemia. Hypoxia can lead to hyperkalemia by diminishing the efficiency of cell membrane active transport, resulting in the escape of potassium to the ECF. Digitalis overdose (toxicity) may cause hyperkalemia by inhibiting the Na^+-K^+ ATPase pump, and thus allowing potassium to remain outside the cell,

Decreased renal excretion of potassium commonly is associated with hyperkalemia. Renal failure that results in oliguria (urine output of 30 ml/hr or less) is accompanied by elevations of serum potassium level. The severity of hyperkalemia is related to the amount of potassium intake, the degree of acidosis, and the rate of renal cell damage. Decreases in the secretion or renal effects of aldosterone also can cause decreases in the urinary excretion of potassium. For example, Addison disease (a disease of adrenal cortical insufficiency) results in decreased production and secretion of aldosterone (and other steroids) and thus contributes to hyperkalemia.

CLINICAL MANIFESTATIONS   Symptoms vary with the severity of hyperkalemia. During mild attacks, increased neuromuscular irritability may be manifested as restlessness, intestinal cramping, and diarrhea. Severe hyperkalemia decreases the resting membrane potential (i.e., from −90 millivolts to −70 millivolts [hyperpolarization]) and causes muscle weakness, loss of muscle tone, and paralysis. In mild states of hyperkalemia, there is more rapid repolarization, reflected in the ECG as narrow and taller T waves with a shortened QT interval. Severe hyperkalemia causes delayed cardiac conduction and prevents repolarization of heart muscle. Severe hyperkalemia depresses the ST segment, prolongs the PR interval, and widens the QRS complex because of decreased conduction velocity from inactivated sodium channels (see Figure 5-8). Bradydysrhythmias and delayed conduction are common in hyperkalemia; severe hyperkalemia can cause ventricular fibrillation or cardiac arrest.[15]

As with hypokalemia, changes in the ratio of intracellular to extracellular potassium concentration contribute to the symptoms of hyperkalemia (see Table 5-6). The neuromuscular effects of hyperkalemia are related to the increase in rate of repolarization and the presence of other contributing factors, such as acidosis and calcium balance. Long-term increases in ECF potassium concentration result in shifts of potassium into the cell, because the tendency is to maintain a normal ratio of ICF to ECF potassium concentrations. Acute elevations of extracellular potassium concentration affect neuromuscular irritability because this ratio is disrupted. Increases in extracellular fluid calcium concentration can override the neuromuscular effects of hyperkalemia because calcium is also a cation and affects the threshold potential (see Chapter 1).

EVALUATION AND TREATMENT   Hyperkalemia should be investigated when there is a history of renal disease, massive trauma, insulin deficiency, Addison disease, use of potassium salt substitutes, or metabolic acidosis. The acuity of the onset of symptoms may be related to the underlying cause.

Management of hyperkalemia includes treating the contributing causes and correcting the potassium excess. When serum potassium levels are dangerously high, calcium gluconate can be administered to restore normal neuromuscular irritability and to stabilize the resting cardiac membrane potential by making the threshold potential less negative. Administration of glucose (which readily stimulates insulin secretion) or administration of both glucose and insulin for diabetic individuals facilitates cellular entry of potassium. Sodium bicarbonate corrects metabolic acidosis and lowers serum potassium concentration. Oral or rectal administration of cation exchange resins, which exchange sodium for potassium in the intestine, can be effective. Dialysis effectively removes potassium when renal failure has occurred.

✔ QUICK CHECK 5-4

1. What role does potassium play in the body? What metabolic dysfunctions occur in potassium deficiency? In potassium excess?
2. Explain how a person can have normal total body potassium levels but still exhibit hypokalemia.
3. What is the most prominent ECG change associated with hyperkalemia? With hypokalemia?

Other Electrolytes—Calcium, Phosphate, and Magnesium

The specifics of balance for the other body electrolytes—calcium (Ca^{++}), phosphate (PO_4^{3-}), and magnesium (Mg^{++})—are summarized in Table 5-7. Parathyroid hormone and vitamin D are important for the regulation of these minerals[16] (see Chapter 18).

ACID-BASE BALANCE

Acid-base balance must be regulated within a narrow range for the body to function normally. Slight changes in amounts of hydrogen and changes in pH can significantly alter biologic processes in cells and tissues.[17] Hydrogen ion is needed to maintain membrane integrity and the speed of metabolic enzyme reactions. Most pathologic conditions disturb acid-base balance, producing circumstances possibly more harmful than the disease process itself.

Hydrogen Ion and pH

The concentration of hydrogen ions in body fluids is very small—approximately 0.0000001 mg/L. This number, which may be expressed as 10^{-7} mg/L, is indicated as pH 7.0. The symbol *pH* represents the acidity or alkalinity of a solution. As the pH changes 1 unit (e.g., from pH 7.0 to pH 6.0), the [H^+] ([H^+] = hydrogen ion concentration) changes tenfold. The greater the [H^+], the more acidic the solution and the lower the pH. The lower the [H^+], the more alkaline or basic the

solution and the higher the pH. In biologic fluids, a pH of less than 7.4 is defined as acidic and a pH greater than 7.4 is defined as alkaline or basic (Table 5-8).

Body acids are formed as end products of protein, carbohydrate, and fat metabolism and acids can release hydrogen ion. Acids must be balanced by the amount of basic substances in the body to maintain normal pH. The lungs, kidneys, and bones are the major organs involved in regulating acid-base balance. The systems work together to regulate short- and long-term changes in acid-base status.

Body acids exist in two forms: volatile (can be eliminated as CO_2 gas) and nonvolatile (can be eliminated by the kidney). The volatile acid is carbonic acid (H_2CO_3), a *weak acid* (i.e., it does not release its hydrogen easily). In the presence of the enzyme carbonic anhydrase, it readily dissociates into carbon dioxide (CO_2) and water (H_2O). The carbon dioxide is then eliminated by pulmonary ventilation.

Nonvolitile acids are sulfuric, phosphoric, and other organic acids. They are *strong acids* (readily release their hydrogens). Nonvolatile acids are secreted into the urine by the renal tubules in amounts of about 60 to 100 mEq of hydrogen per day or about 1 mEq per kilogram of body weight.

Buffer Systems

Buffering occurs in response to changes in acid-base status. Buffers can absorb excessive hydrogen ion (H^+) (acid) or hydroxyl ion (OH^-) (base) and prevent a significant change in pH. The buffer systems are located in both the ICF and the ECF compartments, and they function at different rates (Table 5-9). The most important plasma buffer systems are carbonic acid–bicarbonate and the protein hemoglobin (Figure 5-9). Phosphate and protein are the most important intracellular buffers and provide a first line of defense. Ammonia and phosphate can attach hydrogen ions and are important renal buffers.

Carbonic Acid–Bicarbonate Buffering

The carbonic acid–bicarbonate buffer pair *operates in both the lung and the kidney* and is a major extracellular buffer. The lungs are a second line of defense and can relatively quickly (within seconds to minutes) decrease the amount of carbonic acid by blowing off carbon dioxide and leaving water. The kidneys are a third line of defense (hours to days) and can reabsorb bicarbonate (a type of base) or regenerate new bicarbonate from carbon dioxide and water. The relationship between bicarbonate (HCO_3^-) and carbonic acid (H_2CO_3) is usually expressed as a ratio. Normal bicarbonate level is about 24 mEq/L, and normal carbonic acid level is about 1.2 mEq/L (when the arterial CO_2 partial pressure [$Paco_2$] is 40 mm Hg), producing a 20:1 (24/1.2) ratio and the normal pH of 7.4 (Figure 5-10). These two systems are very effective together because the lungs can adjust acid concentration rapidly by ventilation and bicarbonate is easily reabsorbed or regenerated by the kidney tubules, although more slowly.

Renal and respiratory adjustments to primary changes in pH are known as compensation. The respiratory system compensates for changes in pH by increasing or decreasing the concentration of carbon dioxide (carbonic acid) by changing ventilation. The renal system compensates by producing more acidic or more alkaline urine. The values for $Paco_2$ and bicarbonate will vary from normal levels in an attempt to maintain a ratio of 20:1. Correction occurs when the values for both components of the buffer pair (carbonic acid and bicarbonate) return to normal levels.

Protein Buffering

Both intracellular and extracellular proteins have negative charges and can serve as buffers for hydrogen, but because most proteins are inside cells, they are primarily an intracellular buffer system. Hemoglobin

TABLE 5-7 Alterations in Calcium, Phosphate, and Magnesium

Parameter	Calcium	Phosphate	Magnesium
Normal values	Serum: 8.8-10.5 mg/dl (total), 4.5-5.6 mg/dl (ionized); 99% in bone as hydroxyapatite; remainder in plasma and body cells with 50% bound to plasma proteins; 40% free or ionized; ionized form most important physiologically	Serum: 2.5-5.0 mg/dl, but may be as high as 6.0-7.0 mg/dl in infants and young children; mainly in bone with some in ICF and ECF; exists as phospholipids, phosphate esters, and inorganic phosphate (ionized form)	Serum: 1.8-3.0 mEq/L; 40-60% stored in bone, 33% bound to plasma proteins; primary intracellular divalent cation
Function	Needed for fundamental metabolic processes; major cation for structure of bone and teeth; enzymatic cofactor for blood clotting; required for hormone secretion and function of cell receptors; directly related to plasma membrane stability and permeability, transmission of nerve impulses, and contraction of muscles; parathyroid hormone, vitamin D_3, and calcitonin act together to control calcium absorption and excretion (see Chapter 18)	Intracellular and extracellular anion buffer in regulation of acid-base balance; provides energy for muscle contraction (as ATP); parathyroid hormone, vitamin D_3, and calcitonin act together to control phosphate absorption and excretion (see Chapter 18)	Cofactor in intracellular enzymatic reactions and causes neuromuscular excitability; often interacts with calcium and potassium in reactions at cellular level and has important role in smooth muscle contraction and relaxation; magnesium is absorbed in the intestine and eliminated by the kidney
Excess	**Hypercalcemia** (serum concentrations >10-12 mg/dl)	**Hyperphosphatemia** (serum concentrations >4.7 mg/dl)	**Hypermagnesemia** (serum concentrations >3.0 mEq/L)
Causes	Hyperparathyroidism; bone metastases with calcium resorption from breast, prostate, renal, and cervical cancer; sarcoidosis; excess vitamin D; many tumors that produce PTH	Acute or chronic renal failure with significant loss of glomerular filtration; treatment of metastatic tumors with chemotherapy that releases large amounts of phosphate into serum; long-term use of laxatives or enemas containing phosphates; hypoparathyroidism	Usually renal insufficiency or failure; also excessive intake of magnesium-containing antacids, adrenal insufficiency
Effects	Many nonspecific; fatigue, weakness, lethargy, anorexia, nausea, constipation; impaired renal function, kidney stones; dysrhythmias, bradycardia, cardiac arrest; bone pain, osteoporosis	Symptoms primarily related to low serum calcium levels (caused by high phosphate levels) similar to results of hypocalcemia; when prolonged, calcification of soft tissues in lungs, kidneys, joints	Skeletal smooth muscle contraction; excess nerve function; loss of deep tendon reflexes; nausea and vomiting; muscle weakness; hypotension; bradycardia; respiratory distress
Deficit	**Hypocalcemia** (serum calcium concentration <8.5 mg/dl)	**Hypophosphatemia** (serum phosphate concentration <2.0 mg/dl)	**Hypomagnesemia** (serum magnesium concentration <1.5 mEq/L)
Causes	Related to inadequate intestinal absorption, deposition of ionized calcium into bone or soft tissue, blood administration, or decreases in PTH and vitamin D; nutritional deficiencies occur with inadequate sources of dairy products or green leafy vegetables	Most commonly by intestinal malabsorption related to vitamin D deficiency, use of magnesium- and aluminum-containing antacids, long-term alcohol abuse, and malabsorption syndromes; respiratory alkalosis; increased renal excretion of phosphate associated with hyperparathyroidism	Malnutrition, malabsorption syndromes, alcoholism, urinary losses (renal tubular dysfunction, loop diuretics)
Effects	Increased neuromuscular excitability; tingling, muscle spasm (particularly in hands, feet, and facial muscles), intestinal cramping, hyperactive bowel sounds; severe cases show convulsions and tetany; prolonged QT interval, cardiac arrest	Conditions related to reduced capacity for oxygen transport by red blood cells and disturbed energy metabolism; leukocyte and platelet dysfunction; deranged nerve and muscle function; in severe cases, irritability, confusion, numbness, coma, convulsions; possibly respiratory failure (because of muscle weakness), cardiomyopathies, bone resorption (leading to rickets or osteomalacia)	Behavioral changes, irritability, increased reflexes, muscle cramps, ataxia, nystagmus, tetany, convulsions, tachycardia, hypotension

ATP, Adenosine triphosphate; *PTH*, parathyroid hormone.

(Hb) is an excellent intracellular blood buffer because it can bind with hydrogen ion (H^+) (forming HHb) and carbon dioxide (forming $HHbCO_2$). Hemoglobin bound to hydrogen ion becomes a weak acid. Hemoglobin not saturated with oxygen (venous blood) is a better buffer than hemoglobin saturated with oxygen (arterial blood). The pH control mechanism is illustrated in Figure 5-9.

Renal Buffering

The distal tubule of the kidney regulates acid-base balance by secreting hydrogen into the urine and reabsorbing bicarbonate into the plasma. Dibasic phosphate ($HPO_4^=$) and ammonia (NH_3) are two important renal buffers because they can attach hydrogen ions and be secreted into the urine. The renal buffering of hydrogen ions requires the use of carbon dioxide (CO_2) and water (H_2O) to form carbonic acid (H_2CO_3). The enzyme carbonic anhydrase catalyzes the reaction. The hydrogen in the carbonic acid is then secreted from the tubular cell and buffered in the lumen by phosphate and ammonia (i.e., forms $H_2PO_3^-$ and NH_4^+). The remaining bicarbonate is reabsorbed. The end effect is the addition of new bicarbonate to the plasma, which contributes to the alkalinity of the plasma because the hydrogen ion is excreted from the body (Figure 5-11).

Acid-Base Imbalances

Pathophysiologic changes in the concentration of hydrogen ion in the blood lead to acid-base imbalances.[18,19] In **acidemia** the pH of arterial blood is less than 7.4. A systemic increase in hydrogen ion concentration or a loss of base is termed **acidosis**. In **alkalemia** the pH of arterial blood is greater than 7.4. A systemic decrease in hydrogen ion concentration or an excess of base is termed **alkalosis**. These changes may be caused by metabolic or respiratory processes. Figure 5-10 summarizes the relationship among pH, the partial pressure of carbon dioxide (respiratory regulation), and the concentration of bicarbonate (renal regulation) during alkalosis and acidosis. Acid-base imbalances are assessed using measurement of arterial blood gases, which includes the reporting of pH, $Paco_2$, and HCO_3^-. The medical history and clinical symptoms are important in determining the cause of the disorder.

Figure 5-12 summarizes the relationships among pH, Pco_2, and bicarbonate during different acid-base alterations.

Metabolic Acidosis

In **metabolic acidosis** the concentrations of non–carbonic acids increase or bicarbonate is lost from extracellular fluid or cannot be regenerated by the kidney (Table 5-10). This can occur either quickly, as in lactic acidosis caused by poor perfusion or hypoxemia, or slowly over an extended time, as in renal failure, diabetic ketoacidosis, or starvation (anion gap acidosis).[20] There is a decrease in the 20:1 ratio of HCO_3^- to H_2CO_3.

The buffering systems normally compensate for excess acid and maintain arterial pH within normal range. When acidosis is severe, buffers become depleted and cannot compensate, and the ratio of the concentrations of bicarbonate to carbonic acid decreases to less than 20:1 (see Figure 5-10). An increase in the plasma concentration of chloride out of proportion of sodium causes hyperchloremic acidosis (nonainion gap acidosis). The specific type of acidosis can be determined by examining the serum **anion gap** (see Table 5-10).

Metabolic acidosis is manifested by changes in the function of the neurologic, respiratory, gastrointestinal, and cardiovascular systems. Early symptoms include headache and lethargy, which progress to confusion and coma in severe acidosis. The respiratory system's efforts to compensate for the increase in metabolic acids result in what are termed *Kussmaul respirations* (a form of hyperventilation), which are deep and rapid. This represents the body's attempt to increase pH by expelling carbon dioxide, which decreases carbonic acid concentration. Other symptoms include anorexia, nausea, vomiting, diarrhea, and abdominal discomfort. Death can result in the most severe and prolonged cases preceded by dysrhythmias and hypotension. The underlying condition must be diagnosed to establish effective treatment.

Metabolic Alkalosis

When excessive loss of metabolic acids occurs, bicarbonate concentration increases, causing **metabolic alkalosis**[21] (see Figure 5-12). When acid loss is caused by vomiting, renal compensation is not very effective because loss of chloride (an anion) in hydrochloric acid (HCl) stimulates renal retention of bicarbonate (an anion). The result is known as **hypochloremic metabolic alkalosis**.[21] Hyperaldosteronism also can lead to alkalosis as a result of sodium bicarbonate retention and loss of hydrogen and potassium. Diuretics may produce a mild alkalosis because they promote greater excretion of sodium, potassium, and chloride than of bicarbonate.

TABLE 5-8	pH of Body Fluids	
Body Fluid	**pH**	**Factors Affecting pH**
Gastric juices	1.0-3.0	Hydrochloric acid production
Urine	5.0-6.0	H^+ ion excretion from waste products
Arterial blood	7.35-7.45	pH is slightly higher because there is less carbonic acid (H_2CO_3)
Venous blood	7.37	pH is slightly lower because there is more carbonic acid
Cerebrospinal fluid	7.32	Decreased bicarbonate and higher carbon dioxide content decrease pH
Pancreatic fluid	7.8-8.0	Contains bicarbonate produced by exocrine cells
Bile	7.0-8.0	Contains bicarbonate
Small intestine fluid	6.5-7.5	Contains alkaline fluid from pancreas, liver, and gallbladder

TABLE 5-9	Buffer Systems		
Buffer Pairs	**Buffer System**	**Chemical Reaction**	**Rate**
HCO_3^-/H_2CO_3	Bicarbonate	$H^+ + HCO_3^- \gtrless H_2O + CO_2$	Instantaneously
Hb^-/HHb	Hemoglobin	$HHb \rightleftharpoons H^+ + Hb^-$	Instantaneously
$HPO_4^=/H_2PO_4^-$	Phosphate	$H_2PO_4^- + H^+ + HPO_4^=$	Instantaneously
Pr^-/HPr	Plasma proteins	$HPr \rightleftharpoons H^+ + Pr^-$	Instantaneously
Organs	**Physiologic Mechanism**		**Rate**
Lung ventilation	Regulates retention or elimination of CO_2 and therefore H_2CO_3 concentration		Minutes to hours
Ionic shifts	Exchange of intracellular potassium and sodium for hydrogen		2-4 hours
Kidney tubules	Bicarbonate reabsorption and regeneration, ammonia formation, phosphate buffering		Hours to days
Bone	Exchanges of calcium and phosphate and release of carbonate		Hours to days

CO_2, Carbon dioxide; Hb^-, hemoglobin; HCO_3^-, bicarbonate; H_2CO_3, carbonic acid; HHb, hydrogenated hemoglobin; $HPO_4^=$, dibasic phosphate; $H_2PO_4^-$, monobasic phosphate; HPr, hydrogenated protein; Pr^-, protein.

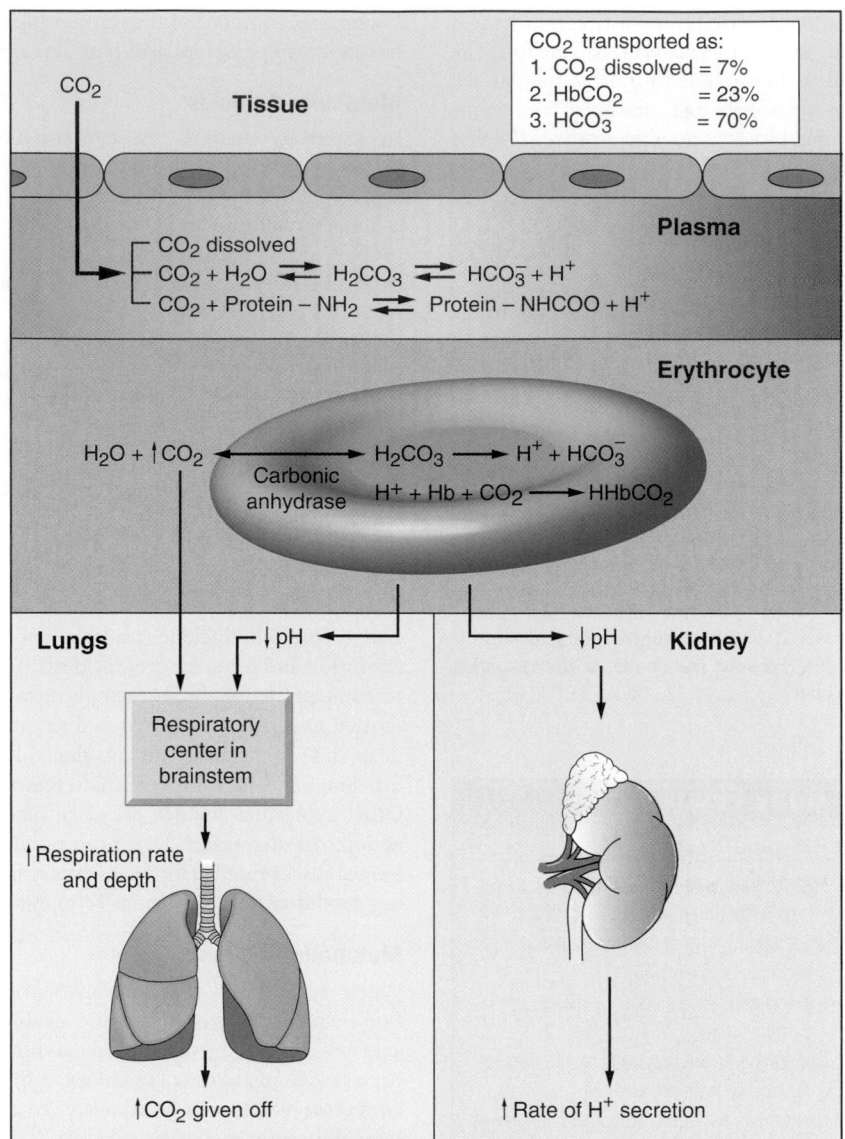

FIGURE 5-9 Integration of pH Control Mechanisms (example for acidosis). CO_2 is produced in tissue cells and diffuses to plasma, where it is transported as dissolved CO_2, or it combines with water to form carbonic acid (H_2CO_3), or it combines with protein from which hydrogen has been released. Most of the CO_2 diffuses into the red blood cells and combines with water to form H_2CO_3. The H_2CO_3 dissociates to form hydrogen ion (H^+) and bicarbonate (HCO_3^-). Hydrogen combines with hemoglobin that has released its oxygen to form HHb, which buffers the hydrogen and makes venous blood slightly more acidic than arterial blood. The increase in H^+ coupled with elevated CO_2 levels results in $HHbCO_3$ and an increase in the respiratory rate and secretion of H^+ by the kidneys.

Some common signs and symptoms of metabolic alkalosis are weakness, muscle cramps, hyperactive reflexes, tetany, confusion, convulsions, and atrial tachycardia. Respirations may be shallow and slow ventilation as the lungs attempt to compensate by increasing carbon dioxide retention. The manifestations vary with the cause and severity of the alkalosis. The symptoms of hyperactive reflexes and tetany occur because alkalosis increases binding of Ca^{++} to plasma proteins, thus decreasing ionized calcium concentration. The decreased ionized calcium concentration causes excitable cells to become hypopolarized, initiating an action potential more easily and causing muscle contraction.

Treatments are related to the underlying cause of the condition. With hypochloremic alkalosis or contraction alkalosis with volume depletion, a sodium chloride solution is required for correction because chloride must be replaced before bicarbonate can be excreted by the kidney.

Respiratory Acidosis

Respiratory acidosis occurs when there is alveolar hypoventilation, resulting in an excess of carbon dioxide in the blood (hypercapnia). The arterial carbon dioxide tension (or pressure) ($Paco_2$) is >45 mm Hg and the pH is less than 7.35 (see Figure 5-12). A decrease in alveolar

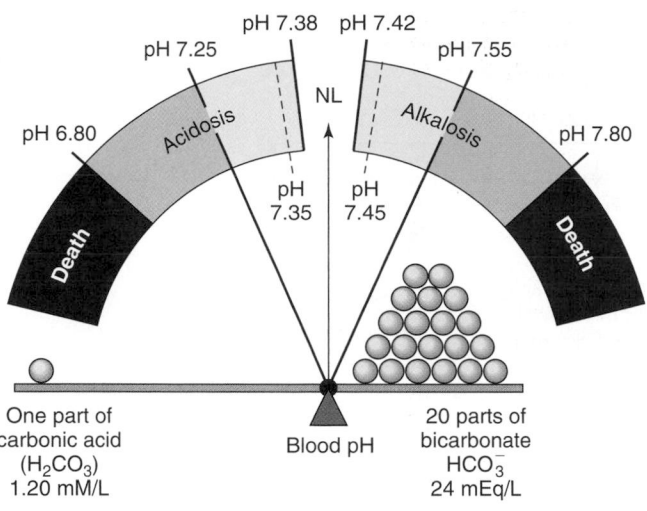

FIGURE 5-10 Ratio of Carbonic Acid and Bicarbonate Concentration in Maintaining pH Within Normal Limits. An increase in H_2CO_3 or decrease in HCO_3^- concentration causes acidosis. A decrease in H_2CO_3 or increase in HCO_3^- concentration causes alkalosis. H_2CO_3, Carbonic acid; HCO_3^-, bicarbonate. (From Monahan FD: *Medical-surgical nursing: health and illness perspectives,* ed 8, St Louis, 2007, Mosby.)

FIGURE 5-11 Renal Excretion of Acid. **1,** Conservation of filtered bicarbonate. Filtered bicarbonate combines with secreted hydrogen ion in the presence of carbon anhydrase *(CA)* to form carbonic acid (H_2CO_3), which then dissociates to water (H_2O) and carbon dioxide (CO_2); both diffuse into the epithelial cell. The CO_2 and H_2O combine to form H_2CO_3 in the presence of CA, and the resulting bicarbonate ion (HCO_3^-) is reabsorbed into the capillary. **2,** Formation of titratable acid. Hydrogen ion is secreted and combines with dibasic phosphate ($HPO_4^=$) to form monobasic phosphate ($H_2PO_4^-$). The secreted hydrogen ion is formed from the dissociation of H_2CO_3, and the remaining HCO_3^- is reabsorbed into the capillary. **3,** Formation of ammonium. Ammonia (NH_3) is produced from glutamine in the epithelial cell and diffuses to the tubular lumen, where it combines with H^+ to form ammonium ion (NH_4^+). Once NH_4^+ has been formed, it cannot return to the epithelial cell (diffusional trapping), and the bicarbonate remaining in the epithelial cell is reabsorbed into the capillary.

TABLE 5-10	Causes of Metabolic Acidosis
Increased Non–Carbonic Acids (Elevated Anion Gap*)	**Bicarbonate Loss or Hyperchloremic Acidosis (Normal Anion Gap)**
Increased H^+ load	Diarrhea
Ketoacidosis (e.g., diabetes mellitus, starvation)	Ureterosigmoidoscopy (chloride absorbed in excess of sodium in small intestine)
Lactic acidosis (e.g., shock, hypoxemia)	Renal failure (loss of bicarbonate)
Ingestion (e.g., ammonium chloride, ethylene glycol, methanol, salicylates, paraldehyde)	Proximal renal tubular acidosis (loss of more renal sodium in relation to chloride)
Decreased renal H^+ excretion	
Uremia	
Distal renal tubule acidosis	

*Anion gap refers to anions not usually measured in laboratory reports (e.g., sulfate, phosphate, and lactate). The anions usually measured are chloride (Cl^-) and bicarbonate (HCO_3^-). When the sum of the concentrations of measured anions (e.g., chloride and bicarbonate) is subtracted from the sum of the concentrations of measured cations (e.g., sodium and potassium), there is a "gap" of approximately 10 to 12 mEq/L; this is the normal anion gap. An elevated anion gap provides clues to the cause of the acidosis (i.e., to the addition of endogenously or exogenously generated acids). In a normal anion gap acidosis, chloride is retained to replace lost bicarbonate.

ventilation in relation to the metabolic production of carbon dioxide produces respiratory acidosis by an increase in the concentration of carbonic acid. Respiratory acidosis can be acute or chronic.[22] Common causes include depression of the respiratory center (e.g., from drugs or head injury), paralysis of the respiratory muscles, disorders of the chest wall (e.g., kyphoscoliosis or broken ribs), and disorders of the lung parenchyma (e.g., pneumonia, pulmonary edema, emphysema, asthma, bronchitis). Renal compensation occurs by elimination of hydrogen ion and retention of bicarbonate.

The signs and symptoms seen often include headache, blurred vision, breathlessness, restlessness, and apprehension followed by lethargy, disorientation, muscle twitching, tremors, convulsions, and coma. Respiratory rate is rapid at first and gradually becomes depressed as the respiratory center adapts to increasing levels of carbon dioxide. The skin may be warm and flushed because the elevated carbon dioxide

FIGURE 5-12 Primary and Compensatory Acid-Base Changes. A systematic approach can be used to interpret the cause of an acid-base imbalance. **1,** Is the pH low or high? **2,** If the pH is low (acidemia), is the cause respiratory (high $PaCO_2$) or metabolic (low HCO_3^-)? **3,** If the pH is high (alkalemia), is the cause respiratory (low $PaCO_2$) or metabolic (high HCO_3^-)? **4,** Is there compensation for the primary acid-base disorder? (a) HCO_3^- will be ≥24 mEq/L if there is renal compensation for a primary respiratory acidosis; (b) $PaCO_2$ will be <40 mm Hg if there is respiratory compensation of a primary metabolic acidosis; (c) HCO_3^- will be <24 mEq/L if there is renal compensation for primary respiratory alkalosis; (d) $PaCO_2$ will be >40 mm Hg if there is respiratory compensation for primary metabolic alkalosis.
NOTE: Examine the pH first to determine if there is acidemia or alkalemia. Then examine the changes in HCO_3^- and $PaCO_2$. **1,** HCO_3^- will be elevated when there is primary metabolic alkalosis or renal compensation for primary respiratory acidosis. **2,** HCO_3^- will be decreased when there is primary metabolic acidosis or renal compensation for primary respiratory alkalosis. **3,** $PaCO_2$ will be elevated when there is primary respiratory acidosis or respiratory compensation for primary metabolic alkalosis. **4,** $PaCO_2$ will be decreased when there is primary respiratory alkalosis or respiratory compensation for metabolic acidosis. *H_2CO_3,* Carbonic acid; *HCO_3^-,* bicarbonate; *$PaCO_2$,* arterial partial pressure of carbon dioxide.

concentration causes vasodilation. The restoration of adequate alveolar ventilation is necessary to remove the excess CO_2 ($\downarrow H_2CO_3$).

Respiratory Alkalosis

Respiratory alkalosis occurs when there is alveolar hyperventilation (deep, rapid respirations). Excessive reduction in plasma carbon dioxide levels (hypocapnia) decrease carbonic acid concentration.[23,24] The $Paco_2$ is <35 mm Hg and the pH is greater than normal (see Figure 5-12). Respiratory alkalosis can be chronic or acute. Hypoxemia (caused by pulmonary disease, congestive heart failure, or high altitudes), hypermetabolic states (e.g., fever, anemia, thyrotoxicosis), early salicylate intoxication, hysteria, cirrhosis, and gram-negative sepsis stimulate hyperventilation. Improper use of mechanical ventilators also can cause iatrogenic (treatment-related) respiratory alkalosis, and secondary alkalosis may develop as a result of hyperventilation stimulated by metabolic or respiratory acidosis. The kidneys compensate by decreasing hydrogen excretion and bicarbonate reabsorption.

The central and peripheral nervous systems are stimulated by respiratory alkalosis, causing dizziness, confusion, tingling of extremities (paresthesias), convulsions, and coma. Cerebral vasoconstriction reduces cerebral blood flow. Carpopedal spasm (spasm of muscles in the fingers and toes), tetany, and other symptoms of hypocalcemia (see Table 5-7, p. 126) are similar to those of metabolic alkalosis. The underlying disturbance must be treated, particularly hypoxemia.

✔**QUICK CHECK 5-5**

1. What is the difference between compensation and correction of acid-base disturbances?
2. What two chemicals are altered in metabolic acid-base disturbances?
3. How do alterations in carbon dioxide concentration influence acid-base status?

PEDIATRIC CONSIDERATIONS
Distribution of Body Fluids

Newborn Infants
At birth TBW represents about 75% to 80% of body weight and decreases to about 67% during the first year of life. Physiologic loss of body water amounting to 5% of body weight occurs as an infant adjusts to a new environment. Infants are particularly susceptible to significant changes in TBW because of a high metabolic rate and greater body surface area, as compared to adults. Consequently, they have a greater fluid intake and output in relation to their body size. Renal mechanisms of fluid and electrolyte conservation may not be mature enough to counter abnormal losses related to vomiting or diarrhea, thereby allowing dehydration to occur. Symptoms of dehydration include increased thirst, decreased urine output, decreased body weight, decreased skin elasticity, sunken fontanels, absent tears, dry mucous membranes, increased heart rate, and irritability.

Children and Adolescents
TBW slowly decreases to 60% to 65% of body weight. At adolescence the percentage of TBW approaches adult levels and differences according to gender appear. Males have a greater percentage of body water because of increased muscle mass, and females have more body fat because of the influence of estrogen and thus less water.

GERIATRIC CONSIDERATIONS
Distribution of Body Fluids

The further decline in the percentage of TBW in the elderly is in part the result of a decreased free fat mass and decreased muscle mass, as well as a reduced ability to regulate sodium and water balance. Kidneys are less efficient in producing either a concentrated or a diluted urine, and sodium-conserving responses are sluggish. Thirst perception also may decline and loss of cognitive function can influence access to beverages. Healthy older adults can adequately maintain their hydration status. When disease is present, a decrease in TBW, dehydration, and hypernatremia can become life-threatening.

▮ DID YOU UNDERSTAND?

Distribution of Body Fluids
1. Body fluids are distributed among functional compartments and are classified as intracellular fluid (ICF) and extracellular fluid (ECF).
2. The sum of all fluids is the total body water (TBW), which varies with age and amount of body fat.
3. Water moves between the ICF and ECF compartments principally by osmosis.
4. Water moves between the plasma and interstitial fluid by osmosis (pulling of water) and hydrostatic pressure (pushing of water), which occur across the capillary membrane.
5. Movement across the capillary wall is called *net filtration* and is described according to Starling law (the balance between hydrostatic and osmotic forces).

Alterations in Water Movement
1. Edema is a problem of fluid distribution that results in accumulation of fluid within the interstitial spaces.
2. The pathophysiologic process that leads to edema is related to an increase in forces favoring fluid filtration from the capillaries or lymphatic channels into the tissues.
3. Edema is caused by arterial dilation, venous or lymphatic obstruction, increased vascular volume, loss of plasma proteins, or increased capillary permeability.
4. Edema may be localized or generalized and usually is associated with weight gain, swelling and puffiness, tighter-fitting clothes and shoes, and limited movement of the affected area.

Sodium, Chloride, and Water Balance
1. There is an intimate relationship between the balance of sodium and water levels; chloride levels are generally proportional to changes in sodium levels.
2. Water balance is regulated by the sensation of thirst and by antidiuretic hormone (ADH), which is secreted in response to an increase in plasma osmolality or a decrease in circulating blood volume.
3. Sodium balance is regulated by aldosterone, which increases reabsorption of sodium from the urine into the blood by the distal tubule of the kidney.
4. Renin and angiotensin are enzymes that promote secretion of aldosterone and thus regulate sodium and water balance.
5. Natriuretic hormones are involved in decreasing tubular reabsorption and promoting urinary excretion of sodium.

Alterations in Sodium, Water, and Chloride Balance
1. Alterations in sodium and water balance may be classified as isotonic, hypertonic, or hypotonic.
2. Isotonic alterations occur when changes in TBW are accompanied by proportional changes in electrolytes.
3. Hypertonic alterations develop when the osmolality of the ECF is elevated above normal, usually because of an increased concentration of ECF sodium or a deficit of ECF water.
4. Hypernatremia (sodium levels more than 145 mEq/L) may be caused by an acute increase in sodium level or a loss of water.
5. Hypernatremia can be isovolemic, hypovolemic, or hypervolemic depending on accompanying changes in the level of body water.
6. Hypernatremia with marked water deficit is manifested by hypovolemia and dehydration.
7. Hyperchloremia is caused by an excess of sodium or a deficit of bicarbonate.
8. Hypotonic alterations occur when the osmolality of the ECF is less than normal.
9. Hyponatremia (serum sodium concentration less than 135 mEq/L) usually causes movement of water into cells.
10. Hyponatremia may be caused by sodium loss, inadequate sodium intake, or dilution of the body's sodium level with excess water.
11. Hyponatremia can be isovolemic, hypervolemic or hypovolemic, or dilutional depending on accompanying changes in the amount of body water.
12. Hypochloremia usually is the result of hyponatremia or elevated bicarbonate concentrations.

Alterations in Potassium and Other Electrolytes

1. Potassium is the predominant ICF ion; it regulates ICF osmolality, maintains the resting membrane potential, and is required for deposition of glycogen in liver and skeletal muscle cells.
2. Potassium balance is regulated by the kidney, by aldosterone and insulin secretion, and by changes in pH.
3. Potassium adaptation allows the body to accommodate slowly to increased levels of potassium intake.
4. Hypokalemia (serum potassium concentration less than 3.5 mEq/L) indicates loss of total body potassium, although ECF hypokalemia can develop without losses of total body potassium, and plasma potassium levels may be normal or elevated when total body potassium is depleted.
5. Hypokalemia may be caused by reduced potassium intake, a shift of potassium from the ECF to the ICF, increased aldosterone secretion, increased renal excretion, and alkalosis.
6. Hyperkalemia (potassium levels that are greater than 5.5 mEq/L) may be caused by increased potassium intake, a shift of potassium from the ICF to the ECF, or decreased renal excretion.
7. Calcium is an ion necessary for bone and teeth formation, blood coagulation, hormone secretion and cell receptor function, and membrane stability.
8. Phosphate acts as a buffer in acid-base regulation and provides energy for muscle contraction.
9. Calcium and phosphate concentrations are rigidly controlled by parathyroid hormone (PTH), vitamin D, and calcitonin.
10. Hypocalcemia (serum calcium concentration less than 8.5 mg/dl) is related to inadequate intestinal absorption, deposition of calcium into bone or soft tissue, blood administration, or decreased PTH and vitamin D levels.
11. Hypercalcemia (serum calcium concentration greater than 12 mg/dl) can be caused by a number of diseases, including hyperparathyroidism, bone metastases, sarcoidosis, and excess vitamin D.
12. Hypophosphatemia is usually caused by intestinal malabsorption and increased renal excretion of phosphate.
13. Hyperphosphatemia develops with acute or chronic renal failure when there is significant loss of glomerular filtration.
14. Magnesium is a major intracellular cation and is regulated principally by PTH.
15. Magnesium functions in enzymatic reactions and often interacts with calcium at the cellular level.
16. Hypomagnesemia (serum magnesium concentrations less than 1.5 mEq/L) may be caused by malabsorption syndromes.
17. Hypermagnesemia (serum magnesium concentrations greater than 2.5 mEq/L) is rare and usually is caused by renal failure.

Acid-Base Balance

1. Hydrogen ions, which maintain membrane integrity and the speed of enzymatic reactions, must be concentrated within a narrow range if the body is to function normally.
2. Hydrogen ion concentration, $[H^+]$, is expressed as pH, which represents the negative logarithm (i.e., 10^{-7}) of hydrogen ions in solution (i.e., 0.0000001 mg/L).
3. Different body fluids have different pH values; values less than 7.4 are more acidic and values greater than 7.4 are more basic.
4. The renal and respiratory systems, together with the body's buffer systems, are the principal regulators of acid-base balance.
5. Buffers are substances that can absorb excessive acid or base without a significant change in pH.
6. Buffers exist as acid-base pairs; the principal plasma buffers are carbonic acid (H_2CO_3), bicarbonate (HCO_3^-), protein (hemoglobin), and phosphate.
7. The lungs and kidneys act to compensate for primary changes in pH by increasing or decreasing ventilation and by producing more acidic or more alkaline urine.
8. Correction is a process different from compensation; correction occurs when the values for both components of the buffer pair return to normal as the primary disorder is treated or resolves.
9. Acid-base imbalances are caused by changes in the concentration of hydrogen ion in the blood; an increase causes acidosis, and a decrease causes alkalosis.
10. An abnormal increase or decrease in bicarbonate concentration causes metabolic alkalosis or metabolic acidosis; changes in the rate of alveolar ventilation and removal of carbon dioxide produce respiratory acidosis or respiratory alkalosis.
11. Metabolic acidosis is caused by an increase in the levels of non–carbonic acids or by the loss of bicarbonate from the extracellular fluid.
12. Metabolic alkalosis occurs with an increase in bicarbonate concentration, which is usually caused by loss of metabolic acids from conditions such as vomiting or gastrointestinal suctioning or by excessive bicarbonate intake, hyperaldosteronism, and diuretic therapy.
13. Respiratory acidosis occurs with decreased alveolar ventilation, which in turn causes hypercapnia (an increase in carbon dioxide concentration) and increased carbonic acid concentration.
14. Respiratory alkalosis occurs with alveolar hyperventilation and excessive reduction of carbon dioxide level, or hypocapnia with decreases in carbonic acid concentration.

KEY TERMS

Acidemia, 127
Acidosis, 127
Aldosterone, 117
Alkalemia, 127
Alkalosis, 127
Angiotensin I, 117
Angiotensin II, 117
Anion gap, 127
Aquaporin, 115
Antidiuretic hormone (ADH), 117
Baroreceptor, 119
Buffer, 125

Buffering, 125
Capillary hydrostatic pressure (blood pressure), 115
Capillary (plasma) oncotic pressure, 115
Carbonic acid–bicarbonate buffer, 125
Chloride (Cl−), 117
Compensation, 125
Correction, 125
Dehydration, 119
Dilutional hyponatremia (water intoxication), 121

Edema, 115
Extracellular fluid (ECF), 114
Hypercapnia, 128
Hyperchloremia, 120
Hyperkalemia, 124
Hypernatremia, 119
Hypertonic fluid alterations, 119
Hypervolemic hypernatremia, 119
Hypervolemic hyponatremia, 121
Hypocapnia, 130
Hypochloremia, 121

Hypochloremic metabolic alkalosis, 127
Hypokalemia, 122
Hyponatremia, 121
Hypotonic fluid imbalance, 121
Hypovolemic hypernatremia, 119
Hypovolemic hyponatremia, 121
Interstitial fluid, 114
Interstitial hydrostatic pressure, 115
Interstitial oncotic pressure, 115
Intracellular fluid (ICF), 114
Intravascular fluid, 114

REFERENCES

1. Day RE et al: Human aquaporins: regulators of transcellular water flow, *Biochim Biophys Acta* 1840(5):1492-1506, 2014.

2. Trayes KP et al: Edema: diagnosis and management, *Am Fam Physician* 88(2):102-110, 2013.

3. Ridner SH: Pathophysiology of lymphedema, *Semin Oncol Nurs* 29(1):4-11, 2013.

4. Motiwala SR, Januzzi JL Jr: The role of natriuretic peptides as biomarkers for guiding the management of chronic heart failure, *Clin Pharmacol Ther* 93(1):57-67, 2013.

5. Cheuvront SN et al: Physiologic basis for understanding quantitative dehydration assessment, *Am J Clin Nutr* 97(3):455-462, 2013.

6. Sam R, Feizi I: Understanding hypernatremia, *Am J Nephrol* 36(1):97-104, 2012.

7. Berend K, van Hulsteijn LH, Gans RO. Chloride: the queen of electrolytes? *Eur J Intern Med* 23(3):203-211, 2012.

8. Sterns RH: Disorders of plasma sodium—causes, consequences, and correction, *N Engl J Med* 372(1):55-65, 2015.

9. Gross P: Clinical management of SIADH, *Ther Adv Endocrinol Metab* 3(2):61-73, 2012.

10. Lehrich RW et al: Role of vaptans in the management of hyponatremia, *Am J Kidney Dis* 62(2):364-376, 2013.

11. Youn JH: Gut sensing of potassium intake and its role in potassium homeostasis, *Semin Nephrol* 33(3):248-256, 2013.

12. Lee Hamm L et al: Acid-base and potassium homeostasis, *Semin Nephrol* 33(3):257-264, 2013.

13. Pepin J, Shields C: Advances in diagnosis and management of hypokalemic and hyperkalemic emergencies, *Emerg Med Pract* 14(2):1-17, 2012.

14. Lim S: Approach to hyperkalemia, *Acta Med Indones* 39(2):99-103, 2007.

15. Maxwell AP et al: Management of hyperkalaemia, *J R Coll Physicians Edinb* 43(3):246-251, 2013.

16. Moe SM: Disorders involving calcium, phosphorus and magnesium, *Prim Care* 35(2):215-237, 2008.

17. Adeva-Andany MM et al: The importance of the ionic product for water to understand the physiology of the acid-base balance in humans, *Biomed Res Int* 2014:695281, 2014.

18. Berend K, de Vries AP, Gans RO: Physiological approach to assessment of acid-base disturbances, *N Engl J Med* 371(15):1434-1445, 2014. Erratum in: *N Engl J Med* 371(20):1948.

19. Carmody JB, Norwood VF: A clinical approach to paediatric acid-base disorders, *Postgrad Med J* 88(1037):143-151, 2012.

20. Kraut JA, Madias NE: Differential diagnosis of nongap metabolic acidosis: value of a systematic approach, *Clin J Am Soc Nephrol* 7(4):671-679, 2012.

21. Soifer JT, Kim HT: Approach to metabolic alkalosis, *Emerg Med Clin North Am* 32(2):453-463, 2014.

22. Bruno CM, Valenti M: Acid-base disorders in patients with chronic obstructive pulmonary disease: a pathophysiological review, *J Biomed Biotechnol* 2012:915150, 2012.

23. Palmer BF: Evaluation and treatment of respiratory alkalosis, *Am J Kidney Dis* 60(5):834-838, 2012.

24. Madias NE: Renal acidification responses to respiratory acid base disorders, *J Nephrol* 16(Suppl 16):S85-S91, 2010.

6

Innate Immunity: Inflammation and Wound Healing

Neal S. Rote

ⓔ EVOLVE WEBSITE

http://evolve.elsevier.com/Huether/
Student Review Questions
Audio Key Points

Case Studies
Animations
Quick Check Answers

The human body is continually exposed to a large variety of conditions that result in damage, such as sunlight, pollutants, agents that can cause physical trauma, and infectious agents (viruses, bacteria, fungi, parasites). Damage can also arise from within, such as cancers. The damage may be at the level of a single cell, which can be easily repaired, or may be at the level of multiple cells or tissues or organs, which can result in disease and potentially the death of the individual. To protect us from these conditions, the body has developed a highly sophisticated, multilevel system of interactive defense mechanisms.

HUMAN DEFENSE MECHANISMS

The human body has developed several means of protecting itself from injury and infection. Innate immunity, also known as natural or native immunity, includes natural barriers (physical, mechanical, and biochemical) and inflammation. Innate barriers form the first line of defense at the body's surfaces and are in place at birth to prevent damage by substances in the environment and thwart infection by pathogenic microorganisms. Surface barriers may also harbor a group of microorganisms known as the "normal flora" that can protect us from pathogens. If the surface barriers are breached, the second line of defense, the inflammatory response, is activated to protect the body from further injury, prevent infection of the injured tissue, and promote healing. The inflammatory response is a rapid activation of

biochemical and cellular mechanisms that are relatively nonspecific, with similar responses being initiated against a wide variety of causes of tissue damage. The third line of defense, adaptive immunity (also known as acquired or specific immunity), is induced in a relatively slower and more specific process and targets particular invading microorganisms for the purpose of eradicating them. Adaptive immunity also involves "memory," which results in a more rapid response during future exposure to the same microorganism. Comparisons among defense mechanisms are described in Table 6-1. The information presented in this chapter introduces the components and processes of innate immunity and sets the stage for Chapter 7, which presents an overview of adaptive immunity, and Chapter 8, which discusses processes of infection and alterations in immune defenses.

INNATE IMMUNITY

Innate immunity includes natural barriers (physical, mechanical, and biochemical) that form the first line of defense at the body's surfaces and are in place at birth. Surface barriers also may harbor a group of frequently benign microorganisms known as the "normal microbiome" that can protect us from pathogenic microorganisms. Innate immunity in the newborn and changes associated with aging are reviewed in the *Pediatric* and *Geriatric Considerations* boxes.

TABLE 6-1 Overview of Human Defenses

Characteristics	Barriers	Innate Immunity	Adaptive (Acquired) Immunity
Level of defense	First line of defense against infection and tissue injury	Second line of defense; occurs as response to tissue injury or infection (inflammatory response)	Third line of defense; initiated when innate immune system signals cells of adaptive immunity
Timing of defense	Constant	Immediate response	Delay between primary exposure to antigen and maximal response; immediate against secondary exposure to antigen
Specificity	Broadly specific	Broadly specific	Response is very specific toward "antigen"
Cells	Epithelial cells Microbiome	Mast cells, granulocytes (neutrophils, eosinophils, basophils), monocytes/ macrophages, natural killer (NK) cells, platelets, endothelial cells	T lymphocytes, B lymphocytes, macrophages, dendritic cells
Memory	No memory involved	No memory involved	Specific immunologic memory by T and B lymphocytes
Active molecules	Defensins, cathelicidins, collectins, lactoferrin, bacterial toxins	Complement, clotting factors, kinins, cytokines	Antibodies, complement, cytokines
Protection	Protection includes anatomic barriers (i.e., skin and mucous membranes), cells and secretory molecules (e.g., lysozymes, low pH of stomach and urine), and ciliary activity	Protection includes vascular responses, cellular components (e.g., mast cells, neutrophils, macrophages), secretory molecules or cytokines, and activation of plasma protein systems	Protection includes activated T and B lymphocytes, cytokines, and antibodies

First Line of Defense: Physical and Biochemical Barriers and the Human Microbiome
Physical Barriers

The physical barriers that cover the external parts of the human body offer considerable protection from damage and infection. These barriers are composed of tightly associated epithelial cells of the skin and of the linings of the gastrointestinal, genitourinary, and respiratory tracts (Figure 6-1). When pathogens attempt to penetrate this physical barrier, they may be removed by mechanical means—sloughed off with dead skin cells as they are routinely replaced, expelled by coughing or sneezing, vomited from the stomach, or flushed from the urinary tract by urine. Epithelial cells of the upper respiratory tract also produce mucus and have hair-like cilia that trap and move pathogens upward to be expelled by coughing or sneezing. Additionally, the low temperature (such as on the skin) and the low pH (such as of the skin and stomach) generally inhibit microorganisms, most of which routinely require temperatures near 37°C (98.6°F) and pH near neutral for efficient growth.

Epithelial Cell–Derived Chemicals

Epithelial cells secrete an array of substances that protect against infection, including mucus, perspiration (or sweat), saliva, tears, and earwax. These can trap potential invaders and contain substances that will kill microorganisms. Perspiration, tears, and saliva contain an enzyme (lysozyme) that attacks the cell walls of gram-positive bacteria. Sebaceous glands in the skin also secrete fatty acids and lactic acid that kill bacteria and fungi. These glandular secretions create an acidic (pH 3 to 5) and inhospitable environment for most bacteria.

Epithelial cell secretions also contain small-molecular-weight antimicrobial peptides that kill or inhibit the growth of disease-causing bacteria, fungi, and viruses.[1] These are generally positively charged polypeptides of approximately 15 to 95 amino acids. More than a thousand antimicrobial peptides have been found, but the best studied are cathelicidins and defensins.

Several cathelicidins have been discovered in other species, but only one is currently known to function in humans. Bacteria have cholesterol-free cell membranes into which cathelicidin can insert and disrupt the membrane, killing the bacteria. Cathelicidin is produced by epithelial cells of the skin, gut, urinary tract, and respiratory tract, and is stored in neutrophils, mast cells, and monocytes and can be released during inflammation.

In contrast, many different human defensins have been identified. Defensin molecules can be further subdivided into α (at least six identified in humans) and β types (at least six identified, but perhaps up to 40 different molecules). The α-defensins often require activation by proteolytic enzymes, whereas the β-defensins are synthesized in active forms. Given the similarity in their chemical charges, defensins may kill bacteria in the same way as cathelicidin. The α-defensins are particularly rich in the granules of neutrophils and may contribute to the killing of bacteria by those cells. They are also found in Paneth cells lining the small intestine, where they protect against a variety of disease-causing microorganisms. The β-defensins are found in epithelial cells lining the respiratory, urinary, and intestinal tracts, as well as in the skin. In addition to antibacterial properties, β-defensins may also help protect epithelial surfaces from infection with adenovirus (one of the causes of the common cold) and human immunodeficiency virus (HIV). Both classes of antimicrobial peptides also can activate cells of the next levels of defense: innate and acquired immunity.

The lung also produces and secretes a family of glycoproteins, collectins, which includes surfactant proteins A through D and mannose-binding lectin. Collectins react with carbohydrates on the surface of a wide array of pathogenic microorganisms and help cells of the innate immune system (macrophages) to recognize and kill the microorganism. Mannose-binding lectin (MBL) recognizes a sugar commonly found on the surface of microbes and is a powerful activator of a plasma protein system (complement) resulting in damage to bacteria or increased recognition by macrophages.

The Normal Microbiome

The body's surfaces are colonized with an array of microorganisms, the normal microbiome previously known as normal flora. Each surface (the skin and the mucous membranes of the eyes, upper and lower

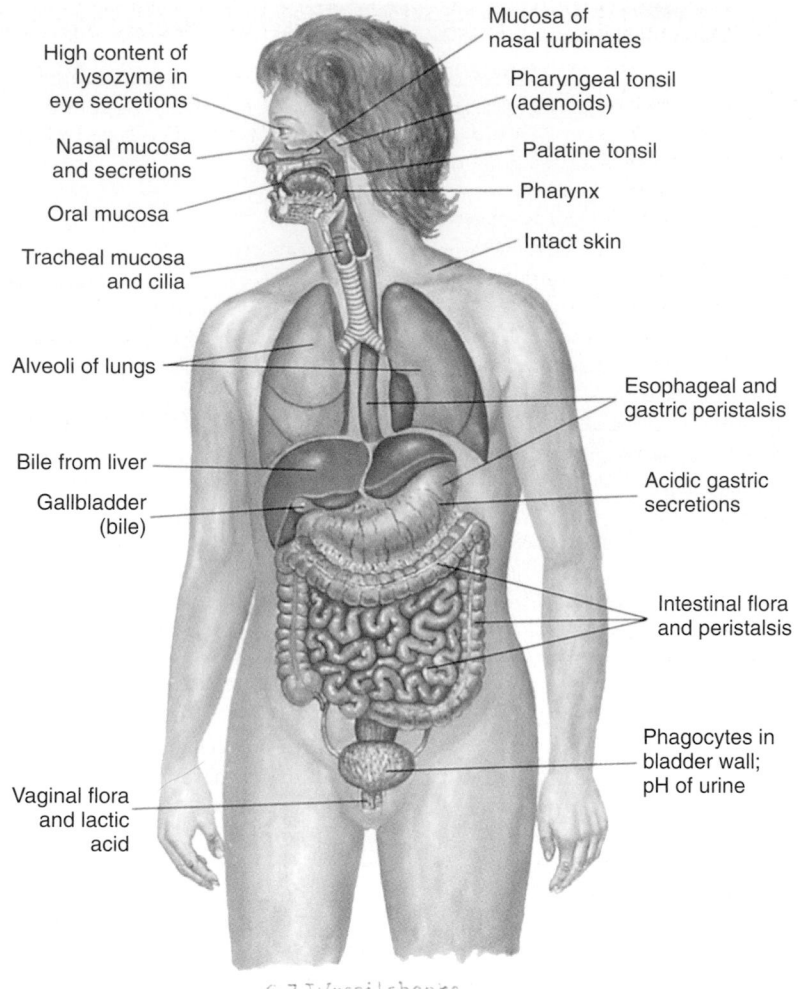

High content of
lysozyme in
eye secretions

Nasal mucosa
and secretions

Oral mucosa

Tracheal mucosa
and cilia

Alveoli of lungs

Bile from liver

Gallbladder
(bile)

Vaginal flora
and lactic
acid

Mucosa of
nasal turbinates

Pharyngeal tonsil
(adenoids)

Palatine tonsil

Pharynx

Intact skin

Esophageal and
gastric peristalsis

Acidic gastric
secretions

Intestinal flora
and peristalsis

Phagocytes in
bladder wall;
pH of urine

G.J.Wassilchenko

FIGURE 6-1 The Closed Barrier. The digestive, respiratory, and genitourinary tracts and skin form closed barriers between the internal organs and the environment. (From Grimes DE: *Infectious diseases*, St. Louis, 1991, Mosby.)

gastrointestinal tracts, upper respiratory tract, urethra, and vagina) is colonized by a combination of bacteria and fungi that is unique to the particular location and individual[2] (Table 6-2). The microorganisms in the microbiome do not normally cause disease, and although their relationship with humans has been referred to as *commensal* (to the benefit of one organism without affecting the other), the relationship may be more *mutualistic* (to the benefit of both organisms). Using the colon for an example, at birth the lower gut is relatively sterile but colonization with bacteria begins quickly, with the number, diversity, and concentration increasing progressively during the first year of life.

The normal microbiome benefits us in many ways; bacteria in the gastrointestinal (GI) tract produce (1) enzymes that facilitate the digestion and utilization of many molecules in the human diet, such as fatty acids and large polysaccharides; (2) usable metabolites (e.g., vitamin K, B vitamins); and (3) antibacterial factors that prevent colonization by pathogenic microorganisms (see Chapter 8) For instance, members of the normal microbiome in the colon produce chemicals (ammonia, phenols, indoles, and other toxic materials) and proteins *(bacteriocins)* that are toxic to more pathogenic microorganisms. They also compete with pathogens for nutrients and block attachment to the epithelium, which is an obligatory first step in the infectious process by most pathogens. Additionally, the normal microbiome of

the gut helps train the adaptive immune system by inducing growth of gut-associated lymphoid tissue (where most cells of the adaptive immune system reside) and the development of both local and systemic adaptive immunity. Bidirectional communication between the brain and GI tract (brain-gut axis) is influenced by GI bacteria with importance for cognitive function, behavior, pain modulation, and stress responses.[3]

Prolonged treatment with broad-spectrum antibiotics can alter the normal microbiome, decreasing its protective activity, and lead to an overgrowth of pathogenic microorganisms. In the intestine, overgrowth of the yeast *Candida albicans* or the bacteria *Clostridium difficile* (a cause of pseudomembranous colitis, an infection of the colon) may occur. The bacterium *Lactobacillus* is a major constituent of the normal gastrointestinal and vaginal microbiome in healthy women.[4] This microorganism produces a variety of chemicals (e.g., hydrogen peroxide, lactic acid, bacteriocins) that help prevent infections of the vagina and urinary tract by other bacteria and yeast. Prolonged antibiotic treatment can diminish colonization with *Lactobacillus* and increase the risk for urologic or vaginal infections, such as vaginosis.

The mutualistic relationship with the microbiome is maintained through the physical integrity of the skin and mucosal epithelium and other mechanisms that protect the microbiome from the immune and inflammatory systems. Some members of the normal bacterial

TABLE 6-2   The Human Microbiome

Location	Microorganisms
Skin	Predominantly gram-positive cocci and rods; *Staphylococcus epidermidis*, corynebacteria, mycobacteria, and streptococci are primary inhabitants; *Staphylococcus aureus* in some people; also yeasts *(Candida, Pityrosporum)* in some areas of skin
	Numerous transient microorganisms may become temporary residents
	In moist areas, gram-negative bacteria
	Around sebaceous glands, *Propionibacterium* and *Brevibacterium*
	Mite *Demodex folliculorum* lives in hair follicles and sebaceous glands around face
Nose	Predominantly gram-positive cocci and rods, especially *S. epidermidis*
	Some people are nasal carriers of pathogenic bacteria, including *S. aureus*, β-hemolytic streptococci, and *Corynebacterium diphtheria*
Mouth	Complex of bacteria that includes several species of streptococci, *Actinomyces*, lactobacilli, and *Haemophilus*
	Anaerobic bacteria and spirochetes colonize gingival crevices
Pharynx	Similar to flora in mouth plus staphylococci, *Neisseria*, and diphtheroids
	Some asymptomatic persons also harbor pathogens: pneumococcus, *Haemophilus influenzae*, *Neisseria meningitidis*, and *C. diphtheria*
Distal small intestine	Enterobacteria, streptococci, lactobacilli, anaerobic bacteria, and *C. albicans*
Colon	Bacteroides, lactobacilli, clostridia, *Salmonella, Shigella, Klebsiella, Proteus, Pseudomonas, enterococci*, and other streptococci, bacilli, and *Escherichia coli*
Distal urethra	Typical bacteria found on skin, especially *S. epidermidis* and diphtheroids; also lactobacilli and nonpathogenic streptococci
Vagina	Birth to 1 month: similar to adult
	1 month to puberty: *S. epidermidis*, diphtheroids, *E. coli*, and streptococci
	Puberty to menopause: *Lactobacillus acidophilus*, diphtheroids, staphylococci, streptococci, and variety of anaerobes
	Postmenopause: similar to prepubescence

Adapted from Bennett JE et al, editors: *Mandell, Douglas, and Bennett's principles and practice of infectious diseases,* ed 8, Philadelphia, 2015, Saunders.

microbiome are opportunistic; opportunistic microorganisms can cause disease if the individual's defenses are compromised. These microorganisms are normally controlled by the innate and adaptive immune systems and contribute to our defenses. For example, *Pseudomonas aeruginosa* is a member of the normal microbiome of the skin and produces a toxin that protects against infections with staphylococcal and other bacteria. However, severe burns compromise the integrity of the skin and may lead to life-threatening systemic infections with *Pseudomonas*.

✔ QUICK CHECK 6-1

1. How do physical and mechanical barriers contribute to defense mechanisms?
2. What are antimicrobial peptides?
3. What two types of defensins contribute to the biochemical barrier?
4. What is the normal bacterial flora? What is its role in defense?
5. What are opportunistic microorganisms?

Second Line of Defense: Inflammation

Whereas the physical and chemical barriers of the innate immune system are relatively static, inflammation is programmed to respond to cellular or tissue damage, whether the damaged tissue is septic or sterile. The response is a rapid initiation of an interactive system of humoral (soluble in the blood) and cellular systems designed to limit the extent of tissue damage, destroy contaminating infectious microorganisms, initiate the adaptive immune response, and begin the healing process.

The inflammatory response (1) occurs in tissues with a blood supply (vascularized); (2) is activated *rapidly* (within seconds) after damage occurs; (3) depends on the activity of both *cellular and chemical components*; and (4) is *nonspecific*, meaning that it takes place in approximately the same way regardless of the type of stimulus or whether exposure to the same stimulus has occurred in the past.

Inflammation will be activated by virtually any injury to vascularized tissues, including infection or tissue necrosis (e.g., ischemia, trauma, physical or chemical injury, foreign bodies, immune reactions). The classic or cardinal signs of acute inflammation were described in the first century by a Roman named Celsus and included rubor (redness), calor (heat), tumor (swelling), and dolor (pain). A fifth sign, functio laesa (loss of function), was added later. Microscopic inflammatory changes occur within seconds in the microcirculation (arterioles, capillaries, and venules) near the site of an injury and include the following processes (Figure 6-2):

1. Vasodilation (increased size of the blood vessels), which causes slower blood velocity and increases blood flow to the injured site
2. Increased vascular permeability (the blood vessels become porous from contraction of endothelial cells) and leakage of fluid out of the vessel (exudation), causing swelling (edema) at the site of injury; as plasma moves outward, blood in the microcirculation becomes more viscous and flows more slowly, and the increased blood flow and increasing concentration of red cells at the site of inflammation cause locally increased redness (erythema) and warmth
3. White blood cell adherence to the inner walls of vessels and their migration through enlarged junctions between the endothelial cells lining the vessels into the surrounding tissue

Each of the characteristic changes associated with inflammation is the direct result of the activation and interactions of a host of chemicals and cellular components found in the blood and tissues. The vascular changes deliver leukocytes (particularly neutrophils), plasma proteins, and other biochemical mediators to the site of injury, where they act in concert. Some of these chemical mediators activate pain fibers. The tissue injury, pain, and swelling contribute to loss of function. Figure 6-3 summarizes the process of inflammation. The lymphatic vessels drain the extravascular fluid to the lymph nodes and

NORMAL

INFLAMED

FIGURE 6-2 The Major Local Changes in the Process of Inflammation. Compared with the normal circulation, inflammation is characterized by (1) dilation of the blood vessels and increased blood flow, leading to erythema and warmth; (2) increased vascular permeability with leakage of plasma from the vessels, leading to edema; and (3) movement of leukocytes from the vessels into the site of injury. (From Kumar V et al: *Robbins and Cotran pathological basis of disease,* ed 8, Philadelphia, 2009, Saunders.)

may, themselves, become secondarily inflamed; lymphangitis of the lymph vessels and lymphadenitis of the nodes, which become hyperplastic, enlarged, and frequently painful.

There are several benefits of inflammation, including the following:

1. Prevents infection and further damage by invading microorganisms. The inflammatory exudate dilutes toxins produced by bacteria and released from dying cells. The activation of plasma protein systems (e.g., complement and clotting systems) helps contain and destroy bacteria. The influx of phagocytes (e.g., neutrophils, macrophages) destroys cellular debris and microorganisms.
2. Limits and controls the inflammatory process. The influx of plasma protein systems (e.g., clotting system), plasma enzymes, and cells (e.g., eosinophils) prevents the inflammatory response from spreading to areas of healthy tissue.

3. Interacts with components of the adaptive immune system to elicit a more specific response to contaminating pathogen(s) through the influx of macrophages and lymphocytes that destroy pathogens.
4. Prepares the area of injury for healing and repair through removal of bacterial products, dead cells, and other products of inflammation (e.g., by way of channels through the epithelium or drainage by lymphatic vessels).

Fluid and debris that accumulate at an inflamed site are drained by lymphatic vessels. This process also facilitates the development of acquired immunity because microbial antigens in lymphatic fluid pass through the lymph nodes, where they encounter lymphocytes.

> ✔ **QUICK CHECK 6-2**
> 1. Why are innate immunity and inflammation described as "nonspecific"?
> 2. How are the five classic superficial symptoms of inflammation related to the process of inflammation?
> 3. Describe the basic steps in acute inflammation.
> 4. What are the benefits of inflammation?

Plasma Protein Systems and Inflammation

Three key **plasma protein systems** are essential to an effective inflammatory response (Figure 6-4). These are the complement system, the clotting system, and the kinin system. Although each system has a unique role in inflammation, they have many similarities. Each system consists of multiple proteins found in the blood, usually in inactive forms; several are enzymes that circulate as proenzymes. Each system contains a few proteins that can be activated early in inflammation. Activation of the first components results in sequential activation of other components of the system, leading to a biologic function that helps protect the individual. This sequential activation is referred to as a *cascade*. Thus, we occasionally refer to the complement cascade, the clotting cascade, or the kinin cascade. In some cases, activation of a particular protein in the system may require that it be enzymatically cut into two pieces of different size. Usually the larger fragment continues the cascade by activating the next component, and the smaller fragment frequently has potent proinflammatory activities.

Complement System

The complement system consists of a large number of proteins (sometimes called complement factors) that together constitute about 10% of the total circulating serum protein. Activation of the complement system produces several factors that can destroy pathogens directly or can activate or increase the activity of many other components of the inflammatory and adaptive immune response. Factors produced during activation of the complement system are among the body's most potent defenders, particularly against bacterial infection.

The most important function of the complement cascade is activation of C3 and C5, which results in a variety of molecules that are (1) opsonins, (2) chemotactic factors, or (3) anaphylatoxins.[5] **Opsonins** coat the surface of bacteria and increase their susceptibility to being phagocytized (eaten) and killed by inflammatory cells, such as neutrophils and macrophages. **Chemotactic factors** diffuse from a site of inflammation and attract phagocytic cells to that site. **Anaphylatoxins** induce rapid degranulation of mast cells (i.e., release of histamine that induces vasodilation and increased capillary permeability), a major cellular component of inflammation. The most potent complement products are C3b (opsonin), C3a (anaphylatoxin), and C5a (anaphylatoxin, chemotactic factor). Activation of terminal complement

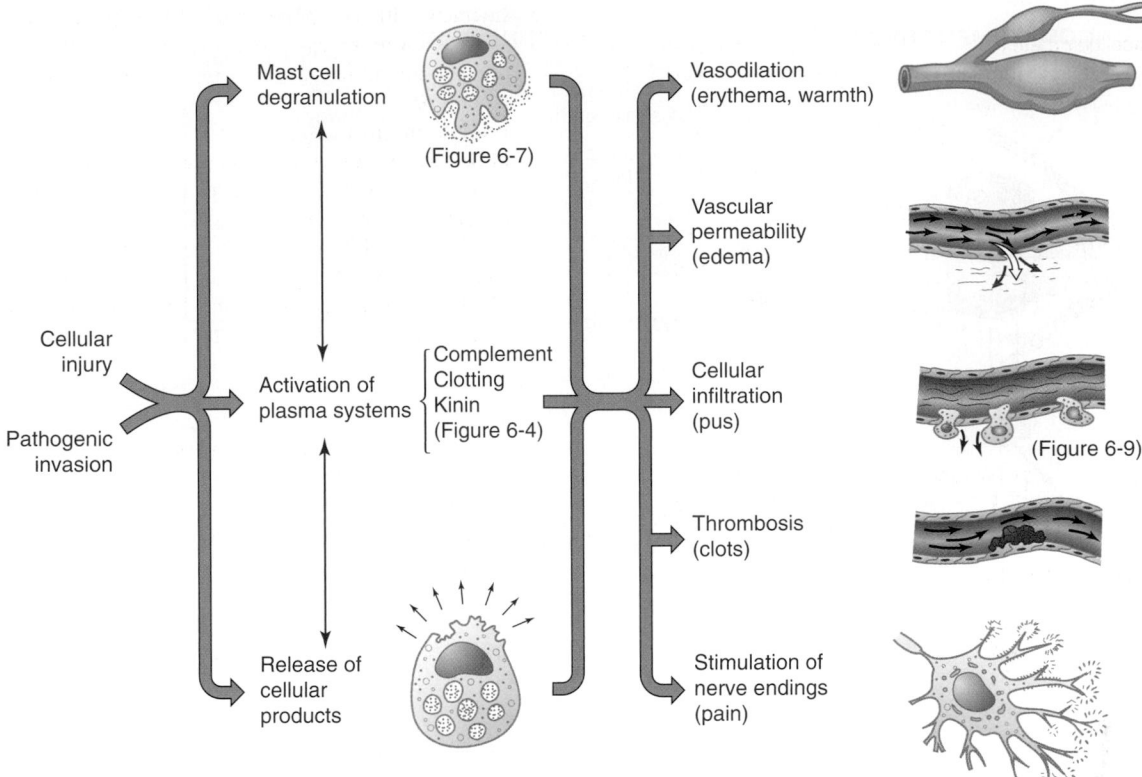

FIGURE 6-3 Acute Inflammatory Response. Inflammation is usually initiated by cellular injury and may be complicated by infection. Mast cell degranulation, the activation of three plasma systems, and the release of subcellular components from the damaged cells occur as a consequence. These systems are interdependent, so that induction of one (e.g., mast cell degranulation) can result in the induction of the other two. The result is the development of the characteristic microscopic and clinical hallmarks of inflammation. The figure numbers refer to additional figures in which more detailed information may be found on that portion of the response.

components C5b through C9 (membrane attack complex, or MAC) results in a complex that creates pores in the outer membranes of cells or bacteria. The pores disrupt the cell's membrane and permit water to enter, causing the death of the cell.

Three major pathways control the activation of complement (see Figure 6-4). The **classical pathway** is primarily activated by antibodies, which are proteins of the acquired immune system. Antibodies must first bind to their targets, called antigens, which can be proteins or carbohydrates from bacteria or other infectious agents. Antibodies activate the first component of complement, C1, which leads to activation of other complement components, leading to activation of C3 and C5. Thus, antibodies of the acquired immune response can use the complement system to kill bacteria and activate inflammation.

The **alternative pathway** is activated by several substances found on the surface of infectious organisms (e.g., lipopolysaccharides [endotoxin] on the bacterial surface or yeast cell wall carbohydrates [zymosan]). This pathway uses unique proteins (factor B, factor D, and properdin) to form a complex that activates C3. C3 activation leads to C5 activation and convergence with the classical pathway. Thus, the complement system can be directly activated by certain infectious organisms without antibody being present.

The **lectin pathway** is similar to the classical pathway but is independent of antibody. It is activated by several plasma proteins, particularly mannose-binding lectin (MBL). MBL binds to bacterial polysaccharides containing the carbohydrate mannose and activates complement through two proteins that are similar to C1—MASP-1 (mannose-binding lectin-associated serine protease) and MASP 2.[6] Thus, infectious agents that do not activate the alternative pathway may be susceptible to complement through the lectin pathway.

In summary, the complement cascade can be activated by at least three different means, and its products have four functions: (1) opsonization (C3b), (2) anaphylatoxic activity resulting in mast cell degranulation (C3a, C5a), (3) leukocyte chemotaxis (C5a), and (4) cell lysis (C5b-C9; membrane attack complex [MAC]).

Clotting System

The **clotting (coagulation) system** is a group of plasma proteins that, when activated sequentially, form a blood clot. A **blood clot** is a meshwork of protein (fibrin) strands that contains platelets (the primary cellular initiator of clotting) and traps other cells, such as erythrocytes, phagocytes, and microorganisms. Clots (1) plug damaged vessels and stop bleeding, (2) trap microorganisms and prevent their spread to adjacent tissues, and (3) provide a framework for future repair and healing. Specific details and illustrations of the clotting system are presented in Chapter 20 (also see Figure 20-18) and only the relationship between clotting and inflammation is presented here.

The clotting system can be activated by many substances that are released during tissue injury and infection, including collagen, proteinases, kallikrein, and plasmin, as well as by bacterial products such as endotoxins. Like the complement cascade, the coagulation cascade can be activated through different pathways that converge and result in the

FIGURE 6-4 Plasma Protein Systems in Inflammation: Complement, Clotting, and Kinin Systems.
Each plasma protein system consists of a family of proteins that are activated in sequence to create potent biologic effects. The complement system can be activated by three mechanisms, each of which results in proteolytic activation of C3. The fragments of C3 activation, C3a and C3b, are major components of inflammation. C3a is a potent anaphylatoxin, which induces degranulation of mast cells. C3b can bind to the surface or cells, such as bacteria, and either serve as an opsonin for phagocytosis or proteolytically activate the next component of the complement cascade, C5. The smaller fragment of C5 activation is C5a, a powerful anaphylatoxin, and is also chemotactic for neutrophils, attracting them to the site of inflammation. The larger fragment, C5b, activates the components of the membrane attack complex (C5-C9), which damage the bacterial membrane and kill the bacteria. The clotting system can be activated by the tissue factor (extrinsic) pathway and the contact activation (intrinsic) pathway. All routes of clotting initiation lead to activation of factor X and thrombin. Thrombin is an enzyme that proteolytically activates fibrinogen to form fibrin and small fibrinopeptides (FPs). Fibrin polymerizes to form a clot, and the FPs are highly active as chemotactic factors and cause increased vascular permeability. The XIIa produced by the clotting system can also be activated by kallikrein of the **kinin system** *(red arrow)*. Prekallikrein is enzymatically converted to kininogen, which activates bradykinin. Bradykinin functions similar to histamine and increases vascular permeability. Bradykinin can also stimulate nerve endings to cause pain. *FP,* Fibrinopeptide; *TF,* tissue factor.

formation of a clot (see Figure 6-4). The **tissue factor (extrinsic) pathway** is activated by **tissue factor (TF)** (also called **tissue thromboplastin**) that is released by damaged endothelial cells in blood vessels and reacts with activated factor VII (VIIa). The **contact activation (intrinsic) pathway** is activated when the vessel wall is damaged and Hageman factor (factor XII) in plasma contacts negatively-charged subendothelial substances. The pathways converge at factor X. Activation of factor X begins a common pathway leading to activation of fibrin that polymerizes to form a fibrin clot.

As with the complement system, activation of the clotting system produces protein fragments known as fibrinopeptides (FPs) A and B that enhance the inflammatory response. Fibrinopeptides are released

from fibrinogen when fibrin is produced. Both fibrinopeptides (especially fibrinopeptide B) are chemotactic for neutrophils and increase vascular permeability by enhancing the effects of bradykinin (formed from the kinin system) on endothelial cells.

Kinin System

The third plasma protein system, the **kinin system** (see Figure 6-4), interacts closely with the coagulation system. Both the clotting and kinin systems can be initiated through activation of **Hageman factor (factor XII)** to factor XIIa. Another name for factor XIIa is *prekallikrein* activator because it enzymatically activates the first component of the kinin system, prekallikrein. The final product of the kinin system is a small-molecular-weight molecule, bradykinin, which is produced from a larger precursor molecule, kininogen. Bradykinin causes dilation of blood vessels, acts with prostaglandins to induce pain, causes smooth muscle cell contraction, and increases vascular permeability.

Control and Interaction of Plasma Protein Systems

The three plasma protein systems are highly interactive so that activation of one results in production of a large number of very potent, biologically active substances that further activate the other systems. Very tight regulation of these processes is essential for the following two reasons.

1. The inflammatory process is critical for an individual's survival; thus efficient activation must be guaranteed regardless of the cause of tissue injury. Interaction among the plasma systems may result in activation of the entire inflammatory response regardless of which system is activated initially.

2. The biochemical mediators generated during these processes are potent and potentially detrimental to the individual, and their actions must be strictly confined to injured or infected tissues.

Therefore, multiple mechanisms are available to either activate or inactivate (regulate) these plasma protein systems. For instance, the plasma that enters the tissues during inflammation (edema) contains enzymes that destroy mediators of inflammation. Carboxypeptidase inactivates the anaphylatoxic activities of C3a and C5a, and kininases degrade kinins. Histaminase degrades histamine and kallikrein and down-regulates the inflammatory response.

The formation of clots also activates a fibrinolytic system that is designed to limit the size of the clot and remove the clot after bleeding has ceased. Thrombin of the clotting system activates plasminogen in the blood to form the enzyme plasmin. The primary activity of plasmin is to degrade fibrin polymers in clots. However, plasmin can also activate the complement cascade through components C1, C3, and C5 and the kinin cascade by activating factor XII and producing prekallikrein activator.

Another example of a common regulator is C1 esterase inhibitor (C1 inh). C1 inh inhibits complement activation through C1 (classical pathway), MASP-2 (lectin pathway), and C3b (alternative pathway). It is also a major inhibitor of the clotting and kinin pathway components (e.g., kallikrein, factor XIIa). A genetic defect in C1 inh (C1 inh deficiency) results in hereditary angioedema, which is a self-limiting edema of cutaneous and mucosal layers resulting from stress, illness, or relative minor or unapparent trauma. The disease is characterized by hyperactivation of all three plasma protein systems, although excessive production of bradykinin appears to be the principal cause of increased vascular permeability.

Many cells are protected from inadvertent complement system damage by factors linked to the external surface of the plasma membrane. Two examples are decay accelerating factor (DAF) and CD59; DAF prevents activation of C3 and CD59 inhibits the membrane attack complex.

✔ **QUICK CHECK 6-3**

1. What are the three most important products of the complement system?
2. How is the coagulation cascade activated? How is it related to the plasma kinin cascade?
3. What factors control the plasma protein systems of inflammation?

Cellular Components of Inflammation

Inflammation is a process in vascular tissue; thus the cellular components can be found in the blood or in tissue surrounding the blood

FIGURE 6-5 **Cellular Components of the Blood.** Cells in the blood can be classified as red blood cells (erythrocytes), cellular fragments (platelets), or white blood cells (leukocytes). Leukocytes consist of lymphocytes, monocytes, and granulocytes (neutrophils, eosinophils, basophils). (Erythrocyte plate from Goldman L, Schafer AI, editors: *Goldman's Cecil medicine,* ed 24, Philadelphia, 2012, Saunders; rest of plates from McPherson RA, editor: *Henry's clinical diagnosis and management by laboratory methods,* ed 22, Philadelphia, 2012, Saunders.)

vessels. The blood vessels are lined with endothelial cells, which under normal conditions actively maintain blood flow. During inflammation the vascular endothelium becomes a principal coordinator of blood clotting and the passage of cells and fluid into the tissue. The tissues close to the vessels contain mast cells, which are probably the most important activators of inflammation, and dendritic cells, which connect the innate and acquired immune responses. The blood contains a complex mixture of cells (Figure 6-5 and see Chapter 20). Blood cells are divided into erythrocytes (red blood cells), platelets, and leukocytes (white blood cells). Erythrocytes carry oxygen to the tissues and platelets are small cell fragments involved in blood clotting. Leukocytes are subdivided into granulocytes (containing many enzyme-filled cytoplasmic granules), monocytes, and lymphocytes. Granulocytes are the most common leukocytes and are classified by the type of stains needed to visualize enzyme-containing granules in their cytoplasm (basophils, eosinophils, and neutrophils). Monocytes are precursors of macrophages that are found in the tissue. Various forms of lymphocytes participate in the innate immune response (e.g., natural killer [NK] cells) and the acquired immune response (B and T cells).

Cells of both innate and acquired immune systems respond to molecules produced at a site of cellular damage and are recruited to that site to augment the protective response. These molecules originate from destroyed or damaged cells, contaminating microbes, activation of the plasma protein systems, or secretions by other cells of the innate or acquired immune systems. Each cell has a set of cell surface receptors that specifically bind these molecules, resulting in activation of

TABLE 6-3   Cellular Source and Microbial Target for Each Toll-like Receptor (TLR)

Receptor	Cellular Expression Pattern	PAMP Recognition
TLR1	Cell surface (ubiquitous): neutrophils, monocytes/macrophages, dendritic cells, T cells, B cells, NK cells	Fungal, bacterial, viral; forms heterodimer with TLR2 (see TLR2 recognition)
TLR2	Cell surface: neutrophils, monocytes/macrophages, dendritic cells	Fungal (yeast zymosan), bacterial (gram-positive bacterial peptidoglycan, lipoproteins), viral (lipoproteins)
TLR3	Intracellular: monocytes/macrophages, dendritic cells, T cells, NK cells, epithelial cells	Double-stranded RNA produced by many viruses
TLR4	Cell surface: granulocytes, monocytes/macrophages, dendritic cells, T cells, B cells, epithelial cells	Bacterial (primarily gram-negative bacterial LPS, lipoteichoic acids), viral (RSV F protein, hepatitis C)
TLR5	Cell surface: granulocytes, monocytes/macrophages, dendritic cells, NK cells, epithelial cells	Bacterial (flagellin); forms heterodimer with TLR4
TLR6	Cell surface: monocytes/macrophages, dendritic cells, B cells, NK cells	Fungal, bacterial, viral; forms heterodimer with TLR2 (see TLR2 recognition)
TLR7	Intracellular: monocytes/macrophages, dendritic cells, B cells	Natural ligand uncertain; may bind viral single-strand RNA
TLR8	Cell surface: monocytes/macrophages, dendritic cells, NK cells	Natural ligand uncertain; may bind fungal PAMPs or viral single-stranded RNA
TLR9	Intracellular: monocytes/macrophages, dendritic cells, B cells	Bacterial (unmethylated DNA [CpG dinucleotides])
TLR10	Cell surface: monocytes/macrophages, dendritic cells, B cells	Natural ligand uncertain; may form heterodimers with TLR2
TLR11	*TLR11* gene does not code a full-length protein in humans	No known immune response

intracellular signaling pathways and activation of the cell itself. Activation may result in the cell gaining a function critical to the inflammatory response or the induction of the release of additional cellular products that increase inflammation, or both. Most of these inflammatory cells and protein systems, along with the substances they produce, act at the site of tissue injury to confine the extent of damage; kill microorganisms; remove the cellular debris; and activate healing, tissue regeneration (a process known as resolution), or repair.

Cellular Receptors

As will be discussed in Chapter 7, B and T lymphocytes of the adaptive immune system have evolved surface receptors (i.e., the T-cell receptor, or TCR, and the B-cell receptor, or BCR) that bind a large spectrum of antigens. Cells involved in innate resistance have evolved a different set of receptors that recognize a much more limited array of specific molecules (ligands). These are referred to as pattern recognition receptors (PRRs). PRRs recognize two types of molecular *patterns:* molecules that are expressed by infectious agents, either found on their surface or released as soluble molecules (pathogen-associated molecular patterns, or PAMPs); or products of cellular damage (damage-associated molecular patterns, or DAMPs). Thus cells of the innate immune system can respond to both sterile (through DAMPs) and septic (through PAMPs and DAMPs) tissue damage. It is estimated that at least 100 different PRRs are expressed that recognize more than 1000 different molecules.

PRRs are generally expressed on cells in tissues near the body's surface (i.e., skin, respiratory tract, gastrointestinal tract, genitourinary tract) where they monitor the environment for products of cellular damage and potentially infectious microorganisms. Classes of cellular PRRs primarily differ in the specificity of ligands they bind. PRRs can be found as cell surface receptors that bind extracellular ligands, in endosomes in contact with ingested microbes and other materials, in the cytosol where they bind intracellular materials resulting from cellular damage, or secreted into the extracellular environment. An example of a secreted PRR is mannose-binding lectin of the lectin pathway of complement activation (see p. 139).

Toll-like receptors (TLRs) primarily recognize a large variety of PAMPs located on the microorganism's cell wall or surface (e.g., bacterial lipopolysaccharide [LPS], peptidoglycans, lipoproteins, yeast zymosan, viral coat proteins), other surface structures (e.g., bacterial flagellin), or microbial nucleic acid (e.g., bacterial DNA, viral double-stranded RNA).[7] Ten different TLRs have been described in humans (Table 6-3). They are expressed on the surface of many cells that have direct and early contact with potential pathogenic microorganisms, including mucosal epithelial cells, mast cells, neutrophils, macrophages, dendritic cells, and some subpopulations of lymphocytes. TLRs are linked to pathways that produce two groups of transcription factors: *NF-κB*, which controls synthesis and release of cytokines; and *interferon regulatory factors (IRFs)*, which control the production of anti-viral type I interferons.[8]

Complement receptors are found on many cells of the innate and acquired immune responses (e.g., granulocytes, monocytes/macrophages, lymphocytes, mast cells, erythrocytes, platelets), as well as some epithelial cells. They recognize several fragments produced through activation of the complement system, particularly C3a, C5a, and C3b.

Scavenger receptors are primarily expressed on macrophages and facilitate recognition and phagocytosis of bacterial pathogens, as well as damaged cells and altered soluble lipoproteins associated with vascular damage (e.g., high-density lipoprotein [HDL], acetylated low-density lipoprotein [LDL], oxidized LDL).[9] More than eight receptors have been identified. Some scavenger receptors (e.g., SR-PSOX) recognize the cell membrane phospholipid phosphatidylserine (PS). PS is normally sequestered on the cytoplasmic surface of the cell membrane, but is externalized under a very limited variety of conditions, including erythrocyte senescence and cellular apoptosis. Thus macrophages, through this receptor, can identify and remove old red blood cells and cells undergoing apoptosis.

NOD-like receptors (NLRs) are cytoplasmic receptors that recognize products of microbes and damaged cells. At least 22 NLRs have been identified in humans. NOD-1 and NOD-2 are cytoplasmic and recognize fragments of peptidoglycans from intracellular bacteria and initiate production of proinflammatory mediators, such as tumor necrosis factor (TNF) and interleukin-6 (IL-6).[10] Other NLRs associate with intracellular multiprotein complexes called inflammasomes. Inflammasomes primarily bind cellular stress-related molecules, a type of DAMP, and control the production of the inflammatory cytokines interleukin-1β (IL-1β) and IL-18.[11]

FIGURE 6-6 Principal Mediators of Inflammatory Processes. *C3b,* Large fragment produced from complement component C3; *C5a,* small fragment produced from complement component C5; *ECF-A,* eosinophil chemotactic factor of anaphylaxis; *FGF,* fibroblast growth factor; *IFN,* interferon; *IgG,* immunoglobulin G (predominant class of antibody in the blood); *IL,* interleukin; *MCF,* monocyte chemotactic factor; *NCF,* neutrophil chemotactic factor; *PAF,* platelet-activating factor; *TGF,* T-cell growth factor; *TNF,* tumor necrosis factor; *VEGF,* vascular endothelial growth factor.

Cellular Products

To elicit an effective inflammatory (or adaptive immune) response, intercellular communication and cooperation are necessary. Cytokines constitute a large family of small-molecular-weight soluble intercellular-signaling molecules that are secreted, bind to specific cell membrane receptors, and regulate innate or adaptive immunity (Figure 6-6). Cytokines may be either *proinflammatory* or *anti-inflammatory* in nature, depending on whether they tend to induce or inhibit the inflammatory response. These molecules usually diffuse over short distances, but some effects occur over long distances, such as the systemic induction of fever by some cytokines (i.e., endogenous pyrogens) that are produced at an inflammatory site. Binding of cytokines to a target cell often induces synthesis of additional cellular products. For example, binding of the cytokine TNF-α to a cell may result in synthesis and release of IL-1.

A large number of cytokines have been described and are classified into several families.[12] The terms lymphokines and monokines refer respectively to cytokines secreted from lymphocytes or monocytes, although cytokines are secreted by many different types of cells. Chemokines are members of a special family of cytokines that are chemotactic and primarily attract leukocytes to sites of inflammation.[13] Chemokines are synthesized by many cell types, including macrophages, fibroblasts, and endothelial cells, in response to proinflammatory cytokines, such as TNF-α. To date, more than 50 different human chemokines have been described. Examples include those that primarily attract macrophages (e.g., monocyte/macrophage chemotactic proteins [MCP-1, MCP-2, and MCP-3]), macrophage inflammatory proteins ([MIP-α and MIP-1β]), or neutrophils (e.g., interleukin-8 [IL-8]).

Interleukins (ILs) are produced predominantly by macrophages and lymphocytes in response to stimulation of PRRs or by other cytokines.[14] More than 30 interleukins have been identified. Their effects include the following:

1. Alteration of adhesion molecule expression on many types of cells
2. Attraction of leukocytes to a site of inflammation (chemotaxis)
3. Induction of proliferation and maturation of leukocytes in the bone marrow
4. General enhancement or suppression of inflammation
5. Development of the acquired immune response

Two major proinflammatory ILs are interleukin-1 and interleukin-6, which cooperate closely with another cytokine, tumor necrosis factor-alpha. Interleukin-1 (IL-1) is produced in two forms, IL-1α and IL-1β, mainly by macrophages.[15] IL-1 activates monocytes, other macrophages, and lymphocytes, thereby enhancing both innate and acquired immunity, and acts as a growth factor for many cells. It has several effects on neutrophils, including induction of proliferation (resulting in an increase in the number of circulating neutrophils), attraction to an inflammatory site (chemotaxis), and increased cellular respiration and lysosomal enzyme activity (both effects resulting in increased cellular killing of bacteria). IL-1 is an endogenous pyrogen (i.e., fever-causing cytokine) that reacts with receptors on cells of the hypothalamus and affects the body's thermostat, resulting in fever.

Interleukin-6 (IL-6) is produced by macrophages, lymphocytes, fibroblasts, and other cells. IL-6 directly induces hepatocytes (liver cells) to produce many of the proteins needed in inflammation (acute-phase reactants, discussed later in this chapter). IL-6 also stimulates growth and differentiation of blood cells in the bone marrow and the growth of fibroblasts (required for wound healing).

Although not classified as an interleukin, tumor necrosis factor-alpha (TNF-α) is secreted by macrophages and other cells (e.g., mast cells) in response to stimulation of TLRs. TNF-α induces a multitude of proinflammatory effects, particularly on the vascular endothelium and macrophages. When secreted in large amounts, TNF-α has systemic effects that include the following:

1. Inducing fever by acting as an endogenous pyrogen
2. Causing increased synthesis of inflammation-related serum proteins by the liver
3. Causing muscle wasting (cachexia) and intravascular thrombosis in cases of severe infection and cancer.

Very high levels of TNF-α can be lethal and are probably responsible for fatalities from shock caused by gram-negative bacterial infections.

Some cytokines are anti-inflammatory and diminish the inflammatory response. The most important are interleukin-10 and transforming growth factor-beta. Interleukin-10 (IL-10) is primarily produced by lymphocytes and suppresses the growth of other lymphocytes and the production of proinflammatory cytokines by macrophages, leading to down-regulation of both inflammatory and acquired immune responses. Transforming growth factors, including transforming growth factor-beta (TGF-β), are produced by many cells in response to inflammation and induce cell division and differentiation of other cell types, such as immature blood cells.

Interferons (IFNs) are members of a family of cytokines that protect against viral infections and modulate the inflammatory response. (Mechanisms of viral infection are described in Chapter 8.) Type I interferons (primarily IFN-α, IFN-β) are produced and released by virally infected cells in response to viral double-stranded RNA and other viral PAMPs. These IFNs do not kill viruses directly but instead are secreted and induce antiviral proteins and protection in neighboring healthy cells. Type II interferon (IFN-γ) is produced primarily by lymphocytes; it activates macrophages, resulting in increased capacity to kill infectious agents (including viruses and bacteria), and enhances the development of acquired immune responses against viruses.

Mast Cells and Basophils

The mast cell is probably the most important cellular activator of the inflammatory response. Mast cells are filled with granules and located in the loose connective tissues close to blood vessels near the body's outer surfaces (i.e., in the skin and lining the gastrointestinal and respiratory tracts). Basophils are found in the blood and probably function in the same way as tissue mast cells.[16] A great number of stimuli activate mast cells to release potent soluble inducers of inflammation. These are released by (1) degranulation (the release of the contents of mast cell granules) and (2) *synthesis* (the new production and release of mediators in response to a stimulus) (Figure 6-7).

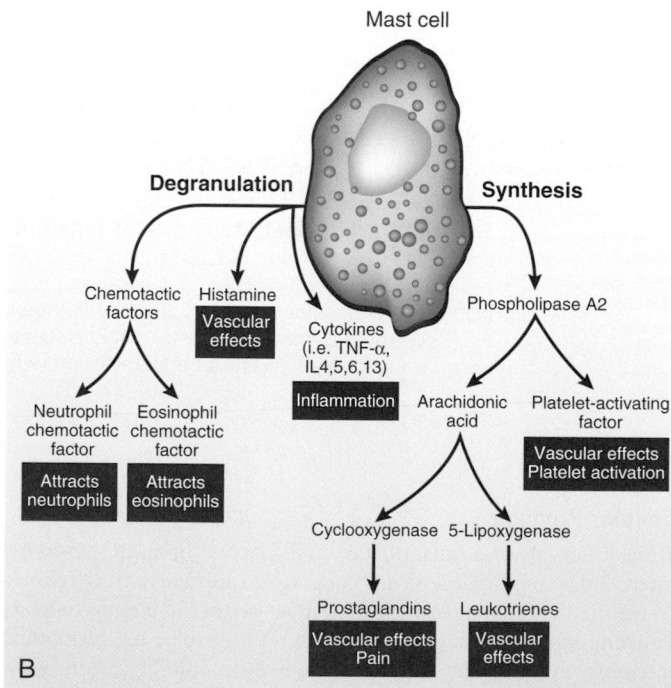

FIGURE 6-7 Mast Cell and Mast Cell Degranulation and Synthesis of Biologic Mediators During Inflammation. A, Colorized photomicrograph of mast cell; dense red granules contain histamine and other biologically active substances. Among these are histamine, which is a major initiator of vascular changes, and a variety of chemotactic factors. **B,** Mast cell degranulation *(left)* and synthesis *(right).* Histamine and other biologically active substances are released immediately after stimulation of mast cells. **(A** from Roitt IM et al: *Immunology,* ed 3, St Louis, 1993, Mosby.)

Degranulation. In response to a stimulus, biochemical mediators in the mast cell granules, including histamine, chemotactic factors, and cytokines (e.g., tumor necrosis factor-alpha [TNF-α], IL-4), are released within seconds and exert their effects immediately. **Histamine** is a small-molecular-weight molecule with potent effects on many other cells, particularly those that control the circulation. Histamine, along with serotonin (found in many cells, but not human mast cells), is called a vasoactive amine. These molecules cause temporary, rapid constriction of smooth muscle and dilation of the postcapillary venules, which results in increased blood flow into the microcirculation. Histamine also causes increased vascular permeability resulting from retraction of endothelial cells lining the capillaries and increased adherence of leukocytes to the endothelium. Histamine affects cells by binding to histamine H1 and H2 receptors on the target cell surface (Figure 6-8). Antihistamines are drugs that block the binding of histamine to its receptors, resulting in decreased inflammation.

Binding of histamine to the *H1 receptor* is essentially proinflammatory; that is, it promotes inflammation. On the other hand, binding to the *H2 receptor* is generally anti-inflammatory because it results in suppression of leukocyte function. The H1 receptor is present on smooth muscle cells, especially those of the bronchi, and causes bronchial smooth muscle to contract (bronchoconstriction) when stimulated. Both types of receptors are distributed among many different cells and are often present on the same cells and may act in an antagonistic fashion. For instance, stimulation of H1 receptors on neutrophils results in augmentation of neutrophil chemotaxis, whereas H2 receptor stimulation results in its inhibition. The H2 receptor is especially abundant on parietal cells of the stomach mucosa and induces the secretion of gastric acid as part of the normal physiology of the stomach. The role of histamine receptors and hypersensitivity is discussed in Chapter 8.

Mast cell granules also contain chemotactic factors, two of which are **neutrophil chemotactic factor (NCF)** and **eosinophil chemotactic factor of anaphylaxis (ECF-A)**. **Chemotaxis** is directional movement of cells along a chemical gradient formed by a chemotactic factor. Neutrophils are the predominant cell needed to kill bacteria in the early stages of inflammation. Eosinophils help regulate the inflammatory response. Both cells are discussed in more detail later in this chapter.

Synthesis of mediators. Activated mast cells initiate synthesis of other mediators of inflammation. These include leukotrienes, prostaglandins, and platelet-activating factor, which are produced from lipids (arachidonic acid) in the plasma membrane. **Leukotrienes (slow-reacting substances of anaphylaxis [SRS-A])** are sulfur-containing lipids produced by lipoxygenase that initiate histamine-like effects: smooth muscle contraction and increased vascular permeability. Leukotrienes appear to be important in the later stages of the inflammatory response because they stimulate slower and more prolonged inflammatory responses than does histamine.

Prostaglandins cause increased vascular permeability, neutrophil chemotaxis, and pain by direct effects on nerves. They are long-chain, unsaturated fatty acids produced by the action of the enzyme cyclooxygenase (COX) on arachidonic acid; prostaglandins are classified into groups (E, D, A, F, and B) according to their structure with numeral subscripts designating the number of double bonds. Prostaglandins E_1 and E_2 cause increased vascular permeability and smooth muscle contraction. COX exists in two different forms: COX-1 is found in most tissues and COX-2 is associated with inflammation. Aspirin and other nonsteroidal anti-inflammatory drugs inhibit both COX-1 and COX-2, but inhibition of COX-1 causes complications, such as gastrointestinal toxicity. Selective COX-2 inhibitors are now available.

Platelet-activating factor (PAF) is produced by removal of a fatty acid from the plasma membrane phospholipids by phospholipase A_2. Although mast cells are a major source of PAF, this molecule also can be produced by neutrophils, monocytes, endothelial cells, and platelets. The biologic activity of PAF is virtually identical to that of leukotrienes, namely, causing endothelial cell retraction to increase vascular permeability, leukocyte adhesion to endothelial cells, and platelet activation.

Endothelium

The lining of blood vessels consists of a layer of endothelial cells that adhere to an underlying matrix of connective tissue that

Target cell	Effect of histamine
Smooth muscle cell	Contraction
Endothelial cell	Contraction (retraction at endothelial junctions)
Neutrophil	Increased chemotaxis
Mast cell	Prostaglandin synthesis
Parietal cell of stomach mucosa	Secretion of gastric acid
Lymphocyte	Decreased activity
Eosinophil	Decreased activity
Neutrophil	Decreased chemotaxis
Mast cell	Decreased degranulation

FIGURE 6-8 Effects of Histamine Through H1 and H2 Receptors. The effects depend on (1) the density and affinity of H1 or H2 receptors on the target cell and (2) the identity of the target cell. *ATP,* Adenosine triphosphate; *cAMP,* cyclic adenosine monophosphate; *cGMP,* cyclic guanosine monophosphate; *GTP,* guanosine triphosphate.

contains a variety of proteins, including collagen, fibronectin, and laminins. Endothelial cells regulate circulating components of the inflammatory system and maintain normal blood flow by preventing spontaneous activation of platelets and members of the clotting system. Nitric oxide (NO) produced from arginine and prostacyclin (PGI_2) from arachidonic acid maintain blood flow and pressure and inhibit platelet activation. PGI_2 and NO are synergistic. NO is released continually to relax vascular smooth muscle and suppress the effects of low levels of cytokines, thus maintaining vascular tone. PGI_2 production varies a great deal and is increased when additional regulation is needed.

Damage to the endothelial cell lining of the vessel exposes the subendothelial connective tissue matrix, which is prothrombogenic and initiates platelet activation and formation of clots (the contact activation [intrinsic] clotting pathway). Proinflammatory mediators (e.g., histamine, prostacyclin, and many others) affect the endothelium, resulting in adherence of leukocytes to the vessel surface, invasion of leukocytes into the tissue, and efflux of plasma from the vessel.

Platelets

Platelets are anucleate cytoplasmic fragments formed from *megakaryocytes*. They circulate in the bloodstream until vascular injury occurs resulting in platelet activation by many products of tissue destruction and inflammation, including collagen, thrombin, and platelet-activating factor. Activated platelets (1) interact with components of the coagulation cascade to stop bleeding; (2) degranulate, releasing biochemical mediators such as serotonin, which has vascular effects similar to those of histamine; and (3) synthesize thromboxane A_2 (TXA_2) from prostaglandin H_2. TXA_2 is a potent vasoconstrictor and inducer of platelet aggregation. Prolonged use of low-dose aspirin preferentially suppresses production of TXA_2 without interfering with the production of anti-inflammatory PGI_2 by the endothelium. Platelets also release growth factors that promote wound healing. (Platelet function is described in detail in Chapter 20.)

Phagocytes

The primary role of most granulocytes (neutrophils, eosinophils, basophils) and monocytes/macrophages is phagocytosis—the process by which a cell ingests and disposes of damaged cells and foreign material, including microorganisms.

Neutrophils. The neutrophil, or polymorphonuclear neutrophil (PMN), is a member of the granulocytic series of white blood cells and is named for the characteristic staining pattern of its granules as well as its multilobed nucleus. Neutrophils are the predominant phagocytes in the early inflammatory site, arriving within 6 to 12 hours after the initial injury. Several inflammatory mediators (e.g., some bacterial proteins, complement fragments C3a and C5a, and mast cell neutrophil chemotactic factor) specifically and rapidly attract neutrophils from the circulation and activate them.[17]

Because the neutrophil is a mature cell that is incapable of division and sensitive to acidic environments, it is short lived at the inflammatory site and becomes a component of the purulent exudate, or pus, which is removed from the body through the epithelium or drained from the infected site via the lymphatic system. (The lymphatic system is described in Chapter 23.) The primary roles of the neutrophil are removal of debris and dead cells in sterile lesions, such as burns, and destruction of bacteria in nonsterile lesions.

Eosinophils. Another population of granulocytes is the eosinophil. Although eosinophils are only mildly phagocytic, they have two specific functions: (1) serve as the body's primary defense against parasites, and (2) help regulate vascular mediators released from mast cells. The role of eosinophils in resistance to parasites occurs in collaboration with specific antibodies produced by the acquired immune system (discussed in Chapter 7).[18]

Regulation of mast cell–derived inflammatory mediators is critical to control inflammation. The acute inflammatory response is needed only in a circumscribed area and for a limited time. Therefore, control mechanisms are necessary to prevent biochemical mediators from evoking more inflammation than necessary. Mast cell eosinophil chemotactic factor–A (ECF-A) attracts eosinophils to the site of inflammation. Eosinophil lysosomal granules contain enzymes that degrade vasoactive molecules, thereby controlling the vascular effects of inflammation. Histaminase degrades histamine, and arylsulfatase B degrades leukotrienes.

Basophils. The basophil is the least prevalent granulocyte in the blood. It is very similar to mast cells in the content of its granules and, in addition, is an important source of the cytokine IL-4, which is a key regulator of the adaptive immune response. Although often associated with allergies and asthma, its primary role is yet unknown.

Monocytes and macrophages. Monocytes are the largest normal blood cells (14 to 20 μm in diameter). Monocytes are produced in the bone marrow, enter the circulation, and migrate to the inflammatory site where they develop into macrophages. Monocytes also appear to be the precursors of macrophages that are found in tissues (tissue macrophages) including Kupffer cells in the liver, alveolar macrophages in the lungs, and microglia in the brain. Macrophages are generally larger (20 to 40 μm) and are more active as phagocytes than their monocytic precursors. Macrophages, particularly those residing in the tissues, are often important cellular initiators of the inflammatory response.

Monocyte-derived macrophages from the circulation may appear at the inflammatory site as soon as 24 hours after the initial neutrophil infiltration, but usually arrive 3 to 7 days later. Neutrophils and monocytes/macrophages differ chiefly in the following ways:

1. *Speed:* Neutrophils arrive at the injury site first, whereas macrophages move more sluggishly.
2. *Active life span:* Macrophages survive and divide in the acidic inflammatory site, whereas neutrophils cannot.
3. *Chemotactic factors:* Neutrophils and macrophages are not attracted by the same factors, such as macrophage chemotactic factor, which is released by neutrophils.
4. *Enzymatic content of their lysosomes, or digestive vacuoles:* Neutrophils have a more active NADPH oxidase and produce more hydrogen peroxide; macrophage phagolysosomes are more acidic, favoring the activity of acidic proteases and other enzymes.
5. *Role in the immune response:* Macrophages, but not neutrophils, are involved in activation of the adaptive immune system.
6. *Role in wound repair:* Macrophages are the primary cells that infiltrate tissue in wounds, remove cells and cellular debris, promote angiogenesis, and produce cytokines and growth factors that suppress further inflammation and initiate healing by promoting epithelial cell division, activating fibroblasts, and promoting synthesis of extracellular matrix and collagen.

The bactericidal activity of macrophages can increase markedly with the help of inflammatory cytokines produced by cells of the acquired immune system (subsets of T lymphocytes) or cells activated through Toll-like receptors (TLRs). Macrophage activation results in two subpopulations of cells.[19] M1 macrophages are activated through TLRs by substances found in sites of inflammation and have greater bacterial killing capacity. M2 macrophages are activated by lymphocyte-produced cytokines and are primarily involved in healing and repair.[20]

Several bacteria are resistant to killing by granulocytes and can even survive inside macrophages. Microorganisms, such as *Mycobacterium tuberculosis* (tuberculosis), *Mycobacterium leprae* (leprosy), *Salmonella typhi* (typhoid fever), *Brucella abortus* (brucellosis), and *Listeria monocytogenes* (listeriosis), can remain dormant or multiply inside the phagolysosomes of macrophages.

Dendritic cells. Dendritic cells provide one of the major links between the innate and acquired immune responses. They are the primary phagocytic cells located in the peripheral organs and skin, where molecules released from infectious agents are encountered, recognized through PRRs, and internalized through phagocytosis. Dendritic cells then migrate through the lymphatic vessels to lymphoid tissue, such as lymph nodes, and interact with T lymphocytes to generate an acquired immune response.[21] Through the production of a family of cytokines, they guide development of a subset of T cells (helper cells) that coordinate the development of functional B and T cells (discussed in Chapter 7).

Phagocytosis. The two most important phagocytes are neutrophils and macrophages. Both cells are circulating in the blood and must first leave the circulation and migrate to the site of inflammation before initiating phagocytosis (Figure 6-9). Many products of inflammation affect expression of surface molecules involved in cell-to-cell adherence. Both leukocytes and endothelial cells begin expressing molecules (selectins and integrins) that increase adhesion, or stickiness, causing the leukocytes to adhere more avidly to the endothelial cells in the walls of the capillaries and venules in a process called margination, or pavementing. Leukocyte-endothelial interactions lead to diapedesis, or emigration of the cells through the inter-endothelial junctions that have loosened in response to inflammatory mediators.[22]

Once inside the tissue, leukocytes undergo a process of directed migration (chemotaxis) by which they are attracted to the inflammatory site by chemotactic factors.[23] The primary chemotactic factors include many bacterial products, neutrophil chemotactic factor produced by mast cells, the chemokine IL-8, complement fragments C3a and C5a, and products of the clotting and kinin systems. Red blood cells cannot repair themselves and are phagocytized by macrophages at the end of their lifespan (Figure 6-10).

At the inflammatory site, the process of phagocytosis involves five steps: (1) recognition and adherence of the phagocyte to its target, (2) engulfment (ingestion or endocytosis), (3) formation of a phagosome, (4) fusion of the phagosome with lysosomal granules within the phagocyte, and (5) destruction of the target. Throughout the process, both the target and the digestive enzymes are isolated within membrane-bound vesicles. Isolation protects the phagocyte itself from the harmful effects of the target microorganisms, as well as its own enzymes.

Most phagocytes can trap and engulf bacteria using PRRs, although the process is relatively slow. Opsonization greatly enhances adherence by acting as a glue to tighten the affinity of adherence between the phagocyte and the target cell. The most efficient opsonins are antibodies and C3b produced by the complement system. Antibodies are made against antigens on the surface of bacteria and are highly specific to that particular microorganism. Certain bacterial and fungal polysaccharide coatings activate the alternative and lectin pathways of complement activation, which deposits C3b on the bacterial surface and increases phagocytosis. The surface of phagocytes contains a variety of specific receptors that will strongly bind to opsonins. These include complement receptors that bind to C3b and Fc receptors that bind to a site on antibody molecules.

Engulfment (endocytosis) is carried out by small pseudopods that extend from the plasma membrane and surround the adherent microorganism, forming an intracellular phagocytic vacuole, or phagosome (see Figures 6-9 and 6-10). After the formation of the phagosome, lysosomes converge, fuse with the phagosome, and discharge their contents, creating a phagolysosome. Destruction of the bacterium takes place within the phagolysosome and is accomplished by both oxygen-dependent and oxygen-independent mechanisms.

Oxygen-dependent killing mechanisms result from the production of toxic oxygen species. Phagocytosis is accompanied by a burst of oxygen uptake by the phagocyte; this is termed the *respiratory burst* and results from a shift in much of the cell's glucose metabolism to the hexose-monophosphate shunt, which produces nicotinamide adenine dinucleotide phosphate (NADPH). A membrane-associated enzyme, NADPH oxidase, uses NADPH to generate superoxide (O_2^-), hydrogen peroxide (H_2O_2), and other reactive oxygen species that can be highly damaging to bacteria. Hydrogen peroxide also can collaborate with the lysosomal enzyme *myeloperoxidase* and halide anions (Cl^- and Br^-) to form acids that kill bacteria and fungi.

Oxygen-independent mechanisms of microbial killing include (1) the acidic pH (3.5 to 4.0) of the phagolysosome, (2) cationic proteins that bind to and damage target cell membranes, (3) enzymatic attack of the microorganism's cell wall by lysozyme and other enzymes, and (4) inhibition of bacterial growth by lactoferrin binding of iron.

When a phagocyte dies at an inflammatory site, it frequently lyses (breaks open) and releases its cytoplasmic contents into the tissue. For instance, contents of neutrophil primary granules (lysozyme, hydrolases, neutral proteases) and secondary granules (lysozyme, collagenase, gelatinase) can digest the connective tissue matrix, causing much of the tissue destruction associated with inflammation.[24] The destructive effects of many enzymes and reactive oxygen molecules released by dying phagocytes are minimized by natural inhibitors found in the blood, such as superoxide dismutase (breaks down superoxide), catalase (breaks down hydrogen peroxide), and the antiproteinases α_1-antitrypsin and α_2-macroglobulin (both produced by the liver). An inherited deficiency of α_1-antitrypsin often leads to chronic lung damage and emphysema as a result of inflammation. (The pulmonary effects of α_1-antitrypsin deficiency are described in Chapter 27.)

Natural Killer Cells and Lymphocytes

The main function of natural killer (NK) cells is recognition and elimination of cells infected with viruses, although they also are somewhat effective at elimination of other abnormal cells, specifically cancer cells.[25] NK cells seem to be more efficient in this role when they encounter an infected cell within the circulatory system as opposed to within tissues. NK cells have inhibitory and activating receptors that allow differentiation between infected or tumor cells and normal cells. If the NK cell binds to a target cell through activating receptors, it produces several cytokines and toxic molecules that can kill the target.[26] NK cells and lymphocytes, which are the principal cells of the adaptive immune response, will be discussed in much more detail in Chapter 7.

> ✔ **QUICK CHECK 6-4**
> 1. What are pattern recognition receptors?
> 2. What are cytokines? How do cytokines promote inflammation?
> 3. What products do the mast cells release during inflammation, and what are their effects?
> 4. What phagocytic cell types are involved in the acute inflammatory response? What is the role of each?
> 5. What are the four steps in the process of phagocytosis?

ACUTE AND CHRONIC INFLAMMATION

Inflammation can be divided into phases of acute and chronic inflammation. The acute inflammatory response is self-limiting—that is, it continues only until the threat to the host is eliminated. This usually takes 8 to 10 days from onset to healing. If the acute inflammatory

A. Tissue

B. Recognition and attachment   **C. Phagocytosis**

FIGURE 6-9 Process of Phagocytosis. The process that results in phagocytosis is characterized by three interrelated steps: adherence and diapedesis, tissue invasion by chemotaxis, and phagocytosis. **A,** *Adherence, margination, diapedesis, and chemotaxis.* The primary phagocyte in the blood is the neutrophil, which usually moves freely within the vessel **(1)**. At sites of inflammation, the neutrophil progressively develops increased adherence to the endothelium, leading to accumulation along the vessel wall (margination or pavementing) **(2)**. At sites of endothelial cell retraction the neutrophil exits the blood by means of diapedesis **(3)**. *Chemotaxis.* In the tissues, the neutrophil detects chemotactic factor gradients through surface receptors **(1)** and migrates towards higher concentrations of the factors **(2)**. The high concentration of chemotactic factors at the site of inflammation immobilizes the neutrophil **(3)**. **B,** *Specific receptors for recognition and attachment.* **C,** *Phagocytosis.* Opsonized microorganisms bind to the surface of a phagocyte through specific receptors **(1)**. The microorganism is ingested into a phagocytic vacuole, or phagosome **(2)**. Lysosomes fuse with the phagosome, resulting in the formation of a phagolysosome **(3)**. During this process the microorganism is exposed to products of the lysosomes, including a variety of enzymes and products of the hexose-monophosphate shunt (e.g., H_2O_2, O_2^-). The microorganism is killed and digested **(4)**. *Ab,* Antibody; *AbR,* antibody receptor; *C3b,* complement component C3b; *C3bR,* complement C3b receptor; *PAMP,* pathogen-associated molecular pattern; *PRR,* pattern recognition receptor.

response proves inadequate, a chronic inflammation may develop and persist for weeks or months. If healing has not been initiated, inflammation may progress to a granulomatous response that is designed to contain the cause of tissue damage so it no longer poses any harm to the individual. The characteristics of the early (i.e., acute) inflammatory response differ from those of the later (i.e., chronic) response, and each phase involves different biochemical mediators and cells that function together. Depending on the successful containment of tissue damage wond infection, the acute and chronic phases may lead to healing without progression to the next phase.

FIGURE 6-10 Phagocytosis of Red Blood Cell. This scanning electron micrographs shows the progressive steps in phagocytosis. **A,** Red blood cells *(R)* attach to the surface of a macrophage *(M)*. **B,** Part of the macrophage *(M)* membrane starts to enclose the red cell *(R)*. **C,** The red blood cells are almost totally engulfed by the macrophage. (Modified from King DW et al: *General pathology: principles and dynamics,* Philadelphia, 1983, Lea & Febiger.)

Local Manifestations of Acute Inflammation

The cells and plasma protein systems of the inflammatory response interact to produce all the characteristics of inflammation, whether local or systemic (discussed in the next section), as well as determine the duration of inflammation, either acute or chronic. All the local characteristics of acute inflammation (i.e., swelling, pain, heat, and redness [erythema]) result from vascular changes and the subsequent leakage of circulating components into the tissue.

The exudate of inflammation results from increased vascular permeability and varies in composition, depending on the stage of the inflammatory response and, to some extent, the injurious stimulus. In early or mild inflammation, the exudate may be watery (serous exudate) with very few plasma proteins or leukocytes, such as the fluid in a blister. In more severe or advanced inflammation, the exudate may be thick and clotted (fibrinous exudate), such as in the lungs of individuals with pneumonia. If a large number of leukocytes accumulate, as in persistent bacterial infections, the exudate consists of pus and is called a purulent (suppurative) exudate. Purulent exudate is characteristic of walled-off lesions (cysts or abscesses). If bleeding occurs, the exudate is filled with erythrocytes and is described as a hemorrhagic exudate.

Systemic Manifestations of Acute Inflammation

The three primary systemic changes associated with the acute inflammatory response are fever, leukocytosis (a transient increase in the levels of circulating leukocytes), and increased levels of circulating plasma proteins.

Fever

Fever is partially induced by specific cytokines (e.g., IL-1, released from neutrophils and macrophages). These are known as endogenous pyrogens to differentiate them from pathogen-produced *exogenous pyrogens.* Pyrogens act directly on the hypothalamus, the portion of the brain that controls the body's thermostat. (Mechanisms of temperature regulation and fever are discussed in Chapter 14.) A fever can be beneficial because some microorganisms (e.g., those that cause syphilis or gonococcal urethritis) are highly sensitive to small increases in body temperature. On the other hand, fever may have harmful side effects because it may enhance the host's susceptibility to the effects of endotoxins associated with gram-negative bacterial infections (bacterial toxins are described in Chapter 8).

Leukocytosis

Leukocytosis is an increase in the number of circulating white blood cells (greater than $11,000/ml^3$ in adults). During many infections, leukocytosis may be accompanied by a *left shift* in the ratio of immature to mature neutrophils, so that the more immature forms of neutrophils, such as band cells, metamyelocytes, and occasionally myelocytes, are present in relatively greater than normal proportions. (Chapter 20 contains a more complete discussion of the development and maturation of blood cells.) Production of immature leukocytes increases primarily from proliferation and release of granulocyte and monocyte precursors in the bone marrow, which is stimulated by several products of inflammation.

Plasma Protein Synthesis

The synthesis of many plasma proteins, mostly products of the liver, is increased during inflammation. These proteins, which can be either proinflammatory or anti-inflammatory in nature, are referred to as acute-phase reactants (Table 6-4). Acute-phase reactants reach maximal circulating levels within 10 to 40 hours after the start of inflammation. IL-1 is indirectly responsible for the synthesis of acute-phase reactants through the induction of IL-6, which directly stimulates liver cells to synthesize most of these proteins.

Common laboratory tests for inflammation measure levels of acute-phase reactants. For example, an increase in blood levels of acute-phase reactants, primarily fibrinogen, is associated with an increased adhesion among erythrocytes and a corresponding increase in the sedimentation rate. The erythrocyte sedimentation rate is a measurement of the rate at which red blood cells sediment in a tube over a prescribed time span (usually an hour). Although increased erythrocyte sedimentation is a nonspecific reaction, it is considered a good indicator of an acute inflammatory response.

Chronic Inflammation

Superficially, the difference between acute and chronic inflammation is duration; chronic inflammation lasts 2 weeks or longer, regardless of cause. Chronic inflammation is sometimes preceded by an unsuccessful acute inflammatory response (Figure 6-11). For example, if bacterial contamination or foreign objects (e.g., dirt, wood splinter, silica, and glass) persist in a wound, an acute response may be prolonged beyond 2 weeks. Pus formation, suppuration (purulent discharge), and incomplete wound healing may characterize this type of chronic inflammation.

Chronic inflammation can occur also as a distinct process without previous acute inflammation. Some microorganisms (e.g., mycobacte-

ria that cause tuberculosis) have cell walls with a very high lipid and wax content, making them relatively insensitive to breakdown by phagocytes. Other microorganisms (e.g., those that cause leprosy, syphilis, and brucellosis) can survive within the macrophage and avoid removal by the acute inflammatory response. Other microorganisms produce toxins that damage tissue and cause persistent inflammation even after the organism is killed. Finally, chemicals, particulate matter, or physical irritants (e.g., inhaled dusts, wood splinters, and suture material) can cause a prolonged inflammatory response.

Chronic inflammation is characterized by a dense infiltration of lymphocytes and macrophages. If macrophages are unable to protect the host from tissue damage, the body attempts to wall off and isolate the infected area, thus forming a granuloma (Figure 6-12). For example, infections caused by some bacteria (listeriosis, brucellosis), fungi (histoplasmosis, coccidioidomycosis), and parasites (leishmaniasis, schistosomiasis, toxoplasmosis) can result in granuloma formation. TNF-α primarily drives granuloma formation.[27] Some macrophages differentiate into large epithelioid cells, which specialize in taking up debris and other small particles. Other macrophages fuse into multinucleated giant cells, which are active phagocytes that can engulf very large particles—larger than those that can be engulfed by a single macrophage. These two types of specialized cells form the center of the granuloma, which is surrounded by a wall of lymphocytes. The granuloma itself is often encapsulated by fibrous deposits of collagen and may become cartilaginous or possibly calcified by deposits of calcium carbonate and calcium phosphate.

The classic granuloma associated with tuberculosis is characterized by a wall of epithelioid cells surrounding a cheeselike proteinaceous center derived from dead and decaying tissue (caseous necrosis) and

TABLE 6-4   Circulating Levels of Acute-Phase Reactants During Inflammation

Function	Increased	Decreased
Coagulation components	Fibrinogen Prothrombin Factor VIII Plasminogen	None
Protease inhibitors	α₁-Antitrypsin α₁-Antichymotrypsin	Inter-α1-antitrypsin
Transport proteins	Haptoglobin Hemopexin Ceruloplasmin Ferritin	Transferrin
Complement components	C1s, C2, C3, C4, C5, C9, factor B, C1 inhibitor	Properdin
Miscellaneous proteins	α₁-Acid glycoprotein Fibronectin Serum amyloid A (SAA) C-reactive protein (CRP)	Albumin Prealbumin α₁-Lipoprotein β-Lipoprotein

FIGURE 6-11 The Chronic Inflammatory Response. Inflammation usually becomes chronic because of the persistence of an infection, an antigen, or a foreign body in the wound. Chronic inflammation is characterized by the persistence of many of the processes of acute inflammation. In addition, large amounts of neutrophil degranulation and death, the activation of lymphocytes, and the concurrent activation of fibroblasts result in the release of mediators that induce the infiltration of more lymphocytes and monocytes/macrophages and the beginning of wound healing and tissue repair. For more detailed information on each portion of the response, see the figures referenced in this illustration.

Langhans giant cell

FIGURE 6-12 Tuberculous Granuloma. A central area of amorphous caseous necrosis *(C)* is surrounded by a zone of lymphocytes *(L)* and enlarged epithelioid cells *(E)*. Activated macrophages frequently fuse to form multinucleated cells (Langhans giant cells). In tuberculoid granulomas the nuclei of the giant cells move to the cellular margins in a horseshoe-like formation.

mycobacteria.[28] Decay of cells within the granuloma results in the release of acids and the enzymatic contents of lysosomes from dead phagocytes. In this inhospitable environment, the cellular debris is broken down into its basic constituents, and a clear fluid may remain (liquefaction necrosis). Eventually, this fluid diffuses out and leaves a hollow, thick-walled structure that has replaced normal tissue and reduced the function of the lung.

✔ **QUICK CHECK 6-5**
1. Describe how acute inflammation differs from chronic inflammation. What characteristics do they share?
2. List the types of exudate produced in inflammation.

WOUND HEALING

The conclusion of inflammation is healing and repair. The most favorable outcome is a return to normal structure and function if damage is minor, no complications occur, and destroyed tissues are capable of regeneration (replacement of damaged tissue with healthy tissue, such as occurs in the epithelia of the skin and intestines and in some organs, such as the liver) (Figure 6-13). This restoration is called resolution and may take up to 2 years, and local production of IL-10 appears to play a critical role.[29] Resolution may not be possible if extensive damage

HEALING BY PRIMARY INTENTION

HEALING BY SECONDARY INTENTION

Coagulation
— Platelets

Inflammation
— Neutrophils

24 hours

Proliferation
— Mitoses
— Granulation tissue
Macrophage
— Lymphocyte
— Fibroblast
— New capillary

3 to 14 days

Remodeling Maturation
— Reepithelialization

— Fibrous union (Scar)

Wound contraction

Weeks to Months

FIGURE 6-13 Wound Healing by Primary and Secondary Intention and Phases of Wound Healing. Phases of wound healing (coagulation, inflammation, proliferation, remodeling, and maturation) and steps in wound healing by primary intention *(left)* and secondary intention *(right)*. Note large amounts of granulation tissue and wound contraction in healing by secondary intention. (From Roberts JR, Custalow CB: *Roberts and Hedges' clinical procedures in emergency medicine,* ed 6, Philadelphia, 2013, Saunders.)

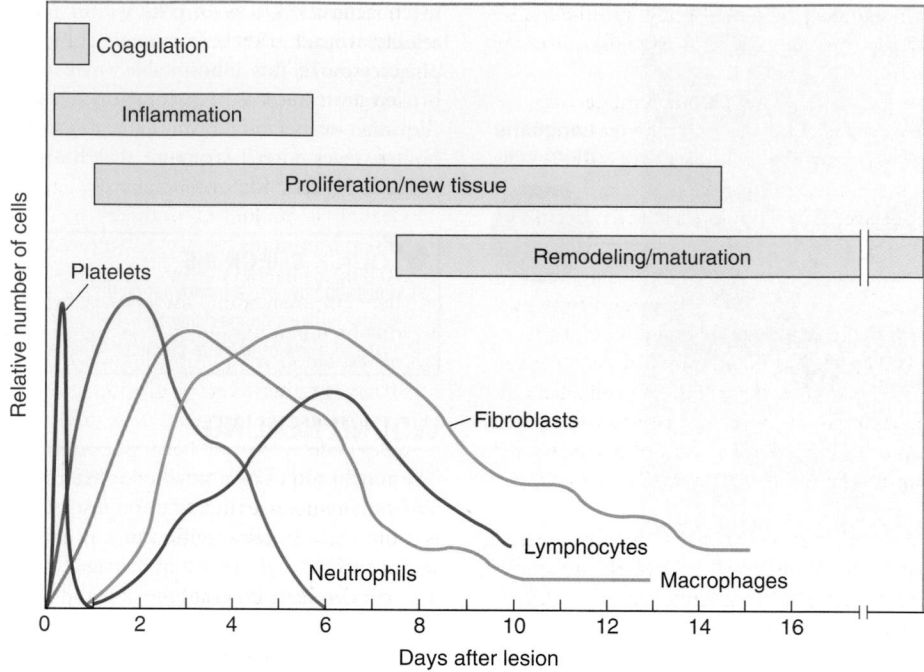

FIGURE 6-14 Time Course of Cells Infiltrating a Wound. Neutrophils and macrophages are the predominant cells that infiltrate a wound during inflammation. Lymphocytes appear later and peak at day 7. Fibroblasts are the predominant cells during the proliferative and remodeling phases of the healing process. (Adapted from Townsend CM et al, editors: *Sabiston textbook of surgery*, ed 19, St Louis, 2012, Elsevier.)

is present, the tissue is not capable of regeneration, infection results in abscess or granuloma formation, or fibrin persists in the lesion. In those cases, repair takes place instead of resolution. **Repair** is the replacement of destroyed tissue with scar tissue. **Scar tissue** is composed primarily of collagen that fills in the lesion and restores strength but cannot carry out the physiologic functions of destroyed tissue, resulting in loss of function.

Wound healing involves processes that (1) fill in, (2) seal, and (3) shrink the wound. These characteristics of healing vary in importance and duration among different types of wounds. A clean incision, such as a paper cut or a sutured surgical wound, heals primarily through the process of collagen synthesis. Because this type of wound has minimal tissue loss and close apposition of the wound edges, very little sealing (**epithelialization**) and shrinkage (**contraction**) are required. Wounds that heal under conditions of minimal tissue loss are said to heal by **primary intention** (see Figure 6-13).

Other wounds do not heal as easily. Healing of an open wound, such as a stage IV pressure ulcer (decubitus ulcer), requires a great deal of tissue replacement so that epithelialization, scar formation, and contraction take longer and healing occurs through **secondary intention** (see Figure 6-13). Healing by either primary or secondary intention may occur at different rates for different types of tissue injury.

Epidermal wounds that heal by secondary intention and unsutured internal lesions are not completely restored by healing. At best, repaired tissue regains 80% of its original tensile strength. Only epithelial, hepatic (liver), and bone marrow cells are capable of the complete mitotic regeneration of the normal tissue known as *compensatory hyperplasia*. In fibrous connective tissue, such as joints and ligaments, normal healing results in replacement of the original tissue with new tissue that does not have exactly the same structure or function as that of the original. Some tissues heal without replacement of cells. For example, damage resulting from myocardial infarction heals with a scar composed of fibrous tissue rather than with cardiac muscle.

Wound healing occurs in three overlapping phases: inflammation, proliferation and new tissue formation, and remodeling and maturation.

Phase I: Inflammation

The early phase of wound healing, the transition from acute inflammation to healing, begins almost immediately. The **inflammatory phase** includes coagulation or hemostasis and the infiltration of cells that participate in wound healing, including platelets, neutrophils, and macrophages (Figure 6-14). The fibrin mesh of the blood clot acts as a scaffold for cells that participate in healing. Platelets contribute to clot formation and, as they degranulate, release growth factors that initiate proliferation of undamaged cells. Neutrophils clear the wound of debris and bacteria and are later replaced by macrophages. Macrophages are essential to wound healing because they clear debris, release wound healing mediators and growth factors, recruit fibroblasts, and help promote formation of a new blood supply (**angiogenesis**) during the proliferative phase of wound healing.

Phase II: Proliferation and New Tissue Formation

The proliferative phase begins 3 to 4 days after the injury and continues for as long as 2 weeks. The wound is sealed and the fibrin clot is replaced by normal tissue or scar tissue during this phase. The **proliferative phase** is characterized by macrophage invasion of the dissolving clot and recruitment and proliferation of fibroblasts (connective tissue cells), followed by fibroblast collagen synthesis, epithelialization, contraction of the wound, and cellular differentiation. Macrophages secrete a variety of biochemical mediators that promote healing, including:

1. Transforming growth factor-beta (TGF-β) stimulates fibroblasts entering the lesion to synthesize and secrete the collagen precursor procollagen.
2. **Angiogenesis factors**, such as vascular endothelial growth factor (VEGF) and fibroblast growth factor-2 (FGF-2), stimulate vascular

endothelial cells to form capillary buds that grow into the lesion; decreased pH and decreased wound oxygen tension also promote angiogenesis.[30]

3. **Matrix metalloproteinases (MMPs)** degrade and remodel extracellular matrix proteins (e.g., collagen and fibrin) at the site of injury.[31]

Granulation tissue grows into the wound from surrounding healthy connective tissue and consists of invasive cells, new lymphatic vessels, and new capillaries derived from capillaries in the surrounding tissue, giving the granulation tissue a red, granular appearance. During this process the healing wound must be protected. Epithelialization is the process by which epithelial cells grow into the wound from surrounding healthy tissue.[32] Epithelial cells migrate under the clot or scab using MMPs to unravel collagen. Migrating epithelial cells contact similar cells from all sides of the wound and seal it. The epithelial cells remain active, undergoing differentiation to give rise to the various epidermal layers (see Chapter 41). Epithelialization of a skin wound can be hastened if the wound is kept moist, preventing the fibrin clot from becoming a scab.

Fibroblasts are important cells during healing because they secrete collagen and other connective tissue proteins. Fibroblasts are stimulated by macrophage-derived TGF-β to proliferate, enter the lesion, and deposit connective tissue proteins in débrided areas about 6 days after the fibroblasts have entered the lesion. Collagen is the most abundant protein in the body.[33] It contains high concentrations of the amino acids glycine, proline, and lysine, many of which are enzymatically modified. Modification of proline and lysine requires several cofactors that are absolutely necessary for proper collagen polymerization and function. These include iron, ascorbic acid (vitamin C), and molecular oxygen (O_2); absence of any of these results in impaired wound healing. As healing progresses, collagen molecules are cross-linked by intermolecular covalent bonds to form collagen fibrils that are further cross-linked to form collagen fibers. The complete process takes several months.

In granulation tissue, TGF-β induces some fibroblasts to transition into myofibroblasts, specialized cells responsible for wound contraction.[34] Myofibroblasts have features of both smooth muscle cells and fibroblasts. They appear microscopically similar to fibroblasts but differ in that their cytoplasm contains bundles of parallel fibers similar to those found in smooth muscle cells. Wound contraction occurs as extensions from the plasma membrane of myofibroblasts establish connections between neighboring cells, contract their fibers, and exert tension on the neighboring cells while anchoring themselves to the wound bed. Wound contraction is necessary for closure of all wounds, especially those that heal by secondary intention. Contraction is noticeable 6 to 12 days after injury.

Phase III: Remodeling and Maturation

Tissue remodeling and maturation begins several weeks after injury and is normally complete within 2 years. During this phase, there is continuation of cellular differentiation, scar formation, and scar remodeling. The fibroblast is the major cell of tissue remodeling with the deposition of collagen into an organized matrix. Tissue regeneration and wound contraction continue in the remodeling and maturation phase—a phase for recovering normal tissue structure that can persist for years. For wounds that heal by scarring, scar tissue is remodeled and capillaries disappear, leaving the scar avascular. Within 2 to 3 weeks after maturation has begun, the scar tissue has gained about two thirds of its eventual maximal strength.

Dysfunctional Wound Healing

Dysfunctional wound healing and impaired epithelialization may occur during any phase of the healing process. The cause of dysfunctional wound healing includes ischemia, excessive bleeding, excessive

fibrin deposition, a predisposing disorder such as diabetes mellitus, obesity, wound infection, inadequate nutrients, numerous drugs, and tobacco smoke.[35]

Oxygen-deprived (ischemic) tissue is susceptible to cellular death and infection, which prolongs inflammation and delays healing. *Ischemia* reduces energy production and impairs collagen synthesis and the tensile strength of regenerating connective tissue.

Healing is prolonged if there is *excessive bleeding*. Large clots increase the amount of space that granulation tissue must fill and serve as mechanical barriers to oxygen diffusion. Accumulated blood is an excellent culture medium for bacteria and promotes infection, thereby prolonging inflammation by increasing exudation and pus formation.[32] Decreased blood volume also inhibits inflammation because of vessel constriction rather than the dilation required to deliver inflammatory cells, nutrients, and oxygen to the site of injury.

Obesity delays wound healing because of impaired leukocyte function and predisposition to infection, decreases in the number of growth factors, and increases in the levels of proinflammatory cytokines. Additionally, there is dysregulation in collagen synthesis and a decrease in angiogenesis.[36]

Excessive fibrin deposition is detrimental to healing. Fibrin released in response to injury must eventually be reabsorbed to prevent organization into fibrous adhesions. Adhesions formed in the pleural, pericardial, or abdominal cavities can bind organs together by fibrous bands and distort or strangulate the affected organ.

Persons with *diabetes* are at risk for prolonged wound healing. Wounds are often ischemic because of the potential for small-vessel diseases that impair the microcirculation and alter (glycosylated) hemoglobin, which has an increased affinity for oxygen and thus does not readily release oxygen in tissues. Consequences of hyperglycemia also include suppression of macrophages and increased risk for wound infection.

Wound infection is caused by the infiltration of pathogens. Pathogens damage cells, stimulate the continued release of inflammatory mediators, consume nutrients, and delay wound healing.

Optimal *nutrition* is important during all phases of healing because metabolic needs increase. Leukocytes need glucose to produce adenosine 5′-triphosphate (5′-ATP) necessary for chemotaxis, phagocytosis, intercellular killing, and initiation of healing; therefore the wounds of persons with diabetes who receive insufficient insulin heal poorly. Hypoproteinemia impairs fibroblast proliferation and collagen synthesis. Prolonged lack of vitamins A and C results in poorly formed connective tissue and greatly impaired healing because they are cofactors required for collagen synthesis.[37] Other nutrients, including iron, zinc, manganese, and copper, are also required as cofactors for collagen synthesis. Malnutrition increases risk for wound infection, delays healing, and reduces wound tensile strength.

Medications, including antineoplastic (anticancer) agents, nonsteroidal anti-inflammatory drugs (NSAIDs), and steroids, delay wound healing. Antineoplastic agents slow cell division and inhibit angiogenesis. Although NSAIDs inhibit prostaglandin production and suppress acute inflammation and relieve pain, they also can delay wound healing, particularly bone formation, and may contribute to the formation of excessive scarring. Steroids prevent macrophages from migrating to the site of injury and inhibit release of collagenase and plasminogen activator. Steroids also inhibit fibroblast migration into the wound during the proliferative phase and delay epithelialization. Toxic agents in *tobacco smoke* (i.e., nicotine, carbon monoxide, and hydrogen cyanide) delay wound healing and increase the risk for wound infection.

Dysfunctional collagen synthesis may involve excessive production of collagen, leading to a hypertrophic scar or keloid.[38] A **hypertrophic scar** is raised but remains within the original boundaries of the wound

FIGURE 6-15 Hypertrophic Scar and Keloid Scar Formation.
Hypertrophic scar (**A**) and keloid scar (**B**) caused by excessive synthesis of collagen at suture sites. (**A** from Flint PW et al: *Cummings otolaryngology: head & neck surgery*, ed 6, Philadelphia, 2015, Mosby; **B** from Damjanov I, Linder J: *Anderson's pathology*, ed 10, St Louis, 1996, Mosby.)

and tends to regress over time (Figure 6-15, *A*). A **keloid** is a raised scar that extends beyond the original boundaries of the wound, invades surrounding tissue, and is likely to recur after surgical removal (Figure 6-15, *B*). A familial tendency to keloid formation has been observed, with a greater incidence in blacks than whites.

Wound Disruption

A potential complication of wounds that are sutured closed is **dehiscence**, in which the wound pulls apart at the suture line. Dehiscence generally occurs 5 to 12 days after suturing, when collagen synthesis is at its peak. Approximately half of dehiscence occurrences are associated with wound infection, but they also may be the result of sutures breaking because of excessive strain. Obesity increases the risk for dehiscence because adipose tissue is difficult to suture. Wound dehiscence usually is heralded by increased serous drainage from the wound and a patient's perception that "something gave way." Prompt surgical attention is required.

Impaired Contraction

Wound contraction, although necessary for healing, may become excessive, resulting in a deformity or **contracture of scar tissue**. Burns of the skin are especially susceptible to contracture development, particularly at joints, resulting in loss of movement around the joints. Internal contractures include duodenal strictures caused by

dysfunctional healing of a peptic ulcer; esophageal strictures caused by chemical burns, such as lye ingestion; or abdominal adhesions caused by surgery, infection, or radiation. Contracture may occur in cirrhosis of the liver, constricting vascular flow and contributing to the development of portal hypertension and esophageal varices. Proper positioning, range-of-motion exercises, and surgery are among the physical means used to overcome excessive skin contractures. Surgery is performed to release internal contractures.

> ✔ **QUICK CHECK 6-6**
> 1. How does regeneration of tissue differ from repair of tissue?
> 2. What does it mean to heal by primary intention?
> 3. What is the role of fibroblasts in wound healing?
> 4. Describe various ways wound healing may be dysfunctional.

PEDIATRIC CONSIDERATIONS

Age-Related Factors Affecting Innate Immunity in the Newborn Child

- Newborn physiologic immunity acquired from mother through placenta and breast milk.
- Newborns have transiently depressed inflammatory responses.
- Neutrophils are incapable of chemotaxis, lacking fluidity in the plasma membrane.
- Complement levels are diminished, especially components of the alternative pathways (e.g., factor B), particularly in premature newborns.
- Monocyte/macrophage numbers are normal but chemotaxis of monocytes is delayed.
- There is a tendency for infections associated with chemotactic defects, for example, cutaneous abscesses caused by staphylococci and cutaneous candidiasis.
- There are diminished oxidative and bacterial responses in those stressed by in utero infection or respiratory insufficiency.
- There is a tendency to develop severe overwhelming sepsis and meningitis when infected by bacteria against which no maternal antibodies are present.
- The establishment of the gut microbiome is facilitated by breast milk.
- Cesarean delivered newborns have reduced gut microbial diversity.

GERIATRIC CONSIDERATIONS

Age-Related Factors Affecting Innate Immunity in the Elderly

- Normal numbers of cells of innate immunity but possible diminished function (e.g., decreased phagocytic activity, decreased antibody production, and altered cytokine synthesis)
- Increased incidence of chronic inflammation, possibly related to increased production of proinflammatory mediators
- At risk for impaired healing and infection associated with chronic illness (e.g., diabetes mellitus, peripheral vascular disease, or cardiovascular disease) and decreased phagocytosis
- Use of medications interfering with healing (e.g., anti-inflammatory steroids)
- Loss of subcutaneous fat, diminishing layers of protection against injury
- Atrophied epidermis, including underlying capillaries, which decreases perfusion and increases risk of hypoxia in wound bed
- Aging of the immune system, diminishing the effectiveness of vaccines

DID YOU UNDERSTAND?

Innate Immunity

1. Neonates often have transiently depressed inflammatory function, particularly neutrophil chemotaxis and alternative complement pathway activity.

2. Elderly persons are at risk for impaired wound healing, usually because of chronic illnesses.

3. There are three layers of human defense: barriers; innate immunity, which includes the inflammatory response; and adaptive (acquired) immunity.

4. Physical barriers are the first lines of defense that prevent damage to the individual and prevent invasion by pathogens; these include the skin and mucous membranes.

5. Antibacterial peptides (cathelicidins, defensins, collectins, and mannose-binding lectin) in mucous secretions, perspiration, saliva, tears, and other secretions provide a biochemical barrier against pathogenic microorganisms.

6. The skin and mucous membranes are colonized by commensal or mutualistic microorganisms that provide protection by releasing chemicals that facilitate immune responses, prevent colonization by pathogens, and facilitate digestion in the gastrointestinal tract.

7. The second line of defense is the inflammatory response, a rapid and nonspecific protective response to cellular injury from any cause. It can occur only in vascularized tissue.

8. The macroscopic hallmarks of inflammation are redness, swelling, heat, pain, and loss of function of the inflamed tissues.

9. The microscopic hallmarks of inflammation are vasodilation, increased capillary permeability, and an accumulation of fluid and cells at the inflammatory site.

10. Inflammation is mediated by three key plasma protein systems: the complement system, the clotting system, and the kinin system. The components of all three systems are a series of inactive proteins that are activated sequentially.

11. The complement system can be activated by antigen-antibody reactions (through the classical pathway) or by other products, especially bacterial polysaccharides (through the lectin pathway or the alternative pathway), resulting in the production of biologically active fragments that recruit phagocytes, activate mast cells, and destroy pathogens.

12. The most biologically potent products of the complement system are C3b (opsonin), C3a (anaphylatoxin), and C5a (anaphylatoxin, chemotactic factor).

13. The clotting system stops bleeding, localizes microorganisms, and provides a meshwork for repair and healing.

14. Bradykinin is the most important product of the kinin system and causes vascular permeability, smooth muscle contraction, and pain.

15. Control of inflammation regulates inflammatory cells and enzymes and localizes the inflammatory response to the area of injury or infection.

16. Carboxypeptidase, histaminase, and C1 esterase inhibitor are inactivating enzymes, and the fibrinolytic system and plasmin facilitate clot degradation after bleeding is stopped.

17. Many different types of cells are involved in the inflammatory process including mast cells, endothelial cells, platelets, phagocytes (neutrophils, eosinophils, monocytes and macrophages, dendritic cells), natural killer (NK) cells, and lymphocytes.

18. Most cells express plasma membrane pattern recognition receptors (PRRs) that recognize molecules produced by infectious microorganisms (pathogen-associated molecular patterns, or PAMPs), or products of cellular damage (damage-associated molecular patterns, or DAMPs). Toll-like receptors (TLRs) and NOD-like receptors are expressed on many inflammatory cells, recognize PAMPs and DAMPs, and promote release of cytokines and inflammatory mediators that eliminate damaged cells and protect against invasion by microbes.

19. The cells of the innate immune system secrete many biochemical mediators (cytokines) that are responsible for activating other cells and regulating the inflammatory response; these cytokines include chemokines, interleukins, interferons, and other molecules.

20. Chemokines induce chemotaxis of leukocytes, fibroblasts, and other cells to promote phagocytosis and wound healing.

21. Interleukins are produced primarily by lymphocytes and macrophages and promote or inhibit inflammation by activating growth and differentiation of leukocytes and lymphocytes.

22. The most important proinflammatory interleukins are interleukin-1 (IL-1), interleukin-6 (IL-6), and tumor necrosis factor-alpha (TNF-α). Interleukins 6 and 10 down-regulate the inflammatory response.

23. Interferons are produced by cells that are infected by viruses. Once released from infected cells, interferons can stimulate neighboring healthy cells to produce substances that prevent viral infection.

24. The most important activator of the inflammatory response is the mast cell, which is located in connective tissue near capillaries and initiates inflammation by releasing biochemical mediators (histamine, chemotactic factors) from preformed cytoplasmic granules and synthesizing other mediators (prostaglandins, leukotrienes, and platelet-activating factor) in response to a stimulus. Basophils are found in the blood and function similar to mast cells.

25. Histamine is the major vasoactive amine released from mast cells. It causes dilation of capillaries and retraction of endothelial cells lining the capillaries, which increases vascular permeability.

26. The endothelial cells lining the circulatory system (vascular endothelium) normally regulate circulating components of the inflammatory system and maintain normal blood flow by preventing spontaneous activation of platelets and members of the clotting system.

27. During inflammation the endothelium expresses receptors that help leukocytes leave the vessel and retract to allow fluid to pass into the tissues.

28. Platelets interact with the coagulation cascade to stop bleeding and release a number of mediators that promote and control inflammation.

29. The polymorphonuclear neutrophil (PMN), the predominant phagocytic cell in the early inflammatory response, exits the circulation by diapedesis through the retracted endothelial cell junctions and moves to the inflammatory site by chemotaxis.

30. Eosinophils release products that control the inflammatory response and are the principal cell that kills parasitic organisms.

31. The macrophage, the predominant phagocytic cell in the late inflammatory response, is highly phagocytic, is responsive to cytokines, and promotes wound healing.

32. Dendritic cells connect the innate and acquired immune systems by collecting antigens at the site of inflammation and transporting them to sites, such as the lymph nodes, where immunocompetent B and T cells reside and are transformed into functional cells.

33. Phagocytosis is a multistep cellular process for the elimination of pathogens and foreign debris. The steps include recognition and attachment, engulfment, formation of a phagosome and

phagolysosome, and destruction of pathogens or foreign debris. Phagocytic cells engulf microorganisms and enclose them in phagocytic vacuoles (phagolysosomes), within which toxic products (especially metabolites of oxygen) and degradative lysosomal enzymes kill and digest the microorganisms.

34. Opsonins, such as antibody and complement component C3b, coat microorganisms and make them more susceptible to phagocytosis by binding them more tightly to the phagocyte.

Acute and Chronic Inflammation

1. Acute inflammation is self-limiting and usually resolves within 8 to 10 days.
2. Local manifestations of inflammation are the result of the vascular changes associated with the inflammatory process, including vasodilation and increased capillary permeability. The symptoms include redness, heat, swelling, and pain.
3. The principal systemic effects of inflammation are fever and increases in levels of circulating leukocytes (leukocytosis) and plasma proteins (acute-phase reactants [i.e., IL-1 and IL-6]).
4. Chronic inflammation can be a continuation of acute inflammation that lasts 2 weeks or longer. It also can occur as a distinct process without much preceding acute inflammation.
5. Chronic inflammation is characterized by a dense infiltration of lymphocytes and macrophages. The body may wall off and isolate the infection to protect against tissue damage by formation of a granuloma.

Wound Healing

1. Resolution (regeneration) is the return of tissue to nearly normal structure and function. Repair is healing by scar tissue formation.
2. Damaged tissue proceeds to resolution (restoration of the original tissue structure and function) if little tissue has been lost or if injured tissue is capable of regeneration. This is called healing by primary intention.
3. Tissues that sustained extensive damage or those incapable of regeneration heal by the process of repair resulting in the formation of a scar. This is called healing by secondary intention.
4. Resolution and repair occur in two separate phases: the reconstructive phase in which the wound begins to heal and the maturation phase in which the healed wound is remodeled.
5. Dysfunctional wound healing can be related to ischemia, excessive bleeding, excessive fibrin deposition, a predisposing disorder (such as diabetes mellitus), wound infection, inadequate nutrients, numerous drugs, or altered collagen synthesis.
6. Dehiscence is a disruption in which the wound pulls apart at the suture line.
7. A contracture is a deformity caused by the excessive shortening of collagen in scar tissue.

KEY TERMS

Abscess, 149
Acute inflammation, 149
Acute-phase reactant, 149
Adaptive immunity, 134
Alternative pathway, 139
Anaphylatoxin, 138
Angiogenesis factor, 152
Antimicrobial peptide, 135
α_1-Antitrypsin, 147
Basophil, 144
Blood clot, 139
Bradykinin, 141
C1 esterase inhibitor
   (C1 inh), 141
C1 inh deficiency, 141
Carboxypeptidase, 141
Cathelicidin, 135
Chemokine, 143
Chemotactic factor, 138
Chemotaxis, 145, 147
Chronic inflammation, 149
Classical pathway, 139
Clotting (coagulation)
   system, 139
Collagen, 153
Collectin, 135
Complement receptor, 142
Complement system, 140
Contact activation (intrinsic)
   pathway, 140
Contraction, 152
Contracture of scar tissue, 154
Cyst, 149
Cytokine, 143

Damage-associated molecular
   pattern (DAMP), 142
Defensin, 135
Degranulation, 144
Dehiscence, 154
Dendritic cell, 147
Diapedesis, 147
Endogenous pyrogen, 149
Endothelial cell, 146
Eosinophil, 146
Eosinophil chemotactic factor of
   anaphylaxis (ECF-A), 145
Epithelialization, 152
Epithelioid cell, 150
Exudate, 149
Fc receptor, 147
Fever, 149
Fibrinolytic system, 141
Fibrinous exudate, 149
Fibroblast, 153
Giant cell, 150
Granulation tissue, 153
Granuloma, 150
Hageman factor
   (factor XII), 140
Hemorrhagic exudate, 149
Hereditary angioedema, 141
Hexose-monophosphate
   shunt, 147
Histaminase, 141
Histamine, 145
Hypertrophic scar, 153
Inflammasomes, 142
Inflammation, 137

Inflammatory phase, 152
Inflammatory response, 134, 137
Innate immunity, 134
Interferon (IFN), 144
Interleukin (IL), 143
Interleukin-1 (IL-1), 144
Interleukin-6 (IL-6), 144
Interleukin-10 (IL-10), 144
Keloid, 154
Kinin system, 140
Lectin pathway, 139
Leukocytosis, 149
Leukotriene (slow-reacting
   substance of anaphylaxis
   [SRS-A]), 145
Lymphocyte, 141
Lysozyme, 135
Macrophage, 146
Mannose-binding lectin
   (MBL), 135
Margination (pavementing), 147
Mast cell, 144
Matrix metalloproteinase
   (MMP), 153
Monocyte, 146
Myofibroblast, 153
Natural killer (NK) cells, 147
Neutrophil (polymorphonuclear
   neutrophil [PMN]), 146
Neutrophil chemotactic factor
   (NCF), 145
Nitric oxide (NO), 146
NOD-like receptors
   (NLRs), 142

Normal flora, 135
Normal microbiome, 135
Opportunistic
   microorganism, 137
Opsonin, 138
Opsonization, 147
Pathogen-associated molecular
   pattern (PAMP), 142
Pattern recognition receptor
   (PRR), 142
Phagocyte, 138
Phagocytosis, 146
Phagolysosome, 147
Phagosome, 147
Plasma protein system, 138
Plasmin, 141
Plasminogen, 141
Platelet, 146
Platelet-activating factor
   (PAF), 145
Primary intention, 152
Proliferative phase, 152
Prostacyclin (PGI$_2$), 146
Prostaglandin, 145
Purulent (suppurative)
   exudate, 149
Pyrogen, 149
Regeneration, 151
Repair, 152
Resolution, 151
Scar tissue, 152
Scavenger receptors, 142
Secondary intention, 152
Serous exudate, 149

REFERENCES

1. Peterson LW, Artis D: Intestinal epithelial cells: regulators of barrier function and immune homeostasis, *Nat Rev Immunol* 14(3):141-153, 2014.
2. Human Microbiome Project Consortium: Structure, function and diversity of the healthy human microbiome, *Nature* 486(7402):207-214, 2012.
3. Mayer EA et al: Gut/brain axis and the microbiota, *J Clin Invest* 125(3):926-938, 2015.
4. Moal VL-L, Servin AL: Anti-infective activities of *Lactobacillus* strains in the human intestinal microbiota: from probiotics to gastrointestinal anti-infectious biotherapeutic agents, *Clin Microbiol Rev* 27(2):167-199, 2014.
5. Ricklin D, Lambris JD: Complement in immune and inflammatory disorders: therapeutic interventions, *J Immunol* 190(8):3839-3847, 2013.
6. Sekine H et al: The role of MASP-1/3 in complement activation, *Adv Exp Med Biol* 735:41-53, 2013.
7. O'Neil LA et al: The history of Toll-like receptors—redefining innate immunity, *Nat Rev Immunol* 13(6):453-460, 2013.
8. Qian C, Cao X: Regulation of Toll-like receptor signaling pathways in innate immune responses, *Ann N Y Acad Sci* 1283(2013):67-74, 2013.
9. Canton J et al: Scavenger receptors in homeostasis and immunity, *Nat Rev Immunol* 13(9):621-634, 2013.
10. Philpott DJ et al: NOD proteins: regulators of inflammation in health and disease, *Nat Rev Immunol* 14(1):9-23, 2014.
11. Saxena M, Yeretssian G: NOD-like receptors: master regulators of inflammation and cancer, *Front Immunol* 5:327, 2014.
12. Schett G et al: Toward a cytokine-based disease taxonomy, *Nat Med* 19(7):822-824, 2013.
13. Martins-Green M et al: Chemokines and their receptors are key players in the orchestra that regulates wound healing, *Adv Wound Care (New Rochelle)* 2(7):327-347, 2013.
14. Akdis M et al: Interleukins, from 1 to 37 and interferon-γ: receptors, functions, and roles in diseases, *J Allergy Clin Immunol* 127(3):701-721, 2011.
15. Ivashkiv LB, Donlin LT: Regulation of type I interferon responses, *Nat Rev Immunol* 14(1):36-49, 2014.
16. Cromheecke JL et al: Emerging role of human basophil biology in health and disease, *Curr Allergy Asthma Rep* 14(1):408, 1-9, 2014.
17. Kolaczkowska E, Kubes P: Neutrophil recruitment and function in health and inflammation, *Nat Rev Immunol* 13(3):159-175, 2013.
18. Melo RC et al: Eosinophil-derived cytokines in health and disease: unraveling novel mechanisms of selective secretion, *Allergy* 68(3):274-284, 2013.
19. Wynn TA et al: Macrophage biology in development, homeostasis and disease, *Nature* 496(7446):445-455, 2013.
20. Van Dyken SJ, Locksley RM: Interleukin-4- and interleukin-13-mediated alternatively activated macrophages: roles in homeostasis and disease, *Annu Rev Immunol* 31(2013):317-343, 2013.
21. Platt AM, Randolph GJ: Dendritic cell migration through the lymphatic vasculature to lymph nodes, *Adv Immunol* 120(2013):51-68, 2013.
22. Herter J, Zarbock A: Integrin regulation during leukocyte recruitment, *J Immunol* 190(9):4451-4457, 2013.
23. Weninger W et al: Leukocyte migration in the interstitial space of non-lymphoid organs, *Nat Rev Immunol* 14(4):232-248, 2014.
24. Wilgus TA et al: Neutrophils and wound repair: positive actions and negative reactions, *Adv Wound Care (New Rochelle)* 2(7):379-388, 2013.
25. Campbell KS, Hasegawa J: Natural killer cell biology: an update and future directions, *J Allergy Clin Immunol* 132(3):536-544, 2013.
26. Long EO et al: Controlling natural killer cell responses: integration of signals for activation and inhibition, *Annu Rev Immunol* 31(2013):227-258, 2013.
27. Dorhoi A, Kaufmann SH: Tumor necrosis factor alpha in mycobacterial infection, *Semin Immunol* 2014 May 9. [Epub ahead of print.]
28. O'Garra A et al: The immune response to tuberculosis, *Annu Rev Immunol* 31(2013):475-527, 2013.
29. King A et al: Regenerative wound healing: the role of interleukin-10, *Adv Wound Care (New Rochelle)* 3(4):315-323, 2014.
30. Raju R et al: A network map of EGF-1/FGFR signaling system, *J Signal Transduct* 2014:962962.
31. Khokha R et al: Metalloproteinases and their natural inhibitors in inflammation and immunity, *Nat Rev Immunol* 13(9):649-665, 2013.
32. Longmate WM, Dipersio CM: Integrin regulation of epidermal function in wounds, *Adv Wound Care (New Rochelle)* 3(3):229-246, 2014.
33. Mienaltowski MJ, Birk DE: Structure, physiology, and biochemistry of collagens, *Adv Exp Med Biol* 802(2014):5-29, 2014.
34. Yang X et al: Reversal of myofibroblast differentiation: a review, *Eur J Pharmacol* Jul 5;734:83-90, 2014.
35. Pierpont YN et al: Obesity and surgical wound healing: a current review, *ISRN Obes* 2014:638936, 2014.
36. Pence BD, Woods JA: Exercise, obesity, and cutaneous wound healing: evidence from rodent and human studies, *Adv Wound Care (New Rochelle)* 3(1):71-79, 2014.
37. Moores J: Vitamin C: a wound healing perspective, *Br J Community Nurs* Suppl:S6, S8-S11, 2013.
38. Monstrey S et al: Updated scar management practical guidelines: non-invasive and invasive measures, *J Plast Reconstr Aesthet Surg* 67(8):1017-1025, 2014.

7

Adaptive Immunity

Neal S. Rote

ⓔ EVOLVE WEBSITE

http://evolve.elsevier.com/Huether/
Student Review Questions
Audio Key Points

Case Studies
Animations
Quick Check Answers

CHAPTER OUTLINE

The third line of defense in the human body is adaptive (acquired) immunity, often called the immune response or immunity, and consists of lymphocytes (Figure 7-1) and serum proteins called antibodies. Once external barriers have been compromised and inflammation (innate immunity, see Chapter 6) has been activated, the adaptive immune response is called into action. Inflammation is the "first responder" that contains the initial injury and slows the spread of infection, whereas adaptive immunity slowly augments the initial defenses against infection and provides long-term security against reinfection.

THIRD LINE OF DEFENSE: ADAPTIVE IMMUNITY

Inflammation and adaptive immunity differ in several key ways. First, the components of inflammation are activated immediately after tissue damage. Adaptive immunity is *inducible;* the effectors of the immune response, lymphocytes and antibodies, do not preexist but must be produced in response to infection. Thus, adaptive immunity develops more slowly than inflammation. Second, the inflammatory response is similar regardless of differences in the cause of tissue damage or whether the inflammatory site is sterile or contaminated with infectious microorganisms. The immune response is exquisitely *specific*. The lymphocytes and antibodies induced in response to infection are extremely specific to the infecting microbe. Third, the residual mediators of inflammation must be removed quickly to limit damage to surrounding healthy tissue and allow healing. The effectors of the immune response are *long-lived* and systemic, providing long-term protection against specific infections. Finally, the inflammatory

response to both recurrent tissue damage and infection is identical. The immune response has *memory*. If reinfected with the same microbe, protective lymphocytes and antibody are produced immediately, thus providing permanent long-term protection against infection.

Despite the differences, the innate and adaptive immune systems are highly interactive and complementary. Many components of innate resistance are necessary for the development of the adaptive immune response. Conversely, products of the adaptive immune response activate components of innate resistance. Thus, both systems are essential for complete protection against infectious disease.

The mechanisms underlying the immune response will be discussed in this chapter. As with Chapter 6, a complete description of all the important components and processes of an effective immune response would require far more space than available. Therefore, this chapter will focus on the basic concepts and the most important, or well-studied, mediators of the immune response.

The adaptive immune response has its own vocabulary (Figure 7-2). Antigens are the molecular targets of antibodies and lymphocytes. Antigens are generally small molecules, usually within proteins, carbohydrates, or lipids, found on the surface of microbes or infected cells, although this definition will be expanded as we discuss immunologic diseases in Chapter 8. In the fetus, well before being exposed to any infectious microorganisms, lymphocytes have undergone extensive differentiation. Some lymphoid stem cells enter the thymus and differentiate into T lymphocytes (T cells, T indicates thymus derived), whereas others enter specific regions of the bone marrow and differentiate into B lymphocytes (B cells, B indicates bone marrow derived).

Each type of cell develops origin-specific cell surface proteins that identify them as T or B cells. Both B and T cells also develop cell surface antigen receptors. The receptors are remarkable because an individual lymphocyte is programmed to recognize only one specific antigen before having encountered that antigen. It is estimated that before birth each individual has produced a population of B and T lymphocytes capable of recognizing at least 10^8 different antigens. This process is called generation of clonal diversity and refers to the process by which the extensive diversity of antigen receptors on B and T cells is established (see Figure 7-2).

Lymphocytes leave the primary lymphoid organs (bone marrow and thymus) as immunocompetent, but naïve, B and T cells. The cells are immunocompetent in that they have the capacity to respond to antigens, but they are naïve in that they have not yet encountered antigen. These cells enter the blood and lymphatic vessels and migrate to the secondary lymphoid organs (e.g., lymph nodes, spleen) of the

FIGURE 7-1 Lymphocytes. A scanning electron micrograph showing lymphocytes (yellow, like cotton candy), red blood cells, and platelets. (Copyright Dennis Kunkel Microscopy, Inc.)

systemic immune system (Figure 7-3). Some take up residence in B cell and T cell rich areas of those organs, and others reenter the circulation. Approximately 60% to 70% of circulating lymphocytes are immunocompetent T cells, and 10% to 20% are immunocompetent B cells.

A second process, clonal selection, is initiated when an infection occurs. This process requires the cooperation among a variety of cells in the secondary lymphoid organs; antigen needs to be processed by phagocytic cells, primarily dendritic cells, which also express the processed antigen on their surfaces and present the antigen to lymphocytes. Thus begins a symphony of cellular interactions, referred to as clonal selection, involving several subsets of B and T cells, intercellular adhesion through antigen receptors and specific intercellular adhesion molecules, the production and response to multiple cytokines, and eventual differentiation of immunocompetent B and T cells into highly specialized effector cells. B cells develop into plasma cells that become factories for the production of antibody. T cells develop into several subsets that can identify and kill a target cell (T-cytotoxic cells, Tc cells), regulate the immune response by helping the clonal selection process (T-helper cells, Th cells), or suppress inappropriate immune responses (T-regulatory cells, Treg cells). Both B and T cells also differentiate into very long-lived memory cells that exist for decades or, in some cases, for the life of the individual. Memory cells are rapidly activated if a second infection occurs with the same microbe.

Antibodies circulate in the blood and defend against extracellular microbes and microbial toxins. This is referred to as the humoral immune response, or humoral immunity. Effector T cells are found in the blood and tissues and defend against intracellular pathogens (e.g., viruses) and cancer cells. This is referred to as the cellular immune response, or cellular immunity (also cell-mediated immunity).

The preceding overview describes what is termed active immunity (active acquired immunity), which develops in response to antigen. In certain clinical situations, preformed antibody or lymphocytes may be administered to an individual, termed passive immunity (passive acquired immunity). Examples include individuals exposed to an infectious agent without having a preexisting vaccine-induced immunity (e.g., hepatitis A virus or rabies virus) (Table 7-1). Passive immunization with specific T cells has been used to treat several forms of

TABLE 7-1 Clinical Use of Antigen or Antibody

	USE OF ANTIGEN OR ANTIBODY			
Antigen Source	Protection: Combat Active Disease	Protection: Vaccination	Diagnosis	Therapy
Infectious agents	Neutralize or destroy pathogenic microorganisms (e.g., antibody response against viral infections)	Induce safe and protective immune response (e.g., recommended childhood vaccines)	Measure circulating antigen from infectious agent or antibody (e.g., diagnosis of hepatitis B infection)	Passive treatment with antibody to treat or prevent infection (e.g., administration of antibody against hepatitis A)
Cancers	Prevent tumor growth or spread (e.g., immune surveillance to prevent early cancers)	Prevent cancer growth or spread (e.g., vaccination with cancer antigens)	Measure circulating antigen (e.g., circulating PSA for diagnosis of prostate cancer)	Immunotherapy (e.g., treatment of cancer with antibodies against cancer antigens)
Environmental substances	Prevent entrance into body (e.g., secretory IgA limits systemic exposure to potential allergens)	No clear example	Measure circulating antigen or antibody (e.g., diagnosis of allergy by measuring circulating IgE)	Immunotherapy (e.g., administration of antigen for desensitization of individuals with severe allergies)
Self-antigens	Immune system tolerance to self-antigens, which may be altered by an infectious agent leading to autoimmune disease (see Chapter 8)	Some cases of vaccination alter tolerance to self-antigens, leading to autoimmune disease	Measure circulating antibody against self-antigen for diagnosis of autoimmune disease (see Chapter 8)	Oral administration of self-antigens to diminish production of autoimmune disease–associated autoantibodies

PSA, Prostate-specific antigen.

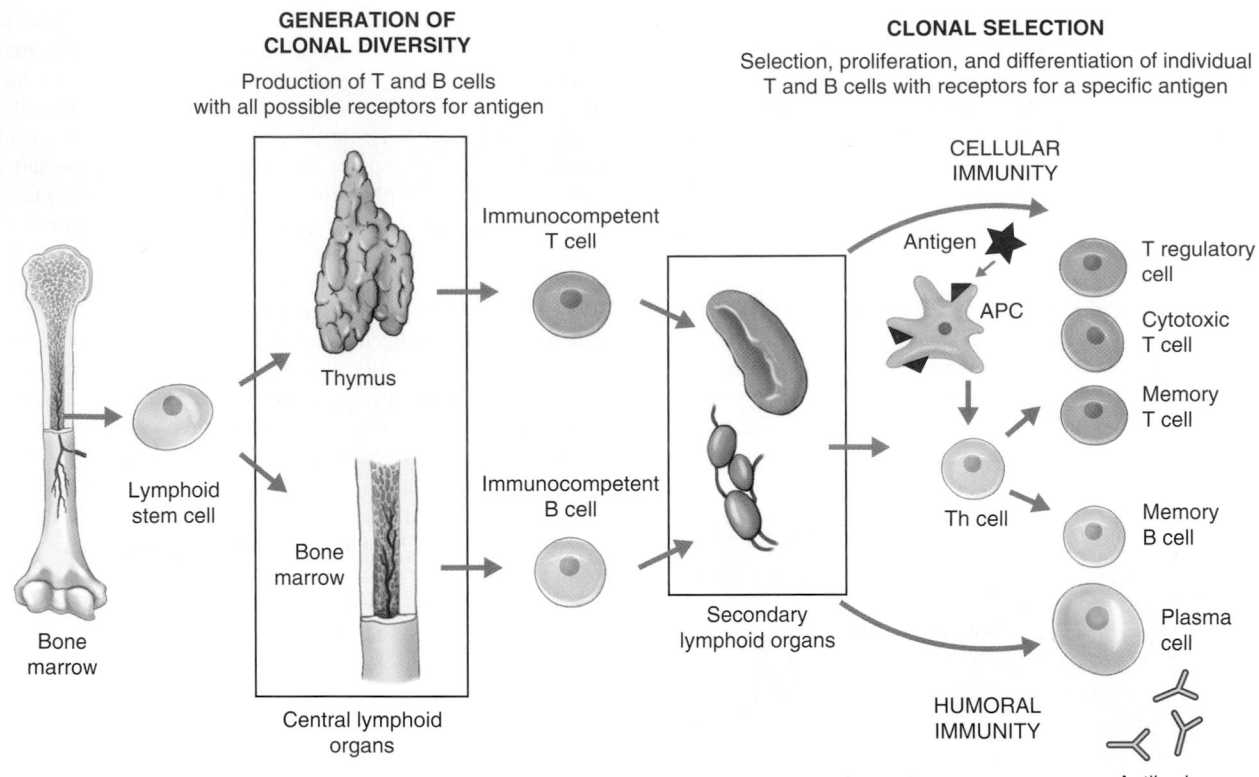

GENERATION OF CLONAL DIVERSITY

Production of T and B cells with all possible receptors for antigen

CLONAL SELECTION

Selection, proliferation, and differentiation of individual T and B cells with receptors for a specific antigen

FIGURE 7-2 Overview of the Immune Response. The immune response can be separated into two phases: the *generation of clonal diversity* and *clonal selection*. During the generation of clonal diversity, lymphoid stem cells from the bone marrow migrate to the central lymphoid organs (the thymus or regions of the bone marrow), where they undergo a series of cellular division and differentiation stages resulting in either immunocompetent T cells from the thymus or immunocompetent B cells from the bone marrow. These cells are still naïve in that they have never encountered foreign antigen. The immunocompetent cells enter the circulation and migrate to the secondary lymphoid organs (e.g., spleen and lymph nodes), where they establish residence in B- and T-cell–rich areas. The clonal selection phase is initiated by exposure to foreign antigen. The antigen is usually processed by antigen-presenting cells (APCs) for presentation to T-helper cells (Th cells). The intercellular cooperation among APCs, Th cells, and immunocompetent T and B cells results in a second stage of cellular proliferation and differentiation. Because antigen has "selected" those T and B cells with compatible antigen receptors, only a small population of T and B cells undergo this process at one time. The result is an active cellular immunity or humoral immunity, or both. Cellular immunity is mediated by a population of *effector* T cells that can kill targets (T-cytotoxic cells) or regulate the immune response (T-regulatory cells), as well as a population of memory cells (T-memory cells) that can respond more quickly to a second challenge with the same antigen. Humoral immunity is mediated by a population of soluble proteins (antibodies) produced by plasma cells and by a population of memory B cells that can produce more antibody rapidly to a second challenge with the same antigen.

cancer. Whereas active acquired immunity is long lived, passive immunity is only temporary because the donor's antibodies or T cells are eventually destroyed.

ANTIGENS AND IMMUNOGENS

We need to initially understand the molecules against which an immune response is directed. Although the terms *antigen* and *immunogen* are commonly used as synonyms, there are clinically important differences between the two. **Antigen** is commonly used to describe a molecule that can *bind with* antibodies or antigen receptors on B and T cells. A molecule that will *induce* an immune response is an **immunogen**. Thus all immunogens are antigens but not all antigens are immunogens. For instance, immunogenicity is frequently related to the size of the antigen. In general, large molecules (those greater than 10,000 daltons), such as proteins and polysaccharides, are most

immunogenic. Many low-molecular-weight molecules can function as **haptens**; they are too small to be immunogens by themselves but become immunogenic after combining with larger molecules that function as carriers for the hapten. Poison ivy contains an oily sap called urushiol (molecular weight approximately 1500 daltons), which upon contact with the skin is chemically altered, binds to large proteins in the skin, and becomes immunogenic, resulting in a T-cell response and onset of a classic poison ivy rash. Similar conditions will be discussed in Chapter 8.

> ✔ **QUICK CHECK 7-1**
> 1. Define acquired immunity.
> 2. Distinguish between innate and acquired immunity.
> 3. Distinguish between humoral and cell-mediated immunity.
> 4. What are the differences among antigens, immunogens, and haptens?

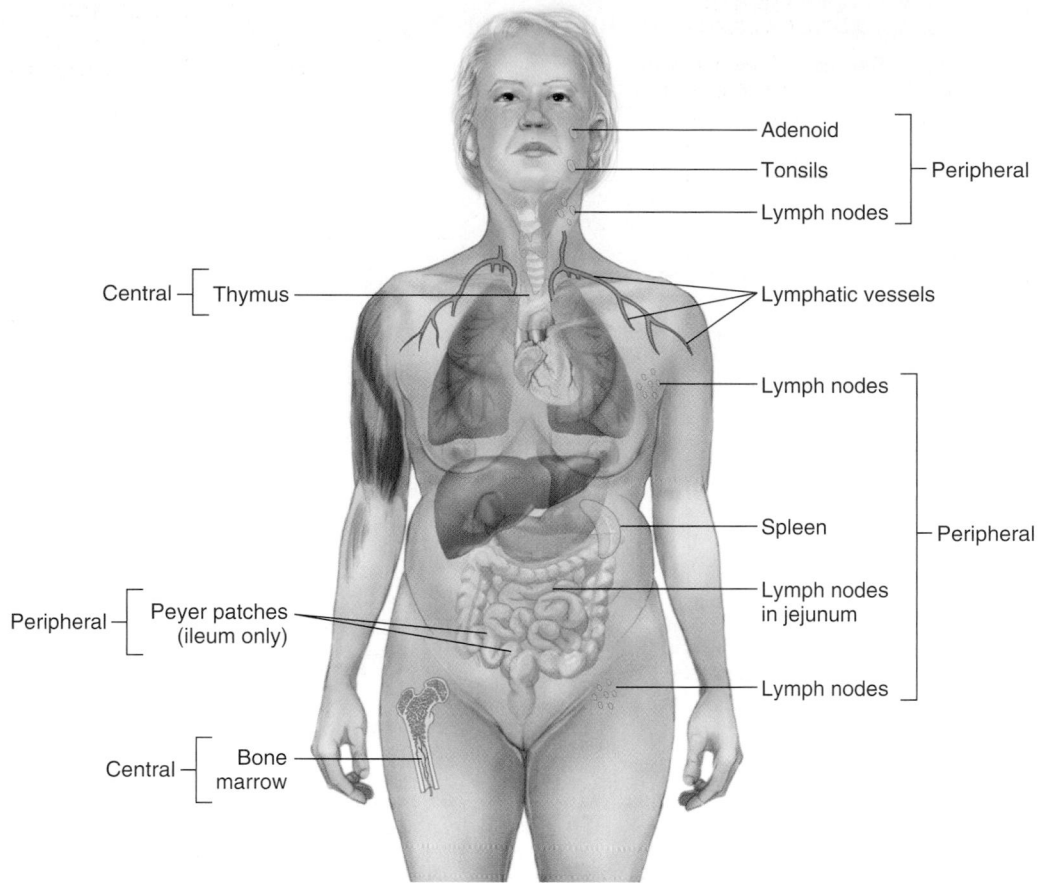

FIGURE 7-3 Lymphoid Tissues: Sites of B-Cell and T-Cell Differentiation. Immature lymphocytes migrate through central (primary) lymphoid tissues: the bone marrow (central lymphoid tissue for B lymphocytes) and the thymus (central lymphoid tissue for T lymphocytes). Mature lymphocytes later reside in the T- and B-lymphocyte–rich areas of the peripheral (secondary) lymphoid tissues.

ANTIBODIES

A basic understanding of antibodies and how they react with antigen provides a foundation for more complex topics, such as the B-cell and T-cell antigen receptors, the generation of clonal diversity, and intercellular collaborations during clonal selection, which are discussed later in this chapter. The terms antibody and immunoglobulin (Ig) are frequently used interchangeably. In general, immunoglobulin is frequently used as a generic description of a general group of antibodies, whereas antibody commonly denotes one particular set of immunoglobulins known to have specificity for a particular antigen.

Classes of Immunoglobulins

There are five classes of immunoglobulins (IgG, IgA, IgM, IgE, and IgD), which are characterized by differences in structure and function (Figure 7-4). Both IgG and IgA have subclasses (Table 7-2).

IgG is the most abundant class of immunoglobulins, constituting 80% to 85% of the immunoglobulins in the blood and accounting for most of the protective activity against infections. During pregnancy maternal IgG is transported across the placenta and protects the newborn child during the first 6 months of life.

IgA is found in the blood and in bodily secretions as secretory IgA (subclass IgA2). Secretory IgA is a *dimer* consisting of two IgA2 molecules held together through a J chain and secretory piece.

The secretory piece is attached to dimeric IgA during transportation through mucosal epithelial cells to protect against degradation by enzymes also found in secretions.

IgM is the largest immunoglobulin and usually exists as a pentamer (a molecule consisting of five identical smaller molecules) that is stabilized by a J chain. It is the first antibody produced during the initial, or primary, response to antigens. IgM is usually synthesized early in neonatal life, but may be increased as a response to infection in utero.

IgD is found in low concentrations in the blood. Its primary function is as an antigen receptor on the surface of early B cells.

IgE is normally at low concentrations in the circulation. It has very specialized functions as a mediator of many common allergic responses (see Chapter 8) and in the defense against parasitic infections.[1]

Molecular Structure

There are three parts to an antibody molecule (Figure 7-5). Two identical fragments have the ability to bind antigen and are termed antigen-binding fragments (Fab). The third fragment is termed the crystalline fragment (Fc). The Fab portions contain the recognition sites (receptors) for antigens and confer the molecule's specificity toward a particular antigen. The Fc portion is responsible for most of the biologic functions of antibodies.

An immunoglobulin molecule consists of four polypeptide chains: two identical light (L) chains and two identical heavy (H) chains. The

TABLE 7-2   Properties of Immunoglobulins

Class	Subclass	Adult Serum Levels (mg/dl)	Present in Secretions	Complement Activation	Opsonin	Agglutinin	Mast Cell Activation	Placental Transfer
IgG	IgG1	800-900	+	++	++	+	−	+++
	IgG2	280-300	+	+	−	+	−	+
	IgG3	90-100	+	+++	++	+	−	+++
	IgG4	50	−	−	−	+	+	++
IgM		120-150	+	++++	−	++++	−	−
IgA	IgA1	280-300	+	−	−	+	−	−
	IgA2	50	+	−	−	+	−	−
	sIgA	5	++++	−	−	+	−	−
IgD		3	−	−	−	−	−	−
IgE		0.03	+	−	−	−	+++	−

sIgA, Secretory immunoglobulin A; − indicates lack of activity; + to ++++ indicate relative activity or concentration.

FIGURE 7-4 **Structures of Different Immunoglobulins.** Secretory IgA, IgD, IgE, IgG, and IgM. The black circles attached to each molecule represent carbohydrate residues.

class of antibody is determined by different amino acid sequences in the heavy chains. The light and heavy chains are held together by noncovalent bonds and covalent disulfide linkages. A set of disulfide bridges between the heavy chains occurs in the hinge region and, in some instances, lends a degree of flexibility at that site.

Each L and H chain is further subdivided structurally into constant (C) and variable (V) regions. The constant regions have relatively stable amino acid sequences within a particular immunoglobulin class. Conversely, among different antibodies, the sequences of the variable regions have a large number of amino acid differences and these are called **complementary determining regions (CDR)**. They determine the specificity of an antibody for a particular antigen. The regions between the CDR's are called framework regions (FR) and they have more stable amino acid sequences (see Figure 7-5).

Antigen-Antibody Binding

Because antigens are relative small, a large molecule (e.g., protein, polysaccharide, nucleic acid) usually contains multiple and diverse antigens. The precise area of the antigen that is recognized by an antibody is called its **antigenic determinant**, or **epitope**. The matching

portion on the antibody is sometimes referred to as the **antigen-binding site**, or **paratope**. The antigen fits into the antigen binding site of the antibody with the specificity of a key into a lock and is held there by noncovalent chemical interactions.

Function of Antibodies

The chief function of antibodies is to protect against infection. The mechanism can be either *direct*—through the action of antibody alone or *indirect*—requiring activation of other components of the innate immune response (Figure 7-6). Directly, antibodies can affect infectious agents or their toxic products by **neutralization** (inactivating or blocking the binding of antigens to receptors), **agglutination** (clumping insoluble particles that are in suspension), or **precipitation** (making a soluble antigen into an insoluble precipitate). For instance, many pathogens initiate infection by attaching to specific receptors on cells. Viruses that cause the common cold or the influenza virus must attach to specific receptors on respiratory tract epithelial cells. Some bacteria, such as *Neisseria gonorrhoeae* that causes gonorrhea, must attach to specific sites on urogenital epithelial cells. Antibodies may protect the host by covering sites on the microorganism that are

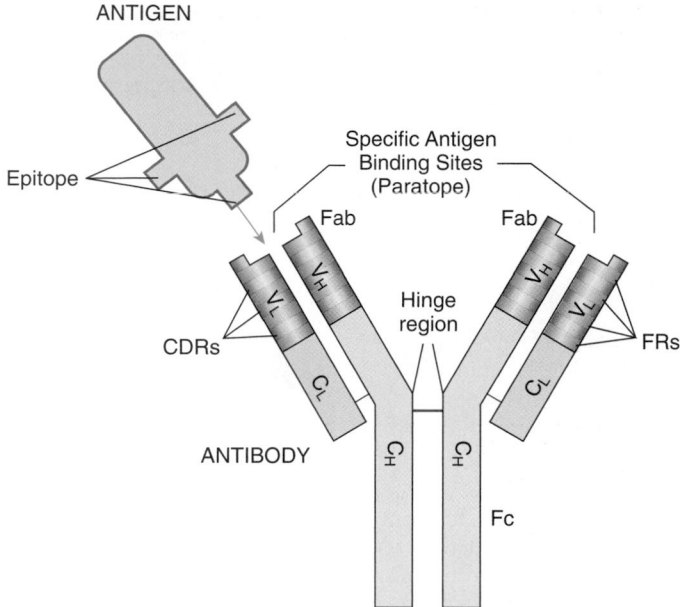

FIGURE 7-5 Antigen-Antibody Binding. C_H, Constant region heavy chain; V_L, Variable region light chain; V_H, Variable region heavy chain; C_L, Constant region light chain; Fab, Fragment antigen binding; Fc, Crystalline fragment; CDR's, Complementary determining regions; FR's, Framework regions; Red lines are disulfide linkages.

needed for attachment, thereby preventing infection. Many viral infections can be prevented by vaccination with inactivated or attenuated (weakened) viruses designed to induce neutralizing antibody production at the site of the entrance of the virus into the body. Vaccination against influenza using an inhaled vaccine particularly induces protective IgA in the respiratory tract.

Some bacteria secrete toxins that harm individuals. For instance, specific bacterial toxins cause the symptoms of tetanus or diphtheria. Most toxins are proteins that bind to surface molecules on cells and damage those cells. Protective antibodies produced against the toxin (referred to as *antitoxins*) can bind to the toxins, prevent their interaction with host cells, and neutralize their biologic effects (see Chapter 8).

Indirectly, through the Fc portion, antibodies activate components of innate resistance, including complement and phagocytes (Figure 7-7). Through the classical pathway, complement component C1 will be activated by binding simultaneously to the Fc regions of two adjacent antibodies bound to a microbe, resulting in activation of the entire cascade. Phagocytic cells express receptors that bind the Fc portion of antibody; thus antibody is an opsonin that facilitates phagocytosis of bacteria.[3] IgM is the best complement-activating antibody, and IgG is the best opsonin. Some antibodies are more protective than others. It is now a common procedure to clone the "best" antibodies (monoclonal antibodies) for use in diagnostic tests and for therapy (Box 7-1).

FIGURE 7-6 Direct and Indirect Functions of Antibody. Protective activities of antibodies can be direct (through the action of antibody alone) or indirect (requiring activation of other components of the innate immune response, usually through the Fc region). *Direct* means include neutralization of viruses or bacterial toxins before they bind to receptors on the surface of the host's cells. *Indirect* means include activation of the classical complement pathway through C1, resulting in formation of the membrane-attack complex (MAC), or increased phagocytosis of bacteria opsonized with antibody and complement components bound to appropriate surface receptors (FcR and C3bR).

FIGURE 7-7 IgE Function. (**1**) Soluble antigens from a parasitic infection cause production of IgE antibody by B cells. (**2**) Secreted IgE binds to IgE-specific receptors on the mast cell. (**3**) Additional soluble parasite antigen cross-links the IgE on the mast cell surface, (**4**) leading to mast cell degranulation and release of many proinflammatory products, including eosinophil chemotactic factor of anaphylaxis (ECF-A). (**5**) ECF-A attracts eosinophils from the circulation. (**6**) The eosinophil attaches to the surface of the parasite and releases potent lysosomal enzymes that damage microorganisms.

IgE

IgE is a special class of antibody that protects the individual from infection with large parasitic worms (helminths).[4] However, when IgE is produced against relatively innocuous environmental antigens, it is also the primary cause of common allergies (e.g., hay fever, dust allergies, bee stings). The role of IgE in allergies is discussed in Chapter 8.

Large multicellular parasites usually invade mucosal tissues. Many antigens from the parasites induce IgE, as well as other antibody classes. IgG, IgM, and IgA bind to the surface of parasites, activate complement, generate chemotactic factors for neutrophils and macrophages, and serve as opsonins for those phagocytic cells. This response, however, does not greatly damage parasites. The only inflammatory cell that can adequately damage a parasite is the eosinophil because of the special contents of its granules, including major basic protein, eosinophil cationic protein, eosinophil peroxidase, and eosinophil neurotoxin, each of which can damage infectious worms. Thus, IgE is designed to specifically initiate an inflammatory reaction that preferentially attracts eosinophils to the site of parasitic infection.

Mast cells in the tissues have Fc receptors that specifically and with high affinity bind IgE. IgE antibodies against antigens of the parasite are rapidly bound to the mast cell surface. Soluble parasite molecules with multiple antigenic determinants diffuse to neighboring mast cells and simultaneously bind to multiple IgE molecules. This reaction initiates a cascade of effects that can ultimately kill the parasite. The steps of the cascade are presented in Figure 7-7.

Secretory Immune System

Immunocompetent lymphocytes migrate among secondary lymphoid organs and tissue as part of the systemic immune system. Another, partially independent, immune system protects the external surfaces of the body through lacrimal and salivary glands and a network of lymphoid tissues residing in the breasts, bronchi, intestines, and genitourinary tract. This system is called the secretory (mucosal) immune system (Figure 7-8). Plasma cells in those sites secrete antibodies in bodily secretions such as tears, sweat, saliva, mucus, and breast milk to prevent pathogenic microorganism from infecting the body's surfaces and possibly penetrating to cause systemic disease.[5] Alternatively, the microorganisms may reside in the membranes without causing disease, be shed, and cause infection for other individuals. Thus, an individual may become a carrier for a particular infectious organism. For instance,

in the 1950s two vaccines were developed to prevent infection with poliovirus, which enters through the gastrointestinal tract. The Sabin vaccine was administered orally as an attenuated (i.e., inactivated so as to render relatively harmless) live virus. This route caused a transient, limited infection and induced effective systemic and secretory immunity that prevented both the disease and the establishment of a carrier state. The Salk vaccine, on the other hand, consisted of killed viruses administered by injection in the skin. It induced adequate systemic protection but did not generally prevent an intestinal carrier state. Thus, recipients of the Salk vaccine were protected from disease but could still shed the virus and infect others.

IgA is the dominant secretory immunoglobulin, although IgM and IgG also are present in secretions. The primary role of IgA is to prevent the attachment and invasion of pathogens through mucosal membranes, such as those of the gastrointestinal, pulmonary, and genitourinary tracts. Dimeric IgA antibodies containing the J chain are produced by plasma cells of the mucosa. Mucosal epithelium expresses a cell surface immunoglobulin receptor that binds and internalizes IgA. The IgA, along with the epithelial receptor (secretory piece), is secreted as secretory IgA (sIgA).

The lymphoid tissues of the secretory immune system are connected; thus many foreign antigens in a mother's gastrointestinal tract (e.g., polio virus) induce secretion of specific antibodies into the breast milk. Colostral antibodies (i.e., those found in the colostrum of breast milk) may protect the nursing newborn against infectious disease agents that enter through the gastrointestinal tract. Although colostral antibodies provide the newborn with passive immunity against gastrointestinal infections, they do not provide systemic immunity because transport across the newborn's gut into the bloodstream is discontinued after the first 24 hours of life. Maternal antibodies that pass across the placenta into the fetus before birth provide passive systemic immunity.

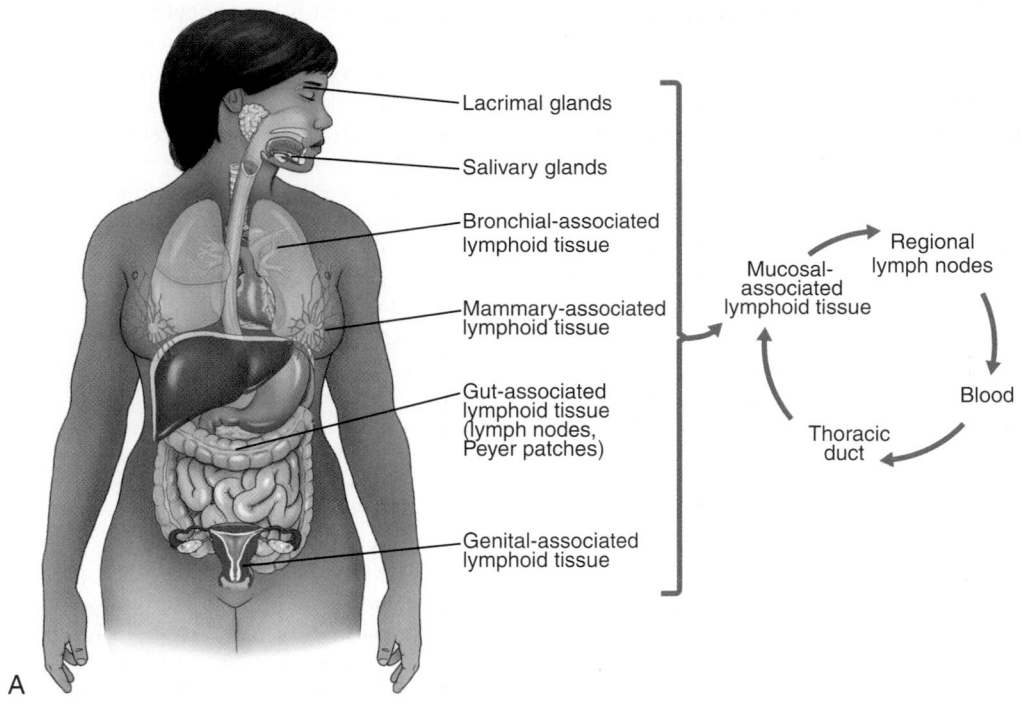

Lacrimal glands

Salivary glands

Bronchial-associated lymphoid tissue

Mammary-associated lymphoid tissue

Gut-associated lymphoid tissue (lymph nodes, Peyer patches)

Genital-associated lymphoid tissue

Mucosal-associated lymphoid tissue → Regional lymph nodes → Blood → Thoracic duct → Mucosal-associated lymphoid tissue

A

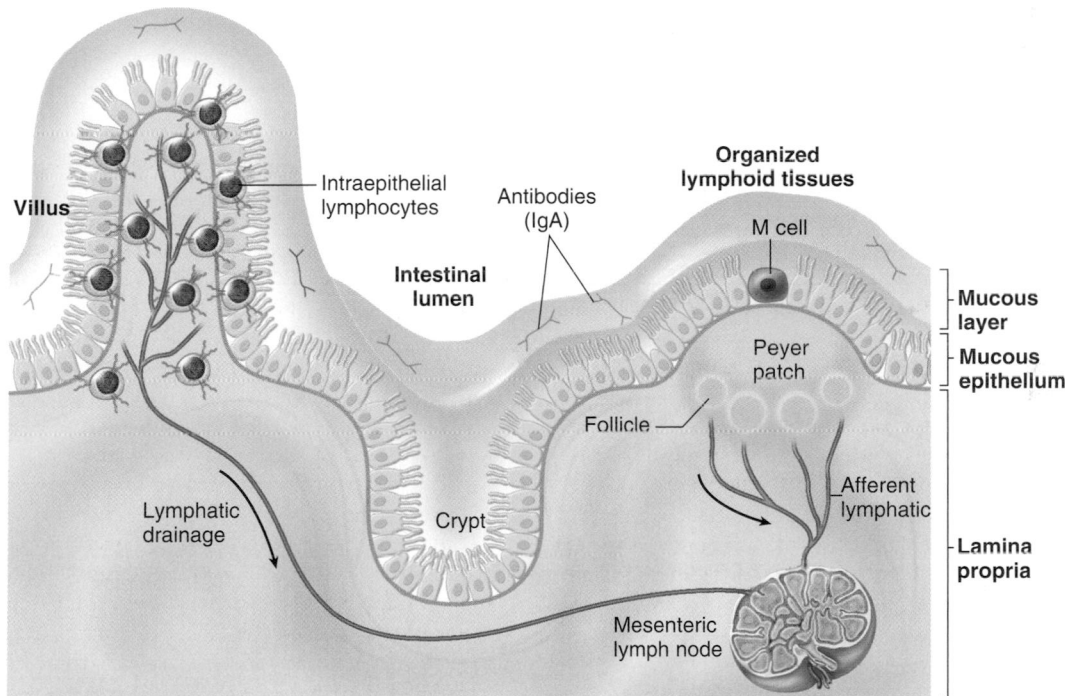

Villus

Intraepithelial lymphocytes

Antibodies (IgA)

Organized lymphoid tissues

M cell

Intestinal lumen

Peyer patch

Mucous layer

Mucous epithelium

Follicle

Afferent lymphatic

Lymphatic drainage

Crypt

Lamina propria

Mesenteric lymph node

B

FIGURE 7-8 Secretory Immune System. A, Lymphocytes from the mucosal-associated lymphoid tissues circulate throughout the body in a pattern separate from other lymphocytes. For example, lymphocytes from the gut-associated lymphoid tissue circulate through the regional lymph nodes, the thoracic duct, and the blood and return to other mucosal-associated lymphoid tissues rather than to lymphoid tissue of the systemic immune system. **B,** Lymphoid tissue associated with mucous membranes is called mucosal-associated lymphoid tissue (MALT).

IMMUNE RESPONSE: COLLABORATION OF B CELLS AND T CELLS

Generation of Clonal Diversity

The immune response occurs in two phases: generation of clonal diversity and clonal selection (Table 7-3 and see Figure 7-2). Clonal diversity is the production of a large population of B cells and T cells before birth that have the capacity to recognize almost any foreign antigen found in the environment. This process mostly occurs in specialized lymphoid organs (the primary [central] lymphoid organs): the bone marrow for B cells and the thymus for T cells.[6] The result is the differentiation of lymphoid stem cells into B and T lymphocytes with the ability to react against almost any antigen that will be encountered throughout life. It is estimated that B and T cells can collectively recognize more than 10^8 different antigenic determinants. Lymphocytes are released from these organs into the circulation as immunocompetent cells that have the capacity to react with antigens and migrate to the circulation and other (secondary) lymphoid organs in the body.

Development of B Lymphocytes

Lymphocytes destined to become B cells circulate through the specialized regions of the bone marrow, where they are exposed to hormones and cytokines that induce proliferation and differentiation into B cells (see Figure 7-2). Lymphoid stem cells in the bone marrow interact with stromal cells through a variety of intercellular adhesion molecules. As the stem cell begins to mature, it progressively develops a variety of necessary surface markers important for the further differentiation and proliferation of the B cell.[7] The next stage in development is formation of the B-cell receptor (BCR).

The B-cell receptor (BCR) is a complex of antibody bound to the cell surface and other molecules involved in intracellular signaling (Figure 7-9). Its role is to recognize an antigen and communicate that information to the cell's nucleus. The BCRs in immunocompetent cells are membrane-associated IgM (mIgM) and IgD (mIgD) immunoglobulins that have identical specificities for antigen. The mIgM is a monomer rather than the pentamer primarily found in the blood.

TABLE 7-3 Generation of Clonal Diversity vs. Clonal Selection

	Generation of Clonal Diversity	Clonal Selection
Purpose?	To produce large numbers of T and B lymphocytes with maximum diversity of antigen receptors	Select, expand, and differentiate clones of T and B cells against specific antigen
When does it occur?	Primarily in fetus	Primarily after birth and throughout life
Where does it occur?	Central lymphoid organs: thymus for T cells, bone marrow for B cells	Peripheral lymphoid organs, including lymph nodes, spleen, and other lymphoid tissues
Is foreign antigen involved?	No	Yes, antigen determines which clones of cells will be selected
What hormones or cytokines are involved?	Thymic hormones, IL-7, others	Many cytokines produced by Th cells and APCs
Final product?	Immunocompetent T and B cells that can react with antigen, but have not seen antigen, and migrate to secondary lymphoid organs	Plasma cells that produce antibody, effector T cells that help (Th cells), kill targets (Tc cells), or regulate immune responses (Treg cells); memory B and T cells

APCs, Antigen-presenting cells; *Tc*, T-cytotoxic cells; *Th*, T-helper cells; *Treg cells*, T-regulatory cells.

A   B

FIGURE 7-9 B-cell Antigen Receptor and T-cell Antigen Receptor. A, The antigen receptor on the surface of B cells (BCR complex) is a monomeric (single) antibody with a structure similar to that of circulating antibody, with an additional transmembrane region *(TM)* that anchors the molecule to the cell surface. The active BCR complex contains molecules (*Igα* and *Igβ*) that are responsible for intracellular signaling after the receptor has bound antigen. **B,** The T-cell receptor *(TCR)* consists of an α- and a β-chain joined by a disulfide bond. Each chain consists of a constant region (*Cα* and *Cβ*) and a variable region (*Vα* and *Vβ*). Each variable region contains CDRs and FRs in a structure similar to that of antibody. The active TCR is associated with several molecules that are responsible for intracellular signaling after antigen binding. These include the CD3, which is a complex of γ (gamma), ξ (epsilon), and δ (delta) subunits and a complex of two ζ (zeta) molecules. The ζ molecules are attached to a cytoplasmic protein kinase (*ZAP70*) that is critical to intracellular signaling.

As described previously, the variable regions of antibodies, as well as the BCR, contain CDR areas. The diversity of these CDRs is responsible for the variety of antigens that can be recognized by immunocompetent B cells.[8] The enormous repertoire of specificities is made possible by rearrangement of existing DNA during B-cell development in the primary lymphoid organs, a process known as somatic recombination. Multiple loci in the DNA that encode for the variable regions of immunoglobulins are recombined to generate receptors that collectively can recognize and bind to any possible antigen.[8] To create the variable region of a light chain, different regions are rearranged using enzymes encoded by *recombination activating genes (RAG-1, RAG-2)*. The DNA is cut and spliced (repaired) so that after this manipulation, the progeny of a single lymphocyte will synthesize immunoglobulins with identical variable regions. Those variable regions, however, are cut and spliced differently from those of another lymphocyte, making each cell unique and therefore able to react with different antigens. The gene for the H chain undergoes similar rearrangement.

Somatic rearrangement of the variable regions will frequently result in a BCR that recognizes the individual's own antigens, which may result in inadvertent attack on "self" antigens expressed on various tissue and organs causing autoimmune disease or hypersensitivites. Many of these "autoreactive" B cells are eliminated in the bone marrow. It is estimated that more than 90% of developing B cells are induced to undergo apoptosis. This process is referred to as central tolerance, so that resultant immunocompetent B cells are against foreign antigens and "tolerant" to *self-antigens*. The process of peripheral tolerance is discussed on p. 173.

B-cell differentiation also is characterized by the development of a variety of important surface molecules that are markers for B cells. These include CD21 (a complement receptor) and CD40 (adhesion molecule required for later interactions with T cells).

Development of T Lymphocytes

The process of T-cell proliferation and differentiation is similar to that for B cells (see Figure 7-2). The primary lymphoid organ for T-cell development is the thymus.[9] Lymphoid stem cells journey through the thymus, where, under influence of thymic hormones and the cytokine IL-7, they are driven to undergo cell division and simultaneously produce receptors (T-cell receptors [TCRs]) against the diversity of antigens the individual will encounter throughout life. They exit the thymus through the blood vessels and lymphatics as mature (immunocompetent) T cells with antigen-specific receptors on the cell surface and establish residence in secondary lymphoid organs.

Production of the TCR proceeds in a manner very similar to that described earlier for B cells. The most common TCR resembles an antibody Fab region and consists of two protein chains, α- and β-chains, each of which has a variable region and a constant region (see Figure 7-9). The variable regions also undergo somatic recombination. As with the BCR, a set of intracellular signaling molecules co-assemble in the membrane with the TCR. The complex of these signaling molecules is called CD3.[10] Thus, all immunocompetent T cells can be identified by the presence of CD3 on the surface.

Differentiation of T cells in the thymus also results in expression in a variety of other important surface molecules. Initially, proteins called CD4 and CD8 are concurrently expressed on the developing cells. CD4 cells develop into T-helper cells (Th cells), whereas CD8 cells become T-cytotoxic cells (Tc cells). Approximately 60% of immunocompetent T cells in the circulation express CD4 and 40% express CD8.

Central tolerance also occurs in the thymus where more than 95% of developing T cells are deleted. Like B-cells, T-cells can also become autoreactive.

✔ QUICK CHECK 7-2
1. What are the major functions of antibodies?
2. What is the difference between the secretory and systemic immune systems?
3. What are the different types of T cells, and what function does each have?

Clonal Selection

Antigens initiate the second phase of the immune response, clonal selection. Clonal selection is the processing of antigen for a specific immune response. This process involves a complex interaction among cells in the secondary lymphoid organs (see Figure 7-2). To initiate an effective immune response, most antigens must be *processed* because they cannot react directly with most cells of the immune system and must be shown or *presented* to the immune cells in a specific manner. This is the job of antigen-processing (antigen-presenting) cells (usually dendritic cells, macrophages, or similar cells), generally referred to as APCs. The interaction among APCs, subpopulations of T cells that facilitate immune responses (T-helper [Th] cells), and immunocompetent B or T cells results in differentiation of B cells into active antibody-producing cells (plasma cells) and T cells into effector cells, such as T-cytotoxic cells. Both lines also develop into memory cells that respond even faster when that antigen enters the body again. Thus, activation of the immune system produces a long-lasting protection against specific antigens (see Figure 7-2). Defects in any aspect of cellular collaboration will lead to defects in cell-mediated immunity, humoral immunity, or both and, depending on the particular defect, potentially the individual's death from infection (see Chapter 8).

Primary and Secondary Immune Responses

The immune response to antigen has classically been divided into two phases—the primary and secondary responses—that are most easily demonstrated by measuring concentrations of circulating antibodies over time (Figure 7-10). After a single initial exposure to most antigens, there is a latent period, or lag phase, during which clonal selection occurs. After approximately 5 to 7 days, IgM antibody is detected in the circulation. This is the primary immune response, characterized typically by initial production of IgM followed by production of IgG against the same antigen. The quantity of IgG may be about equal to or less than the amount of IgM. The amount of antibody in a serum sample is frequently referred to as the titer; a higher titer indicates more antibodies. If no further exposure to the antigen occurs, the circulating antibody is catabolized (broken down) and measurable quantities fall. The individual's immune system, however, has been primed.

A second challenge by the same antigen results in the secondary immune response, which is characterized by the more rapid production of a larger amount of antibody than the primary response. The rapidity of the secondary immune response is the result of memory cells that require less further differentiation. IgM may be transiently produced in the secondary response, but IgG production is increased considerably, making it the predominant antibody class. Natural infection (e.g., rubella) may result in measurable levels of protective IgG for the life of the individual. Some vaccines (e.g., polio) also may produce extremely long-lived protection, although most vaccines require boosters at specified intervals.

Antigen Processing and Presentation

For most antigens, the first step in clonal selection is processing and presentation by APCs. Antigens are usually expressed on large

FIGURE 7-10 Primary and Secondary Immune Responses. The initial administration of antigen induces a primary response during which IgM is initially produced, followed by IgG. Another administration of the antigen induces the secondary response in which IgM is transiently produced and larger amounts of IgG are produced over a longer period of time.

Coded on Chromosome 6 HLA Molecules	
Class I MHC Molecules (HLA-A, HLA-B, HLA-C)	Class II MHC Molecules (HLA-DR, HLA-DP, HLA-DQ)
Expressed on all nucleated cells and platelets	Expressed only on antigen-presenting cells (APC's): Macrophages Dendritic cells B cells
Presents endogenous antigen	Presents exogenous antigen
Recruits CD8+ Tc-Cells	Recruits CD4+ Th-Cells

T cells recognize antigenic fragments complexed to HLA-encoded molecules as "non-self".

FIGURE 7-11 Antigen-Presenting Molecules.

molecules found on microbes, which undergo phagocytosis and destruction by dendritic cells and macrophages. These are referred to as *exogenous antigens.* Other antigens, *endogenous antigens,* originate within a cell that has been infected by a virus or has become cancerous.

Processing results in the release of small antigenic determinants, which are presented on the surface of APCs by specialized molecules, molecules of the major histocompatibility complex (MHC). MHC molecules in humans also are called **human leukocyte antigens (HLA)** (discussed in more detail in Chapter 8) and are related to their role in transplantation. **Major histocompatibility complex (MHC)** molecules are glycoproteins found on the surface of all human cells except red blood cells. They are divided into two general classes, class I and class II, based on their molecular structure, distribution among cell populations, and function in antigen presentation. MHC class I molecules are composed of a large alpha (α) chain along with a smaller chain called β_2-microglobulin. MHC class II molecules are composed of α- and β-chains that differ from the ones used for MHC class I. The α- and β-chains of the MHC molecules are encoded from different genetic loci located as a large complex of genes on human chromosome 6 (Figure 7-11). MHC genes are probably the most polymorphic of any human genes; therefore, no two individuals, except identical twins, will have a complete set of identical MHC molecules.

MHC class I molecules present endogenous antigens, which are primarily recognized by T-cytotoxic (Tc) cells. Because MHC class I molecules are expressed on all cells, except red blood cells, any change in that cell caused by viral infection or malignancy may result in foreign antigens being presented. MHC class II molecules present exogenous antigens (Figure 7-12). Antigen presented by MHC class II molecules is preferentially recognized by T-helper (Th) cells. Thus, antigen presentation to Tc cells is *MHC class I restricted* and presentation to Th cells *is MHC class II restricted.* MHC class II molecules are co-expressed with MHC class I molecules on a limited number of cells that have APC function, including macrophages, dendritic cells, and B lymphocytes.

Thus, the term **antigen processing** relates to the process by which large exogenous and endogenous antigens are cut up by enzymes into small antigenic fragments that are linked with the appropriate MHC molecules and inserted into the membrane of the APC.[11] Lipid antigens are frequently presented by a molecule unrelated to the MHC, CD1, which is not discussed here.

Cellular Interactions in the Immune Response

The second step in clonal selection is a finally tuned set of intercellular collaborations that result in the production of effector cells (plasma cells, Th cells, Tc cells) and memory cells.[12] Each collaboration requires three complementary intracellular signaling events: antigen-specific recognition through the TCR complex, activation of intercellular adhesion molecules, and the response to specific groups of cytokines. Without each signaling event, a protective immune response will not be produced.

T-helper lymphocytes. Regardless of whether an antigen primarily induces a cellular or humoral immune response, APCs usually must present antigens to T-helper cells (Th cells). The APC presents antigen held by the polymorphic regions ($\alpha 1$ and $\beta 1$) of the α- and β-chains of MHC class II molecules.[13] The antigen also binds to the TCR on the Th cell (see Figure 7-9). The strength of the intercellular antigen binding is increased by CD4 on the Th cell, which binds to a nonpolymorphic region of the $\beta 2$ region of the MHC class II molecule. The cytoplasmic portions of CD3 and CD4 interact to activate intracellular signaling pathways. A second co-stimulatory signal results from the interaction of a variety of adhesion molecules; the most critical being B7 on the APC and CD28 on the Th cell.

The third signal occurs through Th-cell cytokine receptors. In the early stages of Th-cell differentiation, IL-1 secreted by the APC provides this signal through the IL-1 receptor on the Th cell (Figure 7-13). The initial differentiation response by the Th cell includes the production of the cytokine IL-2 and up-regulation of IL-2 receptors. IL-2 is secreted and acts in an autocrine (self-stimulating) fashion to induce further maturation and proliferation of the Th cell. Without IL-2 production, the Th cell cannot efficiently mature into a functional helper cell.

At this point and depending on the predominant cytokines in the immediate environment, Th cells undergo differentiation into one of several subsets: Th1, Th2, Th17, or Treg cells.[14] These subsets have different functions: **Th1 cells** preferentially provide help in developing

FIGURE 7-12 Antigen Processing. Antigen processing and presentation are required for initiation of most immune responses. Foreign antigen may be either endogenous (cytoplasmic protein) or exogenous (e.g., bacterium). Endogenous antigenic peptides are transported into the endoplasmic reticulum (ER) **(1)**, where the MHC molecules are being assembled. In the ER, antigenic peptides bind to the α-chains of the MHC class I molecule **(2)**, and the complex is transported to the cell surface **(3)**. The α- and β-chains of the MHC class II molecules are also being assembled in the endoplasmic reticulum **(4)**, but the antigen-binding site is blocked by a small molecule (invariant chain) to prevent interactions with endogenous antigenic peptides. The MHC class II–invariant chain complex is transported to phagolysosomes **(5)**, where exogenous antigenic fragments have been produced as a result of phagocytosis **(6)**. In the phagolysosomes, the invariant chain is digested and replaced by exogenous antigenic peptides **(7)**, after which the MHC class II–antigen complex is inserted into the cell membrane **(8)**.

Tc cells (cell-mediated immunity), Th2 cells provide more help for developing B cells (humoral immunity), Th17 cells are lymphokine-secreting cells that activate macrophages, and Treg cells limit the immune response (these will discussed later in this chapter).[15] The Th subsets differ considerably in the spectrum of cytokines they produce. Additionally, Th1 and Th2 cells may suppress each other so that the immune response may favor either antibody formation, with suppression of a cell-mediated response, or the opposite. For example, antigens derived from viral or bacterial pathogens and those derived from cancer cells seem to induce a greater number of Th1 cells relative to Th2 cells, whereas antigens derived from multicellular parasites and allergens may result in production of more Th2 cells. Many antigens (e.g., tetanus vaccine), however, will produce excellent humoral and cell-mediated responses simultaneously. Th cells are necessary for development of most humoral and cellular immune responses; therefore the virus that causes acquired immune deficiency syndrome (AIDS) results in life-threatening infections because it specifically infects and destroys Th cells (see Chapter 8).

Superantigens. Several pathogenic microorganisms, particularly viruses and bacteria, manipulate the normal interaction between APCs and Th cells to the detriment of the individual and the benefit of the microbe. A group of microbial molecules are called superantigens

(SAGs). SAGs bind to the portion of the TCR outside of its normal antigen-specific binding site, as well as to MHC class II molecules outside of their antigen-presentation sites (Figure 7-14). Some SAGs also react with CD28 on the Th cells and provide a co-stimulatory signal. Thus, SAGs are not processed by an APC to be presented to an immune cell. This binding, which is independent of antigen recognition, provides a signal for Th-cell activation, proliferation, and cytokine production. The normal antigen-specific recognition between Th cells and APCs results in activation of relatively few cells—only those cells with specific TCRs against that antigen. SAGs activate a large population of Th cells, regardless of antigen specificity, and induce excessive production of cytokines, including IL-2, interferon gamma (IFN-γ), and tumor necrosis factor-alpha (TNF-α). The overproduction of inflammatory cytokines results in symptoms of a systemic inflammatory reaction, including fever, low blood pressure, and, potentially, fatal shock. Some examples of SAGs are the bacterial toxins produced by *Staphylococcus aureus* and *Streptococcus pyogenes* (SAGs that cause toxic shock syndrome and food poisoning).[16]

T-cytotoxic lymphocytes. The differentiation of immunocompetent T cells into effector T-cytotoxic cells (Tc cells) requires similar intercellular communications as described for Th cells, with some very important differences. Rather than interacting with an APC, the

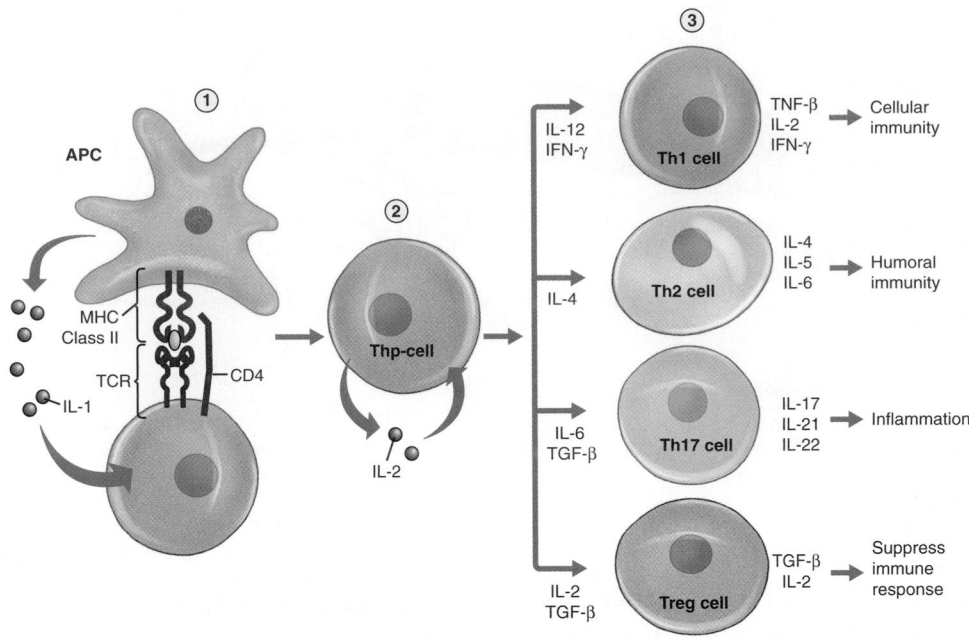

FIGURE 7-13 Development of T-Cell Subsets. The most important step in clonal selection is the production of populations of T-helper (Th) cells (Th1, Th2, and Th17) and T-regulatory (Treg) cells that are necessary for the development of cellular and humoral immune responses. In this model, APCs **(1)** (probably multiple populations) may influence whether a precursor Th cell (Thp cell) **(2)** will differentiate into a Th1, Th2, Th17, or Treg cell **(3)**. Differentiation of the Thp cell is initiated by three signaling events. The antigen signal is produced by the interaction of the T-cell receptor (TCR) and CD4 with antigen presented by MHC class II molecules. A set of co-stimulatory signals is produced from interactions between adhesion molecules (not shown). A third signal is produced by the interactions of cytokines (particularly interleukin-1 [IL-1]) with appropriate cytokine receptors (IL-1R) on the Thp cell. The Thp cell up-regulates IL-2 production and expression of the IL-2 receptor (IL-2R), which acts in an autocrine fashion to accelerate Thp cell differentiation and proliferation. Commitment to a particular phenotype results from the relative concentrations of other cytokines. IL-12 and IFN-γ produced by some populations of APCs favor differentiation into the Th1 cell phenotype; IL-4, which is produced by a variety of cells, favors differentiation into the Th2 cell phenotype; IL-6 and TGF-β (T-cell growth factor) facilitate differentiation into Th17 cells; IL-2 and TGF-β induce differentiation into Treg cells. The Th1 cell is characterized by the production of cytokines that assist in the differentiation of T-cytotoxic (Tc) cells, leading to cellular immunity, whereas the Th2 cell produces cytokines that favor B-cell differentiation and humoral immunity. Th1 and Th2 cells affect each other through the production of inhibitory cytokines: IFN-γ will inhibit development of Th2 cells, and IL-4 will inhibit the development of Th1 cells. Th17 cells produce cytokines that affect phagocytes and increase inflammation. Treg cells produce immunosuppressive cytokines that prevent the immune response from being excessive. *APC,* Antigen-presenting cell; *IFN,* interferon; *MHC,* major histocompatibility complex; *TGF,* transforming growth factor.

immunocompetent Tc cell recognizes antigen presented by MHC class I molecules on the surface of a virus-infected cell or cancerous cell (Figure 7-15). The Tc cell expresses CD8, rather than CD4. CD8 binds to the MHC class I molecule and, as with Th cell differentiation, the proximity of the CD3 and CD8 cytoplasmic portions activates intercellular signaling pathways. Cytokine signals, especially IL-2, are produced by Th1 cells and activate cytokine receptors on the Tc cells.

B-cell clonal selection. A further sequence of cellular interactions is required to produce an effective antibody response. The immunocompetent B cell is also an APC and expresses surface mIgM and mIgD B-cell receptors (BCRs) (Figure 7-16). Unlike the T-cell receptor that can only *see* processed and presented antigens, the BCR can react with soluble antigens that have not been processed. B cells also express surface CD21, which is a receptor for opsonins produced by complement activation. Antigen binding through the BCR and CD21 activates the B cell, resulting in internalization, processing, and presentation of

antigen fragments by MHC class II molecules.[17] The antigen presented on the B-cell surface is recognized by a Th2 cell through the TCR and CD4. The intercellular bridges created through antigen and other intercellular adhesion molecules induce the Th2 cell to secrete cytokines (particularly IL-4) that initiate B-cell proliferation and maturation into plasma cells.[18]

A major component of B-cell maturation is class switch, the process that results in the change in antibody production from one class to another (e.g., IgM to IgG during the primary immune response). Before exposure to antigens and Th2 cells, the B cell produces IgM and IgD, which are used as cell membrane receptors. During the clonal selection process, a B cell proliferates and develops into antibody-secreting plasma cells, and each B cell has the option of becoming a secretor of IgM or changing the class of antibody to a secreted form of IgG, IgA, or IgE. Class switch occurs by another round of somatic recombination with the variable region of the antibody

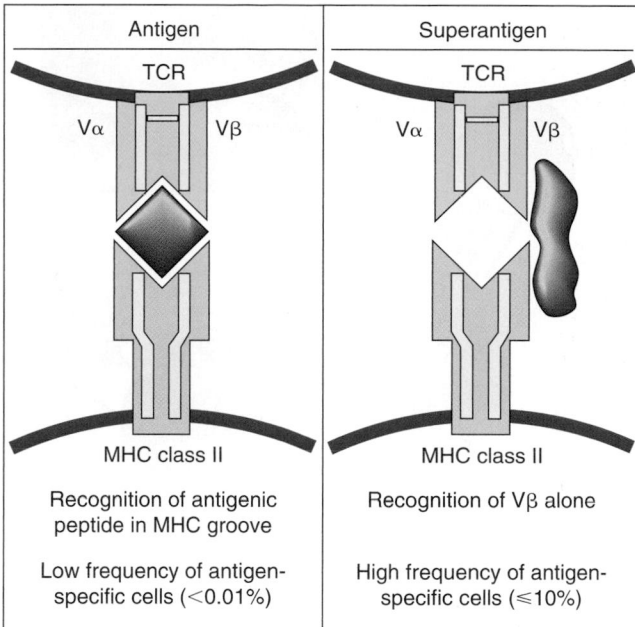

FIGURE 7-14 **Superantigens.** The T-cell receptor (TCR) and major histocompatibility complex (MHC) class II molecule are normally held together by processed antigen. Superantigens, such as some bacterial exotoxins, bind directly to the variable region of the TCR β-chain and the MHC class II molecule. Each superantigen activates sets of Vβ chains independently of the antigen specificity of the TCR.

FIGURE 7-16 **B-Cell Clonal Selection.** Immunocompetent B cells undergo proliferation and differentiation into antibody-secreting plasma cells. Multiple signals are necessary (**1**). The B cell itself can directly bind soluble antigen through the B-cell receptor (BCR) and act as an antigen-processing cell. Antigen is internalized, processed (**2**), and presented (**3**) to the TCR on a Th2 cell by MHC class II molecules (**4**). A cytokine signal is provided by the Th2 cell cytokines (e.g., IL-4) that react with the B cell (**5**). The B cell differentiates into plasma cells that secrete antibody (**6**).

FIGURE 7-17 **Activation of a B Cell by a T-Cell–Independent Antigen.** Molecules containing repeating identical antigenic determinants may interact simultaneously with several receptors on the surface of the B cell and induce the proliferation and production of immunoglobulins. Because Th2 cells do not participate, class switch does not occur and the resultant antibody response is IgM.

FIGURE 7-15 **Tc-Cell Clonal Selection.** The immunocompetent Tc cell can react with antigen but cannot yet kill target cells. During clonal selection, this cell reacts with antigen presented by MHC class I molecules on the surface of a virally infected or cancerous *abnormal* cell. (**1**) The antigen–MHC class I complex is recognized simultaneously by the T-cell receptor (TCR), which binds to antigen, and CD8, which binds to the MHC class I molecule. (**2**) A separate signal is provided by cytokines, particularly IL-2 from Th1 cells. (**3**) In response to these signals, the Tc cell develops into an effector Tc cell with the ability to kill abnormal cells.

heavy chain being combined with a different constant region of the heavy chain. Because the variable region is conserved and the light chain remains unchanged, the antigenic specificity of the antibody also remains unchanged. The particular constant region chosen by each cell during class switch appears to be, at least partially, under the control of specific Th2 cytokines. For instance, IL-4 and IL-13 appear to preferentially stimulate switch to IgE secretion, and transforming growth factor-beta (TGF-β) and IL-5 appear to play major roles in class switch to IgA secretion. Thus, during clonal selection, a B cell may produce a population of plasma cells that are capable of producing many different classes of antibodies against the same antigen.

Although most antigens require B cells to interact with Th cells, a few antigens can bypass the need for cellular interactions and can directly stimulate B-cell maturation and proliferation. These are called *T-cell–independent antigens* (Figure 7-17). They are mostly bacterial products that are large and are likely to have repeating identical antigenic determinants that bind and cross-link several BCRs. The accumulated intracellular signal is adequate to induce differentiation into a plasma cell but is not adequate to induce a change in the class of antibody that will be produced. Therefore, T-cell–independent antigens usually induce relatively pure IgM primary and secondary immune responses.

Memory cells. During the clonal selection process, both B cells and T cells differentiate and proliferate into an extremely large population of long-lived **memory cells.**[19] Memory cells remain inactive until subsequent exposure to the same antigen. Upon reexposure, these memory cells do not require much further differentiation and will therefore rapidly become new plasma cells or effector T cells without the cellular interactions described previously.

CELL-MEDIATED IMMUNITY

The rather straightforward function of antibodies has been discussed earlier in this chapter. The function of effector T cells is more complex and utilizes the principles of intercellular recognition necessary for clonal selection.

T-Lymphocyte Function

The clonal selection process produces several subsets of effector T cells. Th cells and T memory cells have already been discussed. Other effector T cells include T-cytotoxic (Tc) cells that attack and destroy cells expressing antigens from intracellular (endogenous) origins, T-regulatory cells (Treg) that limit (suppress) the immune response, and T-lymphokine producing cells that secrete cytokines that activate other cells.

T-Cytotoxic Lymphocytes

T-cytotoxic (Tc) cells are responsible for the cell-mediated destruction of tumor cells or cells infected with viruses. In a fashion similar to intercellular recognition during the clonal selection process, the Tc cell must directly adhere to the target cell through antigen presented by MHC class I molecules and CD8 (Figure 7-18). Because of the broad cellular distribution of MHC class I molecules, Tc cells can recognize antigens on the surface of almost any type of cell that has been infected by a virus or has become cancerous. Unlike clonal selection, the roles of co-stimulatory signals through adhesion molecules and cytokines are of less importance here. Attachment to a target cell activates multiple killing mechanisms through which the Tc cell induces the target cell to undergo apoptosis.

Various other cells kill targets in a fashion similar to Tc lymphocytes. Prominent among these cells are natural killer cells. **Natural killer (NK) cells** are a special group of lymphoid cells that are similar to T cells but lack antigen-specific receptors. Instead, they express a variety of cell surface activation receptors (similar to pattern recognition receptors, see Chapter 6) that identify protein changes on the surface of cells infected with viruses or that have become cancerous. After attachment, the NK cell kills its target in a manner similar to that of Tc cells. NK cells also have receptors for MHC class I. However, NK cells lack CD8; therefore binding to MHC class I molecules results in inactivation of the NK cell. Thus, NK cells complement the effects of Tc cells. In some instances, a virus-infected or cancerous cell will "protect" itself by down-regulating MHC class I molecule expression. Without surface MHC class I molecules a cell becomes resistant to Tc-cell recognition and killing. NK cells primarily kill target cells that have suppressed the expression of MHC class I.

NK cells, as well as some macrophages, can specifically kill targets through use of antibodies. NK cells express Fc receptors for IgG.

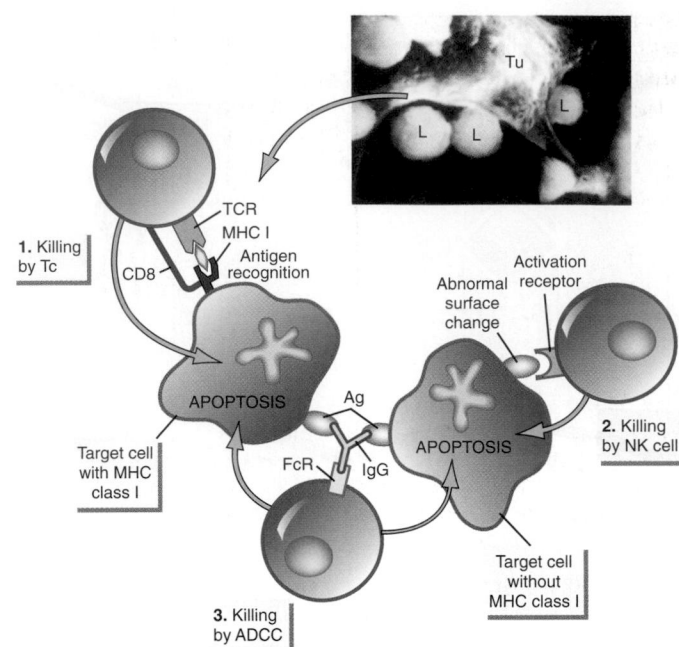

FIGURE 7-18 Cellular Killing Mechanisms. Several cells have the capacity to kill abnormal (e.g., virally infected, cancerous) target cells. **(1)** T-cytotoxic (Tc) cells recognize endogenous antigen presented by MHC class I molecules. The Tc cell mobilizes multiple killing mechanisms that induce apoptosis of the target cell. **(2)** Natural killer (NK) cells identify and kill target cells through receptors that recognize abnormal surface changes. NK cells specifically kill targets that do not express surface MHC class I molecules. **(3)** Several cells, including macrophages and NK cells, can kill by antibody-dependent cellular cytotoxicity (ADCC). IgG antibodies bind to foreign antigen on the target cell, and cells involved in ADCC bind IgG through Fc receptors (FcR) and initiate killing. The insert is a scanning electron microscopic view of Tc cells *(L)* attacking a much larger tumor cell *(Tu)*. (Insert from Abbas A, Lichtman A: *Cellular and molecular immunology*, ed 5, Philadelphia, 2003, Saunders.)

If antigens on the infected or cancerous cell bind IgG, the NK cell can attach through Fc receptors and activate its normal killing mechanisms. This is referred to as **antibody-dependent cellular cytotoxicity (ADCC).**

Lymphokine-Secreting T Cells

Two subsets of Th cells amplify inflammation. Th1 cells, in addition to assisting Tc-cell clonal selection, secrete cytokines that activate M1 macrophages to increase phagocytic and microbial killing functions (described in Chapter 6). The most important cytokine for macrophage activation is interferon-γ (IFN-γ). Th2 cells, in addition to assisting B-cell clonal selection, secrete cytokines (e.g., IL-4, IL-13) that activate M2 macrophages for healing and repair of damaged tissue (described in Chapter 6). Th17 cells secrete a set of cytokines (e.g., IL-17, IL-22, chemokines) that recruit phagocytic cells to a site of inflammation.[20] Th17-cell cytokines also may activate cells, particularly epithelial cells, to produce antimicrobial proteins in defense against certain bacterial and fungal pathogens.

T-Regulatory Lymphocytes

T-regulatory (Treg) cells are a diverse group of T cells that control the immune response, usually suppressing the response and maintaining tolerance against self-antigens.[21] This process occurs in the secondary lymphoid organs and other tissues, known as peripheral tolerance, in contrast to the process of central tolerance described earlier. This population of Treg cells that differentiate from the Th-cell population expresses CD4 and binds to antigens presented by MHC class II molecules. Unlike other Th cells, however, Treg cells express consistently high levels of CD25 (the IL-2 receptor). Differentiation from the Th precursor cell is controlled, primarily by TGF-β and IL-2. Treg cells produce very high levels of immunosuppressive cytokines TGF-β and IL-10, which generally decrease Th1 and Th2 activity by suppressing antigen recognition and Th-cell proliferation.

✔ QUICK CHECK 7-3

1. What are antigen-presenting cells?
2. Define BCR and TCR.
3. What is the role of T-helper cells?
4. Why are cytokines important to the immune response?
5. What is the difference between central tolerance and peripheral tolerance?

Age-related mechanisms of self-defense in the newborn child and in the elderly are listed in the *Pediatric Considerations* and *Geriatric Considerations* boxes.

PEDIATRIC CONSIDERATIONS

Age-Related Factors Affecting Mechanisms of Self-Defense in the Newborn Child

Normal human newborns are immunologically immature; they have deficient antibody production, phagocytic activity, and complement activity, especially components of alternative pathways (e.g., factor B).

The newborn cannot produce all classes of antibody; IgM is produced by the newborn (develops in the last trimester) to in utero infections (e.g., cytomegalovirus, rubella virus, and *Toxoplasma gondii*); only limited amounts of IgA are produced in the newborn; IgG production begins after birth and rises steadily throughout the first year of life.

Maternal antibodies provide protection within the newborn's circulation (see figure below).

Deficits in specific maternal transplacental antibody may lead to a tendency to develop severe, overwhelming sepsis and meningitis in the newborn.

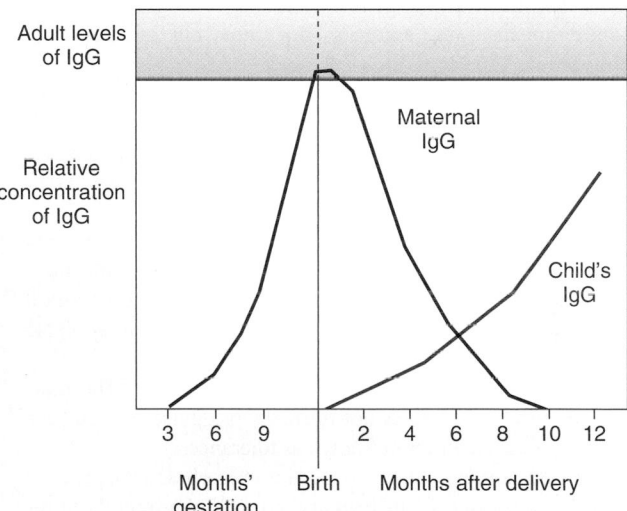

Antibody Levels in Umbilical Cord Blood and in Neonatal Circulation. Early in gestation, maternal IgG begins active transport across the placenta and enters the fetal circulation. At birth, the fetal circulation may contain nearly adult levels of IgG, which is almost exclusively from the maternal source. The fetal immune system has the capacity to produce IgM and small amounts of IgA before birth (not shown). After delivery, maternal IgG is rapidly destroyed and neonatal IgG production increases.

GERIATRIC CONSIDERATIONS

Age-Related Factors Affecting Mechanisms of Self-Defense in the Elderly

Immune function decreases with age; diminished T-cell function and reduced antibody responses to antigenic challenge occur with age.

The thymus reaches maximum size at sexual maturity and then undergoes involution until it is a vestigial remnant by middle age; by 45 to 50 years of age, the thymus is only 15% of its maximum size.

With age there is a decrease in thymic hormone production and the organ's ability to mediate T-cell differentiation.

DID YOU UNDERSTAND?

Third Line of Defense: Adaptive Immunity

1. Adaptive immunity is a state of protection, primarily against infectious agents, that differs from inflammation by being slower to develop, being more specific, and having memory that makes it much longer lived.
2. The adaptive immune response is most often initiated by cells of the innate system. These cells process and present portions of invading pathogens (i.e., antigens) to lymphocytes in peripheral lymphoid tissue.
3. The adaptive immune response is mediated by two different types of lymphocytes—B lymphocytes and T lymphocytes. Each has distinct functions. B cells are responsible for humoral immunity that is mediated by circulating antibodies (immunoglobulins), whereas T cells are responsible for cell-mediated immunity, in which they kill targets directly or stimulate the activity of other leukocytes.
4. Adaptive immunity can be either active or passive depending on whether immune response components originated in the host or came from a donor.

Antigens and Immunogens

1. Antigens are molecules that bind and react with components of the immune response, such as antibodies and receptors on B and T cells. Most antigens can induce an immune response, and these antigens are called immunogens.
2. All immunogens are antigens but not all antigens are immunogens.
3. Some pathogens are successful because they mimic "self" antigens but avoid inducing an immune response.
4. Large molecules, such as proteins, polysaccharides, and nucleic acids, are most immunogenic. Thus molecular size is an important factor for antigen immunogenicity.
5. Haptens are antigens too small to be immunogens by themselves but become immunogenic after combining with larger molecules.
6. The antigenic determinant, or epitope, is the precise chemical structure with which an antibody or B-cell/T-cell receptor reacts.
7. Self-antigens are antigens on an individual's own cells. The individual's immune system does not normally recognize self-antigens as immunogenic, a condition known as tolerance.
8. The response to antigen can be divided into two phases: the primary and secondary responses. The primary response of humoral immunity is usually dominated by IgM, with lesser amounts of IgG. The secondary immune response has a more rapid production of a larger amount of antibodies, predominantly IgG.

Antibodies

1. The humoral immune response consists of molecules (antibodies) produced by B cells. B cells are lymphocytes.
2. Antibodies are plasma glycoproteins that can be classified by chemical structure and biologic activity as IgG, IgM, IgA, IgE, or IgD.
3. A typical antibody molecule is constructed of two identical heavy chains and two identical light chains (either κ or λ) and has two Fab portions that bind antigen and an Fc portion that interacts with complement or receptors on cells.
4. The protective effects of antibodies may be *direct* through the action of antibody alone or *indirect* requiring activation of other components of the innate immune response.

5. IgE is a special class of antibody produced against environmental antigens that are the primary cause of common allergies. It also protects the individual from infection by large parasitic worms (helminthes).
6. The secretory immune system protects the external surfaces of the body through secretion of antibodies in bodily secretions, such as tears, sweat, saliva, mucus, and breast milk. IgA is the dominant secretory immunoglobulin.

Immune Response: Collaboration of B Cells and T Cells

1. The generation of clonal diversity results in production of B and T lymphocytes with receptors against millions of antigens that possibly will be encountered in an individual's lifetime occurs in the fetus in the primary lymphoid organs: the thymus for T cells and portions of the bone marrow for B cells..
2. The generation of clonal diversity is the differentiation of lymphoid stem cells into B and T lymphocytes. Lymphoid stem cells interact with stromal cells through a variety of adhesion factors. As the stem cell matures it develops a variety of surface markers or receptors, one of the earliest is IL-7 receptor. IL-7, produced by stromal cells is critical for driving differentiation and proliferation of the B cell.
3. The next stage in development is formation of the B-cell receptor (BCR). The role of the BCR is to recognize antigen and communicate that information to the cell's nucleus.
4. The variable regions of antibodies, as well as the BCR, contain CDR areas. The diversity of these CDRs is responsible for the variety of antigens recognized by immunocompetent B cells. The enormous repertoire of antibody specificities is made possible by rearrangement of existing DNA during B-cell development in the primary lymphoid organs, a process called somatic recombination.
5. Somatic rearrangement of the antibody variable regions will frequently result in a BCR that recognizes the individual's own antigens, which may result in attack on "self" antigens expressed on various tissue and organs. Many of these "autoreactive" B cells are eliminated in the bone marrow. Most of the developing B cells undergo apoptosis. This entire process is referred to as central tolerance.
6. The process of T-cell proliferation and differentiation is similar to that for B cells. The primary lymphoid organ for T-cell development is the thymus. Lymphoid stem cells travel through the thymus, where thymic hormones and the cytokine IL-7 promote lymphoid stem cell division and the production of receptors. They exit the thymus as mature immunocompetent T cells with antigen-specific receptors on the cell surface.
7. T cell receptor, or TCR, proceeds in a manner similar to BCR. Initially proteins called CD4 and CD8 are expressed on the developing cells. Eventually CD4 cells develop into T-helper cells (Th cells) and CD 8 cells become T-cytotoxic cells. Other mature T cells include T-regulatory cells (Treg) and memory cells.
8. The generation of clonal diversity concludes when immunocompetent T and B cells migrate from the primary lymphoid organs into the circulation and secondary lymphoid organs to await antigen.
9. The induction of an immune response, or clonal selection, begins when antigen enters the individual's body.
10. Most antigens must first interact with antigen-presenting cells (APCs) (e.g., macrophages). Dendritic cells present in the skin, mucosa, and lymphoid tissues also present antigen.

11. Antigen is processed in the APCs and presented on the cell surface by molecules of the MHC. The particular MHC molecule (class I or class II) that presents antigen determines which cell will respond to that antigen. Th cells require that the antigen be presented in a complex with MHC class II molecules. Tc cells require that the antigen be presented by MHC class I molecules.

12. The T cell sees the presented antigen through the T-cell receptor (TCR) and accessory molecules: CD4 or CD8. CD4 is found on Th cells and reacts specifically with MHC class II. CD8 is found on Tc cells and reacts specifically with MHC class I.

13. Th cells consist of Th1 cells, which help Tc cells respond to antigen; Th2 cells, which help B cells develop into plasma cells; and Th17 cells, which help activate macrophages.

14. Tc cells bind to and kill cellular targets such as cells infected with viruses or cancer cells.

15. The natural killer (NK) cell has some characteristics of the Tc cells and is important for killing target cells in which viral infection or malignancy has resulted in the loss of cellular MHC molecules.

Pediatric Considerations: Age-Related Factors Affecting Mechanisms of Self-Defense in the Newborn Child

1. Neonates often have transiently depressed inflammatory function, particularly neutrophil chemotaxis and alternative complement pathway activity.

2. The T-cell–independent immune response is adequate in the fetus and neonate, but the T-cell–dependent immune response develops slowly during the first 6 months of life.

3. Maternal IgG antibodies are transported across the placenta into the fetal blood and protect the neonate for the first 6 months, after which they are replaced by the child's own antibodies.

Geriatric Considerations: Age-Related Factors Affecting Mechanisms of Self-Defense in the Elderly

1. Elderly persons are at risk for impaired wound healing, usually because of chronic illnesses.

2. T-cell function and antibody production are somewhat deficient in elderly persons. Elderly individuals also tend to have increased levels of circulating autoantibodies (antibodies against self-antigens).

KEY TERMS

Active immunity (active acquired immunity), 159
Adaptive (acquired) immunity, 158
Agglutination, 162
Antibody, 161
Antibody-dependent cellular cytotoxicity (ADCC), 172
Antigen, 158, 160
Antigen-binding fragment (Fab), 161
Antigen-binding site (paratope), 162
Antigen processing, 168
Antigen-processing (antigen-presenting) cell (APC), 167
Antigenic determinant (epitope), 162
B-cell receptor (BCR), 166

B lymphocyte (B cell), 158
CD3, 167
CD4, 167
CD8, 167
CDR, 167
Cellular immunity, 159
Central tolerance, 167
Class switch, 170
Clonal diversity, 159, 166
Clonal selection, 159, 167
Complementary-determining region (CDR), 162
Crystalline fragment (Fc), 161
Dendritic cell, 167
Hapten, 160
Human leukocyte antigens (HLA), 168
Humoral immunity, 159
Immune response, 158
Immunity, 158

Immunocompetent, 159
Immunogen, 160
Immunoglobulin (Ig), 161
Lymphocyte, 158
Lymphoid stem cell, 166
Major histocompatibility complex (MHC), 168
Memory cell, 159
Natural killer (NK) cell, 172
Neutralization, 162
Passive immunity (passive acquired immunity), 159
Peripheral tolerance, 173
Plasma cell, 159
Precipitation, 162
Primary immune response, 167
Primary (central) lymphoid organ, 166
Secondary immune response, 167

Secondary lymphoid organ, 159
Secretory (mucosal) immune system, 164
Secretory immunoglobulin, 164
Somatic recombination, 167
Superantigen (SAG), 169
Systemic immune system, 164
T-cell receptor (TCR), 167
T-cytotoxic (Tc) cell, 159
T-helper (Th) cell, 159
T lymphocyte (T cell), 158
T-regulatory (Treg) cell, 159, 169, 172
Th1 cell, 168
Th2 cell, 169
Th17 cell, 169
Titer, 167

REFERENCES

1. Wu LC, Zarrin AA: The production and regulation of IgE by the immune system, *Nat Rev Immunol* 14(4):247-259, 2014.
2. Sela-Culang I et al: The structural basis of antibody-antigen recognition, *Front Immunol* 4:302, 2013.
3. Guilliams M et al: The function of Fcγ receptors in dendritic cells and macrophages, *Nat Rev Immunol* 14(2):94-108, 2014.
4. Fitzsimmons CM et al: Helminth allergens, parasite-specific IgE, and its protective role in human immunity, *Front Immunol* 5:61, 2014.
5. Rescigno M: Mucosal immunology and bacterial handling in the intestine, *Best Pract Res Clin Gastroenterol* 27(1):17-24, 2013.
6. Miyazaki K et al: The establishment of B versus T cell identity, *Trends Immunol* 35(5):205-210, 2014.
7. Clark MR et al: Orchestrating B cell lymphopoiesis through interplay of IL-7 receptor and pre-B cell receptor signalling, *Nat Rev Immunol* 14(2):69-89, 2014.

8. Shih H-Y, Krangel MS: Chromatin architecture, CCCTC-binding factor, and V(D)J recombination: managing long-distance relationships at antigen receptor loci, *J Immunol* 190(10):4915-4921, 2013.
9. Boehm T, Swann JB: Thymus involution and regeneration: two sides of the same coin? *Nat Rev Immunol* 13(11):831-838, 2013.
10. Brownlie RJ, Zamoyska R: T cell receptor signalling networks: branching, diversified and bounded, *Nat Rev Immunol* 13(4):257-269, 2013.
11. Blum JS et al: Pathways of antigen processing, *Annu Rev Immunol* 31(2013):143-473, 2013.
12. Batista FD, Dustin ML: Cell:cell interactions in the immune system, *Immunol Rev* 251(1):7-12, 2013.
13. Fooksman DR: Organizing MHC class II presentation, *Front Immunol* 5:158, 2014.
14. Yamane H, Paul WE: Early signaling events that underlie fate decisions of naïve CD4+ T cells toward distinct T-helper cell subsets, *Immunol Rev* 252(1):12-23, 2013.

15. Jiang S, Dong C: A complex issue on CD4+ T-cell subsets, *Immunol Rev* 252(1):5-11, 2013.
16. Ramachandran G: Gram-positive and gram-negative bacterial toxins in sepsis, *Virulence* 5(1):213-218, 2014.
17. Avalos AM, Ploegh HL: Early BCR events and antigen capture, processing, and loading on MHC class II on B cells, *Front Immunol* 5:92, 2014.
18. Njau MN, Jacob J: The CD28/B7 pathway: a novel regulator of plasma cell function, *Adv Exp Med Biol* 785(2013):67-75, 2013.
19. Farber DL et al: Human memory T cells: generation, compartmentalization and homeostasis, *Nat Rev Immunol* 14(1):24-35, 2014.
20. Annunziato F et al: Main features of human T helper 17 cells, *Ann N Y Acad Sci* 1284(2013):66-70, 2013.
21. Singer BD et al: Regulatory T cells as immunotherapy, *Front Immunol* 5:46, 2014.

8

Infection and Defects in Mechanisms of Defense

Neal S. Rote

℮ EVOLVE WEBSITE

http://evolve.elsevier.com/Huether/
Student Review Questions
Audio Key Points

Case Studies
Animations
Quick Check Answers

CHAPTER OUTLINE

The defensive system protecting the body from infection is a finely tuned network, but it is not perfect. Sometimes infectious agents can inhibit or escape defense mechanisms or the system may break down, leading to inadequate protection or inappropriate activation. An inadequate response (commonly called an immune deficiency) may range from relatively mild defects to life-threatening severity. Inappropriate responses (hypersensitivity reactions) may be (1) exaggerated against noninfectious environmental substances (allergy); (2) misdirected against the body's own cells (autoimmunity); or (3) directed against beneficial foreign tissues, such as transfusions or transplants (alloimmunity). Several of these inappropriate responses can be serious or life-threatening. This chapter provides an overview of conditions under which our protective systems have failed.

INFECTION

Modern health care has shown great progress in preventing and treating infectious diseases. In the United States, heart disease and malignancies greatly surpass infectious disease as major causes of death. However, endemic diseases, such as chronic hepatitis, human immunodeficiency virus (HIV), other sexually transmitted infections, and foodborne infections, remain major challenges.[1] Most deaths related to infections occur in individuals whose protective systems are compromised (children, elderly, and those with chronic disease). Influenza/pneumonia (eighth leading cause of death) and sepsis (eleventh leading cause) accounted for more than 89,000 deaths (3.5% of the total number of deaths) in 2011.[2] Other infections resulted in an additional 27,000 deaths.

Infectious disease remains a significant threat to life in many parts of the world, including India, Africa, and Southeast Asia.[3] The advent of sanitary living conditions, clean water, uncontaminated food, vaccinations, and antimicrobial medications has improved the health of many; but inefficient healthcare systems, endemic poverty, political unrest, and other factors have slowed progress in some regions. As a result of these initiatives, smallpox has been eradicated from the globe (the last reported case was in 1975 in Somalia). Worldwide, polio has declined by more than 99% and eradicated from the Western hemisphere. Measles was decreased by 78% and was nearly eliminated in the Western hemisphere. Although vaccines and antimicrobials have diminished the frequency of some infectious diseases, the emergence of new diseases, such as West Nile virus, severe acute respiratory syndrome (SARS), Middle East respiratory syndrome coronavirus (MERS-CoV), and *Hantavirus,* and the uncontrolled spread of diseases, such as Ebola virus infection, into new regions of Africa, as well as the continued development of many multiple drug–resistant microorganisms, are examples of the current intense challenges in the struggle to prevent and control infectious disease. Some tropical diseases are emerging for the first time in the United States, possibly a result of global warming.

Microorganisms and Humans: A Dynamic Relationship

The increase in antibiotic resistance, in particular, places more importance on maintenance of an intact inflammatory and immune system. Individuals with immune deficiencies become easily infected with opportunistic microorganisms—those that normally would not cause disease but seize the opportunity provided by the person's decreased immune or inflammatory responses.

Unlike opportunistic infections, true pathogens have devised means to circumvent the normal controls provided by the innate and adaptive system. Several factors influence the capacity of a pathogen to cause disease.

- **Communicability**: Ability to spread from one individual to others (e.g., measles and pertussis spread very easily; human immunodeficiency virus [HIV] is of lower communicability)
- **Infectivity**: Ability of the pathogen to invade and multiply in the host (e.g., herpes simplex virus can survive for long periods in a latent stage)
- **Virulence**: Capacity of a pathogen to cause severe disease (e.g., measles virus is of low virulence; rabies and Ebola viruses are highly virulent)
- **Pathogenicity**: Ability of an agent to produce disease—success depends on communicability, infectivity, extent of tissue damage, and virulence (e.g., HIV can kill T lymphocytes)
- **Portal of entry**: Route by which a pathogenic microorganism infects the host (e.g., direct contact, inhalation, ingestion, or bites of an animal or insect)
- **Toxigenicity**: Ability to produce soluble toxins or endotoxins, factors that greatly influence the pathogen's degree of virulence

Infectivity is facilitated by the ability of pathogens to attach to cell surfaces, release enzymes that dissolve protective barriers, multiply rapidly, escape the action of phagocytes, or resist the effect of low pH. After penetrating protective barriers (invasion), pathogens then multiply and spread through the lymph and blood to tissues and organs, where they continue multiplying and cause disease. In humans the route of entrance of many pathogenic microorganisms also becomes the site of shedding of new infectious agents to other individuals, completing a cycle of infection.

Infectious disease can be caused by microorganisms that range in size from 20 nanometers (nm) (poliovirus) to 10 meters (m) (tapeworm). Classes of pathogenic microorganisms and their characteristics are summarized in Table 8-1. Some mechanisms of tissue damage

caused by microorganisms are summarized in Table 8-2. The multiple layers of defense against infection are described in Chapters 6 and 7. Table 8-3 contains examples of microorganisms that defeat our protective systems.

Bacterial Disease

Bacteria are prokaryotes (lacking a discrete nucleus) and are relatively small. They can be aerobic or anaerobic and motile or immotile. Spherical bacteria are called cocci, rodlike forms are called bacilli, and spiral forms are termed *spirochetes*. Gram stain differentiates the microorganisms as gram-positive or gram-negative bacteria. Examples of human diseases caused by specific bacteria are listed in Table 8-4. The general structure of bacteria is reviewed in Figure 8-1.

Bacterial survival and growth depend on the effectiveness of the body's defense mechanisms and on the bacterium's ability to resist

TABLE 8-1 Classes of Microorganisms Infectious to Humans

Class	Size	Site of Reproduction	Example
Virus	20-300 nm	Intracellular	Poliomyelitis
Chlamydiae	200-1000 nm	Intracellular	Urethritis
Rickettsiae	300-1200 nm	Intracellular	Rocky Mountain spotted fever
Mycoplasma	125-350 nm	Extracellular	Atypical pneumonia
Bacteria	0.8-15 mcg	Skin	Staphylococcal wound infection
		Mucous membranes	Cholera
		Extracellular	Streptococcal pneumonia
		Intracellular	Tuberculosis
Fungi	2-200 mcg	Skin	Tinea pedis (athlete's foot)
		Mucous membranes	Candidiasis (e.g., thrush)
		Extracellular	Sporotrichosis
		Intracellular	Histoplasmosis
Protozoa	1-50 mm	Mucosal	Giardiasis
		Extracellular	Sleeping sickness
Helminths	3 mm to 10 m	Intracellular	Trichinosis
		Extracellular	Filariasis

TABLE 8-2 Examples of Microorganisms That Cause Tissue Damage

PATHOGENS THAT DIRECTLY CAUSE TISSUE DAMAGE

Produce Exotoxin

Streptococcus pyogenes	Tonsillitis, scarlet fever
Staphylococcus aureus	Boils, toxic shock syndrome, food poisoning
Corynebacterium diphtheria	Diphtheria
Clostridium tetani	Tetanus
Vibrio cholerae	Cholera

Produce Endotoxin

Escherichia coli	Gram-negative sepsis
Haemophilus influenzae	Meningitis, pneumonia
Salmonella typhi	Typhoid
Shigella	Bacillary dysentery
Pseudomonas aeruginosa	Wound infection
Yersinia pestis	Plague

Cause Direct Damage with Invasion

Variola	Smallpox
Varicella-zoster	Chickenpox, shingles
Hepatitis B virus	Hepatitis
Poliovirus	Poliomyelitis
Measles virus	Measles, subacute sclerosing panencephalitis
Influenza virus	Influenza
Herpes simplex virus	Cold sores

PATHOGENS THAT INDIRECTLY CAUSE TISSUE DAMAGE

Produce Immune Complexes

Hepatitis B virus	Kidney disease
S. pyogenes	Glomerulonephritis
Treponema pallidum	Kidney damage in secondary syphilis
Most acute infections	Transient renal deposits

Cause Cell-Mediated Immunity

Mycobacterium tuberculosis	Tuberculosis
Mycobacterium leprae	Tuberculoid leprosy
Lymphocytic choriomeningitis virus	Aseptic meningitis
Borrelia burgdorferi	Lyme arthritis
Herpes simplex virus	Herpes stromal keratitis

Data modified from Janeway CA et al: *Immunobiology: the system in health and disease*, ed 5, New York, 2001, Garland.

TABLE 8-3   Examples of Mechanisms Used by Pathogens to Resist the Immune System

Mechanisms	Effect on Immunity	Example of Specific Microorganisms
Destroy or Block Component of Immune System		
Produce toxins	Kills phagocyte or interferes with chemotaxis	*Staphylococcus*
	Prevents phagocytosis by inhibiting fusion between phagosome and lysosomal granules	*Streptococcus*
		Mycobacterium tuberculosis
Produce antioxidants (e.g., catalase, superoxide dismutase)	Prevents killing by O$_2$-dependent mechanisms	*Mycobacterium* sp.
	Promotes bacterial attachment	*Salmonella typhi*
Produce protease to digest IgA		*Neisseria gonorrhoeae* (urinary tract infection), *Haemophilus influenzae*, and *Streptococcus pneumoniae* (pneumonia)
Produce surface molecules that mimic Fc receptors and bind antibody	Prevents activation of complement system	*Staphylococcus*
	Prevents antibody functioning as opsonin	Herpes simplex virus
Mimic Self-Antigens		
Produce surface antigens (e.g., M protein, red blood cell antigens) that are similar to self-antigens	Pathogen resembles individual's own tissue; in some individuals, antibodies can be formed against self-antigen, leading to hypersensitivity disease (e.g., antibody to M protein also reacts with cardiac tissue, causing rheumatic heart disease; antibody to red blood cell antigens can cause anemia)	Group A *Streptococcus* (M protein) *Mycoplasma pneumoniae* (red cell antigens)
Change Antigenic Profile		
Undergo mutation of antigens or activate genes that change surface molecules	Immune response delayed because of failure to recognize new antigen	Influenza HIV Some parasites

TABLE 8-4   Examples of Common Bacterial Infections

Microorganism	Gram Stain	Respiratory Pathway	Intracellular or Extracellular
Respiratory Tract Infections			
Upper Respiratory Tract Infections			
Corynebacterium diphtheriae (diphtheria)	Gram +	Facultative anaerobic	Extracellular
Haemophilus influenzae	Gram −	Facultative anaerobic	Extracellular
Streptococcus pyogenes (group A)	Gram +	Facultative anaerobic	Extracellular
Otitis Media			
Haemophilus influenzae	Gram −	Facultative anaerobic	Extracellular
Streptococcus pneumoniae	Gram +	Facultative anaerobic	Extracellular
Lower Respiratory Tract Infections			
Bacillus anthracis (pulmonary anthrax)	Gram +	Facultative anaerobic	Extracellular
Bordetella pertussis (whooping cough)	Gram −	Aerobic	Extracellular
Chlamydia pneumonia	Not stainable	Aerobic	Obligate intracellular
Escherichia coli	Gram −	Facultative anaerobic	Extracellular
Haemophilus influenzae	Gram −	Facultative anaerobic	Extracellular
Legionella pneumophila	Gram −	Aerobic	Facultative intracellular
Mycobacterium tuberculosis	Gram + (weakly)	Aerobic	Extracellular
Mycoplasma pneumoniae	Not stainable	Aerobic	Extracellular
Neisseria meningitidis (develops into meningitis)	Gram −	Aerobic	Extracellular
Pseudomonas aeruginosa	Gram −	Aerobic	Extracellular
Streptococcus agalactiae (group B; develops to meningitis)	Gram +	Facultative anaerobic	Extracellular
Streptococcus pneumoniae	Gram +	Facultative anaerobic	Extracellular
Yersinia pestis (plague)	Gram −	Facultative anaerobic	Extracellular
Gastrointestinal Infections			
Inflammatory Gastrointestinal Infections			
Bacillus anthracis (gastrointestinal anthrax)	Gram +	Facultative anaerobic	Extracellular
Clostridium difficile	Gram +	Anaerobic	Extracellular

TABLE 8-4 Examples of Common Bacterial Infections—cont'd

Microorganism	Gram Stain	Respiratory Pathway	Intracellular or Extracellular
Escherichia coli O157:H7	Gram −	Facultative anaerobic	Extracellular
Vibrio cholerae	Gram −	Facultative anaerobic	Extracellular
Invasive Gastrointestinal Infections			
Brucella abortus (brucellosis, undulant fever, leading to sepsis, heart infection)	Gram −	Aerobic	Intracellular
Helicobacter pylori (gastritis and peptic ulcers)	Gram −	Microaerophilic	Extracellular
Listeria monocytogenes (leading to sepsis and meningitis)	Gram +	Aerobic	Intracellular
Salmonella typhi (typhoid fever)	Gram −	Anaerobic	Extracellular
Shigella sonnei	Gram −	Facultative anaerobic	Extracellular
Food Poisoning			
Bacillus cereus	Gram +	Facultative anaerobic	Extracellular
Clostridium botulinum	Gram +	Anaerobic	Extracellular
Clostridium perfringens	Gram +	Anaerobic	Extracellular
Staphylococcus aureus	Gram +	Facultative anaerobic	Extracellular
Sexually Transmitted Infections			
Chlamydia trachomatis (pelvic inflammatory disease)	Not stainable	Aerobic	Intracellular
Neisseria gonorrhoeae (urethritis)	Gram −	Aerobic	Facultative intracellular
Treponema pallidum (spirochete; syphilis)	Gram −	Aerobic	Extracellular
Skin and Wound Infections			
Bacillus anthracis (cutaneous anthrax)	Gram +	Facultative anaerobic	Extracellular
Borrelia burgdorferi (Lyme disease; spirochete)	Gram −	Aerobic	Extracellular
Clostridium tetani (tetanus)	Gram +	Anaerobic	Extracellular
Clostridium perfringens (gas gangrene)	Gram +	Anaerobic	Extracellular
Mycobaterium leprae (leprosy)	Gram + (weakly)	Aerobic	Extracellular
Pseudomonas aeruginosa	Gram −	Aerobic	Extracellular
Rickettsia prowazekii (rickettsia; typhus)	Gram −	Aerobic	Obligate intracellular
Staphylococcus aureus	Gram +	Facultative anaerobic	Extracellular
Streptococcus pyogenes (group A)	Gram +	Facultative anaerobic	Extracellular
Eye Infections			
Chlamydia trachomatis (conjunctivitis)	Not stainable	Aerobic	Obligate intracellular
Haemophilus aegyptius (pink eye)	Gram −	Facultative anaerobic	Extracellular
Zoonotic Infections			
Bacillus anthracis (anthrax)	Gram +	Facultative anaerobic	Extracellular
Brucella abortus (brucellosis, also called undulant fever)	Gram −	Aerobic	Intracellular
Borrelia burgdorferi (spirochete; Lyme disease)	Gram −	Aerobic	Extracellular
Listeria monocytogenes	Gram +	Aerobic	Intracellular
Rickettsia rickettsii (rickettsia; Rocky Mountain spotted fever)	Gram −	Aerobic	Obligate intracellular
Rickettsia prowazekii (rickettsia; typhus)	Gram −	Aerobic	Obligate intracellular
Yersinia pestis (plague)	Gram −	Facultative anaerobic	Extracellular
Nosocomial Infections			
Enterococcus faecalis	Gram +	Facultative anaerobic	Extracellular
Enterococcus faecium	Gram +	Facultative anaerobic	Extracellular
Escherichia coli (cystitis)	Gram −	Facultative anaerobic	Extracellular
Pseudomonas aeruginosa	Gram −	Obligate anaerobic	Extracellular
Staphylococcus aureus	Gram +	Facultative anaerobic	Extracellular
Staphylococcus epidermidis	Gram +	Facultative anaerobic	Extracellular

FIGURE 8-1 General Structure of Bacteria. A, The structure of the bacterial cell wall determines its staining characteristics with Gram stain. A gram-positive bacterium has a thick layer of peptidoglycan *(left).* A gram-negative bacterium has a thick peptidoglycan layer and an outer membrane *(right).* **B,** Example of a gram-positive (darkly stained microorganisms, *arrow)* group A *Streptococcus.* This microorganism consists of cocci that frequently form chains. **C,** Example of a gram-negative (pink microorganisms, *arrow) Neisseria meningitides* in cerebrospinal fluid. *Neisseria* form complexes of two cocci (diplococci). (**A** from Murray PR et al: *Medical microbiology,* ed 7, Philadelphia, 2013, Saunders; **B, C** from Murray PR et al: *Medical microbiology,* ed 4, St Louis, 2002, Mosby.)

these defenses. A vast amount of information has been published about bacterial pathogenesis. The main aspects of how bacteria cause disease may be illustrated in how one particular microorganism, *Staphylococcus aureus,* has adapted to become a life-threatening pathogen.

Staphylococcus aureus has become a major cause of hospital-acquired (nosocomial) infections and is now spreading throughout the community. This microorganism is a common commensal inhabitant of normal skin and nasal passages (estimates depict that from 30% to 80% of individuals may be nasal carriers) and can be transmitted by direct skin-to-skin contact or by contact with shared items or surfaces that have become contaminated by another person (e.g., towels, used bandages).[4]

Although a relatively benign commensal microorganism under normal conditions, *S. aureus* is well equipped to act as a life-threatening pathogen when the opportunity arises; thus it is an opportunistic microorganism. Skin infections may occur at sites of trauma, such as

cuts and abrasions, and at areas of the body covered by hair (e.g., back of neck, groin, buttock, armpit, beard area of men). Most infections are relatively mild and localized, appearing as red and swollen pustules on the skin, containing pus or other drainage. They can develop into abscesses, boils, carbuncles, cellulitis, or furunculosis. Invasive disease may originate from wound infections (e.g., trauma, surgical wounds, indwelling medical devices, prosthetic joints) and lead to fatal septicemia and abscesses in internal organs (e.g., lungs, kidney, bones, skeletal muscle, meninges, or heart) (Figure 8-2).

Microscopically, staphylococci are gram-positive cocci that generally grow in grapelike clusters. However, this microorganism possesses a myriad of potential virulence factors that determine the severity, location, and clinical features of infection. It should be noted that individual strains of this opportunistic pathogen utilize only some of the entire array of virulence factors.

Microorganisms frequently exist as part of complex multicellular masses called biofilms. Biofilms consist of mixed species of microorganisms, including bacteria, fungi, and viruses. Growth of bacteria in biofilms offers survival advantage by protection from the host's responses and exposure to antibiotics. These structures are associated with otitis media; urinary tract infections secondary to indwelling catheters; foot ulcers in diabetic persons; infected burn wounds; vaginitis; osteomyelitis; pneumonia secondary to cystic fibrosis; and diseases of the oral cavity related to dental plaque, such as dental caries and periodontitis. *S. aureus* biofilms are associated with persistent nasopharyngeal colonization and colonization of implanted devices.[5]

A variety of surface proteins mediate adherence among microorganisms in biofilms and to connective tissue (laminin, fibrin, fibronectin) and endothelium. Attachment to collagen occurs in strains causing osteomyelitis and septic arthritis. The capsular polysaccharide mediates attachment to prosthetic devices and also protects against phagocytosis. One surface protein, protein A, binds IgG by the Fc portion so that the Fab regions are facing outward.

Thus, the bacteria appear coated with a self-protein, and, with the Fc bound directly to protein A, the IgG cannot activate complement or act as an opsonin.[6] A coagulase that induces fibrin clotting on the bacterial surface also masks bacterial antigens under a surface of self-proteins. Staphylococcal protein A and also a protein called staphylococcal binder of immunoglobulin are secreted and bind and neutralize IgG. *Staphylococcus* produces proteins that inhibit complement activity, including activation of C3 and C5, preventing production of C3b, C3a, and C5a.[7]

Some strains of *S. aureus* are programmed to avoid innate immunity. They can produce inhibitors of antimicrobial peptides and avoid recognition by Toll-like receptors.[8] Even when engulfed by a phagocyte, *S. aureus* may resist intracellular oxidative killing by inactivating hydrogen peroxide and other reactive oxygen species. They also resist lysozyme by changing the chemistry of the cell wall.[9]

Many bacteria use toxins as virulence factors, including exotoxins and endotoxins. Exotoxins are secreted molecules and are immunogenic eliciting production of antibodies known as antitoxins (important for vaccine development, see page 187). The most poisonous yet discovered is botulinum neurotoxin produced by *Clostridium botulinum;* less than 1 ng/kg is toxic to humans. Strains of *S. aureus* are capable of producing a wide array of secreted toxic molecules or exotoxins. These include those that damage the cell membrane (α-toxin, which forms pores in membranes; hemolysin, which destroys erythrocytes; β-toxin, which is a sphingomyelinase; δ-toxin, a detergent-like toxin; and leukocidin, which lyses phagocytes). Other toxins include coagulase, which causes blood clots; staphylokinase, which breaks down clots; exfoliative toxins, which cause separation of the epidermis resulting in scalded skin syndrome; lipase, which degrades lipids on

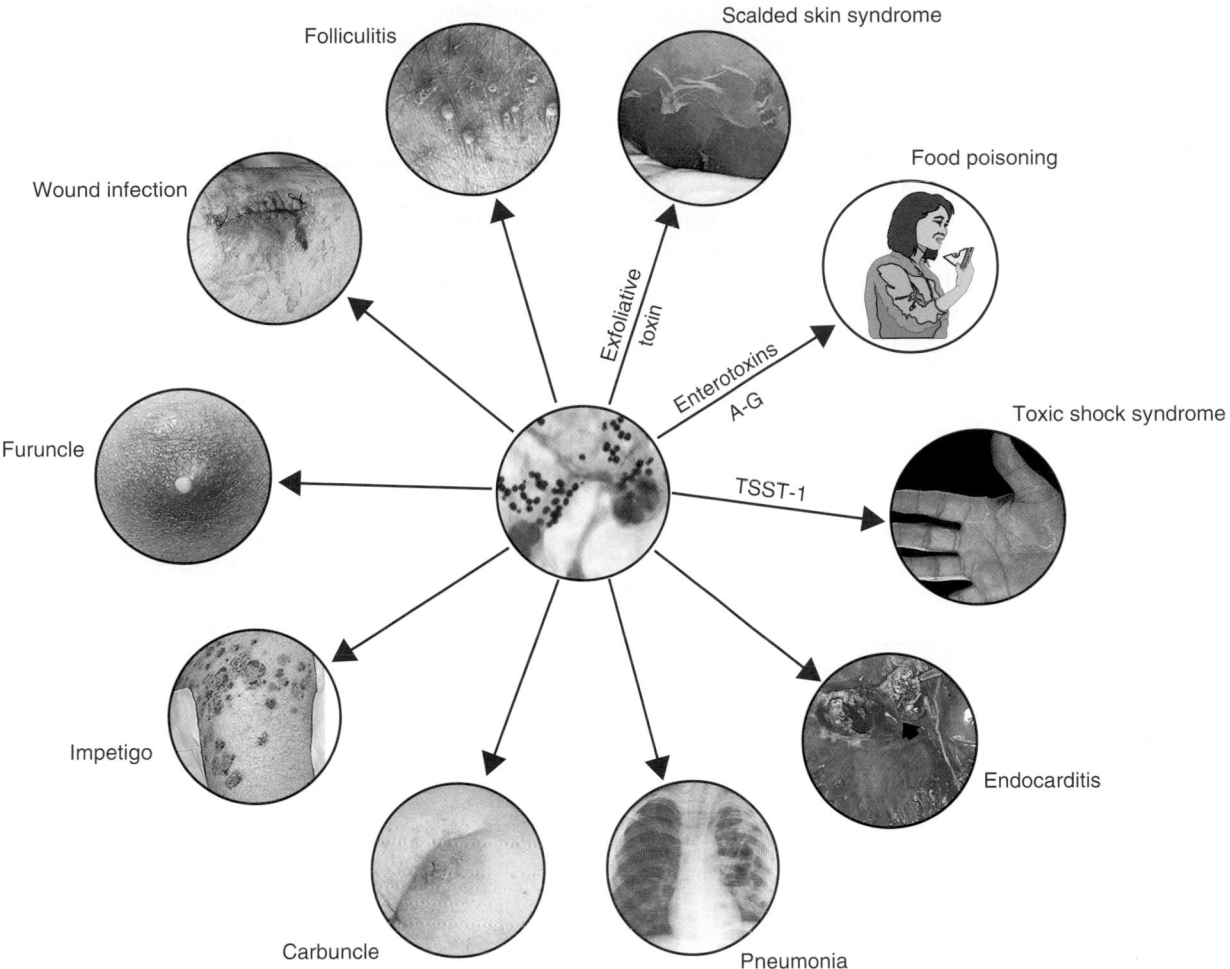

FIGURE 8-2 *Staphylococcus aureus* **Infections.** Different strains of *S. aureus* (gram-positive cocci in sputum from an individual with pneumonia *[center photograph])* cause a variety of infections. The particular infection may depend on the toxin produced: exfoliative toxin (scalded skin syndrome), enterotoxins A-G (food poisoning), or toxic shock syndrome toxin-1 *(TSST-1)*. (Toxic shock syndrome, carbuncle, impetigo, and wound infection photos from Cohen J, Powderly WG: *Infectious diseases,* ed 3, St Louis, 2010, Mosby; folliculitis photo from Goldman L, Ausiello D: *Cecil medicine,* ed 24, Philadelphia, 2012, Saunders; center photo and photos of food poisoning and endocarditis from Kumar V et al: *Robbins and Cotran pathologic basis of disease,* ed 8, Philadelphia, 2010, Saunders; furuncle photo from Long S et al: *Principles and practice of pediatric infectious diseases,* ed 4, Philadelphia, 2012, Saunders; scalded skin syndrome and pneumonia photos from Mandell G et al: *Principles and practice of infectious diseases,* ed 7, Philadelphia, 2010, Churchill Livingstone.)

the skin surface and facilitates abscess formation; enterotoxins, which cause food poisoning; and superantigens (discussed in Chapter 7).[10] Each infectious strain of *S. aureus* may produce a few of these toxins so that strains differ in their capacities to cause particular diseases; thus, different strains may cause purulent dermal infections, food poisoning, or toxic shock syndrome.

Antibiotic resistance has become a major problem with *S. aureus*. For several decades pathogenic strains have commonly produced β-lactamase, an enzyme that destroys penicillin. More recently, staphylococci have developed resistance to broad-spectrum antibiotics, including methicillin-like antibiotics (methicillin-resistant *Staphylococcus aureus* [MRSA]), which were widely used to treat penicillin-resistant microorganisms.

It is clear that *S. aureus* succeeds as an opportunistic pathogen because of a wide array of virulence factors that neutralize important components of the innate and adaptive immune systems, destroy tissue, and resist much of our repertoire of antibiotics. The major remaining option is the development of an effective vaccine, a task that is sometimes difficult.[11] As mentioned in the beginning of this section, *S. aureus* is only one of many bacteria that have developed similar characteristics.

Gram-negative microbes produce an **endotoxin (lipopolysaccharide [LPS])** that is a structural portion of the cell wall and is released during growth, lysis, or destruction of the bacteria or during treatment with antibiotics. Therefore, antibiotics cannot prevent the toxic effects of the endotoxin. Bacteria that produce endotoxins are called pyrogenic bacteria because they activate the inflammatory process and produce fever. The innermost part of the lipopolysaccharide, lipid A, consists of polysaccharide and fatty acids and is responsible for the substance's toxic effects.

Bacteremia occurs when bacteria are present in the blood. Gram-negative sepsis (**sepsis** or **septicemia**) occurs when bacteria are growing in the blood and release large amounts of endotoxin, which can cause endotoxic shock with up to 50% mortality.[12] Released endotoxin, as well as other bacterial products, reacts with pattern recognition receptors (PRRs) and induces the overproduction of proinflammatory cytokines, particularly tumor necrosis factor-alpha (TNF-α), interleukin-1 (IL-1), and interleukin-6 (IL-6), which may secondarily be immunosuppressive.[13] Endotoxin also is a potent activator of the complement and clotting systems, leading to a degree of capillary permeability sufficient to permit escape of large volumes of plasma into surrounding tissue, contributing to hypotension and, in severe cases, cardiovascular shock (see Chapter 24). Activation of the coagulation cascade leads to the syndrome of disseminated (or diffuse) intravascular coagulation (see Chapter 21).

Viral Disease

Viral diseases are the most common afflictions of humans and range from the common cold, caused by many viruses, and the "cold sore" of herpes simplex virus to cancers and acquired immunodeficiency syndrome (AIDS). Examples of human diseases caused by specific viruses are listed in Table 8-5. Viruses are very simple microorganisms consisting of nucleic acid protected from the environment by a layer or layers of proteins (capsid). The viral genome can be double-stranded DNA (dsDNA), single-stranded DNA (ssDNA), double-stranded RNA (dsRNA), or single-stranded RNA (ssRNA). A select group of viruses (e.g., human immunodeficiency virus [HIV], herpesviruses, influenza virus) bud from the surface of an infected cell, retaining a portion of the cell's plasma membrane (envelope) as added protection. Viral replication depends totally on their ability to infect a permissive host cell—a cell that cannot resist viral invasion and replication. Thus,

TABLE 8-5   Examples of Human Diseases Caused by Specific Viruses

Baltimore Classification	Family	Virus	Envelope	Main Route of Transmission	Disease
dsDNA	Adenoviruses	Adenovirus	No	Droplet contact	Acute febrile pharyngitis
	Herpesviruses	Herpes simplex type 1 (HSV-1)	Yes	Direct contact with saliva or lesions	Lesions in mouth, pharynx, conjunctivitis
		Herpes simplex type 2 (HSV-2)	Yes	Sexually, contact with lesions during birth	Sores on labia, meningitis in children
		Herpes simplex type 8 (HSV-8)	Yes	Sexually?, body fluids	Kaposi sarcoma
		Epstein-Barr virus (EBV)	Yes	Saliva	Mononucleosis, Burkitt lymphoma
		Cytomegalovirus (CMV)	Yes	Body fluids, mother's milk, transplacental	Mononucleosis, congenital infection
		Varicella-zoster virus (VZV)	Yes	Droplet contact	Chickenpox, shingles
ssDNA	Papovaviruses	Papillomavirus	No	Direct contact	Warts, cervical carcinoma
dsRNA	Reoviruses	Rotavirus	No	Fecal-oral	Severe diarrhea
ssRNA+	Picornaviruses	Coxsackievirus	No	Fecal-oral, droplet contact	Nonspecific febrile illness, conjunctivitis, meningitis
		Hepatitis A virus	No	Fecal-oral	Acute hepatitis
		Poliovirus	No	Fecal-oral	Poliomyelitis
		Rhinovirus	No	Droplet contact	Common cold
	Flaviviruses	Hepatitis C virus	Yes	Blood, sexually	Acute or chronic hepatitis, hepatocellular carcinoma
		Yellow fever virus	Yes	Mosquito vector	Yellow fever
		Dengue virus	Yes	Mosquito vector	Dengue fever
		West Nile virus	Yes	Mosquito vector	Meningitis, encephalitis
	Togaviruses	Rubella virus	Yes	Droplet contact, transplacental	Acute or congenital rubella
	Coronaviruses	SARS	Yes	Droplets in aerosol or direct contact	Severe respiratory tract disease
	Caliciviruses	Norovirus	No	Fecal-oral	Gastroenteritis
ssRNA−	Orthomyxoviruses	Influenza virus	Yes	Droplet contact	Influenza
	Paramyxoviruses	Measles virus	Yes	Droplet contact	Measles
		Mumps virus	Yes	Droplet contact	Mumps
		Parainfluenza virus	Yes	Droplet contact	Croup, pneumonia, common cold
		Respiratory syncytial virus (RSV)	Yes	Droplet contact, hand-to-mouth	Pneumonia, influenza-like syndrome
	Rhabdoviruses	Rabies virus	Yes	Animal bite, droplet contact	Rabies
	Bunyaviruses	Hantavirus	Yes	Aerosolized animal fecal material	Viral hemorrhagic fever
	Filoviruses	Ebola virus	Yes	Direct contact with body fluids	Viral hemorrhagic fever
		Marburg virus	Yes	Direct contact with body fluids	Viral hemorrhagic fever
	Arenavirus	Lassa virus	Yes	Aerosolized animal fecal material	Viral hemorrhagic fever
ssRNA+ with RT	Retroviruses	HIV	Yes	Sexually, blood products	AIDS
dsDNA with RT	Hepadnaviruses	Hepatitis B virus	Yes	All body fluids	Acute or chronic hepatitis, hepatocellular carcinoma

viruses are obligatory intracellular microbes. Transmission is usually from one infected individual to an uninfected individual by aerosols of respiratory tract fluids, contact with infected blood, sexual contact, or transmission from an animal reservoir (**zoonotic infection**) usually through a vector, such as mosquitoes.[14]

To understand the basic concepts of viral pathogenicity, it may be best to look closely at a single virus. Influenza is a ssRNA virus with a segmented genome (eight pieces of ssRNA). It is transmitted through aerosols or body fluids and is highly infectious. Symptoms begin 1 to 4 days after infection and may include chills, fever, sore throat, muscle aches, severe headaches, coughing, weakness, generalized discomfort, nausea, and vomiting and may lead to pneumonia. It can be fatal, particularly in young children and older adults.[15] The normal rate of infectivity is about 5% to 15%, with a mortality of about 0.1%, and in most cases recovery occurs in 1 to 2 weeks. Yearly seasonal influenza outbreaks result in about 250,000 to 500,000 deaths worldwide.

The life cycle of every virus is completely intracellular and involves several steps, the first being *attachment* to a receptor on the target cell (Figure 8-3). The influenza virion expresses two surface proteins that are essential to virulence. The hemagglutinin (HA) protein is a glycoprotein that is necessary for entrance into cells by binding to glycan receptors on the surface of respiratory tract epithelium. The viral surface neuraminidase (NA) is an enzyme that is necessary for release of new virions from infected cells by cleaving cellular sialic acids (a common component of mammalian cell membranes). The specificity of this virus-receptor interaction (**tropism**) dictates the range of host cells that a particular virus will infect and, therefore, the clinical symptoms that reflect the alteration of the function of the infected cells. Other viruses also use specific receptors; for example, HIV attaches to CD4 on T-helper cells, Epstein-Barr virus (EBV, a cause of mononucleosis and Burkitt lymphoma) attaches to complement receptor 2 (CR2) on B lymphocytes, and *Rhinovirus* (a group of viruses that cause the common cold) attaches to intracellular adhesion molecule-1 (ICAM-1) on respiratory tract epithelium.

Attachment is followed by *penetration* (entrance into the cell by endocytosis or membrane fusion), *uncoating* (release of viral nucleic acid from the viral capsid by viral or host enzymes), *replication* (synthesis of mRNA and viral proteins), *assembly* (formation of new virions), and *release* (exit from the cell by lysis or budding). The influenza virus enters the respiratory tract epithelial cells by endocytosis. Low pH leads to intermembrane fusion between the endosome and viral envelop and uncoating.[16] The viral ssRNA is transported to the nucleus where transcription and replication occur using the viral RNA-dependent RNA polymerase.[17] Viral proteins assemble in the cytoplasm to form the matrix around the viral genome, and the virion buds from the cell surface. Infected cells usually die as a direct effect of the virus. The severity of clinical symptoms is usually secondary to the level of cytokines produced by the infected cells or in response to death of the cells.

The effects of virus on the infected cell vary greatly. Some viruses, such as herpesviruses, will initiate a latency phase during which the host cell is transformed (i.e., herpes simplex viruses 1 and 2 establish latency in neurons). During this phase, the viral DNA may be integrated into the DNA of the host cell and become a permanent passenger in that cell and its progeny. In response to stimuli, such as stress, hormonal changes, or disease, the virus may exit latency and enter a productive cycle. Herpesviruses 1 and 2 are released from the neurons and infect skin epithelium, where lesions in the skin are a result of the immune response against the infected epithelium.

Cytopathic effects caused by other viruses include the following:

1. Cessation of DNA, RNA, and protein synthesis (e.g., herpesvirus)
2. Disruption of lysosomal membranes, resulting in release of digestive lysosomal enzymes that can kill the cell (e.g., herpesvirus)
3. Fusion of host cells, producing multinucleated giant cells (e.g., respiratory syncytial virus)
4. Alteration of the antigenic properties, or identity, of the infected cell, causing the individual's immune system to attack the cell as if it were foreign (e.g., hepatitis B virus)
5. Transformation of host cells into cancerous cells, resulting in uninhibited and unregulated growth (e.g., human papillomavirus)
6. Promotion of secondary bacterial infection in tissues damaged by viruses

The principal method by which influenza virus eludes the immune system is by changing viral surface antigens, a process known as **antigenic variation**. Antibodies against the HA and NA antigens are responsible for protection against influenza infection. Infections are seasonal and protection gained from the previous year's infection does not totally protect against influenza in the following year because the HA and NA antigens undergo yearly change. Usually antigenic variation is relatively minor (**antigenic drift**) and results from mutations. Individuals frequently have partial protection resulting from the previous year's infection, which lessens the clinical effects of the disease. Two groups of influenza virus, influenza A and influenza B, infect humans and the yearly vaccine against influenza is a trivalent mixture of inactivated proteins from two influenza A subtypes and one influenza B subtype. Influenza B almost exclusively infects humans and mutates at a much lower rate than influenza A. Influenza A has antigenically distinct subtypes based on HA (17 forms) and NA (10 forms) antigens. Currently, subtypes H1N1, H1N2, and H3N2 are the primary causes of influenza worldwide.

Influenza A periodically undergoes major antigenic changes (**antigenic shifts**) (Figure 8-4). Influenza A can infect birds and mammals and shifts occur in animals coinfected by a human and an avian strain of influenza. The genome is segmented and the segments can undergo recombination, during which the human virus obtains a new HA or NA antigen. Without a shift occurring, clinical influenza is usually

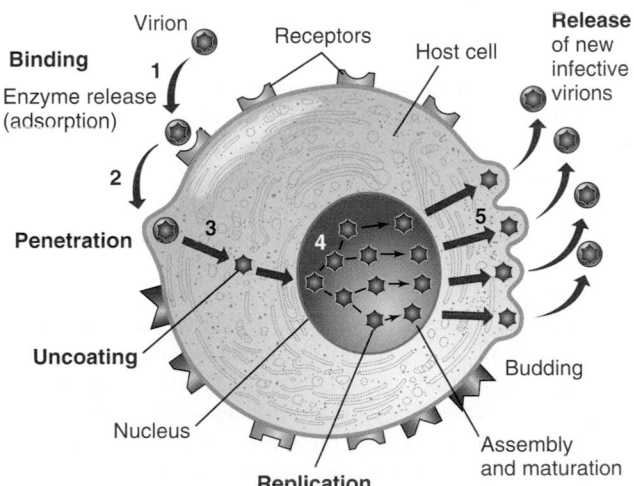

FIGURE 8-3 Stages of Viral Infection of a Host Cell. The virion (**1**) becomes attached to the cell's plasma membrane by absorption; (**2**) releases enzymes that weaken the membrane and allow it to penetrate the cell; (**3**) uncoats itself; (**4**) replicates; and (**5**) matures and escapes from the cell by budding from the plasma membrane. The infection then can spread to other host cells.

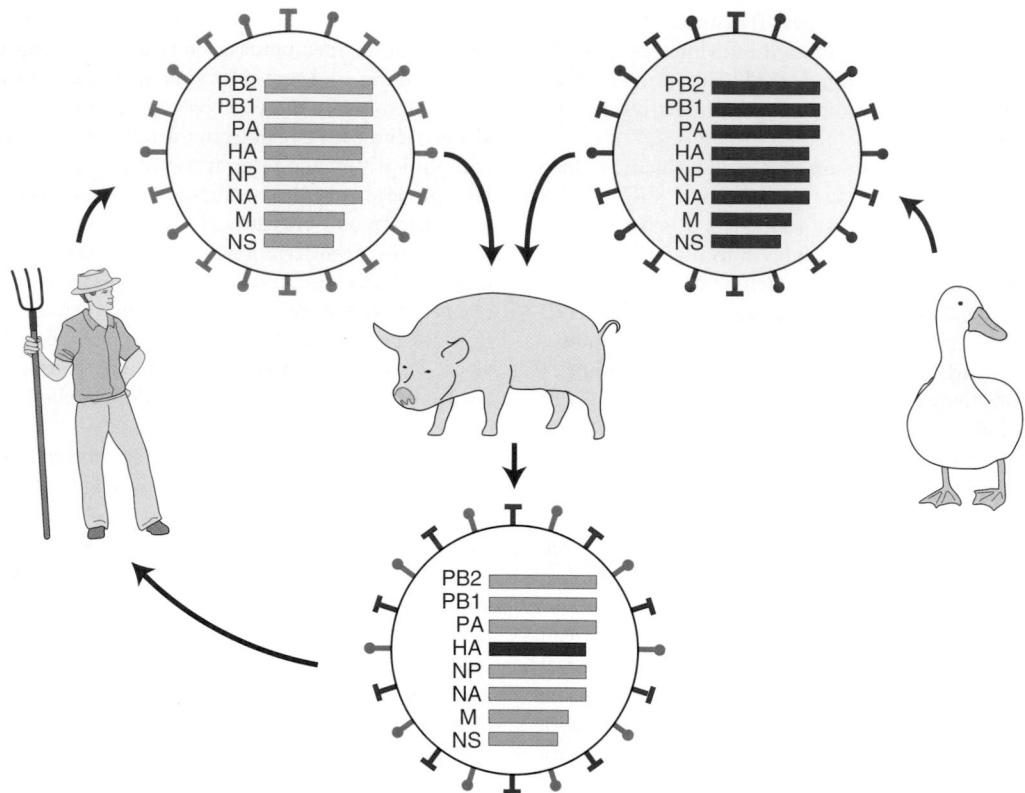

FIGURE 8-4 Antigenic Shifts in Influenza Virus. One theory proposes that antigenic shifts occur when a human influenza virus *(blue)* and an avian influenza virus *(red)* coinfect a species that is permissive for both. The eight ssRNA strands are co-expressed in the same infected cell, resulting in mixing of the strands so that a hybrid virus can be produced. The hybrid virus indicated here contains all the genetic information of the original virus that infected humans, but contains a new hemagglutinin *(HA)*-containing stand from the avian virus. This virus expresses a new HA antigen and will be less susceptible to residual immunity that normally provides partial protection against yearly influenza infections.

considered epidemic (the number of new infections exceeds the number usually observed at other times of the year). When major antigenic changes occur, previous protection may not exist, resulting in a major pandemic (an epidemic that spreads over a large area, such as a continent or worldwide) and much more severe disease.

A major worry regards zoonotic influenza during which a lethal influenza virus that infects birds or other animals suddenly develops the capacity to infect humans.[14] These infections are monitored closely by agencies, such as the Centers for Disease Control and Prevention (CDC) in Atlanta. The CDC is currently monitoring human cases of several zoonotic influenza outbreaks, including swine influenza virus (H1N1), a pathogenic H5N1 avian influenza virus, and a new strain of avian influenza (H7N9) that recently appeared.

Viral pathogens bypass many defense mechanisms by hiding within cells and away from normal inflammatory or immune responses. Some viruses spread from cell-to-cell through the bloodstream (e.g., influenza, rubella) and are highly sensitive to neutralizing antibodies that block viral spread and eventually cure the infection; therefore the disease is described as self-limiting. Other viruses (e.g., measles, herpes) are inaccessible to antibodies after initial infection because they remain inside infected cells, spreading by direct cell-to-cell contact. Most viruses have developed additional defense mechanisms. For instance, influenza virus produces NS1 protein (viral non-structural protein-1) that blocks the antiviral effects of type I interferon.

Fungal Disease

Fungi are relatively large eukaryotic microorganisms with thick walls that have two basic structures: single-celled yeasts (spheres) or multicellular molds (filaments or hyphae) (Figure 8-5). Some fungi can exist in either form and are called dimorphic fungi. The cell walls of fungi are rigid and multilayered and composed of polysaccharides different from the peptidoglycans of bacteria. The lack of peptidoglycans allows fungi to resist the action of bacterial cell wall inhibitors such as penicillin and cephalosporin. Molds are aerobic, and yeasts are facultative anaerobes, which adapt to, but do not require, anaerobic conditions. They usually reproduce by simple division or budding.

Diseases caused by fungi are called mycoses. Mycoses can be superficial, deep, or opportunistic. Superficial mycoses occur on or near skin or mucous membranes and usually produce mild and superficial disease. Fungi that invade the skin, hair, or nails are known as dermatophytes. The diseases they produce are called *tineas* (ringworm), for example, tinea capitis (scalp), tinea pedis (feet), and tinea cruris (groin). Chapter 41 discusses the various skin disorders caused by fungi.

Pathologic fungi cause disease by adapting to the host environment. Fungi that colonize the skin can digest keratin. Other fungi can grow with wide temperature variations in lower oxygen environments. Still other fungi have the capacity to suppress host immune defenses. Phagocytes and T lymphocytes are important in controlling fungi. Low

MOLDS
Filamentous fungi grow as multinucleate, branching hyphae, forming a mycelium (i.e., ringworm)

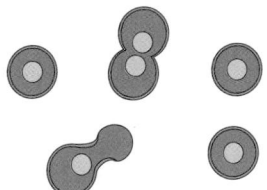

YEASTS
Yeasts grow as ovoid or spherical; single cells multiply by budding and division (i.e., *Histoplasma*)

A

FIGURE 8-5 Morphology of Fungi. (A) Fungi may be either mold or yeast forms, or dimorphic. **(B)** Photograph showing *Candida albicans* with both the mycelial and the yeast forms. **(C)** Oral infection with *C. albicans* (candidiasis, i.e., thrush). **(D)** Gram stain of sputum showing that clinical isolates of *C. albicans* present as chains of elongated budding yeasts (× 1000). (**A, B** from Goering R et al: *Mims' medical microbiology*, ed 5, London, 2013, Saunders. **C** from McPherson R, Pincus M: *Henry's clinical diagnosis and management by laboratory methods*, ed 22, Philadelphia, 2012, Saunders; **D** courtesy Dr. Stephen Raffanti.)

white blood cell counts promote fungal infection and infection control is particularly important for individuals who are immunosuppressed. Common pathologic fungi are summarized in Table 8-6.

Candida albicans is the most common cause of fungal infections in humans. It is an opportunistic yeast that is a commensal inhabitant in the normal microbiome of many healthy individuals, residing in the skin, gastrointestinal tract, mouth (30% to 55% of healthy individuals), and vagina (20% of healthy women). *Candida albicans* is normally under the control of local defense mechanisms, including members of the bacterial microbiome that produce antifungal agents. In healthy individuals antibiotic therapy can diminish the microbiome (e.g., diminished levels of *Lactobacillus* in the gastrointestinal or vaginal microbiome). *Candida* overgrowth may occur, resulting in localized infection such as vaginitis or oropharyngeal infection (thrush).

In immunocompromised individuals, particularly those with diminished levels of neutrophils (neutropenia), disseminated infection may occur. *Candida* is the most common fungal infection in people with cancer (particularly acute leukemia and other hematologic cancers), transplantation (bone marrow and solid organ), and HIV/AIDS. Invasive candidiasis also may be secondary to indwelling catheters, intravenous lines, or peritoneal dialysis, which provides direct entrance into the bloodstream.

Disseminated candidiasis may involve deep infections of several internal organs, including abscesses in the kidney, brain, liver, and heart, and is characterized by persistent or recurrent fever, gram-negative shock-like symptoms (hypotension, tachycardia), and disseminated intravascular coagulation (DIC). The death rates of septic or disseminated candidiasis are in the range of 30% to 40%.

Parasitic Disease

Parasitic microorganisms establish a relationship in which the parasite benefits at the expense of the other species. Parasites range from a unicellular protozoan to large worms. Parasitic worms (helminths) include intestinal and tissue nematodes (e.g., hookworm, roundworm), flukes (e.g., liver fluke, lung fluke), and tapeworms. A protozoan is a eukaryotic, unicellular microorganism with a nucleus and cytoplasm. Pathogenic protozoa include malaria (*Plasmodium*), amoebae (e.g., *Entamoeba histolytica*, which causes amoebic dysentery), and flagellates (e.g., *Giardia lamblia*, which causes diarrhea; *Trypanosoma*, which causes sleeping sickness). Although less common in the United States, parasites and protozoa are common causes of infections worldwide, with a significant effect on the mortality and morbidity of individuals in developing countries. Important parasites of humans are listed in Table 8-7.

Malaria is one of the most common infections worldwide. In 2012, the World Health Organization (WHO) estimated that there were 207 million cases of malaria with an estimated 627,000 deaths; 90% were in Africa where 82% of the deaths were children younger than age 5 years.[18] Malaria is caused by *Plasmodium falciparum*, a protozoan (unicellular) parasite.

TABLE 8-6 Common Pathogenic Fungi

Primary Site of Infection	Fungus	Disease (Primary)	Symptoms
Superficial (no tissue invasion, little inflammation)	*Malassezia furfur*	Tinea versicolor, seborrheic dermatitis, dandruff	Red rash on body
Cutaneous (no tissue invasion, inflammatory response)	Dermatophytes	Tinea pedis (athlete's foot)	Scaling, fissures, pruritus
	Trichophyton mentagrophytes	Tinea cruris (jock itch)	Rash, pruritus
	Trichophyton rubrum	Tinea corporis (ringworm)	Lesion, raised border, scaling
	Microsporum canis		
	Candida albicans	Cutaneous candidiasis	Lesions in most areas of skin, mucous membranes, thrush, vaginal infection
Subcutaneous (tissue invasion)	*Sporothrix schenckii*	Sporotrichosis	Ulcers or abscesses on skin and other organ systems
Systemic (dimorphic; causes disease in healthy individuals)	*Stachybotrys chartarum,* or "black mold"	Black mold disease	Rash, headaches, nausea, pain
	Coccidioides immitis	Coccidioidomycosis	Valley fever, flulike symptoms
	Histoplasma capsulatum	Histoplasmosis	Lung, flulike symptoms, disseminates to multiple organs, eye
	Blastomyces dermatitidis	Blastomycosis	Flulike symptoms, chest pains
Systemic (opportunistic)	*Aspergillus fumigatus, Aspergillus flavus*	Aspergillosis	Invasive to lungs and other organs
	Pneumocystis jiroveci	Pneumocystis pneumonia (PCP)	Pneumonia
	Cryptococcus neoformans	Cryptococcosis	Pneumonia-like illness, skin lesions, disseminates to brain, meningitis
	Candidia albicans	Systemic candidiasis	Sepsis, endocarditis, meningitis

AIDS, Acquired immunodeficiency syndrome; *DNA,* deoxyribonucleic acid; *ds,* double-stranded; *HIV,* human immunodeficiency virus; *RNA,* ribonucleic acid; *RT,* reverse transcriptase; *SARS,* severe acute respiratory syndrome; *ss,* single-stranded.

TABLE 8-7 Examples of Parasites That Are Important in Humans

Category	Subgroup	Species	Disease	Organs Affected/Symptoms
Protozoa	Ameboid	*Entamoeba histolytica*	Amebiasis	Dysentary, liver abscess
	Flagellate	*Giardia lamblia*	Giardiasis*	Diarrhea
		Trichomonas vaginalis	Trichomoniasis	Inflammation of reproductive organs
		Trypanosoma cruzi, T. brucei	Chagas disease: African sleeping sickness	Generalized, blood and lymph nodes, progressing to cardiac and CNS
	Ciliate	*Balantidium coli*	Balantidiasis	Small intestines, invasion of colon, diarrhea
	Sporozoa (nonmotile)	*Cryptosporidium parvum, C. hominis*	Cryptosporidiosis*	Intestine, diarrhea
		Plasmodium spp.	Malaria	Blood, liver
		Toxoplasma gondii	Toxoplasmosis*	Intestine, eyes, blood, heart, liver
Helminths	Flukes (trematodes)	*Fasciola hepatica*	Fasciolosis	Liver destruction
		Schistosoma mansoni	Schistosomiasis	Blood, diarrhea, bladder, generalized symptoms
	Tapeworms (cestodes)	*Taenia solium*	Pork tapeworm	Encysts in muscle, brain, liver
	Roundworms (nematodes)	*Ascaris lumbricoides*	Ascariasis	Intestinal obstruction, bile duct obstruction
		Necator americanus (hookworm)	Hookworm disease	Intestinal parasite
		Trichinella spiralis	Trichinosis*	Intestine, diarrhea, muscle, CNS, death
		Wuchereria bancrofti	Filariasis, elephantiasis	Lymphatics
		Enterobius vermicularis (pinworm)	Pinworm infection	Intestines
		Onchocerca volvulus	Onchocerciasis	Blindness, dermatitis

*Most common in the United States.

Many protozoan parasites are transmitted through vectors or ingested. Vectors include the tsetse fly (*Trypanosoma cruzi,* which causes Chagas disease in South America; *Trypanosoma brucei,* which causes sleeping sickness in Africa) and sand fleas (leishmaniasis). Water and food can be contaminated with protozoal parasites (e.g., *E. histolytica, G. lamblia*). Transmission of *Plasmodium* is through the bite of an infected female *Anopheles* mosquito, where the parasite grows in the salivary gland.

The initial attachment to cells depends on the presence of the microorganism in the bloodstream or gastrointestinal tract. Microorganisms in the bloodstream have surface proteins that allow them to attach to various receptors to infect macrophages, red blood cells, or organ cells such as the liver. For example, multiplication of *Plasmodium* occurs in erythrocytes and results in the release of additional parasites that infect other erythrocytes. Periodic (48 to 72 hours) lysis of the erythrocytes results in anemia and induction of cytokines (e.g.,

TABLE 8-8 Reduction in Vaccine-Preventable Diseases in the United States as of 2009

Disease	Baseline 20th Century Annual Cases*	2011* Cases	% Reduction
Diphtheria	175,885	0	100
Measles	503,282	212	99.9
Mumps	152,209	370	99.4
Pertussis	147,271	15,216	90.8
Smallpox	48,164	0	100
Polio	16,316	0	100
Rubella	47,745	4	99.9
Tetanus	1,314	9	99.9
Haemophilus influenzae type b, invasive	20,000	1,170	94.2

*Average number of reported cases over multiple years before initiation of vaccine.
From Centers for Disease Control and Prevention: *2012 data from provisional cases of selected notifiable diseases, *MMWR Morb Mortal Wkly Rep* 60(51):1762-1765, 2011. Available at: http://www.cdc.gov/vaccines/pubs/pinkbook/downloads/appendices/G/cases-deaths.pdf.

TABLE 8-9 Chemicals or Antimicrobials Identified That Prevent Growth of or Destroy Microorganisms

Mechanism of Action	Agents
Inhibits synthesis of cell wall	Penicillins, cephalosporins, monobactams, carbapenems, vancomycin, bacitracin, cycloserine, fosfomycin
Cell membrane inhibitors	Amphotericin, ketoconazole, polymycin
Damages cytoplasmic membrane	Polymyxins, polyene antifungals, imidazoles
Alters metabolism of nucleic acid	Quinolones, rifampin, nitrofurans, nitroimidazoles
Inhibits protein synthesis	Aminoglycosides, tetracyclines, chloramphenicol, macrolides, clindamycin, spectinomycin
Inhibits folic acid synthesis (needed for protein synthesis)	Sulfonamides, trimethoprim
Alters energy metabolism	Trimethoprim, dapsone, isoniazid

Adapted from Brenner GM, Stevens CW: *Pharmacology*, ed 4, Philadelphia, 2013, Saunders.

TNF-α, IFN-γ, IL-1) that provoke fever, chills, sweating, headache, muscle pains, and vomiting, Severe symptoms include anemia, pulmonary edema, and other complications causing death. Neurologic complications may result from infected red blood cells adhering to endothelium in capillaries of the brain.

Countermeasures Against Infectious Microorganisms

The body's innate and adaptive responses against microorganisms are numerous and involve an interaction between the immune and inflammatory systems. Pathogenic microorganisms, however, have developed means of circumventing the individual's protective defenses. Therefore prophylactic or interventive procedures have been developed either to prevent the pathogen from initiating disease (vaccines, public health measures) or to destroy the pathogen once the disease process has started (antimicrobials). Most vaccine development has focused on preventing the most severe and common infections (Table 8-8). With the initial success of antibiotic therapy, there was no perceived need for vaccination against many common and non–life-threatening infections. The increasing problem of antibiotic-resistant pathogens, however, has forced a reappraisal of that strategy, and a greater emphasis now is being placed on the development of new vaccines.

Infection Control Measures

Although effective means of safeguarding populations from exposure to infectious disease are well-known, lack of implementation or breakdowns in application of these initiatives has led to the reemergence of some infectious diseases, particularly in less developed countries. The following are some examples of environmental infection control measures:

1. Sanitary disposal of sewage, garbage, and animal waste
2. Provision of water treatment and prevention of water contamination
3. Maintenance of sanitation practices for the transport, preparation, and serving of food
4. Control of insect vectors by draining standing water and implementation of mosquito eradication programs
5. Support of research to develop safe agents for insecticide-resistant insect vectors

Antimicrobials

Since initiation of the widespread use of penicillin during World War II, antibiotics have significantly prevented the spread of infections. Antibiotics are natural products of fungi, bacteria, and related microorganisms that affect the growth of other microorganisms. Some antibacterial antibiotics are *bactericidal* (kill the microorganism), whereas others are *bacteriostatic* (inhibit growth until the microorganism is destroyed by the individual's own protective mechanisms). The mechanisms of action of most antibiotics are (1) inhibition of the function or production of the cell wall/membrane, (2) prevention of protein synthesis, (3) blockage of DNA replication, or (4) interference with folic acid metabolism (Table 8-9). Because viruses use the enzymes of the host's cells, there has been far less success in developing antiviral antibiotics.

Immediately after antibiotics became widely used, antibiotic-resistant microorganisms were observed. By 1944 an adequate supply of penicillin allowed its widespread use to treat infections. In 1946 a hospital in Britain reported that 14% of all *Staphylococcus aureus* infections were penicillin resistant, producing β-lactamase, an enzyme that destroys penicillin. The same hospital reported an increase to 59% by 1950 and to greater than 89% in the 1990s.

More than 2 million individuals develop antibiotic-resistant infections yearly, resulting in more than 23,000 deaths. Antibiotic resistance to a single antibiotic has rapidly progressed to multiple-antibiotic resistance. The CDC released a lengthy document on *Antibiotic Resistance Threats in the United States, 2013*, in which 18 pathogens were sorted into "Urgent Threats," "Serious Threats," and "Concerning Threats."[19] The most urgent threats are *Clostridium difficile (C. difficile)*, carbapenem (an "antibiotic of last resort" against penicillin-resistant organisms) resistant Enterobacteriaceae species (i.e., *Klebsiella* and *E. coli*), and drug-resistant *Neisseria gonorrhoeae (N. gonorrhoeae)*.

Many other infections considered routine and easily treatable are now resistant to almost all currently available antibiotics, including methicillin-resistant *Staphylococcus aureus* [MRSA] and *Streptococcus pneumoniae*, which causes pneumonia, meningitis, and acute otitis media (middle ear infection), which were once routinely susceptible to penicillin. Additionally, there are major increases in resistant *Salmonella typhi* (typhoid fever), *Shigella* (bloody diarrhea), *Acinetobacter* (pneumonia), *Campylobacter* (bloody diarrhea), *Enterococcus* (sepsis, wound infection, urinary tract infection), *Pseudomonas aeruginosa* (burn infection, sepsis), and *Mycobacterium tuberculosis* (tuberculosis).[20] Antibiotic-resistant fungi (e.g., fluconazole-resistant *Candida albicans*) have evolved and malarial parasites have recently developed broad drug resistance, including to chloroquine—the previous mainstay of the preventive and therapeutic arsenal of antimalarial drugs.

Antibiotic resistance is usually a result of *genetic mutations* that can be transmitted directly to neighboring microorganisms by plasmid exchange or incorporation of free DNA. Some microorganisms can *inactivate antibiotics,* penicillin resistance being the classic example. Other forms of resistance result from *modification of the target molecule.* Azidothymidine (AZT) is a family of antivirals that suppresses the enzymatic activity of reverse transcriptase, a viral-specific enzyme responsible for the replication of viral RNA and production of a DNA copy. HIV frequently mutates and produces an AZT-resistant reverse transcriptase. Multidrug transporters in the microorganism's membrane mediate a third mechanism of resistance. These transporters affect the rate of intracellular accumulation of the antimicrobial by *preventing entrance* or, more commonly, by *increasing active efflux of the antibiotic.* Antibiotic-resistant strains of *M. tuberculosis* are protected from aminoglycosides and tetracycline by a multidrug pump that increases efflux.

Why have multiple antibiotic–resistant microorganisms appeared? Lack of compliance in completing the therapeutic regimen with antibiotics allows the selective resurgence of microorganisms that are more relatively resistant to the antibiotic. Overuse of antibiotics can lead to the destruction of the normal microbiome, allowing the selective overgrowth of antibiotic-resistant strains or pathogens that had previously been controlled. There also is concern that overuse of antibiotics to promote growth in cattle results in ingestion of antibiotic-containing meat.[21]

Active Immunization

Recovery from an infection generally results in the strongest resistance to a future infection with the same microbe. Vaccines are biologic preparations of antigens that when administered stimulate production of protective antibodies or cellular immunity against a specific pathogen without causing potentially life-threatening disease. The purpose of vaccination is to induce long-lasting protective immune responses under safe conditions. The primary immune response from vaccination is generally short lived; therefore booster injections are used to push the immune response through multiple secondary responses that result in large numbers of memory cells and sustained protective levels of antibody or T cells, or both.

Mass vaccination programs have been tremendously successful and have led to major changes in the health of the world's population.[22] In the early 1950s an estimated 50 million cases of smallpox occurred each year, with about 15 million deaths. The World Health Organization (WHO) conducted an aggressive immunization campaign from 1967 to 1977 that resulted in the global eradication of smallpox by 1979. Many vaccines are used in the United States and the Centers for Disease Control and Prevention (CDC) provides updated

vaccine schedules at their website: www.cdc.gov/vaccines/recs/schedules/default.htm.

Development of a successful vaccine is costly and depends on several factors. These include identification of the protective immune response and the appropriate antigen to induce that response. For instance, individuals with ongoing HIV infection produce a great deal of antibody against several HIV antigens. But, for development of a successful vaccine, we must first understand which antibody, if any, will protect against an initial infection.

Once a good candidate antigen is identified, it must be developed into an effective, cost-efficient, stable, and safe vaccine. Most vaccines against viral infection (measles, mumps, rubella, varicella [chickenpox]) contain live viruses that are weakened (attenuated virus) so they continue to express appropriate antigens but establish only a limited and easily controlled infection. Limited replication of the virus appears to afford better long-term protection than using viral antigen. Current exceptions are the hepatitis B vaccine, which uses a recombinant viral protein, and the hepatitis A vaccine, which is an inactivated (killed) virus and normally should not cause an infection.

Even attenuated viruses can establish life-threatening infections in individuals whose immune systems are deficient or suppressed. The risk of infection by the vaccine strain of virus is extremely small, but it may affect the choice of recommended vaccines. For instance, the Sabin polio vaccine was an attenuated virus that was administered orally. It provided systemic protection and induced a secretory immune response to prevent growth of the poliovirus in the intestinal tract. Being a live virus, the vaccine could cause polio in some children who had unsuspected immune deficiencies (about 1 case in 2.4 million doses). The Salk vaccine was a completely inactivated virus administered by injection. It induced protective systemic immunity but did not provide adequate secretory immunity. Therefore even if the individual was protected from systemic infection by poliovirus, the virus could establish a limited infection in the individual's intestinal mucosa, be shed, and infect others. When polio was epidemic, the oral vaccine was preferred. However, the live attenuated vaccine itself caused about eight cases of paralytic polio per year in the United States in individuals with inadequate immune systems. As a result, the current recommendation of the CDC is vaccination with the killed virus.

Some common bacterial vaccines are killed microorganisms or extracts of bacterial antigens. The vaccine against pneumococcal pneumonia consists of a mixture of capsular polysaccharides from 23 strains of *Streptococcus pneumoniae*. Of the more than 90 known strains of this microorganism, these 23 cause the most severe illnesses. However, the capsular vaccine is not very immunogenic in young children. A *conjugated* vaccine is available that contains capsular polysaccharides from 13 strains conjugated to carrier proteins in order to increase immunogenicity. A similar vaccine is available for *Haemophilus influenzae* type b (Hib).

Some bacterial pathogens are not invasive, but colonize mucosal membranes or wounds and release potent exotoxins that act locally or systemically. Vaccination against systemic exotoxins (e.g., diphtheria, tetanus, pertussis) has been achieved using toxoids—purified exotoxins that have been chemically detoxified without loss of immunogenicity. Pertussis (whooping cough) vaccine has been changed from a killed whole-cell vaccine to cellular extract (acellular) vaccine that contains the pertussis toxoid and additional bacterial antigens. This change has dramatically reduced adverse side effects (fever, local inflammatory reactions, and others) of vaccination.

With so many recommended vaccines, there has been an effort to combine vaccines in order to minimize the number of required injections. One of the first licensed vaccine mixtures was DPT, which now usually contains diphtheria (D) and tetanus (T) toxoids and acellular pertussis vaccine (aP). More recent mixtures include DTaP with inactivated poliovirus, either with Hib conjugate to tetanus toxoid or with hepatitis B antigen.

Common problems confronting vaccination programs include access to the programs in less developed countries or lack of compliance of the susceptible population even when vaccination programs are available. A certain percentage of the population will be genetically unresponsive or less responsive to a particular vaccine and therefore will not produce a protective immune response. As many as 10% of the population may not respond adequately to the recommended series of injections. With most vaccines, the percentage of unresponsive individuals is low, and they will benefit from successful immunization of the rest of the population. Depending on the microorganism, a certain percentage of the population (usually about 85%) should be immunized in order to achieve protection of the total population. This is referred to as herd immunity. If this level of immunization is not achieved, outbreaks of infection can occur. More recently resistance to immunization with measles has increased, and in early 2008 the number of measles cases in the United States increased by about fourfold. In several European countries antivaccine groups have disrupted immunization programs. As a result the incidence of pertussis (whooping cough) increased by 10 to 100 times in those countries compared with neighboring countries that maintained a high incidence of immunization. Immunizations should be complete before children start school.

The reluctance to vaccinate has generally been based on potential vaccine dangers.[23] As with any medicine, complications can arise. In the case of vaccines, these include pain and redness at the injection site, fever, allergic reactions to vaccine ingredients, infection associated with attenuated viruses in immune-deficient individuals, and others. More severe dangers do exist, although they are extremely rare. More commonly the reluctance to vaccination is based on inadequate information.[24] A common fear related to the presence of the preservative thimerosal in vaccines. Thimerosal is a mercury-containing compound that had been used as a preservative since the 1930s. Although no cases of mercury toxicity have been reported secondary to vaccination, thimerosal was removed from all vaccines in 2001, with the exception of some inactivated influenza vaccines. In 2003 groups in northern Nigeria claimed that the oral vaccine was unsafe and were tainted with antifertility drugs (estradiol), HIV, and cancer-causing agents.[25] The reasoning appeared to be secondary to mounting distrust of Western nations because of conflicts in the Middle East. The effect was suspension of polio immunization for almost 1 year in two Nigerian states and reduction of immunization in three other states. The incidence of polio rose dramatically, and more than 27,000 cases of paralysis resulted. The goal of the WHO is to eradicate polio worldwide by 2022. As of November 2014, the total global number of wild polio (naturally occurring) cases was 291; the highest number of cases were in Pakistan (246).[26]

Passive Immunotherapy

Passive immunotherapy is a form of countermeasure against pathogens in which preformed antibodies are given to the individual. Passive immunotherapy with human immunoglobulin has been approved for several infections, including hepatitis A and hepatitis B. Treatment of potential rabies infection after a bite combines passive and active immunization. The rabies virus proliferates very slowly.[27] Individuals who have been bitten receive a onetime injection with human rabies immunoglobulin, or, more recently, with monoclonal antibody to

slow further viral proliferation, followed by multiple injections with a killed viral vaccine to induce greater protective immunity. More specific therapy with monoclonal antibodies is being evaluated for other infectious diseases. A monoclonal antibody against respiratory syncytial virus has been approved for therapy, and recently an experimental monoclonal antibody preparation seems to have neutralized the Ebola virus.

In the past, vaccines and therapeutic antibodies were developed only for the most deadly pathogens. With the increase in antibiotic-resistant microorganisms, the development and widespread use of new vaccines and antibodies against these microorganisms must be considered.[28]

> ✔ **QUICK CHECK 8-1**
> 1. How do antigenic changes in viral pathogens promote disease?
> 2. What are three mechanisms pathogens use to block the immune system?
> 3. What is the difference between an endotoxin and an exotoxin?
> 4. How do bacteria develop antibiotic resistance?

DEFICIENCIES IN IMMUNITY

An immune deficiency is the failure of the immune or inflammatory response to function normally, resulting in increased susceptibility to infections. Primary (congenital) immune deficiency is caused by a genetic defect, whereas secondary (acquired) immune deficiency is caused by another condition, such as cancer, infection, or normal physiologic changes, such as aging. Acquired forms of immune deficiency are far more common than the congenital forms.

Initial Clinical Presentation

The clinical hallmark of immune deficiency is a tendency to develop unusual or recurrent, severe infections. The most severe primary immune deficiencies develop in young children, 2 years old and younger. Preschool and school-age children normally may have 6 to 12 infections per year, and adults may have 2 to 4 infections per year. Most of these are not severe and are limited to viral infections of the upper respiratory tract, recurrent streptococcal pharyngitis, or mild otitis media (middle ear infections).

Potential immune deficiencies should be considered if the individual has experienced severe, documented bouts of pneumonia, otitis media, sinusitis (sinus infection), bronchitis, septicemia (blood infection), or meningitis or infections with rare opportunistic microorganisms (e.g., *Pneumocystis carinii*).[29] Infections are generally recurrent with only short intervals of relative health, and multiple simultaneous infections are common. Individuals with immune deficiencies often have eight or more purulent ear infections, two or more serious sinus infections, and two or more pneumonias, recurrent abscesses, or persistent fungal infections (particularly thrush) within a year. Invasive fungal infections are rare in healthy individuals and strongly indicate a defective immune system. Recurrent internal infections, such as meningitis, osteomyelitis, or sepsis, are common. Prolonged antibiotic use is commonly ineffective by oral or injected routes and may necessitate intravenous administration. Children frequently present with failure to thrive because of chronic diarrhea and other chronic symptoms. A familial history of immune deficiency may be found in some types of primary deficiency.

Routine care of individuals with immune deficiencies must be tempered with the knowledge that the immune system may be totally

TABLE 8-10   Examples of Primary Immune Deficiencies

Classification	Example	Immune Deficiency	Outcome
Combined Immune Deficiencies: Without Nonimmune Defects			
Defective development of both B and T cells	Severe combined immunodeficiencies (SCIDs)	Lack of both T and B cells, little or no antibody production or cellular immunity	Recurrent, life-threatening infections with variety of microorganisms
	X-linked SCID	Defective interleukin receptors needed for lymphocyte maturation	Recurrent, life-threatening infections with variety of microorganisms
Defects in cooperation among B cells, T cells, and antigen-presenting cells	Bare lymphocyte syndrome	No antigen presentation because of lack of MHC class I or MHC class II molecules on cell surface	Recurrent, life-threatening infections with variety of microorganisms
Combined Immune Deficiencies: With Nonimmune Defects			
Defect in actin cytoskeleton	Wiskott-Aldrich syndrome (WAS)	Decreased IgM antibody	Recurrent infections with encapsulated bacteria; thrombocytopenia; eczema
Defective development of T cells in central lymphoid organ (thymus)	DiGeorge syndrome	Lack of T cells	Recurrent, life-threatening fungal and viral infections; defective parathyroid gland; abnormal facial development
Predominantly Antibody Deficiencies			
Defect in class-switch to IgA	Selective IgA deficiency	Diminished or absent IgA	Asymptomatic or recurrent mild sinus, pulmonary, and gastrointestinal infections
Defect in development of B cells in the bone marrow	Bruton agammaglobulinemia	Few B cells	Recurrent bacterial infections
Phagocytic Defects			
Defects in production of neutrophils	Severe congenital neutropenia	Lack of neutrophils	Recurrent, life-threatening bacterial infections
Defects in bacterial killing	Chronic granulomatous disease	Lack of production of oxygen products (e.g., hydrogen peroxide)	Recurrent infections with bacteria that are sensitive to killing by oxygen-dependent mechanisms
Defects in Innate Immunity			
Defect in development of cellular immunity against specific antigen	Chronic mucocutaneous candidiasis	Lack of T-cell response to *Candida*	Recurrent and disseminated infections with fungus *Candida albicans*
Complement Deficiencies			
Defective production of C3	C3 deficiency	Little or no C3 produced	Recurrent, life-threatening bacterial infections
Defective production of component of membrane attack complex	C6, C7, C8, or C9 deficiency	Little or no C6, C7, C8, or C9 produced	Recurrent disseminated infections with *Neisseria gonorrhoeae* or *N. meningitides*
Defective production of component of lectin pathway	Mannose-binding lectin (MBL) deficiency	Little or no activation of lectin pathway	Recurrent infections with bacteria and yeast with mannose-containing capsules

ineffective. It is unsafe to administer conventional immunizing agents or blood products to many of these individuals because of the risk of causing an uncontrolled infection. Infection is a particular problem when attenuated vaccines that contain live but weakened microorganisms are used (e.g., live polio vaccine; vaccines against measles, mumps, and rubella).

The type of recurrent infections may indicate the type of immune defect. Deficiencies in T-cell immune responses are associated with recurrent infections caused by certain viruses (e.g., varicella herpes, cytomegalovirus), fungi, and yeasts (e.g., *Candida, Histoplasma*), or atypical microorganisms (e.g., *P. carinii*). B-cell deficiencies and phagocyte deficiencies, however, are suggested if the individual has documented, recurrent infections with microorganisms that require opsonization (e.g., encapsulated bacteria) or with viruses against which humoral immunity is normally effective (e.g., rubella). Some complement deficiencies resemble defects in antibody or phagocyte function, but others are associated with disseminated infections with

bacteria of the genus *Neisseria* (*Neisseria meningitides* and *Neisseria gonorrhoeae*).

Primary (Congenital) Immune Deficiencies

Most primary immune deficiencies are the result of *single gene defects* (Table 8-10). Generally, the mutations are sporadic and not inherited: a family history exists in only about 25% of individuals. The sporadic mutations occur before birth, but the onset of symptoms may be early or later, depending on the particular syndrome. In some instances, symptoms of immune deficiency appear within the first 2 years of life. Other immune deficiencies are progressive, with the onset of symptoms appearing in the second or third decade of life.

Individually, primary immune deficiencies are rare. For instance, only 30 to 50 new cases of severe combined immunodeficiency (SCID) are diagnosed in the United States yearly. However, more than 250 different deficiencies have been identified, and the number is growing rapidly.[30] Together, primary immune deficiencies are more common than cystic fibrosis, hemophilia, childhood leukemia, or many other well-known diseases. Many are subtle with minor deficiencies, but several result from major defects and lead to recurrent life-threatening infections. The distribution between genders is about even, although some specific diseases have a male or female predominance. The three most commonly diagnosed deficiencies are common variable immune deficiency (34% of individuals with primary immune deficiencies), selective immunoglobulin A (IgA) deficiency (24%), and IgG subclass deficiency (17%).

Primary immune deficiencies have recently been reclassified into nine groups, based on the principal component of the immune or inflammatory systems that is defective.[31] The major groups include combined with or without nonimmune defects (both B and T lymphocytes are deficient, although this group contains some diseases previously classified as T-cell defects), predominantly antibody deficiencies, immune dysregulation (defects in control of lymphocyte proliferation, T-regulatory cells defects), phagocytic defects (inadequate numbers or function), defects in innate immunity, and complement defects. To provide a better understanding of the diversity and severity of primary immune deficiencies, a few select examples will be discussed.

Combined Deficiencies

Combined deficiencies include the most life-threatening disorders and result from defects that directly affect the development of both T and B lymphocytes. However, the severity depends upon the degree to which B and T cells are affected.[32] The most severe disorders are called severe combined immunodeficiencies (SCIDs). Most individuals with SCIDs have few detectable lymphocytes in the circulation and secondary lymphoid organs (spleen, lymph nodes). The thymus usually is underdeveloped because of the absence of T cells. Immunoglobulin levels, especially IgM and IgA, are absent or greatly reduced. Several forms of SCID are caused by autosomal recessive enzymatic defects that result in the accumulation of toxic metabolites, and rapidly dividing cells, such as lymphocytes, are especially sensitive. For instance, deficiency of adenosine deaminase (ADA deficiency) results in the accumulation of toxic purines. X-linked SCID results from a common defect in most of the important interleukin (IL) receptors needed for lymphocyte maturation (e.g., IL-2, IL-4, IL-7, and others).

Even if nearly adequate numbers of B and T cells are produced, their cooperation may be defective. The bare lymphocyte syndrome is an immune deficiency characterized by an inability of lymphocytes and macrophages to produce major histocompatibility complex (MHC) class I or class II molecules. Without MHC molecules, antigen presentation and intercellular cooperation cannot occur effectively. Children with this deficiency develop serious, life-threatening infections and usually die before the age of 5 years.

Some combined immune deficiencies result in depressed development of a small portion of the immune system. For instance, an individual can be unable to produce a certain class of antibody, as in Wiskott-Aldrich syndrome (WAS, an X-linked recessive disorder), where IgM antibody production is greatly depressed. Antibody responses against antigens that elicit primarily an IgM response, such as polysaccharide antigens from bacterial cell walls (e.g., *P. aeruginosa*, *S. pneumoniae, Haemophilus influenzae*, and other microorganisms with polysaccharide outer capsules), are deficient.

Many combined immune deficiencies also are associated with other characteristic defects, some of which appear to be unrelated to the immune system yet may be life-threatening by themselves. These associated symptoms can be useful diagnostically and can clarify the pathophysiology of the disease. WAS results from a mutation in the *WAS*

FIGURE 8-6 Facial Anomalies Associated with DiGeorge Syndrome. Note the wide-set eyes, low-set ears, and shortened structure of the upper lip. (From Male D et al: *Immunology*, ed 8, Philadelphia, 2013, Mosby.)

gene that affects the actin cytoskeleton, which is important for platelet function. Thus, WAS has an associated major defect in platelet function and is classified as a combined deficiency with nonimmune defects. Clinical manifestations include bleeding secondary to thrombocytopenia (low platelet counts), eczema, and recurrent infections (e.g., otitis media, pneumonia, herpes simplex, cytomegalovirus).

DiGeorge syndrome (congenital thymic aplasia or hypoplasia and diminished parathyroid gland development) is caused by the lack or partial lack of the thymus, resulting in greatly decreased T-cell numbers and function. Defective development of the third and fourth pharyngeal pouches during embryonic development results in the thymic defects and the lack of the parathyroid gland (causing an inability to regulate calcium concentration). Low blood calcium levels cause the development of tetany or involuntary rigid muscular contraction. DiGeorge syndrome is frequently associated with abnormal development of facial features that are controlled by the same embryonic pouches; these include low-set ears, fish-shaped mouth, and other altered features (Figure 8-6). Other examples of combined immune deficiencies include defects in CD3 resulting in the loss of T-cell receptor intracellular signaling, defective somatic gene rearrangement of variable region genes or constant region genes, IL-2 receptor defects, and defects in DNA repair.

Predominantly Antibody Deficiencies

Predominantly antibody deficiencies result from defects in B-cell maturation or function and are the most common of immune deficiencies.[33] T-cell immune responses are not affected in pure B-lymphocyte deficiencies. The results are lower levels of circulating immunoglobulins (hypogammaglobulinemia) or occasionally totally or nearly absent immunoglobulins (agammaglobulinemia).

Some defects may involve a particular class of antibody, such as selective IgA deficiency, in which only IgA is suppressed. This occurs in 1 in 700 to 1 in 400 individuals and may result from a failure to class-switch to IgA and mature into IgA-producing plasma cells. Many individuals are asymptomatic, although others have a history of recurring sinus, pulmonary, and gastrointestinal infections. Individuals with IgA deficiency often have chronic intestinal candidiasis (infection with *C. albicans*). Complications of IgA deficiency include severe allergic disease and autoimmune diseases. Secretory IgA normally may prevent the uptake of allergens from the environment; therefore IgA deficiency may lead to a more intense challenge to the immune system by environmental antigens.

Bruton agammaglobulinemia is caused by blocked development of mature B cells in the bone marrow. There are few or no circulating B cells, although T-cell number and function are normal, resulting in repeated bacterial infections, such as otitis media, streptococcal sore throat, and conjunctivitis, and more serious conditions, such as septicemia.

Other predominantly antibody deficiencies include severe reduction in particular classes or subclasses of antibody; defects in B-cell surface receptors, such as CD21 and CD40; and defects in class-switch, which may result in a hyper-IgM syndrome.

Phagocyte Defects

Phagocyte defects range from inadequate numbers of phagocytes (e.g., severe congenital neutropenia) to defects in phagocyte function that can result in recurrent infections with the same group of microorganisms (encapsulated bacteria) associated with antibody, and complement deficiencies. Chronic granulomatous disease (CGD) is a severe defect in the myeloperoxidase–hydrogen peroxide system—a major means of bacterial destruction using the enzyme myeloperoxidase, halides (e.g., chloride ion), and hydrogen peroxide (H_2O_2).[34] As a result of phagocytosis, neutrophils and other phagocytes switch much of their glucose metabolism to the hexose-monophosphate shunt. A byproduct of this pathway is the conversion of molecular oxygen by nicotinamide adenine dinucleotide phosphate (NADPH) oxidase into highly reactive oxygen derivatives, including hydrogen peroxide. Mutations in NADPH oxidase result in deficient production of hydrogen peroxide and other oxygen products needed for phagocytic killing. Thus, affected individuals have adequate myeloperoxidase and halide but lack the necessary hydrogen peroxide. This results in recurrent severe pneumonias; tumor-like granulomata in lungs, skin, and bones; and other infections with some opportunistic microorganisms, such as *Staphylococcus aureus*, *Serratia marcescens*, and *Aspergillus* species. Other phagocytic deficiencies include defects in various leukocyte adhesion molecules, defects in the phagocytosis process or bacterial killing, and defects in cytokine receptors.

Defects in Innate Immunity

Some immune deficiencies are characterized by a defect in the capacity to produce an immune response against a particular antigen. In chronic mucocutaneous candidiasis, interaction between the Th17 lymphocytes and macrophages is ineffective related to a specific infectious agent, *C. albicans*. Thus the macrophage cannot be activated and these individuals usually have mild to extremely severe recurrent *Candida* infections involving the mucous membranes and skin. Other defects in innate immunity include defects in Toll-like receptors and natural killer cells.

Complement Deficiencies

Many complement deficiencies have been described. C3 deficiency is the most severe defect because of its central role in the complement cascade. Loss of C3b and C3a production and the inability to activate C5 result in recurrent life-threatening infections with encapsulated bacteria (e.g., *Haemophilus influenzae* and *Streptococcus pneumoniae*) at an early age. Deficiencies of any of the terminal components of the complement cascade (C5, C6, C7, C8, or C9 deficiencies) are associated with increased infections with only one group of bacteria—those of the genus *Neisseria* (*Neisseria meningitides* or *N. gonorrhoeae*). *Neisseria* bacteria usually cause localized infections (meningitis or gonorrhea), but terminal pathway defects result in an 8000-fold increased risk for systemic infections with atypical strains of these microorganisms.

Mannose-binding lectin (MBL) deficiency is the primary defect of the lectin pathway of complement activation. This defect, as well as defects in the alternative pathway, results in increased risk of infection with microorganisms that have polysaccharide capsules rich in mannose, particularly the yeast *Saccharomyces cerevisiae* and encapsulated bacteria such as *N. meningitidis* and *S. pneumoniae*. Other complement deficiencies include defects in components C1, C4, C2, C5, C1 inhibitor, factor B, factor D, properdin, complement control factors, MASP, or complement receptors.

Secondary (Acquired) Immune Deficiencies

Secondary, or acquired, immune deficiencies are far more common than primary deficiencies. These deficiencies are complications of other physiologic or pathophysiologic conditions. Some conditions that are known to be associated with acquired deficiencies are summarized in Box 8-1.

Although secondary deficiencies are common, many are not clinically relevant. In many cases, the degree of the immune deficiency is

---

BOX 8-1 Some Conditions Known to Be Associated with Acquired Immunodeficiencies

Normal Physiologic Conditions
Pregnancy
Infancy
Aging

Psychologic Stress
Emotional trauma
Eating disorders

Dietary Insufficiencies
Malnutrition caused by insufficient intake of large categories of nutrients, such as protein or calories
Insufficient intake of specific nutrients, such as vitamins, iron, or zinc

Infections
Congenital infections, such as rubella, cytomegalovirus, hepatitis B
Acquired infections, such as AIDS

Malignancies
Malignancies of lymphoid tissues, such as Hodgkin disease, acute or chronic leukemia, or myeloma
Malignancies of nonlymphoid tissues, such as sarcomas and carcinomas

Physical Trauma
Burns

Medical Treatments
Stress caused by surgery
Anesthesia
Immunosuppressive treatment with corticosteroids or antilymphocyte antibodies
Splenectomy
Cancer treatment with cytotoxic drugs or ionizing radiation

Other Diseases or Genetic Syndromes
Diabetes
Alcoholic cirrhosis
Sickle cell disease
Systemic lupus erythematosus (SLE)
Chromosome abnormalities, such as trisomy 21

relatively minor and without any apparent increased susceptibility to infection. Alternatively, the immune system may be substantially suppressed, but only for a short duration, thus minimizing the incidence of clinically relevant infections. Some secondary immune deficiencies (e.g., AIDS or immunosuppression by cancer), however, are extremely severe and may result in recurrent life-threatening infections.

Evaluation and Care of Those with Immune Deficiency

A review of clinical characteristics can help select the appropriate tests. A basic screening test is a complete blood count (CBC) with a differential. The CBC provides information on the numbers of red blood cells, white blood cells, and platelets, and the differential indicates the quantities of lymphocytes, granulocytes, and monocytes in the blood. Quantitative determination of immunoglobulins (IgG, IgM, IgA) is a screening test for antibody production, and an assay for total complement (total hemolytic complement, CH_{50}) is useful if a complement defect is suspected. Further testing is described in Table 8-11.

Replacement Therapies for Immune Deficiencies

Many immune deficiencies can be successfully treated by replacing the missing component of the immune system. Individuals with B-cell deficiencies that cause hypogammaglobulinemia or agammaglobulinemia usually are treated by administration of intravenous immune globulin (IVIg), antibody-rich fractions prepared from plasma pooled from large numbers of donors.[35] Administration of IVIg replaces the individual's antibodies temporarily; these antibodies have a half-life of 3 to 4 weeks. Thus individuals must be treated repeatedly to maintain a protective level of antibodies in the blood.

Defects in lymphoid cell development in the primary lymphoid organs (e.g., SCID, Wiskott-Aldrich syndrome) can sometimes be treated by replacement of stem cells through transplantation of bone marrow, umbilical cord cells, or other cell populations that are rich in stem cells. Thymic defects (e.g., DiGeorge syndrome, chronic mucocutaneous candidiasis) may be treated by transplantation of fetal thymus tissue or thymic epithelial cells (the cells that produce thymic hormones). However, in most cases improvement is only temporary.

Enzymatic defects that cause SCID (e.g., adenosine deaminase deficiency) have been treated successfully with transfusions of glycerol frozen-packed erythrocytes. The donor erythrocytes contain the needed enzyme and can, at least temporarily, provide sufficient enzyme for normal lymphocyte function.

Bone marrow transplants containing hematopoietic stem cells are routinely used to treat SCID. However, as discussed later in this chapter, the donor and recipient should be matched as closely as possible for HLA antigens. Individuals with SCID are at risk for graft-versus-host disease (GVHD). This occurs if T cells in a transplanted graft (e.g., transfused blood, bone marrow transplants) are mature and therefore capable of cell-mediated immunity against the recipient's HLA. The primary targets for GVHD are the skin (e.g., rash, loss or increase of pigment, thickening of skin), liver (e.g., damage to bile duct, hepatomegaly), mouth (e.g., dry mouth, ulcers, infections), eyes (e.g., burning, irritation, dryness), and gastrointestinal tract (e.g., severe diarrhea), and the disease may lead to death from infections. The risk of GVHD can be diminished by removing mature T cells from tissue used to treat individuals with immune deficiencies.[36]

Injection of mesenchymal stem cells (MSCs) may be useful in these individuals. Stem cells are relatively undifferentiated cells and can be obtained from a variety of sources (e.g., embryos, bone marrow, adult tissues). MSCs are present in all adult tissues. These particular stem cells undergo differentiation into other cell types and, more importantly, have potent immunosuppressive properties.[37] Several clinical trials have demonstrated complete suppression of GVHD in a large number of recipients of MSCs.[38]

TABLE 8-11 Laboratory Evaluation of Immune Deficiencies

Function Tested	Laboratory Test	Significance of Test
Tests of Humoral Immune Function		
Antibody production	Total immunoglobulin levels, including IgG, IgM, and IgA	Decrease or absence of total antibody production or of specific classes of antibody, which is associated with many B-cell and combined deficiencies
	Levels of isohemagglutinins	Production of specific IgM antibodies, which is decreased in some combined deficiencies; not useful with persons who are blood type AB and do not have naturally occurring isohemagglutinins
	Levels of antibodies against vaccines—especially diphtheria and tetanus toxoids	Production of specific IgG antibodies, which is decreased when B cells are deficient or class-switch is blocked
B-cell numbers	Numbers of lymphocytes with surface immunoglobulin	Production of circulating B cells, which is decreased in many severe B-cell or combined deficiencies
Antibody subclasses	Level-specific subclasses, particularly IgG1, IgG2, and IgG3	Decrease or absence of a particular subclass, which is characteristic of several immune deficiencies
Tests of Cellular Immune Function		
Delayed hypersensitivity skin test	Skin test reaction against previously encountered antigens, especially *Candida albicans* or tetanus toxoid	Defects in antigen-responsive T cells and skin test cellular interactions (e.g., lymphokine activity and macrophage function)
T-cell numbers	Numbers of T cells expressing characteristic membrane antigens (CD3 or CD11)	Defects in production of circulating T cells
T-cell proliferation in vitro	Proliferative response to nonspecific mitogens (e.g., phytohemagglutinin)	General T-cell defects in response to nonspecific stimulation (mitogens)
	Proliferative response to antigens (e.g., tetanus toxoid)	Defects in response of T cells to specific antigens
T-cell subpopulations	Quantify percentage of T cells with specific markers for total T cells (CD3), Th cells (CD4), Tc cells (CD8)	Decrease in numbers of CD4 cells, which is related to AIDS progression

The first successful therapeutic replacement of defective genes was performed in two girls with SCID caused by an ADA deficiency.[39] The normal gene for ADA was cloned and inserted into a retroviral vector.[40] The gene for ADA replaced some retroviral genes, resulting in a virus that carried the normal human gene but did not cause disease. The virus was used to infect bone marrow stem cells from these children. The retrovirus inserted the normal *ADA* gene into the individuals' genetic material. The genetically altered stem cells were infused into the children, resulting in reconstitution of their immune systems. Gene therapy trials have verified immune reconstitution in individuals with ADA deficiency, X-linked SCID, CGD, and WAS.[41] However, the treatment trials have not been without some major complications, such as leukemia, that raise questions concerning the use of retroviral vectors for the insertion of new genes.

Acquired Immunodeficiency Syndrome (AIDS)

Acquired immunodeficiency syndrome is a secondary immune deficiency that develops in response to viral infection. The human immunodeficiency virus (HIV) infects and destroys the CD4-positive (CD4+) Th cells, which are necessary for the development of both plasma cells and cytotoxic T cells. Therefore HIV suppresses the immune response against itself and secondarily creates a generalized immune deficiency by suppressing the development of immune responses against other pathogens and opportunistic microorganisms, leading to the development of acquired immunodeficiency syndrome (AIDS).

Despite major efforts by healthcare agencies around the world, the number of cases and deaths from HIV infection and AIDS (HIV/AIDS) remains a major health concern. The WHO estimated that at the end of 2013, 35.3 million people were living with HIV/AIDS worldwide and more than 2.5 million were newly infected.[42] Approximately 3 million deaths occur each year from AIDS. Since 1980 it is estimated that more than 36 million individuals have died from AIDS worldwide. The majority of cases are in sub–Saharan Africa where about 1 in 20 adults is living with HIV, but the epidemic is worldwide and the number of new cases is increasing rapidly, particularly in Asia.

In the United States the spread of HIV/AIDS remains somewhat stable. The CDC estimated in 2013 (the most recent data) that approximately 47,352 people were newly infected with HIV.[43] Although new infections remain at about 50,000 per year, both encouraging and discouraging trends were apparent. Although new HIV infections in black women decreased by 12% between 2008 and 2010, new infections in young gay and bisexual men increased by 21%. Men who had sex with men accounted for 78% of new HIV infections in 2010. Heterosexual transmission accounted for about 25% of new HIV infections. with two thirds of those cases occurring in women, with the highest number among black women. Deaths related to HIV/AIDS were 13,712 in 2012, and appear to be decreasing. The cumulative number of HIV/AIDS-related deaths in the United States is in excess of 658,507, and more than 1,201,100 persons age 13 years and older are currently living with HIV/AIDS.

Before the implementation of massive public health campaigns and the use of antiviral drugs in the United States, the progression from HIV infection to AIDS and death was unrelenting. In 1995 AIDS became the number one killer of individuals between the ages of 25 and 44 years and remains the eighth most common cause of death in that age group. With the advent of effective therapy to stabilize progression of the disease in the mid-1990s, HIV infection has become a chronic disease in the United States, with many fewer deaths.

Epidemiology of AIDS

HIV is a blood-borne pathogen with the typical routes of transmission: blood or blood products, intravenous drug abuse, both heterosexual and homosexual activity, and maternal-child transmission before or during birth. Although the disease first gained attention in the United States related to sexual transmission between males, the most common route worldwide is through heterosexual activity (see *Health Alert:* Risk of HIV Transmission Associated with Sexual Practices). Worldwide, women constitute more than half of those living with HIV/AIDS. In the United States, as in the rest of the world, the predominant means of transmission to women is through heterosexual contact. Hundreds of thousands of cases of HIV/AIDS have been reported in children who contracted the virus from their mothers across the placenta, through contact with infected blood during delivery, or through the milk during breast-feeding.

HEALTH ALERT

Risk of HIV Transmission Associated with Sexual Practices

High Risk (in descending order of risk)
Receptive anal intercourse with ejaculation (no condom)
Receptive vaginal intercourse with ejaculation (no condom)
Insertive anal intercourse (no condom)
Insertive vaginal intercourse (no condom)
Receptive anal intercourse with withdrawal before ejaculation
Insertive anal intercourse with withdrawal before ejaculation
Receptive vaginal intercourse (with spermicidal foam but no condom)
Insertive vaginal intercourse (with spermicidal foam but no condom)
Receptive anal or vaginal intercourse (with a condom)
Insertive anal or vaginal intercourse (with a condom)

Some Risk (in descending order of risk)
Oral sex with men with ejaculation
Oral sex with women
Oral sex with men with preejaculation fluid (precum)
Oral sex with men, no ejaculation or precum
Oral sex with men (with a condom)

Some Risk (depending on situation, intactness of mucous membranes, etc.)
Mutual masturbation with external or internal touching
Sharing sex toys
Anal or vaginal fisting

No Risk
Masturbating with another person without touching one another
Hugging/massage/dry kissing
Frottage (rubbing genitals while remaining clothed)
Masturbating alone
Abstinence

Unresolved Issues
The role of precum in transmission
The protection offered by covering female genitals with a dental dam during oral sex on the women
The risk of transmission from wet kissing

Pathogenesis of AIDS

HIV is a member of a family of viruses called retroviruses, which carry genetic information in the form of RNA rather than DNA (Figure 8-7). Retroviruses use a viral enzyme, reverse transcriptase, to convert RNA into double-stranded DNA. Using a second viral enzyme, HIV integrase, the new DNA is inserted into the infected cell's genetic material, where it may remain dormant. If the cell is activated, translation of the viral information may be initiated, resulting in the formation of new

gag
Large protein processed by viral protease into Matrix protein (p17), Capsid protein (p24), and others.

pol
Polymerase
Encodes viral enzymes Protease, Reverse transcriptase, Integrase, and RNAse H

Env
Envelope (gp160)
Large protein processed by cellular protease into Transmembrane protein (gp41) and Surface protein (gp120) that binds to CD4 and chemokine receptors

LTR
Long Terminal Repeat Required for the initiation of transcription

vif, vpr, vpu, tat, rev, nef
Regulatory Proteins
Affect transcription activity, rate of the release of new virions, integration of viral DNA, and other activities

FIGURE 8-7 **The Structure and Genetic Map of HIV-1.** The HIV-1 virion consists of a core of two identical strands of viral RNA molecules of viral enzymes (reverse transcriptase [RT], protease [PR], integrase [IN]) encoated in a core capsid structure consisting primarily of the structural viral protein p24. The capsid is further encased in a matrix consisting primarily of viral protein p17. The outer surface is an envelope consisting of the plasma membrane of the cell from which the virus budded (lipid bilayer) and two viral glycoproteins: a transmembrane glycoprotein, gp41, and a noncovalently attached surface protein, gp120. The HIV-1 genome contains regions that encode the structural proteins (*gag*), the viral enzymes (*pol*), and the envelope proteins (*env*). The genome of complex retroviruses, like HIV-1, often contains a variety of small regions that regulate expression of the virus. (Modified from Kumar V et al, editors: *Robbins and Cotran pathologic basis of disease,* ed 9, Philadelphia, 2015, Saunders.)

virions, lysis and death of the infected cell, and shedding of infectious HIV particles. During that process, HIV protease is essential in processing proteins needed from the viral internal structure (capsid). If, however, the cell remains relatively dormant, the viral genetic material may remain latent for years and is probably present for the life of the individual.

The primary surface receptor on HIV is the envelope protein gp120, which binds to the molecule CD4 on the surface of Th cells. Several other necessary co-receptors, particularly the chemokine receptor CCR5, have been identified on target cells. Thus the major immunologic finding in AIDS is the striking decrease in the number of CD4+ Th cells (Figure 8-8).

Clinical Manifestations of AIDS

Depletion of CD4+ cells has a profound effect on the immune system, causing a severely diminished response to a wide array of infectious pathogens and cancers (Box 8-2). At the time of diagnosis, the individual may present with one of several different conditions: serologically negative (no detectable antibody), serologically positive (positive for antibody against HIV proteins) but asymptomatic, early stages of HIV disease, or AIDS (Figure 8-9).

The presence of circulating antibody against the HIV protein p24 followed by more complex tests for antibodies against additional HIV proteins (e.g., Western blot analysis) or for HIV DNA (e.g., polymerase chain reaction) indicates infection by the virus, although many of these

FIGURE 8-8 Life Cycle and Possible Sites of Therapeutic Intervention of Human Immunodeficiency Virus (HIV). The HIV virion consists of a core of two identical strands of viral RNA encoated in a protein structure with viral proteins gp41 and gp120 on its surface (envelope). HIV infection begins when a virion binds to CD4 and chemokine co-receptors on a susceptible cell and follows the process described here. The provirus may remain latent in the cell's DNA until it is activated (e.g., by cytokines). The HIV life cycle is susceptible to blockage at several sites (see the text for further information), including entrance inhibitors, reverse transcriptase inhibitors, integrase inhibitors, and protease inhibitors. (Modified from Kumar V et al, editors: *Robbins and Cotran pathologic basis of disease,* ed 9, Philadelphia, 2015, Saunders.)

BOX 8-2   AIDS-Defining Opportunistic Infections and Neoplasms Found in Individuals with HIV Infection

Infections

Protozoal and Helminthic Infections

Cryptosporidiosis or isosporiasis (enteritis)

Pneumocystosis (pneumonia or disseminated infection)

Toxoplasmosis (pneumonia or CNS infection)

Fungal Infections

Candidiasis (esophageal, tracheal, or pulmonary)

Coccidioidomycosis (disseminated)

Cryptococcosis (CNS infection)

Histoplasmosis (disseminated)

Bacterial Infections

Mycobacteriosis ("atypical," e.g., *Mycobacterium avium-intracellulare*, disseminated or extrapulmonary

M. tuberculosis, disseminated or extrapulmonary)

Nocardiosis (pneumonia, meningitis, disseminated)

Salmonella infections (septicemia, recurrent)

Viral Infections

Cytomegalovirus (pulmonary, intestinal, retinitis, or CNS)

Herpes simplex virus (localized or disseminated)

Progressive multifocal leukoencephalopathy

Varicella-zoster virus (localized or disseminated)

Neoplasms

Invasive cancer of the uterine cervix

Kaposi sarcoma

Non-Hodgkin lymphomas (Burkitt, immunoblastic)

Primary lymphoma of brain

CNS, Central nervous system.

From Kumar V et al: *Robbins and Cotran pathologic basis of disease*, ed 9, Philadelphia, 2015, Saunders.

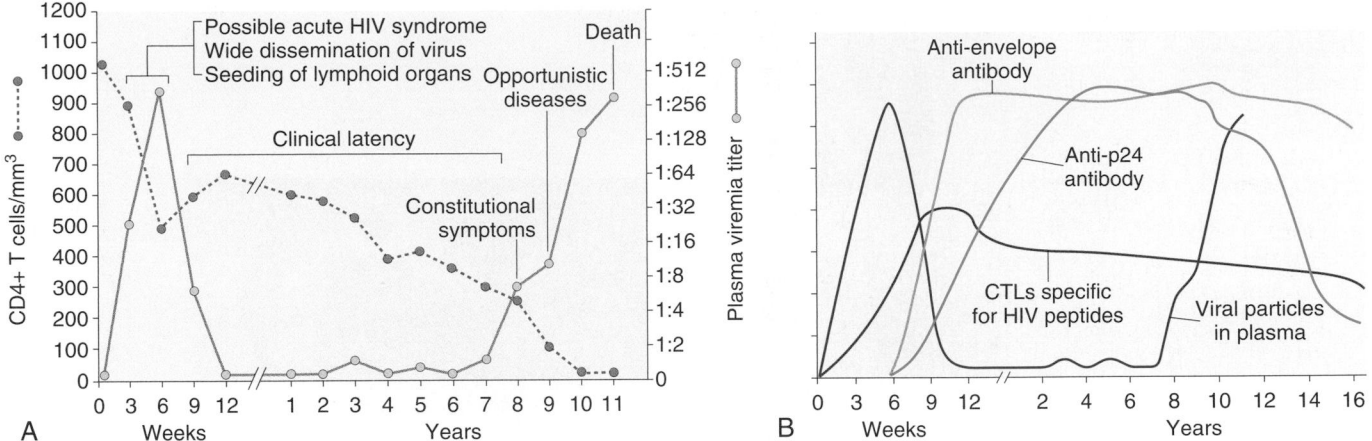

FIGURE 8-9 Typical Progression from HIV Infection to AIDS in Untreated Persons. A, Clinical progression begins within weeks after infection; the person may experience symptoms of acute HIV syndrome. During this early period, the virus progressively infects T cells and other cells and spreads to the lymphoid organs, with a sharp decrease in the number of circulating CD4+ T cells. During a period of clinical latency, the virus replicates and T-cell destruction continues, although the person is generally asymptomatic. The individual may develop HIV-related disease (constitutional symptoms)—a variety of symptoms of acute viral infection that do not involve opportunistic infections or malignancies. When the number of CD4+ cells is critically suppressed, the individual becomes susceptible to a variety of opportunistic infections and cancers with a diagnosis of AIDS. The length of time for progression from HIV infection to AIDS may vary considerably from person to person. **B,** Laboratory tests are changing throughout infection. Antibody and Tc cell (cytotoxic T lymphocytes [CTLs]) levels change during the progression to AIDS. During the initial phase antibodies against HIV-1 are not yet detectable (window period), but viral products, including proteins and RNA, and infectious virus may be detectable in the blood a few weeks after infection. Most antibodies against HIV are not detectable in the early phase. During the latent phase of infection antibody levels against p24 and other viral proteins, as well as HIV-specific CTLs, increase, and then remain constant until the development of AIDS. (**A** redrawn from Fauci AS, Lane HC: Human immunodeficiency virus disease: AIDS and related conditions. In Fauci AS et al, editors: *Harrison's principles of internal medicine,* ed 14, New York, 1997, McGraw-Hill; **B** from Kumar V et al: *Robbins and Cotran pathologic basis of disease,* ed 9, Philadelphia, 2015, Saunders.)

individuals are asymptomatic. Antibody appears rather rapidly after infection through blood products, usually within 4 to 7 weeks, although some individuals have been seronegative for longer periods. The period between infection and the appearance of antibody is referred to as the window period. Although a person does not have antibody against HIV, he or she may have virus growing, have virus in the blood and body fluids, and be infectious to others.

Those with the early stages of HIV disease (early-stage disease) usually initially present with relatively mild and nonspecific symptoms resembling influenza, such as headaches, fever, or fatigue. These symptoms disappear after 1 to 6 weeks, and although individuals appear to be in clinical latency the virus is actively proliferating in lymph nodes.

The currently accepted definition of AIDS relies on both laboratory tests and clinical symptoms. If the individual is positive for antibodies against HIV, the diagnosis of AIDS is made in association with various clinical symptoms (Figure 8-10; also see Box 8-2). The symptoms include atypical or opportunistic infections and cancers, as well as indications of debilitating chronic disease (e.g., wasting syndrome, recurrent fevers). Most commonly, new cases of AIDS are diagnosed initially by decreased CD4+ T cell numbers. Individuals who are not HIV infected typically have 800 to 1000 CD4+ cells per cubic millimeter of blood, with a range from 600/mm³ to 1200/mm³. A diagnosis of AIDS can be made if the CD4+ T cell numbers decrease to less than 200/mm³. Without treatment, the average time from infection to development of AIDS is just over 10 years. Some estimates are that approximately 99% of untreated HIV-infected individuals would eventually progress to AIDS.

Treatment and Prevention of AIDS

Approved AIDS medications are classified by mechanism of action: nucleoside and non-nucleoside inhibitors of reverse transcriptase (**reverse transcriptase inhibitors**), inhibitors of the viral protease (**HIV protease inhibitors**), inhibitors of the viral integrase (**HIV integrase inhibitors**), inhibitors of viral entrance into the target cell (**HIV fusion inhibitors**), and a **CCR5 antagonist** (inhibitor of viral attachment) (see Figure 8-8). The current regimen for treatment of HIV infection is a combination of drugs, termed **antiretroviral therapy** (**ART**). ART protocols require a combination of synergist drugs from different classes and specific regimens (e.g., timing of drug administration, doses, drug combinations) are adapted based on age of the individual, secondary clinical symptoms (renal or hepatic insufficiency), CD4+ T cell levels, viral load, specific coinfections, pre-existing cardiac risk factors, past history of treatment failure, suspected drug resistance, and other parameters.[44,45] The clinical benefits of ART are profound. Death from AIDS-related diseases has been reduced significantly since the introduction of ART. However, resistant variants to these drugs have been identified. Drug therapy for AIDS is not curative because HIV incorporates into the genetic material of the host, particularly CD4+ T memory cells, and may never be removed by antimicrobial therapy.[46] Therefore drug administration to control the virus may have to continue for the lifetime of the individual. Additionally, HIV may persist in regions where the antiviral drugs are not as effective, such as the CNS.

The chronic nature of HIV/AIDS resulting from successful ART has led to additional concerns. Long-term toxicity of ART drugs has

FIGURE 8-10 Clinical Symptoms of AIDS. A, Severe weight loss and anorexia. B, Kaposi sarcoma lesions. C, Perianal lesions of herpes simplex infection. D, Deterioration of vision from cytomegalovirus retinitis leading to areas of infection, which can lead to blindness. (A and D from Taylor PK: *Diagnostic picture tests in sexually transmitted diseases,* London, 1995, Mosby; B and C from Morse SA et al, editors: *Atlas of sexually transmitted diseases and AIDS,* ed 4, London, 2011, Saunders.)

resulted in increased risk for cardiovascular disease, metabolic disorders, and organ failure. Treated individuals frequently fail to reconstitute their immune system and develop chronic immune activation characterized by activation of monocytes and T cells, production of pro-inflammatory cytokines (e.g., interferon- γ [IFN-γ], interleukin-6 [IL-6]), and depletion of Th17 cells.[47] Chronic immune activation tends to exacerbate clinical disease in adults and neonates.[48]

Vaccine development should be the most effective means of preventing HIV infection and may be useful in treating preexisting infection. Most of the common viral vaccines (e.g., rubella, mumps, influenza) induce protective antibodies that block the initial infection. Only one vaccine (rabies) is used after the infection has occurred. The rabies vaccine is successful because the rabies virus proliferates and spreads very slowly. However, the ability of an HIV vaccine to either successfully prevent or treat HIV infection is questionable for several reasons.[49] First, the AIDS virus is genetically and antigenically variable, like the influenza virus, so that a vaccine created against one variant may not provide protection against another variant. Second, although individuals with HIV/AIDS have high levels of circulating antibodies against the virus, these antibodies do not appear to be protective. Therefore even if a circulating antibody response can be induced by vaccination, that response might not be effective. A vaccine may have to induce both circulating and secretory (to prevent initial infection of the mucosal T cell) antibody and Tc cells.

Pediatric AIDS and Central Nervous System Involvement

HIV can be transmitted from mother to child during pregnancy, at the time of delivery, or through breast-feeding, although the risk of mother-to-child transmission has dropped precipitously since the use of anti-retroviral drugs in pregnant women. The clinical diagnosis of HIV infection in young children born of HIV-infected mothers is very often a difficult task because the presence of maternal antibodies may result in a misleading false-positive test for antibodies against HIV for as long as 18 months after birth. Testing for antibody against HIV can be performed recurrently from birth until 18 months; if the test results

TABLE 8-12   Relative Incidence and Examples of Hypersensitivity Diseases*

| | MECHANISM | | | |
Target Antigen	Type I (IgE Mediated)	Type II (Tissue Specific)	Type III (Immune Complex Mediated)	Type IV (Cell Mediated)
Allergy Environmental antigens	++++ Hay fever	+ Hemolysis in drug allergies	+ Gluten (wheat) allergy	++ Poison ivy allergy
Autoimmunity Self-antigens	+ May contribute to some type III reactions	++ Autoimmune thrombocytopenia	+++ Systemic lupus erythematosus	++ Hashimoto thyroiditis
Alloimmunity Another person's antigens	+ May contribute to some type III reactions	++ Hemolytic disease of the newborn	+ Individuals who do not make their own IgA may have an anaphylactic response against IgA in human immune globulin	++ Graft rejection

*The frequency of each reaction is indicated in a range from rare (+) to very common (++++). An example of each reaction is given.

become negative and remain so after 12 months, the child can be considered uninfected.

The 2008 revised surveillance case definition for HIV infection in children younger than 18 months, which remains in effect today, recommends testing for HIV or viral components in two separate specimens, not including cord blood.[50] These include detection of HIV nucleic acid or p24 antigen, or direct isolation of HIV in viral cultures.

HIV infection of babies is generally more aggressive than in adults; on average an untreated child will die by his or her second birthday. Neurologic involvement occurs more commonly in children than in adults and results from CNS involvement, rather than effects on peripheral portions of the nervous system. HIV encephalopathy occurs with varying degrees of severity and is a clinical component in the diagnosis of AIDS in children. Most HIV-infected newborns appear normal, but may progressively develop signs of CNS involvement. These usually appear as failure to attain, or loss of, developmental milestones or loss of intellectual ability, verified by standard developmental scale or neuropsychologic tests; acquired symmetric motor deficits, seen in children older than age 1 month; impaired brain growth or acquired microcephaly, demonstrated by head circumference measurements; or brain atrophy, demonstrated by computed tomography (CT) or magnetic resonance imaging (MRI) with serial imaging and required in children younger than 2 years of age.

It may be difficult to completely differentiate the effect of HIV infection on the CNS from other risk factors, including prenatal drug exposure, prematurity, chronic illness, and a chaotic social atmosphere. The pathogenesis of HIV encephalopathy in children is poorly understood, but the presence of inflammatory mediators may be a contributing factor.

Because HIV infection in infants progresses very rapidly, treatment must begin at the diagnosis of infection. In older children the criteria for treatment are similar to those used in adults. A growing number of investigational protocols are available for treatment of children with HIV. In general, treatment is focused on the preservation and maintenance of the immune system, aggressive response to opportunistic infections, support and relief of symptomatic occurrences, and administration of ART.

HYPERSENSITIVITY: ALLERGY, AUTOIMMUNITY, AND ALLOIMMUNITY

Allergy, autoimmunity, and alloimmunity are classified as *hypersensitivity reactions*. **Hypersensitivity** is an altered immunologic response

---

✔ QUICK CHECK 8-2

1. Why is the development of recurrent or unusual infections the clinical hallmark of immunodeficiency?
2. Compare and contrast the most common infections in individuals with defects in cell-mediated immune response and those with defects in humoral immune response.
3. What are the new treatments for HIV?

---

to an antigen that results in disease or damage to the individual. Allergy, autoimmunity, and alloimmunity (also termed *isoimmunity*) can be most easily understood in relationship to the source of the antigen against which the hypersensitivity response is directed (Table 8-12). **Allergy** refers to a hypersensitivity to environmental antigens. These can include medicines, natural products (e.g., pollens, bee stings), infectious agents, and any other antigen that is not naturally found in the individual.

Autoimmunity is a disturbance in the immunologic tolerance of self-antigens. The immune system normally does not strongly recognize the individual's own antigens. Healthy individuals of all ages, but particularly the elderly, may produce low quantities of antibodies against their own antigens (*autoantibodies*) without developing overt autoimmune disease. Therefore the presence of low quantities of autoantibodies does not necessarily indicate a disease state. Autoimmune diseases occur when the immune system reacts against self-antigens to such a degree that autoantibodies or autoreactive T cells damage the individual's tissues. Many clinical disorders are associated with autoimmunity and are generally referred to as **autoimmune diseases** (Table 8-13). Autoimmune diseases are more prevalent in women and the overall prevalence is rising.[51]

Alloimmune diseases occur when the immune system of one individual produces an immunologic reaction against tissues of another individual. **Alloimmunity** can be observed during immunologic reactions against transfusions, transplanted tissue, or the fetus during pregnancy.

The mechanism that initiates the onset of hypersensitivity, whether allergy, autoimmunity, or alloimmunity, is not completely understood. It is generally accepted that genetic, infectious, and possibly environmental factors contribute to the development of hypersensitivity reactions.

Mechanisms of Hypersensitivity

Hypersensitivity reactions can be characterized also by the particular immune mechanism that results in the disease (Table 8-14). These

TABLE 8-13   Examples of Autoimmune Disorders

System Disease	Organ or Tissue	Probable Self-Antigen
Endocrine System		
Hyperthyroidism (Graves disease)	Thyroid gland	Receptors for thyroid-stimulating hormone on plasma membrane of thyroid cells
Hashimoto hypothyroidism	Thyroid gland	Thyroid cell surface antigens, thyroglobulin
Insulin-dependent diabetes	Pancreas	Islet cells, insulin, insulin receptors on pancreatic cells
Addison disease	Adrenal gland	Surface antigens on steroid-producing cells; microsomal antigens
Male infertility	Testis	Surface antigens on spermatozoa
Skin		
Pemphigus vulgaris	Skin	Intercellular substances in stratified squamous epithelium
Bullous pemphigoid	Skin	Basement membrane
Vitiligo	Skin	Surface antigens on melanocytes (melanin-producing cells)
Neuromuscular Tissue		
Multiple sclerosis	Neural tissue	Surface antigens of nerve cells
Myasthenia gravis	Neuromuscular junction	Acetylcholine receptors; striations of skeletal and cardiac muscle
Rheumatic fever	Heart	Cardiac tissue antigens that cross-react with group A streptococcal antigen
Cardiomyopathy	Heart	Cardiac muscle
Gastrointestinal System		
Ulcerative colitis	Colon	Mucosal cells
Pernicious anemia	Stomach	Surface antigens of parietal cells; intrinsic factor
Primary biliary cirrhosis	Liver	Cells of bile duct
Chronic active hepatitis	Liver	Surface antigens of hepatocytes, nuclei, microsomes, smooth muscle
Eye		
Sjögren syndrome	Lacrimal gland	Antigens of lacrimal gland, salivary gland, thyroid, and nuclei of cells
Connective Tissue		
Ankylosing spondylitis	Joints	Sacroiliac and spinal apophyseal joint
Rheumatoid arthritis	Joints	Collagen, IgG
Systemic lupus erythematosus	Multiple sites	Numerous antigens in nuclei, organelles, and extracellular matrix
Renal System		
Immune complex glomerulonephritis	Kidney	Numerous immune complexes
Goodpasture syndrome	Kidney	Glomerular basement membrane
Hematologic System		
Idiopathic neutropenia	Neutrophil	Surface antigens on polymorphonuclear neutrophils
Idiopathic lymphopenia	Lymphocytes	Surface antigens on lymphocytes
Autoimmune hemolytic anemia	Erythrocytes	Surface antigens on erythrocytes
Autoimmune thrombocytopenic purpura	Platelets	Surface antigens on platelets
Respiratory System		
Goodpasture syndrome	Lung	Septal membrane of alveolus

TABLE 8-14   Immunologic Mechanisms of Tissue Destruction

Type	Name	Rate of Development	Class of Antibody Involved	Principal Effector Cells Involved	Participation of Complement	Examples of Disorders
I	IgE-mediated reaction	Immediate	IgE	Mast cells	No	Seasonal allergic rhinitis Asthma
II	Tissue-specific reaction	Immediate	IgG IgM	Macrophages in tissues	Frequently	Autoimmune thrombocytopenic purpura, Graves disease, autoimmune hemolytic anemia
III	Immune complex–mediated reaction	Immediate	IgG IgM	Neutrophils	Yes	Systemic lupus erythematosus
IV	Cell-mediated reaction	Delayed	None	Lymphocytes Macrophages	No	Contact sensitivity to poison ivy, metals (jewelry), and latex

mechanisms are apparent in most hypersensitivity reactions and have been divided into four distinct types: *type I* (IgE-mediated reactions), *type II* (tissue-specific reactions), *type III* (immune complex–mediated reactions), and *type IV* (cell-mediated reactions). This classification is artificial and seldom is a particular disease associated with only a single mechanism. The four mechanisms are interrelated, and in most hypersensitivity reactions several mechanisms can be functioning simultaneously or sequentially.

As with all immune responses, hypersensitivity reactions require sensitization against a particular antigen that results in a primary immune response. Disease symptoms appear after an adequate secondary immune response occurs. Hypersensitivity reactions are immediate or delayed, depending on the time required to elicit clinical symptoms after reexposure to the antigen. Reactions that occur within minutes to a few hours after exposure to antigen are termed immediate hypersensitivity reactions. Delayed hypersensitivity reactions may take several hours to appear and are at maximal severity days after reexposure to the antigen. Generally, immediate reactions are caused by antibody, whereas delayed reactions are caused by cells (e.g., T cells, NK cells, macrophages).

The most rapid and severe immediate hypersensitivity reaction is anaphylaxis. Anaphylaxis occurs within minutes of reexposure to the antigen and can be either systemic (generalized) or cutaneous (localized). Symptoms of systemic anaphylaxis include pruritus, erythema, vomiting, abdominal cramps, diarrhea, and breathing difficulties, and the most severe reactions may include contraction of bronchial smooth muscle, edema of the throat, and decreased blood pressure that can lead to shock and death.[52] Examples of systemic anaphylaxis are allergic reactions to bee stings (see p. 206), peanuts, shellfish, or eggs. Cutaneous anaphylaxis results in local symptoms, such as pain, swelling, and redness, which occur at the site of exposure to an antigen (e.g., a painful local reaction to an injected vaccine or drug).

Type I: IgE-Mediated Hypersensitivity Reactions

Type I hypersensitivity reactions are mediated by antigen-specific IgE and the products of tissue mast cells (Figure 8-11). Most common allergic reactions are type I reactions. In addition, most type I reactions occur against environmental antigens and are therefore allergic. Because of this strong association, many healthcare professionals use the term *allergy* to indicate only IgE-mediated reactions. However, IgE

FIGURE 8-11 Mechanism of Type I, IgE-Mediated Reactions. First exposure to an allergen leads to antigen processing and presentation of antigen by an antigen-presenting cell (APC) to B lymphocytes, which is under the direction of T-helper 2 (Th2) cells. Th2 cells produce specific cytokines (e.g., IL-4, IL-13, and others) that favor maturation of the B lymphocytes into plasma cells that secrete IgE. The IgE is adsorbed to the surface of the mast cell by binding with IgE-specific Fc receptors. When an adequate amount of IgE is bound the mast cell is sensitized. During a reexposure, the allergen cross-links the surface-bound IgE and causes degranulation of the mast cell. Contents of the mast cell granules, primarily histamine, induce local edema, smooth muscle contraction, mucous secretion, and other characteristics of an acute inflammatory reaction. (See Chapter 6 for more details on the role of mast cells in inflammation.)

can contribute to some autoimmune and alloimmune diseases, and many common allergies (e.g., poison ivy) are not mediated by IgE.

IgE has a relatively short life span in the blood because it rapidly binds to Fc receptors on mast cells.[53] Unlike Fc receptors on phagocytes, which bind IgG that has previously reacted with antigen, the Fc receptors on mast cells specifically bind IgE that has not previously interacted with antigen. After a large amount of IgE has bound to the mast cells, an individual is considered *sensitized*. Further exposure of a sensitized individual to the allergen results in degranulation of the mast cell and the release of mast cell products (see Chapter 6).

Mechanisms of IgE-mediated hypersensitivity. The most potent mediator of IgE-mediated hypersensitivity is histamine, which affects several key target cells. Acting through H1 receptors, histamine contracts bronchial smooth muscles (bronchial constriction), increases vascular permeability (edema), and causes vasodilation (increased blood flow) (see Chapter 6). The interaction of histamine with H2 receptors results in increased gastric acid secretion. Blocking histamine receptors with antihistamines can control some type I responses.

Clinical manifestations of IgE-mediated hypersensitivity. The clinical manifestations of type I reactions are attributable mostly to the biologic effects of histamine. The tissues most commonly affected by type I responses contain large numbers of mast cells and are sensitive to the effects of histamine released from them. These tissues are found in the gastrointestinal tract, the skin, and the respiratory tract (Figure 8-12 and Table 8-15).

Gastrointestinal allergy is caused by allergens that enter through the mouth—usually foods or medicines. Symptoms include vomiting,

diarrhea, or abdominal pain. Foods most often implicated in gastrointestinal allergies are milk, chocolate, citrus fruits, eggs, wheat, nuts, peanut butter, and fish.[54] The most common food allergy in adults is a reaction to shellfish, which may initiate an anaphylactic response and death.[55] When food is the source of an allergen, the active immunogen may be an unidentifiable product of how the food is processed during manufacture or broken down by digestive enzymes.[56] Sometimes the allergen is a drug, an additive, or a preservative in the food. For example, cows treated for mastitis with penicillin yield milk containing trace amounts of this antibiotic. Thus hypersensitivity apparently caused by milk proteins may instead be the result of an allergy to penicillin.

Urticaria, or hives, is a dermal (skin) manifestation of allergic reactions (see Figure 8-12). The underlying mechanism is the localized release of histamine and increased vascular permeability, resulting in limited areas of edema. Urticaria is characterized by white fluid-filled blisters (wheals) surrounded by areas of redness (flares). This wheal and flare reaction is usually accompanied by pruritus. Not all urticarial symptoms are caused by immunologic reactions. Some, termed *nonimmunologic urticaria*, result from exposure to cold temperatures, emotional stress, medications, systemic diseases, or malignancies (e.g., lymphomas).

Effects of allergens on the mucosa of the eyes, nose, and respiratory tract include conjunctivitis (inflammation of the membranes lining the eyelids) (see Figure 8-12), rhinitis (inflammation of the mucous membranes of the nose), and asthma (constriction of the bronchi). Symptoms are caused by vasodilation, hypersecretion of mucus,

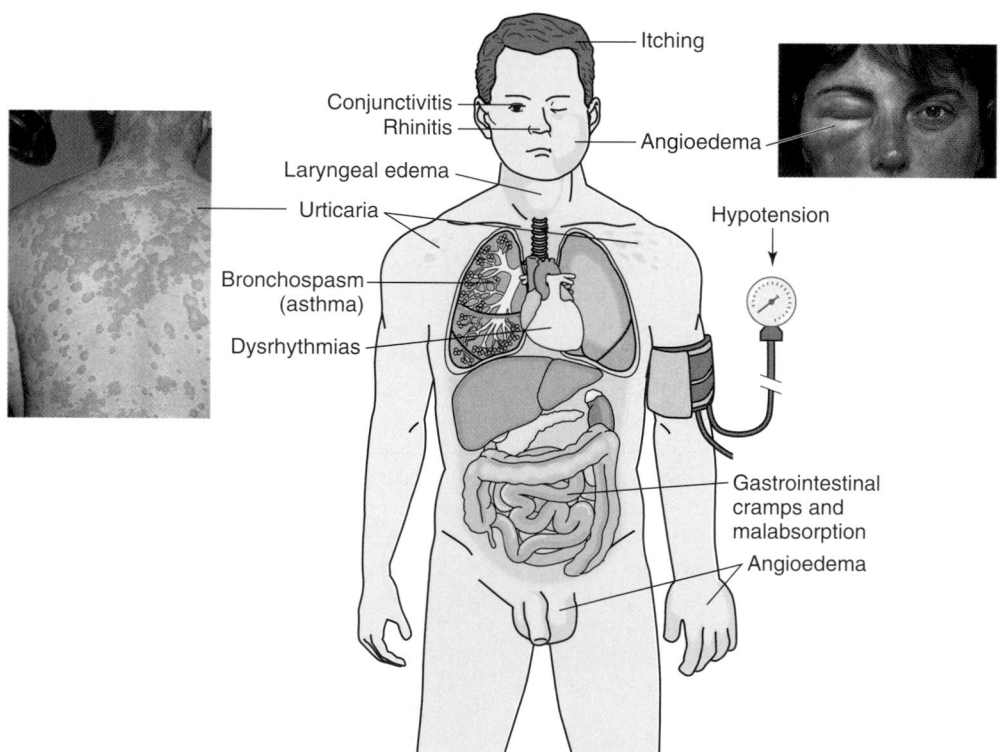

FIGURE 8-12 Type I Hypersensitivity Reactions. Manifestations of allergic reactions as a result of type I hypersensitivity include pruritus, angioedema (swelling caused by exudation), edema of the larynx, urticaria (hives), bronchospasm (constriction of airways in the lungs), hypotension (low blood pressure), and dysrhythmias (irregular heartbeat) because of anaphylactic shock, and gastrointestinal cramping caused by inflammation of the gastrointestinal mucosa. Photographic inserts show a diffuse allergic-like eye and skin reaction on an individual. The skin lesions have raised edges and develop within minutes or hours, with resolution occurring after about 12 hours. (Inserts from Male D et al: *Immunology*, ed 8, St Louis, 2013, Mosby.)

TABLE 8-15 Causes of Clinical Allergic Reactions

Typical Allergen	Mechanism of Hypersensitivity	Clinical Manifestation
Ingestants		
Foods	Type I	Gastrointestinal allergy
Drugs	Types I, II, III	Urticaria, immediate drug reaction, hemolytic anemia, serum sickness
Inhalants		
Pollens, dust, molds	Type I	Allergic rhinitis, bronchial asthma
Aspergillus fumigatus	Types I, III	Allergic bronchopulmonary aspergillosis
Thermophilic actinomycetes*	Types III, IV	Extrinsic allergic alveolitis
Injectants		
Drugs	Types I, II, III	Immediate drug reaction, hemolytic anemia, serum sickness
Bee venom	Type I	Anaphylaxis
Vaccines	Type III	Localized Arthus reaction
Serum	Types I, III	Anaphylaxis, serum sickness
Contactants		
Poison ivy, metals	Type IV	Contact dermatitis
Latex	Type I, IV	Contact dermatitis, anaphylaxis

*An order of fungi that grows best at high temperatures (between 45° and 80°C [113° and 176°F]).

Modified from Bellanti JA: *Immunology III*, Philadelphia, 1985, Saunders.

edema, and swelling of the respiratory mucosa. Because the mucous membranes lining the respiratory tract are continuous, they are all adversely affected. The degree to which each is affected determines the symptoms of the disease; most anaphylactic reactions are type I hypersensitivities.

The central problem in allergic diseases of the lung is obstruction of the large and small airways (bronchi) of the lower respiratory tract by bronchospasm (constriction of smooth muscle in airway walls), edema, and thick secretions. This leads to ventilatory insufficiency, wheezing, and difficult or labored breathing (see Chapter 27).

Certain individuals are genetically predisposed to develop allergies and are called **atopic**. In families in which one parent has an allergy, allergies develop in about 40% of the offspring. If both parents have allergies, the incidence may be as high as 80%. Atopic individuals tend to produce higher quantities of IgE and have more Fc receptors for IgE on their mast cells. The airways and the skin of atopic individuals have increased responsiveness to a wide variety of both specific and non-specific stimuli.

Evaluation and treatment of IgE hypersensitivity. Allergic reactions can be life-threatening; therefore it is essential that severely allergic individuals be informed of the specific allergen against which they are sensitized and instructed to avoid contact with that material. Several tests are available to evaluate allergic individuals. These include food challenges, skin tests with allergens, and laboratory tests for total IgE and allergen-specific IgE.

Type II: Tissue-Specific Hypersensitivity Reactions

Type II hypersensitivities are generally reactions against a specific cell or tissue. Cells express a variety of antigens on their surfaces, some of which are called tissue-specific antigens because they are expressed on the plasma membranes of only certain cells. Platelets, for example, have groups of antigens that are found on no other cells of the body. The symptoms of many type II diseases are determined by which tissue or organ expresses the particular antigen. Environmental antigens (e.g., drugs or their metabolites) may bind to the plasma membranes of specific cells (especially erythrocytes and platelets) and function as targets of type II reactions. The five general mechanisms by which type II hypersensitivity reactions can affect cells are shown in Figure 8-13. Each mechanism begins with antibody binding to tissue-specific antigens or antigens that have attached to particular tissues.

The cell may be destroyed by antibody and complement (see Figure 8-13, *A*). The antibody (IgM or IgG) reacts with an antigen on the surface of the cell, causing activation of the complement cascade through the classical pathway. Formation of the membrane attack complex (C5-9) damages the membrane and may result in lysis of the cell. For example, erythrocytes are destroyed by complement-mediated lysis in individuals with autoimmune hemolytic anemia (see Chapters 21 and 22) or as a result of an alloimmune reaction to mismatched transfused blood cells.

Antibody may cause cell destruction through phagocytosis by macrophages (see Figure 8-13, *B*). The antibody may additionally activate complement, resulting in the deposition of C3b on the cell surface. Receptors on the macrophage recognize and bind opsonins (e.g., antibody or C3b) and increase phagocytosis of the target cell. For example, antibodies against platelet-specific antigens or against red blood cell antigens of the Rh system cause their removal by phagocytosis in the spleen.

Tissue damage may be caused by *toxic products produced by neutrophils* (see Figure 8-13, *C*). Soluble antigens such as medications, molecules released from infectious agents, or molecules released from an individual's own cells may enter the circulation. In some instances, the antigens are deposited on the surface of tissues, where they bind antibody. The antibody may activate complement, resulting in the release of C3a and C5a, which are chemotactic for neutrophils, and the deposition of complement component C3b. Neutrophils are attracted, bind to the tissues through receptors for the Fc portion of antibody (Fc receptor) or for C3b, and release their granules onto the healthy tissue. The components of neutrophil granules, as well as the toxic oxygen products produced by these cells, will damage the tissue.

Antibody-dependent cell-mediated cytotoxicity (ADCC) involves natural killer (NK) cells (see Figure 8-13, *D*). Antibody on the target cell is recognized by Fc receptors on the NK cells, which release toxic substances that destroy the target cell.

The last mechanism does not destroy the target cell but rather *causes the cell to malfunction* (see Figure 8-13, *E*). The antibody is usually directed against antigenic determinants associated with specific cell surface receptors. The antibody changes the function of the receptor by preventing interactions with their normal ligands, replacing the ligand and inappropriately stimulating the receptor, or destroying the receptor. For example, in the hyperthyroidism (excessive thyroid activity) of Graves disease, autoantibody binds to and activates receptors for thyroid-stimulating hormone (TSH) (a pituitary hormone that controls the production of the hormone thyroxine by the thyroid). In this way, the antibody stimulates the thyroid cells to produce thyroxine. Under normal conditions, the increasing levels of thyroxine in the blood would signal the pituitary to decrease TSH production, which would result in less stimulation of the TSH receptor in the thyroid and a concomitant decrease in thyroxine production. Increasing amounts

FIGURE 8-13 Mechanisms of Type II, Tissue-Specific Reactions. Antigens on the target cell bind with antibody and are destroyed or prevented from functioning by one of the following mechanisms: **(A)** complement-mediated lysis (an erythrocyte target is illustrated here); **(B)** clearance (phagocytosis) by macrophages in the tissue; **(C)** neutrophil-mediated immune destruction; **(D)** antibody-dependent cell-mediated cytotoxicity (ADCC) (apoptosis of target cells is induced by natural killer [NK] cells by two mechanisms: by the release of granzymes and perforin, which is a molecule that creates pores in the plasma membrane, and enzymes [granzymes] that enter the target through the perforin pores; by the interactions of Fas ligand [FasL; a molecule similar to TNF-α] on the surface of NK cells with Fas [the receptor for FasL] on the surface of target cells); or **(E)** modulation or blocking of the normal function of receptors by antireceptor antibody. This example of mechanism **(E)** depicts myasthenia gravis in which acetylcholine receptor antibodies block acetylcholine from attaching to its receptors on the motor end plates of skeletal muscle, thereby impairing neuromuscular transmission and causing muscle weakness. *C1,* Complement component C1; *C3b,* complement fragment produced from C3, which acts as an opsonin; *C5a,* complement fragment produced from C5, which acts as a chemotactic factor for neutrophils; *Fcγ receptor,* cellular receptor for the Fc portion of IgG; *FcR,* Fc receptor.

FIGURE 8-14 Mechanism of Type III, Immune Complex–Mediated Reactions. Immune complexes form in the blood from circulating antigen and antibody. Both small and large immune complexes are removed successfully from the circulation and do not cause tissue damage. Intermediate-sized complexes are deposited in certain target tissues in which the circulation is slow or filtration of the blood occurs. The complexes activate the complement cascade through C1 and generate fragments including C5a and C3b. C5a is chemotactic for neutrophils, which migrate into the inflamed area and attach to the IgG and C3b in the immune complexes. The neutrophils attempt unsuccessfully to phagocytose the tissue and in the process release a variety of degradative enzymes that destroy the healthy tissues. Fcγ receptor is the cellular receptor for the Fc portion of IgG.

of thyroxine in the blood have no effect on anti-TSH receptor antibodies, which continue to stimulate despite decreasing amounts of TSH (see Chapter 19).

Type III: Immune Complex–Mediated Hypersensitivity Reactions

Mechanisms of type III hypersensitivity. Most type III hypersensitivity diseases reactions are caused by antigen-antibody (immune) complexes that are formed in the circulation and deposited later in vessel walls or other tissues (Figure 8-14). The primary difference between type II and type III mechanisms is that in type II hypersensitivity antibody binds to antigen on the cell surface, whereas in type III antibody binds to soluble antigen that was released into the blood or body fluids, and the complex is then deposited in the tissues. Type III reactions are not organ specific, and symptoms are mostly unrelated to the particular antigenic target of the antibody. The harmful effects of immune complex deposition are caused by complement activation, particularly through the generation of chemotactic factors for neutrophils. The neutrophils bind to antibody and C3b contained in the complexes and attempt to ingest the immune complexes. They are often unsuccessful because the complexes are bound to large areas of tissue. During the attempted phagocytosis, large quantities of lysosomal enzymes are released into the inflammatory site instead of into phagolysosomes. The attraction of neutrophils and the subsequent release of lysosomal enzymes cause most of the resulting tissue damage.

Immune complex disease. Two prototypic models of type III hypersensitivity help explain the variety of diseases in this category. Serum sickness is a model of systemic type III hypersensitivities, and the Arthus reaction is a model of localized or cutaneous reactions.

Serum sickness–type reactions are caused by the formation of immune complexes in the blood and their subsequent generalized deposition in target tissues. Typically affected tissues are the blood vessels, joints, and kidneys. Symptoms include fever, enlarged lymph nodes, rash, and pain at sites of inflammation. Serum sickness was initially described as a complication of therapeutic administration of horse serum that contained antibody against tetanus toxin. Foreign serum is not administered to individuals today, although serum sickness reactions can be caused by the repeated intravenous administration of other antigens, such as drugs, and the characteristics of serum sickness are observed in systemic type III autoimmune diseases.

A form of serum sickness is Raynaud phenomenon, a condition caused by the temperature-dependent deposition of immune complexes in the capillary beds of the peripheral circulation. Certain immune complexes precipitate at temperatures below normal body temperature, particularly in the tips of the fingers, toes, and nose, and are called cryoglobulins. The precipitates block the circulation and cause localized pallor and numbness, followed by cyanosis (a bluish tinge resulting from oxygen deprivation) and eventually gangrene if the circulation is not restored.

An Arthus reaction is caused by repeated local exposure to an antigen that reacts with preformed antibody and forms immune complexes in the walls of the local blood vessels. Symptoms of an Arthus reaction begin within 1 hour of exposure and peak 6 to 12 hours later. The lesions are characterized by a typical inflammatory reaction, with increased vascular permeability, an accumulation of neutrophils, edema, hemorrhage, clotting, and tissue damage.

Arthus reactions may be observed after injection, ingestion, or inhalation of allergens. Skin reactions can follow subcutaneous or intradermal inoculation with drugs, fungal extracts, or antigens used

FIGURE 8-15 Mechanism of Type IV, Cell-Mediated Reactions. Antigens from target cells stimulate T cells to differentiate into T-cytotoxic cells *(Tc cells),* which have direct cytotoxic activity, and T-helper cells *(Th1 cells)* involved in delayed hypersensitivity. The Th1 cells produce lymphokines (especially interferon-γ [*IFN-γ*]) that activate the macrophage through specific receptors (e.g., IFN-γ receptor [*IFNγR*]). The macrophages can attach to targets and release enzymes and reactive oxygen species that are responsible for most of the tissue destruction.

in skin tests. Gastrointestinal reactions, such as gluten-sensitive enteropathy (celiac disease), follow ingestion of antigen, usually gluten from wheat products (see Chapter 37). Allergic alveolitis (farmer lung, pigeon breeder disease) is an Arthus-like acute hemorrhagic inflammation of the air sacs (alveoli) of the lungs resulting from inhalation of fungal antigens, usually particles from moldy hay or pigeon feces (see Chapter 27).

Type IV: Cell-Mediated Hypersensitivity Reactions

Whereas types I, II, and III hypersensitivity reactions are mediated by antibody, type IV hypersensitivity reactions are mediated by T lymphocytes and do not involve antibody (Figure 8-15). Type IV mechanisms occur through either cytotoxic T lymphocytes (Tc cells) or lymphokine-producing Th1 and Th17 cells. Tc cells attack and destroy cellular targets directly. Th1 and Th17 cells produce cytokines that recruit and activate phagocytic cells, especially macrophages. Destruction of the tissue is usually caused by direct killing by Tc cells or the release of soluble factors, such as lysosomal enzymes and toxic reactive oxygen species, from activated macrophages.

Clinical examples of type IV hypersensitivity reactions include graft rejection, the skin test for tuberculosis, and allergic reactions resulting from contact with such substances as poison ivy and metals. A type IV component also may be present in many autoimmune diseases. For example, T cells against type II collagen (a protein present in joint tissues) contribute to the destruction of joints in rheumatoid arthritis; T cells against a thyroid cell–surface antigen contribute to the destruction of the thyroid in autoimmune thyroiditis (Hashimoto disease); and T cells against an antigen on the surface of pancreatic beta cells (the cell that normally produces insulin) are responsible for beta-cell destruction in insulin-dependent (type 1) diabetes mellitus.

In 1891 Ehrlich was the first to thoroughly describe a type IV hypersensitivity reaction in the skin, leading to the development of a diagnostic skin test for tuberculosis. The reaction follows an intradermal injection of tuberculin antigen into a suitably sensitized individual and is called a delayed hypersensitivity skin test because of its slow onset—24 to 72 hours to reach maximal intensity. The reaction site is infiltrated with T lymphocytes and macrophages, resulting in a clear hard center (induration) and a reddish surrounding area (erythema).

Allergic type IV reactions are elicited by some environmental antigens that are haptens (Chapter 7) and become immunogenic after binding to larger (carrier) proteins in the individual. In allergic contact dermatitis, the carrier protein is in the skin. The best-known example is poison ivy (Figure 8-16). The antigen is a plant catechol, urushiol, which reacts with normal skin proteins and evokes a cell-mediated immune response. Skin reactions to industrial chemicals, cosmetics, detergents, clothing, food, metals, and topical medicines (such as penicillin) are elicited by the same mechanism. Contact dermatitis consists of lesions only at the site of contact with the allergen, such as a metal allergy to jewelry.

✔ **QUICK CHECK 8-3**
1. Distinguish among the four types of hypersensitivity mechanisms.
2. What is the mechanism of anaphylaxis?
3. What are some clinical examples of type IV hypersensitivity?

Antigenic Targets of Hypersensitivity Reactions
Allergy

Allergens. Allergies are the most common hypersensitivity reactions. The majority of allergies are type I reactions that lead to annoying symptoms, including rhinitis, sneezing, and other relatively mild reactions. In some individuals, however, these reactions can be excessive and life-threatening (anaphylaxis). Antigens that cause allergic responses are called allergens. It is not known why some antigens are allergens and others are not. Typical allergens include pollens (e.g., ragweed), molds and fungi (e.g., *Penicillium chrysogenum*), foods (e.g., milk, eggs, fish), animals (e.g., cat dander, dog dander), cigarette smoke, and components of house dust (e.g., fecal pellets of house mites). Often the allergen is contained within a particle that is too large to be phagocytosed or is surrounded by a protective nonallergenic coat. The actual allergen is released after enzymatic breakdown (e.g., by lysozyme in secretions) of the larger particle.

Allergic disease: bee sting allergy. Bee venoms contain a mixture of enzymes and other proteins that may serve as allergens and cause a type I hypersensitivity reaction. About 1% of children may have an anaphylactic reaction to bee venom.[57] Within minutes they may develop excessive swelling (edema) at the bee sting site, followed by generalized hives, pruritus, and swelling in areas distal from the sting (e.g., eyes, lips), and other systemic symptoms including flushing, sweating, dizziness, and headache. The most severe symptoms may include gastrointestinal (e.g., stomach cramps, vomiting), respiratory (e.g., tightness in the throat, wheezing, difficulty breathing), and vascular (e.g., low blood pressure, shock) reactions. Severe respiratory tract and vascular reactions may lead to death.

For an individual with known bee sting hypersensitivity, lifestyle changes include avoidance of stinging or biting insects. If a child has experienced a previous anaphylactic reaction, the chance of having another is about 60%. The primary life-threatening symptoms result from contraction of respiratory tract smooth muscle. Autonomic nervous system mediators, such as epinephrine, bind to specific receptors on smooth muscle and reverse the effects of histamine, resulting in muscle relaxation. Thus most individuals with bee sting allergies

FIGURE 8-16 Development of Allergic Contact Dermatitis. A, The development of type IV hypersensitivity to poison ivy. The first (primary) contact with allergen sensitizes (produces reactive T cells) the individual but does not produce a rash (dermatitis). Secondary contact activates a type IV cell-mediated reaction that causes dermatitis. **B,** Contact dermatitis caused by a delayed hypersensitivity reaction leading to vesicles and scaling at the sites of contact. (From Damjanov I, Linder J: *Anderson's pathology,* ed 10, St Louis, 1996, Mosby.)

carry self-injectable epinephrine. The administration of antihistamines has little effect because histamine has already bound H1 receptors and initiated severe bronchial smooth muscle contraction.

Clinical **desensitization** to allergens can be achieved in some individuals. Minute quantities of the allergen are injected in increasing doses over a prolonged period. The procedure may reduce the severity of the allergic reaction in the treated individual. However, this form of therapy may trigger systemic anaphylaxis, which can be severe and life-threatening. This approach works best for routine respiratory tract allergens and biting insect allergies (80% to 90% rate of desensitization over 5 years of treatment).[58] Food allergies have been very difficult to suppress, but some promising trials are underway to evaluate desensitization by oral or sublingual administration of increasing amounts of allergen.

Autoimmunity

Autoimmune diseases originate from an initiating event in a genetic predisposed individual. Current models of factors related to autoimmune diseases include genetic factors, environmental factors, and random or stochastic changes.[59] Some autoimmune diseases can be familial and attributed to the presence of a very small number of susceptibility genes; affected family members may not all develop the same disease, but have different disorders characterized by a variety of hypersensitivity reactions, including autoimmune and allergic. For instance, the HLA antigen B27 (HLA is discussed further under transplant rejection, p. 209) is a risk factor for developing **ankylosing spondylitis (AS)**, an autoimmune inflammatory disease of the spine; 95% of individuals diagnosed with AS express HLA-B27 whereas only 4% to 8% of the general population expresses this antigen.[60] Although most autoimmune diseases appear as isolated events without a positive family history, susceptibility for developing such diseases appears to be linked to a combination of multiple genes.

Breakdown of tolerance. An individual is usually tolerant to his or her own antigens. Tolerance is a state of immunologic control so that the individual does not make a detrimental immune response against his or her own cells and tissues. Autoimmune disease results from a breakdown of this tolerance.

The initiating event that breaks tolerance is unclear for most autoimmune diseases. It is also unclear as to the bodily site initially involved to cause autoimmunity.[59] Potential infectious initiators of autoimmune disease are being investigated,[61] but only one example is known: acute rheumatic fever. In a small number of individuals with group A streptococcal sore throats, the M proteins in the bacterial capsule mimic *(antigenic mimicry)* normal heart antigens and induce antibodies that also react with proteins in the heart valve, damaging the valve.[62] Thus acute rheumatic fever is a type II autoimmune hypersensitivity. Additionally, some streptococcal skin or throat infections release bacterial antigens into the blood that form circulating immune complexes. The complexes may deposit in the kidneys and initiate an immune complex–mediated glomerulonephritis (inflammation of the kidney).[63] Thus streptococcal antigens (an environmental antigen) may also cause a type III allergic hypersensitivity (poststreptococcal glomerulonephritis).

Autoimmune disease: systemic lupus erythematosus. Systemic lupus erythematosus (SLE) is the most common, complex, and serious of the autoimmune disorders. SLE is characterized by the production of a large variety of antibodies (autoantibodies) against self-antigens, including nucleic acids, erythrocytes, coagulation proteins, phospholipids, lymphocytes, platelets, and many other self-components. The most characteristic autoantibodies are against nucleic acids (e.g., single-stranded DNA, double-stranded DNA), histones, ribonucleoproteins, and other nuclear materials. Approximately 98% of persons with SLE have detectable antibodies against nuclear antigens. The blood normally contains many of these products of cellular turnover and breakdown so that autoantibodies react with the circulating antigen and form circulating immune complexes. The deposition of circulating DNA/anti-DNA complexes in the kidneys can cause severe kidney inflammation. Similar reactions can occur in the brain, heart, spleen, lung, gastrointestinal tract, peritoneum, and skin. Thus some of the symptoms of SLE result from a type III hypersensitivity reaction. Other symptoms, such as destruction of red blood cells (anemia), lymphocytes (lymphopenia), and other cells, may be type II hypersensitivity reactions.

SLE, like most autoimmune diseases, occurs more often in women (approximately a 9:1 predominance of females), especially in the 20- to 40-year-old age group.[64] Blacks are affected more often than whites (about an eightfold increased risk). A genetic predisposition for the disease has been implicated on the basis of increased incidence in twins and the existence of autoimmune disease in the families of individuals with SLE.

As with many autoimmune diseases, clinical manifestations of SLE may wax and wane; the individual may go through periods of remission and be relatively disease free until the onset of a *flare* (exacerbated disease activity). Symptoms include arthralgias or arthritis (90% of individuals), vasculitis and rash (70% to 80% of individuals), renal disease (40% to 50% of individuals), hematologic abnormalities (50% of individuals, with anemia being the most common complication), and cardiovascular diseases (30% to 50% of individuals) (see discoid lupus erythematosus in Chapter 41). Because the signs and symptoms affect almost every body system and tend to vacillate, SLE is extremely difficult to diagnose. This has led to the development of a list of 11

common clinical findings,[65] which has been modified slightly to increase sensitivity of the diagnosis.[66] The serial or simultaneous presence of at least four of these findings indicates that the individual has SLE. The findings are as follows:

1. Facial rash confined to the cheeks (malar rash)
2. Discoid rash (raised patches, scaling)
3. Photosensitivity (development of skin rash as a result of exposure to sunlight)
4. Oral or nasopharyngeal ulcers
5. Nonerosive arthritis of at least two peripheral joints
6. Serositis (inflammation of membranes of lung [pleurisy] or heart [pericarditis])
7. Renal disorder (persistent proteinuria of >0.5 g/day or >3 on dipstick, or cellular casts)
8. Neurologic disorders (seizures or psychosis in the absence of known causes)
9. Hematologic disorders (hemolytic anemia, leukopenia, lymphopenia, or thrombocytopenia)
10. Immunologic disorders (anti–double-stranded DNA (dsDNA), anti–Smith [Sm] antigen, false-positive serologic test for syphilis, or antiphospholipid antibodies [anticardiolipin antibody or lupus anticoagulant])
11. Presence of antinuclear antibody (ANA)

Laboratory diagnosis is usually based on a positive ANA screening test; about 98% of individuals with SLE are positive, but a substantial number of false-positives occur in healthy individuals and those with other diseases. Because SLE is a progressive and slowly developing disease, some laboratory tests, including the ANA, may be positive years before the onset of clinical symptoms.[64] Detection of a positive ANA is usually followed by one or more specific tests (e.g., antibodies against Sm, dsDNA) that are complicated by low sensitivity (only a portion of individuals with SLE will be positive, although the number of false-positives is low).

There is no cure for SLE or most other autoimmune diseases. Fatalities resulting from SLE are usually related to infection, organ failure, or cardiovascular disease. The goals of treatment are to control symptoms and prevent further damage by suppressing the autoimmune response. Nonsteroidal anti-inflammatory drugs, such as aspirin, ibuprofen, or naproxen, reduce inflammation and relieve pain. Corticosteroids are often prescribed for more serious active disease. Immunosuppressive drugs (e.g., methotrexate, azathioprine, or cyclophosphamide) are used to treat severe symptoms involving internal organs. Antimalarial medications (e.g., hydroxychloroquine) are preferred treatments for individuals with stable disease.[64] Ultraviolet light may initiate flares and protection from sun exposure is helpful. Prolonged use of certain drugs can cause transient SLE-like symptoms, and the medication history is important for differential diagnosis.

Alloimmunity

Alloantigens. Genetic diversity is the norm in humans. Diversity also is observed among self-antigens, so that two individuals may have different antigens on their tissues and, therefore, make an immune response against each other's tissues. Some self-antigens, such as the ABO blood group, have limited diversity with very few different antigens being expressed in the population, whereas others, such as the HLA system, have tremendous diversity.

Alloimmune disease: transfusion reactions. Red blood cells (erythrocytes) express several important surface antigens, which are known collectively as the blood group antigens and can be targets of alloimmune reactions. More than 80 different red cell antigens are grouped into several dozen blood group systems. The most important

Blood Type

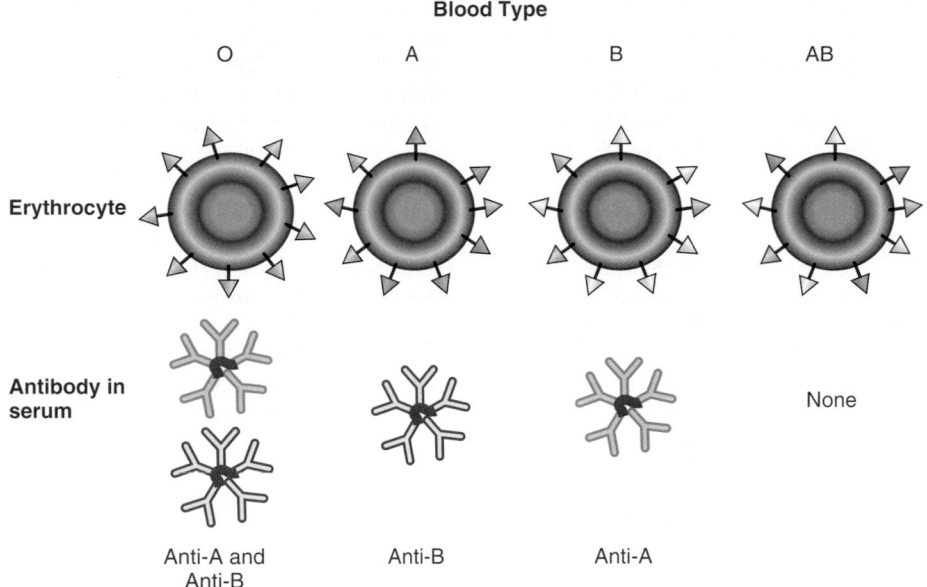

FIGURE 8-17 ABO Blood Types. This figure shows the relationship of antigens and antibodies associated with the ABO blood groups. The surfaces of erythrocytes of individuals with blood group O have a core carbohydrate that is present on cells of all ABO blood groups (H antigen). The sera of blood group O individuals contain IgM antibodies against both A and B carbohydrates. In individuals of the blood group A, some of the H antigens have been modified into A antigens. The sera of these individuals have IgM antibodies against the B antigen. In individuals with blood group B, some of the H antigens have been modified into B antigens. These individuals have IgM antibodies against the A antigen in their sera. In individuals of the blood group AB, some of the H antigens have been modified into both the A and B antigens. These individuals do not have antibody to either A or B antigens.

of these, because they provoke the strongest humoral alloimmune response, are the ABO and Rh systems.

The ABO blood group consists of two major carbohydrate antigens, labeled A and B (Figure 8-17), that are expressed on virtually all cells. These are codominant so that both A and B can be simultaneously expressed, resulting in an individual having any one of four different blood types. The erythrocytes of blood type A express the type A carbohydrate antigen, those with blood type B express the B antigen, those with blood type AB express both A and B antigens on the same cell, and those of blood type O express neither the A nor the B antigen. A person with type A blood also has circulating antibodies to the B carbohydrate antigen. If this person receives blood from a type AB or B individual, a severe transfusion reaction occurs, and the transfused erythrocytes are destroyed by agglutination or complement-mediated lysis. Similarly, a type B individual (whose blood contains anti-A antibodies) cannot receive blood from a type A or AB donor. Type O individuals, who have neither antigen but have both anti-A and anti-B antibodies, cannot accept blood from any of the other three types. These naturally occurring antibodies, called isohemagglutinins, are IgM immunoglobulins and are induced early in life against similar antigens expressed on naturally occurring bacteria in the intestinal tract.

Because individuals with type O blood lack both types of antigens, they are considered universal donors, meaning that anyone can accept their red blood cells. Similarly, type AB individuals are considered universal recipients because they lack both anti-A and anti-B antibodies and can be transfused with any ABO blood type. Harmful transfusion reactions can be prevented only by complete and careful ABO matching between donor and recipient.

The Rh blood group is a group of antigens expressed only on red blood cells. This is the most diverse group of red cell antigens, consisting of at least 45 separate antigens, although only 1 is considered of major importance: the D antigen. Individuals who express the D antigen on their red cells are Rh-positive, whereas individuals who do not express the D antigen are Rh-negative. When discussing the gene for the Rh antigen, the letter *d* is used to indicate lack of D. Rh-positive individuals can have either a *DD* or *Dd* genotype, whereas Rh-negative individuals have the *dd* genotype. About 85% of North Americans are Rh-positive. Rh-negative individuals can make an IgG antibody to the D antigen (anti-D) if exposed to Rh-positive erythrocytes.

A disease called *hemolytic disease of the newborn* was most commonly caused by IgG anti-D alloantibody produced by Rh-negative mothers against erythrocytes of their Rh-positive fetuses (see Chapter 22). The mother's antibody crossed the placenta and destroyed the red blood cells of the fetus. The occurrence of this particular form of the disease has decreased dramatically because of the use of prophylactic anti-D immunoglobulin (i.e., RhoGAM). By mechanisms that are still not completely understood, administration of anti-D antibody within a few days of exposure to RhD-positive erythrocytes completely prevents sensitization against the D antigen. Because hemolytic disease of the newborn related to the D antigen has been controlled, alloantibodies against the other Rh antigens have become more important. In general, these alloantibodies are associated with a less severe hemolytic disease.

Alloimmune disease: transplant rejection. Molecules of the major histocompatibility complex (MHC) were discussed in Chapter 7 as antigen-presenting molecules. MHC molecules are also a major target of transplant rejection. As a result of studies of transplantation, the human MHC molecules are also referred to as **human leukocyte antigens (HLAs)** and the different MHC genetic loci are commonly called HLA-A, HLA-B, HLA-C, HLA-DR, HLA-DQ, and HLA-DP (Figure 8-18). Additional genes for complement components (e.g., C4, factor B) are also contained in the MHC region and are referred to as class III loci. The class I (HLA-A, -B, and -C) and class II MHC loci (HLA-DR, -DQ, and -DP) are the most genetically diverse (polymorphic) of any human genetic loci. Within the human population, the number of possible different alleles (i.e., forms of the gene) expressed by each locus is astounding. For example, more than 300 different HLA-A molecules are expressed in the population. These numbers are based on the polymorphism of observed DNA sequences and may not reflect differences in function.

Clearly, not every allele is expressed in the same individual. Humans have two copies of each MHC locus (one inherited from each parent) that are codominant so that molecules encoded by each parent's genes are expressed on the surface of every cell, except erythrocytes. Within an individual, each locus will express only one allele. For instance, each person will have at most two different HLA-A proteins (one from each parent). However, with the tremendous number of possible alleles that can be expressed throughout the population, it is likely that any two unrelated individuals will have different MHC antigens.

The diversity of MHC molecules becomes clinically relevant during organ transplantation. The recipient of a transplant can mount an immune response against the foreign HLA antigens on the donor tissue, resulting in rejection. To minimize the chance of tissue rejection, the donor and recipient are often tissue-typed beforehand to identify differences in HLA antigens. Because of the large number of different alleles, it is highly unlikely that a perfect match can be found between someone who needs a transplant and a potential donor from the general population. The more similar two individuals are in their HLA tissue type, the more likely a transplant from one to the other will be successful. Clearly, the most successful transplants would be between identical twins because they are identical genetically.

The specific combination of alleles at the six major HLA loci on one chromosome (A, B, C, DR, DQ, and DP) is termed a haplotype. Each individual has two HLA haplotypes, one from the paternal chromosome 6 and another from the maternal chromosome (Figure 8-19). Each parent passes on one set of HLA antigens to each of his or her offspring, meaning that children usually share half their HLA antigens with each parent. Odds dictate that children will share one haplotype with half their siblings and either no haplotypes or both haplotypes with a quarter of their siblings. Thus the chance of finding a match among siblings is much higher (25%) than the general population.

Transplant rejection may be classified as hyperacute, acute, or chronic, depending on the amount of time that elapses between transplantation and rejection. **Hyperacute rejection** is immediate and rare. When the circulation is reestablished to the grafted area, the graft may immediately turn white (the so-called *white graft*) instead of a normal pink color. Hyperacute rejection usually occurs because of preexisting antibody (type II reaction) to HLA antigens on the vascular endothelial cells in the grafted tissue.

Acute rejection is a cell-mediated immune response that occurs within days to months after transplantation. This type of rejection occurs when the recipient develops an immune response against unmatched HLA antigens after transplantation. A biopsy of the rejected organ usually shows an infiltration of lymphocytes and macrophages characteristic of a type IV reaction.

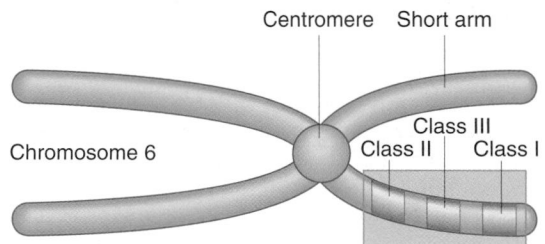

FIGURE 8-18 Human Leukocyte Antigens (HLAs). The major histocompatibility complex *(MHC)* is located on the short arm of chromosome 6 and contains genes that code for class I antigens, class II antigens, and class III proteins (i.e., complement proteins and cytokines). (From Peakman M, Vergani D: *Basic and clinical immunology,* ed 2, London, 2009, Churchill Livingstone.)

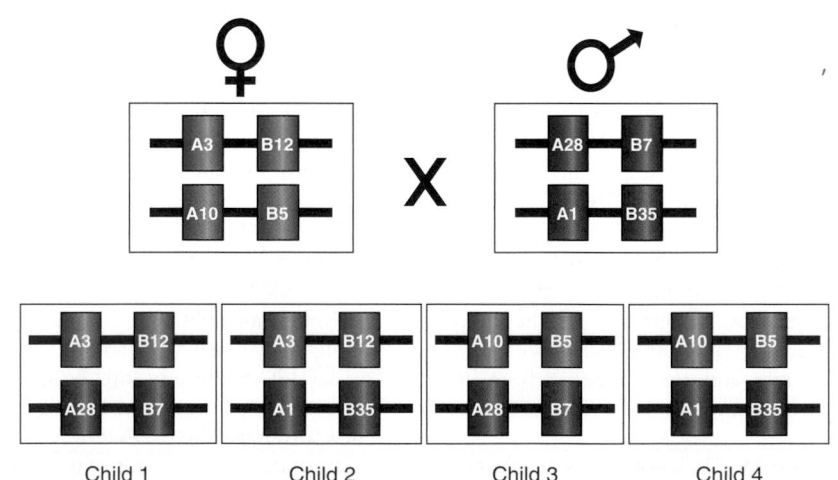

FIGURE 8-19 Inheritance of HLA. HLA alleles are inherited in a codominant fashion; both maternal and paternal antigens are expressed. Specific HLA alleles are commonly given numbers to indicate different antigens. In this example, the mother has linked genes for HLA-A3 and HLA-B12 on one chromosome 6 and genes for HLA-A10 and HLA-B5 on the second chromosome 6. The father has HLA-A28 and HLA-B7 on one chromosome and HLA-A1 and HLA-B35 on the second chromosome. The children from this pairing may have one of four possible combinations of maternal and paternal HLA.

Chronic rejection may occur after a period of months or years of normal function. It is characterized by slow, progressive organ failure. Chronic rejection usually results from a weak cell-mediated (type IV) reaction against minor histocompatibility antigens on the grafted tissue. However, antibodies against HLA and other antigens also may cause chronic rejection through activation of complement or antibody-dependent cellular cytotoxicity (ADCC) with NK cells.

✔ QUICK CHECK 8-4
1. Why do certain drugs become immunogenic to the host?
2. Why is SLE considered an autoimmune disease?
3. Define the different types of graft rejection.

DID YOU UNDERSTAND?

Infection

1. Infectious disease is a significant cause of morbidity and mortality in the United States and worldwide.
2. Pathogens have unique characteristics that influence their ability to cause disease.
3. Bacteria injure cells by producing exotoxins or endotoxins. Exotoxins are enzymes that can damage the plasma membranes of host cells or can inactivate enzymes critical to protein synthesis, and endotoxins activate the inflammatory response and produce fever.
4. Septicemia is the proliferation of bacteria in the blood. Endotoxins released by blood-borne bacteria cause the release of vasoactive enzymes that increase the permeability of blood vessels. Leakage from vessels causes hypotension that can result in septic shock.
5. Viruses enter host cells and use the metabolic processes of host cells to proliferate and cause disease.
6. Viruses that have invaded host cells may decrease protein synthesis, disrupt lysosomal membranes, form inclusion bodies where synthesis of viral nucleic acids is occurring, fuse with host cells to produce giant cells, alter antigenic properties of the host cell, transform host cells into cancerous cells, and promote bacterial infection.
7. Diseases caused by fungi are called mycoses, and they occur in two forms: yeasts (spheres) and molds (filaments or hyphae).
8. Dermatophytes are fungi that infect skin, hair, and nails with diseases such as ringworm and athlete's foot.
9. Fungi release toxins and enzymes that are damaging to tissue. *Candida albicans* is the most common cause of fungal infections in humans.
10. Parasitic microorganisms range from unicellular protozoa to large worms. Although less common in the United States, parasites and protozoa are common causes of infection worldwide.
11. Parasitic and protozoal infections are rarely transmitted from human to human. Infection mainly spreads through vectors (e.g., by mosquito bites) or through contaminated water or food (i.e., malaria, Chagas disease, sleeping sickness, and leishmaniasis).
12. Infection control measures include implementation of clean food and water, management of sewage and waste, control of insects that transmit disease, vaccination, appropriate use of antimicrobials, and passive immunotherapy.

Deficiencies in Immunity

1. Immunodeficiency is the failure of mechanisms of self-defense to function in their normal capacity.
2. Immunodeficiencies are either congenital (primary) or acquired (secondary). Congenital immunodeficiencies are caused by genetic defects that disrupt lymphocyte development, whereas acquired immunodeficiencies are secondary to disease or other physiologic alterations.

3. The clinical hallmark of immunodeficiency is a propensity to unusual or recurrent severe infections. The type of infection usually reflects the immune system defect.
4. The most common infections in individuals with defects of cell-mediated immune response are fungal and viral, whereas infections in individuals with defects of the humoral immune response or complement function are primarily bacterial.
5. Severe combined immunodeficiency (SCID) is a total lack of T-cell function and a severe (either partial or total) lack of B-cell function.
6. Wiskott-Aldrich syndrome is caused by decreased production of IgM antibody.
7. DiGeorge syndrome (congenital thymic aplasia or hypoplasia) is characterized by complete or partial lack of the thymus (resulting in depressed T-cell immunity), frequently associated with diminished or absent parathyroid gland activity (resulting in hypocalcemia) and cardiac anomalies.
8. Antibody deficiencies result from defects in B-cell maturation or function and range from a complete lack of the human bursal equivalent, the lymphoid organs required for B-cell maturation (as in Bruton agammaglobulinemia), to deficiencies in a single class of immunoglobulins (e.g., selective IgA deficiency).
9. Phagocyte defects include inadequate numbers or alteration in function, such as inadequate adhesion to bacteria or ineffective killing.
10. Complement and mannose-binding lectin deficiencies also are rare causes of increased risk for infection.
11. Acquired immunodeficiencies are caused by superimposed conditions, such as malnutrition, medical therapies, physical or psychologic trauma, or infections.
12. Immunodeficiency syndromes usually are treated by replacement therapy. Deficient antibody production is treated by replacement of missing immunoglobulins with commercial gamma-globulin preparations. Lymphocyte deficiencies are treated by the replacement of host lymphocytes with transplants of bone marrow, fetal liver, or fetal thymus from a donor. There are ongoing trials for gene therapy.
13. AIDS is an acquired dysfunction of the immune system caused by a retrovirus (HIV) that infects and destroys CD4+ lymphocytes (T-helper cells).

Hypersensitivity: Allergy, Autoimmunity, and Alloimmunity

1. Hypersensitivity is an immune response misdirected against the host's own tissues (autoimmunity) or directed against beneficial foreign tissues, such as transfusions or transplants (alloimmunity); or it can be exaggerated responses against environmental antigens (allergy).
2. Mechanisms of hypersensitivity are classified as type I (IgE-mediated) reactions, type II (tissue-specific) reactions, type III

(immune complex–mediated) reactions, and type IV (cell-mediated) reactions.

3. Hypersensitivity reactions can be immediate (developing within seconds or hours) or delayed (developing within hours or days).

4. Anaphylaxis, the most rapid immediate hypersensitivity reaction, is an explosive reaction that occurs within minutes of reexposure to the antigen and can lead to cardiovascular shock.

5. Type I (IgE-mediated) reactions occur after antigen reacts with IgE on mast cells, leading to mast cell degranulation and the release of histamine and other inflammatory substances.

6. Type II (tissue-specific) reactions are caused by four possible mechanisms: complement-mediated lysis, opsonization and phagocytosis, antibody-dependent cell-mediated cytotoxicity, and modulation of cellular function.

7. Type III (immune complex–mediated) reactions are caused by the formation of immune complexes that are deposited in target tissues, where they activate the complement cascade, generating chemotactic fragments that attract neutrophils into the inflammatory site.

8. Immune complex disease can be a systemic reaction, such as serum sickness (e.g., Raynaud phenomenon), or localized, such as the Arthus reaction.

9. Type IV (cell-mediated) reactions are caused by specifically sensitized T cells, which either kill target cells directly or release lymphokines that activate other cells, such as macrophages.

10. Allergens are antigens that cause allergic responses, usually a type I hypersensitivity response.

11. Autoimmune disease is loss of tolerance to self-antigens. There can be a genetic predisposition and the diseases can be a type II or type III hypersensitivity reaction.

12. Alloimmunity is the immune system's reaction against antigens on the tissues of other members of the same species.

13. Alloimmune disorders include transient neonatal disease, in which the maternal immune system becomes sensitized against antigens expressed by the fetus; and transplant rejection and transfusion reactions, in which the immune system of the recipient of an organ transplant or blood transfusion reacts against foreign antigens on the donor's cells.

KEY TERMS

ABO blood group, 209
Acquired immunodeficiency syndrome (AIDS), 194
Acute rejection, 210
Adenosine deaminase (ADA) deficiency, 191
Agammaglobulinemia, 191
Allergen, 206
Allergy, 199
Alloimmune disease, 199
Alloimmunity, 199
Anaphylaxis, 201
Ankylosing spondylitis, 207
Antibiotic resistance, 181, 187
Antibody-dependent cell-mediated cytotoxicity (ADCC), 203
Antigenic drift, 183
Antigenic shift, 183
Antiretroviral therapy (ART), 197
Antitoxin, 180
Arthus reaction, 205
Atopic, 203
Attenuated virus, 188
Autoimmune disease, 199, 208
Autoimmunity, 199
β-lactamase, 181
Bacteremia, 182
Bare lymphocyte syndrome, 191
Biofilms, 180
Blood group antigen, 208
Bruton agammaglob-ulinemia, 192
C3 deficiency, 192

CCR5 antagonist, 197
Chronic granulomatous disease (CGD), 192
Chronic mucocutaneous candidiasis, 192
Chronic rejection, 211
Communicability, 177
Complement deficiency, 192
Contact dermatitis, 206
Cryoglobulins, 205
Defects in innate immunity, 191
Delayed hypersensitivity reaction, 201
Delayed hypersensitivity skin test, 206
Dermatophyte, 184
Desensitization, 207
DiGeorge syndrome, 191
Dimorphic fungus (pl., fungi), 184
Endotoxic shock, 182
Endotoxin (lipopolysaccharide [LPS]), 181
Erythema, 206
Exotoxin, 180
Graft-versus-host disease (GVHD), 193
Herd immunity, 189
HIV integrase, 194
HIV integrase inhibitor, 197
HIV fusion inhibitor, 197
HIV protease, 195
HIV protease inhibitor, 197
Human immunodeficiency virus (HIV), 194

Human leukocyte antigen (HLA), 210
Hyperacute rejection, 210
Hypersensitivity, 199
Hypogammaglobulinemia, 191
Immediate hypersensitivity reaction, 201
Immune deficiency, 189
Immunogenicity, 188
Induration, 206
Infectivity, 177
Isohemagglutinin, 209
Major histocompatibility complex (MHC), 209
Mannose-binding lectin deficiency, 192
Mesenchymal stem cell (MSC), 193
Methicillin-resistant *Staphylococcus aureus* (MRSA), 188
Multiple-antibiotic resistance, 187
Mycosis (pl., mycoses), 184
Parasitic microorganisms, 185
Passive immunotherapy, 189
Pathogenicity, 177
Phagocytic defects, 192
Portal of entry, 177
Predominantly antibody deficiency, 191
Primary (congenital) immune deficiency, 189
Raynaud phenomenon, 205
Reverse transcriptase, 194

Reverse transcriptase inhibitor, 197
Rh blood group, 209
Secondary (acquired) immune deficiency, 189
Selective IgA deficiency, 191
Septicemia, 182
Serum sickness, 205
Severe combined immunodeficiency (SCID), 191
Severe congenital neutropenia, 192
Systemic lupus erythematosus (SLE), 208
Tissue-specific antigen, 203
Tolerance, 208
Toxigenicity, 177
Toxoid, 188
Type I hypersensitivity, 201
Type II hypersensitivity, 203
Type III hypersensitivity, 205
Type IV hypersensitivity, 206
Universal donor, 209
Universal recipient, 209
Urticaria (hives), 202
Vaccination, 188
Vaccine, 188
Virulence, 177
Wheal and flare reaction, 202
Wiskott-Aldrich syndrome, 191
X-linked SCID, 191

REFERENCES

1. Khabbaz RF et al: Challenges of infectious diseases in the USA, *Lancet* 384(9937):53-63, 2014.
2. Hoyert DL, Xu J: *Deaths: preliminary data for 2011, national vital statistics reports*, vol 61, no. 6, Hyattsville, Md, 2012, National Center for Health Statistics.
3. Murthy S et al: Infections of the developing world, *Crit Care Clin* 29(3):485-507, 2013.
4. Brown AF et al: *Staphylococcus aureus* colonization: modulation of host immune response and impact on human vaccine design, *Front Immunol* 4:507, 2014.
5. Scherr TD et al: Hiding in plain sight: interplay between staphylococcal biofilms and host immunity, *Front Immunol* 5:37, 2014.
6. Foster TJ et al: Adhesion, invasion and evasion: the many functions of the surface proteins of *Staphylococcus aureus*, *Nat Rev Microbiol* 12(1): 49-62, 2014.
7. Zecconi A, Scali F: *Staphylococcus aureus* virulence factors in evasion from innate immune defenses in human and animal diseases, *Immunol Lett* 150: 12-22, 2013.
8. Monack DM, Hultgren SJ: The complex interactions of bacterial pathogens and host defenses, *Curr Opin Microbiol* 16(1):1-3, 2013.
9. Baxt LA et al: Bacterial subversion of host innate immune pathways, *Science* 340(6133):697-701, 2013.
10. Alonzo F 3rd, Torres VJ: The bicomponent pore-forming leucocidins of *Staphylococcus aureus*, *Microbiol Mol Biol Rev* 78(2):199-230, 2014.
11. Scully IL et al: Covering all the bases: preclinical development of an effective *Staphylococcus aureus* vaccine, *Front Immunol* 5:109, 2014.
12. Huet O, Chin-Dusting JPF: Septic shock: desperately seeking treatment, *Clin Sci* 126(1): 31-39, 2014.
13. Hotchkiss RS et al: Sepsis-induced immunosuppression: from cellular dysfunctions to immunotherapy, *Nat Rev Immunol* 13(12):862-874, 2013.
14. Bean AGD et al: Studying immunity to zoonotic diseases in the natural host—keeping it real, *Nat Rev Immunol* 13(12):851-861, 2013.
15. Ramsey CD, Kumar A: Influenza and endemic viral pneumonia, *Crit Care Clin* 29:1069-1086, 2013.
16. Sun X, Whittaker GR: Entry of influenza virus, *Adv Exp Med Biol* 790:72-82, 2014.
17. Schrauwen EJA et al: Determinants of virulence of influenza A virus, *Eur J Clin Microbiol Infect Dis* 33(4):479-490, 2014.
18. World Health Organization (WHO): *Malaria Fact Sheet No 94 Reviewed April 2015*, Geneva Switzerland, 2015, Author. Available at: http://www.who.int/mediacentre/factsheets/fs094/en/
19. Centers for Disease Control and Prevention (CDC): *Antibiotic resistance threats in the United States, 2013*. Available at: www.cdc.gov/drugresistance/threat-report-2013/pdf/ar-threats-2013-508.pdf, 2013. Accessed to May 12, 2015.
20. Rubinstein E, Keynan Y: Vancomycin-resistant enterococci, *Crit Care Clin* 29:841-852, 2013.
21. Kennedy D: Time to deal with antibiotics, *Science* 342(6160):776-777, 2013.
22. Rappuoli R et al: Vaccines, new opportunities for a new society, *Proc Natl Acad Sci U S A* 111(34): 12288-12293, 2014.
23. Larson HJ et al: Measuring vaccine confidence: analysis of data obtained by a media surveillance system used to analyse public concerns about vaccines, *Lancet Infect Dis* 13(7):606-613, 2013.
24. Smith JC et al: Building confidence in vaccines, *Adv Exp Med Biol* 764:81-98, 2013.

25. Centers for Disease Control and Prevention (CDC): Progress toward poliomyelitis eradication—Nigeria, January 2009–June 2010, *MMWR Morb Mortal Wkly Rep* 59(26):802-807, 2010.
26. Global Polio Eradication Initiative: *Data and monitoring, November 19, 2014*. Available at http://polioeradication.org/Dataandmonitoring/Poliothisweek.aspx.
27. Hemachudha T et al: Human rabies: neuropathogenesis, diagnosis, and management, *Lancet Neurol* 12(5):498-513, 2013.
28. Graham BS: Advances in antiviral vaccine development, *Immunol Rev* 255(1):230-242, 2013.
29. Cant A, Battersby A: When to think of immunodeficiency, *Adv Exp Med Biol* 764:167-177, 2013.
30. Milner JD, Holland SM: The cup runneth over: lessons from the ever-expanding pool of primary immunodeficiency diseases, *Nat Rev Immunol* 13(9):635-648, 2013.
31. Al-Herz W et al: Primary immunodeficiency diseases: an update on the classification from the International Union of Immunological Societies Expert Committee for Primary Immunodeficiency, *Front Immunol* 5:162, 2014.
32. van der Burg M, van Zelm MC: Clinical spectrum of SCID: the key is the thymus? *Front Immunol* 5:111, 2014.
33. Durandy A et al: Primary antibody deficiencies, *Nat Rev Immunol* 13(7):510-533, 2013.
34. Holland SM: Chronic granulomatous disease, *Hematol Oncol Clin N Am* 27:89-99, 2013.
35. Schwab I, Nimmerjahn F: Intravenous immunoglobulin therapy: how does IgG modulate the immune system, *Nat Rev Immunol* 13(3): 176-189, 2013.
36. Horn B, Cowan MJ: Unresolved issues in hematopoietic stem cell transplantation for severe combined immunodeficiency: need for safer conditioning and reduced late effects, *J Allergy Clin Immunol* 131(5):1306-1311, 2013.
37. Eggenhofer E et al: The life and fate of mesenchymal stem cells, *Front Immunol* 55:148, 2014.
38. Toubai T et al: Mesenchymal stem cells for treatment and prevention of graft-versus-host disease after allogeneic hematopoietic cell transplantation, *Curr Stem Cell Res Therapy* 4(4): 252-259, 2009.
39. Blaese RM: Development of gene therapy for immunodeficiency: adenosine deaminase deficiency, *Pediatr Res* 33(1 Suppl):S49-S53, 1993.
40. Onodera M et al: Gene therapy for severe combined immunodeficiency caused by adenosine deaminase deficiency: improved retroviral vectors for clinical trials, *Acta Haematol* 101(2):89-96, 1999.
41. Mukherjee S, Thrasher AJ: Gene therapy for PIDs: progress, pitfalls, and prospects, *Gene* 525:174-181, 2013.
42. World Health Organization (WHO): *Towards universal access: scaling up priority HIV/AIDS interventions in the health sector: progress report 2009*, Geneva Switzerland, 2009, Author.
43. Centers for Disease Control and Prevention (CDC): *Diagnosis of HIV infection in the United States and dependent areas, 2013*, HIV Surveillance Report, Volume 25. Available at: http://www.cdc.gov/hiv/library/reports/surveillance/2013/surveillance_Report_vol_25.html Last updated: February 23, 2015 Accessed March 27, 2015.
44. World Health Organization (WHO): *Patient evaluation and antiretroviral treatment for adults and adolescents clinical protocol for the WHO European Region 2012, revision*, Geneva, Switzerland, 2012, Author.

45. National Institutes of Health (NIH): *Guidelines for the use of antiretroviral agents in HIV-1-infected adults and adolescents*. Available at: http://aidsinfo.nih.gov/guidelines. Accessed August 11, 2014.
46. Archin NM, Margolis DM: Emerging strategies to deplete the HIV reservoir, *Curr Opin Infect Dis* 27(1):29-35, 2014.
47. Smith PL et al: Developments in HIV-1 immunotherapy and therapeutic vaccination, *F1000Prime Reports* 6:43, 2014.
48. Roff SR et al: The significance of interferon-γ in HIV-1 pathogenesis, therapy, and prophylaxis, *Front Immunol* 4:498, 2014.
49. Chiodi F, Weiss RA: Human immunodeficiency virus antibodies and the vaccine problem, *J Intern Med* 275(5):444-455, 2014.
50. Schneider E et al: Revised surveillance case definitions for HIV infection among adults, adolescents, and children aged <18 months and for HIV infection and AIDS among children aged 18 months to <13 years—United States, 2008, *MMWR Morb Mortal Wkly Rep* 57(RR10):1-8, 2008.
51. Ngo ST et al: Gender differences in autoimmune disease, *Front Endocrinol* 35(3):347-369, 2014.
52. Brown SGA et al: Anaphylaxis: clinical patterns, mediator release, and severity, *J Allergy Clin Immunol* 132(11):1141-1149, 2013.
53. Eckl-Dorna J, Niederberger V: What is the source of serum allergen-specific IgE? *Curr Allergy Asthma Rep* 13(3):281-287, 2013.
54. Longo G et al: IgE-mediated food allergy in children, *Lancet* 382(9905):1656-1664, 2013.
55. Lopata AL, Jeebhay MF: Airborne seafood allergens as a cause of occupational allergy and asthma, *Curr Allergy Asthma Rep* 13(3):288-297, 2013.
56. Mueller GA et al: The molecular basis of peanut allergy, *Curr Allergy Asthma Rep* 14(5):429-438, 2014.
57. Golden DBK: Advances in diagnosis and management of insect sting allergy, *Ann Allergy Asthma Immunol* 111(4):84-89, 2013.
58. Burks AW et al: Update on allergy immunotherapy: American Academy of Allergy, Asthma & Immunology/European Academy of Allergy and Clinical Immunology/PRACTALL consensus report, *J Allergy Clin Immunol* 131(5):1288-1296, 2013.
59. Deane KD, El-Gabalawy H: Pathogenesis and prevention of rheumatic disease: focus on preclinical RA and SLE, *Nat Rev Rheumatol* 10(4): 212-228, 2014.
60. Sorrentino R et al: HLA-B27 and antigen presentation: at the crossroads between immune defense and autoimmunity, *Mol Immunol* 57(1): 22-27, 2014.
61. Root-Bernstein R, Fairweather D: Complexities in the relationship between infection and autoimmunity, *Curr Allergy Asthma Rep* 14(1): 407-414, 2014.
62. Alam J et al: Potential role of bacterial infection in autoimmune diseases: a new aspect of molecular mimicry, *Immune Netw* 14(1):7-13, 2014.
63. Kurts C et al: The immune system and kidney disease: basic concepts and clinical implications, *Nat Rev Immunol* 13(10):738-753, 2013.
64. Kirtakidou M et al: Systemic lupus erythematosus, *Ann Int Med* 159(1):ITC4-1-ITC4-16, 2013.
65. Hochberg MC: Updating the American College of Rheumatology revised criteria for the classification of systemic lupus erythematosus, *Arthritis Rheum* 40(9):1725, 1997.
66. Petri M et al: Deviation and validation of the Systemic Lupus International Collaborating Clinics classification for systemic lupus erythematosus, *Arthritis Rheum* 64(8):2677-2686, 2012.

9

Stress and Disease

Margaret F. Clayton, Kathryn L. McCance, and Lorey K. Takahashi

EVOLVE WEBSITE

http://evolve.elsevier.com/Huether/

Student Review Questions
Audio Key Points

Case Studies
Animations
Quick Check Answers

CHAPTER OUTLINE

Stress is broadly defined as a perceived or anticipated threat that disrupts a person's well-being or homeostasis. Stress involves a complex interaction between the body and brain in the face of random and constant external and internal challenges called stressors.[1,2] A stressor may stem from psychologic/emotional (fear, social rejection), physical (dramatic temperature changes, abuse), or physiologic (infection, inflammation) stimuli that trigger the stress response. Many physical and physiologic stressors also are discussed in various chapters. This chapter highlights the effects of psychologic and emotional stressors on modulating the onset of human diseases.

Exposure to acute stress activates defensive neural, autonomic, and immune systems to facilitate adaptation and survival.[3-5] However, unremitting or toxic stress induces adverse effects by promoting pathophysiology in the very systems that function to meet the challenges of acute stress. For example, whereas acute stress enhances the immune system to protect the individual, adverse situations that cannot be resolved and are accompanied by prolonged activation of the body's stress systems may lead to immunosuppression that impairs the body's ability to fight diseases.[6]

Although modern society offers many positive opportunities, events perceived as especially stressful and uncontrollable, such as loss of a family member, loss of a job, cancer diagnosis, physical abuse, social neglect, or financial hardships, may induce unhealthy coping strategies (e.g., smoking, drinking alcohol, drug abuse) and poor decisions, such as foregoing sleep, eating high calorie comfort foods, and withdrawing from physical activity. Continued engagement in these behavioral activities is linked to a number of serious illnesses, such as hypertension, depression, diabetes, and obesity (Figure 9-1).[4,7,8] Thus, information should be made widely available to inform people of the positive benefits of coping behavior (e.g., mindfulness, yoga, exercise) or to seek social support from others and healthcare professionals to maintain a healthy behavioral and physiologic profile.

HISTORICAL BACKGROUND AND GENERAL CONCEPTS

Walter B. Cannon used the term *stress* in both a physiologic and a psychologic sense as early as 1914, and coined the term "fight-or flight response" to describe the body's preparation to deal with threat.[9] He applied the engineering concepts of stress and strain in a physiologic context and believed that emotional stimuli also were capable of causing stress. The physiologic reactions to stress included increased heart rate and blood supply of oxygen and glucose to muscles and the brain, elevated respiration, dilation of pupils, and inhibition of gastric secretions.

In 1946, Hans Selye further popularized and advanced the concept of stress in terms of a chemical or physical change (i.e., physiologic stress, in response either to the external environment or within the body itself). His work showed that physiologic stress involved: (1) enlargement of the adrenal gland, (2) decreased lymphocyte levels in the blood from damage to lymphatic structures of the immune system, and (3) development of bleeding ulcers in the stomach and duodenal lining. Selye concluded physiologic stress will impair the ability of the organism to resist future stressors and represented the hallmark pattern of a nonspecific stress response that was labeled the general adaptation syndrome (GAS).[10]

The GAS involved three successive stages: the alarm, the resistance or adaptation, and the exhaustion stages. The alarm stage is the emergency reaction that prepares the body to fight or flee from threat. This stage involves the secretion of hormones and catecholamines to

Environmental stressors (work, home, neighborhood)	Major life events	Trauma, abuse

FIGURE 9-1 Physiologic and Behavioral Stress Responses. Stress processes arise from bidirectional communication patterns between the brain and other physiologic systems (autonomic, immune, neural, and endocrine). Importantly, these bidirectional mechanisms are protective, promoting short-term adaptation (allostasis). Chronic stress mechanisms, however, can lead to long-term dysregulation and promote behavioral responses and physiologic responses that lead to stress-induced disorders/diseases (allostatic load), compromising health. (From McEwen BS: *Eur J Pharmacol* 583[2-3]:174-185, 2008.)

support physiologic/metabolic activity (Figures 9-2 and 9-3) and boosts the immune system to thwart infection and disease. The ensuing resistance or adaptation stage requires continued mobilization of the body's resources to cope and overcome a sustained challenge. The exhaustion stage (currently described as allostatic overload; discussed later) occurs then the body's physiologic and immune systems no longer effectively cope with the stressor and marks the onset of diseases (diseases of adaptation). That is, when stress continues unabated and adaptation is not successful, body organs that are weak, such as the heart and kidney, may no longer function and lead to death.

Although the GAS is considered a cornerstone of stress research, the concept that stress is entirely the result of a physical disturbance is an oversimplification. In the mid-1950s, studies emerged demonstrating that psychologic stressors were highly effective in activating adrenal hormone secretion. For example, stress hormone levels increased when monkeys were reexposed to a clicking sound previously paired with electric shock.[11] Similarly, stress hormone secretion in humans increased when exposed to psychologic stressors,[12] such as a stressful interview.[13] According to Mason a number of psychologic factors, such as degree of comfort, unpleasantness, or suddenness of an unanticipated stimulus, could modulate the magnitude of the stress response.[14]

Research from the 1970s has demonstrated a remarkable sensitivity of the central nervous system and endocrine system to emotional, psychologic, and social influences. Psychologic stressors can elicit a reactive or anticipatory stress response. For example, an examination with no physical stressor may elicit a reactive response involving physiologic changes, such as increased heart rate and dry mouth. Anticipatory responses occur when physiologic responses develop in anticipation of psychologic stress or threat. Anticipatory responses can be generated by the fear of a potential encounter with a dangerous, unconditioned stimulus (such as a predator) or in conditioned situations when a person learns that a specific event was associated with an aversive situation.[15] Anticipation of reexposure to these unwanted events produces a physiologic stress response. For example, a child with

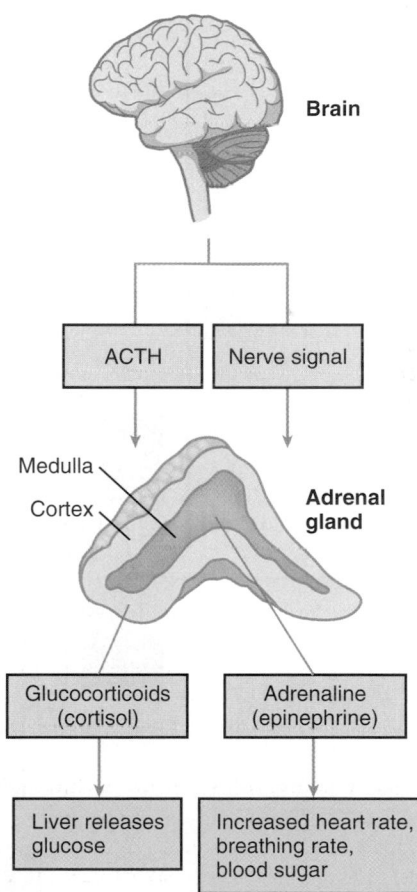

FIGURE 9-2 The Alarm Reaction. The alarm reaction includes increased secretion of glucocorticoids (cortisol) by the adrenal cortex and increased secretion of epinephrine and small amounts of norepinephrine from the adrenal medulla. The response to the release of cortisol and sympathetic nerve activation is summarized in Figure 9-3. *ACTH,* Adrenocorticotropic hormone. (Adapted from Thibodeau GA, Patton KT: *Anatomy & physiology,* ed 9, St Louis, 2016, Mosby.)

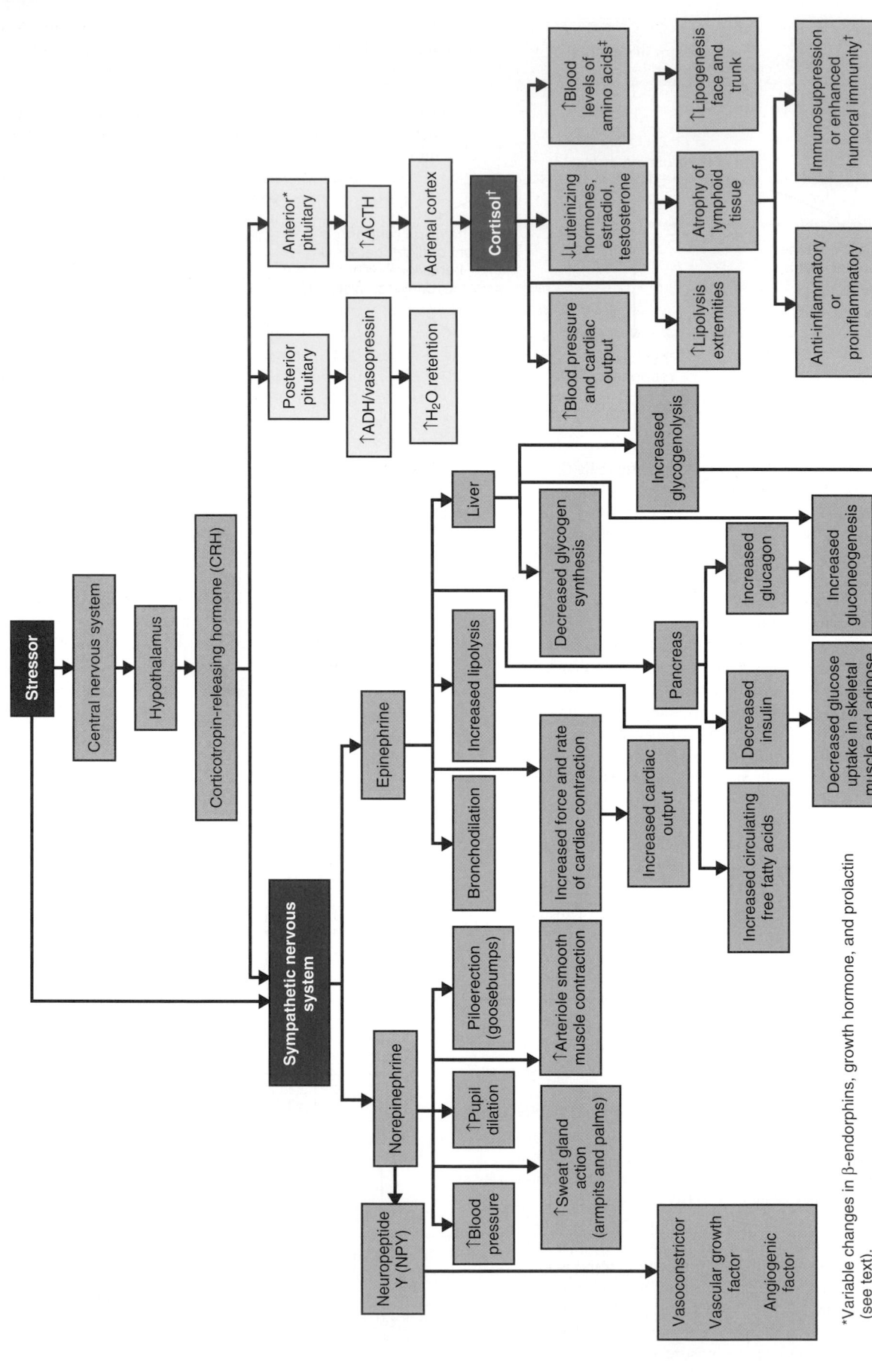

FIGURE 9-3 The Stress Response.

*Variable changes in β-endorphins, growth hormone, and prolactin (see text).
†Effects may be dependent on *amount* of cortisol and nature of the stressor.
‡Caused by protein catabolism in muscle, adipose tissue, skin, bones, lymphoid tissue.
ADH, Antidiuretic hormone; *ACTH,* adrenocorticotropic hormone.

a history of parental abuse may experience a physiologic stress response in anticipation of further abuse when that parent enters the room. Another well-known example of a conditioned emotional response is the development of posttraumatic stress disorder (PSTD) in some military veterans and survivors of natural disasters.

Psychoneuroimmunology (PNI) is the study of how consciousness (*psycho*), mediated by the CNS (*neuro*), interacts with the immune system (*immunology*) to defend the body against infection. Psychoneuroimmunology assumes that immune-mediated diseases result from complex interrelationships among psychosocial, emotional, genetic, neurologic, endocrine, immunologic, and behavioral factors.[16-18] The immune system is integrated with other physiologic processes and sensitive to changes in CNS and endocrine functioning linked to psychologic states. Stressors include a broad range of physical and emotional sources—for example, infection, noise, decreased oxygen supply, pain, malnutrition, heat, cold, trauma, prolonged exertion, radiation, responses to life events (including anxiety, depression, anger, fear, loss, and excitement), obesity, advanced age, drugs, disease, surgery, and medical treatment.

The study of PNI has generated broad scientific debate, especially with respect to the causal role of personality and emotional factors in cancer mortality and morbidity. For example, mouse models suggest a strong link between stress and breast cancer progression, but this effect is not consistently found in humans.[19,20] What is becoming increasingly clear is that secretion of stress hormones influences many metabolic systems and physiologic events in both adults and children.[21,22] Furthermore, studies now point to a strong association between modulation of the immune system by psychosocial stressors and health outcomes.[3,23-25] With increased understanding of the relationship between stress and human diseases, new strategies are emerging to treat stress-related disorders.

Stress Overview: Allostasis, Multiple Mediators, and Systems

Increased knowledge of the link between stress and disease is supported by the concept of **allostasis**, introduced by Sterling and Eyer,[26] and refers to "stability through change." This concept differs from the "fixed homeostasis model" in which physiologic regulation revolves around an unchanging set point. For example, after exposure to a challenging stressor, heighted physiologic secretion of stress hormones (e.g., cortisol) must return to basal levels. By contrast, allostasis involves a dynamic strategy with the brain continuously monitoring many parameters to anticipate what is required from the neuroendocrine and autonomic systems to meet the challenges of future events.[3,27,28] Hence, return to initial basal hormone levels may not be the most adaptive strategy to cope with anticipated stress encounters. However, when chronic activation of regulatory systems taxes the body and brain, diseases and disorders may emerge. **Allostatic overload** is the term used to describe overactivation of adaptive regulatory physiologic systems that may lead to clinical pathophysiology and increase susceptibility of disease.

Research suggests that allostasis and allostatic overload are highly individualized; that is, an event or situation that is considered normal in one person may be stressful to another.[29,30] In people experiencing allostatic overload, this load exacts a "wear and tear" toll on our bodies. Because the brain is a key player in perceiving stress, it is influential in determining when we have reached allostatic overload. Thus, psychologic stress is increasingly recognized both as a precipitating factor for some diseases as well as a contributor that worsens symptoms and negative outcomes in anxiety, chronic pain and fatigue syndromes, ulcers, asthma, obesity, metabolic syndrome, essential hypertension, and type 2 diabetes. In addition, stress disrupts the biologic process of sleep and growth and reproductive functions.[24,31-34] Some of these disorders are the leading causes of death in the United States (Table 9-1).

In response to acute and chronic stress, brain regions, including the hippocampus, amygdala, and prefrontal cortex, may respond by undergoing structural remodeling that alters behavioral and physiologic responses to increase the risk of developing cognitive impairments and depression.[1,28] Key physiologic systems involved in allostatic overload include exaggerated secretion of cortisol, catecholamines of the sympathetic nervous system, and proinflammatory cytokines, as well as a decline in parasympathetic activity. A prevalent example is sleep deprivation from being "stressed out." Sleep deprivation and disturbances, such as sleep apnea, short sleep duration, and insomnia,

TABLE 9-1	**Examples of Stress-Related Diseases and Conditions**		
Target Organ or System	**Disease or Condition**	**Target Organ or System**	**Disease or Condition**
Cardiovascular system	Coronary artery disease	Gastrointestinal system	Ulcer
	Hypertension		Irritable bowel syndrome
	Stroke		Diarrhea
	Disturbances of heart rhythm		Nausea and vomiting
			Ulcerative colitis
Muscle	Tension headaches	Genitourinary system	Diuresis
	Muscle contraction backache		Impotence
			Frigidity
Connective tissues	Rheumatoid arthritis (autoimmune disease)	Skin	Eczema
			Neurodermatitis
	Related inflammatory diseases of connective tissue		Acne
Pulmonary system	Asthma (hypersensitivity reaction)	Endocrine system	Type 2 diabetes mellitus
	Hay fever (hypersensitivity reactions)		Amenorrhea
Immune system	Immunosuppression or deficiency	Central nervous system	Fatigue and lethargy
	Autoimmune diseases		Type A behavior
			Overeating
			Depression
			Insomnia

have significant associations with allostatic load, leading to damaging effects including elevated evening cortisol concentration; elevated insulin and blood glucose levels; increased blood pressure; reduced parasympathetic activity; increased levels of proinflammatory cytokines; and increased secretion of the hormone ghrelin (primarily by cells of the stomach and pancreas), which increases appetite.[35,36] Overall, the dynamic and damaging effects of allostatic overload can induce sleep deprivation, which then facilitates increased caloric intake, depressed mood, cognitive deficits, and a host of other unhealthy responses.

✔ **QUICK CHECK 9-1**
1. How is stress related to unhealthy coping behaviors?
2. Briefly describe the three stages of the general adaptation syndrome.
3. Define allostatic load and allostatic overload.

THE STRESS RESPONSE

Because evidence points to the important role that stress plays in many disease processes, research has begun to focus on physiologic mechanisms underlying mind-body interactions in order to understand and prevent stress-related diseases. Using a multidisciplinary approach involving molecular biology, immunology, neurology, endocrinology, and behavioral science, researchers are investigating how stressful life events occurring over a prolonged period of time impair immune functions. Knowledge emerging from the various disciplines offers a holistic and complex model of the biochemical relationships among the central nervous system (CNS), autonomic nervous system (ANS), endocrine system, and immune system.

Regulation of the Hypothalamic-Pituitary-Adrenal System

A key stress hormone relationship is the regulation of the hypothalamic-pituitary-adrenal (HPA) system (Figure 9-4). In sequence, the perception of stress activates the hypothalamus to secrete corticotropin-releasing hormone (CRH), which binds to specific receptors on anterior pituitary cells that, in turn, produce adrenocorticotropic hormone (ACTH). ACTH is then transported through the blood to the adrenal glands located on the top of the kidneys. After binding to specific receptors on the cortex of the adrenal glands, glucocorticoid hormones (primarily cortisol) are released.

Physiologic Effects of Cortisol

During stress, the secretion of glucocorticoid hormones, primarily cortisol (cortisol is known outside the body as hydrocortisone), reaches all tissues, including the brain, easily penetrates cell membranes, and reacts with numerous intracellular glucocorticoid receptors (see Figure 9-3). Because they spare almost no tissue or organ and influence a large proportion of the human genome, glucocorticoids exert significant diverse biologic actions.[24] They regulate many functions of the CNS, including arousal, cognition, mood, sleep, metabolism, maintenance of cardiovascular tone, the immune and inflammatory reaction, and growth and reproduction.

Cortisol mobilizes substances needed for cellular metabolism and stimulates gluconeogenesis or the formation of glucose from noncarbohydrate sources, such as amino acids or free fatty acids in the liver. In addition, cortisol enhances the elevation of blood glucose levels that is promoted by other hormones, such as epinephrine, glucagon, and growth hormone. Cortisol also inhibits the uptake and oxidation of glucose by many body cells. Overall, cortisol's actions on

FIGURE 9-4 Hypothalamic-Pituitary-Adrenal (HPA) Axis. The response to stress begins in the brain. The hypothalamus is the control center in the brain for many hormones including corticotropin-releasing hormone (CRH).

carbohydrate metabolism result in increased blood glucose levels, thereby energizing the body to combat the stressor. The effects of cortisol are summarized in Table 9-2.

Cortisol also affects protein metabolism. It has an anabolic effect by increasing the rate of protein synthesis and ribonucleic acid (RNA) in the liver. This is countered by its catabolic effect on protein stores in other tissues. Protein catabolism acts to increase levels of circulating amino acids; therefore chronic exposure to excess cortisol can severely deplete protein stores in muscle, bone, connective tissue, and skin.

Another important adaptive function of cortisol is to enhance immunity during acute stress.[37] Cortisol exerts beneficial effects by inhibiting initial inflammatory effects, for example, vasodilation and increased capillary permeability. Cortisol also promotes resolution and repair. These actions are mainly accomplished by facilitating the effects of glucocorticoid receptor (GR), namely, the transcription of genetic material (through DNA binding) within leukocytes.[38]

Pathophysiologic Effects of Cortisol

Chronic dysregulation of the HPA axis, especially abnormal elevated levels of cortisol, has been linked to a wide variety of disorders, including obesity, sleep deprivation, lipid abnormalities, hypertension, diabetes, atherosclerosis, and loss of bone density.[3,24,30,39] In the brain, chronic glucocorticoid secretion may reduce hippocampal volume, enlarge the ventricles, and modulate reversible cortical atrophy.[1,24]

TABLE 9-2   **Physiologic Effects of Cortisol**

Functions Affected	Physiologic Effects
Carbohydrate and lipid metabolism	Diminishes peripheral uptake and utilization of glucose; promotes gluconeogenesis in liver metabolism cells; enhances gluconeogenic response to other hormones; promotes lipolysis in adipose tissue
Protein metabolism	Increases protein synthesis in liver and decreases protein synthesis (including immunoglobulin synthesis) in muscle, lymphoid tissue, adipose tissue, skin, and bone; increases plasma level of amino acids; stimulates deamination in liver
Anti-inflammatory effects (systemic effects)	High levels of cortisol used in drug therapy suppress inflammatory response and inhibit proinflammatory activity of many growth factors and cytokines; however, over time some individuals may develop tolerance to glucocorticoids, causing an increased susceptibility to both inflammatory and autoimmune diseases
Proinflammatory effects (possible local effects)	Cortisol levels released during stress response may increase proinflammatory effects
Lipid metabolism	Lipolysis in extremities and lipogenesis in face and trunk
Immune effects	*Treatment* levels of glucocorticoids are immunosuppressive; thus they are valuable agents used in numerous diseases/conditions; T-cell or innate immune system is particularly affected by these larger doses of glucocorticoids, with suppression of Th1 function or innate immunity; *stress* can cause a different pattern of immune response; these nontherapeutic levels can suppress innate (Th1) and increase adaptive (Th2) immunity—the so-called Th2 shift; several factors influence this complex physiology and include long-term adaptations, reproductive hormones (i.e., overall, androgens suppress and estrogens stimulate immune responses), defects of the hypothalamic-pituitary-adrenal axis, histamine-generated responses, and acute versus chronic stress; thus stress seems to cause a Th2 shift *systemically*, whereas *locally*, under certain conditions, it can induce proinflammatory activities and by these mechanisms may influence onset or course of infections, autoimmune/inflammatory, allergic, and neoplastic diseases
Digestive function	Promotes gastric secretion
Urinary function	Enhances excretion of calcium
Connective tissue function	Decreases proliferation of fibroblasts in connective tissue (thus delaying healing)
Muscle function	Maintains normal contractility and maximal work output for skeletal and cardiac muscle
Bone function	Decreases bone formation
Vascular system/myocardial function	Maintains normal blood pressure; permits increased responsiveness of arterioles to constrictive action of adrenergic stimulation; optimizes myocardial performance
Central nervous system function	Somehow modulates perceptual and emotional functioning; essential for normal arousal and initiation of daytime activity
Possible synergism with estrogen in pregnancy?	May suppress maternal immune system to prevent rejection of fetus

These CNS changes may contribute to cognitive impairments and emotional disorders.

In the periphery, heightened stress-induced cortisol levels promote gastric secretion in the stomach and intestines, potentially causing gastric ulcers, which may account for the gastrointestinal ulceration observed by Selye. Furthermore, glucocorticoids contribute to the development of metabolic syndrome and the pathogenesis of obesity (see *Health Alert:* Glucocorticoids, Insulin, Inflammation, and Obesity) by directly causing insulin resistance and influencing genetic variations that predispose to obesity.[40-42]

The impact of cortisol on fetal development and subsequent risk for future disease also has been investigated. Reynolds offers convincing data associating high maternal cortisol levels during pregnancy with low birth weight.[43] The consequences of cortisol-induced low birth weight have now extended to disease risk in later life, for example, obesity; cardiovascular conditions, such as hypertension; and behavioral disorders attributed to altered brain structure.[43-45] Thus, glucocorticoids dramatically affect human pathophysiology and, consequently, longevity.[3,24,39]

The feedback mechanisms of the HPA axis sense and determine the circulating glucocorticoid levels, whereas other tissues passively accept the actions of circulating glucocorticoids.[24] Thus, discrepancy in the glucocorticoid sensing network between the HPA axis and peripheral tissues could possibly produce peripheral tissue hypercortisolism or hypocortisolism. For example, both high HPA axis reactivity to stress and increased peripheral tissue sensitivity to glucocorticoids are associated with the severity of coronary artery disease (see *Health Alert: Psychosocial Stress and Progression to Coronary Heart Disease*).[46,47]

Cortisol secretion during stress exerts beneficial effects by inhibiting initial inflammatory effects, for example, vasodilation and increased capillary permeability.[38] Cortisol also promotes resolution and repair. These actions are mainly accomplished by facilitating the effects of glucocorticoid receptor (GR), namely, the transcription of genetic material (through DNA binding) within leukocytes.[38] Because glucocorticoids are so widely expressed, they influence virtually all immune cells. The adaptiveness or destructiveness of cortisol-induced effects may depend on the intensity, type, and duration of the stressor; the tissue involved; and the subsequent concentration and length of cortisol exposure. Finally, glucocorticoids have been shown to induce T-cell apoptosis.[38,48]

Effects of Exogenous Glucocorticoids

Stress hormones, especially glucocorticoids (cortisol), are used therapeutically as powerful anti-inflammatory/immunosuppressive agents. The synthetic forms of glucocorticoid hormones (exogenous types of anti-inflammatory glucocorticoids administered for a pharmaceutical reaction) are poorly metabolized when compared with endogenous glucocorticoids, leading to a longer half-life and no circadian rhythm for these compounds. Moreover, these synthetic compounds bind with different targets, so each has a unique effect.[49]

Elevated levels of glucocorticoids and catecholamines (epinephrine and norepinephrine), both endogenous and exogenously administered,

HEALTH ALERT

Glucocorticoids, Insulin, Inflammation, and Obesity

The signs and symptoms of Cushing syndrome (e.g., excess glucocorticoids [GCs]) include truncal obesity, relatively thin extremities, a "moon face," and a "buffalo [neck] hump." In such individuals the possibility of associated hypertension is high as well as increased risk of infection and metabolic syndrome or frank type 2 diabetes. In addition, the likelihood of an elevated ratio of intraabdominal subcutaneous fat mass to nonabdominal fat mass is high because the glucocorticoids mediate the redistribution of stored calories into the abdominal region. The specific increase in abdominal fat stores is a consequence of elevated levels of glucocorticoids combined with increased insulin action. However, the increased levels of glucocorticoids need not be present in the circulation; instead, they can be generated locally in fat by conversion of inactive cortisone to active cortisol through the action of the isoenzyme 11β-hydroxysteroid dehydrogenase (11β-HSD) type 1. This conversion is referred to as "pre-receptor" metabolism of cortisol. The active steroid is secreted directly to the liver through the portal vein. In vitro insulin synthesis and secretion from the pancreas are inhibited by the glucocorticoids. However, increasing levels of glucocorticoids in vivo are associated with increasing insulin secretion, possibly because of an anti-insulin effect on the liver, which appears to be vulnerable to the negative effects of glucocorticoids on insulin action. Hepatic insulin resistance is strongly associated with abdominal obesity.

Recent data reveal that the plasma concentration of inflammatory mediators, such as tumor necrosis factor-alpha (TNF-α) and interleukin-6 (IL-6), is increased in the insulin-resistant states of obesity and type 2 diabetes. Two mechanisms might be involved in the pathogenesis of inflammation: (1) glucose and macronutrient intake (i.e., which can be mediated through chronic stress) causes oxidative stress; and (2) the increased concentrations of TNF-α and IL-6 associated with obesity and type 2 diabetes might interfere with insulin signal transduction. This interference might promote inflammation. Chronic overnutrition (obesity) might thus be a proinflammatory state with oxidative stress.

Stress, Inflammation, Obesity, and Type 2 Diabetes. The induction of reactive oxygen species (ROS) generation and inflammation through the proinflammatory transcription factor, NF-κβ, activates most proinflammatory genes. Macronutrient intake, obesity, free fatty acids, infection, smoking, psychologic stress, and genetic factors increase the production of ROS. Interference with insulin signaling (insulin resistance) leads to hyperglycemia and proinflammatory changes. Proinflammatory changes increase levels of TNF-α and IL-6, and also lead to the inhibition of insulin signaling and insulin resistance. Inflammation in pancreatic beta cells leads to beta-cell dysfunction, which in combination with insulin resistance leads to type 2 diabetes. *CRP,* C-Reactive protein.

Data from Dallman MF et al: *Endocrinology* 145(6):2633-2638, 2004; Dandona P et al: *Trends Immunol* 25(1):4-7, 2004; Kim SP et al: *Diabetes* 52:2453-2460, 2003; Masuzaki H et al: *Science* 94:2166-2170, 2001; Padgett DA, Glaser R: *Trends Immunol* 24(8):444-448, 2003; Spencer SJ, Tilbrook A: *Stress* 14(3), 2011; Strack AM et al: *Am J Physiol* 268:R142-R149, 1995; Wagen Knecht LE et al: *Diabetes* 52:2490-2496, 2003; Shimanoe C et al: *PLoS* 10(2):e0118105, 2015; Khadir A et al: *Mediators Inflamm* 2015:512-603, 2015.

may decrease innate immunity and increase autoimmune responses. In addition, prolonged effects of cortisol may accentuate inflammation and potentially increase neuronal death (e.g., in stroke victims)[49] and induce T-cell apoptosis.[38,48]

Initially, immune responses are regulated by cells of innate immunity called antigen-presenting cells (APCs), such as monocytes/macrophages (see Chapter 7), dendritic cells, and other phagocytic cells, and by Th1 and Th2 lymphocytes (cells involved in adaptive immunity; see Chapter 7). These cells secrete cytokines, the chemical messengers that regulate innate and adaptive immune responses.

Antigen-presenting cells also release cytokines that induce T cells to differentiate into Th1 cells. Th1 cells and APC cytokines work together to stimulate the activity of cytotoxic T cells, natural killer (NK) cells, and activated macrophages—the major components of innate immunity (see Chapter 6).

Cytokines secreted by Th2 cells also act to inhibit Th1 cells and can promote adaptive immunity by stimulating growth and activating mast cells and eosinophils, as well as the differentiation of B-cell immunoglobulins. Thus, these cytokines are considered to be the major anti-inflammatory cytokines (Figure 9-5).[25] The decrease in

HEALTH ALERT

Psychosocial Stress and Progression to Coronary Heart Disease

The link between stress and coronary heart disease was proposed as early as the 1970s; however, it was only recently that conclusive evidence and proposed mechanisms for development of the disease were identified. Much work continues to focus on elucidating the interaction between stress and cardiovascular disease.

One of the primary risk factors for coronary heart disease is hypertension. A new designation of prehypertension was recently created and found to be a good predictor for future cardiovascular events. Prehypertension is defined as a systolic blood pressure of 120 to 139 mm Hg or a diastolic blood pressure of 80 to 90 mm Hg. Individuals with prehypertension are much more likely to develop frank hypertension and, eventually, coronary heart disease.

Studies show that persons with a highly reactive personality type who experience high levels of anxiety with stress are much more likely to progress from prehypertension to hypertension and then to develop cardiac disease, specifically coronary heart disease, than those who have better coping abilities. Further long-term psychologic stress, such as that experienced in a strained marriage or an unhappy work environment, not only was shown to accelerate the progression of hypertension and coronary heart disease but also is correlated with higher mortality rates from coronary heart disease.

Trait anger, defined as a stable personality trait characterized by frequency, intensity, and duration of anger, also was shown to be a factor in the development of coronary heart disease at higher rates than the general population. Individuals with trait anger also experienced more strokes. Hostile individuals with advanced cardiovascular disease may be particularly susceptible to stress-induced increases in sympathetic activity and inflammation.

One popular mechanism for the interaction between psychosocial stress and cardiovascular disease suggests that stress triggers an inflammatory response that, over time, increases the chances of developing coronary heart disease. The primary mechanisms proposed are chronically elevated cortisol levels and dysregulation of the circadian rhythm for cortisol release. Further, chronic stress alters hypothalamic-pituitary-adrenal (HPA) function, resulting in an abnormal stress response pattern. This alteration in HPA activity was found in persons with coronary heart disease along with increased inflammatory markers. A newer and emerging mechanism is the involvement of regulatory T cells (Tregs). Tregs play an important role in maintaining peripheral tolerance of tissue antigens, preventing autoimmune diseases, and decreasing chronic inflammatory diseases. Studies have shown that naturally occurring CD4+CD25+ Tregs are down-regulated in individuals with acute coronary syndrome (ACS). Additionally, the sympathetic nervous system plays an important role in immune homeostasis by maintaining the number of Tregs in the periphery and this may be affected by psychologic stress. The Treg lineage, however, is heterogenous.

Because coronary heart disease is one of the major causes of death in industrialized countries, development of successful interventional programs is of high priority. Programs in which dietary changes, exercise, stress management, and positive support systems are implemented continue to show positive results for slowing the progression of heart disease and decreasing the risk factors for disease development. Further, individuals in these programs report decreased levels of depression and stress as well as overall improvement in mental health.

Data from Bhowmick S et al: *J Leukoc Biol* 86:1275-1283, 2009; Brydon L et al: *J Psychosom Res* 68(2):109-116, 2010; Cheng X et al: *Clin Immunol* 127:89-97, 2008; Davidson KW: *Cleve Clin J Med* 75(Suppl 2):S15-S19, 2008; Miyara M, Sakaguchi S: *Trends Mol Med* 13:108-116, 2007; Mor A et al: *Eur Heart J* 27:2530-2537, 2006; Nijm J et al: *J Int Med* 262(3):375-384, 2007; Sawant DV, Vignali DA, *Immunol Rev* 259(1):173-191, 2014; Sakaguchi S et al: *Cell* 33:775-787, 2008; Sardella G et al: *Thromb Res* 120:631-634, 2007; Shamaei-Tousi A et al: *Cell Stress Chaperons* 12(4):384-382, 2007; Shevach EM: *Annu Rev Immunol* 18:423-449, 2000; Steptoe A, Brydon L: *Neurosci Biobehav Rev* 33:63-70, 2009; Vignali DA et al: *Nat Rev Immunol* 8:523-532, 2008; Vizza J et al: *J Cardiopulm Rehabil Prev* 27(6):378-383, 2007; Zhu Z et al: *PloS* 9(2):e88775, 2014.

Th1 activity and increase in Th2 activity is sometimes called a Th1 to Th2 shift.

Neuroendocrine Regulation: Autonomic Nervous System

Sympathetic Nervous System

The sympathetic nervous system is aroused, simultaneously with the HPA system during stress, to release norepinephrine (adrenergic stimulation) and stimulate the medulla of the adrenal gland to release catecholamines (80% epinephrine and 20% norepinephrine) into the bloodstream. Sympathetic nerves also contain nonadrenergic mediators that amplify or antagonize the effects of adrenal catecholamines.

Circulating catecholamines essentially mimic direct sympathetic stimulation. Catecholamines cannot cross the blood-brain barrier and are synthesized locally in the brain. The physiologic effects of the catecholamines on organs and tissues are summarized in Table 9-3. Norepinephrine regulates blood pressure, promotes arousal, and increases vigilance, anxiety, and other protective emotional responses.

The catecholamines stimulate two major classes of receptors: α-adrenergic receptors (α_1 and α_2) and β-adrenergic receptors (β_1 and β_2). Table 13-7 summarizes the actions of the two subclasses of adrenergic receptors. (A discussion of receptors can be found in Chapters 1, 18, and 23.) Epinephrine binds with and activates both α and β receptors whereas norepinephrine binds primarily with α receptors.

Epinephrine in the liver and skeletal muscles is rapidly metabolized. Epinephrine influences cardiac action by enhancing myocardial contractility (inotropic effect), increasing heart rate (chronotropic effect), and increasing venous return to the heart, ultimately increasing both cardiac output and blood pressure. Epinephrine dilates blood vessels supplying skeletal muscles, allowing for greater oxygenation. Metabolically, it causes transient hyperglycemia (high blood sugar), reduces glucose uptake in the muscles and other organs, and decreases insulin release from the pancreas, thus preventing glucose uptake by peripheral tissue and preserving it for the CNS. Epinephrine also mobilizes free fatty acids and cholesterol.

Catecholamine secretion also increases proinflammatory cytokine production, which elevates heart rate and blood pressure and impairs wound healing.[50] Recent research further indicates that chronic stress-induced increases in norepinephrine levels ultimately result in increased production of inflammatory leukocytes that adhere to vessel walls and promote the development of plaque.[47,51] Proteases released from these inflammatory leukocytes further promote risk of myocardial infarction and stroke by weakening the fibrous cap of the plaque, which can promote plaque rupture.[47] In addition to a stress-induced increased risk of cardiovascular disease, the effects of stress on inflammatory cytokine secretion also influence depression, autoimmune disorders, and virally-mediated cancers,[52,53] and may be important in functional decline that leads to frailty, disability, and untimely death.[32,54] Finally, stress-induced excessive levels of inflammatory cytokines during

FIGURE 9-5 Stress Interactions Are Nonlinear and Complex. Nonlinearity means that when one mediator is increased or decreased, the subsequent compensatory changes in other mediators depend on time and level of change, causing multiple interacting variables. The inevitable consequences from adapting to daily life over time include changes in behavioral responses. For example, these changes include sleeping patterns, smoking, alcohol consumption, physical activity, and social interactions. These behavioral patterns are a part of the allostatic overload with chronic elevations in cortisol level, sympathetic activity, and levels of proinflammatory cytokines, and a decrease in parasympathetic activity. (From McEwen BS: *Eur J Pharmacol* 583[2-3]:174-185, 2008.)

TABLE 9-3	**Physiologic Effects of Catecholamines***
Organ/Tissue	**Process or Result**
Brain	Increased blood flow; increased glucose metabolism
Cardiovascular system	Increased rate and force of contraction
	Peripheral vasoconstriction
Pulmonary system	Bronchodilation
Skeletal muscle	Increased glycogenolysis
	Increased contraction
	Increased dilation of muscle vasculature
	Decreased glucose uptake and utilization (decreases insulin release)
Liver	Increased glucose production
	Increased glycogenolysis
Adipose tissue	Increased lipolysis
	Decreased glucose uptake
Skin	Decreased blood flow
Gastrointestinal and genitourinary tracts	Decreased protein synthesis
	Decreased smooth muscle contraction
	Increased renin release
	Increased gastrointestinal sphincter tone
Lymphoid tissue	Acute and chronic stress inhibits several components of innate immunity, particularly decreasing natural killer cells
Macrophages	Inhibit and stimulate macrophage activity
	Depends on availability of type 1/proinflammatory cytokines, presence or absence of antigenic stressors, and peripheral corticotropin-releasing hormone (CRH)

Data from Elenkov IJ, Chrousos GP: *Ann N Y Acad Sci* 966:290-303, 2002; Granner DK: Hormones of the adrenal medulla. In Murray RK et al, editors: *Harper's biochemistry,* ed 25, New York, 2000, McGraw-Hill.
*Some of these responses require glucocorticoids (e.g., cortisol) for maximal activity (see text for explanation).

infection or inflammatory illness may activate a collection of nonspecific symptoms called the "sickness syndrome."

Parasympathetic Nervous System

The parasympathetic system balances the sympathetic nervous system and thus also influences adaptation or maladaptation to stressful events. The parasympathetic system generally opposes the sympathetic system; for example, the parasympathetic nervous system slows the heart rate. The parasympathetic system also has anti-inflammatory effects.[49] Under conditions of allostatic overload, the parasympathetic system may decrease its containment of the sympathetic system, resulting in increased or prolonged inflammatory responses.[3] Researchers evaluate the relative balance of the parasympathetic and sympathetic nervous systems using a technique known as heart rate variability (the measurement of R wave variability from heartbeat to heartbeat).

Histamine and Other Hormones

The immune system is integrated with other physiologic processes and is sensitive to changes in CNS and endocrine functioning, such as those that accompany psychologic states.[55,56] Stressors can elicit the stress response through the action of the nervous and endocrine systems, specifically CRH from the hypothalamus and from peripheral inflammatory sites (called peripheral or immune CRH).[57,58] **Peripheral (immune) CRH** is proinflammatory, causing an increase in vasodilation and vascular permeability. Therefore it appears that mast cells are the target of peripheral CRH. Mast cells release histamine, which is a well-known mediator of acute inflammation and allergic reactions (Figure 9-6). Histamine induces acute inflammation and allergic reactions while suppressing Th1 activity (decreasing innate immunity) and promoting Th2 activity (increasing adaptive immunity).[59-62]

Thyroid hormone synthesis, which is involved in growth and reproduction, is suppressed during stress, which may conserve energy. **Neuropeptide Y (NPY)**, a sympathetic neurotransmitter, has recently been shown to be a stress mediator. Because NPY is a growth factor for many cells, it is implicated in atherosclerosis and tissue remodeling. Other hormones that influence the stress response are listed in Table 9-4.

Locally, stress can exert proinflammatory or anti-inflammatory effects. Moreover, some evidence indicates that stress is not a uniform, nonspecific reaction.[63] Different types of stressors might have variable

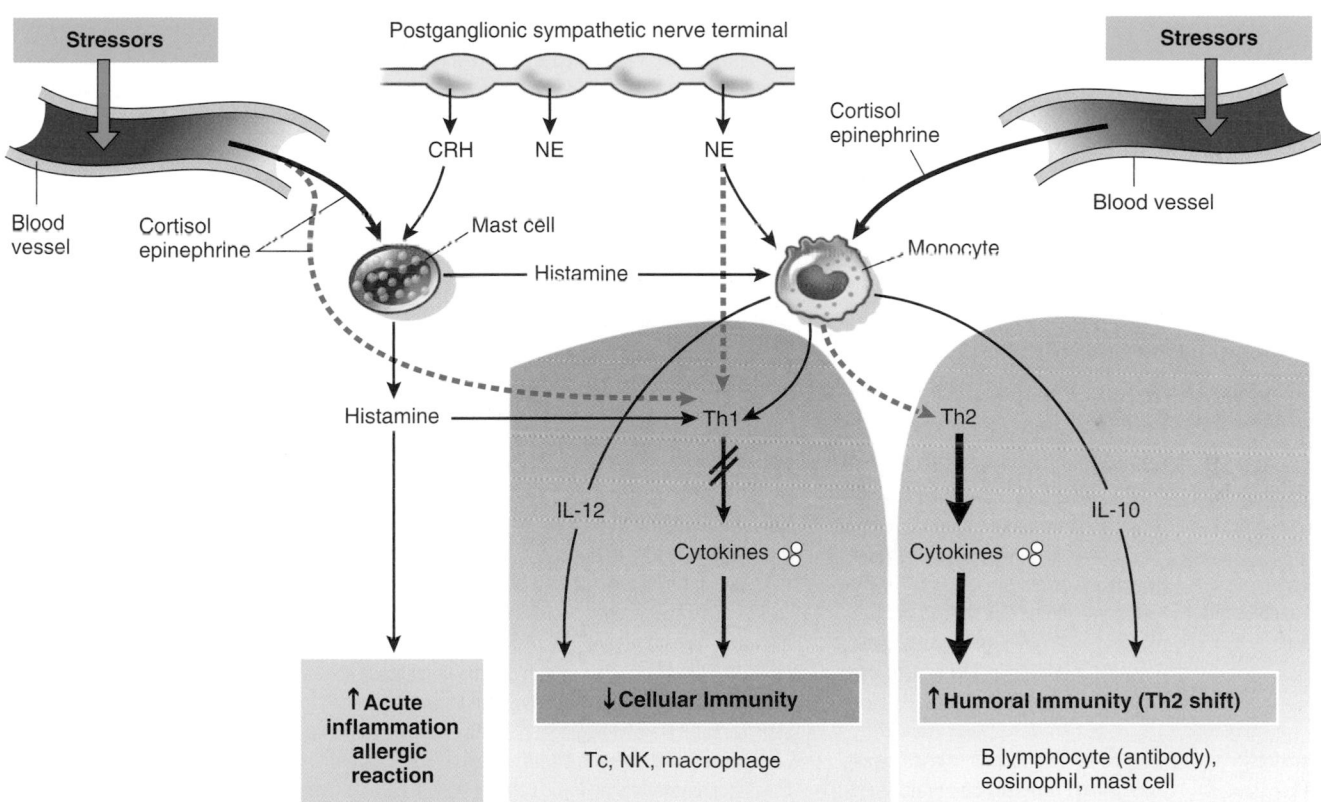

FIGURE 9-6 Effect of Corticotropin-Releasing Hormone (CRH)–Mast Cell–Histamine Axis, Cortisol, and Catecholamines on the Th1/Th2 Balance—Innate and Adaptive Immunity. Adaptive immunity provides protection against multicellular parasites, extracellular bacteria, some viruses, soluble toxins, and allergens. Innate immunity provides protection against intracellular bacteria, fungi, protozoa, and several viruses. Type 1 cytokines or proinflammatory cytokines include IL-12, interferon-gamma (IFN-γ), and tumor necrosis factor-alpha (TNF-α). Type 2 cytokines or anti-inflammatory cytokines include IL-10 and IL-4. Solid lines (black) represent stimulation, whereas dashed lines (blue) represent inhibition (i.e., Th1 and Th2 are mutually inhibitory, IL-12 and IFN-γ inhibit Th2, and vice versa; IL-4 and IL-10 inhibit Th1 responses). Stress and CRH modulate inflammatory/immune and allergic responses by stimulating cortisol (glucocorticoid), catecholamines, and peripheral (immune) CRH secretion and by changing the production of regulatory cytokines and histamines. CRH (peripheral, immune), corticotropin-releasing hormone; IL, interleukin; NE, norepinephrine; Tc, cytotoxic T cell; Th, helper T cell; NK, natural killer cell; dashed lines, decreased (inhibited); solid lines, increased (stimulation). (Redrawn from Elenkov IJ, Chrousos GP: Trends Endocrinol Metab 10[9]:359-368, 1999.)

TABLE 9-4 Other Hormones That Influence the Stress Response

Hormone	Source	Action
β-Endorphins (endogenous opiates)	Pituitary and hypothalamus	Activates endorphin (opiate) receptors on peripheral sensory nerves, leading to pain relief or analgesia Hemorrhage increases levels to inhibit blood pressure or delay compensatory changes that would increase blood pressure[1]
Growth hormone (GH, somatotropin)	Anterior pituitary gland	Affects protein, lipid, and carbohydrate metabolism Counters effects of insulin Involved in tissue repair May participate in growth and function of immune system[2] Levels increase after variety of stressful stimuli (cardiac catheterization, electroshock therapy, gastroscopy, surgery, fever, physical exercise) Increased levels associated with psychologic stimuli (taking examinations, viewing violent or sexually arousing films, participating in certain psychologic performance tests) Prolonged stress (chronic stress) suppresses growth hormone
Prolactin	Anterior pituitary gland; numerous extrapituitary tissue sites[12]	Increases in response to many stressful stimuli (including procedures such as gastroscopy, proctoscopy, pelvic examination, and surgery)[3]; increased for insitu breast cancer[3A] Requires more intense stimuli than those leading to increases in catecholamine or cortisol levels Levels show little change after exercise
Oxytocin	Hypothalamus	Promotes bonding and social attachment[4] In animals associated with reduced hypothalamic-pituitary-adrenal (HPA) activation levels and reduced anxiety[4]
Testosterone	Leydig cells in testes	Regulates male secondary sex characteristics and libido Levels decrease after stressful stimuli (anesthesia, surgery, marathon running, mountain climbing)[5] Decreased by psychologic stimuli; however, some data indicate that psychologic stress associated with competition (e.g., pistol shooting) increases both testosterone and cortisol levels, especially in athletes older than 45 years[6] Markedly reduced in individuals with respiratory failure, burns, and congestive heart failure[7] Decreased levels occur during aging and are associated with lowered cortisol responsiveness to stress-induced inflammation[8]
Estrogen	Ovaries	Works in concert with oxytocin, exerting calming effect during stressful situations[9]
Melatonin	Produced by pineal gland	Increases during stress response; release is suppressed by light and increased in dark; receptors have been identified on lymphoid cells, possibly higher density of receptors on T cells than on B cells; suppression of lymphocyte function by trauma was reversed by melatonin[10]
Somatostatin (SOM)	Produced by sensory nerve terminals found in and released from lymphoid cells and hypothalamus	Natural killer (NK) function and immunoglobulin synthesis decreased by SOM; growth hormone secretion decreased by SOM
Vasoactive intestinal peptide (VIP)	Found in neurons of CNS and in peripheral nerves	VIP increases during stress; VIP-containing nerves are located in both primary and secondary lymphoid tissues, around blood vessels, and in gastrointestinal tract; VIP receptors are on both T and B cells; VIP may influence lymphocyte maturation; cytokine production by T cells is modified by VIP; B-cell and antibody production is influenced by VIP
Calcitonin gene–related peptide (CGRP)	Found in spinal cord motor neurons and in sensory neurons near dendritic cells of skin and in primary and secondary lymphoid tissues	CGRP receptors are present on T and B lymphocytes; thus it is likely that CGRP can modulate immune function; CGRP may enhance acute inflammatory response because it is vasodilator; maturation of immune B lymphocytes is inhibited by CGRP; IL-1 is inhibited by CGRP, which is important for activation of T cells; it has been shown to interfere with lymphocyte activation
Neuropeptide Y (NPY)	Present in neurons of CNS and in neurons throughout body; colocalized in nerve terminals in lymphatic tissues with norepinephrine	Lymphocytes have receptors for NPY and thus may modulate their function[11]; several lines of evidence suggest that NPY is neurotransmitter and neurohormone involved in stress response; increased levels of NPY occur in plasma in response to severe or prolonged stress; may be responsible for stress-induced regional vasoconstriction (splanchnic, coronary, and cerebral); may also increase platelet aggregation.[2] May be important in preventing depression.
Substance P (SP)	Produced by neuropeptide classified as tachykinin (increases heart rate subsequent to lowering blood pressure) found in brain, as well as nerves innervating secondary lymphoid tissues	SP increases in response to stress; receptors for SP are found on membranes of both T and B cells, mononuclear phagocytic cells, and mast cells; proinflammatory activity induces release of histamine from mast cells during stress response; causes smooth muscle contraction, causes macrophages and T cells to release cytokines, and increases antibody production

1. Amico JA et al: *J Neuroendocrinol* 16(4):319-324, 2004.
2. Rabin BS: The nervous system—immune system connection. In *Stress, immune function, and health: the connection,* New York, 1999, Wiley-Liss.
3. Rohleder N et al: *J Neuroimmunol* 126(1-2):69-77, 2002.
3A. Tikk K et al: *Breast Cancer Research* 17(1):49, 2015.
4. Lieberwirth C, Wang Z: *Front Neurosci* 8:171, 2014.
5. Chesnokova V, Melmed S: *Endocrinology* 143(5):1571-1574, 2002.
6. Guezennec CY et al: *Int J Sports Med* 16(6):368-372, 1995.
7. Volterrani M et al: *Endocrine* 42(2):272-277, 2012.
8. Bauer-Wu SM: *Clin J Oncol Nurs* 6(4):243-246, 2002.
9. Kudwa AE et al: *Physiol Behav* 129:287-296, 2014.
10. Maestroni GJ: *Adv Exp Med Biol* 460:396, 1999.
11. Petito JM et al: *J Neuroimmunol* 54:81, 1994.
12. Cacioppo JT et al: *Ann N Y Acad Sci* 840:664-673, 1998.

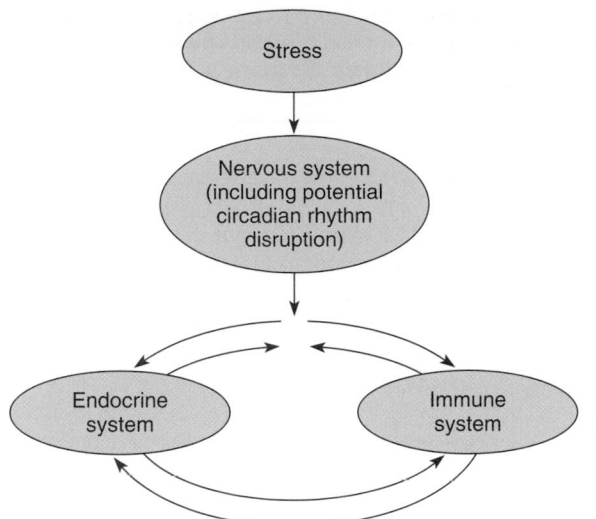

FIGURE 9-7 Nervous System/Endocrine System/Immune System Interactions. Interconnections or pathways of communication among the immune, nervous, and endocrine systems.

effects on the immune response. Thus, stress may systemically cause a decrease in innate immunity and enhance adaptive immunity, whereas locally, under certain conditions, it can induce proinflammatory activities that may influence the onset and cause of infection, autoimmune/inflammatory, and allergic responses. In summary, stress can activate an excessive immune response and, through cortisol and the catecholamines, suppress Th1 responses while enhancing Th2 responses.

Role of the Immune System

The immune, nervous, and endocrine systems communicate through similar (and highly complex) pathways using hormones, neurotransmitters, neuropeptides, and immune cell products.[38] Various components of immune system responses are affected by neuroendocrine-produced factors involved in the stress reaction. Conversely, immune cell–derived cytokines and other products affect neurocrine and endocrine cells.[55,64,65] Several pathways regulate communication among these systems (Figure 9-7).

Stress-induced secretion of HPA hormones and catecholamines of the ANS sympathetic branch directly influences the immune system. Immune cells have receptors for ACTH, CRH, endorphins, norepinephrine, growth hormone, steroids, and other products of the stress response.[56] In addition, cholinergic, adrenergic, and peptidergic nerves innervate lymphoid organs, such as the thymus, spleen, lymph nodes, and bone marrow.[64] Exposure to stress increases endogenous opiate secretion to enhance or suppress immune cell functions in a concentration-dependent manner (see Table 9-4).[64,66-69]

Lymphocytes also produce ACTH and endorphins in small amounts that influence the immune response in an autocrine (same cell stimulation) or paracrine (cell to cell) manner in ongoing immune and memory cytotoxic responses.[64,70,71] The T-cell growth factor interleukin-2 (IL-2) can up-regulate pituitary ACTH. Immune-derived cytokines have direct and indirect effects on HPA and adrenal cell functions. Thus, the immune system has an adaptive role as a signal organ to alert other systems of internally threatening stimuli (e.g., infection, tissue damage, tumor cells). The release of immune inflammatory mediators (IL-6, tumor necrosis factor-beta [TNF-β], interferon) is triggered by bacterial or viral infections, cancer, tissue injury, and other stressors that in turn initiate a stress response through the

HPA pathway. Enhanced systemic production of these cytokines also induces other CNS and behavior changes during an acute infectious episode.[72-75]

Although acute stress activates HPA hormone secretion and immune system products, such as interleukin-1 (IL-1), continued stress-induced secretion of glucocorticoids (GCs) inhibits production of IL-1 by activated macrophages and monocytes.[64,76] Prolonged severe stress may lead to enlargement of the adrenal gland with simultaneous involution of the thymus and lymph nodes. Increased secretion of GCs may be an important mechanism underlying stress-related immune structure alterations and suppression of the immune response.[55]

In addition to the HPA and sympathetic nervous system, the pineal gland regulates the immune response and mediates the effects of circadian rhythm on immunity. When melatonin production by the pineal gland is blocked (by continuous light or by pharmacologic means), the immune response is suppressed, whereas administration of melatonin reverses these effects.[77] This immunomodulation pathway may effect immune changes found with sleep disturbance and dysregulated circadian rhythm,[78] which are common among acutely ill, stressed persons.

In summary, neuropeptides and hormones have significant effects on the immune system. Whether this impact on immune system functions is suppressive or potentiating depends on the type of factor secreted (some factors enhance, some suppress, and some both enhance and suppress), the concentration and length of exposure, and the target cell.[75] Neuropeptides and neuroendocrine hormones may directly control biochemical events affecting cell proliferation, differentiation, and function or may indirectly control immune cell behavior by affecting the production or activity of cytokines.[64,65] Chronic stress affects many immune cell functions, including decreased natural killer cell and T-cell cytotoxicity and impaired B-cell function.[33,71] Importantly, these impairments in the immune system may have negative health consequences for stressed individuals, such as increased risk of infection and some types of cancer.[79,80] Common pathophysiologic origins relating to chronic inflammatory processes include cardiovascular disease, osteoporosis, arthritis, type 2 diabetes mellitus, chronic obstructive pulmonary disease (COPD), other diseases associated with aging, and some cancers; all are characterized by the prolonged presence of proinflammatory cytokines.[15,81]

It is important to note that although inflammation is a normal response and considered beneficial, excessive inflammation can damage tissue. Stress and negative emotions are associated directly with the production of increased levels of proinflammatory cytokines, providing a link between stress, immune function, and disease.[82-84]

STRESS, PERSONALITY, COPING, AND ILLNESS

Extreme physiologic stressors, such as severe burn injury, represent a predictable stimulus for stress responses. A less severe and defined event or situation, however, can be a stressor for one person and not for another. As discussed previously, stress itself is not an independent entity but a system of interdependent processes moderated by the nature, intensity, and duration of the stressor and the perception, appraisal, and coping efficacy of the affected individual, all of which in turn mediate the psychologic and physiologic response to stress. Further, adjustment to repetitive stressors is known to be individualized, based on a person's appraisal of a situation.[3,29] Illustrating the influence of an individualized stress appraisal on physiologic processes, a meta-analysis of the relationship between stressors and immunity found that a higher perception of stress was associated with reduced Tc-cell cytotoxicity, although not with levels of circulating T-helper or Tc lymphocytes.

Psychosocial distress may be predictive of psychologic, social, and physical health outcomes (see *Health Alert: Acute Emotional Stress and Adverse Heart Effects*). A psychologically distressed individual may experience a general stress-induced state of unpleasant arousal that manifests as physiologic, emotional, cognitive, and behavior changes.[85] Periods of depression and emotional upheaval associated with adverse life events may place the affected individual at increased risk for immunologic deficits accompanied by ill health.[55] For example, studies showed a relationship between depression and reduction in lymphocyte proliferation and NK-cell activity.[86] Multiple moderating factors may be important in immune modulation in depressed individuals, including alcoholism and other lifestyle factors, such as social support. Examples of triggering circumstances include bereavement, academic pressures, and marital conflict. Aging also may increase psychosocial distress and is associated with immune changes (see *Health Alert: Partner's Survival and Spouse's Hospitalizations and/or Death*).[81,82]

HEALTH ALERT
Acute Emotional Stress and Adverse Heart Effects

Myocardial Ischemia
- Individuals with coronary heart disease may develop myocardial ischemia during mental or acute emotional stress even though their exercise or chemical nuclear test results are negative.
- Systemic vascular resistance increases during periods of mental or acute emotional stress with concomitant increased myocardial oxygen demand.

Left Ventricular Dysfunction
- More evidence for left ventricular dysfunction exists in older women.
- After acute emotional stress or trauma, there is an increase in sudden chest pain and shortness of breath.
- Left ventricular dysfunction is more common in the cardiac apex.
- Alterations are possibly a result of increased levels of catecholamines.

Ventricular Dysrhythmias
- Intense or unusual acute stress precipitates about 20% of serious ventricular dysrhythmias or sudden cardiac death.
- Altered brain activity may lead to changes in ventricular repolarization and electrical instability of the cardiac muscle.

Data from Pimple P et al: *Am Heart J* 169(1):115-121, 2015; Ramadan R et al: *J Am Heart Assoc* 2(5):e000321, 2013; Wei J et al: *Am J Cardiol* 114(2):187-192, 2014; Wittstein IS et al: *N Engl J Med* 352(6):539-548, 2005; Ziegelstein RC: *JAMA* 298(3):324-329, 2007.

Personality characteristics are associated with differences in appraisal and response to stressors. Specific personality characteristics, such as academic achievement, motivation, optimism, and aggression, are correlated with immunologic alterations. For example, aggression is positively associated with changes in T- and B-cell numbers in male military personnel. In addition, optimism, perceived stress, and anxiety enhance responses to influenza vaccinations after age 50.[69,87]

Stressful life events and mood are important factors that exacerbate symptoms in acquired immunodeficiency syndrome (AIDS) infection, diabetes, and multiple sclerosis.[65,88,89] In addition, the interaction with healthcare providers in a clinical setting, the diagnosis of a major illness, and the process of undergoing various clinical procedures (e.g., blood sampling, injections, examinations, surgical procedures) may represent significant negative life events to many individuals (Figure 9-8). These additional stresses may interfere with the efficacy of the

---

HEALTH ALERT
Partner's Survival and Spouse's Hospitalizations and/or Death

A Harvard study shows that a spouse's chances of dying increase not only when the partner dies but also when that partner becomes seriously ill. The 9-year follow-up study consisted of 518,240 elderly couples. Mortality after the partner's hospitalization varied according to the spouse's diagnosis. For elderly people whose spouse had been hospitalized, the short-term risk of dying approaches that of an elderly person after his or her spouse's death. A wife's hospitalization increased her husband's chances of dying within 1 month by 35%; a husband's hospitalization increased his wife's chances of dying by 44%. Likewise, a wife's death increased her partner's 1-month mortality risk by 53%, and a husband's death raised his partner's risk by 61%. The researchers commented that a spouse's illness or death can increase a partner's mortality by causing severe stress and removing a primary source of emotional, psychologic, practical, and financial support.

Data from Christakis NA, Allison PD: *N Engl J Med* 354(7):719-730, 2006; Carey FM et al: *JAMA Int Med* 174(4):598-605, 2014.

---

medical intervention. Identifying and reducing stress in the clinical setting have particular applicability for both preventing disease and managing illness.

Many studies have linked severe psychosocial stress resulting from negative life events to chronic disorders with mental and physical consequences. A life-threatening event may lead to the development of posttraumatic stress disorder (PTSD).[90-93] Early research with breast cancer survivors demonstrated a link between sympathetic activity and HPA axis activation, noting that some women reported symptoms of PTSD (heart palpitations, panic, shakiness, nausea) when they thought about cancer recurrence or when they found themselves near the hospital where treatment began.[94] Furthermore, the threat of cancer recurrence (using a simulated mammography event as a stressor to elicit thoughts of cancer recurrence) elicited greater alterations in heart rate variability when compared with another simulated controlled stressor.[95] These studies show a connection between reexposure to mammography, which occurred repeatedly throughout breast cancer survivorship, and activation of the autonomic nervous system.

These uncontrolled stressful events may negatively affect the course of illness and interfere with the efficacy of the medical intervention. Identifying and reducing stress in the clinical setting have particular applicability in both disease prevention and illness management. In addition to medical procedures, patient-provider communication provides an important area for future research. Recent studies of cancer communication and patient-provider interaction indicate a link between communication events and emotional outcomes, such as uncertainty and mood state in breast cancer survivors.[96,97]

Coping

Coping is the process of managing stressful challenges that tax the individual's resources.[68] Coping responses may be adaptive or maladaptive and the extent to which an individual responds to distress, using effective positive coping strategies, determines the degree of successful moderation of the stress challenge. For example, studies are beginning to support a role for stress reduction in slowing human immunodeficiency virus (HIV) progression.[43,47,52,98] Other investigations are underway to determine the benefits offered by exercise and mindfulness, as well as others such as inclusion of green space in urban environments.[32] Studies also are focusing on mediating factors that influence stress susceptibility or resilience, such as age, socioeconomic

POTENTIAL EFFECTS IN HEALTHY INDIVIDUALS

POTENTIAL EFFECTS DURING MEDICAL INTERVENTION

POTENTIAL EFFECTS IN SYMPTOMATIC INDIVIDUALS

FIGURE 9-8 Health Outcome Determination in Stressful Life Situations Is Moderated by Numerous Factors. Whether a life-challenged individual experiences distress or illness depends on the subject's appraisal of the event and the coping strategies used during the stressful period. Models **(A)** and **(B)** reflect possible outcomes in stressed healthy and symptomatic individuals. Model **(C)** illustrates the dynamic clinical setting in which the diagnosis of a serious illness and subsequent medical interventions may be perceived as stressful challenges and have potentially detrimental influences on physical outcome.

status, gender, social support, religious or spiritual factors, personality, self-esteem, genetics, past experiences, and current health status (Figure 9-9).[39,99,100]

Coping strategies are especially beneficial when they are problem-focused and individuals seek social support.[68,77] Evidence suggests that effective interventions may result in greater stress resilience and improved psychologic and physiologic outcomes.[101] For example, women with recurrent metastatic breast cancer and provided weekly group counseling in conjunction with routine medical treatment lived an average of 19 months longer than control subjects, suggesting a positive influence of group support for these women.[75,77]

Maladaptive coping can result in a change in behavior contributing to potentially adverse health effects (e.g., increased smoking, change in eating habits). Serious disturbances of the sleep-wake cycle observed in many stressed people and in experimental and many clinical settings[35,102] may exacerbate the pathophysiologic status of some individuals.[103-105] Sleep deprivation and circadian disruption, even in young otherwise healthy individuals, have detrimental influences on respiratory and immune system function. Even partial sleep deprivation was associated with reduced NK-cell activity in healthy subjects, and only recently have seriously ill individuals been assessed for adequacy and structure of sleep during recovery.[103]

Behavioral styles, such as overcommitment to employment-related tasks, repression, denial, escape-avoidance, and concealment, are associated with altered immune functions.[56,106] Repression is associated with lower monocyte counts, higher eosinophil counts, higher serum glucose levels, and more self-reported medication reactions in medical outpatients,[78] and with higher Epstein-Barr virus (EBV) antibody titers in students.[76] A prospective long-term study also found increased markers of accelerated human immunodeficiency virus (HIV) infection in gay men who concealed their homosexual identity.[65] School teachers who devoted long hours without reward and who were unable

to disengage from work-related tasks were found to have lowered innate immune responses.[106]

The importance of social support for seriously ill individuals also has focused attention on the health of caregivers. Significant stress manifested as depression, anxiety, and fatigue has been noted in family caregivers of those with cancer, Alzheimer disease, and burn trauma.[107] Enhanced social support of caregivers improves measures of immune function.[66,67,77,108,109]

Interventions to potentially prevent or manage stress-related psychologic or physical problems include both short- and long-term education on evaluating and adopting effective coping strategies. Approaches may be used or investigated on an individual or group basis. Incorporation of effective stress management approaches into clinical education facilitates their use in the clinical arena. Future research could focus on the efficacy of such approaches with different populations because it is clear one size does not fit all (coping of cancer survivors may be vastly different from coping of combat veterans).

In summary, the mind and body are connected through a multitude of complex physical and emotional interactions. Understanding the complexity of these interactions is a challenge for researchers. Areas of promise include investigating relationships between the effects of stress on illness, as well as developing effective stress management techniques and approaches that improve health outcomes.

✔ **QUICK CHECK 9-2**
1. Define the HPA axis.
2. Define psychoneuroimmunology.
3. How does the immune system participate in stress-related diseases?
4. Why do stress-related diseases occur?
5. What intervention or prevention activities reduce stress-related diseases?

Staying on the Good Side of the Stress Spectrum

FIGURE 9-9 Staying on the Good Side of the Stress Spectrum. GOOD stress is shown on the left of the spectrum and involves a rapid biologic response to the stressor, followed by a rapid shutdown of the response upon cessation of the stressor. These responses support physiologic conditions that are likely to enhance protective immunity, cognitive and physical performance, and overall health. BAD stress, represented on the right of the spectrum, involves exposure to chronic or long-term biologic changes that are likely to result in dysregulation or suppression of immune function, a decrease in cognitive and physical performance, and an increased likelihood of disease. Short- and/or long-term stress is generally superimposed on a psychophysiologic RESTING ZONE of low/no stress that also represents a state of health maintenance/restoration. To maintain health, one needs to optimize GOOD stress, maximize the RESTING ZONE, and minimize BAD stress. Achieving psychologic and physiologic resilience involves a multi-pronged approach. Sleep of a quality and duration that helps one feel rested in the morning, a moderate and healthy diet, and consistent and moderate exercise or physical activity are three LIFESTYLE FACTORS that are likely to enable one to stay on the "good" side of the stress spectrum. Effective appraisal and coping mechanisms, genuine gratitude, social support, and compassion toward others and oneself are likely to provide PSYCHO-SOCIAL BUFFERS against bad stress and enable one to stay on the "good" side of the stress spectrum. Additionally, depending on individual preferences, ACTIVITIES, such as, meditation, yoga, being in nature, exercise/physical activity, music, art, craft, dance, fishing, painting, also may reduce BAD stress, extend The RESTING ZONE, and optimize GOOD stress. Such personal activities are likely to involve different strokes for different folks and need not always be meditative or reflective in nature. (Adapted from Dhabhar FS, McEwen BS. Bidirectional effects of stress on immune function: possible explanations for salubrious as well as harmful effects. In Ader R, editor. Psychoneuroimmunology IV, San Diego, 2007, Elsevier.)

GERIATRIC CONSIDERATIONS

Aging & the Stress-Age Syndrome

With aging, sometimes a set of neurohormonal and immune alterations, as well as tissue and cellular changes, develops. These changes have been defined as stress-age syndrome and include the following:

- Alterations in the excitability of structures of the limbic system and hypothalamus
- Increase of the blood concentrations of catecholamines, ADH, ACTH, and cortisol
- Decrease of the concentrations of testosterone, thyroxine, and others
- Alterations of opioid peptides
- Immunodepression and pattern of chronic inflammation
- Alterations in lipoproteins
- Hypercoagulation of the blood
- Free radical damage of cells

Some of the alterations are adaptational, whereas others are potentially damaging. These stress-related alterations of aging can influence the course of developing stress reactions and lower adaptive reserve and coping capacity.

Data from Frolkis VV: *Mech Ageing Dev* 69(1-2)93-107, 1998.
ACTH, Adrenocorticotropic hormone; *ADH,* antidiuretic hormone.

DID YOU UNDERSTAND?

Concepts of Stress

1. Stress is broadly defined as a threat that is perceived or anticipated, resulting in interactions between the body and the brain (the stress response).

2. Originally proposed by Cannon in 1914, the idea that stressful events could cause physiologic responses was further developed by Selye in 1946. Selye's work demonstrated that internal or external stressors could result in adrenal gland enlargement, immune alterations (increased leukocytes), and gastrointestinal manifestations (ulcers). These global physiologic responses were labeled the General Adaptation Syndrome (GAS).

3. The GAS occurs in three stages: the alarm stage; the stage of resistance or adaptation; and the stage of exhaustion, which is now referred to as allostatic overload. Diseases of adaptation develop if the stage of resistance or adaptation does not restore homeostasis. Although important, this approach is now thought to be greatly oversimplified.

4. Continuing the evolution of this research, adrenal gland hormone responses to stressors were suggested in the 1950s and CNS and endocrine responses were proposed in the 1970s. The study of the body's response to stressors continues to evolve and has become known by the term Psychoneuroimmunology (PNI).

5. Psychologic stressors can be anticipatory and triggered by expectations of an upcoming stressor or can be reactive to a stressor. Both of these psychologic stressors are capable of eliciting a physiologic stress response.

The Stress Response

1. The concepts of allostasis (stability through change; monitoring the environment for adaptive response) and homeostasis (return to base levels reflecting an unchanging set point) both indicate physiologic responses. Allostatic overload can occur when there is overactivation of adaptive responses that may in turn increase susceptibility to disease.

2. The stress response involves the nervous system (sympathetic branch of the autonomic nervous system), the endocrine system (pituitary and adrenal glands), and the immune system. More simply, these relationships are often cited together as the hypothalamic-pituitary-adrenal (HPA) axis.

3. The stress response is initiated when a stressor is present in the body or perceived by the mind. Psychologic stress may cause or worsen several diseases or disorders including anxiety, depression, insomnia, chronic pain and fatigue syndromes, obesity, metabolic syndrome, essential hypertension, type 2 diabetes, atherosclerosis and its cardiovascular consequences, osteoporosis, and autoimmune inflammatory and allergic disorders. A classic example of stress and allostatic overload is sleep alteration and the associated damaging effects of elevated evening cortisol, insulin, and glucose.

4. The physiology of managing stressful events is complex, involving mechanisms of both protection and injury. The two major stress systems include the autonomic and hypothalamic-pituitary-adrenal (HPA) system.

5. Activation of the autonomic nervous system consists of sympathetic stimulation of the adrenal medulla and nerve endings to rapidly secrete catecholamines (norepinephrine, epinephrine, neuropeptide Y).

6. Activation of the HPA system involves sequential secretion of corticotropin-releasing hormone from the hypothalamus, which stimulates receptors in the anterior pituitary to secrete ACTH that, in turn, stimulates the adrenal cortex to secrete glucocorticoids, particularly cortisol.

7. Chronic dysregulation of the HPA axis, especially abnormal elevated levels of cortisol, has been linked to a wide variety of disorders, including obesity, sleep deprivation, lipid abnormalities, hypertension, diabetes, atherosclerosis, and loss of bone density.

8. Glucocorticoids from the adrenal cortex, in response to ACTH from the pituitary gland, comprise the major stress hormones along with the catecholamines epinephrine and norepineprine.

9. In general, catecholamines of the sympathetic system prepare the body to act; for example, cortisol mobilizes glucose (for energy) and other substances. The parasympathetic system balances or restrains the sympathetic system, resulting in slowed heart rates, and anti-inflammatory effects. During prolonged stress (allostatic overload) the parasympathetic system is less effective in opposing the sympathetic system.

10. Epinephrine exerts its chief effects on the cardiovascular system. Epinephrine increases cardiac output and increases blood flow to the heart, brain, and skeletal muscles by dilating vessels that supply these organs. It also dilates the airways, thereby increasing delivery of oxygen to the bloodstream.

11. Norepinephrine's chief effects complement those of epinephrine. Norepinephrine constricts blood vessels of the viscera and skin; this has the effect of shifting blood flow to the vessels dilated by epinephrine. Norepinephrine also increases mental alertness.

12. Glucocorticoids reach all tissues, including the brain, easily penetrate cell membranes, and react with numerous intracellular glucocorticoid receptors. Because they spare almost no tissue or organ and influence a large proportion of the human genome, they broadly exert diverse biologic actions. For example, glucocorticoids have an important modulatory role in the CNS. These hormones regulate memory, cognition, mood, and sleep and influence many other body systems.

13. Cortisol is the primary glucocorticoid produced during stress.

14. Cortisol's chief effects involve metabolic processes. By inhibiting the use of metabolic substances while promoting their formation, cortisol mobilizes glucose, amino acids, lipids, and fatty acids and delivers them to the bloodstream. As an example, anabolic effects of cortisol increase the rate of protein synthesis in the liver, whereas the catabolic effects of cortisol increase levels of amino acids, ultimately depleting protein stores in muscle, bone, skin, and connective tissue.

15. Cortisol contributes to elevated blood glucose and inhibits glucose uptake by body cells providing energy to combat perceived or anticipated stressors.

16. Glucocorticoids contribute to the development of metabolic syndrome and the pathogenesis of obesity. They can directly cause insulin resistance and influence genetic variations that predispose to obesity.

17. Elevated levels of glucocorticoids and catecholamines (epinephrine and norepinephrine), both endogenous and exogenous (synthetic pharmaceuticals), may decrease innate immunity and increase autoimmune responses. However, prolonged effects of cortisol may accentuate inflammation. Overall, stress activates an excessive immune response and, through cortisol and the catecholamines, suppresses Th1 responses while enhancing Th2 responses.

18. The impact of cortisol on fetal development and subsequent risk of future disease is being considered.

19. Other hormones, including β-endorphins, growth hormone, prolactin, oxytocin, the steroid sex hormones, and antidiuretic hormone, influence the stress response by their diverse actions.

Stress, Personality, Coping, and Illness

1. Stress is a system of interdependent processes that are moderated by the nature, intensity, and duration of the stressor and the coping efficacy of the affected individual, all of which in turn mediate the psychologic and physiologic response to stress.

2. Personality characteristics are associated with individual differences in appraisal and response to stressors. Further, the appraisal of events as distressful may be predictive of psychological, social, and physical health outcomes (maladaptive coping, depression, PTSD, heart disease, altered immunity).

3. Coping styles associated with altered immunity include repression, denial, escape-avoidance, and concealment. Coping strategies are more beneficial when they are problem-focused and may result in improved resilience and better psychological and physiologic outcomes.

Geriatric Considerations: Aging & the Stress-Age Syndrome

1. With aging, often a set of neurohormonal and immune alterations, including tissue and cellular changes, occur. These changes are collectively called stress-age syndromes.

2. The changes are numerous, with some being adaptive whereas others are potentially damaging.

3. Coping techniques for managing stress may mitigate the effects of stress on maladaptive behaviors such as excessive alcohol ingestion and smoking, and by extension impact the effects of existing chronic illness.

KEY TERMS

Adrenocorticotropic hormone (ACTH), 218
Alarm stage, 214
Allostasis, 217
Allostatic overload, 217
Anticipatory response, 215
Coping, 226
Corticotropin-releasing hormone (CRH), 218

Cortisol, 218
Diseases of adaptation, 215
Exhaustion stage, 215
General adaptation syndrome (GAS), 214
Homeostasis, 214
Hypothalamic-pituitary-adrenal (HPA) system, 218
Neuropeptide Y (NPY), 223

Peripheral (immune) CRH, 223
Physiologic stress, 214
Psychoneuroimmunology (PNI), 217
Reactive response, 215
Resistance or adaptation stage, 215
Stress response, 214

Stressor, 214
Th1 to Th2 shift, 221

REFERENCES

1. McEwen BS: Brain on stress: how the social environment gets under the skin, *Proc Natl Acad Sci U S A* 109:17180-17185, 2012.
2. Nicolaides NC et al: Circadian endocrine rhythms: the hypothalamic-pituitary-adrenal axis and its actions, *Ann N Y Acad Sci* 1318:71-80, 2014.
3. McEwen BS: Central effects of stress hormones in health and disease: understanding the protective and damaging effects of stress and stress mediators, *Eur J Pharmacol* 583(2-3):174-185, 2008.
4. Dhbhar FS et al: Stress induced redistribution of immune cells—from barracks to boulevards to battlefields: a tale of three hormones, *Psychoneuroendocrinology* 37:1345-1368, 2012.
5. Ulrich-Lai YM, Herman JP: Neural regulation of endocrine and autonomic stress responses, *Nat Rev Neurosci* 10:397-409, 2009.
6. Dhabhar FS, McEwen BS: Enhancing versus suppressive effects of stress hormones on skin immune function, *Proc Natl Acad Sci U S A* 96(3):1059-1064, 1999.
7. Compare A et al: Emotional regulation and depression: a potential mediator between heart and mind, *Cardiovasc Psychiatry Neurol* 2014 Jun 22. [Epub ahead of print.]
8. Peskind ER et al: Influence of lifestyle modifications on age-related free radical injury to brain, *J Am Med Assoc Neurol* 2014 Jul 21. [Epub ahead of print.]
9. Cannon WB et al: Experimental hyperthyroidism, *Am J Physiol* 36:363, 1914.
10. Selye H: The general adaptation syndrome and the diseases of adaptation, *J Clin Endocrinol* 6:117-230, 1946.
11. Mason JW, Brady JV: Plasma 17-hydroxycorticosteroid changes related to reserpine effects on emotional behaviors, *Science* 124:983, 1956.
12. Hill SR et al: Studies on adrenocortical and psychological responses to stress in man, *Arch Intern Med* 97:269, 1956.
13. Hetzel BS et al: Changes in urinary 17-hydroxycorticosteroid excretion during stressful life experiences in man, *J Clin Endocrinol Metab* 15(9):1057-1068, 1955.
14. Mason JW: Organization of psychoendocrine mechanisms: a review and reconsideration of research. In Greenfield NS, Steinbach RA, editors: *Handbook of psychophysiology*, New York, 1972, Holt, Rinehart, & Winston.
15. Herman JP et al: Central mechanisms of stress integration: hierarchical circuitry controlling hypothalamo-pituitary-adrenocortical responsiveness, *Front Neuroendocrinol* 24(3):151-158, 2003.
16. Bauer-Wu SM: Psychoneuroimmunology. Part I: physiology, *Clin J Oncol Nurs* 6(3):167-170, 2002.
17. Bauer-Wu SM: Psychoneuroimmunology. Part II: Mind-body interventions, *Clin J Oncol Nurs* 6(4):243-246, 2002.
18. Irwin MR: Human psychoneuroimmunology: 20 years of discovery, *Brain Behav Immun* 22(2):129-139, 2008.
19. Ranchor AV et al: Invited commentary: personality as a causal factor in cancer risk and mortality—time to retire a hypothesis? *Am J Epidemiol* 172(4):386-388, 2010.
20. Sloan EK et al: The sympathetic nervous system induces a metastatic switch in primary breast cancer, *Cancer Res* 70(18):7042-7052, 2010.
21. O'Connor TG et al: Annual research review: the neuroinflammation hypothesis for stress and psychopathology in children—developmental psychoneuroimmunology, *J Child Psychol Psychiatry* 55(6):615-631, 2014.
22. Rector JL et al: Consistent associations between measures of psychological stress and CMV antibody levels in a large occupational sample, *Brain Behav Immun* 38:133-141, 2014.
23. Cacioppo JT et al: Autonomic, neuroendocrine, and immune responses to psychological stress: the reactivity hypothesis, *Ann N Y Acad Sci* 840:664-673, 1998.
24. Chrousos GP, Kino T: Glucocorticoid signaling in the cell: expanding clinical complications to complex human behavioral and somatic disorders, *Ann N Y Acad Sci* 1179:153-166, 2009.
25. Elenkov IJ et al: Cytokine dysregulation, inflammation, and well-being, *Neuroimmunomodulation* 12(5):255-269, 2005.
26. Sterling P, Eyer, J: Allostasis: a new paradigm to explain arousal pathology. In Fisher S, Reason J, editors: *Handbook of life stress, cognition, and health*, pp 629-649, New York, 1988, John Wiley and Sons.
27. Sterling P: Allostasis: A model of predictive regulation, *Physiol Behav* 106:5-15, 2012.
28. Schulkin J: Social allostasis: anticipatory regulation of the internal milieu, *Front Evol Neurosci* 2:e111, 2011,
29. Dich N et al: A non-linear association between self-reported negative emotional response to stress and subsequent allostatic load: prospective results from the Whitehall II cohort study, *Psychoneuroendocrinology* 49C:54-61, 2014.
30. Seeman T et al: Socio-economic differentials in peripheral biology: cumulative allostatic load, *Ann N Y Acad Sci* 1186:223-239, 2010.
31. Everson-Rose SA et al: Chronic stress, depressive symptoms, anger, hostility, and risk of stroke and transient ischemic attack in the multi-ethnic study of atherosclerosis, *Stroke* 45(8):2318-2323, 2014.
32. Jonker MF et al: The effect of urban green on small-area (healthy) life expectancy, *J Epidemiol Community Health* 2014 Jul 22. [Epub ahead of print.]

33. Kiecolt-Glaser JK et al: Psychoneuroimmunology: psychological influences on immune function and health, *J Consult Clin Psychol* 70(3):537-547, 2002.

34. Liu LY et al: School examinations enhance airway inflammation to antigen challenge, *Am J Respir Crit Care Med* 165(8):1062-1067, 2002.

35. Chen X et al: Associations of allostatic load with sleep apnea, insomnia, short sleep duration, and other sleep disturbances: findings from the National Health and Nutrition Examination Survey 2005 to 2008, *Ann Epidemiol* 24(8): 612-619, 2014.

36. McEwen BS: Sleep deprivation as neurobiologic and physiologic stressor, allostasis and allostatic load, *Metabolism* 55:S20-S23, 2006.

37. Dhabhar FS: Effects of stress on immune function: the good, the bad, and the beautiful, *Immunol Res* 58:193-210, 2014.

38. Coutinho AE, Chapman KE: The anti-inflammatory and immunosuppressive effects of glucocorticoids, recent developments and mechanistic insights, *Mol Cell Endocrinol* 335(1): 2-13, 2011.

39. Monaghan P: Organismal stress, telomeres and life histories, *J Exp Biol* 217(Pt 1):57-66, 2014.

40. Martinac M et al: Metabolic syndrome, activity of the hypothalamic-pituitary-adrenal axis and inflammatory mediators in depressive disorder, *Acta Clin Croat* 25(1):55-71, 2014.

41. Nakamura A: Genotypes of the renin-angiotensin system and glucocorticoid complications, *Pediatr Int* 2014 Jul 1. [Epub ahead of print.]

42. Paredes S, Ribiero L: Cortisol: the villain in metabolic syndrome? *Rev Assoc Med Bras* 60(1): 84-92, 2014.

43. Reynolds RM: Glucocorticoid excess and the developmental origins of disease: two decades of testing the hypothesis—2012 Curt Richter award winner. *Psychoneuroendocrinology* 38(1):1-11, 2013.

44. Kajantie E et al: Body size at birth predicts hypothalamic-pituitary-adrenal axis response to psychosocial stress at 60 to 70 years, *J Clin Endocrinol Metab* 92(11):4094-4100, 2007.

45. Painter RC et al: Long-term effects of prenatal stress and glucocorticoid exposure, *Birth Defects Res C Embryo Today* 96(4):315-324, 2012.

46. Alevizaki M et al: High anticipatory stress plasma cortisol levels and sensitivity to glucocorticoids predict severity of coronary artery disease in subjects undergoing coronary angiography, *Metabolism* 56:222-226, 2007.

47. Hanna RN, Hedrick CC: Stressing out stem cells: linking stress and hematopoiesis in cardiovascular disease, *Nat Med* 20(7):707-708, 2014.

48. Liddicoat DR et al: The glucocorticoid receptor 1A3 promoter correlates with high sensitivity to glucocorticoid-induced apoptosis in human lymphocytes, *Immunol Cell Biol* 2014 Jul 22. [Epub ahead of print.]

49. Sorrells SF et al: The stressed CNS: when glucocorticoids aggravate inflammation (review), *Neuron* 64(1):33-39, 2009.

50. Kim MH et al: Catecholamine stress alters neutrophil trafficking and impairs wound healing by β2-adrenergic receptor-mediated upregulation of IL-6, *J Invest Dermatol* 134(3): 809-817, 2014.

51. Heidt T et al: Chronic variable stress activates hematopoietic stem cells, *Nat Med* 20(7):754-758, 2014.

52. Chhatre S et al: Effects of behavioral stress reduction transcendental meditation intervention in persons with HIV, *AIDS Care* 25(10): 1291-1297, 2013.

53. Heinzelmann-Schwarz VA et al: Management of human papillomavirus-related gynecological malignancies, *Curr Probl Dermatol* 45:216-224, 2014.

54. Bruunsgard H, Pedersen BK: Age-related inflammatory cytokines and disease, *Immunol Allergy Clin North Am* 23(1):15-39, 2003.

55. Shelby J et al: Neurohormone and neuropeptide regulation of the post-traumatic immune response. In Faist E, editor: *Host defense alterations of trauma, shock, and sepsis: multi-organ failure/ immunotherapy of sepsis*, Berlin, 1996, Pabst.

56. Sundar SK et al: Brain IL-1–induced immunosuppression occurs through activation of both pituitary-adrenal axis and sympathetic nervous system by corticotropin-releasing factor, *J Neurosci* 10(11):3701-3706, 1990.

57. Calcagni E, Elenkov I: Stress system activity, innate and T helper cytokines, and susceptibility to immune-related diseases (review), *Ann N Y Acad Sci* 1069:62-76, 2006.

58. Lagier B et al: Different modulation by histamine of IL-4 and interferon-gamma (IFN-gamma) release according to the phenotype of human Th0, Th1, and Th2 clones, *Clin Exp Immunol* 108(3): 545-551, 1997.

59. Jochem J et al: Endogenous opioid peptides system in haemorrhagic shock—central cardiovascular regulation, *Med Sci Monit* 7(3): 545-549, 2001.

60. Molina PE: Opiate modulation of hemodynamic, hormonal, and cytokine responses to hemorrhage, *Shock* 15(6):471-478, 2001.

61. Molina PE: Stress-specific opioid modulation of haemodynamic counter-regulation, *Clin Exp Pharmacol Physiol* 29(3):248-253, 2002.

62. Rocklin RE, editor: *Histamine and H2 antagonists in inflammation and immunodeficiency*, New York, 1990, Marcel Dekker.

63. Burguera B et al: Dual and selective actions of glucocorticoid upon basal and stimulated growth hormone release in man, *Neuroendocrinology* 51(1):51-58, 1990.

64. Reiche EMV et al: Stress, depression, the immune system, and cancer (review), *Lancet Oncol* 5(10): 617-625, 2004.

65. Coyle PK: The neuroimmunology of multiple sclerosis, *Adv Neuroimmunol* 6(2):143-154, 1996.

66. Baron RS et al: Social support and immune function among spouses of cancer patients, *J Pers Soc Psychol* 59(2):344-352, 1990.

67. Fawzy FI et al: Malignant melanoma: effects of an early structured psychiatric intervention, coping, and affective state on recurrence and survival 6 years later, *Arch Gen Psychiatry* 50(9):681-689, 1993.

68. Folkman S, Lazarus RS: The relationship between coping and emotion: implications for theory and research, *Soc Sci Med* 26(3):309-317, 1988.

69. Granger DA et al: Human aggression and enumerative measures of immunity, *Psychosom Med* 62(4):583-590, 2000.

70. Cole SW et al: Accelerated course of human immunodeficiency virus infection in gay men who conceal their homosexual identity, *Psychosom Med* 58(3):219-231, 1996.

71. Johnson EW et al: ACTH enhancement of T-lymphocyte cytotoxic responses, *Cell Mol Neurobiol* 25(3-4):743-757, 2005.

72. Busbridge NJ, Grossman AB: Stress and the single cytokine: interleukin modulation of the pituitary-adrenal axis, *Mol Cell Endocrinol* 82(2-3):C209-C214, 1991.

73. Hori T et al: Immune cytokines and regulation of body temperature, food intake, and cellular immunity, *Brain Res Bull* 27(3-4):309-313, 1991.

74. Navarra P et al: Interleukins-1 and -6 stimulate the release of corticotropin releasing hormone-41 from rat hypothalamus in vitro via the eicosanoid cyclooxygenase pathway, *Endocrinology* 128(1): 37-44, 1991.

75. Spiegel D: Psychosocial aspects of breast cancer treatment, *Semin Oncol* 24(1 Suppl 1):S1-47, 1997.

76. Esterling B et al: Emotional repression, stress disclosure responses, and Epstein-Barr viral capsid antigen titers, *Psychosom Med* 52(4):397-410, 1990.

77. Spiegel D et al: Effects of psychosocial treatment in prolonging cancer survival may be mediated by neuroimmune pathways, *Ann N Y Acad Sci* 840:674-683, 1998.

78. Jamner LD et al: The relationship between repressive and defensive coping styles and monocyte, eosinophil, and serum glucose levels: support for the opioid peptide hypothesis of regression, *Psychosom Med* 50(6):567-575, 1988.

79. Imia K et al: Natural cytotoxic activity of peripheral-blood lymphocytes and cancer incidence: an 11-year follow-up study of a general population, *Lancet* 356(9244):1795-1799, 2000.

80. Teicher MH et al: Developmental neurobiology of childhood stress and trauma, *Psych Clin North Am* 25(2):297-426, 2002.

81. Frolkis VV: Stress-age syndrome, *Mech Ageing Dev* 69(1-2):93-107, 1993.

82. Hirokawa K: Reversing and restoring immune functions, *Mech Ageing Dev* 93(1-3):119-124, 1997.

83. Kopnisky KL et al: Workshop report: the effects of psychological variables on the progression of HIV-1 disease, *Brain Behav Immun* 18(3):246-261, 2004.

84. Wellen KE, Hotamisligil GS: Inflammation, stress, and diabetes, *J Clin Invest* 115(5):1111-1119, 2005.

85. Thoits PA: Dimensions of life events that influence psychological distress: an evaluation and synthesis of the literature. In Kaplan HB, editor: *Psychosocial stress: trends in theory and research*, Orlando, Fla, 1983, Academic Press.

86. Irwin M: Immune correlates of depression, *Adv Exp Med Biol* 461:1-24, 1999.

87. Hayney MS et al: Age and psychological influences on immune responses to trivalent inactivated influenza vaccine in the Meditation or Exercise for Preventing Acute Respiratory Infection (MEPARI) trial, *Hum Vaccin Immunother* 10(1):83-91, 2014.

88. Solomon GF et al: Psychoneuroimmunologic aspects of human immunodeficiency virus infection. In Alder R et al, editors: *Psychoneuroimmunology*, ed 2, New York, 1991, Academic Press.

89. Surwit RS, Schneider MS: Role of stress in the etiology and treatment of diabetes mellitus, *Psychosom Med* 55(4):380-393, 1993.

90. Bremner JD et al: Neural correlates of memories of childhood sexual abuse in women with and without posttraumatic stress disorder, *Am J Psychiatry* 156(11):1787-1795, 1999.

91. Busso DS et al: Media exposure and sympathetic nervous system reactivity predict PTSD symptoms after the Boston marathon bombings, *Depress Anxiety* 31(7):551-558, 2014.

92. Clohessy S, Ehlers A: PTSD symptoms, response to intrusive memories and coping in ambulance service workers, *Br J Clin Psychol* 38(Pt 3): 251-265, 1999.

93. Donnelly CL et al: Psychopharmacology of pediatric posttraumatic stress disorder, *J Child Adolesc Psychopharmacol* 9(3):203-220, 1999.

94. Cordova MJ et al: Frequency and correlates of posttraumatic stress-disorder-like symptoms after treatment for breast cancer, *J Consult Clin Psychol* 63(6):981-986, 1995.

95. Ma Z et al: Exploring women's psychoneuroendocrine responses to cancer threat: insights from a computer-based guided imagery task, *Can J Nurs Res* 39(1):98-115, 2007.

96. Clayton MF et al: Communication with breast cancer survivors, *Health Commun* 23(3):207-221, 2008.

97. Porter LS et al: Cortisol levels and responses to mammography screening in breast cancer survivors: a pilot study, *Psychosom Med* 65(5): 842-848, 2003.

98. Vedhara K, Irwin M, editors: *Human psychoimmunology*, Oxford, England, 2005, Oxford University Press.

99. Childs E et al: Personality traits modulate emotional and physiological responses to stress, *Behav Pharmacol* 25(5-6):493-502, 2014.

100. Jodczyk S et al: No association between mean telomere length and life stress observed in a 30 year birth cohort, *PLoS One* 9(5):e97102, 2014.

101. Lazar JS: Mind-body medicine in primary care. Implications and applications, *Prim Care* 23(1):169-182, 1996.

102. Jiang Y, Zhu J: Effects of sleep deprivation on behaviors and abnormal hippocampal BDNF/miR-10B expression in rats with chronic stress depression, *Int J Clin Exp Pathol* 8(1):586-593, 2015.

103. Irwin M et al: Partial sleep deprivation reduces natural killer cell activity in humans, *Psychosom Med* 56(6):493-498, 1994.

104. Pollmacher T et al: Influence of host defense activation on sleep in humans, *Adv Neuroimmunol* 5(2):155-169, 1995.

105. White D et al: Sleep deprivation and the control of ventilation, *Am Rev Respir Dis* 128(6):984-986, 1983.

106. Bellingrath S et al: Healthy working school teachers with high effort-reward-imbalance and overcommitment show increased pro-inflammatory immune activity and a dampened innate immune defence, *Brain Behav Immun* 24(8):1332-1339, 2010.

107. Pinquart M, Sörensen S: Differences between caregivers and noncaregivers in psychological health and physical health: a meta-analysis, *Psychol Aging* 18(2):250-267, 2003.

108. Kiecolt-Glaser J et al: Chronic stress and immunity in family caregivers of Alzheimers disease victims, *Psychosom Med* 49(5):523-535, 1987.

109. Shelby J et al: Severe burn injury: effects on psychologic and immunologic function in noninjured close relatives, *J Burn Care Rehabil* 13(1):58-63, 1992.

10

Biology of Cancer

Neal S. Rote and David M. Virshup

EVOLVE WEBSITE

http://evolve.elsevier.com/Huether/
Student Review Questions
Audio Key Points

Case Studies
Animations
Quick Check Answers

CHAPTER OUTLINE

Cancer is a leading cause of suffering and death in the developed world. Over the past 35 years, intensive research has led to a significantly enhanced understanding of this complex and frightening disease. We now understand that cancer is a collection of more than 100 different diseases, each caused by a specific and often unique age-related accumulation of genetic and epigenetic alterations. Environment, heredity, and behavior interact to modify the risk of developing cancer and the response to treatment. Improvements in treatment strategies and supportive care, coupled with new, often individualized therapies based on advances in our fundamental understanding of the basic pathophysiology of malignancy, have contributed to an increasing number of effective options for these diverse, often lethal, disorders collectively called cancer.

CANCER TERMINOLOGY AND CHARACTERISTICS

Any discussion of cancer must start with a definition of what it is and what it is not. Although most readers may have an intuitive understanding of this disorder, composing an exact definition that encompasses this broad category is more challenging. The National Cancer Institute (NCI) of the National Institutes of Health (NIH) defines cancer as "diseases in which abnormal cells divide without control and are able to invade other tissues."[1]

The term *cancer* comes from the Latin translation of the Greek word for crab, *karkinoma*, which the physician Hippocrates used to describe the appendage-like projections extending from tumors into adjacent tissue. The word *tumor* originally referred to any swelling that is caused by inflammation but is now generally reserved for describing a new growth, or *neoplasm*.

Tumor Classification and Nomenclature

The careful evaluation of each cancer is important for many reasons. Different cancers will have different causes, different rates and patterns of progression, and different responses to treatment. The classification starts with knowing the tissue and organ of origin, the extent of distribution to other sites, and the microscopic appearance of the lesion. Increasingly, it also includes a detailed description of the critical genetic changes in the cancer.

Benign and Malignant

Not all tumors or neoplasms, however, are cancer; they can be benign or malignant (cancerous). *Benign tumors* are usually encapsulated

Endometrium

Fallopian tube

Ovary

Tumor

Vein

BENIGN
(Leiomyoma)

MALIGNANT
(Leiomyosarcoma)

Small	Noninvasive	Large	Locally invasive
Well demarcated	Nonmetastatic	Poorly demarcated	Metastatic
Slow growing	Well differentiated	Rapidly growing with	Poorly differentiated
		hemorrhage and necrosis	

FIGURE 10-1 Comparison Between a Benign Tumor and a Malignant Tumor of the Same Origin.
(From Kumar V et al: *Robbins and Cotran pathologic basis of disease,* ed 9, Philadelphia, 2015, Saunders.)

with connective tissue and contain fairly well-differentiated cells and well-organized stroma (Figure 10-1). They retain recognizable normal tissue structure and do not invade beyond their capsule, nor do they spread to regional lymph nodes or distant locations. Mitotic cells are very rarely present during microscopic analysis. Benign tumors are generally named according to the tissues from which they arise with the suffix "-oma," which indicates a tumor or mass. For example, a benign tumor of the smooth muscle of the uterus is a *leiomyoma,* and a benign tumor of fat cells is a *lipoma.* It is important to understand that benign tumors can become extremely large and, depending on their location in the body, can cause morbidity or be life-threatening. For example, a benign meningioma at the base of the skull may cause symptoms by compressing adjacent normal brain tissue.

Some tumors initially described as benign can progress to cancer and then are referred to as malignant tumors, which are distinguished from benign tumors by more rapid growth rates and specific microscopic alterations, including loss of differentiation and absence of normal tissue organization (Figure 10-2). One of the microscopic hallmarks of cancer cells is anaplasia, the loss of cellular differentiation. Malignant cells are also pleomorphic, with marked variability of size and shape. They often have large darkly stained nuclei and mitotic cells are common. Malignant tumors may have a substantial amount of stroma, but it is disorganized, with loss of normal tissue structure. Malignant tumors lack a capsule and grow to invade nearby blood vessels, lymphatics, and surrounding structures. The most important and most deadly characteristic of malignant tumors is their ability to spread far beyond the tissue of origin, a process known as *metastasis.*

Unlike benign tumors, which are named related to the tissue of origin, cancers generally are named according to the cell type from which they originate. Cancers arising in epithelial tissue are called carcinomas, and if they arise from or form ductal or glandular structures are named adenocarcinomas. Hence, a malignant tumor arising from breast glandular tissue is a mammary adenocarcinoma, whereas an example of a benign breast tumor is a fibroadenoma. Cancers arising from mesenchymal tissue (including connective tissue, muscle, and bone) usually have the suffix sarcoma. For example, malignant cancers of skeletal muscle are known as rhabdomyosarcomas. Cancers of lymphatic tissue are called lymphomas, whereas cancers of blood-forming cells are called leukemias. However, many cancers, such as Hodgkin disease and Ewing sarcoma, are named for historical reasons that do not follow this nomenclature convention.

Carcinoma in Situ

Carcinoma in situ (often abbreviated CIS) refers to preinvasive epithelial tumors of glandular or squamous cell origin. Cancers develop incrementally, as they accumulate specific genetic lesions. Careful surveillance for cancer often detects abnormal growths in epithelial tissues that have atypical cells and increased proliferation rate compared with normal surrounding tissues. These early-stage cancers are localized to the epithelium and have not penetrated the local basement membrane or invaded the surrounding stroma. Based on these characteristics, they are not malignant. CIS occurs in a number of sites, including the cervix, skin, oral cavity, esophagus, and bronchus. In glandular epithelium, in situ lesions occur in the stomach, endometrium, breast, and large bowel. In the breast, ductal carcinoma in situ (DCIS) fills the mammary ducts but has not progressed to local tissue invasion.[2] DCIS lesions are readily treatable, although the optimal therapeutic approach is controversial. CIS lesions can have one of the following three fates: (1) they can remain stable for a long time, (2) they can progress to invasive and metastatic cancers, or (3) they can regress and disappear. CIS can vary from low-grade to high-grade dysplasia, with the high-grade lesions having the highest likelihood of becoming invasive cancers. The time that such preinvasive lesions remain in situ before becoming invasive is unknown. Some carcinomas of the cervix appear

FIGURE 10-2 Loss of Cellular and Tissue Differentiation During the Development of Cancer. The cells of a benign neoplasm (B) resemble those of the normal colonic epithelium (A), in that they are columnar and have an orderly arrangement. Loss of some degree of differentiation is evident in that the neoplastic cells do not show much mucin vacuolization (large, clear cytoplasmic vacuoles in A). Cells of the well-differentiated malignant neoplasm (C) of the colon have a haphazard arrangement, and although gland lumina are formed they are architecturally abnormal and irregular. Nuclei vary in shape and size, especially when compared with those illustrated in (A). Cells in the poorly-differentiated malignant neoplasm (D) have an even more haphazard arrangement, with very poor formation of gland lumina. Nuclei show greater variation in shape and size compared with the well-differentiated malignant neoplasm (C). Cells in anaplastic malignant neoplasms (E) bear no relation to the normal epithelium, with no recognizable gland formation. Tremendous variation is found in the size of cells and their nuclei, with very intense staining (hyperchromatic nuclei). Not knowing the site of origin makes it impossible to classify this tumor by microscopic appearance alone. Well-differentiated tumors often resemble their cell of origin, as shown in the example of a benign tumor of smooth muscles (F). (From Stevens A, Lowe J: *Pathology,* ed 2, London, 2000, Mosby.)

| NORMAL EPITHELIUM | LOW-GRADE INTRAEPITHELIAL NEOPLASIA | HIGH-GRADE INTRAEPITHELIAL NEOPLASIA | INVASIVE CARCINOMA |

50 µm

FIGURE 10-3 Progression from Normal to Neoplasm in the Uterine Cervix. A sequence of cellular and tissue changes progressing from low-grade to high-grade intraepithelial neoplasms (also called carcinoma in situ) and then to invasive cancer is seen often in the development of cancer. In this example of the early stages of cervical neoplastic changes, the presence of anaplastic cells and loss of normal tissue architecture signify the development of cancer. The high rate of cell division and the presence of local mutagens and inflammatory mediators all contribute to the accumulation of genetic abnormalities that lead to cancer. (From Alberts B et al: *Molecular biology of the cell*, ed 5, New York, 2008, Garland.)

as preinvasive lesions in situ for several years before they progress to invasive carcinoma and metastatic tumors (Figure 10-3). Knowing how to best treat low-grade CIS lesions is challenging, because the proportion that progress to cancer versus the proportion that will never cause clinical problems is usually not known. Although most persons prefer removal of any CIS as opposed to "watchful waiting," this topic continues to be a source of great debate.

✓ QUICK CHECK 10-1
1. What is cancer?
2. Identify the major differences between benign and malignant tumors.
3. What is carcinoma in situ?

THE BIOLOGY OF CANCER CELLS

In two seminal publications, Drs. Douglas Hanahan and Robert Weinberg[3,4] described what they considered the hallmarks of cancer. Both articles stimulated considerable discussion and, especially, debate. The original publication contained six hallmarks, but with time and new research findings, increased to eight hallmarks and two traits that enable cancer progression. Their analysis remains the leading overview of why a cell is malignant. The following discussion is organized in the context of those ten hallmarks/enablers (Figure 10-4). Two fundamental concepts are the foundation for understanding the

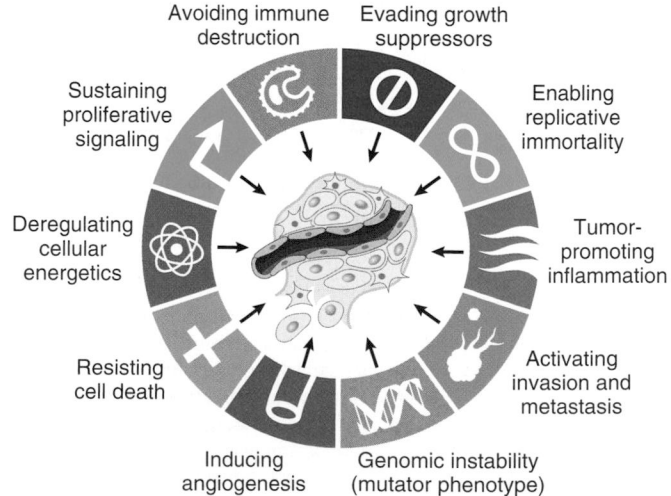

Avoiding immune destruction

Evading growth suppressors

Sustaining proliferative signaling

Enabling replicative immortality

Deregulating cellular energetics

Tumor-promoting inflammation

Resisting cell death

Activating invasion and metastasis

Inducing angiogenesis

Genomic instability (mutator phenotype)

FIGURE 10-4 Hallmarks of Cancer. (Adapted from Hanahan D, Weinberg RA. *Cell* 2011; 144:646. Found in Kumar V et al: *Robbins and Cotran pathologic basis of disease*, ed 9, Philadelphia, 2015, Saunders.)

FIGURE 10-5 Oncogene Activation Mechanisms. Cellular genes may become cancerous oncogenes as a result of (**A**) point mutations that alter one or a few nucleotide base pairs, causing the production of a protein that is activated as a result of the altered sequence (e.g., RAS); (**B**) amplification of the cellular gene, resulting in higher levels of protein expression (e.g., MYCN in neuroblastoma); or (**C**) chromosomal transloca-tions that either (1) lead to the juxtaposition of a strong promoter, causing increased protein expression (MYC in Burkitt lymphoma), or (2) produce a novel fusion protein that is derived from gene fragments normally present on different chromosomes (BCR-ABL in chronic myeloid leukemia). (From Haber DA: *Molecular genetics of cancer.* In *ACP medicine,* Danbury, Conn, 2004, WebMD.)

biology of cancer. Cancer is a complex genetic disease, and the micro-environment of a tumor is a heterogeneous mixture of cells, both cancerous and benign. These concepts affect every stage of cancer development and evolve during that development. **Tumor initiation,** the process that produces the initial cancer cells, is dependent on spe-cific mutations and characteristics of the microenvironment. **Tumor promotion,** the process during which the population of cancer cells expands with diversity of cancer cell phenotypes, is dependent on additional mutations and a changing tumor microenvironment. **Tumor progression,** the process leading to spread of the tumor to adjacent and distal sites (metastasis), is governed by further mutations and changing microenvironments at the primary tumor and at sites of metastasis.

Cancer is a disease of cumulative genetic changes during aging. The fraction of individuals who develop cancer increases dramatically with age. Genetic changes may occur by both mutational and epigenetic mechanisms. Mutation generally means an alteration in the DNA sequence affecting expression or function of a gene (Figure 10-5). Mutations include small-scale changes in DNA, such as **point muta-tions;** the alteration of one or a few nucleotide base pairs (see Chapter 2). This type of mutation can have profound effects on the activity of resultant proteins. **Chromosome translocations** are large changes in chromosome structure in which a piece of one chromosome is trans-located to another chromosome. **Gene amplification** is the result of repeated duplication of a region of a chromosome, so that instead of the normal two copies of a gene, tens or even hundreds of copies are present. Gene expression also may be altered indirectly by epigenetic effects including **DNA methylation,** histone acetylation, or altered expression of **non–coding RNA** (see Chapter 3). Some mutations,

referred to as *driver mutations,* "drive" the progression of cancer. There may be as many as 140 different driver mutations, although some are more critical than others, and each cancer only has a relatively small number of these.[5] Not all mutations in cancer contribute to the malig-nant phenotype. Some are just random events and are referred to as *passenger mutations;* they are just along for the ride. After a critical number of driver mutations have occurred, the cell becomes cancer-ous. The cancer cell has a selective advantage over its neighbors; its progeny can accumulate faster than its nonmutant neighbors. This is referred to as **clonal proliferation** or **clonal expansion** (Figure 10-6). As a clone with mutations proliferates, it may become an early-stage tumor, for example, a carcinoma in situ or a benign colonic polyp. The increasingly rapid cell division and impaired DNA repair mechanisms of cancer cells result in a continuing accumulation of mutations throughout the progression to the most aggressive metastatic lesion. Thus, **transformation,** the process by which a normal cell becomes a cancer cell, is directed by progressive accumulation of genetic changes that alter the basic nature of the cell and drive it to malignancy. The process of tumor development is a form of darwinian evolution; cells with a heritable change that confers a survival advantage out-compete their neighbors. Each cancer cell may develop its own set of mutations resulting in a genomically heterogeneous mixture of cells with subsets that have accumulated more and more mutations that increase the cell's malignant potential.[6] Thus many cancer cells that do not accu-mulate a critical set of mutations lose the competition and die during this process.

The processes occurring during the development of cancer are, in many ways, analogous to wound healing. The initial proliferation of cancer cells and enlargement of the tumor elicit the synthesis of

Genetic Event	Cell Behavior
Inactivation of APC	Cell seems normal but is predisposed to proliferate excessively
Mutational activation of K-ras	Cell begins to proliferate too much but is otherwise normal
Loss of DCC, over-expression of COX-2	Cell proliferates more rapidly; it also undergoes structural changes
Loss of *TP53*, activation of telomerase	Cell grows uncontrollably and looks obviously abnormal

FIGURE 10-6 Clonal Proliferation Model of Neoplastic Progression in the Colon. During clonal proliferation, progressively altered populations of colon cells (colonocytes) arise over time. As genetic and epigenetic changes occur, different subclones (indicated by different color cells) coexist for a time. Clones that grow the fastest out-compete other clones, producing even more malignant, and abnormal-appearing, growths. The sequential accumulation of mutations has been well studied in the progression from a normal colon cell to a benign intestinal polyp to a malignant colon cancer. One of the earliest mutations in colon cancer is loss of the tumor-suppressor gene *APC.* Additional mutations (often in the oncogene *RAS*), activation of COX-2, and loss of the tumor suppressors *DCC* and *TP53* occur as the lesion progresses from a benign polyp to an invasive carcinoma. *APC,* Adenomatous polyposis coli; *COX-2,* cyclooxygenase-2; *DCC,* deleted in colon cancer; *TP53,* p53 gene. (Modified from Mendelsohn I et al: *The molecular basis of cancer,* ed 2, Philadelphia, 2001, Saunders; and Kumar V et al: *Basic pathology,* ed 6, Philadelphia, 1997, Saunders.)

pro-inflammatory mediators by the cancer cells and adjacent nonmalignant cells. As with wound healing, mediators recruit inflammatory/immune cells (primarily T lymphocytes and macrophages, but also B cells and neutrophils) and cells normally associated with tissue repair (fibroblasts, adipocytes, mesenchymal stem cells, endothelial cells, and pericytes). These cells form the stroma (tumor microenvironment) that surrounds and infiltrates the tumor (Figure 10-7).[7] In some conditions, stromal cells may make up 90% of the tumor mass.[8] Extensive paracrine signaling among the stromal and cancer cells affects both populations; cancer cells increase proliferation and become more heterogeneous during tumor growth, and several populations of stromal cells undergo evolution to phenotypes that promote cancer progression and metastatic potential.[9] Cancer heterogeneity arises from ongoing proliferation and mutation. Tumor-associated endothelial cells, fibroblasts, and inflammatory cells develop different and distinct gene expression profiles with unique cell surface molecules and patterns of secreted molecules. During this process there is generally a great deal of cancer cell death, but the surviving cells are more aggressive and many take on a metastatic phenotype. Because continuing somatic mutations may be random, cancer cells in different regions of the tumor may be genetically diverse. Additionally, a population of cancer stem cells may arise, the origin of which is still unclear. Many of the hallmarks of cancer are consequences of cancer-stromal interactions (discussed later).

Several of the hallmarks/enablers are primarily genomic alterations that initiate and maintain development of cancer. These will be discussed first and include sustained proliferative signaling, evading growth suppression, genomic instability, and replicative immortality (see Figure 10-4). Other hallmarks/enablers are secondary to genomic change and include inducing angiogenesis and reprogramming energy metabolism. A third group, tumor resistance to destruction by the

host's protective mechanisms, includes resistance to apoptotic cell death, tumor-promoting inflammation, and avoiding immune destruction. The last hallmark is the culmination of the previous nine: activating invasion and metastasis.

 QUICK CHECK 10-2

1. Describe the differences between point mutations, chromosomal translocations, and gene amplification in the process of cancer.
2. Why is the tumor microenvironment important to cancer progression?

Sustained Proliferative Signaling

The first and foremost hallmark of cancer is uncontrolled cellular proliferation. Normal cells generally only enter proliferative phases in response to growth factors that bind to specific receptors on the cell surface. The cytoplasmic components of the receptors are associated with signaling molecules that undergo activation and in turn activate intracellular signaling pathways leading to induction/activation of regulatory factors affecting DNA synthesis, entrance into the cell cycle, and changes in expression of other genes related to cell metabolism for optimal growth (Figure 10-8). One example is initiation of proliferation by epidermal growth factor (EGF). EGF binds and cross-links two EGF receptors on the cell surface. The cytoplasmic portions of the receptors are tyrosine kinases that attach phosphorus to tyrosine in neighboring proteins, including each other (autophosphorylation). Phosphorylation allows the receptor to attach to bridging protein, which links the EGF receptors to plasma membrane–associated inactive RAS. RAS is an acronym for "rat sarcoma," where it was found originally. Inactive RAS is associated with guanine diphosphate (GDP).

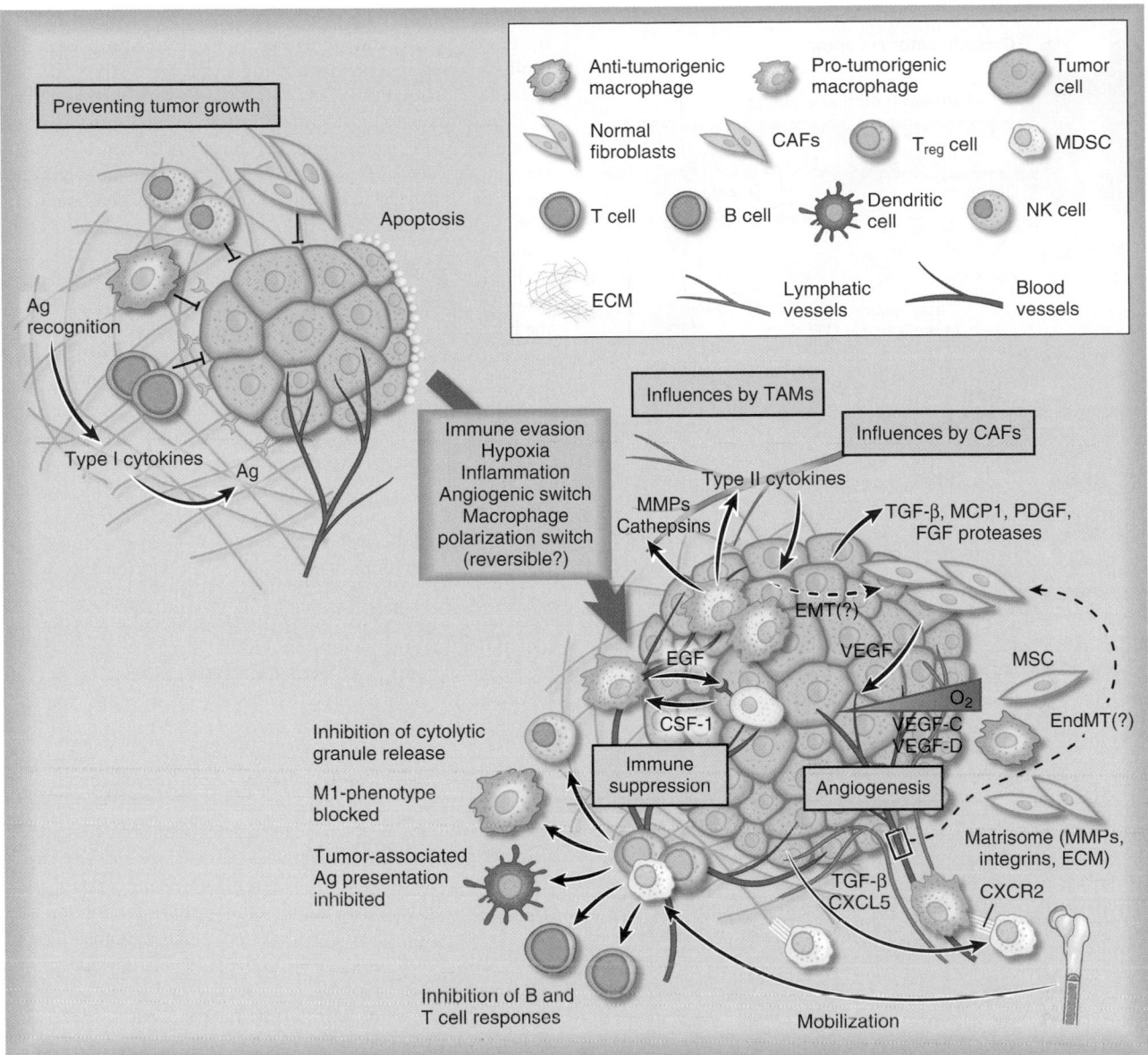

FIGURE 10-7 Cancers Live in a Complex Microenvironment. Cancer cells express tumor-specific antigens that ideally can be recognized by cells of the immune system and inflammatory systems (natural killer cells, antitumor M1 macrophages, T-cytotoxic cells) and destroyed by apoptosis or undergo growth suppression by type I cytokines. However, successful cancers produce a variety of cytokines and chemokines that are chemoattractants for stromal cells that infiltrate the tumor and undergo change to pro-tumor phenotypes. These include tumor-associated M2 macrophages (TAMs), cancer-associated fibroblasts (CAFs), mesenchymal stem cells (MSCs), and immune suppressor cells of T-cell origin (T-regulatory cells) and myeloid origin (myeloid-derived suppressor cells). Through multiple receptor-mediated interactions between other stromal cells and the cancer cells, the stromal cells, as well as the cancer cells, collectively produce a battery of additional cytokines (e.g., TGF-β, type II cytokines), chemokines (e.g., CXCL5), growth factors (e.g., VEGF, EGF, CSF-1, FGF, PDGF), and proteases (e.g., MMPs) and secrete components of the extracellular matrix (ECM). The stromal reaction promotes tumor progression, including new blood vessel growth (angiogenesis), tumor cell proliferation and differentiation, suppression of immune rejection and tumor cell apoptosis, invasion, and commitment to metastasis. *CAF,* Cancer-associated fibroblast; *CSF-1,* colony-stimulating factor-1; *CXCL5,* C-X-C motif chemokine 5; *ECM,* extracellular matrix; *EGF,* epidermal growth factor; *FGF,* fibroblast growth factor; *MSC,* mesenchymal stem cell; *MMP,* matrix metalloproteinase; *NK,* natural killer cell; *PDGF,* platelet-derived growth factor; *TAM,* tumor-associated macrophage; *TGF-β,* tumor growth factor-beta; *Treg,* T-regulatory cell; *VEGF,* vascular endothelial cell growth factor. (Modified from Quail DF, Joyce JA: Microenvironmental regulation of tumor progression and metastasis, *Nat Med* 19[11]:1423-1437, 2013.)

FIGURE 10-8 Growth Factor Signaling Pathways in Cancer. Growth factor receptors, RAS, PI3K, MYC, and D cyclins are oncoproteins that are activated by mutations in various cancers. GAPs apply brakes to RAS activation, and PTEN serves the same function for PI3K. *GAP,* GTPase-activating protein; *GDP,* guanosine diphosphate; *GTP,* guanosine triphosphate; *MAPK,* mitogen-activated protein kinase; *PI3K,* phosphoinositidyl-3-kinase; *PTEN,* phosphatase and tensin homolog. (From Kumar V et al: *Robbins and Cotran pathologic basis of disease,* ed 9, Philadelphia, 2015, Saunders.)

Oncogenes are independent of normal regulatory mechanisms; thus the cell is driven into a state of unregulated constitutive expression of proliferation signals and uncontrolled cell growth. Oncogenes can affect any portion of the growth factor pathways, such as described for EGF. For instance, most growth factors originate from neighboring cells, but some cancers acquire the ability to secrete growth factors that stimulate their own growth, a process known as **autocrine stimulation.** As described later in this chapter, noncancerous stromal cells within a tumor are frequently modified to benefit the cancer. In some instances, stromal cells produce excessive growth factors that drive the proliferation of cancer cells. Other cancers increase the expression of growth factor receptors; for example, in breast cancer production of the human epidermal growth factor receptor 2 (HER2, also known as the epidermal growth factor receptor gene *[ERBB-2])* is up-regulated and is hyperresponsive to low levels of EGF. Some breast and lung cancers are effectively treated by inhibitors of HER2 and other EGF receptors that block this pathway.[10]

Oncogenes may lead to constant activation of the signal cascade from the cell surface receptor to the nucleus. Up to a third of all cancers have an activating mutation in the *RAS* gene resulting in a continuous cell growth signal even when growth factors are missing (see Figure 10-8). Other mutations in the EGF receptor pathway include excessive proliferation signaling by hyperactivation of the PI3 kinase.

Several types of genetic events can activate oncogenes. A point mutation that is frequently observed in lung cancer results in continuous activation of the EGF **receptor tyrosine kinase.** A point mutation in the *RAS* gene converts it from a regulated proto-oncogene to an unregulated oncogene. Activating point mutations in *RAS* are found in many cancers, especially pancreatic and colorectal cancer. Specialized tests, such as direct DNA sequencing, can detect such point mutations in clinical samples.

Translocations can activate oncogenes in one of two distinct mechanisms (Figure 10-9). First, a translocation can cause excess and inappropriate production of a proliferation factor. One of the best examples is the t(8;14) translocation found in many Burkitt lymphomas; t(8;14) designates a chromosome that has a piece of chromosome 8 fused to a piece of chromosome 14 (see Chapter 21).[11] Burkitt lymphoma is an aggressive cancer of B lymphocytes. The *MYC* proto-oncogene found on chromosome 8 is normally activated at low levels in proliferating lymphocytes and is inactivated in mature lymphocytes. If the t(8;14) translocation occurs, the *MYC* gene is aberrantly placed under the control of a B-cell immunoglobulin gene *(IG)* present on chromosome 14. The *IG* gene is very active in maturing B lymphocytes. The t(8;14) translocation alters the control of *MYC;* its normal low level expression is switched to high levels, as directed by an *IG* gene promoter. Hyperproduction of MYC protein drives proliferation and blocks differentiation.

Second, chromosome translocations can lead to production of novel proteins with growth-promoting properties. In chronic myeloid leukemia (CML) a specific chromosome translocation is almost always present (see Figure 10-9). This translocation, t(9;22), was first identified in association with CML in Philadelphia in 1960 and is often referred to as the *Philadelphia chromosome.*[12] Translocation fuses two chromosomes in the middle of two different genes: *BCR* (break point cluster region gene) on chromosome 9 and *ABL* (Abelson gene) on chromosome 22. The result is production of a BCR-ABL fusion protein containing the first half of *BCR* and the second half of *ABL* (a nonreceptor tyrosine kinase). BCR-ABL is an unregulated protein tyrosine kinase that promotes growth of myeloid cells. Imatinib, a drug that specifically targets this tyrosine kinase, represents the first successful chemotherapy targeted against the product of a specific oncogenic

Association between the EGF receptor and inactive RAS modifies the binding of GDP, which is replaced with guanine triphosphate (GTP). GTP activates RAS, which is a GTPase that converts GTP to GDP, during which it can activate signaling pathways such as the mitogen-activated protein kinase (MAPK) pathway and the phosphatidylinosityl-3-kinase (PI3K) pathway. These signaling pathways phosphorylate other cytoplasmic proteins and affect activity and nuclear localization of transcription factors, such as MYC (myelocytomatosis viral oncogene homolog), that govern the transcription of cell cycle regulators, such as cyclins, and entrance into cellular proliferation. Proliferation can be discontinued through this pathway by decreased levels of growth factors in the environment or inactivation of signaling pathway components.

The genes that encode components of receptor-mediated pathways designed to regulate normal cellular proliferation are collectively called **proto-oncogenes.** Cancerous cells characteristically express mutated or overexpressed proto-oncogenes, which are referred to as **oncogenes.**

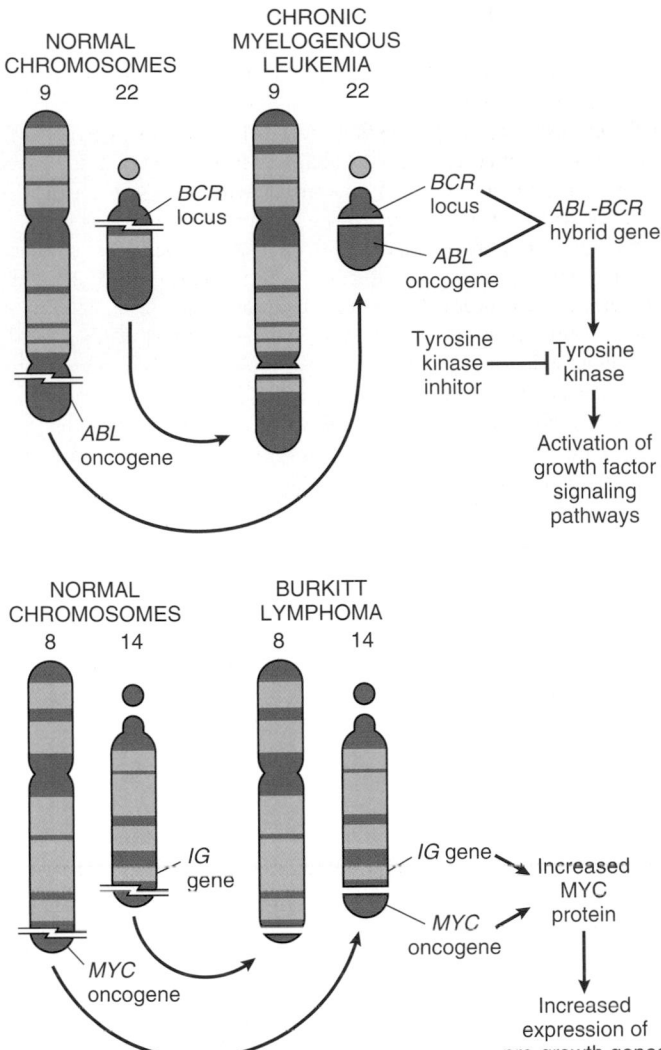

FIGURE 10-9 Examples of Chromosomal Translocations and Associated Oncogenes. See text for further explanation. (From Kumar V et al: *Robbins and Cotran pathologic basis of disease*, ed 9, Philadelphia, 2015, Saunders.)

mutation. Imatinib and related tyrosine kinase inhibitors (TKIs) are highly effective in the treatment of CML and, because of their specificity, lack the toxic side effects noted with nonspecific anticancer drugs. However, imatinib is not effective in cancers that do not have the t(9;22) translocation or related mutations. In modern personalized cancer therapy, knowledge of the specific genetic alteration can dictate the optimal drugs for the individual.

Oncogenes also may be activated by gene amplification (Figure 10-10). Gene amplification results in increased expression of an oncogene, or in some cases drug resistance genes. The N-*MYC* oncogene, a member of the *MYC* family, is amplified in 25% of childhood neuroblastoma and confers a poor prognosis. The HER2 gene (*ERBB2*) is amplified in 20% of breast cancers.

Evading Growth Suppressors

Uncontrolled cancer cell proliferation also is related to inactivation of tumor-suppressor genes. Tumor-suppressor genes normally regulate the cell cycle, inhibit proliferation resulting from growth signals, stop

cell division when cells are damaged, and prevent mutations. Hence, they also have been referred to as anti-oncogenes. Whereas oncogenes are *activated* in cancers, tumor suppressors must be *inactivated* to allow cancer to occur (Table 10-1 and Figure 10-11). A single genetic event can activate an oncogene because it can act in a dominant manner in the cell. However, we have two copies of each tumor-suppressor gene, one from each parent. Both copies must be inactivated; therefore two mutations are necessary.

A prototypical tumor-suppressor gene is the retinoblastoma *(RB)* gene. Normal cells receive diverse "antigrowth" signals from their normal environment. Contact with other cells, with basement membranes, and with some soluble factors normally signal cells to stop proliferating. Tumor-suppressor genes, such as *RB*, monitor antigrowth cellular signals and block activation of the growth/division phase in the cell cycle; thus mutations in *RB* lead to persistent cell growth. Anti-proliferative activity of *RB* depends on the degree of protein phosphorylation.[13] Low levels of phosphorylation (hypophosphorylation) result in *RB* binding to and inhibiting transcription factors that regulate genes controlling passage through the cell cycle. Growth factor–regulated kinases increase phosphorylation (hyperphosphorylation) and inactivation of *RB*. A variety of genetic mutations in cancers also inactivate *RB*, resulting in unregulated and continuous cellular proliferation. *RB* is mutated in childhood retinoblastoma, and in many lung, breast, and bone cancers as well. The *RB* gene resides on chromosome 13, in a region referred to as q14 (13q14). Most individuals with *RB* mutations have a subtle mutation, such as a point mutation, in one allele. The *RB* gene in the other chromosome may be inactivated through loss of the 13q14 region or epigenetic mechanisms.

Another classic tumor suppressor gene is tumor protein p53 *(TP53)*. The protein p53 has been called the *guardian of the genome*. TP53 monitors intracellular signals related to stress and activates caretaker genes—genes that are responsible for the maintenance of genomic integrity (Figure 10-12). Many types of cellular stress (e.g., anoxia, oncogene expression, nuclear damage) produce intracellular signals (e.g., levels of nucleotides and glucose, degree of oxygenation, DNA damage, and other indicators of cellular abnormalities) detectable by p53. Normally p53 is in an inactive complex with inhibitor molecules. Stress activates kinases that phosphorylate p53 into an active suppressor of cell division and activator of caretaker genes. Caretaker genes encode proteins that are involved in repairing damaged DNA, such as occurs with errors in DNA replication, mutations caused by ultraviolet or ionizing radiation, and mutations caused by chemicals and drugs. The p53 protein also controls initiation of cellular senescence or apoptosis, and suppresses cell division until DNA repair is complete or other effects of stress are corrected. If not corrected, the cell enters senescence or apoptosis, thus preventing further DNA damage and mutations. Loss of function of *TP53* or caretaker genes leads to increased mutation rates and cancer.[14]

Because inactivation of tumor-suppressor genes requires at least two mutations (one in each allele), a single **germ cell mutation** (sperm or egg) results in the transmission of cancer-causing genes from one generation to the next, producing families with a high risk for specific cancers. These inherited mutations that predispose to cancer are almost invariably in tumor-suppressor genes because only a single additional mutation in any other cell (**somatic cell mutation**) is needed to inactivate completely the tumor-suppressor gene (Table 10-2).[15]

An example of increased risk for cancer that can be inherited is the familial form of retinoblastoma. A mutation in one *RB* allele is inherited so that only one additional mutation in the normal allele will lead

FIGURE 10-10 N-*MYC* Gene Amplification in Neuroblastoma. (A) The N-*MYC* gene is present on chromosome 2, becomes amplified, and is seen either as extra chromosomal double minutes or as a chromosomal homologous staining region. The N-*MYC* gene is detected in human neuroblastoma cells using a technique called FISH (fluorescent in situ hybridization). **(B)** A single pair of N-*MYC* genes is detected in normal cells and in low-grade neuroblastoma. **(C)** Multiple, amplified copies of the N-*MYC* gene are detected in some cases of neuroblastoma. Amplification of the N-*MYC* gene is strongly associated with a poor prognosis in childhood neuroblastoma. (**A** from Kumar V et al: *Robbins and Cotran pathologic basis of disease,* ed 9, Philadelphia, 2015, Saunders. **B, C** courtesy Arthur R. Brothman, PhD, FACMG, University of Utah School of Medicine, Salt Lake City, Utah.)

TABLE 10-1   Comparison of Cancer Gene Types

Gene Type	Normal Function	Mutation Effect
Caretaker	DNA and chromosome stability	Chromosome instability and increased rates of mutation
Dominant oncogenes*	Encode proteins that promote growth (e.g., growth factors)	Overexpression or amplification causes gain of function
Tumor suppressors (recessive oncogenes)	Encode proteins that inhibit proliferation and prevent or repair mutations	Requires loss of function of both alleles to increase cancer risk

*Nonmutant state referred to as proto-oncogene.

TABLE 10-2   Some Familial Cancer Syndromes Caused by Tumor-Suppressor Gene Function Loss

Syndrome	Gene
Retinoblastoma	*RB1*
Li-Fraumeni syndrome	*p53 (TP53)*
Familial melanoma	$p16^{INK\alpha}$ *(CDKN2A)*
Neurofibromatosis	*Neurofibromin (NF1)*
Familial adenomatous polyps	*APC*
Breast cancer	*BRCA1*

to cancer (see Table 10-2). Approximately half of children with retinoblastoma have the inheritable form and most will develop tumors in both eyes (bilateral retinoblastoma). Also, Li-Fraumeni syndrome is a very rare inheritable loss-of-function mutation in *TP53* in one allele resulting in a 25-fold increase of developing malignancy at early age (<50 years of age). These malignancies may include breast cancer, brain tumors, acute leukemia, soft tissue sarcomas, bone sarcoma, and adrenal cortical carcinoma. Other familial cancers with inheritable mutations in tumor-suppressor genes include Wilms tumor, a childhood cancer of the kidney *(WT1* gene); neurofibromatosis *(NF1* gene); and familial polyposis coli or adenomas of the colon *(APC* gene). Characterization of cancer-causing genes and other genetic factors helps identify individuals prone to developing cancer and contributes to our understanding of sporadic cancers. Individuals known to carry mutations in tumor-suppressor genes are offered targeted cancer screening to facilitate early cancer detection and therapy.

Genomic Instability

Genomic instability refers to an increased tendency of alterations—mutability—in the genome during the life cycle of cells. Inherited and acquired mutations in caretaker genes that protect the integrity of the genome and DNA repair increase the level of genomic instability and risk for developing cancer. Acquired mutations in "guardians of the genome," such as *TP53*, that detect DNA damage and activate repair mechanisms result in an increasing accumulation of mutations. Xeroderma pigmentosum is a defect in the repair of DNA pyrimidine dimers created by ultraviolet (UV) light that increases the risk for skin cancers. Hereditary nonpolyposis colorectal cancer results from an inherited defect in repairing DNA base pair mismatches that occur

FIGURE 10-11 Silencing Tumor-Suppressor Genes. Tumor-suppressor genes can be deactivated by a variety of mechanisms. **(A)** In this example, the first hit is a point mutation in a tumor-suppressor gene (white box), followed by either epigenetic silencing or chromosome loss of the second allele (red box). **(B)** Genes can normally be silenced by a variety of interacting processes including DNA methylation, histone modification, nucleosomal remodeling, and microRNA changes (not shown). A number of cellular enzymes contribute to these modifications, including DNA methyltransferases *(DNMTs)*, histone deacetylases *(HDACs)*, histone methyltransferases *(HMTs)*, and complex nucleosomal remodeling factors *(NURFs)*. Gene silencing is essential for normal development and differentiation. **(C)** Histone modification and promoter methylation regulate gene expression. Genes are transcribed when chromatin is modified by addition of acetyl *(Ac)* groups to specific lysine groups in histones. Gene expression can be turned off when specific acetyl groups are removed (by HDACs) or when the CpG-rich promoter regions of genes are modified by direct DNA methylation (by DNA methyltransferase). In addition, small endogenous RNA molecules (microRNAs or miRNA) can bind to mRNA and reduce gene expression. **(D)** Changes in promoter methylation turn cancer genes off and on. Oncogenes can be turned on by promoter hypomethylation, and tumor-suppressor genes can be turned off by promoter hypermethylation. Each of these changes can produce selective growth and survival advantages for the cancer cell. *Me,* Methylation; *TF,* transcription factor. (**B** adapted from Jones PA, Baylin SB: The epigenomics of cancer, *Cell* 128:683-692, 2007; **C** from Gluckman PD et al: *N Engl J Med* 359[1]:66, 2008; **D** from Shames DS et al: *Curr Mol Med* 7:85-102, 2007.)

FIGURE 10-12 The Role of p53 in Maintaining the Integrity of the Genome. Activation of normal p53 by DNA-damaging agents or by hypoxia leads to cell cycle arrest in G₁ by up-regulation of the cell cycle inhibitor p21 and induction of DNA repair transcriptional up-regulation of the cyclin-dependent kinase inhibitor *CDKN1A* (encoding the cyclin-dependent kinase inhibitor p21) and the *GADD45* genes. Successful repair of DNA allows cells to proceed with the cell cycle. If DNA repair fails, *p53* triggers either apoptosis or senescence. In cells with loss or mutation of the *p53* gene, DNA damage does not induce cell cycle arrest or DNA repair, and genetically damaged cells proliferate, giving rise eventually to malignant neoplasms. (From Kumar V et al: *Robbins and Cotran pathologic basis of disease*, ed 9, Philadelphia, 2015, Saunders.)

occasionally during DNA replication. Affected individuals have an increased rate of small insertions and deletions in DNA, leading to a high rate of colon and other cancers. Some inherited mutations threaten the integrity of entire chromosomes. Bloom syndrome, caused by mutations in a DNA helicase, presents with an increased risk of several forms of cancer, and those with Fanconi aplastic anemia, caused by loss of function for repairing DNA double-strand breaks, have a particularly increased risk of acute myelogenous leukemia. These examples are autosomal recessive disorders in which affected individuals demonstrate marked chromosomal instability.

Genomic instability also may result from increased epigenetic silencing or modulation of gene function (Chapter 3). Many cancers have increased methylation of DNA in the promoter region of tumor-suppressor genes. They also have associated changes in the modification of histones in the chromatin, often correlated with methylation

of DNA. These changes alter the promoter regions of genes, leading to their silencing or altered gene expression.

Changes in gene regulation can affect not just single genes, but also entire intracellular signaling networks. Gene expression networks can be regulated by changes in microRNAs (miRNAs, or miRs) and other non–coding RNAs (ncRNAs).[16] miRs regulate diverse signaling pathways; the miRs that stimulate cancer development and progression are termed oncomirs.[17] miRs decrease the stability and expression of other genes by pairing with mRNA.

Mutations in *BRCA1* and *BRCA2* (breast cancer 1 and 2, early onset genes) are currently of clinical importance. Both are tumor-suppressors and caretaker genes that repair double-stranded DNA breaks. Inherited mutations in either gene greatly increase the risk for a variety of tumors, especially breast cancer in both women and men, and ovarian or prostate cancers. Approximately 12% of women generally will develop breast cancer within their lifetime, whereas about 60% of women with a high-risk *BRCA1* mutation and 45% with a *BRCA2* mutation will develop cancer by age 70.[18] Ovarian cancer occurs in approximately 1.4% of the general population, but about 39% of women with an inherited mutation in *BRCA1* and about 15% with a mutation in *BRCA2* will develop ovarian cancer by age 70. At-risk women are currently offered prophylactic surgery to reduce the risk of cancer.

In addition to specific gene mutations and abnormal epigenetic silencing, chromosome instability also appears to be increased in malignant cells, resulting in a high rate of chromosome loss, as well as loss of heterozygosity and chromosome amplification. The underlying mechanism of this instability is not clear but may be caused by malfunctions in the cellular machinery that regulates chromosome segregation at mitosis.

Enabling Replication Immortality

A hallmark of cancer cells is their immortality, in that they seem to have an unlimited life span and will continue to divide for years under appropriate laboratory conditions. One of the most commonly used laboratory cell lines, HeLa cells, was derived from a cervical cancer specimen obtained in 1951 that continues to grow and divide in laboratories around the world.[19] Most normal cells are not immortal and can divide only a limited number of times (known as the Hayflick limit) before they either enter senescence (cease dividing) or enter crisis (apoptosis) and die. One major block to unlimited cell division (i.e., immortality) is the size of a specialized structure called the *telomere*. Telomeres are protective ends, or caps, of repeating hexanucleotides (six nucleotide units) on each chromosome and are placed and maintained by a specialized enzyme called telomerase (Figure 10-13).[20] As one might expect, telomerase is usually active only in germ cells (in ovaries and testes) and in stem cells. All other cells of the body lack telomerase activity. Therefore, when non–germ cells begin to proliferate abnormally their telomere caps shorten with each cell division. Short telomeres normally signal the cell to cease cell division. If the telomeres become critically small, the chromosomes become unstable and fragment, and the cells die.

Cancer cells are very heterogeneous and many cells die as the cancer develops. When they reach a critical age, most cancer cells activate telomerase to restore and maintain their telomeres, thereby allowing continuous division.[21] The trigger for reexpression of telomerase activity remains unclear, but seems to require expression of specific oncogenes, such as *RAS* or *MYC*, and loss of function of certain tumor-suppressor molecules, such as p53 and RB. Telomerase activity is restored in about 90% of cancers. The remaining cancers appear to recruit or originate from stem cells, becoming cancer stem cells that maintain levels of telomerase activity characteristically found in somatic stem cells.[22] Because telomerase is specifically activated in cancer cells, and potentially in cancer stem cells, it is an attractive therapeutic target.

FIGURE 10-13 Control of Immortality: Telomeres and Telomerase. Normal adult somatic cells cannot divide indefinitely because the ends of their chromosomes are capped by telomeres. In the absence of the telomerase enzyme, telomeres become progressively shorter with each division until, when they are critically short, they signal to the cell to stop dividing. In germ cells, adult stem cells, and cancer cells the telomerase gene is "switched on," producing an enzyme that rebuilds the telomeres. Thus, like germ cells, the cancer cell becomes immortal and able to divide indefinitely without losing its telomeres.

Inducing Angiogenesis

A major component of wound healing is the process of establishing new blood vessels within the tissue undergoing repair (called neovascularization or angiogenesis). Access to a blood supply also is obligatory to the growth and spread of cancer. Without a blood supply to deliver oxygen and nutrients, growth of a tumor is limited to about a millimeter in diameter.

Angiogenic factors and angiogenic inhibitors normally control development of new vessels. In cancerous tumors several mechanisms increase and maintain secretion of angiogenic factors by the cancer cells, as well as prevent release of angiogenic inhibitors. **Hypoxia-inducible factor-1α (HIF-1α)**, an oxygen-sensitive transcription factor, is a major regulator of angiogenesis in normal tissue; HIF-1α is stabilized under hypoxic conditions and induces expression of pro-angiogenic factors, such as vascular endothelial growth factor (VEGF) and basic fibroblast growth factor (bFGF). Inactivation of tumor-suppressor genes (e.g., *p53*) or increased expression of oncogenes (e.g., *HER2*) leads to increased expression of HIF-1α–regulated angiogenic factors and increased vascularization. Increased expression of HIF-1α also is related to increased resistance to chemotherapy, increased tumor cell glycolysis, increased metastasis, and a poor prognosis. These effects may likely occur through an autocrine mechanism by which VEGF activates tumor-associated VEGF receptors. For instance, in soft tissue sarcomas VEGF induces increased expression of anti-apoptotic proteins (e.g., Bcl-2) and activation of intracellular survival signal pathways. The use of angiogenic inhibitors targeting VEGF signaling can inhibit angiogenesis and diminish tumor growth.

Other routes of angiogenic factor induction include mutations in cancer oncogenes (e.g., *RAS*, *MYC*) that increase transcription of

---

✔ QUICK CHECK 10-3

1. What are the heritable changes in cells that contribute to cancer development?
2. Define oncogene, proto-oncogene, and tumor-suppressor gene.
3. Biologically, why do tumor-suppressor genes have to be inactivated to cause cancer?
4. Define epigenetics and epigenetic silencing.
5. Distinguish between mutations in somatic cells versus in germ cells.
6. Define telomeres, telomerase, and senescence and describe their effects on cancer.

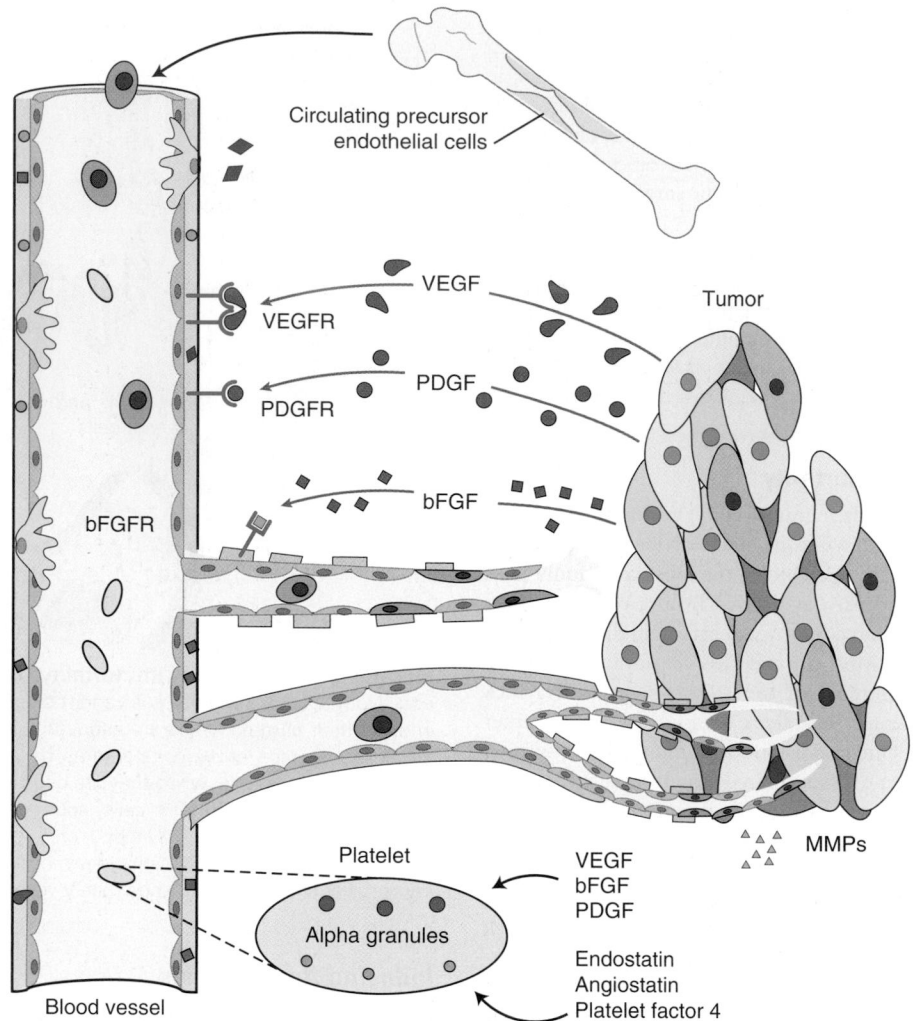

FIGURE 10-14 Tumor-Induced Angiogenesis. Malignant tumors secrete angiogenic factors and tissue-remodeling matrix metalloproteinases (MMPs) that actively induce formation of new blood vessels. New blood vessels are formed from both local endothelial cells and circulating precursor cells recruited from the bone marrow. Circulating platelets can also release regulatory proteins into the tumor. *bFGF* and *bFGFR*, Basic fibroblast growth factor and its receptor, respectively; *MMPs*, matrix metalloproteinases; *PDGF* and *PDGFR*, platelet-derived growth factor and its receptor, respectively; *VEGF* and *VEGFR*, vascular endothelial growth factor and its receptor, respectively. (Adapted from Folkman J: Angiogenesis: an organizing principle for drug discovery? *Nat Rev Drug Discov* 6[4]:273-286, 2007.)

VEGF by cancer cells. Most cells in the tumor microenvironment also secrete VEGF, including tumor-infiltrating monocytes, endothelial cells, adipocytes, and cancer-associated fibroblasts. Angiogenesis inhibitors, such as thrombospondin-1 (TSP-1), normally bind to cellular surface receptors on inflammatory cells and negatively regulate angiogenesis in wound healing and tissue remodeling. The expression of angiogenesis inhibitors is under the control of p53, which is suppressed in cancer cells, thus diminishing the control of stromal inflammatory cell secretion of angiogenic factors.

Cancer cells and stromal cells may increase production of matrix metalloproteinases (e.g., MMP-9) (Figure 10-14). **MMPs** are zinc-dependent proteases that digest the surrounding extracellular matrix (ECM). The ECM contains stored latent (inactive) forms of some angiogenic factors (e.g., bFGF, transforming growth factor-beta [TGF-β]). MMPs activate the stored forms into functional angiogenic factors.

The vessels formed within tumors differ from those in healthy tissue. They originate from endothelial sprouting from existing capillaries and irregular branching, rather than regular branching seen in healthy tissue. The interendothelial cell contact is less tight so the vessels are more porous and prone to hemorrhage, as well as allowing passage of tumor cells into the vascular system.

Reprograming Energy Metabolism

Cancer cells live in a distinct environment from normal cells and have different nutritional requirements from nonproliferating cells. The successful cancer cell divides rapidly, with the consequent requirement for the building blocks to construct new cells. Nonmalignant cells in the presence of adequate oxygen normally generate adenosine triphosphate (ATP) by mitochondrial oxidative phosphorylation (OXPHOS), generating 36 ATP molecules from each glucose molecule that is broken down to water and carbon dioxide. In the absence of sufficient oxygen (hypoxia) normal cells perform glycolysis (anaerobic glycolysis), generating only two ATP molecules per molecule of glucose, with lactic acid and pyruvate as byproducts.

FIGURE 10-15 Cancers Have Altered Metabolism. Normal tissues use oxidative phosphorylation (OXPHOS) to turn glucose into CO_2 and energy (in the form of ATP). Cancers take a different approach; even in the presence of oxygen, they do not use OXPHOS. Instead, they consume large quantities of glucose to make cellular building blocks, supporting rapid proliferation. (From Van der Heiden MG et al: Understanding the Warburg effect: the metabolic requirements of cell proliferation, *Science* 324:1029-1033, 2009.)

Even in the presence of adequate oxygen, cancer cells may not use OXPHOS, but are reprogrammed to glycolysis (Warburg effect) (Figure 10-15). Thus, the Warburg effect is the use of glycolysis under normal oxygen conditions, hence the name **aerobic glycolysis**. Although aerobic glycolysis was postulated to arise from cancer-specific mitochondrial dysfunction, it is now apparent that this is instead a highly regulated and beneficial adaptation for cancer cells.[73] The shift from OXPHOS to glycolysis allows lactate and other products of glycolysis to be used for the more efficient production of lipids, nucleosides, amino acids, and other molecular building blocks needed for rapid cell growth.

A new model, the reverse Warburg effect, may play a role in certain cancers. Cancer cells may continue using the OXPHOS to generate large amounts of ATP. However, they also may manipulate the cancer-associated fibroblasts (CAFs), perhaps by inducing oxidative stress, to undergo aerobic glycolysis and secrete metabolites (e.g., lactate, pyruvate) that the cancer cells can use in the citric acid cycle (Krebs cycle) to feed OXPHOS and produce ATP.[24] A secondary consequence would be induction of autophagy in the CAFs, resulting in consumption of the CAFs and release of materials needed by the cancer cell in the synthesis of new organelles.

Promoters of aerobic glycolysis are activated by oncogenes and mutated tumor-suppressor molecules. Up-regulation of GLUT1 (glucose transporter 1) under the control of oncogenes (e.g., *RAS*, *MYC*) and mutant tumor suppressors (e.g., *TP53*) increases transport of glucose into the cytoplasm. These and other oncogenes or mutant tumor-suppressor genes inhibit OXPHOS and promote the aerobic glycolytic pathway and related metabolic pathways that support the rapid growth of cancers.[25]

Clinically the high glucose utilization of a cancer can be exploited for its detection.[26] ^{18}F-Fluorodeoxyglucose (FDG) is incorporated into cells in the same way as glucose, with two key differences. Because it is missing a key hydroxyl group it cannot be broken down by glycolysis and, thus, FDG accumulates in cells. Because it is tagged with ^{18}F, it can be imaged by a positron emission tomography (PET) scan. Small metastatic tumor masses that are consuming huge amounts of glucose can readily be detected with this imaging method (Figure 10-16).

Resisting Apoptotic Cell Death

Programmed cell death (apoptosis) is a mechanism by which individual cells can self-destruct under conditions of tissue remodeling or as a protection against aberrant cell growth that may lead to malignancy. Two pathways may trigger apoptosis (Figure 10-17). The intrinsic pathway (mitochondrial pathway) monitors cellular stress. Cellular stress may include DNA damage, genomic instability, aberrant proliferation, loss of adhesion to extracellular matrix or to adjacent cells, and other causes and characteristics of abnormal cellular physiology. The extrinsic pathway is activated through a plasma membrane receptor complex linked to intracellular activators of apoptosis (known as the death receptor).

The balance between pro-apoptotic (e.g., Bcl-2–associated X protein [BAX] and Bcl-2–homologous antagonist/killer [BAK]) and anti-apoptotic (e.g., BCL2 [B-cell lymphoma 2]) members of the Bcl-2 family regulates apoptosis. Both groups regulate mitochondrial release of pro-apoptotic molecules (e.g., cytochrome *c*). As mentioned previously, expression of the tumor-suppressor gene *TP53* is affected by intracellular stress, particularly DNA damage. If DNA damage is irreparable, p53 is activated by phosphorylation and induces transcription of pro-apoptotic factors.

The extrinsic pathway is relatively dormant until the death receptor is activated. The principal apoptotic receptor is called Fas/CD95 (the CD95 nomenclature is an alternative for Fas) (see Figure 10-17). Fas is a receptor for Fas ligand (FasL) and similar molecules, such as tumor necrosis factor (TNF). Cytotoxic T lymphocytes and NK cells express

FIGURE 10-16 The Intense Glucose Requirement of Cancer Aids in Diagnosis. This 54-year-old woman had a non–small cell lung cancer (NSCLC) surgically removed. Five years later, these images were obtained. The positron emission tomography (PET) scan using ^{18}F-deoxyglucose shows metastatic lesions in the brain, right shoulder, and mediastinal and cervical lymph nodes as well as the liver, left pelvis, and proximal femur. *(Left)* PET whole-body image. *(Right)* Representative coronal image from the whole-body FDG-PET/CT–fused image of the same patient. The fused image consists of the CT image with the metabolic information superimposed in color. The pattern of distribution is most likely from the primary tumor to the large mediastinal lymph nodes, followed by lymphatic spread to cervical lymph nodes. Blood-borne dissemination produced the bone, brain, and liver metastases. Normally, only the heart, brain, and bladder show a strong signal on PET scan. *CT,* Computed tomography; *FDG,* fluorodeoxyglucose. (Images courtesy John Hoffman, MD, Huntsman Cancer Institute, Salt Lake City, Utah.)

FIGURE 10-17 Extrinsic and Intrinsic Pathways of Apoptosis and Mechanisms Used by Tumor Cells to Evade Cell Death. **(1)** Loss of p53 leading to reduced function of pro-apoptotic factors, such as BAX. **(2)** Reduced egress of cytochrome *c* from mitochondria as a result of up-regulation of anti-apoptotic factors, such as BCL-2. **(3)** Loss of apoptotic peptidase-activating factor 1 (APAF1). **(4)** Up-regulation of inhibitors of apoptosis (IAP). **(5)** Reduced CD95 levels. **(6)** Inactivation of death domain signaling complex (FADD). (From Kumar V et al: *Robbins and Cotran pathologic basis of disease,* ed 9, Philadelphia, 2015, Saunders.)

surface and soluble FasL and can produce TNF, thus inducing apoptosis in target cells. The Fas receptor is linked to a complex of intracellular proteins (FADD, the Fas-associated death domain signaling complex) that triggers apoptosis.

Both pathways activate a series of intracellular effector enzymatic molecules (caspases). Pro-apoptotic molecules released by mitochondria in the intrinsic pathway activate caspase 9, which in turn activates caspase 3. Caspase 3 cuts DNA and other substrates, leading to cell death. Activation of the extrinsic pathway activates caspase 8, which can directly activate caspase 3.

Apoptotic pathways are dysregulated in most cancers. Most commonly, loss-of-function mutations to the *TP53* gene suppress activation of apoptosis during DNA damage. The balance between pro- and anti-apoptotic molecules also can be affected by overexpression of anti-apoptotic molecules or diminished expression of anti-apoptotic molecules resulting from mutations. Overexpression of Bcl-2 occurs in the vast majority of follicular B-cell lymphomas. Excess expression of other anti-apoptotic members of the Bcl-2 family also may provide increased resistance to chemotherapeutic drugs, many of which act through induction of apoptosis. Other mechanisms of providing resistance to apoptosis include down-regulation of caspases or production of caspase inhibitors. By whatever mechanism, or combination of mechanisms, successful cancers suppressed apoptotic pathways and increased resistance to cell death.

Tumor-Promoting Inflammation

Historically, an immune/inflammatory response to cancer was considered a detrimental condition that successful tumors evolved methods of evading. We now realize that the relationship between a cancer and the inflammatory system is much more complex.[27] The inflammatory response may contribute to the onset of cancer and be manipulated throughout the process to benefit tumor progression and spread.[28]

Chronic inflammation has been recognized for close to 150 years as being an important factor in the development of cancer.[29] Chronic inflammations may result from many causes, for example, solar irradiation, asbestos exposure (mesothelioma), pancreatitis, and infection (Table 10-3). Additionally, some organs appear to be more susceptible to the oncogenic effects of chronic inflammation (e.g., the

TABLE 10-3 Chronic Inflammatory Conditions and Infectious Agents Associated with Neoplasms

Inflammatory Condition	Associated Neoplasm(s)
Asbestosis, silicosis	Mesothelioma, lung carcinoma
Bronchitis	Lung carcinoma
Cystitis, bladder inflammation	Bladder carcinoma
Gingivitis, lichen planus	Oral squamous cell carcinoma
Inflammatory bowel disease, Crohn disease, chronic ulcerative colitis	Colorectal carcinoma
Lichen sclerosus	Vulvar squamous cell carcinoma
Chronic pancreatitis, hereditary pancreatitis	Pancreatic carcinoma
Reflux esophagitis, Barrett esophagus	Esophageal carcinoma
Sialadenitis	Salivary gland carcinoma
Sjögren syndrome, Hashimoto thyroiditis	MALT lymphoma
Skin inflammation	Melanoma

Infectious Agent (Nonviral)	Associated Neoplasm(s)
Helicobacter pylori	Gastric adenocarcinoma, MALT lymphoma
Chronic bacterial cholecystitis	Gallbladder cancer
Schistosomiasis	Bladder, liver, rectal carcinoma; follicular lymphoma of spleen
Liver flukes	Cholangiocarcinoma

Infectious Agent (Viral)	Associated Neoplasm(s)
Human immunodeficiency virus type 1 (HIV-1)	Non-Hodgkin lymphoma, squamous cell carcinomas, Kaposi sarcoma
Hepatitis B and hepatitis C	Hepatocellular carcinoma
Epstein-Barr virus	B-cell non-Hodgkin lymphoma, Burkitt lymphoma, nasopharyngeal carcinoma
KSHV/HHV8 and immunodeficiency	Kaposi sarcoma
HPV-16, -18, -31, others	Cervical, anogenital
HTLV-1	Adult T-cell leukemia/lymphoma

From Kuper H et al: Infections as a major preventable cause of human cancer, *J Intern Med* 248(3):171-183, 2000.

gastrointestinal [GI] tract, prostate, thyroid gland). Individuals who have suffered with ulcerative colitis for 10 years or more have up to a 30-fold increase in the risk of developing colon cancer.[30] Chronic viral hepatitis caused by hepatitis B virus (HBV) or hepatitis C virus (HCV) infection markedly increases the risk of liver cancer.

A specific example is the association between gastric inflammation induced by infection with the bacterium *Helicobacter pylori* (H. pylori) and the risk for gastric cancer. *H. pylori* is a bacterium that infects more than half of the world's population. Chronic infection with *H. pylori* is an important cause of peptic ulcer disease and is strongly associated with gastric carcinoma, a leading cause of cancer deaths worldwide. It also is associated with a less common cancer, gastric mucosa–associated lymphoid tissue (MALT) lymphomas.[31] *H. pylori* infection is often acquired in childhood and disproportionately affects lower socioeconomic classes. Although most infections are asymptomatic, prolonged chronic inflammation can lead to increased gastric acid secretion, atrophic gastritis, and duodenal ulcers, or benign cellular proliferation that can in a small fraction of individuals progress to dysplastic changes

and finally gastric adenocarcinoma. *H. pylori* infection can both directly and indirectly produce genetic and epigenetic changes in cells of infected stomachs, including mutations in *TP53* and alterations in the methylation of specific genes. Eradication of *H. pylori* from infected individuals before the development of dysplasia may prevent the development of cancer. However, there is no expert consensus on the value of population screening and treatment strategies. The MALT lymphomas associated with chronic *H. pylori* infections may depend on chronic inflammation and antigenic stimulation associated with infections, and therefore treatment with antibiotics may be useful even in cases of early lymphoma.

Once cells with malignant phenotypes have developed, additional complex interactions occur between the tumor and the surrounding stroma and cells of the immune and inflammatory systems. Cancers disrupt the environment, initiate or enhance inflammation, and in turn recruit local and distant cells (macrophages, lymphocytes, and other cellular components of inflammation). The acute inflammatory response is initially designed to eliminate infection, but evolves to initiate and direct the healing process (see Chapter 6). Successful tumors appear capable of manipulating cells of the inflammatory response from a rejection response towards the phenotypes associated with wound healing and tissue regeneration; a process that includes induction in the damaged tissue of cellular proliferation, neovascularization, and local immune suppression.[32] These activities benefit cancer progression, as well as increase resistance to chemotherapeutic agents.

One of the key cells that promote tumor survival is the **tumor-associated macrophage (TAM)**. Tumors commonly produce cytokines and chemokines that are chemotactic factors for monocytes/macrophages (e.g., colony-stimulating factor-1 [CSF1; also known as macrophage colony stimulating factor or M-CSF], the chemokine ligand 2 [CCL2; also known as monocyte chemotactic protein-1 or MCP-1]). Levels of CCL2 in human breast cancer and cancers of the esophagus are related to the degree of macrophage infiltration and progression of the tumor. Most tumors have large numbers of TAMs, whose presence frequently correlates with a worse prognosis. Thus, monocytes are attracted from the blood and into the tumor, where they mature into macrophages. Monocytes have the capacity to differentiate into several macrophage phenotypes, depending upon the conditions in the microenvironment. The classic proinflammatory macrophage (M1) is the primary macrophage in the acute inflammatory response and is responsible for removal and destruction of infectious agents. During healing, however, a different phenotype (M2) produces antiinflammatory mediators to suppress ongoing inflammation and induce cellular proliferation, angiogenesis, and wound healing.[33] TAMs appear to phenotypically mimic the M2 phenotype.

TAMs have diminished cytotoxic response, and develop the capacity to block T-cytotoxic cell and NK-cell functions and produce cytokines that are advantageous for tumor growth and spread. TAMs secrete cellular growth factors (e.g., TGF-β and fibroblast growth factor-2 [FGF-2]) that favor tumor cell proliferation, angiogenesis, and tissue remodeling, similar to their activities in wound healing. They also secrete angiogenesis factors (e.g., VEGF) that induce neovascularization and matrix metalloproteinases (MMPs) that degrade intercellular matrix. The overall effect is increased tumor growth, invasion of the blood vessels, increased oxygen to the tumor, and invasion through the degraded matrix into the local tissue.

Cancer-associated fibroblasts (CAFs) synthesize the extracellular matrix that surrounds and permeates the tumor.[34] Cytokines and growth factors stored in the matrix as well as growth factors, metalloproteases, proteoglycans, and other molecules secreted by CAFs contribute greatly to cancer progression, local spread, and metastasis.

Evading Immune Destruction

Many cancers express cell surface antigens that are not generally found on normal cells from the same tissue. Tumor-associated antigens include products of oncogenes, antigens from oncogenic viruses, oncofetal antigens (expressed in embryonic tissues and tumors), and altered glycoproteins and glycolipids.[35] Viral and tumor antigens are processed by the tumor cell and presented on the cell surface by MHC class I molecules and are targets of CD8+ T-cytotoxic cells (Tcyto) (see Chapter 7). NK cells recognize altered cell surface glycoproteins and glycolipids. Thus, cancer cells should be recognized as foreign and destroyed by the immune system. In the laboratory, T lymphocytes and NK cells recognize and kill cancer cells. This observation gave rise to two hypotheses—immune surveillance and immunotherapy. The immune surveillance hypothesis predicts that most developing malignancies are suppressed by an efficient immune response against tumor-associated antigens. The immunotherapy hypothesis predicts that the immune system could be used to target tumor-associated antigens and destroy tumors clinically. Immunotherapy could be either active, by immunization with tumor antigens to elicit or enhance the immune response against a particular cancer, or passive, by injecting the cancer patient with antibodies or lymphocytes directed against the tumor antigens. However, the interactions between cancer and the immune system are more complex than originally envisioned and both hypotheses remain controversial.

What is the role of the immune system in protecting against cancer? The most clearly documented effective immune response is prophylactic and directed against oncogenic viruses. Several viruses have been associated with human cancer; human papillomavirus (HPV), Epstein-Barr virus (EBV; also known as HHV4), Kaposi sarcoma herpesvirus (KSHV; also known as HHV8), and hepatitis B and C viruses (HBV, HCV) are associated with about 15% of all human cancers worldwide (see Table 10-3).[36] Cancer of the cervix and hepatocellular carcinoma account for approximately 80% of virus-linked cancer cases.

Virtually all cervical cancer is caused by infection with specific types of HPV, which infects basal skin cells and commonly causes warts. There are more than 120 HPV types, but only about 40 can infect human mucosal tissue, and only a few (HPV-16, -18, -31, and -45) are associated with the highest risk for developing cervical, anogenital, and penile cancer. Most HPV infection is handled effectively and rapidly by the immune system and does not cause cancer. Cancer is more common in people with prolonged infection with HPV (a decade or more), during which the viral DNA becomes integrated into the genomic DNA of the infected basal cell of the cervix and directs the persistent production of viral oncogenes. Early oncogenic HPV infection is readily detected by the Papanicolaou (Pap) test, an examination of cervical epithelial scrapings. Early detection of atypical cells in a Pap test alerts healthcare providers to the possibility of cervical carcinoma in situ, which can be effectively treated. The Pap test is probably the most effective cancer-screening test developed to date. For women age 30 to 65 years old, additional testing for HPV infection of cervical cells (HPV test) should be added.[37] Vaccines protecting against the common oncogenic HPV types (HPV-16 and HPV-18 [types that cause 70% of cervical cancers] and HPV-6 and HPV-11 [types that cause 90% of genital warts]) were approved for clinical use beginning in 2006; if these vaccines are administered to young women and men before an initial HPV infection, this is likely to prevent many cases of cervical cancer.

Chronic hepatitis B infections are common in parts of Asia and Sub-Saharan Africa and confer up to a 200-fold increased risk of developing liver cancer. Chronic hepatitis C infections have become increasingly recognized in Western countries. Up to 80% of liver cancer cases worldwide are associated with chronic hepatitis caused either by HBV or by HCV. The initial infection with hepatitis B or C is not associated with cancer; instead, it is acquisition of a chronic viral hepatitis that markedly increases cancer risk. In both cases, it appears that a lifetime of chronic liver inflammation predisposes to the development of hepatocellular carcinoma. Widespread use of the HBV vaccine is expected to significantly decrease the incidence of chronic hepatitis B and hence hepatocellular carcinoma. Unfortunately, a vaccine for HCV is not yet available.

For most other human tumor viruses, immunoprophylaxis is not yet available. EBV and HHV8 are members of the Herpesviridae family. More than 90% of adults have been infected with EBV, usually as children and without symptoms. EBV infection during adolescence may cause infectious mononucleosis. The virus infects B lymphocytes and stimulates their limited proliferation and usually becomes latent throughout the individual's life. If the individual is immunosuppressed because of HIV infection or because of drugs given for an organ transplant, persistent EBV infection can lead to the development of B-cell lymphomas. EBV infection also is associated with Burkitt lymphoma in areas of endemic malaria and with nasopharyngeal carcinoma, a cancer endemic in Chinese populations in Southeast Asia. HHV8 is linked to the development of Kaposi sarcoma, a cancer that was once seen primarily in older men but now occurs in a markedly more virulent form in immunosuppressed individuals, especially those with acquired immunodeficiency syndrome (AIDS). HHV8 also has been linked to several rare lymphomas. **Human T-cell lymphotropic virus type 1 (HTLV-1)** is an oncogenic retrovirus linked to the development of adult T-cell leukemia and lymphoma (ATLL). HTLV is transmitted vertically (that is, inherited by children from infected parents) and horizontally (e.g., by breast-feeding, sexual intercourse, blood transfusions, and exposure to infected needles). Infection with HTLV may be asymptomatic, and only a small fraction of infected individuals develop ATLL, often many years after acquiring the virus.

Thus immunization has proven beneficial in preventing viral-induced cancers. The immune surveillance hypothesis, however, would predict that components of the immune system, especially T cells, monitor the body and destroy most nascent tumors, even those not caused by viruses. If the immune surveillance hypothesis is correct, compromise of the immune system by immunosuppressive drugs or development of genetic or acquired immune deficiencies would result in increased incidences of all types of cancer.[38] However, defective immune responses generally only increase the risk for lymphoid cancers, many of which are associated with viral infections. For instance, individuals taking chronic powerful immunosuppressive drugs, such as those given for kidney, heart, or liver transplant, have a much higher risk of developing viral-associated cancers, with a 10-fold increased risk of non-Hodgkin lymphoma (caused by EBV) and up to a 1000-fold increased risk of Kaposi sarcoma (caused by HHV8). The same immunosuppressed individuals, however, have only a slight increase in the risk of common cancers such as lung and colon cancer (and this could well be because of increased inflammation at those sites), and no increase in the risk of breast or prostate cancer.

However, many tumors have an abundance of tumor-infiltrating lymphocytes (TILs). Although the immune cells frequently found in tumors were once thought to be futile attempts at an antitumor response, instead it appears that cancers actively recruit an immune and stromal response to assist in remodeling of tissues, formation of new blood vessels, and promotion of metastasis.[39] NK cells are generally in low amounts in tumors. The predominant TILs are T-regulatory (Treg) cells. Treg cells are CD4+ cells that differentiate under the control of specific cytokines, primarily TGF-β. The role of Treg cells during wound healing is to control or limit the immune response to protect the host's own tissues against autoimmune reactions. Their role in tumors is manipulated to prevent a destructive antitumor immune response and provide cytokines that facilitate tumor cell proliferation and spread. Treg cells and TAMs, as well as other stromal cells, produce very high levels of TGF-β and interleukin-10 (IL-10). IL-10 is an immunosuppressive cytokine, which generally decreases T-helper cell 1 (Th1) and Th2 activity, suppresses antigen recognition and cell proliferation by Th cells, and suppresses the capacity of CD8+ T-cytotoxic (Tcyto) cells to recognize, proliferate, and kill tumor cells.[40] The goal of current immunotherapy regimens is to reverse this relationship and facilitate T-cell–mediated cancer cell death (discussed later in this chapter).

The release of immunosuppressive factors into the tumor microenvironment also increases resistance of the tumor to chemotherapy and radiotherapy. Increased levels of Treg cells in blood and lymph nodes and infiltrating the tumor correlate with poor outcomes in breast and GI tumors. In advanced non–small cell lung cancer, an elevated ratio of Treg to Tcyto cells is related to a poor response to platinum-based chemotherapy. Immunosuppressive cytokines additionally lower the cancer cell's sensitivity to immune-mediated death (Figure 10-18). With increasing heterogeneity of cells within the tumor, subpopulations of antigen-negative cancer cell variants may selectively outgrow more immune-sensitive cells.[41] Variants may suppress the production of particular antigens or suppress levels of

antigen-presenting MHC class I. Other cytokines appear to increase the cancer cells' resistance to apoptosis. For example, the Th2 cytokine IL-4 increases the resistance of thyroid cancer to chemotherapy; IL-6 produced by Th cells, adipocytes, and fibroblasts activates survival pathways in breast cancer leading to resistance to radiotherapy; and adipocytes enhance the transcription of the anti-apoptotic factor Bcl-2 in leukemia cells.

Activating Invasion and Metastasis

Metastasis is the spread of cancer cells from the site of the original tumor to distant tissues and organs through the body. Metastasis is a defining characteristic of cancer and is the major cause of death from cancer. Cancer that has not metastasized can often be cured by a combination of surgery, chemotherapy, and radiation. These same therapies are frequently ineffective against cancer that has metastasized. For example, in appropriately treated women with localized low-stage breast cancer, the 5-year survival rate is often greater than 90%. Tragically, less than 30% of women with metastatic breast cancer are still alive 5 years after diagnosis. A growing body of basic and clinical research is defining the biologic principles of metastasis, with the hope that this improved understanding will lead to novel diagnostic approaches and better therapies to prevent and treat metastatic cancers.

How do cancer cells develop the ability to metastasize? Metastasis is a highly inefficient process. Cancer cells must surmount multiple physical and physiologic barriers in order to spread, survive, and proliferate in distant locations, and the destination must be receptive to the growth of the cancer. Changes in the tumor microenvironment initiate the metastatic process and may include stromal cell adaptation to increase tumor mass and intratumor hypoxia.[42] As this diversity increases within the changing tumor microenvironment, some cancer cells evolve with multiple new abilities that can facilitate metastasis. The model for transition to metastatic cancer cells is called epithelial-mesenchymal transition.[43]

Epithelial-mesenchymal transition (EMT) has been most extensively described for carcinomas, which originate from highly differentiated and polarized epithelial cells that form structured sheets stabilized by multiple adherences to neighboring cells and to a basement membrane (an extracellular meshwork of collagens and other connective tissue proteins) along the cell's basal surface. Although the degree of malignant transformation resulting in a primary carcinoma may be adequate for local expansion of the tumor, neoplastic cells usually retain some epithelial-like characteristics that prevent dissociation from the extracellular matrix and preclude successful metastasis to distal sites. A greater degree of cellular "dedifferentiation" is necessary to produce the phenotype that can separate from the primary tumor and flourish in a potentially hostile secondary site. This results from a programmed transition of the still partially epithelial-like carcinoma to a more undifferentiated mesenchymal-like phenotype (Figure 10-19). A similar process occurs with tumors of endothelial origin (endothelial-mesenchymal transition).

EMT is a process that occurs normally in embryonic development, as well as wound healing and tissue repair. Generally, cells that have transitioned into a mesenchymal-like phenotype have suppressed expression of adhesion molecules with a loss of polarity, increased migratory capacity, elevated resistance to apoptosis, and demonstrated the potential to redifferentiate into other cell types.[44] The transition to a mesenchymal-like phenotype is, in most cases, driven by cytokines and chemokines produced within the tumor microenvironment.[45] IL-8 is an effective driver of carcinoma cells into EMT.

Invasion, or local spread, is a prerequisite for metastasis. In its earliest stages local invasion may occur by direct tumor extension. Eventually, however, cells migrate away from the primary tumor and

FIGURE 10-18 Mechanisms by Which Tumor Cells Evade the Immune System. Tumors may evade the immune response by losing expression of antigens or major histocompatibility complex (MHC) molecules or by producing immunosuppressive cytokines or ligands for inhibitory receptors on T cells. (From Kumar V et al: *Robbins and Cotran pathologic basis of disease,* ed 9, Philadelphia, 2015, Saunders.)

The figure labels include:

ANTITUMOR IMMUNITY

Tumor cell — T cell specific for tumor antigen — Tumor antigen — MHC molecule — **T cell recognition of tumor antigen leading to T cell activation**

IMMUNE EVASION BY TUMORS

Failure to produce tumor antigen
Antigen-loss variant of tumor cell — **Lack of T cell recognition of tumor**

Mutations in MHC genes or genes needed for antigen processing
Class I MHC-deficient tumor cell — **Lack of T cell recognition of tumor**

Production of immunosuppressive proteins or expression of inhibitory cell surface proteins
Inhibitory ligand — Inhibitory receptor — Immunosuppressive cytokines — **Inhibition of T cell activation**

FIGURE 10-19 Epithelial-mesenchymal Transition and Metastasis. The microenvironment supports metastatic dissemination and colonization at secondary sites. Stromal cells (e.g., mesenchymal stem cells [MSC]) possibly facilitated by a relative decrease in oxygen levels in the tumor, contribute to the epithelial-to-mesenchymal transition (EMT) through which tumor cells develop a metastatic phenotype characterized by suppression of adhesion molecules and reduced adherence to adjacent cells and extracellular matrix, increased local invasion, and access to the blood and lymphatic circulations. One major mediator of this process is TGF-β, which is secreted by the tumor stroma. Intravascularization of tumor cells into the circulation is facilitated by protumorigenic TAMs, and CAFs tend to cluster at the leading edge of the invading cancer cells and secrete matrix metalloproteinases that promote digestion and remodeling of the surrounding ECM. Survival in the circulation is promoted by association with platelets and clotting factors that shield the cancer cells from cytotoxic immune cells (T-cytotoxic cells and NK cells) that also are suppressed by myeloid-derived suppressor cells (MDSC). Potential metastatic sites are prepared by induction of fibronectin, which provides a site for the influx of hematopoietic progenitor cells (HPC) that have receptors for VEGF. HPC appear essential for establishment of a metastatic site. At a metastatic site, cancer cells will adhere to local vascular endothelium, undergo extravascularization facilitated by the effects of ATP on the endothelium, and undergo mesenchymal-to-epithelial transition (MET). The premetastatic niche may have been prepared by molecular signaling from the cancer and initiation of a favorable microenvironment. *CAF,* Cancer-associated fibroblast; *ECM,* extracellular matrix; *NK,* natural killer cell; *PDGF,* platelet-derived growth factor; *TAM,* tumor-associated macrophage; *TGF-β,* tumor growth factor-beta; *Treg,* T-regulatory cell; *VEGF,* vascular endothelial cell growth factor. (Modified from Quail DF, Joyce JA: Microenvironmental regulation of tumor progression and metastasis, *Nat Med* 19[11]:1423-1437, 2013.)

invade the surrounding tissues (see Figure 10-19). Invasion is a multistep process within EMT that includes diminished cell-to-cell adhesion, digestion of the surrounding extracellular matrix, and increased motility of individual cancer cells. TGF-β induces changes in expression of E-cadherin (an integral component of tight junctions) and of β₄-integrin in mammary gland tumor cells. The loss of E-cadherin in particular allows cells to detach from extracellular matrix and migrate more readily.

Recruitment of TAMs and other cell types is critical for invasion. Cells are normally attached to the extracellular matrix (ECM). TAMs and other stromal cells secrete proteases and protease activators, such as the MMPs and plasminogen activators, which promote digestion of connective tissue capsules and other structural barriers. Degradation of the surrounding ECM creates pathways through which cells can move, while releasing bioactive peptides as digestion products that further stimulate tumor growth and mobility.

Normal cells, when separated from their ECM, undergo *anoikis,* a form of apoptosis. Tumor cells adapted to a hypoxic environment have already been selected for resistance to apoptosis, often by loss of normal cell death pathways. The process of EMT frequently increases resistance to apoptosis. For example, neuroblastomas with loss of the pro-apoptotic caspase 8 genes are able to avoid apoptosis after loss of integrins and are more able to metastasize than the same cells with normal levels of caspase 8. Accordingly, individuals whose neuroblastomas have low levels of caspase 8 have a poor prognosis (see Chapter 1).

To transition from local to distant metastasis, the cancer cells must also be able to invade local blood and lymphatic vessels, a task facilitated by stimulation of neoangiogenesis and lymphangiogenesis by factors such as VEGF. After release from the ECM and digestion of basement membranes, mobile cancer cells gain access to the circulation, perhaps facilitated by the leaky newly made vessels and attraction of the cells because of chemoattractants coming from these new vessels. Once in the circulation, metastatic cells must be able to withstand the physiologic stresses of travel in the blood and lymphatic circulation, including high shear rates and exposure to immune cells. One mechanism is for tumor cells to bind to blood platelets, giving them a protective coat of nonmalignant blood cells that both shields the tumor cells and creates a small tumor embolus, or cancer clot, that can promote cancer cell survival in distant locations (see Figure 10-19).

Cancer cells spread through vascular and lymphatic pathways. The **neovascularization** of a cancer offers malignant cells direct access into the venous blood and draining lymphatic vessels. The venous and lymphatic drainage networks associated with the primary tumor frequently determine the pattern of metastasis. Single cells, clumps, and even tumor fragments can disseminate by these routes. Anatomic patterns of lymphatic and venous blood flow help determine how colon cancers spread to the liver, liver cancers spread through the portal vein to the lungs, lung cancers spread through the systemic circulation to the brain, and breast cancer spreads through the lymphatics to axillary lymph nodes. Cancers often spread first to regional lymph nodes through the lymphatics and then to distant organs through the bloodstream.

There also is a major yet poorly understood selectivity of different cancers for different sites. Metastatic breast cancer often spreads through the bloodstream to bones but rarely to kidney or spleen, whereas lymphomas often spread to the spleen but uncommonly spread to bone. In a key study, different types of cancer cells were injected into the carotid artery of mice.[46] In spite of identical blood flow–mediated distribution of the cancer cells, each cell type produced cancers in very different parts of the brain. This tissue selectivity is likely caused by specific interactions between the cancer cells and specific receptors on the small blood vessels in different organs. Experimental metastasis studies in mice are beginning to reveal additional molecular reasons for this tissue specificity. Examples include interaction between α3β1 integrins binding to laminin-5 receptors in the lung, and the chemokine receptor CXCR4 on breast cancer cells promoting homing to lung tissues expressing the ligand CXCL12.[47]

A cancer's ability to establish a metastatic lesion in a new location requires that the cancer survive in the specific environment and be capable of forming complex and heterogeneous tumors. In some cases, these tumor-initiating cells are very rare. Human cancers transplanted into special immune-deficient mice will grow and can metastases. Experiments have been performed to determine how few cancer cells are capable of establishing a tumor; only 1 in 10,000 human colon cancer cells are able to re-form a complex and heterogeneous colon cancer in mice; however, in human melanomas 1 in 4 cells can initiate a complex tumor in the appropriate mouse model. Thus, the number of potentially metastatic cells may vary greatly with the particular cancer.

The degree of dedifferentiation may be variable, but most cells undergoing EMT acquire stem cell traits that facilitate initial growth in a new microenvironment.[48] The EMT is not a stable transition; after taking residence in the metastatic site, the tumor tends to regain some characteristics of the primary tumor, thus reverting to some extent to its epithelial origins. Because metastasis requires successful completion of each and every step, there may be many opportunities to interrupt this potentially lethal pathway.

However, metastasis does not universally result in proliferation at a new site. Some cancer cells survive at a new site but do not proliferate to form a clinically relevant metastatic site. These cancer cells appear to exist in a state of *dormancy*. Dormancy is cellular quiescence—a stable, nonproliferative state that is reversible. Cells may remain quiescent for years before initiating proliferation. About two thirds of breast cancer deaths occur after a 5-year disease-free interval. In other conditions, solitary tumor cells can be detected in the blood years after a complete clinical remission in individuals, and many people with detectable micrometastases will not develop clinically obvious metastases. Cancer cell dormancy may be extremely common, even without a history of clinical cancer. Studies of deceased individuals without any history of cancer suggest that most of us have dormant cancer cells that never adjusted to form a malignant tumor.[49]

The causes of dormancy and, more importantly, escape from dormancy and development of a malignant cancer are unknown. Dormancy may result from features of the cell or the environmental niche, or both. Individuals with clinical cancers may shed disseminated tumor cells very early from premetastatic lesions.[50] These early cells may have developed inadequately to a metastatic phenotype and thus cannot recruit cells into a supportive stroma or initiated angiogenesis. Another consideration is the niche itself. It is not clear whether a developing cancer secretes factors that enter the bloodstream and prepare potential metastatic niches.[51] If so, early disseminated cancer cells may encounter nonsupportive niches that foster dormancy. A clear understanding of dormancy is needed because existing cancer therapies do not address this condition (also see p. 871).

✔ **QUICK CHECK 10-4**
1. Why is the stroma important for cancer growth and invasion?
2. Identify cancers that are the result of chronic inflammation.
3. Why does inflammation fuel cancer development/invasion?
4. Identify common viruses that can cause cancer.
5. How do cancers protect themselves from cell death?
6. Why is angiogenesis important to cancer development?

CLINICAL MANIFESTATIONS OF CANCER

The clinical manifestations of cancer are numerous and depend on the localization and type of tumor, and some are apparent before actual diagnosis of a malignancy. Generally, the variety and intensity of symptoms will increase as the malignancy progresses.

Paraneoplastic Syndromes

Paraneoplastic syndromes are symptom complexes that are triggered by a cancer but are not caused by direct local effects of the tumor mass. They are most commonly caused by biologic substances released from the tumor (e.g., hormones, cytokines) or by an immune response triggered by the tumor. For example, a small fraction of carcinoid tumors release substances, including serotonin, into the bloodstream that cause flushing, diarrhea, wheezing, and rapid heartbeat. A number of cancers trigger an antibody response that attacks the nervous system, causing a variety of neurologic disorders that can precede other symptoms of cancer by months.

Although infrequent, paraneoplastic syndromes are significant because they may be the earliest symptom of an unknown cancer and, in affected individuals, can be serious, often irreversible, and sometimes life-threatening. Table 10-4 presents the classifications of paraneoplastic syndromes.

TABLE 10-4 Paraneoplastic Syndromes

Clinical Syndromes	Major Forms of Underlying Cancer	Causal Mechanism
Endocrinopathies		
Cushing syndrome	Small cell carcinoma of lung	ACTH or ACTH-like substance
	Pancreatic carcinoma	
	Neural tumors	
Syndrome of inappropriate antidiuretic hormone (SIAH) secretion	Small cell carcinoma of lung; intracranial neoplasms	Antidiuretic hormone or atrial natriuretic hormones
Hypercalcemia	Squamous cell carcinoma of lung	PTHRP, TGF-α, TNF, IL-1
	Breast carcinoma	
	Renal carcinoma	
	Adult T-cell leukemia/lymphoma	
	Ovarian carcinoma	
Hypoglycemia	Fibrosarcoma	Insulin or insulin-like substance
	Other mesenchymal sarcomas	
	Hepatocellular carcinoma	
Carcinoid syndrome	Bronchial adenoma (carcinoid)	Serotonin, bradykinin
	Pancreatic carcinoma	
	Gastric carcinoma	
Polycythemia	Renal carcinoma	Erythropoietin
	Cerebellar hemangioma	
	Hepatocellular carcinoma	
Nerve and Muscle Syndromes		
Myasthenia	Bronchogenic carcinoma	Immunologic
Disorders of central and peripheral nervous systems	Breast carcinoma	Unknown
Dermatologic Disorders		
Acanthosis nigricans	Gastric carcinoma	Immunologic; secretion of epidermal growth factor
	Lung carcinoma	
	Uterine carcinoma	
Dermatomyositis	Bronchogenic, breast carcinoma	Immunologic
Osseous, Articular, and Soft Tissue Changes		
Hypertrophic osteoarthropathy and clubbing of fingers	Bronchogenic carcinoma	Unknown
Vascular and Hematologic Changes		
Venous thrombosis (Trousseau phenomenon)	Pancreatic carcinoma	Tumor products (mucins that activate clotting)
	Bronchogenic carcinoma	
	Other cancers	
Nonbacterial thrombotic endocarditis	Advanced cancers	Hypercoagulability
Anemia	Thymic neoplasms	Unknown
Others		
Nephrotic syndrome	Various cancers	Tumor antigens, immune complexes

From Kumar V et al: *Pathologic basis of disease,* ed 7, Philadelphia, 2005, Saunders.
ACTH, Adrenocorticotropic hormone; *IL,* interleukin; *PTHRP,* parathyroid hormone–related protein; *TGF,* transforming growth factor; *TNF,* tumor necrosis factor.

Pain

Pain is one of the most feared complications of advanced cancer. Although pain can be one of the presenting symptoms of cancer, most commonly there is little or no pain during the early stages of malignant disease. Significant pain, however, occurs in a large fraction of those individuals who are terminally ill with cancer. Pain is strongly influenced by fear, anxiety, sleep loss, fatigue, and overall physical deterioration. It occurs through an interaction among physiologic, cultural, and psychologic components. (The neurophysiology of pain is discussed in Chapter 14.)

Cancer-associated pain can arise from a variety of direct and indirect mechanisms. Direct pressure, obstruction, invasion of a sensitive structure, stretching of visceral surfaces, tissue destruction, infection, and inflammation all can cause pain. Pain can occur at the site of the primary tumor or can result from a distant metastatic lesion. Furthermore, pain may be referred away from the involved site and manifest, for example, as back pain.

Specific sites are more prone to cancer-associated pain. Bone metastases, common in advanced breast and prostate cancer, can cause significant pain because of periosteal irritation, medullary pressure, vertebral collapse, and pathologic fractures. Brain tumors (primary or metastatic) can, depending on the location, cause headache, seizures, or neurologic deficits. Pain in the abdomen may be caused by bowel obstruction, or inflammation and infection. Hepatic malignancies can stretch the liver, resulting in a dull pain or a feeling of fullness over the right upper abdominal quadrant. Mucosal surfaces can develop painful ulcerative lesions from the cancer, chemotherapy, and radiation or leukopenia (or both).

The diagnosis and treatment of pain is one of the primary responsibilities of the medical team. The individual's perception and, hence, reporting of pain can vary widely and be affected by such factors as age and cultural background. The first priority of treatment is to control pain rapidly and completely as judged by the individual. The second priority is to prevent recurrence of pain. Objective measurements of pain are increasingly being included along with the reporting of more traditional vital signs. Many institutions are using specialized pain management teams that are trained to recognize different types of acute and chronic pain, as well as the individual's response to that pain. Many modalities are available to treat pain, ranging from combinations of nonsteroidal anti-inflammatory drugs (NSAIDs) and narcotics to palliative surgery and radiation therapy. Individual-controlled analgesia provides many benefits, not the least of which is regaining some control over one's own body. Although cancer pain is a complex problem arising from multiple sources, individuals should be assured that suffering is not inevitable and that relief is attainable.

Fatigue

Fatigue is the most frequently reported symptom of cancer and cancer treatment. The exact mechanisms that produce fatigue are poorly understood. Suggested causes include sleep disturbances, various biochemical changes secondary to disease and treatment, numerous psychosocial factors, and environmental and physical factors.

The physiologic understanding of fatigue probably includes mechanisms for decreased muscle contractility. Overall, studies of muscle function suggest that some individuals with cancer may lose portions of muscle function needed to perform normal physical activities. Other areas of research include muscle function consequences from metabolic products of cancer treatment and associated muscle loss from circulating cytokines (e.g., tumor necrosis factor [TNF] and interleukin-1 [IL-1]). Similar to pain, fatigue is a subjective clinical manifestation. Individuals with cancer describe fatigue in many ways (e.g., weakness, lack of energy, depression). Some of these symptoms

have been termed "chemo brain," or mild cognitive impairment. The changes in cognitive function can be caused by the cancer itself or by the stress associated with the diagnosis of cancer, because symptoms similar to "chemo brain" also occur in individuals who have not received chemotherapy.

Cachexia

The multiorgan syndrome of cachexia includes a constellation of clinical manifestations, including anorexia; wasting, thermogenesis; altered heart and liver function; gut malabsorption; early satiety (filling); taste alterations; and altered protein, lipid, and carbohydrate metabolism (Figure 10-20).

Although several definitions of cachexia exist two factors are significant: weight loss and inflammation. Severe weight loss is primarily from loss of skeletal muscle and body fat.[52] The wasting that occurs in muscle may be dependent on alterations in other organs or tissues including white adipose tissue.[52] Important is that cachexia is multifactorial, involving changes in many metabolic pathways. The cachectic syndrome involves abnormalities in heart function, alterations in liver protein synthesis, changes in hypothalamic mediators, and activation of brown adipose tissue and gastrointestinal function.[52] All of these changes result in a major decrease in quality of life and indirectly result in death in some individuals. The incidence of the syndrome among individuals with cancer is very high and varies by tumor type.[52]

Molecular Basis of Cachexia

Cachexia has been discussed as a type of energy balance disorder where energy intake is decreased and energy expenditure is increased.[52] Energy intake and expenditure depends on the tumor type and its growth phase. Because individuals who are being administered total parenteral nutrition still lose weight, increased resting energy expenditure may be the cause of the wasting syndrome.[52] Investigators are studying the role of both mitochondria and sarcoplasmic reticulum (SR) in muscle function and its relationship to cachexia. Hypotheses related to these functions include increased production of peroxisome-proliferator–activated receptor-γ co-activator-1α (PGC1α), which can activate a mitochondrial protein (mitofusin-2 [MFN2]) that interacts with muscle SR and controls interorganelle calcium (Ca^{2+}) signaling. Therefore, one hypothesis is the overexpression of PGC1α can activate MFN2 expression, leading to Ca^{2+} deregulation, which is closely associated with muscle wasting.[52] Muscle weakness and fatigue is related to loss of myofibrillar proteins in muscle cells. Abnormalities in protein and amino acid metabolism are noted in cachetic muscle (Figure 10-21).

Contributing further to muscle wasting is an increase in apoptosis and an impaired capacity for regeneration.[52] Many signaling pathways are involved in protein turnover leading to the wasting process and are activated by inflammatory mediators including cytokines, myostatin, and tumor-derived factors. In addition to muscle wasting, miRNAs may be involved in stimulating the breakdown of adipose tissue.[53,54] In cancer cachexia, skeletal muscle loss includes major loss of *white adipose tissue (WAT)*. The WAT loss is thought to be caused by (1) increased lipolysis, (2) decreased activity of lipoprotein lipase (LPL), and (3) decreased new or de novo lipogenesis in adipose tissue.[52] New data show that WAT cells undergo a "browning" process during cancer cachexia where they change to beige cells called BAT-like cells.[55,56] Browning is associated with increased thermogenesis. Tumor-derived compounds, such as IL-6 (which also may be released by immune cells) and parathyroid-hormone–related protein (PTHRP), may be the drivers of thermogenesis.[55]

An unusual and frustrating component of cancer care is the person's early satiety, or a sense of being full after only a few mouthfuls

FIGURE 10-20 Cachexia: A Multiorgan Syndrome. Loss of skeletal muscle and adipose tissue are major contributors to cachexia. But many other organs have a role in the cachexia syndrome and the wasting that takes place in muscle may be dependent on alterations in these other organs or tissues. Changes in hypothalamic function and activation of brown adipose tissue, as well as alterations in liver and heart function, also are involved in the syndrome. Recent studies support a role for gut microbiota in cancer cachexia and the possibility of a gut-microbiota-skeletal muscle relationship. Recent data suggest that the conversion of white adipose tissue to brown adipose tissue is triggered by both humoral inflammatory mediators, such as interleukin-6 (IL-6), and tumor derived compounds, such as parathyroid-hormone–related protein (PTHRP). (From Bindels LB, Delzenne NM: Muscle wasting: the gut microbiota as a new therapeutic target? *Int J Biochem Cell Biol* 45:2186-2190, 2013; Bindels LB et al: Restoring specific lactobacilli levels decreases inflammation and muscle atrophy markers in an acute leukemia mouse model, *PLoS One* 7[6]:e37971, 2012.)

of food. Brain mediators are involved in the regulation of food intake and include appetite, satiation, taste, and smell of food. Therefore, the brain is an important organ in anorexia and consequently altered energy balance. Profoundly altered are both *orexigenic* (appetite-stimulating) and *anorexigenic* (appetite-suppressing) brain pathways.[57] (Cytokines are discussed in detail in Chapters 6 and 7.)

Anemia

Anemia is commonly associated with malignancy; 20% of persons diagnosed with cancer have hemoglobin concentrations less than 9 g/dl (normal value = 15 g/dl). Mechanisms that cause anemia include chronic bleeding (resulting in iron deficiency), severe malnutrition, cytotoxic chemotherapy, and malignancy in blood-forming organs. Chronic bleeding and iron deficiency can accompany colorectal or genitourinary malignancy. Iron also is malabsorbed in persons with gastric, pancreatic, or upper intestinal cancer. Often there is a defect in the reutilization of iron because of lack of transfer of iron from the storage pool to blood cell precursors. This defect may be caused by increased secretion of IL-6 and hepcidin (a hormone secreted by the

liver that regulates the body's iron distribution) (see Chapter 20). Defects in erythropoietin production and shortened duration of red cell survival also have been documented. In addition, anorexia can cause both iron and folate deficiency. Megaloblastic (large red cell) anemias also may develop after methotrexate treatment.

Administration of erythropoietin, which stimulates production of erythrocytes, has been effective in correcting anemia in persons with cancer; fewer red blood cell transfusions were required in most of the studied subjects. In addition, anemias occurring after chemotherapy or radiotherapy have been treated successfully with erythropoietin. However, recent studies have shown that aggressive use of erythropoietin increases the risk of blood clots and can decrease cancer survival.

Leukopenia and Thrombocytopenia

Direct tumor invasion of the bone marrow causes both leukopenia (a decreased total white blood cell count) and thrombocytopenia (a decreased number of platelets). More commonly, many chemotherapeutic drugs, which primarily affect rapidly dividing cells, are toxic to

TABLE 10-5 Factors Predisposing Individuals with Cancer to Infection

Factor	Basis
Age	Many common malignancies occur mostly in older age. Immunologic functions decline with age. General debility reduces immunocompetence. Immobility predisposes to infection. Far-advanced cancer often results in immobility and general debility that worsen with age. Elderly persons are predisposed to nutritional inadequacies. Malnutrition impairs immunocompetence.
Tumor	Nutritional derangements can result. Sites and circumstances favorable to growth of microorganisms (obstruction, serous or blood effusion, ulceration) can be created. Far-advanced disease predisposes individuals to debility and immobility. Humoral or cellular immune defects may result. Metastasis to bone marrow may cause leukopenia or other defects in immunity.
Leukemias	Inadequate granulocyte production (impaired phagocytosis) results. Thrombocytopenia (bleeding) can occur. Late effect: chronic lung disease from *Pneumocystis carinii* pneumonia can develop during therapy.
Lymphomas and other mononuclear phagocyte malignancies	Humoral and cellular immune defects (anergy, altered immunoglobulin production) result. Late effect: splenectomy in children can cause increased susceptibility to infection.
Surgical treatment	Invasive procedure interrupts first lines of defense. Radical nature of surgery (removal of large blocks of tissue in lengthy procedures) causes hemorrhage, decreased tissue perfusion, creation of dead spaces, devitalization of tissues. Procedure may be "dirty" surgery (bowel, infected or contaminated areas). Surgery patients are often older and at poor risk. Long preoperative hospitalization often precedes surgery. Patients may have received previous adrenocorticosteroid therapy. Patients may have infections at sites remote from operative area. Nutritional derangements (especially important in head and neck surgery) may result. Lymph node dissection may predispose patient to local infection and impair containment to area. Gynecologic surgery may result in fistulae. Lung surgery may cause bronchopleural fistulae. Debility and immobility may result.

Data from Donovan MI, Girton SF: *Cancer care nursing,* ed 2, New York, 1984, Appleton-Century-Crofts; Murphy GP et al: *Clinical oncology,* ed 2, New York, 1994, American Cancer Society.

FIGURE 10-21 Wasting of Skeletal Muscle. Inflammation plays a major role in muscle wasting and is linked to alterations in protein and amino acid metabolism, activation of muscle cell apoptosis, and decreased regeneration. (Adapted from Argilés JM et al: Cancer cachexia: understanding the molecular basis, *Nat Rev Cancer* 14[11]:754-762, 2014.)

the bone marrow, often causing granulocytopenia and thrombocytopenia. Granulocytopenia also can result from radiation therapy if it encompasses significant areas of the bone marrow. The duration of granulocytopenia and hence the risk of serious infection can be lessened by treatment with recombinant human granulocyte colony–stimulating factor (rhG-CSF, filgrastim). rhG-CSF stimulates white blood cell precursors in the marrow to proliferate and differentiate rapidly. Thrombocytopenia is a major cause of hemorrhage in persons with cancer and is often treated with platelet transfusions. Thrombocytopenia also is an accompanying disorder of disseminated intravascular coagulation that occurs in persons with acute promyelocytic leukemia (see Chapter 21) and severe infections.

Infection

Infection is the most significant cause of complications and death in persons with malignant disease. Advanced malignancies are highly immunosuppressive, as well as the radiotherapy and chemotherapy used to treat it. (Factors that predispose persons with cancer to infection are summarized in Table 10-5.) When the absolute granulocyte count falls below 500 cells per microliter, the risk of serious microbial (bacterial and fungal) infection increases. Surgery also can lower resistance to infection because removal of large quantities of tissue, together with hemorrhage, dead spaces, and poor tissue perfusion, can create favorable sites for infection. Hospital-related (nosocomial) infections increase because of indwelling medical devices, inadequate wound care, and the introduction of microorganisms from visitors and other individuals.

Gastrointestinal Tract

The entire gastrointestinal (GI) tract relies on rapidly growing cells to produce an effective barrier to trauma and infection and to provide an absorptive surface for nutrients. Both chemotherapy and radiation therapy may cause a decreased cell turnover, thereby leading to oral ulcers (stomatitis), malabsorption, and diarrhea. The disruption of barrier defenses also increases the risk for infection, especially invasion by a person's own GI microbiome.

Therapy-induced nausea, thought to be caused by an agent's direct action upon the central nervous system's vomiting centers, historically has been a major obstacle for continuing therapy. Aggressive antinausea (antiemetic) therapy, including the centrally acting serotonin 5-hydroxytryptamine (5-HT3) antagonists (such as ondansetron or dolasetron), has allowed better tolerance of highly emetogenic protocols. Other popular antiemetics include steroids and phenothiazines. Synthetic cannabinoids, the active ingredients in marijuana, increase appetite in addition to having antinausea properties. Analgesia often includes opiate agents, vital in treating severe cases of mucosal lesions. Supplemental nutrition through enteral or parenteral routes may be needed to combat malnutrition. Good oral hygiene may help prevent complications arising from mucosal membrane breakdown.

Hair and Skin

Alopecia (hair loss) results from chemotherapy effects on hair follicles. Alopecia is usually temporary, although hair may regrow with a different texture initially. Not all chemotherapeutic agents cause alopecia. Decreased renewal rates of the epidermal layers in the skin may lead to skin breakdown and dryness, altering the normal barrier protection against infection. Radiation therapy may cause skin erythema (redness) and contribute to breakdown.

DIAGNOSIS, CHARACTERIZATION, AND TREATMENT OF CANCER

The diagnosis of cancer has a profound effect on individuals and their families. Responses range from depression to resigned fatalism to an aggressive no-holds-barred pursuit of therapy. The choice of therapy should be based on full consideration by the individual, the family, and the medical team of the individual's diagnosis, prognosis, and therapeutic options. Many types of cancer can be effectively treated with chemotherapy, radiotherapy, surgery, and combinations of these modalities. Caregivers must recognize that many individuals seek additional non–science-based explanations and therapies and often use these therapies, either concurrently or sequentially.

Diagnosis and Staging
Histologic Staging

Cancer can be discovered in many ways: after screening tests, from routine exams, and after investigation of symptoms. The symptoms a cancer produces are as diverse as the types of cancer. The location of the cancer can determine symptoms by physical pressure, obstruction, and loss of normal function, or a cancer can cause problems far away from its source by pressing on nerves or secreting bioactive compounds. Whatever the initial complaint, once the diagnosis is suspected and a tumor has been identified, it is essential that tumor tissue be obtained to establish a definitive diagnosis and correctly classify the disease. Various methods of obtaining tissue are described in Table 10-6.

Once tissue is obtained, it is examined microscopically by the pathologist for the histologic hallmarks of cancer detailed in the beginning of this chapter. The classification of the cancer can be further facilitated by a variety of clinically available tests, including immunohistochemical stains, flow cytometry, electron microscopy, chromosome analysis, and genetic studies.

If the diagnosis of cancer is established, it is critical to determine if the cancer has spread, known as the stage of the cancer. Staging initially involves determining the size of the tumor, the degree to which it has locally invaded, and the extent to which it has spread

TABLE 10-6	Obtaining Tissue—The Biopsy	
Procedure	**Purpose**	**Example**
Excisional biopsy	Complete removal, usually with margin of normal tissue	Full resection (e.g., mastectomy, partial colectomy)
Incisional biopsy	Removal of portion of lesion	Lymph node biopsy, muscle mass biopsy
Core needle biopsy	Often performed with direct vision, or guided with ultrasound or CT	Needle biopsy of prostate or liver mass
Fine needle aspirate	Obtains dissociated cells for cytologic study but does not preserve tissue structure	Thyroid, breast mass
Exfoliative cytology	Cells shed from surface (e.g., from cervix, sputum [lung], or urine)	Brushings from lung or colon endoscopy

(metastasized) (Figure 10-22). Specific molecular tests are increasingly used in staging as well. Diverse schemes are used for staging different tumors. In general, a four-stage system is used, with carcinoma in situ regarded as a special case. Cancer confined to the organ of origin is stage 1; cancer that is locally invasive is stage 2; cancer that has spread to regional structures, such as lymph nodes, is stage 3; and cancer that has spread to distant sites, such as a liver cancer spreading to lung or a prostate cancer spreading to bone, is stage 4. One common scheme for standardizing staging is the World Health Organization's TNM system: *T* indicates tumor spread, *N* indicates node involvement, and *M* indicates the presence of distant metastasis (see Figure 10-22). The prognosis generally worsens with increasing tumor size, lymph node involvement, and metastasis. Staging also may alter the choice of therapy, with more aggressive therapy being delivered to more invasive disease.

Tumor Markers

During surveillance or diagnosis of cancer as well as following therapy, specific biochemical markers of tumors have proven to be helpful. These tumor markers are substances produced by both benign and malignant cells that are either present in or on tumor cells or found in blood, spinal fluid, or urine. Some tumor markers have been known for many decades. Tumor markers include hormones, enzymes, genes, antigens, and antibodies (Table 10-7). If the tumor marker itself has biologic activity, then it can cause symptoms, such as those described in Table 10-7. For example, the adrenal medulla normally secretes the catecholamine epinephrine (adrenaline). Benign tumors of the adrenal medulla (pheochromocytoma) can produce catecholamines (e.g., adrenaline) in vast excess, leading to rapid pulse rate, high blood pressure, diaphoresis (i.e., sweating), and tremors. Detection of elevated blood or urine levels of catecholamines helps to confirm the diagnosis, and treatment of the disease relieves the symptoms. Tumor markers can be used in three ways: (1) to screen and identify individuals at high risk for cancer; (2) to help diagnose the specific type of tumor in individuals with clinical manifestations relating to their tumor, as in adrenal tumors or enlarged liver or prostate; and (3) to follow the clinical course of a tumor.

To date, no tumor marker has proven satisfactory to screen populations of healthy individuals for cancer.[58] Testing large populations will always detect a few normal individuals with test results at the high end of the normal distribution (the "false positives"), which can lead to

T = Primary tumor; the number equals size of tumor and its local extent. The number can vary according to site.
T0 = Breast free of tumor
T1 = Lesion <2 cm in size
T2 = Lesion 2-5 cm
T3 = Skin and/or chest wall involved by invasion

N = Lymph node involvement; a higher number means more nodes are involved.
N0 = No axillary nodes involved
N1 = Mobile nodes involved
N2 = Fixed nodes involved

M = Extent of distant metastases
M0 = No metastases
M1 = Demonstrable metastases
M2 = Suspected metastases

FIGURE 10-22 Tumor Staging by the TNM System. Example of staging for breast cancer. (See figure for explanation of the abbreviations.)

TABLE 10-7 Examples of Tumor Markers

Marker Name	Nature	Type of Tumor
Adrenocorticotropic hormone (ACTH)	Peptide hormone	Pituitary adenomas
Alpha fetoprotein (AFP)	70-kDa protein	Hepatic, germ cell
Beta-human chorionic gonadotropin (β-HCG)	Glycopeptide hormone	Germ cell
CA15-3/CA27.29	Protein antigen	Breast
CA-125	Glycoprotein antigen	Ovary
Carcinoembryonic antigen (CEA)	200-kDa glycoprotein	GI, pancreas, lung, breast, etc.
Catecholamines	Epinephrine and precursors	Pheochromocytoma (adrenal medulla)
Estrogen receptor (ER)/ progesterone receptor (PR)	Extracted receptor	Breast
Homovanillic acid/ vanillylmandelic acid (HVA/VMA)	Catecholamine metabolites	Neuroblastoma
Prostate-specific antigen (PSA)	33-kDa glycoprotein	Prostate
Urinary Bence Jones protein	Ig light chain	Multiple myeloma

GI, Gastrointestinal; *Ig,* immunoglobulin; *kDa,* kilodalton(s).

expensive and invasive additional tests, and unnecessary concern. Similarly, some individuals with disease will have test results in the normal range ("false negatives"). More importantly, some nonmalignant conditions also can produce tumor markers. The presence of an elevated tumor marker therefore may suggest a specific diagnosis, but it is not used alone as a definitive diagnostic test. For instance, prostate tumors secrete *prostate specific antigen (PSA)* into the blood. But, enthusiasm has waned for routine testing for PSA levels. Most men

BOX 10-1 Types of Genetic Lesions in Cancer

1. Point mutations
2. Subtle alterations (insertions, deletions)
3. Chromosome changes (aneuploidy and loss of heterozygosity)
4. Amplifications
5. Gene silencing (DNA methylation, histone modification, microRNAs)
6. Exogenous sequences (tumor viruses)

(approximately 75%) with elevated levels of PSA do not have cancer upon biopsy.[59] A taskforce to study the use of PSA detection concluded that for every 1000 men (ages 55 to 69) screened repeatedly, only zero to 1 prostate cancer–related death would be avoided, 100 to 120 men would undergo unnecessary biopsies with some complications, and 110 men would be diagnosed with prostate cancer (frequently slow growing and not life-threatening) and 50 of these would have major complications related to treatment.[60] However, falling levels of PSA after radiation or surgical therapy may indicate successful treatment for prostate cancer, and a later rise may indicate a recurrence. Identification of ideal sensitive and specific tumor markers that are elevated early in the course of common cancers remains a high priority because the early detection of cancer often improves the treatment outcome.

Classification of Tumors—Classic Histology and Modern Genetics

Because our knowledge about the cellular and molecular alterations in individual cancers can influence the choices of therapy, it becomes increasingly important for clinicians to accurately classify each cancer (Box 10-1). The classification, and hence the treatment decisions, of cancers was originally based on gross and light microscopic appearance and is now commonly accompanied by immunohistochemical analysis of protein expression. Increasingly, this is supplemented by a more extensive genetic analysis of the tumors. The range of genetic analysis is expanding rapidly. A single gene may be examined (for example, to determine if there is a characteristic chromosomal translocation diagnostic of chronic myelogenous leukemia [CML]), or a panel of genes and proteins may be examined (e.g., in breast cancer) to determine if the tumor expresses estrogen receptor, progesterone receptor, and the epidermal growth factor (EGF) receptor HER2, or if there are mutations in specific genes that modify response to therapy. In a research setting and increasingly in clinical settings, global gene expression and mutation analysis can be measured using polymerase chain reaction (PCR), microarray, or advanced DNA sequencing technology. These analyses can be used to classify tumors more precisely and may predict the most effective therapy. This detailed analysis of each tumor is a form of personalized medicine that offers therapy based on a very detailed knowledge of the characteristics of each individual's specific cancer.[61] This enhanced molecular characterization subdivides cancers into therapeutically and prognostically relevant smaller groups. As an example, breast cancers can now be subclassified into over four types (luminal A, luminal B, basal-like, and others) based on their expression of specific markers, such as estrogen receptor, HER2/Neu, and other specific genes and proteins. Each subtype has a different response to therapy and a different prognosis.

Treatment

Until late in the last century the mainstays of cancer therapy have been surgery, chemotherapy, and radiation therapy. These approaches have been highly successful for certain types of cancer, but have many limitations. Immunotherapy has been the Holy Grail of cancer therapists, but successes have been few. Cancer therapy is now in a process of rapid evolution. Armed with a more clear understanding that cancer is in fact multiple diseases that share general hallmarks/enablers and that the specific mechanisms underlying each hallmark may vary considerably among cancers (e.g., the large variety of oncogenes that may be used to differentiate cancers), modern cancer therapy is reaching a stage where complete genetic analysis of an individual cancer may determine the appropriate combination of therapies. Thus, effective therapy may include a combination of reagents targeting several hallmarks and under constant modification to target the evolving cancer cells.

Surgery

Surgery plays many roles in the care of individuals with cancer. The multiple approaches to obtaining tissue for diagnosis have been discussed. Surgery is often the definitive treatment of cancers that do not spread beyond the limits of surgical excision. It also is indicated for the relief of symptoms, for instance, those caused by tumor mass obstruction. In selected high-risk diseases, surgery plays a role in the prevention of cancer. For example, individuals with familial adenomatous polyposis because of germline mutations of the *APC* gene have close to a 100% lifetime risk of colon cancer, so a prophylactic colectomy is indicated. Similarly, women with *BRCA1/2* mutations have a markedly increased risk of breast and ovarian cancer, and often choose prophylactic mastectomy or bilateral salpingo-oophorectomy (removal of ovaries and fallopian tubes), or both.

Key principles apply specifically to cancer surgery, including obtaining adequate surgical margins during a resection to prevent local recurrences, placing needle tracks and biopsy incision scars (that may be contaminated with cancer cells) carefully so they can be removed in subsequent incisions, avoiding the spread of cancer cells during surgical procedures through careful technique, and paying attention to obtaining adequate tissue specimens during biopsies so that the

pathologist can be confident of the diagnosis. Additionally, the surgeon provides critical staging information by inspection, sampling, and removal of local and region lymph nodes during procedures.

Radiation Therapy

Radiation therapy is used to kill cancer cells while minimizing damage to normal structures. Ionizing radiation damages cells by imparting enough energy to cause molecular damage, especially to DNA. The damage may be lethal, in which the cell is killed by radiation; potentially lethal, in which the cell is so severely affected by radiation that modifications in its environment will cause it to die; or sublethal, in which the cell can subsequently repair itself. Cellular compartments with rapidly renewing cells are, in general, more radiosensitive. Effective cell killing by radiation also requires good local delivery of oxygen, something not always present in large cancers. Radiation produces slow changes in most cancers and irreversible changes in normal tissues as well. Because of these irreversible changes, each tissue has a maximum lifetime dose of radiation it can tolerate. Radiation is well suited to treat localized disease in areas that are hard to reach surgically, for example, in the brain and pelvis. A number of radiation delivery methods are available, with external beam being the most common. Radiation sources, such as small ^{125}I-labeled capsules (also called seeds), can also be temporarily placed into body cavities, a delivery method termed brachytherapy. Brachytherapy is useful in the treatment of cervical, prostate, and head and neck cancers.

Chemotherapy

The era of modern chemotherapy began with the observation in World War II that mustard gas exposure caused suppression of the bone marrow. Related compounds, such as nitrogen mustard and cyclophosphamide, were then tested and produced clinical responses in hematologic malignancies, including lymphomas. Also in the late 1940s, based on the remarkable clinical observation that the vitamin folic acid could *increase* leukemia growth, antifolate drugs were developed (leading ultimately to methotrexate) that produced remissions in previously untreatable leukemia.

All chemotherapeutic agents take advantage of specific vulnerabilities in target cancer cells. Antimetabolites, such as methotrexate and L-asparaginase, block normal growth pathways in all cells, but leukemia and other cancer cells are exquisitely sensitive to folic acid and asparagine deprivation, whereas nonmalignant cells are far less sensitive. Similarly, some cancer cells are highly sensitive to DNA-damaging agents, such as cyclophosphamide and anthracyclines, because of the oncogenic mutations that accelerate the cell cycle and DNA synthesis. Cellular checkpoints prevent normal cells treated with microtubule-directed drugs, such as vincristine and the taxanes, from undergoing mitosis, whereas cancer cells treated with these agents lack normal checkpoints, continue through mitosis, and undergo mitotic catastrophe (see Chapter 1).

Single chemotherapeutic agents often shrink cancers, but these drugs given alone rarely, if ever, provide a cure. Hence, chemotherapy drugs are usually given in combinations designed to attack a cancer from many different weaknesses at the same time and to limit the dose and therefore the toxicity of any single agent. Cancers contain a very large number of cells, and commonly a small fraction of those cells may be resistant to a particular drug. However, those cells are likely to be sensitive to the second or third drug in a chemotherapy cocktail. Scheduling of drug administration is also very important, with many studies showing cancers are more likely to develop drug resistance if there are significant delays between planned courses of chemotherapy.

Chemotherapy can be used for several distinct purposes. Induction chemotherapy seeks to cause shrinkage or disappearance of tumors.

In Hodgkin disease, for example, chemotherapy alone can be used in some cases to cure the disease. In other settings, chemotherapy may shrink the tumor and improve symptoms without ultimately providing a cure. Adjuvant chemotherapy is given after surgical excision of a cancer with the goal of eliminating micrometastases. Neoadjuvant chemotherapy is given before localized (surgical or radiation) treatment of a cancer. As with induction chemotherapy, the effectiveness, or lack thereof, of neoadjuvant therapy can be measured (for example, with follow-up scans). Neoadjuvant therapy can shrink a cancer so that surgery may spare more normal tissue. For example, in the bone cancer osteogenic sarcoma, neoadjuvant therapy often converts a large tumor mass into a much smaller mass, allowing the surgeon to perform a limb-sparing excision rather than an amputation.

Immunotherapy

The expression of unique antigens on cancer cells that can be targeted by T cells has driven the quest for effective therapies to initiate an immune response, boost a currently inadequate immune response, or convert a tumor-protective immune response to a destructive one. Since the 1950s this quest has been characterized by promises and frustrations.

Vaccines have been extremely effective in protecting us against infective agents. Although they generally induce a prophylactic immune response, at least one vaccine (against rabies) is administered after the infection. Vaccines against oncogenic viruses provide protection and prevent the onset of viral-induced tumors. For approximately 50 years, numerous potential therapeutic vaccines have been tested with little success. Initially, whole tumor cell vaccines prepared from an individual's own cancer (autologous) or from cancers from other individuals (allogeneic) were used, with or without adjuvants that induced inflammatory responses (e.g., BCG) or augmented the vaccine's immunogenicity. Several allogeneic cancer cell vaccines continue to be tested. So far, none has been shown to be effective enough to be licensed. Other approaches included immunization with the following:

- Protein extracts from cancers
- Peptides that represented the epitope from these proteins
- Dendritic cells that have processed and present cancer antigens
- DNA containing the genetic sequence for cancer antigens that transfects the recipient's cells and expresses that antigen
- Viral vectors that contain the genetic information for cancer antigens[62]

Several trials are underway, and one approach has been approved by the FDA. Sipuleucel-T (Provenge®) has been approved for the treatment of metastatic prostate cancer that is resistant to conventional therapy. Dendritic cells are obtained from an individual with prostate cancer and incubated with a protein resulting from the fusion of prostatic acid phosphatase, a cancer antigen found in 95% of prostate cancers, and granulocyte-macrophage colony–stimulating factor (GM-CSF), an immune cell stimulating cytokine. The dendritic cells process and present the antigen and are infused back into the patient. In clinical trials treatment with sipuleucel-T extended the lives of patients by 4.1 months. These results may not seem spectacular, but were meaningful in this group of patients with very advanced and terminal disease. Other vaccine approaches against B-cell lymphoma and melanoma have shown promising results.[63]

Passive immunotherapy using lymphocytes against cancer cell antigens has been attempted, with limited success, since the early 1970s. In recent years, passive administration of tumor-targeting lymphocytes (adoptive cell therapy, ACT) has developed more promise as a result of various pretreatment ex vivo techniques that improve treatment efficacy. A major source of patient's lymphocytes is those that have infiltrated the tumor (tumor-infiltrating lymphocytes, TIL).[64] The efficacy of these cells is increased by depleting the Treg cells within the population or by engineering the T-cell receptor for greater specificity against the tumor.[65]

A family of monoclonal antibodies, called checkpoint inhibitors, is under investigation. These antibodies are directed against co-stimulatory molecules involved in repressing T-cell immune responses (see Chapter 7). By blocking inhibitory signals, T-cytotoxic cells may retain tumor-killing capacity.

Targeted Disruption of Cancer

As discussed previously, cancers appear to share a variety of hallmarks that contribute to the malignant phenotype. Recent molecular and genetic analyses of groups of cancer can classify an individual's cancer by the spectrum of mutations underlying the cancer phenotype.[66] However, each of the therapeutic approaches described previously generally treats specific vulnerabilities of the cancer rather than a variety of contributing factors. That approach is not successful in most invasive cancers because some cancer cells may undergo further mutation leading to therapeutic resistance.

Exceptions include targeted drugs, used in combination with conventional chemotherapy, against very specific characteristics of selected cancers. For example, imatinib is a competitive inhibitor of tyrosine kinases, primarily the BCR-ABL tyrosine kinase (Table 10-8). It is highly effective in treating CML but ineffective in virtually all other cancers. Monoclonal antibodies against the CD20 antigen expressed on some B-cell lymphomas, the epidermal growth factor (EGF) receptor on colon cancers and head and neck cancers, and the HER2 EGF receptor on breast cancer are relatively successful.[67] These drugs are so tightly targeted they have much less toxicity than conventional chemotherapies that have targets in virtually all cells.

Tumor growth and progression is dependent on a variety of mutations leading to expression of oncogenes, inactivation of tumor-suppressor molecules, and interactions with inflammatory cells in the

TABLE 10-8	**Examples of Molecular-Era Anticancer Drugs**		
Drug (Trade Name)	**Type of Drug**	**Molecular Target**	**Disease**
Imatinib (Gleevec)	Small molecule TKI	BCR-ABL tyrosine kinase, FGF receptor tyrosine kinase	Chronic myeloid leukemia (CML), gastrointestinal stromal tumor (GIST)
Erlotinib (Tarceva)	Small molecule TKI	FGF receptor tyrosine kinase	Subset of lung cancer
Trastuzumab (Herceptin)	Monoclonal antibody	HER2 receptor tyrosine kinase	HER2-positive breast cancer
Bevacizumab (Avastin)	Monoclonal antibody	VEGF receptor	Advanced colorectal cancer
Rituximab (Rituxan)	Monoclonal antibody	CD20 antigen on B lymphocytes	B-cell malignancies

EGF, Endothelial growth factor; *FGF,* fibroblast growth factor; *HER2,* human epidermal growth factor receptor 2; *TKI,* tyrosine kinase inhibitor; *VEGF,* vascular endothelial growth factor.

tumor microenvironment that foster angiogenesis, resistance to apoptosis and immune-mediated cancer cell death, altered tumor cell metabolism, and metastasis. A more efficacious therapeutic approach, therefore, may be a combination of drugs highly targeted to cancer hallmarks.[68]

More than 25 drugs are listed at the National Cancer Institute as cancer-targeting agents that inactivate oncogenes, block angiogenesis, and affect cancer cell metabolism.[69] Monoclonal antibodies are available that induce apoptosis in tumor-infiltrating cells such as TAM, Treg cells, and tumor endothelium.[70] Additionally, specific antagonists may neutralize the effects of cytokines, chemokines, and

other tumor-enhancing mediators produced in the tumor microenvironment.[71] These are usually in the form of monoclonal antibodies, which are available against TNF-α, VEGF, HER-2, and other ligands and their receptors. Such highly specific targeting would minimize secondary toxic effects.

> ### ✔ QUICK CHECK 10-5
> 1. Describe the major clinical manifestations of cancer.
> 2. How is cancer diagnosed?
> 3. What are the most common treatments of cancer?

◼ DID YOU UNDERSTAND?

Cancer Terminology and Characteristics

1. Benign tumors are usually encapsulated and well differentiated and do not spread to distant locations.
2. Malignant tumors, compared with benign tumors, have more rapid growth rates, specific microscopic alterations (anaplasia, loss of differentiation), absence of normal tissue organization, and no capsule. They invade blood vessels and lymphatics and have distant metastases.
3. Carcinomas arise from epithelial tissue, and leukemias are cancers of blood-forming cells. Carcinoma in situ (CIS) refers to noninvasive epithelial tumors of glandular or squamous cell origin.

The Biology of Cancer Cells

1. Genetic changes are the basis of cancer. These changes include small and large DNA mutations that alter genes, chromosomes, and non–coding RNAs, as well as epigenetic changes because of altered chemical modifications of DNA and histones.
2. The incidence of cancer increases with age as the individual acquires genetic hits or mutations with time. Mutations activate growth-promotion pathways, block antigrowth signals, prevent apoptosis, stimulate telomerase and new blood vessel growth, and allow tissue invasion and distant metastasis.
3. Key genetic mechanisms have a role in human carcinogenesis: (1) mutations of proto-oncogenes, resulting in hyperactivity of growth-related gene products (such genes are called *oncogenes*); (2) mutation of genes, resulting in loss or inactivity of gene products that normally would inhibit growth (such genes are called *tumor-suppressor genes*); and (3) mutation of caretaker genes that normally prevent mutations.
4. Some mutations are more important for cancer progression. These mutations can be called driver mutations. Passenger mutations are random mutations that presumably do not contribute to cancer progression.
5. Cancerous cells characteristically express mutated or overexpressed proto-oncogenes, referred to as oncogenes, which are independent of normal regulatory mechanisms and signal uncontrolled proliferation.
6. Some oncogenes, such as *RAS*, result from point mutations.
7. Oncogenes can result from genetic translocations. The Philadelphia chromosome in chronic myeloid leukemias (CML) results from a translocation that creates a novel protein fusion of the *BCR* and *ABL* genes and expression of an unregulated promoter of cell growth.
8. Tumor-suppressor genes must be inactivated in cancer cells by mutations to each allele, one from each parent.

9. A common mutation in cancer cells is inactivation of the tumor-suppressor gene tumor protein p53 *(TP53)*, which controls expression of many genes that repair DNA damage, suppression of cellular proliferation during genomic repair, and initiation of apoptosis. Inactivation of p53 results in increased mutation rates and cancer.
10. In rare families, an initial inheritable mutation in a tumor-suppressor gene, such as *TP53*, the retinoblastoma gene *(RB)*, or the breast cancer genes *(BRCA1* and *BRCA2)*, may lead to a greatly increased risk for developing particular cancers.
11. Caretaker genes are responsible for maintaining genomic integrity. Inherited mutations can disrupt caretaker genes and cause chromosome instability.
12. Abnormal gene silencing is emerging as a major factor in cancer progression. Gene expression can be regulated in a heritable manner (i.e., passed from a parent to a child or from a single cell to its progeny) by an "epigenetic" mechanism called silencing.
13. Changes in gene regulation can affect not just single genes, but entire networks of signaling. Gene expression networks can be regulated by changes in microRNAs (miRNAs or miRs) and other non–coding RNAs (ncRNAs).
14. Cancer cells are immortal.
15. When they reach a critical age, cancer cells activate telomerase to restore and maintain their telomeres, thereby allowing cancer cells to divide repeatedly or become immortal.
16. Like many normal adult tissues, cancers can contain rare stem cells that provide a source of immortal cells. To fully eradicate a cancer, it may be necessary to target the cancer stem cell.
17. Most of the genetic and epigenetic alterations that cause cancer occur within the somatic tissues during the lifetime of the individual.
18. Access to the vascular system is essential for tumor growth.
19. Stromal cells and cancer cells can secrete multiple factors, such as vascular endothelial growth factor (VEGF), that stimulate new blood vessel growth (called neovascularization or angiogenesis).
20. The successful cancer cell divides rapidly, with the consequent requirement for the building blocks of new cells; cancer cell division often occurs in a hypoxic and acidic environment. Many cancer genes also encourage aerobic glycolysis and promote high glucose utilization of a cancer.
21. In cancer, defects in the intrinsic or extrinsic pathways, or both, provide resistance to apoptotic cell death.
22. Overexpression of BCL-2 blocks apoptosis in most follicular B-cell lymphomas.

23. Some conditions of chronic inflammation increase the risk of developing cancer. A prime example is the association between gastric cancer and infection with *Helicobacter pylori*.

24. Cells recruited to the tumor microenvironment are essential to the growth and spread of cancer and are active participants in induction of cellular proliferation, angiogenesis, degradation of extracellular matrix, suppression of infiltrating immune cells, and the development and spread of metastatic cells.

25. Defects in the immune system increase the risk of viral-associated cancers but have a minimal effect on the risk of other cancers.

26. Antibodies induced by vaccines against oncogenic viruses, such as human papillomavirus (HPV) and hepatitis B virus (HBV), protect against initial infection and development of cervical and liver tumors, respectively.

27. Unique antigens and other markers on tumor cells can be recognized by T cells and NK cells of the immune system, leading to destruction of the tumor cell.

28. Cancer cells can evade rejection by the immune system by production of immunosuppressive factors, induction of immunosuppressive T-regulator cells, evolution of tumor-antigen negative variants, or suppressed expression of antigen-presenting MHC class I molecules.

29. Metastasis is the major cause of death from cancer.

30. Metastasis is a complex process that requires cells to have many new abilities, including the ability to invade, survive, and proliferate in a new environment.

31. Invasion consists of loss of cell-to-cell contact, degradation of the extracellular matrix (ECM), and migration of tumor cells to the vascular or lymphatic systems. Stromal cells, particularly tumor-associated macrophages (TAMs), are essential to this process.

32. Carcinomas undergo a process of epithelial-mesenchymal transition (EMT) during which many epithelial-like characteristics are lost (e.g., polarity, adhesion to basement membrane), resulting in increased migratory capacity, increased resistance to apoptosis, and a dedifferentiated stem cell–like state that favors growth in foreign microenvironments and establishment of metastatic disease.

33. Some cancers appear to selectively home to particular metastatic sites, which may be a result of expression of particular receptors for ligands expressed by cells at the site.

Clinical Manifestations of Cancer

1. Paraneoplastic syndromes are rare symptom complexes, often caused by biologically active substances released from a tumor or by an immune response triggered by a tumor, that manifest as symptoms not directly caused by the local effects of the cancer.

2. Clinical manifestations of cancer include pain, cachexia, anemia, leukopenia, thrombocytopenia, and infection.

3. Pain is generally associated with the late stages of cancer. It can be caused by pressure, obstruction, invasion of a structure sensitive to pain, stretching, tissue destruction, and inflammation.

4. Fatigue is the most frequently reported symptom of cancer and cancer treatment.

5. Cachexia is a multiorgan syndrome with many clinical manifestations including anorexia; muscle wasting; thermogenesis; altered heart and liver function; gut malabsorption; early satiety; taste alterations; and altered protein, lipid, and carbohydrate metabolism. Two factors are most significant: muscle loss and inflammation. Muscle wasting involves many protein signaling pathways

and inflammatory mediators. Profoundly altered are both appetite-stimulating and appetite-suppressing brain pathways.

6. Anemia associated with cancer usually occurs because of malnutrition, chronic bleeding and resultant iron deficiency, chemotherapy, radiation, and malignancies in the blood-forming organs.

7. Leukopenia is usually a result of chemotherapy (which is toxic to bone marrow) or radiation (which kills circulating leukocytes).

8. Thrombocytopenia is usually the result of chemotherapy or malignancy in the bone marrow.

9. Infection may be caused by leukopenia, immunosuppression, or debility associated with advanced disease. It is the most significant cause of complications and death.

10. The gastrointestinal tract relies on rapidly growing cells to provide an absorptive surface for nutrients. Both chemotherapy and radiation therapy may cause decreased cell turnover, thereby leading to oral ulcers (stomatitis), malabsorption, and diarrhea.

11. Alopecia (hair loss) results from chemotherapy effects on hair follicles. Alopecia is usually temporary, although hair may initially regrow with a different texture. Not all chemotherapeutic agents cause alopecia. Decreased renewal rates of the epidermal layers in the skin may lead to skin breakdown and dryness, altering the normal barrier protection against infection.

Diagnosis, Characterization, and Treatment of Cancer

1. The diagnosis of cancer requires a biopsy and examination of tumor tissue by a pathologist. Cancer classification is established by a variety of tests.

2. Tumor staging involves the size of the tumor, the degree to which it has locally invaded, and the extent to which it has spread. A standard scheme for staging is the T (tumor spread), N (node involvement), and M (metastasis) system.

3. The classification, and hence the treatment decisions, of cancers was originally based on gross and light microscopic appearance, and is now commonly accompanied by immunohistochemical analysis of protein expression. Increasingly, this is supplemented by a more extensive molecular analysis of the tumors.

4. Tumor markers are substances (i.e., hormones, enzymes, genes, antigens, antibodies) found in cancer cells and in blood, spinal fluid, or urine. They are used to screen and identify individuals at high risk for cancer, to help diagnose specific types of tumors, and to follow the clinical course of cancer.

5. Cancer is treated routinely with surgery, radiation therapy, chemotherapy, and combinations of these modalities.

6. Surgical therapy is used for nonmetastatic disease (in which cure is possible by removing the tumor) and as a palliative measure to alleviate symptoms.

7. Ionizing radiation causes cell damage; therefore the goal of radiation therapy is to damage the tumor without causing excessive toxicity or damage to nondiseased structures.

8. The theoretic basis of chemotherapy is the vulnerability of tumor cells in various stages of the cell cycle.

9. Modern chemotherapy uses combinations of drugs with different targets and different toxicities.

10. Immunotherapy attempts to modify the immune system from a cancer-protective state to a destructive condition.

11. Future treatment of tumors will, most likely, use a careful histologic and genetic analysis of individual cancers that prescribes a combination of tumor-targeting drugs to simultaneously disrupt multiple hallmarks of that particular cancer.

KEY TERMS

Adenocarcinoma, 234
Adjuvant chemotherapy, 261
Anaplasia, 234
Angiogenesis, 245
Angiogenic factor, 245
Apoptosis, 247
Autocrine stimulation, 240
Benign tumor, 233
Brachytherapy, 260
Cachexia, 255
Cancer, 233
Cancer-associated fibroblasts (CAFs), 249
Carcinoma, 234
Carcinoma in situ (CIS), 234
Caretaker gene, 241
Chromosome instability, 245

Chromosome translocation, 237
Clonal expansion, 237
Clonal proliferation, 237
DNA methylation, 237
Dormancy, 253
Epigenetic silencing, 244
Epithelial-mesenchymal transition (EMT), 251
Gene amplification, 237
Human T-cell lymphotropic virus type 1 (HTLV-1), 250
Induction chemotherapy, 260
Leukemia, 234
Lymphoma, 234
Malignant tumor, 234
Matrix metalloproteinases, 246
Metastasis, 251

MicroRNA (miRNA, miR), 244
Neoadjuvant chemotherapy, 261
Neoplasm, 233
Neovascularization, 245
Non–coding RNA, 237
Oncogene, 240
Oncomir, 244
Paraneoplastic syndrome, 254
Personalized medicine, 260
Pleomorphic, 234
Point mutation, 237
Proto-oncogene, 240
RAS, 238
Receptor tyrosine kinase, 240
Retinoblastoma (RB) gene, 241
Reverse Warburg effect, 247
Sarcoma, 234

Silencing, 244
Stage of cancer, 258
Stroma, 234
Telomerase, 245
Telomere, 245
Thrombospondin-1 (TSP-1), 246
Tumor, 233
Tumor initiation, 237
Tumor marker, 258
Tumor progression, 237
Tumor promotion, 237
Tumor protein p53 (TP53), 241
Tumor-associated macrophage (TAM), 249
Tumor-suppressor gene, 241

REFERENCES

1. National Cancer Institute (NCI): *Fact sheet: what is cancer?* Available at: www.cancer.gov/cancertopics/cancerlibrary/what-is-cancer. Accessed November 30, 2014.
2. Pieri A et al: Pleomorphic lobular carcinoma in situ of the breast: can the evidence guide practice? *World J Clin Oncol* 5(3):546-553, 2014.
3. Hanahan D, Weinberg RA: Hallmarks of cancer, *Cell* 100(1):57-70, 2000.
4. Hanahan D, Weinberg RA: Hallmarks of cancer: the next generation, *Cell* 144(5):646-674, 2011.
5. Vogelstein B et al: Cancer genome landscapes, *Science* 339(6127):1546-1558, 2013.
6. Alexandrov LB, Stratton MR: Mutational signatures: the patterns of somatic mutations hidden in cancer genomes, *Curr Opin Genet Dev* 24:52-60, 2014.
7. Hanahan D, Coussens LM: Accessories to the crime: functions of cells recruited to the tumor microenvironment, *Cancer Cell* 21(3):309-322, 2012.
8. Berns A, Pandolfi PP: Tumor microenvironment revisited, *EMBO Rep* 15(5):458-459, 2014.
9. Quail DF, Joyce JA: Microenvironmental regulation of tumor progression and metastasis, *Nat Med* 19(11):1423-1437, 2013.
10. Perez EA et al: HER2 testing: current status and future directions, *Cancer Treat Rev* 40(2):276-284, 2014.
11. Ott G et al: Understanding MYC-driven aggressive B-cell lymphomas: pathogenesis and classification, *Hematol Am Soc Hematol Educ Program* 2013:575-583, 2013.
12. Jabbour E, Kantarjian H: Chronic myeloid leukemia: 2014 update on diagnosis, monitoring, and management, *Am J Hematol* 89(5):547-556, 2014.
13. Rubin SM: Deciphering the retinoblastoma protein phosphorylation code, *Trends Biochem Sci* 38(1):12-19, 2013.
14. Muller PAJ, Vousden KH: Mutant p53 in cancer: new functions and therapeutic opportunities, *Cancer Cell* 25(3):304-317, 2014.
15. Rahman N: Realizing the promise of cancer predisposition genes, *Nature* 505(7483):302-308, 2014.
16. Kim E-W et al: Differential microRNA expression signatures and cell type-specific association with Taxol resistance in ovarian cancer cells, *Drug Des Develop Therapy* 8:293-314, 2014.
17. Jerónimo C, Henrique R: Epigenetic biomarkers in urological tumors: a systemic review, *Cancer Lett* 342(2):264-274, 2014.

18. National Cancer Institute (NCI): *Fact Sheet: BRCA1 and BRCA2: cancer risk and genetic testing.* Available at: www.cancer.gov/cancertopics/factsheet/Risk/BRCA. Accessed November 30, 2014.
19. Lucey BP et al: HeLa cells, and cell culture contamination, *Arch Pathol Lab Med* 133(9):1463-1467, 2009.
20. Azzalin CM, Lingner J: Telomere functions grounding on TERRA firma, *Trends Cell Biol* 25(1):29-36, 2014.
21. Shay JW, Wright WE: Role of telomeres and telomerase in cancer, *Semin Cancer Biol* 21(6):349-353, 2011.
22. Beck B, Blanpain C: Unravelling cancer stem cell potential, *Nat Rev Cancer* 13(10):727-738, 2013.
23. Xie J et al: Beyond Warburg effect—dual metabolic nature of cancer cells, *Sci Rep* 4:4927, 2014.
24. Morandi A, Chiarugi P: Metabolic implication of tumor: stroma crosstalk in breast cancer, *J Mol Med (Berlin)* 92(2):117-126, 2014.
25. Zhao Y et al: Targeting cellular metabolism to improve cancer therapeutics, *Cell Death Dis* 4:e532, 2013.
26. Parks SK et al: Disrupting proton dynamics and energy metabolism for cancer therapy, *Nat Rev Cancer* 13(9):611-623, 2013.
27. Okada F: Inflammation-related carcinogenesis: current findings in epidemiological trends, causes and mechanisms, *Yonago Acta Med* 57(2):65-72, 2014.
28. Coffelt SB, De Visser KE: Cancer: inflammation lights the way to metastasis, *Nature* 507(7490):48-49, 2014.
29. Elinav E et al: Inflammation-induced cancer: crosstalk between tumours, immune cells and microorganisms, *Nat Rev Cancer* 13(11):759-771, 2013.
30. Rogler G: Chronic ulcerative colitis and colorectal cancer, *Cancer Lett* 345(2):235-241, 2014.
31. Pasechnikov V et al: Gastric cancer: prevention, screening and early diagnosis, *World J Gastroenterol* 20(38):13842-13862, 2014.
32. Goubran H et al: Regulation of tumor growth and metastasis: the role of tumor microenvironment, *Cancer Growth Metastasis* 7:9-18, 2014.
33. Van Overmeire E et al: Mechanisms driving macrophage diversity and specialization in distinct tumor microenvironments and parallelisms with other tissues, *Front Immunol* 5:127, 2014.
34. Miles FL, Sikes RA: Insidious changes in stromal matrix fuel cancer progression, *Mol Cancer Res* 12(3):297-312, 2014.

35. Coulie PG et al: Tumour antigens recognized by T lymphocytes: at the core of cancer immunotherapy, *Nat Rev Cancer* 14(2):135-146, 2014.
36. Mesri EA et al: Human viral oncogenesis: a cancer hallmarks analysis, *Cell Host Microbe* 15(3):266-282, 2014.
37. Volerman A, Cifu AS: Cervical cancer screening, *J Am Med Assoc* 312(21):2279-2280, 2014.
38. Corthay A: Does the immune system naturally protect against cancer? *Front Immunol* 5:197, 2014.
39. Stockmann C et al: The impact of the immune system on tumor: angiogenesis and vascular remodeling, *Front Oncol* 4:69, 2014.
40. Talmadge JE, Gabrilovich DI: History of myeloid-derived suppressor cells, *Nat Rev Cancer* 13(10):739-752, 2013.
41. Jamal-Hanjani M et al: Tumour heterogeneity and immune-modulation, *Curr Opin Pharmacol* 13(4):497-503, 2013.
42. Gilkes DM et al: Hypoxia and the extracellular matrix: drivers of tumour metastasis, *Nat Rev Cancer* 14(6):430-439, 2014.
43. Kothari AN et al: Novel clinical therapeutics targeting the epithelial to mesenchymal transition, *Clin Transl Med* 3(35):1-14, 2014.
44. De Craene B, Berx G: Regulatory networks defining EMT during cancer initiation and progression, *Nat Rev Cancer* 13(2):97-110, 2013.
45. Smith HA, Kang Y: The metastasis-promoting roles of tumor-associated immune cells, *J Mol Med* 91(2013):411-429, 2013.
46. Fidler IJ et al: The biology of melanoma brain metastasis, *Cancer Metastasis Rev* 18(3):387-400, 1999.
47. Domanska UM et al: A review on CXCR4/CXCL12 axis in oncology: no place to hide, *Eur J Cancer* 49(1):219-230, 2013.
48. Barcellos-de-Souza P et al: Tumor microenvironment: bone marrow-mesenchymal stem cells as key players, *Biochim Biophys Acta* 1836(2):321-335, 2013.
49. Benzekry S et al: Global dormancy of metastases due to systemic inhibition of angiogenesis, *PLoS ONE* 9(1):e84249, 2014.
50. Sosa MS et al: Mechanisms of disseminated cancer dormancy: an awakening field, *Nat Rev Cancer* 14(9):611-622, 2014.
51. Klein-Goldberg A et al: The role played by the microenvironment in site-specific metastasis, *Cancer Lett* 352(1):54-58, 2014.

52. Argilés JM et al: Cancer cachexia: understanding the molecular basis, *Nat Rev Cancer* 14(11): 754-762, 2014.

53. He WA et al: Microvesicles containing miRNAs promote muscle cell death in cancer cachexia via TLR7, *Proc Natl Acad Sci U S A* 111(12): 4525-4529, 2014.

54. Hitachi K, Tsuchida K: Role of microRNAs in skeletal muscle hypertrophy, *Front Physiol* 4:408, 2013.

55. Kir S et al: Tumour-derived PTH-related protein triggers tissue browning and cancer cachexia, *Nature* 513(7516):100-104, 2014.

56. Petruzzelli M et al: A switch from white to brown fat increases energy expenditure in cancer-associated cachexia, *Cell Metab* 20(3):433-447, 2014.

57. Ramos EJ et al: Cancer anorexia-cachexia syndrome: cytokines and neuropeptides, *Curr Opin Clin Nutr Metab Care* 7(4):427-434, 2004.

58. American Cancer Society (ACS): *Tumor markers.* Available at: www.cancer.org/acs/groups/cid/ documents/webcontent/003189-pdf.pdf. Accessed November 30, 2014.

59. National Cancer Institute (NCI): *Fact sheet: prostate-specific antigen (PSA) test.* Available at: www.cancer.gov/cancertopics/factsheet/detection/ PSA. Accessed November 30, 2014.

60. Moyer VA, U.S. Preventive Services Task Force: Screening for prostate cancer: U.S. Preventive Services Task Force recommendation statement, *Ann Intern Med* 157(2):120-134, 2012.

61. Shames DS, Wistuba II: The evolving genomic classification of lung cancer, *J Pathol* 232(2):121-133, 2014.

62. National Cancer Institute (NCI): *Fact sheet: immunotherapy: using the immune system to treat cancer.* Available at: www.cancer.gov/ researchandfunding/progress/immunotherapy -using-immune-system-to-treat-cancer. Accessed November 30, 2014.

63. Gao J et al: Advances in the development of cancer immunotherapies, *Trends Immunol* 34(2):90-98, 2013.

64. Hinrichs CS, Rosenberg SA: Exploiting the curative potential of adoptive T-cell therapy for cancer, *Immunol Rev* 257(1):56-71, 2014.

65. Phan GQ, Rosenberg SA: The potential and promise of cancer immunotherapy, *Cancer Control* 20(4):289-297, 2013.

66. Hoadley KA et al: Multiplatform analysis of 12 cancer types reveals molecular classification within and across tissues of origin, *Cell* 158(4):929-944, 2014.

67. Sliwkowski MX, Mellman I: Antibody therapeutics in cancer, *Science* 341(6151):1192-1198, 2013.

68. Hanahan D: Rethinking the war on cancer, *Lancet* 383(9916):558-563, 2014.

69. Nero TL et al: Oncogenic protein interfaces: small molecules, big challenges, *Nat Rev Cancer* 14(4): 248-262, 2014.

70. Tan J: Waging war on cancer with the sword of immunity, *Cell* 158:233-234, 2014.

71. O'Shea JJ et al: In search of magic bullets: the golden age of immunotherapeutics, *Cell* 157(1): 227-240, 2014.

Cancer Epidemiology

Kathryn L. McCance

CHAPTER OUTLINE

Although cancer arises from a complicated and an interacting web of multiple etiologies, avoiding high-risk behaviors and exposure to **individual carcinogens,** or cancer-causing substances, will prevent many types of cancer (Figure 11-1). Research has shown that lifestyle behaviors, dietary and environmental factors, and occupational exposure contribute to the number of cancer cases and deaths.[1-3] In this context, any of the following factors can contribute to the development of cancer[4-6]:

- Lifestyle choices, such as smoking, alcohol use, nutritional intake
- Lack of physical exercise and overweight/obesity
- Infections, sexual practices
- Environmental conditions, including exposure to sunlight, natural and medical radiation, workplace exposures, and involuntary or unknown exposures
- Prescribed and illicit medications
- Socioeconomic factors that affect exposures and susceptibility
- Carcinogenic substances present in air, water, and soil

Estimates of environmental factors and their attributable risk for cancer vary. The International Agency for Research on Cancer (IARC) completed a review of the more than 100 chemicals, occupations, physical agents, biologic agents, and other agents classified as carcinogenic to humans.[4] Simplified tables with a list of classifications by cancer sites with sufficient or limited evidence in humans are contained in Table 11-1.

GENETICS, EPIGENETICS, AND TISSUE

Cancers are caused by environmental-lifestyle factors and genetic factors (Figure 11-2). *Patterns* of cancer incidence around the world

are environmental in origin—and not primarily genetic. At the level of the cell, cancer is *driven* by genetic alterations and epigenetic abnormalities with included variations in detoxifying enzymes or DNA repair genes. Interacting factors causing cancer risk are weaker immune systems and differences in hormone levels and metabolic factors (see Chapter 10). These interacting factors are influenced by the greater external environment and the cell's immediate environment. The biologic environment surrounding cells includes metabolic and hormonal factors, for example, excess estrogen production, inflammation, and disordered glucose and lipid metabolism. Thus, the biologic environment is modified by metabolic requirements, physical activity, infections, nutrition, occupational carcinogens, air pollution, and many other environmental factors. Investigators are challenged to connect the complex web between genotype, phenotype, and the environment to understand a person's chances of developing cancer.

Cancer development and progression involves the tissue microenvironment, or stroma. Emerging is the importance of the microenvironment's interaction with environmental factors because stromal tissue has various immune cells that can promote inflammation. Chronic inflammation is at the interface of environmental factors and genetics. Inflammation caused by environmental factors includes, for example, inhaled tobacco smoke, asbestos fibers, or fine particles in the air from diesel engine exhaust and other industrial sources. These sources are major factors in lung and other respiratory tract cancers.[7,8] In summary, once malignant phenotypes have developed, complex interactions occur between the tumor, the surrounding stroma, and the cells of the immune and inflammatory systems (see Chapter 10).

Text continued on p. 272

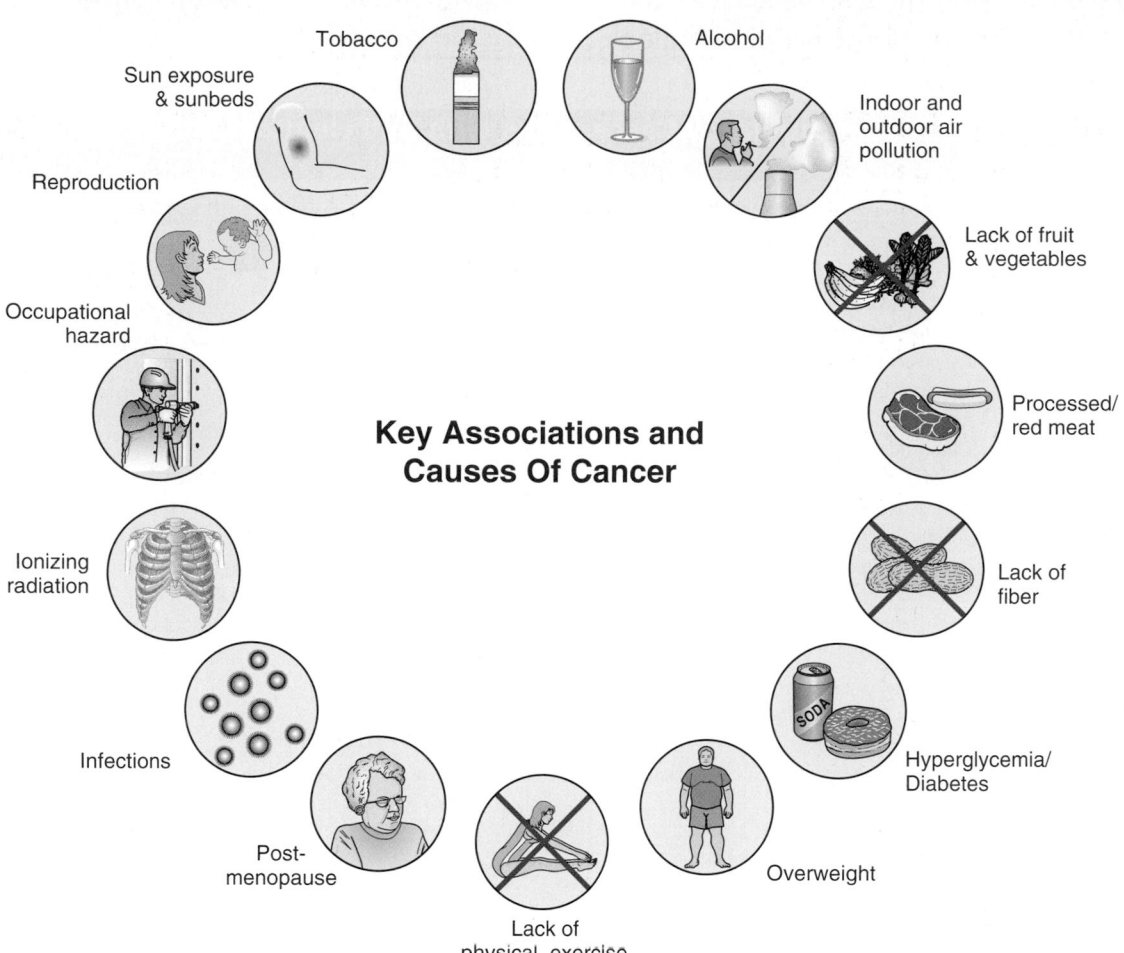

Key Associations and Causes Of Cancer

Tobacco

Alcohol

Indoor and outdoor air pollution

Sun exposure & sunbeds

Lack of fruit & vegetables

Reproduction

Processed/red meat

Occupational hazard

Lack of fiber

Ionizing radiation

Hyperglycemia/Diabetes

Infections

Overweight

Post-menopause

Lack of physical exercise

FIGURE 11-1 Key Associations and Causes of Cancer. Tobacco, diet and alcohol, obesity, lack of physical activity, hormones, infections, ionizing radiation, occupational hazards, reproductive factors, and ultraviolet light are key factors for cancer. Although diet is key and known to affect cancer risk, determining specific dietary factors has been very difficult and is emerging.

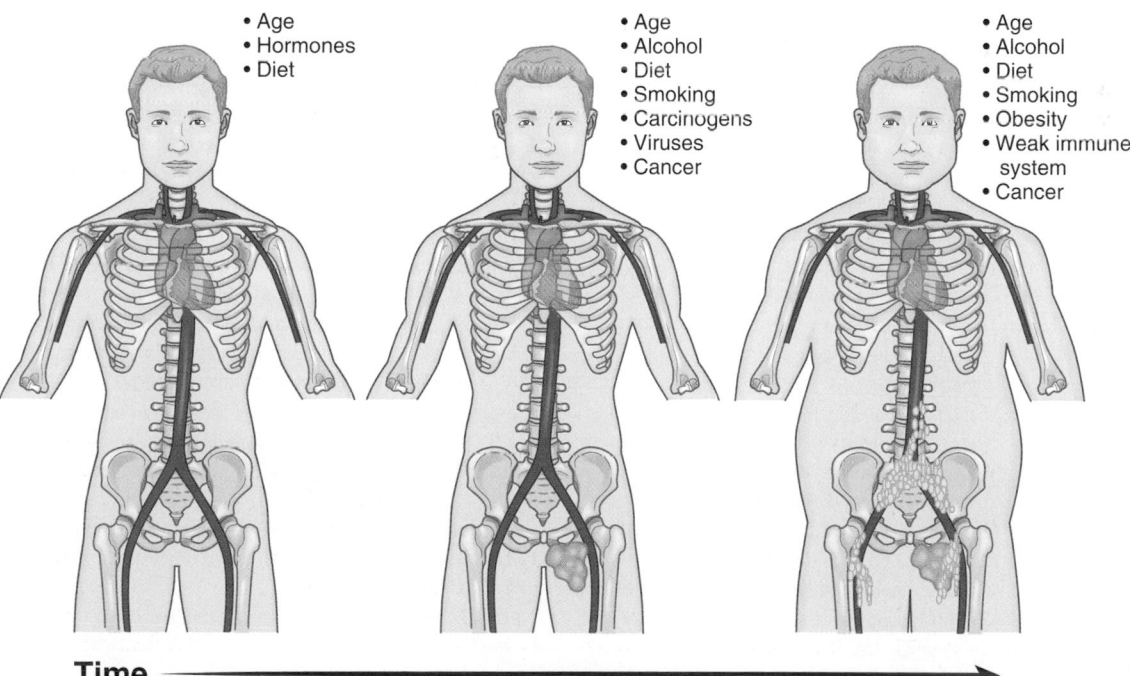

- Age
- Hormones
- Diet

- Age
- Alcohol
- Diet
- Smoking
- Carcinogens
- Viruses
- Cancer

- Age
- Alcohol
- Diet
- Smoking
- Obesity
- Weak immune system
- Cancer

Time

FIGURE 11-2 Environmental Factors and Genetic, Epigenetic, and Other Host Factors. Over time a person's internal genetic makeup persistently interacts with external or environmental factors. Environmental factors (e.g., diet, smoking, alcohol use, hormones, certain viruses, chemical carcinogens) collectively interact with internal epigenetic factors and genetic mutations to destabilize normal biologic factors including immune factors for balancing growth and maturation. (Adapted from NCI: *Understanding cancer series: cancer: inside and outside factors,* Washington, DC, National Cancer Institute, National Institutes of Health, 2007.)

TABLE 11-1   List of Classifications by Cancer Sites with Sufficient or Limited Evidence in Humans*

Cancer Site	Carcinogenic Agents with Sufficient Evidence in Humans	Agents with Limited Evidence in Humans
Lip, Oral Cavity, and Pharynx		
Lip		Solar radiation
Oral cavity	Alcoholic beverages	
	Betel quid with tobacco	
	Betel quid without tobacco	
	Human papillomavirus type 16	
	Tobacco, smokeless	
	Tobacco smoking	
Salivary gland	X-radiation, γ-radiation	Radioiodines, including iodine-131
Tonsil	Human papillomavirus type 16	
Pharynx	Alcoholic beverages	Asbestos (all forms)
	Betel quid with tobacco	Mate drinking, hot
	Human papillomavirus type 16	Printing presses
	Tobacco smoking	Tobacco smoke, secondhand
Nasopharynx	Epstein-Barr virus	
	Formaldehyde	
	Salted fish, Chinese style	
	Wood dust	
Digestive tract, upper	Acetaldehyde associated with consumption of alcoholic beverages	
Digestive Organs		
Esophagus	Acetaldehyde associated with consumption of alcoholic beverages	Dry cleaning
	Alcoholic beverages	Mate drinking, hot
	Betel quid with tobacco	Pickled vegetables (traditional Asian)
	Betel quid without tobacco	Rubber production industry
	Tobacco, smokeless	Tetrachloroethylene
	Tobacco smoking	
	X-radiation, γ-radiation	
Stomach	*Helicobacter pylori*	Asbestos (all forms)
	Rubber production industry	Epstein-Barr virus
	Tobacco smoking	Lead compounds, inorganic
	X-radiation, γ-radiation	Nitrate or nitrite (ingested) under conditions that result in endogenous nitrosation
		Pickled vegetables (traditional Asian)
		Salted fish (Chinese style)
Colon and rectum	Alcoholic beverages	Asbestos (all forms)
	Tobacco smoking	*Schistosoma japonicum*
	X-radiation, γ-radiation	
Anus	Human immunodeficiency virus type 1	Human papillomavirus types 18, 33
	Human papillomavirus type 16	
Liver and bile duct	Aflatoxins	Androgenic (anabolic) steroids
	Alcoholic beverages	Arsenic and inorganic arsenic compounds
	Clonorchis sinensis	Betel quid without tobacco
	Estrogen-progestogen contraceptives	Human immunodeficiency virus type 1
	Hepatitis B virus	Polychlorinated biphenyls
	Hepatitis C virus	*Schistosoma japonicum*
	Opisthorchis viverrini	Trichloroethylene
	Plutonium	X-radiation, γ-radiation
	Thorium-232 and its decay products	
	Tobacco smoking (in smokers and in smokers' children)	
	Vinyl chloride	
Gallbladder	Thorium-232 and its decay products	
Pancreas	Tobacco, smokeless	Alcoholic beverages
	Tobacco smoking	Thorium-232 and its decay products
		X-radiation, γ-radiation
Digestive Tract, Unspecified		Radioiodines, including iodine-131

TABLE 11-1 **List of Classifications by Cancer Sites with Sufficient or Limited Evidence in Humans—cont'd**

Cancer Site	Carcinogenic Agents with Sufficient Evidence in Humans	Agents with Limited Evidence in Humans
Respiratory Organs		
Nasal cavity and paranasal sinus	Isopropyl alcohol production Leather dust Nickel compounds Radium-226 and its decay products Radium-228 and its decay products Tobacco smoking Wood dust	Carpentry and joinery Chromium (VI) compounds Formaldehyde Textile manufacturing
Larynx	Acid mists, strong inorganic Alcoholic beverages Asbestos (all forms) Tobacco smoking	Human papillomavirus type 16 Mate drinking, hot Rubber production industry Sulfur mustard Tobacco smoke, secondhand
Lung	Aluminum production Arsenic and inorganic arsenic compounds Beryllium and beryllium products Bis(chloromethyl) ether; chloromethyl methyl ether (technical grade) Cadmium and cadmium compounds Chromium (VI) compounds Coal, indoor emissions from household combustion Coal gasification Coal-tar pitch Coke production Hematite mining (underground) Iron and steel founding MOPP (vincristine-prednisone-nitrogen mustard-procarbazine mixture) Nickel compounds Painting Plutonium Radon-222 and its decay products Rubber production industry Silica dust, crystalline Soot Sulfur mustard Tobacco smoke, secondhand Tobacco smoking X-radiation, γ-radiation	Acid mists, strong inorganic Art glass, glass containers, and pressed ware (manufacture of) Biomass fuel (primarily wood), indoor emissions from household combustion of Bitumens, oxidized, and their emissions during roofing Bitumens, hard, and their emissions during mastic asphalt work Carbon electrode manufacture α-Chlorinated toluenes and benzyl chloride (combined exposure) Cobalt metal with tungsten carbide Creosotes Engine exhaust, diesel Frying, emissions from high-temperature Insecticides, nonarsenical (occupational exposures in spraying and application) Printing processes 2,3,7,8-Tetrachlorodibenzo-*para*-dioxin Welding fumes
Bone, Skin, Mesothelium, Endothelium, and Soft Tissue		
Bone	Plutonium Radium-224 and its decay products Radium-226 and its decay products Radium-228 and its decay products X-radiation, γ-radiation	Radioiodines, including iodine-131
Skin (melanoma)	Solar radiation Ultraviolet-emitting tanning devices	
Skin (other malignant neoplasms)	Arsenic and inorganic arsenic compounds Azathioprine Coal-tar distillation Coal-tar pitch Cyclosporine Methoxypsoralen plus ultraviolet A Mineral oils, untreated or mildly treated Shale oils Solar radiation Soot X-radiation, γ-radiation	Creosotes Human immunodeficiency virus type 1 Human papillomavirus types 5 and 8 (in individuals with epidermodysplasia verruciformis) Nitrogen mustard Petroleum refining (occupational exposures) Ultraviolet-emitting tanning devices Merkel cell polyomavirus (MCV)

Continued

TABLE 11-1   List of Classifications by Cancer Sites with Sufficient or Limited Evidence in Humans—cont'd

Cancer Site	Carcinogenic Agents with Sufficient Evidence in Humans	Agents with Limited Evidence in Humans
Mesothelium (pleura and peritoneum)	Asbestos (all forms) Erionite Painting	
Endothelium (Kaposi sarcoma)	Human immunodeficiency virus type 1 Kaposi sarcoma herpesvirus	
Soft tissue		Polychlorophenols or their sodium salts (combined exposures) Radioiodines, including iodine-131 2,3,7,8-Tetrachlorodibenzo-*para*-dioxin
Breast and Female Genital Organs		
Breast	Alcoholic beverages Diethylstilbestrol Estrogen-progestogen contraceptives Estrogen-progestogen menopausal therapy X-radiation, γ-radiation	Estrogen menopausal therapy Ethylene oxide Shiftwork that involves circadian disruption Tobacco smoking
Vulva	Human papillomavirus 16	Human immunodeficiency virus type 1
Vagina	Diethylstilbestrol (exposure in utero) Human papillomavirus 16	Human immunodeficiency virus type 1
Uterine cervix	Diethylstilbestrol (exposure in utero) Estrogen-progestogen contraceptives Human immunodeficiency virus type 1 Human papillomavirus types 16, 18, 31, 33, 35, 39, 45, 51, 52, 56, 58, 59 Tobacco smoking	Human papillomavirus types 26, 53, 66, 67, 68, 70, 73, 82 Tetrachloroethylene
Endometrium	Estrogen menopausal therapy Estrogen-progestogen menopausal therapy Tamoxifen	Diethylstilbestrol
Ovary	Asbestos (all forms) Estrogen menopausal therapy Tobacco smoking	Talc-based body powder (perineal use) X-radiation, γ-radiation
Male Genital Organs		
Penis	Human papillomavirus type 16	Human immunodeficiency virus type 1 Human papillomavirus type 18
Prostrate		Androgenic (anabolic) steroids Arsenic and inorganic arsenic compounds Cadmium and cadmium compounds Rubber production industry Thorium-232 and its decay products X-radiation, γ-radiation
Testis		Diethylstilbestrol exposure in utero
Urinary Tract		
Kidney	Tobacco smoking X-radiation, γ-radiation	Arsenic and inorganic arsenic compounds Cadmium and cadmium compounds Printing processes
Renal pelvis and ureter	Aristolochic acids, plants containing phenacetin Phenacetin, analgesic mixtures containing Tobacco smoking	Aristolochic acids
Urinary bladder	Aluminum production 4-Aminobiphenyl Arsenic and inorganic arsenic compounds Auramine production Benzidine Chlornaphazine Cyclophosphamide Magenta production 2-Naphthylamine	4-Chloro-*ortho*-toluidine Coal-tar pitch Coffee Dry cleaning Engine exhaust, diesel Hairdressers and barbers (occupational exposure) Printing processes Soot Textile manufacturing

TABLE 11-1　**List of Classifications by Cancer Sites with Sufficient or Limited Evidence in Humans—cont'd**

Cancer Site	Carcinogenic Agents with Sufficient Evidence in Humans	Agents with Limited Evidence in Humans
	Painting	
	Rubber production industry	
	Schistosoma haematobium	
	Tobacco smoking	
	ortho-Toluidine	
	X-radiation, γ-radiation	

Eye, Brain, and Central Nervous System

Cancer Site	Carcinogenic Agents with Sufficient Evidence in Humans	Agents with Limited Evidence in Humans
Eye	Human immunodeficiency virus type 1	Solar radiation
	Ultraviolet-emitting tanning devices	
	Welding	
Brain and central nervous system	X-radiation, γ-radiation	Radiofrequency electromagnetic fields (including from wireless phones)

Endocrine Glands

Cancer Site	Carcinogenic Agents with Sufficient Evidence in Humans	Agents with Limited Evidence in Humans
Thyroid	Radioiodines, including iodine-131	
	X-radiation, γ-radiation	

Lymphoid, Hematopoietic, and Related Tissue

Cancer Site	Carcinogenic Agents with Sufficient Evidence in Humans	Agents with Limited Evidence in Humans
Leukemia and/or lymphoma	Azathioprine	Bis(chloroethyl)nitrosourea
	Benzene	Chloramphenicol
	Busulfan	Ethylene oxide
	1,3-Butadiene	Etoposide
	Chlorambucil	Hepatitis B virus
	Cyclophosphamide	Magnetic fields, extremely low frequency (childhood leukemia)
	Cyclosporine	
	Epstein-Barr virus	Mitoxantrone
	Etoposide with cisplatin and bleomycin	Nitrogen mustard
	Fission products, including strontium-90	Painting (childhood leukemia from maternal exposure)
	Formaldehyde	Petroleum refining (occupational exposures)
	Helicobacter pylori	Polychlorophenols or their sodium salts (combined exposures)
	Hepatitis C virus	
	Human immunodeficiency virus type 1	Radioiodines, including iodine-131
	Human T-cell lymphotropic virus type 1	Radon-222 and its decay products
	Kaposi sarcoma herpesvirus	Styrene
	Melphalan	Teniposide
	MOPP (vincristine-prednisone-nitrogen mustard-procarbazine mixture)	Tetrachloroethylene
	Phosphorus-32	Trichloroethylene
	Rubber production industry	2,3,7,8-Tetrachlorodibenzo-*para*-dioxin
	Semustine (methyl-CCNU)	Tobacco smoking (childhood leukemia in smokers' children)
	Thiotepa	
	Thorium-23 and its decay products	Malaria (caused by infection with *Plasmodium falciparum* in holoendemic areas)
	Tobacco smoking	
	Treosulfan	
	X-radiation, γ-radiation	

Multiple or Unspecific Sites

Cancer Site	Carcinogenic Agents with Sufficient Evidence in Humans	Agents with Limited Evidence in Humans
Multiple sites (unspecified)	Cyclosporine	Chlorophenoxy herbicides
	Fission products, including strontium-90	Plutonium
	X-radiation, γ-radiation (exposure in utero)	
All cancer sites (combined)	2,3,7,8-Tetrachlorodibenzo-*para*-dioxin	

Adapted from Cogliano VJ et al: *J Natl Cancer Inst* 103:1-13, 2011. Available at: http://jnci.oxfordjournals.org/content/early/2011/12/11/jnci.djr483.short?rss=1.

***NOTE:** This table does not include factors not covered in the IARC Monographs, notably genetic traits, reproductive status, and some nutritional factors.

Incidence and Mortality Trends

Incidence Trends

Globally, cancer is reported to become a major cause of morbidity and mortality in the coming decades in all regions of the world[9] (see *Health Alert:* Global Cancer Statistics and Risk Factors Associated with Causes of Cancer Death). According to a report by GLOBACAN, an estimated 14.1 million new cancer cases and 8.2 million cancer deaths were reported and 32.6 million people were found to be living with cancer (diagnosed in the past 5 years) in 2012 worldwide.[10] The global cancer burden is shifting from the more developed countries to economically disadvantaged countries.[11] In the 2013 annual report to the nation, the National Cancer Institute, American Cancer Society, the Centers for Disease Control and Prevention, and the North American Association of Central Cancer Registries collaborated to provide updates on cancer incidence, death rates, and trends in these rates for the United States.[12] Incidence rates were calculated for all cancer sites combined, childhood cancers (ages 0 to 14 and 0 to 19 years), and the 17 most common cancers among men and 18 most common cancers among women to enable the overall 15 most common cancers for all races and ethnicities combined and for the 5 major racial and ethnic groups (black, white, Asian and Pacific Islander [API], American Indian/Alaska Native [AI/AN], and Hispanic) by gender.[12] Overall, cancer incidence rates in all racial and ethnic groups and genders combined were stable from 2000 to 2009.

Among men, overall cancer incidence decreased on average by 0.6% annually from 1994 to 2009. For women, overall cancer incidence rates decreased 0.5% annually from 1998 to 2006, but rates were stable from 2006 to 2009.[12] For children, overall cancer incidence rates increased by 0.6% per year aged 0 to 14 years and by 0.7% per year among children aged 0 to 19 years from 2000 to 2009, a trend continuing from 1992. Among men, incidence rates from 2000 to 2009 decreased for 5 of the 17 most common cancers: prostate, lung and bronchus (lung), colon and rectum (colorectal), stomach, and larynx. In contrast, rates among men during the same time period increased for 6 cancers: kidney and renal pelvis (kidney), pancreas, liver and intrahepatic bile duct (liver), thyroid, melanoma of the skin (melanoma), and myeloma. Incidence rates among women decreased from 2000 to 2009 for 7 of the 18 most common cancers: lung, colorectal, urinary bladder (bladder), cervix uteri (cervix), oral cavity and pharynx, ovary, and stomach. Among women, incidence rates increased for 7 cancers from 2000 to 2009: thyroid, melanoma, kidney, pancreas, leukemia, liver, and corpus and uterus (uterus). Incidence rates were stable for the remaining cancers from 2000 to 2009, including breast cancer and non-Hodgkin lymphoma in men and women.[12]

From 2005 to 2009 for all cancer sites combined and all racial and ethnic groups, cancer incidence rates were higher among men than women.[12] For all racial and ethnic groups black men had the highest overall cancer incidence rate. The highest incidence rates among men were reported for prostate cancer, followed by lung and colorectal cancer in each group, except for Hispanics, and for them colorectal cancer ranked second.[12] For the same time period, among women the highest incidence rates were in whites followed by blacks. Breast cancer had the highest incidence rate, followed by lung and colorectal cancers, except among API and Hispanic women, for them colorectal cancer was more common than lung cancer.[12] Uterine cancer ranked fourth among women for each group except API women, for them thyroid cancer was the fourth most common cancer. During the period 2000 to 2009, incidence rates for all cancers declined among men of each racial and ethnic group except the decline for AI/AN men that was not statistically significant.[12] In contrast, rates for all cancers combined among women decreased only in whites and Hispanics.[12] Among children 0 to 19 years of age, cancer incidence rates increased for black and Hispanic children and were stable for children of all other racial and ethnic groups; however, blacks had the lowest rates of any racial and ethnic group.[12]

Mortality Trends

Overall cancer death rates have been declining since the early 1990s, with rates decreasing approximately 1.8% per year in men and by 1.4% per year in women from 2000 to 2009. Rates in children have continued to decrease since 1975 with a brief interruption in the decrease from 1998 to 2003.[12] From the period 2000 to 2009 and the period from 2005 to 2009, death rates among men decreased for 10 of the 17 most common cancers (lung, prostate, colorectal, leukemia, non-Hodgkin lymphoma, kidney, stomach, myeloma, oral cavity and pharynx, and larynx). Rates increased for men for cancers of the pancreas, liver, and melanoma. For the same time periods, death rates among women decreased for 15 of the 18 most common cancers (lung, breast, colorectal, ovary, leukemia, non-Hodgkin lymphoma, brain and central nervous system, myeloma, kidney, stomach, cervix, bladder, esophagus, oral cavity and pharynx, and gallbladder). Death rates increased for women for cancers of the pancreas, liver, and uterus.[12]

For all racial and ethnic groups, for both genders, and children for the time period 2000 to 2009, overall cancer death rates declined.[12] Among men, death rates for the most common cancers (lung, colorectal, and prostate) decreased in all racial and ethnic groups, except among AI/AN men, where the decreases for lung and colorectal cancers were not statistically significant. Among women, death rates for lung, breast, and colorectal cancers decreased in all racial and ethnic groups, except among AI/AN women for all three cancers and among API women for lung cancer.[12] Increased death rates occurred for liver cancer in white, black, and Hispanic men and among white and Hispanic women, but rates decreased among API men and women. Death rates for pancreatic cancer were stable among population groups except they increased among white men and women and API men. Melanoma death rates increased only among white men.[12]

IN UTERO AND EARLY LIFE CONDITIONS

From studies of the etiology of certain cancers, it is widely accepted that a long latency period precedes the onset of adult cancers. Accumulating data suggest early life events influence later susceptibility to certain chronic diseases (Figure 11-3).[13] Developmental plasticity is the degree to which an organism's development is contingent (external cues) on its environment. Specifically, the developmental origins' hypothesis postulates that nutrition and other environmental factors affect cellular pathways during gestation, enabling a single genotype to produce a broad range of adult phenotypes.[14] Plasticity refers to the ability of genes to organize physiologically or structurally in response to environmental conditions during fetal development. The hypothesis also postulates that persistent epigenetic adaptations that occur early in development in response to maternal nutrition and the environment are associated with increased susceptibility to cancer and other adult-onset chronic diseases.[15] Throughout in utero development, the placenta plays a major role in controlling growth and development.[16] Because the placenta is a regulator of the intrauterine environment and can be influenced by exposures throughout pregnancy,[16] much research

Global Cancer Statistics and Risk Factors Associated with Causes of Cancer Death

The growth of an aging population and increasing prevalence of established risk factors—smoking, overweight, physical inactivity, changing reproductive patterns associated with urbanization, and economic development—are increasing the occurrence of cancer In 2012 worldwide, based on GLOBOCAN, about 14.1 million new cancer cases and 8.2 million deaths occurred. Lung cancer is the leading cause of cancer death among males in both developed and developing countries and lung cancer has surpassed breast cancer as the leading cause of cancer death among females in more developed countries. Breast cancer is the leading cause of cancer death among females in less developed countries. In developed countries, other leading causes of cancer death include colorectal cancer among males and females and prostate cancer among males. In less developed countries, the leading causes of cancer death are liver and stomach cancer among males and cervical cancer among females. Of concern is that cancer incidence rates for all cancers combined are nearly twice as high in more developed countries in both genders, but mortality rates are only 8% to 15% higher in more developed countries. This disparity reflects many factors including geographic regional differences in the mix of types of cancer, which is effected by risk factors, detection practices, and availability of treatment. Risk factors associated with leading causes of cancer death include tobacco use (lung, colorectal, stomach, and liver cancer), overweight/obesity and physical inactivity (breast and colorectal cancer), and infection (liver, stomach, and cervical cancer). Effective application of tobacco control, vaccination, and use of early detection tests could prevent a substantial portion of cancer cases and deaths.

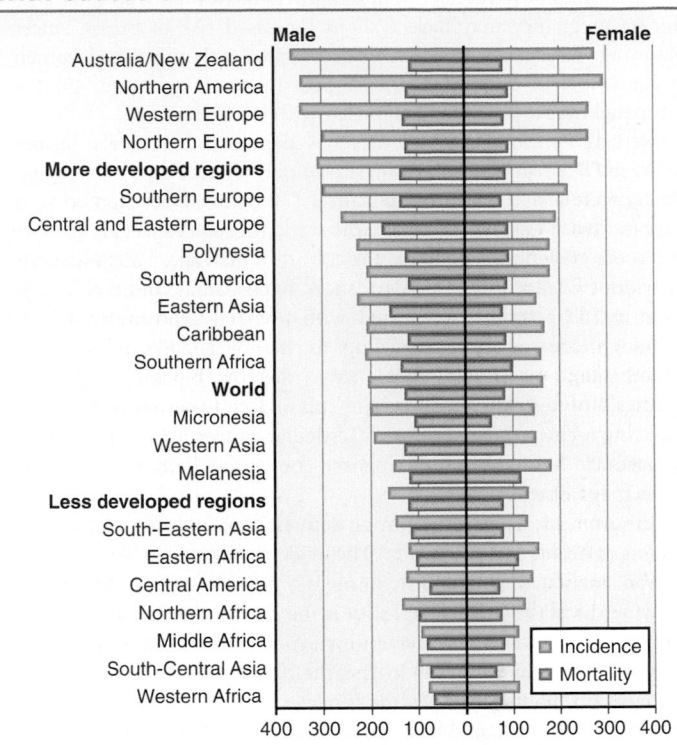

Data from Torre LA et al: *Cancer J Clin* 65(2):87-108, 2015.

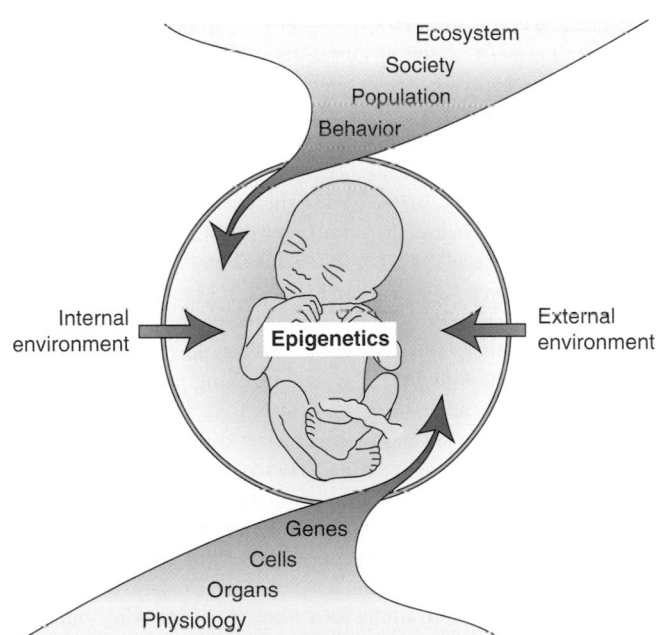

FIGURE 11-3 Fetal Vulnerability to External and Internal Environments. The fetus is particularly vulnerable to changes in the external and internal environments, which can have immediate and lifelong consequences. Such environmentally induced changes can occur at multiple levels, including molecular and behavioral. Ultimately these alterations may be epigenetic, inducing mitotically heritable alterations in gene expression without changing the DNA. (Adapted from Crews E, McLachlan JA: *Endocrinology* 147[6 suppl]:S4-S10, 2006.)

is being done with DNA methylation linking environmental cues to placental pathologies and adult life. The Dutch Famine Birth Cohort is a well-known study of the effects of prenatal undernutrition in humans. Undernutrition was linked to increased heart disease, metabolic disorders, and a possible link with breast cancer decades later.[17] Early versus late undernutrition in pregnancy indicated that the first trimester of pregnancy is particularly vulnerable to disease outcome in adulthood.[18] Much research is needed to understand nutrition in pregnancy and child vulnerabilities later in life. Recently, a striking experiment in mice demonstrated how extra vitamin doses during pregnancy in the mother's diet changed the fur color of pups.[19] This was the first study to show maternal nutrition and subsequent phenotype changes. The nutrients (B_{12}, folic acid, choline, and betaine) silenced the gene that rendered mice fat and yellow but did not alter its DNA sequence. Silencing, or switching the gene off, linked prenatal diet to such diseases as diabetes, obesity, and cancer. These concepts, called the *developmental basis of health and disease,* are defining the hypothesis of disease onset. Subsequently, the focus of disease prevention and intervention needs to include the decades before onset—that is, in utero and neonatal periods. Emerging studies on epigenetic mechanisms in dietary-associated transgenerational human disease will, hopefully, lead to beneficial health outcomes in the next generation.[18]

Perhaps one of the best examples of early life events and future cancer is the chemical exposure to diethylstilbestrol (DES), a synthetic nonsteroidal estrogen. This medication was prescribed between 1938 and 1971 to attempt to prevent multiple pregnancy-related problems, such as miscarriage, premature birth, and abnormal bleeding.[20] By the 1950s it became clear that DES interfered with the *development* of the reproductive system in the fetus and did not prevent miscarriage. Data suggest that a DES-associated increase in cancer of the female genital tract is elevated throughout a woman's reproductive years.[21,22] More recent studies have revealed that daughters of women who took DES during pregnancy may have a slight increased risk of breast cancer before age 40 (i.e., 1.9 times the risk compared with unexposed women at age 40).[23] For every 1000 DES-exposed women ages 45 to 49, it is estimated that four will be diagnosed with breast cancer.

Research from animal studies has demonstrated a relationship between DES exposure and an increased rate of a rare type of testicular cancer (rete testis) and prostate cancer.[24] Whether DES-exposed sons have increased risks of testicular cancer and prostate cancer are unclear and more evidence is needed as the cohort of men age.[22] Meta-analysis provides evidence that testicular cancer, hypospadias, and cryptorchidism are all positively associated with prenatal exposure to DES.[25] Although controversial, according to the NCI, DES inhibits the hypothalamic-pituitary-gonadal axis, thereby blocking testicular synthesis of testosterone, lowering plasma testosterone levels, and inducing a chemical castration.[22] Testicular cancer is becoming more common in low- and middle-income countries where optimal treatment may not exist.[26]

In summary, fetal programming defines, in part, the developmental origins of health and disease.[27,28] The evidence for specific DNA methylation marks, in utero environments, and future phenotypes is growing. Increasing the complexity is the recent report that genotype and gene-environmental interactions explain substantial proportions of interindividual variation in the methylome (set of nucleic acid methylation modifications in the genome or cell) at birth.[29] This new report suggests the possible importance in both fixed genetic variation and environmental factors in understanding epigenetic variation. In addition, epigenetic effects may help explain transgenerational effects[30] (Tables 11-2 and 11-3). For example, Newbold and colleagues[31] demonstrated that DES-related reproductive cancers in mice also occurred in the grandsons and granddaughters of mothers treated with DES.

TABLE 11-2 Differences Between Multigenerational and Transgenerational Phenotypes

Phenotype	Exposure	Definition
Multigenerational	Direct	Simultaneous exposure of multiple generations to an environmental factor
Transgenerational	Initial germline exposure (ancestral)	Transgenerational phenotype is transmitted to future generations via germline inheritance

TABLE 11-3 Somatic Versus Germ Cell Inheritance

Cell Type	Biologic Response
Somatic cells	Critical for adult-onset disease in exposed individual; not transmitted to future generations as transgenerational effect
Germ cells	Allows transmission between generations; promotes transgenerational phenotype

✔ QUICK CHECK 11-2
1. Discuss briefly the incidence rates and death rates of common cancers among racial and ethnic groups
1. Define developmental plasticity.
2. Discuss how epigenetic processes can be modified by environmental factors.
3. Define the developmental basis of health and disease.

ENVIRONMENTAL-LIFESTYLE FACTORS

Tobacco Use

Cigarette smoking is carcinogenic and remains the most important cause of cancer. Tobacco smoking causes cancer in more than 15 organ sites, and exposure to secondhand smoke and parental smoking causes cancer in daughters and sons and in other nonsmokers.[32,33] The largest preventable cause for cancer is tobacco use. More than 20 million premature deaths are attributable to smoking and exposure to secondhand smoke.[34] The risk is greatest in those who begin to smoke when young and continue throughout life, but tobacco smoking is pandemic, affecting more than 1 billion people of all ages.[32] Importantly, the eradication of tobacco use can only be achieved by preventing children and adolescents from starting tobacco use. Globally, tobacco use is greatest in developing countries, where 84% of 1.3 billion current smokers live.[35] Asia is now considered the largest tobacco producer and consumer in the world.[36] The World Health Organization (WHO) reports tobacco use causes more than 6 million deaths per year from cancer, chronic lung disease, cardiovascular disease, and stroke.[37] On average, smokers die 13 to 14 years earlier than nonsmokers[38]; about 25% will die prematurely during middle age (35 to 69 years).[39]

Cigarette smoking is the leading cause of preventable death in the United States, accounting for more than 480,000 deaths or 1 of every 5 deaths each year.[40] About 18.1% of all U.S. adults smoke cigarettes. Estimates of cigarette smoking by age are as follows: 17.3%, ages 18 to 24; 21.6%, ages 25 to 44; 19.5%, ages 45 to 64; and 8.9%, ages 65 and older.[40] Cigarette smoking is more common among men (20.5%) than women (15.8%), and the prevalence varies by race or ethnicity, or both, with American Indians/Alaska Natives (21.8%) having the highest prevalence and Asians (10.7%) having the lowest. It is more common among adults living below the poverty level (27.9%) than those at or above the poverty level (17.0%); it is significantly higher in the South (19.7%) and Midwest (20.6%) than in the West (14.2%) and Northeast (16.5%); and it is more prevalent in those having a disability/limitation (22.7%) than in those without a disability/limitation (16.5%).[40] During the period from 2005 to 2012, cigarette smoking prevalence declined among U.S. adults and the quit ratio increased.[41] Although the incidence of smoking is lower in women, the disease risks have risen sharply and are now equal to those in men for lung cancer, chronic obstructive pulmonary disease, and cardiovascular disease.[34]

Smoking affects nearly every organ of the body[34,42] (Figure 11-4). Since the first Surgeon General's report on smoking and health in 1964, more than 20 million Americans have died as a result of smoking.[34] Most of these deaths were adults with a history of smoking, but about 2.5 million were nonsmokers who died from lung cancer and heart disease from secondhand smoke[34] (see Figure 11-4). Secondhand smoke, also called environmental tobacco smoke (ETS), is the combination of sidestream smoke (burning end of a cigarette, cigar, or pipe) and mainstream smoke (exhaled by the smoker). More than 7000 chemicals have been identified in mainstream tobacco smoke. Nonsmokers who live with smokers are at greatest risk for lung cancer as well as numerous noncancerous conditions.[43] Additionally, another

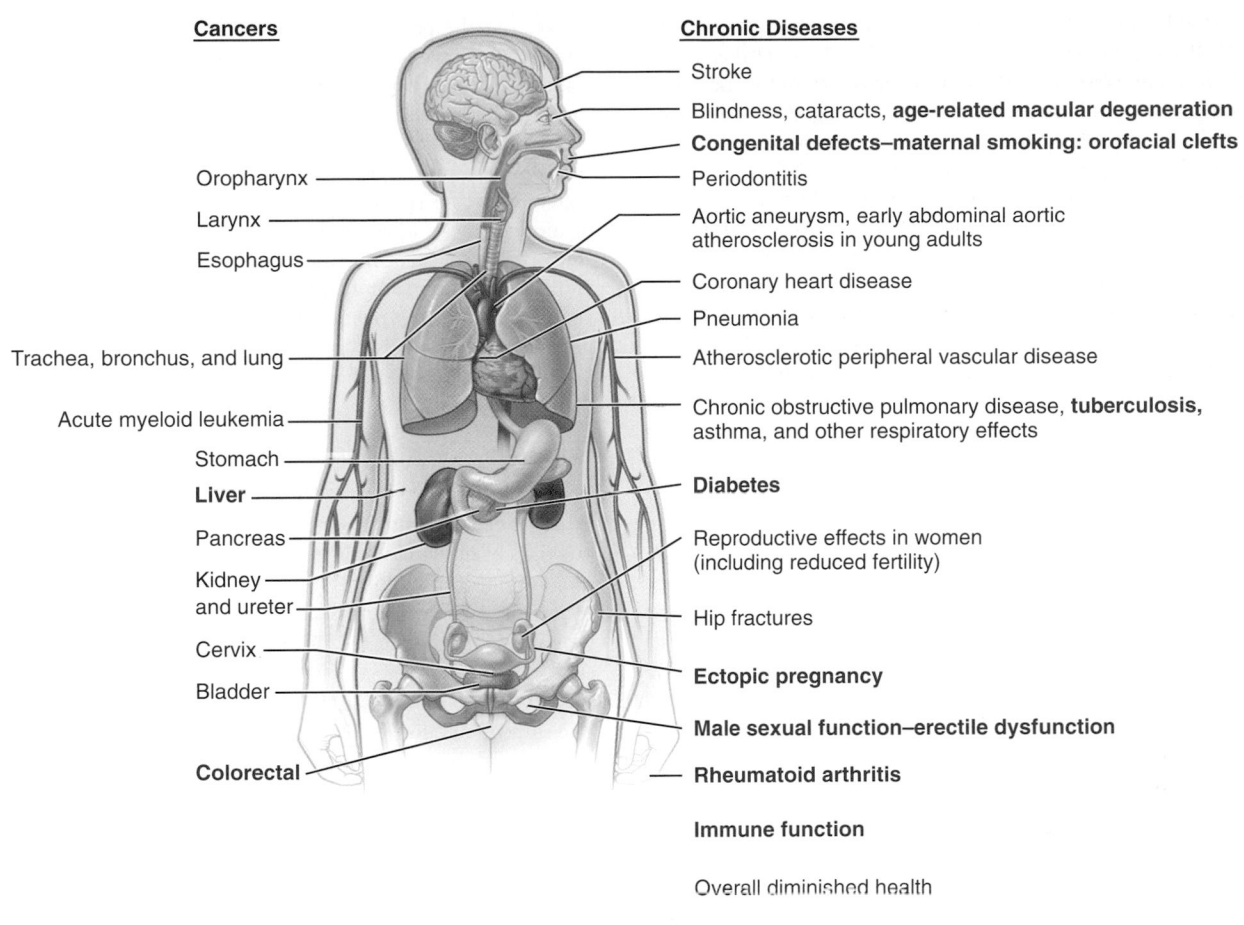

Cancers
- Oropharynx
- Larynx
- Esophagus
- Trachea, bronchus, and lung
- Acute myeloid leukemia
- Stomach
- **Liver**
- Pancreas
- Kidney and ureter
- Cervix
- Bladder
- **Colorectal**

Chronic Diseases
- Stroke
- Blindness, cataracts, **age-related macular degeneration**
- **Congenital defects–maternal smoking: orofacial clefts**
- Periodontitis
- Aortic aneurysm, early abdominal aortic atherosclerosis in young adults
- Coronary heart disease
- Pneumonia
- Atherosclerotic peripheral vascular disease
- Chronic obstructive pulmonary disease, **tuberculosis,** asthma, and other respiratory effects
- **Diabetes**
- Reproductive effects in women (including reduced fertility)
- Hip fractures
- **Ectopic pregnancy**
- **Male sexual function–erectile dysfunction**
- **Rheumatoid arthritis**
- **Immune function**
- Overall diminished health

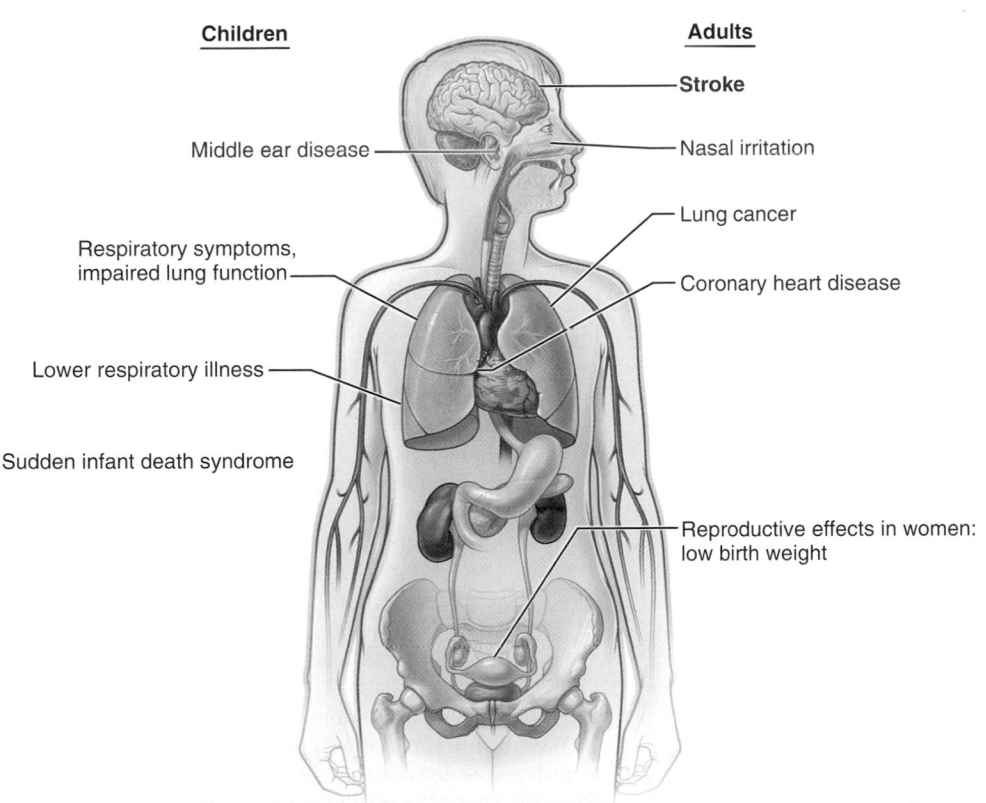

Children
- Middle ear disease
- Respiratory symptoms, impaired lung function
- Lower respiratory illness
- Sudden infant death syndrome

Adults
- **Stroke**
- Nasal irritation
- Lung cancer
- Coronary heart disease
- Reproductive effects in women: low birth weight

FIGURE 11-4 The Health Consequences Linked to Smoking. NOTE: The conditions in red are new diseases that have causally been linked to smoking. See text for discussion.

100,000 fatalities were babies who died of sudden infant death syndrome (SIDS) or complications from low birth weight or other conditions as a result of parental smoking, particularly from the mother.[34]

Smoking tobacco is linked to cancers of the lung, upper aerodigestive tract (oral cavity, pharynx, larynx, nasal cavity, paranasal sinuses, esophagus, and stomach), lower urinary tract (renal pelvis, penis, and bladder), kidney, pancreas, cervix, and uterus, as well as myeloid leukemia (see Figure 11-4). The new list of disease risks includes liver cancer and colorectal cancer. Secondhand smoke is a cause of stroke; increases the risk of death in people with cancer and cancer survivors as well as those with age-related macular degeneration, tuberculosis, ectopic pregnancy, and diabetes mellitus; increases inflammation; impairs immunity; and is a cause of rheumatoid arthritis. Smoking causes even more deaths from vascular, respiratory, and other diseases than from cancer. The epidemic of smoking ranks among the greatest health catastrophes of the century and has caused an enormous avoidable public health tragedy.[34]

Cigar or pipe smoking, or both, is strongly and causally related to cancers of the oral cavity, oropharynx, hypopharynx, larynx, esophagus, and lung. Cigar smokers who inhale deeply may be at increased risk for developing coronary heart disease and chronic obstructive pulmonary disease.[44] Pipe smokers have an increased risk of dying from cancers of the lung, lip, throat, esophagus, larynx, pancreas, and colon and rectum.[45] Consumption of loose tobacco (i.e., roll-your-own cigarette tobacco and pipe tobacco) changed substantially from 2000 to 2011.[46] Roll-your-own cigarette equivalent consumption decreased by 56.3%, whereas pipe tobacco consumption increased by 482.1%. Changes also were observed with cigars whereby consumption of small cigars decreased 65% and consumption of large cigars increased 233.1%. Consumption of pipe smoking and large cigars has increased substantially since the federal tobacco excise tax was increased for cigarettes in 2009, making these products less expensive.[46] Bidi smoking, a small amount of tobacco wrapped in the leaf of another plant (used in South Asia), delivers higher amounts of nicotine per gram of tobacco and comparable or greater amounts of tar compared with cigarettes.[47] Case-controlled studies indicate bidi smoking can cause cancers of the respiratory and digestive sites. A recent study in India show esophageal cancer is associated with smoking (including bidi) and alcohol.[48] The IARC reports *sufficient evidence* in humans that smokeless tobacco is associated with oral cavity, esophageal, and pancreatic cancers.[4]

The U.S. Department of Health and Human Services and the WHO Framework Convention on Tobacco Control (WHO FCTC) are the national and global tobacco control organizations for reducing both demand for and supply of tobacco products. Control policies enforce bans on tobacco advertising, promotion, and sponsorship and provide evidence that calls for dramatic action.

Diet

Understanding dietary factors that increase the risk for cancer is most important but can be difficult. The ways in which diet affects one's likelihood of developing cancer are complicated by the variety of foods consumed, the many constituents of foods, the metabolic consequences of eating, and the temporal changes in the patterns of food use. Cancer risks in older adults may depend as much on diet in early life as on current eating practices.[49] In addition, studies in humans targeting diet and disease associations face a variety of challenges including measurements of specific nutrients, food types, and dietary patterns.

Dietary sources of carcinogenic substances include compounds produced in the cooking of fat, meat, or protein and naturally occurring carcinogens associated with plant food substances, such as alkaloids or mold byproducts.[50] Figure 11-5 is a summary of convincing and probable judgments related to food and physical activity risk factors and the prevention of cancer.[50] Dietary components can act directly as mutagens or interfere with mutagen elimination. Abundant evidence exists that nutritional factors in many processes are related to cancer development (Figure 11-6).

Research is ongoing to understand the complexity of genomics, epigenomics, transcription factors (transcriptomics), proteomics, and metabolic factors (metabolomics) and the way that modifying any one or more of these factors influences cancer risk. Nutrigenomics is the study of the effects of nutrition on the phenotypic variability of individuals based on genomic differences (see Figure 11-6). Investigators are focusing on the sequence and functions of genes, single nucleotide polymorphisms (SNPs), and amplifications and deletions within the DNA sequences as modifiers of the response to foods and drinks and their components.[50]

Nutrition, Obesity, Alcohol Consumption, and Physical Activity: Impacts on Cancer

What we eat, how much we weigh, and how much we move influence our risks of developing cancer. Mounting evidence is clear—everyday *choices* impact our chances of getting or preventing cancer. Ongoing tedious and comprehensive investigative work is linking diet, body weight, and exercise to risk of specific cancers.

Nutrition

The implementation of dietary patterns (e.g., Mediterranean dietary pattern) and the promotion of specific dietary recommendations (e.g., dietary approaches to lower blood pressure) are becoming more widespread for fostering lifelong health.[51] The results of decades of research activity on the association of *specific* nutrients and foods and many forms of cancer have been controversial. Although so much in the cancer literature regarding nutrition is argued, it is difficult to ignore the data showing changes in cancer risk among migrants in low-risk countries compared with those in high-risk countries. For example, much of the geologic variation in incidence across the world for colorectal cancer has been attributed to differences in diet, particularly the consumption of red and processed meat, fiber, and alcohol, as well as body weight and physical activity.[52,53] With migration, these changes in risk are rapid and the most plausible determinants of such changes are the so-called adoption of the "Western" diet. Japan has seen a rapid increase in the incidence of colorectal cancer with westernization of diet.[54] It seems clear that focusing on dietary patterns, as well as meaningful biomarkers reflecting specific nutritional factors relevant to carcinogenesis, may be a more successful approach. The following important cellular processes are affected by nutrition (Figure 11-7):

- The cell cycle
- The balance between cell proliferation and cell death (e.g., apoptosis)
- Cell differentiation
- Genes, including oncogenes and tumor-suppressor genes
- Cell signaling
- Gene expression
- Cellular microenvironment that influences gene expression
- Epigenetic regulation
- Hormonal regulation
- DNA damage and repair
- Carcinogen metabolism
- Inflammation and immunity

Gene expression is influenced by epigenetic processes such as DNA methylation or acetylation (addition of an acetyl group) (see Chapters 3 and 10). Dietary sources of methyl groups, including folate, methionine, betaine, serine, and choline, are primary potential donors as modulators of DNA methylation[55] (Figure 11-8). A recent report from

FIGURE 11-5 Summary of Convincing and Probable Judgments. (From World Cancer Research Fund/American Institute for Cancer Research: *Food, nutrition, physical activity, and the prevention of cancer: a global perspective*, Washington, DC, 2007, AICR.)

FIGURE 11-6 Basis for the Study of Food, Nutrition, Obesity, Physical Activity, and the Cancer Process. The genetic message in the DNA code is translated to RNA, and then into protein synthesis, and so determines metabolic processes. Research methods, called "-omics," address these different stages. (Adapted from World Cancer Research Fund/American Institute for Cancer Research: *Food, nutrition, physical activity, and the prevention of cancer: a global perspective*, Washington, DC, 2007, AICR.)

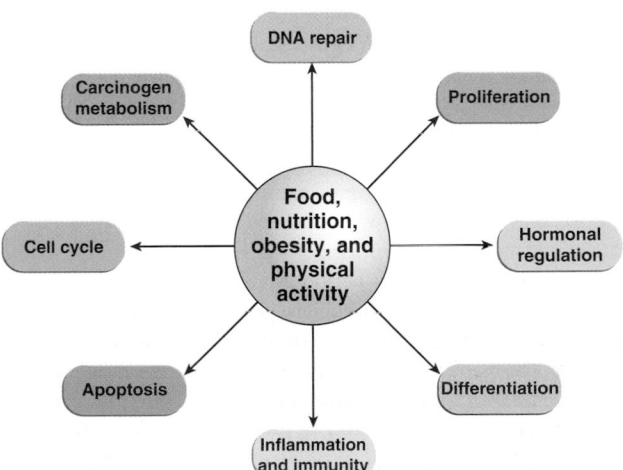

FIGURE 11-7 Food, Nutrition, Obesity, Physical Activity, and Cellular Processes Linked to Cancer. Food, nutrition, and physical activity can influence fundamental processes shown here, which may promote or inhibit cancer development and progression. (Adapted from World Cancer Research Fund/American Institute for Cancer Research: *Food, nutrition, physical activity, and the prevention of cancer: a global perspective*, Washington, DC, 2007, AICR.)

Bioactive Food Substances in Epigenetics

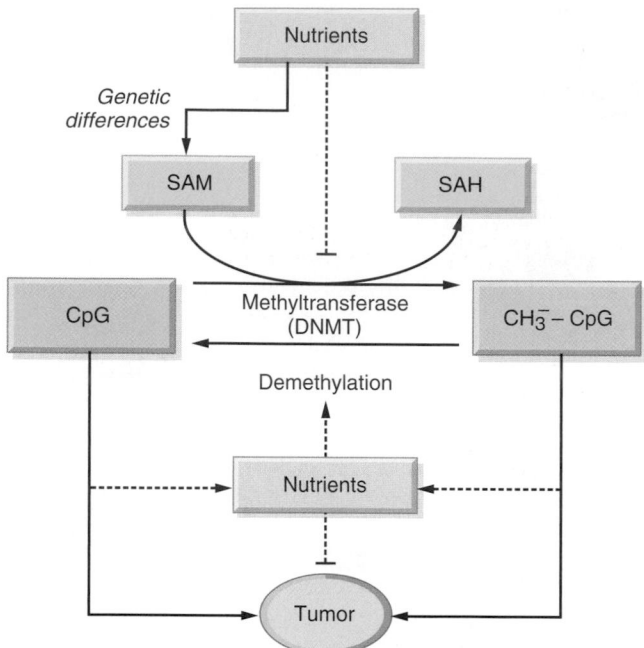

FIGURE 11-8 Dietary Factors, DNA Methylation, and Cancer. Certain dietary factors (see Table 11-5) may supply methyl groups (+CH₃) that can be donated through *S*-adenosylmethionine *(SAM)* to many acceptors in the cell (DNA, proteins, lipids, and metabolites). Donation and removal (demethylation) are affected by numerous enzymes, including DNA methyltransferase *(DNMT)*. Increased DNMT activity occurs in many tumor cells. Hypermethylation can inhibit or silence tumor-suppressor genes (see Chapter 10), and DNA methylation inhibitors as anticancer agents can block DNMT, thus reactivating tumor-suppressor genes. DNA hypomethylation can reactivate and mutate genes, including cancer-causing oncogenes. *SAH, S*-Adenosylhomocysteine.

the European Prospective Investigation into Cancer and Nutrition (EPIC) found individuals with high plasma concentrations of methionine, choline, and betaine may be at reduced risk of colorectal cancer.[56]

B vitamins, coenzymes in one-carbon metabolism (vitamins B₂, B₆, B₁₂), also are modulators of DNA methylation.[57] To date there are limited human studies of the effects of methyl donor supply on methylation of specific genomic sequences.[55] However, a study[58] found that periconceptional maternal supplementation with 400 micrograms (mcg) of folic acid per day was associated with increased methylation in offspring aged 17 months. In experimental animals, maternal diet during the periconceptional period established DNA methylation in the offspring with permanent phenotypic changes.[59] In the Waterland study,[60] methylation effects were found to be similar in all tissues examined, suggesting that the mechanism may alter markings in stem cells early in embryogenesis before tissue differentiation, and persist into adult life. Choline deficiency in pregnancy results in hypermethylation of genomic DNA and of the *IGF2* gene.[61] Several studies have reported that severe folate deficiency (which increases the risk of hepatocellular cancer) induces hypomethylation of the *p53* tumor-suppressor gene.[62-64] In vitro studies have shown that several bioactive food components, including tea polyphenols and bioflavonoids, inhibit DNA methyltransferase (DNMT)-mediated DNA methylation in a dose-dependent manner[65] (see Figure 11-8). Acetylation and deacetylation are mediated by enzyme histones, histone acetyl transferase

(HAT), and histone deacetylation (HDAC). Dietary components have been identified that act as regulators of gene expression by epigenetic mechanisms.[66,67] For example, there is strong evidence for the epigenetic effects of organosulfur compounds from garlic and of isothiocyanates from cruciferous vegetables.[66] Butyrate produced in the colon by bacterial fermentation of non–starch polysaccharide (fiber), diallyl disulfide from garlic and other allium vegetables, and sulforaphane from cruciferous vegetables can act as histone deacetylase inhibitors to maintain DNA stability or modify transcription.[50] A recent laboratory study found sulforaphane to inhibit modulators of inflammation in human mammary epithelial cells.[68]

Studies involving cultured cancer cells and animal models have illustrated the potential protective role of dietary polyphenols, such as curcumin, resveratrol, genistein, epigallocatechin-3-gallate, and indole-3-carbinol and its derivative 3,3′-diindolylmethane. The effects of these dietary agents may include antiproliferation and pro-apoptosis through the epigenetic regulation of miRNAs.[69] Because of the promising results from these in vitro and in vivo studies, the efficacies of these natural agents in cancer therapies are being investigated in clinical trials (see www.clinicaltrials.gov/). Interest in resveratrol, a polyphenolic compound with anti-inflammatory, antioxidant, and anticancer activities, is growing because of its demonstrable role in possibly delaying age-related diseases, including cancers.[70] Feeding mice a diet supplemented with human equivalent doses of 105 and 210 mg of resveratrol daily resulted in inhibition of colorectal tumors through an epigenetic mechanism (miR-96, a miRNA).[70] Yet, a recent prospective cohort study in older community-dwelling adults found total urinary resveratrol metabolite concentration was not associated with inflammatory markers, cardiovascular disease, or cancer or predictive of all-cause mortality.[71] More research needs to be done with resveratrol.

MicroRNA (miRNA) expression in response to diet may be involved in several cancers.[50] Several dietary factors, including macronutrients (fat, protein, and alcohol) and micronutrients (folate and vitamin E, curcumin), alter the expression of many miRNAs in animals and humans[55,72] (see Chapter 10). Curcumin analogs (compared with just curcumin) with increased anticancer activity and solubility, such as EF24 (3,5-bis(2-fluorobenzylidene)piperidin-4-one), show enhanced expression of potential tumor-suppressor miRNAs.[73]

Bioactive components have a profound effect on differentiation and a major area of investigation is on the differentiation of cancer stem cells. Cancer stem cells have been isolated and identified in hematopoietic and epithelial cancers, including cancers of the brain, breast, ovary, prostate, colon, and stomach.[50,74] Stem cells are found among most adult tissues, where they maintain and regenerate tissues. Stem cells can remodel organs in response to physiologic triggers—*adaptive resizing*.[75] Cancer stem cells utilize several developmental mechanisms for self-renewal and these mechanisms appear to be fundamental to the initiation and recurrence of tumors. Even if chemotherapy or radiation eliminates cancer cells, it is only when the cancer stem cells are destroyed that a full recovery is achievable.[74] Repopulation with radioresistant or chemoresistant stem cells may significantly contribute to therapy resistance. Evidence from both drug and bioactive food constituents shows modifications in cancer stem cell self-renewal capabilities; for example, retinoic acid may promote differentiation of breast cancer stem cells.[76] Adequate consumption of specific food compounds, including vitamins A and D, genistein, green tea, epigallocatechin gallate (EGCG), sulforaphane, theanine, curcumin, choline, and possibly many others, may suppress cancer stem renewal.[74] An uncontrolled self-renewal process may be initiated by abnormal developmental signals that come from the extracellular microenvironment known as "niches." The loss of regulation in self-renewal signals,

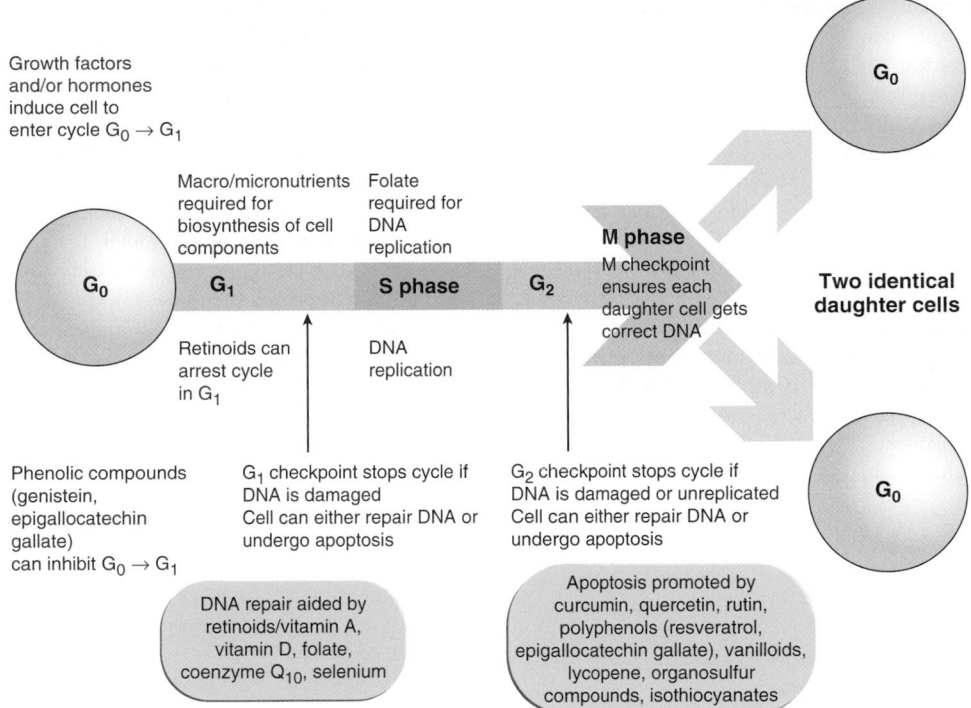

FIGURE 11-9 Cell Cycle and Nutrition Regulation. Nutrition may influence the regulation of the normal cell cycle, which ensures correct DNA replication. G_0 represents the resting phase, G_1 the growth and preparation of the chromosome for replication, S the synthesis of DNA, G_2 the preparation of the cell for division, and M mitosis. (Adapted from World Cancer Research Fund/American Institute for Cancer Research: *Food, nutrition, physical activity, and the prevention of cancer: a global perspective,* Washington, DC, 2007, AICR.)

including Wnt, Notch, and hedgehog pathways, is a characteristic of cancer stem cells.[74] Various food bioactive components can modulate the signaling pathway.

A variety of food constituents may influence DNA repair[50,77] (Figure 11-9). Observational studies suggest that malnutrition can reduce DNA repair from damage.[78] In vivo studies have demonstrated that healthy adults consuming kiwi fruits, cooked carrots, or supplemental coenzyme Q_{10} improved their DNA repair.[50] Consumption of lycopene-rich vegetable juice was associated with significantly decreased damage to the DNA of lung epithelial cells in healthy adults.[79]

Humans are constantly exposed to a variety of compounds termed **xenobiotics** (the Greek word *xenos* means "foreign"; *bios* means "life") that include toxic, mutagenic, and carcinogenic chemicals. Many of these chemicals are found in the human diet. Most xenobiotics are transported in the blood by lipoproteins and penetrate lipid membranes (see Chapter 4). The body has two main defense systems for counteracting these effects: (1) detoxification enzymes and (2) antioxidant systems (see Chapter 4). Enzymes that activate xenobiotics are called **phase I activation enzymes**. **Phase II detoxification enzymes** then protect further against a large array of reactive intermediates and nonactivated xenobiotics.[50] These enzymes are located predominantly in the liver and provide clearance of compounds through the portal circulation, thereby preventing the potentially carcinogenic agent(s) from entering the body through the gastrointestinal tract and portal circulation. They also occur in the skin epithelia and can be induced in other extrahepatic tissue, such as the lung. They represent a potential target to influence carcinogen metabolism. Isothiocyanates from cruciferous vegetables induce the expression of phase II detoxification enzymes. Food and nutrition modify carcinogen metabolism and may modify carcinogenesis.

Glutathione-*S*-transferases (GSTs) are enzyme housekeepers involved in the metabolism of environmental carcinogens and reactive oxygen species. Individuals who lack these enzymes may be at higher risk for cancers because of decreased capacity to dispose of activated carcinogens. For example, the fungi that produce aflatoxins can grow on certain crops such as peanuts and some cereals (e.g., grains). Aflatoxins are carcinogens activated by phase I enzymes in the liver that can produce DNA adducts. Individuals lacking these enzymes are at higher risk of colon cancer. Diets high in isothiocyanates (from cruciferous vegetables) may decrease this risk.[80] Individuals who consume diets high in red meat and processed meat and who carry certain genetic polymorphisms have an increased risk of developing colorectal cancer.[50,81-83] Processed meats include those treated by preservatives or by smoking, curing, or salting. The European Prospective Investigation into Cancer and Nutrition (EPIC) study, which included 478,040 people from 10 countries, reports that the most convincing data are from meats, including sausages, bratwursts, frankfurters, and hot dogs, all of which have nitrites, nitrates, or other preservatives. These *N*-nitroso compounds can increase nitrogenous residues in the colon and cause DNA damage.[50] Dietary components either can be activated into potential carcinogens through metabolic processes or can be inactivated and prevent DNA damage.[50] High intake of red meat may result in the synthesis of higher levels of heme iron; iron can activate oxidative stress and inflammation in the colon. Meat may have certain thermoresistant oncogenic bovine viruses (e.g., polyoma-papilloma) or possible single-stranded DNA viruses.[84] Certain single nucleotide polymorphisms (SNPs) in the *N*-acetyltransferase gene alter the activity of the enzyme involved in the activation of heterocyclic amines from cooking meat at high temperatures and may increase the risk of colon cancer.[50]

Red cabbage leads to changes in meat-derived mutagens in urine.[50] Flavonoids found in plants may alter carcinogen metabolism, and dietary indole-3-carbinol inhibited spontaneous occurrence of endometrial adenocarcinomas in rats.[50]

Chronic inflammation and immune function may help explain patterns of cancer around the world. People who are undernourished or live in poverty may have impaired immune status, which can be a factor in cancers caused by infectious agents, for example, cancers of the liver and cervix.[50]

Diet affects many pathways to cancer (see p. 276) and many of these processes are likely influenced, if not regulated, by DNA methylation, an epigenetic mechanism that affects gene function (also see Chapter 3). As illustrated in Figure 11-10, it is possible that many environmental factors interact with the genome to produce altered epigenetic markers that change the expression of cancer-causing genes, tumor-suppressor genes, and oncogenes. Future research is needed to define robust biomarkers of cancer risk.

Obesity

Obesity in most developed countries (and in urban areas of many developing countries) has been increasing rapidly over the past 20 years. Obesity in the United States is an epidemic and constitutes a startling setback to major improvements in other areas of health during the past century.[85] In 2012, more than one third of children and adolescents were overweight or obese.[86] Numerous health conditions are linked to obesity and physical inactivity. The substantial suffering and long-term human and societal costs of obesity underlie the urgency to accelerate progress in obesity prevention.[85] Studies have significantly improved the understanding of the relationship between overweight/obesity, energy balance and cancer risk, cancer recurrence, and survival.[50,87,88] Consensus now exists that obesity is a risk factor for cancers of the endometrium, colorectum, kidney, esophagus, breast (postmenopausal), and pancreas. Evidence is evolving of the association between obesity and cancers of the thyroid, gallbladder, liver, and ovary, as well as aggressive types of prostate cancer and non-Hodgkin

FIGURE 11-10 Epigenetic Modulation and Modifications. **A,** Overview of the potential role of epigenetic modulation by dietary and other environmental factors in cancer development. **B,** Epigenetic modulation model according to current knowledge. The different types of chemical modifications, such as methylation or acetylation, of promoter regions and/or other regulatory DNA sequences outside the gene can have a severe impact on gene transcription and translation and a resultant high modulation of gene expression and product (protein) functionality. (**B,** Adapted from Nowsheen S, et al.: *Cancer Letters* 342(3):213-222, 2014.)

lymphoma.[50,87] Importantly, obesity is recognized as a poor prognostic factor for several cancers.[89-91]

The only globally accepted criteria for overweightness and obesity are based on the body mass index (BMI). Widely accepted standards based on BMI criteria for overweightness and obesity are recommended by the WHO[50] (Table 11-4) and supported by other panels and federal agencies. According to the WHO, worldwide obesity has doubled since 1980 and more than 1.4 billion adults, 20 years of age and older, were overweight. Of these, more than 200 million men and 300 million women were obese. Worldwide, more than 40 million children younger than age 5 years were overweight or obese in 2012.[92]

The mechanisms of obesity-associated cancer risks are unclear and may vary by type of tumor and distribution of body fat. Emerging, however, are three main factors related to obesity and cancer: (1) the insulin–insulin-like growth factor 1 (IGF-1) axis, (2) sex hormones, and (3) adipokines or adipocyte-derived cytokines.[93] These three factors are linked to metabolic dysregulation of adipose tissue and endocrine and paracrine altered signaling of adipose tissue in obesity.[93,94] Metabolic changes in adipose tissue from obesity result in several alterations and include insulin resistance, hyperglycemia, dyslipidemia, hypoxia, and chronic inflammation.[93,95] Because tumor growth is regulated by interactions between tumor cells and their tissue microenvironment or stromal compartments that are rich in adipose tissue, adipocytes function as endocrine cells and critically shape the tumor microenvironment. Dysfunctional adipose tissue can create altered signaling pathways that involve proinflammatory mediators, macrophages, and cancer-associated fibroblasts. All of these cells are tumor-promoting cell types and, with insulin resistance and hypoxia, can trigger compensatory angiogenesis and an energy reservoir for the embedded cancer cells.[93] The cancer-associated adipocytes (CAAs) undergo both structural and functional alterations during cancer progression that altogether create an environment toward increased cancer invasiveness and aggression[93] (Figure 11-11).

Alcohol Consumption

Alcohol is classified by the International Agency for Cancer Research as a human carcinogen. Excessive alcohol plays a contributory role in several common cancers.[50] Overall, there are strong data linking alcohol with cancers of the mouth, pharynx, larynx, esophagus, liver, colorectum, and breast[4,50,55,96] (Table 11-5). The evidence does not show any "safe limit" of intake, and the effect is from ethanol regardless of the type of drink.[50]

Mechanisms involved in alcohol-related carcinogenesis include the effect of acetaldehyde, the first metabolite of ethanol oxidation; the induction of cytochrome P-450 2E1 (genetic variant CYP2E1) leading to the generation of reactive oxygen species (ROS); increased pro-carcinogen activation (e.g., nitrosamines); modulation of cellular regeneration (cell cycle); nutritional deficiencies (retinol, retinyl esters, folic acid, other vitamins) that may predispose to altered mucosal integrity and enzyme and metabolic dysfunction; and other structural abnormalities. Inherited factors also put some individuals at increased risk in DNA repair ability, carcinogen metabolism, and cell cycle control.[84] Recent investigation is concerned with epigenetic mechanisms and alcohol metabolism.[97,98] Figure 11-12 summarizes some of these epigenetic mechanisms and the effects of alcohol metabolism that may be important for cancer pathogenesis.

TABLE 11-4 WHO Classification of Body Mass Index (BMI)

BMI (kg/m²)*	WHO Classification	Other Descriptions
<18.5	Underweight	Thin
18.5-24.9	Normal range	"Healthy," "normal," or "acceptable" weight
25-29.9	Preobese	Overweight
30-34.9	Obese class I	Obesity
35-39.9	Obese class II	—*
>40	Obese class III	Morbidly overweight

Data available at: http://apps.who.int/bmi/index.jsp?introPage=intro_3 .html.

WHO, World Health Organization.

*The cutoffs are somewhat arbitrary, although they are derived from epidemiologic studies of BMI and overall mortality. It is important to understand that within each category of BMI there can be substantial individual variation in total and visceral adiposity and in related metabolic factors. These variations are also true for the normal range BMI.

TABLE 11-5 Alcoholic Drinks and Risk of Cancer*

	DECREASES RISK		INCREASES RISK	
	Exposure	Cancer Site	Exposure	Cancer Site
Convincing			Alcoholic drinks	Mouth, pharynx and larynx, esophagus
				Colorectum (men)†
				Breast (pre- and postmenopause)
Probable			Alcoholic drinks	Liver‡
				Colorectum (women)†
Limited—suggestive				
Substantial effect on risk unlikely	Alcoholic drinks (adverse effect): kidney§			

Adapted from World Cancer Research Fund/American Institute for Cancer Research (WCRF/AICR): *Second expert report: food, nutrition, physical activity, and the prevention of cancer: a global perspective*, London, 2007, Author.

*In the judgment of the Panel (WCRF/AICR), the factors listed modify the risk of cancer. Judgments are graded according to the strength of the evidence.

†The judgments for men and women are different because there are fewer data for women. Increased risk is only apparent above a threshold of 30 g/day of ethanol for both genders.

‡Cirrhosis is an essential precursor of liver cancer caused by alcohol. The International Agency for Research on Cancer has graded alcohol as a class 1 carcinogen for liver cancer. Alcohol alone only causes cirrhosis in the presence of other factors.

§The evidence was sufficient to judge that alcoholic drinks are unlikely to have an adverse effect on the risk of kidney cancer; it was inadequate to draw a conclusion regarding the protective effect.

FIGURE 11-11 Structural and Functional Changes in Adipocytes and Interaction with the Microenvironment Contribute to Cancer Progression and Metastases: A Working Model. **A,** Signaling interactions occur between cancer cells and cancer-associated adipocytes. This interaction within the tumor microenvironment creates a place or *niche* permissive for cancer growth. Cancer cells stimulate the breakdown of lipids in adipocytes, leading to *delipidation* and the emergence of a fibroblast-like phenotype in adipocytes. The continuing alterations are associated with functional changes in the cells and include increased secretion of inflammatory mediators (cytokines) and proteases, and increased release of free fatty acids. All of these changes can support tumor growth and invasiveness. **B,** Obesity leads to excessive levels of proinflammatory cytokines, sex hormones, lipid metabolites, and altered adipokines. The altered adipose tissue becomes a source of various extracellular matrix proteins, cancer stem cells, and cancer-associated adipokines. Collectively these alterations contribute to tumor initiation, growth, and recurrence. The systemic metabolic changes of obesity—hyperinsulinemia and hyperglycemia—can further contribute to a tumor-permissive environment. (Adapted from Park J et al: *Nat Rev Endocrinol* 10[8]:455-465, 2014.)

Interactions Between Alcohol Metabolism and Epigenetics

FIGURE 11-12 Alcohol Metabolism and Epigenetics. Chronic alcohol intake leads to decreased methylation called hypomethylation by decreasing S-adenosylmethionine *(SAM)* that is used by DNA enzymes called methyltransferases *(DNMTs)* and histone enzymes called methyl transferases *(HMTs)* to methylate DNA and histones. Additionally, alcohol metabolism increases the ratio of the coenzyme reduced nicotinamide adenine dinucleotide *(NADH)* to the oxidized nicotinamide adenine dinucleotide *(NAD+)*; this step inhibits the sirtuin enzyme SIRT1, which interferes with normal histone acetylation patterns. (Adapted from Zakhari S: Alcohol metabolism and epigenetic changes, *Alcohol Res* 35[1]:6-16, 2013.)

Physical Activity

Physical activity reduces the risk of breast and colon cancers and may reduce the risk of other cancers including endometrial, lung, and prostate cancers.[99] Several biologic mechanisms causing this effect have been proposed and include decreasing insulin and IGF levels; decreasing obesity; increasing free radical scavenger systems; altering inflammatory mediators; decreasing levels of circulating sex hormones and metabolic hormones; improving immune function; enhancing cytochrome P-450, thus modifying carcinogen activation; and increasing gut motility.[100-102] For colon cancer, physical activity increases gut motility, which reduces the length of time (transit time) that the bowel lining is exposed to potential mutagens.[103] For breast cancer, vigorous physical activity may decrease exposure of breast tissue to ovarian hormones, insulin, and IGF. A randomized trial found that after 12 months of moderate-intensity exercise, postmenopausal women had significantly decreased levels of serum estrogens.[104] Physical activity also helps prevent type 2 diabetes, which has been associated with risk of cancer of the colon and pancreas.[103,105]

Many questions are unanswered regarding frequency, intensity, and duration of exercise. Much of the literature suggests that between 3.5 and 4 hours of vigorous activity per week are necessary to optimize protection for colon cancer.[102] There is likely a dose-response relationship for colon cancer and breast cancer, and 30 to 60 minutes per day of moderate to vigorous intensity activity is proposed to decrease breast cancer risk.[106] A randomized controlled trial (12 months) recently supported the Institute of Medicine and Department of Agriculture guidelines of 60 minutes per day of moderate to vigorous physical activity for decreasing weight, BMI, and percent of body fat and intra-abdominal fat.[107] A Cochrane review found that aerobic exercise was beneficial for adults with cancer-related fatigue during and after cancer treatment.[108] Another Cochrane review found exercise in children with cancer was associated with improved body composition, flexibility, and cardiorespiratory fitness.[109] More research on exercise for adults and children for prevention of cancer, postcancer treatment, and survivors of cancer is needed.

Ionizing Radiation

Much of the knowledge of the effects of ionizing radiation on human cancer has stemmed from observations of the Hiroshima and Nagasaki atomic bomb exposures, particularly the Life Span Study. These data provide the best estimate of human cancer risk over the dose range from 20 to 250 centigray (cGy) for low linear energy transfer (LET) radiation, such as x-rays or γ-rays. Other evidence is derived from groups exposed for medical reasons, underground miners exposed to radon gas, and other occupational exposures (Table 11-6). The atomic bomb exposures in Japan caused acute leukemias in adults and children and increased frequencies of thyroid and breast carcinomas. Lung, stomach, colon, esophageal, and urinary tract cancers and multiple myeloma have been added to the list. At Nagasaki and Hiroshima, leukemia incidence in individuals 15 years or younger reached its peak 6 to 7 years after the explosions and has steadily declined since 1952. People 45 years and older at the time of exposure had a latent period of 20 years before developing acute leukemia.

Recently, standard models and evaluations of age of exposure to radiation and radiation-induced cancer risks have been questioned.[110-112] Epidemiologic data from Japanese atomic bomb survivors and from children exposed to radiation for medical intervention suggest that excess relative risks (ERRs) for radiation-induced cancers at a given age are exceptionally higher for individuals exposed during childhood than for those exposed at older ages.[113] These data also are published by the International Commission on Radiological Protection (ICRP) and the National Academy of Sciences Committee on the Biological Effects of Ionizing Radiation (BEIR Committee).[114] What is at question is the ERRs of radiation exposure in *adulthood* and radiation-induced cancer risk. Recent analyses of Japanese bomb survivors suggest that the ERR for cancer induction decreases with increasing age at exposure only until exposure ages of 30 to 40 years; with radiation exposure at older ages, the ERR does not decrease further and for many individual cancer sites (liver, colon, lung, stomach, and bladder) the EER may actually increase in all solid cancers combined.[110,112,115] These new data present a challenge to conceptual understanding of the mechanisms of cancer induction.[112] Biologic models of cancer development all predict that ERRs should decrease continuously with increasing age of radiation exposure. Recent models,

however, of radiation carcinogenesis show ionizing radiation acts not only as an *initiator* of premalignant cell clones but also as a *promoter* of preexisting premalignant cell alterations.[110,112,115] Promotion is used here to mean the process by which an initiated cell clonally expands. Therefore, promotional processes from radiation can result in increasing excess lifetime cancer risks with increasing age at exposure. From these new data investigators propose that radiation-induced cancer risks after exposure in middle age may be almost twice as high as previously estimated.[112]

Human exposure to ionizing radiation includes emissions from the environment (e.g., radon), x-rays, CT scans, radioisotopes, and other radioactive sources (Figure 11-13). Health risks involve not only neoplastic diseases but also cardiovascular disease and stroke following high doses in therapeutic medicine and lower doses in A-bomb survivors (BEIR VII).[114,116] Late effects of radiation in A-bomb survivors show persistent elevations of inflammatory markers, implying immunologic damage may be the cause of later cardiovascular effects.[117] For the first time, investigators using a model of umbilical vein endothelial cells showed that low doses (0.05 Gy) of x-rays induce DNA damage and apoptosis in endothelial cells. These findings will need continued research.[118] Cardiac and blood vessel damage may manifest years after completion of radiation therapy.[119] Other risks include somatic mutations that may contribute to other diseases (e.g., birth defects and eye maladies) and, from animal studies, inherited mutations that may affect the incidence of diseases in future generations. Exposure to diagnostic radiography in utero has been associated with childhood cancer, particularly leukemia.[120-122] The link or association between in utero irradiation and childhood cancer is, however, controversial and varies with study methodology.[123] Heritable mutations are of particular concern for women because the number of oocytes is presumably fixed at birth and mutations, if not repaired, are cumulative.[124] An important summary point in BEIR VII[114] is the concern from high-dose medical

TABLE 11-6   Cancer Associated with Exposure to Ionizing Radiation

Cancer Type	AB	AS	PM	TC	TH	RP	UM	RD
Leukemia	X	X			X			X
Thyroid	X			X				
Breast	X		X					
Lung	X	X			X		X	
Bone						X		
Stomach	X	X						
Esophagus	X	X						
Lymphoma	X	X						X
Brain				X			X	
Liver					X			
Skin					X		X	X

Data from Jones JA et al: Ionizing radiation as a carcinogen. In McQueen E, editor: *CA comprehensive toxicology*, ed 2, St Louis, 2010, Elsevier.

AB, Atomic bomb survivors; *AS,* ankylosing spondylitis patients; *PM,* postpartum mastitis patients; *TC,* tinea capitis patients; *TH,* individuals receiving Thorotrast; *RD,* radiologists; *RP,* radium dial painters; *UM,* underground miners.

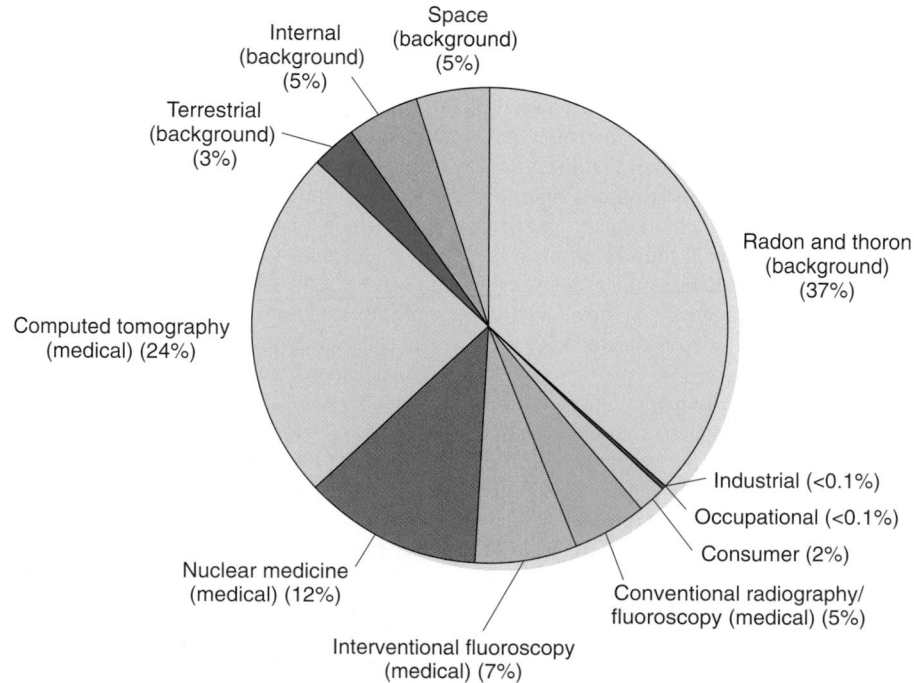

FIGURE 11-13 Pie Chart Showing Sources of Exposure to Ionizing Radiation. Percent contribution of various sources of exposure to the total collective effective dose (1,870,000 person-Sv) and the total effective dose per individual in the U.S. population (6.2 mSv) for 2006. Percent values have been rounded to the nearest 1%, except those <1%. *Sv,* Sievert. (From NCRP: *2009 Ionizing radiation exposure of the population of the United States,* NCRP Report No. 160, Bethesda, Md, 2009, Author.)

exposure, for example, computed tomography (CT) scans (see *Health Alert: Increasing Use of Computed Tomography Scans and Risks*). In 2009 the National Council on Radiation Protection and Measurements (NCRP)[125] reported Americans were exposed to more than seven times as much ionizing radiation from medical procedures as compared with that in the 1980s. The increased exposure is mostly because of the rapid increase in the use of CT imaging.[126] The increase in imaging is likely driven by several factors, including improvements in the technology, that have led to increased clinical applications, patient demand, physician demand, defensive medical practices, and medical uncertainty.[127]

The risks of low-dose radiation are being debated among radiobiologists, geneticists, physicists, and others because of the potential effect on the health of current and future generations.[128] The expression of radiation-induced damage depends not only on dose, fractionation, and protraction but also on repair mechanisms; bystander effects; radioprotective substances, such as antioxidants; and the mechanism of radiation delivery.[124]

Radiation-Induced Cancer

Ionizing radiation (IR) is a mutagen and carcinogen and can penetrate cells and tissues and deposit energy in tissues at random in the form of ionizations (e.g., excitation or removal of an electron from the target atom). These ionizations can lead to irreversible or indirect damage from formation and attack by water-based free radicals (radiolysis).[128] The *general* characteristics of IR-induced carcinogenesis are well established.[129] The past two decades have focused on *specific* cellular and

molecular mechanisms that relate to the induction of cancer, including dose-response relationships for chromosome aberrations, cell transformation, gene expression (genetic and epigenetic), alternative targets, mutagenesis in somatic cells, the biologic effects that occur in nonirradiated cells (i.e., **nontargeted effects**), and effects on the microenvironment.[130] IR is a potent DNA-damaging agent causing cross-linking, nucleotide base damage, and single- and double-strand breaks[131] to DNA and disrupted cellular regulation processes can lead to carcinogenesis.[131] The double-strand break (DSB) (Figure 11-14) is considered the characteristic lesion observed for the effects of IR. In certain experimental systems, a single DSB may lead to cell cycle arrest and possible further repair. Yet many DSBs appear to result from clustered damage, a consequence of the pattern of distribution of ionizations with DNA. These patterns of clustered damage may be more difficult to accurately repair.[132] Importantly, DSBs are mostly repaired by the nonhomologous end joining (NHEJ) pathway. This pathway is efficient for joining the DNA broken ends; however, errors can occur and repair may decline with age.[133] Irradiated human cells unable to execute the NHEJ pathway are supersensitive to the introduction of large-scale mutations and chromosomal aberrations.[128]

Although evidence suggests that interindividual differences in radiation responses may be attributed to certain genes, IR can activate oncogenes, resulting in uncontrolled cell growth[130,134] (see Chapter 10). Tumor-suppressor genes also are sensitive to IR. Several tumor-suppressor genes have been identified that are deactivated by IR that promotes carcinogenesis.[130,134] Recent research has shown that cells can detect and respond epigenetically, altering gene expression after low

HEALTH ALERT

Increasing Use of Computed Tomography Scans and Risks

A review article in the *New England Journal of Medicine* on computed tomography (CT) and radiation exposure has received much media attention. The article was written by radiology researchers at Columbia University. In short, the numbers of CT scans have greatly increased in the United States. This increase has occurred both as a diagnostic treatment for individuals with symptoms and as a diagnostic modality for individuals without symptoms (heart, lung, colon, and whole-body screening). Faster scanning times are partly responsible for increased CT use in pediatric populations. Typical doses are larger from CT scans than for a conventional examination (e.g., 50 times more radiation to stomach than an x-ray). Based on data correlations from Japanese survivors of atomic bombs, the authors estimated that 1.5% to 2.0% of cancers in the United States might be attributable to CT radiation. The authors note that CT scans are sometimes ordered excessively and repeated unnecessarily because of defensive medicine. They also include three ways to reduce radiation exposure from CT: (1) reduce radiation doses in individual studies (i.e., use modern scanners), (2) substitute ultrasonography with magnetic resonance imaging (MRI) for CT whenever possible, and (3) order CT scans only when absolutely necessary.

CT scans in the United States

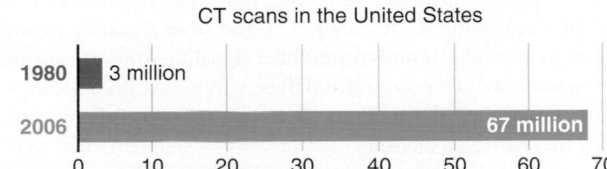

NCRP estimates that 67 million CT scans (compared with 3 million in 1980), 18 million nuclear medicine procedures, 17 million interventional fluoroscopy procedures, and 18 million nuclear medicine procedures were performed in the United States in 2006.

Median Effective Radiation Dose for Each Type of CT Study

Anatomic Area, Study Type	Median (mSv)	Range (mSv)	Dose Equivalent (No. of Chest X-rays)
Head and Neck			
Routine head	2	0.3-6	30
Routine neck	4	0.7-9	55
Suspected stroke	14	4-56	199
Chest			
Chest, no contrast	8	2-24	117
Chest, with contrast	8	2-19	119
Suspected pulmonary embolus	10	2-30	137
Coronary angiogram	22	7-39	309
Abdomen-Pelvis			
Routine abdomen-pelvis, no contrast	15	3-43	220
Routine abdomen-pelvis, with contrast	16	4-45	234
Multiphase abdomen-pelvis	31	6-90	442
Suspected aneurysm or dissection	24	4-68	347

Data from Brenner DJ, Hall E: *N Engl J Med* 357:2277, 2007; Brett AS: *J Watch* 28(1):3, 2008; Food and Drug Adminmistration Public Health Notification: *Reducing radiation risk from computed tomography for pediatric and small adult patients*, Silver Spring, Md, 2001, FDA.

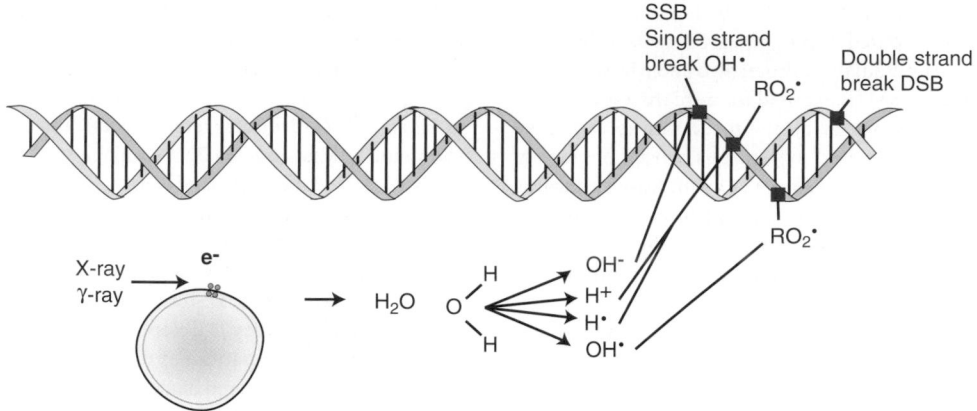

FIGURE 11-14 Free Radicals. Free radicals formed by water nearby and around DNA cause indirect effects. These effects have a short life of single free radicals. Oxygen can modify the reaction, enabling longer lifetimes of oxidative free radicals.

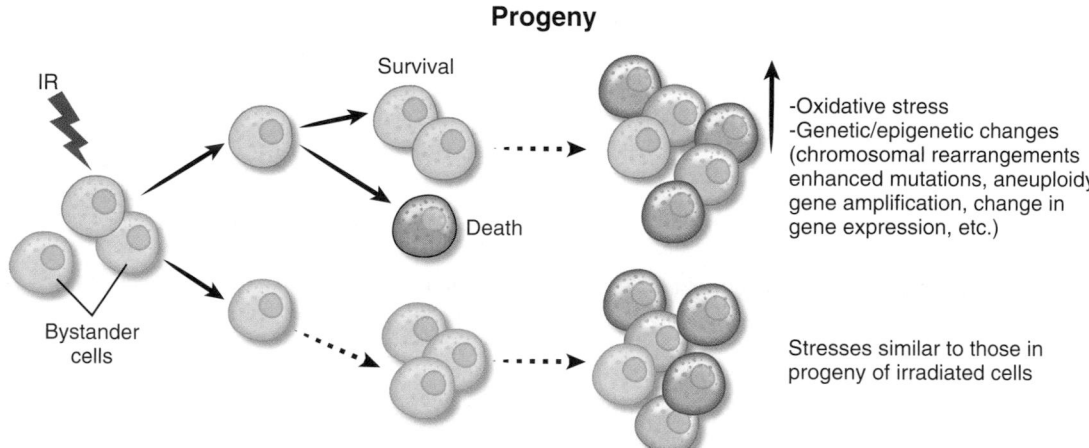

FIGURE 11-15 Radiation: Targeted and Nontargeted or Bystander Effects. Signaling from cells exposed to irradiation causes stressful effects, including oxidative stress, to those cells not directly radiated called bystander cells and their progeny. These induced effects may be similar to those reported in the progeny of irradiated cells. (Adapted from Azzam EI et al: Ionizing radiation-induced metabolic oxidative stress and prolonged cell injury, *Cancer Lett* 327[1-2]:48-60, 2012.)

doses of radiation.[130] Gene expression can change as a function of radiation dose and radiation type.[130]

Nontargeted Effects

A long-held assumption is that cellular alterations—mutations and malignant transformation—occur only in cells directly radiated. It is now known that cells not directly exposed to radiation, but instead the progeny of cells that were irradiated many cell divisions previously, may express a high level of gene mutations, cell lethality, and chromosomal aberration. Altogether these effects are called genomic instability. Investigators are studying genomic instability as it may contribute to secondary cancers. The directly irradiated cells also can lead to genetic effects in so-called bystander cells or innocent cells (called bystander effects) even though they themselves received no direct radiation exposure.[128] For example, using an in vivo mouse model, investigators found that localized radiation to the head led to induced bystander effects in the lead-shielded distant spleen tissue.[135] These radiosensitive mice showed unexpected enhancement of medulloblastoma in their cerebellum. The bystander effect has

been demonstrated in three-dimensional human tissues and recently in other whole animal organisms.[101] Both double-strand DNA breaks and apoptotic cell death were induced by bystander effects, supporting the role of signaling between the irradiated cells (the targeted cells) and unirradiated cells (the nontargeted or bystander cells) (Figure 11-15). Such communication is thought to occur from direct physical connection between cells or gap junctions, called gap junctional intercellular communication (GJIC, see p. 12), and from signaling pathways. Numerous intercellular and intracellular signaling pathways are implicated in the bystander response and these effects have been shown to be transmitted to their descendants. These various effects demonstrated in vivo may reflect an ongoing inflammatory response (oxidative stress response) to the initial radiation-induced injury[136] (Box 11-1). One hypothesis is the stress response is due to elevated reactive oxygen species (ROS) affecting genomic instability. Importantly, by therapeutic interference with specific signaling pathways (e.g., p38MAPK) may result in genome stabilization.[137] Both the bystander and the genomic instability effects have been termed "nontargeted" effects (see pp. 285-287).

BOX 11-1 A Paradigm Shift? Responses to Ionizing Radiation Mediated by Inflammatory Mechanisms

Many observations have not been supportive of the conventional paradigm of biologic responses to ionizing radiation (IR). The conventional paradigm is that the consequences of exposure to IR have been attributed solely to mutational DNA damage or cell death induced in irradiated cells at the time of exposure. The challenges to this paradigm come from three types of published data: (1) abscopal, or "out-of-field," effects, where radiation treatment to one local area of the body results in an antitumor effect distant to the radiation site; (2) detection of plasma factors in vivo (clastogenic [or capable of chromosome damage] factors) that can affect the survival and function of irradiated cells; and (3) effects in nonirradiated cells that are in the vicinity of irradiated cells (bystander effects) or in the descendants of irradiated cells several generations after the initial radiation exposure (genomic instability). These nontargeted effects are different than the targeted effects that arise in cells upon immediate deposition of energy at the time of radiation exposure. The nontargeted effects arise as a result of intracellular signaling and appear to represent a genotype-dependent balance (and various epigenetic influences) of toxic factors and cellular responses that may involve both oxidative stress and inflammatory type processes (see Figure 11-15).

Data from Azzam E, Jay-Gerin JP: *Cancer Lett* 327(1-2):48-60, 2012; Mukherjee D et al: *J Pathol* 232(3):289-299, 2014.

Acute, Latent, and Microenvironmental Effects

IR causes acute and persistent short- and long-term effects.[102-104] Acute exposure to IR can cause damage to several organ systems, especially those with highly proliferative cells such as the hematopoietic system, the skin, and the gastrointestinal system[105] (see Chapter 4). Investigators have postulated that radiation's carcinogenic potential persists because of nontargeted radiation effects that alter cell and tissue signaling and change the microenvironment.[106,107] Investigators report the brain's innate immune system is very vulnerable to cranial irradiation, altering the microenvironment and causing the recruitment and infiltration of macrophages.[138] With improvement in cancer survival, the long-term risks of a second cancer developing from treatment become more important.[139]

Radiation-induced cancer in humans has latent periods, usually 5 to 10 years, but can be decades.[130] British investigators reported the following results: for solid cancers, radiation-related excess risk starts to appear about 5 years after exposure in therapeutically irradiated groups; and for leukemia, it starts to appear within 5 years of exposure.[140] Using U.S. Surveillance Epidemiology and End Results (SEER) data, the estimated excess of second cancers that could be related to radiotherapy is about 8%; data from the United Kingdom, which included diagnostic procedures and excluded therapeutic irradiation, yielded an estimation of 15%.[139,140]

Low Dose and Dose Rate

Recent events, including the 2011 Fukushima nuclear accident, terrorist attacks, and exposure to radiation from medical procedures, have increased the need to understand the human health effects of exposure to low-level ionizing radiation.[141] Risk estimates for human exposure at low-dose, low-LET ionizing radiation (0 to 100 millisieverts [mSv], or less than 0.1 gray [Gy]) are constantly debated. Although investigators have reported that accurate measurements of risks from low doses of radiation are statistically difficult because they require such large populations, researchers have developed an in silico simulation model of a population-based cohort study for conducting future

epidemiologic studies of excess cancer risks in CT-exposed individuals.[142] Simulation models may provide reasonable approximations and theoretic models are still used to estimate response curves (Box 11-2).

Ultraviolet Radiation

Ultraviolet radiation, called UV radiation, comes from sunlight. Other sources of UV radiation include electric lights, black lights, and tanning lamps.[143] UV radiation is divided into three major wavelengths: UVA, UVB, and UVC radiation. Most of the UV radiation received on earth is UVA and some UVB.[143] UVA radiation is weaker than UVB, but UVA penetrates deeper into the skin and is more constant throughout the year despite the weather.[143] UVB affects the outer layer of the skin and UVC radiation does not increase health risks as much as UVB.[143] UV radiation also can be important to health and produces vitamin D that helps in the absorption of calcium and phosphorus from food, which are all important for bone development. The WHO recommends 5 to 15 minutes of sun exposure two to three times a week; however, overexposure can result in acute and chronic health effects on the skin, eye, and immune system.[144]

There are three main types of skin cancer: cancer that forms in melanocytes (pigment cells) called melanoma, cancer in the lower part of the epidermis or outer layer of the skin called basal cell carcinoma (BCC), and cancer in the flat cells that form the surface of the skin called squamous cell carcinoma (SCC) (see Chapter 41). Melanoma, the most lethal form of skin cancer, can occur on any skin surface; however, in men it is often found on the skin on the head, the neck, between the shoulders, and the hips. In women it is more commonly found on the skin on the lower legs, between the shoulders, and the hips. Although rare in people with dark skin, melanoma is usually found under the fingernails, under the toenails, on the palms of the hands, or on the soles of the feet.[145] Basal cell carcinoma commonly occurs on the head and neck. Squamous cell carcinoma is found more commonly in men who work outdoors, but can occur in anyone. SCC occurs on sun-exposed areas of the skin including the nose, ears, lower lip, and dorsa of the hand. SCCs are composed of keratinizing cells and are more aggressive then BCC, but the development into invasive SCC is low.[146] For a more complete discussion about these skin cancers see Chapter 41.

The incidence of basal cell carcinoma and squamous cell carcinoma is strongly correlated with lifetime sunlight exposure (i.e., photocarcinogenesis). Specific patterns of sunlight exposure, intermittent or chronic, confer different host effects, acute or cumulative. Intense intermittent recreational sun exposure has been associated with melanoma and BCC. Chronic occupational sun exposure has been associated with SCC. Tanning bed use also has been associated with an increased risk of BCC. The risk was higher in females and with higher use of indoor tanning facilities.[147] For other occupational factors linked to skin cancers, see Chapter 41. Depending on the time of day and a person's skin type, acute sun exposure may result in sunburn.[145] From epidemiologic studies, a sunburn is defined as a burn or pain and/or blistering that lasts for 2 or more days.[145] Cumulative sun exposure is the additive effects of intermittent sun exposure, chronic sun exposure, or both. Other skin cancer risk factors include ionizing radiation, chronic arsenic ingestion, immunosuppression, and genetic factors. These skin cancers have a higher incidence among people with a light or fair skin tone, but they can occur in anyone and in those who do not burn from sunlight.[148]

UV radiation is known to cause specific gene mutations; for example, squamous cell carcinoma involves mutation in the *TP53* gene, basal cell carcinoma in the patched 1 tumor-suppressor gene (*PTCH1*), and melanoma in the *p16* gene.[149] The patched/hedgehog intracellular signaling pathway plays a central role in both sporadic BCCs and

BOX 11-2   Theoretical Models to Understand Low-Dose Radiation

Several models include the linear no-threshold (LNT) relationship, in which any dose, including very low doses, has the potential to cause mutations (see **A**). Another model, the linear-quadratic relationship, proposes there is a risk mathematical term that is directly proportional to the dose (linear term) and another term proportional to the square of the dose (quadratic term) (see **B**). The threshold model proposes a threshold dose below which radiation may not cause cancer in humans (see **C**). Proponents of this model argue that such thresholds

are derived, for example, from the ability to repair damage caused by lower doses of radiation. There is some evidence that low doses may actually produce a higher level of risk per unit of dose, which is called the supralinear hypothesis (see **D**). **E**, Stochastic or random probability is a major model for understanding low-dose radiation. Currently, the shape of the response curve for the low-dose region is really unknown.

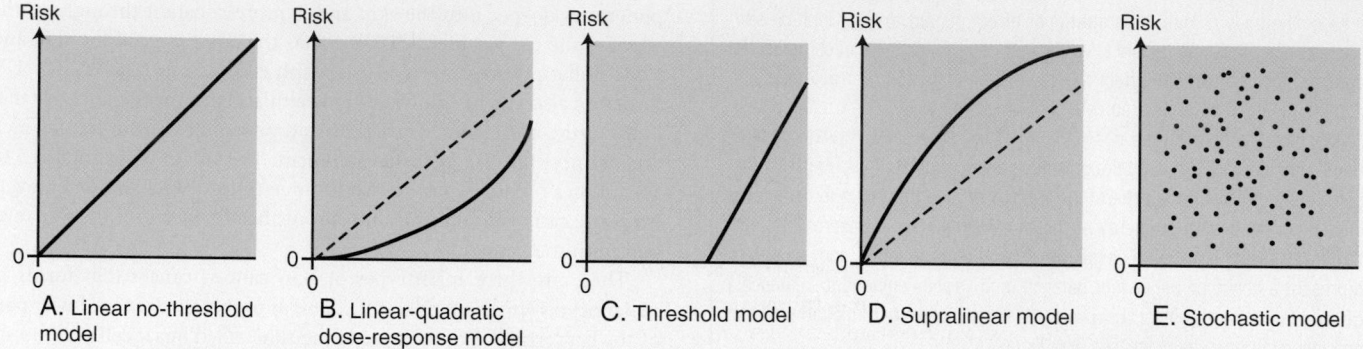

A. Linear no-threshold model

B. Linear-quadratic dose-response model

C. Threshold model

D. Supralinear model

E. Stochastic model

Theoretic Models for Estimating Risk of Low-Dose Ionizing Radiation. Collective population dose is expressed as a person-rem (roentgen equivalent, man). Estimating a collective dose then enables an application of a "constant risk factor" to obtain a statistical estimate of the number of additional cancers (above background radiation) from that exposure. These computations apply to low doses–low dose rates only (**A**). Many propose the best fit is the linear no-threshold (LNT) model (**B**). The most common alternative to the LNT model is the linear-quadratic model. The quadratic term is the square of the dose. The linear term is equal to zero (**C**). The threshold model is a threshold below which there is *no* increase in cancer risk. Proponents of this model argue that because some toxic chemicals/materials exhibit such thresholds, radiation must also have a threshold. Their arguments are related to repair of the radiation damage caused by lower doses of radiation (**D**). Some evidence exists that low levels of radiation produce a higher level of risk per unit dose, which is called the supralinear model. The stochastic model describes effects that are random and the events cannot be predicted (**E**). (Adapted from Makhijani A et al: *Science for the vulnerable: setting radiation and multiple exposure environmental health standards to protect those at most risk,* Takoma Park, Md, 2006, Institute for Energy and Environmental Research.)

---

nevoid BCC syndrome (Gorlin syndrome) tumor growth.[150] Investigators are identifying aberrant DNA methylation and histone modifications in tumor tissues and cell lines for skin cancers.[151-153] In addition, UV light induces the release of tumor necrosis factor-alpha (TNF-α) in the epidermis, which may reduce immune surveillance against skin cancer.[154] The identification of transcription factors and chemokine receptors suggests a critical role of inflammation in skin carcinogenesis.[155]

Skin exposure to UVR and ionizing radiation, as well as chemical (xenobiotic) agents/drugs, produces ROS in large quantities.[156] Uncontrolled release of ROS is an important contributor to skin carcinogenesis.[156] Imbalances in ROS and antioxidants can lead to oxidative stress, tissue injury, and direct DNA damage (Figure 11-16). ROS can induce a number of transcription factors (e.g., activator protein-1 [AP-1] and NF-κβ)[157] and increase regulating genes that induce inflammation.[156,158] Inflammation is a critical component of tumor progression.

The incidence of melanoma has been increasing annually at rates of 2% to 7% for white populations.[159] The increasing incidence is worldwide and in the United States the incidence has been increasing for about 30 years. From 2007 to 2011 incidence rates were stable in men and women younger than 50 years but increased by 2.6% per year in women aged 50 years and older. Mortality rates decreased by 2.6% in people younger than 50 years but increased in those aged 50 years and older.[160] Although pediatric melanoma is rare, most studies have

indicated that incidence has been increasing.[161] A new study has found that the incidence of pediatric melanoma in the United States actually has decreased from 2004 to 2010, but only in those children (with melanoma) with good prognostic indicators.[161] Therefore, health programs need to continue to encourage sun protective behavior (protective clothing, sunscreen use, decreased time spent outside, decreased indoor tanning) to reduce melanoma incidence. Because death rates from melanoma have not risen as rapidly as incidence rates, controversy still exists about whether some of the incidence is a result of overdiagnosis.[162,163] Melanomas can appear suddenly without warning and can arise from or near a mole (melanocytic nevus) and freckles.[164] Complex interactions between UV exposure profiles and genotype combinations determine nevus numbers and size, as well as facial freckling.[164] When detected in the early stages, melanoma is highly curable.[165] Early stage melanoma is classified as radial growth phase (RGP). Later stage melanoma, called vertical growth phase (VGP), is characterized by invasion into the dermal layer and is frequently metastatic.[166] Much research is ongoing to understand the mechanisms that promote progression from less invasive RGP melanoma to aggressive VGP melanoma. Recent progress in understanding the molecular alterations in melanoma will likely advance its diagnosis, prognosis, and treatment.

The pathogenesis of melanoma is very complex, involving genetic and environmental factors. The genetic factors can be inherited, for

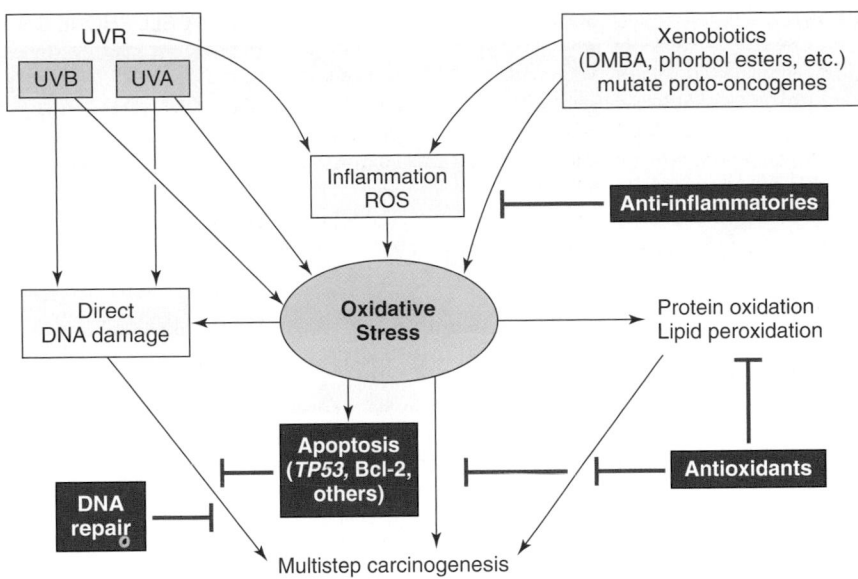

FIGURE 11-16 Theoretic Scheme of Multistep Skin Carcinogenesis. Ultraviolet radiation *(UVR)*, inflammation, and xenobiotics (see p. 279) lead to oxidative stress, resulting in direct DNA damage, protein oxidation, lipid peroxidation, and apoptosis. The protective mechanisms shown in *red* include apoptosis, DNA repair, and antioxidants. *DMBA,* Dimethylbenz[a]anthracene; *ROS,* reactive oxygen species; *UVA,* ultraviolet A; *UVB,* ultraviolet B. (Adapted from Sander CD et al: *Int J Dermatol* 43[5]:326-340, 2004.)

example, in high-susceptibility genes (i.e., *cyclin-dependent kinase inhibitor 2A [CDKN2A]*) or in low-susceptibility genes (i.e., *melanocortin-1*). About 10% to 15% of melanomas are inherited as an autosomal dominant trait with variable penetrance.[167] The majority of melanomas are sporadic and seem to involve ultraviolet radiation (UVR) damage.[167] UVR is correlated with DNA damage. Epidemiologic and case-control studies suggest that UVR exposure is the most significant factor for the development of melanoma (episodes of intense, intermittent exposure [measured as history of sunburn]). Other evidence, however, reports rates of melanoma are uncommon in persons with outdoor occupations. Furthermore, because melanomas sometimes occur in dark-skinned individuals, other environmental factors may be important. Recent analyses in Iceland and Italy and a previous large prospective study in Norway and Sweden suggest sunbed use as a reason for increased melanoma, especially in women.[168-170] Indoor tanning (sunbed use) is a risk factor for melanoma[171] (i.e., frequent indoor tanning increases melanoma risk). Certain skin conditions also are treated with UVA and UVB light therapy. Family history (i.e., genetic factors), skin type, and the density of moles are important in determining the risk of developing melanoma. Traits associated with a high risk of melanoma are light-colored hair, eyes, and skin; an inability to tan; and a tendency to freckle, sunburn, and develop nevi.

The emerging molecular changes associated with melanoma emphasize that melanoma, like many other cancers, is not a single disease but a diverse group of disorders. The most frequent driver mutations in melanoma involve cell cycle control, pro-growth pathways, and telomerase.[167] Although other genes may be involved, melanoma progression is often associated with a mutation in the *BRAF* oncogene.[166] The most common mutation in *BRAF*[V600E] promotes the progression of melanoma through activation of the mitogen-activated protein kinase (MAPK) signaling cascade.[166] Investigators report disease progression may involve factors secreted by the melanoma cells that activate extracellular matrix enzymes (matrix metalloproteinase-1 [MMP-1]) and adjacent stromal fibroblasts in the tumor microenvironment.[166]

Although avoiding sunlight by keeping in the shade and covering up is very important for protection, more data are needed to understand if sunscreen prevents melanoma. A significant benefit from regular sunscreen use has not yet demonstrated primary prevention for basal cell carcinoma and melanoma.[172] Increased knowledge of the intricate cellular interactions in melanoma will increase understanding of melanoma etiology and pathogenesis. This knowledge is essential for early detection and treatment.

Electromagnetic Radiation

Health risks associated with radiofrequency electromagnetic radiation (RF-EMR) are very controversial. RF-EMR is in the frequency range of 30 kHz to 300 GHz. Electromagnetic fields (EMFs) generated by RF sources couple with the body and result in induced electric and magnetic fields with associated currents inside tissue.[173] Exposure to electric and magnetic fields is widespread. Microwaves, radar, mobile and cell phones, mobile phone base stations, power frequency radiation associated with electricity and radio waves, fluorescent lights, computers, and other electric equipment create EMRs of varying strength. Despite the breadth of literature on microwaves (MW), the impact of EMR on human health has not been fully assessed. Scientific evidence is accumulating although it has been hampered by the scarcity of methods to accurately measure exposure, the lack of a clear dose-response relationship, and the difficulty in reproducing effects. In addition, with competing priorities such as convenience, financial interest, and health necessity, a consensus of the risk/benefit ratio of EMR exposure may be difficult to achieve, and safety standards vary significantly, up to 1000 times among countries.[174,175] The National Institute of Environmental Health Sciences Electric and Magnetic Fields Working Group[176] recommended that low-frequency electromagnetic fields (EMFs) be classified as possible carcinogens. Overall, there is limited evidence that magnetic fields cause childhood leukemia and insufficient evidence for other cancers in children.[177-180] A recent large census-cohort study from Switzerland did not suggest an association between predicted RF-EMF exposure from broadcast transmitters

BRAIN SCAN · BOTH CELL PHONES OFF · RIGHT CELL PHONE ON

Area of scan

Phone

Note: Images are from a single participant

Rate of brain glucose metabolism

Low · High

FIGURE 11-17 Electromagnetic Radiation from a Cell Phone Can Penetrate the Skull. EMR from a cell phone can penetrate the skull and deposit energy 4 to 6 cm into the brain. 50-minute cell phone exposure was associated with increased brain glucose metabolism in the region closest to the antenna. This finding is of unknown clinical significance. (From Volkow ND et al: Effects of cell phone radiofrequency signal exposure on brain glucose metabolism, *JAMA* 305[8]:808-813, 2011.)

and childhood leukemia.[181] Studies of magnetic field exposure from power lines and electric blankets in adults reveal little evidence of an association with leukemia, brain tumors, or breast cancer.[177]

The most extensively studied exposure is from use of wireless telephones (mobile and cordless); other exposures include occupational settings and sources from the general environment.[173] One cohort study and five case-control studies did not show an increased rate of brain tumors after the increase in mobile phone use. However, these studies had limitations because most of the analyses examined trends only in the early 2000s.[173] The INTERPHONE study,[182] a multicenter case-control study, is the largest study so far that studies the relationship between mobile phone use and brain tumors—glioma, acoustic neuroma, and meningioma. Results for cordless phones are lacking in the INTERPHONE study.[183] The pooled analyses included 2708 glioma cases and 2972 controls. The odds ratios (ORs) in terms of time spent on the phone showed that the highest time spent on the phone (>1640 hours of use) was related to glioma risk (OR 1.40; 95% confidence interval [CI] 1.03-1.89). There was a suggestion of increased risk of tumors on the same side of the head as the phone use (ipsilateral exposure) in the temporal lobe, where radiofrequency (RF) EMF exposure is highest.[173] The OR for glioma increased with increasing RF dose for exposure 7 years or more before diagnosis, and there was no association with estimated dose for exposure less than 7 years before diagnosis.[173] A Swedish investigative group performed a pooled analysis of two similar studies between the relationship of glioma, acoustic neuroma, and meningioma manifestation and mobile and cordless phone use.[184] Study participants who used a mobile phone for more than 1 year had an OR for glioma of 1.3 (95% CI 1.1-1.6). The OR increased with increasing time since first use and with total call time, 3.2 (2.0-5.1) for more than 2000 hours of use.[173] Ipsilateral use of the phone was associated with higher risk.[173] Similar findings were reported for cordless phones.[173] Although the INTERPHONE and Swedish studies were judged susceptible to bias, the Working Group concluded that the findings could not be dismissed because of bias alone and a causal relationship between phones and glioma is possible.[173] The Working Group concluded that there is "limited evidence in humans" for the carcinogenicity of RF-EMF based on associations between glioma and acoustic neuroma and exposure to RF-EMF from wireless phones.[173]

The Working Group reviewed numerous mechanisms of carcinogenicity from RF-EMF.[173] The mechanisms included genotoxicity,

effects on immune function, gene and protein expression, cell signaling, oxidative stress, apoptosis, and the blood-brain barrier. Other suggested mechanisms may include altered DNA repair mechanisms and epigenetic changes to DNA.[183] The Working Group classified RF-EMF as "possibly carcinogenic to humans" (Group 2B).

EMR from a cell phone can penetrate the skull and deposit energy 4 to 6 cm into the brain (Figure 11-17).[185] Investigators found a 50-minute cell phone exposure was associated with increased brain glucose metabolism in the region closest to the antenna.[186] Children have a smaller head and thinner skull bone than adults, and investigators have reported higher conductivity and higher absorption from RF-EMF than for adults.[187-189] Concern is for children in whom the effects may be compounded because of increased vulnerability to radiation and their longer use of cell phones into adulthood. Advice about reducing exposures through simple precautions is increasing; for example, don't hold a cell phone directly to your head, pregnant women should keep cell phones away from their abdomen, and don't allow children to play with or use your cell phone. Mobile phone manufacturers themselves are issuing advice on reducing exposures.[190] Ongoing unbiased research is desperately needed. Absolute proof of causation may be hindered because of the ethical questions of exposing individuals to potentially harmful interventions.

> ✔ **QUICK CHECK 11-3**
> 1. What are the cancers associated with cigarette smoking?
> 2. How are dietary components related to cancer?
> 3. What are the possible pathophysiologic mechanisms of obesity-associated cancer risk?
> 4. How does ionizing radiation contribute to carcinogenesis? UV radiation?
> 5. Discuss the difficulty in determining cancer risks with electromagnetic radiation.

Infection, Sexual and Reproductive Behavior

Infection is an important contributor to cancer worldwide. Of cancers diagnosed in 2008, about 2 million new cases were caused by infections.[191] Infection and cancer rates vary widely by region: with a 7.4% rate for more developed regions and a 22.9% rate for less developed regions.[191] The highest rate, 32.7%, is found in sub-Saharan Africa.[191] Cancer-causing agents classified by the IARC were used in this

TABLE 11-7   Number of New Cancer Cases* in 2008 Attributable to Infection, by Infectious Agent, and Development Status†

	Less Developed Regions	More Developed Regions	World
Hepatitis B and C viruses	520,000 (32.0%)	80,000 (19.4%)	600,000 (29.5%)
Human papillomavirus	490,000 (30.2%)	120,000 (29.2%)	610,000 (30.0%)
Helicobacter pylori	470,000 (28.9%)	190,000 (46.2%)	660,000 (32.5%)
Epstein-Barr virus	96,000 (5.9%)	16,000 (3.9%)	110,000 (5.4%)
Human herpesvirus type 8	39,000 (2.4%)	4,100 (1.0%)	43,000 (2.1%)
Human T-cell lymphotropic virus type 1	660 (0.0%)	1,500 (0.4%)	2,100 (0.1%)
Opisthorchis viverrini and *Clonorchis sinensis*	2,000 (0.1%)	0 (0.0%)	2,000 (0.1%)
Schistosoma haematobium	6,000 (0.4%)	0 (0.0%)	6,000 (0.3%)
TOTAL	**1,600,000 (100.0%)**	**410,000 (100.0%)**	**2,000,000 (100.0%)**

Data from de Martel C et al: *Lancet Oncol* 13(6):607-615, 2012.
*Numbers are rounded to two significant digits.
†Data are number of new cancer cases attributed to a particular infectious agent (proportion of the total number of new cases attributed to infection that is due to a specific agent).

report because the strength of published evidence is controversial. The four top notable infections and new cancer cases include human papillomavirus (HPV), *Helicobacter pylori (H. pylori)*, hepatitis B virus (HBV), and hepatitis C virus (HCV) (Table 11-7). According to investigators, these results are probably conservative and underestimate the true burden of infection-associated cancers.[191] Hepatitis B and hepatitis C can infect the liver and together account for the large majority of liver cancer cases (see Chapter 36). It has been estimated that *H. pylori* accounted for about 75% of all stomach cancers;[192] however, updated estimates using both enzyme-linked immunosorbent assay (ELISA) and Western blot for detection of anti–*H. pylori* antibodies include an additional 120,000 cases of gastric cancer for a total percentage of 89.0%.[193] Epstein-Barr virus (EBV) is linked to cancers of the nasopharynx, Hodgkin disease, and non-Hodgkin lymphoma. Human herpesvirus type 8 is linked to Kaposi sarcoma, and human T-cell lymphotropic virus type 1 is linked to leukemia and lymphoma. The following discussion will concern human papillomavirus (HPV).

Human papillomavirus (HPV) is the most common sexually transmitted virus in the United States. At least 50% of sexually active people will have genital HPV at some time in their lives.[194] HPVs are a group of more than 150 related viruses. More than 40 of these viruses can easily spread from direct skin contact or through vaginal, rectal, or oral sex.[195] *Low-risk HPVs* do not cause cancer but can cause skin warts, called condylomata acuminata. *High-risk*, or oncogenic, *HPVs* can cause cancer. Even though about a dozen HPVs are identified, HPV types 16 and 18 are responsible for the majority of cancers.[195] However, most high-risk HPV infections may cause cytologic abnormalities or abnormal cell changes that disappear unexpectedly. According to the National Cancer Institute, most infections will be suppressed by the immune system.[196] Persistence of infection with high-risk HPV is a prerequisite for the development of cervical intraepithelial neoplasia (CIN) (see Figure 33-19), lesions, and invasive cervical cancers.[12,196] HPV infection has been identified as a definite carcinogen for six types of cancer: cervix, penis, vulva, anus, and some oropharynx (including the base of the tongue and tonsils).[196,197] The incidence of HPV-associated oropharyngeal cancer has increased during the past 20 years, especially among men. Factors that may increase the risk of developing cancer following a high-risk HPV infection include smoking, decreased immunity, having many children (for increased risk of cervical cancer), long-term oral contraceptive use (for increased risk of cervical cancer), poor oral hygiene (for increased risk of oropharyngeal cancer), and chronic inflammation.[198] Although the main mode of HPV transmission occurs through sexual contact, HPV has been found in virginal women before first intercourse.[199] Consensus is that newborn babies can be exposed to cervical HPV infection from the mother.[199] The possible modes of transmission in children, however, are controversial.[200] The *Health Alert:* Rising Incidence of HPV-Associated Oropharyngeal Cancers contains information on the rising incidence of HPV-associated oropharyngeal cancers.

HEALTH ALERT

Rising Incidence of HPV-Associated Oropharyngeal Cancers

The incidence of head and neck cancers has fallen with a decrease in smoking in the United States; however, the incidence of HPV-associated oropharyngeal cancers (tonsil and tongue base) appears to be rising—especially in young white men. The two classes of oropharyngeal squamous cell carcinoma seem to have different causes: HPV-positive oral cancers are possibly associated with sex-related risk factors, whereas HPV-negative cancers are associated with tobacco and alcohol consumption. Epidemiologic studies support little interaction between the two sets of risk factors, suggesting that HPV-positive cancer and HPV-negative cancer have *distinct* pathogenesis. Tobacco use and alcohol use are known etiologic factors in head and neck cancers; it is surprising that most cases of oropharyngeal cancers in non-smokers are HPV-related. Not yet known is whether this increase is attributed to changes in sexual norms (from past generations), with more oral sex partners or oral sex at an earlier age. Smoking, however, has an adverse effect on both HPV-positive and HPV-negative oral cancers. In Sweden the incidence of oropharyngeal cancers caused by HPV increased from 23% in the 1970s to 57% in the 1990s to 93% in 2007. Emerging data indicate that HPV is now the primary cause of tonsillar cancer in North America and Europe. The mechanism of HPV-oropharyngeal cancer is different than that related to tobacco use: *P53* degradation occurs (i.e., *P53* helps direct genetic repair and cell death [see Chapter 10]), the retinoblastoma *RB* pathway is inactivated (cell signaling pathway), and the risk of HPV-16 (i.e., *P16*) is increased. Tobacco-related oropharyngeal cancers are characterized by *TP53* mutation and a decrease in the *CDKN2A* mutation (cell cycle gene), and thus a decrease in *P16*. Individuals with *P16*-positive tumors have a better prognosis than those with *P16*-negative tumors.

Data from Chaturvedi AK et al: *J Clin Oncol* 29(32):4294-4301, 2011; Lowy DR, Munger K: *N Engl J Med* 363(1):82-84, 2010; Marur S et al: *Lancet Oncol* 11(8):781-789, 2010; Nasman A et al: *Int J Cancer* 125:362-366, 2009.

Current guidelines recommend that women should have a Papanicolaou smear (Pap test) every 3 years beginning at age 21. Guidelines also specify that women ages 30 to 65 should have HPV and Pap co-testing every 5 years or a Pap test alone every 3 years. Women with certain risk factors may need more frequent screening or to continue screening beyond age 65. Women who have received the HPV vaccine still need regular cervical screening[196,201] (see Chapter 33 for a discussion on the HPV vaccine). HPV vaccines protect males and females against diseases, including cancers, when given in the recommended age groups. HPV vaccines are given in three shots over 6 months.[202]

Other Viruses and Microorganisms

A discussion of the relationship between viruses, bacteria, and cancer is contained in Chapter 10 and appropriate chapters in Unit II. Other microorganisms involved in carcinogenesis include parasites such as *Opisthorchis viverrini* (bile duct cancer) and *Schistosoma haematobium* (bladder cancer). Their specific roles in carcinogenesis are reported to be related to cofactors or carcinogens, or both.

Air Pollution

Outdoor air pollution is a complex mixture of many known carcinogens and its relationship to lung cancer has been studied for more than 50 years.[203] Past reviews of outdoor and household air pollution indicated that both were associated with increased rates of lung cancer, most particularly with exposures to increased levels of particles called particulate matter (PM). Particulate matter, also known as *particle pollution,* is a mixture of extremely small particles and liquid droplets. Particle pollution consists of a complex mix of acids (such as nitrates and sulfates), organic chemicals, metals, and soil or dust particles. The International Agency for Research on Cancer (IARC) recently concluded that exposure to outdoor air pollution and to particulate matter (PM) in outdoor air is carcinogenic to humans (IARC Group 1) and causes lung cancer.[204,205] The IARC's evaluation came from long-term epidemiologic studies of residential exposure to air pollution. Specifically, focused reviews of lung cancer risk are with prominent components of PM in outdoor air ($PM_{2.5}$ particles with aerodynamic diameter ≤ 2.5 μm, or fine particles and PM_{10} [≤ 10 μm, or inhalable particles]) (Figure 11-18).

$PM_{2.5}$ includes a higher proportion of mutagenic agents.[206] Importantly, analyses by continent of study (including North America, Europe, and others) yielded consistent, positive associations between $PM_{2.5}$ and lung cancer.[203] *Primary particles* are emitted directly from a source, for example, construction sites, unpaved roads, fields, smokestacks, or fires. *Secondary particles* are emitted from power plants, industries, and automobiles. These particles are a complex of chemicals including sulfur dioxide and nitrogen oxides and make up most of the fine particle pollution in the United States.[207] Fine or ultrafine particles are easily absorbed by the lungs and phagocytosed by macrophages and neutrophils that release tissue-damaging inflammatory mediators. Acute exposure to diesel exhaust that contains fine particles is linked to lung, throat, and eye irritations; asthma attacks; and myocardial ischemia (Figure 11-19).[208] Importantly, according to the WHO, diesel exhaust is carcinogenic and causes lung cancer.[209] The central hypothesis, based on rat studies, for the mechanisms related to particle-induced lung carcinogenesis is that insoluble particles cause pulmonary inflammation (e.g., cytokine release, ROS), which leads to oxidative stress and oxidation of DNA, proliferative response, and tissue remodeling progressing toward fibrosis and tumor development.

The Global Burden of Disease collaboration estimated that approximately 3.22 million deaths were caused by exposure to air pollution in 2010, an increase from 2.91 million deaths attributed to air pollution in 1990.[210] From data in 2010, cancers of the trachea, bronchus, or lung represent about 7% of total mortality attributable to $PM_{2.5}$.[210] So far, data have not allowed the clear relationships of air pollution on lung cancer risk between former heavy smokers versus light smokers.[203]

Living close to certain industries is a recognized cancer risk factor.[211] Overall, fine particle pollution also is linked to other health problems and includes (1) premature death in people with heart or lung disease, (2) nonfatal heart attacks, (3) irregular heartbeat, (4) aggravated asthma, (5) decreased lung function, and (6) respiratory symptoms, including irritation of the airways, coughing, and shortness of breath.[207] Additionally, other effects of particle pollution include reduced visibility (haze); environmental damage in lakes and streams, coastal waters, and river basins; depletion of nutrients in soil; and damage to forests and food crops.[207]

Indoor pollution is generally considered worse than outdoor pollution, partly because of cigarette smoke. Environmental tobacco smoke (ETS; passive smoking) can cause the formation of reactive oxygen free radicals and thus DNA damage. The IARC has classified ETS as a human carcinogen. Another significant indoor air pollutant

FIGURE 11-18 Particle Sizes and Pollution. (From Environmental Protection Agency: *Particulate matter updated March 18, 2013,* Washington, DC, 2013, Author.)

FIGURE 11-19 Exhaust Particulate Matter. Diesel exhaust is carcinogenic and causes lung cancer. (From Science Photo Laboratory.)

is radon gas. Radon is a natural radioactive gas derived from the radioactive decay of uranium that is ubiquitous in rock and soil; it can become trapped in houses and form radioactive decay products known to be carcinogenic to humans. The most hazardous houses can be identified by testing and then be modified to prevent further radon contamination. Exposure levels are greater from underground mines than from houses. Most of the lung cancers associated with radon are bronchogenic; however, small cell carcinoma does occur with greater frequency in underground miners. Radon increases the risk of lung cancer in underground miners in spite of their smoking status.

In China, some regions report very high levels of lung cancer in women who spend much of their time indoors. Exposures from heating and cooking combustion sources (e.g., oil vapors) and asbestos are identified as risk factors for lung cancer.[212] In addition, domestic coal use and ETS increase the risk of lung cancer in women and men.[213,214]

Inorganic arsenic, found principally in underground water (at levels ranging from 1000 to 4000 mcg/L), is found in many regions of the world. According to the IARC, strong evidence indicates an increased risk of bladder, skin, and lung cancers following consumption of water with high levels of arsenic (generally greater than 200 mcg/L).[215] Evidence for cancers of the liver, colon, and kidney is weaker. Other sources of inorganic arsenic are related to occupational exposures (see Table 11-1).

Chemical and Occupational Hazards as Carcinogens

An estimated 100,000 synthetic chemicals are used in the United States.[216] Of those, only about 7% have been tested for their health effects[217]; another 1000 chemicals are added each year.[216] Exposure to chemicals occurs every day—they are present in air, soil, food, water, household products, toys, personal care products, workplaces, and homes. The number of known carcinogens in experimental animals is large. It is suspected that most of these chemical carcinogens are potentially carcinogenic in humans but documentation is lacking. Table 11-1 (pp. 268-271) provides a summary of the chemicals according to sufficient or limited evidence in humans by cancer site. Known and probable carcinogenic agents are updated by the International Agency for Research on Cancer (IARC).

Chemical carcinogenesis involves the classic genotoxic mechanisms, and exposure to genotoxic carcinogens also might involve a variety of nongenotoxic effects in cells.[218] A number of studies reported that the carcinogenic effects induced by several chemicals, including 2-acetylaminofluorene, tamoxifen, trichloroethylene, aflatoxin B₁, ochratoxin, nickel, and chromium, do not follow a classic genotoxic carcinogenesis model, but rather involve a spectrum of cellular alterations encompassing epigenetic alterations.[219] These epigenetically reprogrammed cells show an epigenetic profile similar to that frequently observed in cancer cells, including altered histone patterns, hypomethylation of DNA repetitive elements, alterations in proto-oncogenes, and hypermethylation of tumor-suppressor genes. Altered epigenetic status confers genome instability and loss of controlled

growth signals, typically observed in cancer cells.[220] According to the director of the National Institute of Environmental Health Sciences, "… exposure to gene-altering substances, particularly in the womb and shortly after birth can lead to increased susceptibility to disease. There is a huge potential impact from these exposures, partly because the changes maybe inherited across generations."[221]

A substantial percentage of cancers of the upper respiratory passages, lung, bladder, and peritoneum are attributed to occupational factors; however, fewer studies of nonsmokers exist.[222] One notable occupational factor is asbestos-silicate mineral woven into fabrics, used in fire-resistant, insulating materials, and many other industrial sources. Chrysotile asbestos, more than any other type, accounts for a majority of asbestos in buildings in the United States. Asbestos increases the risk of mesothelioma and lung cancer and possibly other cancers. Benign conditions of asbestos exposures include pleural plaques, diffuse pleural thickening, and pulmonary fibrosis. The asbestos-related disorders (ARDs) are currently of significant occupational and public health concern.[223] Asbestos was used in homes and buildings built before the 1970s to insulate ceiling tiles, flooring, and pipe covers. In Western Europe, the epidemic of mesothelioma in building workers and other workers born after 1940 did not become apparent until the 1990s because of long latency. Asbestos usage has been banned in most developed countries, but is still used in many developing countries and the incidence of cases of ARDs is rising.[223] No exposure to asbestos is without risk.

Carcinoma of the bladder has been linked with the manufacture of dyes, rubber, paint, and aromatic amines, especially β-naphthylamine and benzidine. Benzol inhalation is linked to leukemia in shoemakers and in workers in the rubber cement, explosives, and dyeing industries. Other notable occupational hazards include heavy metals (e.g., high-nickel alloy, chromium VI compounds, inorganic arsenic), silica, polycyclic aromatic hydrocarbons, sulfuric acid, and chloromethyl ether. Data from the Nurse's Health Study in the United States showed increased lung cancer associated with particulate matter air pollution exposure.[224] Data from the European Study of Cohorts for Effects report particulate matter contributes to lung cancer incidence in Europe.[225] Studies of occupational exposure to diesel exhaust indicate an increased risk of lung cancer.[226] Other important exposures are included in Table 11-1 (pp. 268-271). Disentangling data related to lung cancer, air pollution, and occupational risks is complex, especially in combination with active and passive smoking and the interplay of environmental factors and genetic polymorphisms at multiple loci.

✔ **QUICK CHECK 11-4**

1. Identify the high-risk types of HPV that are carcinogenic.
2. What components of air pollution are considered most important for carcinogenesis?
3. Why do certain chemicals present a notable challenge to the environment and cancer?

▮ DID YOU UNDERSTAND?

1. Cancer arises from a complicated and interacting web of multiple etiologies. Avoiding high-risk behaviors and exposure to individual carcinogens will prevent many types of cancers.
2. Lifestyle behaviors, dietary and environmental factors and occupational exposure contribute to the number of cancer cases and deaths.
3. Cancers are caused by environmental-lifestyle factors and genetic/epigenetic factors. Driven by genetic alterations and epigenetic

abnormalities, biologic processes also include variations in detoxifying enzymes or DNA repair genes. Interacting factors are weaker immune systems, differences in hormone levels, and metabolic factors. These factors are influenced by the surrounding microenvironment or stroma.

4. Altogether the biologic environment is modified by metabolic and hormonal factors, inflammation, and disordered glucose and lipid metabolism. Once malignant phenotypes have developed, complex

interactions occur between the tumor, the surrounding stroma, and the cells of the immune and inflammatory systems.

Incidence and Mortality Trends

1. Globally cancer is reported to become a major cause of morbidity and mortality in the coming decades.
2. The global cancer burden is shifting from the more developed countries to economically disadvantaged countries.
3. In the United States, cancer incidence rates in all racial and ethnic groups and genders combined were stable from 2000 to 2009. Cancer incidence rates have increased in children 0 to 19 years of age for black (overall lowest rates) and Hispanic children and stable for all other racial and ethnic groups.
4. Overall, cancer death rates have been declining since the early 1990s in both men and women. Death rates for men, however, increased for cancers of the pancreas, liver, and melanoma. Death rates increased for women for cancers of the pancreas, liver, and uterus. For all racial and ethnic groups, for both genders and children for the time period 2000 to 2009, overall cancer death rates declined.

In Utero and Early Life Conditions

1. Emerging data suggest early life events influence later susceptibility to chronic diseases.
2. Developmental plasticity is the degree to which an organism's development is contingent on its environment. Plasticity refers to the ability of genes to organize physiologically or structurally in response to environmental conditions during fetal development.
3. Early versus late undernutrition in pregnancy indicated that the first trimester of pregnancy is particularly vulnerable to disease outcome in adulthood.
4. Research on DNA methylation marks, in utero environments, and future phenotypes is growing.

Environmental-Lifestyle Factors

Tobacco Use

1. Cigarette smoking is carcinogenic and the most important cause of cancer. Tobacco smoking causes cancer in more than 15 organ sites, and exposure to secondhand smoke and parental smoking causes cancer in daughters and sons and in other nonsmokers. The risk is greatest in those who begin to smoke when young and continue throughout life. Smoking is, however, pandemic affecting all ages.
2. Cigarette smoking causes more than 6 million deaths per year from cancer, chronic lung disease, cardiovascular disease, and stroke.
3. Smoking tobacco is linked to cancers of the lung, upper aerodigestive tract, lower urinary tract, kidney, pancreas, cervix, uterus, and myeloid leukemia. Recently added to the list are liver cancer and colorectal cancer.
4. Secondhand smoke is a cause of stroke; increases the risk of death in people with cancer and cancer survivors as well as those with macular degeneration, tuberculosis, ectopic pregnancy, and diabetes mellitus. Smoking increases inflammation, impairs immunity, and is a cause of rheumatoid arthritis. Smoking causes even more deaths from vascular and respiratory diseases.
5. Cigar or pipe smoking is causally related to cancers of the oral cavity, oropharynx, hypopharynx, larynx, esophagus, and lung. Pipe smokers have an increased risk of dying from cancers of lung, lip, throat, esophagus, larynx, pancreas, and colon and rectum.
6. Bidi smoking can cause cancers of the respiratory and digestive sites.

Diet

1. Understanding diet as a factor for increasing the risk of cancer is difficult and essential. The complexity is because of the variety of foods consumed, the many constituents of foods, the metabolic consequences of eating, and the temporal changes in the patterns of food use.
2. Nutrigenomics is the study of the effects of nutrition on the phenotypic variability of individuals based on genomic differences. Investigators are focused on genes, SNPs, amplifications, and deletions within the DNA sequences as modifiers of the response to foods and drinks.
3. Decades of research on specific nutrients and foods and cancers have been controversial. Less controversial are the implementation of dietary patterns, for example, the Mediterranean dietary pattern, and the promoting of specific dietary recommendations, for example, approaches to lower blood pressure.
4. The importance of diet has been illustrated by data showing changes in cancer risk among migrants in low-risk countries compared with those in high-risk countries. With migration these changes (low risk becomes high risk) are rapid and a plausible determinant of such changes is the adoption of the Western diet.
5. Most relevant to carcinogenesis, because many cellular functions are affected by nutrition (i.e., cell cycle, cell differentiation, proliferation, miRNA expression, self-renewal, DNA repair, hormonal axes), is focusing on dietary patterns and meaningful biomarkers specific to nutritional factors.
6. Carcinogenic substances from diet can develop from the cooking of fat, meat, or protein (e.g., heterocyclic aromatic amines), and from naturally occurring compounds associated with plant foods.
7. Nutrition may directly influence epigenetic factors that silence genes that should be active or activate genes that should be silent.
8. Dietary components can act directly as mutagens or interfere with their elimination.

Nutrition, Obesity, Alcohol Consumption, and Physical Activity: Impacts on Cancer

1. Obesity has been increasing in developed countries and in urban areas of developing countries. Obesity in the United States is an epidemic. Studies have significantly improved the understanding of the relationship between overweight/obesity, energy balance and cancer risk, cancer recurrence, and survival.
2. Obesity is a risk factor for cancers of the endometrium, colorectum, kidney, esophagus, breast (postmenopausal), and pancreas. Evidence is evolving for other cancers.
3. The mechanisms of obesity-associated cancer risks are unclear and vary by type of tumor and distribution of body fat. Emerging are three main factors: (1) insulin-insulin-like growth factor (IGF-1) axis, (2) sex hormones, and (3) adipokines.
4. Metabolic changes in adipose tissue from obesity result in several alterations and include insulin resistance, hyperglycemia, dyslipidemia, hypoxia, and chronic inflammation. Tumor growth is regulated by interactions between tumor cells and stromal compartments that are rich in adipose tissue, adipocytes function as endocrine cells and shape the tumor microenvironment.
5. Alcohol plays a contributory role in several common cancers. Strong data link alcohol with cancers of the mouth, pharynx, larynx, esophagus, liver, colorectum, and breast.
6. Evidence does not show any safe limit of alcohol and the health effects are from ethanol regardless of the type of drink.

7. Alcohol-related carcinogenesis involves acetaldehyde, ROS, pro-carcinogen activation, cellular regeneration, nutritional deficiencies, altered mucosal integrity, and enzyme and metabolic dysfunction. Under investigation are epigenetic alterations and the effects of alcohol metabolism.

8. Physical activity reduces the risk for breast and colon cancers and may reduce the risk for other cancers.

9. Biologic mechanisms for the protective effects of physical activity include decreasing insulin and IGF levels, decreasing obesity, increasing free radical scavenger systems, altering inflammatory mediators, decreasing levels of circulating sex hormones and metabolic hormones, improving immune function, enhancing cytochrome P-450 activity (thus modifying carcinogen activation), and increasing gut motility.

10. Physical activity helps to prevent type 2 diabetes, which has been associated with cancer of the pancreas and colon. Exercise in children with cancer was associated with improved body composition, flexibility, and cardiorespiratory fitness.

11. Many unanswered questions remain regarding frequency of exercise, intensity, and duration.

12. Recent data encourage 60 minutes of vigorous activity daily for decreasing BMI, body fat, and intra-abdominal fat.

Ionizing Radiation (IR)

1. Much of the knowledge of the effects of ionizing radiation on human cancer has come from Hiroshima and Nagasaki atomic bomb exposures, particularly the Life Span Study. Other evidence is from exposure to radiation for medical reasons, underground miners, and other occupational exposures. Human exposure includes emissions from the environment, x-rays, CT scans, radio isotopes, and other radioactive sources.

2. From the exposures in Japan increased frequencies of cancers occurred in thyroid and breast tissue, and lung, stomach, colon, esophageal, urinary tract, and multiple myeloma.

3. Excess relative risks (ERRs) for radiation-induced cancers at a given age are much higher for individuals exposed during childhood. What is at question now is the ERRs of radiation exposure in adulthood.

4. New models of carcinogenesis identify ionizing radiation not only as an initiator of premalignant cell clones but also as a promoter of preexisting-premalignant damage.

5. Other health risks from radiation include cardiovascular effects and somatic mutations that may contribute to other diseases. These effects may manifest years after completion of radiation therapy.

6. A summary point from BEIR VII and the NCRP is concern about the increased IR exposure from medical procedures, particularly CT scans and nuclear medicine procedures.

7. The risks from low-dose radiation are being debated among radiobiologists, geneticists, physicists, and others because of the potential effect on the health of current and future generations.

8. IR is a mutagen and carcinogen; it can penetrate cells and tissues and deposit energy in tissues at random in the form of ionizations.

9. IR affects many cellular processes, including gene expression, mitochondrial function, nucleotide base damage, and single- and double-strand DNA breaks. These changes can lead to carcinogenesis.

10. It is now known that radiation may induce a type of genomic instability to the progeny of the directly irradiated cells over many generations of cell divisions and can affect so-called innocent bystander cells. Investigators are studying genomic instability as it may contribute to secondary cancers.

11. Epigenetic events after radiation include alterations in pathways affecting cell adhesion, extracellular matrix interactions, and cell-to-cell communication.

Ultraviolet Radiation (UVR)

1. Ultraviolet (UV) radiation comes from sunlight. Other sources of UV radiation include electric lights, black lights, and tanning lamps. Most of the UV radiation received on earth is UVA and some UVB. UVA radiation is weaker than UVB, but UVA penetrates deeper into the skin and is more constant throughout the year despite the weather.

2. The incidence of basal cell carcinoma (BCC) and squamous cell carcinoma (SCC) is strongly correlated with lifetime sunlight exposure. Intense intermittent recreational sun exposure has been associated with melanoma and BCC. Tanning bed use has been associated with an increased risk of BCC and data suggest sunbed use as a reason for increased melanoma, especially in women. Chronic occupational sun exposure has been associated with SCC.

3. Cumulative sun exposure is the additive effects of intermittent sun exposure, chronic sun exposure, or both.

4. UV radiation is known to cause specific gene mutations: for example, squamous cell carcinoma involves mutation in the *TP53* gene, basal cell carcinoma in the *patched* gene, and melanoma in the *p16* gene. Investigators are identifying epigenetic alterations in tumor tissues and cell lines for skin cancers.

5. Skin exposure to UV radiation produces ROS in large quantities that can overwhelm tissue antioxidants and other oxygen-degrading pathways. Imbalances in ROS can lead to oxidative stress, tissue injury, and direct DNA damage.

6. UV radiation can activate the transcription factor NF-$\kappa\beta$ and other free radicals important in regulating genes that induce inflammation. Inflammation is a critical component of tumor progression.

7. Melanoma is the most lethal skin cancer and the incidence of melanoma has been increasing worldwide. The pathogenesis of melanoma is complex, including genetic and environmental factors.

Electromagnetic Radiation (EMR)

1. Radiofrequency electromagnetic radiation (RF-EMR) is a type of nonionizing and low-frequency radiation. Health risks associated with RF-EMR are controversial. Exposure to electric and magnetic fields is widespread.

2. RF-EMRs of varying strength include microwaves, radar, power frequency radiation associated with electricity and radio waves, fluorescent lights, computers, electric equipment, cell and cordless phones, and others.

3. Data regarding the effects of RF-EMR have been slow to emerge because of methods to accurately measure exposure, the lack of clear dose-response relationships, reproducing effects, financial interests, and other priorities such as convenience.

4. Overall there is limited evidence that magnetic fields cause childhood leukemia and insufficient evidence for other cancers in children.

5. The Working Group classified RF-EMF as "possibly carcinogenic to humans" (Group 2B).

Infection, Sexual and Reproductive Behavior

1. Infection is an important contributor to cancer worldwide. The four top infections and new cancer cases include HPV, *H. pylori*, HBV, and HCV.

2. HPV is the most common sexually transmitted virus in the United States. Although a dozen HPVs are identified, HPV types 16 and 18 are responsible for the majority of cancers. Persistence of infection with high-risk HPV is a prerequisite for the development of cervical intraepithelial neoplasia (CIN) lesions, and invasive cancer.

3. HPV infection has been identified as a definite carcinogen for 6 types of cancer: cervix, penis, vulva, anus, and some oropharynx (including the base of the tongue and tonsils).

4. The incidence of HPV-associated oropharyngeal cancer has increased during the past 20 years, especially among men.

5. Biologic factors that may interact with HPV infection to increase cancer risk include long-term oral contraceptive use, smoking, decreased immunity, having many children, poor oral hygiene (for increased risk of oropharyngeal cancer), and chronic inflammation.

6. HPV may be transmitted by genital contact (oral, touching, or sexual intercourse). The possible modes of transmission in children are controversial, newborn babies can be exposed to cervical HPV infection from the mother. A second peak of high-risk HPV prevalence occurs in postmenopausal women.

7. The incidence of oropharyngeal cancers caused by HPV is increasing worldwide.

8. HPV vaccination programs have made it possible to eliminate the majority of all invasive cervical cancer worldwide.

Air Pollution

1. Indoor and outdoor air pollution are both associated with increased rates of lung cancer. The IARC concluded that exposure to outdoor air pollution and to particulate matter (PM) in outdoor air is carcinogenic to humans.

2. $PM_{2.5}$ includes a higher proportion of mutagenic agents. Primary particles are emitted directly from a source, for example, construction sites, unpaved roads, or smokestacks. Secondary particles are emitted from power plants, industries, and automobiles. Diesel exhaust is carcinogenic and causes lung cancer.

3. Acute exposure to diesel exhaust that contains fine particles is linked to lung, throat and eye irritations, asthma attacks, and myocardial ischemia.

4. Fine particle pollution also is linked to premature death in people with heart or lung disease, nonfatal heart attacks, irregular heartbeat, and decreased lung function.

5. Mechanisms related to particle-induced lung carcinogenesis include soluble particles cause pulmonary inflammation, which leads to oxidative stress and oxidation of DNA, proliferative response, tissue remodeling toward fibrosis, and tumor development.

6. Indoor air pollution is generally considered worse than outdoor pollution. Sources of indoor air pollution include tobacco smoke, heating and cooking combustion sources, radon, and coal use.

Chemicals and Occupational Hazards as Carcinogens

1. The International Agency for Research on Cancer (IARC) has classified carcinogenic agents as known and probable.

2. An estimated 100,000 synthetic chemicals are used in the United States. Only 7% have been fully tested for their impact on health and another 1000 are added each year.

3. Exposure to chemicals occurs from air, soil, food, water, personal care products, toys, household products, medications, workplaces, and homes

4. Chemical carcinogenesis involves genotoxic and epigenetic alterations. Other mechanisms include hormonal disruption, interference with cell signaling mechanisms and other unknown effects.

5. Exposure to gene-altering substances, particularly in the womb and shortly after birth, can lead to increased susceptibility to disease.

6. Asbestos is linked to an epidemic of mesothelioma and asbestos usage has been banned in most developed countries.

7. A substantial percentage of cancers of the upper respiratory passages, lung, bladder, and peritoneum are attributed to occupational factors.

KEY TERMS

Abscopal, 287
Asbestos-silicate mineral, 293
Basal cell carcinoma (BCC), 287
Bystander effect, 286
Developmental plasticity, 272
Environmental tobacco smoke (ETS), 274

Genomic instability, 286
Individual carcinogen, 266
Melanoma, 287
Methylome, 274
"Nontargeted" effect, 286
Nutrigenomics, 276
Particulate matter (PM), 292

Phase I activation enzymes, 279
Phase II detoxification enzymes, 279
Radiofrequency electromagnetic radiation (RF-EMR), 289
Radon, 293

Squamous cell carcinoma (SCC), 287
UV radiation, 287
Xenobiotics, 279

REFERENCES

1. Clapp RW et al: Environmental and occupational causes of cancer: a call to act on what we know, *Biomed Pharmacother* 61(10):631-639, 2007.
2. Clapp RW et al: Environmental and occupational causes of cancer; new evidence 2005-2007, *Rev Environ Health* 23(1):1-37, 2008.
3. World Health Organization: *World cancer report 2014*, Geneva, Switzerland, 2014, Agency for Research on Cancer, World Health Organization.
4. Cogliano VJ et al: Preventable exposures associated with human cancers, *J Natl Cancer Inst* 103(24):1827-1839, 2011.
5. Institute of Medicine (IOM): *Rebuilding the unity of health and the environment: a new vision of environmental health for the 21st century. Workshop*

summary, Washington, DC, 2001, National Academy Press.
6. National Toxicology Program: *Report on carcinogens*, ed 12, Washington, DC, 2011, U.S. Department of Health and Human Services.
7. International Agency for Research on Cancer (IARC): *Special report: policy—a review of human carcinogens—part C: metals, arsenic, dusts, and fibres*, 2012. Available at: http://monographs.iarc.fr/ENG/Monographs/vol100C/index.php. Accessed July 2012.
8. Straif K et al: A review of human carcinogens—part C: metals, arsenic, dusts, and fibres, *Lancet Oncol* 10(5):453-454, 2009.

9. Bray F et al: Global cancer transitions according to the Human Development Index (2008–2030): a population-based study, *Lancet Oncol* 13(8):790-801, 2012.
10. Ferlay J et al: Cancer incidence and mortality worldwide: sources, methods, and major patterns in GLOBOCAN 2012, *Int J Cancer* 136(5):E359-E386, 2015.
11. National Cancer Institute: *Epidemiology and genomics research global health and cancer epidemiology*, Bethesda MD, 2014, Author.
12. Jemal A et al: Annual report to the nation on the status of cancer, 1975-2009, featuring the burden and trends in human papillomavirus (HPV)-associated cancers and HPV vaccination

coverage levels, *J Natl Cancer Inst* 105(3):175-201, 2013.

13. Gluckman PD et al: Developmental origins of health and disease: reducing the burden of chronic disease in the next generation, *Genome Med* 2(2):14, 2010.

14. Bateson P et al: Developmental plasticity and human health, *Nature* 430:419-421, 2004.

15. Waterland RA, Jirtle RJ: Early nutrition, epigenetic changes at transposons and imprinted genes, and enhanced susceptibility to adult chronic disease, *Nutrition* 20:63-68, 2004.

16. Koukoura O et al: DNA methylation in the human placenta and fetal growth, *Mol Med Rep* 5:883-889, 2012.

17. Painter RC et al: Early onset of coronary artery disease after prenatal exposure to the Dutch famine, *Am J Clin Nutr* 84:322-327, 2006.

18. Jang H, Serra C: Nutrition, epigenetics, and diseases, *Clin Nutr Res* 3(1):1-8, 2014.

19. Waterland RA: Early environmental effects on epigenetic regulation in humans, *Epigenet* 4(8): 523-525, 2009.

20. Rubin MM: Antenatal exposure to DES: lessons learned … future concerns, *Obstet Gynecol Surv* 62(8):548-555, 2007.

21. Park SK et al: Intrauterine environments and breast cancer risk: meta-analysis and systematic review, *Breast Cancer Res* 10(1):R8, 2008.

22. National Cancer Institute (NCI): *Diethylstibestrol (DES) and cancer*, Washington, DC, 2011, National Institutes of Health. Available at: www.cancer.gov/cancertopics/factsheet/Risk/DES. Accessed May 7, 2014.

23. Palmer JR et al: Prenatal diethylstilbestrol exposure and risk of breast cancer, *Cancer Epidemiol Biomarkers Prev* 15(8):1509-1514, 2006.

24. Newbold RR: Prenatal exposure to diethylstilbestrol (DES), *Fertil Steril* 89(2 suppl): e55-e56, 2008.

25. Martin O et al: Testicular dysgenesis syndrome and the estrogen hypothesis: a quantitative meta-analysis, *Ciên Saúde Colet* 13(5):1601-1618, 2008. Available at: www.scielo.br/scielo.php?script=sci_arttext&pid=S1413-81232008000500024&lng=en&nrm=iso>. Accessed April 30, 2014.

26. Znaor A et al: International variations and trends in testicular cancer incidence and mortality, *Eur Urol* 65(6):1095-1106, 2014.

27. Gluckman PD et al: Effect of in utero and early-life conditions on adult health and disease, *N Engl J Med* 359(1):61-73, 2008.

28. Gluckman PD et al: Epigenetic mechanisms that underpin metabolic and cardiovascular diseases, *Nat Rev Endocrinol* 5(7):401-408, 2009.

29. Teh AL et al: The effect of genotype and in utero environment on inter-individual variation in neonate DNA methylomes, *Genome Res* 24(7): 1064-1074, 2014.

30. Luteijn MJ, Ketting RF: PIWI-interacting RNAs: from generation to transgenerational epigenetics, *Nat Rev Genet* 14(8):523-534, 2013.

31. Newbold RR et al: Adverse effects of the model environmental estrogen diethylstilbestrol are transmitted to subsequent generations, *Endocrinology* 147(6 suppl):S11-S17, 2006.

32. International Agency for Research on Cancer (IARC): *IARC handbooks of cancer prevention. Tobacco control: effectiveness of tax and price policies for tobacco*, Geneva, Switzerland, 2011, IARC World Health Organization.

33. Secretan B et al: A review of human carcinogens—part E: tobacco, areca nut, alcohol, coal smoke, and salted fish, *Lancet Oncol* 10(11): 1033-1034, 2009.

34. Office of the Surgeon General: *The health consequences of smoking—50 years of progress. A report of the Surgeon General executive summary*, Rockville, Md, 2014, U.S. Department of Health and Human Services.

35. Centers for Disease Control and Prevention: Global youth tobacco surveillance, 2000–2007, *MMWR Morb Mortal Wkly Rep* 57(5501):1-21, 2008.

36. Zeng W et al: Burden of total and cause-specific mortality related to tobacco smoking among adults aged ≥45 years in Asia: a pooled analysis of 21 cohorts, *PLoS Med* 11(4):e1001631, 2014.

37. World Health Organization: *WHO report on the global tobacco epidemic, 2011. Warning about the dangers of tobacco, executive summary*, Geneva, Switzerland, 2011, Author.

38. Centers for Disease Control and Prevention: Annual smoking-attributable mortality, years of potential life lost, and productivity losses—United States, 1995–1999, *MMWR Morb Mortal Wkly Rep* 51(14):300-303, 2002.

39. World Health Organization (WHO): *World cancer report: global cancer rates could increase by 50% to 15 million by 2020*. Available at: www.WHO.int/mediacentre/news/release/2003/pr27/en/. Accessed July 2008.

40. Centers for Disease Control and Prevention: Current cigarette smoking among adults—United States, 2005–2012, *MMWR Morb Mortal Wkly Rep* 63(02):29-34, 2014.

41. Agaku IT et al: Current cigarette smoking among adults—United States, 2005–2012, *MMWR Morb Mortal Wkly Rep* 63(2):29-34, 2014.

42. Lushniak BD: A historic moment: the 50th anniversary of the first Surgeon General's Report on smoking and health, *Public Health Rep* 129(1):5-6, 2014.

43. Centers for Disease Control and Prevention: *Smoking and secondhand smoke*. Available at: www.cdc.gov/cancer/lung. Accessed July 2010.

44. Centers for Disease Control and Prevention: *Cigar smoking and cancer*. Available at: www.cancer.gov/cancertopics/factsheet/Tobacco/cigars. Accessed July 2010.

45. American Cancer Society (ACS): *What are the health risks of smoking pipes or cigars?* Atlanta, Ga, 2014, Author. Accessed October 11, 2014.

46. Centers for Disease Control and Prevention: Consumption of cigarettes and combustible tobacco—United States, 2000–2011, *MMWR Morb Mortal Wkly Rep* 61(30), 2012.

47. Taioli E: Gene-environment interaction in tobacco-related cancers, *Carcinogenesis* 29(8): 1467-1474, 2008.

48. Giri PA et al: Study of socio-demographic determinants of esophageal cancer at a tertiary care teaching hospital of Western Maharashtra, India, *South Asian J Cancer* 3(1):54-56, 2014.

49. Farvid MS et al: Dietary protein sources in early adulthood and breast cancer incidence: prospective cohort study, *Br J* 348:g3437, 2014.

50. World Cancer Research Fund/American Institute for Cancer Research (WCRF/AICR): *Second expert report: food, nutrition, physical activity, and the prevention of cancer: a global perspective*, London, 2007, Author.

51. Kiefte-de Jong JC et al: Nutrition and healthy aging: the key ingredients, *Proc Nutr Soc* 73(2):249-259, 2014.

52. Cancer Research UK: *Bowel cancer incidence statistics*, London, U.K., 2013, Registered Charity in England, Wales, Scotland, and the Isle of Man.

53. Hjartaker A et al: Subsite-specific dietary risk factors for colorectal cancer: a review of cohort studies, *J Oncol*, Article ID 703854, 14 pp, 2014.

54. Center MM et al: International trends in colorectal cancer incidence rates, *Cancer Epidemiol Biomarkers Prev* 18(6):1688-1694, 2009.

55. Mathers JC et al: Induction of epigenetic alterations by dietary and other environmental factors, *Adv Genet* 71:3-39, 2010.

56. Nitter M et al: Plasma methionine, choline, betaine, and dimethylglycine, in relation to colorectal cancer risk in the European Prospective Investigation into Cancer and Nutrition (EPIC), *Ann Oncol* 25(8):1609-1615, 2014.

57. Choi S-W et al: Nutrients and DNA methylation. In Choi S-W, Frisco S, editors: *Nutrients and epigenetics*, Boca Raton, Fla, 2009, pp 105-126, CRC Press Taylor & Francis Group.

58. Steegers-Theunissen RP et al: Periconceptional maternal folic acid use of 4000 microg per day is related to increased methylation of the IGF2 gene in the very young child, *PLoS One* 4(11):e7845, 2009.

59. Dominguez-Salas P et al: Maternal nutrition at conception modulates DNA methylation of human metastable epialleles, *Nat Comm* 5:3746, 2014.

60. Waterland RA, Jirtle RL: Transposable elements: targets for early nutritional effects on epigenetic gene regulation, *Mol Cell Biol* 23:5293-5300, 2003.

61. Kovacheva VP et al: Gestational choline deficiency causes global and Igf2 gene DNA hypermethylation by up-regulation of Dnmt1 expression, *J Biol Chem* 282(43):31777-31788, 2007.

62. Kim YI et al: Folate deficiency in rats induces DNA strand breaks and hypomethylation within the p53 tumor suppressor gene, *Am J Clin Nutr* 65(1):46-52, 1997.

63. Persson EC et al: Alcohol consumption, folate intake, hepatocellular carcinoma, and liver disease mortality, *Cancer Epidemiol Biomarkers Prev* 22(3):415-421, 2013.

64. Wu MY et al: Lymphocytic mitochondrial DNA deletions, biochemical folate status and hepatocellular carcinoma susceptibility in a case-control study, *Br J Nutr* 102(5):715-721, 2009.

65. Lee WJ et al: Mechanisms for the inhibition of DNA methyltransferases by tea catechins and bioflavonoids, *Mol Pharmacol* 68(4):1018-1030, 2005.

66. Delage B, Dashwood RH: Dietary manipulation of histone structure and function, *Annu Rev Nutr* 28:347-366, 2008.

67. Miozzo M et al: Epigenetic alterations in cancer and personalized cancer treatment, *Future Oncol* 11(2):333-348, 2015.

68. Kim HN et al: Sulforaphane inhibits phorbol ester-stimulated IKK-NK-κB signaling and COX-2 expression in human mammary epithelial cells by targeting NF-κB activating kinase and ERK, *Cancer Lett* 351(1):41-49, 2014.

69. Phuah NH, Nagoor NH: Regulation of microRNAs by natural agents: new strategies in cancer therapies, *Biomed Res Int* 2014:804510, 2014.

70. Saud SM et al: Resveratrol prevents tumorigenesis in mouse model of Kras activated colorectal cancer by suppressing oncogenic Kras expression, *Carcinogenesis* 35(12):2778-2786, 2014.

71. Semba RD et al: Resveratrol levels and all-cause mortality in older community-welling adults, *J Am Med Assoc Intern Med* 174(7):1077-1084, 2014.

72. Dahmke IN et al: Curcumin intake affects miRNA signature in murine melanoma with mmu-miR-205-5p most significantly altered, *PLoS One* 8(12):e81122, 2013.

73. Yang CH et al: The curcumin analog EF24 targets NF-κB and miRNA-21, and has potent anticancer activity in vitro and in vivo, *PLoS One* 8(8):e71130, 2013.

74. Kim YS et al: Cancer stem cells: potential target for bioactive food components, *J Nutr Biochem* 23:691-698, 2012.

75. O'Brien LE et al: Altered modes of stem cell division drive adaptive intestinal growth, *Cell* 147:603-614, 2011.

76. Ginestier C et al: Retinoid signaling regulates breast cancer stem cell differentiation, *Cell Cycle* 8:3297-3302, 2009.

77. Slyskova J et al: Both genetic and dietary factors underlie individual differences in DNA damage levels and DNA repair capacity, *DNA Repair (Amst)* 16:66-73, 2014.

78. Gonzalez C et al: Hydrogen peroxide-induced DNA damage and DNA repair in lymphocytes from malnourished children? *Environ Mol Mutagen* 39:33-42, 2002.

79. Arab L et al: Lycopene and the lung, *Exp Biol Med (Maywood)* 227:894-899, 2002.

80. Yang G et al: Isothiocyanate exposure, glutathione S-transferase polymorphisms, and colon cancer risk, *Am J Nutr* 91(3):704-711, 2010.

81. Corpet DE: Epidemiological evidence for the association between red and processed meat intake and colorectal cancer, *Science* 98:115, 2014.

82. Eicholzer M et al: Polymorphisms in heterocyclic aromatic amines metabolism-related genes are associated with colorectal adenoma risk, *Int J Mol Epidemiol Genet* 3(2):96-106, 2012.

83. World Cancer Research Fund/American Institute for Cancer Research: *WCRF/AICR systematic literature review continuous update project report,* 2011. Available from www.wcrf.org/PDFs/Colorectal-cancer-CUP-report-2010.pdf.

84. zur Hausen H: Red meat consumption and cancer: reasons to suspect involvement of bovine infectious factors in colorectal cancer, *Int J Cancer* 130(11):2475-2483, 2012.

85. Glickman D et al: *Accelerating progress in obesity prevention: solving the weight of the nation,* Washington, DC, 2012, The National Academies Press.

86. Ogden CL et al: Prevalence of childhood and adult obesity in the United States, 2011-2014, *J Am Med Assoc* 311(8):806-814, 2014.

87. Demark-Wahnefried W et al: The role of obesity in cancer survival and recurrence, *Cancer Epidemiol Biomarkers Prev* 21(8):1244-1259. 2012.

88. Haslam D: Obesity: a medical history, *Obes Rev* 8(Suppl 1):31-36, 2007.

89. Cao Y, Ma J: Body mass index, prostate cancer-specific mortality, and biochemical recurrence: a systematic review and meta-analysis, *Cancer Prev Res (Phila)* 4:486-501, 2011.

90. Ewertz M et al: Effect of obesity on prognosis after early-stage breast cancer, *J Clin Oncol* 29:25-31, 2011.

91. Sinicrope FA et al: Obesity is an independent prognostic variable in colon cancer survivors, *Clin Cancer Res* 16:1884-1893, 2010.

92. World Health Organization: *Obesity and overweight,* World Health Organization, Geneva, 2014, Author.

93. Park J et al: Obesity and cancer—mechanisms underlying tumor progression and recurrence, *Nat Rev Endocrinol* 10(8):455-465, 2014.

94. Park J et al: Paracrine and endocrine effects of adipose tissue on cancer development and progression, *Endocr Rev* 32(4):550-570, 2011.

95. Pérez-Hernández AI et al: Mechanisms linking excess adiposity and carcinogenesis promotion, *Front Endocrinol (Lausanne)* 5:65, 2014.

96. American Cancer Society (ACS): *Cancer treatment and survivorship facts & figures 2012-2013,* Atlanta, Ga, 2012, Author.

97. Mandrekar P: Epigenetic regulation in alcoholic liver disease, *World J Gastroenterol* 17(20):2456-2464, 2011.

98. Zakhari S: Alcohol metabolism and epigenetic changes, *Alcohol Res* 35(1):6-16, 2013.

99. National Cancer Institute (NCI): *Physical activity and cancer,* Washington, DC, 2009, National Institutes of Health. Available at: www.cancer.gov/cancertopics/factsheet/prevention/physicalactivity. Accessed September 17, 2014.

100. Soria G et al: Prime, repair, restore: the active role of chromatin in the DNA response, *Mol Cell* 46(6):722-734, 2012.

101. Bertucci A et al: Microbeam irradiation of the *C. elegans* nematode, *J Radiat Res* 50:A49-A54, 2009.

102. Mancuso M et al: Oncogeneic bystander radiation effects in patched heterozygous mouse cerebellum, *Proc Natl Acad Sci U S A* 105(34):12445-12450, 2008.

103. Nguyen DH et al: Radiation acts on the microenvironment to affect breast carcinogenesis by distinct mechanisms that decrease cancer latency and affect tumor type, *Cancer Cell* 19:640-651, 2011.

104. Ojima M et al: Persistence of DNA double-strand breaks in normal human cells induced by radiation-induced bystander effect, *Radiat Res* 175:90-96, 2011.

105. Chute JP: To survive radiation injury, remember you're APCs, *Nat Med* 18(7):1013-1014, 2012.

106. Barcellos-Hoff MH, Nguyen DH: Radiation carcinogenesis in context: how do irradiated tissues become tumors? *Health Phys* 97(5):446-457, 2009.

107. Wright EG: Manifestations and mechanisms of non-targeted effects of ionizing radiation, *Mutat Res* 687(1-2):28-33, 2010.

108. Cramp F, Byron-Daniel J: Exercise for the management of cancer-related fatigue in adults, *Cochrane Database Syst Rev* 11:CD006145, 2012.

109. Braam KI et al: Physical exercise training interventions for children and young adults during and after treatment for childhood cancer, *Cochrane Database Syst Rev* 4:CD008796, 2013.

110. Little MP: Heterogeneity of variation of relative risk by age at exposure in the Japanese atomic bomb survivors, *Radiat Environ Biophys* 48(3):253-262, 2009.

111. Shuryak I et al: A new view of radiation-induced cancer: integrating short- and long-processes. Part I: Approach, *Radiat Environ Biophys* 48(3):263-274, 2009.

112. Shuryak I et al: Cancer risks after radiation exposure in middle age, *J Natl Cancer Inst* 102(21):1606-1609, 2010.

113. Preston DL et al: Solid cancer incidence in atomic bomb survivors: 1958–1998, *Radiat Res* 168(1):1-64, 2007.

114. Committee on the Biological Effects of Ionizing Radiation: *Health risks from exposure to low levels of ionizing radiation, BEIR VII Phase 2,* Washington, DC, 2006, National Academies Press.

115. Walsh L: Heterogeneity of variation of relative risk by age at exposure in Japanese atomic bomb survivors, *Radiat Environ Biophys* 48(3):345-347, 2009.

116. Preston DL et al: Studies of mortality of atomic bomb survivors. Report 13: solid cancer and noncancer disease mortality: 1950–1997, *Radiat Res* 160:381-407, 2003.

117. Hoel DG: Ionizing radiation and cardiovascular disease, *Ann N Y Acad Sci* 1076:309-317, 2006.

118. Rombouts C et al: Differential response to acute low dose radiation in primary and immortalized endothelial cells, *Int J Radiat Biol* 89(10):841-850, 2013.

119. Yusuf SW et al: Radiation-induced heart disease: a clinical update, *Cardiol Res Pract* 317659:2011, 2011.

120. Linet MS et al: Children's exposure to diagnostic medical radiation and cancer risk: epidemiologic and dosimetric considerations, *Pediatr Radiol* 39(Suppl 1):S4-S26, 2009.

121. Schulze-Rath R et al: Are pre- or postnatal diagnostic X-rays a risk factor for childhood cancer? A systematic review, *Radiat Environ Biophys* 47:301-312, 2008.

122. Wakeford R: Childhood leukaemia following medical diagnostic exposure to ionizing radiation in utero or after birth, *Radiat Prot Dosimetry* 132:166-174, 2008.

123. Harbron RW: Cancer risks from low dose exposure to ionising radiation—is the linear no-threshold model still relevant? *Radiography* 18:28-33, 2012.

124. Prasad KN et al: Health risks of low dose ionizing radiation in humans: a review, *Exp Biol Med* 229(5):378-382, 2004.

125. National Council on Radiation Protection and Measurement (NCRP): *1929–2009 medical radiation exposure of the U.S. population greatly increased since the early 1980s,* March 2009. Available at: http://NCRPonline%2Corg.

126. Brenner DJ, Hall EJ: Computed tomography—an increasing source of radiation exposure, *N Engl J Med* 357(22):2277-2284, 2007.

127. Smith-Bendman R et al: Use of diagnostic imaging studies and associated radiation exposure for patients enrolled in large integrated health care system, 1996-2010, *J Am Med Assoc* 307(22):2400-2409, 2012.

128. Little JB: Cellular radiation effects and the bystander response, *Mutat Res* 597:113-118, 2006.

129. Little JB: Radiation carcinogenesis, *Carcinogenesis* 21(3):397-404, 2000.

130. Jones JA et al: Ionizing radiation as a carcinogen. In McQueen CA, editor: *Comprehensive toxicology,* ed 2, St Louis, 2010, Elsevier.

131. Kovalchuk O, Baulch JE: Epigenetic changes and nontargeted radiation effects—is there a link? *Environ Mol Mutagen* 49(1):16-25, 2008.

132. Cunniffe S et al: Reduced repair capacity of a DNA clustered damage site comprised of 8-oxo-7,8-dihydro-2″-deoxyguanosine and 2-deoxyribonolactone results in an increased mutagenic potential of these lesions, *Mutat Res Fundam Mol Mech Mutagen* 762:32-39, 2014.

133. Vaidya A et al: Knock-in reporter mice demonstrate that DNA repair by non-homologous end joining declines with age, *PLoS Genet* 10(7):e1004511, 2014.

134. Nag S et al: The MDM2-p53 pathway revisited, *J Biomed Res* 27(4):254-271, 2013.

135. Koturbash I et al: In vivo bystander effects: cranial x-irradiation leads to elevated DNA damage, altered cellular proliferation and apoptosis, and increased p53 levels in shielded spleen, *Int J Radiat Oncol Biol Phys* 70(2):554-562, 2008.

136. Mukherjee D et al: Responses to ionizing radiation mediated by inflammatory mechanisms, *J Pathol* 232(3):289-299, 2014.

137. Werner E et al: Opposite roles for p38MAPK-driven responses and reactive oxygen species in the persistence and resolution of radiation-induced genomic instability, *PLoS One* (10):e108234, 2014.

138. Morganti JM et al: Cranial irradiation alters the brain's microenvironment and permits CCR2+ macrophage infiltration, *PLoS One* 9(4):e93650, 2014.

139. Barrington de Gonzalez A et al: Proportion of second cancers attributable to radiotherapy treatment in adults: a prospective cohort study in the US SEER cancer registries, *Lancet Oncol* 12(4):353-360, 2011.

140. Parkin DM, Darby SC: Cancers in 2010 attributable to ionising radiation exposure in the UK, *BJ Cancer* 105:S57-S65, 2011.

141. Institute of Medicine: *Findings from research on health effects of low-level ionizing radiation exposure: opportunities for the Armed Forces Radiobiology Research Institute,* Washington DC, June 2014, Author.

142. Shuryak I et al: Potential for adult-based epidemiological studies to characterize overall cancer risks associated with a lifetime of CT scans, *Radiat Res* 181(6):584-591, 2014.

143. Centers for Disease Control and Treatment (CDC): *Radiation and your health,* Atlanta, Ga, 2014, Author. Available at: www.cdc.gov/nceh/radiation/. Accessed August 17, 2014.

144. World Health Organization (WHO): *Ultraviolet radiation and the INTERSUN,* Geneva, 2014, Programme World Health Organization.

145. National Cancer Institute (NCI): *Types of skin cancer,* Washington, DC, 2011, National Institutes of Health. Available at: www.cancer.gov/cancertopics/wyntk/skin/page4. Accessed August 20, 2014.

146. National Cancer Institute (NCI): *Cellular classification of skin cancer,* Washington, DC, 2013, National Institutes of Health.

147. National Cancer Institute (NCI): *Genetics of skin cancer,* Washington, DC, 2014, National Institutes of Health. Accessed August 20, 2014.

148. National Cancer Institute (NCI): *Anyone can get skin cancer,* Washington, DC, 2011, National Institutes of Health. Accessed August 20, 2014.

149. Cleaver JE, Crowley E: UV damage, DNA repair, and skin carcinogenesis, *Front Biosci* 7:d1024-d1043, 2002.

150. Atwood SX et al: Advanced treatment for basal cell carcinomas, *Cold Spring Harb Perspect Med* 4(7):a013581, 2014.

151. Besaratinia A, Tommasi S: Epigenetics of human melanoma: promises and challenges, *J Mol Cell Biol* 6(5):356-367, 2014.

152. Stamatelli A et al: Epigenetic alterations in sporadic basal cell carcinomas, *Arch Dermatol Res* 306(6):561-569, 2014.

153. Wu Y et al: Clinical significance of methylation of E-cadherin and p14ARF gene promoters in skin squamous cell carcinoma tissues, *Int J Clin Exp Med* 7(7):1808-1812, 2014.

154. Streilein JW et al: Immune surveillance and sunlight-induced skin cancer, *Immunol Today* 15(4):174-179, 1994

155. Maru GB et al: The role of inflammation in skin cancer, *Adv Exp Med Biol* 816:437-469, 2014.

156. Bickers DR, Ather M: Oxidative stress in the pathogenesis of skin disease, *J Invest Dermatol* 126:2562-2575, 2006.

157. Dhar A et al: The role of AP-1, NF-kappaB, and ROS/NOS in skin carcinogenesis: the JB6 model is predictive, *Mol Cell Biochem* 234(1-2):185-193, 2002.

158. Sander CD et al: Role of oxidative stress and the antioxidant network in cutaneous carcinogenesis, *Int J Dermatol* 43(5):326-335, 2004.

159. Lin J et al: Genetics of melanoma, *Br J Dermatol* 159(2):286-291, 2008.

160. American Cancer Society: *Cancer facts and figures 2015*, Atlanta, Ga: 2015, Author. Accessed April 1, 2015.

161. Campbell LB et al: Melanoma incidence in children and adolescents: decreasing trends in the United States, *J Pediatr* 2015 Apr 9. [Epub ahead of print.]

162. Frangos JE et al: Increased diagnosis of thin superficial spreading melanomas: a 20-year study, *J Am Academy Dermatol* 67(3):387-394, 2012.

163. Welch HG, Black WC: Overdiagnosis in cancer, *J Natl Cancer Inst* 102:605-613, 2010.

164. Baron AE et al: Interactions between ultraviolet light and MC1R and OCA2 variants are determinants of childhood nevus and freckle phenotypes, *Cancer Epidemiol Biomarkers Prev* 23(12):2829-2839, 2014.

165. Heymann WR: Screening for melanoma, *J Am Acad Dermatol* 56(1):144-145, 2007.

166. Whipple CA, Brinkerhoff CE: BRAFv600E melanoma cells secrete factors that activate stromal fibroblasts and enhance tumorigenicity, *Br J Cancer* 111(8):1625-1633, 2014.

167. Kumar V et al: *Robbins and Cotran pathologic basis of disease*, ed 9, Philadelphia, 2014, Saunders.

168. Dore JF, Chignol MC: Tanning salons and skin cancer, *Photochem Photobiol* 11(1):30-37, 2012.

169. Gandini S et al: Melanoma attributable to sunbed use and tan seeking behaviors: an Italian survey, *Eur J Dermatol* 24(1):35-40, 2014.

170. Héry C et al: A melanoma epidemic in Iceland: possible influence of sunbed use, *Am J Epidemiol* 172(7):762-767, 2010.

171. Lazovich D et al: Indoor tanning and risk of melanoma: a case-control study in a highly exposed population, *Cancer Epidemiol Biomarkers Prev* 19(60):1557-1568, 2010.

172. Bens G: Sunscreens, *Adv Exp Med Biol* 810:429-463, 2014.

173. Baan R et al: Carcinogenicity of radiofrequency electromagnetic fields, *Lancet Oncol* 12(7):624-626, 2011.

174. Genuis SJ: Fielding a current idea: exploring the public health impact of electromagnetic radiation, *Public Health* 122(2):113-124, 2008.

175. Belyaev IY: Dependence of non-thermal biological effects of microwaves on physical and biological variables: implications for reproducibility and safety standards, *Eur J Oncol Library* 5:187-219, 2010.

176. National Institute of Environmental Health Sciences (NIEHS) Working Group Report: *Assessment of health effects from exposure to power-line frequency electric and magnetic fields*, Washington, DC, 1998, U.S. Government Printing Office.

177. National Cancer Institute (NCI): *Fact sheet: magnetic field exposure and cancer*, Washington,

DC, 2005, National Institutes of Health, National Cancer Institute. Available at: www.cancer.gov/cancertopics/factsheet/Risk/magnetic-fields. Accessed July 2012.

178. UK Childhood Cancer Study Investigators: Exposure to power-frequency magnetic fields and the risk of childhood cancer, *Lancet* 354(9194):1925-1931, 1999.

179. UK Childhood Cancer Study Investigators: Childhood cancer and residential proximity to power lines, *Br J Cancer* 83(11):1573-1580, 2000.

180. Bunch KJ et al: Residential distance at birth from overhead high-voltage powerlines: childhood cancer risk in Britain 1962-2008, *Br J Cancer* 110:1402-1408, 2014.

181. Hauri DD et al: Exposure to radio-frequency electromagnetic fields from broadcast transmitters and risk of childhood cancer: a census-based cohort study, *Am J Epidemiol* 179(7):843-851, 2014.

182. INTERPHONE Study Group: Brain tumour risk in relation to mobile telephone use: results of the INTERPHONE International Case-control Study, *Int J Epidemiol* 39:675-694, 2010.

183. Hardell L et al: Use of mobile phones and cordless phones is associated with increased risk for glioma and acoustic neuroma, *Pathophysiology* 20:85-110, 2013.

184. Hardell L et al: Pooled analysis of case-control studies on malignant brain tumours and the use of mobile and cordless phones including living and deceased subjects, *Int J Oncol* 38:1465-1474, 2011.

185. Christensen HC et al: Cellular telephone use and risk of acoustic neuroma, *Am J Epidemiol* 159(3):277-283, 2004.

186. Volkow ND et al: Effects of cell phone radiofrequency signal exposure on brain glucose metabolism, *J Am Med Assoc* 305(8):808-813, 2011.

187. Cardis E et al: Distribution of RF energy emitted by mobile phones in anatomical structures of the brain, *Phys Med Biol* 53(11):2771-2783, 2008.

188. Christ A et al: Age-dependent tissue-specific exposure of cell phone users, *Phys Med Biol* 55(7):1767-1783, 2010.

189. Gandhi OP et al: Exposure limits: the underestimation of absorbed cell phone radiation, especially in children, *Electromagn Biol Med* 31(1):34-51, 2012.

190. Davis DL et al: Swedish review strengthens grounds for concluding that radiation from cellular and cordless phones is a probable human carcinogen, *Pathophysiology* 20(2):123-129, 2013.

191. de Martel C et al: Global burden of cancers attributable to infections in 2008: a review and synthetic analysis, *Lancet Oncol* 13(6):607-615, 2012.

192. Dart H et al: Commentary: eight ways to prevent cancer: a framework for effective prevention messages for the public, *Cancer Causes Control* 23(4):601-608, 2012.

193. Plummer M et al: Global burden of gastric cancer attributable to *Helicobacter pylori*, *Int J Cancer* 136(2):487-490, 2014.

194. Centers for Disease Control and Prevention (CDC): *Human papillomavirus (HPV)*, Atlanta, Ga, 2012, Author.

195. National Cancer Institute (NCI): *HPV and cancer*, Washington, DC, 2012, Author.

196. National Cancer Institute (NCI): *Pap and HPV testing*, National Cancer Institute, National Institutes of Health updated 09/09/2014. Available at: www.cancer.gov/cancertopics/factsheet/detection/Pap-HPV-testing. Accessed September 16, 2014.

197. International Agency for Research on Cancer (IARC): *IARC monographs on the evaluation of carcinogenic risks to humans, Biological agents 100B: a review of human carcinogens*, Lyon, France, 2012, Author. Available at: http://monographs.iarc.fr/ENG/Monographs/vol100B/index.php.

198. Schiffman M et al: Human papillomavirus and cervical cancer, *Lancet* 370(9590):890-907, 2007.

199. Smith EM et al: Evidence for vertical transmission of HPV from mothers to infants, *Infect Dis Obstet Gynecol* 2010:326369, 2010. Available at: http://dx.doi.org/10.1155/2010/326369.

200. Syrjanen S, Puranen M: Human papillomavirus infections in children: the potential role of maternal transmission, *Crit Rev Oral Biol Med* 11(2):259-274, 2000.

201. Moyer VA: U.S. Preventive Services Task Force screening for cervical cancer: U.S. Preventive Services Task Force recommendation statement, *Ann Intern Med* 156(12):880-891, 2012.

202. Centers for Disease Control and Prevention (CDC): *Genital HPV infection-fact sheet*, Atlanta GA, 2015, Author.

203. Hamra GB et al: Outdoor particulate matter exposure and lung cancer: a systematic review and meta-analysis, *Environ Health Perspect* 122(9):906-911, 2014.

204. International Agency for Research on Cancer (IARC): *Outdoor air pollution, IARC Monogr Eval Carcinog Risks Hum* Volume 109, Lyon, France 2013.

205. Loomis D et al: The carcinogenicity of outdoor air pollution, *Lancet Oncol* 14:1262-1263, 2013.

206. Buschini A et al: Urban airborne particulate: genotoxicity evaluation of different size fractions by mutagenesis tests on microorganisms and comet assay, *Chemosphere* 44:1723-1736, 2001.

207. Environmental Protection Agency (EPA): *Particulate matter, updated March 18, 2013*, Washington, DC, 2013, Author.

208. Puett RC et al: Chronic fine and course particulate exposure, mortality, and coronary heart disease in the Nurses' Health Study, *Environ Health Perspect* 117(11):1697-1701, 2009.

209. Gulland A: Diesel engine exhaust causes lung cancer, says WHO, *Br Med J* 344:e4174, 2012.

210. Lim SS et al: A comparative risk assessment of burden of disease and injury attributable to 67 risk factors and risk factor clusters in 21 regions, 1990-2010: a systematic analysis for the Global Burden of Disease Study 2010, *Lancet* 380:2224-2260, 2012.

211. Boffetta P et al: Mortality among workers employed in the titanium dioxide production industry in Europe, *Cancer Causes Control* 15(7):697-706, 2004.

212. Hecht SS et al: Elevated levels of volatile organic carcinogen and toxicant biomarkers in Chinese women who regularly cook at home, *Cancer Epidemiol Biomarkers Prev* 19(5):1185-1192, 2010.

213. Barone-Adesi F et al: Risk of lung cancer associated with domestic use of coal in Xuanwei, China: retrospective cohort study, *Br Med J* 345:e5411, 2012.

214. Zhao Y et al: Air pollution and lung cancer risks in China—meta-analysis, *Sci Total Environ* 366(2-3):500-513, 2006.

215. Borm PJ et al: Inhaled particles and lung cancer, part B: paradigms and risk assessment, *Int J Cancer* 110(1):3-14, 2004.

216. Agency for Toxic Substances and Disease Registry (ATSDR): *Chemicals, cancer, and you*, Atlanta, Ga, Agency for Toxic Substances and Disease Registry, Division of Health Assessment and Consultation, U.S. Department of Health and Human Services. Available at: www.atsdr.cdc.gov/.../Chemicals,%20Cancer,%20and%20You%20FS.pdf. Accessed September 18, 2014.

217. Gray J: *State of the evidence 2008: the connection between breast cancer and the environment*, San Francisco, 2008, Breast Cancer Fund.

218. Tryndyak VP et al: Effect of long-term tamoxifen exposure on genotoxic and epigenetic changes in rat liver: implications for tamoxifen-induced hepatocarcinogenesis, *Carcinogenesis* 27:1713-1720, 2006.

219. Karpinets TV, Foy BD: Tumorigenesis: the adaptation of mammalian cells to sustained stress

environment by epigenetic alterations and succeeding matched mutations, *Carcinogenesis* 26:1323-1334, 2005.

220. Tabish AM et al: Epigenetic factors in cancer risk: effect of chemical carcinogens on global DNA methylation pattern in human TK6 cells, *PLoS One* 7(4):e34674, 2012.

221. Hileman B: *Chemicals can turn genes on and off; new tests needed, scientists say, Environmental Health News,* Charlottesville, Va, August 3, 2009,

National Institute of Environmental Health Sciences.

222. Neuberger JS, Field RW: Occupation and lung cancer in nonsmokers, *Rev Environ Health* 18(4):251-267, 2003.

223. Prazakova S et al: Asbestos and the lung in the 21st century: an update, *Clin Respir J* 8(1):1-10, 2014.

224. Puett RC et al: Particulate matter air pollution exposure, distance to road, and incident lung

cancer in the nurses' health study cohort, *Environ Health Perspect* 122(9):926-932, 2014.

225. Raaschou-Nielsen O et al: Air pollution and lung cancer incidence in 17 European cohorts: prospective analyses from the European Study of Cohorts for Air Pollution Effects (ESCAPE), *Lancet Oncol* 14(9):813-822, 2013.

226. Vineis P et al: Outdoor air pollution and lung cancer: recent epidemiologic evidence, *Int J Cancer* 111(5):647-652, 2004.

12

Cancer in Children and Adolescents

Lauri A. Linder and Nancy E. Kline

CHAPTER OUTLINE

Cancer in children and adolescents is rare; however, it remains the leading cause of death that is attributable to disease for this age group.[1] Survival rates among children and adolescents with cancer have dramatically improved since the 1960s. Among the factors leading to improved cure rates include the use of combination chemotherapy, the incorporation of research data obtained from clinical trials, and the utilization of multimodal treatment for solid tumors.

INCIDENCE, ETIOLOGY, AND TYPES OF CHILDHOOD CANCER

More than 15,500 children and adolescents 19 years of age and younger were estimated to be diagnosed with cancer in the United States in 2014.[2] The overall incidence of childhood and adolescent cancer is 17.2 per 100,000 children (Figure 12-1).[3] This incidence, however, demonstrates a bimodal distribution across age groups with peaks among children less than 5 years of age and adolescents 15 to 19 years of age. Childhood cancer in the United States also is slightly more common in boys than in girls. The male/female ratio for childhood cancers is 1.2 : 1.0.[3]

In 2011, the death rates of children from birth to 14 years of age with cancer were 2.3 per 100,000 for males and 2.1 per 100,000 for females. Death rates for adolescents 15 to 19 years of age were 3.4 per 100,000 for males and 2.5 per 100,000 for females.[3] By comparison, cancer had an overall mortality of 163.2 per 100,000 adults in 2013.[4]

The types of malignancies occurring in children are vastly different from those that affect adults. The most common types of cancer among adults include prostate, breast, lung, and colon. In contrast, children tend to develop leukemias, brain tumors, and sarcomas. Although many adult cancers have associated lifestyle factors that could theoretically be avoided, such as smoking and exposure to sun, very few environmental factors have been linked to pediatric malignancies. More data are emerging that the developing child may be affected by epigenetic modifications resulting from parental exposures before conception, exposures in utero, and nutrition during early life.[5,6]

Most childhood cancers originate from the mesodermal germ layer, which develops into connective tissue, bone, cartilage, muscle, blood, blood vessels, gonads, kidney, and the lymphatic system (Figure 12-2). Thus the more common childhood cancers are leukemias, sarcomas, and embryonic tumors.

Embryonic tumors originate during intrauterine life and contain abnormal cells that appear to be immature embryonic tissue unable to mature or differentiate into fully developed functional cells. Embryonic tumors are most often diagnosed early in life (usually by 5 years of age) and are rare in older children, adolescents, and adults. The names of these tumors often include the root term *blast* (e.g., neuroblastoma, retinoblastoma), which indicates the embryonic stage of development.

Sarcomas, leukemias, and lymphomas are cancers observed in childhood and also may occur in adults. Most adult cancers, however, involve epithelial tissue and are, therefore, carcinomas. Carcinomas rarely occur in children because these cancers most commonly result from environmental carcinogens and require a long period from exposure to the appearance of the carcinoma. Carcinomas begin to increase in incidence between the ages of 15 and 19 years, becoming the most common cancer tissue type observed after adolescence.[3]

Childhood cancers are often diagnosed during peak times of physical growth and maturation, accounting for the bimodal distribution in their incidence. In general, they are extremely fast-growing cancers, resulting in a relatively short latency period—that is, the time from the initial exposure to the onset of symptoms. The distribution of cancer types also changes during childhood and adolescence. Leukemias and embryonal tumors have a peak incidence before the child is 5 years of age. Brain tumors, the second leading type of childhood cancer overall, have a peak incidence among children less than 15 years of age. The incidence of specific subtypes of brain tumors does, however, vary across childhood and adolescence. Lymphomas, both Hodgkin and non-Hodgkin, represent the third most common type of childhood cancer. Lymphoma is rare in children less than 5 years of age and occurs with increasing frequency in children and adolescents 10 years

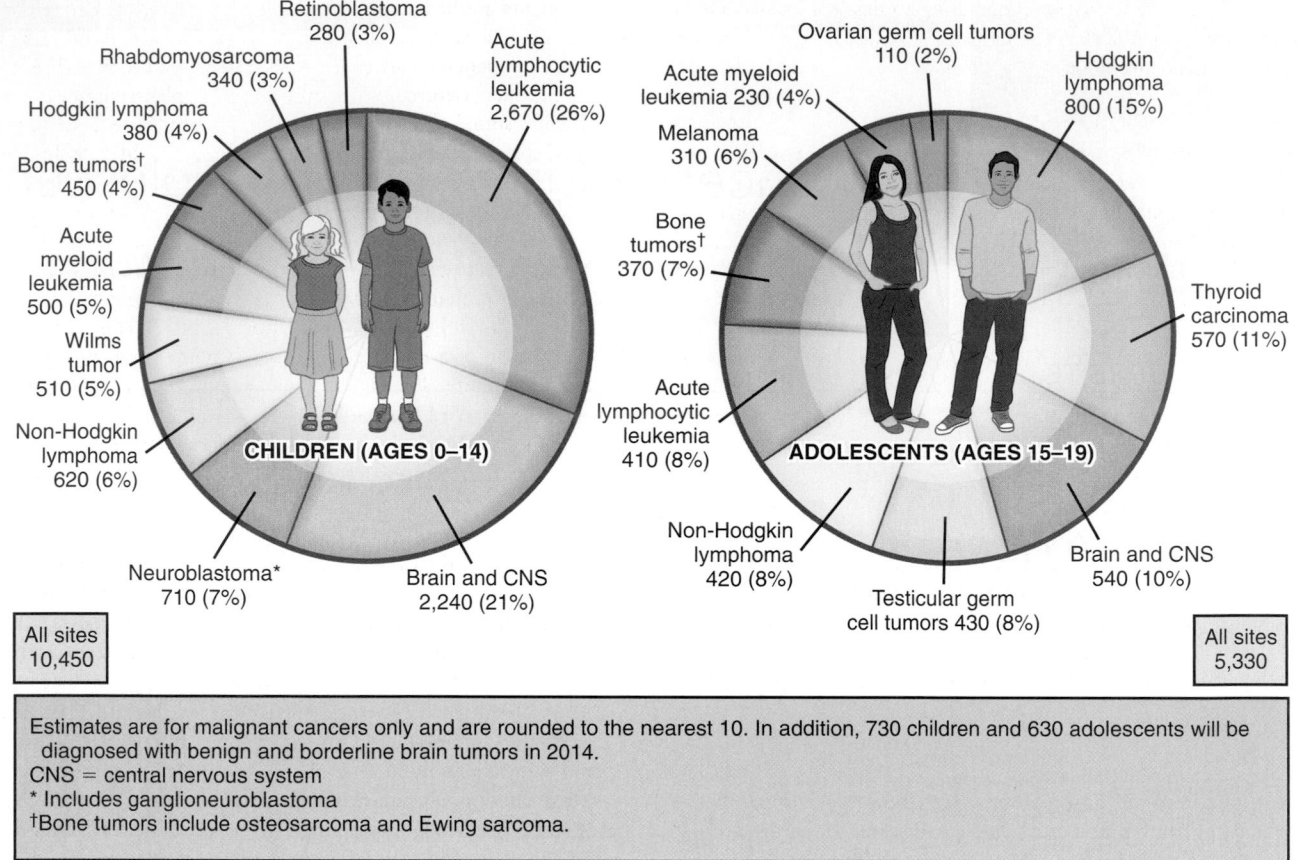

Retinoblastoma
280 (3%)

Rhabdomyosarcoma
340 (3%)

Acute lymphocytic leukemia
2,670 (26%)

Hodgkin lymphoma
380 (4%)

Bone tumors†
450 (4%)

Acute myeloid leukemia
500 (5%)

Wilms tumor
510 (5%)

Non-Hodgkin lymphoma
620 (6%)

CHILDREN (AGES 0–14)

Neuroblastoma*
710 (7%)

Brain and CNS
2,240 (21%)

All sites
10,450

Ovarian germ cell tumors
110 (2%)

Acute myeloid leukemia 230 (4%)

Hodgkin lymphoma
800 (15%)

Melanoma
310 (6%)

Bone tumors†
370 (7%)

Thyroid carcinoma
570 (11%)

Acute lymphocytic leukemia
410 (8%)

ADOLESCENTS (AGES 15–19)

Non-Hodgkin lymphoma
420 (8%)

Testicular germ cell tumors 430 (8%)

Brain and CNS
540 (10%)

All sites
5,330

Estimates are for malignant cancers only and are rounded to the nearest 10. In addition, 730 children and 630 adolescents will be diagnosed with benign and borderline brain tumors in 2014.
CNS = central nervous system
* Includes ganglioneuroblastoma
†Bone tumors include osteosarcoma and Ewing sarcoma.

FIGURE 12-1 Estimated Cases for Childhood and Adolescent Cancers, United States, 2014.
(Data from American Cancer Society, Atlanta, Ga, 2014.)

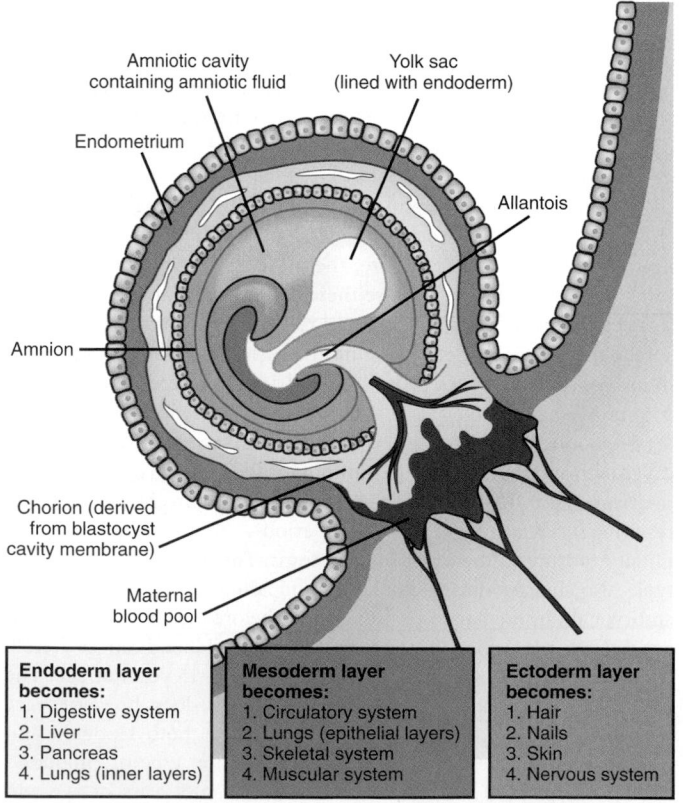

Amniotic cavity containing amniotic fluid

Yolk sac (lined with endoderm)

Endometrium

Allantois

Amnion

Chorion (derived from blastocyst cavity membrane)

Maternal blood pool

Endoderm layer becomes:	**Mesoderm layer becomes:**	**Ectoderm layer becomes:**
1. Digestive system	1. Circulatory system	1. Hair
2. Liver	2. Lungs (epithelial layers)	2. Nails
3. Pancreas	3. Skeletal system	3. Skin
4. Lungs (inner layers)	4. Muscular system	4. Nervous system

FIGURE 12-2 Mesodermal Germ Layer.

of age and older. Rhabdomyosarcoma is the most common soft tissue sarcoma of childhood. Rhabdomyosarcoma has a bimodal age distribution with two thirds of cases occurring in children less than 6 years of age and one third occurring in children and adolescents 10 years of age and older. The two most common types of bone tumors are osteosarcoma and Ewing sarcoma. These cancers are more likely to occur in adolescents ages 15 and older (Table 12-1). Cancer also is more common in white children relative to other racial groups (Table 12-2).

Etiology

The causes of cancer in children are largely unknown. A few environmental factors are known to predispose a child to cancer, but causal factors have not been established for most childhood cancers. A number of host factors, many of which are genetic risk factors or congenital conditions, have been implicated in the development of childhood cancer (Table 12-3).

Because of their relatively short latency period, most childhood cancers do not lend themselves to early cancer warning signs. Certainly the American Cancer Society's seven warning signs of cancer do not apply because they describe adult, environmentally caused carcinomas. Likewise, efforts to establish early screening strategies for childhood cancers have not been effective. Although host factors are important in identifying populations of children at risk for cancer, most children who are diagnosed with cancer do not have known predisposing environmental or host factors.

Multiple causation theory provides a useful framework for interpreting the results of epidemiologic studies. For example, laboratory and epidemiologic studies may indicate that exposure to a certain chemical can cause leukemia, but not all children exposed to that chemical will develop leukemia. Additional studies will be needed to determine what other host and environmental factors must interact with chemical exposure to cause the disease.

Genetic and Genomic Factors

Acquired or inherited mutations in individual genes may contribute to the development of cancer in children and adolescents. Mutations in more than 150 oncogenes and tumor-suppressor genes have been associated with the subsequent development of both childhood and adult cancers (Table 12-4). Fanconi anemia and Bloom syndrome are two autosomal recessive conditions that result in impaired DNA repair and are risk factors for the development of acute leukemia.[7] Retinoblastoma, a malignant embryonic tumor of the eye, occurs either as an inherited defect in the *RB1* gene or as an acquired mutation (see Chapter 17).

Although leukemia is not inherited as a genetic condition, siblings of children with leukemia have a two to four times increased risk for the development of leukemia relative to that of siblings of healthy children. The occurrence of leukemia in monozygous twins is estimated to be as high as 25%.

Li-Fraumeni syndrome (LFS) is an autosomal dominant disorder involving the *TP53* tumor-suppressor gene. For individuals with a mutation in the *TP53* gene, the risk of developing cancer as a child or adult is significantly higher than the risk in the unaffected population.

Children and adults in families affected by LFS are at risk for soft tissue sarcoma, breast cancer, leukemia, osteosarcoma, melanoma, and cancer of the colon, pancreas, adrenal cortex, and brain. Individuals with LFS also are at increased risk for developing multiple primary cancers.[8]

Chromosomal abnormalities also may contribute to the development of childhood cancer. Chromosome abnormalities include aneuploidy, deletions, amplifications, translocations, and fragility (see Chapter 2). These abnormalities may occur within the affected cancer cells as a consequence of malignant transformation or may be present as the consequence of a congenital syndrome.

A chromosomal translocation results from the rearrangement of two nonhomologous chromosomes. Translocations may result in the creation of a fusion gene in which the two previously separate gene regions unite. Two fusion genes associated with acute lymphocytic leukemia (ALL) in children are the *BCR-ABL* gene, resulting from a translocation between chromosomes 9 and 22, and the *TEL-AML1* gene, resulting from a translocation between chromosomes 12 and 21.[9,10]

Several syndromes associated with specific congenital malformations are associated with a higher incidence of cancer development. In some cases, these children may be carefully followed and screened for tumor development. One of the more recognized syndromes is trisomy 21 (Down syndrome), which has an increased susceptibility to acute leukemia. The risk of developing leukemia is 10 to 20 times greater among children with Down syndrome than in healthy children. The age distribution for developing ALL among children with Down syndrome is similar to that of children without Down syndrome.[11,12]

Wilms tumor, a malignant tumor of the kidney, is particularly recognized for its association with a number of congenital anomalies, including genitourinary anomalies, aniridia (congenital absence of the iris), hemihypertrophy (muscular overgrowth of half of the body or face), and intellectual disabilities. Identifiable malformations and congenital predisposition syndromes are present in approximately 17% of children diagnosed with Wilms tumor.[13]

Environmental Factors

Finding the cause of any disease is typically a long, slow process. Epidemiologic studies require many years to determine whether a risk factor is possibly related to the development of childhood cancer. No single factor determines whether an individual will develop cancer, even if a specific environmental exposure explains a high proportion of the occurrence of a specific cancer (Box 12-1).

Prenatal Exposure

Prenatal exposure to some drugs and to ionizing radiation has been linked to childhood cancers. The most well-described drug is diethylstilbestrol (DES), which was prescribed by physicians to prevent

---

TABLE 12-1 Childhood Age-Adjusted Invasive Cancer Incidence Rates by Primary Site and Age, United States*

Site	Birth to 14 Years	Birth to 19 Years
All sites	15.7	17.9
Leukemia (all types)	5.1	4.6
Acute lymphocytic leukemia	4.3	3.7
Brain and other nervous system	3.3	2.9
Soft tissue	1.1	1.2
Kidney and renal	0.9	0.7
Bones and joints	0.7	0.9
Non-Hodgkin lymphoma	0.9	1.1
Hodgkin lymphoma	0.6	1.3

Data modified from Howlader N et al, editors: *SEER cancer statistics review, 1975-2011*, Bethesda, Md, 2013, National Cancer Institute. Available at http://seer.cancer.gov/csr/1975_2011/.
*Rates are per 100,000 persons and are age-adjusted to the 2000 U.S. standard population (19 age groups—Census P25-1130).

TABLE 12-2 Childhood Age-Adjusted Cancer Incidence Rates for Children <19 Years of Age by Primary Site, Race, and Ethnicity, United States*

Cancer Site	White	Black	Asian/Pacific Islander	American Indian/Alaska Native	Hispanic[†]
All cancer sites combined	19.5	13.0	12.4	16.6	16.6
Brain and other nervous systems	4.8	3.4	3.2	3.0	3.6
Leukemia	5.4	3.1	4.0	4.0	6.0
Lymphoma	2.6	2.1	1.9	1.3	2.1
Other	7.7	5.6	5.8	4.8	6.7

Data modified from Howlader N et al, editors: *SEER cancer statistics review, 1975-2011*, Bethesda, Md, 2013, National Cancer Institute. Available at http://seer.cancer.gov/csr/1975_2011/.
*Rates are per 100,000 persons and are age-adjusted to the 2000 U.S. standard population (19 age groups—Census P25-1130).
[†]Hispanic origin is not mutually exclusive from race categories (white, black, Asian/Pacific Islander, American Indian/Alaska Native).

TABLE 12-3 Congenital Factors Associated with Childhood Cancer

Syndrome	Associated Childhood Cancer
Chromosome Alterations	
Down syndrome	Acute leukemia
13q syndrome	Retinoblastoma
Chromosome Instability	
Ataxia-telangiectasia	Lymphoma
Bloom syndrome	Acute leukemia, lymphoma, Wilms tumor
Fanconi anemia	Acute myelogenous leukemia, myelodysplastic syndrome, hepatic tumors
Hereditary Syndromes	
Beckwith-Wiedemann syndrome	Wilms tumor, sarcoma, brain tumors, neuroblastoma, hepatoblastoma
Neurofibromatosis type I	Brain tumor, sarcomas, neuroblastomas, Wilms tumor, nonlymphocytic leukemia
Neurofibromatosis type II	Meningioma (malignant or benign), acoustic neuroma/schwannoma, gliomas, ependymomas
Tuberous sclerosis	Glial tumors
Li-Fraumeni syndrome	Sarcoma, adrenocortical carcinoma
Von Hippel-Lindau disease	Cerebellar hemangioblastoma, retinal angioma, renal cell carcinoma, pheochromocytomas
Ataxia-telangiectasia	Leukemia, lymphoma, brain tumors
Gorlin syndrome	Medulloblastoma, skin tumors
Immunodeficiency Disorders	
Congenital	
Agammaglobulinemia	Lymphoma, leukemia, brain tumors
Immunoglobulin A (IgA) deficiency	Lymphoma, leukemia, brain tumors
Wiskott-Aldrich syndrome	Leukemia, lymphoma
Acquired	
Aplastic anemia	Leukemia
HIV/AIDS	
Organ transplantation	Leukemia, lymphoma
Congenital Malformation Syndromes	
Aniridia, hemihypertrophy, hamartoma, genitourinary anomalies	Wilms tumor
Cryptorchidism	Testicular tumor
Gonadal dysgenesis	Gonadoblastoma
Family Susceptibility	
Twin or sibling with leukemia	Leukemia

TABLE 12-4 Selected Oncogenes and Tumor-Suppressor Genes Associated with Childhood Cancer

Gene	Associated Pediatric Tumor
Oncogenes	
ABL	Acute lymphoblastic leukemia
MYCN	Neuroblastoma
MYB	Neural tumors, leukemia, lymphoma, rhabdomyosarcoma, Wilms tumor, neuroblastoma
erbB	Glioblastomas
NRAS	Neuroblastoma, leukemia
HRAS/KRAS	Neuroblastoma, rhabdomyosarcoma, leukemia
ATM	Lymphoma, leukemia
Tumor-Suppressor Genes	
RB1	Retinoblastoma, sarcoma
WT1, WT2	Wilms tumor, leukemia
NF-1	Sarcoma, primitive neuroectodermal tumor, juvenile chronic myelocytic leukemia
NF-2	Brain tumors, melanoma, meningiomas
p16	Brain tumors, leukemia
TP53	Sarcoma, leukemia, brain tumors, lymphoma
DCC	Ewing sarcoma, rhabdomyosarcoma
CDKN2A	Glioblastoma, acute lymphoblastic leukemia
CDC2L1	Non-Hodgkin lymphoma, neuroblastoma

Data from Esparza SD et al: *Medscape, 2009.* Available at http://emedicine.medscape.com/article/989983-overview. Accessed January 27, 2015. Beamer LC et al: *Nurs Clin North Am* 48(4):585-626, 2013.

BOX 12-1 Factors That May Contribute to the Development of Childhood and Adolescent Cancer

- Genetic and epigenetic factors
- Diet
- Immune function
- Occupational exposure
- Ionizing radiation
- Hormonal variations
- Viral illnesses
- Individual characteristics, such as the biologic, social, and physical environment

An association between antenatal x-ray exposure and childhood brain tumors has not been identified.[15] Other current areas of research include exploring epigenetic modifications resulting from prenatal exposures and their role in future cancer development.[6]

Childhood Exposure

Childhood exposure to ionizing radiation, drugs, electromagnetic fields, or viruses has been associated with the risk of developing cancer. Retrospective research has shown a significant correlation between radiation-induced malignancies and either radiotherapy (cancer treatment) or radiation exposure from diagnostic imaging[16] (see *Health Alert:* Radiation Risks and Pediatric Computed Tomography [CT]: Data from the National Cancer Institute). In addition to the drug and environmental agents that are known to cause cancer in adults and therefore also are risks for exposure during childhood, a few drugs may particularly increase cancer risk during childhood (Table 12-5).

spontaneous miscarriage (in women with previous miscarriage). In 1971 DES was identified as a transplacental chemical carcinogen because a small percentage of the daughters of women who took DES developed adenocarcinomas of the vagina. Since then, other studies have attempted to identify other drugs taken by pregnant women that may cause cancer in their offspring, but no other drugs have been found. Current evidence suggests an increased risk of childhood leukemia is associated with low levels of exposure to antenatal x-rays.[14]

TABLE 12-5 Drugs That May Increase Risk of Childhood Cancer

Drug Class	Uses	Cancer Risk
Anabolic androgenic steroids	Stimulate bone growth and appetite; induce puberty; increase muscle mass and physical strength	Hepatocellular carcinoma
Epipodophyllotoxin and anthracycline chemotherapy agents	Cancer treatment	Leukemia
Immunosuppressive agents	Prevent organ rejection following transplantation surgery	Lymphoma

HEALTH ALERT

Radiation Risks and Pediatric Computed Tomography (CT): Data from the National Cancer Institute

Emerging is the concern of radiation risks in children because the use of pediatric CT has been increasing rapidly. Pediatric CT is now a public health concern. Children are more sensitive to radiation than adults as demonstrated in epidemiologic studies. Children have a longer life expectancy than adults, increasing the window of opportunity to express radiation damage, and children may receive higher radiation dose than necessary if CT is not adjusted for their smaller size. Although CT scans comprise up to about 12% of diagnostic radiologic procedures in large U.S. hospitals, it is estimated that they account for approximately 49% of the U.S. population's collective radiation dose from all medical x-ray examinations. CT is the largest contributor to medical radiation exposure among the U.S. population. It is important to stress that the absolute cancer risks associated with CT scans are small. The lifetime risks of cancer because of CT scans, which have been estimated in the literature using projection models based on atomic bomb survivors, are about 1 case of cancer for every 1000 people who are scanned, with a maximal incidence of about 1 case of cancer for every 500 people who are scanned. The benefits of properly performed and clinically justified CT examinations should always outweigh the risks for an individual child; unnecessary exposure is associated with unnecessary risk. Minimizing radiation exposure from pediatric CT, whenever possible, will reduce the projected number of CT-related cancers.

Data from National Cancer Institute, National Institutes of Health: *NCI radiation risks and pediatric computed tomography (CT): a guide for health care workers*, Bethesda, Md, 2012, National Cancer Institute. Accessed January 26, 2015.

The relationship between childhood cancer and other environmental factors (e.g., electromagnetic fields, small appliances, radon) has been the focus of many epidemiologic studies. Although associations between some environmental exposures and acute leukemia have been demonstrated, no conclusive causal evidence has been reported[17-19] (see *Health Alert:* Magnetic Fields and Development of Pediatric Cancer).

The strongest association between viruses and the development of cancer in children has been the Epstein-Barr virus (EBV), which is linked to Burkitt lymphoma, nasopharyngeal carcinoma, and Hodgkin disease.[20] Children with acquired immunodeficiency syndrome (AIDS), caused by human immunodeficiency virus (HIV), have an increased risk of developing non-Hodgkin lymphoma and Kaposi sarcoma.

HEALTH ALERT

Magnetic Fields and Development of Pediatric Cancer

Several recent reports have suggested an association between environmental sources and the development of cancer in children. The presence of low-frequency magnetic fields has been a concern for many years as causing leukemia in children. The World Health Organization (WHO) research agenda identified the importance of such an analysis as a high research priority in 2007. A recent meta-analysis evaluated 9 case-control studies, representing 8 different countries, conducted between 1997 and 2013 and involving 11,699 cases of children with leukemia and 13,194 controls. This meta-analysis identified an increased risk of childhood leukemia associated with high levels of magnetic field exposure (≥ 0.4 μT). For additional perspective, the WHO estimates that only about 1% to 4% of children worldwide live in conditions that exceed this level of exposure. Ongoing research needs to be done in this area because environmental factors may require many years of exposure to cause disease. Additionally, an association between an environmental factor and childhood cancer does not establish causality. Ongoing research is needed to better understand the relationships between environmental factors and other factors associated with the childhood cancer, as well as potential underlying mechanisms by which environmental factors may contribute to the development of childhood cancer.

Data from World Health Organization: *Fact sheet: electromagnetic fields and public health: exposure to extremely low frequency fields,* available at www.who.int/peh-emf/publications/facts/fs322/en/. Accessed January 30, 2015. Zhao L et al: *Leuk Res* 38(3):269-274, 2014.

However, with the use of highly active antiretroviral therapy in the developed world, the incidence of AIDS-related malignancies has declined dramatically.[21]

PROGNOSIS

More than 70% of children diagnosed with cancer are cured. Some of the factors leading to improved cure rates in pediatric oncology include the use of combination chemotherapy or multimodal treatment for solid childhood tumors and improvements in nursing and supportive care. The development of research centers for comprehensive childhood cancer treatment and cooperative study groups also have facilitated refinements in treatment protocols and data sharing, leading to improved survival rates.

Survival rates for children younger than 15 years of age have increased at a rate of 1.5% per year, which is similar to increases in survival for adults older than 50 years of age. Adolescents and young adults between 15 and 24 years of age, however, have experienced increases in survival of less than 0.5% per year.[3] A partial explanation for the relative lack of progress in curing the adolescent population at the same rate as that realized in the younger pediatric population is the lack of participation in clinical trials. Between 1997 and 2003, the percentage of 15- to 19-year-olds with cancer participating in clinical trials was estimated at 10% to 15%. This value is approximately one fourth the clinical trial participation rate of children younger than 15 years and is likely due to the fact that fewer trials are available for young adolescents. The National Cancer Institute (NCI) and pediatric and adult cooperative groups sponsored by the NCI have launched a national initiative to increase the numbers of adolescents and young adults in clinical trials.[22]

Survivors of childhood cancer are at increased risk of developing a second malignancy later in life. This risk may be associated with a variety of factors, including previous chemotherapy or radiotherapy, genetic factors, and type of primary cancer (e.g., soft tissue sarcoma, neuroblastoma).

Because childhood cancer should be viewed as a chronic disease instead of a fatal illness, treatment includes attention to quality of life and symptom management. Even those cancers that cannot be cured generally can be treated, resulting in significantly improved quality of life. Children and adolescents whose cancers are regarded as cured still face residual and late effects of their treatment. These late effects are more significant in children than in adults because treatment given during childhood occurs in a physically immature, growing individual. Late effects that need further study include physical impairments, reproductive dysfunction, soft tissue and bone atrophy, learning disabilities, secondary cancers, and psychologic sequelae. More must be

learned about the genetic factors associated with childhood malignancies and about the genetic consequences of treatment. A referral to genetic services is appropriate for families of children whose cancer is known to be transmitted genetically (e.g., retinoblastoma, Li-Fraumeni syndrome).

✔QUICK CHECK 12-1

1. What are the most common childhood cancers, and how do they differ from adult cancers?
2. Why are children less likely to develop carcinomas?
3. Compare and contrast different etiologic factors associated with the development of childhood cancer.

DID YOU UNDERSTAND?

Incidence and Types of Childhood Cancers

1. Childhood cancer is a rare disease, but it remains the second leading cause of death in children.
2. The most common type of childhood cancer is leukemia, and the second most common type of pediatric malignancy is a tumor involving the brain or central nervous system.

Etiology

1. Because most carcinomas are caused by environmental exposure, these cancers are extremely rare in children because they have not lived long enough to be exposed to carcinogens.
2. Children with immunodeficiencies are at increased risk for developing cancer because of an ineffective immune system.
3. Children with Down syndrome are at increased risk for developing leukemia.

4. Risk factors that may be associated with the development of childhood cancer include inherited and acquired genetic and genomic changes, nutrition and diet, immune function, occupational exposure, hormonal variations, and viral illnesses, as well as other individual characteristics such as biologic, social, or physical environments.

Prognosis

1. Survivors of childhood cancer are at increased risk for developing a second cancer during their lifetime, compared with the general population.
2. Improved survival for children and adolescents with cancer has been facilitated, in part, by research aimed at identifying less toxic treatments that minimize residual effects.

KEY TERMS

Embryonic tumor, 301
Li-Fraumeni syndrome (LFS), 303

Mesodermal germ layer, 301

Multiple causation, 302

Wilms tumor, 303

REFERENCES

1. Heron M: Deaths: leading causes for 2010, *Natl Vital Stat Rep* 62(6):1-96, 2013. Available at: www.cdc.gov/nchs/data/nvsr/nvsr62/nvsr62_06.pdf. Accessed January 26, 2015.
2. Ward E et al: Childhood and adolescent cancer statistics, *CA Cancer J Clin* 64(2):83-103, 2014.
3. Howlader N et al, editors: *SEER cancer statistics review, 1975-2011,* Bethesda, Md, 2013, National Cancer Institute. Available at: http://seer.cancer.gov/csr/1975_2011/.
4. Kochanek KD et al: *Mortality in the United States, 2013,* data brief no. 178, National Center for Health Statistics (NCHC), 2014. Available at: www.cdc.gov/nchs/data/databriefs/db178.pdf. Accessed January 26, 2015.
5. Burdge GC et al: Nutrition in early life, and risk of cancer and metabolic disease: alternative endings in an epigenetic tale? *Br J Nutr* 101(5):619-630, 2009.
6. Kaur P et al: The epigenome as a potential mediator of cancer prevention by dietary phytochemicals: the fetus as a target, *Nutr Rev* 71(7):441-457, 2013.
7. Seif AE: Pediatric leukemia predisposition syndromes: clues to understanding leukemogenesis, *Cancer Genet* 204(5):227-244. 2011.
8. McBride KA et al: Li-Fraumeni syndrome: cancer risk assessment and clinical management, *Nat Rev Clin Oncol* 11(5):260-271, 2014.

9. Izraeli S: Beyond Philadelphia: "ph-like" B cell precursor acute lymphoblastic leukemia–diagnostic challenges and therapeutic promises, *Curr Opin Hematol* 21(4):289-296, 2014.
10. Linka Y et al: The impact of TEL-AML1 (ETV6-RUNX1) expression in precursor B cells and implications for leukaemia using three different genome-wide screening methods, *Blood Cancer J* 3:e151, 2013.
11. Maloney KW: Acute lymphoblastic leukaemia in children with Down syndrome: an updated review, *Br J Haematol* 155(4):420-425, 2011.
12. Whitlock JA et al: Clinical characteristics and outcome of children with Down syndrome and acute lymphoblastic leukemia: a Children's Cancer Group study, *Blood* 106(13):4043-4049, 2005.
13. Dumoucel S et al: Malformations, genetic abnormalities, and Wilms tumor, *Pediatr Blood Cancer* 61(1):140-144, 2014.
14. Wakeford R: The risk of childhood leukaemia following exposure to ionising radiation, *J Radiol Prot* 33(1):1-25, 2013.
15. Milne E et al: Childhood and parental diagnostic radiological procedures and risk of childhood brain tumors, *Cancer Causes Control* 25(3):375-383, 2014.
16. Miglioretti DL et al: Pediatric computed tomography and associated radiation exposure and

estimated cancer risk, *JAMA Pediatr* 167(8):700-707, 2013.
17. Heck JE et al: Risk of leukemia in relation to exposure to ambient air toxins in pregnancy and early childhood, *Int J Hyg Environ Health* 217(6):662-668, 2014.
18. Sermage-Faure C et al: Childhood leukemia close to high-voltage power lines—the Geocap study, 2002-2007, *Br J Cancer* 108(9):1899-1906, 2013.
19. Zhao L et al: Magnetic fields exposure and childhood leukemia risk: a meta-analysis based on 11,699 cases and 13,194 controls, *Leuk Res* 38(3):269-274, 2014.
20. Houldcroft CJ, Kellam P: Host genetics of Epstein-Barr virus infection, latency and disease, *Rev Med Virol* 25(2):71-84, 2015.
21. Simard EP et al: Mortality due to cancer among people with AIDS: a novel approach using registry-linkage data and population attributable risk methods, *AIDS* 26(10):1311-1318, 2012.
22. Adolescent and Young Adult Oncology Press Review Group, LiveStrong Young Adult Alliance: *Closing the gap: research and care imperatives for adolescents and young adults with cancer,* Bethesda, Md, 2006, National Cancer Institute. Available at: http://planning.cancer.gov/library/AYAO_PRG _Report_2006_FINAL.pdf. Accessed January 28, 2014.

13

Structure and Function of the Neurologic System

Lynne M. Kerr, Sue E. Huether, and Richard A. Sugerman*

ⓔ EVOLVE WEBSITE

http://evolve.elsevier.com/Huether/

Student Review Questions
Audio Key Points

Case Studies
Animations
Quick Check Answers

CHAPTER OUTLINE

The human nervous system is a remarkable structure responsible for decision making, for the body's ability to interact with the environment, and for the regulation and control of activities involving our internal organs. It is a network composed of complex structures that transmit electrical and chemical signals between the brain and the body's many organs and tissues. Aging changes occur throughout life and vary among individuals (see *Geriatric Considerations:* Aging & the Nervous System). This chapter provides a basic overview of the structure and function of the nervous system and supports the understanding of nervous system pathophysiology in the following chapters.

OVERVIEW AND ORGANIZATION OF THE NERVOUS SYSTEM

Although the nervous system functions as a unified whole, structures and functions have been divided here to facilitate understanding. Structurally, the nervous system is divided into the central nervous system and the peripheral nervous system. The central nervous system (CNS) consists of the brain and spinal cord, enclosed within the protective cranial vault and vertebrae, respectively. The peripheral nervous system (PNS) is composed of the cranial nerves and the spinal nerves and their ganglia. Peripheral nerve pathways are differentiated into afferent pathways (ascending pathways), which carry sensory impulses toward the CNS, and efferent pathways (descending pathways), which innervate skeletal muscle or effector organs by transmitting motor impulses away from the CNS.

Functionally, the PNS can be divided into the somatic nervous system and the autonomic nervous system. The somatic nervous system consists of pathways that regulate voluntary motor control (e.g., skeletal muscle). The autonomic nervous system (ANS) is involved with regulation of the body's internal environment (viscera) through involuntary control of organ systems. The ANS is further divided into sympathetic and parasympathetic divisions. Organs innervated by specific components of the nervous system are called effector organs.

CELLS OF THE NERVOUS SYSTEM

Two basic types of cells constitute nervous tissue: neurons and supporting nonneuronal cells. The neuron is the primary cell of the nervous system. It is an electrically excitable cell and transmits information. Cells, such as neuroglial cells (astrocytes, microglia, and oligodendrocytes in the CNS) and Schwann (neurilemma) and satellite cells (in the PNS), provide structural support, protection, and nutrition for the neurons.

The Neuron

Working alone or in units, neurons detect environmental changes and initiate body responses to maintain a dynamic steady state. Neuronal size and structure vary markedly, so that each neuron is adapted to

---

*Dr. Richard A. Sugerman contributed to this chapter in the previous edition.

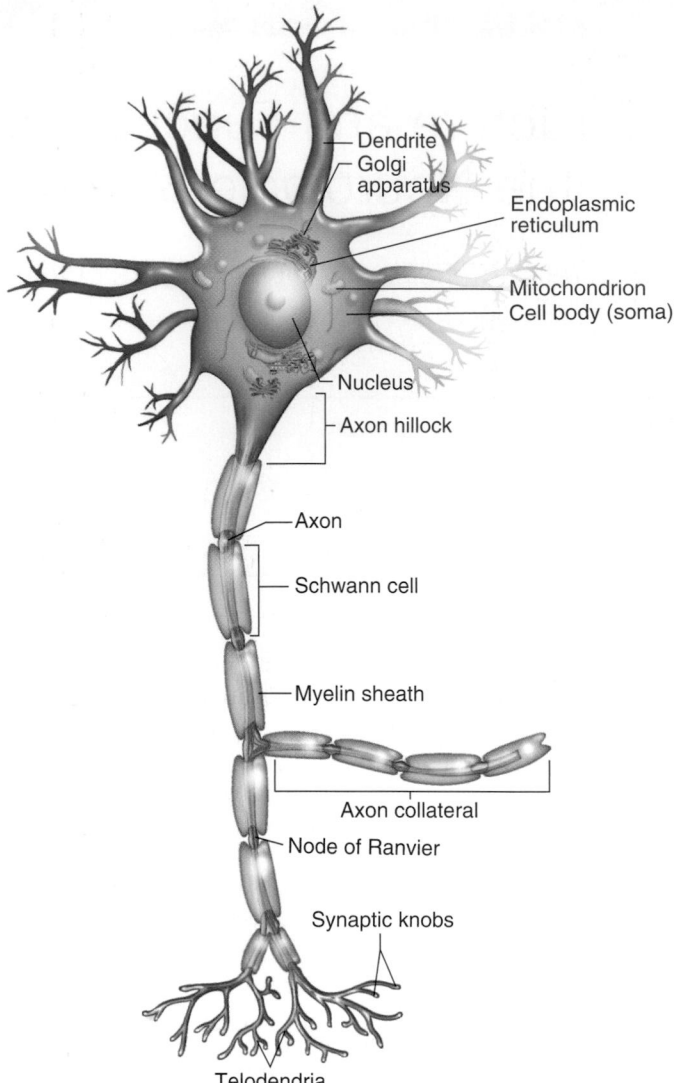

FIGURE 13-1 Neuron with Composite Parts. Multipolar neuron: PNS neuron with multiple extensions from the cell body. *PNS,* Peripheral nervous system. (Modified from Patton KT, Thibodeau GA, Douglas MM: *Essentials of anatomy & physiology,* St Louis, 2012, Mosby.)

Labels in figure: Dendrite; Golgi apparatus; Endoplasmic reticulum; Mitochondrion; Cell body (soma); Nucleus; Axon hillock; Axon; Schwann cell; Myelin sheath; Axon collateral; Node of Ranvier; Synaptic knobs; Telodendria

with a segmented layer of lipid material called myelin, an insulating substance that speeds impulse propagation. This entire membrane is referred to as the myelin sheath (see Figures 13-2 and 13-25, *B*). The myelin sheaths are interrupted at regular intervals by the nodes of Ranvier. Axons can branch at the nodes of Ranvier. In the CNS myelin is produced by oligodendrocytes. In the PNS myelin is produced by Schwann cells. Telodendria form presynaptic vesicles for neurotransmission.

The principle of *divergence* refers to the ability of axonal branches to influence many different neurons. *Convergence* applies when branches of various numbers of neurons "converge" on and influence a single neuron. Nutrient exchange is not possible through the myelin sheath, although it can occur at the nodes of Ranvier where the axon is not insulated. Where there is myelin, the velocity of nerve impulses increases. Myelin acts as an insulator that allows an action potential to leap between segments rather than flow along the entire length of the membrane, yielding the increased velocity. This mechanism is referred to as saltatory conduction. Disorders of the myelin sheath (demyelinating diseases), such as multiple sclerosis and Guillain-Barré syndrome, demonstrate the important role myelin plays in nerve conduction (see Chapter 16). Conduction velocities depend not only on the myelin coating but also on the diameter of the axon. Larger axons transmit impulses at a faster rate.

Neurons are structurally classified on the basis of the number of processes (projections) extending from the cell body. There are four basic types of cell configuration: (1) unipolar, (2) pseudounipolar, (3) bipolar, and (4) multipolar. Unipolar neurons have one process that branches shortly after leaving the cell body. One example is found in the retina. Pseudounipolar neurons (some authors call them *unipolar*) also have one process; the dendritic portion of each of these neurons extends away from the CNS and the axon portion projects into the CNS (Figure 13-2). This configuration is typical of sensory neurons in both cranial and spinal nerves. Bipolar neurons have two distinct processes arising from the cell body. This type of neuron connects the rod and cone cells of the retina. Multipolar neurons are the most common and have multiple processes capable of extensive branching. A motor neuron is typically multipolar (see Figure 13-2).

Functionally, there are three types of neurons (their direction of transmission and typical configuration are noted in parentheses): (1) sensory (afferent, mostly pseudounipolar), (2) associational (interneurons, multipolar), and (3) motor (efferent, multipolar). Sensory neurons carry impulses from peripheral sensory receptors to the CNS. Associational neurons (interneurons) transmit impulses from neuron to neuron—that is, sensory to motor neurons. They are located solely within the CNS. Motor neurons transmit impulses away from the CNS to an effector (i.e., skeletal muscle or organs). In skeletal muscle the end processes form a neuromuscular (myoneural) junction (see Figure 13-15).

Neuroglia and Schwann Cells

Neuroglia ("nerve glue") are the general classification of nonneuronal cells that support the neurons of the CNS. They comprise approximately half of the total brain and spinal cord volume and are 5 to 10 times more numerous than neurons. Different types of neuroglia serve different functions. Astrocytes, for example, surround blood vessels, fill the spaces between neurons, and contribute to synaptic function in the CNS.[1] Oligodendroglia (oligodendrocytes) form myelin sheaths within the CNS. Ependymal cells line the cerebrospinal fluid (CSF)-filled cavities of the CNS. Microglia remove debris (phagocytosis) in the CNS. Schwann cells form the myelin sheath around axons and direct axonal regrowth and functional recovery in the PNS.[2] Nonmyelinating Schwann cells provide metabolic support. (Characteristics

perform specialized functions. The fuel source for the neuron is predominantly glucose; insulin, however, is not required for cellular glucose uptake in the CNS. The cellular constituents of neurons include microtubules (transport substances within the cell), neurofibrils (very thin supportive fibers that extend throughout the neuron), microfilaments (thought to be involved in transport of cellular products), and Nissl substances (endoplasmic reticulum and ribosomes) involved in protein synthesis.

A neuron (Figure 13-1) has three components: a cell body (soma), the dendrites (thin branching fibers of the cell), and the axons. Most cell bodies are located within the CNS; those in the PNS usually are found in groups called ganglia (or plexuses—a group of relay nerves). The dendrites are extensions that carry nerve impulses toward the cell body. Axons are long, conductive projections that carry nerve impulses away from the cell body. The axon hillock is the cone-shaped process where the axon leaves the cell body. The first part of the axon hillock has the lowest threshold for stimulation, so action potentials begin there. A typical neuron has only one axon, which may be wrapped

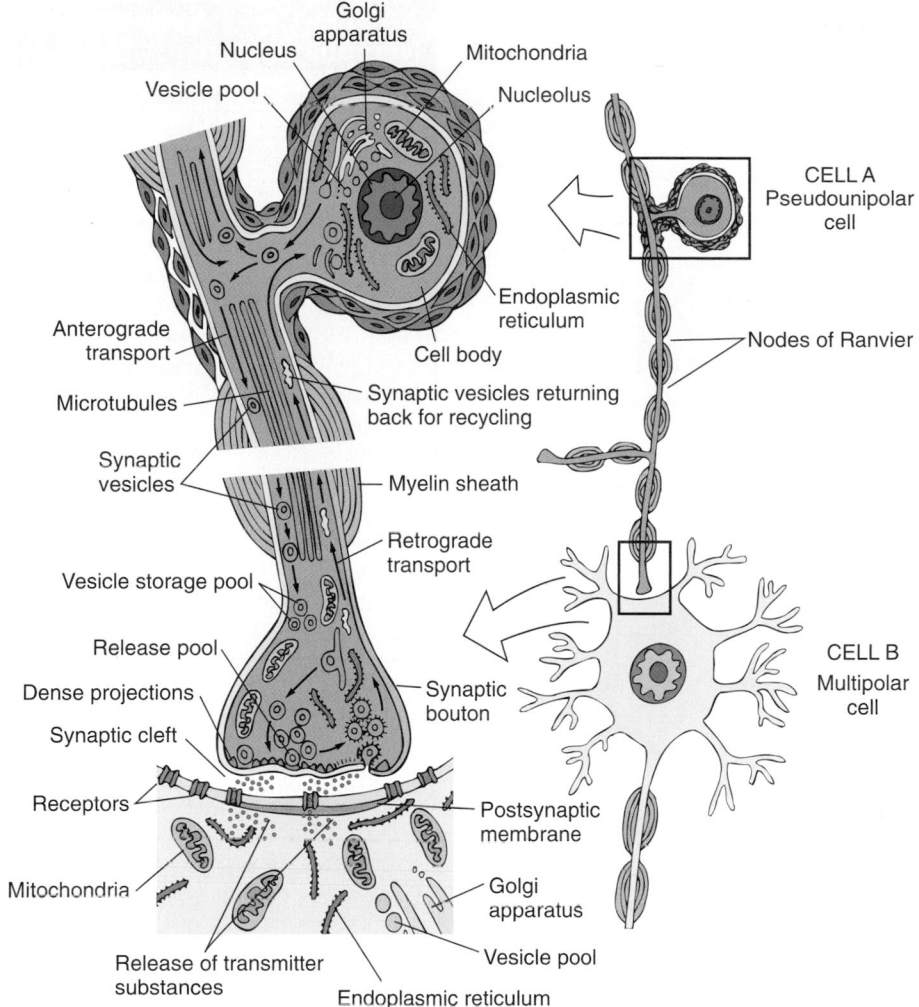

FIGURE 13-2 Neuronal Transmission and Synaptic Cleft. Electrical impulse travels along axon of first neuron (presynaptic cell) to synapse. Chemical transmitter is secreted into synaptic space to depolarize membrane (dendrite or cell body) of next neuron (postsynaptic cell) in pathway. *Cell A* represents pseudounipolar cell; *cell B* represents multipolar cell.

of neuroglia and Schwann cells are summarized in Figure 13-3 and Table 13-1.)

Nerve Injury and Regeneration

Mature nerve cells do not divide, and injury can cause permanent loss of function. When an axon is severed, Wallerian degeneration occurs in the distal axon: (1) a characteristic swelling appears within the portion of the axon distal to the cut; (2) the neurofilaments hypertrophy; (3) the myelin sheath shrinks and disintegrates; and (4) the axon degenerates and disappears. The myelin sheaths re-form into Schwann cells that align in a column between the severed part of the axon and the effector organ.

At the proximal end of the injured axon, similar changes occur but only back to the next node of Ranvier. The cell body responds to trauma by swelling and dying by chromatolysis (dispersing the Nissl substance) or apoptosis. During the repair process, the cell increases protein synthesis and mitochondrial activity. Approximately 7 to 14 days after the injury, new terminal sprouts project from the proximal segment and may enter the remaining Schwann cell pathway. (Figure 13-4 contains a more detailed representation of these events.) This process, however, is limited to myelinated fibers and generally occurs only in the PNS. The regeneration of axonal constituents in the CNS is limited by an increased incidence of scar formation and the different nature of myelin formed by the oligodendrocyte.

Nerve regeneration depends on many factors, such as location of the injury, the type of injury, the presence of inflammatory responses, and the process of scarring. The closer to the cell body of the nerve, the greater the chances that the nerve cell will die and not regenerate. A crushing injury allows recovery more fully than does a cut injury. Crushed nerves sometimes recover fully, whereas cut nerves form connective tissue scars that block or slow regenerating axonal branches. Peripheral nerves injured close to the spinal cord recover poorly and slowly because of the long distance between the cell body and the peripheral termination of the axon.[3]

THE NERVE IMPULSE

Neurons generate and conduct electrical and chemical impulses by selectively changing the electrical potential of the plasma membrane and influencing other nearby neurons by releasing chemicals (neurotransmitters). An unexcited neuron maintains a resting membrane potential. When the membrane potential is sufficiently raised, an

CENTRAL NERVOUS SYSTEM NEUROGLIA

TABLE 13-1 Support Cells of the Nervous System

Cell Type	Primary Functions
Astrocytes	Form specialized contacts between neuronal surfaces and blood vessels
	Provide rapid transport for nutrients and metabolites
	Thought to form an essential component of blood-brain barrier
	Appear to be scar-forming cells of CNS, which may be foci for seizures
	Appear to work with neurons in processing information and memory storage
Oligodendroglia (oligodendrocytes)	Formation of myelin sheath in CNS
Schwann cells	Formation of myelin sheath in PNS
Nonmyelinating Schwann cells	Provide neuronal metabolic support and regeneration in PNS
Microglia	Responsible for clearing cellular debris (phagocytic properties)
Ependymal cells	Serve as a lining for ventricles and choroid plexuses involved in production of cerebrospinal fluid

Some data from Martinez Banaclocha MA: *Int J Neurosci* 115(3):329-337, 2005; Sofroniew MV, Vinters HV: *Acta Neuropathol* 119(1):7-35, 2010; Vanderah T, Gould D: *Nolte's The Human Brain: An Introduction to its Functional Anatomy*, ed 7, St Louis, 2015, Mosby. *CNS*, Central nervous system; *PNS*, peripheral nervous system.

PERIPHERAL NERVOUS SYSTEM NEUROGLIA

FIGURE 13-3 Types of Neuroglial Cells. Neuroglia of the CNS: **A,** Astrocytes attached to the outside of a capillary blood vessel in the brain. **B,** A phagocytic microglial cell. **C,** Ciliated ependymal cells forming a sheet that usually lines fluid cavities in the brain. **D,** An oligodendrocyte with processes that wrap around nerve fibers in the CNS to form myelin sheaths. Neuroglia of the peripheral nervous system (PNS): **E,** A Schwann cell supporting a bundle of nerve fibers in the PNS. **F,** Another type of Schwann cell encircling a peripheral nerve fiber to form a thick myelin sheath. (From Patton KT, et al: *Essentials of anatomy & physiology*, St Louis, 2012, Mosby.)

FIGURE 13-4 Repair of a Peripheral Nerve Fiber. When cut, a damaged motor axon can regrow to its distal connection only if the Schwann cells remain intact (to form a guiding tunnel) and if scar tissue does not block its way. (From Patton KT, Thibodeau GA: *Anatomy & physiology*, ed 8, St Louis, 2013, Mosby.)

action potential is generated and the nerve impulse then flows to all parts of the neuron. The action potential response occurs only when the stimulus is strong enough; if it is too weak, the membrane remains unexcited. This property is termed the *all-or-none response* (see Chapter 1 for a discussion of electrical impulse conduction).

✔ QUICK CHECK 13-1

1. How do the functions of the somatic and autonomic nervous systems differ?
2. What are the three components of a neuron?
3. How does myelin affect nerve impulses?
4. Name the process through which injured axons are repaired, and describe the process.

Synapses

Neurons are not physically continuous with one another. The region between adjacent neurons is called a synapse (see Figure 13-2). Impulses are transmitted across the synapse by chemical and electrical conduction (see Figure 13-2); only chemical conduction is discussed here. Chapter 1 contains information on electrical conduction (see Figure 1-29). The neurons that conduct a nerve impulse are named according to whether they relay impulses toward (presynaptic neurons) or away from (postsynaptic neurons) the synapse. When an impulse originates in a presynaptic neuron, the impulse reaches the vesicles, where chemicals (neurotransmitters) are stored in the synaptic bouton. Once released from the vesicles, the neurotransmitters diffuse across the synaptic cleft (the space between the neurons) and bind to specific neurotransmitter (protein) receptor sites on the plasma membrane of the postsynaptic neuron, relaying the impulse (see Figure 13-2). Brain synapses can change in strength and number throughout life and this is known as synaptic plasticity or neuroplasticity (see *Health Alert:* Neuroplasticity).

HEALTH ALERT

Neuroplasticity

Neuroplasticity is the lifelong ability of the brain to adapt to new conditions by reorganizing neural pathways and forming new synapses, resulting in development, learning, and memory or recovery from injury. The process is complex and the underlying mechanisms include environmental influences, genetics, neurochemical alterations, functional changes in excitatory and inhibitory synapses, and axonal and dendritic sprouting and turnover. Research is currently in progress to identify the sequence of molecular and structural processes involved, and ways of delivering agents and therapies to promote neurorestoration and enhance brain or spinal cord reorganization of motor and sensory function following injury or disease. The new clinical area of neuro-optometry provides an example of neuroplasticity within the brain. The utilization of external prisms and computerized vision programs for visual rehabilitation can modify the visual processing system in children and adults to significantly improve visual performance.

From Hübener M, Bonhoeffer T: *Cell* 159(4):727-737, 2014; Sale A et al: *Physiol Rev* 94(1):189-234, 2014; Srivastava DP et al: *Pharmacol Rev* 65(4):1318-1350, 2013; Tononi G, Cirelli C: *Neuron* 81(1):12-34, 2014.

Neurotransmitters

Neurotransmitters are chemicals synthesized in the neuron and localized in the presynaptic terminal (synaptic bouton). Neurotransmitters are then released into the synaptic cleft and bind to a receptor site (binding site) on the postsynaptic membrane of another neuron or effector, where they affect ion channels (see Figure 13-2). Each neurotransmitter is removed by a specific mechanism from its site of action. Many substances are neurotransmitters, including norepinephrine, acetylcholine, dopamine, histamine, and serotonin. Many of these transmitters have more than one function.[4] Neurotransmitter and neuromodulator substances are summarized in Table 13-2.

Because the neurotransmitter is normally stored on one side of the synaptic cleft and the receptor sites are on the other side, chemical synapses operate in one direction. Therefore action potentials are transmitted along a multineuronal pathway in one direction. The binding of the neurotransmitter at the receptor site changes the permeability of the postsynaptic neuron and, consequently, its membrane potential. Two possible scenarios can then follow: (1) the postsynaptic neuron may be excited (depolarized; excitatory postsynaptic potentials [EPSPs]) or (2) the postsynaptic neuron's plasma membrane may be inhibited (hyperpolarized; inhibitory postsynaptic potentials [IPSPs]). Cannabinoid transmitters have been discovered that are released from postsynaptic neurons and modulate neurotransmitter release from the presynaptic neurons (retrograde transmission).[5,6] (Chapter 1 reviews electrical impulses and membrane potentials.)

Usually a single EPSP cannot induce a neuron's action potential and the propagation of the nerve impulse. Whether this occurs depends on the number and frequency of potentials the postsynaptic neuron receives—a concept known as summation. Temporal summation (time relationship) refers to the effects of successive, rapid impulses received from a single neuron at the same synapse. Spatial summation (spacing effect) is the combined effects of impulses from a number of neurons onto a single neuron at the same time. Facilitation refers to the effect of EPSP on the plasma membrane potential. The plasma membrane is facilitated when summation brings the membrane closer to the threshold potential and decreases the stimulus required to induce an action potential. The effect that a chemical neurotransmitter has on the plasma membrane potential depends on the balance of these effects. The mechanisms of convergence (many neurons firing and converging on one neuron), divergence (one neuron firing and diverging on many neurons), summation, and facilitation allow for the integrative processes of the nervous system.

✔ QUICK CHECK 13-2

1. Explain the process of the chemical conduction of impulses.
2. What are neurotransmitters? Give two examples.
3. Compare summation and facilitation.

THE CENTRAL NERVOUS SYSTEM

The Brain

The brain is a functionally integrated circuit of millions of neurons with different genomes, structures, molecular composition, networks, and connections. It weighs approximately 3 pounds and receives 15% to 20% of the total cardiac output. The brain enables a person to reason, function intellectually, express personality and mood, and perceive and interact with the environment.

The three major structural divisions of the brain are (1) the forebrain (prosencephalon), which includes the telencephalon and diencephalon; (2) the midbrain (mesencephalon), which connects the pons to the diencephalon; and (3) the hindbrain (rhombencephalon), which includes the cerebellum, pons, and medulla (Table 13-3 and Figure 13-5). The midbrain, medulla, and pons comprise the brainstem, which connects the hemispheres of the brain, cerebellum, and

TABLE 13-2   Substances That Are Neurotransmitters or Neuromodulators

Substance	Location	Effect	Clinical Example
Acetylcholine	Many parts of brain, spinal cord, neuromuscular junction of skeletal muscle, and many ANS synapses	Excitatory or inhibitory	Alzheimer disease (a type of dementia) is associated with a decrease in acetylcholine-secreting neurons. Myasthenia gravis (weakness of skeletal muscles) results from a reduction in acetylcholine receptors.
Monoamines			
Norepinephrine	Many areas of brain and spinal cord; also in some ANS synapses	Excitatory or inhibitory	Cocaine and amphetamines,* resulting in overstimulation of postsynaptic neurons.
Serotonin	Many areas of brain and spinal cord	Generally inhibitory	Involved with mood, anxiety, and sleep induction. Levels of serotonin are elevated in schizophrenia (delusions, hallucinations, withdrawal).
Dopamine	Some areas of brain and ANS synapses	Generally excitatory	Parkinson disease (depression of voluntary motor control) results from destruction of dopamine-secreting neurons. Drugs used to increase dopamine production induce vomiting and schizophrenia.
Histamine	Posterior hypothalamus	Excitatory (H1 and H2 receptors) and inhibitory (H3 receptors)	No clear indication of histamine-associated pathologic conditions. Histamine is involved with arousal and attention and links to other brain transmitter systems.
Amino Acids			
Gamma-aminobutyric acid (GABA)	Most neurons of CNS have GABA receptors	Majority of postsynaptic inhibition in brain	Drugs that increase GABA function have been used to treat epilepsy by inhibiting excessive discharge of neurons.
Glycine	Spinal cord	Most postsynaptic inhibition in spinal cord	Glycine receptors are inhibited by strychnine.
Glutamate and aspartate	Widespread in brain and spinal cord	Excitatory	Drugs that block glutamate or aspartate, such as riluzole, used to treat amyotrophic lateral sclerosis. These drugs might prevent overexcitation from seizures and neural degeneration.
Neuropeptides			
Endorphins and enkephalins	Widely distributed in CNS and PNS	Generally inhibitory	Morphine and heroin bind to endorphin and enkephalin receptors on presynaptic neurons and reduce pain by blocking release of neurotransmitter.
Substance P	Spinal cord, brain, and sensory neurons associated with pain, GI tract	Generally excitatory	Substance P is a neurotransmitter in pain transmission pathways. Blocking release of substance P by morphine reduces pain.

From Daroff RB et al: *Bradley's neurology in clinical practice*, ed 6, Philadelphia, 2012, Saunders.
ANS, Autonomic nervous system; *CNS*, central nervous system; *GI*, gastrointestinal; *PNS*, peripheral nervous system.
*Increase the release and block the reuptake of norepinephrine.

TABLE 13-3   Divisions of the Central Nervous System

Primary Brain Vesicles	Secondary Vesicles	Structures in Secondary Vesicles
Forebrain (prosencephalon)	Telencephalon	Cerebral hemispheres
		Cerebral cortex
		Basal ganglia
	Diencephalon	Epithalamus
		Thalamus
		Hypothalamus
		Subthalamus
Midbrain (mesencephalon)	Mesencephalon	Corpora quadrigemina (tectum— superior and inferior colliculi)
		Cerebral peduncles
Hindbrain (rhombencephalon)	Metencephalon	Cerebellum
		Pons
	Myelencephalon	Medulla oblongata
Spinal cord	Spinal cord	Spinal cord

FIGURE 13-5 Structural Divisions of the Brain. (From Standring S: *Gray's anatomy: the anatomical basis of clinical practice*, ed 40, Philadelphia, 2008, Elsevier.)

Auditory and
visual information

Reticular activating
system

Ascending sensory
information

FIGURE 13-6 Reticular Activating System (RAS). The RAS consists of nuclei in the brainstem reticular formation plus fibers that conduct sensory information to the nuclei and fibers that conduct from the nuclei to widespread areas of the cerebral cortex. Functioning of the reticular activating system is essential for consciousness.

BOX 13-1 Brain Networks

The architecture and integrated function of neural nodes, networks, and interconnected pathways within the brain are being mapped in the advancing field of human connectomics. Imaging techniques include positron emission tomography (PET, measures pairs of gamma rays emitted by an introduced positron-emitting radionuclide), tracer diffusion tensor magnetic resonance imaging (MRI, measures diffusion of water in tissue), functional MRI (measures changes in blood flow), magnetoencephalography (MEG, measures magnetic fields produced by electric currents generated by neurons), and electroencephalography (EEG, measures voltage changes in brain neurons), which are combined with mathematical and computational models.

The figure below provides an illustration of brain connectivity showing interconnecting cortical pathways using diffusion tensor imaging tracking technology. Such mapping of the brain contributes to an understanding of the commonalities and individual differences of the normally functioning brain and changes associated with aging and disease (i.e., degenerative brain disease, epilepsy, schizophrenia, and brain tumors).

(From Filippi M et al: *Lancet Neurol* 12[12]:1189-1199, 2013.)

From Park HJ, Friston K: *Science* 342(6158):1238411, 2013; Pollock JD et al: *Trends Neurosci* 37(2):106-123, 2014; Sporns O: *Neuroimage* 80:53-61, 2013; also see the *Human Connectome Project* at http://humanconnectome.org/about/project/.

---

spinal cord. A collection of nerve cell bodies (nuclei) within the brainstem makes up the **reticular formation** (Figure 13-6). The reticular formation is a large network of diffuse nuclei that connect the brainstem to the cortex and control vital reflexes, such as cardiovascular function and respiration. It is essential for maintaining wakefulness and attention and, therefore, is referred to as the **reticular activating system** (see Figure 13-6). Some nuclei within the reticular formation cause specific motor movements, such as balance and posture.[4]

Divisions of the brain are associated with different functions, but attributing specific functions to definite regions of the brain is not entirely accurate. However, for clinical considerations functional specificity is very useful for localizing pathologic conditions in various nervous system regions. A neuropsychiatrist (Brodmann) is credited with postulating that various activities are correlated to many regions of the cerebral cortex.[7] (Figure 13-7, *C* illustrates these regions and describes some of the areas). The mapping of **brain networks** is also helpful in discovering how varying parts of the brain are interconnected when performing a specific function[8,9] (Box 13-1).

Forebrain

Telencephalon. The **telencephalon (cerebral hemispheres)** consists of the cerebral cortex (the largest portion of the brain) and the basal ganglia (composed of several *nuclei*). The surface of the cerebral cortex is covered with convolutions called *gyri* (see Figure 13-7), which greatly increase the cortical surface area and the number of neurons. Grooves between adjacent gyrus are termed **sulci**; deeper grooves are fissures. The **cerebral cortex** contains an outer layer of cell bodies of neurons (**gray matter**). **White matter** lies beneath the cerebral cortex and is composed of myelinated nerve fibers.

The two cerebral hemispheres are separated by a deep groove known as the **longitudinal fissure**. The surface of each hemisphere is divided into lobes named after the region of the skull under which each

lobe lies. The posterior margin of the **frontal lobe** is on the **central sulcus (fissure of Rolando)**, and it borders inferiorly on the **lateral sulcus (sylvian fissure, lateral fissure)** (see Figure 13-7). The **prefrontal area** is responsible for goal-oriented behavior (e.g., ability to concentrate), short-term or recall memory, the elaboration of thought, and inhibition of the limbic areas of the CNS. The **premotor area (Brodmann area 6)** (see Figure 13-7, *C*) is involved in programming motor movements. This area contains the cell bodies that form part of the **basal ganglia system (extrapyramidal system**—efferent pathways outside the pyramids of the medulla oblongata). The frontal eye fields (the lower portion of Brodmann area 8), which are involved in controlling eye movements, are located on the middle frontal gyrus.

The **primary motor area (Brodmann area 4)** is located along the **precentral gyrus** forming the **primary voluntary motor area**, which has a somatotopic organization that is often referred to as a *homunculus* (little man) (Figure 13-8). Electrical stimulation of specific areas of this cortex causes specific muscles of the body to move. For example, stimulation of Brodmann area 4 in the medial longitudinal fissure affects the lower limb and foot, whereas stimulation of the superior lateral surface of the precentral gyrus affects the torso and arm, the middle third of the hand, and the lower third of the face and mouth/

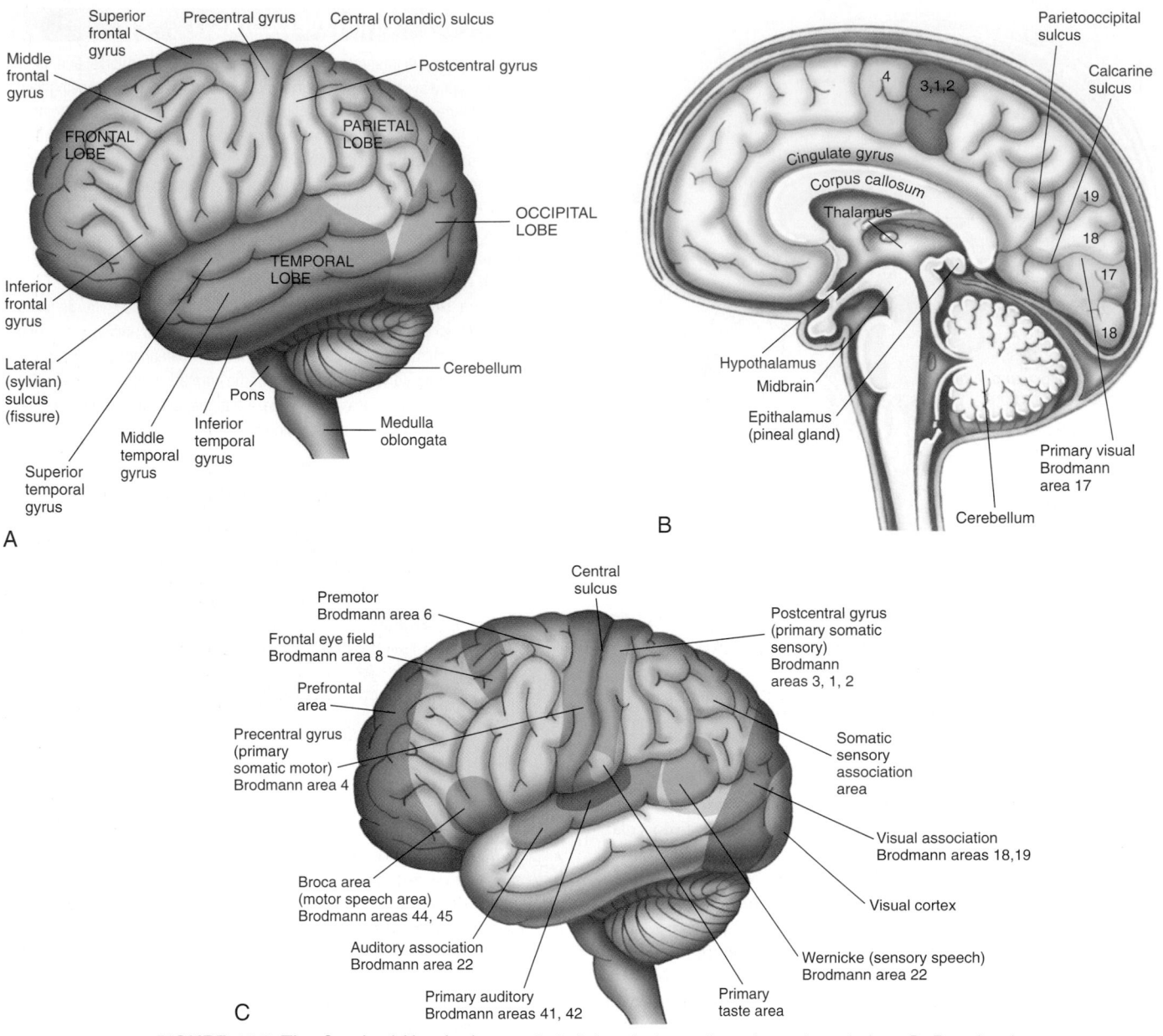

FIGURE 13-7 The Cerebral Hemispheres. A, Left hemisphere of cerebrum, lateral view. **B,** Functional areas of the cerebral cortex, midsagittal view. **C,** Functional areas of the cerebral cortex, lateral view.

throat. The axons traveling from the cell bodies in and on either side of this gyrus project fibers (axons) that form the **pyramidal system.** This system includes the **corticobulbar tract** that synapses in the brainstem and provides voluntary control of muscles in the head and neck, and the **corticospinal tracts (pyramidal system)** that descend into the spinal cord and provide voluntary control of muscles throughout the body. Cerebral impulses control function on the opposite side of the body, a phenomenon called **contralateral control** (Figure 13-9, *A*). The **Broca speech area (Brodmann areas 44, 45)** is rostral on the inferior frontal gyrus. It is usually on the left hemisphere and is responsible for the motor aspects of speech. Damage to this area, commonly as a result of a cerebrovascular accident (stroke), results in the inability to form words or at least some difficulty in forming words (expressive aphasia or dysphasia) (see Chapter 15).

The **parietal lobe** lies within the borders of the central, parietooccipital, and lateral sulci. This lobe contains the major area for somatic

sensory input, located primarily along the **postcentral gyrus** (Brodmann areas 3, 1, 2) (see Figure 13-7), which is adjacent to the primary motor area. Communication between the motor and sensory areas (and among other regions in the cortex) is provided by **association fibers.** Much of this region is involved in sensory association (storage, analysis, and interpretation of stimuli). (shows the distribution of functions associated with both the primary motor area and the primary sensory area of the cerebral cortex.)

The **occipital lobe** lies caudal to the parietooccipital sulcus and is superior to the cerebellum. The primary visual cortex (Brodmann area 17) is located in this region and receives input from the retinas. Much of the remainder of this lobe is involved in visual association (Brodmann areas 18, 19). The **temporal lobe** lies inferior to the lateral fissure and is composed of the superior, middle, and inferior temporal gyri. The primary auditory cortex (Brodmann area 41) and its related association area (Brodmann area 42) lie deep within the lateral sulcus on

A Motor   B Sensory

FIGURE 13-8 Primary Somatic Sensory (A) and Motor (B) Areas of the Cortex. A, The motor homunculus shows proportional somatotopical representation in the main motor area. **B,** The sensory homunculus shows proportional somatotopical representation in the somaesthetic cortex. (From Standring S, et al. (eds): *Gray's Anatomy,* ed 40, Edinburgh, Churchill Livingstone, 2008.)

the superior temporal gyrus. The Wernicke area, along with adjacent portions of the parietal lobe, constitutes a *sensory speech area*. This area is responsible for reception and interpretation of speech, and dysfunction may result in receptive aphasia or dysphasia. The temporal lobe also is involved in memory consolidation and smell.

Another lobe, the insula (insular lobe), lies hidden from view in the lateral sulci between the temporal and frontal lobes of each hemisphere. The insula processes sensory and emotional information and routes the information to other areas of the brain. Lying directly beneath the longitudinal fissure is a mass of white matter pathways called the corpus callosum (transverse or commissural fibers). This structure connects the two cerebral hemispheres through sensory and motor contralateral projection of axons and is essential in coordinating activities between hemispheres (see Figure 13-7).

Inside the cerebrum are numerous tracts (white matter) and nuclei (gray matter). The major cerebral nuclei are called the basal ganglia (basal nuclei) system. The basal ganglia system is a group of nuclei that includes the caudate nucleus, putamen, and globus pallidus. The putamen and globus pallidus together are called the lentiform nucleus. The caudate nucleus and **putamen** together are called the striatum[7] (Figure 13-10). Other structures in the basal ganglia include the *substantia nigra,* the *nucleus accumbens,* and the *subthalamic nucleus.* The nuclei of the basal ganglia are important for voluntary movement and cognitive and emotional functions.

The internal capsule is a thick layer of white matter in which axons of afferent (sensory) and efferent (motor) pathways pass to and from the cerebral cortex through the center of the cerebral hemispheres and between the caudate and lentiform nuclei (see Figure 13-10, *B*).

The basal ganglia plus their direct and indirect interconnections with the thalamus, premotor cortex, red nucleus, reticular formation, and spinal cord have been considered part of the extrapyramidal system. The extrapyramidal system is a part of the motor control system that causes involuntary reflexes and movement and has a stabilizing effect on motor control. Parkinson disease (substantia nigra) and Huntington disease (striatum) are characterized by various involuntary or exaggerated motor movements (see Chapter 15).

The limbic system is a group of interconnected structures located between the telencephalon and diencephalon and surrounding the corpus callosum. It is composed of the amygdala, hippocampus, fornix, hypothalamus, and related autonomic nuclei (see Figure 13-10). It is an extension or modification of the olfactory system and influences the autonomic and endocrine systems. The limbic system mediates emotion and long-term memory through connections in the prefrontal cortex (limbic cortex). Its principal effects are involved in primitive behavioral responses, visceral reaction to emotion, motivation, mood, feeding behaviors, biologic rhythms, and the sense of smell.

Diencephalon. The diencephalon (interbrain), surrounded by the cerebrum and sitting on top of the brainstem, has four divisions: epithalamus, thalamus, hypothalamus, and subthalamus (see Table 13-3 and Figure 13-7). The epithalamus forms the roof of the third ventricle (a brain cavity) and composes the most superior portion of the diencephalon. The diencephalon controls vital functions and visceral activities and is closely associated with those of the limbic system.

The thalamus borders and surrounds the third ventricle. It is a major integrating center for afferent impulses to the cerebral cortex. Various sensations are perceived at this level, but cortical processing is required for interpretation. The thalamus serves also as a relay center for information from the basal ganglia and cerebellum to the appropriate motor area.

FIGURE 13-9 Examples of Somatic Motor and Sensory Pathways. A, Motor tracts. The pyramidal pathway through the lateral corticospinal tract and the extrapyramidal pathways through the rubrospinal, reticulospinal and vestibulospinal tracts. **B,** Sensory tracts. **1,** The dorsal column-medial lemniscal pathway for transmitting critical types of tactile signals: touch/proprioception. Note the lateral corticospinal tract decussation is in the lower medulla. **2,** Anterior and lateral divisions of the anterolateral sensory pathway: pain/temperature. Note the decussation is in the spinal cord. (**A,** from Compston A, et al: *McAlpine's multiple sclerosis,* ed 4, London, 2006, Churchill Livingstone. **B,** from Hall JE: *Guyton and Hall textbook of medical physiology,* ed 13, Philadelphia, 2016, Saunders.)

The hypothalamus forms the base of the diencephalon. The hypothalamus functions to (1) maintain a constant internal environment and (2) implement behavioral patterns. Integrative centers control autonomic nervous system (ANS) function, regulate body temperature and endocrine function, and adjust emotional expression. The hypothalamus exerts its influence through the endocrine system, as well as through neural pathways (Box 13-2). The subthalamus flanks the hypothalamus laterally. It serves as an important basal ganglia center for motor activities.

Midbrain

Mesencephalon. The **midbrain (mesencephalon)** is composed of three structures: the **corpora quadrigemina** (located on the tectum, the ceiling of the midbrain), which is composed of the two pairs of

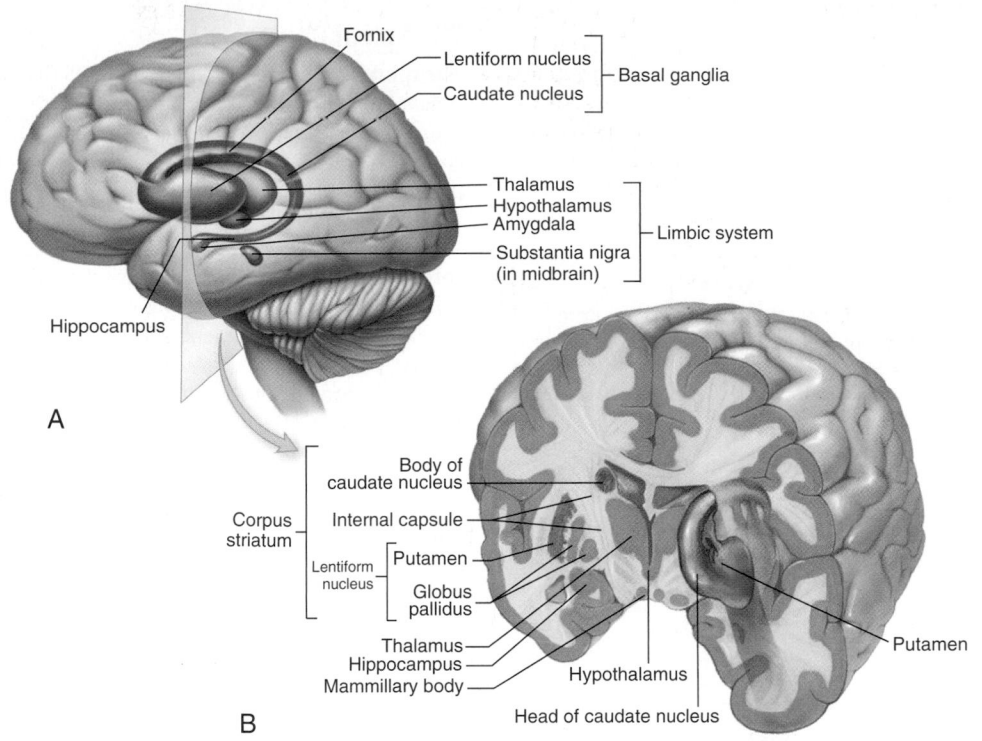

FIGURE 13-10 Basal Ganglia. A, The basal ganglia seen through the cortex of the left cerebral hemisphere. **B,** The basal ganglia seen in a frontal (coronal) section of the brain. (From Patton KT, Thibodeau GA: *Anatomy & physiology,* ed 9, St Louis, 2016, Mosby.)

BOX 13-2   Functions of the Hypothalamus

- Visceral and somatic responses
- Affectual responses
- Hormone synthesis
- Sympathetic and parasympathetic activity
- Temperature regulation
- Fluid balance
- Appetite and feeding responses
- Physical expression of emotions
- Sexual behavior
- Pleasure-punishment centers
- Level of arousal or wakefulness

---

superior colliculi and two pairs of inferior colliculi; the **tegmentum** (the floor of the midbrain), which is composed of the red nucleus, substantia nigra, and the basis pedunculi. The tegmentum and basis pedunculi are collectively called the **cerebral peduncles.**

The **superior colliculi** are involved with voluntary and involuntary visual motor movements (e.g., the ability of the eyes to track moving objects in the visual field). The **inferior colliculi** accomplish similar motor activities but involve movements affecting the auditory system (e.g., positioning the head to improve hearing). The **red nucleus** receives ascending sensory information from the cerebellum and projects a minor motor pathway, the rubrospinal tract, to the cervical spinal cord. The last portion of the basal ganglia is the **substantia nigra,** which synthesizes **dopamine,** a neurotransmitter and precursor of norepinephrine. Its dysfunction is associated with Parkinson disease and schizophrenia. The **basis pedunculi** are made up of efferent fibers of the corticospinal, corticobulbar, and corticopontocerebellar tracts.

Other notable structures of this region are the nuclei of the third and fourth cranial nerves. The **cerebral aqueduct (aqueduct of Sylvius),** which carries cerebrospinal fluid, also traverses this structure. Obstruction of this aqueduct is often the cause of hydrocephalus.

Hindbrain

Metencephalon. The major structures of the **metencephalon** are the cerebellum and the pons. The **cerebellum** (see Figure 13-7) is composed of gray and white matter, and its cortical surface is convoluted like the surface of the cerebrum. It also is divided by a central fissure into two lobes connected by the **vermis.**

The cerebellum is responsible for reflexive, involuntary fine-tuning of motor control and for maintaining balance and posture through extensive neural connections with the medulla (through the inferior cerebellar peduncle) and with the midbrain (through the superior cerebellar peduncle). The two hemispheres are connected to the pons by the middle cerebellar peduncles. These connections allow extensive sampling of visual, vestibular, and proprioceptive data from other regions of the CNS and periphery.

The **pons** (bridge) is easily recognized by its bulging appearance below the midbrain and above the medulla. Primarily it transmits information from the cerebellum to the brainstem and between the two cerebellar hemispheres. The nuclei of the fifth through eighth cranial nerves are located in this structure.

Myelencephalon. The **myelencephalon** usually is called the medulla oblongata and forms the lowest portion of the brainstem. Reflex activities, such as heart rate, respiration, blood pressure, coughing, sneezing, swallowing, and vomiting, are controlled in this area. The nuclei of cranial nerves IX through XII are located in this region.

A major portion of the descending motor pathways (i.e., corticospinal tracts) cross to the other side, or decussate, at the medulla (see Figure 13-9). These pathways, together with other areas of decussation in the CNS, are the basis for the phenomenon of *contralateral control.* Sleep-wake rhythms also are processed by neural influences from lower brain centers and are associated with a complex group of diffuse structures and functions (see Chapter 14), including the reticular activating system (cells that receive collateral signals from the afferent sensory pathways and project the signals to the higher brain centers, thus controlling CNS activity) (see Figure 13-6).

✔ **QUICK CHECK 13-3**
1. Name the three major divisions of the brain and their component parts.
2. Describe the limbic system's functions.
3. What are the two major functions of the hypothalamus?

The Spinal Cord

The spinal cord is the portion of the CNS that lies within the vertebral canal and is surrounded and protected by the vertebral column. The spinal cord has many functions, which include a long nerve cable that connects the brain and body, somatic and autonomic reflexes, motor pattern control centers, and sensory and motor modulation. It originates in the medulla oblongata and ends at the level of the first or second lumbar vertebra in adults (Figure 13-11). The end of the spinal cord, the conus medullaris, is cone shaped. Spinal nerves continue from the end of the spinal cord and form a nerve bundle called the cauda equina. The filament anchor from the conus medullaris to the coccyx is the filum terminale (see Figure 13-11). The coverings of the spinal cord are illustrated in Figure 13-12.

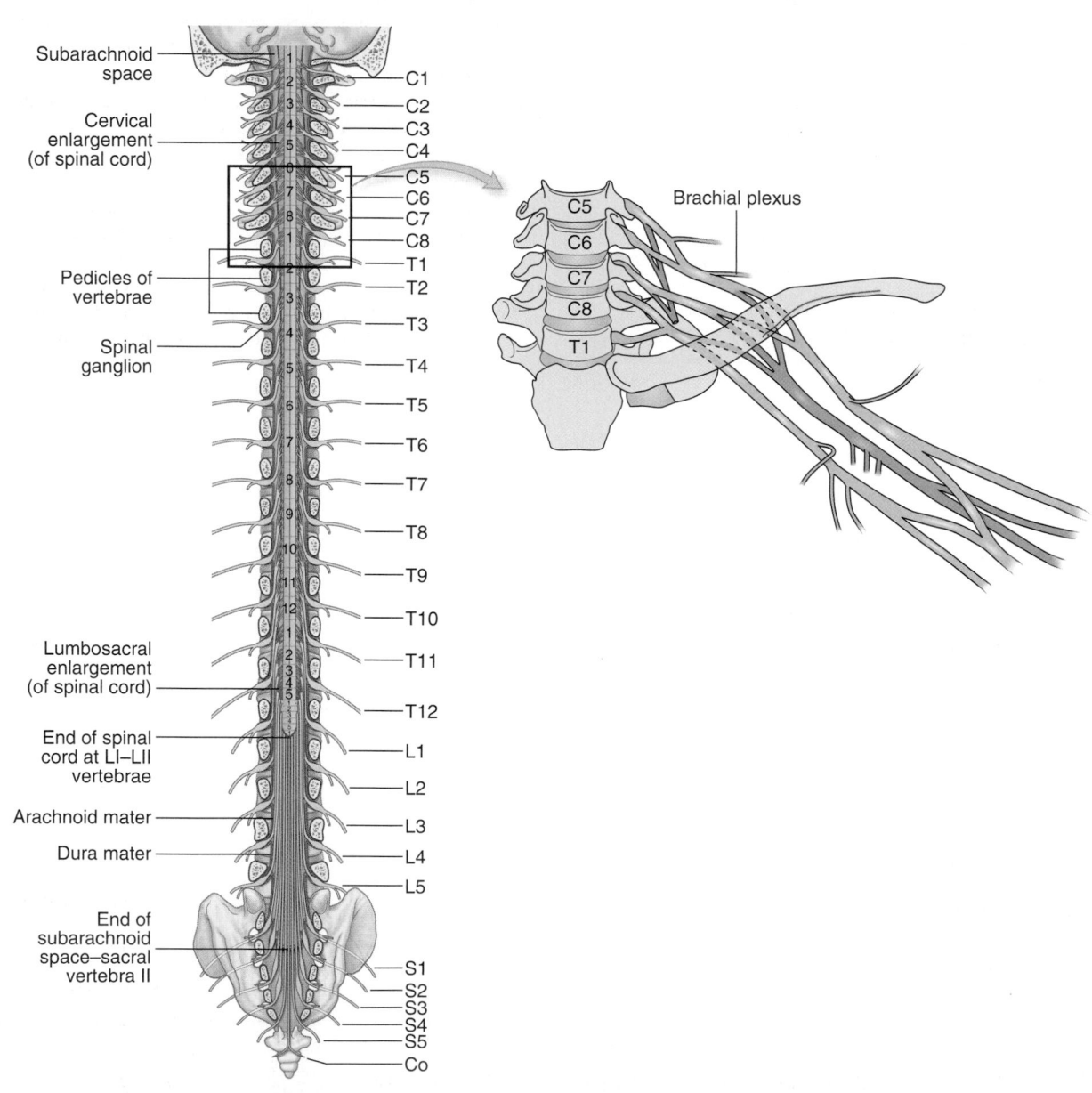

FIGURE 13-11 Vertebral Canal, Spinal Cord, and Spinal Nerves. Enlarged schematic of the brachial plexus is shown. (From Drake R, et al: *Gray's anatomy for students,* ed 3, London, 2015, Churchill Livingstone. **Inset,** from Chung KC, et al: *Practical management of pediatric and adult brachial plexus palsies,* London, 2012, Saunders.)

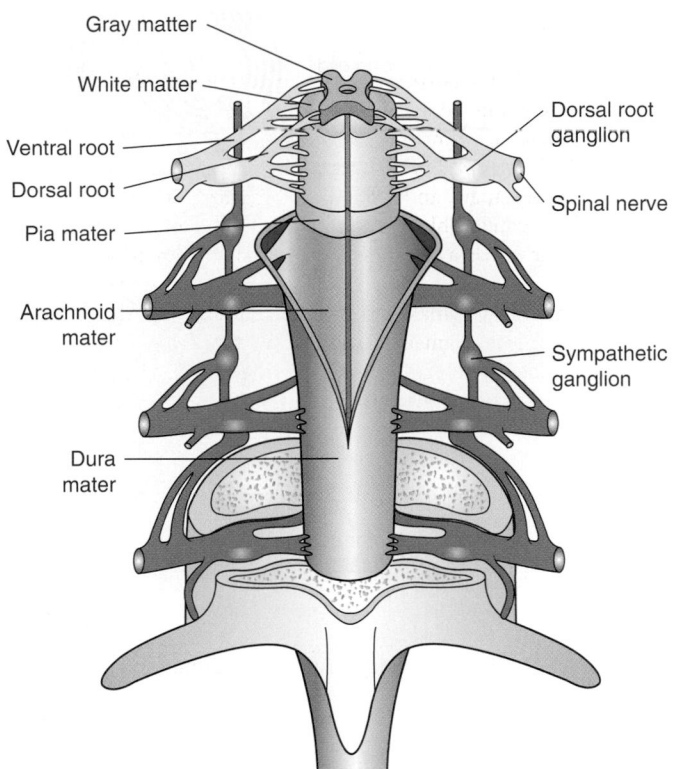

Gray matter
White matter
Ventral root
Dorsal root
Pia mater
Arachnoid mater
Dura mater

Dorsal root ganglion
Spinal nerve
Sympathetic ganglion

FIGURE 13-12 Coverings of the Spinal Cord. The dura mater is shown in natural color. Note how it extends to cover the spinal nerve roots and nerves. The arachnoid is highlighted in blue and the pia mater in pink. (From Patton KT, Thibodeau GA: *Structure and function of the body,* ed 15, St Louis, 2016, Mosby.)

Grossly, the spinal cord is divided into vertebral sections (8 cervical, 12 thoracic, 5 lumbar, 5 sacral, and 1 coccygeal) that correspond to paired nerves (see Figure 13-11). A cross section of the spinal cord (Figure 13-13) is characterized by a butterfly-shaped inner core of gray matter (containing nerve cell bodies). The **central canal** lies in the center of this region and extends through the spinal cord from its origin in the fourth ventricle. The gray matter of the spinal cord is divided into three regions and displays specific functional characteristics. These regions include the **posterior horn**, or dorsal horn (composed primarily of interneurons and axons from sensory neurons whose cell bodies lie in the **dorsal root ganglion**). At the tip of the posterior horn is the **substantia gelatinosa**, a structure involved in pain transmission (see Chapter 14). The **lateral horn** contains cell bodies involved with the ANS. The **anterior horn**, or **ventral horn**, contains the nerve cell bodies for efferent pathways that leave the spinal cord by way of spinal nerves.

Surrounding the gray matter is white matter that forms ascending and descending pathways called **spinal tracts**. Spinal tracts are named to denote their beginning and ending points. For example, the **spinothalamic tract** (see Figure 13-9, *B*, and Figure 13-13) carries nerve impulses from the spinal cord to the thalamus in the diencephalon. Numerous spinal tracts are grouped into columns according to their location within the white matter. These include the **anterior columns**, **lateral columns**, and posterior (dorsal) columns (see Figure 13-13).

Neural circuits in the spinal cord, when activated, display specific sets of motor responses. **Reflex arcs** form basic units that respond to stimuli and provide protective circuitry for motor output. Structures needed for a reflex arc are a receptor, an **afferent (sensory) neuron**, an **efferent (motor) neuron**, and an effector muscle or gland. A simple reflex arc may contain only two neurons (Figure 13-14). Interneurons are usually present and provide a link between sensory and motor

Posterior (dorsal)

Ascending tracts | Descending tracts

Fasciculus gracilis
Fasciculus cuneatus
Dorsal spinocerebellar tract
Ventral spinocerebellar tract
Spinothalamic tract

Fasciculus proprius
Lissauer's tract
Lateral corticospinal tract
Rubrospinal tract
Medial longitudinal fasciculus
Medullary reticulospinal tract
Lateral vestibulospinal tract
Pontine reticulospinal tract
Tectospinal tract
Ventral corticospinal tract

Anterior (ventral)

FIGURE 13-13 Ascending and Descending Tracts of the Spinal Cord. All ascending *(sensory)* and descending *(motor)* tracts are present bilaterally. In this figure, ascending tracts are emphasized on the left side and descending tracts are emphasized on the right side. The location of Lissauer's tract and the fasciculus proprius (which contain both ascending and descending fibers) are also shown. (From Crossman AR, Neary D: *Neuroanatomy: an illustrated colour text,* ed 4, London, 2015, Churchill Livingstone.)

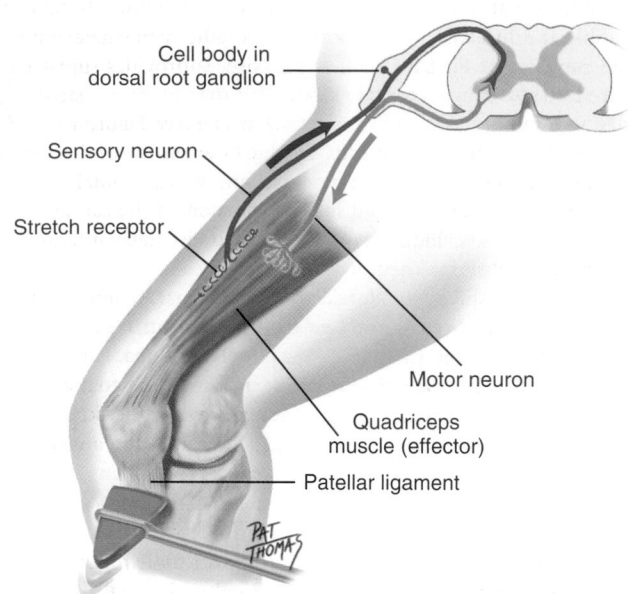

FIGURE 13-14 Cross Section of Spinal Cord Showing Simple Reflex Arc. (From Jarvis C: *Physical examination & health assessment,* ed 7, St Louis, 2016, Saunders.)

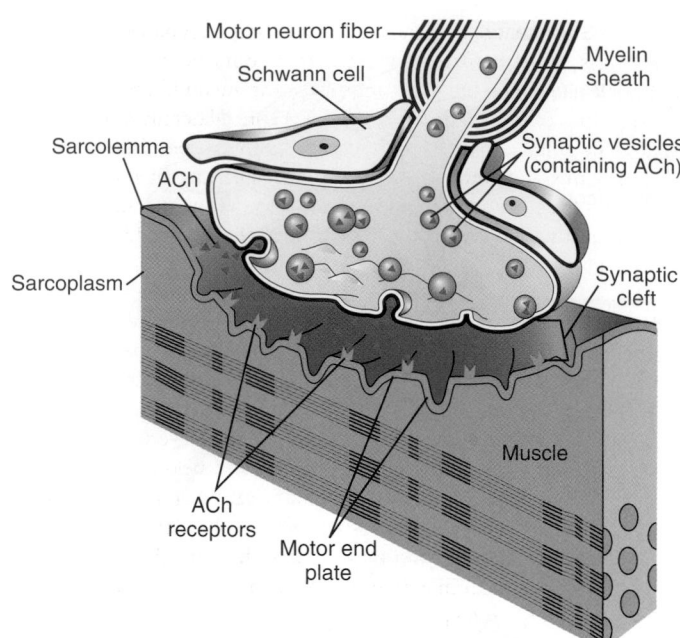

FIGURE 13-15 Normal Neuromuscular Junction. This figure shows how the distal end of a motor neuron fiber forms a synapse, or "chemical junction," with an adjacent muscle fiber. Neurotransmitters (specifically, acetylcholine) are released from the neuron's synaptic vesicles and diffuse across the synaptic cleft. There, they stimulate receptors in the motor end-plate region of the sarcolemma. (From Damjanov I: *Pathology for the health professions,* ed 4, St Louis, 2012, Saunders.)

neurons. The motor effects of reflex arcs generally occur before the event is perceived in the brain's higher centers. Much internal environmental regulation is mediated by reflex activity involving the ANS.

Afferent pathways transmit information from peripheral receptors and eventually it terminates in the cerebral or cerebellar cortex, or both. Efferent pathways primarily relay information from the cerebrum to the brainstem or spinal cord. Upper motor neurons are completely contained within the CNS. Their primary roles are controlling fine motor movement and influencing/modifying spinal reflex arcs and circuits. Generally, upper motor neurons form synapses with interneurons, which then form synapses with lower motor neurons that project into the periphery. Lower motor neurons directly influence muscles. Their cell bodies lie in the gray matter of the brainstem and spinal cord, but their processes extend out of the CNS and into the PNS. Destruction of upper motor neurons usually results in initial paralysis followed within days or weeks by partial recovery, whereas destruction of the *lower motor neurons* leads to paralysis unless peripheral nerve damage is followed by nerve regeneration and recovery (see Figure 13-4).

Muscle activity (i.e., stimulation and contraction) is regulated by nerve impulses. Motor neurons innervate one or more muscle cells, forming motor units, which consist of a neuron and the skeletal muscles it stimulates. The junction between the axon of the motor neuron and the plasma membrane of the muscle cell is called the neuromuscular (myoneural) junction (Figure 13-15). (Injury to motor neurons is discussed in Chapter 16.)

Motor Pathways

Clinically relevant motor pathways are the lateral corticospinal and corticobulbar pyramidal tracts; and the extrapyramidal reticulospinal, vestibulospinal, and rubrospinal tracts. The corticospinal and corticobulbar pathways are essentially the same tract and consist of a two-neuron chain. The cell bodies (upper motor neurons) originate in and around the precentral gyrus; pass through the corona radiata of the cerebrum, the internal capsule, middle three fifths of the cerebral

pedunculus, pons, and pyramid; and decussate (cross contralaterally) in the medulla oblongata and form the lateral corticospinal tract of the spinal cord (see Figures 13-9A and 13-13) and thus control the opposite side of the body. The corticobulbar tract axons synapse on motor cranial nuclei within the brainstem that control muscles of the face, head, and neck. The lateral corticospinal tract axons leave the tract to go to specific interneurons or motor neurons in the anterior horn. The lateral corticospinal tract has the same somatotopic organization as the body (see Figures 13-8 and 13-9, *A*). These lower motor neurons project through nerves to specific muscles. These tracts are involved in precise motor movements. The reticulospinal tract (see Figure 13-13) modulates motor movement by inhibiting and exciting spinal activity. The vestibulospinal tract arises from a vestibular nucleus in the pons and causes the extensor muscles of the body to rapidly contract, most dramatically witnessed when a person starts to fall backward. The rubrospinal tract originates in the red nucleus, decussates, and terminates in the cervical spinal cord. It is important for muscle movement and fine muscle control in the upper extremities.

Sensory Pathways

The three clinically important spinal afferent pathways are the posterior column, anterior spinothalamic tract, and lateral spinothalamic tract (see Figures 13-8, *B*, 13-9, *B*, and 13-13). The posterior (dorsal) column (fasciculus gracilis and fasciculus cuneatus) carries fine-touch sensation, two-point discrimination, and proprioceptive information (i.e., epicritic information). The posterior column is formed by a three-neuron chain. The first neuron of the chain is the primary afferent neuron. It also is the sensory neuron of the reflex arc. After entering the spinal cord it sends its axon ipsilaterally up the spinal cord to a specific part of the posterior column and synapses in the three posterior column nuclei in the medulla oblongata. A basketball playing center has primary afferent neurons that could be more than 6 feet long, running from the great toe up to the medulla oblongata. The axon of the second-order neuron crosses contralaterally at the medial lemniscus and ascends and synapses with a specific nucleus of the thalamus. The third-order neuron, originating in the thalamus, continues the tract into the internal capsule, corona radiata, and postcentral gyrus (Brodmann areas 3, 1, 2) (see Figures 13-7, 13-8, *A,* and 13-9, *B*).

The anterior and lateral spinothalamic tracts are responsible for vague touch sensation and for pain and temperature perception, respectively (see Figure 13-9, *B*). These modalities are referred to as protopathic. These tracts also form a three-neuron chain. However, their primary afferent neurons synapse in the posterior horn of the spinal cord, not just at the level they enter the intervertebral foramen but in a number of spinal segments above and below their point of entry. This is an example of divergence. The axons of the second-order neurons in the posterior horn cross to the contralateral side in the spinal cord in the lateral column, ascend to the same thalamic nucleus as the posterior column pathway, and continue with the posterior column pathway to the postcentral gyrus.

Protective Structures of the Central Nervous System
Cranium

The cranium is composed of eight bones. The cranial vault encloses and protects the brain and its associated structures. The galea aponeurotica, which is a thick, fibrous band of tissue overlying the cranium between the frontal and occipital muscles, affords added protection to the skull. The subgaleal space has venous connections with the dural sinuses, and with increased intracranial pressure, blood can be shunted to the space, thus reducing pressure in the intracranial cavity. The subgaleal space is also a common site for wound drains after intracranial surgery.

The floor of the cranial vault is irregular and contains many foramina (openings) for cranial nerves, blood vessels, and the spinal cord to exit. The cranial floor is divided into three fossae (depressions). The frontal lobes lie in the anterior fossa, the temporal lobes and base of the diencephalon lie in the middle fossa (temporal fossa), and the cerebellum lies in the posterior fossa. These terms are commonly used anatomic landmarks to describe the location of intracranial lesions.

Meninges

Surrounding the brain and spinal cord are three protective membranes: the dura mater, the arachnoid, and the pia mater. Collectively they are called the meninges (Figure 13-16, *C*). The dura mater (meaning literally "hard mother") is composed of two layers, with the venous sinuses formed between them. The outermost layer forms the periosteum (endosteal layer) of the skull. The inner dura (meningeal layer) is responsible for forming rigid membranes that support and separate various brain structures.

One of these membranes, the falx cerebri, dips between the two cerebral hemispheres along the longitudinal fissure. The falx cerebri is anchored anteriorly to the base of the brain at the crista galli of the ethmoid bone. The tentorium cerebelli, a common landmark, is a membrane that separates the cerebellum below from the cerebral structures above. Internal to the dura mater is the location of the arachnoid, a spongy, weblike structure that loosely follows the contours of the cerebral structures.

The subdural space lies between the dura and arachnoid. Many small bridging veins that have little support traverse the subdural space. Their disruption results in a subdural hematoma (see Chapter 16). The subarachnoid space lies between the arachnoid and the pia

mater and contains cerebrospinal fluid (CSF) (see Figure 13-16, *A* and *C*). Unlike the dura mater and arachnoid, the delicate pia mater adheres to the contours of the brain and spinal cord. It provides support for blood vessels serving brain tissue. The choroid plexuses, structures that produce CSF, arise from the pial membrane (see Figure 13-16, *B*). The spinal cord is anchored to the vertebrae by extension of the meninges. The meninges continue beyond the end of the spinal cord (at vertebrae levels L1 and L2) to the lower portion of the sacrum. CSF contained within the subarachnoid space also circulates inferiorly to about the second sacral vertebra.

The meninges form potential and real spaces important to understanding functional and pathologic mechanisms. For example, between the dura mater and skull lies a potential space termed the epidural space (see Figure 13-16, *C*). The arterial supply to the meninges consists of blood vessels that lie within grooves in the skull. A skull fracture can severe one of these vessels and produce an epidural hematoma.

Cerebrospinal Fluid and the Ventricular System

Cerebrospinal fluid (CSF) is a clear, colorless fluid similar to blood plasma and interstitial fluid. The intracranial and spinal cord structures float in CSF and are thereby partially protected from jolts and blows. The buoyant properties of the CSF also prevent the brain from tugging on meninges, nerve roots, and blood vessels. (Constituents of CSF are listed in Table 13-4.) Between 125 and 150 ml of CSF is circulating within the ventricles (small cavities) and subarachnoid space at any given time. Approximately 600 ml of CSF is produced daily.

The choroid plexuses in the lateral, third, and fourth ventricles produce the major portion of CSF. (Ventricles are illustrated in Figure 13-16.) These plexuses are characterized by a rich network of blood vessels, supplied by the pia mater, that lie close to the ependymal cells of the ventricles. The tight junctions of the choroid blood vessel provide a limiting barrier between the CSF and blood that functions similarly to the blood-brain barrier (see p. 324).

The CSF exerts pressure within the brain and spinal cord. When a person is supine, CSF pressure is about 80 to 180 mm of water pressure, or approximately 5 to 14 mm of mercury pressure, but doubles when the person moves to an upright position. CSF flow results from the pressure gradient between the arterial system and the CSF-filled cavities. Beginning in the lateral ventricles, the CSF flows through the interventricular foramen (foramen of Monro) into the third ventricle and then passes through the cerebral aqueduct (aqueduct of Sylvius)

TABLE 13-4 Composition of Cerebrospinal Fluid	
Constituent	**Normal Value**
Na^+	148 mM
K^+	2.9 mM
Cl^-	125 mM
HCO_3^-	22.9 mM
Glucose (fasting)	50-75 mg/dl (60% of serum glucose)
pH	7.3
Protein	15-45 mg/dl
Albumin	80%
Globulin	6-10%
Cells	
White (lymphocyte)	0-6/mm^3
Red	0

FIGURE 13-16 Flow of Cerebrospinal Fluid and Meninges of the Brain. A, Ventricles highlighted in blue within a translucent brain in a left lateral view. **B,** Flow of cerebral spinal fluid. The fluid produced by filtration of blood by the choroid plexus of each ventricle flows inferiorly through the lateral ventricles, interventricular foramen, third ventricle, cerebral aqueduct, fourth ventricle, and subarachnoid space to the blood. **C,** Meninges of the brain in relation to CSF and venous blood flow. (**A, B,** from Waugh A, Grant A: *Ross and Wilson anatomy and physiology in health and illness,* ed 12, London, 2012, Churchill Livingstone. **C,** from Drake R, et al: *Gray's anatomy for students,* ed 3, London, 2015, Churchill Livingstone.)

into the fourth ventricle. From the fourth ventricle the CSF may pass through either the paired lateral apertures (foramen of Luschka) or the median aperture (foramen of Magendie) before communicating with the subarachnoid spaces of the brain and spinal cord. The CSF does not, however, accumulate. Instead, it is reabsorbed into the venous circulation through the arachnoid villi. The arachnoid villi protrude from the arachnoid space, through the dura mater, and lie within the blood flow of the venous sinuses (see Figure 13-16, *B*). CSF is reabsorbed through a pressure gradient between the arachnoid villi and the cerebral venous sinuses. The villi function as one-way valves directing CSF outflow into the blood but preventing blood flow into the subarachnoid space. Thus CSF is formed from the blood, and after circulating throughout the CNS, it returns to the blood.

Vertebral Column

The vertebral column (Figure 13-17) is composed of 33 vertebrae: 7 cervical, 12 thoracic, 5 lumbar, 5 fused sacral, and 4 fused coccygeal. Between each interspace (except for the fused sacral and coccygeal vertebrae) is an intervertebral disk (Figure 13-18). At the center of the intervertebral disk is the nucleus pulposus, a pulpy mass of elastic fibers. The intervertebral disk absorbs shocks, preventing damage to the vertebrae. The intervertebral disk is also a common source of back

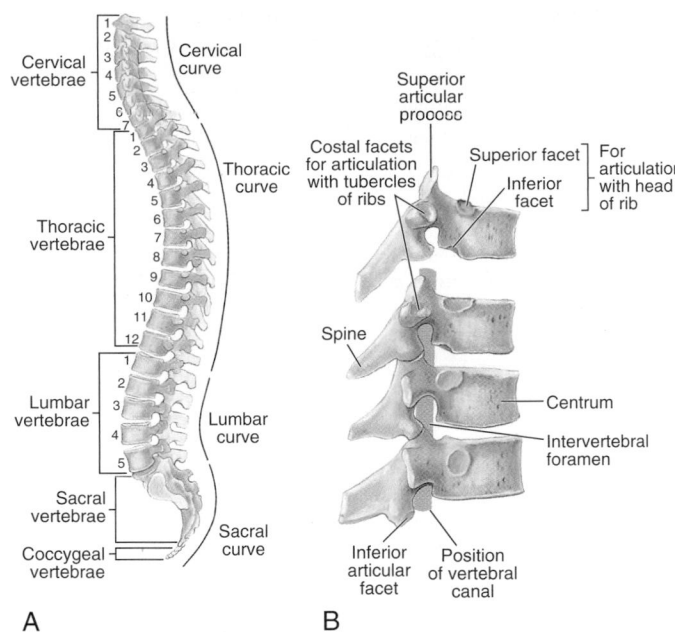

FIGURE 13-17 Vertebral Column. A, The normal curves and regions of the vertebral column. The vertebrae in each region are numbered. **B,** Lateral view of several vertebrae showing how they articulate. (From Solomon E: *Introduction to human anatomy and physiology,* ed 4, St Louis, 2016, Saunders.)

problems. If too much stress is applied to the vertebral column, the disk contents may rupture and protrude into the spinal canal, causing compression of the spinal cord or nerve roots.

✔ **QUICK CHECK 13-4**

1. What information is conveyed in the ascending and descending spinal tracts?
2. Contrast the functions of upper and lower motor neurons.
3. Name the protective structures of the central nervous system, and briefly describe each one.

Blood Supply of the Central Nervous System
Blood Supply to the Brain

The brain receives approximately 20% of the cardiac output, or 800 to 1000 ml of blood flow per minute. Carbon dioxide is a primary regulator for blood flow within the CNS. It is a potent vasodilator, and its effects ensure an adequate blood supply.

The brain derives its arterial supply from two systems: the internal carotid arteries and the vertebral arteries (Figure 13-19). The internal carotid arteries supply a proportionately greater amount of blood flow. They originate at the common carotid arteries, enter the cranium through the base of the skull, and pass through the cavernous sinus. After forming some small branches, these arteries divide into the anterior and middle cerebral arteries. The vertebral arteries originate at the subclavian arteries and pass through the transverse foramina of the cervical vertebrae, entering the cranium through the foramen magnum. They join at the junction of the pons and medulla to form the basilar artery (Figure 13-20). The basilar artery divides at the level of the midbrain to form paired posterior cerebral arteries.

The circle of Willis (see Figure 13-20) provides an alternative route for blood flow when one of the contributing arteries is obstructed

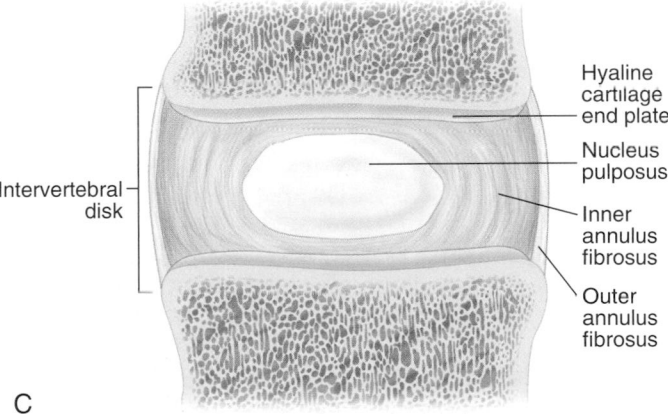

FIGURE 13-18 Intervertebral Disc. A, Sagittal illustration. **B,** Superior view of the structures of a typical vertebra. **C,** Magnified illustration. (**A** and **B,** from Drake R, Vogl AW, Mitchell AWM: *Gray's anatomy for students,* ed 3, London, 2015, Churchill Livingstone. **C,** from Lawry GV, et al: *Fam's musculoskeletal examination and joint injection techniques,* ed 2, Philadelphia, 2010, Mosby.)

(collateral blood flow). The circle of Willis is formed by the posterior cerebral arteries, posterior communicating arteries, internal carotid arteries, anterior cerebral arteries, and anterior communicating artery. The anterior cerebral, middle cerebral, and posterior cerebral arteries leave the circle of Willis and extend to various brain structures. The border zone is the area between the major arterial territories

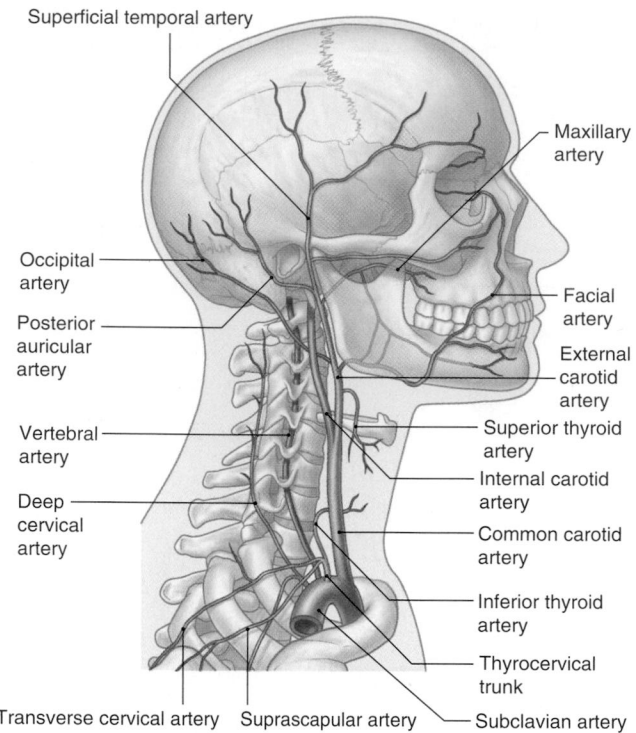

FIGURE 13-19 Major Arteries of the Head and Neck. (From Moses KP, et al: *Atlas of clinical gross anatomy,* ed 2, Philadelphia, 2013, Saunders.)

(Table 13-5 and Figure 13-21 illustrate structures served, functional relationships, and pathologic considerations related to occlusion of cerebral arteries).

Cerebral venous drainage does not parallel its arterial supply, whereas the venous drainage of the brainstem and cerebellum does parallel the arterial supply of these structures. The cerebral veins are classified as superficial and deep veins. The veins drain into venous plexuses and dural sinuses (formed between the dural layers) and eventually join the internal jugular veins at the base of the skull (Figure 13-22). Adequacy of venous outflow can significantly affect intracranial pressure. For example, head-injured individuals who turn or let their heads fall to the side partially occlude venous return, and the intracranial pressure can increase then because of decreased flow through the jugular veins.

Blood-Brain Barrier

The **blood-brain barrier (BBB)** describes cellular structures that selectively inhibit certain potentially harmful substances in the blood from entering the interstitial spaces of the brain or CSF allowing neurons to function normally. Endothelial cells in brain capillaries with their intracellular tight junctions are the site of the BBB. Supporting cells include astrocytes, pericytes, and microglia[10] (Figure 13-23 and see Chapter 1). The exact nature of this mechanism is controversial, but it appears that certain metabolites, electrolytes, and chemicals can cross into and out of the brain to varying degrees. This has substantial implications for drug therapy because certain types of antibiotics and chemotherapeutic drugs show a greater propensity than others for crossing this barrier. Breakdown of the BBB can contribute to neuroinflammation and neurodegeneration.

A

B

FIGURE 13-20 Arteries at the Base of the Brain. The arteries that compose the circle of Willis are the two anterior cerebral arteries, joined to each other by the anterior communicating artery and two short segments of the internal carotids, off of which the posterior communicating arteries connect to the posterior cerebral arteries. (**A,** from Moses KP, et al: *Atlas of clinical gross anatomy,* ed 2, Philadelphia, 2013, Saunders. **B,** from Hagen-Ansert S: *Textbook of diagnostic sonography,* ed 7, St Louis, 2012, Mosby.)

TABLE 13-5   Arterial Systems Supplying the Brain

Arterial Origin	Structures Served	Conditions Caused by Occlusion
Anterior cerebral artery	Basal ganglia; corpus callosum; medial surface of cerebral hemispheres; superior surface of frontal and parietal lobes	Hemiplegia on contralateral side of body, greater in lower than in upper extremities
Middle cerebral artery	Frontal lobe; parietal lobe; temporal lobe (primarily cortical surfaces)	Aphasia in dominant hemisphere and contralateral hemiplegia (see Chapter 15)
Posterior cerebral artery	Part of diencephalon (thalamus, hypothalamus) and temporal lobe; occipital lobe	Visual loss; sensory loss; contralateral hemiplegia if cerebral peduncle affected

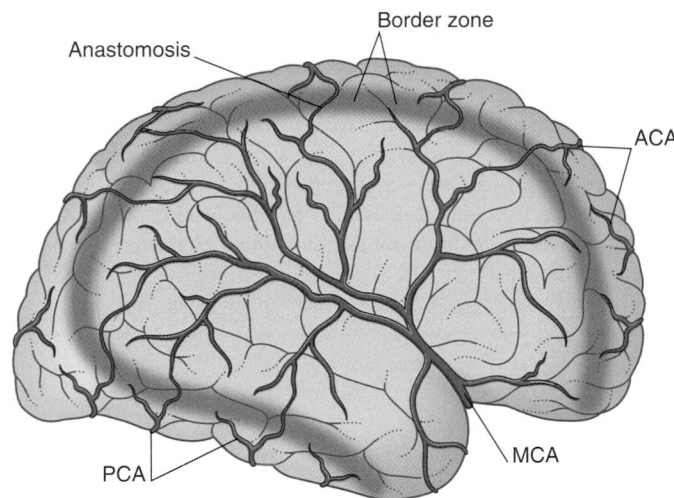

FIGURE 13-21 Areas of the Brain Affected by Occlusion of the Anterior, Middle, and Posterior Cerebral Artery Branches. *ACA,* Gray area affected by occlusion of branches of anterior cerebral artery; *PCA,* orange area affected by occlusion of branches of posterior cerebral artery; *MCA,* pink area affected by occlusion of branches of middle cerebral artery. Occlusions can occur in the cortical or deep areas of the border zone. (From Fitzgerald MJT et al: *Clinical neuroanatomy and neuroscience,* ed 6, Philadelphia, 2012, Saunders.)

Blood Supply to the Spinal Cord

The spinal cord derives its blood supply from branches off the vertebral arteries and from branches from various regions of the aorta (Figure 13-24). The anterior spinal artery and the paired posterior spinal arteries branch from the vertebral artery at the base of the cranium and descend alongside the spinal cord. Arterial branches from vessels exterior to the spinal cord follow the spinal nerve through the intervertebral foramina, pass through the dura, and divide into the anterior and posterior radicular arteries.

The radicular arteries eventually connect to the spinal arteries. Branches from the radicular and spinal arteries form plexuses whose branches penetrate the spinal cord, supplying the deeper tissues. Venous drainage parallels the arterial supply closely and drains into venous sinuses located between the dura and periosteum of the vertebrae.

THE PERIPHERAL NERVOUS SYSTEM

The cranial and spinal nerves, including their branches and ganglia, constitute the peripheral nervous system (PNS). A peripheral nerve (cranial or spinal) is composed of individual axons wrapped in a myelin sheath. These individual fibers are arranged in bundles called fascicles (Figure 13-25, *B*).

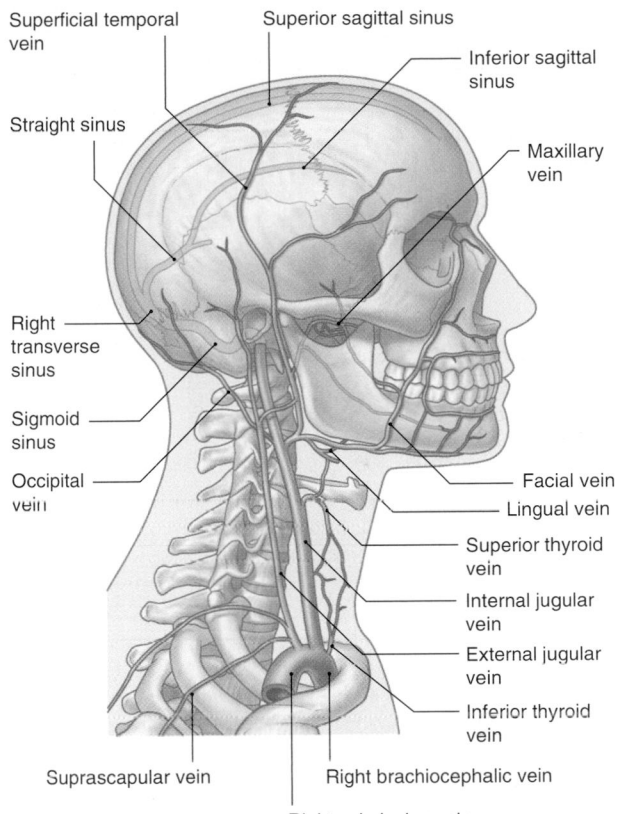

FIGURE 13-22 Veins of the Head and Neck. Deep veins and dural sinuses are projected on the skull. Note two superficial veins in the face are tributaries that send blood through emissary veins in the skull foramen into deep veins inside the skull terminating in the internal jugular vein. (From Moses KP, et al: *Atlas of clinical gross anatomy,* ed 2, Philadelphia, 2013, Saunders.)

The 31 pairs of spinal nerves derive their names from the vertebral level from which they exit. There are 8 cervical, 12 thoracic, 5 lumbar, 5 sacral pair of spinal nerves, and 1 coccygeal. The first cervical nerve exits above the first cervical vertebra, and the rest of the spinal nerves exit below their corresponding vertebrae. From the thoracic region (and inferiorly), nerves correspond to the vertebral level above their exit.

Spinal nerves contain both sensory and motor neurons and are called mixed nerves. They arise as rootlets lateral to anterior and posterior horns of the spinal cord. These two spinal nerve roots converge in the region of the intervertebral foramen to form the spinal nerve trunk. Shortly after converging, the spinal nerve divides into anterior and posterior rami (branches). The anterior rami (except the thoracic) initially form **plexuses** (networks of nerve fibers), which then branch into the peripheral nerves. Instead of forming plexuses, the thoracic nerves pass through the intercostal spaces and innervate regions of the thorax.

The main spinal nerve plexuses innervate the skin and the underlying muscles of the limbs. The **brachial plexus**, for example, is formed by the last four cervical nerves (C5 to C8) and the first thoracic nerve (T1) (see Figure 13-11). The brachial plexus innervates the nerves of the arm, wrist, and hand. The **lumbar plexus** (L1 to L4) and **sacral plexus** (L5 to S5) contain nerves that innervate the anterior and posterior portions of the lower body, respectively.

The posterior rami of each spinal nerve, with their many processes, are distributed to a specific area in the body. Sensory signals thus arise from specific sites associated with a specific spinal cord segment. Specific areas of cutaneous innervation at these spinal cord segments are called **dermatomes** (Figure 13-25, *C*).

Like spinal nerves, cranial nerves are categorized as peripheral nerves. Most of these are mixed nerves (like the spinal nerves), although some are purely sensory or purely motor. Cranial nerves (see Figure 13-25, *A*) connect to nuclei in the brain and brainstem. Table 13-6 describes structural and functional characteristics of the cranial nerves.

FIGURE 13-23 Blood-Brain Barrier. Cell membranes with tight junctions create a physical barrier between capillary blood and the cytoplasm of astrocytes. (From Bradley WG, editor: *Neurology in clinical practice*, ed 5, London, 2007, Butterworth-Heinemann.)

> ✔ **QUICK CHECK 13-5**
> 1. Describe the circle of Willis and explain its role in supplying blood to the brain.
> 2. What is the source of the spinal cord's blood supply?
> 3. What are the plexuses? Give two examples in the PNS.
> 4. What are the cranial nerves? Give three examples.
> 5. Describe the anatomy and function of the PNS.

THE AUTONOMIC NERVOUS SYSTEM

The structure and function of the autonomic nervous system (ANS) are complex and still not well understood. Components of the ANS

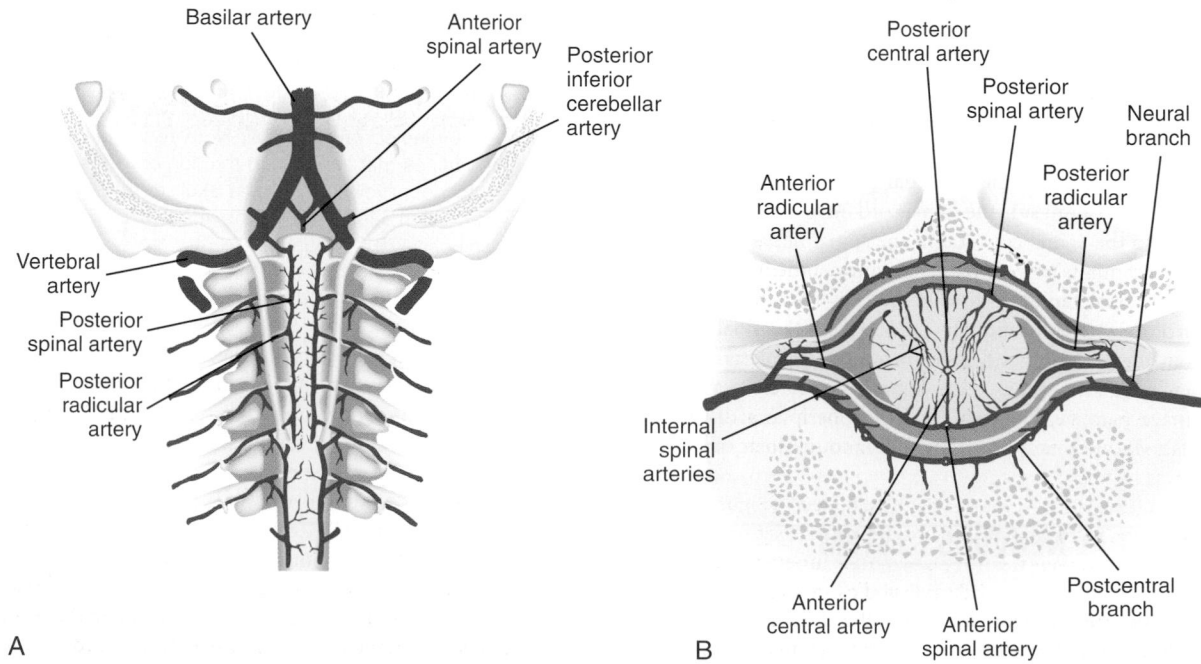

FIGURE 13-24 Arteries of the Spinal Cord. A, Arteries of cervical cord exposed from the rear. **B,** Arteries of spinal cord diagrammatically shown in horizontal section. (Redrawn from Rudy EB, editor: *Advanced neurological and neurosurgical nursing*, St Louis, 1984, Mosby.)

FIGURE 13-25 Cranial and Peripheral Nerves and Skin Dermatomes. A, Ventral surface of the brain showing attachment of the cranial nerves. The red lines indicate motor function, and the blue lines indicate sensory function. **B,** Peripheral nerve trunk and coverings. **C,** Dermatome map, anterolateral view (left) and posterolateral view (right). (**A,** from Applegate E: *The anatomy and physiology learning system,* ed 4, St Louis, 2011, Saunders. **C,** from Salvo SG: *Mosby's pathology for massage therapists,* ed 3, St Louis, 2014, Mosby.)

are located in both the CNS and the PNS; however, the ANS is considered to be part of the efferent division of the PNS, even though visceral afferent neurons are certainly an important part of this system. Many neurons of the ANS travel in the spinal nerves and certain cranial nerves. The widespread activity of this system indicates that its components are distributed all over the body. The peripheral autonomic nerves carry mainly efferent fibers. The motor component of the ANS is a two-neuron system consisting of **preganglionic neurons** (myelinated) and **postganglionic neurons** (unmyelinated) (Figure 13-26). This arrangement contrasts with the somatic nervous system, where a single motor neuron travels from the CNS to the innervated structure. Visceral afferent neurons have their cell bodies in some sensory and cranial ganglia and their fiber processes traveling in peripheral nerves.

The CNS has autonomic areas in the intermediolateral horns of the spinal cord, the cardiovascular and respiratory centers in the reticular formation, and both sympathetic and parasympathetic areas in the hypothalamus. CNS pathways interconnect all these areas.

The ANS coordinates and maintains a steady state among visceral (internal) organs, such as regulation of cardiac muscle, smooth muscle, and the glands of the body. This system is considered an involuntary system because one generally cannot *will* these functions to happen. The ANS is separated both structurally and functionally into two divisions: (1) the **sympathetic nervous system** and (2) the **parasympathetic nervous system** (Figure 13-27).

Anatomy of the Sympathetic Nervous System

The sympathetic nervous system mobilizes energy stores in times of need (e.g., in the "fight or flight" or stress response) (see Figure 9-3; see also Chapter 9). The sympathetic division is innervated by cell bodies located from the first thoracic (T1) through the second lumbar (L2) regions of the spinal cord and therefore is called the **thoracolumbar division**. The preganglionic axons of the sympathetic division form synapses shortly after leaving the spinal cord in the **sympathetic (paravertebral) ganglia**. These preganglionic axons travel several

TABLE 13-6   The Cranial Nerves

Number and Name	Origin and Course	Function	How Tested
I. Olfactory	Fibers arise from nasal olfactory epithelium and form synapses with olfactory bulbs, which transmit impulses to temporal lobe	Purely sensory; carries impulses for sense of smell	Person is asked to sniff aromatic substances, such as oil of cloves and vanilla, and to identify them
II. Optic	Fibers arise from retina of eye to form optic nerve, which passes through sphenoid bone; two optic nerves then form optic chiasma (with partial crossover of fibers) and eventually end in occipital cortex	Purely sensory; carries impulses for vision	Vision and visual field tested with an eye chart and by testing point at which person first sees an object (finger) moving into visual field; inside of eye is viewed with ophthalmoscope to observe blood vessels of eye interior
III. Oculomotor	Fibers emerge from midbrain and exit from skull to run to eye	Contains motor fibers to inferior oblique and to superior, inferior, and medial rectus extraocular muscles that direct eyeball; levator muscles of eyelid; smooth muscles of iris and ciliary body; and proprioception (sensory) to brain from extraocular muscles	Pupils examined for size, shape, and equality; pupillary reflex tested with a penlight (pupils should constrict when illuminated); ability to follow moving objects
IV. Trochlear	Fibers emerge from posterior midbrain and exit from skull to run to eye	Proprioceptor and motor fibers for superior oblique muscle of eye (extraocular muscle)	Tested in common with cranial nerve III relative to ability to follow moving objects
V. Trigeminal	Fibers emerge from pons and form three divisions that exit from skull and run to face and cranial dura mater	Both motor and sensory for face; conducts sensory impulses from mouth, nose, surface of eye, and dura mater; also contains motor fibers that stimulate chewing muscles	Sensations of pain, touch, and temperature tested with safety pin and hot and cold objects; corneal reflex tested with a wisp of cotton; motor branch tested by asking subject to clench teeth, open mouth against resistance, and move jaw from side to side
VI. Abducens	Fibers leave inferior pons and exit from skull to run to eye	Contains motor fibers to lateral rectus muscle and proprioceptor fibers from same muscle to brain	Tested in common with cranial nerve III relative to ability to move each eye laterally
VII. Facial	Fibers leave pons and travel through temporal bone to reach face	Mixed: (1) supplies motor fibers to muscles of facial expression and to lacrimal and salivary glands and (2) carries sensory fibers from taste buds of anterior part of tongue	Anterior two thirds of tongue tested for ability to taste sweet (sugar), salty, sour (vinegar), and bitter (quinine) substances; symmetry of face checked; subject asked to close eyes, smile, whistle, and so on; tearing tested with ammonia fumes
VIII. Vestibulocochlear (acoustic)	Fibers run from inner ear (hearing and equilibrium receptors in temporal bone) to enter brainstem just below pons	Purely sensory; vestibular branch transmits impulses for sense of equilibrium; cochlear branch transmits impulses for sense of hearing	Hearing checked by air and bone conduction by use of a tuning fork; vestibular tests: Bárány and caloric tests
IX. Glossopharyngeal	Fibers emerge from medulla and leave skull to run to throat	Mixed: (1) motor fibers serve pharynx (throat) and salivary glands, and (2) sensory fibers carry impulses from pharynx, posterior tongue (taste buds), and pressure receptors of carotid artery	Gag and swallow reflexes checked; subject asked to speak and cough; posterior one third of tongue may be tested for taste
X. Vagus	Fibers emerge from medulla, pass through skull, and descend through neck region into thorax and abdominal region	Fibers carry sensory and motor impulses for pharynx; a large part of this nerve is parasympathetic motor fibers, which supply smooth muscles of abdominal organs; receives sensory impulses from viscera	Same as for cranial nerve IX (IX and X are tested in common) because they both serve muscles of throat
XI. Spinal accessory	Fibers arise from medulla and superior spinal cord and travel to muscles of neck and back	Provides sensory and motor fibers for sternocleidomastoid and trapezius muscles and muscles of soft palate, pharynx, and larynx	Sternocleidomastoid and trapezius muscles checked for strength by asking subject to rotate head and shrug shoulders against resistance
XII. Hypoglossal	Fibers arise from medulla and exit from skull to travel to tongue	Carries motor fibers to muscles of tongue and sensory impulses from tongue to brain	Subject asked to stick out tongue, and any position abnormalities are noted

FIGURE 13-26 Preganglionic and Postganglionic Fibers of the Autonomic Nervous System. (From Applegate E: *The anatomy and physiology learning system,* ed 4, St Louis, 2011, Saunders.)

different ways: (1) directly synapsing with postganglionic neurons in the sympathetic chain ganglion at their level; (2) up or down the sympathetic chain ganglion before forming synapses with a higher or lower postganglionic neuron; or (3) through the sympathetic chain ganglion, postganglionic neurons within collateral ganglia (see Figure 13-27). Some preganglionic axons form pathways called splanchnic nerves, which lead to collateral ganglia on the front of the aorta. The collateral ganglia are named according to the branches of the aorta nearest them, namely, the celiac, superior mesenteric, and inferior mesenteric. The preganglionic neurons synapse with postganglionic neurons within the collateral ganglia. These postganglionic neurons leave the collateral ganglia and innervate the viscera below the diaphragm.

Preganglionic sympathetic neurons that innervate the adrenal medulla also travel in the splanchnic nerves and *do not* synapse before reaching the gland. The secretory cells in the adrenal medulla are considered modified postganglionic neurons. Because preganglionic sympathetic fibers are all myelinated, travel to the adrenal medulla is quick, and innervation causes the rapid release of epinephrine and norepinephrine. Epinephrine and norepinephrine are mediators of the fight or flight response (see Chapter 9).

Anatomy of the Parasympathetic Nervous System

The parasympathetic nervous system conserves and restores energy. The nerve cell bodies of this division are located in the cranial nerve nuclei and in the sacral region of the spinal cord and therefore constitute the craniosacral division. Unlike the sympathetic branch, the preganglionic fibers in the parasympathetic division travel close to the organs they innervate before forming synapses with the relatively short postganglionic neurons (see Figure 13-27). Parasympathetic nerves arising from nuclei in the brainstem travel to the viscera of the head, thorax, and abdomen within cranial nerves—including the oculomotor (III), facial (VII), glossopharyngeal (IX), and vagus (X) nerves.

Preganglionic parasympathetic nerves that originate from the sacral region of the spinal cord run either separately or together with some spinal nerves. The preganglionic axons unite to form the pelvic nerve, which innervates the viscera of the pelvic cavity. These preganglionic axons synapse with postganglionic neurons in terminal ganglia located close to the organs they innervate.

Neurotransmitters and Neuroreceptors

Sympathetic preganglionic fibers and parasympathetic preganglionic and postganglionic fibers release acetylcholine—the same neurotransmitter released by somatic efferent neurons (see Figure 13-26). These fibers are characterized by cholinergic transmission. Most postganglionic sympathetic fibers release norepinephrine (adrenaline) and thus are considered to function by adrenergic transmission. A few postganglionic sympathetic fibers, such as those that innervate the sweat glands, release acetylcholine.

The action of catecholamines varies with the type of neuroreceptor stimulated. It should be remembered that catecholamines also are released by the adrenal medulla gland that physiologically and biochemically resembles the sympathetic nervous system. Two types of adrenergic receptors exist, α and β. Cells of the effector organs may have only one or both types of adrenergic receptors. The α-adrenergic receptors have been further subdivided according to the action produced. α_1-Adrenergic activity is associated mostly with excitation or stimulation; α_2-adrenergic activity is associated with relaxation or inhibition. Most of the α-adrenergic receptors on effector organs belong to the α_1 class. The β-adrenergic receptors are classified as β_1-adrenergic receptors (which facilitate increased heart rate and contractility and cause the release of renin from the kidney) and β_2-adrenergic receptors (which facilitate all remaining effects attributed to β receptors).[11] Norepinephrine stimulates all α_1 and β_1 receptors and only certain β_2 receptors. The primary response from norepinephrine, however, is stimulation of the α_1-adrenergic receptors that cause vasoconstriction. Epinephrine strongly stimulates all four types of receptors and induces general vasodilation because of the predominance of β receptors in muscle vasculatures. (Table 13-7 summarizes the effects of neuroreceptors on their effector organs.)

Functions of the Autonomic Nervous System

Many body organs are innervated by both the sympathetic and parasympathetic nervous systems. The two divisions often cause opposite responses; for example, sympathetic stimulation of the stomach causes decreased peristalsis, whereas parasympathetic stimulation of the intestine increases peristalsis. In general, sympathetic stimulation promotes responses for the protection of the individual. For example, sympathetic activity increases blood glucose levels and

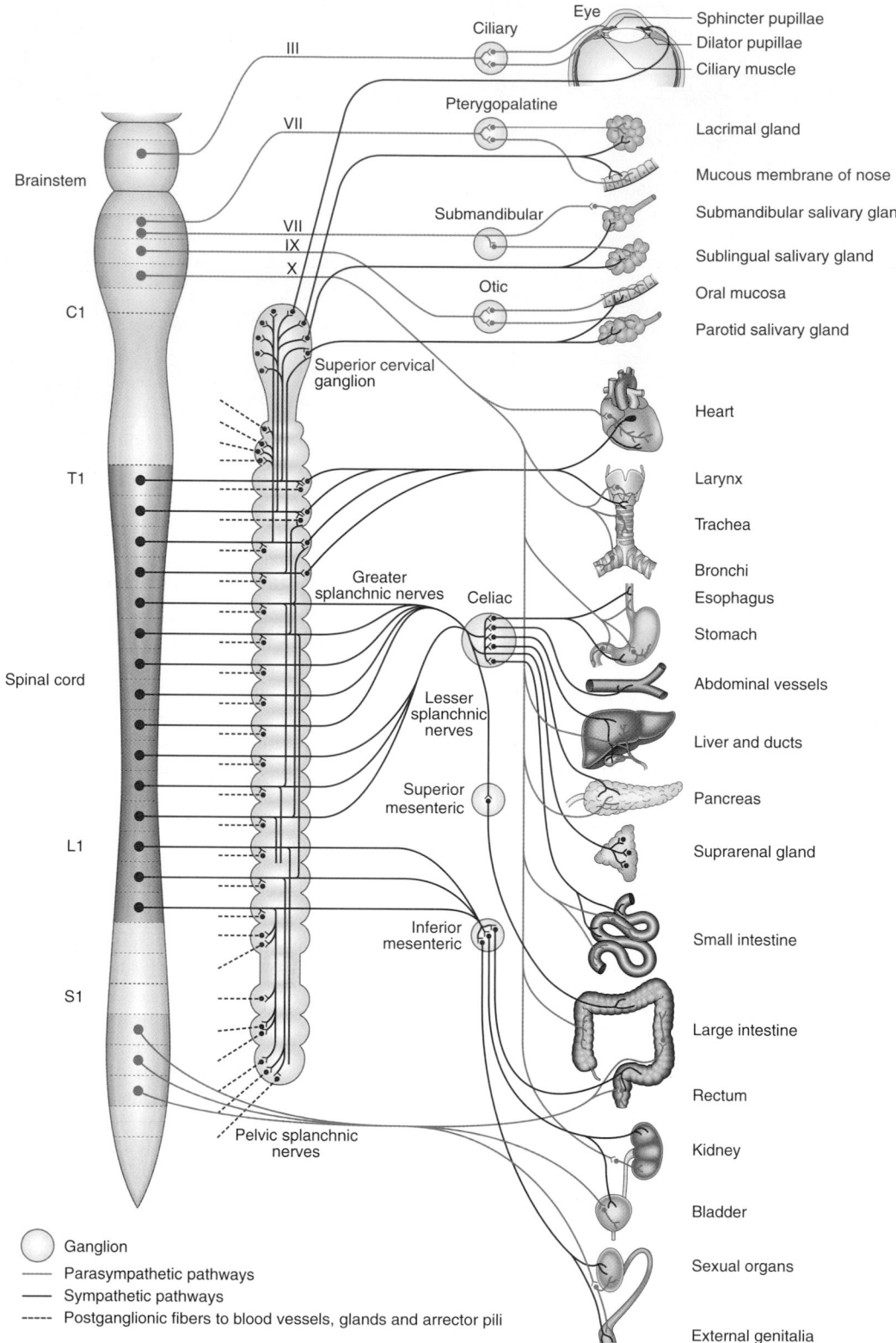

FIGURE 13-27 Sympathetic and Parasympathetic Divisions of the Autonomic Nervous System.
Preganglionic neuron cell bodies are located in the brainstem and sacral cord segments (parasympathetic or "cranio-sacral" division) and thoracic and upper lumbar cord segments (sympathetic or "thoraco-lumbar" division). The axons of these neurons synapse with postganglionic neurons, which innervate smooth muscle, cardiac muscle, and glands of the body. The postganglionic neuron cell bodies may be located in distinct autonomic ganglia (represented with circles), or in or very near the wall of the innervated visceral organ. Note that sympathetic fibers provide the only innervation to peripheral effectors (sweat glands, arrector pili muscles, adipose tissue, and blood vessels). (From Cramer D et al: *Basic and clinical anatomy of the spine, spinal cord, and ANS*, ed 2, St Louis, 2005, Elsevier Mosby.)

TABLE 13-7   Actions of Autonomic Nervous System Neuroreceptors

Effector Organ or Tissue	Adrenergic Receptors	Adrenergic Effects	Cholinergic Effects (Nicotine and Muscarinic* Receptors)
Eye, iris			
Radial muscle	α_1	Dilation	—
Sphincter muscle	—	—	Constriction
Eye, ciliary muscle	β_2	Relaxation for far vision	Contraction for near vision
Lacrimal glands	α_1	Secretion	Secretion
Nasopharyngeal glands	—	—	Secretion
Salivary glands	α_1	Secretion of potassium and water	Secretion of potassium and water
	β	Secretion of amylase	—
Heart			
SA node	β_1, β_2	Increase heart rate	Decrease heart rate; vagus arrest
Atrial	β_1, β_2	Increase contractility and conduction velocity	Decrease contractility; shorten action potential duration
AV junction	β_1, β_2	Increase automaticity and propagation velocity	Decrease automaticity and propagation velocity
Purkinje system	β_1, β_2	Increase automaticity and propagation velocity	—
Ventricles	β_1, β_2	Increase contractility	Slight decrease in contraction
Arterioles			
Coronary	$\alpha_1, \alpha_2, \beta_2$	Constriction, dilation	Dilation
Skin and mucosa	α_1, α_2	Constriction	Dilation
Skeletal muscle	α, β_2	Dilation, constriction	Dilation
Cerebral	α_1	Constriction (slight)	Dilation
Pulmonary	α_1, β_2	Constriction, dilation	Dilation
Mesenteric	α_1	Constriction	Dilation
Renal	$\alpha_1, \beta_1, \beta_2$	Constriction, dilation	Dilation
Salivary glands	α_1, α_2	Constriction	Dilation
Veins, systemic	$\alpha_1, \alpha_2, \beta_2$	Constriction, dilation	—
Lung			
Bronchial muscle	α_2	Relaxation	Contraction
Bronchial glands	α_1, β_2	Decrease secretion; increase secretion	Stimulation
Stomach			
Motility	$\alpha_1, \alpha_2, \beta_1, \beta_2$	Decrease (usually)	Increase
Sphincters	α_1	Contraction (usually)	Relaxation (usually)
Secretion	α_2	Inhibition	Stimulation
Liver	α_1, β_2	Glycogenolysis and gluconeogenesis	—
Gallbladder and ducts	β_2	Relaxation	Contraction
Pancreas			
Acini	α	Decrease secretion	Secretion
Islet cells	α_2, β_2	Decrease secretion; increase secretion	—
Intestine			
Motility and tone	$\alpha_1, \alpha_2, \beta_1, \beta_2$	Decrease	Increase
Sphincters	α_1	Contraction	Relaxation (usually)
Secretion	α_2	Inhibition	Stimulation
Adrenal medulla	—	Secretion of epinephrine and norepinephrine (nicotinic effect)	
Kidney			
Renin secretion	α_1, β_1	Decrease; increase	—
Ureter			
Motility and tone	β_1	Increase	Increase (?)
Urinary bladder			
Detrusor	β_2	Relaxation	Contraction
Trigone and sphincter	α_1	Contraction	Relaxation
Sex organs, male	α_1	Ejaculation	Erection

Continued

TABLE 13-7 Actions of Autonomic Nervous System Neuroreceptors—cont'd

Effector Organ or Tissue	Adrenergic Receptors	Adrenergic Effects	Cholinergic Effects (Nicotine and Muscarinic* Receptors)
Skin			
Pilomotor muscles	α_1	Contraction	—
Sweat glands	α_1	Localized secretion	—
Fat cells	$\alpha_2, \beta_1, \beta_2, \beta_3$	Inhibition of lipolysis; stimulation of lipolysis	—
Pineal gland	β	Melatonin synthesis	—

Modified from Brunton LL et al, editors: *Goodman & Gilman's the pharmacological basis of therapeutics,* ed 12, New York, 2010, McGraw-Hill; Yagiela JA et al: *Pharmacology and therapeutics for dentistry,* ed 6, St Louis, 2011, Mosby.
*Muscarinic receptors respond to circulating muscarinic antagonists.

temperature and raises the blood pressure. In emergency situations, a generalized and widespread discharge of the sympathetic system occurs and is known as the "fight or flight" reflex or acute stress response (see Chapter 9). This is accomplished by an increased firing frequency of sympathetic fibers and by activation of sympathetic fibers normally silent and at rest (fibers to the sweat glands, pilomotor muscles, and the adrenal medulla, as well as vasodilator fibers to muscle). Regulation of vasomotor tone is considered the single most important function of the sympathetic nervous system. (Figure 13-28 illustrates some of the most important functions of the sympathetic nervous system.)

Increased parasympathetic activity promotes rest and tranquility and is characterized by reduced heart rate and enhanced visceral functions concerned with digestion. Stimulation of the vagus nerve (cranial nerve X) in the gastrointestinal tract increases peristalsis and secretion, as well as the relaxation of sphincters. Activation of parasympathetic fibers in the head, provided by cranial nerves III, VII, and IX, causes constriction of the pupil, tear secretion, and increased salivary secretion. Stimulation of the sacral division of the parasympathetic system contracts the urinary bladder and facilitates the process of genital erection.

The parasympathetic system lacks the generalized and widespread response of the sympathetic system. Specific parasympathetic fibers are activated to regulate particular functions. Although the actions of the parasympathetic and sympathetic systems are usually antagonistic, there are exceptions. Peripheral vascular resistance, for example, is increased dramatically by sympathetic activation but is not altered appreciably by activity of the parasympathetic system. Most blood vessels involved in the control of blood pressure are innervated by sympathetic nerves. To decrease blood pressure, therefore, it is more important to block or paralyze the continuous (tonic) discharge of the sympathetic system than to promote parasympathetic activity.

QUICK CHECK 13-6
1. What are the structural and functional divisions of the ANS?
2. Compare cholinergic and adrenergic transmission.
3. What are the functions of the ANS?

GERIATRIC CONSIDERATIONS
Aging & the Nervous System

Structural Changes with Aging
Decreased brain weight and size, particularly frontal regions
Increase in ventricular volume
Fibrosis and thickening of the meninges
Narrowing of gyri and widening of sulci
Increase in size of ventricles

Cellular Changes with Aging
Decrease in number of neurons not consistently related to changes in mental function
Decreased myelin
Lipofuscin deposition (a pigment resulting from cellular autodigestion)
Decreased number of dendritic processes and synaptic connections
Intracellular neurofibrillary tangles; significant accumulation in cortex associated with Alzheimer dementia
Imbalance in amount and distribution of neurotransmitters
Decrease in glucose metabolism

Cerebrovascular Changes with Aging
Arterial atherosclerosis (may cause infarcts and scars)
Increased permeability of blood-brain barrier
Decreased vascular density

Functional Changes with Aging
Decreased tendon reflexes
Progressive deficit in taste and smell
Decreased vibratory sense
Decrease in accommodation and color vision
Decrease in neuromuscular control with change in gait and posture
Sleep disturbances
Memory impairments
Cognitive alterations associated with chronic disease
Functional changes and nervous system aging have significant individual variation

Data from Chételat G et al: *Neuroimage* 76:167-177, 2013; Fjell AM, Walhovd KB: *Rev Neurosci* 21(3):187-221, 2010; Fjell AM et al: *Prog Neurobiol* 117:20-40, 2014; Xekardaki A et al: *Adv Exp Med Biol* 821:11-17, 2015.

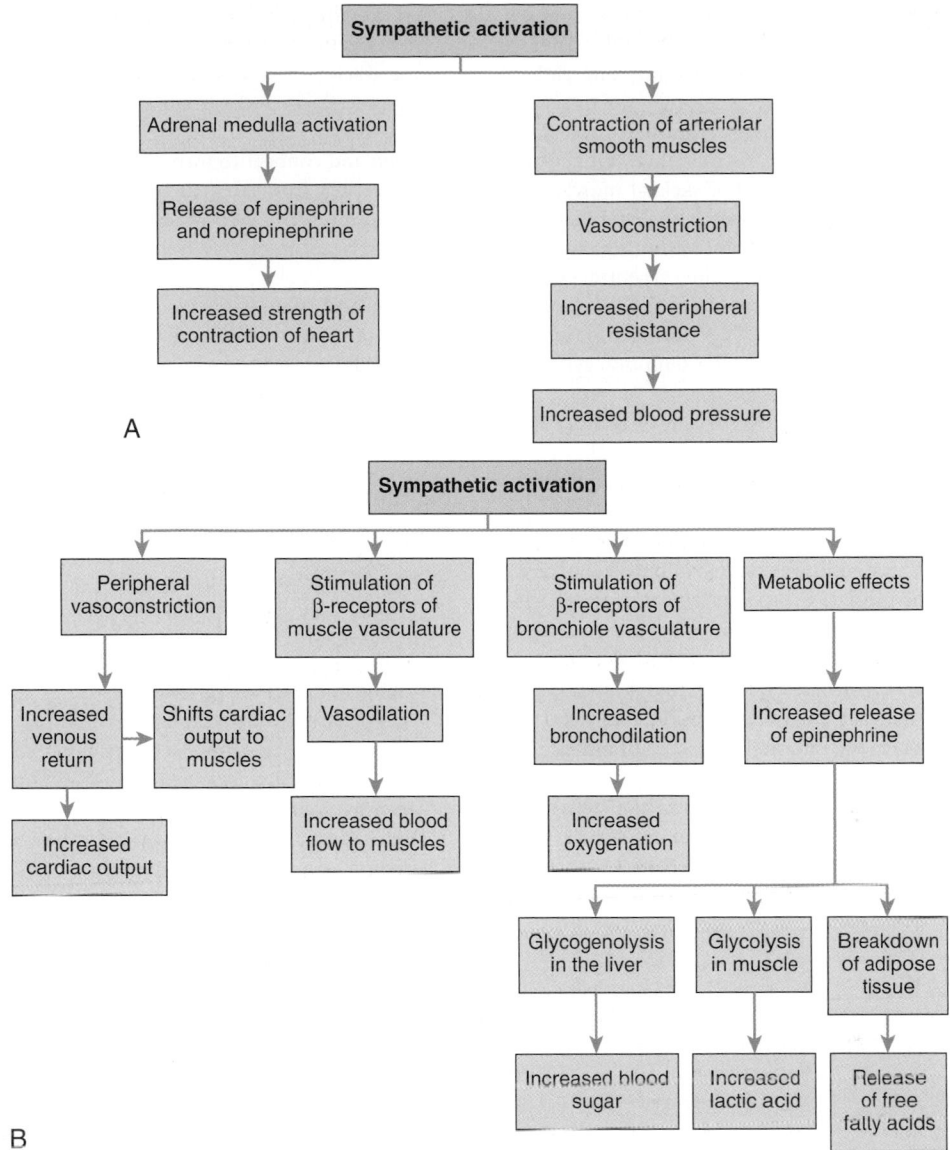

FIGURE 13-28 Examples of Important Functions of the Sympathetic Nervous System. **A**, Regulation of vasomotor tone. **B**, Regulation of strenuous muscular exercise ("fight or flight" or stress response). (See also Chapter 9 and Figure 9-3 for more detail on the stress response.)

DID YOU UNDERSTAND?

Overview and Organization of the Nervous System

1. The divisions of the nervous system have been categorized as either structural (central nervous system [CNS] and peripheral nervous system [PNS]) or functional (somatic nervous system and autonomic nervous system [ANS]).
2. The CNS is contained within the brain and spinal cord.
3. The PNS is composed of cranial and spinal nerves, which carry impulses toward the CNS (afferent—sensory) and away from the CNS (efferent—motor) to and from target organs or skeletal muscle.

Cells of the Nervous System

1. The neuron and neuroglial cells (nonnerve cells) constitute nervous tissue. The neuron is specialized to transmit and receive electrical and chemical impulses, whereas the neuroglial cell provides supportive and maintenance functions. The neuron is further divided

into unipolar, pseudounipolar, bipolar, and multipolar categories, according to its structure and particular mechanics of impulse transmission.
2. The neuron is composed of a cell body, dendrite(s), and an axon. A myelin sheath around selected axons forms insulation that allows faster nerve impulse conduction.

The Nerve Impulse

1. The region between the neurons is the synapse, and the region between the neuron and muscle is the myoneural junction.
2. Neurotransmitters are responsible for chemical conduction across the synapse, and the myoneural junction nerve impulse is regulated predominantly by a balance of inhibitory postsynaptic potentials (IPSPs) and excitatory postsynaptic potentials (EPSPs), temporal and spatial summation, and convergence and divergence.

The Central Nervous System

1. The brain is contained within the cranial vault and is divided into three distinct regions: (1) forebrain, (2) hindbrain, and (3) midbrain.
2. The forebrain comprises the two cerebral hemispheres and allows conscious perception of internal and external stimuli, thought and memory processes, and voluntary control of skeletal muscles. The deep portion of the forebrain is termed the *diencephalon* and processes incoming sensory data. The center for voluntary control of skeletal muscle movements is located along the precentral gyrus in the frontal lobe, whereas the center for perception is along the postcentral gyrus in the parietal lobe. The Broca area (inferior frontal gyrus) and the Wernicke area (superior temporal gyrus) are major speech centers.
3. The hindbrain allows sampling and comparison of sensory data, which are received from the periphery and motor impulses of the cerebral hemispheres, for the purpose of coordination and refinement of skeletal muscle movement.
4. The midbrain is primarily a relay center for motor and sensory tracts, as well as a center for auditory and visual reflexes.
5. The spinal cord contains most of the nerve fibers that connect the brain with the periphery. The corticospinal tracts are descending pyramidal (motor) pathways from the motor cortex. The rubrospinal and reticulospinal tracts are descending extrapyramidal tracts that coordinate movement. The anterior, posterior, and lateral spinothalamic tracts carry sensory information to the brainstem and thalamus, where information is relayed to the sensory cortex. Reflex arcs are sensory and motor circuits completed in the spinal cord and influenced by the higher centers in the brain.
6. The CNS is protected by the scalp, bony cranium, meninges (dura mater, arachnoid, membrane, and pia mater), vertebral column,

and cerebrospinal fluid (CSF). CSF is formed from blood components in the choroid plexuses of the ventricles and is reabsorbed in the arachnoid villi (located in the dural venous sinuses) after circulating through the brain and subarachnoid space.

7. The paired carotid and vertebral arteries supply blood to the brain and connect to form the circle of Willis. The major branches projecting from the circle of Willis are the anterior, middle, and posterior cerebral arteries. Drainage of blood from the brain is accomplished through the venous sinuses and jugular veins.
8. The blood-brain barrier is provided by tight junctions between the cells of brain capillary endothelial cells and surrounding supporting cells.
9. Blood supply to the spinal cord originates from the vertebral arteries and branches arising from the aorta.

The Peripheral Nervous System

1. The cranial and spinal nerves constitute the PNS. The PNS relays information from the CNS to muscle and effector organs through cranial and spinal nerve tracts arranged in fascicles (multiple fascicles bound together form the peripheral nerve).

The Autonomic Nervous System

1. The ANS is responsible for maintaining a steady state in the internal environment. Two opposing systems make up the ANS: (1) the sympathetic nervous system (thoracolumbar division) responds to stress by mobilizing energy stores and prepares the body to defend itself, and (2) the parasympathetic nervous system (craniosacral division) conserves energy and the body's resources. Both systems function, more or less, at the same time.

▮ KEY TERMS

Acetylcholine, 329
α-Adrenergic receptor, 329
β-Adrenergic receptor, 329
Adrenergic transmission, 329
Afferent (sensory) neuron, 319
Afferent pathway (ascending pathway), 307
Anterior column, 319
Anterior fossa, 321
Anterior horn (ventral horn), 319
Anterior spinal artery, 325
Anterior spinothalamic tract, 321
Arachnoid, 321
Arachnoid villi, 322
Association fiber, 314
Associational neuron (interneuron), 308
Astrocyte, 308
Autonomic nervous system (ANS), 307
Axon, 308
Axon hillock, 308
Basal ganglia (basal nuclei), 315
Basal ganglia system (extrapyramidal system), 313
Basilar artery, 323

Basis pedunculi, 317
Bipolar neuron, 308
Blood-brain barrier (BBB), 324
Brachial plexus, 326
Brain network, 313
Brainstem, 311
Broca speech area (Brodmann areas 44, 45), 314
Cauda equina, 318
Caudate nucleus, 315
Cavernous sinus, 323
Celiac, 329
Central canal, 319
Central nervous system (CNS), 307
Central sulcus (fissure of Rolando), 313
Cerebellum, 317
Cerebral aqueduct (aqueduct of Sylvius), 317
Cerebral cortex, 313
Cerebral nuclei, 315
Cerebral peduncle, 317
Cerebrospinal fluid (CSF), 321
Cholinergic transmission, 329
Choroid plexus, 321
Circle of Willis, 323

Collateral ganglia, 329
Contralateral control, 314
Conus medullaris, 318
Convergence, 311
Corpora quadrigemina, 316
Corpus callosum (transverse fibers or commissural fibers), 315
Corticobulbar tract, 314
Corticobulbar tract axon, 320
Corticospinal tract (pyramidal system), 314
Cranial nerve, 307
Craniosacral division, 329
Dendrite, 308
Dermatome, 326
Diencephalon (interbrain), 315
Divergence, 311
Dopamine, 317
Dorsal root ganglion, 319
Dura mater, 321
Efferent (motor) neuron, 319
Effector organ, 307
Efferent pathway (descending pathway), 307
Ependymal cell, 308
Epicritic information, 320

Epidural space, 321
Epithalamus, 315
Excitatory postsynaptic potential (EPSP), 311
Extrapyramidal system, 313
Facilitation, 311
Falx cerebri, 321
Fascicle, 325
Filum terminale, 318
Frontal lobe, 313
Galea aponeurotica, 321
Ganglia (plexus), 308
Globus pallidus, 315
Gray matter, 313
Hypothalamus, 315
Inferior colliculi, 317
Inferior mesenteric, 329
Inhibitory postsynaptic potential (IPSP), 311
Inner dura (meningeal layer), 321
Insula (insular lobe), 315
Internal capsule, 315
Internal carotid artery, 323
Interventricular foramen (foramen of Monro), 321
Intervertebral disk, 322

REFERENCES

1. Bernardinelli Y et al: Astrocyte-synapse structural plasticity, *Neural Plast* 2014:232105, 2014.
2. Kim HA et al: Plastic fantastic: Schwann cells and repair of the peripheral nervous system, *Stem Cells Transl Med* 2(8):553-557, 2013.
3. Sulaiman W, Gordon T: Neurobiology of peripheral nerve injury, regeneration, and functional recovery: from bench top research to bedside application, *Ochsner J* 13(1):100-108, 2013.
4. Kolb B, Whishaw IQ: *An introduction to brain and behavior*, ed 3, New York, 2011, Worth.
5. Elphick MR: The evolution and comparative neurobiology of endocannabinoid signalling, *Philos Trans R Soc Lond B Biol Sci* 367(1607):3201-3215, 2012.
6. Vaughan CW, Christie MJ: Retrograde signalling by endocannabinoids, *Handb Exp Pharmacol* (168):367-383, 2005.
7. Vanderah T, Gould D: *Nolte's The human brain: an introduction to its functional anatomy*, ed 7, St Louis, 2015, Mosby.
8. Meehan TP, Bressler SL: Neurocognitive networks: findings, models, and theory, *Neurosci Biobehav Rev* 36(10):2232-2247, 2012.
9. Stam CJ, van Straaten EC: The organization of physiological brain networks, *Clin Neurophysiol* 123(6):1067-1087, 2012.
10. Obermeier B et al: Development, maintenance and distribution of the blood-brain barrier, *Nat Med* 19:1584-1596, 2013.
11. Siegel R et al: *Basic neurochemistry: molecular, cellular, and medical aspects*, ed 8, Philadelphia, 2012, Academic Press.

14

Pain, Temperature, Sleep, and Sensory Function

*George W. Rodway, Sue E. Huether, and Jan Belden**

ⓔ EVOLVE WEBSITE

http://evolve.elsevier.com/Huether/
Student Review Questions
Audio Key Points

Case Studies
Animations
Quick Check Answers

CHAPTER OUTLINE

Alterations in sensory function may involve dysfunctions of the general or the special senses. Dysfunctions of the general senses include chronic pain, abnormal temperature regulation, and tactile or proprioceptive dysfunction. Pain is an unpleasant but protective phenomenon that is uniquely experienced by each individual, and it cannot be adequately defined, identified, or measured by an observer. Like pain, variations in temperature can signal disease. Fever is a common manifestation of dysfunction and is often the first symptom observed in an infectious or inflammatory condition.

Sleep is a normal cyclic process that restores the body's energy and maintains normal functioning. Sleep is so essential to both physiologic and psychologic function that sleep deprivation causes a wide range of clinical manifestations. The special senses of vision, hearing, touch, smell, and taste are the means by which individuals perceive stimuli that are essential in interacting with the environment. Dysfunctions of the special senses include visual, auditory, vestibular, olfactory, and gustatory (taste) disorders.

PAIN

Pain is a complex experience. It is comprised of dynamic interactions between physical, cognitive, spiritual, emotional, and environmental factors and cannot be characterized as only a response to injury. McCaffery defined pain as "whatever the experiencing person says it is, existing whenever he says it does."[1] The International Association for the Study of Pain and the American Pain Society defined pain as "an unpleasant sensory and emotional experience associated with actual or potential tissue damage or described in terms of such damage."[2] Acute pain is protective and promotes withdrawal from painful stimuli, allows the injured part to heal, and teaches avoidance of painful stimuli.

Neuroanatomy of Pain

Three portions of the nervous system are responsible for the sensation, perception and response to pain:

1. The *afferent pathways*, which begin in the peripheral nervous system (PNS), travel to the spinal gate in the dorsal horn and then ascend to higher centers in the central nervous system (CNS)
2. The *interpretive centers* located in the brain stem, midbrain, diencephalon, and cerebral cortex
3. The *efferent pathways* that descend from the CNS back to the dorsal horn of the spinal cord

The processing of potentially harmful (noxious) stimuli through a normally functioning nervous system is called nociception.[2] Nociceptors, or pain receptors, are free nerve endings in the afferent peripheral nervous system. When they are stimulated they cause nociceptive pain. The cell bodies of nociceptors are located in the dorsal root ganglia

*Jan Belden contributed to this chapter in the previous edition.

336

(DRG) for the body and in the trigeminal ganglion for the face. Nociceptors have a peripheral and central axonal branch that innervates their target organ and the spinal cord, respectively. Nociceptors are unevenly distributed throughout the body so the relative sensitivity to pain differs according to their location (Table 14-1). Nociceptors respond to different types of noxious stimuli: mechanical (pressure or mechanical distortion), thermal (extreme temperatures), or chemical (acids or chemicals of inflammation such as bradykinin, histamine,

leukotrienes, or prostaglandins). Nociception involves four phases: transduction, transmission, perception, and modulation.[3,4]

Pain transduction begins when nociceptors are activated by a noxious stimulus, causing ion channels (sodium, potassium, calcium) on nociceptors to open, creating electrical impulses that travel through axons of two primary types of nociceptors that are transmitted to the spinal cord, brainstem, thalamus, and cortex (see Figure 13-9).[5] There are two primary types of nociceptors: A-delta (Aδ) fibers and C fibers. Aδ fibers are larger myelinated fibers that rapidly transmit sharp, well-localized "fast" pain sensations such as a burn or pinprick to the skin. Activation of these fibers causes a spinal reflex withdrawal of the affected body part from the stimulus, before a pain sensation is perceived.[6] C fibers are the most numerous, are smaller and unmyelinated, and are located in muscle, tendons, body organs, and in the skin. They slowly transmit dull, aching, or burning sensations that are poorly localized and often constant.[3,6,7]

Pain transmission is the conduction of pain impulses along the Aδ and C fibers (primary order neurons) into the dorsal horn of the spinal cord (Figure 14-1). Here they form synapses with excitatory or inhibitory interneurons (second order neurons) in the substantia gelatinosa of the dorsal horn. The impulses then synapse with projection neurons (third order neurons), cross the midline of the spinal cord, and ascend to the brain through two lateral spinothalamic tracts. The neospinothalamic tract (anterior spinal thalamic tract) carries fast impulses for acute sharp pain. The paleospinothalamic tract (lateral spinothalamic tract) carries slow impulses for dull or chronic pain. The fast sharp pain is perceived first, followed by dull, throbbing pain. These tracts connect to the reticular formation, hypothalamus, thalamus (the major relay station of sensory information), and limbic system. The impulses are then projected to the somatosensory cortex for interpretation of

TABLE 14-1	Stimuli That Activate Nociceptors (Pain Receptors)
Location of Receptor	**Provoking Stimuli**
Skin	Pricking, cutting, crushing, burning, freezing
Gastrointestinal tract	Engorged or inflamed mucosa, distention or spasm of smooth muscle, traction on mesenteric attachment
Skeletal muscle	Ischemia, injuries of connective tissue sheaths, necrosis, hemorrhage, prolonged contraction, injection of irritating solutions
Joints	Synovial membrane inflammation
Arteries	Piercing, inflammation
Head	Traction, inflammation, or displacement of arteries, meningeal structures, and sinuses; prolonged muscle contraction
Heart	Ischemia and inflammation
Bone	Periosteal injury: fractures, tumor, inflammation

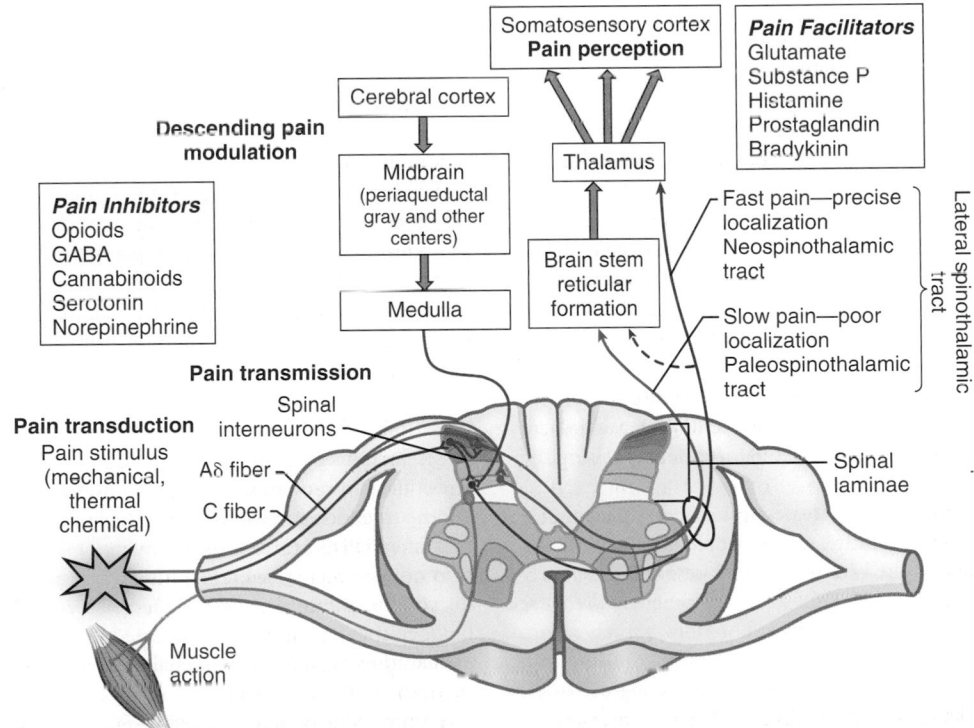

FIGURE 14-1 Transmission of Pain Sensations. The Aδ and C fibers synapse in the laminae of the dorsal horn, cross over to the contralateral spinothalamic tract, and then ascend to synapse in the midbrain through the neospinothalamic and paleospinothalamic tracts. Impulses are then conducted to the sensory cortex. Descending pain inhibition is initiated in the cerebral cortex or from the midbrain and medulla.

TABLE 14-2 Pain Perception in Infants, Children, and Elderly Persons

	Infants	Children	Elderly Persons
Pain threshold	Painful neonatal experiences increase pain sensitivity (lower threshold); pain may be increased with future procedures	Lower or same as adults	Individual responses may vary but pain threshold may be lower
Physiologic symptoms	Increased heart rate, blood pressure, and respiratory rate; flushing or pallor, sweating, and decreased oxygen saturation	Same as infants; nausea and vomiting	Same as infants and children; nausea and vomiting; may be decreased in individuals with cognitive impairment
Behavioral responses	Changes in facial expression, crying, and body movements, with lowered brows drawn together; vertical bulge and furrows in forehead between brows; broadened nasal root; tightly closed eyes; angular, square-shaped mouth, chin quiver; withdrawal of affected limbs, rigidity, flailing	Individual responses vary	Individual responses vary and may be influenced by presence of painful chronic diseases and decline in renal, intestinal, hepatic, cardiovascular, and neurologic function; individuals with cognitive impairment may demonstrate changes in behavior (e.g., combative or withdrawn, increased confusion)

Data from Maxwell LG et al: *Clin Perinatol* 40(3):457-469, 2013; Molton IR, Terrill AL: *Am Psychol* 69(2):197-207, 2014; Tracy B, Sean Morrison R: *Clin Ther* 35(11):1659-1668, 2013; Walker SM: *Paediatr Anaesth* 24(1):39-48, 2014.

location and intensity of pain (see Figure 14-1), and to other areas of the brain for an integrated response to pain.

Pain perception is the conscious awareness of pain, which occurs primarily in the reticular and limbic systems and the cerebral cortex. Interpretation of pain is influenced by many factors including genetics, cultural preferences, gender roles, and life experience, including past pain experiences and level of health.[8] Three systems interact to produce the perception of pain.[9] The **sensory-discriminative system** is mediated by the somatosensory cortex and is responsible for identifying the presence, character, location, and intensity of pain. The **affective-motivational system** determines an individual's conditioned avoidance behaviors and emotional responses to pain. It is mediated through the reticular formation, limbic system, and brainstem. The **cognitive-evaluative system** overlies the individual's learned behavior concerning the experience of pain and therefore can modulate perception of pain. It is mediated through the cerebral cortex. The integration of these three systems is referred to as the "pain matrix."[10]

Pain threshold and tolerance are subjective phenomena that influence an individual's perception of pain. They can be influenced by genetics, gender, cultural perceptions, expectations, role socialization, physical and mental health, and age[11,12] (Table 14-2).

Pain threshold is defined as the lowest intensity of pain that a person can recognize.[2] Intense pain at one location may increase the threshold in another location. For example, a person with severe pain in one knee is more likely to experience less intense chronic back pain (this is called **perceptual dominance**). Because of perceptual dominance, pain at one site may mask other painful areas. Stress, excessive physical exertion, acupuncture, sexual activity, and other factors can increase the levels of circulating neuromodulators, thereby raising the pain threshold.

Pain tolerance is defined as the greatest intensity of pain that a person can endure.[2] It varies greatly among people and in the same person over time because of the body's ability to respond differently to noxious stimuli (see Table 14-2). Pain tolerance generally *decreases* with repeated exposure to pain, fatigue, anger, boredom, apprehension, and sleep deprivation and may *increase* with alcohol consumption, persistent use of opioid medications, hypnosis, distracting activities, and strong beliefs or faith.

Pain Modulation

Pain modulation involves many different mechanisms that increase or decrease the transmission of pain signals throughout the nervous system. Depending on the mechanism, modulation can occur before, during, or after pain is perceived.[7]

Neurotransmitters of Pain Modulation

A wide variety of neurotransmitters act to modulate control over transmission of pain impulses in the periphery, spinal cord, and brain.[13,14] The peripheral triggering mechanisms that initiate release of **excitatory neurotransmitters** include tissue injury (prostaglandins, histamine, bradykinin) and chronic inflammatory lesions (lymphokines). Glutamate, aspartate, substance P, and calcitonin are common excitatory neurotransmitters in the brain and spinal cord. These substances sensitize nociceptors by reducing the activation threshold, leading to increased responsiveness of nociceptors.[15]

Inhibitory neurotransmitters in the spinal cord include gamma-aminobutyric acid (GABA) and glycine. Norepinephrine and 5-hydroxytryptamine (serotonin) contribute to pain inhibition in the medulla and pons, but can excite peripheral nerves.[4]

Endogenous opioids are a family of morphine-like neuropeptides that inhibit transmission of pain impulses in the periphery, spinal cord, and brain by binding with specific opioid receptors (mu [μ], kappa [κ], and delta [δ]) on neurons. They inhibit ion channels, preventing the release of excitatory neurotransmitters, such as substance P and glutamate, in the dorsal horn. In the midbrain they influence descending inhibitory pathways[16] (Figure 14-2). In peripheral inflamed tissue, opioids are produced and released from immune cells and activate opioid receptors on sensory nerve terminals.[17] Opioid receptors are widely distributed throughout the body and are responsible for general sensations of well-being and modulation of many physiologic processes including control of respiratory and cardiovascular functions, stress and immune responses, gastrointestinal function, reproduction, and neuroendocrine control.[18,19]

Enkephalins are the most prevalent of the natural opioids and bind to δ opioid receptors. **Endorphins** (endogenous morphine) are produced in the brain. The best studied endorphin is β-endorphin, which binds to μ receptors and is purported to produce the greatest sense of exhilaration as well as substantial natural pain relief. **Dynorphins** are the most potent of the endogenous opioids, binding strongly with κ receptors to impede pain signals. Paradoxically, they play a role in neuropathic pain and in mood disorders and drug addiction.[20] **Endomorphins** bind with μ receptors and have potent analgesic effects.[21] **Nociceptin/orphanin FQ** is an opioid that *induces* pain or hyperalgesia but does not interact with opioid receptors. The nociceptin receptor is

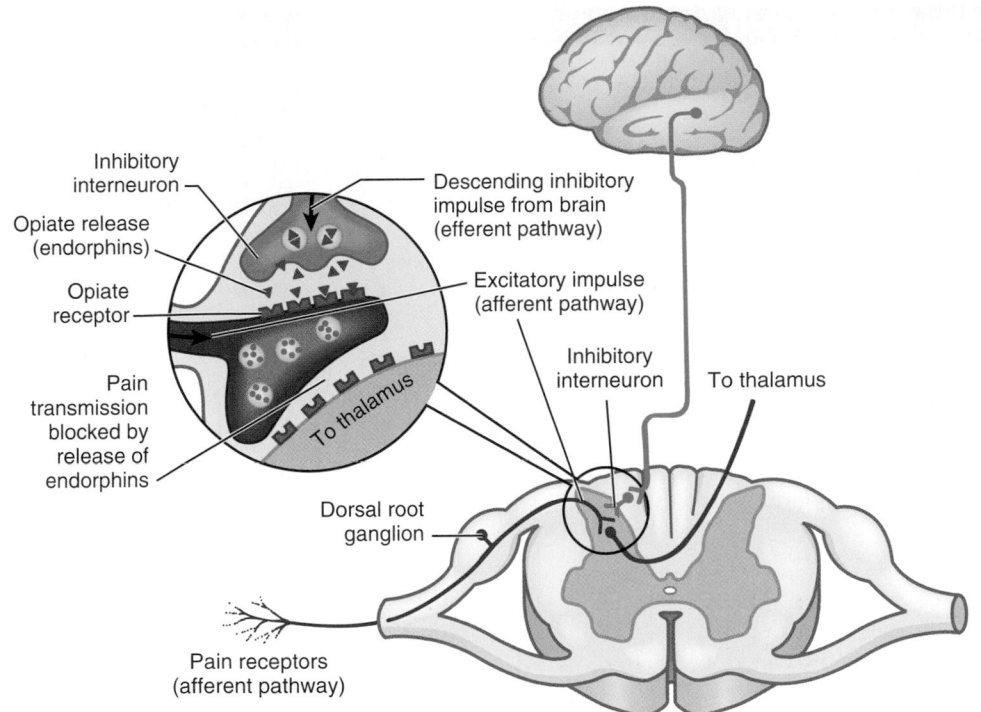

FIGURE 14-2 Descending Pathway and Endorphin Response. In this figure, a descending inhibitory impulse is transmitted from the brain to an inhibitory interneuron in the dorsal horn stimulating the release of endorphin. The endorphin activates a mu opioid receptor and results in inhibition of pain transmission to ascending pathways.

widely distributed throughout the peripheral and central nervous system and is also associated with inflammation, immune regulation, mood, and emotion.[22]

Synthetic and natural opiates have pharmacologic actions similar to morphine and bind as direct agonists to the opioid receptors. Morphine has a 50 times higher affinity for μ receptors in comparison with other opioids. Naloxone is the only clinically used opioid receptor antagonist, with a higher affinity for the μ receptors than for the other receptors.[23]

Endocannabinoids are synthesized from phospholipids and are classified as eicosanoids. They activate cannabinoid CB₁ (primarily in the central nervous system [CNS]) and CB₂ receptors (primarily in immune tissue [e.g., the spleen]) to modulate pain and other functions including memory, appetite, immune function, sleep, stress response, thermoregulation, and addiction. CB₁ receptors decrease pain transmission by inhibiting release of excitatory neurotransmitters in the spinal dorsal horn, periaqueductal gray, thalamus, rostral ventromedial medulla, and amygdala. Cannabis (marijuana) produces a resin containing cannabinoids. Cannabinoids are analgesic in humans, but their use is limited by their psychoactive and addictive properties. Work is in progress to develop cannabinoid receptor agonists that do not have addictive side effects.[24-26]

Pathways of Modulation

Descending inhibitory and facilitatory pathways and nuclei inhibit or facilitate pain. Afferent stimulation of particularly the ventromedial medulla and periaqueductal gray (PAG) (gray matter surrounding the cerebral aqueduct) in the midbrain stimulates efferent pathways, which inhibit afferent pain signals at the dorsal horn.[27] The rostroventromedial medulla (RVM) stimulates efferent pathways that facilitate or inhibit pain in the dorsal horn.[28] Inhibitory pathways can activate

opioid receptors and inhibit release of excitatory neurotransmitters, facilitate release of inhibitory neurotransmitters, or stimulate inhibitory interneurons.

Segmental pain inhibition occurs when A-beta (Aβ) fibers (large myelinated fibers that transmit touch and vibration sensations) are stimulated and the impulses arrive at the same spinal level as impulses from Aδ or C fibers. They stimulate an inhibitory interneuron and decrease pain transmission. An example is rubbing an area that has been injured to relieve pain.[7]

Diffuse noxious inhibitory control (DNIC) is an inhibitory pain system that involves a spinal-medullary-spinal pathway. Pain is relieved when two noxious stimuli occur at the same time from different sites (pain inhibiting pain). This also is known as heterosegmental pain inhibition and is the basis for pain relief with acupuncture, deep massage, or intense cold or heat.[29]

Expectancy-related cortical activation (placebo effect [beneficial expectations] or nocibo effect [adverse expectations]) can exert control over analgesic systems to attenuate or intensify pain.[30] In other words, cognitive expectations can cause real, measurable physiologic effects that share some of the same descending pain pathways as the pain modulatory systems.

Clinical Descriptions of Pain

Pain can be described in a variety of ways. Because of the complex nature of pain, however, many terms overlap and more than one description is often used. The broad categories of pain are summarized in Box 14-1. Some of the most common clinical pain presentations are summarized below.

Acute pain (nociceptive pain) is a normal protective mechanism that alerts the individual to a condition or experience that is immediately harmful to the body and mobilizes the individual to take prompt

BOX 14-1 Categories of Pain

I. Neurophysiologic Pain
  A. Nociceptive pain
    1. Somatic (e.g., skin, muscle, bone)
    2. Visceral (e.g., intestine, liver, stomach)
    3. Referred
  B. Neuropathic (non-nociceptive)
    1. Central pain (lesion in brain or spinal cord)
    2. Peripheral pain (lesion in PNS)

II. Neurogenic Pain
  A. Neuralgia (pain in the distribution of a nerve)
  B. Constant
    1. Sympathetically independent
    2. Sympathetically dependent

III. Temporal Pain (time related, duration)
  A. Acute pain
    1. Somatic
    2. Visceral
    3. Referred
  B. Chronic

IV. Pain Location
  A. Abdominal pain
  B. Chest pain
  C. Headache
  D. Low back pain
  E. Orofacial pain
  F. Pelvic pain

V. Etiologic Pain
  A. Cancer pain
  B. Dental pain
  C. Inflammatory pain
  D. Ischemic pain
  E. Vascular pain

Adapted from Mersky H: Taxonomy and classification of chronic pain syndromes. In Benzon HT et al, editors: *Practical management of pain*, ed 5, pp 13-18, St Louis, 2014, Mosby.

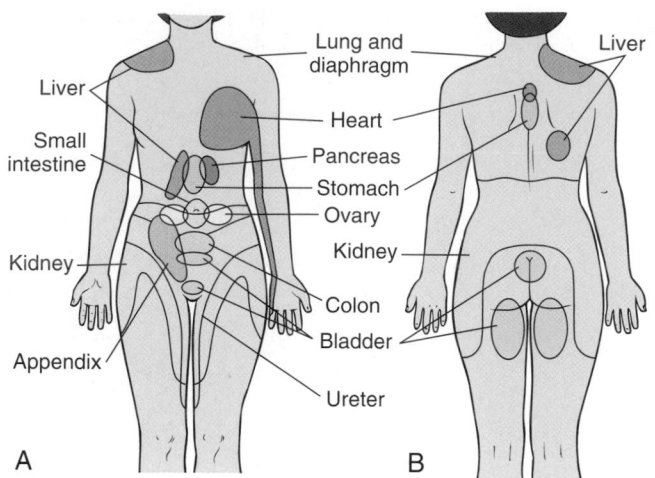

FIGURE 14-3 Sites of Referred Pain. **A,** Anterior view. **B,** Posterior view.

Visceral pain often radiates (spreads away from the actual site of the pain) or is referred. Referred pain is felt in an area removed or distant from its point of origin—the area of referred pain is supplied by the same spinal segment as the actual site of pain. Referred pain can be acute or chronic. Impulses from many cutaneous and visceral neurons converge on the same ascending neuron, and the brain cannot distinguish between the different sources of pain. Because the skin has more receptors, the painful sensation is experienced at the referred site instead of at the site of origin.[33] Referred pain can be acute or chronic. Figure 14-3 illustrates common areas of referred pain and their associated sites of origin.

Chronic or persistent pain has been defined as lasting for more than 3 to 6 months and is pain lasting well beyond the expected normal healing time. It varies with type of injury.[34] Chronic or persistent pain serves no purpose and is poorly understood and causes suffering. It often appears to be out of proportion to any observable tissue injury. It may be ongoing (e.g., low back pain) or intermittent (e.g., migraine headaches). Changes in the peripheral and central nervous systems that cause dysregulation of nociception and pain modulation processes (peripheral and central sensitization) are thought to lead to chronic pain[35,36] (see neuropathic pain, described later in this section).

Neuroimaging studies have demonstrated brain changes in individuals with chronic pain, which may lead to cognitive deficits and decreased ability to cope with pain.[37] These negative manifestations of chronic pain are thought to be due, in part, to the stress of coping with continuous pain and may be reversible when pain is controlled.[38-40] Because it is not yet possible to predict when acute pain will develop into chronic pain, early treatment of acute pain is encouraged.[41]

Physiologic responses to intermittent chronic pain are similar to those for acute pain, whereas persistent pain allows for physiologic adaptation, producing normal heart rate and blood pressure. This leads many to mistakenly conclude that people with chronic pain are malingering because they do not appear to be in pain. As chronic pain progresses, certain behavioral and psychologic changes often emerge, including depression, difficulty eating and sleeping, preoccupation with the pain, and avoidance of pain-provoking stimuli.[42] The desire to relieve pain and the need to hide it become conflicting drives for those with chronic pain, who fear being labeled complainers.[43] Chronic pain is perceived as meaningless and is often associated with a sense of hopelessness as more time elapses and no cure seems possible. Some of the chronic pain syndromes are listed in Table 14-3. Comparison of

action to relieve it. Acute pain is transient, usually lasting seconds to days, sometimes up to 3 months.[31] It begins suddenly and is relieved after the chemical mediators that stimulate pain receptors are removed.[32] Stimulation of the autonomic nervous system results in physical manifestations including increased heart rate, hypertension, diaphoresis, and dilated pupils. Anxiety related to the pain experience, including its cause, treatment, and prognosis, is common as is the hope of recovery and expectation of limited duration.[8]

Acute pain arises from cutaneous, deep somatic, or visceral structures and can be classified as (1) somatic, (2) visceral, or (3) referred. Somatic pain arises from the skin, joints, and muscles. It is either sharp and well localized (especially fast pain carried by Aδ fibers) or dull, aching, throbbing, and poorly localized as seen in polymodal C fiber transmissions. Visceral pain is transmitted by C fibers and refers to pain in internal organs and the lining of body cavities; it tends to be poorly localized with an aching, gnawing, throbbing, or intermittent cramping quality. It is carried by sympathetic fibers and is associated with nausea and vomiting, hypotension, and, in some cases, shock.

TABLE 14-3 Chronic Pain Syndromes

Condition	Description
Persistent low back pain	Most common chronic pain condition
	Results from poor muscle tone, inactivity, muscle strain, or sudden, vigorous exercise
Myofascial pain syndromes	Pain results from muscle spasm, tenderness, stiffness, or injury to muscle and fascia with peripheral and central sensitization
	Examples include myositis, fibrositis, myalgia, fibromyalgia, and muscle strain
	Trigger points—small hypersensitive regions in muscle or connective tissues that, when stimulated, produce pain in a specific area
	As disorder progresses, pain becomes increasingly generalized
Chronic postoperative pain	Persistent pain that can occur with disruption or cutting of sensory nerves; examples include post-thoracotomy, postmastectomy; risk factors may include preexisting pain and genetic susceptibility
Cancer pain	Attributed to advance of disease, treatment, or coexisting disease entities
Deafferentation pain	Pain due to loss of sensory input into CNS caused by lesion in peripheral nerves (e.g., brachial plexus injury) or pathology of CNS (e.g., complex regional pain syndrome); described as constant, vicelike ache with paroxysms of burning or shocklike sensations
	Common types include severe burning pain triggered by various stimuli, such as cold, light touch, or sound, and complex regional pain syndromes (occur after peripheral nerve injury and are characterized by continuous, severe, burning pain associated with vasomotor changes and muscle wasting)
Hyperalgesia	Increased sensitivity and decreased pain threshold to tactile and painful stimuli
	Pain is diffuse, modified by fatigue and emotion, and mixed with other sensations
	May result from chronic irritation of CNS areas
Hemiagnosia	Loss of ability to identify source of pain on one side of body
	Painful stimuli on that side produce discomfort, anxiety, moaning, agitation, and distress but no attempt to withdraw from stimulus
	Associated with stroke
Phantom limb pain	Pain experienced in amputated limb after stump has completely healed; may be immediate or occur months later; associated with preamputation pain, acute postoperative pain
	Exact cause is unknown, thought to originate in brain; can be influenced by emotions/sympathetic stimulation

From c.p.van.wilgen@sport.umcg.nl.

TABLE 14-4 Comparison of Acute and Chronic Pain

Characteristic	Acute Pain	Chronic Pain
Experience	An event	A situation; state of existence
Source	External agent or internal disease, injury, or inflammation	Unknown; if known, treatment is prolonged or ineffective
Onset	Usually sudden	May be sudden or develop insidiously
Duration	Transient (up to 3 months); usually of short duration	Prolonged (months to years); lasts beyond expected normal healing time
	Resolves with treatment and healing	
Pain identification	Painful and nonpainful areas generally well identified	Painful and nonpainful areas less easily differentiated; change in sensations becomes more difficult to evaluate
Clinical signs	Typical response pattern with more visible signs	Response patterns vary; fewer overt signs (adaptation)
	Anxiety and emotional distress common	Can interfere with sleep, productivity, and quality of life
Significance	Significant (informs person something is wrong); protective	Person looks for significance and meaning; serves no useful purpose
Pattern	Self-limiting or readily corrected	Continuous or intermittent; intensity may vary or remain constant
Course	Suffering usually decreases over time	Suffering usually increases over time
Actions	Leads to actions to relieve pain	Leads to actions to modify pain experience
Prognosis	Likelihood of eventual complete relief	Complete relief usually not possible

acute and chronic pain is summarized in Table 14-4. Chronic pain associated with specific organ systems is discussed in later chapters. Neuropathic pain is presented next.

Neuropathic pain is chronic pain initiated or caused by a primary lesion or dysfunction in the nervous system and leads to long-term changes in pain pathway structures (neuroplasticity) and abnormal processing of sensory information.[44] There is amplification of pain without stimulation by injury or inflammation. Neuropathic pain is often described as burning, shooting, shocklike, or tingling. It is characterized by increased sensitivity to painful or nonpainful stimuli with hyperalgesia, allodynia (the induction of pain by normally nonpainful stimuli), and the development of spontaneous pain.[45] Neuropathic pain is classified as either peripheral or central and is associated with central and peripheral sensitization.[46] Peripheral neuropathic pain is caused by peripheral nerve lesions and an increase in the sensitivity and excitability of primary sensory neurons and cells in the dorsal root ganglion (peripheral sensitization). Examples include nerve entrapment, diabetic neuropathy, or chronic pancreatitis.

Central neuropathic pain is caused by a lesion or dysfunction in the brain or spinal cord. A progressive repeated stimulation of group C neurons (wind-up) in the dorsal horn leads to increased sensitivity of central pain signaling neurons (central sensitization). This results in pathologic changes in the CNS that cause chronic pain.[47] Examples include brain or spinal cord trauma, tumors, vascular lesions, multiple sclerosis, Parkinson disease, postherpetic neuralgia, and phantom limb pain.[35,36]

The following mechanisms have been implicated in the cause of neuropathic pain[45,48,49]:

- Changes in sensitivity of neurons—lower threshold with peripheral and central sensitization
- Spontaneous impulses from regenerating peripheral nerves
- Alterations in the dorsal root ganglion and spinothalamic tract in response to peripheral nerve injury (i.e., deafferentation pain—loss of pain-related afferent information to the brain)
- Loss of pain inhibition and stimulation of pain facilitation by excitatory neurotransmitters in the dorsal horn (e.g., release of glutamate by stimulation of N-methyl-D-aspartate [NMDA] receptors)
- Loss of descending inhibitory pain modulation
- Hyperexcitable spinal interneurons stimulated by Aβ fibers (nonpainful stimulation of pain)
- Release of nociceptive inflammatory cytokines, chemokines, and growth factors by activated glial cells
- Structural and functional alterations in brain processing neural networks

Because of the complexity of the causes of neuropathic pain syndromes, they are difficult to treat. Multimodal therapy is often needed including nondrug treatment.[50]

✔ QUICK CHECK 14-1

1. What is the difference between A-delta and C fibers?
2. Give two examples of pain excitatory and inhibitory neurotransmitters.
3. How do A-beta fibers inhibit pain and cause pain?
4. What are two differences between nociceptive pain and neuropathic pain?

TEMPERATURE REGULATION

Human **thermoregulation** is achieved through precise balancing of heat production, heat conservation, and heat loss The normal range of body temperature is considered to be 36.2° to 37.7° C (96.2° to 99.4° F) overall, but a person's individual body parts will vary in temperature. Body temperature rarely exceeds 41° C. The extremities are generally cooler than the trunk and the temperature at the core of the body (as measured by rectal temperature) is generally 0.5° C higher than the surface temperature (as measured by oral temperature). Internal temperature varies in response to activity, environmental temperature, and daily fluctuation (circadian rhythm). Oral temperatures fluctuate within 0.2° to 0.5° C during a 24-hour period. Women tend to have wider fluctuations that follow the menstrual cycle, with a sharp rise in temperature just before ovulation. The daily fluctuating temperature in both genders peaks around 6 PM and is at its lowest during sleep. Maintenance of body temperature within the normal range is necessary for life.

Control of Body Temperature

Temperature regulation (thermoregulation) is mediated primarily by the hypothalamus and endocrine system. Peripheral thermoreceptors in the skin and abdominal organs (unmyelinated C fibers and thinly myelinated A-delta fibers) and central thermoreceptors in the hypothalamus, spinal cord, abdominal organs, and other central locations provide the hypothalamus with information about skin and core temperatures. If these temperatures are low or high, the hypothalamus triggers heat production and heat conservation or heat loss mechanisms.

Body heat is produced by the chemical reactions of metabolism and skeletal muscle tone and contraction. The heat-producing mechanism (chemical or nonshivering thermogenesis) begins with hypothalamic thyrotropin-stimulating hormone-releasing hormone (TSH-RH); it stimulates the anterior pituitary to release thyroid-stimulating hormone (TSH), which acts on the thyroid gland and stimulates the release of thyroxine. Thyroxine then acts on the adrenal medulla, causing the release of epinephrine into the bloodstream. Epinephrine causes vasoconstriction, stimulates glycolysis, and increases metabolic rate, thus increasing body heat. Norepinephrine and thyroxine activate brown fat thermogenesis where energy is released as heat instead of as adenosine triphosphate (ATP). Heat is distributed by the circulatory system.[51]

The hypothalamus also triggers heat conservation by stimulating the sympathetic nervous system, which stimulates the adrenal cortex and results in increased skeletal muscle tone, initiating the shivering response and producing vasoconstriction. By constricting peripheral blood vessels, centrally warmed blood is shunted away from the periphery to the core of the body where heat can be retained. This involuntary mechanism takes advantage of the insulating layers of the skin and subcutaneous fat to protect core temperature. The hypothalamus relays information to the cerebral cortex about cold and voluntary responses result. Individuals typically bundle up, keep moving, or curl up in a ball. These types of voluntary physical activities respectively provide insulation, increase skeletal muscle activity, and decrease the amount of skin surface available for heat loss through radiation, convection, and conduction.[52]

The hypothalamus responds to warmer core and peripheral temperatures by reversing the same mechanisms resulting in heat loss. Heat loss is achieved through (1) radiation, (2) conduction, (3) convection, (4) vasodilation, (5) evaporation (sweating), (6) decreased muscle tone, (7) increased respiration, (8) voluntary measures, and (9) adaptation to warmer climates (i.e., increasing or decreasing the volume of sweat). Table 14-5 summarizes further information about heat production and loss.

Temperature Regulation in Infants and Elderly Persons

Infants (particularly low birth weight infants) and elderly persons require special attention to maintenance of body temperature. Term infants produce sufficient body heat, primarily through metabolism of brown fat, but cannot conserve heat produced because of their small body size, greater ratio of body surface to body weight, and inability to shiver. Infants also have little subcutaneous fat and thus are not as well insulated as adults.[53] Children also have a greater ratio of body surface to body weight, lower sweating rate, higher peripheral blood flow in the heat, and a greater extent of vasoconstriction in the cold than adults. They can acclimatize to changes in environmental temperatures, but do so at a lower rate than adults.[54]

Elderly persons respond poorly to environmental temperature extremes because of their slowed blood circulation, structural and functional skin changes, overall decreased heat-producing activities, and the presence of disease (i.e., congestive heart failure, chronic lung disease, diabetes mellitus, or peripheral vascular disease). Cold stress in older adults also decreases coronary perfusion.[55] In addition, elderly persons have a decreased shivering response (delayed onset and decreased effectiveness), slowed metabolic rate, decreased vasoconstrictor response, diminished or absent ability to sweat, decreased peripheral sensation, desynchronized circadian rhythm, decreased perception of heat and cold, decreased thirst, decreased nutritional reserves, and decreased brown adipose tissue.[56]

Pathogenesis of Fever

Fever (febrile response) is a temporary resetting of the hypothalamic thermostat to a higher level in response to exogenous or endogenous

TABLE 14-5 Mechanisms of Heat Production and Heat Loss

Condition	Description
Heat Production	
Chemical reactions of metabolism	Occur during ingestion and metabolism of food and while maintaining body at rest (basal metabolism); occur in body core (e.g., liver)
Skeletal muscle contraction	Gradual increase in muscle tone or rapid muscle oscillations (shivering)
Chemical thermogenesis	Epinephrine is released and produces rapid, transient increase in heat production by raising basal metabolic rate; quick, brief effect that counters heat lost through conduction and convection; involves brown adipose tissue, which decreases markedly in older adults; thyroid hormone increases metabolism
Heat Loss	
Radiation	Heat loss through electromagnetic waves emanating from surfaces with temperature higher than surrounding air
Conduction	Heat loss by direct molecule-to-molecule transfer from one surface to another, so that warmer surface loses heat to cooler surface
Convection	Transfer of heat through currents of gases or liquids; exchanges warmer air at body's surface with cooler air in surrounding space
Vasodilation	Diverts core-warmed blood to surface of body, with heat transferred by conduction to skin surface and from there to surrounding environment; occurs in response to autonomic stimulation under control of hypothalamus
Evaporation	Body water evaporates from surface of skin and linings of mucous membranes; major source of heat reduction connected with increased sweating in warmer surroundings
Decreased muscle tone	Exhausted feeling caused by moderately reduced muscle tone and curtailed voluntary muscle activity
Increased respiration	Air is exchanged with environment through normal process; minimal effect
Voluntary mechanisms	"Stretching out" and "slowing down" in response to high body temperatures; increasing body surface area available for heat loss; dressing in light-colored, loose-fitting garments
Adaptation to warmer climates	Gradual process beginning with lassitude, weakness, and faintness; proceeding through increased sweating, lowered sodium content, decreased heart rate, and increased stroke volume and extracellular fluid volume; and terminating in improved warm weather functioning and decreased symptoms of heat intolerance (work output, endurance, and coordination increase; subjective feelings of discomfort decrease)

pyrogens. Exogenous pyrogens (endotoxins produced by pathogens; see Chapter 8) stimulate the release of endogenous pyrogens from phagocytic cells, including tumor necrosis factor-alpha (TNF-α), interleukin-1 (IL-1), interleukin-6 (IL-6), and interferon (IFN). These pyrogens raise the thermal set point by inducing the hypothalamic synthesis of prostaglandin E_2 (PGE_2). This produces an integrated response that raises body temperature through an increase in heat production and conservation (Figure 14-4). The individual feels colder, dresses more warmly, decreases body surface area by curling up, and may go to bed in an effort to get warm. Body temperature is maintained at the new level until the fever "breaks," when the set point begins to return to normal with decreased heat production and increased heat reduction mechanisms. The individual feels very warm, dons cooler clothes, throws off the covers, and stretches out. Once the body has returned to a normal temperature the individual feels more comfortable and the hypothalamus adjusts thermoregulatory mechanisms to maintain the new temperature.

Fever of unknown origin (FUO) is a body temperature of greater than 38.3° C (101° F) for longer than 3 weeks' duration that remains undiagnosed after 3 days of hospital investigation, 3 outpatient visits, or 1 week of ambulatory investigation. The clinical categories of FUO include infectious, rheumatic/inflammatory, neoplastic, HIV-associated, and miscellaneous disorders.[57]

Benefits of Fever

Moderate fever helps the body respond to infectious processes through several mechanisms[58,59]:

1. Raising of body temperature kills many microorganisms and adversely affects their growth and replication.
2. Higher body temperatures decrease serum levels of iron, zinc, and copper—minerals needed for bacterial replication.
3. Increased temperature causes lysosomal breakdown and autodestruction of cells, preventing viral replication in infected cells.

PATHOPHYSIOLOGY MAP

FIGURE 14-4 Production of Fever. When monocytes/macrophages are activated, they secrete cytokines such as interleukin-1 (*IL-1*), interleukin-6 (*IL-6*), and tumor necrosis factor (*TNF*), which reach the hypothalamic temperature-regulating center. These cytokines promote the synthesis and secretion of prostaglandin E_2 (*PGE_2*) in the anterior hypothalamus. PGE_2 increases the thermostatic set point, and the autonomic nervous system is stimulated, resulting in shivering, muscle contraction, peripheral vasoconstriction and increased metabolism mediated by thyroid hormone. (From Lewis SM et al: *Medical-surgical nursing: assessment and management of clinical problems*, ed 9, St Louis, 2014, Mosby.)

4. Heat increases lymphocytic transformation and motility of polymorphonuclear neutrophils, facilitating the immune response.
5. Phagocytosis is enhanced, and production of antiviral interferon is augmented.

Suppression of fever with antipyrogenic medications can be effective but should be used with caution.[60,61] Infection and fever responses in elderly persons and children may vary from those in normal adults. Box 14-2 lists the principal features associated with fever at these extremes of age.[62]

Disorders of Temperature Regulation
Hyperthermia

Hyperthermia is elevation of the body temperature without an increase in the hypothalamic set point. Hyperthermia can produce nerve damage, coagulation of cell proteins, and death. At 41° C (105.8° F), nerve damage produces convulsions in the adult. Death results at 43° C (109.4° F). Hyperthermia may be therapeutic, accidental, or associated with stroke or head trauma. Prevention of hyperthermia in stroke and head trauma assists in limiting brain injury.[63]

Therapeutic hyperthermia is a form of local, regional, or whole-body hyperthermia used to destroy pathologic microorganisms or tumor cells by facilitating the host's natural immune process or tumor blood flow.[64]

The forms of **accidental hyperthermia** are summarized as follows[65]:
1. **Heat cramps**—severe, spasmodic cramps in the abdomen and extremities that follow prolonged sweating and associated sodium loss. Usually occur in those not accustomed to heat or those performing strenuous work in very warm climates. Fever, rapid pulse rate, and increased blood pressure accompany the cramps.
2. **Heat exhaustion**—results from prolonged high core or environmental temperatures, which cause profound vasodilation and profuse sweating, leading to dehydration, decreased plasma volumes, hypotension, decreased cardiac output, and tachycardia. Symptoms include weakness, dizziness, confusion, nausea, and fainting.
3. **Heat stroke**—a potentially lethal result of an overstressed thermoregulatory center. Heat stroke can be caused by exertion, by overexposure to environmental heat, or from impaired physiologic mechanisms for heat loss. With very high core temperatures (>40° C; 104° F), the regulatory center ceases to function and the body's heat loss mechanisms fail. Symptoms include high core temperature, absence of sweating, rapid pulse rate, confusion, agitation, and coma. Complications include cerebral edema, degeneration of the CNS, swollen dendrites, renal tubular necrosis, and hepatic failure with delirium, coma, and eventually death if treatment is not undertaken.[66]
4. **Malignant hyperthermia**—a potentially lethal hypermetabolic complication of a rare inherited muscle disorder that may be triggered by inhaled anesthetics and depolarizing muscle relaxants.[67]

The syndrome involves altered calcium function in muscle cells with hypermetabolism, uncoordinated muscle contractions, increased muscle work, increased oxygen consumption, and a raised level of lactic acid production. Acidosis develops, and body temperature rises, with resulting tachycardia and cardiac dysrhythmias, hypotension, decreased cardiac output, and cardiac arrest. Signs resemble those of coma—unconsciousness, absent reflexes, fixed pupils, apnea, and occasionally a flat electroencephalogram. Oliguria and anuria are common. It is most common in children and adolescents.

Hypothermia

Hypothermia (core body temperature less than 35° C [95° F]) produces depression of the central nervous and respiratory systems, vasoconstriction, alterations in microcirculation and coagulation, and ischemic tissue damage. Hypothermia may be accidental or therapeutic (Box 14-3). Most tissues can tolerate low temperatures in controlled situations, such as surgery. However, in severe hypothermia, ice crystals form on the inside of the cell, causing cells to rupture and die. Tissue hypothermia slows cell metabolism, increases the blood viscosity, slows microcirculatory blood flow, facilitates blood coagulation, and stimulates profound vasoconstriction (also see Frostbite, Chapter 41).

Trauma and Temperature

Major body trauma can affect temperature regulation through various mechanisms. Damage to the CNS, inflammation, increased intracranial pressure, or intracranial bleeding typically produces a body temperature of greater than 39° C (102.2° F). This sustained noninfectious fever, often referred to as a "**central fever**," appears with or without bradycardia. A central fever does not induce sweating and is very resistant to antipyretic therapy.[68] Other traumatic mechanisms that produce temperature alterations include accidental injuries, hemorrhagic shock, major surgery, and thermal burns. The severity and type of alteration (hyperthermia or hypothermia) vary with the severity of the cause and the body system affected.

SLEEP

Sleep is an active multiphase process that provides restorative functions and promotes memory consolidation. Complex neural circuits, interacting hormones, and neurotransmitters involving the hypothalamus, thalamus, brainstem, and cortex control the timing of the sleep-wake cycle and coordinate this cycle with circadian rhythms (24-hour rhythm cycles).[69] Normal sleep has two phases that can be documented by electroencephalogram (EEG): rapid eye movement (REM) sleep (20% to 25% of sleep time) and slow-wave (non-REM) sleep. Non-REM sleep is further divided into three stages (N1, N2, N3) from light to deep sleep followed by REM sleep. Four to six cycles of REM and non-REM sleep occur each night in an adult.[70]

The hypothalamus is a major sleep center and the hypocretins (orexins), acetylcholine, and glutamate are neuropeptides secreted by the hypothalamus that promote wakefulness. Prostaglandin D$_2$,

BOX 14-3 Defining Characteristics of Hypothermia

Accidental Hypothermia

The unintentional decrease in core temperature to less than 35° C (95° F) results from sudden immersion in cold water, prolonged exposure to cold environments, diseases that diminish the ability to generate heat, or altered thermoregulatory mechanisms. It is most common among young and elderly persons.

Factors That Increase Risk
1. Hypothyroidism
2. Hypopituitarism
3. Malnutrition
4. Parkinson disease
5. Rheumatoid arthritis
6. Chronic increased vasodilation
7. Failure of thermoregulatory control resulting from cerebral injury, ketoacidosis, uremia, sepsis, and drug overdose

Response Mechanisms
1. Peripheral vasoconstriction—shunts blood away from cooler skin to core to decrease heat loss and produces peripheral tissue ischemia
2. Intermittent reperfusion of extremities (Lewis phenomenon) helps preserve peripheral oxygenation until core temperature drops dramatically
3. Hypothalamic center induces shivering; thinking becomes sluggish, and coordination is depressed
4. Stupor; heart rate and respiratory rate decline; cardiac output diminishes; metabolic rate falls; acidosis; eventual ventricular fibrillation and asystole occur at 30° C (86° F) and lower

Treatment
1. Most changes are reversible with rewarming
2. Core temperature greater than 30° C (86° F)—active rewarming (external)
3. Core temperature less than 30° C (86° F) or with severe cardiovascular problems—active core rewarming (internal)

Therapeutic Hypothermia

Used to slow metabolism and preserve ischemic tissue during surgery (e.g., limb reimplantation), after cardiac arrest, or following neurologic injury

Effects and Cautions
1. Stresses the heart, leading to ventricular fibrillation and cardiac arrest (may be desired outcome in open heart surgery when heart must be stopped)
2. Exhausts liver glycogen stores by prolonged shivering
3. Surface cooling may cause burns, frostbite, and fat necrosis
4. Immunosuppression with increased infection risk
5. Slows drug metabolism

From Corneli HM: *Pediatr Emerg Care* 28(5):475-480, 2012; Frink M et al: *Mediators Inflamm* 2012:762840, 2012; Lantry J et al: *Br J Hosp Med (Lond)* 73(1):31-37, 2012.

BOX 14-4 Sleep Characteristics of Infants and Elderly Persons

Infants
- Sleep 10 to 16 hours per day: 50% REM (active) sleep, 25% non-REM (inactive) sleep.
- Infant sleep cycles are 50 to 60 minutes in length; 10 to 45 minutes of REM sleep accompanied by movement of the arms, legs, and facial muscles followed by about 20 minutes of non-REM sleep.
- At 1 year, REM and non-REM sleep cycles are about equal in length and infants sleep through the night with about two naps per day.

Elderly Persons
- Total sleep time is decreased with a longer time to fall asleep and poorer quality sleep.
- Total time in slow-wave and final phase of non-REM sleep decreases by 15% to 30%.
- Increases in stage 1 and 2 non-REM sleep, attributable to an increased number of spontaneous arousals.
- Elderly individuals tend to go to sleep earlier in the evening and wake earlier in the morning because of a phase advance in their normal circadian sleep cycle.
- Alterations in sleep patterns occur about 10 years later in women than in men.
- Sleep disorders more likely in elderly and increase risk of morbidity and mortality.

From Edwards BA et al: *Semin Respir Crit Care Med* 31(5):618-633, 2010; Galland BC et al: *Sleep Med Rev* 16(3):213-222, 2012; Neikrug AB, Ancoli-Israel S: *Gerontology* 56(2):181-189, 2010; Ng DK, Chan CH: *Pediatr Neonatol* 2013 Apr;54(2):82-87, 2013.

---

pattern is similar to that of the normal awake pattern and the brain is very active with dreaming. REM and non-REM sleep alternate throughout the night, with lengthening intervals of REM sleep and fewer intervals of deeper stages of non-REM sleep toward morning. The changes associated with REM sleep include increased parasympathetic activity and variable sympathetic activity associated with rapid eye movement; muscle relaxation; loss of temperature regulation; altered heart rate, blood pressure, and respiration; penile erection in men and clitoral engorgement in women; release of steroids; and many memorable dreams. Respiratory control appears largely independent of metabolic requirements and oxygen variation. Loss of normal voluntary muscle control in the tongue and upper pharynx may produce some respiratory obstruction. Cerebral blood flow increases.

Non-REM sleep (NREM) accounts for 75% to 80% of sleep time in adults and is initiated when inhibitory signals are released from the hypothalamus. Sympathetic tone is decreased and parasympathetic activity is increased during NREM sleep, creating a state of reduced activity. The basal metabolic rate falls by 10% to 15%; temperature decreases 0.5° to 1.0° C (0.9° to 1.8° F); heart rate, respiration, blood pressure, and muscle tone decrease; and knee jerk reflexes are absent. Pupils are constricted. During the various stages, cerebral blood flow to the brain decreases and growth hormone is released, with corticosteroid and catecholamine levels depressed. Box 14-4 summarizes sleep characteristics in infants and elderly persons.

Sleep Disorders

Because classification of sleep disorders is complex, a system has been established by the American Academy of Sleep Medicine and includes six classifications: (1) insomnia, (2) sleep related breathing disorders,

---

adenosine, melatonin, serotonin, L-tryptophan, gamma-aminobutyric acid (GABA), and growth factors promote sleep. The pontine reticular formation is primarily responsible for generating REM sleep, and projections from the thalamocortical network produce non-REM sleep.[71]

REM (rapid eye movement) sleep is initiated by *REM-on* and *REM-off* neurons in the pons and mesencephalon. REM sleep occurs about every 90 minutes beginning 1 to 2 hours after non-REM sleep begins. This sleep is known as *paradoxical sleep* because the EEG

(3) central disorders of hypersomnolence, (4) circadian rhythm sleep-wake disorders, (5) parasomnias, (6) sleep related movement disorders.[72] The most common disorders are summarized here.

Common Dyssomnias

Insomnia is the inability to fall or stay asleep; it is accompanied by fatigue during wakefulness and may be mild, moderate, or severe. It may be transient, lasting a few days or months (primary insomnia), and related to travel across time zones or caused by acute stress.[73] Chronic insomnia can be idiopathic, start at an early age, and be associated with drug or alcohol abuse, chronic pain disorders, chronic depression, the use of certain drugs, obesity, aging, genetics, and environmental factors that result in hyperarousal.[74]

Obstructive sleep apnea syndrome (OSAS) is the most commonly diagnosed sleep disorder. An estimated 1% to 5% of children, 9% of women, and 24% of men younger than 65 years of age in the United States have diagnosable sleep-disordered breathing. The incidence increases in those older than 65 years. Major risk factors include obesity, male gender, older age, and postmenopausal status (not on hormone therapy) in women.[75] A lack of daytime sleepiness often lessens awareness of a potential sleep disorder and many persons are never properly diagnosed and treated.[76] OSAS results from partial or total upper airway collapse with obstruction to airflow recurring during sleep with excessive loud snoring, gasping, and multiple apneic episodes that last 10 seconds or longer. The periodic breathing eventually produces arousal, which interrupts the sleep cycle, reducing total sleep time and producing sleep and REM deprivation. Associated conditions include decreased sensitivity to carbon dioxide and oxygen tensions, upper airway obstruction, a small airway, and decreased airway dilator muscle activation. **Obesity hypoventilation syndrome** may be related to leptin resistance because leptin also is a respiratory stimulant. Sleep apnea produces hypercapnia and low oxygen saturation and eventually leads to polycythemia, pulmonary hypertension, systemic hypertension, stroke, right-sided congestive heart failure, dysrhythmias, liver congestion, cyanosis, and peripheral edema.[77] Hypersomnia (excessive daytime sleepiness) is associated with OSAS. Individuals may fall asleep while driving a car, working, or even while conversing, with significant safety concerns.[78] Sleep deprivation also can result in impaired mood and cognitive function characterized by impairments of attention, episodic memory, working memory, and executive functions.[79]

Polysomnography is needed to diagnose OSAS in addition to the history and physical examination. Treatments include use of nasal continuous positive airway pressure and dental devices, surgery of the upper airway and jaw in selected individuals, and management of obesity.[80] Adenotonsillar hypertrophy is the major cause of obstructive sleep apnea in children and obesity increases risk. Adenotonsillectomy is the treatment of choice.[81,82]

Narcolepsy is a primary hypersomnia characterized by hallucinations, sleep paralysis, and, rarely, cataplexy (brief spells of muscle weakness). Narcolepsy is usually sporadic or can occur in families. Narcolepsy without cataplexy is associated with immune-mediated destruction of hypocretin (orexin)-secreting cells in the hypothalamus. Orexins stimulate wakefulness.[83]

Circadian rhythm sleep disorders are common disorders of the 24-hour sleep-wake schedule (circadian rhythm sleep disorders). They can result from having rapid time-zone changes (or jet-lag syndrome), alternating the sleep schedule (rotating work shifts) involving 3 hours or more in sleep time, changing the total sleep time from day to day, or being diagnosed either with advanced sleep phase disorder (early morning waking–early evening sleeping), resulting in sleep loss if social requirements are for late sleeping, or with delayed sleep phase disorder (late morning waking–late night to early morning sleeping), with loss of sleep because of required early morning rising (common in adolescents). These changes desynchronize the circadian rhythm, which can depress the degree of vigilance, performance of psychomotor tasks, and arousal.[84,85] A circadian rhythm sleep disorder known as shift work sleep disorder affects many shift workers who rotate or swing long shifts (such as nurses), particularly between the hours of 2200 (10:00 AM) and 0600 (6:00 AM).[86,87] Our sleep-wake cycle is driven by circadian rhythms and the disruption of this circadian influence may cause problems in the short term, such as cognitive deficits and difficulty concentrating. However, long-term health consequences of shift work sleep disorder may be quite serious and include depression/anxiety, increased risk for cardiovascular disease, and increased all-cause mortality.[84] Sleep cycle phenotype also has a genetic basis and influences the timing and cycles of sleep and can affect advances or delays in sleep-wake times.[88,89]

Common Parasomnias

Parasomnias are unusual behaviors occurring during NREM stage 3 (slow wave) sleep.[90] These behaviors include sleepwalking, having night terrors, rearranging furniture, eating food, and exhibiting sleep sex or violent behavior, and having restless legs syndrome. REM sleep behavior disorder is manifested by loss of REM paralysis, leading to potentially injurious dream enactment.[91,92]

Two dysfunctions of sleep (somnambulism and night terrors) are common in children and may be related to central nervous system immaturity. Somnambulism (sleepwalking) is a disorder primarily of childhood and appears to resolve within a few years. Sleepwalking is therefore not associated with dreaming, and the child has no memory of the event on awakening. Sleepwalking in adults is often associated with sleep disordered breathing. Night terrors are characterized by sudden apparent arousals in which the child expresses intense fear or emotion. However, the child is not awake and can be difficult to arouse. Once awakened, the child has no memory of the night terror event. Night terrors are not associated with dreams. Although this problem occurs most often in children, adults also may experience it with corresponding daytime anxiety.

Restless Leg Syndrome

Restless legs syndrome (RLS)/Willis Ekbom disease is a common sensorimotor disorder associated with unpleasant sensations (prickling, tingling, crawling) and nonvolitional periodic leg movements that occurs at rest and is worse in the evening or at night. There is a compelling urge to move the legs for relief with a significant effect on sleep and quality of life. The disorder is more common in women, during pregnancy, the elderly, and individuals with iron deficiency. RLS has a familial tendency and is associated with a circadian fluctuation of dopamine in the substantia nigra. Iron is a cofactor in dopamine production and some individuals respond to iron administration as well as dopamine agonists.[93] Diagnostic and treatment guidelines have been established to assist with disease management.[94]

> ✔ **QUICK CHECK 14-3**
> 1. Describe REM and non-REM sleep.
> 2. What is the major difference between the dyssomnias and parasomnias?

THE SPECIAL SENSES

Vision

The eyes are complex sense organs responsible for vision. Within a protective casing, each eye has receptors, a lens system for focusing light on the receptors, and a system of nerves for conducting impulses from the receptors to the brain. Visual dysfunction may be caused by abnormal ocular movements or alterations in visual acuity, refraction, color vision, or accommodation. Visual dysfunction also may be the secondary effect of another neurologic disorder.

The Eye

The wall of the eye consists of three layers: (1) sclera, (2) choroid, and (3) retina (Figure 14-5). The sclera is the thick, white, outermost layer. It becomes transparent at the cornea—the portion of the sclera in the central anterior region that allows light to enter the eye. The choroid is the deeply pigmented middle layer that prevents light from scattering inside the eye. The iris, part of the choroid, has a round opening, the pupil, through which light passes. Smooth muscle fibers control the size of the pupil so that it adjusts to bright light or dim light and to close or distant vision.

The retina is the innermost layer of the eye, and contains millions of rods and cones—special photoreceptors that convert light energy into nerve impulses. Rods mediate peripheral and dim light vision and

are densest at the periphery. Cones, densest in the center of the retina, are color and detail receptors. There are no photoreceptors where the optic nerve leaves the eyeball; this creates the optic disc, or blind spot. Lateral to each optic disc is the macula lutea, the area of most distinct vision, and in the center is the fovea centralis, a tiny area that contains only cones and provides the greatest visual acuity (see Figure 14-5).

As shown in Figure 14-8 (p. 350), nerve impulses pass through the optic nerves (second cranial nerve) to the optic chiasm. The nerves from the inner (nasal) halves of the retinas cross to the opposite side and join fibers from the outer (temporal) halves of the retinas to form the optic tracts. The fibers of the optic tracts synapse in the dorsal lateral geniculate nucleus and pass by way of the optic radiation (or geniculocalcarine tract) to the primary visual cortex in the occipital lobe of the brain. Some fibers terminate in the suprachiasmatic nucleus (SCN) (located above the optic chiasm) and are involved in regulating the sleep-wake cycle. Light entering the eye is focused on the retina by the lens—a flexible, biconvex, crystal-like structure. The flexibility of the lens allows a change in curvature with contraction of the ciliary muscles, called accommodation, and allows the eye to focus on objects at different distances. The lens divides the anterior chamber into (1) the aqueous chamber and (2) the vitreous chamber. Aqueous humor fills the aqueous chamber and helps maintain pressure inside the eye, as well as provide nutrients to the lens and cornea. Aqueous humor is secreted by the ciliary processes and reabsorbed into the canal of Schlemm. If drainage is blocked, intraocular pressure increases (causing glaucoma). The vitreous chamber is filled with a gel-like substance called vitreous humor. Vitreous humor helps to prevent the eyeball from collapsing inward.

The central retinal artery provides blood to the inner retinal surface, and the choroid supplies nutrients to the outer surface of the retina. Six extrinsic eye muscles allow gross eye movements and permit eyes to follow a moving object (Figure 14-6).

Visual Dysfunction

Alterations in ocular movements. Abnormal ocular movements result from oculomotor, trochlear, or abducens cranial nerve dysfunction (see Table 13-6). The three types of eye movement disorders are (1) strabismus, (2) nystagmus, and (3) paralysis of individual extraocular muscles.

In strabismus, one eye deviates from the other when the person is looking at an object. This is caused by a weak or hypertonic muscle in

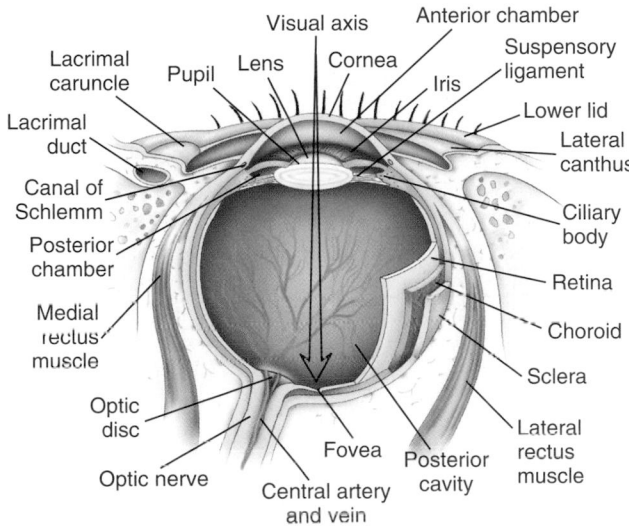

FIGURE 14-5 Internal Anatomy of the Eye. (Adapted from Patton KT, Thibodeau GA: *Structure & function of the human body,* ed 13, St Louis, 2008, Mosby.)

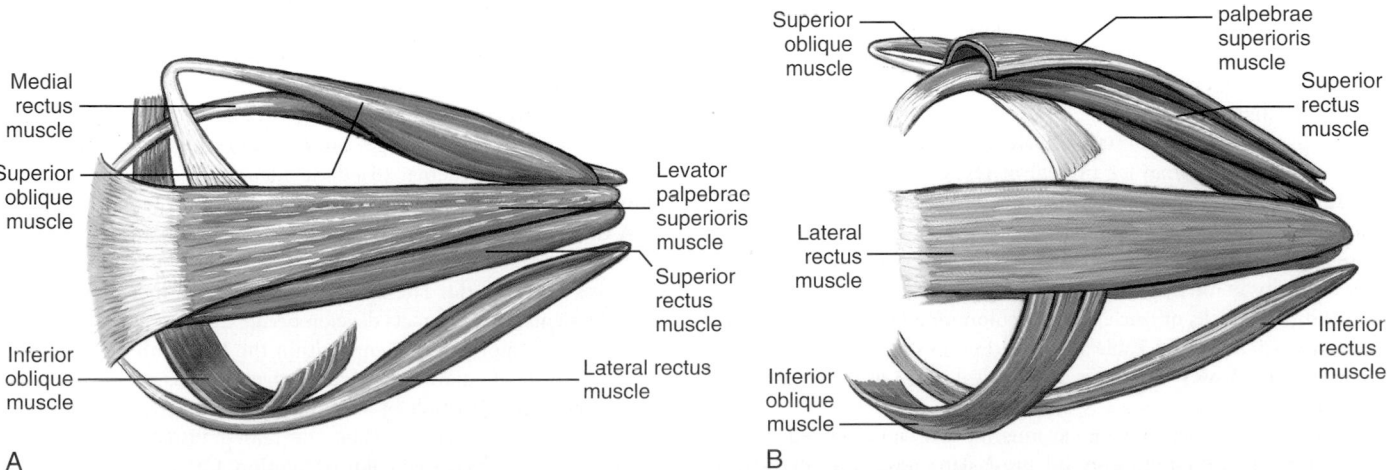

FIGURE 14-6 Extrinsic Muscles of the Right Eye. A, Superior view. B, Lateral view. (From Dutton JJ: *Atlas of clinical and surgical orbital anatomy,* ed 2, Philadelphia, 2011, Saunders.)

TABLE 14-6 Changes in the Eye Caused by Aging

Structure	Change	Consequence
Cornea	Thicker and less curved	Increase in astigmatism
Formation of gray ring at edge of cornea (arcus senilis)	Not detrimental to vision	
Anterior chamber	Decrease in size and volume caused by thickening of lens	Occasionally exerts pressure on Schlemm canal and may lead to increased intraocular pressure and glaucoma
Lens	Increase in opacity	Decrease in refraction with increased light scattering (blurring) and decreased color vision (green and blue); can lead to cataracts
Ciliary muscles	Reduction in pupil diameter, atrophy of radial dilation muscles	Persistent constriction (senile miosis); decrease in critical flicker frequency*
Retina	Reduction in number of rods at periphery, loss of rods and associated nerve cells	Increase in minimum amount of light necessary to see an object

*The rate at which consecutive visual stimuli can be presented and still be perceived as separate.

TABLE 14-7 Causes of Visual Acuity Changes

Disorder	Description
Amblyopia	Reduced or dimmed vision; cause unknown
	Associated with strabismus
	Accompanies such diseases as diabetes mellitus, renal failure, and malaria and use of drugs such as alcohol and tobacco
Scotoma	Circumscribed defect of central field of vision
	Often associated with retrobulbar neuritis and multiple sclerosis, compression of optic nerve by tumor, inflammation of optic nerve, pernicious anemia, methyl alcohol poisoning, and use of tobacco
Cataract	Cloudy or opaque area in ocular lens
	Incidence increases with age because most commonly a result of degeneration; other causes are congenital
Papilledema	Edema and inflammation of optic nerve where it enters eyeball
	Caused by obstruction of venous return from retina by one of three main sources: increased intracranial pressure, retrobulbar neuritis, or changes in retinal blood vessels
Dark adaptation	With age, eye does not adapt as readily to dark
	Also, changes in quantity and quality of rhodopsin are causative; vitamin A deficiencies can produce this at any age
Glaucoma	Increased intraocular pressures (>12-20 mm Hg)
	Loss of acuity results from pressure on optic nerve, which blocks flow of nutrients to optic nerve fibers, leading to their death; sixth leading cause of blindness
Retinal detachment	Tear or break in retina with accumulation of fluid and separation from underlying tissue; seen as floaters, flashes of light, or a curtain over visual field; risks include extreme myopia, diabetic retinopathy, sickle cell disease

one eye. The deviation may be upward, downward, inward (entropia), or outward (extropia). Strabismus in children requires early intervention to prevent amblyopia (reduced vision in the affected eye caused by cerebral blockage of the visual stimuli). The primary symptom of strabismus is diplopia (double vision). Causes include neuromuscular disorders of the eye muscle, diseases involving the cerebral hemispheres, or thyroid disease.

Nystagmus is an involuntary unilateral or bilateral rhythmic movement of the eyes. It may be present at rest or when the eye moves. Pendular nystagmus is characterized by a regular back and forth movement of the eyes. In jerk nystagmus, one phase of the eye movement is faster than the other. Nystagmus may be caused by imbalanced reflex activity of the inner ear, vestibular nuclei, cerebellum, medial longitudinal fascicle, or nuclei of the oculomotor, trochlear, and abducens cranial nerves (see Table 13-6 and Figure 13-25). Drugs, retinal disease, and diseases involving the cervical cord also may produce nystagmus.

Paralysis of specific extraocular muscles may cause limited abduction, abnormal closure of the eyelid, ptosis (drooping of the eyelid), or diplopia (double vision) as a result of unopposed muscle activity. Trauma or pressure in the area of the cranial nerves or diseases such

as diabetes mellitus and myasthenia gravis also paralyze specific extraocular muscles.

Alterations in visual acuity. Visual acuity is the ability to see objects in sharp detail. With advancing age, the lens of the eye becomes less flexible and adjusts slowly, and there is altered refraction of light by the cornea and lens. Thus, visual acuity declines with age. Table 14-6 contains a summary of changes in the eye caused by aging. Specific causes of visual acuity changes are (1) amblyopia, (2) scotoma, (3) cataracts, (4) papilledema, (5) dark adaptation, (6) glaucoma, (7) retinal detachment, and (8) macular degeneration (Table 14-7).

A cataract is a cloudy or opaque area in the ocular lens and leads to visual loss when located on the visual axis. It is the leading cause of blindness in the world. The incidence of cataracts increases with age as the lens enlarges. Cataracts develop because of alterations of metabolism and transport of nutrients within the lens. Although the most common form of cataract is degenerative, cataracts also may occur congenitally or as a result of infection, radiation, trauma, drugs, or diabetes mellitus. Cataracts cause decreased visual acuity, blurred vision, glare, and decreased color perception. Cataracts are treated by removal of the entire lens and replacement with an intraocular artificial lens.[95]

Glaucomas are the second leading cause of blindness and are characterized by intraocular pressures greater than 12 to 20 mm Hg with death of retinal ganglion cells and their axons.[96]

There are three primary types of glaucoma.[97]

1. *Open angle.* This type of glaucoma is characterized by outflow obstruction of aqueous humor at the trabecular meshwork or canal of Schlemm even though there is adequate space for drainage; often this is an inherited disease and is a leading cause of blindness with few preliminary symptoms.

2. *Angle closure.* In this type of glaucoma there is displacement of the iris toward the cornea with obstruction of the trabecular meshwork and obstruction of outflow of aqueous humor from the anterior chamber; it may occur acutely with a sudden rise in intraocular pressure, causing pain and visual disturbances.

3. *Congenital closure.* This is a rare disease associated with congenital malformations and other genetic anomalies.

Glaucoma is often asymptomatic and diagnosis may not occur until a late stage of disease. Both medical and surgical therapies are available.[98]

Age-related macular degeneration (AMD) is a severe and irreversible loss of vision and a major cause of blindness in older individuals. Hypertension, cigarette smoking, diabetes mellitus, and family history of AMD are risk factors. The degeneration usually occurs after the age of 60 years. There are two forms: atrophic (dry, nonexudative) and neovascular (wet, exudative). The atrophic form is more common and is slowly progressive with inflammation and accumulation of lipofuscin (a lysosomal pigmented residue) and drusen (waste products from photoreceptors) in the retina and may include limited night vision and difficulty reading. The neovascular form includes accumulation of drusen and lipofuscin, abnormal choroidal blood vessel growth, leakage of blood or serum, retinal detachment, fibrovascular scarring, loss of photoreceptors, and more severe and rapid loss of central vision. Treatment includes antivascular endothelial growth factor (anti-VEGF) injection for wet macular degeneration and antioxidant vitamins for dry macular degeneration.[99] Two carotenoids, lutein and zeaxanthin, are antioxidants that selectively accumulate in the retina and may protect the eye from AMD.[100]

Alterations in accommodation. Accommodation refers to changes in the thickness of the lens. Accommodation is needed for clear vision and is mediated through the oculomotor nerve. Pressure, inflammation, age, and disease of the oculomotor nerve may alter accommodation, causing diplopia, blurred vision, and headache.

Loss of accommodation with advancing age is termed **presbyopia**, a condition in which the ocular lens becomes larger, firmer, and less elastic. The major symptom is reduced near vision, causing the individual to hold reading material at arm's length. Treatment includes corrective forward, contact, and intraocular lenses or laser refractive surgery for monovision.[101,102]

Alterations in refraction. Alterations in refraction are the most common visual problem. Causes include irregularities of the corneal curvature, the focusing power of the lens, and the length of the eye. The major symptoms of refraction alterations are blurred vision and headache. Three types of refraction are as follows (Figure 14-7):

Myopia—nearsightedness: Light rays are focused in front of the retina when the person is looking at a distant object.

Hyperopia—farsightedness: Light rays are focused behind the retina when a person is looking at a near object.

Astigmatism—unequal curvature of the cornea: Light rays are bent unevenly and do not come to a single focus on the retina. Astigmatism may coexist with myopia, hyperopia, or presbyopia.

Alterations in color vision. Normal sensitivity to color diminishes with age because of the progressive yellowing of the lens that

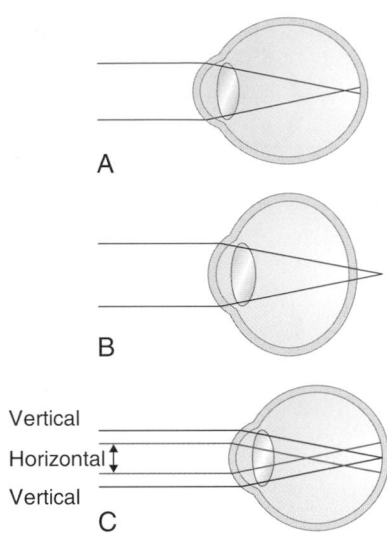

FIGURE 14-7 Alterations in Refraction. **A,** Myopic eye. Parallel rays of light are brought to a focus in front of the retina. **B,** Hyperopic eye. Parallel rays of light come to a focus behind the retina in the unaccommodative eye. **C,** Simple myopic astigmatism. The vertical bundle of rays is focused on the retina; the horizontal rays are focused in front of the retina. (From Stein HA et al: *The ophthalmic assistant: a text for allied and associated ophthalmic personnel*, ed 9, Philadelphia, 2013, Saunders.)

occurs with aging. All colors become less intense, although color discrimination for blue and green is greatly affected. Color vision deteriorates more rapidly for individuals with diabetes mellitus than for the general population.

Abnormal color vision also may be caused by **color blindness** and is an X-linked genetic trait. Color blindness affects 6% to 8% of the male population and about 0.5% of the female population. Although many forms of color blindness exist, most commonly the affected individual cannot distinguish red from green.[103] In the most severe form individuals see only shades of gray, black, and white.

Neurologic disorders causing visual dysfunction. Vision may be disrupted at many points along the visual pathway, causing various defects in the visual field. Visual changes may cause defects or blindness in the entire visual field or in half of a visual field (hemianopia). (Figure 14-8 illustrates the many areas along the visual pathway that may be damaged and the associated visual changes.) Injury to the optic nerve causes same-side blindness. Injury to the **optic chiasm** (the X-shaped crossing of the optic nerves) can cause various defects, depending on the location of the injury.

External Eye Structure and Disorders

Protective external eye structures include the eyelids (palpebrae), conjunctivae, and lacrimal apparatus. The eyelids control the amount of light reaching the eyes, and the conjunctiva lines the eyelids. Tears released from the lacrimal apparatus bathe the surface of the eye and prevent friction, maintain hydration, and wash out foreign bodies and other irritants (Figure 14-9).

Infection and inflammatory responses are the most common conditions affecting the supporting structures of the eyes. **Blepharitis** is an inflammation of the eyelids caused by *Staphylococcus* or seborrheic dermatitis. A **hordeolum (stye)** is an infection (usually staphylococcal) of the sebaceous glands of the eyelids usually centered near an eyelash. A **chalazion** is a noninfectious lipogranuloma of the meibomian (oil-secreting) gland that often occurs in association with a hordeolum and

1. Lesion of right optic nerve and right eye blindness

2. Lesion in optic chiasm and bitemporal hemianopia

3. Left optic tract lesion and bilateral right hemianopia

FIGURE 14-8 Visual Pathways and Defects. (Modified from Thompson JM et al: *Mosby's clinical nursing,* ed 5, St Louis, 2002, Mosby.)

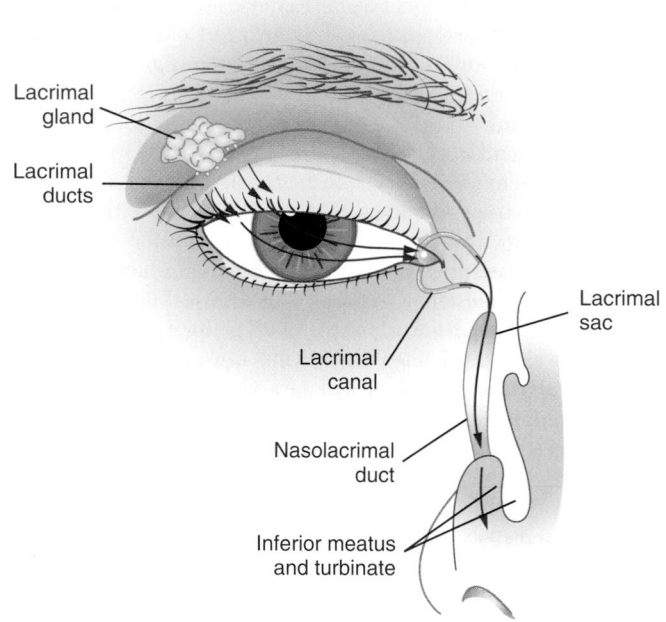

FIGURE 14-9 Lacrimal Apparatus. Fluid produced by lacrimal glands (tears) streams across the eye surface, enters the canals, and then passes through the nasolacrimal duct to enter the nose. (From Applegate E: *The anatomy and physiology learning system,* ed 4, St Louis, 2011, Saunders.)

appears as a deep nodule within the eyelid. These conditions present with redness, swelling, and tenderness and are treated symptomatically. **Entropion** is a common eyelid malposition in which the lid margin turns inward against the eyeball. There are both surgical and nonsurgical treatments to reposition the lid margin.

Conjunctivitis is an inflammation of the conjunctiva (mucous membrane covering the front part of the eyeball) caused by viruses (most common), bacteria, allergies, or chemical irritants.[104] **Acute bacterial conjunctivitis (pinkeye)** is highly contagious and often caused by *Staphylococcus, Haemophilus, Streptococcus pneumoniae,* and *Moraxella catarrhalis,* although other bacteria may be involved. In children younger than 6 years, *Haemophilus* infection often leads to otitis media (conjunctivitis-otitis syndrome). Preventing the spread of the microorganism with meticulous handwashing and use of separate towels is important. The disease also is treated with antibiotics.

Viral conjunctivitis is caused by an adenovirus. Again, it is contagious, with symptoms of watering, redness, and photophobia. **Allergic conjunctivitis** is associated with a variety of antigens, including pollens. **Chronic conjunctivitis** results from any persistent conjunctivitis. **Trachoma** (chlamydial conjunctivitis) is caused by *Chlamydia trachomatis* and often is associated with poor hygiene. It is the leading cause of preventable blindness in the world.

Keratitis is an infection of the cornea caused by bacteria or viruses. Bacterial infections can cause corneal ulceration, and type 1 herpes simplex virus can involve both the cornea and the conjunctiva. *Acanthamoeba* keratitis can occur from contact lens wear because of poor hygiene. Severe ulcerations with residual scarring require corneal transplantation.

Hearing

The external auditory canal is surrounded by the bones of the cranium. The opening (meatus) of the canal is just above the **mastoid process**. The air-filled sinuses, called **mastoid air cells**, of the mastoid process promote conductivity of sound between the external and the middle ear.

The Normal Ear

The ear is divided into three areas: (1) the external ear, involved only with hearing; (2) the middle ear, involved only with hearing; and (3) the inner ear, involved with both hearing and equilibrium.

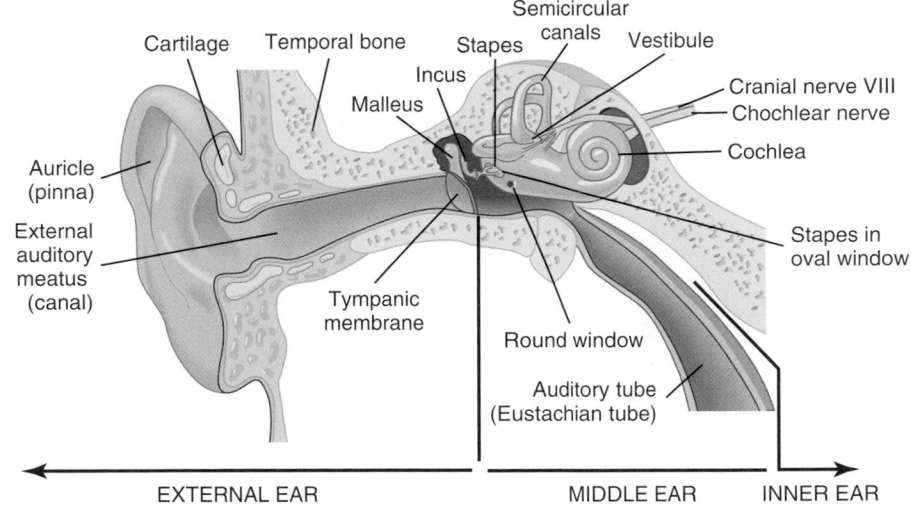

FIGURE 14-10 The Ear. External, middle, and inner ears. (Anatomic structures are not drawn to scale.) (From Applegate E: *The anatomy and physiology learning system,* ed 4, St Louis, 2011, Saunders.)

The external ear is composed of the **pinna** (auricle), which is the visible portion of the ear, and the **external auditory canal,** a tube that leads to the middle ear (Figure 14-10). The external auditory canal is surrounded by the bones of the cranium. The opening (meatus) of the canal is just above the **mastoid process.** The air-filled sinuses, called mastoid air cells, of the mastoid process promote conductivity of sound between the external and the middle ear. The **tympanic membrane** separates the external ear from the middle ear. Sound waves entering the external auditory canal hit the tympanic membrane (eardrum) and cause it to vibrate.

The middle ear is composed of the **tympanic cavity,** a small chamber in the temporal bone. Three ossicles (small bones known as the **malleus [hammer], incus [anvil],** and **stapes [stirrup]**) transmit the vibration of the tympanic membrane to the inner ear. When the tympanic membrane moves, the malleus moves with it and transfers the vibration to the incus, which passes it on to the stapes. The stapes presses against the **oval window,** a small membrane of the inner ear. The movement of the oval window sets the fluids of the inner ear in motion (Figure 14-11).

The **eustachian (pharyngotympanic) tube** connects the middle ear with the thorax. Normally flat and closed, the eustachian tube opens briefly when a person swallows or yawns, and it equalizes the pressure in the middle ear with atmospheric pressure. Equalized pressure permits the tympanic membrane to vibrate freely. Through the eustachian tube the mucosa of the middle ear is continuous with the mucosal lining of the throat.

The inner ear is a system of osseous labyrinths (bony, mazelike chambers) filled with **perilymph.** The bony labyrinth is divided into the **cochlea,** the **vestibule,** and the **semicircular canals** (see Figure 14-10). Suspended in the perilymph is the endolymph-filled membranous labyrinth that basically follows the shape of the bony labyrinth.

Within the cochlea is the **organ of Corti,** which contains **hair cells** (hearing receptors). Sound waves that reach the cochlea through vibrations of the tympanic membrane, ossicles, and oval window set the cochlear fluids into motion. Receptor cells on the basilar membrane are stimulated when their hairs are bent or pulled by fluid movement. Once stimulated, hair cells transmit impulses along the cochlear nerve (a division of the vestibulocochlear nerve) to the auditory cortex of the temporal lobe in the brain (see Figure 14-11 and view an animation

at https://www.youtube.com/watch?v=46aNGGNPm7s). This is where interpretation of the sound occurs.

The semicircular canals and vestibule of the inner ear contain **equilibrium receptors.** In the semicircular canals the dynamic equilibrium receptors respond to changes in direction of movement. Within each semicircular canal is the **crista ampullaris,** a receptor region composed of a tuft of hair cells covered by a gelatinous cupula. When the head is rotated, the endolymph in the canal lags behind and moves in the direction opposite to the head's movement. The hair cells are stimulated, and impulses are transmitted through the vestibular nerve (a division of the vestibulocochlear nerve) to the cerebellum.

The vestibule in the inner ear contains **maculae**—receptors essential to the body's sense of static equilibrium. As the head moves, **otoliths** (small pieces of calcium salts) move in a gel-like material in response to changes in the pull of gravity. The otoliths pull on the gel, which in turn pulls on the hair cells in the maculae. Nerve impulses in the hair cells are triggered and transmitted to the brain (see Figure 14-11). Thus the ear not only permits the hearing of a large range of sounds but also assists with maintaining balance through the sensitive equilibrium receptors (see animation at https://www.youtube.com/watch?v=YMIMvBa8XGs).

Auditory Dysfunction

Between 5% and 10% of the general population have impaired hearing, and it is the most common sensory defect. The major categories of auditory dysfunction are conductive hearing loss, sensorineural hearing loss, mixed hearing loss, and functional hearing loss. Hearing loss may range from mild to profound. Auditory changes caused by aging are common and incremental (see the *Geriatric Considerations: Aging & Changes in Hearing* box).

Conductive hearing loss. A **conductive hearing loss** occurs when a change in the outer or middle ear impairs conduction of sound from the outer to the inner ear. Conditions that commonly cause a conductive hearing loss include impacted cerumen, foreign bodies lodged in the ear canal, benign tumors of the middle ear, carcinoma of the external auditory canal or middle ear, eustachian tube dysfunction, otitis media, acute viral otitis media, chronic suppurative otitis media, cholesteatoma (accumulation of keratinized epithelium), and otosclerosis.

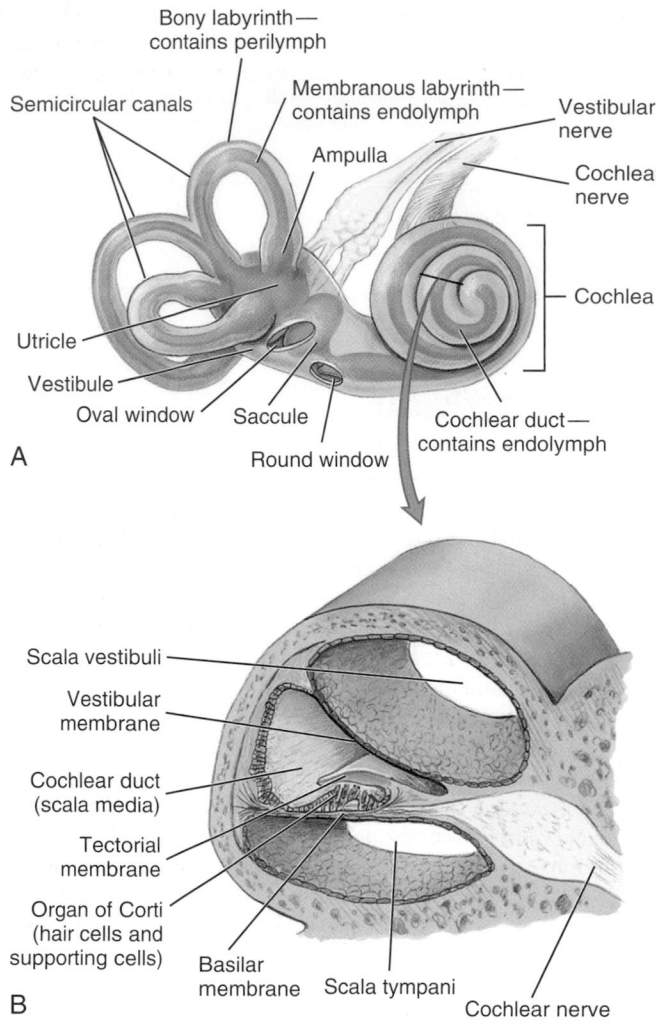

FIGURE 14-11 The Inner Ear. A, The bony labyrinth *(tan)* is the hard outer wall of the entire inner ear and includes the semicircular canals, vestibule, and cochlea. Within the bony labyrinth is the membranous labyrinth *(purple),* which is surrounded by perilymph and filled with endolymph. Each ampulla in the vestibule contains a crista ampullaris that detects changes in head position and sends sensory impulses through the vestibular nerve to the brain. **B,** Section of the membranous cochlea. Hair cells in the organ of Corti detect sound and send the information through the cochlear nerve. The vestibular and cochlear nerves join to form the eighth cranial nerve. (From Applegate E: *The anatomy and physiology learning system,* ed 4, St Louis, 2011, Saunders.)

Symptoms of conductive hearing loss include diminished hearing and soft speaking voice. The voice is soft because often the individual hears his or her voice, conducted by bone, as loud.

Sensorineural hearing loss. A sensorineural hearing loss is caused by impairment of the organ of Corti or its central connections. The loss may occur gradually or suddenly. Conditions causing sensorineural loss include congenital and hereditary factors, noise exposure, aging, Ménière disease, ototoxicity, systemic disease (syphilis, Paget disease, collagen diseases, diabetes mellitus), neoplasms, and autoimmune processes.[105] Congenital and neonatal sensorineural hearing loss may be caused by maternal rubella, ototoxic drugs, prematurity, traumatic delivery, erythroblastosis fetalis, bacterial meningitis, and congenital hereditary malfunction. Diagnosis often is made when delayed

speech development is noted. Sudden onset bilateral sensorineural hearing loss is a medical emergency.[106]

Presbycusis is the most common form of sensorineural hearing loss in elderly people. Its cause may be atrophy of the basal end of the organ of Corti, loss of auditory receptors, changes in vascularity, or stiffening of the basilar membranes. Drug ototoxicities (drugs that cause destruction of auditory function) have been observed after exposure to various chemicals; for example, antibiotics such as streptomycin, neomycin, gentamicin, and vancomycin; diuretics such as ethacrynic acid and furosemide; and chemicals such as salicylate, quinine, carbon monoxide, nitrogen mustard, arsenic, mercury, gold, tobacco, and alcohol. In most instances, the drugs and chemicals listed initially cause tinnitus (ringing in the ear), followed by a progressive high-tone sensorineural hearing loss that is permanent.

Mixed and functional hearing loss. A mixed hearing loss is caused by a combination of conductive and sensorineural losses. With functional hearing loss, which is rare, the individual does not respond to voice and appears not to hear. It is thought to be caused by emotional or psychologic factors.

Ménière disease. Ménière disease (endolymphatic hydrops) is an episodic disorder of the middle ear with an unknown etiology that can be unilateral or bilateral. There is excessive endolymph and pressure in the membranous labyrinth that disrupts both vestibular and hearing functions. There are four symptoms: recurring episodes of vertigo (often accompanied by severe nausea and vomiting), hearing loss, ringing in the ears (tinnitus), and a feeling of fullness in the ear. Treatment is symptomatic with medical management or surgical management when medications fail.[107]

Ear Infections

Otitis externa. Otitis externa is the most common inflammation of the outer ear and may be acute or chronic, infectious or noninfectious. The most common origins of acute infections are bacterial microorganisms including *Pseudomonas, Staphylococcus aureus,* and, less commonly, *Escherichia coli.* Fungal infections are less common. Infection usually follows prolonged exposure to moisture (swimmer's ear). The earliest symptoms are inflammation with pruritus, swelling, and clear drainage progressing to purulent drainage with obstruction of the canal. Tenderness and pain with earlobe retraction accompany inflammation. Acidifying solutions are used for early treatment and topical antimicrobials usually provide effective treatment for later stages of disease.[108] Chronic infections are more often related to allergy or skin disorders.

Otitis media. Otitis media is a common infection of infants and children. Most children have one episode by 3 years of age. The most common pathogens are *Streptococcus pneumoniae, Haemophilus influenzae,* and *Moraxella catarrhalis.* Predisposing factors include allergy, sinusitis, submucosal cleft palate, adenoidal hypertrophy, eustachian tube dysfunction, and immune deficiency. Breast-feeding is a protective factor. Recurrent acute otitis media may be genetically determined.[109]

Acute otitis media (AOM) is associated with ear pain, fever, irritability, inflamed tympanic membrane, and fluid in the middle ear. The appearance of the tympanic membrane progresses from erythema to opaqueness with bulging as fluid accumulates. There is an increasing prevalence of AOM caused by penicillin-resistant microorganisms. Otitis media with effusion (OME) is the presence of fluid in the middle ear without symptoms of acute infection.

Treatment includes symptom management, particularly of pain, with watchful waiting, antimicrobial therapy for severe illness, and placement of tympanostomy tubes when there is persistent bilateral effusion and significant hearing loss. Complications include

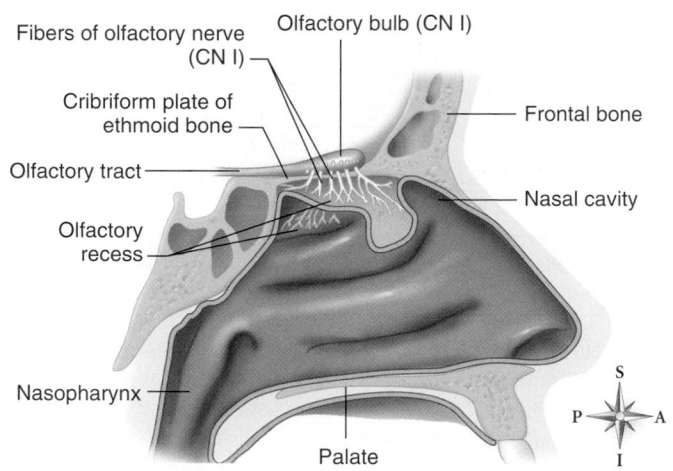

Fibers of olfactory nerve (CN I)
Olfactory bulb (CN I)
Cribriform plate of ethmoid bone
Frontal bone
Olfactory tract
Nasal cavity
Olfactory recess
Nasopharynx
Palate

FIGURE 14-12 Olfaction. Midsagittal section of the nasal area shows the location of major olfactory sensory structures. (From Patton KT, Thibodeau GA, Douglas MM: *Essentials of anatomy & physiology,* St Louis, 2012, Mosby.)

mastoiditis, brain abscess, meningitis, and chronic otitis media with hearing loss. Persistent middle ear effusions may affect speech, language, and cognitive abilities. Multivalent vaccines for prevention of otitis media are effective for reducing disease incidence.[110,111]

Olfaction and Taste

Olfaction (smell) is a function of cranial nerve I and part of cranial nerve V. Taste (gustation) is a function of multiple nerves in the tongue, soft palate, uvula, pharynx, and upper esophagus innervated by cranial nerves VII and IX. Both of these cranial nerves are influenced by hormones within the sensory cells. Dysfunctions of smell and taste may occur separately or jointly. The strong relationship between smell and taste creates the sensation of flavor. If either sensation is impaired, the perception of flavor is altered. Olfactory structures are illustrated in Figure 14-12.

Olfactory cells, located in the olfactory epithelium, are the receptor cells for smell. Seven different primary classes of olfactory stimulants have been identified: (1) camphoraceous, (2) musky, (3) floral, (4) peppermint, (5) ethereal, (6) pungent, and (7) putrid. The primary sensations of taste are (1) sour, (2) salty, (3) sweet, (4) bitter, and (5) umami (savoriness). Taste buds (fungiform, foliate, and circumvallate) sensitive to each of the primary sensations are located in specific areas of the tongue.[112]

Sensitivity to odors declines steadily with aging. See the *Geriatric Considerations:* Aging & Changes in Olfaction and Taste box for a summary of changes in olfaction and taste with aging.

Olfactory and Taste Dysfunctions

Olfactory dysfunctions include the following:
1. Hyposmia—impaired sense of smell
2. Anosmia—complete loss of sense of smell
3. Olfactory hallucinations—smelling odors that are not really present
4. Parosmia—abnormal or perverted sense of smell

The sense of taste can be impaired by injury. Altered taste may be attributed to impaired smell associated with injury near the hippocampus.

Hypogeusia is a decrease in taste sensation, whereas ageusia is an absence of the sense of taste. These disorders result from cranial nerve injuries and can be specific to the area of the tongue innervated. Dysgeusia is a perversion of taste in which substances possess an unpleasant flavor (i.e., metallic). Alterations in taste may compromise adequate nutrition or cause anorexia.[113]

> **✔ QUICK CHECK 14-4**
> 1. List the major structures of the eye.
> 2. Visual disorders fall into several categories; name them.
> 3. How does fluid accumulate in the middle ear during otitis media?
> 4. What factors are involved in the sensation of flavor?

SOMATOSENSORY FUNCTION

Touch

The sensation of touch involves four afferent fiber types that mediate tactile sensation and there may be an additional sensory nerve that transmits pleasurable touch.[114] Receptors sensitive to touch are present in the skin with high densities in the fingers and lips. Meissner and pacinian corpuscles are fast adapting receptors and sense movement across the skin and vibration, respectively. The slowly adapting Merkel disks sense sustained light touch, and Ruffini endings respond to deep sustained pressure, stretch, and joint position. Specific sensory input is carried to the higher levels of the CNS by the dorsal column of the spinal cord and the anterior spinothalamic tract.

The cutaneous senses develop before birth, but structural growth continues into early adulthood. Then a gradual decline occurs, with loss in tactile discrimination with advancing age.[115] Abnormal tactile perception may be caused by alterations at any level of the nervous system, from the receptor to the cerebral cortex. Factors that interrupt or impair reception, transmission, perception, or interpretation of touch—including trauma, tumor, infection, metabolic changes, vascular changes, and degenerative diseases—may cause tactile dysfunction. In addition, most tactile sensations evoke affective responses that determine whether the sensation is unpleasant, pleasant, or neutral.

Proprioception

Proprioception is the awareness of the position of the body and its parts. It depends on impulses from the inner ear and from receptors in joints and ligaments. Sensory data are transmitted to higher centers, primarily through the dorsal columns and the spinocerebellar tracts, with some data passing through the medial lemnisci and thalamic radiations to the cortex. These stimuli are necessary for the coordination of movements, the grading of muscular contraction, and the maintenance of equilibrium.

A progressive loss of proprioception has been reported in elderly persons with increased risk for falls and injury.[116] As with tactile dysfunction, any factor that interrupts or impairs the reception, transmission, perception, or interpretation of proprioceptive stimuli also alters proprioception and increases risk for falls and injury. Two common causes are vestibular dysfunction and neuropathy.

Specific vestibular dysfunctions are vestibular nystagmus and vertigo. Vestibular nystagmus is the constant, involuntary movement of the eyeball and develops when the semicircular canal system is overstimulated. Vertigo is the sensation of spinning that occurs with inflammation of the semicircular canals in the ear. The individual may feel either that he or she is moving in space or that the world is revolving. Vertigo often causes loss of balance, and nystagmus may occur. Ménière disease can cause loss of proprioception during an acute attack, so that standing or walking is impossible.

Peripheral neuropathies also can cause proprioceptive dysfunction. They may be caused by several conditions and commonly are associated with renal disease and diabetes mellitus. Although the exact sequence of events is unknown, neuropathies cause a diminished or absent sense of body position or position of body parts. Gait changes often occur.

QUICK CHECK 14-5
1. How are different touch receptors distributed over the body?
2. What are two causes of alterations in proprioception?

GERIATRIC CONSIDERATIONS
Aging & Changes in Hearing*

Changes in Structure	Changes in Function
Cochlear hair cell degeneration	Inability to hear high-frequency sounds (presbycusis, sensorineural loss); interferes with understanding speech; hearing may be lost in both ears at different times
Loss of auditory neurons in spiral ganglia of organ of Corti	Inability to hear high-frequency sounds (presbycusis, sensorineural loss); interferes with understanding speech; hearing may be lost in both ears at different times
Degeneration of basilar (cochlear) conductive membrane of cochlea	Inability to hear at all frequencies but more pronounced at higher frequencies (cochlear conductive loss)
Decreased vascularity of cochlea	Equal loss of hearing at all frequencies (strial loss); inability to disseminate localization of sound
Loss of cortical auditory neurons	Equal loss of hearing at all frequencies (strial loss); inability to disseminate localization of sound

Data from Frisina RD: *Ann N Y Acad Sci* 1170:708-717, 2009; Roth TN: Aging of the auditory system, *Handb Clin Neurol* 129:357-373, 2015.
*Hearing loss affects about 33% of older people.

GERIATRIC CONSIDERATIONS
Aging & Changes in Olfaction and Taste

- Decline in sensitivity to odors, usually after age 80, occurs.
- Loss of olfaction may diminish appetite, taste, and food selection and may affect nutrition.
- Inability to smell toxic fumes or gases can pose a safety hazard.

- Decline in taste sensitivity is more gradual than decline in sense of smell.
- Higher concentrations of flavors required to stimulate taste.
- Taste may be influenced by decreased salivary secretion.

DID YOU UNDERSTAND?

Pain

1. Pain (nociception) is a complex, unpleasant sensory experience involving emotion, cognition, and motivation. Pain is protective.
2. Three portions of the nervous system are responsible for the sensation, perception, and response to pain: (1) the afferent pathways, (2) the central nervous system, and (3) the efferent pathways.
3. There are two types of nociceptors. Mylinated Aδ fibers transmit sharp, "fast" pain. Smaller, unmyelinated C fibers more slowly transmit dull, less localized pain.
4. Nociception involves four phases: transduction, transmission, perception, and modulation.
5. The somatosensory cortex mediates localization and intensity of pain. The reticular formation, limbic system, and brain stem control emotional and affective responses to pain. The cortex coordinates the meaning an experience of pain.
6. Pain threshold is the least experience of pain that a person can recognize. Pain tolerance is the greatest level of pain that an individual is prepared to tolerate. Both are subjective and influenced by many factors.
7. Neuromodulators of pain include substances that (1) stimulate pain nociceptors (e.g., prostaglandins, bradykinins, lymphokines, substance P, glutamate) and (2) suppress pain (e.g., GABA, endogenous opioids, endocannabinoids). Some substances excite peripheral nerves but inhibit central nerves (e.g., serotonin, norepinephrine).

8. Descending inhibitory and facilitatory pathways and nuclei inhibit or facilitate pain. Efferent pathways from the ventromedial thalamus and periaqueductal gray inhibit pain impulses at the dorsal horn. The rostroventromedial medulla (RVM) stimulates efferent pathways that facilitate or inhibit pain in the dorsal horn
9. Segmental pain inhibition occurs when impulses from Aβ fibers (touch and vibration sensations) arrive at the same spinal level as impulses from Aδ or C fibers.
10. Diffuse noxious inhibitory control occurs when pain signals from two different sites are transmitted simultaneously and inhibit pain through a spinal-medullary-spinal pathway.
11. Endogenous opioids inhibit pain transmission and include enkephalins, endorphins, dynorphins, and endomorphins. They are produced in the central nervous system.
12. Classifications of pain include nociceptive pain (with a known physiologic cause), non-nociceptive pain (neurologic pain), acute pain (signal to the person of a harmful stimulus), and chronic pain (persistence of pain of unknown cause or unusual response to therapy).
13. Acute pain may be (1) somatic (superficial), (2) visceral (internal), or (3) referred (present in an area distant from its origin). The area of referred pain is supplied by the same spinal segment as the actual site of pain.
14. Chronic pain is pain lasting well beyond the expected normal healing time and may be intermittent (e.g., low back pain) or persistent (e.g., migraine headaches).

15. Psychologic, behavioral, and physiologic responses to chronic pain include depression, sleep disorders, preoccupation with pain, lifestyle changes, and physiologic adaptation.

16. Neuropathic pain is increased sensitivity to painful stimuli and results from abnormal processing of pain information in the peripheral or central nervous system.

Temperature Regulation

1. Temperature regulation is achieved through precise balancing of heat production, heat conservation, and heat loss. Body temperature is maintained in a range around 37° C (98.6° F).

2. Temperature regulation is mediated by the hypothalamus through thermoreceptors in the skin, hypothalamus, spinal cord, and abdominal organs.

3. Heat is produced through chemical reactions of metabolism and skeletal muscle contraction.

4. Heat is lost through radiation, conduction, convection, vasodilation, decreased muscle tone, evaporation of sweat, increased respiration, and voluntary mechanisms.

5. Heat is conserved through vasoconstriction and voluntary mechanisms.

6. Infants do not conserve heat well because of their greater body surface/mass ratio and decreased amounts of subcutaneous fat. Elderly persons have poor responses to environmental temperature extremes as a result of slowed blood circulation, structural and functional changes in the skin, and overall decrease in heat-producing activities.

7. Fever is triggered by the release of exogenous pyrogens from bacteria or the release of endogenous pyrogens (cytokines) from phagocytic cells. Fever is both a normal immunologic mechanism and a symptom of disease.

8. Fever involves the "resetting of the hypothalamic thermostat" to a higher level. When the fever breaks, the set point returns to normal.

9. Fever production aids responses to infectious processes. Higher temperatures kill many microorganisms, promote immune responses, and decrease serum levels of iron, zinc, and copper, which are needed for bacterial replication.

10. Fever of unknown origin is a body temperature greater than 38.3° C (101° F) for longer than 3 weeks that remains undiagnosed after 3 days of investigation.

11. Hyperthermia (marked warming of core temperature) can produce nerve damage, coagulation of cell proteins, and death. Forms of accidental hyperthermia include heat cramps, heat exhaustion, heat stroke, and malignant hyperthermia. Heat stroke and malignant hyperthermia are potentially lethal.

12. Hypothermia (marked cooling of core temperature) slows the rate of chemical reaction (tissue metabolism), increases the viscosity of the blood, slows blood flow through the microcirculation, facilitates blood coagulation, and stimulates profound vasoconstriction. Hypothermia may be accidental or therapeutic.

Sleep

1. Sleep is an active process and is divided into REM and non-REM stages, each of which has its own series of stages. While asleep, an individual progresses through REM and non-REM (slow wave) sleep in a predictable cycle.

2. REM sleep is controlled by mechanisms in the pons and mesencephalon. Non-REM sleep is controlled by release of inhibitory signals from the hypothalamus and accounts for 75% to 80% of sleep time.

3. The sleep patterns of the newborn and young child vary from those of the adult in total sleep time, cycle length, and percentage of time spent in each sleep cycle. Elderly persons experience a total decrease in sleep time.

4. The restorative, reparative, and growth processes occur during slow-wave (non-REM) sleep. Sleep deprivation can cause profound changes in personality and functioning.

5. Sleep disorders include (1) dyssomnias (disorders of initiating sleep [i.e., insomnia, sleep disordered breathing, hypersomnia, or disorders of the sleep-wake schedule]) and (2) parasomnias (i.e., sleepwalking or night terrors and restless legs syndrome).

The Special Senses

1. The wall of the eye has three layers: sclera, choroid, and retina. The retina contains millions of baroreceptors known as rods and cones that receive light through the lens and then convey signals to the optic nerve and subsequently to the visual cortex of the brain.

2. The eye is filled with vitreous and aqueous humor, which prevent it from collapsing.

3. The eyelids, conjunctivae, and lacrimal apparatus protect the eye. Infections are the most common disorders; they include blepharitis, conjunctivitis, chalazion, and hordeolum.

4. Structural eye changes caused by aging result in decreased visual acuity.

5. The major alterations in ocular movement include strabismus, nystagmus, and paralysis of the extraocular muscles.

6. Alterations in visual acuity can be caused by amblyopia, scotoma, cataracts, papilledema, glaucoma, and macular degeneration.

7. A cataract is a cloudy or opaque area in the ocular lens and leads to visual loss when located on the visual axis.

8. Glaucomas are characterized by intraocular pressures greater than 12 to 20 mm Hg with death of retinal ganglion cells and their axons.

9. Age-related macular degeneration is irreversible loss of vision with dry or wet forms.

10. Alterations in accommodation develop with increased intraocular pressure, inflammation, and disease of the oculomotor nerve. Presbyopia is loss of accommodation caused by loss of elasticity of the lens with aging.

11. Alterations in refraction, including myopia, hyperopia, and astigmatism, are the most common visual disorders.

12. Alterations in color vision can be related to yellowing of the lens with aging and color blindness, an inherited trait.

13. Trauma or disease of the optic nerve pathways, or optic radiations, can cause blindness in the visual fields. Homonymous hemianopsia is caused by damage of one optic tract.

14. Blepharitis is an inflammation of the eyelid; a hordeolum (stye) is an infection of the eyelid's sebaceous gland; and a chalazion is an infection of the eyelid's meibomian gland.

15. Conjunctivitis can be acute or chronic, bacterial, viral, or allergic. Redness, edema, pain, and lacrimation are common symptoms. Chlamydial conjunctivitis is the leading cause of blindness in the world and is associated with poor sanitary conditions.

16. Keratitis is a bacterial or viral infection of the cornea that can lead to corneal ulceration. Photophobia, pain, and tearing are common symptoms.

17. The ear is composed of external, middle, and inner structures. The external structures are the pinna, auditory canal, and tympanic membrane. The tympanic cavity (containing three bones: the malleus, the incus, and the stapes), oval window, eustachian tube,

and fluid compose the middle ear and transmit sound vibrations to the inner ear.

18. The inner ear includes the bony and membranous labyrinths that transmit sound waves through the cochlea to the acoustic division of the eighth cranial nerve. The semicircular canals and vestibule help maintain balance through the equilibrium receptors.

19. Approximately one third of all people older than 65 years have hearing loss.

20. Hearing loss can be classified as conductive, sensorineural, mixed, or functional.

21. Conductive hearing loss occurs when sound waves cannot be conducted through the middle ear.

22. Sensorineural hearing loss develops with impairment of the organ of Corti or its central connections. Presbycusis is the most common form of sensorineural hearing loss in elderly people.

23. A combination of conductive and sensorineural loss is a mixed hearing loss.

24. Loss of hearing with no known organic cause is a functional hearing loss.

25. Ménière disease is a disorder of the middle ear that affects hearing and balance.

26. Otitis externa is an infection of the outer ear associated with prolonged exposure to moisture.

27. Otitis media is an infection of the middle ear that is common in children. Accumulation of fluid (effusion) behind the tympanic membrane is a common finding.

28. The perception of flavor is altered if olfaction or taste dysfunctions occur. Sensitivity to odor and taste decreases with aging.

29. Hyposmia is a decrease in the sense of smell, and anosmia is the complete loss of the sense of smell. Inflammation of the nasal mucosa and trauma or tumors of the olfactory nerve lead to a diminished sense of smell.

30. Hypogeusia is a decrease in taste sensation, and ageusia is the absence of the sense of taste. Loss of taste buds or trauma to the facial or glossopharyngeal nerves decreases taste sensation.

Somatosensory Function

1. Tactile sensation is a function of receptors present in the skin (pacinian corpuscles), and the sensory response is conducted to the brain through the dorsal column and anterior spinothalamic tract.

2. Alterations in touch can result from disruption of skin receptors, sensory transmission, or central nervous system perception.

3. Proprioception is the position and location of the body and its parts. Proprioceptors are located in the inner ear, joints, and ligaments. Proprioceptive stimuli are necessary for balance, coordinated movement, and grading of muscular contraction.

4. Disorders of proprioception can occur at any level of the nervous system and result in impaired balance and lack of coordinated movement.

KEY TERMS

A-beta (Aβ) fiber, 339
Accidental hyperthermia, 344
Accommodation, 347
Acute bacterial conjunctivitis (pinkeye), 350
Acute otitis media (AOM), 352
Acute pain, 339
A-delta (Aδ) fiber, 337
Affective-motivational system, 338
Age-related macular degeneration (AMD), 349
Ageusia, 353
Allergic conjunctivitis, 350
Allodynia, 341
Amblyopia, 348
Anosmia, 353
Aqueous humor, 347
Astigmatism, 349
Blepharitis, 349
Cannabinoid, 339
Cannabis, 339
Cataract, 348
Central fever, 344
Central neuropathic pain, 341
Central sensitization, 341
C fiber, 337
Chalazion, 349
Choroid, 347
Chronic conjunctivitis, 350
Chronic pain, 340

Circadian rhythm sleep disorder, 346
Cochlea, 351
Cognitive-evaluative system, 338
Color blindness, 349
Conductive hearing loss, 351
Cone, 347
Conjunctivitis, 350
Cornea, 347
Crista ampullaris, 351
Descending inhibitory pathway, 339
Diffuse noxious inhibitory control (DNIC), 339
Diplopia, 348
Dynorphin, 338
Dysgeusia, 353
Endocannabinoid, 339
Endogenous opioid, 338
Endogenous pyrogen, 343
Endomorphin, 338
Endorphin, 338
Enkephalin, 338
Entropion, 350
Equilibrium receptor, 351
Eustachian (pharyngotympanic) tube, 351
Excitatory neurotransmitter, 338
Exogenous pyrogen, 343
Expectancy-related cortical activation, 339
External auditory canal, 351

Facilitatory pathway, 339
Fever, 342
Fever of unknown origin (FUO), 343
Fovea centralis, 347
Functional hearing loss, 352
Glaucoma, 349
Hair cell, 351
Heat cramp, 344
Heat exhaustion, 344
Heat stroke, 344
Heterosegmental pain inhibition, 339
Hordeolum (stye), 349
Hyperopia, 349
Hypersomnia, 346
Hyperthermia, 344
Hypogeusia, 353
Hyposmia, 353
Hypothermia, 344
Incus (anvil), 351
Inhibitory neurotransmitter, 338
Insomnia, 346
Iris, 347
Jerk nystagmus, 348
Keratitis, 350
Lens, 347
Macula lutea, 347
Maculae, 351
Malignant hyperthermia, 344
Malleus (hammer), 351
Mastoid air cell, 350

Mastoid process, 350
Meissner corpuscle, 353
Ménière disease (endolymphatic hydrops), 352
Merkel disk, 353
Mixed hearing loss, 352
Myopia, 349
Narcolepsy, 346
Neuropathic pain, 341
Night terrors, 346
Nociception, 336
Nociceptin/orphanin FQ, 338
Nociceptive pain, 336
Nociceptor, 336
Non-REM sleep (NREM), 345
Nystagmus, 348
Obstructive sleep apnea syndrome (OSAS), 346
Olfaction, 353
Olfactory hallucination, 353
Optic chiasm, 349
Optic disc, 347
Optic nerve, 347
Organ of Corti, 351
Otitis externa, 352
Otitis media, 352
Otitis media with effusion (OME), 352
Otolith, 351
Oval window, 351
Pacinian corpuscle, 353
Pain modulation, 338

REFERENCES

1. McCaffery M: Nursing practice theories related to cognition, bodily pain and nonenvironment interactions, Los Angeles, Calif, 1968, University of California at Los Angeles Students' Store.
2. International Association for the Study of Pain (IASP): IASP pain terminology. Available at wwwiasp-pain.org/AM/Template.cfm?Section=pain_Definitions&;Template=/CM/HTMLDisplay.cfm&ContentIK=1728#Pain. Accessed April 2011.
3. Arnstein P: Clinical coach for effective pain management, Philadelphia, 2010, FA Davis.
4. Pasero C, McCaffery M: Pain assessment and pharmacologic management, St Louis, 2011, Mosby.
5. Basbaum AI et al: Cellular and molecular mechanisms of pain, Cell 139(2):267-284, 2009.
6. Helms JF, Barone CP: Physiology and treatment of pain, Crit Care Nurs 28:38-40, 2004.
7. Marchand S: The physiology of pain mechanisms: from the periphery to the brain, Rheum Dis Clin North Am 34:285-309, 2008.
8. Argoff CE et al: Multimodal analgesia for chronic pain: rationale and future directions, Pain Med 10(S2):S53-S66, 2009.
9. Casey KL: Forebrain mechanisms of nociception and pain: analysis through imaging, Proc Natl Acad Sci U S A 96(14):7668-7674, 1999.
10. Garcia-Larrea L, Peyron R: Pain matrices and neuropathic pain matrices: a review, Pain 154(Suppl 1):S29-S43, 2013.
11. Wandner LD et al: The perception of pain in others: how gender, race, and age influence pain expectations, J Pain 13(3):220-227, 2013.
12. Bartley EJ, Fillingim RB: Sex differences in pain: a brief review of clinical and experimental findings, Br J Anaesth 111(1):52-58, 2013.
13. Ossipov MH et al: Central modulation of pain, J Clin Invest 120(11):3779-3787, 2010.
14. Fields HL et al: Central nervous system mechanism of pain modulation. In McMahon S, Koltzenburg M, editors: Wall and Melzack's textbook of pain, ed 5, Edinburgh, Scotland, 2005, Churchill Livingstone.
15. Gangadharan V, Kuner R: Pain hypersensitivity mechanisms at a glance, Dis Model Mech 6(4):889-895, 2013.
16. Lau BK, Vaughan CW: Descending modulation of pain: the GABA disinhibition hypothesis of analgesia, Curr Opin Neurobiol 29C:159-164, 2014.
17. Ninkovic J, Roy S: Role of the mu-opioid receptor in opioid modulation of immune function, Amino Acids 45(1):9-24, 2013.
18. Bodnar RJ: Endogenous opiates and behavior: 2009, Peptides 31(12):2325-2359, 2010.
19. Busch-Dienstfertig M, Stein C: Opioid receptors and opioid peptide-producing leukocytes in inflammatory pain—basic and therapeutic aspects, Brain Behav Immun 24(5):683-694, 2010.
20. Lutz PE, Kieffer BL: The multiple facets of opioid receptor function: implications for addiction, Curr Opin Neurobiol 23(4):473-479, 2013.
21. Perlikowska R, Janecka A: Bioavailability of endomorphins and the blood-brain barrier—a review, Med Chem 10(1):2-17, 2014.
22. Tariq S et al: Deciphering intracellular localization and physiological role of nociceptin and nocistatin, Peptides 43:174-183, 2013.
23. Koob GF et al: Opioids, Chapter 5. In Koob GF et al, editors: Drugs, addiction and the brain, pp 133-171, Amsterdam, 2014, Academic Press.
24. Davis MP: Cannabinoids in pain management: CB1, CB2 and non-classic receptor ligands, Exp Opin Investig Drugs 23(8):1123-1140, 2014.
25. Guindon J, Hohmann AG: The endocannabinoid system and pain, CNS Neurol Disord Drug Targets 8(6):403-421, 2009.
26. Ulugöl A: The endocannabinoid system as a potential therapeutic target for pain modulation, Balkan Med J 31(2):115-120, 2014.
27. Mason P: Deconstructing endogenous pain modulations, J Neurophysiol 94(3):1659-1663, 2005.
28. Dogrul A et al: Differential mediation of descending pain facilitation and inhibition by spinal 5HT-3 and 5HT-7 receptors, Brain Res 1280:52-59, 2009.
29. van Wijk G, Veldhuijzen DS: Perspective on diffuse noxious inhibitory controls as a model of endogenous pain modulation in clinical pain syndromes, J Pain 11(5):408-419, 2010.
30. Colloca L, Grillon C: Understanding placebo and nocebo responses for pain management, Curr Pain Headache Rep 18(6):419, 2014.
31. American Pain Society: Principles of analgesic use in the treatment of acute pain and cancer pain, ed 6, Glenview, Ill, 2008, Author.
32. Costigan M et al: Neuropathic pain: a maladaptive response of the nervous system to damage, Annu Rev Neurosci 32:1-32, 2009.
33. Thibodeau GA, Patton KT: Anatomy & physiology, ed 5, St Louis, 2003, Mosby.
34. Apkarian AV et al: Towards a theory of chronic pain, Prog Neurobiol 87(2):8197, 2009.
35. Mifflin KA, Kerr BJ: The transition from acute to chronic pain: understanding how different biological systems interact, Can J Anaesth 61(2):112-122, 2014.
36. Fornasari D: Pain mechanisms in patients with chronic pain, Clin Drug Investig 32(Suppl 1):45-52, 2012.
37. Attal N et al: Does cognitive functioning predict chronic pain? Results from a prospective surgical cohort, Brain 137(Pt 3):904-917, 2014.
38. May A: Chronic pain may change the structure of the brain, Pain 137:7-15, 2008.
39. Rodriguez-Raecke R et al: Brain gray matter decrease in chronic pain is the consequence and not the cause of pain, J Neurosci 29(44):12746-12750, 2009.
40. Tracey I, Bushnell MC: How neuroimaging studies have challenged us to rethink: is chronic pain a disease? J Pain 10(11):1113-1120, 2009.
41. McGreevy K et al: Preventing chronic pain following acute pain: risk factors, preventive strategies, and their efficacy, Eur J Pain Suppl 5(2):365-372, 2011.
42. Garland EL: Pain processing in the human nervous system: a selective review of nociceptive and biobehavioral pathways, Prim Care 39(3):561-571, 2012.
43. Miles A et al: Managing constraint: the experience of people with chronic pain, Soc Sci Med 61(2):431-441, 2005.
44. Nickel FT et al: Mechanisms of neuropathic pain, Eur Neuropsychopharmacol 22(2):81-91, 2012.
45. Jensen TS, Finnerup NB: Allodynia and hyperalgesia in neuropathic pain: clinical manifestations and mechanisms, Lancet Neurol 13(9):924-935, 2014.
46. Smith HS, Meek PD: Pain responsiveness to opioids: central versus peripheral neuropathic pain, J Opioid Manag 7(5):391-400, 2011.
47. Woolf CJ: Central sensitization: implications for the diagnosis and treatment of pain, Pain 152(3 Suppl):S2-S15, 2011.
48. Cohen SP, Mao J: Neuropathic pain: mechanisms and their clinical implications, Br Med J 348:f7656, 2014.
49. Gold MS, Miroslav MB: Chapter 41, Pain: from neurobiology to disease. In Zigmond MJ et al, editors: Neurobiology of brain disorders: biological basis of neurological and psychiatric disorders, pp 674-692, London, 2015, Academic Press.
50. Vranken JH: Elucidation of pathophysiology and treatment of neuropathic pain, Cent Nerv Syst Agents Med Chem 12(4):304-314, 2012.
51. Clapham JC: Central control of thermogenesis, Neuropharmacol 63(1):111-123, 2012.
52. Rothwell NJ: CNS regulation of thermogenesis, Crit Rev Neurobiol 8(1-2):1-10, 1994.
53. Baumgart S: Iatrogenic hyperthermia and hypothermia in the neonate, Clin Perinatol 35(1):183-197, 2008:ix-x.
54. Falk B, Dotan R: Temperature regulation and elite young athletes, Med Sport Sci 56:126-149, 2011.
55. Gao Z et al: Altered coronary vascular control during cold stress in healthy older adults, Am J Physiol Heart Circ Physiol 302(1):H312-H318, 2012.

56. Saely CH et al: Brown versus white adipose tissue: a mini-review, *Gerontology* 58(1):15-23, 2012.

57. Kaya A et al: The management and the diagnosis of fever of unknown origin, *Exp Rev Anti Infect Ther* 11(8):805-815, 2013.

58. Barone JE: Fever: fact and fiction, *J Trauma* 67(2):406-409, 2009.

59. Cannon JG: Perspective on fever: the basic science and conventional medicine, *Complement Ther Med* 21(Suppl 1):S54-S60, 2013.

60. Purssell E, While AE: Does the use of antipyretics in children who have acute infections prolong febrile illness? A systematic review and meta-analysis, *J Pediatr* 163(3):822-827, 2013.

61. Wing R et al: Fever in the pediatric patient, *Emerg Med Clin North Am* 31(4):1073-1096, 2013.

62. Roghmann MC et al: The relationship between age and fever magnitude, *Am J Med Sci* 322(2):68-70, 2001.

63. Wang H et al: Brain temperature and its fundamental properties: a review for clinical neuroscientists, *Front Neurosci* 8:307, 2014.

64. Ahmed K, Zaidi SF: Treating cancer with heat: hyperthermia as promising strategy to enhance apoptosis, *J Pak Med Assoc* 63(4):504-508, 2013.

65. Gomez CR: Disorders of body temperature, *Handb Clin Neurol* 120:947-957, 2014.

66. Atha WF: Heat-related illness, *Emerg Med Clin North Am* 31(4):1097-1108, 2013.

67. Bandschapp O, Girard T: Malignant hyperthermia, *Swiss Med Wkly* 142:w13652, 2012.

68. Hocker SE et al: Indicators of central fever in the neurologic intensive care unit, *JAMA Neurol* 70(12):1499-1504, 2013.

69. Albrecht U: Timing to perfection: the biology of central and peripheral circadian clocks, *Neuron* 74(2):246-260, 2012.

70. Iber C et al: *The AASM manual for the scoring of sleep and associated events*, Westchester Ill, 2007, American Academy of Sleep Medicine.

71. España RA, Scammell TE: Sleep neurobiology from a clinical perspective, *Sleep* 34(7):845-858, 2011.

72. American Academy of Sleep Medicine: *International Classification of Sleep Disorders, Third Edition: Diagnostic and Coding Manual*, Westchester, Ill, 2014, Author.

73. Ellis JG et al: Acute insomnia: current conceptualizations and future directions, *Sleep Med Rev* 16(1):5-14, 2012.

74. Buysse DJ: Insomnia, *J Am Med Assoc* 309(7):706-716, 2013.

75. Badran M et al: Insights into obstructive sleep apnea research, *Sleep Med* 15(5):485-495, 2014.

76. Berry RB: *Fundamentals of sleep medicine*, Philadelphia, 2012, Elsevier.

77. Ayas NT et al: New frontiers in obstructive sleep apnea, *Clin Sci (Lond)* 127(4):209-216, 2014.

78. De Backer W: Obstructive sleep apnea/hypopnea syndrome, *Panminerva Med* 55(2):191-195, 2013.

79. Gagnon K et al: Cognitive impairment in obstructive sleep apnea, *Pathol Biol (Paris)* 62(5):233-240, 2014.

80. Freedman N: Improvements in current treatments and emerging therapies for adult obstructive sleep apnea, *F1000Prime Rep* 6:36, 2014.

81. Carter KA et al: Common sleep disorders in children, *Am Fam Physician* 89(5):368-377, 2014.

82. Mannarino MR et al: Obstructive sleep apnea syndrome, *Eur J Intern Med* 23(7):586-593, 2012.

83. Mignot EJ: A practical guide to the therapy of narcolepsy and hypersomnia syndromes, *Neurotherapeutics* 9(4):739-752, 2012.

84. Baron KG, Reid KJ: Circadian misalignment and health, *Int Rev Psychiatry* 26(2):139-154, 2014.

85. Nesbitt AD, Dijk DJ: Out of synch with society: an update on delayed sleep phase disorder, *Curr Opin Pulm Med* 20(6):581-587, 2014.

86. Morrissette DA: Twisting the night away: a review of the neurobiology, genetics, diagnosis, and treatment of shift work disorder, *CNS Spectr* 18(Suppl 1):45-53, 2013.

87. Thorpy M: Understanding and diagnosing shift work disorder, *Postgrad Med* 123(5):96-105, 2011.

88. Hida A et al: Pathophysiology and pathogenesis of circadian rhythm sleep disorders, *J Physiol Anthropol* 31:7, 2012.

89. Jones CR et al: Genetic basis of human circadian rhythm disorders, *Exp Neurol* 243:28-33, 2013.

90. Matwiyoff G, Lee-Chiong T: Parasomnias: an overview, *Indian J Med Res* 131:333-337, 2010.

91. Howell MJ: Parasomnias: an updated review, *Neurotherapeutics* 9(4):753-775, 2012.

92. Zadra A, Pilon M: NREM parasomnias, *Handb Clin Neurol* 99:851-868, 2011.

93. Wijemanne S, Jankovic J: Restless legs syndrome: clinical presentation diagnosis and treatment, *Sleep Med* 16(6):678-690, 2015.

94. Allen RP: Restless legs syndrome/Willis Ekbom disease: evaluation and treatment, *Int Rev Psychiatry* 26(2):248-262, 2014.

95. Voleti VB, Hubschman JP: Age-related eye disease, *Maturitas* 75(1):29-33, 2013.

96. Casson RJ et al: Definition of glaucoma: clinical and experimental concepts, *Clin Exp Ophthalmol* 40(4):341-349, 2012.

97. Agarwal R et al: Current concepts in the pathophysiology of glaucoma, *Indian J Ophthalmol* 57(4):257-266, 2009.

98. Weinreb RN et al: The pathophysiology and treatment of glaucoma: a review, *J Am Med Assoc* 311(18):1901-1911, 2014.

99. Khan M et al: Present and possible therapies for age-related macular degeneration, *ISRN Ophthalmol* 2014:608390, 2014.

100. Hampton BM et al: Pharmacogenetics and nutritional supplementation in age-related macular degeneration, *Clin Ophthalmol* 9:873-876, 2015.

101. Liu HH, Hu Y, Cui HP: Femtosecond laser in refractive and cataract surgeries, *Int J Ophthalmol* 8(2):419-426, 2015.

102. Lichtinger A, Rootman DS: Intraocular lenses for presbyopia correction: past, present, and future, *Curr Opin Ophthalmol* 23(1):40-46, 2012.

103. Neitz J, Neitz M: The genetics of normal and defective color vision, *Vision Res* 51(7):633-651, 2011.

104. Azari AA, Barney NP: Conjunctivitis: a systematic review of diagnosis and treatment, *J Am Med Assoc* 310(16):1721-1729, 2013.

105. Kozak AT, Grundfast KM: Hearing loss, *Otolaryngol Clin North Am* 42(1):79-85, 2009.

106. Sara SA et al: Bilateral sudden sensorineural hearing loss: review, *J Laryngol Otol* 128(Suppl 1):S8-S15, 2014.

107. Foster CA, Breeze RE: The Meniere attack: an ischemia/reperfusion disorder of inner ear sensory tissues, *Med Hypotheses* 81(6):1108-1115, 2013.

108. Wipperman J: Otitis externa, *Prim Care* 41(1):1-9, 2014.

109. Rye MS et al: Genetic susceptibility to otitis media in childhood, *Laryngoscope* 122(3):665-675, 2012.

110. Pichichero ME: Otitis media, *Pediatr Clin North Am* 60(2):391-407, 2013.

111. Principi N et al: Prevention of acute otitis media using currently available vaccines, *Future Microbiol* 7(4):457-465, 2012.

112. Roper SD: Taste buds as peripheral chemosensory processors, *Semin Cell Dev Biol* 24(1):71-79, 2013.

113. Visvanathan R, Chapman IM: Undernutrition and anorexia in the older person, *Gastroenterol Clin North Am* 38(3):393-409, 2009.

114. McGlone F, Reilly D: The cutaneous sensory system, *Neurosci Biobehav Rev* 34(2):148-159, 2010.

115. Norman JF et al: Aging and curvature discrimination from static and dynamic touch, *PLoS One* 8(7):e68577, 2013.

116. Proske U, Gandevia SC: The proprioceptive senses: their roles in signaling body shape, body position and movement, and muscle force, *Physiol Rev* 92(4):1651-1697, 2012.

15

Alterations in Cognitive Systems, Cerebral Hemodynamics, and Motor Function

Barbara J. Boss and Sue E. Huether

CHAPTER OUTLINE

A person achieves cognitive and behavioral functional competence by integrated processes of cognitive systems, sensory systems, and motor systems. The purpose of this chapter is to present the concepts and processes of alterations in these systems as an approach to understanding the manifestations of neurologic dysfunction and disease.

The neural systems that are essential to cognitive function are: (1) attentional systems that provide arousal and maintenance of attention over time; (2) memory and language systems by which information is communicated; and (3) affective or emotive systems that mediate mood, emotion, and intention. These core systems are fundamental to the processes of abstract thinking and reasoning. The products of abstraction and reasoning are organized and made operational through the executive attentional networks. The normal functioning of these networks manifests through the motor network in a behavioral array viewed by others as appropriate to human activity and successful living.

ALTERATIONS IN COGNITIVE SYSTEMS

Full **consciousness** is a state of awareness both of oneself and of the environment, and a set of responses to that environment. The fully conscious individual initiates spontaneous, purposeful activity independently to a perceived stimulus. Any decrease in this state of awareness and varied responses is a decrease in consciousness.

Consciousness has two distinct components: arousal (state of awakeness) and awareness (content of thought). **Arousal** is mediated by the reticular activating system, which regulates aspects of attention and information processing and maintains consciousness. Awareness encompasses all cognitive functions and is mediated by attentional systems, memory systems, language systems, and executive systems.

Alterations in Arousal

Alterations in level of arousal may be caused by structural, metabolic, or psychogenic (functional) disorders.

PATHOPHYSIOLOGY Structural alterations in arousal are divided according to the original location of the pathologic condition. Causes include infection, vascular alterations, neoplasms, traumatic injury, congenital alterations, degenerative changes, polygenic traits, and metabolic disorders.

Supratentorial disorders (above the tentorium cerebelli) produce changes in arousal by either diffuse or localized dysfunction. Diffuse dysfunction may be caused by disease processes affecting the cerebral cortex or the underlying subcortical white matter (e.g., encephalitis). Disorders outside the brain but within the cranial vault (extracerebral) can produce diffuse dysfunction, including neoplasms, closed-head trauma with subsequent subdural bleeding, and accumulation of pus in the subdural space. Disorders within the brain substance (intracerebral)—bleeding, infarcts, emboli, and tumors—function primarily as masses. Such localized destructive processes directly impair function of the thalamic or hypothalamic activating systems or secondarily compress these structures in a process of herniation.

Infratentorial disorders (below the tentorium cerebelli) produce a decline in arousal by (1) direct destruction or compression of the reticular activating system and its pathways (e.g., accumulations of blood or pus, neoplasms, and demyelinating disorders) or (2) the brainstem (midbrain, pons, medulla) may be destroyed either by direct invasion or by indirect impairment of its blood supply.

Metabolic disorders produce a decline in arousal by alterations in delivery of energy substrates as occurs with hypoxia, electrolyte disturbances, or hypoglycemia. Metabolic disorders caused by liver or renal failure cause alterations in neuronal excitability because of failure to metabolize or eliminate drugs and toxins. All the systemic diseases that eventually produce nervous system dysfunction are part of this metabolic category.

Psychogenic alterations in arousal (unresponsiveness), although uncommon, may signal general psychiatric disorders. Despite apparent unconsciousness, the person actually is physiologically awake and the neurologic examination reflects normal responses.

CLINICAL MANIFESTATIONS AND EVALUATION Five patterns of neurologic function are critical to the evaluation process: (1) level of consciousness, (2) pattern of breathing, (3) pupillary reaction, (4) oculomotor responses, and (5) motor responses. Patterns of clinical manifestations help in determining the extent of brain dysfunction and serve as indexes for identifying increasing or decreasing central nervous system (CNS) function. Distinctions are made between metabolic and structurally induced manifestations (Table 15-1). The types of manifestations suggest the cause of the altered arousal state (Table 15-2).

Level of consciousness is the most critical clinical index of nervous system function, with changes indicating either improvement or deterioration of the individual's condition. A person who is alert and

TABLE 15-1 Clinical Manifestations of Metabolic and Structural Causes of Altered Arousal

Manifestations	Metabolically Induced	Structurally Induced
Blink to threat (cranial nerves II, VII)	Equal	Asymmetric
Optic discs (cranial nerve II)	Flat, good pulsation	Papilledema
Extraocular movement (cranial nerves III, IV, VI)	Roving eye movements; normal doll's eyes and calorics	Gaze paresis, nerve palsy
Pupils (cranial nerves II, III)	Equal and reactive; may be dilated (e.g., atropine), pinpoint (e.g., opiates), or midposition and fixed (e.g., glutethimide [Doriden])	Asymmetric or nonreactive; may be midposition (midbrain injury), pinpoint (pons injury), large (tectal injury)
Corneal reflex (cranial nerves V, VII)	Symmetric response	Asymmetric response
Grimace to pain (cranial nerve VII)	Symmetric response	Asymmetric response
Motor function movement	Symmetric	Asymmetric
Muscle tone	Symmetric	Paratonic (rigid), spastic, flaccid, especially if asymmetric
Posture	Symmetric	Decorticate, especially if symmetric; decerebrate, especially if asymmetric (see Figure 15-6)
Deep tendon reflexes	Symmetric	Asymmetric
Babinski sign	Absent or symmetric response	Present
Sensation	Symmetric	Asymmetric

TABLE 15-2 Differential Characteristics of States Causing Altered Arousal

Mechanism	Manifestations
Supratentorial mass lesions compressing or displacing diencephalon or brainstem	Initiating signs usually of focal cerebral dysfunction: vomiting, headache, hemiparesis, ocular signs, seizures, coma
	Signs of dysfunction progress rostral to caudal
	Neurologic signs at any given time point to one anatomic area (e.g., diencephalon, mesencephalon, medulla)
	Motor signs often asymmetric
Infratentorial mass of destruction causing coma	History of preceding brainstem dysfunction or sudden onset of coma
	Localizing brainstem signs precede or accompany onset of coma and always include oculovestibular abnormality
	Cranial nerve palsies usually manifest "bizarre" respiratory patterns that appear at onset
Metabolic coma	Confusion and stupor commonly precede motor signs
Exogenous toxins (drugs)	Motor signs usually are symmetric
Endogenous toxins (organ system failure)	Pupillary reactions usually are preserved
	Asterixis, myoclonus, tremor, and seizures are common
	Acid-base imbalance with hyperventilation or hypoventilation is common
Psychiatric unresponsiveness	Lids close actively; pupils reactive or dilated (cycloplegics)
	Oculocephalic reflexes are unpredictable; oculovestibular reflexes are physiologic (nystagmus is present)
	Motor tone is inconsistent or normal
	Eupnea or hyperventilation is usual
	No pathologic reflexes are present
	Electroencephalogram (EEG) is normal

oriented to self, others, place, and time is considered to be functioning at the highest level of consciousness, which implies full use of all the person's cognitive capacities. From this normal alert state, levels of consciousness diminish in stages from confusion and disorientation (can occur simultaneously) to coma, each of which is clinically defined (Table 15-3).

Patterns of breathing help evaluate the level of brain dysfunction and coma (Figure 15-1). Rate, rhythm, and pattern should be evaluated. Breathing patterns can be categorized as hemispheric or brainstem patterns (Table 15-4).

With normal breathing, a neural center in the forebrain (cerebrum) produces a rhythmic pattern. When consciousness decreases, lower brainstem centers regulate the breathing pattern by responding only to changes in $Paco_2$ levels; this is called *posthyperventilation apnea*. *Cheyne-Stokes respiration* is an abnormal rhythm of ventilation with alternating periods of tachypnea and apnea (crescendo-decrescendo pattern). Increases in $Paco_2$ levels lead to tachypnea. The $Paco_2$ level then decreases to below normal and breathing stops (apnea) until the carbon dioxide reaccumulates and again stimulates tachypnea (see Figure 15-1). In cases of opiate or sedative drug overdose, the respiratory center is depressed so the rate of breathing gradually decreases until respiratory failure occurs.

Pupillary changes indicate the presence and level of brainstem dysfunction because brainstem areas that control arousal are adjacent to areas that control the pupils (Figure 15-2). For example, severe ischemia and hypoxia usually produce dilated, fixed pupils. Hypothermia may cause fixed pupils.

Some drugs affect pupils and must be considered in evaluating individuals in comatose states. Large doses of atropine and scopolamine fully dilate and fix pupils. Doses of sedatives (e.g., glutethimide) in sufficient amounts to produce coma cause the pupils to become midposition or moderately dilated, unequal, and commonly fixed to light. Opiates cause pinpoint pupils. Severe barbiturate intoxication may produce fixed pupils.

Oculomotor responses (resting, spontaneous, and reflexive eye movements) change at various levels of brain dysfunction in comatose individuals. Persons with metabolically induced coma, except with barbiturate-hypnotic and phenytoin poisoning, generally retain ocular reflexes even when other signs of brainstem damage are present. Destructive or compressive injury to the brainstem causes specific abnormalities of the oculocephalic and oculovestibular reflexes (Figures 15-3 and 15-4). Injuries that involve an oculomotor nucleus or nerve cause the involved eye to deviate outward, producing a resting dysconjugate lateral position of the eye.

Assessment of motor responses helps to evaluate the level of brain dysfunction and determine the most severely damaged side of the brain. The pattern of response noted may be (1) purposeful; (2) inappropriate, generalized motor movement; or (3) not present.

TABLE 15-3 Levels of Altered Consciousness

State	Definition
Confusion	Loss of ability to think rapidly and clearly; impaired judgment and decision making
Disorientation	Beginning loss of consciousness; the person may exhibit restlessness, anxiety, and irritation; disorientation to time occurs first, followed by disorientation to place and familiar others (family members) and impaired memory; recognition of self is lost last
Lethargy	Limited spontaneous movement or speech; easy arousal with normal speech or touch; may or may not be oriented to time, place, or person
Obtundation	Mild to moderate reduction in arousal (awakeness) with limited response to environment; falls asleep unless stimulated verbally or tactilely; answers questions with minimal response
Stupor	Condition of deep sleep or unresponsiveness from which person may be aroused or caused to open eyes only by vigorous and repeated stimulation; response is often withdrawal or grabbing at stimulus
Light coma	Associated with purposeful movement on stimulation
Coma	Associated with nonpurposeful movement only on stimulation
Deep coma	Associated with unresponsiveness or no response to any stimulus

FIGURE 15-1 Abnormal Respiratory Patterns with Corresponding Level of Central Nervous System Activity. (From Urden LD et al: *Critical care nursing: diagnosis and management*, ed 6, St Louis, 2010, Mosby.)

TABLE 15-4 Patterns of Breathing

Breathing Pattern	Description	Location of Injury
Hemispheric Breathing Patterns		
Normal	After a period of hyperventilation that lowers arterial carbon dioxide pressure (PaCO₂), individual continues to breathe regularly but with reduced depth.	Response of nervous system to an external stressor—not associated with injury to CNS
Posthyperventilation apnea	Respirations stop after hyperventilation has lowered PCO₂ level below normal. Rhythmic breathing returns when PCO₂ level returns to normal.	Associated with diffuse bilateral metabolic or structural disease of cerebrum
Cheyne-Stokes respirations	Breathing pattern has a smooth increase (crescendo) in rate and depth of breathing (hyperpnea), which peaks and is followed by a gradual smooth decrease (decrescendo) in rate and depth of breathing to point of apnea, when cycle repeats itself. Hyperpneic phase lasts longer than apneic phase.	Bilateral dysfunction of deep cerebral or diencephalic structures; seen with supratentorial injury and metabolically induced coma states
Brainstem Breathing Patterns		
Central neurogenic hyperventilation	A sustained, deep, rapid, but regular pattern (hyperpnea) occurs, with a decreased PaCO₂ and a corresponding increase in pH and PO₂.	May result from CNS damage or disease that involves midbrain and upper pons; seen after increased intracranial pressure and blunt head trauma
Apneusis	A prolonged inspiratory cramp (a pause at full inspiration) occurs; a common variant of this is a brief end-inspiratory pause of 2 or 3 sec, often alternating with an end-expiratory pause.	Indicates damage to respiratory control mechanism located at pontine level; most commonly associated with pontine infarction but documented with hypoglycemia, anoxia, and meningitis
Cluster breathing	A cluster of breaths has a disordered sequence with irregular pauses between breaths.	Dysfunction in lower pontine and high medullary areas
Ataxic breathing	Completely irregular breathing occurs, with random shallow and deep breaths and irregular pauses. Rate is often slow.	Originates from a primary dysfunction of medullary neurons controlling breathing
Gasping breathing pattern (agonal gasps)	A pattern of deep "all-or-none" breaths is accompanied by a slow respiratory rate.	Indicative of a failing medullary respiratory center

CNS, Central nervous system.

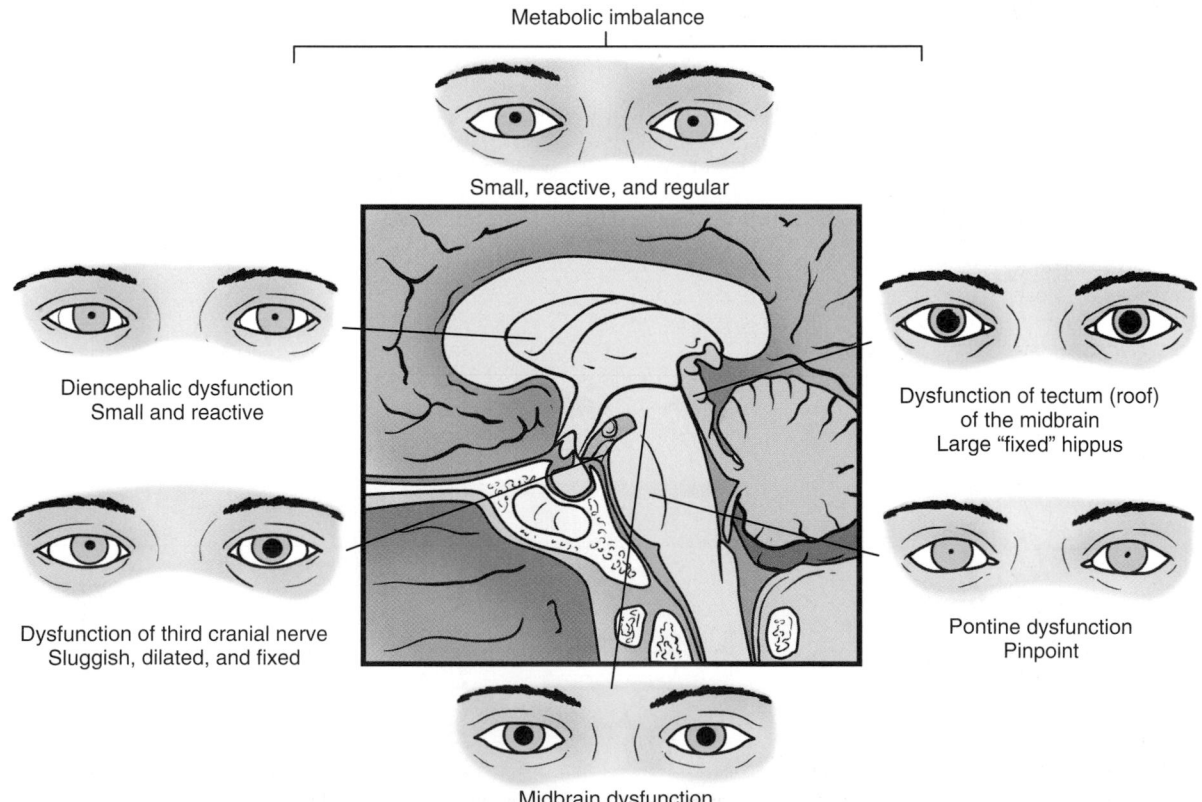

Metabolic imbalance
Small, reactive, and regular

Diencephalic dysfunction
Small and reactive

Dysfunction of third cranial nerve
Sluggish, dilated, and fixed

Dysfunction of tectum (roof) of the midbrain
Large "fixed" hippus

Pontine dysfunction
Pinpoint

Midbrain dysfunction
Midposition and fixed

FIGURE 15-2 Appearance of Pupils at Different Levels of Consciousness.

Motor signs indicating loss of cortical inhibition that are commonly associated with decreased consciousness include primitive reflexes and rigidity (paratonia) (Figure 15-5). Primitive reflexes include grasping, reflex sucking, snout reflex, and palmomental reflex, all of which are normal in the newborn but disappear in infancy. Abnormal flexor and extensor responses in the upper and lower extremities are defined in Table 15-5 and illustrated in Figure 15-6.

Vomiting, yawning, and hiccups are complex reflex-like motor responses that are integrated by neural mechanisms in the lower brainstem. These responses may be produced by compression or diseases involving tissues of the medulla oblongata (e.g., infection, neoplasm, infarction) but also occur relative to other more benign stimuli to the vagal nerve. Most CNS disorders produce nausea and vomiting. Vomiting without nausea indicates direct involvement of the central neural mechanism (or pyloric obstruction; see Chapters 36 and 37). Vomiting often accompanies CNS injuries that (1) involve the vestibular nuclei or its immediate projections, particularly when double vision (diplopia) also is present; (2) impinge directly on the floor of the fourth ventricle; or (3) produce brainstem compression secondary to increased intracranial pressure.

> ✔ **QUICK CHECK 15-1**
> 1. Why are structural as well as metabolic factors capable of producing coma?
> 2. Why is level of consciousness the most critical index of central nervous system function?
> 3. Why do Cheyne-Stokes respirations appear in coma?
> 4. Why are oculomotor changes associated with levels of brain injury?

FIGURE 15-3 Test for Oculocephalic Reflex Response (Doll's Eyes Phenomenon). A, Normal response—eyes turn together to side opposite from turn of head. **B,** Abnormal response—eyes do not turn in conjugate manner. **C,** Absent response—eyes move in direction of head movement (brainstem injury). (From Rudy EB: *Advanced neurological and neurosurgical nursing,* St Louis, 1984, Mosby.)

FIGURE 15-5 Pathologic Reflexes. A, Grasp reflex. **B,** Snout reflex. **C,** Palmomental reflex. **D,** Suck reflex.

FIGURE 15-4 Test for Oculovestibular Reflex (Caloric Ice Water Test). A, Ice water is injected into the ear canal. Normal response—conjugate eye movements. **B,** Abnormal response—dysconjugate or asymmetric eye movements. **C,** Absent response—no eye movements.

TABLE 15-5 Abnormal Motor Responses with Decreased Responsiveness

Motor Response	Description	Location of Injury
Decorticate posturing/rigidity: upper extremity flexion, lower extremity extension	Slowly developing flexion of arm, wrist, and fingers with adduction in the upper extremity and extension, internal rotation, and plantar flexion of lower extremity	Hemispheric damage above midbrain releasing medullary and pontine reticulospinal systems
Decerebrate posturing/rigidity: upper and lower extremity extensor responses	Opisthotonos (hyperextension of vertebral column) with clenching of teeth; extension, abduction, and hyperpronation of arms; and extension of lower extremities	Associated with severe damage involving midbrain or upper pons
	In acute brain injury, shivering and hyperpnea may accompany unelicited recurrent decerebrate spasms	Acute brain injury often causes limb extension regardless of location
Extensor responses in upper extremities accompanied by flexion in lower extremities		Pons
Flaccid state with little or no motor response to stimuli		Lower pons and upper medulla

FIGURE 15-6 Decorticate and Decerebrate Posture/Responses. **A,** Decorticate posture/response. Flexion of arms, wrists, and fingers with adduction in upper extremities. Extension, internal rotation, and plantar flexion in lower extremities. Both sides. **B,** Decerebrate posture/response. All four extremities in rigid extension, with hyperpronation of forearms and plantar extension of feet. (From deWit SC, Kumagai CK: *Medical-surgical nursing,* ed 2, St Louis, 2013, Saunders.)

Outcomes of Alterations in Arousal

Outcomes of alterations in arousal fall into two categories: *extent of disability (morbidity)* and *mortality*. Outcomes depend on the cause and extent of brain damage and the duration of coma. Some individuals may recover consciousness and an original level of function, some may have permanent disability, and some may never regain consciousness and experience neurologic death. Two forms of neurologic death—brain death and cerebral death—result from severe pathologic conditions and are associated with irreversible coma. Other possible outcomes are a vegetative state, a minimally conscious state, or locked-in syndrome. The extent of disability has four subcategories: recovery of consciousness, residual cognitive function, psychologic function, and vocational function.

Brain death (total brain death) occurs when the brain is damaged so completely that it can never recover (irreversible) and cannot

BOX 15-1 Criteria for Brain Death

1. Completion of all appropriate diagnostic and therapeutic procedures with no possibility of brain function recovery
2. Unresponsive coma (no motor or reflex movements)
3. No spontaneous respiration (apnea)
4. No brainstem functions (ocular responses to head turning or caloric stimulation; dilated, fixed pupils; no gag or corneal reflex [see Figures 15-3 and 15-4])
5. Isoelectric (flat) EEG (electrocerebral silence)
6. Persistence of these signs for an appropriate observation period

Summarized from Wijdicks EF et al: *Neurology* 74(23):1911-1918, 2010.

maintain the body's internal homeostasis. State laws define brain death as irreversible cessation of function of the entire brain including the brainstem and cerebellum. On postmortem examination, the brain is autolyzing (self-digesting) or already autolyzed. Brain death has occurred when there is no evidence of brain function for an extended period.[1] The abnormality of brain function must result from structural or known metabolic disease and must *not* be caused by a depressant drug, alcohol poisoning, or hypothermia. An isoelectric, or flat, electroencephalogram (EEG) (electrocerebral silence) for 6 to 12 hours in a person who is not hypothermic and has not ingested depressant drugs indicates brain death. The clinical criteria used to determine brain death are noted in Box 15-1. A task force for determination of brain death in children recommended the same criteria as for adults, but with a longer observation period.[2]

Cerebral death, or irreversible coma, is death of the cerebral hemispheres exclusive of the brainstem and cerebellum. Brain damage is permanent, and the individual is forever unable to respond behaviorally in any significant way to the environment. The brainstem may continue to maintain internal homeostasis (i.e., body temperature, cardiovascular functions, respirations, and metabolic functions). The survivor of cerebral death may remain in a coma or emerge into a persistent vegetative state (VS) or a minimally conscious state (MCS). In coma, the eyes are usually closed with no eye opening. The person does not follow commands, speak, or have voluntary movement.[3]

A persistent vegetative state is complete unawareness of the self or surrounding environment and complete loss of cognitive function. The individual does not speak any comprehensible words or follow commands. Sleep-wake cycles are present, eyes open spontaneously, and blood pressure and breathing are maintained without support. Brainstem reflexes (pupillary, oculocephalic, chewing, swallowing) are intact but cerebral function is lost. There is bowel and bladder incontinence. Recovery is unlikely if the state persists for 12 months. In a minimally conscious state (MCS) individuals may follow simple commands, manipulate objects, gesture or give yes/no responses, have intelligible speech, and have movements such as blinking or smiling.[4]

With locked-in syndrome there is complete paralysis of voluntary muscles with the exception of eye movement. Content of thought and level of arousal are intact, but the efferent pathways are disrupted (injury at the base of the pons with the reticular formation intact, often caused by basilar artery occlusion).[5] Thus, the individual cannot communicate through speech or body movement but is fully conscious, with intact cognitive function. Vertical eye movement and blinking are a means of communication.

Alterations in Awareness

Awareness (content of thought) encompasses all cognitive functions, including awareness of self, environment, and affective states (i.e., moods). Awareness is mediated by all of the core networks under the guidance of executive attention networks including selective attention and memory. Executive attention networks involve abstract reasoning, planning, decision making, judgment, error correction, and self-control. Each attentional function is a network of interconnected brain areas and not localized to a single brain area.

Selective attention (orienting) refers to the ability to select specific information to be processed from available, competing environmental and internal stimuli, and to focus on that stimulus (i.e., to concentrate on a specific task without being distracted).[6] Selective visual attention is the ability to select objects from multiple visual stimuli and process them to complete a task. Selective auditory or hearing attention is the ability to select or filter specific sounds and process them to complete a task. Multiple areas of the brain are involved in selective attention including cortical areas, thalamic nuclei, and the limbic system. Selective attention deficits can be temporary, permanent, or progressive. Disorders associated with selective attention deficits include seizure activity, parietal lobe contusions, subdural hematomas, stroke, gliomas or metastatic tumor, late Alzheimer dementia, frontotemporal dementia, and psychotic disorders.

Memory is the recording, retention, and retrieval of information. Amnesia is the loss of memory and can be mild or severe. Two types of amnesia are retrograde amnesia and anterograde amnesia. The person experiencing retrograde amnesia has difficulty retrieving past personal history memories or past factual memories. Anterograde amnesia is the inability to form new personal or factual memories but memories of the distant past are retained and retrieved. Image processing is a higher level of memory function and includes the ability to use sensory data and language to form concepts, assign meaning, and make abstractions. Alterations in image processing include an inability to form concepts and generalizations or to reason. Thinking is very concrete. These memory disorders may be temporary (e.g., after a seizure) or permanent (e.g., after severe head injury or in Alzheimer disease). There may be only the memory disorder, or the memory disorder may be associated with other cognitive disorders.

Executive attention deficits include the inability to maintain sustained attention and a working memory deficit. Sustained attention deficit is an inability to set goals and recognize when an object meets a goal. A working memory deficit is an inability to remember instructions and information needed to guide behavior. Executive attention deficits may be temporary, progressive, or permanent. Attention-deficit/hyperactivity disorder (ADHD) is a common disorder of

---

> ### BOX 15-2   Attention-Deficit/Hyperactivity Disorder (ADHD)
>
> Initially ADHD was viewed as a neurodevelopmental disorder of childhood. It is now recognized that 50% to 75% of persons diagnosed in childhood have continuing symptoms into adulthood. Often the diagnosis is first made in adolescence or young adulthood when behavioral control and self-organization are expected of the person. The ability to function at work, at home, and in social situations is often impaired because of inattentiveness, hyperactivity, impulsivity, and problems with executive function. Continued treatment including medications for symptomatic adults is supported; substance abuse, which is more common in persons with ADHD, is reduced with continued treatment. The multifactorial patterns of inheritance and gene-environment interactions are under investigation as are the pathogenesis and pathophysiology of this complex disorder. Findings from structural and functional neuroimaging suggest the involvement of developmentally abnormal brain networks related to cognition, attention, emotion, and sensorimotor functions. Hopefully new findings will lead to improved prevention, diagnosis, treatment options and functional outcomes.

Data from Baroni A, Castellanos FX: *Curr Opin Neurobiol* 30:1-8, 2015; Harstad E, Levy S: *Pediatrics* 134(1):e293-e301, 2014; Sharma A, Couture J: *Ann Pharmacother* 48(2):209-225, 2014; Matthews M et al: *Curr Top Behav Neurosci* 16:235-266, 2014.

childhood that can continue through adulthood (Box 15-2). Table 15-6 summarizes alterations in memory and attention.

PATHOPHYSIOLOGY   Very generally, the primary pathophysiologic mechanisms that operate in disorders of awareness are (1) direct destruction caused by ischemia and hypoxia or indirect destruction resulting from compression and (2) the effects of toxins and chemicals or metabolic disorders. Disorders of selective attention, at least as they relate to visual orienting behavior, are produced by disease that involves portions of the midbrain. Disease affecting the superior colliculi manifests as a slowness in orienting attention. Parietal lobe disease may produce *unilateral neglect syndrome* or lack of awareness of one side of the body or lack of response to stimuli on one side of the body and can occur after a stroke. An individual may groom or dress on only one side or eat food from only one side of the plate. Sensory inattentiveness is a form of neglect. The person is able to recognize individual sensory input from the dysfunctional side when asked, but ignores the sensory input from the dysfunctional side when stimulated from both sides (extinction). The entire complex of denial of dysfunction, loss of recognition of one's own body parts, and extinction sometimes is referred to as hemineglect or neglect syndrome. A disorder in vigilance may be produced by disease in the prefrontal areas. Dysfunction in the right anterior cingulate gyrus and basal ganglia may cause detection problems, whereas problems with working memory may be produced with left lateral frontal injury. Anterograde amnesia originates from pathologic conditions in the hippocampus and related temporal lobe structures; the diencephalic region including the thalamus; and the basal forebrain. Retrograde amnesia and higher level memory deficits originate from pathologic conditions in the widely distributed association areas of the cerebral cortex (see Figure 13-7, C). Executive attention deficits are associated with alterations in the frontal and prefrontal cortex including the anterior cingulate gyrus, supplementary motor area, and portions of the basal ganglia.

CLINICAL MANIFESTATIONS   Clinical manifestations of selective attention deficits, memory deficits, and executive attention function deficits are presented in Table 15-6.

TABLE 15-6   Clinical Manifestations of Alterations in Attention and Memory

Deficit	Clinical Signs	Symptoms
Attention		
Selective attention (orienting)	Inability to focus attention; decreased eye, head, and body movements associated with focusing on stimuli; decreased search and scanning; faulty orientation to stimuli, causing safety problems	Person reports inability to focus attention, failure to perceive objects and other stimuli (history of injuries, falls, safety problems); can exhibit neglect syndrome (i.e., unilateral neglect with failure to groom or recognize one side of the body)
Memory		
Antegrade amnesia (inability to form new memories)	*Left hemisphere:* disorientation to time, situation, place, name, person (verbal identification); impaired language memory (e.g., names of objects); impaired semantic memory *Right hemisphere:* disorientation to self, person (visual), place (visual); impaired episodic memory (personal history); impaired emotional memory *Either or both hemispheres:* confusion; behavioral change	Person reports disorientation, confusion, "not listening," "not remembering"; reports by others of person being disoriented, not able to remember, not able to learn new information
Retrograde amnesia (loss of past memories)	*Left hemisphere:* inability to retrieve personal history, past medical history; unaware of recent current events *Right hemisphere:* inability to recognize persons, places, objects, music, and so on from past	Person reports remote memory problems; others report that person cannot recall formerly known information
Image processing	Inability to categorize (identify similarities and differences) or sort; inability to form concepts; inability to analyze relationships; misinterpretations; inability to interpret proverbs	Reports by others of frequent misinterpretation of data, failure to conceptualize or generalize information
	Inability to perform deductive reasoning (convergent reasoning); inability to perform inductive reasoning (divergent reasoning); inability to abstract; concrete reasoning demonstrated; delusions	Reports by others of predominantly concrete thinking; lack of understanding of everyday situations, healthcare regimens, and such; delusional thinking
Executive Attention Deficits		
Vigilance	Failure to stay alert and orient to stimuli	Person reports decreased alertness or ability to orient
Detection	Lack of initiative (anergy); lack of ambition; lack of motivation; flat affect; no awareness of feelings; appears depressed, apathetic, and emotionless; fails to appreciate deficit; disinterested in appearance; lacks concern about childish or crude behavior	Reports by others of laziness or apathy, flat affect, or lack of emotional expression; failure to exhibit or be aware of feelings
Mild	Responds to immediate environment but no new ideas; grooming and social graces are lacking	Reports by others of lack of ambition, motivation, or initiative; failure to carry out adult tasks; lack of social graces and new ideas
Severe	Motionless; lack of response to even internal cues; does not respond to physical needs; does not interact with surroundings	Reports by others of failure to groom or toilet self, unawareness of surroundings and own physical needs
	Inability to use feedback regarding behavior; failure to recognize omissions and errors in self-care, speech, writing, and arithmetic; impaired cue utilization; overestimation of performance	Reports by others of not changing behavior when requested; unawareness of limitations; does not recognize and correct errors in dressing, grooming, toileting, eating, and such; fails to recognize speech and arithmetic errors; careless speech
	Failure to shift response set; failure to change behavior when conditions change; cue utilization may be impaired	Reports by others of failure to use feedback; inability to incorporate feedback (does not correct when feedback is given)
Working memory (recent or short-term memory)	Inability to set goals or form goals; indecisiveness	Reports by others of failure to set goals, indecisiveness
	Failure to make plans; inability to produce a complete line of reasoning; inability to make up a story; appears impulsive	Reports by others of failure to plan, impulsiveness, "does not think things through"
	Failure to initiate behavior; failure to maintain behavior; failure to discontinue behavior; slowness to alternate response for the next step; motor perseveration	Reports by others of not knowing where to begin, inability to carry out sequential acts (maintain a behavior), inability to cease a behavior

EVALUATION AND TREATMENT   Immediate medical management is directed at diagnosing the cause and treating reversible factors. Rehabilitative measures generally focus on compensatory or restorative activities and recently have been greatly facilitated by computer technology and other electronic devices.

✔ QUICK CHECK 15-2
1. Why is irreversible coma different from brain death?
2. What is the difference between anterograde and retrograde amnesia?
3. What is an example of neglect syndrome?

Data Processing Deficits

Data processing deficits are problems associated with recognizing and processing sensory information and include agnosia, dysphasia, and acute confusional states.

Agnosia

Agnosia is a defect of pattern recognition—a failure to recognize the form and nature of objects. Agnosia can be tactile, visual, or auditory, but generally only one sense is affected. For example, an individual may be unable to identify a safety pin by touching it with a hand but is able to name it when looking at it. Agnosia may be as minimal as a finger agnosia (failure to identify by name the fingers of one's hand) or more extensive, such as a color agnosia. Although agnosia is associated most commonly with cerebrovascular accidents, it may arise from any pathologic process that injures specific areas of the brain.

Dysphasia

Dysphasia is impairment of comprehension or production of language with impaired communication. Comprehension or use of symbols, in either written or verbal language, is disturbed or lost. Aphasia is a more severe form of dysphasia and an inability to communicate using language. Often the terms *dysphasia* and *aphasia* are used interchangeably. The term *dysphasia* is used here. Dysphasia results from dysfunction in the left cerebral hemisphere (i.e., Broca area [inferior frontal gyrus] and Wernicke area [superior temporal gyrus]) and the subcortical and cortical connecting networks (Figure 15-7 and see Figure 13-7). Dysphasias usually are associated with a cerebrovascular accident involving the middle cerebral artery or one of its many branches. Language disorders, however, may arise from a variety of injuries and diseases including vascular, neoplastic, traumatic, degenerative, metabolic, or infectious causes. Most language disorders result from acute processes or a chronic residual deficit of the acute process.

Dysphasias have been classified anatomically (i.e., Wernicke or Broca area dysphasias) or functionally as disorders of fluency (quality and content of speech). *Expressive dysphasia,* also known as Broca, motor, or nonfluent dysphasia, involves loss of ability to produce spoken or written language with slow or difficult speech. Verbal comprehension is usually present. Expressive dysphasia is differentiated from *dysarthria,* in which words cannot be articulated clearly as a result of cranial nerve damage or muscle impairment. *Receptive dysphasia,* also known as Wernicke, sensory, or fluent dysphasia, involves an inability to understand written or spoken language. Speech is fluent, flowing at a normal rate, but words and phrases have no meaning. *Anomic aphasia* is a sensory aphasia distinguished by difficulty finding words and naming a person or object. Circumlocution, or describing an object as a way of trying to name something, is common in anomic aphasia. Auditory comprehension is present in *conductive dysphasia,* but there is impaired verbatim repetition. Naming also can be impaired. The person recognizes the errors and tries to correct them. Speech is fluent but words and sounds may be transposed. Damage is in the left hemisphere to networks that connect Broca and Wernicke areas. *Transcortical dysphasias* are rare and can be motor, sensory, or mixed. They involve areas of the brain that connect into the language centers. *Global dysphasia* is the most severe dysphasia and involves both expressive and receptive dysphasia. The individual is nonfluent or mute; cannot read or write; and has impaired comprehension, naming, reading, and writing. Global dysphasia is usually associated with a cerebrovascular accident involving the middle cerebral artery. Table 15-7 compares types of dysphasias, and Table 15-8 illustrates some of the language disturbances. Pure dysphasias are rare and are often mixed, making diagnosis difficult. All types of dysphasia usually improve with speech rehabilitation.

Acute Confusional States and Delirium

Acute confusional states (also may be known as acute organic brain syndromes) are transient disorders of awareness and may have either a sudden or a gradual onset. Delirium can be considered as a type of acute confusional state, but for this discussion acute confusional states and delirium are considered to be synonymous. There are many medical conditions associated with delirium, and they are summarized in Box 15-3.

PATHOPHYSIOLOGY Acute confusional states arise from disruption of a widely distributed neural network involving the reticular activating system of the upper brainstem and its projections into the thalamus, basal ganglion, and specific association areas of the cortex and limbic areas. Delirium (hyperactive confusional state) is associated with autonomic nervous system overactivity and typically develops over 2 to 3 days. It most commonly occurs in critical care units, following surgery, or during withdrawal from central nervous system depressants (i.e., alcohol or narcotic agents). Delirium is associated with right-upper middle-temporal gyrus or left temporal-occipital

FIGURE 15-7 Right Cortical, Subcortical, and Brainstem Areas of the Brain Mediating Cognitive Function. (From Boss GJ, Wilkerson R: Communication: language and pragmatics. In Hoeman SP, editor: *Rehabilitation nursing; prevention, intervention & outcomes,* ed 4, p 508, St Louis, 2008, Mosby.)

BOX 15-3 Conditions Causing Acute Confusional States or Delirium

Drug intoxication
Alcohol or drug withdrawal
Metabolic disorders (e.g., hypoglycemia, thyroid storm)
Brain trauma or surgery
Postanesthesia
Febrile illnesses or heat stroke
Electrolyte imbalance, dehydration
Heart, kidney, or liver failure

TABLE 15-7 Major Types of Dysphasia

Type	Expression	Verbal Comprehension	Repetition	Reading Comprehension	Writing	Location of Lesion	Cause of Lesion
Expressive							
Broca, nonfluent or motor aphasia	Cannot find words, difficulty writing	Relatively intact	Impaired	Variable	Impaired	Left posteroinferior frontal lobe (Broca area)	Occlusion of one or several branches of left middle cerebral artery supplying inferior frontal gyrus
Transcortical motor, nonfluent dysphasia	Halting speech	Intact	Intact	Impaired	Impaired	Anterior superior frontal lobe	Occlusion at the border zone between two arterial territories
Receptive							
Wernicke, receptive fluent or sensory dysphasia	Meaningless verbal language, inappropriate words or unable to monitor language for correctness so errors are not recognized. Intonation, accent, cadence, rhythm, and articulation normal	Impaired; disturbance in understanding all language	Impaired	Impaired	Impaired	Left posterosuperior temporal lobe (Wernicke area)	Occlusion of inferior division of left middle cerebral artery
Conductive dysphasia	Difficulty repeating words, phrases spoken to them; naming is impaired	Intact	Severely impaired	Variable	Variable	Inferior and posterior temporal lobe; parietotemporal junction	Occlusion in distributions of left middle cerebral artery
Anomic dysphasia	Hesitancy, difficulty recalling names, objects, or numbers	Intact	Impaired	Variable	Intact except for anomia	Left temporoparietal zones; arcuate fasciculus	Diffuse left hemisphere brain disease
Transcortical sensory, fluent dysphasia	Repeats words and phrases spoken to them	Poor	Intact	Impaired	Impaired	Posterior temporal lobe	Occlusion at the border zone between two cerebral arterial territories
Other							
Transcortical mixed motor and sensory, nonfluent	Repeats words and phrases spoken to them	Impaired	Intact	Impaired	Impaired	Left cerebral hemisphere; spares the perisylvian cortex	Occlusion at the border zone between two cerebral arterial territories
Global or nonfluent; summation of motor and sensory aphasia	Mute	Impaired	Impaired	Impaired	Impaired	Large areas of the left cortex and subcortical regions	Occlusion of left middle cerebral artery of left internal carotid artery, tumors, other mass lesions, hemorrhage, embolic occlusion of ascending parietal or posterior temporal branch of middle cerebral artery

junction disruption and several neurotransmitters (i.e., acetylcholine and dopamine) are involved.[7] **Excited delirium syndrome (ExDS)**, also known as agitated delirium, is a type of hyperkinetic delirium that can lead to sudden death. Its symptoms include altered mental status, combativeness, aggressiveness, tolerance to significant pain, rapid breathing, sweating, severe agitation, elevated temperature, noncompliance or poor awareness to direction from police or medical personnel, inability to become fatigued, unusual or superhuman strength, and inappropriate clothing for the current environment. **Hypoactive delirium (hypoactive confusional state)** is more likely to be associated with right-sided frontal-basal ganglion disruption.

Most metabolic disturbances (i.e., hypoglycemia, thyroid disorders, liver or kidney disease) that produce delirium interfere with neuronal metabolism or synaptic transmission. Many drugs and toxins also interfere with neurotransmission function at the synapse.

CLINICAL MANIFESTATIONS Delirium initially manifests as difficulty in concentrating, restlessness, irritability, insomnia, tremulousness, and poor appetite. Some persons experience seizures. Unpleasant, even terrifying, dreams or hallucinations may occur. In a fully developed delirium state, the individual is completely inattentive and perceptions are grossly altered, with extensive misperception and misinterpretation. The person appears distressed and often perplexed; conversation is incoherent. Frank tremor and high levels of restless movement are common. Violent behavior may be present. The individual cannot sleep, is flushed, and has dilated pupils, a rapid pulse rate (tachycardia), elevated temperature, and profuse sweating (diaphoresis). Delirium typically abates suddenly or gradually in 2 to 3 days, although occasionally delirium states persist for weeks.

Hypoactive delirium is associated with underactivity and may occur in individuals who have fevers or metabolic disorders (i.e., chronic liver or kidney failure), or who are under the influence of central nervous system depressants. The individual exhibits decreases in mental function, specifically alertness, attention span, accurate perception, interpretation of the environment, and reaction to the environment. Forgetfulness and apathy are prominent, speech may be slow and the individual dozes frequently.

EVALUATION AND TREATMENT The initial goals are to (1) establish that the individual is confused and (2) determine the cause of the confusion (organic or functional) (Table 15-9). The next step is to differentiate whether the confusion is delirium or an underlying dementia. Individuals with dementia are at increased risk for developing delirium. A complete history, physical examination and laboratory tests (electrocardiogram and blood, urine, cerebrospinal fluid, and radiologic studies) are needed. Several assessment scales are available to guide evaluation (such as Clinical Assessment of Confusion A and B, Confusion State Evaluation, Confusion Assessment Method for the Intensive Care Unit [CAM-ICU], and Intensive Care Delirium Screening Checklist).[8-11] Once the cause is established, treatment is directed at controlling the primary disorder with supportive measures used as appropriate. Delirium is preventable in some individuals.[12] Table 15-10

TABLE 15-8 Examples of Dysphasia

Disorder	Example
Wernicke/Fluent/Sensory Dysphasia	
Verbal paraphasia	*Question:* What did the car do?
	Patient: The car would spit sweetly down the road.
	(The car sped swiftly down the road.)
Wernicke/Fluent/Sensory Dysphasia	
Literal paraphasia	*Request:* Say, "Persistence is essential to success."
	Patient: Mesastence is instans to success.
Wernicke/Fluent/Sensory Dysphasia	
Neologism	*Question:* What do you call this? (Pointing to a plant.)
	Patient: It's a logper.
Anomic dysphasia (circumlocution example)	*Question:* What do you call this? (Pointing to a plant.)
	Patient: Something that grows.
	Patient: It's…
	Or
	Question: What did you do this morning?
	Patient: Reading.
	Question: Were you reading a book or newspaper?
	Patient: One of those.
Broca or Motor Dysphasia	
Telegraphic style	*Question:* Where is your daughter?
	Patient: New Orleans … home … Monday.

From Boss BJ: *J Neurosurg Nurs* 16(3):151-160, 1984.

TABLE 15-9 Differences Between Organic and Functional Confusion

Factor	Organic Confusion	Functional Confusion
Memory impairment	Recent more impaired than remote	No consistent difference between recent and remote
Disorientation		
Time	Within own lifetime or reasonably near future	May not be related to person's lifetime
Place	Familiar place or one where person might easily be found	Bizarre or unfamiliar places
Person	Sense of identity usually preserved	Sense of identity diminished
	Misidentification of others as familiar	Misidentification of others based on delusion system
Hallucinations	Visual, vivid	Auditory more frequent
	Animals and insects common	Bizarre and symbolic
Illusions	Common	Not prominent
Delusions	Concern everyday occurrences and people	Bizarre and symbolic
Confused	Spotty confusion	More consistent
	Clear intervals mixed with confused episodes	No tendency to become worse at night
	Worse at night	

From Morris M, Rhodes M: *Am J Nurs* 72(9):1632, 1972.

TABLE 15-10 Comparison of Delirium and Dementia

Feature	Delirium	Dementia
Age	Usually older	Usually older
Onset	Acute—common during hospitalization	Usually insidious; acute in some cases of strokes/trauma
Associated conditions	Urinary tract infection, thyroid disorders, hypoxia, hypoglycemia, toxicity, fluid-electrolyte imbalance, renal insufficiency, trauma, postsurgical anesthesia	May have no other conditions Brain trauma
Course	Fluctuating/reversible with treatment	Chronic slow decline
Duration	Hours to weeks	Months to years
Attention	Impaired	Intact early; often impaired late
Sleep-wake cycle	Disrupted	Usually normal
Alertness	Impaired	Normal
Orientation	Impaired	Intact early; impaired late
Behavior	Agitated, withdrawn/depressed	Intact early
Speech	Incoherent, rapid/slowed	Word-finding problems
Thoughts	Disorganized, delusions	Impoverished
Perceptions	Hallucinations/illusions	Usually intact early

Adapted from Caplan JP, Rabinowitz T: *Med Clin North Am* 94(6):1103-1116, ix, 2010.

TABLE 15-11 Clinical Manifestations of the Major Degenerative Dementias

Disease	First Symptom	Mental Status	Neurobehavior	Neurologic Examination
Alzheimer disease	Memory loss; impaired learning	Episodic memory loss	Initially normal, progressive cognitive impairment	Initially normal
Creutzfeldt-Jakob disease	Dementia, mood, anxiety, movement disorders	Variable, frontal/executive, focal cortical, memory	Depression, anxiety	Myoclonus, rigidity, parkinsonism
Dementia with Lewy body	Visual hallucinations; delusions that family members/friends are someone else; REM sleep disorder; delirium; parkinsonism	Drawing and frontal/executive; spares memory; delirium prone	Visual hallucinations, depression, sleep disorder, delusions	Parkinsonism
Frontotemporal dementia	Apathy; poor judgment/reasoning, speech/language	Frontal/executive, language; spares drawing	Apathy, decline in person or social conduct, euphoria, depression	Due to PSP/CBD overlap; vertical gaze palsy, axial rigidity, dystonia, alien hand
Vascular dementia	Often but not always sudden, usually within 3 months of a stroke; variable: apathy, falls, focal weakness	Frontal/executive, cognitive slowing; memory can be intact	Apathy, delusions, anxiety	Usually motor slowing; can be normal

Adapted from Bird TD, Miller BL: Dementia. In Fauci AS et al, editors: *Harrison's principles of internal medicine,* ed 15, p 2538, New York, 2008, McGraw-Hill.
CBD, Cortical basal degeneration; *PSP,* progressive supranuclear palsy; *REM,* rapid eye movement.

contains a comparison of the features differentiating delirium and dementia.

QUICK CHECK 15-3
1. What are two types of dysphasia?
2. How does dysphasia differ from dysarthria?
3. What are some causes of delirium?

Dementia

Dementia is an acquired deterioration and a progressive failure of many cerebral functions that includes impairment of intellectual processes with a decrease in orienting, memory, language, judgment, and decision making. Because of declining intellectual ability, the individual may exhibit alterations in behavior, for example, agitation, wandering, and aggression.

PATHOPHYSIOLOGY Mechanisms leading to dementia include neuron degeneration, compression of brain tissue, atherosclerosis of cerebral vessels, and brain trauma. Genetic predisposition is associated with the neurodegenerative diseases, including Alzheimer, Huntington, and Parkinson diseases. CNS infections, including the human immunodeficiency virus (HIV) and slow-growing viruses associated with Creutzfeldt-Jakob disease, also lead to nerve cell degeneration and brain atrophy.

CLINICAL MANIFESTATIONS Clinical manifestations of the major dementias are presented in Table 15-11.

EVALUATION AND TREATMENT Establishing the cause for dementia may be complicated, but individuals with clinical manifestations of dementia should be evaluated with laboratory and neuropsychologic testing to identify underlying conditions that may be treatable. Unfortunately, no specific cure exists for most progressive dementias.

Therapy is directed at maintaining and maximizing use of the remaining capacities, restoring functions if possible, and accommodating to lost abilities. Helping the family to understand the process and to learn ways to assist the individual is essential.

Alzheimer Disease

Alzheimer disease (AD) (dementia of Alzheimer type [DAT], senile disease complex) is the leading cause of severe cognitive dysfunction in older persons. The three forms of AD are nonhereditary sporadic or late-onset AD (70% to 90%), early-onset familial AD (FAD), and early-onset AD (very rare). Approximately 5.2 million Americans have AD and the numbers are expected to be 7.1 million by 2015.[13]

PATHOPHYSIOLOGY The exact cause of Alzheimer disease is unknown. Early-onset FAD has been linked to three genes with mutations on chromosome 21 (abnormal amyloid precursor protein 14 [APP14], abnormal presenilin 1 [PSEN1], and abnormal presenilin 2 [PSEN2]). Late-onset AD may be related to the involvement of chromosome 19 with the apolipoprotein E gene-allele 4 (APOE4). Studies are ongoing to classify the genetic variations of AD.[14] DNA methylation is an epigenetic marker for Alzheimer disease.[15] Sporadic late-onset AD is the most common, and does not have a specific genetic association; however, the cellular pathology is the same as that for gene-associated early- and late-onset AD.[16] Pathologic alterations in the brain include accumulation of extracellular neuritic plaques containing a core of amyloid beta protein, intraneuronal neurofibrillary tangles, and degeneration of basal forebrain cholinergic neurons with loss of acetylcholine. Failure to process and clear amyloid precursor protein results in the accumulation of toxic fragments of amyloid beta protein that leads to formation of diffuse neuritic plaques, disruption of nerve impulse transmission, and death of neurons. The tau protein, a microtubule-binding protein, in neurons detaches and forms an insoluble filament called a neurofibrillary tangle, contributing to neuronal death (Figure 15-8). Neuritic plaques and neurofibrillary tangles are more concentrated in the cerebral cortex and hippocampus. The loss of neurons results in brain atrophy with widening of sulci and shrinkage of gyri (see Figure 15-8). Loss of synapses, acetylcholine and other neurotransmitters contributes to the decline of memory and attention and the loss of other cognitive functions associated with AD.[17]

CLINICAL MANIFESTATIONS AD has a long preclinical and prodromal course, and pathophysiologic changes can occur decades before the appearance of the clinical dementia syndrome. The disease progresses from mild short-term memory deficits culminating in total loss of cognitive and executive functions. Initial clinical manifestations are insidious and often are attributed to forgetfulness, emotional upset, or other illness. The individual becomes progressively more forgetful over time, particularly in relation to recent events. Memory loss increases as the disorder advances, and the person becomes disoriented and confused and loses the ability to concentrate. Abstraction, problem solving, and judgment gradually deteriorate with failure in mathematic calculation ability, language, and visuospatial orientation. Dyspraxia may appear. The mental status changes induce behavioral changes, including irritability, agitation, and restlessness. Mood changes also result from the deterioration in cognition. The person may become anxious, depressed, hostile, emotionally labile, and prone to mood swings. Motor changes may occur if the posterior frontal lobes are involved, causing rigidity and flexion posturing. Weight loss can be significant. Great variability in age of onset, intensity and sequence of symptoms, and location and extent of brain abnormalities is common. Stages for the progression of Alzheimer disease are summarized in Table 15-12.

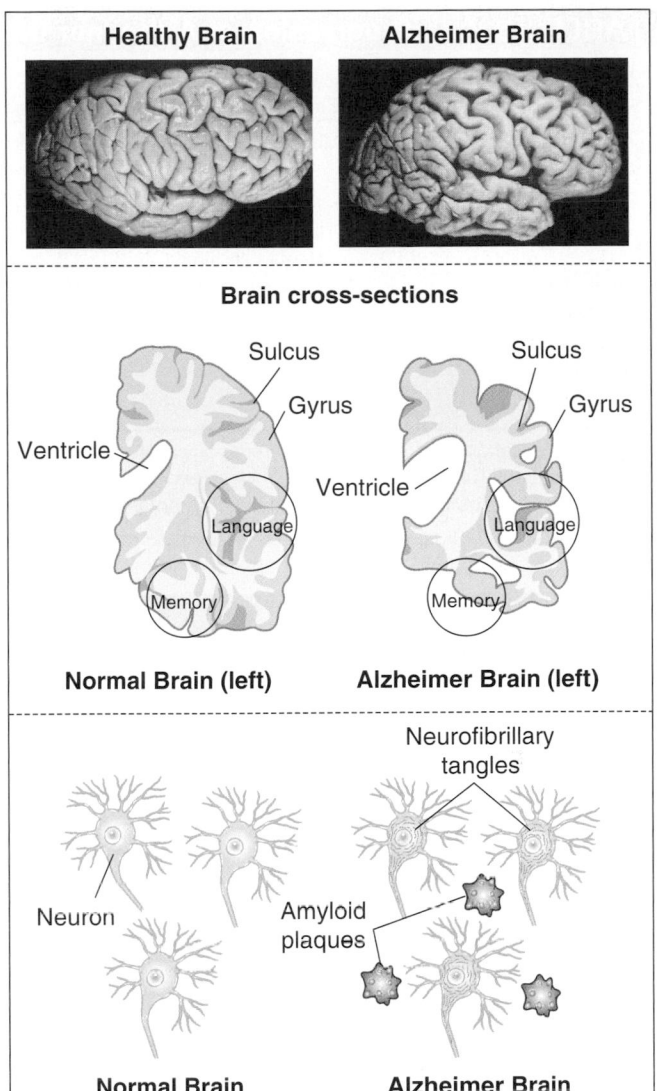

FIGURE 15-8 Common Pathologic Findings in Alzheimer Disease. The middle panel represents coronal slices through the left brain (facing anterior).

EVALUATION AND TREATMENT The diagnosis of Alzheimer disease is made by ruling out other causes. Clinical criteria have been developed to assist diagnosis.[18] The clinical history, including mental status examinations (mini–mental status examination, clock drawing, and geriatric depression scale), laboratory tests, brain imaging of structure, blood flow and metabolism, and the course of the illness (which may span 5 years or more), is used to assess progression of the disease. Efforts are in progress to identify imaging and biochemical markers for risk assessment and early diagnosis and progression of Alzheimer type and other neurodegenerative causes of dementia (see Health Alert: Biomarkers and Neurodegenerative Dementia).[19]

Treatment is directed at using devices to compensate for the impaired cognitive function, such as memory aids; maintaining unimpaired cognitive functions; and maintaining or improving the general state of hygiene, nutrition, and health. Cholinesterase inhibitors have shown a modest effect on cognitive function in mild to moderate Alzheimer disease. An N-methyl-D-aspartate (NMDA) receptor antagonist blocks glutamate activity and may slow progression of disease in

TABLE 15-12   Progression of Alzheimer Disease

Stage	Mild Cognitive Impairment	Early Stage	Middle Stage	Late Stage	End Stage
Cognitive	Mild memory loss	Measurable short-term memory loss; difficulty with word finding; other cognition problems compared with previous behavior	Moderate to severe cognitive problems: impaired reasoning, judgment, and problem solving; disorientation to time, place, and person; difficulty planning and organizing; progressive memory loss	Little cognitive ability; language not clear	No significant cognitive function; loss of orientation to self
Functional	Possibly depression (vs. apathy); mild anxiety	Mild IADL problems	IADL-dependent; some ADL problems	ADL-dependent; incontinent	Nonambulatory/bedbound; unable to eat related to failure to sense hunger or thirst, difficulty swallowing

Adapted from National Conference of Gerontological Nurse Practitioners and the National Gerontological Nursing Association: *Counseling Points* 1(1):6, 2008; Peña-Casanova J et al: *Arch Med Res* 43(8):686-693, 2012.
ADL, (Basic) activities of daily living; *IADL,* instrumental activities of daily living.

HEALTH ALERT

Biomarkers and Neurodegenerative Dementia

Neurodegenerative disease processes that lead to dementia begin many years before clinical manifestations are evident for Alzheimer disease, Huntington disease, and Parkinson disease. Efforts are under way to identify neuroimaging techniques and predictive biomarkers in the brain, spinal fluid, and blood that will guide a more comprehensive understanding of the etiology and biologic pathways that mediate neurodegeneration. Identification and profiling of such molecules and images will promote early identification of risk factors, enhance preventive and protective measures, provide alerts for progression from mild to advanced stages, and accelerate development of presymptomatic treatment for these diseases.

Data from Anstey KJ et al: *J Alzheimers Dis* 42(0):S463-S473, 2014; Cummings J, Zhong K: *Clin Pharmacol Ther* 95(1):67-77, 2014; Wurtman R: *Metabolism* 64(3 Suppl 1):S47-50, 2015.

moderate to severe AD. Treatments, beginning in the preclinical stage, are being developed to prevent, modify, or halt disease pathology.[20]

Frontotemporal Dementia

Frontotemporal dementia (FTD), previously known as Pick disease, is the second most common form of dementia and is a degenerative disease of the frontal and anterior frontal lobes. There is a familial association with an age of onset less than 60 years and an estimated incidence of 15 per 100,000. The majority of cases involve mutations of genes encoding tau protein. Three distinct clinical syndromes are presented in frontotemporal degeneration, depending on the site of atrophy: behavioral variant of frontotemporal dementia, progressive nonfluent aphasia, and semantic dementia. Differentiating pathologic and clinical diagnostic criteria are in development.[21] There is no specific treatment.

Seizure Disorders

Seizure disorders represent a manifestation of disease and not a specific disease entity. A seizure is a sudden, transient disruption in brain electrical function caused by abnormal excessive discharges of cortical neurons. Epilepsy is the recurrence of seizures and a type of seizure disorder for which no underlying, correctable cause for the seizure can be found. The term convulsion is sometimes applied to seizures and

TABLE 15-13   Structural/Metabolic Causes of Recurrent Seizures in Adults

Age at Onset	Probable Cause
Young adults (18 to 35 yr)	Alcohol or drug withdrawal (e.g., barbiturates, benzodiazepines)
	Brain tumor
	Idiopathic
	Illicit drug use (e.g., cocaine, amphetamine)
	Posttraumatic brain injury
	Perinatal insults
Older adults (>35 yr)	Alcohol or drug withdrawal (e.g., barbiturates, benzodiazepines)
	Brain tumor
	Cerebrovascular disease (e.g., stroke, aneurysm, arteriovenous malformations, infection)
	CNS degenerative diseases (e.g., Alzheimer disease, multiple sclerosis)
	Idiopathic
	Metabolic disorders (e.g., uremia, hepatic failure, electrolyte abnormalities, hypoglycemia)
	Posttraumatic brain injury

Data from Daroff RB et al: *Bradley's neurology in clinical practice,* ed 6, Saunders, 2012, Philadelphia.
CNS, Central nervous system.

refers to the tonic-clonic (jerky, contract-relax) movement associated with some seizures. Seizures in children are presented in Chapter 17.

Conditions Associated with Seizure Disorders

Any disorder that alters the neuronal environment may cause seizure activity. Conditions that may produce a seizure are metabolic disorders, congenital malformations, genetic predisposition, perinatal injury, postnatal trauma, myoclonic syndromes, infection, brain tumor, vascular disease, and drug or alcohol abuse. The onset of seizures also may indicate the presence of an ongoing primary neurologic disease. Metabolic and structural causes of recurrent seizures in adults are summarized in Table 15-13. The cause of seizures is often unknown.

The threshold for seizures may be lowered by hypoglycemia, fatigue or lack of sleep, emotional or physical stress, fever, large amounts of

TABLE 15-14 Terminology Applied to a Seizure Disorder

Term	Definition
Preictal Phase	
Prodroma	Early clinical manifestation (such as malaise, headache, or sense of depression) that may occur a few days to hours before onset of a seizure
Aura	A partial seizure experienced as a peculiar sensation preceding onset of generalized seizure that may take the form of gustatory, visual, or auditory experience or a feeling of dizziness, numbness, or just "a funny feeling"
Ictal Phase	The event of the seizure
Tonic phase	A state of muscle contraction in which there is excessive muscle tone
Clonic phase	A state of alternating contraction and relaxation of muscles
Postictal Phase	Time period immediately following cessation of seizure activity

water ingestion, constipation, use of antipsychotic drugs (i.e., chlorpromazine and clozapine) especially when combined with alcohol, withdrawal from depressant drugs (including alcohol), or hyperventilation (respiratory alkalosis). Some environmental stimuli, such as blinking lights, a poorly adjusted television screen, loud noises, certain music, certain odors, or merely being startled, have been known to initiate a seizure. Women may have increased seizure activity immediately before or during menses.

Types of Seizure

Seizures are classified in different ways: by clinical manifestations, site of origin, EEG correlates, or response to therapy. Types of seizures and clinical manifestations are presented in Chapter 17 (see Table 17-6). Terms used to describe seizure activity are defined in Table 15-14.

Epilepsy now is considered to be the result of the interaction of complex genetic mutations with environmental effects that cause abnormalities in synaptic transmission, an imbalance in the brain's neurotransmitters, or the development of abnormal nerve connections after injury.[22] A group of neurons may exhibit a paroxysmal depolarization shift and function as an **epileptogenic focus**. These neurons are hypersensitive and are more easily activated by hyperthermia, hypoxia, hypoglycemia, hyponatremia, repeated sensory stimulation, and certain sleep phases. Epileptogenic neurons fire more frequently and with greater amplitude. When the intensity reaches a threshold point, cortical excitation spreads. Excitation of the subcortical, thalamic, and brainstem areas corresponds to the **tonic phase** (muscle contraction with increased muscle tone) and is associated with loss of consciousness. The **clonic phase** (alternating contraction and relaxation of muscles) begins when inhibitory neurons in the cortex, anterior thalamus, and basal ganglia react to the cortical excitation. The seizure discharge is interrupted, producing intermittent muscle contractions that gradually decrease and finally cease. The epileptogenic neurons are exhausted.

During seizure activity, oxygen is consumed at a high rate—about 60% greater than normal. Although cerebral blood flow also increases, oxygen is rapidly depleted, along with glucose, and lactate accumulates in brain tissue. Continued, severe seizure activity has the potential for

progressive brain injury and irreversible damage. In addition, if a seizure focus in the brain is active for a prolonged period, a **mirror focus** may develop in contralateral normal tissue and cause seizure activity.

CLINICAL MANIFESTATIONS The clinical manifestations associated with seizure depend on its type (see Table 17-6). Two types of symptoms signal the **preictal phase** of a generalized tonic-clonic seizure: **prodroma**, early manifestations occurring hours to days before a seizure and may include anxiety, depression, or inability to think clearly; and a partial seizure that immediately precedes the onset of a generalized tonic-clonic seizure. Both may become familiar to the person experiencing recurrent generalized seizures and may enable the person to prevent injuries during the seizure. The **ictus** is the episode of the epileptic seizure with tonic-clonic activity. Relaxation of urinary and bowel sphincters may occur, leading to bladder and bowel incontinence. Airway maintenance needs to be ensured. **Status epilepticus** in adults is a state of continuous seizures lasting more than 5 minutes, or rapidly recurring seizures before the person has fully regained consciousness from the preceding seizure, or a single seizure lasting more than 30 minutes. The **postictal state** follows an epileptic seizure and can include signs of headache, confusion, dysphasia, memory loss, and paralysis that may last hours or a day or two. Deep sleep also is common.[23]

EVALUATION AND TREATMENT The health history, physical examination, and laboratory tests of blood and urine (concentrations of blood glucose, serum calcium, blood urea nitrogen, and urine sodium; and creatinine clearance time) can identify systemic diseases known to promote seizures. Brain imaging and cerebrospinal fluid (CSF) examination help identify neurologic diseases associated with seizures. The EEG is used to assess the type of seizure and determine its focus in brain tissue.

Treatment for a seizure disorder is to first correct or control its cause if possible. If this is not possible, the major means of management is the judicious administration of antiseizure medications. Dietary treatments (e.g., ketogenic and Adkins diet) are effective for some individuals. Surgical interventions can improve seizure control and quality of life in people with drug-resistant epilepsy.[24,25]

✔ **QUICK CHECK 15-4**
1. What is an eliptogenic focus?
2. Why can so many conditions precipitate seizures?
3. Why is continued seizing dangerous?

ALTERATIONS IN CEREBRAL HEMODYNAMICS

An injured brain reacts with structural, chemical, and pathophysiologic changes. Primary brain injury is the original trauma and secondary brain injury is a consequence of alterations in cerebral blood flow, intracranial pressure, and oxygen delivery (Box 15-4 and see Chapter 16).

Alterations in cerebral blood flow (CBF) may be related to three injury states: inadequate cerebral perfusion, normal cerebral perfusion but with an elevated intracranial pressure, and excessive cerebral blood volume (CBV). Treatments for these injury states are directed at improving or maintaining **cerebral perfusion pressure** (CPP), as well as controlling intracranial pressure.

Increased Intracranial Pressure

Increased intracranial pressure (IICP) may result from an increase in intracranial content (as occurs with tumor growth), edema, excess CSF, or hemorrhage. It necessitates an equal reduction in volume of the other cranial contents. The most readily displaced content is CSF. If intracranial pressure remains high after CSF displacement out of the cranial vault, cerebral blood volume and blood flow are altered.

In *stage 1 of intracranial hypertension,* vasoconstriction and external compression of the venous system occur in an attempt to further decrease the intracranial pressure. Thus, during the first stage of intracranial hypertension, intracranial pressure (ICP) may not change because of the effective compensatory mechanisms, and there may no detectable symptoms (Figure 15-9). Small increases in volume, however, cause an increase in pressure, and the pressure may take longer to return to baseline. This pressure change can be detected with ICP monitoring.

In *stage 2 of intracranial hypertension,* there is continued expansion of intracranial contents. The resulting increase in ICP may exceed the

ability of the brain's compensatory mechanisms to adjust. The pressure begins to compromise neuronal oxygenation, and systemic arterial vasoconstriction occurs in an attempt to elevate the systemic blood pressure sufficiently to overcome the IICP. Clinical manifestations at this stage usually are subtle and transient, including episodes of confusion, restlessness, drowsiness, and slight pupillary and breathing changes (see Figure 15-9). Interventions at this stage reduce ICP and promote better clinical outcomes.

In *stage 3 of intracranial hypertension,* ICP begins to approach arterial pressure, the brain tissues begin to experience hypoxia and hypercapnia, and the individual's condition rapidly deteriorates. Clinical manifestations include decreasing levels of arousal or central neurogenic hyperventilation, widened pulse pressure, bradycardia, and small, sluggish pupils (see Figure 15-9).

Dramatic sustained rises in ICP are not seen until all compensatory mechanisms have been exhausted. Then dramatic rises in ICP occur over a very short period. Autoregulation, the compensatory alteration in the diameter of the intracranial blood vessels designed to maintain a constant blood flow during changes in cerebral perfusion pressure, is lost with progressively increased ICP. Accumulating carbon dioxide may still cause vasodilation locally, but without autoregulation this vasodilation causes the blood pressure in the vessels to drop and the blood volume to increase. The brain volume is thus further increased and ICP continues to rise. Small increases in volume cause dramatic increases in ICP, and the pressure takes much longer to return to baseline. As the ICP begins to approach systemic blood pressure, cerebral perfusion pressure falls and cerebral perfusion slows dramatically. The brain tissues experience severe hypoxia, hypercapnia, and acidosis.

In *stage 4 of intracranial hypertension,* brain tissue shifts (herniates) from the compartment of greater pressure to a compartment of lesser pressure and IICP in one compartment of the cranial vault is not evenly distributed throughout the other vault compartments

---

BOX 15-4 Cerebral Hemodynamics

Cerebral blood flow (CBF) to the brain is normally maintained at a rate that matches local metabolic needs of the brain.

Cerebral perfusion pressure (CPP) (70-90 mm Hg) is the pressure required to perfuse the cells of the brain.

Cerebral blood volume (CBV) is the amount of blood in the intracranial vault at a given time.

Cerebral blood oxygenation is measured by oxygen saturation in the internal jugular vein.

Intracranial pressure (ICP) normally is 1 to 15 mm Hg, or 60 to 180 cm H_2O.

FIGURE 15-9 Clinical Correlates of Compensated and Uncompensated Stages of Intracranial Hypertension. (From Beare PG, Myers JL: *Principles and practice of adult health nursing,* ed 3, St Louis, 1998, Mosby.)

FIGURE 15-10 Brain Herniation Syndromes. Herniations can occur both above and below the tentorial membrane. Supratentorial: **1**, uncal (transtentorial); **2**, central; **3**, cingulate; **4**, transcalvarial (external herniation through an opening in the skull). Infratentorial: **5**, upward herniation of cerebellum; **6**, cerebellar tonsillar move down through foramen magnum.

FIGURE 15-11 Brain Edema. This coronal section of the cerebrum demonstrates marked compression in the lateral ventricles *(long arrows)* and flattening of gyri *(short arrows)* from extensive bilateral cerebral edema. Edema increases intracranial pressure, leading to herniation. (From Klatt EC: *Robbins and Cotran atlas of pathology,* ed 2, Philadelphia, 2010, Saunders.)

(see Figures 15-9 and 15-10). With this shift in brain tissue, the herniating brain tissue's blood supply is compromised, causing further ischemia and hypoxia in the herniating tissues. The volume of content within the lower pressure compartment increases, exerting pressure on the brain tissue that normally occupies that compartment, and thus impairs its blood supply. For example, herniation into the brainstem impairs the vital cardiovascular and respiratory regulatory centers and can cause death. The herniation process markedly and rapidly increases intracranial pressure. Mean systolic arterial pressure soon equals ICP, and cerebral blood flow ceases at this point. The types of herniation syndromes are outlined in Box 15-5.

Cerebral Edema

Cerebral edema is an increase in the fluid content of brain tissue (Figure 15-11). The result is increased extracellular or intracellular tissue volume. It occurs after brain insult from trauma, infection, hemorrhage, tumor, ischemia, infarction, or hypoxia. The harmful effects of cerebral edema are caused by distortion of blood vessels, displacement of brain tissues, increase in intracranial pressure, and eventual herniation of brain tissue to a different brain compartment.

Three types of cerebral edema are (1) vasogenic edema, (2) cytotoxic (metabolic) edema, and (3) interstitial edema. **Vasogenic edema** is clinically the most important type and is caused by the increased permeability of the capillary endothelium of the brain after injury to the vascular structure. The selective permeability of capillaries that comprise the blood-brain barrier is disrupted. Plasma proteins leak into the extracellular spaces, drawing water to them and increasing the water content of the brain parenchyma. Vasogenic edema begins in the area of injury and spreads, with fluid accumulating in the white matter of the ipsilateral side because the parallel myelinated fibers separate more easily. Edema promotes more edema because of ischemia from the increasing ICP.

Clinical manifestations of vasogenic edema include focal neurologic deficits, disturbances of consciousness, and a severe increase in ICP. Vasogenic edema resolves by slow diffusion.

BOX 15-5 Brain Herniation Syndrome

Supratentorial Herniation

1. *Uncal herniation.* Occurs when the uncus or hippocampal gyrus, or both, shifts from the middle fossa through the tentorial notch into the posterior fossa, compressing the ipsilateral third cranial nerve, the contralateral third cranial nerve, and the mesencephalon. Uncal herniation generally is caused by an expanding mass in the lateral region of the middle fossa. The classic manifestations of uncal herniation are a decreasing level of consciousness, pupils that become sluggish before fixing and dilating (first the ipsilateral, then the contralateral pupil), Cheyne-Stokes respirations (which later shift to central neurogenic hyperventilation), and the appearance of decorticate and then decerebrate posturing.

2. *Central herniation.* Occurs when there is a straight downward shift of the diencephalon through the tentorial notch. It may be caused by injuries or masses located around the outer perimeter of the frontal, parietal, or occipital lobes; extracerebral injuries around the central apex (top) of the cranium; bilaterally positioned injuries or masses; and unilateral cingulate gyrus herniation. The individual rapidly becomes unconscious; moves from Cheyne-Stokes respirations to apnea; develops small, reactive pupils and then dilated, fixed pupils; and passes from decortication to decerebration.

3. *Cingulate gyrus herniation.* Occurs when the cingulate gyrus shifts under the falx cerebri. Little is known about its clinical manifestations.

4. *Transcalvarial.* The brain shifts through a skull fracture or a surgical opening in the skull. This type of external herniation may occur during a craniectomy—surgery in which a flap of skull is removed. This type of herniation prevents the piece of skull from being replaced.

Infratentorial Herniation

1. The most common syndrome is *cerebellar tonsillar.* The cerebellar tonsil shifts through the foramen magnum because of increased pressure within the posterior fossa. The clinical manifestations are an arched stiff neck, paresthesias in the shoulder area, decreased consciousness, respiratory abnormalities, and pulse rate variations. Occasionally the force produces an *upward transtentorial* herniation of a cerebellar tonsil or the lower brainstem. There is increased ICP but no specific set of clinical manifestations associated with infratentorial herniation (see Figure 15-10).

In cytotoxic (metabolic) edema, toxic factors directly affect the cellular elements of the brain parenchyma (neuronal, glial, and endothelial cells), causing failure of the active transport systems. The cells lose their potassium and gain larger amounts of sodium. Water follows by osmosis into the cells, so that the cells swell. Cytotoxic edema occurs principally in the gray matter and may increase vasogenic edema.

Interstitial edema is seen most often with noncommunicating hydrocephalus. The edema is caused by transependymal movement of CSF from the ventricles into the extracellular spaces of the brain tissues. The brain fluid volume increases predominantly around the ventricles, with increased hydrostatic pressure within the white matter. The size of the white matter is reduced because of the rapid disappearance of myelin lipids.

Hydrocephalus

The term hydrocephalus refers to various conditions characterized by excess fluid in the cerebral ventricles, subarachnoid space, or both. Hydrocephalus occurs because of interference with CSF flow caused by increased fluid production, obstruction within the ventricular system, or defective reabsorption of the fluid. A tumor of the choroid plexus may, in rare instances, cause overproduction of CSF. The types of hydrocephalus are reviewed in Table 15-15.

Hydrocephalus may develop from infancy through adulthood. Communicating hydrocephalus is defective resorption of CSF from the cerebral subarachnoid space and is found more often in adults. Noncommunicating hydrocephalus (internal hydrocephalus, intraventricular hydrocephalus) is obstruction within the ventricular system and is seen more often in children (see Figure 17-6). Congenital hydrocephalus is ventricular enlargement before birth and is rare.

PATHOPHYSIOLOGY   The obstruction of CSF flow associated with hydrocephalus produces increased pressure and dilation of the ventricles proximal to the obstruction. The increased pressure and dilation cause atrophy of the cerebral cortex and degeneration of the white matter tracts. Selective preservation of gray matter occurs. When excess CSF fills a defect caused by atrophy, a degenerative disorder, or a surgical excision, this fluid is not under pressure; therefore atrophy and degenerative changes do not occur.

CLINICAL MANIFESTATIONS   Most cases of hydrocephalus develop gradually and insidiously over time. Acute hydrocephalus presents with signs of rapidly developing IICP. The person quickly deteriorates into a deep coma if not promptly treated. Normal-pressure hydrocephalus (dilation of the ventricles without increased pressure) develops slowly, with the individual or family noting declining memory and cognitive function. The triad symptoms of an unsteady, broad-based gait with a history of falling; incontinence; and dementia is common and may be treated surgically.[26]

EVALUATION AND TREATMENT   The diagnosis is based on physical examination, computed tomography (CT) scan, and magnetic resonance imaging (MRI). A radioisotopic cisternogram may be performed to diagnose normal-pressure hydrocephalus. Hydrocephalus can be treated by surgery to resect cysts, neoplasms, or hematomas or by ventricular bypass into the normal intracranial channel or into an extracranial compartment using a shunting procedure, one of the three most common neurosurgical procedures. Excision or coagulation of the choroid plexus occasionally is needed when a papilloma is present. In normal-pressure hydrocephalus, reduction in CSF is achieved through diuresis or placement of a ventriculoperitoneal shunt.[27]

✓**QUICK CHECK 15-5**
1. What are the four stages of increased intracranial pressure?
2. How does supratentorial herniation differ from infratentorial herniation?
3. What are the different types of cerebral edema?
4. How is communicating hydrocephalus different from noncommunicating hydrocephalus?

ALTERATIONS IN NEUROMOTOR FUNCTION

Movements are complex patterns of activity controlled by the cerebral cortex, the pyramidal system, the extrapyramidal system, and the motor units. Dysfunction in any of these areas can cause motor dysfunction. General neuromotor dysfunctions are associated with changes in muscle tone, movement, and complex motor performance.

Alterations in Muscle Tone

Normal muscle tone involves a slight resistance to passive movement. Throughout the range of motion, the resistance is smooth, constant, and even. The alterations of muscle tone and their characteristics and causes are presented in Table 15-16.

Hypotonia

In hypotonia (decreased muscle tone), passive movement of a muscle occurs with little or no resistance. Causes include cerebellar damage and pure pyramidal tract damage (a rare occurrence). The hypotonia contributes to the ataxia and intention tremor in cerebellar damage and manifests with minimal weakness and normal or slightly exaggerated reflexes. A pure pyramidal tract injury produces hypotonia and weakness. Hypotonia also occurs when the nerve impulses needed for muscle tone are lost, such as in spinal cord injury or cerebrovascular accident.

Individuals with hypotonia tire easily or are weak. They may have difficulty rising from a sitting position, sitting down without using arm support, and walking up and down stairs, as well as an inability to stand

TABLE 15-15   Types of Hydrocephalus

Type	Mechanism	Cause
Noncommunicating	Obstruction of CSF flow between ventricles	Congenital abnormality
	Aqueduct stenosis	
	Arnold-Chiari malformation (brain extension through foramen magnum)	
	Compression by tumor	
Communicating	Impaired absorption of CSF within subarachnoid space	Infection with inflammatory adhesions
	Compression of subarachnoid space by a tumor	
	High venous pressure in sagittal sinus	
	Head injury	
	Congenital malformation	
	Increased CSF secretion by choroid plexus	Secreting tumor

CSF, Cerebrospinal fluid.

TABLE 15-16 Alterations in Muscle Tone

Alterations	Characteristics	Cause
Hypotonia	Passive movement of a muscle mass with little or no resistance Muscles may be moved rapidly without resistance	Thought to be caused by decreased muscle spindle activity as a result of decreased excitability of neurons (e.g., muscular dystrophy, cerebral palsy)
Flaccidity	Associated with limp, atrophied muscles, and paralysis	Occurs typically when nerve impulses necessary for muscle tone are lost
Hypertonia	Increased muscle resistance to passive movement May be associated with paralysis May be accompanied by muscle hypertrophy	Results when lower motor unit reflex arc continues to function but is not mediated or regulated by higher centers (e.g., stroke, brain tumors, multiple sclerosis)
Spasticity	A gradual increase in tone causing increased resistance until tone suddenly diminishes, which results in clasp-knife phenomenon; increased deep tendon reflexes (hyperreflexia); clonus (spread of reflexes)	Exact mechanism unclear; appears to arise from an increased excitability of alpha motor neurons to any input because of absence of descending inhibition of pyramidal systems (e.g., multiple sclerosis, brain trauma, cerebral palsy)
Paratonia (gegenhalten)	Resistance to passive movement, which varies in direct proportion to force applied	Exact mechanism unclear; associated with frontal lobe injury (e.g., progressive Alzheimer dementia)
Dystonia	Sustained involuntary muscle contraction with twisting movement	Produced by slow muscular contraction; lack of reciprocal inhibition of muscle (e.g., neuroleptic drug side effects, meningitis)
Rigidity	Muscle resistance to passive movement of a rigid limb that is uniform in both flexion and extension throughout the motion	Occurs as a result of constant, involuntary contraction of muscle—usually involves extrapyramidal tracts (e.g., Parkinson disease)
Plastic or lead-pipe rigidity	Increased muscular tone relatively independent of degree of force used in passive movement; does not vary throughout the passive movement	Associated with basal ganglion damage (e.g., Parkinson disease)
Cogwheel rigidity	Uniform resistance may be interrupted by a series of brief jerks, resulting in movements much like a ratchet, "cogwheel" phenomenon	Associated with basal ganglion damage
Gamma rigidity	Characterized by extensor posturing (decerebrate rigidity)	Loss of excitation of extensor inhibitory areas by cerebral cortex decreasing inhibition of alpha and gamma motor neurons
Alpha rigidity	Impaired relaxation characterized by extensor rigidity of skeletal muscle after contraction	Loss of cerebellum input to lateral vestibular nuclei

on their toes. Because of their weakness, accidents during ambulatory and self-care activities are common. The joints become hyperflexible, so persons with hypotonia may be able to assume positions that require extreme joint mobility. The joints may appear loose. The muscle mass atrophies because of decreased input entering the motor unit, and muscles appear flabby and flat. Muscle cells are gradually replaced by connective tissue and fat. Fasciculations may be present in some cases.

Hypertonia

In hypertonia (increased muscle tone), passive movement of a muscle occurs with resistance to stretch and is caused by upper motor neuron damage (see p. 381). The four types of hypertonia are spasticity (usually corticospinal in origin) (Figures 15-12 and 15-13), paratonia (gegenhalten), dystonia (Figure 15-14), and rigidity (usually extrapyramidal in origin). Four types of rigidity are described: plastic or lead-pipe, cogwheel, gamma (independent of stretch reflex pathways), and alpha (dependent on stretch reflex pathways) (see Table 15-16).

Individuals with hypertonia tire easily or are weak. Passive movement and active movement are affected equally, except in paratonia, in which more active than passive movement is possible. As a result of hypertonia and weakness, accidents occur during ambulatory and self-care activities.

The muscles may atrophy because of decreased use. However, hypertrophy occasionally occurs as a result of the overstimulation of muscle fibers. Overstimulation occurs when the motor unit reflex arc remains intact and functioning but is not inhibited by higher centers. This causes continual muscle contraction, resulting in enlargement of the muscle mass and the development of firm muscles.

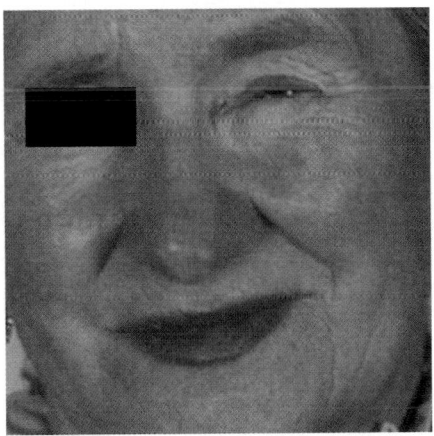

FIGURE 15-12 Paroxysm of Left-Sided Hemifacial Spasm. (From Perkin GD: *Mosby's color atlas and text of neurology,* ed 2, London, 2002, Mosby.)

Alterations in Muscle Movement

Movement requires a change in the contractile state of muscles. Abnormal movements occur when CNS dysfunction alters muscle innervation. The neurotransmitter *dopamine* has a role in several movement disorders. Some movement disorders (e.g., the akinesias) result from too little dopaminergic activity, whereas others (e.g., chorea, ballism, tardive dyskinesia) result from too much dopaminergic activity. Still others are not primarily related to dopamine function. Movement

FIGURE 15-13 Dystonic Posturing of the Hand and Foot. (From Perkin GD: *Mosby's color atlas and text of neurology*, ed 2, London, 2002, Mosby.)

FIGURE 15-14 Spasmodic Torticollis. A characteristic head posture related to spasticity. (From Perkin GD: *Mosby's color atlas and text of neurology*, ed 2, London, 2002, Mosby.)

Tardive dyskinesia is the involuntary movement of the face, lip, tongue, trunk, and extremities. Although the condition occurs occasionally in individuals with Parkinson disease, it usually occurs as a side effect of prolonged antipsychotic drug therapy. The most common symptom of tardive dyskinesia is rapid, repetitive, stereotypic movements, such as continual chewing with intermittent protrusions of the tongue, lip smacking, and facial grimacing. The symptoms also are called extrapyramidal symptoms because the extrapyramidal system controls involuntary reflexes and coordination of movement and posture (see p. 386).

Other movement disorders in this category are (1) complex repetitive movements, including automatism (unconscious behavior), stereotypy (ritualistic behavior such as rocking), complex tics such as Tourette syndrome (see *Health Alert:* Tourette Syndrome), compulsions, perseverations, and mannerisms; (2) excessive reactions to certain stimuli; and (3) paroxysmal excessive activity, including cataplexy and excessive startle reaction.

HEALTH ALERT
Tourette Syndrome

There is growing evidence that Tourette syndrome (TS) occurs worldwide and has common features across all races and cultures. The hallmark of TS is the presence of motor tics (sudden, rapid, repetitive nonrhythmic movements) and vocal tics. The tics may be either simple, involving only an individual muscle group (e.g., eye blinking or grunting), or complex, requiring coordinated movement of muscle groups (e.g., head banging or repeating of another person's words). Sensory tics involve unpleasant sensations in the face, head, and neck areas. Probably underdiagnosed, the onset of TS is typically between the ages of 2 and 15 years, with the tics lessening in adulthood. The syndrome has a complex multifactorial etiology with undetermined genetic, environmental, immune, and hormonal factors. The pathophysiology of TS is unclear and currently under study. There is evidence of cortico-striato-thalamocortical dysfunction and, in some cases, altered dopaminergic neurotransmission. TS is often diagnosed in association with anxiety, depression, attention-deficit/hyperactivity disorder (ADHD), and obsessive-compulsive disorder. Habit reversal therapy is the most common behavioral therapy and all behavioral therapy needs further investigation. Pharmacologic treatments target symptoms and have significant side effects. New drugs are being evaluated to identify the best outcomes. Deep brain stimulation is under investigation.

Data from Cohen SC et al: *Neurosci Biobehav Rev* 37(6):997-1007, 2013; Frank M, Cavanna AE: *Behav Neurol* 27(1):105-117, 2013; Ganos C et al: *Neurosci Biobehav Rev* 37(6):1050-1062, 2013; Hirschtritt ME et al *J Am Med Assoc Psychiatry* 72(4):325-333, 2015; Paschou P: *Neurosci Biobehav Rev* 37(6):1026-1039, 2013; Plessen KJ: *Eur Child Adolesc Psychiatry* 22(Suppl 1):S55-60, 2013; Schrock LE et al: *Mov Disord* 30(4):448-471, 2015; Thomas R, Cavanna AE: *J Neural Transm* 120(4):689-694, 2013.

disorders are not necessarily associated with muscle mass, strength, or tone but are neurologic dysfunctions resulting in insufficient or excessive movement or involuntary movement.

Hyperkinesia is excessive, purposeless movement and represents the second broad category of abnormal movements. Within this category are a number of specific dysfunctions including tremors (Table 15-17). Also included under the general category of hyperkinesias are *dyskinesias* and abnormal involuntary movements. Huntington disease symptoms are the hallmark of hyperkinesia.

Paroxysmal dyskinesias are abnormal, involuntary movements that occur as spasms. The type of dyskinesia varies depending on the specific disorder.

Hypokinesia is decreased amplitude of movement, bradykinesia is decreased speed of movement, and akinesia is absence of voluntary movement. These are all terms that represent a deficit of voluntary movement. Parkinson disease symptoms are the hallmark of a lack of voluntary movement.

Huntington Disease

Huntington disease (HD), also known as *chorea*, is a relatively rare, hereditary, degenerative hyperkinetic movement disorder diffusely involving the basal ganglia and cerebral cortex. The onset of Huntington disease is usually between 25 and 45 years of age, when the trait

TABLE 15-17 Types of Hyperkinesia and Tremor

Type	Characteristics	Causes
Hyperkinesia		
Chorea*	Nonrepetitive muscular contractions, usually of extremities of face; random pattern of irregular, involuntary rapid contractions of groups of muscles; disappears with sleep, decreases with resting; increases with emotional stress and attempted voluntary movement	Associated with excess concentration of or supersensitivity to dopamine within basal ganglia
Athetosis*	Disorder of distal muscle postural fixation; slow, sinuous, irregular movements most obvious in distal extremities, more rhythmic than choreiform movements and always much slower; movements accompany characteristic hand posture; slowly fluctuating grimaces	Occurs most commonly as result of injury to putamen of basal ganglion; exact pathophysiologic mechanism is not known
Ballism	Disorder of proximal muscle postural fixation with wild flinging movement of limbs; movement is severe and stereotyped, usually lateral; does not lessen with sleep; ballism is most common on one side of body, a condition termed *hemiballism*	Results from injury to subthalamic nucleus (one of nuclei that comprise basal ganglia); thought to be caused by reduced inhibitory influence in nucleus, a release phenomenon; hemiballism results from injury to contralateral subthalamic nucleus
Hyperactivity	State of prolonged, generalized, increased activity that is largely involuntary but may be subject to some voluntary control; not highly stereotyped but rather manifests as continuous changes in total body posture or in excessive performance of some simple activity, such as pacing under inappropriate circumstances	May be caused by frontal and reticular activating system injury
Wandering	Tendency to wander without regard for environment	"Release phenomenon" associated with bilateral injury to globus pallidus or putamen
Akathisia	Special type of hyperactivity; mild compulsion to move (usually more localized to legs); severe, frenzied motion possible; movements are partly voluntary and may be transiently suppressed; carrying out movement brings sense of relief; frequent complication of antipsychotic drugs	Dopaminergic transmission may be involved
Tremor at Rest		
Parkinsonian tremor	Rhythmic, oscillating movement affecting one or more body parts Regular, rhythmic, slower flexion-extension contraction; involves principally metacarpophalangeal and wrist joints; alternating movements between thumb and index finger described as "pill rolling"; disappears during voluntary movement	Caused by regular contraction of opposing groups of muscles Loss of inhibitory influence of dopamine in the basal ganglia, causing instability of basal ganglial feedback circuit within cerebral cortex
Postural Tremor		
Asterixis (tremor of hepatic encephalopathy)	Irregular flapping movement of hands accentuated by outstretching arms	Exact mechanisms responsible unknown; thought to be related to accumulation of products normally detoxified by liver (e.g., ammonia)
Metabolic	Rapid, rhythmic tremor affecting fingers, lips, and tongue; accentuated by extending body part; enhanced physiologic tremor	Occurs in conditions associated with disturbed metabolism or toxicity, as in thyrotoxicosis (hyperthyroidism), alcoholism, and chronic use of barbiturates, amphetamines, lithium, or amitriptyline (Elavil); exact mechanism responsible unknown
Essential (familial)	Tremor of fingers, hands, and feet; absent at rest but accentuated by extension of body part, prolonged muscular activity, and stress	Not associated with any other neurologic abnormalities; cause unknown
Intention Tremor		
Cerebellar	Tremor initiated by movement, maximal toward end of movement	Occurs in disease of dentate nucleus (one of deep cerebellar nuclei responsible for efferent output) and superior cerebellar peduncle (stalklike structure connected to pons); caused by errors in feedback from periphery and errors in preprogramming goal-directed movement
Rubral	Rhythmic tremor of limbs that originates proximally by movement	Results from lesions involving dentatorubrothalamic tract (a spinothalamic tract connecting red nucleus in reticular formation and dentate nucleus in cerebellum)
Myoclonus	Series of shocklike, nonpatterned contractions of portion of a muscle, entire muscle, or group of muscles that cause throwing movements of a limb; usually appear at random but frequently triggered by sudden startle; do not disappear during sleep	Associated with an irritable nervous system and spontaneous discharge of neurons; structures associated with myoclonus include cerebral cortex, cerebellum, reticular formation, and spinal cord

*Choreoathetosis involves both chorea and athetosis; precise pathophysiology is unknown.

may already have been passed to the person's children. The disorder has a prevalence rate of approximately 5 to 10 per 100,000 persons and occurs in all races.[28]

PATHOPHYSIOLOGY HD is inherited from one or both parents who have the autosomal dominant trait with high penetrance. The genetic defect of HD is on the short arm of chromosome 4. There is an abnormally long polyglutamine tract in the huntingtin (htt) protein that is toxic to neurons caused by a cytosine-adenine-guanine (CAG) trinucleotide repeat expansion (40 to 70 repeats instead of 9 to 34) with abnormal protein folding. Age of symptom onset is related to the length of the repeat sequences and mechanisms of toxicity. Repeat lengths greater than 60 cause the juvenile form of the disease.[29] Fathers, but not mothers, with high normal alleles do not develop HD but are at risk of transmitting potentially penetrant HD alleles (≥36) to their offspring, who can develop HD.[30]

The principal pathologic feature of Huntington disease is severe degeneration of the basal ganglia, particularly the caudate nucleus. Tangles of protein (huntingtin protein) collect in the brain cells and chains of glutamine on the abnormal molecules stick to each other and contribute to neuronal loss. Basal ganglia and nigral depletion of gamma-aminobutyric acid (GABA), an inhibitory neurotransmitter, is the principal biochemical alteration in Huntington disease. It alters the integration of motor and mental function.[31]

CLINICAL MANIFESTATIONS Symptoms of Huntington disease progress slowly and include involuntary fragmentary movements, such as chorea, athetosis, and ballism (see Table 15-17). Chorea, the most common type of abnormal movement, begins in the face and arms, eventually affecting the entire body. There is emotional lability and progressive dysfunction of intellectual and thought processes (dementia). Any one of these features may mark the onset of the disease. Cognitive deficits include loss of working memory and reduced capacity to plan, organize, and sequence. Thinking is slow, and apathy is present. Restlessness, disinhibition, and irritability are common. Euphoria or depression may be present.

EVALUATION AND TREATMENT The diagnosis of Huntington disease is based on family history and clinical presentation of the disorder. Neuroradiologic abnormalities can be demonstrated up to 15 years before clinical symptoms. No known treatment is effective in halting the degeneration or progression of symptoms and the disease is fatal. Symptomatic drug therapies are available.[32]

Hypokinesia

Hypokinesia (decreased movement) is loss of voluntary movement despite preserved consciousness and normal peripheral nerve and muscle function. Types of hypokinesia include akinesia, bradykinesia, and loss of associated movement.

Akinesia and bradykinesia. Akinesia is a decrease in voluntary and associated movements. It is related to dysfunction of the extrapyramidal system and caused by either a deficiency of dopamine or a defect of the postsynaptic dopamine receptors, which occurs in parkinsonism. Bradykinesia is slowness of voluntary movements. All voluntary movements become slow, labored, and deliberate, with difficulty in (1) initiating movements, (2) continuing movements smoothly, and (3) performing synchronous (at the same time) and consecutive tasks. Both akinesia and bradykinesia involve a delay in the time it takes to start to perform a movement.

Loss of associated movement. In hypokinesia, the normal, habitually associated movements that provide skill, grace, and balance to voluntary movements are lost. Decreased associated movements

accompanying emotional expression cause an expressionless face, a statue-like posture, absence of speech inflection, and absence of spontaneous gestures. Decreased associated movements accompanying locomotion cause reduction in arm and shoulder movements, hip swinging, and rotary motion of the cervical spine.

Parkinson Disease

Parkinson disease (PD) is a complex motor disorder accompanied by systemic nonmotor and neurologic symptoms. Etiologic classification of parkinsonism includes primary parkinsonism and secondary parkinsonism. Primary PD begins after the age of 40 years, with the incidence increasing after 60 years. It is more prevalent in males and a leading cause of neurologic disability in individuals older than 60 years. Approximately 60,000 new cases are diagnosed in the United States each year.[33] The familial form represents about 10% of PD; however, the majority of cases are sporadic or idiopathic. Secondary parkinsonism is parkinsonism caused by disorders other than Parkinson disease (i.e., head trauma, infection, neoplasm, atherosclerosis, toxins, drug intoxication). Drug-induced parkinsonism, caused by neuroleptics, antiemetics, and antihypertensives, is the most common secondary form and usually is reversible.

PATHOPHYSIOLOGY The pathogenesis of primary PD is unknown. Several gene mutations have been identified that influence nerve function in PD. Gene-environment interactions are probable causes of neurodegeneration in PD. The primary pathology is degeneration of the basal ganglia (see Figure 13-10) with dysfunctional or misfolded α-synuclein protein and loss of dopamine-producing neurons in the substantia nigra and dorsal striatum. The resulting depletion of dopamine, an inhibitory neurotransmitter, and relative excess of cholinergic (excitatory) activity in the feedback circuit are manifested by hypertonia (tremor and rigidity) and akinesia, producing a syndrome of abnormal movement called parkinsonism (Parkinson syndrome, parkinsonian syndrome, paralysis agitans) (Figure 15-15). Neuroimaging shows degeneration of dopaminergic neurons preceding the

FIGURE 15-15 Pathophysiology of Parkinson Disease.

onset of motor symptoms by as long as 3 to 6 years.[34] Dementia may develop over decades with infiltration of Lewy bodies (accumulation of abnormal protein in nerve cells) and plaque formation similar to Alzheimer disease.[35] Loss of cholinergic subcortical input into the cortex is associated with nonmotor symptoms of PD.[36]

CLINICAL MANIFESTATIONS The classic manifestations of Parkinson disease are resting tremor, rigidity, bradykinesia/akinesia, postural disturbance, dysarthria, and dysphagia. They may develop alone or in combination, but as the disease progresses, all are usually present. There is no true paralysis. The symptoms are always bilateral but usually involve one side early in the illness. Because the onset is insidious, the beginning of symptoms is difficult to document. Early in the disease, reflex status, sensory status, and mental status usually are normal. Loss of smell can be an early nonmotor symptom. Postural abnormalities (flexed, forward leaning), difficulty walking, and weakness develop as neurodegeneration progresses (Figure 15-16). Speech may be slurred.

Disorders of equilibrium result from postural abnormalities. The person with Parkinson disease cannot make the appropriate postural adjustment to tilting or falling and falls like a post when starting to tilt. The festinating gait (short, accelerating steps) of the individual with Parkinson disease is an attempt to maintain an upright position while walking. Individuals are also unable to right themselves when changing from a reclining or crouching position to a standing position and when rolling over from a supine to a lateral or prone position. Sleep disorders and excessive daytime sleepiness are commonly experienced. Sensory disturbances (pain and impaired smell and vision), urinary urgency, difficulty concentrating, depression, and hallucinations are some of the nonmotor symptoms of Parkinson disease.[37,38] Autonomic-neuroendocrine changes also contribute to nonmotor symptoms and include inappropriate diaphoresis, orthostatic hypotension, drooling, gastric retention, constipation, and urinary retention.

Progressive dementia is more common in persons older than 70 years. Mental status may be further compromised by the side effects of the medication taken to control symptoms.

EVALUATION AND TREATMENT The diagnosis of Parkinson disease is based on the history and clinical features of the disease. Causes of secondary parkinsonism are first excluded. Specific gene panels and imaging studies are evolving for early diagnosis.[39] Treatment of Parkinson disease is symptomatic with drug therapy to decrease akinesia. Because of troublesome side effects and loss of effectiveness, however, drug therapy may not be started until the symptoms become incapacitating. Deep brain stimulation (i.e., subthalamic neurostimulation) is replacing surgery to treat persons unresponsive to drug therapy. Implants of stem cells and fetal cells, as well as gene therapy, are strategies for future treatments.[40] Dysphagia and general immobility are special problems of the individual with PD requiring interdisciplinary efforts to improve functional status.[41]

Upper and Lower Motor Neuron Syndromes

Paresis and paralysis are symptoms of upper and lower motor neuron syndromes (Table 15-18). Paresis (weakness) is partial paralysis with incomplete loss of muscle power. Paralysis is loss of motor function so that a muscle group is unable to overcome gravity.

Upper Motor Neuron Syndromes

Upper motor neuron syndromes are the result of damage to descending motor pathways at cortical, brainstem, or spinal cord levels. Upper motor neuron paresis/paralysis is known also as *spastic paresis/paralysis*, and different terms are used to describe the specific disorders (Box 15-6).

Upper motor neuron paresis/paralysis is associated with a pyramidal motor syndrome, which involves a series of motor dysfunctions resulting from interruption of the pyramidal system (Figures 15-17 and 15-18). The injury may be in the cerebral cortex, the subcortical

FIGURE 15-16 Stooped Posture of Parkinson Disease. (From Perkin DG: *Mosby's color atlas and text of neurology,* ed 2, London, 2002, Mosby.)

Labels on figure:
Tremor
Masked facies
Stooped posture
Rigidity
Arms and wrists flexed, reduced swing
Tremor
Slow movement, poor balance
Hips and knees slightly flexed
Tremor
Short shuffling steps

TABLE 15-18 Upper and Lower Motor Neuron Syndromes Signs and Symptoms	
Upper Motor Neuron (Pyramidal Cells—Motor Cortex)	**Lower Motor Neuron (Cranial Nerve Nuclei—Brainstem; Ventral Horn—Spinal Cord)**
Muscle groups are affected	Individual muscles may be affected
Mild weakness	Mild weakness
Minimal disuse muscle atrophy	Marked muscle atrophy
No fasciculations	Fasciculations
Increased muscle stretch reflexes (clasp-knife spasticity; resistance to passive flexion that releases abruptly to allow easy flexion)	Decreased muscle stretch reflexes
Clonus may be present	Clonus not present
Hypertonia, spasticity	Hypotonia, flaccidity Hyporeflexia
Pathologic reflexes (Babinski and Hoffmann signs, loss of abdominal reflexes)	No Babinski sign
Often initial impairment of only skilled movements	Asymmetric and may involve one limb only in beginning to become generalized as disease progresses

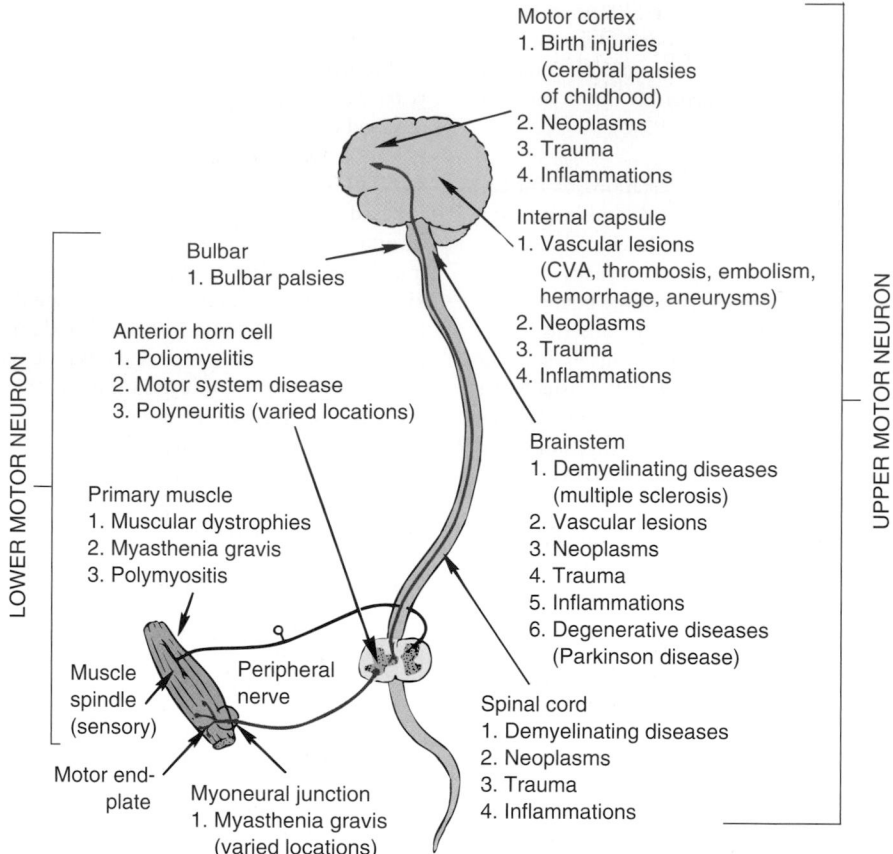

FIGURE 15-17 Motor Function Syndromes. Disturbances in motor function are classified pathologically along upper and lower motor neuron structures. It should be noted that the same pathologic condition occurs at more than one site in an upper motor neuron *(top right)*. A few pathologic conditions involve both upper and lower motor neuron structures, as in amyotrophic lateral sclerosis, for example. Other lesion sites include myoneural junction and primary muscle, making it possible to classify conditions as neuromuscular and muscular, respectively.

BOX 15-6 **Upper Motor Neuron Paralysis**

Hemiparesis/hemiplegia is paresis/paralysis of the upper and lower extremities on one side.

Diplegia is paralysis of corresponding parts of both sides of the body as a result of cerebral hemisphere injuries.

Paraparesis/paraplegia is weakness/paralysis of the lower extremities as a result of lower spinal cord injury.

Quadriparesis/quadriplegia is paresis/paralysis of all four extremities as a result of upper spinal cord injury (spinal cord injury is discussed in Chapter 16).

white matter, the internal capsule, the brainstem, or the spinal cord. The clinical manifestations reflect muscle overactivity and include excessive movements, such as clonus and spasms, occurring regularly as a result of loss of higher motor center control. There is great variation depending on the suddenness of onset and the age of the individual.

Spinal shock is the temporary loss of all spinal cord functions below the lesion (below the level of the pons). It is characterized by complete flaccid paralysis, absence of reflexes, and marked disturbances of bowel and bladder function. Hypotension can occur from loss of sympathetic tone at higher levels of spinal cord injury. A major factor in spinal shock is the sudden destruction of the efferent pathways. If destruction occurs more slowly, spinal shock may not develop (see Chapter 16).

If the pyramidal system is interrupted above the level of the pons, the hand and arm muscles are greatly affected. Paralysis rarely involves all the muscles on one side of the body, even when the hemiplegia results from complete damage to the internal capsule. Bilateral movements, such as those of the eye, jaw, and larynx, as well as those of the trunk, are affected only slightly, if at all. Predominantly the limbs are influenced.

Paralysis associated with a pyramidal motor syndrome rarely remains flaccid for a prolonged time. After a few days or weeks, a gradual return of spinal reflexes marks the end of spinal shock. Reflexes then become hyperactive, and muscle tone increases significantly, particularly in antigravity muscles. *Spasticity* is common, although rigidity occasionally occurs (see p. 377). Most often, passive range-of-motion movements cause "clasp-knife" rigidity, probably by activating the stretch receptors in the muscle spindles and the Golgi tendon organ. (Muscle function is discussed in Chapter 38.) With pyramidal motor syndrome, predominantly the flexors of the arms and the extensors of the legs are affected.

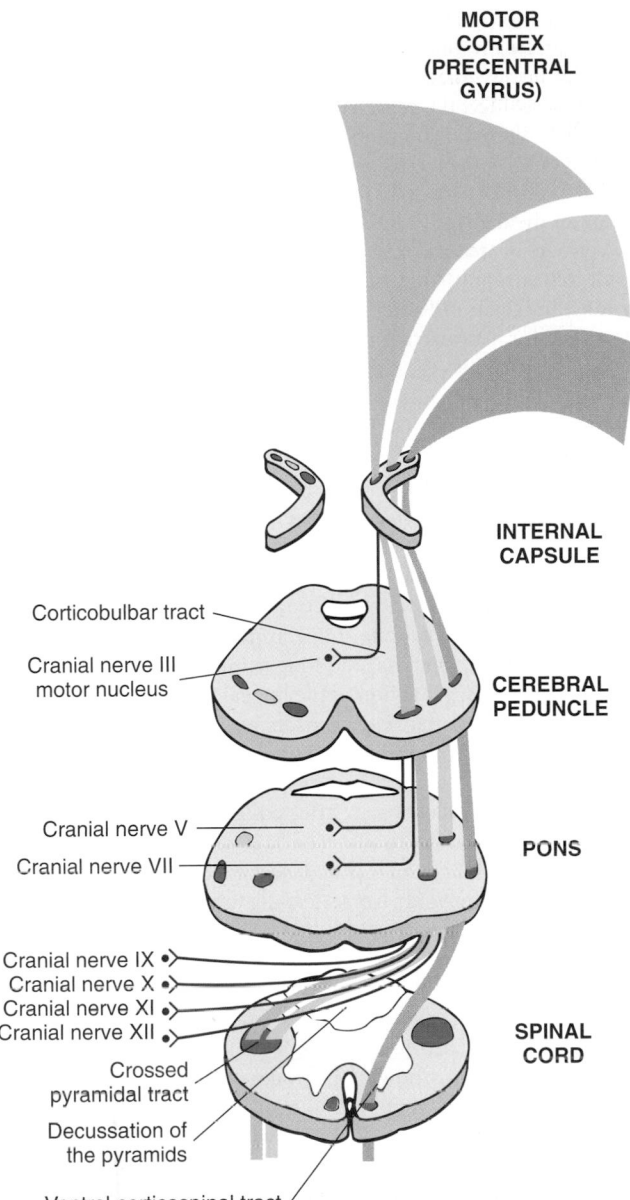

FIGURE 15-18 Structures of the Upper Motor Neuron, or Pyramidal, System. Pyramidal system fibers are shown to originate primarily in cells in the precentral gyrus of the motor cortex; to converge at the internal capsule; to descend to form the central third of the cerebral peduncle; to descend further through the pons, where small fibers supply cranial nerve motor nuclei along the way; to form pyramids at the medulla, where most of the fibers decussate; and then to continue to descend in the lateral column of white matter of the spinal cord. A few fibers descend without crossing at the level of the medulla (i.e., the ventral (anterior) corticospinal tract).

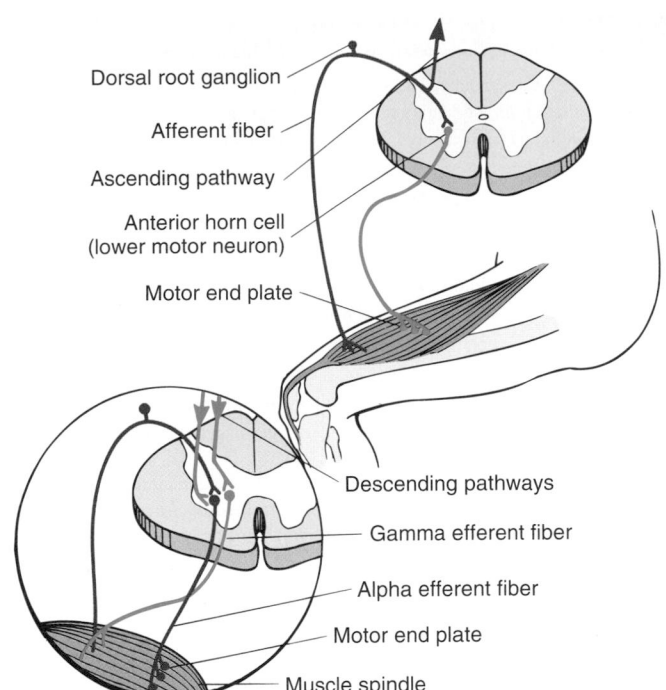

FIGURE 15-19 Structures Composing Lower Motor Neuron, Including Motor (Efferent) and Sensory (Afferent) Elements. *(Top)* Anterior horn cell (in anterior gray column of spinal cord and its axon), terminating in motor end plate as it innervates extrafusal muscle fibers in quadriceps muscle. *(Detailed enlargement)* Sensory and motor elements of gamma loop system. Gamma efferent fibers shown innervating the muscle spindle (sensory receptor of skeletal muscle). Contraction of muscle spindle fibers stretches the central portion of the spindle and causes the gamma afferent spindle fiber to transmit impulse centrally to the cord. Muscle spindle gamma afferent fibers in turn synapse on the anterior horn cell, and impulses are transmitted by way of alpha efferent fibers to skeletal (extrafusal) muscle, causing it to contract. Muscle spindle discharge is interrupted by active contraction of skeletal muscle fibers.

Lower Motor Neuron Syndromes

Lower (primary, alpha) motor neurons are the large motor neurons in the anterior (or ventral) horn of the spinal cord and the motor nuclei of the brainstem. The axons from these nerve cell bodies bring nerve impulses from upper motor neurons to the skeletal muscles through the anterior spinal roots or cranial nerves (Figure 15-19). **Lower motor neuron syndromes** impair both voluntary and involuntary movement. The degree of paralysis or paresis is proportional to the number of lower motor neurons affected. If only some of the motor units that supply a muscle are affected, only partial paralysis (or paresis) results. If all motor units are affected, complete paralysis results. Other clinical manifestations also are proportional to the degree of dysfunction, but the precise manifestations depend on the location of the dysfunction in the motor unit and in the CNS.

Small motor (gamma) neurons, which maintain muscle tone and protect the muscle from injury, are needed for normal motor movement. They depend on input from the muscle spindle (arriving through an afferent limb rising to the cord). Dysfunction in this motor system (the gamma loop) impairs tone and reduces tendon reflexes, causing hyporeflexia. The muscles become susceptible to damage from hyperextensibility.

Generally, the large and small motor neuron systems are equally affected. Therefore the muscle has reduced or absent tone and is accompanied by hyporeflexia or **areflexia** (loss of tendon reflexes) and **flaccid paresis/paralysis**.

Denervated muscles (i.e., muscles that have lost their nervous system input) atrophy over weeks to months, mostly from disuse, and demonstrate **fasciculations** (muscle rippling or quivering under the skin). Occasionally, denervated muscles cramp. **Fibrillation** is isolated contraction of a single muscle fiber because of metabolic changes in denervated muscle and is not clinically visible.

BOX 15-7 Bell Palsy

The etiology of Bell palsy (unilateral facial nerve palsy) remains unknown. There is usually an inflammatory reaction compressing the facial nerve, particularly in the narrowest segment, followed by demyelinating neural change. The most distressing signs are unilateral facial weakness and the inability to smile or whistle. Bell palsy may be caused by reactivation of herpesviruses in cranial nerve VII (facial), geniculate ganglia, or an autoimmune response. The signs usually have an acute onset (within 72 hours). Herpes simplex type 1 has been detected in up to 78% of cases and herpes zoster in 30% of cases. Severe pain with facial palsy and a vesicular rash in the ear or mouth suggest herpes zoster infection. Ramsay Hunt syndrome (herpes zoster oticus) is rare, but complete recovery is less than 50%. Recovery from Bell palsy is usually complete. Both disorders may be treated with combination antivirals and oral steroids. Treatment should be individualized according to severity of symptoms.

Data from Baugh RF et al: *Otolaryngol Head Neck Surg* 149(3 Suppl):S1-S27, 2013 (available at: http://oto.sagepub.com/content/149/3_suppl/S1.full); De Ru JA, Van Benthem PP: *Evid Based Med* 19(1):15, 2014; Glass GE, Tzafetta K: *Fam Pract* 31(6):631-642, 2014; Greco A et al: *Autoimmun Rev* 12(2):323-328, 2012.

Motor Neuron Diseases

Motor neuron diseases result from progressive degeneration of upper or lower motor neurons in the spinal cord, brainstem, or cortex. Amyotrophic lateral sclerosis and paralytic poliomyelitis (see Chapter 8) are examples of these diseases.

Several pathologic processes may give rise to motor neuron diseases that can be sporadic or inherited. A virally induced or postinfectious or postvaccination inflammatory process may injure or destroy anterior horn cells or cranial nerve cell bodies. Most of these inflammatory processes are mild and are followed by rapid cellular recovery (Box 15-7).

In motor neuron disease muscle strength, muscle tone, and muscle bulk are affected in the muscles innervated by the involved motor neurons. The paresis and paralysis associated with anterior horn cell injury are segmental, but because each muscle is supplied by two or more roots, the segmental character of the weakness may be difficult to recognize. When cranial nerve motor nuclei are affected (these lack nerve roots and have only small rootlets near the point of exit from the brainstem), the distribution of the motor weakness follows that of the peripheral nerve. The weakness may involve distal muscles, proximal muscles, and the muscles of midline structures. Hypotonia and hyporeflexia or areflexia are present.

The atrophy associated with motor neuron disease is segmental when the anterior horn cells of the spinal cord are involved and follows the distribution of the peripheral nerve when the motor nuclei of the cranial nerves are affected. The atrophy may be in distal, proximal, or midline muscles. Fasciculations are particularly associated with primary motor neuron injury, and muscle cramps are common. Mild fatigue is a common complaint. If the pathologic process is limited to the primary motor neuron, no sensory changes are evident.

Because degenerative disorders can cause loss of nerve cells in the anterior horn or motor nuclei, the surviving cells are small, shrunken, and filled with lipofuscin. Lost neurons are replaced by astrocytes. The roots or rootlets are thin, and the muscles show denervation and atrophy.

Several brainstem syndromes involve damage to one or more of the cranial nerve nuclei. These are called *cranial nerve palsy* and may be caused by vascular occlusion, tumor, aneurysm, tuberculosis, or hemorrhage.

The anterior horn cells and the motor nuclei of the cranial nerves may be affected secondarily in many severe pathologic processes that primarily involve the peripheral nerves. The condition may extend proximally to affect the nerve roots or rootlets and the motor neurons themselves, a process commonly seen, for example, in **Guillain-Barré syndrome** (see Chapter 16). If sufficient numbers of motor neurons are destroyed, permanent loss of motor function results because regeneration of the damaged axons requires a living neuronal cell body.

A group of degenerative disorders principally cause progressive motor cell atrophy. One of these is **progressive spinal muscular atrophy**, in which the anterior horn cells of the spinal cord are the affected motor neurons that degenerate. This disorder occurs in adults and closely resembles the familial progressive muscular atrophies that occur in infants and children and are considered inherited metabolic disorders (see Chapter 40). If the motor nuclei of the cranial nerves are affected instead of the anterior horn cells, the disorder is labeled **progressive bulbar palsy**, so named because the myelencephalon originally was called the *bulb* and a degenerative process causes a progressively more serious condition. When any lower motor neuron syndrome involves the cranial nerves that arise from the bulb (i.e., cranial nerves IX, X, and XII), the dysfunction is called a **bulbar palsy**.

The clinical manifestations of bulbar palsy include paresis or paralysis of the jaw, face, pharynx, and tongue musculature. Articulation is affected, especially articulation of the lingual *(r, n, l)*, labial *(b, m, p, f)*, dental *(d, t)*, and palatal *(k, g)* consonants. Modulation is impaired, making the voice rasping or nasal. Pharyngeal reflexes are diminished or lost. Palate and vocal cord movement during phonation is impaired, and chewing and swallowing are affected. The facial muscles are weak, and the face appears to droop. The jaw jerk is decreased. Atrophy eventually becomes apparent, as do fasciculations. All these manifestations become progressively worse, leading to aspiration, malnutrition, possible dehydration, and an inability to communicate verbally.

Amyotrophic Lateral Sclerosis

Amyotrophic lateral sclerosis (ALS, sporadic motor neuron disease, sporadic motor system disease, motor neuron disease [MND], Lou Gehrig disease) is a worldwide neurodegenerative disorder that diffusely involves lower and upper motor neurons, resulting in progressive muscle weakness. *Amyotrophic* (without muscle nutrition or progressive muscle wasting) refers to the predominant lower motor neuron component of the syndrome. *Lateral sclerosis*, scarring of the corticospinal tract in the lateral column of the spinal cord, refers to the upper motor neuron component of the syndrome.

ALS may begin at any time from the fourth decade of life; its peak occurrence is between 60 and 69 years, with about 3.9 cases per 100,000 population in the United States. The prevalence is higher in males.[42] Most cases of ALS are sporadic. A subset (about 10%) of persons has a familial form with genetic mutations in superoxide dismutase (SODI) that contribute to the neurotoxicity affecting motor neurons. Mutated TAR RNA-binding protein 43 (TDP-43) is a major constituent of the neuronal protein inclusions in ALS. Gene and environmental interactions are being evaluated as a cause of ALS.[43]

PATHOPHYSIOLOGY The cause of ALS is unknown. Oxidative stress, mitochondrial dysfunction, defects in axonal transport, excitotoxicity and glutamate transport, neuronal cytoplasmic inclusions (i.e., TDP-43 protein), and neuroinflammation as causes of neuron degeneration are under investigation.[44]

The principal pathologic feature of ALS is degeneration of lower and upper motor neurons. There is a decrease in large motor neurons in the spinal cord, brainstem, and cerebral cortex (premotor and motor areas), with ongoing degeneration in the remaining motor neurons.

Death of the motor neuron results in axonal degeneration and secondary demyelination with glial proliferation and sclerosis (scarring). Widespread neural degeneration of nonmotor neurons in the spinal cord and motor cortices, as well as in the premotor, sensory, and temporal cortices, has been found.

Lower motor neuron degeneration denervates motor units. Adjacent, still viable lower motor neurons attempt to compensate by distal intramuscular sprouting, reinnervation, and enlargement of motor units.

CLINICAL MANIFESTATIONS   The initial symptoms of the disease are heterogeneous and may be related to lower or upper motor neuron dysfunction or both. About 60% of individuals have a spinal form of the disease with focal muscle weakness beginning in the arms and legs and progressing to muscle atrophy, spasticity, and loss of manual dexterity and gait. No associated mental, sensory, or autonomic symptoms are present. ALS with progressive bulbar palsy presents with difficulty speaking and swallowing, and peripheral muscle weakness and atrophy usually occur within 1 to 2 years. These individuals have a poorer response to treatment with mechanical ventilation.[45] Frontotemporal dementia may occur concurrently.[46]

EVALUATION AND TREATMENT   Diagnosis of the syndrome is based predominantly on the history and physical examination with no evidence of other neuromuscular disorders. Electromyography and muscle biopsy results verify lower motor neuron degeneration and denervation. Imaging studies and cerebrospinal fluid biomarkers can assist in making the diagnosis. Little treatment is available to alter the overall course of the ALS syndrome. The drug riluzole (Rilutek), an antiglutamate, has extended the length of time patients do not require ventilatory assistance. Supportive and rehabilitative management are directed toward preventing complications of immobility. Psychologic support of the affected individual and the family is extremely important.[47] ALS is fatal from respiratory failure usually within 3 years of diagnosis. A small percentage of individuals live 5 to 10 years or longer.[48]

ALTERATIONS IN COMPLEX MOTOR PERFORMANCE

The alterations in complex motor performance include disorders of posture (stance), disorders of gait, and disorders of expression.

Disorders of Posture (Stance)

An inequality of tone in muscle groups, because of a loss of normal postural reflexes, results in a posturing of limbs. Equilibrium and balance are disrupted. Many reflex systems govern tone and posture, but the most important factor in posture control is the stretch reflex, in which extensor (antigravity) muscle stretching causes increased extensor tone and inhibited flexor tone. Four types of disorders of posture are (1) dystonic posture, (2) decerebrate posture/response, (3) basal ganglion posture, and (4) **basal ganglion posture**.

Dystonia is the maintenance of an abnormal posture through muscular contractions. When muscular contractions are sustained for several seconds, they are called **dystonic movements**; when contractions last for longer periods, they are called **dystonic postures**. Dystonic postures may last for weeks, causing permanent, fixed contractures. Dystonia has been associated with basal ganglia abnormality, but the exact pathophysiologic mechanisms are unknown. One dystonic posture is decorticate posture/response (striatal posture or upper motor neuron dysfunction posture), which may be unilateral or bilateral.

Decorticate posture/response (also referred to as **antigravity posture** or **hemiplegic posture**) is characterized by upper extremities flexed at the elbows and held close to the body and by lower extremities that are externally rotated and extended (see Figure 15-6). Decorticate posture/response is thought to occur when the brainstem is not inhibited by the cerebral cortex motor area. Upper motor neuron posture is more commonly described as the arm flexed at the elbow with a wrist drop, the leg inadequately bent at the knee, the hip excessively circumabducted, and the presence of footdrop.

Decerebrate posture/response refers to increased tone in extensor muscles and trunk muscles, with active tonic neck reflexes. When the head is in a neutral position, all four limbs are rigidly extended (see Figure 15-6). The decerebrate posture is caused by severe injury to the brain and brainstem, resulting in overstimulation of the postural righting and vestibular reflexes.

Basal ganglion posture refers to a stooped, hyperflexed posture with a narrow-based, short-stepped gait. This posture abnormality results from the loss of normal postural reflexes and not from defects in proprioceptive, labyrinthine, or visual function. Dysfunctional equilibrium results when the individual loses stability and cannot make the appropriate postural adjustment to tilting or loss of balance, falling instead. Dysfunctional righting is the inability to right oneself when changing from a lying or crouching to a standing position or when rolling from the supine to the lateral or prone position. Dysfunctional postural fixation is the involuntary flexion of the head and neck, causing the person difficulty in maintaining an upright trunk position while standing or walking. Basal ganglion dysfunction accounts for this posture.

Disorders of Gait

Four predominant types of gait associated with neurologic disorders are (1) upper motor neuron dysfunction gait, (2) cerebellar (ataxic) gait, (3) basal ganglion gait, and (4) frontal lobe ataxic gait. As with posture, equilibrium and balance are affected with gait disturbances.[49]

Several **upper motor neuron gaits** exist. With mild forms, the individual may have footdrop with fatigue and hip and leg pain. A spastic gait, which is associated with unilateral injury, manifests by a shuffling gait with the leg extended and held stiff, causing a scraping over the floor surface. The leg swings improperly around the body rather than being appropriately lifted and placed. The foot may drag on the ground, and the person tends to fall to the affected side. A scissors gait is associated with bilateral injury and spasticity. The legs are adducted so they touch each other. As the person walks, the legs are swung around the body but then cross in front of each other because of adduction. Injury to the pyramidal system accounts for these gaits (e.g., stroke, cerebral palsy, multiple sclerosis, spinal cord tumor).

A **cerebellar (ataxic) gait** is wide-based with the feet apart and often turned outward or inward for greater stability. The pelvis is held stiff, and the individual staggers when walking. Cerebellar dysfunction with loss of coordination accounts for this particular gait.

A **basal ganglion gait** is a broad-based gait in which the person walks with small steps and a decreased arm swing. The head and body are flexed and the arms semiflexed and abducted, whereas the legs are flexed and rigid in more advanced states. Basal ganglion dysfunction accounts for this gait and is associated with Parkinson disease.

A **frontal lobe ataxic gait** is wide-based with increased body sway and falls, loss of control of truncal motion, gait ignition failure, start hesitation, shuffling, and freezing. The gait is associated with frontal lobe damage or degeneration. The pattern may change as the frontal disease progresses. The slowness of walking, lack of heel-shin or upper limb ataxia, dysarthria, or nystagmus distinguishes the wide stance from cerebellar gait ataxia.[50]

TABLE 15-19   Pyramidal vs. Extrapyramidal Motor Syndrome

Manifestations	Pyramidal Motor Syndrome	Extrapyramidal Motor Syndrome
Unilateral movement	Paralysis of voluntary movement	Little or no paralysis of voluntary movement
Tendon reflexes	Increased tendon reflexes	Normal or slightly increased tendon reflexes
Babinski sign	Present	Absent
Involuntary movements	Absence of involuntary movements	Presence of tremor, chorea, athetosis, or dystonia
Muscle tone	Spasticity in muscles (e.g., clasp-knife phenomenon)	Plastic rigidity (equal throughout movement) or intermittent—cogwheel rigidity (generalized but predominantly in flexors of limbs and trunk)
	Hypertonia present in flexors of arms and extensors of legs	Hypotonia, weakness and gait disturbances in cerebellar disease

Gait disorders are often accompanied by balance, coordination, and sensory dysfunction that further alter mobility and increase risk for falls. Assessment and intervention strategies are important for prevention of injury.

Disorders of Expression

Disorders of expression involve the motor aspects of communication and include (1) hypermimesis, (2) hypomimesis, and (3) apraxia/dyspraxia. Hypermimesis commonly manifests as pathologic laughter or crying. Pathologic laughter is associated with right hemisphere injury, and pathologic crying is associated with left hemisphere injury. The exact pathophysiology is not known. Hypomimesis manifests as *aprosody*—the loss of emotional language. *Receptive aprosody* involves an inability to understand emotion in speech and facial expression. *Expressive aprosody* involves the inability to express emotion in speech and facial expression. Aprosody is associated with right hemisphere damage.

Apraxia/dyspraxia is a disorder of learned skilled movements with difficulty planning and executing coordinated motor movements. The term is often used interchangeably with *dyspraxia*. It can be developmental, beginning at birth (developmental apraxia), or associated with vascular disorders (common in stroke), trauma, tumors, degenerative disorders, infections, or metabolic disorders. People with apraxia have difficulty performing tasks requiring motor skills including speaking, writing, using tools or utensils, playing sports, following instructions, and focusing.[51]

True apraxias occur when the connecting pathways between the left and right cortical areas are interrupted. Apraxias may result from any pathologic process that disrupts the cortical areas necessary for the conceptualization and execution of a complex motor act or the communication pathways within the left hemisphere or between the hemispheres.[51,52]

EXTRAPYRAMIDAL MOTOR SYNDROMES

Because the extrapyramidal system encompasses all the motor pathways except the pyramidal system, two types of motor dysfunction make up the extrapyramidal motor syndromes: (1) the basal ganglia motor syndromes and (2) the cerebellar motor syndromes. Unlike pyramidal motor syndromes, both extrapyramidal motor syndromes result in movement or posture disturbance without significant paralysis, along with other distinctive symptoms (Table 15-19).

Basal ganglia motor syndromes are caused by an imbalance of dopaminergic and cholinergic activity in the corpus striatum. A relative excess of cholinergic activity produces akinesia and hypertonia. A relative excess of dopaminergic activity produces hyperkinesia and hypotonia. Symptoms associated with Parkinson and Huntington diseases are exemplary of disorders of the basal ganglia. Cerebellar motor syndromes are associated with ataxia and other symptoms affecting coordinated movement. Cerebellar disorders primarily influence the same side of the body, so that damage to the right cerebellum generally causes symptoms on the right side of the body.

QUICK CHECK 15-6
1. Why are there so many causes of hypertonia?
2. How is chorea different from athetosis?
3. Why is paresis/paralysis a type of hypokinesia?
4. What structures are involved in alterations of complex motor performance?

DID YOU UNDERSTAND?

Alterations in Cognitive Systems

1. Full consciousness is an awareness of oneself and the environment with an ability to respond to external stimuli with a wide variety of responses.
2. Consciousness has two components: arousal (level of awakeness) and awareness (content of thought).
3. An altered level of arousal occurs by diffuse bilateral cortical dysfunction, bilateral subcortical (reticular formation, brainstem) dysfunction, localized hemispheric dysfunction, and metabolic disorders.
4. An alteration in breathing pattern and the level of consciousness reflect the level of brain dysfunction.
5. Pupillary changes reflect changes in level of brainstem function, drug action, and response to hypoxia and ischemia.
6. Abnormal eye movements, including nystagmus and divergent gaze, reflect alterations in brainstem function.
7. Level of brain function manifests by changes in generalized motor responses or no responses.
8. Loss of cortical inhibition associated with decreased consciousness produces abnormal flexor and extensor movements.
9. Cerebral death or irreversible coma represents permanent brain damage, with an ability to maintain cardiac, respiratory, and other vital functions.
10. Brain death results from irreversible brain damage, with an inability to maintain internal homeostasis.
11. Arousal returns in vegetative states, but awareness is absent.
12. Alterations in awareness include alterations in executive attention (abstract reasoning, planning, decision making, judgment, error correction, and self-control) and memory.
13. With a deficit in selective attention, mediated by midbrain, thalamus, and parietal lobe structures, the individual cannot focus on selective stimuli and thus neglects those stimuli.

14. In amnesia, some past memories are lost and new memories cannot be stored.
15. Frontal areas mediate vigilance, detection, and working (short-term) memory.
16. With vigilance deficits, the person cannot maintain sustained concentration.
17. With detection deficits, the person is unmotivated and unable to set goals and plan.
18. Data processing deficits include agnosias, dysphasias, acute confusional states, and dementias.
19. Agnosias are defects of recognition and may be tactile, visual, or auditory. They are caused by dysfunction in the primary sensory area or the interpretive areas of the cerebral cortex.
20. Dysphasia (aphasia) is an impairment of comprehension or production of language. Dysphasia may be expressive or receptive.
21. Acute confusional states are characterized chiefly by a loss of detection and, in the case of delirium, intense autonomic nervous system hyperactivity.
22. Alzheimer disease is a chronic irreversible dementia that is related to altered production or failure to clear amyloid from the brain with plaque formation, formation of neurofibrillary tangles, and loss of basal forebrain cholinergic neurons.
23. Frontotemporal dementias are rare early-onset degenerative diseases similar to Alzheimer disease.
24. Seizures represent a sudden, chaotic discharge of cerebral neurons with transient alterations in brain function. Seizures may be generalized or focal and can result from cerebral lesions, biochemical disorders, trauma, or epilepsy.

Alterations in Cerebral Hemodynamics

1. Alterations in cerebral blood flow are related to changes in cerebral perfusion pressure, changes in cerebral blood volume, and cerebral blood oxygenation.
2. Increased intracranial pressure (IICP) may result from edema, excess cerebrospinal fluid, hemorrhage, or tumor growth. When intracranial pressure approaches arterial pressure, hypoxia and hypercapnia produce brain damage.
3. Cerebral edema is an increase in the fluid content of the brain resulting from infection, hemorrhage, tumor, ischemia, infarction, or hypoxia. Cerebral edema can cause IICP.
4. The shifting or herniation of brain tissue from one compartment to another disrupts the blood flow of both compartments and damages brain tissue.
5. Supratentorial herniation involves the temporal lobe and hippocampal gyrus shifting from the middle fossa to posterior fossa; transtentorial herniation involves a downward shift of the diencephalon through the tentorial notch; and shifting of the cingulate gyrus can occur under the falx cerebri.
6. The most common infratentorial herniation is a shift of the cerebellar tonsils through the foramen magnum.
7. Hydrocephalus comprises a variety of disorders characterized by an excess of fluid within the ventricles, subarachnoid space, or both. Hydrocephalus occurs because of interference with cerebrospinal fluid flow caused by increased fluid production or obstruction within the ventricular system or by defective reabsorption of the fluid.

Alterations in Neuromotor Function

1. Motor dysfunction may be characterized as alterations of motor tone, movement, and complex motor performance.

Alterations in Muscle Tone

1. Hypotonia and hypertonia are the main categories of altered tone.
2. Hypotonia is associated with pyramidal tract or cerebellar injury. Muscles are flaccid and weak with atrophy.
3. The four types of hypertonia are spasticity paratonia (gegenhalten), dystonia, and rigidity.

Alterations in Muscle Movement

1. Paresis, paraplegia, hyperkinesia, and hypokinesia are the main categories of altered movement.
2. Two subtypes of paresis/paralysis are described: upper motor neuron spastic paresis/paralysis and lower motor neuron flaccid paresis/paralysis.
3. An upper motor neuron syndrome is characterized by paresis/paralysis, hypertonia, and hyperreflexia.
4. Interruption of the pyramidal tract below the pons results in spinal shock.
5. Lower motor neuron syndromes manifest by impaired voluntary and involuntary movements and flaccid paralysis.
6. Partial paralysis occurs with only partial loss of alpha motor neurons, and total paralysis is complete loss of alpha motor neurons. Loss of gamma motor neurons impairs muscle tone and decreases tendon reflexes.
7. Included in the category of hyperkinesia are chorea, athetosis, ballism, akathisia, tremor, and myoclonus.
8. Huntington disease (chorea) is a rare hereditary disease involving the basal ganglia and cerebral cortex that commonly manifests between 25 and 45 years of age.
9. The major pathologic feature of Huntington disease is severe degeneration of the basal ganglia and the frontal cerebral cortex with an excess of dopaminergic activity that causes involuntary, fragmentary hyperkinetic movements.
10. Types of hypokinesia include akinesia, bradykinesia, and loss of associated movements.
11. Parkinson disease is a commonly occurring degenerative disorder of the basal ganglia (corpus striatum) involving degeneration of the dopamine-secreting nigrostriatal pathway.
12. Dopamine depletion in the basal ganglia and excess cholinergic activity in the cortex, basal ganglia, and thalamus cause tremor and rigidity in Parkinson disease. Progressive dementia may be associated with an advanced stage of the disease.
13. Upper motor neuron syndromes are the result of damage to descending motor pathways at cortical, brainstem, or spinal cord levels and result in spastic paralysis.
14. Spinal shock is temporary loss of all spinal cord functions below the lesion (below the level of the pons). It is characterized by complete flaccid paralysis, absence of reflexes, and marked disturbances of bowel and bladder function.
15. Lower (primary, alpha) motor neuron syndromes involve the large motor neurons in the anterior (or ventral) horn of the spinal cord and the motor nuclei of the brainstem and cause flaccid paralysis.
16. Amyotrophic lateral sclerosis involves degeneration of both upper and lower motor neurons with progressive muscle weakness and atrophy.

Alterations in Complex Motor Performance

1. Alterations in complex motor performance include disorders of posture (stance), disorders of gait, and disorders of expression.
2. Disorders of posture include dystonic posture, decerebrate posture/response, basal ganglion posture, and senile posture.
3. Disorders of gait include upper motor neuron gait, cerebellar (ataxic) gait, basal ganglion gait, and frontal lobe ataxic gait.

Disorders of Expression

1. Disorders of expression include hypermimesis, hypomimesis, and apraxia (dyspraxia).
2. Apraxia is an impairment of the conceptualization or execution of a complex motor act.

Extrapyramidal Motor Syndromes

1. Extrapyramidal motor syndromes include basal ganglia and cerebellar motor syndromes.

2. Basal ganglia disorders manifest by alterations in muscle tone and posture, including rigidity, involuntary movements, and loss of postural reflexes.
3. Cerebellar motor syndromes result in loss of muscle tone, difficulty with coordination, and disorders of equilibrium and gait.

KEY TERMS

Acute confusional state (ACS), 367
Acute hydrocephalus, 376
Agnosia, 367
Akinesia, 380
Alzheimer disease (AD) (dementia of Alzheimer type [DAT], senile disease complex), 371
Amnesia, 365
Amyotrophic lateral sclerosis, 384
Anterograde amnesia, 365
Aphasia, 367
Apraxia/dyspraxia, 386
Areflexia, 383
Arousal, 359
Autoregulation, 374
Awareness (content of thought), 365
Basal ganglia motor syndrome, 386
Basal ganglion gait, 385
Basal ganglion posture, 385
Bradykinesia, 380
Brain death (total brain death), 364
Bulbar palsy, 384
Cerebellar (ataxic) gait, 385
Cerebellar motor syndrome, 386
Cerebral blood flow (CBF), 374
Cerebral blood volume (CBV), 374
Cerebral death (irreversible coma), 364
Cerebral edema, 375
Cerebral blood oxygenation, 374
Cerebral perfusion pressure (CPP), 373

Clonic phase, 373
Communicating hydrocephalus, 376
Consciousness, 359
Convulsion, 372
Cytotoxic (metabolic) edema, 376
Decerebrate posture/response, 385
Decorticate posture/response (antigravity posture, hemiplegic posture), 385
Delirium (hyperactive confusional state), 367
Dementia, 370
Diplegia, 382
Dysphasia, 367
Dyspraxia, 386
Dystonia, 385
Dystonic movement, 385
Dystonic posture, 385
Epilepsy, 372
Epileptogenic focus, 373
Executive attention deficit, 365
Extinction, 365
Extrapyramidal motor syndrome, 386
Fibrillation, 383
Flaccid paresis/paralysis, 383
Frontal lobe ataxic gait, 385
Frontotemporal dementia (FTD) (Pick disease), 372
Guillain-Barré syndrome, 384
Hemiparesis, 382
Hemiplegia, 382
Hiccup, 363
Huntington disease (HD), 378
Hydrocephalus, 376
Hyperkinesia, 378
Hypermimesis, 386

Hypertonia, 377
Hypokinesia, 380
Hypoactive delirium (hypoactive confusional state), 369
Hypomimesis, 386
Hypotonia, 376
Ictus, 373
Image processing, 365
Intracranial pressure, 374
Increased intracranial pressure (IICP), 374
Interstitial edema, 376
Level of consciousness, 360
Locked-in syndrome, 365
Lower motor neuron syndromes, 383
Memory, 365
Memory disorder, 365
Minimally conscious state (MCS), 365
Mirror focus, 373
Motor response, 361
Neglect syndrome, 365
Neurofibrillary tangle, 371
Noncommunicating hydrocephalus (internal hydrocephalus, intraventricular hydrocephalus), 376
Normal-pressure hydrocephalus, 376
Oculomotor response, 361
Paralysis, 381
Paraparesis, 382
Paraplegia, 382
Paratonia, 377
Paresis, 381
Parkinson disease, 380
Parkinsonism (Parkinson syndrome, parkinsonian

syndrome, paralysis agitans), 380
Paroxysmal dyskinesia, 378
Patterns of breathing, 361
Persistent vegetative state, 364
Postictal state, 373
Preictal phase, 373
Prodroma, 373
Progressive bulbar palsy, 384
Progressive spinal muscular atrophy, 384
Psychogenic alterations in arousal (unresponsiveness), 360
Pupillary change, 361
Pyramidal motor syndrome, 381
Quadriparesis, 382
Quadriplegia, 382
Retrograde amnesia, 365
Rigidity, 377
Secondary parkinsonism, 380
Seizure, 372
Selective attention, 365
Selective attention deficit, 365
Sensory inattentiveness, 365
Spasticity, 377
Spinal shock, 382
Status epilepticus, 373
Structural alterations in arousal, 359
Tardive dyskinesia, 378
Tonic phase, 373
Upper motor neuron gait, 385
Upper motor neuron paresis/ paralysis, 381
Vasogenic edema, 375
Vomiting, 363
Yawning, 363

REFERENCES

1. Wijdicks EF et al: Evidence-based guideline update: determining brain death in adults: report of the Quality Standards Subcommittee of the American Academy of Neurology, *Neurology* 74(23): 1911-1918, 2010.
2. Nakagawa TA et al: Guidelines for the determination of brain death in infants and children: an update of the 1987 task force recommendations, *Crit Care Med* 39(9):2139-2155, 2011.
3. Overgaard M: How can we know if patients in coma, vegetative state or minimally conscious state are conscious? *Prog Brain Res* 177:11-19, 2009.
4. Hirschberg R, Giacino JT: The vegetative and minimally conscious states: diagnosis,

prognosis and treatment, *Neurol Clin* 29(4):773-786, 2011.

5. Lacroix G et al: Transient locked-in syndrome and basilar artery vasospasm, *Neurocrit Care* 16(1):145-147, 2012.

6. Carrasco M: Visual attention: the past 25 years, *Vision Res* 51(13):1484-1525, 2011.

7. Zaal IJ, Slooter AJ: Delirium in critically ill patients: epidemiology, pathophysiology, diagnosis and management, *Drugs* 72(11):1457-1471, 2012.

8. Barr J et al: Clinical practice guidelines for the management of pain, agitation, and delirium in adult patients in the intensive care unit, *Crit Care Med* 41(1):263-306, 2013. Also available at: www.learnicu.org/pages/guidelines.aspx.

9. Devlin JW et al: Optimising the recognition of delirium in the intensive care unit, *Best Pract Res Clin Anaesthesiol* 26(3):385-393, 2012.

10. Grover S, Kate N: Assessment scales for delirium: a review, *World J Psychiatry* 2(4):58-70, 2012.

11. Morandi A et al: Tools to detect delirium superimposed on dementia: a systematic review, *J Am Geriatr Soc* 60(11):2005-2013, 2012. Erratum in *J Am Geriatr Soc* 61(1):174, 2013.

12. Zhang H et al: Strategies for prevention of postoperative delirium: a systematic review and meta-analysis of randomized trials, *Crit Care* 17(2):R47, 2013.

13. Alzheimer's Association: *Alzheimers disease facts and figures, 2014*. Available at: www.alz.org/alzheimers_disease_facts_and_figures.asp#quickFacts.

14. Reitz C, Mayeux R: Alzheimer disease: epidemiology, diagnostic criteria, risk factors and biomarkers, *Biochem Pharmacol* 88(4):640-651, 2014.

15. Coppieters N et al: Global changes in DNA methylation and hydroxymethylation in Alzheimer's disease human brain, *Neurobiol Aging* 35(6):1334-1344, 2014.

16. Loy CT et al: Genetics of dementia, *Lancet* 383(9919):828-840, 2014.

17. Bloom GS: Amyloid-β and tau: the trigger and bullet in Alzheimer disease pathogenesis, *J Am Med Assoc Neurol* 71(4):505-508, 2014.

18. Cummings JL et al: International Work Group criteria for the diagnosis of Alzheimer disease, *Med Clin North Am* 97(3):363-368, 2013.

19. Wurtman R: Biomarkers in the diagnosis and management of Alzheimer's disease, *Metabolism* 64(3 Suppl 1):S47-S50, 2015.

20. Kumar A, Singh A, Ekavali: A review on Alzheimer's disease pathophysiology and its management: an update, *Pharmacol Rep* 67(2):195-203, 2015.

21. Rohan Z, Matej R: Current concepts in the classification and diagnosis of frontotemporal lobar degenerations: a practical approach, *Arch Pathol Lab Med* 138(1):132-138, 2014.

22. Casillas-Espinosa PM et al: Regulators of synaptic transmission: roles in the pathogenesis and treatment of epilepsy, *Epilepsia* 53(Suppl 9):41-58, 2012.

23. Rémi J, Noachtar S: Clinical features of the postictal state: correlation with seizure variables, *Epilepsy Behav* 19(2):114-117, 2010.

24. Kumar A et al: Preoperative estimation of seizure control after resective surgery for the treatment of epilepsy, *Seizure* 22(10):818-826, 2013.

25. Payne NE et al: The ketogenic and related diets in adolescents and adults—a review, *Epilepsia* 52(11):1941-1948, 2011.

26. Kiefer M, Unterberg A: The differential diagnosis and treatment of normal-pressure hydrocephalus, *Dtsch Arztebl Int* 109(1-2):15-25, 2012.

27. Ziebell M et al: Flow-regulated versus differential pressure-regulated shunt valves for adult patients with normal pressure hydrocephalus, *Cochrane Database Syst Rev* 5:CD009706, 2013.

28. Agostinho LA et al: A systematic review of the intergenerational aspects and the diverse genetic profiles of Huntington's disease, *Genet Mol Res* 12(2):1974-1981, 2013.

29. Labbadia J, Morimoto RI: Huntington's disease: underlying molecular mechanisms and emerging concepts, *Trends Biochem Sci* 38(8):378-385, 2013.

30. Ross CA, Tabrizi SJ: Huntington's disease: from molecular pathogenesis to clinical treatment, *Lancet Neurol* 10(1):83-98, 2011.

31. Kumar P et al: Huntington's disease: pathogenesis to animal models, *Pharmacol Rep* 62(1):1-14, 2010.

32. Dayalu P, Albin RL: Huntington disease: pathogenesis and treatment, *Neurol Clin* 33(1):101-114, 2015.

33. Parkinson Disease Foundation, 2014. Available at: www.pdf.org/en/parkinson_statistics.

34. Gaig C, Tolosa E: When does Parkinson's disease begin? *Mov Disord* 24(Suppl 2):S656-S664, 2009.

35. Hirsch EC et al: Pathogenesis of Parkinson's disease, *Mov Disord* 28(1):24-30, 2013.

36. Yarnall A et al: The interplay of cholinergic function, attention, and falls in Parkinson's disease, *Mov Disord* 26(14):2496-2503, 2011.

37. Chaudhuri KR, Odin P: The challenge of non-motor symptoms in Parkinson's disease, *Prog Brain Res* 184:325-341, 2010.

38. Sprenger F, Poewe W: Management of motor and non-motor symptoms in Parkinson's disease, *CNS Drugs* 27(4):259-272, 2013.

39. Miller DB, O'Callaghan JP: Biomarkers of Parkinson's disease: present and future, *Metabolism* 64(3 Suppl 1):S40-S46, 2015.

40. Buttery PC, Barker RA: Treating Parkinson's disease in the 21st century: can stem cell transplantation compete? *J Comp Neurol* 522(12):2802-2816, 2014.

41. Giugni JC, Okun MS: Treatment of advanced Parkinson's disease, *Curr Opin Neurol* 27(4):450-460, 2014.

42. Mehta P et al: Prevalence of amyotrophic lateral sclerosis—United States, 2010-2011, *MMWR Surveill Summ* 63(Suppl 7):1-14, 2014.

43. Al-Chalabi A, Hardiman O: The epidemiology of ALS: a conspiracy of genes, environment and time, *Nat Rev Neurol* 9(11):617-628, 2013.

44. Turner MR et al: Mechanisms, models and biomarkers in amyotrophic lateral sclerosis, *Amyotroph Lateral Scler Frontotemporal Degener* 14(Suppl 1):19-32, 2013.

45. Radunovic A et al: Mechanical ventilation for amyotrophic lateral sclerosis/motor neuron disease, *Cochrane Database Syst Rev* 3:CD004427, 2013.

46. Bennion Callister J, Pickering-Brown SM: Pathogenesis/genetics of frontotemporal dementia and how it relates to ALS, *Exp Neurol* 262(PtB):84-90, 2014.

47. Gordon PH: Amyotrophic lateral sclerosis: an update for 2013 Clinical Features, Pathophysiology, Management and Therapeutic Trials, *Aging Dis* 4(5):295-310, 2013.

48. Wijesekera LC, Leigh PN: Amyotrophic lateral sclerosis, *Orphanet J Rare Dis* 4:3, 2009.

49. Snijders AH et al: Neurological gait disorders in elderly people: clinical approach and classification, *Lancet Neurol* 6(1):63-74, 2007.

50. Thompson PD: Frontal lobe ataxia, *Handb Clin Neurol* 103:619-622, 2012.

51. Foundas AL: Apraxia: neural mechanisms and functional recovery, *Handb Clin Neurol* 110:335-345, 2013.

52. Zadikoff C, Lang AE: Apraxia in movement disorders, *Brain* 128(Pt 7):1480-1497, 2005.

16

Disorders of the Central and Peripheral Nervous Systems and Neuromuscular Junction

Barbara J. Boss and Sue E. Huether

Alterations in central nervous system (CNS) function are caused by traumatic injury, vascular disorders, tumor growth, infectious and inflammatory processes, and metabolic derangements (including those arising from nutritional deficiencies and drugs or chemicals). Alterations in peripheral nervous system function involve the nerve roots, a nerve plexus or the nerves themselves, or the neuromuscular junction.

CENTRAL NERVOUS SYSTEM DISORDERS

Traumatic Brain and Spinal Cord Injury

Traumatic Brain Injury

Traumatic brain injury (TBI) is an alteration in brain function or other evidence of brain pathology caused by an external force. Those at highest risk for TBI are children 14 years and younger and adults 65 years and older. The most common causes are motor vehicle accidents for children and falls for older adults. Males have the highest incidence in every age group. The incidence of traumatic brain injury is highest among American Indian/Alaska Natives and blacks and in lower- and median-income families.[1]

In recent years, individuals with traumatic brain injury have shown improved survival outcomes. Advancements have been made in enhanced safety measures (e.g., passive seat restraints, air bags, protective head gear), reduced transport time to hospitals or trauma centers, improved on-scene medical management, and prevention and management of secondary brain injury.

TBI can be classified as primary or secondary. Primary brain injury is caused by direct impact and can be focal, affecting one area of the brain, or diffuse (diffuse axonal injury [DAI]), involving more than one area of the brain.[2] Focal brain injury and diffuse axonal injury each account for half of all injuries. Focal brain injury accounts for more than two thirds of head injury deaths. DAI accounts for less than one third of deaths. More severely disabled survivors, including those surviving in an unresponsive state or reduced level of consciousness, have DAI. Secondary injury is an indirect consequence of the primary injury and includes systemic responses and a cascade of cellular and molecular cerebral events. TBI can be mild, moderate, or severe. The Glasgow Coma Scale (GCS) is used to grade severity of injury (Table 16-1). Most TBIs are mild. The hallmark of a severe TBI is loss of consciousness for 6 hours or more.[3]

Primary brain injury

Focal brain injury. Focal brain injury can be caused by closed (blunt) trauma or open (penetrating) trauma. Closed injury is more common and involves either the head striking a hard surface or a rapidly moving object striking the head, or by blast waves. The dura remains intact, and brain tissues are not exposed to the environment. Blunt trauma may result in both focal brain injuries and diffuse axonal injuries, and they can occur at the same time (Table 16-2). Open injury occurs with penetrating trauma or skull fracture. A break in the dura results in exposure of the cranial contents to the environment.[3]

Closed brain injuries are specific, grossly observable brain lesions that occur in a precise location; 75% to 90% of blunt trauma injuries are mild. Injury to the vault, vessels, and supporting structures can produce more severe damage, including contusions and epidural, subdural, and intracerebral hematomas. The injury may be coup (injury at site of impact) or contrecoup (injury from brain rebounding and hitting opposite side of skull) (Figure 16-1). Compression of the skull at the point of impact produces contusions or brain bruising from blood leaking from an injured vessel. The severity of contusion varies with the amount of energy transmitted by the skull to underlying brain tissue. The smaller the area of impact, the more severe the injury because of the concentration of force. Brain edema forms around and in damaged neural tissues, contributing to increasing intracranial pressure (see Chapter 15). Multiple hemorrhages, edema, infarction, and

necrosis can occur within the contused areas. The tissue has a pulpy quality. The maximal effects of these injuries peak 18 to 36 hours after severe head injury.

Contusions are found most commonly in the frontal lobes, particularly at the poles and along the inferior orbital surfaces; in the temporal lobes, especially at the anterior poles and along the inferior surface; and at the frontotemporal junction. They cause changes in attention, memory, executive attention functions (see Chapter 15), affect, emotion, and behavior. Less commonly, contusions occur in the parietal and occipital lobes. Focal cerebral contusions are usually superficial, involving just the gyri. Hemorrhagic contusions may coalesce into a large confluent intracranial hematoma.

A contusion may be evidenced by immediate loss of consciousness (generally accepted to last no longer than 5 minutes), loss of reflexes (individual falls to the ground), transient cessation of respiration, brief period of bradycardia, and decrease in blood pressure (lasting 30 seconds to a few minutes). Increased cerebrospinal fluid (CSF) pressure and electrocardiogram (ECG) and electroencephalogram (EEG) changes occur on impact. Vital signs may stabilize to normal values in a few seconds; reflexes then return and the person regains consciousness over minutes to days. Residual deficits may persist and some persons never regain a full level of consciousness.

Evaluation is based on results of the health history, level of consciousness according to the Glasgow Coma Scale (see Table 16-1), outcomes of imaging studies (e.g., computed tomography [CT], magnetic resonance imaging [MRI], and positron emission tomography [PET] scans), and assessment of vital parameters (e.g., intracranial pressure [ICP] and EEG). Large contusions and lacerations with hemorrhage may be surgically excised. Treatment is otherwise directed at controlling intracranial pressure and managing symptoms.

Epidural (extradural) hematomas (bleeding between the dura mater and the skull) represent 1% to 2% of major head injuries and occur in all age groups, but most commonly in those 20 to 40 years old. An artery is the source of bleeding in 85% of epidural hematomas, usually accompanied by a skull fracture; 15% of these injuries result from injury to the meningeal vein or dural sinus (Figure 16-2). The temporal fossa is the most common site of epidural hematoma

TABLE 16-1 Glasgow Coma Scale (GCS)*

Score[†]	Best Eye Response Score (4)	Best Verbal Response Score (5)	Best Motor Response Score (6)
1	No eye opening	No verbal response	No motor response
2	Eye opening to pain	Incomprehensible sounds	Extension to pain
3	Eye opening to verbal command	Inappropriate words	Flexion to pain
4	Eyes open spontaneously	Confused	Withdrawal from pain
5	NA	Oriented	Localizing pain
6	NA	NA	Obeys commands

Data from Teasdale G, Jennett B: *Lancet* 2:81-84, 1974; Salottolo K et al: *J Am Med Assoc Surg* 149(7):727-734, 2014.

*The GCS is scored between 3 and 15, with 3 being the worst and 15 the best. It is composed of the sum of three parameters: Best Eye Response, Best Verbal Response, and Best Motor Response. Mild Brain Injury = 13 or higher; Moderate Brain Injury = 9 to 12; Severe Brain Injury = 8 or less.

[†]NOTE: It is important to break the scoring report into its components, for example, E3V3M5 = GCS 11. A total score is meaningless without this information. Age affects the GCS. Elderly individuals with TBI have better GCS scores than younger individuals with TBI with similar TBI severity (i.e., elderly individuals have higher GCS scores than younger individuals with TBI with similar anatomic TBI severity).

TABLE 16-2 Classification of Brain Injuries

Type of Injury	Mechanism
Primary Brain Injury	
Focal Brain Injury	Localized injury from impact
Closed injury	Blunt trauma
Coup	Injury is directly below site of forceful impact
Contrecoup	Injury is on opposite side of brain from site of forceful impact
Epidural (extradural) hematoma	Vehicular accidents, minor falls, sporting accidents
Subdural hematoma	Forceful impact: vehicular accidents or falls, especially in elderly persons or persons with chronic alcohol abuse
Subarachnoid hemorrhage	Bleeding caused by forceful impact, usually vehicular accidents or long distance falls
Open injury	Penetrating trauma: missiles (bullets) or sharp projectiles (knives, ice picks, axes, screwdrivers)
Compound fracture	Objects strike head with great force or head strikes object forcefully; temporal blows, occipital blows, upward impact of cervical vertebrae (basilar skull fracture)
Diffuse Axonal Injury (can occur with focal injury)	Traumatic shearing forces; tearing of axons from twisting and rotational forces with injury over widespread brain areas; moving head strikes hard, unyielding surface or moving object strikes stationary head; torsional head motion without impact
Secondary Brain Injury	
Secondary brain injury	Decrease in CBF caused by edema, hemorrhage, IICP; neuroinflammation
Cell death	Release of excitatory neurotransmitters (glutamate); failure of cell ion pumps, mitochondrial failure

CBF, Cerebral blood flow; *IICP,* increased intracranial pressure.

FIGURE 16-1 Coup and Contrecoup Focal Injury with Acceleration/Deceleration Axonal Sheering. A, Sagittal force causing coup *(c)* and contrecoup injury *(cc)*. **B,** Lateral force causing coup *(c)* and contrecoup *(cc)* injury. **C,** Axial or rotational injury with shearing of axons, particularly at base of brain. Acceleration/deceleration axonal shearing injury occurs throughout the brain (red and blue directional arrows in all three images). (Borrowed from Pascual JM, Preito R: Chapter 133: Surgical management of severe closed head injury in adults. In Quinones-Hinojosa A, editor: *Schmidek and Sweet operative neurosurgical techniques,* ed 6, vol 2, pp 1513-1538, Philadelphia, 2012, Saunders. Originally redrawn from Adams JH: Brain damage in fatal non-missile head injury in man. In Braakman R, editor: *Handbook of clinical neurology, head injury,* vol 13, pp 43-63, Amsterdam, 1990, Elsevier Science Publishers BV; Gennarelli TA et al: *Ann Neurol* 12:564-574, 1982.)

caused by injury to the middle meningeal artery or vein. The temporal lobe shifts medially, precipitating uncal and hippocampal gyrus herniation through the tentorial notch. Epidural hemorrhages are found occasionally in the subfrontal area, especially in the young and elderly populations, caused by injury to the anterior meningeal artery or a venous sinus; and in the occipital-suboccipital area, resulting in herniation of the posterior fossa contents through the foramen magnum (see Figure 15-10).

Individuals with temporal epidural hematomas lose consciousness at injury; one third of those affected then become lucid for a few minutes to a few days (if a vein is bleeding). As the hematoma

accumulates, a headache of increasing severity, vomiting, drowsiness, confusion, seizure, and hemiparesis may develop. Because temporal lobe herniation occurs, the level of consciousness is rapidly lost, with ipsilateral pupillary dilation and contralateral hemiparesis. A CT scan or MRI usually is needed to diagnose epidural hematoma. The prognosis is good if intervention is initiated before bilateral dilation of the pupils occurs. Epidural hematomas are almost always medical emergencies requiring monitoring and evaluation or surgical evacuation of the hematoma.[4]

Subdural hematomas (bleeding between the dura mater and the brain) arise in 10% to 20% of persons with traumatic brain injury.

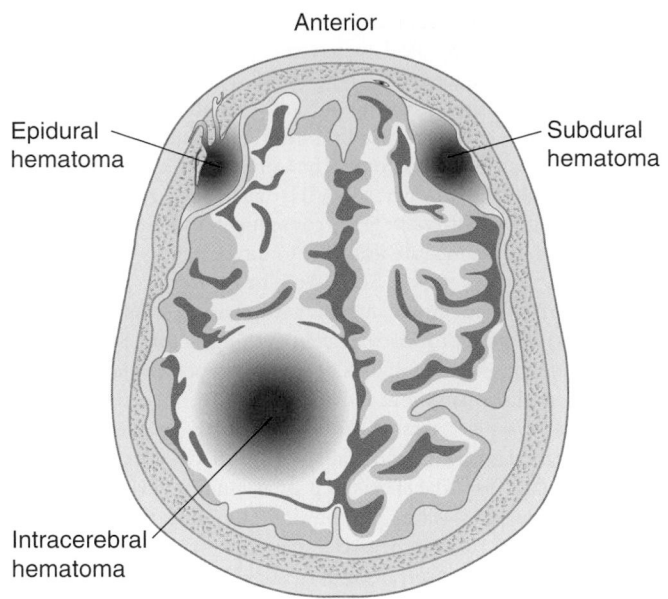

Anterior

Epidural hematoma

Subdural hematoma

Intracerebral hematoma

Posterior

FIGURE 16-2 Brain Hematomas.

Acute subdural hematomas develop rapidly, commonly within hours, and usually are located at the top of the skull (the cerebral convexities). Bilateral hematomas occur in 15% to 20% of persons. Subacute subdural hematomas develop more slowly, often over 48 hours to 2 weeks. *Chronic subdural hematomas* (commonly found in elderly persons and persons who abuse alcohol and have some degree of brain atrophy with a subsequent increase in extradural space) develop over weeks to months. Bridging veins tear, causing both rapidly and subacutely developing subdural hematomas, although torn cortical veins or venous sinuses and contused tissue also may be the source. These subdural hematomas act like expanding masses, increasing intracranial pressure that eventually compresses the bleeding vessels (see Figure 16-2). Brain herniation can result. With a chronic subdural hematoma, the existing subdural space gradually fills with blood. A vascular membrane forms around the hematoma in approximately 2 weeks. Further enlargement may take place.

In acute, rapidly developing subdural hematomas, the expanding clots directly compress the brain. As intracranial pressure rises, bleeding veins are compressed. Thus, bleeding is self-limiting, although cerebral compression and displacement of brain tissue can cause temporal lobe herniation.

An acute subdural hematoma classically begins with headache, drowsiness, restlessness or agitation, slowed cognition, and confusion. These symptoms worsen over time and progress to loss of consciousness, respiratory pattern changes, and pupillary dilation (i.e., the symptoms of temporal lobe herniation). Homonymous hemianopia (defective vision in either the right or the left field [see Figure 14-8]), dysconjugate gaze, and gaze palsies also may occur.

Of those individuals affected by chronic subdural hematomas, 80% have chronic headaches and tenderness over the hematoma on palpation. Most persons appear to have a progressive dementia with generalized rigidity (paratonia). Chronic subdural hematomas require a craniotomy to evacuate the gelatinous blood. Percutaneous drainage for chronic subdural hematomas has proven successful. However, reaccumulation often occurs unless the surrounding membrane is removed.

Intracerebral hematomas (bleeding within the brain) occur in 2% to 3% of persons with head injuries, may be single or multiple, and are associated with contusions. Although most commonly located in the frontal and temporal lobes, they may occur in the hemispheric deep white matter. Penetrating injury or shearing forces traumatize small blood vessels. The intracerebral hematoma then acts as an expanding mass, increasing intracranial pressure, compressing brain tissues, and causing edema (see Figure 16-2). Delayed intracerebral hematomas may appear 3 to 10 days after the head injury. Intracerebral hematomas also can occur with nontraumatic brain injury, such as hemorrhagic stroke (see p. 404).

Intracerebral hematomas cause a decreasing level of consciousness. Coma or a confusional state from other injuries, however, can make the cause of this increasing unresponsiveness difficult to detect. Contralateral hemiplegia also may occur and, as intracranial pressure rises, temporal lobe herniation may appear. In delayed intracerebral hematoma, the presentation is similar to that of a hypertensive brain hemorrhage—sudden, rapidly progressive decreased level of consciousness with pupillary dilation, breathing pattern changes, hemiplegia, and bilateral positive Babinski reflexes.

History and physical examination help to establish the diagnosis, and CT scan, MRI, and cerebral angiography confirm it. Evacuation of a singular intracerebral hematoma has only occasionally been helpful, mostly for subcortical white matter hematomas. Otherwise, treatment is directed at reducing the intracranial pressure and allowing the hematoma to reabsorb slowly.

Open brain injury (trauma that penetrates the dura mater) produces both focal and diffuse injuries and includes compound skull fractures and missile injuries (e.g., bullets, rocks, shell fragments, knives, and blunt instruments). A **compound skull fracture** opens a communication between the cranial contents and the environment and should be investigated whenever lacerations of the scalp, tympanic membrane, sinuses, eye, or mucous membranes are present. Such fractures may involve the cranial vault or the base of the skull (basilar skull fracture). Cranial nerve damage and spinal fluid leak may occur with a basilar skull fracture.

The mechanisms of open brain trauma are crush injury (laceration and crushing of whatever the missile touches) and stretch injury (blood vessels and nerves damaged without direct contact as a result of stretching). The tangential injury is to the coverings and the brain (scalp and brain lacerations) and may also include skull fractures and meningeal or cerebral lacerations from projectiles and debris driven into the brain substance.

Most persons lose consciousness with open brain injury. The depth and duration of the coma are related to the location of injury, extent of damage, and amount of bleeding. Open brain injury often requires débridement of the traumatized tissues to prevent infection and to remove blood clots, thereby reducing intracranial pressure. Intracranial pressure also is managed with steroids, dehydrating agents, osmotic diuretics, or a combination of these drugs. Broad-spectrum antibiotics are administered to prevent infection.

A compound fracture may be diagnosed through physical examination, skull x-ray films, or both. Basilar skull fracture is determined on the basis of clinical findings, such as spinal fluid leaking from the ear or nose. Skull x-rays often do not demonstrate the fracture, although intracranial air or air in the sinuses on x-ray film, CT scan, or MRI is indirect evidence of a basilar skull fracture. Bed rest and close observation for meningitis and other complications are prescribed for a basilar skull fracture.

Diffuse brain injury. Diffuse brain injury (**diffuse axonal injury [DAI]**) involves widespread areas of the brain. Mechanical effects from high levels of acceleration and deceleration, such as whiplash, or rotational forces cause shearing of delicate axonal fibers and white matter tracts that project to the cerebral cortex (see Figure 16-1).

The most severe axonal injuries are located more peripheral to the brainstem, causing extensive cognitive and affective impairments, as seen in survivors of traumatic brain injury from motor vehicle crashes. Axonal damage reduces the speed of information processing and responding and disrupts the individual's attention span.[5]

Pathophysiologically, axonal damage can be seen only with an electron microscope and involves numerous axons, either alone or in conjunction with actual tissue tears. Advanced imaging techniques assist in defining areas of injury. Areas where axons and small blood vessels are torn appear as small hemorrhages, particularly in the corpus callosum and dorsolateral quadrant of the rostral brainstem at the superior cerebellar peduncle. More damaged axons are visible 12 hours to several days after the initial injury. The severity of diffuse injury correlates with how much shearing force was applied to the brainstem. DAI is not associated with intracranial hypertension immediately after injury; however, acute brain swelling caused by increased intravascular blood flow within the brain, vasodilation, and increased cerebral blood volume is seen often and can result in death.

Several categories of diffuse brain injury exist: mild concussion, classic concussion, mild DAI, moderate DAI, and severe DAI.

Mild concussion (mild traumatic brain injury) is characterized by immediate but transitory clinical manifestations. CSF pressure rises, and ECG and EEG changes occur without loss of consciousness.[6] Approximately 75% to 90% of blunt trauma injuries cause mild concussion. The Glasgow Coma Scale score for mild concussion is 13 to 15. The initial confusional state lasts for 1 to several minutes, possibly with amnesia for events preceding the trauma (retrograde amnesia). Anterograde amnesia (lack of memories) may also exist transiently. Persons may experience headache and complain of nervousness and "not being themselves" for up to a few days.

Classic cerebral concussion is any loss of consciousness lasting less than 6 hours accompanied by retrograde and anterograde amnesia with a confusional state lasting for hours to days. Transient cessation of respiration can occur with brief periods of bradycardia and a decrease in blood pressure lasting 30 seconds or less. Vital signs stabilize within a few seconds to within normal limits. Reflexes fail and are regained as responsiveness returns.

DAI is a severe brain injury and produces coma lasting more than 6 hours because of axonal disruption. Three forms of DAI exist: mild, moderate, and severe. In mild diffuse axonal injury, coma lasts 6 to 24 hours with 30% of persons displaying decerebrate or decorticate posturing (see Figure 15-6). They may experience prolonged periods of stupor or restlessness.

In moderate diffuse axonal injury, the score on the Glasgow Coma Scale (GCS) is 4 to 8 initially and 6 to 8 by 24 hours. Thirty-five percent of victims have transitory decerebration or decortication, with unconsciousness lasting days or weeks. On awakening, the person is confused and suffers a long period of posttraumatic anterograde and retrograde amnesia. There is often permanent deficit in memory, attention, abstraction, reasoning, problem solving, executive functions, vision or perception, and language. Mood and affect changes range from mild to severe.

In severe diffuse axonal injury, injury involves both hemispheres and the brainstem. Coma may last days to months. The person experiences immediate autonomic dysfunction (hypertension, tachycardia, tachypnea, extensor posturing) that disappears in a few weeks. Increased intracranial pressure appears 4 to 6 days after injury. Pulmonary complications occur often. Profound sensorimotor and cognitive system deficits are present, including spastic paralysis, dysarthria, dysphagia, memory loss, inability to learn and reason, and failure to modulate behavior. Irreversible coma and death can occur.

High-resolution CT scan and MRI assist in the diagnosis of focal and diffuse injuries. Medical management must address endocrine and metabolic derangements. The goal of treatment is to maintain cerebral perfusion and oxygenation, and promote neuroprotection. Implementation of traumatic brain injury guidelines decreases death and improves neurologic outcome. The Corticosteroid Randomization After Significant Head Injury (CRASH) trial showed corticosteroids increase mortality with acute TBI; consequently, these drugs are no longer used.[3,7] Guidelines are available to direct treatment.[8]

Secondary brain injury. Secondary brain injury is an indirect result of primary brain injury, including trauma and stroke syndromes. Systemic and cerebral processes are contributing factors. Systemic processes include hypotension, hypoxia, anemia, hypercapnia, and hypocapnia. Cerebral contributions include inflammation, cerebral edema, increased intracranial pressure (IICP), decreased cerebral perfusion pressure, cerebral ischemia, and brain herniation. Cellular and molecular brain damage from the effects of primary injury develops hours to days later. Astrocyte swelling and proliferation alter the blood-brain barrier and cause IICP. Ischemia contributes to excitotoxicity with release of excitatory neurotransmitters, such as glutamate and aspartate. They cause cellular influx of calcium, damage mitochondria, and cause neuronal hyperexcitability. A hypermetabolic state, poor perfusion, influx of inflammatory mediators, fluctuations in cellular sodium and potassium ion channels, and mitochondrial failure all contribute to cytotoxic edema, axonal swelling, and neuronal death.[2]

The management of secondary brain injury is related to prevention and includes removal of hematomas and management of hypotension, hypoxemia, anemia, intracranial pressure, fluid and electrolyte balance, body temperature, and ventilation. Thyrotropin-releasing hormone, statins, and other agents are under investigation and may be neuroprotective by decreasing excitotoxicity, neuroinflammation, and other mechanisms of secondary injury.[2,9] Progress is difficult because of the lack of predictive biomarkers and drugs that can cross the blood-brain barrier. Fluid and nutrition management has emerged as critically important in the care of individuals with severe brain injury.[10] Long-term recovery can be influenced by systemic complications, such as pneumonia, fever, infections, and immobility that contribute to further brain injury, and delays in repair and recovery.

Complications of Traumatic Brain Injury

Many complications are associated with TBI and are related to the severity of injury and the parts of the brain that are affected. Altered states of consciousness can range from confusion to deep coma (see Table 15-3). Cognitive deficits; hydrocephalus; sensory-motor disorders, including pain, paresis, and paralysis; and loss of coordination may be present. Three of the most common posttraumatic brain syndromes are summarized below.

Postconcussion syndrome, including headache, dizziness, fatigue, nervousness or anxiety, irritability, insomnia, depression, inability to concentrate, and forgetfulness, may last for weeks to months after a concussion. Treatment entails reassurance and symptomatic relief in addition to 24 hours of close observation after the concussion in the event bleeding or swelling in the brain occurs. Symptoms requiring further evaluation and treatment include drowsiness or confusion, nausea or vomiting, severe headache, memory deficit, seizures, drainage of cerebrospinal fluid from the ear or nose, weakness or loss of feeling in the extremities, asymmetry of the pupils, and double vision. Guidelines for the management of pediatric and adult concussion are available.[11-13] Guidelines have been published for the management of sports-related concussion.[14]

Posttraumatic seizures occur in about 2% to 16% of TBIs, with the highest risk among open brain injuries. Seizures can occur early, within days, and up to 2 to 5 years or longer after the trauma. Causal mechanisms are poorly understood and cellular and molecular changes in the brain associated with injury and repair, such as sprouting of new neurons with hyperexcitability and decreases in GABAergic inhibition, may cause the hyperexcitable state that leads to epileptogenesis. Seizure prevention using drugs, such as phenytoin, is initiated for moderate to severe TBI at the time of injury. Clinical trials are ongoing to test drugs that prevent the development of posttraumatic seizures.[15]

Chronic traumatic encephalopathy (CTE) (previously called *dementia pugilistica*) is a progressive dementing disease that develops with repeated brain injury associated with sporting events, blast injuries in soldiers, or work-related head trauma. Tau neurofibrillary tangles are present in the brain and research is in progress to discover the mechanistic link between neurotrauma and CTE. It is diagnosed from history and clinical evaluation, and at autopsy.[16,17]

> **QUICK CHECK 16-1**
> 1. How is a concussion different from a contusion?
> 2. Why do epidural, subdural, and intracerebral hematomas act like expanding masses?
> 3. Why is head motion the principal causative mechanism of diffuse brain injury?

Spinal Cord and Vertebral Injury

Each year 12,000 persons experience serious spinal cord injury. Male gender and ages 16 to 30 years are strong risk factors. Motor vehicle accidents are the leading cause of injury (36.5%); falls are the next most common cause (28.5%) followed by violence, other events, and sports activities.[18] Elderly people are particularly at risk for trauma that results in serious spinal cord injury because of preexisting degenerative vertebral disorders.

PATHOPHYSIOLOGY Primary spinal cord injury occurs with the initial mechanical trauma and immediate tissue destruction. Injuries to the cord are summarized in Table 16-3. Primary spinal cord injury occurs if an injured spine is not adequately immobilized immediately following injury. Primary spinal cord injury also may occur in the absence of vertebral fracture or dislocation from longitudinal

stretching of the cord with or without flexion or extension of the vertebral column, or both. The stretching causes altered axon transport, edema, myelin degeneration, and retrograde or wallerian degeneration (see Chapter 13).

Secondary spinal cord injury is a pathophysiologic cascade of vascular, cellular, and biochemical events that begins within a few minutes after injury and continues for weeks. Edema, ischemia, excitotoxicity (excessive stimulation by excitatory neurotransmitters such as glutamate), inflammation, oxidative damage, and activation of necrotic and apoptotic cell death signal events similar to those previously described for traumatic brain injury (see p. 390).[19]

With secondary spinal cord injury, microscopic hemorrhages appear in the central gray matter and pia-arachnoid, increasing in size until the entire gray matter is hemorrhagic and necrotic. Edema in the white matter occurs, impairing the microcirculation of the cord. Hemorrhages and edema are followed by reduced vascular perfusion and development of ischemic areas, which are maximal at the level of injury and two cord segments above and below it. Cellular and subcellular alterations and tissue necrosis occur. Cord swelling increases the individual's degree of dysfunction, making it difficult to distinguish functions permanently lost from those temporarily impaired. In the cervical region, cord swelling may be life-threatening. Diaphragm function may be impaired because phrenic nerves exit at C3 to C5. Cardiovascular and respiratory functions mediated by the medulla oblongata can be lost.

Circulation in the white matter tracts of the spinal cord returns to normal in about 24 hours, but gray matter circulation remains altered. Phagocytes appear 36 to 48 hours after injury, and microglia proliferate with altered astrocytes. Red blood cells then begin to disintegrate, and resorption of hemorrhages and edema begins. Degenerating axons are engulfed by macrophages in the first 10 days after injury. The traumatized cord is replaced by acellular collagenous tissue, usually in 3 to 4 weeks. Meninges thicken as part of the scarring process.

Vertebral injuries result from acceleration, deceleration, or deformation forces occurring at impact. These forces cause vertebral fractures, dislocations, and bone fragments that can cause compression to the tissues, pull or exert traction (tension) on the tissues, or cause shearing of tissues so they slide into one another (Figures 16-3 to 16-6). Vertebral injuries can be classified as (1) simple fracture—a single break usually affecting transverse or spinous processes; (2) compressed (wedged) vertebral fracture—vertebral body compressed anteriorly;

TABLE 16-3 Spinal Cord Injuries

Injury	Description
Cord concussion	Results in temporary disruption of cord-mediated functions
Cord contusion	Bruising of neural tissue causes swelling and temporary loss of cord-mediated functions
Cord compression	Pressure on cord causes ischemia to tissues; must be relieved (decompressed) to prevent permanent damage to spinal cord
Laceration	Tearing of neural tissues of spinal cord; may be reversible if only slight damage sustained by neural tissues; may result in permanent loss of cord-mediated functions if spinal tracts are disrupted
Transection	Severing of spinal cord causes permanent loss of function
Complete	All tracts in spinal cord are completely disrupted; all cord-mediated functions below transection are completely and permanently lost
Incomplete	Some tracts in spinal cord remain intact, together with functions mediated by those tracts; has potential for recovery although function is temporarily lost
Preserved sensation only	Some demonstrable sensation below level of injury
Preserved motor nonfunctional	Preserved motor function without useful purpose; sensory function may or may not be preserved
Preserved motor functional	Preserved voluntary motor function that is functionally useful
Hemorrhage	Bleeding into neural tissue as a result of blood vessel damage; usually no major loss of function
Damage or obstruction of spinal blood supply	Causes local ischemia

(3) comminuted (burst) fracture—vertebral body shattered into several fragments; and (4) dislocation.

The vertebrae fracture readily with both direct and indirect trauma. When the supporting ligaments are torn, the vertebrae move out of alignment and dislocations occur. A horizontal force moves the vertebrae straight forward; if the individual is in a flexed position at the time of injury, the vertebrae are then angulated. Flexion and extension injuries may result in dislocations. (Bone, ligament, and joint injuries are presented in Table 16-4.)

Vertebral injuries in adults occur most often at vertebrae C1 to C2 (cervical), C4 to C7, and T10 (thoracic) to L2 (lumbar) (see Figure 13-11), the most mobile portions of the vertebral column. The spinal cord occupies most of the vertebral canal in the cervical and lumbar regions, so it can be easily injured in these locations.

CLINICAL MANIFESTATIONS Spinal shock develops immediately after injury because of loss of continuous tonic discharge from the brain or brainstem and inhibition of suprasegmental impulses caused by cord hemorrhage, edema, or anatomic transection. Normal activity of spinal cord cells at and below the level of injury ceases with complete loss of reflex function, flaccid paralysis, absence of sensation, loss of bladder and rectal control, transient drop in blood pressure, and poor venous circulation. The condition also results in disturbed thermal control because the sympathetic nervous system is damaged. The hypothalamus cannot regulate body heat through vasoconstriction and increased metabolism; therefore the individual assumes the temperature of the air (poikilothermia). Spinal shock generally lasts 7 to 20 days, with a range of a few days to 3 months. It terminates with the reappearance of reflex activity, hyperreflexia, spasticity, and reflex emptying of the bladder. Table 16-5 summarizes the clinical manifestations of spinal cord injury.

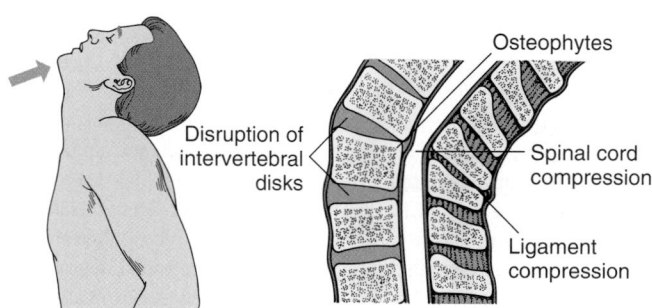

FIGURE 16-3 Hyperextension Injuries of the Spine. Hyperextension injuries of the spine can result in fracture or nonfracture injuries with spinal cord damage.

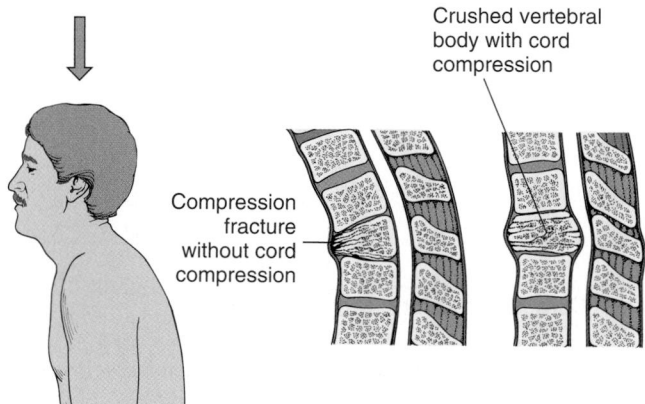

FIGURE 16-5 Axial Compression Injuries of the Spine. In axial compression injuries of the spine, the spinal cord is contused directly by retropulsion of bone or disk material into the spinal canal.

FIGURE 16-4 Flexion Injury of the Spine. Hyperflexion produces translation (subluxation) of vertebrae that compromises the central canal and compresses spinal cord parenchyma or vascular structures.

FIGURE 16-6 Flexion-Rotation Injuries of the Spine.

TABLE 16-4	Mechanisms of Vertebral Injury Involving Bone, Ligaments, and Joints		
Mechanism of Injury	**Location of Vertebral Injury**	**Forces of Injury**	**Location of Injury**
Hyperextension	Fracture and dislocation of posterior elements, such as spinous processes, transverse processes, laminae, pedicles, or posterior ligaments	Results from forces of acceleration-deceleration and sudden reduction in anteroposterior diameter of spinal cord	Cervical area
Hyperflexion	Fracture or dislocation of vertebral bodies, disks, or ligaments	Results from sudden and excessive force that propels neck forward or causes an exaggerated lateral movement of neck to one side	Cervical area
Vertical compression (axial loading)	Shattering fractures	Results from a force applied along an axis from top of cranium through vertebral bodies	T12 to L2
Rotational forces (flexion-rotation)	Rupture support ligaments in addition to producing fractures	Add shearing force to acceleration forces	Cervical area

TABLE 16-5   Clinical Manifestations of Spinal Cord Injury

Stage	Manifestations
Spinal Shock Stage Complete spinal cord transection	Loss of motor function 　　1. Quadriplegia with injuries of cervical spinal cord 　　2. Paraplegia with injuries of thoracic spinal cord Muscle flaccidity Loss of all reflexes below level of injury Loss of pain, temperature, touch, pressure, and proprioception below level of injury Pain at site of injury caused by zone of hyperesthesia above injury Atonic bladder and bowel Paralytic ileus with distention Loss of vasomotor tone in lower body parts; low and unstable blood pressure Loss of perspiration below level of injury Loss or extreme depression of genital reflexes such as penile erection and bulbocavernous reflex Dry and pale skin; possible ulceration over bony prominences Respiratory impairment
Partial spinal cord transection	Asymmetric flaccid motor paralysis below level of injury Asymmetric reflex loss Preservation of some sensation below level of injury Vasomotor instability less severe than that seen with complete cord transection Bowel and bladder impairment less severe than that seen with complete cord transection Preservation of ability to perspire in some portions of body below level of injury *Brown-Séquard syndrome* (associated with penetrating injuries, hyperextension and flexion, locked facets, and compression fractures) 　　1. Ipsilateral paralysis or paresis below level of injury 　　2. Ipsilateral loss of touch, pressure, vibration, and position sense below level of injury 　　3. Contralateral loss of pain and temperature sensations below level of injury *Central cervical cord syndrome* (acute cord compression between bony bars or spurs anteriorly and thickened ligamentum flavum 　　posteriorly associated with hyperextension) 　　1. Motor deficits in upper extremities, especially hands, more dense than in lower extremities 　　2. Varying degrees of bladder dysfunction *Burning hand syndrome* (variant of central cord syndrome; in 50% of cases an underlying spine fracture/dislocation is present) 　　1. Severe burning paresthesias and dysesthesias in the hands or feet *Anterior cord syndrome* (compromise of anterior spinal artery by occlusion or pressure effect of disk) 　　1. Loss of motor function below level of injury 　　2. Loss of pain and temperature sensations below level of injury 　　3. Touch, pressure, position, and vibration senses intact *Posterior cord syndrome* (associated with hyperextension injuries with fractures of vertebral arch) 　　1. Impaired light touch and proprioception *Conus medullaris syndrome* (compression injury at T12 from disk herniation or burst fracture of body of T12) 　　1. Flaccid paralysis of legs 　　2. Flaccid paralysis of anal sphincter 　　3. Variable sensory deficits *Cauda equina syndrome* (compression of nerve roots below L1 caused by fracture and dislocation of spine or large posterocentral 　　intervertebral disk herniation) 　　1. Lower extremity motor deficits 　　2. Variable sensorimotor dysfunction 　　3. Variable reflex dysfunction 　　4. Variable bladder, bowel, and sexual dysfunction *Syndrome of neuropraxia* (postathletic injury, associated with congenital spinal stenosis) 　　1. Dramatic but transient neurologic deficits including quadriplegia *Horner syndrome* (injury to preganglionic sympathetic trunk or postganglionic sympathetic neurons of superior cervical ganglion) 　　1. Ipsilateral pupil smaller than contralateral pupil 　　2. Sunken ipsilateral eyeball 　　3. Ptosis of affected eyeball 　　4. Lack of perspiration on ipsilateral side of face

Continued

TABLE 16-5   Clinical Manifestations of Spinal Cord Injury—cont'd

Stage	Manifestations
Heightened Reflex Activity Stage	Emergence of Babinski reflexes, possibly progressing to a triple reflex; possible development of still later flexor spasms Reappearance of ankle and knee reflexes, which become hyperactive Contraction of reflex detrusor muscle leading to urinary incontinence Appearance of reflex defecation Mass reflex with flexion spasms, profuse sweating, piloerection, and bladder and occasional bowel emptying may be evoked by autonomic stimulation of skin or from full bladder Episodes of hypertension Defective heat-induced sweating Eventual development of extensor reflexes, first in muscles of hip and thigh, later in leg Possible paresthesias below level of transection: dull, burning pain in lower back, abdomen, buttocks, and perineum

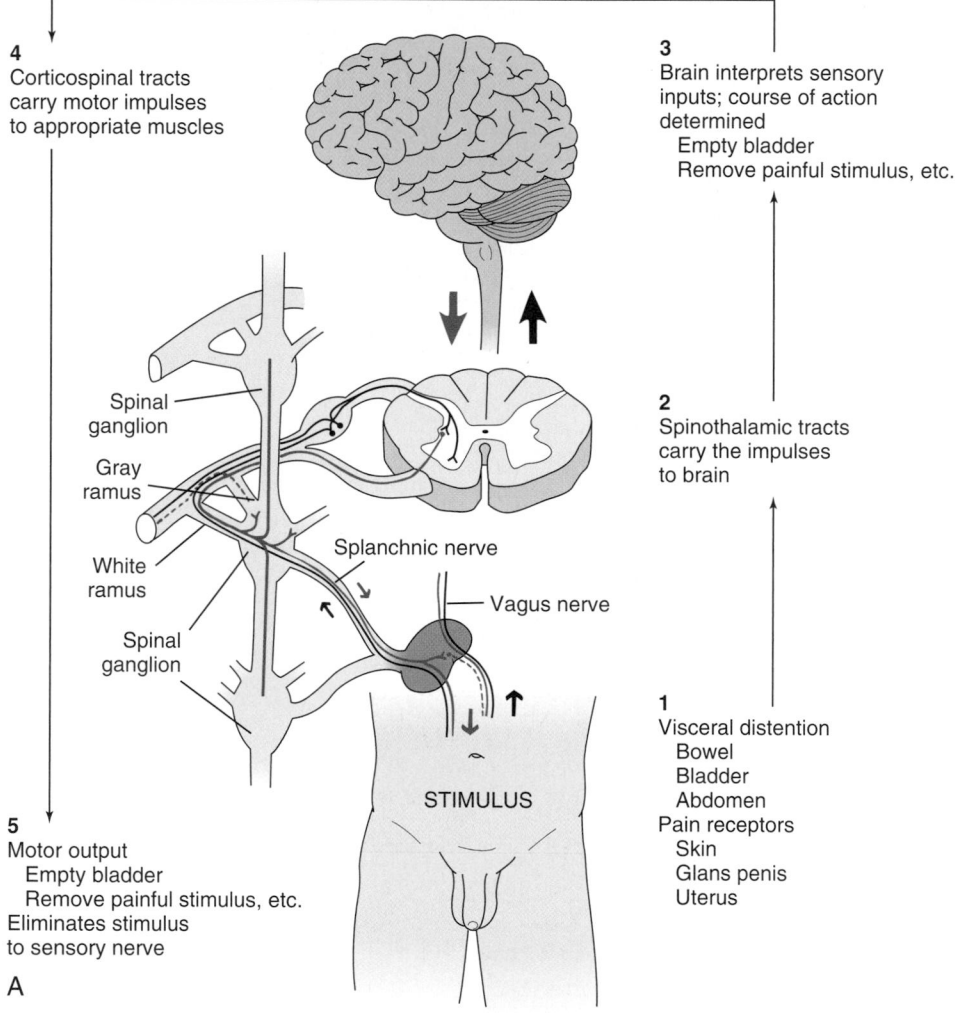

4
Corticospinal tracts carry motor impulses to appropriate muscles

3
Brain interprets sensory inputs; course of action determined
  Empty bladder
  Remove painful stimulus, etc.

Spinal ganglion
Gray ramus
White ramus
Spinal ganglion

Splanchnic nerve

Vagus nerve

2
Spinothalamic tracts carry the impulses to brain

1
Visceral distention
  Bowel
  Bladder
  Abdomen
Pain receptors
  Skin
  Glans penis
  Uterus

STIMULUS

5
Motor output
  Empty bladder
  Remove painful stimulus, etc.
Eliminates stimulus to sensory nerve

A

FIGURE 16-7 Autonomic Hyperreflexia. **A,** Normal response pathway.

Neurogenic shock, also called vasogenic shock, occurs with cervical or upper thoracic cord injury above T5 and may be seen in addition to spinal shock. Neurogenic shock is caused by the absence of sympathetic activity through loss of supraspinal control and unopposed parasympathetic tone mediated by the intact vagus nerve. Symptoms include vasodilation, hypotension, bradycardia, and failure of body temperature regulation. Neurogenic shock may be complicated by hypovolemic or cardiogenic shock if there is concurrent heart failure or blood loss (see Chapter 24).

Autonomic hyperreflexia (dysreflexia) is a syndrome of sudden, massive reflex sympathetic discharge associated with spinal cord injury at level T6 or above where descending inhibition is blocked (Figure 16-7). It may occur after spinal shock resolves and be a recurrent complication. Characteristics include paroxysmal hypertension (up to 300 mm Hg, systolic), a pounding headache, blurred vision, sweating above the level of the lesion with flushing of the skin, nasal congestion, nausea, piloerection caused by pilomotor spasm, and bradycardia (30 to 40 beats/min). The symptoms may develop singly or in

5
Ninth cranial nerve stimulated by carotid; receptors send message to vasomotor center of medulla, vagus nerve stimulated; impulse sent to SA node; results in bradycardia

Carotid sinuses

Glossopharyngeal nerve (IX)

4
Increased blood pressure stimulates carotid sinus receptors

Medulla

Carotid sinus nerve
Vagus nerve (X)

SA node

6
Autonomic response to hypertension down to level of cord lesion
  Arterial dilation
  Flushed skin
  Headache
  Sweating

Loss of descending Inhibition below T6

Lesion at T6

3
Reflex stimulus to major sympathetic outflow resulting in:
  Vasoconstriction
  Hypertension
  Pallor of skin
  Pilomotor spasms

2
Spinothalamic tracts carry sensory impulses to level of lesion (T6 and above)

STIMULUS

1
Visceral distention
  Bowel
  Bladder
  Abdomen
Pain receptors
  Skin
  Glans penis
  Uterus

B

FIGURE 16-7, cont'd B, Autonomic dysreflexia pathway. *SA,* Sinoatrial. (Modified from Rudy EB: *Advanced neurological and neurosurgical nursing,* St Louis, 1984, Mosby.)

combination. The condition can cause serious complications (stroke, seizures, myocardial ischemia, and death) and requires immediate treatment.

In autonomic hyperreflexia, sensory receptors below the level of the cord lesion are stimulated. The intact autonomic nervous system reflexively responds with an arteriolar spasm that increases blood pressure. Baroreceptors in the cerebral vessels, the carotid sinus, and the aorta sense the hypertension and stimulate the parasympathetic system. The heart rate decreases, but the visceral and peripheral vessels do not dilate because efferent impulses cannot pass through the cord.

The most common cause is a distended bladder or rectum; however, any sensory stimulation (i.e., skin or pain receptors) can elicit

autonomic hyperreflexia. Intravenous fluids may be required to maintain blood pressure. Drug therapy, may be required to lower blood pressure and reduce complications. Bladder, bowel, and skin care management are important preventive strategies. Education of the individual and family regarding triggers and acute management is important as is wearing a medic alert tag.[20]

EVALUATION AND TREATMENT Diagnosis of spinal cord injury is based on physical examination and imaging studies. Neurogenic shock must be differentiated from other kinds of shock (i.e., hypovolemic shock). For a suspected or confirmed vertebral fracture or dislocation, regardless of the presence or absence of spinal cord injury, the immediate intervention is immobilization of the spine to prevent further injury. Decompression and surgical fixation may be necessary. Corticosteroids may be given at the time of injury to decrease secondary cord injury from inflammation and thereafter for several days.[21] Therapeutic hypothermia has shown some encouraging evidence for improved outcomes, particularly for cervical cord injuries; however, more research is needed.[22] Clinical trials are in progress to treat acute spinal cord injury, including cell-based therapies, immune modulators, vasculature selective treatments, and functional electrical stimulation.[23] Nutrition; lung function; skin integrity; prevention of pressure ulcers, in particular; and bladder and bowel management must be addressed. Plans for rehabilitation need early consideration.

Degenerative Disorders of the Spine
Low Back Pain

Low back pain (LBP) affects the area between the lower rib cage and gluteal muscles and often radiates into the thighs. The percentage of the population affected with LBP is about 29%, with a higher percentage among older individuals, particularly women older than age 60.[24] LBP is the primary cause of disability worldwide.[25] The burdens of disability include psychologic, financial, occupational, and social effects on the person and family members.

Risk factors include occupations that require repetitive lifting in the forward bent-and-twisted position; exposure to vibrations caused by vehicles or industrial machinery; obesity; and cigarette smoking. Some people have a genetic predisposition for low back pain.

PATHOGENESIS Most cases of LBP are idiopathic or nonspecific, and no precise diagnosis is possible. Acute LBP is often associated with muscle or ligament strain and is more common in individuals younger than 50 years of age without a history of cancer. Common causes of chronic LBP include degenerative disk disease, spondylolysis, spondylolisthesis (vertebra slides forward or slips in relation to a vertebra below), spinal osteochondrosis, spinal stenosis, and lumbar disk herniation. Other causes include tension caused by tumors or disk prolapse, bursitis, synovitis, rising venous and tissue pressures (found in degenerative joint disease), abnormal bone pressures, spinal immobility, inflammation caused by infection (as in osteomyelitis), and pain referred from viscera or the posterior peritoneum. Systemic causes of LBP include bone diseases, such as osteoporosis or osteomalacia, and hyperparathyroidism. Anatomically, low back pain must originate from innervated structures, but deep pain is widely referred and varies. The nucleus pulposus has no intrinsic innervation, but when extruded or herniated through a prolapsed disk, it irritates the spinal nerve dural membranes and causes pain referred to the segmental area[26] (Figure 16-8).

The interspinous bursae can be a source of pain between L3, L4, L5, and S1 but also may affect L1, L2, and L3 spinous processes. The anterior and posterior longitudinal ligaments of the spine and the interspinous and supraspinous ligaments are abundantly supplied with pain receptors, as is the ligamentum flavum. All of these ligaments are vulnerable to traumatic tears (sprains) and fracture. Diskogenic pain also may be related to inflammation and nerve sprouting within the disk.[27]

CLINICAL MANIFESTATIONS About 1% of individuals with acute low back pain have pain along the distribution of a lumbar nerve root (radicular pain), most commonly involving the sciatic nerve (sciatica). Sciatica is often accompanied by neurosensory and motor deficits, such as tingling, numbness, and weakness in various parts of the leg and foot. Major or progressive motor or sensory deficit, cauda equina syndrome (new-onset bowel or bladder incontinence or urinary

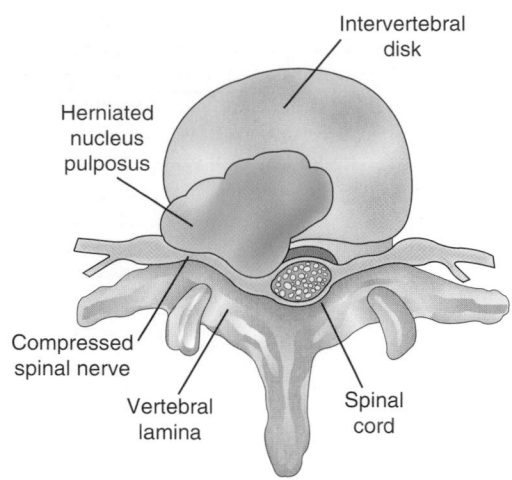

FIGURE 16-8 Herniated Nucleus Pulposus.

retention, loss of anal sphincter tone, and saddle anesthesia), history of cancer metastasis to bone, and suspected spinal infection can be associated with chronic low back pain.

EVALUATION AND TREATMENT Diagnosis of low back pain is based on the history and physical examination. Imaging and nerve conduction studies are obtained with severe neurologic deficit or serious underlying disease. Diagnosis and treatment guidelines are available to plan therapy.[28] Most individuals with acute low back pain benefit from a nonspecific short-term treatment regimen of bed rest, analgesic medications, exercises, physical therapy, and education. Surgical treatments, specifically diskectomy and spinal fusions, are used for individuals not responding to medical management or for emergency management of cauda equina syndrome. Individuals with chronic low back pain may benefit from anti-inflammatory and muscle relaxant medications, exercise programs, massage, topical heat, spinal manipulation, acupuncture, cognitive-behavioral therapies, and interdisciplinary care.[29] There is scant evidence for efficacy of opioids for chronic low back pain, but a high risk for addiction.[30] The complexity of causes contributes to the difficulty in defining pathogenesis and clearly defining the most effective therapies.

Degenerative Joint Disease (DJD)

Degenerative disk disease. Degenerative disk disease (DDD) is common in individuals 30 years of age and older. It is, in part, a process of normal aging as a response to continuous vertical compression of the spine (axial loading). DDD includes a genetic component, involving genes that code the cartilage intermediate layer protein (CILP). The combination of environmental interactions and genetic predisposition increases susceptibility to lumbar disk disease by disrupting normal building and maintenance of cartilage.[27] Causes include biochemical (e.g., inflammatory mediators) and biomechanical alterations (e.g., mechanical loading and compression) of the intervertebral disk tissue. For example, loss of disk proteoglycans and collagen with disk dehydration and loss of hydrostatic pressure alters disk structure and function. The annulus can tear and the disk can herniate, pinching nerves or placing strain on the spine. The pathologic findings in DDD include disk protrusion, spondylolysis and/or subluxation (spondylolisthesis), degeneration of vertebrae, and spinal stenosis. Lumbar disk disease causes one third of all back pain that affects 70% to 90% of adults at some point in their lives. However, only a small percentage of people with degenerative disk disease have any functional incapacity because of pain.

Spondylolysis. Spondylolysis is a structural defect (degeneration, fracture, or developmental defect) in the pars interarticularis of the vertebral arch (the joining of the vertebral body to the posterior structures). The lumbar spine at L5 is affected most often. Mechanical pressure may cause an anterior or posterior displacement of the deficient vertebra (spondylolisthesis). Heredity plays a significant role, and spondylolysis is associated with an increased incidence of other congenital spinal defects. Symptoms include lower back and lower limb pain.

Spondylolisthesis. Spondylolisthesis, an osseous defect of the pars interarticularis, allows a vertebra to slide anteriorly in relation to the vertebra below, commonly occurring at L5-S1. Spondylolisthesis is graded from 1 to 4 based on the percentage of slip that occurs. Grades 1 and 2 have symptoms of pain in the lower back and buttocks, muscle spasms in the lower back and legs, and tightened hamstrings. Conservative management includes exercise, rest, and back bracing. Vertebral slippage in grades 3 and 4 usually requires surgical decompression, stabilization, or both.

Spinal stenosis. Spinal stenosis is a narrowing of the spinal canal that causes pressure on the spinal nerves or cord and can be congenital or acquired (more common) and associated with trauma or arthritis. It is categorized by the area of the spine affected: cervical, thoracic, or lumbar. Acquired conditions include a bulging disk, facet hypertrophy, or a thick ossified posterior longitudinal ligament. Symptoms are related to the area of the spine affected and can produce pain; numbness; and tingling in the neck, hands, arms, or legs with weakness and difficulty walking. Surgical decompression is recommended for those with chronic symptoms and those who do not respond to medical management.

Herniated Intervertebral Disk

Herniation of an intervertebral disk is a displacement of the nucleus pulposus or annulus fibrosus beyond the intervertebral disk space (see Figure 16-8). Rupture of an intervertebral disk usually is caused by trauma, degenerative disk disease, or both. Risk factors are weight-bearing sports, light weight lifting, and certain work activities, such as repeated lifting. Men are affected more often than women, with the highest incidence in the 30- to 50-year age group. Most commonly affected are the lumbosacral disks L4-L5 and L5-S1. Herniation is typically at higher vertebrae in older persons. Disk herniation occasionally occurs in the cervical area, usually at C5-C6 and C6-C7. Herniations at the thoracic level are extremely rare. The herniation may occur immediately, within a few hours, or months to years after injury.

PATHOPHYSIOLOGY In a herniated disk, the ligament and posterior capsule of the disk are usually torn, allowing the nucleus pulposus to extrude and compress the nerve root. The vascular supply may be compromised and cause inflammatory changes in the nerve root (radiculitis). Occasionally, the injury tears the entire disk loose, causing the disk capsule and nucleus pulposus to protrude onto the nerve root or compress the spinal cord. Multiple nerve root compression may be found at the L5-S1 level, where the cauda equina may be compressed, causing cauda equina syndrome (see Table 16-5).

CLINICAL MANIFESTATIONS The location and size of the herniation into the spinal canal, together with the amount of space in the canal, determine the clinical manifestations associated with the injury (Figure 16-9). Compression or inflammation, or both, of a spinal nerve resulting from disk herniation follows a dermatomal distribution called radiculopathy (Figure 16-10). A herniated disk in the lumbosacral area is associated with pain that radiates along the sciatic nerve course over the buttock and into the calf or ankle. The pain occurs with straining, including coughing and sneezing, and usually on straight leg raising.

FIGURE   16-9 Clinical Features of a Herniated Nucleus Pulposus.

Other clinical manifestations include limited range of motion of the lumbar spine; tenderness on palpation in the sciatic notch and along the sciatic nerve; impaired pain, temperature, and touch sensations in the L4-L5 or L5-S1 dermatomes of the leg and foot; decreased or absent ankle jerk reflex; and mild weakness of the foot. More rarely, there is development of cauda equina syndrome.

With the herniation of a lower cervical disk, paresthesias and pain are present in the upper arm, forearm, and hand along the affected nerve root distribution. Neck motion and straining, including coughing and sneezing, may increase neck and nerve root pain. Neck range of motion is diminished. Slight weakness and atrophy of biceps or triceps muscles may occur; the biceps or triceps reflex may decrease. Occasionally, signs of corticospinal and sensory tract impairments appear, including motor weakness of the lower extremities, sensory disturbances in the lower extremities, and presence of a Babinski reflex.

EVALUATION AND TREATMENT Diagnosis of a herniated intervertebral disk is made through the history and physical examination, spinal x-ray films, electromyelography, CT scan, MRI, myelography, diskography, and nerve conduction studies. Evidenced-based practice guidelines have been published to guide treatment options.[31] Most herniated disks heal spontaneously over time and do not require surgery. A surgical approach is indicated if there is evidence of severe compression (weakness or decreased deep tendon, bladder, or bowel

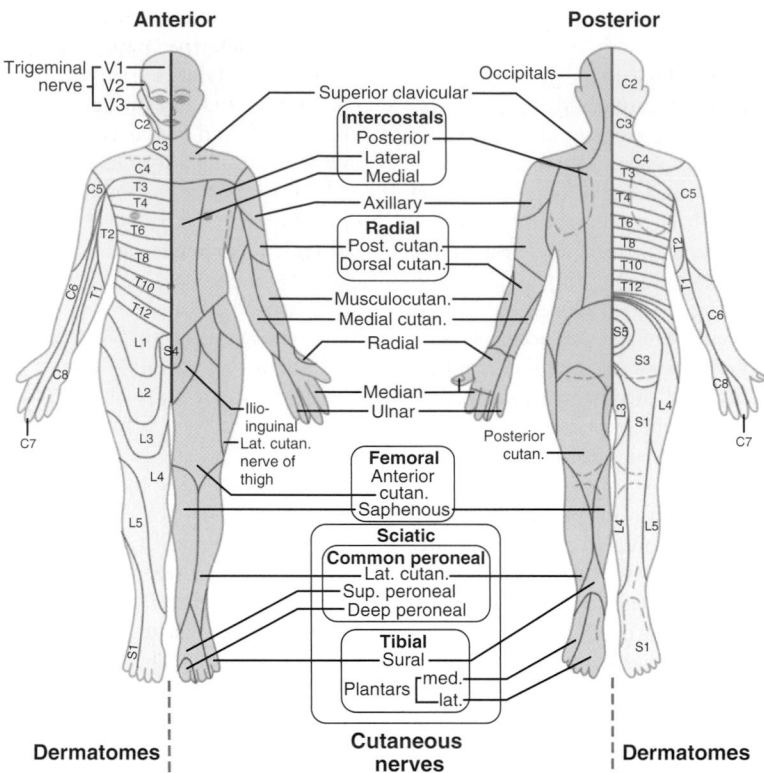

FIGURE 16-10 Sensory Nerve Distribution of Skin Dermatomes. (Redrawn from Patton HD et al, editors: *Introduction to basic neurology*, Philadelphia, 1976, WB Saunders. Borrowed from Canale ST, Beaty JH: *Campbell's operative orthopaedics*, ed 12, St Louis, 2013, Mosby.)

reflexes) or if a conservative approach is unsuccessful.[32] Cauda equina syndrome requires emergency surgical evaluation.[33]

Cerebrovascular Disorders

Cerebrovascular disease is the most frequently occurring neurologic disorder, accounting for more than 50% of the persons admitted to general hospitals with neurologic problems. Any abnormality of the brain caused by a pathologic process in the blood vessels is referred to as a *cerebrovascular disease.* Included in this category are lesions of the vessel wall, occlusion of the vessel lumen by thrombus or embolus, rupture of the vessel, and alteration in blood quality such as increased blood viscosity.

The brain abnormalities induced by cerebrovascular disease are either (1) ischemia with or without infarction (death of brain tissues) or (2) hemorrhage. The common clinical manifestation of cerebrovascular disease is a cerebrovascular accident or stroke. The symptoms occur suddenly and are focal (i.e., slurred speech, difficulty swallowing, limb weakness, or paralysis). In its mildest form, a cerebrovascular accident is so minimal that it is almost unnoticed. In its most severe form, hemiplegia, coma, and death result.

Cerebrovascular Accidents (Stroke Syndromes)

Cerebrovascular accidents (CVAs) are the leading cause of disability and the third cause of death in women and the fifth leading cause of death in men in the United States (see *Health Alert:* Prevention of Stroke in Women). About 75% of CVAs occur among those older than 65 years. The incidence is about 150% greater in blacks than whites.[34] Blacks between the ages of 55 and 64 who live in the southern states are about 50% more likely to die of stroke than blacks of the same age who live in the North.[35] In addition, persons with both hypertension

and type 2 diabetes mellitus have a fourfold increase in stroke incidence and an eightfold increase in stroke mortality.[36] The incidence of stroke decreased 35.8% from 2000 to 2010 and is associated with hypertension, diabetes and high cholesterol control and smoking cessation.[34]

Cerebrovascular accidents (stroke syndromes) are classified pathophysiologically as ischemic, hemorrhagic, or associated with hypoperfusion. Risk factors for stroke include the following:
- Poorly or uncontrolled arterial hypertension
- Smoking, which increases the risk of stroke by 50%
- Insulin resistance and diabetes mellitus
- Polycythemia and thrombocythemia
- High total cholesterol or low high-density lipoprotein (HDL) cholesterol, elevated lipoprotein-a
- Congestive heart disease and peripheral vascular disease
- Hyperhomocysteinemia
- Atrial fibrillation
- *Chlamydia pneumoniae* infection

Ischemic stroke. Ischemic stroke occurs when there is obstruction to arterial blood flow to the brain from thrombus formation, an embolus, or hypoperfusion related to decreased blood volume or heart failure. The inadequate blood supply results in ischemia (inadequate cellular oxygen) and can progress to infarction (death of tissue).

Transient ischemic attacks (TIAs) are episodes of neurologic dysfunction lasting no more than 1 hour and resulting from focal cerebral ischemia. The clinical manifestations of a TIA may include weakness, numbness, sudden confusion, loss of balance, or a sudden severe headache. The use of brain imaging modalities often reveals a brain infarction. About 3% to 17% of individuals experiencing a TIA will have a stroke within 90 days.[37]

HEALTH ALERT

Prevention of Stroke in Women

Stroke is the third leading cause of death in women and the fifth leading cause of death in men. The number of women with stroke will increasingly outnumber men in the future. Guidelines have been developed by the American Heart Association/American Stroke Association Council on Stroke to reduce stroke risk in women considering genetic differences in immunity, coagulation, hormonal factors, reproductive factors including pregnancy and childbirth, and social factors. A summary of these guidelines is presented below:

- Women should be informed about stroke risk factors (e.g., obesity, hypertension, and diabetes) at an early age.
- Women with a history of high blood pressure before pregnancy should be considered for low-dose aspirin or calcium supplement therapy, or both, to lower preeclampsia risks.
- Women who have preeclampsia have twice the risk of stroke and a fourfold increased risk of high blood pressure later in life. Therefore, preeclampsia should be recognized as a risk factor well after pregnancy and other risk factors such as smoking, high cholesterol, and obesity in these women should be treated early.
- Pregnant women with moderately high blood pressure (150-159 mm Hg/100-109 mm Hg) may be considered for safe and effective antihypertensive medication, whereas expectant mothers with severe high blood pressure (160/110 mm Hg or higher) should be treated.
- Women at risk for central venous thrombosis require prothrombotic screening, consideration for antithrombotic therapy, and careful management during pregnancy.
- Women should be screened for high blood pressure before taking birth control pills because the combination raises stroke risks.
- Hormone therapy (conjugated equine estrogen) with or without medroxyprogesterone should not be used for primary or secondary prevention of stroke in postmenopausal women.
- Women who have migraine headaches with aura should stop smoking to avoid higher stroke risks.
- Women with cardiovascular risk factors should engage in regular physical activity, moderate alcohol consumption (<1 drink per day for nonpregnant women), abstention from cigarette smoking, and a diet rich in fruit, vegetables, grains, nuts, olive oil, and low saturated fat.
- Women older than age 75 should be screened for atrial fibrillation risks because of its link to higher stroke risk.

The guidelines are available at: https://my.americanheart.org/idc/groups/ahamah-public/@wcm/@sop/@smd/documents/downloadable/ucm_460480.pdf. Further information is available from Data from Bushnell C, McCullough L: *Ann Intern Med* 160(12):853-857, 2014.

Thrombotic strokes (cerebral thromboses) arise from arterial occlusions caused by thrombi formation in arteries supplying the brain or intracranial vessels. Conditions causing increased coagulation or inadequate cerebral perfusion (e.g., dehydration, hypotension, prolonged vasoconstriction from malignant hypertension) increase the risk of thrombosis. Cerebral thrombosis develops most often from atherosclerosis and inflammatory disease processes that damage arterial walls. It may take as long as 20 to 30 years for obstruction to develop at the branches and curvature found in the cerebral circulation (see Chapter 24 for a discussion of atherogenesis). The smooth stenotic area can degenerate, forming an ulcerated area of the vessel wall. Platelets and fibrin adhere to the damaged wall, and a clot forms, gradually occluding the artery. The clot may enlarge both distally and proximally. Thrombotic strokes also occur when parts of a clot detach, travel upstream, and obstruct blood flow, causing acute ischemia.

Embolic stroke involves fragments that break from a thrombus formed outside the brain, usually in the heart, aorta, or common carotid artery. Other sources of embolism include fat, air, tumor, bacterial clumps, and foreign bodies. The embolus usually involves small brain vessels and obstructs at a bifurcation or other point of narrowing, thus causing ischemia. An embolus may plug the lumen entirely and remain in place or shatter into fragments and become part of the vessel's blood flow. Risk factors for an embolic stroke include atrial fibrillation, left ventricular aneurysm or thrombus, left atrial thrombus, recent myocardial infarction, endocarditis, rheumatic valve disease, mechanical valvular prostheses, atrioseptal defects, patent foramen ovale, and primary cardiac tumors. In persons who experience an embolic stroke, a second stroke usually follows because the source of emboli continues to exist. Embolization is usually in the distribution of the middle cerebral artery (the largest cerebral artery). Ischemic strokes in children are associated with congenital heart disease, cerebral arteriovenous malformations, and sickle cell disease (see Chapter 17).

Lacunar strokes (lacunar infarcts or **small vessel disease)** are usually caused by occlusion of a single, deep perforating artery that supplies small penetrating subcortical vessels, causing ischemic lesions (0.5 to 15 mm, or lacunes) predominantly in the basal ganglia, internal capsules, and pons. These strokes are rare and, because of the location and small area of infarction, they may have pure motor or sensory deficits.[38]

Hypoperfusion, or hemodynamic stroke, is associated with *systemic* hypoperfusion caused by cardiac failure, pulmonary embolism, or bleeding that results in inadequate blood supply to the brain. Stroke may occur more readily if there is carotid artery occlusion. Symptoms are usually bilateral and diffuse.[39]

PATHOPHYSIOLOGY   Cerebral infarction results when an area of the brain loses its blood supply because of vascular occlusion. Causes include (1) abrupt vascular occlusion (e.g., embolus or thrombi), (2) gradual vessel occlusion (e.g., atheroma), and (3) partial occlusion of stenotic vessels. Cerebral thrombi and cerebral emboli most commonly produce occlusion, but atherosclerosis and hypertension are the dominant underlying processes.

There is a central core of irreversible ischemia and necrosis with cerebral infarction. The central core is surrounded by a zone of borderline ischemic tissue, the ischemic penumbra. Ischemia in the penumbra is not severe enough to result in structural damage. Prompt restoration of perfusion in the penumbra by injection of thrombolytic agents promotes perfusion and may prevent necrosis and loss of neurologic function. The window of opportunity for protecting the penumbra is about 3 hours.

Cerebral infarctions are ischemic or hemorrhagic. In *ischemic infarcts,* the affected area becomes pale and softens 6 to 12 hours after the occlusion. Necrosis, swelling around the insult, and mushy disintegration appear by 48 to 72 hours after infarction. There is infiltration of macrophages and phagocytosis of necrotic tissue. The necrosis resolves by about the second week, ultimately leaving a cavity surrounded by glial scarring.

In *hemorrhagic infarcts,* bleeding occurs into the infarcted area through leaking vessels when the embolic fragments resolve and reperfusion begins to occur. Hemorrhagic transformation of ischemic stroke may be exacerbated by thrombolytic therapy.[40]

CLINICAL MANIFESTATIONS   Clinical manifestations of thrombotic and embolic stroke vary, depending on the artery obstructed. Different sites of obstruction create different occlusion syndromes (e.g., carotid artery, dysphasia and contralateral motor [i.e., paresis] sensory [i.e., numbness] deficits, conjugate ipsilateral eye deviation), middle cerebral artery syndromes (dysphasia and contralateral motor and sensory deficits), or vertebrobasilar system syndromes (dizziness and ataxia, can progress to quadriplegia and coma).[41] Contralateral sensory and motor manifestations occur on the opposite side of the body from the location of the brain lesion because motor tracts originate in the cortex and most cross over in the medulla. Sensory tracts originate in the periphery and cross over in the spinal cord. Ipsilateral manifestations occur on the same side as the brain lesion.

EVALUATION AND TREATMENT Imaging is used to diagnose stroke. Treatment of ischemic stroke is focused on (1) restoring brain perfusion in a timeframe that does not contribute to reperfusion injury, (2) counteracting the ischemic cascade pathways, (3) lowering cerebral metabolic demand so that the susceptible brain tissue is protected against impaired perfusion, (4) preventing recurrent ischemic events, and (5) promoting tissue restoration. Thrombolysis, using tissue-type plasminogen activator (tPA), is given within 3 and up to 4.5 hours of onset of symptoms. Endovascular intraarterial thrombolysis may be used to treat those who cannot receive tPA.[42] Supportive management is given to control cerebral edema and increased intracranial pressure and to provide neuroprotection. Arresting the disease process by control of risk factors is critical and antiplatelet therapy may be instituted. Scales and guidelines are available for the assessment and management of acute ischemic stroke.

In embolic strokes, treatment is directed at preventing further embolization by instituting anticoagulation therapy and correcting the primary problem. Rehabilitation is indicated for ischemic strokes and recovery of function is often possible.

Hemorrhagic stroke. Hemorrhagic stroke (intracranial hemorrhage) is the third most common cause of cerebrovascular accident. They can occur within the brain tissue (intraparenchymal) or in the subarachnoid or subdural spaces. The primary cause of intraparenchymal hemorrhagic stroke is hypertension with other causes including tumors, coagulation disorders, trauma, or illicit drug use, particularly cocaine. Prevention or control of hypertension reduces the incidence of hemorrhagic stroke.

Subarachnoid hemorrhage is associated with ruptured aneurysms or arteriovenous malformations (see p. 405) or brain trauma. Subdural hemorrhage (hematoma) is usually associated with brain trauma (see p. 390). Hypertensive causes of hemorrhagic stroke involve primarily smaller arteries and arterioles, resulting in thickening of the vessel walls and increased cellularity of the vessels. Necrosis may be present. Microaneurysms in these smaller vessels or arteriolar necrosis may precipitate the bleeding.

PATHOPHYSIOLOGY A mass of blood is formed as bleeding continues into the brain tissue. Adjacent brain tissue is deformed, compressed, and displaced, producing ischemia, edema, and increased intracranial pressure and necrosis. Rupture or seepage of blood into the ventricular system often occurs and is associated with higher mortality. Hemorrhages are described as massive, small, slit, or petechial. Massive hemorrhages are several centimeters in diameter, small hemorrhages are 1 to 2 cm in diameter, a slit hemorrhage lies in the subcortical area, and a petechial hemorrhage is the size of a pinhead bleed. The most common sites for hypertensive hemorrhages are in the putamen of the basal ganglia, the thalamus, the cortex and subcortex, the pons, the caudate nucleus, and the cerebellar hemispheres. Because neurons surrounding the ischemic or infarcted areas undergo changes that disrupt plasma membranes, cellular edema results, causing further compression of capillaries. Maximal cerebral edema develops in approximately 72 hours and takes about 2 weeks to subside. Most persons survive an initial hemispheric ischemic stroke unless there is massive cerebral edema, which is nearly always fatal. The cerebral hemorrhage resolves through reabsorption. Macrophages and astrocytes clear blood from the area. A cavity forms, surrounded by a dense gliosis (glial scar) after removal of the blood.

CLINICAL MANIFESTATIONS The clinical manifestations of hemorrhagic stroke are similar to those for embolic and thrombotic stroke, and depend on the location and size of the bleed. Symptoms can occur suddenly and with activity. Once a deep unresponsive state occurs, the person rarely survives. The immediate prognosis is grave; however, if the person survives, recovery of function is often possible.

It is difficult to differentiate ischemic from hemorrhagic stroke based on symptoms. Individuals experiencing intracranial hemorrhage from a ruptured or leaking aneurysm have one of three sets of symptoms: (1) onset of an excruciating generalized headache with an almost immediate lapse into an unresponsive state, (2) headache but with consciousness maintained, and (3) sudden lapse into unconsciousness. If the hemorrhage is confined to the subarachnoid space, there may be no local signs. If bleeding spreads into the brain tissue, hemiparesis/paralysis, dysphasia, or homonymous hemianopia may be present. Warning signs of an impending aneurysm rupture include headache, transient unilateral weakness, transient numbness and tingling, and transient speech disturbance. However, such warning signs are often absent.

EVALUATION AND TREATMENT Treatment of an intracranial bleed, regardless of cause, focuses on stopping or reducing the bleeding, controlling the increased intracranial pressure, preventing a rebleed, and preventing vasospasm. There are some attempts to drain blood in a cerebral bleed but the benefit is not documented in studies. Microsurgical interventions are under investigation.[45] Surgical treatments are options for ruptured aneurysms, vascular malformations, and subarachnoid hemorrhage.

Intracranial aneurysm. Intracranial aneurysms may result from arteriosclerosis, congenital abnormality, cocaine use, trauma, inflammation, and vascular sheer wall stress. The size may vary from 2 mm to 2 or 3 cm. Most aneurysms are located at bifurcations in or near the circle of Willis, in the vertebrobasilar arteries, or within the carotid system where there is higher wall sheer stress and flow turbulence (see Figures 13-19 and 13-20). Aneurysms may be single, but in 20% to 25% of the cases, more than one is present. In these instances, the aneurysms may be unilateral or bilateral. Peak incidence of rupture occurs in persons 50 to 59 years of age, with the incidence in postmenopausal women slightly higher than that in men.

PATHOPHYSIOLOGY No single pathologic mechanism exists. Aneurysms may be classified on the basis of shape and form. *Saccular aneurysms (berry aneurysms)* occur frequently (in approximately 2% of the population) and likely result from congenital abnormalities in the tunica media of the arterial wall and hemodynamic and molecular changes.[46] The sac gradually grows over time. A saccular aneurysm may be (1) round with a narrow stalk connecting it to the parent artery, (2) broad-based without a stalk, or (3) cylindrical (Figure 16-11). Saccular aneurysms are rare in childhood; their highest incidence of rupturing or bleeding (subarachnoid hemorrhage) is among persons 20 to 50 years of age (Figure 16-12).

Fusiform aneurysms (giant aneurysms) are less common, occur as a result of diffuse arteriosclerotic changes, and are found most commonly in the basilar arteries or terminal portions of the internal carotid arteries (see Figure 16-11). They act as space-occupying lesions.

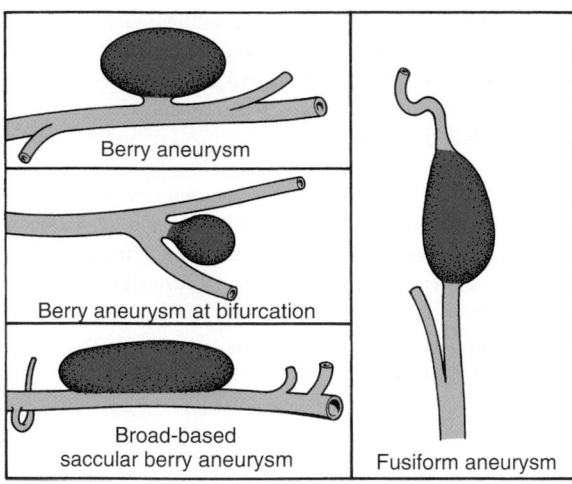

FIGURE 16-11 Types of Aneurysms.

FIGURE 16-12 Berry Aneurysm, Angiogram. In this lateral view with contrast filling a portion of the cerebral arterial circulation can be seen as a berry aneurysm *(arrow)* involving the middle cerebral artery of the circle of Willis at the base of the brain. (From Klatt EC: *Robbins and Cotran atlas of pathology*, ed 3, Philadelphia, 2015, Saunders.)

Aneurysms rupture through thin areas often at bifurcation sites, causing hemorrhage into the subarachnoid space that spreads rapidly, producing localized changes in the cerebral cortex and focal irritation of nerves and arteries (see the discussion of the Laplace law in Chapter 23). Bleeding ceases when a fibrin-platelet plug forms at the point of rupture and as a result of compression. Blood undergoes reabsorption through arachnoid villi within 3 weeks.

CLINICAL MANIFESTATIONS Aneurysms often are asymptomatic. Of all persons undergoing routine autopsy, 5% are found to have one or more intracranial aneurysms. Clinical manifestations include dizziness or headache and cranial nerve compression, but the signs vary depending on the location and size of the aneurysm. Cranial nerves III, IV, V, and VI (see Table 13-6) are affected most often. Unfortunately, the most common first indication of the presence of an aneurysm is an acute subarachnoid hemorrhage, intracerebral hemorrhage, or combined subarachnoid-intracerebral hemorrhage (see Hemorrhagic Stroke, p. 404).

EVALUATION AND TREATMENT Diagnosis before a bleeding episode is made through arteriography. After a subarachnoid or intracerebral hemorrhage, a tentative diagnosis of an aneurysm is based on clinical manifestations, history, and imaging. Treatments for intracranial aneurysm are both medical (i.e., control of hypertension) and surgical (i.e., microvascular clipping or placement of endovascular coils).[47]

Vascular malformation. Vascular malformations are rare congenital vascular lesions. An arteriovenous malformation (AVM) is a mass of dilated vessels between the arterial and venous systems (arteriovenous fistula) without an intervening capillary bed, may occur in any part of the brain and vary in size from a few millimeters to large malformations extending from the cortex to the ventricle. AVMs occur equally in males and females and occasionally occur in families. Although AVMs are usually present at birth, symptoms exhibit a delayed age of onset and commonly occur before 30 years of age.

PATHOPHYSIOLOGY AVMs have abnormal blood vessel structure, are abnormally thin, and have complex growth and remodeling patterns.[48] There is direct shunting of arterial blood into the venous vasculature without the dissipation of the arterial blood pressure with increased risk for rupture. One or several arteries may feed the AVM and, over time, they become tortuous and dilated. With moderate to large AVMs, sufficient blood is shunted into the malformation to deprive surrounding tissue of adequate blood perfusion.

CLINICAL MANIFESTATIONS Twenty percent of persons with an AVM have a characteristic chronic, nondescript headache, although some experience migraine. Fifty percent of persons experience seizures. The other 50% experience an intracerebral, subarachnoid, or subdural hemorrhage with progressive neurologic deficits. Bleeding from an AVM into the subarachnoid space causes symptoms identical to those associated with a ruptured aneurysm. If bleeding is into the brain tissue, focal signs that develop resemble a stroke that is progressing in severity. Ten percent of persons experience hemiparesis or other focal signs. At times, noncommunicating hydrocephalus (see Chapter 15) develops with a large AVM that extends into the ventricular lining.

EVALUATION AND TREATMENT A systolic bruit over the carotid artery in the neck, the mastoid process, or the eyeball in a young person is almost always diagnostic of an AVM. Confirming diagnosis is made by CT and MRI followed by MRA. Treatment options include direct surgical excision, endovascular embolization, or radiotherapy.[49]

Subarachnoid hemorrhage. Subarachnoid hemorrhage (SAH) is the escape of blood from a defective or injured vessel into the subarachnoid space. Individuals at risk for a subarachnoid hemorrhage are those with intracranial aneurysm, intracranial arteriovenous malformation, hypertension, or a family history of SAH, and those who have sustained head injuries. Subarachnoid hemorrhages often recur, especially from a ruptured intracranial aneurysm.

PATHOPHYSIOLOGY When a vessel is leaking, blood oozes into the subarachnoid space. When a vessel tears, blood under pressure is pumped into the subarachnoid space. The blood increases the intracranial volume, and it is also extremely irritating to the neural tissues and produces an inflammatory reaction. In addition, the blood coats nerve roots, clogs arachnoid granulations (impairing CSF reabsorption), and obstructs foramina within the ventricular system (impairing CSF circulation). Intracranial pressure immediately increases to almost diastolic levels but returns to near baseline in about 10 minutes. Cerebral blood flow and cerebral perfusion pressure decrease. Autoregulation of blood flow is impaired, and there is a compensatory increase in systolic blood pressure.[50] The expanding hematoma acts like a space-occupying lesion, compressing and displacing brain tissue with increased intracranial pressure, decreased cerebral blood flow, blood-brain barrier breakdown, brain edema, inflammation, and cell death. Secondary brain injury can occur as described for traumatic brain injury (see p. 390). Granulation tissue is formed, and meningeal scarring with impairment of CSF reabsorption and secondary hydrocephalus often results. Mortality in subarachnoid hemorrhage is 50% at 1 month.

Delayed cerebral ischemia, a syndrome of progressive neurologic deterioration, is associated with *cerebral artery vasospasm*. From 40% to 60% of persons with a subarachnoid hemorrhage experience vasospasms in adjacent and, occasionally, in nonadjacent vessels. Vasospasm may occur because of leukocyte–endothelial cell interactions or the effects of vasoactive substances (e.g., calcium, prostaglandins, serotonin, catecholamines) on the arteries of the subarachnoid space. Edema, medial necrosis, and proliferation of the tunica intima in cerebral arterioles have been found. Vasospasm causes decreased cerebral blood flow, ischemia, and possibly infarct and can lead to delayed ischemic injury and death 3 to 14 days after the initial hemorrhage.[51]

CLINICAL MANIFESTATIONS Early manifestations associated with leaking vessels are episodic and include headache, changes in mental status or level of consciousness, nausea or vomiting, and focal neurologic defects. A ruptured vessel causes a sudden, throbbing, "explosive" headache, accompanied by nausea and vomiting, visual disturbances, motor deficits, and loss of consciousness related to a dramatic rise in intracranial pressure. Meningeal irritation and inflammation often occur, causing neck stiffness (nuchal rigidity), photophobia, blurred vision, irritability, restlessness, and low-grade fever. A positive **Kernig sign** (straightening the knee with the hip and knee in a flexed position produces pain in the back and neck regions) and a positive **Brudzinski sign** (passive flexion of the neck produces neck pain and increased rigidity) may appear. No localizing signs are present if the bleed is confined completely to the subarachnoid space.

The Hunt and Hess subarachnoid hemorrhage (SAH) grading system is based on description of the clinical manifestations (Table 16-6).[52] Rebleeding is a significant risk with a high mortality (up to 70%). The period of greatest risk is during the first 72 hours and up to 2 weeks after the initial bleed. Rebleeding is manifested by a sudden increase in blood pressure and intracranial pressure, along with a deteriorating neurologic status.[53]

Seizures occur in 25% of persons with an SAH, and hydrocephalus after a bleed occurs in 20% of cases. Hypothalamic dysfunction, manifested by salt wasting, hyponatremia, and ECG changes, is common.

EVALUATION AND TREATMENT The diagnosis of an SAH is based on the clinical presentation, imaging, and cerebrospinal fluid evaluation. Treatment is directed at controlling intracranial pressure, improving cerebral perfusion pressure, preventing ischemia and hypoxia of neural tissues, and avoiding rebleeding episodes. Surgical intervention is common. Treatment guidelines are available to direct therapy.[47]

✔**QUICK CHECK 16-2**
1. Why is atherosclerosis a risk factor for thrombotic stroke?
2. Why do the signs and symptoms of a TIA resolve completely?
3. Why do lacunar strokes involve small infarcts?
4. How is an AVM different from an aneurysm?

Headache

Headache is a common neurologic disorder and is usually a benign symptom. However, it can be associated with serious disease such as brain tumor, meningitis, or cerebrovascular disease (e.g., giant cell arteritis, cerebral aneurysm, or cerebral bleeds). The headache syndromes discussed here are the chronic, recurring type not associated with structural abnormalities or systemic disease and include migraine, cluster, and tension headaches. Characteristics of the major types of headache syndromes are summarized in Table 16-7.

Migraine

Migraine is an episodic neurologic disorder characterized by a headache lasting 4 to 72 hours. It is diagnosed when any two of the following features occur: unilateral head pain, throbbing pain, pain worsens with activity, moderate or severe pain intensity; *and* at least one of the following: nausea and/or vomiting, or photophobia and phonophobia.[54] Migraine is broadly classified as (1) *migraine with aura* with visual, sensory, or motor symptoms; and, more commonly, (2) *migraine without aura*.

Migraine occurs in 18% of women and 6% of men in the United States and can occur in children. It is more common in those 25 to 55 years of age. There often is a family history of migraine. In susceptible women, migraine occurs most frequently before and during menstruation and is decreased during pregnancy and menopause. The cyclic withdrawal of estrogen and progesterone may trigger attacks of migraine.[55,56]

Migraine is caused by a combination of multiple genetic and environmental factors. Persons with migraine have an increased risk for epilepsy, depression, anxiety disorders, cardiovascular disease, and stroke. Migraine may be precipitated by triggers. Individuals with migraine are likely to have a genetically determined reduced threshold for triggers. Triggers can include becoming tired or oversleeping, missed meals, overexertion, weather change, stress or relaxation from stress, hormonal changes (menstrual periods), excess afferent stimulation (bright lights, strong smells), and chemicals (alcohol or nitrates).

The pathophysiologic basis for migraine is complex and not clearly established. There is no identifiable pathology but there are associated changes in brain metabolism and blood flow. Current theories includes neurologic, vascular, hormonal, and neurotransmitter components. Migraine aura is associated with cortical spreading depression (CSD). CSD is a spontaneous self-propagating wave of glial and neuronal depolarization resulting in hyperactivity that starts in the occipital

---

TABLE 16-6 Subarachnoid Hemorrhage Classification Scale

Category	Description
Grade I	Neurologic status intact; mild headache, slight nuchal rigidity
Grade II	Neurologic deficit evidenced by cranial nerve involvement; moderate to severe headache with more pronounced meningeal signs (e.g., photophobia, nuchal rigidity)
Grade III	Drowsiness and confusion with or without focal neurologic deficits; pronounced meningeal signs
Grade IV	Stuporous with pronounced neurologic deficits (e.g., hemiparesis, dysphasia); nuchal rigidity
Grade V	Deep coma state with decerebrate posturing and other brainstem functioning

From Tateshima S, Duckwiler G: Vascular diseases of the nervous system. In Daroff RB et al, editors: *Bradley's neurology in clinical practice*, Philadelphia, 2012, Saunders.

TABLE 16-7 Characteristics of Common Headaches

| | MIGRAINE | | Cluster Headache/ | |
	Without Aura	With Aura (25%-30%)	Proximal Hemicrania	Tension-Type Headache
Age of onset	Childhood, adolescence, or young adulthood	Childhood, adolescence, or young adulthood	Young adulthood, middle age	Young adulthood, middle age
Gender	Higher in females	Higher in females	Male	Not gender specific
Family history of headaches	Yes	Yes	No	Yes
Onset and evolution	Slow to rapid	Slow to rapid	Rapid	Slow to rapid
Time course	Episodic	Episodic	Clusters in time	Episodic, may become constant
Quality	Usually throbbing	Usually throbbing	Steady	Steady
Location	Variable, unilateral to bilateral	Variable, unilateral to bilateral	Orbit, temple, cheek	Variable
Associated features	Prodrome, vomiting	Aura: visual, sensory, language, and motor disturbance Prodrome, vomiting	Lacrimation, rhinorrhea, Horner syndrome	None

region and spreads across the cortex.[57] CSD initiates the release of neurotransmitters that activate the trigeminal vascular system (afferent projections from cranial nerve V), stimulating vasodilation of dural blood vessels, activation of inflammation, peripheral and central sensitization of pain receptors (hypersensitivity to pain), and activation of areas of the brainstem and forebrain that modulate pain. Release of inflammatory mediators with sterile meningeal inflammation and edema of blood vessels may be an important component of migraine pain. Vasodilation of blood vessels is not sufficient to account for the pain of migraine. Calcitonin gene–related peptide (CGRP) release by the trigeminal vascular system is related to migraine pain. The mechanism is not clear, but CGRP antagonists stop the headache. Glutamate (an excitatory neurotransmitter) concentration is increased and 5-hydroxytryptamine (5-HT, serotonin) concentration is decreased. 5-HT causes vasoconstriction and antagonizes CGRP. Consequently, 5-HT(1B/1D) receptor agonists (i.e., triptans) and CGRP receptor and glutamate receptor antagonists have been used for the acute treatment of migraine.[58-60]

The clinical phases of a migraine attack are as follows:

1. *Premonitory phase:* Up to one third of persons have premonitory symptoms hours to days before onset of aura or headache. These symptoms may include tiredness, irritability, loss of concentration, stiff neck, and food cravings.
2. *Migraine aura:* Up to one third of persons have aura symptoms at least some of the time that may last up to 1 hour. Symptoms can be visual, sensory, or motor.
3. *Headache phase:* Throbbing pain usually begins on one side and spreads to include the entire head. Headache may be accompanied by fatigue, nausea, and vomiting or dizziness. There may be hypersensitivity to anything touching the head. Symptoms may last from 4 to 72 hours (usually about a day).
4. *Recovery phase:* Irritability, fatigue, or depression may take hours or days to resolve.

Differentiation of types of migraine headache is summarized in Table 16-7. The diagnosis of migraine is made from medical history and physical examination. Differential diagnosis is confirmed by imaging and EEG. Functional neuroimaging and genetic studies are advancing the understanding of the mechanisms involved in migraine attacks and individual variants involved with disease susceptibility.[61] The management of migraine includes avoidance of triggers (e.g., darkening the room, applying ice). Sleeping can provide some relief with the onset of acute migraine. Pharmacologic management for the treatment and prevention of migraine is available.[62,63] A transcutaneous electrical stimulation device providing trigeminal neurostimula-

tion has been approved by the Food and Drug Administration for the prevention of migraine.[64]

Chronic migraines usually begin as episodic migraines that increase in frequency over time. Chronic migraine occurs at least 15 days in a month (can occur daily or on a near-daily basis) for more than 3 months. Chronic migraines are associated with overuse of analgesic migraine medications (sometimes called rebound headaches), obesity, and caffeine overuse. Treatment is similar to that for episodic migraine. Individuals with chronic migraine unresponsive to medical treatment should be evaluated for intracranial hypertension without papilledema and the possibility of sinus venous stenosis.[65]

Cluster Headache

Cluster headaches are one of a group of disorders referred to as trigeminal autonomic cephalagias (headaches involving the autonomic division of the trigeminal nerve).[66] They occur in one side of the head primarily in men between 20 and 50 years of age. The pain may alternate sides with each headache episode and is severe, stabbing, and throbbing. These uncommon headaches occur in clusters (up to 8 attacks per day) and last for minutes to hours for a period of days, followed by a long period of spontaneous remission. Cluster headache has an episodic and a chronic form with extreme pain intensity and short duration. If the cluster of attacks occurs more frequently without sustained spontaneous remission, they are classified as *chronic cluster headaches* (10% to 20% of cases) (see Table 16-7). Triggers are similar to those that cause migraine headache.

Trigeminal activation occurs but the mechanism is unclear. Functional imaging indicates a role for concomitant posterior hypothalamic and pain neuromatrix activation with opioid system involvement.[67] The pathogenic mechanism for pain is related to the release of vasoactive substances and the formation of neurogenic inflammation. Autonomic dysfunction is characterized by sympathetic underactivity and parasympathetic activation. There is unilateral trigeminal distribution of severe pain with ipsilateral autonomic manifestations, including tearing on affected side, ptosis of the ipsilateral eye, and congestion of the nasal mucosa. Prophylactic drugs are used to treat cluster headache, as well as avoidance of triggers. Acute attacks are managed with oxygen inhalation, sumatriptan or inhaled ergotamine administration, and nerve stimulation.[68] New drugs are under investigation.

Tension-Type Headache

Tension-type headache (TTH) is the most common type of headache. The average age of onset is during the second decade of life. It is a mild to moderate bilateral headache with a sensation of a tight band or pressure around the head with gradual onset of pain. The headache occurs in episodes and may last for several hours or several days. It is not aggravated by physical activity. Chronic tension-type headache (CTTH) evolves from episodic tension-type headache and represents headache that occurs at least 15 days per month for at least 3 months.

Both central and peripheral mechanisms operate in causing tension headache. The central pain mechanism is associated with chronic tension headache and a peripheral mechanism with episodic tension headache. The central mechanism probably involves hypersensitivity of pain fibers from the trigeminal nerve that leads to central sensitization. The peripheral sensitization of myofascial sensory nerves may contribute to muscular hypersensitivity and the development of chronic CTTH. Headache sufferers have more localized pain and tenderness of pericranial muscles. Many individuals have both tension-type and migraine headaches.

Mild tension-type headaches are treated with ice, and more severe forms are treated with aspirin or nonsteroidal anti-inflammatory drugs. CTTHs are best managed with a tricyclic antidepressant and behavioral and relaxation therapy. Some individuals benefit from injection of botulinum toxin A. Long-term use of analgesics or other drugs, such as muscle relaxants, antihistamines, tranquilizers, caffeine, and ergot alkaloids, should be avoided.[69]

Infection and Inflammation of the Central Nervous System

The CNS may be infected by bacteria, viruses, fungi, parasites, and mycobacteria. The invading organisms enter the nervous system either by spreading through arterial blood vessels (Figure 16-13) or by directly invading the nervous tissue from another site of infection. Neurologic infections produce disease by several mechanisms: direct neuronal or glial infection, mass lesion formation, inflammation with subsequent edema, interruption of cerebrospinal fluid pathways, neuronal or vascular damage, and secretion of neurotoxins. An immune process may initiate an inflammatory reaction.

Meningitis

Meningitis is inflammation of the brain or spinal cord. Infectious meningitis may be caused by bacteria, viruses, fungi, parasites, or toxins. The infection may be acute, subacute, or chronic with the pathophysiology, clinical manifestations, and treatment differing for each type of microorganism.

Fungal meningitis is a chronic, much less common condition than bacterial or viral meningitis. The infection most often occurs in persons with impaired immune responses or alterations in normal body flora. It develops insidiously, usually over days or weeks. Fungi in the nervous system usually produce a granulomatous reaction, forming granulomata or gelatinous masses in the meninges at the base of the brain. Fungi also may extend along the perivascular sites in the subarachnoid space and into the brain tissue, producing arteritis with thrombosis, infarction, and communicating hydrocephalus. Meningeal fibrosis develops later in the inflammatory process. Cranial nerve dysfunction, caused by compression, often results from the granulomata and fibrosis. The first manifestations are often those of dementia (see Chapter 15) or communicating hydrocephalus (see Chapter 15). The individual is characteristically afebrile.

Viral meningitis (aseptic or nonpurulent meningitis) is thought to be limited to the meninges. An identifiable bacterium cannot be found in the cerebrospinal fluid. The most common viruses are enteroviral viruses (echovirus, coxsackievirus, and nonparalytic poliomyelitis), arboviruses, and herpes simplex type 2. Viruses enter the nervous system by crossing the blood-brain barrier, by direct spread

Neuron: HSV-1, 2, rabies West Nile, Nipah equine encephalitides mumps, VZV measles (SSPE), CMV

Oligodendrocyte: JCV, CMV

Microglia, perivascular macrophages: HIV, CMV

Astrocyte: Equine encephalitis viruses, HIV, JCV, CMV, HTLV-1

Blood-brain barrier

Endothelia: Nipah virus, CMV

FIGURE 16-13 Viral Infection in the Central Nervous System (CNS). Viruses infect specific cell types within the CNS depending on the particular properties of the virus together with individual cell membrane proteins expressed on permissive cell types. Normally the brain is protected from circulating pathogens and toxins by the blood-brain barrier. *CMV,* Cytomegalovirus; *HIV,* human immunodeficiency virus; *HSV,* herpes simplex virus; *HTLV-1,* human T-cell lymphotropic virus (causes T-cell leukemia); *JCV,* John Cunningham virus (a polyomavirus causing progressive multifocal leukoencephalopathy); *SSPE,* subacute sclerosing panencephalitis; *VZV,* varicella-zoster virus. (Adapted from Power C, Noorbakhsh G: Central nervous system viral infections: clinical aspects and pathogenic mechanisms. In Gilman S, editor: *Neurobiology of disease,* p 488, Burlington, Mass, 2007, Elsevier.)

along peripheral nerves, or through the choroid plexus epithelium. Recognition of viral antigens by immune cells activates the inflammatory response. The clinical manifestations of viral meningitis are similar to those of bacterial meningitis but milder. Viral meningitis is managed pharmacologically with antiviral drugs and steroids.

Bacterial meningitis is primarily an infection of the pia mater and arachnoid, the subarachnoid space, the ventricular system, and the CSF. Meningococci (*Neisseria meningitidis*) and pneumococci (*Streptococcus pneumoniae*) are the most common pathogens. An increase of drug-resistant strains of *S. pneumoniae* is an emerging problem worldwide. About 1 in 100,000 persons are affected annually.[70] Meningococcus has been identified worldwide and there are six serogroups: A, B, C, W-135, X, and Y. Most cases are sporadic and occur predominantly in children younger than 1 year of age and adolescents. Local outbreaks may occur in dormitories, military bases, or sub-Saharan Africa. With pneumococcal meningitis, young persons and those more than 40 years of age are mostly affected. Predisposing conditions are otitis or sinusitis (25%), immunocompromised status (16%), and pneumonia (12%). The disease is spread by respiratory droplets and contact with contaminated saliva or respiratory tract secretions (kissing, coughing, sneezing, or sharing utensils, food, and drink).[71] Carriers of the meningococcal bacteria do not develop meningitis but may pass it on to others.

PATHOPHYSIOLOGY Meningococci and pneumococci are inhaled and attach to epithelial cells in the nasopharynx where they cross the mucosal barrier, enter the bloodstream, travel to cerebral blood vessels, cross the blood-brain barrier, and infect the meninges. With bacterial infection, large numbers of neutrophils are recruited to the subarachnoid space. Release of cytotoxic inflammatory agents and bacterial toxins alter the blood-brain barrier, cause cerebral edema, and damage brain tissue. The inflammatory exudate thickens the CSF and interferes with normal CSF flow around the brain and spinal cord, possibly obstructing arachnoid villi and producing hydrocephalus. Meningeal cells become edematous, and the combined exudate and edematous cells increase intracranial pressure. Engorged blood vessels and thrombi can disrupt blood flow, causing further injury.[72] Acute infectious *purpura fulminans* is a rare rapidly progressive syndrome of hemorrhagic infarction of the skin and disseminated intravascular coagulation that can lead to multiple organ failure, ischemic necrosis of digits and limbs with amputation required, and death. It is caused by bacterial endotoxin and inflammatory cytokines.

CLINICAL MANIFESTATIONS The clinical manifestations of bacterial meningitis can be grouped into infectious signs, meningeal signs, and neurologic signs. The clinical manifestations of systemic infection include fever, tachycardia, and chills. The clinical manifestations of meningeal irritation are a severe throbbing headache, severe photophobia, nuchal rigidity, and positive Kernig and Brudzinski signs. The neurologic signs include a decrease in consciousness, cranial nerve palsies, focal neurologic deficits (such as hemiparesis/hemiplegia and ataxia), and seizures. Often there is projectile vomiting. As intracranial pressure increases, papilledema develops and delirium may progress to unconsciousness and death. With meningococcal meningitis, a petechial or purpuric rash covers the skin and mucous membranes.

EVALUATION AND TREATMENT Rapid diagnosis, antibiotic administration, and supportive treatment are important to prevent morbidity and mortality from bacterial meningitis. Diagnosis is based on physical examination, blood cultures, and the results of nasopharyngeal smear and antigen tests. CSF analysis and cultures are required for differential diagnosis.[72,73] Serious complications, including septic shock, disseminated intravascular coagulation, purpura fulminans, limb damage, and multiple organ failure, require intensive multidisciplinary care.

Vaccinations are available to prevent meningococcal, pneumococcal, and *Haemophilus influenzae* meningitis.[74] Meningococcal vaccine promotes antibody protection within 7 to 14 days.[75] Vaccination of children ages 11 or 12 years is recommended with a booster to be given between ages 16 and 18 years or older, particularly college students living in a dormitory.

Brain or Spinal Cord Abscess

Abscesses, localized collections of pus, may form within the parenchyma of the brain or spinal cord but are rare.

Brain abscesses are classified as epidural, subdural, or intracerebral. *Epidural brain abscesses (empyemas)* are associated with osteomyelitis in a cranial bone. *Subdural brain abscesses* (empyemas) arise from a sinus infection or a vascular source. *Intracerebral brain abscesses* arise from a vascular source. Spinal cord abscesses are classified as epidural or intramedullary. Epidural spinal abscesses usually originate as osteomyelitis in a vertebra; the infection then spreads into the epidural space. (Osteomyelitis is discussed in Chapter 39.)

PATHOPHYSIOLOGY Microorganisms gain entrance to the CNS by direct extension or distribution along the wall of a vein. Infective emboli carry organisms from distant sites. Illegal drug users who share needles are at risk as are immunosuppressed persons. For example. *Toxoplasma gondii* is producing an ever-increasing number of CNS abscesses in persons with acquired immunodeficiency syndrome (AIDS).[76] Streptococci, staphylococci, and *Bacteroides,* often combined with anaerobes, are the most common bacteria that cause abscesses; however, yeast and fungi also may be involved.[77]

Brain abscesses progress from localized inflammation to a necrotic core with the formation of a connective tissue capsule, usually within 14 days or longer.[78] Existing abscesses also tend to spread and form daughter abscesses.

CLINICAL MANIFESTATIONS Early manifestations include low-grade fever, headache (most common symptom), nausea and vomiting, neck pain and stiffness, confusion, drowsiness, sensory deficits, and communication deficits. Later manifestations are associated with an expanding mass and include decreased attention span, memory deficits, decreased visual acuity and narrowed visual fields, papilledema, ocular palsy, ataxia, dementia, and seizures. The development of symptoms may be very insidious, often making an abscess difficult to diagnose.[79]

Extradural brain abscesses are associated with localized pain, purulent drainage from the nasal passages or auditory canal, fever, localized tenderness, and neck stiffness. Clinical manifestations of spinal cord abscesses have four stages: (1) spinal aching; (2) severe root pain, accompanied by spasms of the back muscles and limited vertebral movement; (3) weakness caused by progressive cord compression; and (4) paralysis.

EVALUATION AND TREATMENT The diagnosis is suggested by clinical features and confirmed by imaging studies. Antibiotics and surgical aspiration or excision is usually indicated. Intracranial pressure may have to be managed. Spinal cord abscesses are treated with surgical decompression or aspiration, antibiotic therapy, and supportive therapy.

Encephalitis

Encephalitis is an acute febrile illness, usually of viral origin, with nervous system involvement. The most common forms are caused by bites of mosquitos, ticks, or flies. Herpes simplex type 1 is the most common sporadic cause of encephalitis. Viruses infect specific cell types in the CNS as shown in Figure 16-13. Referred to as infectious viral encephalitides, encephalitis may occur as a complication of systemic viral diseases such as poliomyelitis, rabies, or mononucleosis, or it may arise after recovery from viral infections such as rubella, varicella, rubeola, or yellow fever. Encephalitis also may follow vaccination with a live attenuated virus vaccine if the vaccine has an encephalitis component, for example, measles, mumps, and rubella. Typhus, trichinosis, malaria, and schistosomiasis also are associated with encephalitis. Toxoplasmosis may acutely reactivate in immunosuppressed persons when the once-dormant parasite in cyst form disseminates in brain tissues.[80]

With the exception of the California viral encephalitis, which is endemic, the arthropod-borne encephalitides occur in epidemics, varying in geographic and seasonal incidence (Table 16-8 and *Health Alert:* West Nile Virus). Eastern equine encephalitis is the most serious but least common of the encephalitides.

PATHOPHYSIOLOGY Viruses gain access to the CNS through the bloodstream, olfactory bulb, or choroid plexus, or through an intraneuronal route from peripheral nerves. Meningeal involvement is present in all encephalitides. The various encephalitides may cause

TABLE 16-8 **Classification and Characteristics of Arboviruses Causing Encephalitis**

Viruses	Incubation Period (Days)	Family/Genus	Location	Vector	Season	Affected Population
Eastern equine encephalitis	5-10	Togaviridae/*Alphavirus* (formerly group A arbovirus)	Swampy areas of eastern United States and Michigan	Mosquito	June to October	Infants, children, and adults >50 years
Western equine encephalitis	5-10	Same as above	All parts of United States: eastern, central, and western	Mosquito	July to October	All ages
Venezuelan equine encephalitis	2-5	Same as above	Texas, Florida, Mexico; Central and South America	Mosquito	All year	Infants and young children
St. Louis encephalitis	4-21	Flaviviridae/*Flavivirus*	All parts of United States: eastern, central, and western	Mosquito	June to October	Adults >40 years; older adults more often affected than younger ages
La Crosse encephalitis including California	5-15	Bunyaviridae/*Bunyavirus* (California virus serogroup)	Midwestern United States, eastern seaboard, and Canada	Woodland mosquito	July to September	Children <15 years
West Nile encephalitis	3-14	Flaviviridae/*Flavivirus*	Lower 48 states of United States	Mosquito	Summer and fall	Older adults most seriously

HEALTH ALERT

West Nile Virus

West Nile virus (WNV), a *Flavivirus* transmitted predominantly by the *Culex* mosquito, emerged in New York State in 1999. It is the most common cause of epidemic meningoencephalitis in North America and the leading cause of arboviral encephalitis in the United States. By the end of 2004, human cases had been found in the 48 contiguous states. Humans and horses, as well as other mammals, are incidental hosts. Birds and mosquitoes are life cycle hosts. Summer and fall are peak times of infection incidence. The greatest amount of virus is carried by mosquitos in early fall. Besides mosquito transmission, WN virus can be transmitted through blood transfusions and organ transplants. Health experts think that transmission from mother to unborn child and through breast milk is possible.

The human incubation period is 2 to 14 days. Most individuals develop no symptoms. About 20% of those infected have mild symptoms that last 4 to 6 days and generally include fever, headache, skin rash, and lymphadenopathy. Less than 1% of affected persons develop severe illness, including WN encephalitis marked by headache, disorientation, stupor, coma, seizures, and movement disorders including tremor, ataxia, extrapyramidal signs, and paralysis. WN meningitis is characterized by meningeal signs of severe headache, high fever, and nuchal rigidity. Myelitis and polyradiculitis also may be present. Abnormalities in the thalamus, basal ganglia, and cerebellum are often seen on MRI in people with severe infection. Identifiable risk factors are very young or advanced in age, immunocompromised, and pregnancy.

A preliminary diagnosis is made if IgM for the virus is found in serum or CSF. A rapid test became available in 2007. Plaque reduction neutralization assay (PRNA) is the confirmatory test. Treatment is supportive care. No West Nile vaccine has been developed for humans. Environmental control and prevention of mosquito bites is the best protection. Since 2003 all blood banks use blood-screening tests for West Nile virus.

Data from Brandler S, Tangy F: *Viruses* 5(10):2384-2409, 2013; Centers for Disease Control and Prevention: *West Nile virus,* updated January 13, 2015, available at: www.cdc.gov/westnile/index.html; Petersen LR et al: *J Am Med Assoc* 310(3):308-315, 2013; Reisen WK: *Viruses* 5(9):2079-210, 2013.

widespread nerve cell degeneration. Edema, necrosis with or without hemorrhage, and increased intracranial pressure develop.

CLINICAL MANIFESTATIONS Encephalitis ranges from a mild infectious disease to a life-threatening disorder. Mild symptoms include malaise, headache, body aches, nausea, and vomiting. Dramatic clinical manifestations include fever, delirium or confusion progressing to unconsciousness, difficulty with word finding, seizure activity, cranial nerve palsies, paresis and paralysis, involuntary movement, and abnormal reflexes. Signs of marked intracranial pressure may be present.

EVALUATION AND TREATMENT Diagnosis is made by history and clinical presentation aided by CSF examination and culture, serologic studies, white blood cell count, CT scan, or MRI. Empirical treatment is specific to the type of virus and may include antiviral agents, antibiotics, and steroids. Herpes encephalitis is treated with antiviral agents, such as acyclovir. Measures to control intracranial pressure are paramount.[81]

Neurologic Complications of Acquired Immunodeficiency Syndrome (AIDS)

From 40% to 60% of all persons with AIDS (see Chapter 8) have neurologic complications. The most common neurologic disorder is HIV-associated neurocognitive disorder. Others are peripheral neuropathies, vacuolar (spongy softening) myelopathy, opportunistic infections of the CNS, neoplasms, and, less commonly, stroke syndromes.[82]

Human immunodeficiency virus–associated neurocognitive disorder (HAND). A variety of names have been used for **HAND,** including HIV-associated cognitive dysfunction, HIV encephalopathy, subacute encephalitis, HIV-associated dementia complex, HIV cognitive motor complex, AIDS encephalopathy, AIDS dementia complex, and AIDS-related dementia. Both adults and children may be affected by progressive cognitive dysfunction with motor and behavioral alterations. The syndrome typically develops later in the disease but may be an early or singular manifestation in some persons. The syndrome is more prevalent in drug users with HIV. Highly active antiretroviral therapy (HAART) with more efficient CNS drug penetration has reduced the prevalence and improved survival for severe HAND, but milder forms of the disease may persist because of longer life.

The neurologic syndromes develop from properties of the virus, genetic characteristics of the host, and interactions with the environment (including treatment). At the time of primary HIV infection, HIV infects the perivascular macrophages, microglial cells, and astrocytes, particularly the basal ganglia and deep white matter. Affected macrophages, macrophage-derived multinucleated cells, and microglia cause an immune-mediated demyelination process in white matter. Focal and diffuse demyelination of white matter and spongy changes of the spinal cord are present.

HAND is insidious in onset and unpredictable in its course. Most persons experience a steady progression of mental decline characterized by abrupt accelerations of signs over several months to more than 1 year. The triad of clinical manifestations are neurocognitive impairment, behavioral disturbance, and motor abnormalities. Specific manifestations can include an organic psychosis with agitation, inappropriate behavior, and hallucinosis. Motor signs include difficulty speaking; progressive loss of balance; gait ataxia; spastic paraparesis or paralysis; and generalized hyperreflexia sometimes accompanied by decreased writing ability, tremor, myoclonus, and seizure.

Diagnosis is difficult, especially in early stages, and CSF analysis, CT scan, and MRI data help establish the diagnosis. HIV antiretroviral treatment is continued. Although CNS drug penetration is reduced there is decreased prevalence and improved survival for individuals with severe HAND.[83]

HIV myelopathy. HIV myelopathy involves diffuse degeneration of the spinal cord in persons with HIV. *Vacuolar myelopathy* is thought to be a direct consequence of HIV. The lateral and posterior columns of the lumbar spinal cord are affected. Progressive spastic paraparesis with ataxia is the predominant clinical manifestation. Leg weakness, upper motor neuron signs, incontinence, and posterior column sensory loss may be present. Diagnosis is made on the basis of history, physical findings, and supporting data from diagnostic procedures. Treatment is supportive.

HIV-associated peripheral neuropathy. HIV may directly infect nerves and cause HIV distal symmetric polyneuropathy, most commonly sensory neuropathy.[84] Persons experience neuropathic pain including pain burning sensations and numbness commonly in the extremities. Weakness and decreased or absent distal reflexes may be present. Diagnosis is established through history and physical findings, laboratory data, and nerve conduction and electromyogram (EMG) studies.

Viral meningitis and HIV. Some persons develop acute viral meningitis at approximately the time of seroconversion. This may represent the initial infection of the nervous system by the virus. Symptoms include headache, fever, and meningismus (headache, photophobia, nuchal rigidity). Cranial nerve involvement, especially V and VII, may appear, but the disease is self-limiting and requires only symptomatic treatment.

Opportunistic infections and HIV. Opportunistic infections may be bacterial, fungal, or viral in origin and may produce neurologic disease. Typically, bacterial infections are caused by unusual microorganisms. Cryptococcal infection is the most common fungal disorder and the third leading cause of neurologic disease in persons with AIDS. The symptoms are vague, such as fever, headache, malaise, and meningismus. Herpes encephalitis and herpes varicella-zoster radiculitis may develop. Papovavirus may produce a demyelinating disorder. Cytomegalovirus encephalitis, toxoplasmosis (a protozoal infection), and tuberculosis meningitis have a high incidence in African countries.[85,86]

CNS neoplasms and HIV. The incidence of HIV-associated CNS neoplasms has declined significantly with HAART, particularly primary CNS lymphoma. Other neoplasms associated with HIV include systemic non-Hodgkin lymphoma and metastatic Kaposi sarcoma. Primary CNS lymphoma is a large-cell tumor that presents as rapidly developing and expanding multicentric intracranial mass lesions. The meninges and, possibly, the cranial nerves and spinal cord are invaded in systemic non-Hodgkin lymphoma. Metastasis of a Kaposi sarcoma to the CNS is uncommon.[87]

Demyelinating Disorders

Demyelinating disorders result from damage to the myelin nerve sheath and affect neural transmission. They can occur in either the central (i.e., multiple sclerosis) or the peripheral (i.e., Guillain-Barré syndrome) nervous system. Contributing factors include genetics, infections, autoimmune reactions, environmental toxins, and unknown factors.

Multiple Sclerosis

Multiple sclerosis (MS) is a chronic inflammatory disease involving degeneration of CNS myelin, scarring (sclerosis or plaque formation), and loss of axons. MS is caused by an autoimmune response to self or microbial antigens in genetically susceptible individuals. The onset of MS is usually between 20 and 40 years of age and is more common in women. Men may have a more severe progressive course. The prevalence rate is higher in northern latitudes. Risk factors that may be involved include smoking, vitamin D deficiency, and Epstein-Barr virus infection.[88] The etiology of MS is unknown.

PATHOPHYSIOLOGY MS is a diffuse and progressive disease with patches of damage that can occur throughout the brain and spinal cord. Autoreactive T and B cells cross the blood-brain barrier and recognize myelin and oligodendrocyte autoantigens, triggering inflammation and loss of oligodendrocytes (myelin producing cells). Activation of microglia cells (brain macrophages) contributes to inflammation and injury with plaque formation and axonal degeneration. Loss of myelin disrupts nerve conduction with subsequent death of neurons and brain atrophy. Normal appearing white matter can be microscopically very abnormal and gray matter lesions and atrophy have been documented during later stages of the disease process.[89] These degenerative processes begin before symptom onset and progress throughout a person's life (Figure 16-14).[90] Myelin degeneration also can present as *optic neuritis* or involve the spinal cord. *Spinal MS* can occur concurrently or independently of brain lesions. The multifocal, multistaged features of MS lesions in established disease produce symptoms that are multiple and variable.

CLINICAL MANIFESTATIONS The most common initial symptoms of MS are paresthesias of the face, trunk, or limbs; weakness; impaired gait; visual disturbances; or urinary incontinence, indicating diffuse CNS involvement. Cerebellar and corticospinal involvement presents as nystagmus, ataxia, and weakness with all four limbs involved. Intention tremor and slurred speech may also occur.

The onset, duration, and severity of symptoms are different for each person. Disease exacerbations (also known as relapses or flares) are the temporary occurrence or worsening of symptoms. The symptoms may be mild or serious, may last for several days or weeks, and may be followed by progressive symptoms, including include paresthesias, difficulty speaking, ataxia, or visual changes. The mechanism of these exacerbations is related to delayed or blocked conduction caused by inflammation and demyelination. Various events can occur immediately before the exacerbation of symptoms and are regarded as

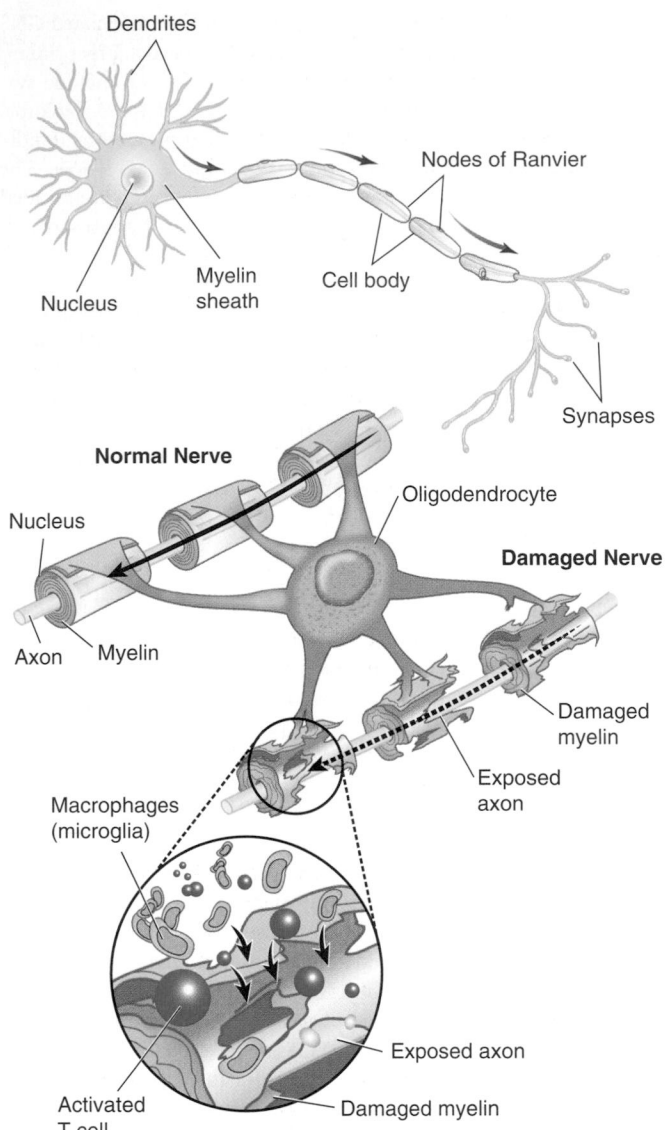

FIGURE 16-14 Pathogenesis of Multiple Sclerosis.

clinical examination in combination with MRI (most sensitive test), CSF findings, and evoked potentials.[92] Persistently elevated levels of CSF immunoglobulin G (IgG) are found in about two thirds of individuals with MS, and oligoclonal IgG bands on electrophoresis are found in more than 90% of MS patients. Evoked potential studies aid diagnosis by detecting decreased conduction velocity in visual, auditory, and somatosensory pathways. MRI is the most sensitive available method of detecting demyelinated plaques and monitoring disease.

The treatment goal in MS is prevention of exacerbations, prevention of permanent neurologic damage, and control of symptoms. Disease-modifying drugs are initiated with diagnosis and include corticosteroids, immunosuppressants, and immune system modulators. Continuous monitoring is important because of the increased risk for infection when taking these drugs. Plasma exchange may be used in persons who do not respond to steroids. Drugs are also available for symptom control. The long-term benefit of these drugs is under investigation.[93] Supportive care includes participation in a regular exercise program, cessation of smoking, and avoidance of overwork, extreme fatigue, and heat exposure. The administration of vitamin D to prevent disease progression is being evaluated.[94] Stem cell therapy is under investigation.[95]

Guillain-Barré Syndrome

Guillain-Barré syndrome is a rare demyelinating disorder caused by a humoral and cell-mediated immunologic reaction directed at the peripheral nerves. It usually occurs after a respiratory tract or gastrointestinal infection. The clinical manifestations can vary from paresis of the legs to complete quadriplegia, respiratory insufficiency, and autonomic nervous system instability. Intravenous immunoglobulin or plasmapheresis is used during the acute phase and followed by aggressive rehabilitation.[96] Recovery occurs within weeks to months or up to 2 years. About 30% of individuals have residual weakness.

✔ **QUICK CHECK 16-3**
1. What are two differences between the symptoms of migraine and cluster headaches?
2. How can bacterial meningitis lead to an amputation?
3. What are the autoimmune mechanisms that cause MS lesions?

---

precipitating factors or triggers, including trauma, emotional stress, and pregnancy. Painful sensory events, spastic paralysis, and bowel and bladder incontinence are common with spinal involvement.[91] Recovery from symptoms during remissions is caused by down-regulation of inflammation and the restoration of axonal function, either by remyelination, the resolution of inflammation, or the restoration of conduction to demyelinated axons.

The subtypes of MS are based on the clinical course: (1) *remitting-relapsing,* initial onset of symptoms followed by remission and exacerbations; (2) *primary-progressive,* a steady decline from onset; (3) *secondary-progressive,* initial remitting and relapsing symptoms with a steady decline in function; and (4) *progressive-relapsing,* a progressive course from onset with superimposed relapses. Initially, 85% to 90% of persons present with a remitting-relapsing course and without treatment transition to the progressive types with insidious neurologic decline. Early cognitive changes are common and may include poor judgment, apathy, emotional lability, and depression.

EVALUATION AND TREATMENT There is no single test available to diagnose or rule out MS. Diagnostic criteria include the history and

PERIPHERAL NERVOUS SYSTEM AND NEUROMUSCULAR JUNCTION DISORDERS

Peripheral Nervous System Disorders

Disease processes may injure the axons traveling to and from the brainstem and spinal cord neuronal cell bodies. The injury may affect a distinct anatomic area on the axon, or the spinal nerves may be injured at the roots, at the **plexus (plexus injuries)** before peripheral nerve formation, or at the nerves themselves. The cranial nerves do not have roots or plexuses and are affected only within themselves. Autonomic nerve fibers may be injured as they travel in certain cranial nerves and emerge through the ventral root and plexuses to pass through the peripheral nerves of the body. Peripheral nervous system disorders are summarized in Table 16-9.

Neuromuscular Junction Disorders

Transmission of the nerve impulse at the neuromuscular junction requires the release of adequate amounts of neurotransmitter from the presynaptic terminals of the axon and effective binding of the released transmitter to the receptors on the membranes of muscle cells (see

TABLE 16-9 Peripheral Nervous System Disorders

Disorder	Pathology	Clinical Manifestations
Radiculopathies	Injury to spinal roots as they exit or enter vertebral canal; caused by compression, inflammation, direct trauma	Affects strength, tone, and bulk of muscles innervated by involved roots; pattern similar to that seen in amyotrophies, with tone and deep tendon reflexes decreased, rarely absent; fasciculations; mild fatigue; sensory alterations, pain
Plexus injuries	Involve nerve plexus distal to spinal roots but proximal to formation of peripheral nerves; caused by trauma, compression, infiltration, or iatrogenic (positioning or intramuscular injection)	Motor weakness, muscle atrophy, sensory loss in affected areas; paralysis common
Neuropathies	Called sensorimotor if sensory, motor, and reflex effects; pure sensory caused by leprosy, industrial solvents, chloramphenicol, and hereditary mechanisms; motor caused by Guillain-Barré syndrome, infectious mononucleosis, viral hepatitis, acute porphyria, or lead, mercury, and triorthocresylphosphate (TCP) poisoning	Affects muscle strength, tone, and bulk; whole muscles or groups may be paretic or paralyzed; muscles of feet and legs first, then hands and arms; tone and deep tendon reflexes generally decreased with atrophy and fasciculation; mild fatigue; some specific symptoms of paresthesia and dysesthesia; altered reflexes; autonomic disturbances; deformities; metabolic changes
Guillain-Barré syndrome (several antibody subtypes have been identified)	Acute onset of motor, sensory, or autonomic symptoms caused by autoimmune inflammatory response, resulting in axonal demyelination; most commonly manifests as ascending motor paralysis; often preceded by respiratory tract or gastrointestinal viral infection	Clinical manifestations are related to antibody subtypes; manifestations can include paresis of legs to complete quadriplegia, paralysis of eye muscles, respiratory insufficiency, autonomic nervous system instability; sensory symptoms (pain, numbness, paresthesias); may progress to respiratory arrest or cardiovascular collapse

From Vucic S et al: *J Clin Neurosci* 16(6):733-741, 2009.

Figure 13-15). [Myasthenia gravis is the most prevalent of the neuromuscular junction disorders and is presented next.]

Myasthenia Gravis

Myasthenia gravis is an acquired chronic autoimmune disease mediated by antibodies against the acetylcholine receptor (AChR) at the postsynaptic membrane of the neuromuscular junction. The incidence is about 9 to 21 per million population[97] and it is more common in women. Thymic tumors, pathologic changes in the thymus, and other autoimmune diseases are associated with the disorder. (Autoimmune mechanisms are discussed in Chapter 8.) Ocular myasthenia, more common in males, involves weakness of the eye muscles and eyelids, and may include swallowing difficulties and slurred speech.

PATHOPHYSIOLOGY Myasthenia gravis results from a defect in nerve impulse transmission at the neuromuscular junction. The postsynaptic AChRs on the muscle cell's plasma membrane are no longer recognized as "self" and elicit T-cell–dependent formation of IgG autoantibodies. The autoantibodies fix onto ACh receptor sites, blocking the binding of acetylcholine. Eventually the antibody action destroys receptor sites. This loss of AChR sites causes diminished transmission of the nerve impulse across the neuromuscular junction and decreased muscle depolarization. Symptomatic individuals without anti-AChR antibodies may have antibodies against muscle-specific kinase (MuSK) with similar symptoms. Why this autosensitization occurs is unknown.

CLINICAL MANIFESTATIONS Myasthenia gravis has an insidious onset. The variable distribution of ACh receptor sites or the number of and different isoforms of antibodies may determine when and which muscle groups are affected first. The muscles of the eyes, face, mouth, throat, and neck usually are affected first. There can be drooling and difficulty chewing and swallowing food. These problems can affect nutrition and put the person as risk for respiratory aspiration.

The muscles of the neck, shoulder girdle, and hip flexors are less frequently affected but muscle fatigue is common after exercise and there can be progressive weakness. The respiratory muscles of the diaphragm and chest wall can become weak with impaired ventilation. Clinical manifestations may first appear during pregnancy, during the postpartum period, or in conjunction with the administration of certain anesthetic agents. The progression of myasthenia gravis varies, appearing first as a mild case that spontaneously remits, with a series of relapses and symptom-free intervals ranging from weeks to months. Over time, the disease can progress. Myasthenic crisis can develop as the disease progresses and occurs when severe muscle weakness causes extreme quadriparesis or quadriplegia, respiratory insufficiency with shortness of breath, and extreme difficulty in swallowing. The individual in myasthenic crisis is in danger of respiratory arrest.

Cholinergic crisis may arise from anticholinesterase drug toxicity with increased intestinal motility, episodes of diarrhea and complaints of intestinal cramping, bradycardia, pupillary constriction, increased salivation, and diaphoresis. These symptoms are caused by the smooth muscle hyperactivity secondary to excessive accumulation of acetylcholine at the neuromuscular junctions and excessive parasympathetic-like activity. As in myasthenic crisis, the individual is in danger of respiratory arrest.

EVALUATION AND TREATMENT The diagnosis of myasthenia gravis is made on the basis of a response to edrophonium chloride (Tensilon), results of EMG studies, and detection of anti-AChR or MuSK antibodies. With the intravenous administration of the drug, immediate demonstrable improvement in muscle strength usually persists for several minutes. Mediastinal tomography and MRI help determine whether a thymoma is present. Current treatments for myasthenia gravis have improved prognosis, including in those who have ocular myasthenia.

Anticholinesterase drugs, steroids, and immunosuppressant drugs (e.g., azathioprine and cyclosporine) are used to treat myasthenia gravis and prevent myasthenic crisis. For individuals with cholinergic crisis, anticholinergic drugs are withheld until blood levels are nontoxic; in addition, ventilatory support is provided and respiratory complications are prevented. Plasmapheresis may be lifesaving. Thymectomy is the treatment of choice in individuals with a thymoma and those with anti-AChR antibodies because this terminates the production of self-reactive T cells and B cells that produce the antibodies.[98,99]

✔ QUICK CHECK 16-4

1. Where in the peripheral nervous system can disease occur?
2. Why do antibodies contribute to the symptoms of myasthenia gravis?
3. How do myasthenic crisis and cholinergic crisis differ in terms of cause and treatment?

TUMORS OF THE CENTRAL NERVOUS SYSTEM

CNS tumors include both brain and spinal cord tumors. Primary CNS tumors had an estimated 22,850 new cases and 15,320 deaths in the United States in 2015.[100] The incidence of CNS tumors increases to age 70 years and then decreases. CNS tumors are the second most common group of tumors occurring in children. Approximately 70%

to 75% of all intracranial tumors in children are located infratentorially (see Chapter 17), and in adults 70% are located supratentorially. Peripheral nerve tumors are rare in children and common in adults. Carcinogenesis is discussed in Chapter 10, pituitary tumors are discussed in Chapter 19, and cerebral tumors in children are discussed in Chapter 17.

Brain Tumors

Tumors within the cranium can be either primary or metastatic. *Primary brain tumors* originate from brain substance, including neuroglia, neurons, cells of blood vessels, and connective tissue. *Extracerebral tumors* originate outside substances of the brain and include meningiomas, acoustic nerve tumors, and tumors of pituitary and pineal glands. *Metastatic (secondary) brain tumors* arise in organ systems outside the brain and spread to the brain. Sites of intracranial tumors are illustrated in Figure 16-15.

Local effects of cranial tumors are caused by the destructive action of the tumor itself on a particular site in the brain and by compression causing decreased cerebral blood flow. Generalized effects result from increased intracranial pressure caused by growth of the tumor, obstruction of the ventricular system, hemorrhages in and around the tumor, or cerebral edema (Figure 16-16). Manifestations include seizures, visual disturbances, unstable gait, and cranial nerve dysfunction.

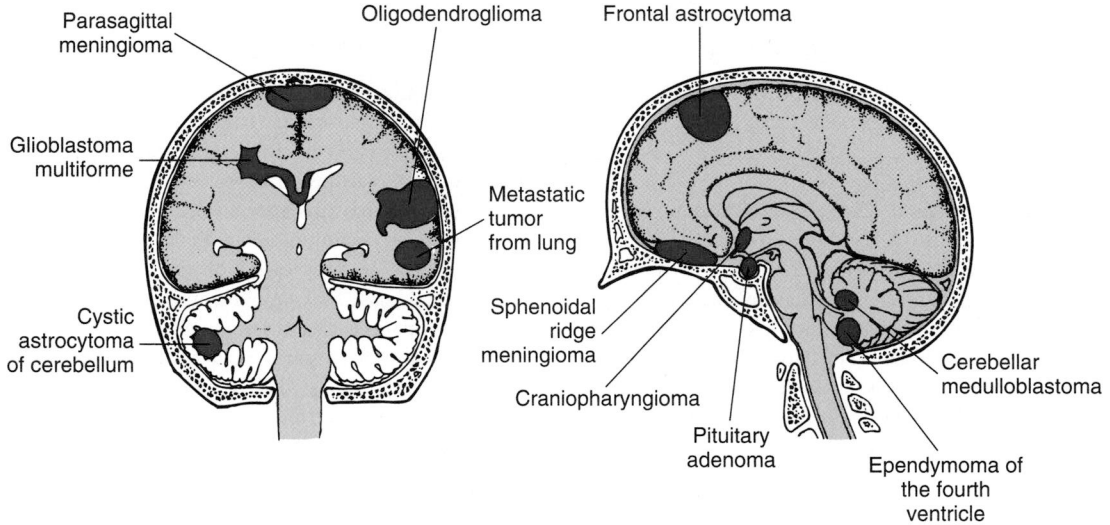

FIGURE 16-15 Common Sites of Intracranial Tumors.

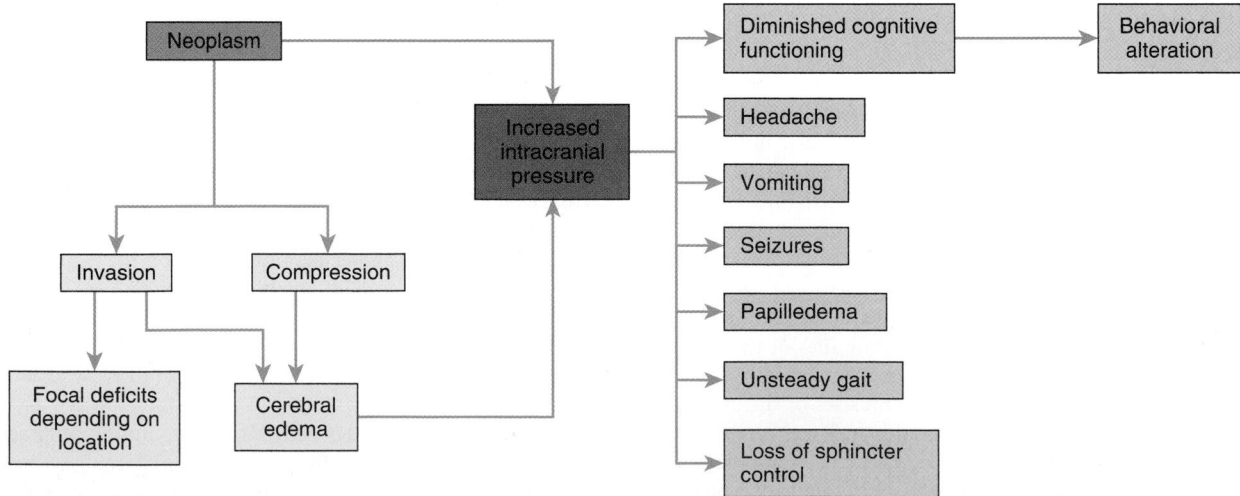

FIGURE 16-16 Origin of Clinical Manifestations Associated with an Intracranial Neoplasm.

Intracranial brain tumors do not metastasize as readily as tumors in other organs because there are no lymphatic channels within the brain substance. If metastasis does occur, it is usually through seeding of cerebral blood or CSF during cranial surgery or through artificial shunts.

Primary Brain (Intracerebral) Tumors

Primary brain (intracerebral) tumors, also called gliomas, include astrocytomas, oligodendrogliomas, and ependymomas. They make up 50% to 60% of all adult brain tumors and about 2% of all cancers in the United States (Table 16-10). The World Health Organization (WHO) divides gliomas into four grades based on histopathologic features, cellular density, atypia, mitotic activity, microvascular proliferation, and necrosis (Table 16-11). Grades I and II are generally benign or slow growing. Grades III and IV are malignant tumors. Etiology for primary brain tumors is not clearly known. Ionizing radiation is the only known environmental risk factor. There may be an association between mobile phone use and gliomas and acoustic neuromas.[101,102]

TABLE 16-10   Brain and Spinal Cord Tumors

Neoplasm	Location	Characteristics	Cell of Origin
Gliomas			
Astrocytoma	Anywhere in brain or spinal cord	Slow growing, invasive	Astrocytes
Glioblastoma multiforme	Predominantly in cerebral hemispheres	Highly invasive and malignant	Thought to arise from mature astrocytes
Oligodendrocytoma	Most commonly in frontal lobes deep in white matter; may arise in brainstem, cerebellum, and spinal cord	Relatively avascular; tends to be encapsulated; more malignant form called *oligodendroblastoma*	Oligodendrites
Ependymoma	Intramedullary: wall of ventricles; may arise in caudal tail of spinal cord	More common in children, variable growth rates; more malignant, invasive form is called *ependymoblastoma;* may extend into ventricle or invade brain tissue	Ependymal cells
Neuronal Cell			
Medulloblastoma	Posterior cerebellar vermis, roof of fourth ventricle	Well demarcated but infiltrating, rapid growing; fills fourth ventricle	Embryonic cells
Mesodermal Tissue			
Meningioma	Intradural, extramedullary: sylvian fissure region, superior parasagittal surface of frontal and parietal lobes, olfactory groove, wing of sphenoid bone, superior surface of cerebellum, cerebellopontine angle, spinal cord	Slow growing, circumscribed, encapsulated, sharply demarcated from normal tissues, compressive in nature	Arachnoid cells; may be from fibroblasts
Choroid Plexus			
Papillomas	Choroid plexus of ventricular system, lateral ventricle in children, fourth ventricle in adults	Usually benign; slow expansion inducing hemorrhage and hydrocephalus; malignant tumor is rare	Epithelial cells
Cranial Nerves and Spinal Nerve Roots			
Neurilemmoma	Cranial nerves (most commonly vestibular division of cranial nerve VIII)	Slow growing	Schwann cells
Neurofibroma	Extramedullary—spinal cord	Slow growing	Neurilemma, Schwann cells
Pituitary Tumors			
	Pituitary gland; may extend to or invade floor of third ventricle	Age linked, several types, slow growing, macroadenomas and microadenomas	Pituitary cells, pituitary chromophobes, basophils, eosinophils
Germ Cell Tumors			
	Neurohypophysis, hypothalamus, pineal region Primarily in adolescents Male > female Variable prognosis	Rare, 0.5% of all primary brain tumors	Several types—germinoma, embryonal carcinoma, yolk sac tumor, choriocarcinoma, teratoma, mixed germ cell tumor—with different cell origins
Pineal region	Pineal region; pineal parenchyma	Several types (germinoma, pineocytoma, teratoma)	Several types with different cell origins
Blood Vessel Tumors			
Angioma	Predominantly in posterior cerebral hemispheres	Slow growing	Arising from congenitally malformed arteriovenous connections
Hemangioblastomas	Predominantly in cerebellum	Slow growing	Embryonic vascular tissue

TABLE 16-11   Grades of Astrocytomas

Grade*	Type	Description	Characteristics
I	Pilocytic astrocytoma	Common in children and young adults and people with neurofibromatosis type 1; common in cerebellum	Least malignant, well differentiated; grows slowly; near-normal microscopic appearance, noninfiltrating
II	Diffuse, low-grade astrocytoma (fibrillary, gemistocytic, protoplasmic) Oligodendroglioma	Common in young adults; more common in cerebrum but can occur in any part of brain	Abnormal microscopic appearance; grows slowly; infiltrates to adjacent tissue; may recur at higher grade
III	Anaplastic (malignant) astrocytoma Anaplastic oligodendroglioma	Common in young adults	Malignant; many cells undergoing mitosis; infiltrates adjacent tissue; frequently recurs at higher grade
IV	Glioblastoma (glioblastoma multiforme)	Common in older adults, particularly men Predominant in cerebral hemispheres	Poorly differentiated; increased number of cells undergoing mitosis; bizarre microscopic appearance; widely infiltrates; neovascularization; central necrosis

Data from American Brain Tumor Association: *Brain tumor primer,* ed 9, Chicago, Ill, 2010, Author, available at: http://neurosurgery.mgh.harvard .edu/abta/; Louis DN et al: *Acta Neuropathol* 114(2):97-109, 2007.
*World Health Organization Grading of Central Nervous System Tumors.

Surgical or radiosurgical excision, surgical decompression, chemotherapy, radiotherapy, and hyperthermia are treatment options for these tumors. Supportive treatment is directed at reducing edema. New treatment options are emerging. (Cancer treatment is discussed in Chapter 10.)

Astrocytoma. Astrocytomas are the most common glioma (about 35% to 50% of all tumors of the brain and spinal cord)[100] and are graded by two classification systems (see Table 16-11). These tumor cells are thought to have lost normal growth restraint and thus proliferate uncontrollably. Astrocytomas are graded I through IV, with grades I and II being slow-growing tumors that are most common in children. Grade I and II astrocytomas commonly progress to a higher grade, faster growing tumor. They may occur anywhere in the brain or spinal cord, and are generally located in the cerebrum, hypothalamus, or pons. Low-grade astrocytomas tend to be located laterally or supratentorially in adults and in a midline or near-midline position in children.

Headache and subtle neurobehavioral changes may be early signs with other neurologic symptoms evolving slowly and increased intracranial pressure occurring late in the tumor's course. Onset of a focal seizure disorder between the second and sixth decade of life suggests an astrocytoma. Low-grade astrocytomas are treated with surgery or by external radiation, and at least 50% of persons survive 5 years when surgery is followed by radiation therapy (RT).[100,103]

Grades III and IV astrocytomas are found predominantly in the frontal lobes and cerebral hemispheres, although they may occur in the brainstem, cerebellum, and spinal cord. Men are twice as likely to have astrocytomas as women; in the 15- to 34-year-old age group they are the third most common brain cancer, whereas in the 35- to 54-year-old age group they are the fourth most common.

Grade IV astrocytoma, glioblastoma multiforme, is the most lethal and common type of primary brain tumor. They are highly vascular and extensively irregular and infiltrative, making them difficult to remove surgically. Fifty percent of glioblastomas are bilateral or at least occupy more than one lobe at the time of death. The typical clinical presentation for a glioblastoma multiforme is that of diffuse, nonspecific clinical signs, such as headache, irritability, and "personality changes" that progress to more clear-cut manifestations of increased intracranial pressure, including headache on position change, papilledema, vomiting, or seizure activity. Symptoms may progress to include definite focal signs, such as

hemiparesis, dysphasia, dyspraxia, cranial nerve palsies, and visual field deficits.

Higher grade astrocytomas are treated surgically and with radiotherapy and chemotherapy. Recurrence is common and survival time is less than 5 years.[104]

Oligodendroglioma. Oligodendrogliomas constitute about 2% of all brain tumors and 10% to 15% of all gliomas. They are typically slow-growing tumors, and most oligodendrogliomas are macroscopically indistinguishable from other gliomas and may be a mixed type of oligodendroglioma and astrocytoma. Most are found in the frontal and temporal lobes, often in the deep white matter, but they are found also in other parts of the brain and spinal cord. Many are found in young adults with a history of temporal lobe epilepsy. Malignant degeneration occurs in approximately one third of persons with oligodendrogliomas, and the tumors are then referred to as oligodendroblastomas.

More than 50% of individuals experience a focal or generalized seizure as the first clinical manifestation. Only half of those with an oligodendroglioma have increased intracranial pressure at the time of diagnosis and surgery, and only one third develop focal manifestations. Treatment includes surgery, radiotherapy, and chemotherapy.

Ependymoma. Ependymomas are nonencapsulated gliomas that arise from ependymal cells; they are rare in adults, usually occurring in the spinal cord.[105] However, in children ependymomas are typically located in the brain. They constitute about 6% of all primary brain tumors in adults and 10% in children and adolescents. Approximately 70% of these tumors occur in the fourth ventricle, with others found in the third and lateral ventricles and caudal portion of the spinal cord. Approximately 40% of infratentorial ependymomas occur in children younger than 10 years. Cerebral (supratentorial) ependymomas occur at all ages.

Fourth ventricle ependymomas present with difficulty in balance, unsteady gait, uncoordinated muscle movement, and difficulty with fine motor movement. The clinical manifestations of a lateral and third ventricle ependymoma that involves the cerebral hemispheres are seizures, visual changes, and hemiparesis. Blockage of the CSF pathway produces hydrocephalus and presents with headache, nausea, and vomiting.

The interval between first manifestations and surgery may be as short as 4 weeks or as long as 7 or 8 years. Ependymomas are treated with radiotherapy, radiosurgery, and chemotherapy. About 20% to

50% of persons survive 5 years. Some persons benefit from a shunting procedure when the ependymoma has caused a noncommunicating hydrocephalus.

Primary Extracerebral Tumors

Meningioma. Meningiomas constitute about 34% of all intracranial tumors. These tumors usually originate from the arachnoidal (meningeal) cap cells in the dura mater and rarely from arachnoid cells of the choroid plexus of the ventricles. Meningiomas are located most commonly in the olfactory grooves, on the wings of the sphenoid bone (at the base of the skull), in the tuberculum sellae (next to the sella turcica), on the superior surface of the cerebellum, and in the cerebellopontine angle and spinal cord. Rarely, they can involve the optic nerve sheath with loss of visual acuity.[106] The cause of meningiomas is unknown.

A meningioma is sharply circumscribed and adapts to the shape it occupies. It may extend to the dural surface and erode the cranial bones or produce an osteoblastic reaction. A few meningiomas exhibit malignant, invasive qualities.

Meningiomas are slow growing and clinical manifestations occur when they reach a certain size and begin to indent the brain parenchyma. Focal seizures are often the first manifestation and increased intracranial pressure is less common than with gliomas.

There is a 20% recurrence rate even with complete surgical excision. If only partial resection is possible, the tumor recurs. Radiation therapies also are used to slow growth.

Nerve sheath tumors. Neurofibromas (benign nerve sheath tumors) are a group of autosomal dominant disorders of the nervous system. They include neurofibromatosis type 1 (NF1, previously known as von Recklinghausen disease) and neurofibromatosis type 2 (NF2); NF1 and NF2 are also known as peripheral and central neurofibromatosis, respectively.

Neurofibromatosis type 1 is the most prevalent with an incidence of about 1 in 3500 people and causes multiple cutaneous neurofibromas, cutaneous macular lesions (café-au-lait spots and freckles), and less commonly bone and soft tissue tumors. Inactivation of the *NF1* gene results in loss of function of neurofibromin in Schwann cells and promotes tumorigenesis (neurofibromas). Learning disabilities are present in about 50% of affected individuals.[107]

Neurofibromatosis type 2 is rare and occurs in about 1 in 60,000 people. The *NF2* gene product is neurofibromin 2 (merlin), a tumor-suppressor protein, and mutations promote development of central nervous system tumors, particularly schwannomas, although other tumor types can occur (meningiomas, ependymomas, astrocytomas, and neurofibromas). Schwannomas of the vestibular nerves present with hearing loss and deafness. Other symptoms may include loss of balance and dizziness. Schwannomas also may develop in other cranial, spinal, and peripheral nerves, and cutaneous signs are less prominent.

Genetic testing is available for the management of families susceptible to NF, and prenatal diagnosis is possible. Diagnosis is based on clinical manifestations and neuroimaging studies, and diagnostic criteria have been established for NF1.[109] Surgery is the major treatment. Individuals with NF2 have extensive morbidity and reduced life expectancy, particularly with early age of onset. Genetically tailored drugs are likely to provide personalized therapy for both of these devastating conditions.

Metastatic brain tumors. Metastatic brain tumors from systemic cancers are 10 times more common than primary brain tumors and 20% to 40% of persons with cancer have metastasis to the brain.[110] Common primary sites include lung, breast, and skin (e.g., melanomas), as well as kidney, colorectal, and other types of cancer.

Metastasis to the brain is thought to be through vascular channels (see Chapter 10).

Metastatic brain tumors produce signs resembling those of glioblastomas, although several unusual syndromes do exist. Carcinomatous (metastatic cancer) encephalopathy causes headache, nervousness, depression, trembling, confusion, forgetfulness, and gait disorder. In carcinomatosis of the cerebellum, headache, dizziness, and ataxia are found. Carcinomatosis of the craniospinal meninges (also called carcinomatous meningitis) manifests with headache, confusion, and symptoms of cranial or spinal nerve root dysfunction. Metastatic brain tumors carry a poor prognosis. Treatment is guided by the pathology of the original tumor; number, size and location of the brain metastasis; and prior cancer treatments. With the development of new drugs that cross the blood-brain barrier, chemotherapy is increasingly recommended.[111] Survival is about 1 year.

Spinal Cord Tumors

Primary spinal cord tumors are rare and represent about 2% of CNS tumors. They may be extramedullary extradural, intradural extramedullary, or intradural intramedullary. Intramedullary tumors, originate within the neural tissues of the spinal cord. Extramedullary tumors, originate from tissues outside the spinal cord. Intramedullary tumors are primarily gliomas (astrocytomas and ependymomas). Gliomas are difficult to resect completely and radiotherapy is required. Spinal ependymomas may be completely resected and are more common in adults. Extramedullary tumors are either peripheral nerve sheath tumors (neurofibromas or schwannomas) or meningiomas. Neurofibromas are generally found in the thoracic and lumbar region, whereas meningiomas are more evenly distributed through the spine. Complete resection of these tumors can be curative. Other extramedullary tumors are sarcomas, vascular tumors, chordomas, and epidermoid tumors. Intramedullary tumors include ependymoma, astrocytoma and hemangioblastoma.

Metastatic spinal cord tumors are usually carcinomas (i.e., from breast, lung, or prostate cancer), lymphomas, or myelomas. Their location is often extradural, having proliferated to the spine through direct extension from tumors of the vertebral structures or from extraspinal sources extending through the interventricular foramen or bloodstream.

PATHOPHYSIOLOGY Intramedullary spinal cord tumors produce dysfunction by both invasion and compression. Extramedullary spinal cord tumors produce dysfunction by compressing adjacent tissue, not by direct invasion. Metastases from spinal cord tumors occur from direct extension or seeding through the CSF or bloodstream.

CLINICAL MANIFESTATIONS An acute onset of clinical manifestations suggests a vascular occlusion of vessels supplying the spinal cord whereas gradual and progressive symptoms suggest compression. The compressive syndrome (sensorimotor syndrome) involves both the anterior and the posterior spinal tracts, and motor function and sensory function are affected as the tumor grows. Pain is usually a presenting symptom.

The irritative syndrome (radicular syndrome) combines the clinical manifestations of a cord compression with radicular pain that occurs in the sensory root distribution and indicates root irritation. The segmental manifestations include segmental sensory changes, such as paresthesias and impaired pain and touch perception; motor disturbances, including cramps, atrophy, fasciculations, and decreased or absent deep tendon reflexes; and continuous spinal pain.

EVALUATION AND TREATMENT The diagnosis of a spinal cord tumor is made through bone scan, PET, CT-guided needle biopsy, or open biopsy. Involvement of specific cord segments is established. Any metastases also are identified. Treatment varies depending on the nature of the tumor and the person's clinical status, but surgery is essential for all spinal cord tumors.[112]

✔**QUICK CHECK 16-5**
1. How is an encapsulated CNS tumor different from a nonencapsulated CNS tumor?
2. What are three types of spinal cord tumors?
3. What are some common signs and symptoms of compressive and irritative spinal cord tumor syndromes?

■ DID YOU UNDERSTAND?

Central Nervous System Disorders

1. Motor vehicle crashes in children and falls in older adults are major risk factors for traumatic brain injury.
2. Causes of TBI include closed-head trauma (blunt) or open-head trauma (penetrating). Closed-head trauma is more common. Open-head trauma involves a skull fracture with exposure of the cranial vault to the environment.
3. Primary brain injury is caused by direct impact and involves neural injury, primary glial injury, and vascular responses.
4. Primary brain injuries can be focal or diffuse.
5. Focal brain injury includes contusion, laceration, extradural hematoma, subdural hematoma, intracerebral hematoma, and open-head trauma.
6. Diffuse brain injury (diffuse axonal injury [DAI]) results from shearing forces that result in axonal damage ranging from concussion to a severe DAI state.
7. Secondary brain injury develops from systemic and intracranial responses to primary brain trauma that result in further brain injury and neuronal death.
8. Spinal cord injury involves damage to neural tissues by compressing tissue, pulling or exerting tension on tissue, or shearing tissues so that they slide into one another. Vertebral fracture occurs with direct or indirect trauma.
9. Spinal cord injury may cause spinal shock with cessation of all motor, sensory, reflex, and autonomic functions below the transected area. Loss of motor and sensory function depends on the level of injury.
10. Neurogenic shock occurs with cervical or upper thoracic cord injury (above T5) and can occur concurrently with spinal shock.
11. Autonomic hyperreflexia (dysreflexia) is a syndrome of sudden, massive reflex sympathetic discharge associated with spinal cord injury at level T6 or above. Flexor spasms are accompanied by profuse sweating, piloerection, and automatic bladder emptying.
12. Complete cord transection results in paralysis. Paralysis of the lower half of the body with both legs involved is called *paraplegia*. Paralysis involving all four extremities is called *quadriplegia*.
13. Return of spinal neuron excitability occurs slowly. Reflex activity can return in 1 to 2 weeks in most persons with acute spinal cord injury. A pattern of flexion reflexes emerges, involving first the toes, then the feet and the legs. Eventually, reflex voiding and bowel elimination appear.
14. Low back pain is pain between the lower rib cage and gluteal muscles and often radiates into the thigh.
15. Most causes of low back pain are unknown; however, some secondary causes are disk prolapse, tumors, bursitis, synovitis, degenerative joint disease, osteoporosis, fracture, inflammation, and sprain.
16. Degenerative disk disease is an alteration in intervertebral disk tissue and can be related to normal aging.
17. Spondylolysis is a structural defect of the spine with displacement of the vertebra.
18. Spondylolisthesis involves forward slippage of the vertebra and can include a crack or fracture of the pars interarticularis, usually at the L5-S1 vertebrae.
19. Herniation of an intervertebral disk is a protrusion of part of the nucleus pulposus. Herniation most commonly affects the lumbo-sacral disks (L5-S1 and L4-5). The extruded pulposus compresses the nerve root, causing pain that radiates along the sciatic nerve course.
20. Cerebrovascular disease is the most frequently occurring neurologic disorder. Any abnormality of the blood vessels of the brain is referred to as a cerebrovascular disease.
21. Cerebrovascular disease is associated with two types of brain abnormalities: (1) ischemia with or without infarction and (2) hemorrhage.
22. Transient ischemic attacks (TIAs) are temporary decreases in brain blood flow.
23. Cerebrovascular accidents (stroke syndromes) are classified pathophysiologically as ischemic (thrombotic or embolic), hemorrhagic (intracranial hemorrhage), or associated with hypoperfusion.
24. Intracranial aneurysms result from defects in the vascular wall and are classified on the basis of form and shape. They are often asymptomatic, but the signs vary depending on the location and size of the aneurysm.
25. An arteriovenous malformation (AVM) is a mass of dilated blood vessels. Although usually present at birth, symptoms are delayed and usually occur before age 30.
26. A subarachnoid hemorrhage occurs when blood escapes from defective or injured vasculature into the subarachnoid space. When a vessel tears, blood under pressure is pumped into the subarachnoid space. The blood produces an inflammatory reaction in these tissues and increased intracranial pressure.
27. Migraine headache is an episodic headache that can be associated with triggers, and may have an aura associated with a cortical spreading depression that alters cortical blood flow. Pain is related to overactivity in the trigeminal vascular system.
28. Cluster headaches are a group of disorders known as trigeminal autonomic cephalalgias and occur primarily in men. They occur in clusters over a period of days with extreme pain intensity and short duration, and are associated with trigeminal activation.
29. Tension-type headache is the most common headache. Episodic-type headaches involve a peripheral pain mechanism and the chronic type involves a central pain mechanism and may be related to hypersensitivity to pain in craniocervical muscles.
30. Infection and inflammation of the CNS can be caused by bacteria, viruses, fungi, protozoa, and rickettsiae. Bacterial infections are pyogenic or pus producing.

31. Meningitis (infection of the meninges) is classified as bacterial (i.e., meningococci), aseptic (viral or nonpurulent), or fungal. Bacterial meningitis primarily is an infection of the pia mater, the arachnoid, and the fluid of the subarachnoid space. Aseptic meningitis is thought to be limited to the meninges. Fungal meningitis is a chronic, less common type of meningitis.

32. Brain abscesses often originate from infections outside the CNS. Organisms gain access to the CNS from adjacent sites or spread along the wall of a vein. A localized inflammatory process develops with formation of exudate. After a few days, the infection becomes delimited with a center of pus and a wall of granular tissue.

33. Encephalitis is an acute, febrile illness of viral origin with nervous system involvement. The most common encephalitides are caused by arthropod-borne (mosquito-borne) viruses and herpes simplex type 1. Meningeal involvement appears in all encephalitides.

34. Herpes encephalitis is treated with antiviral agents. No definitive treatment exists for the other encephalitides.

35. The common neurologic complications of AIDS are HIV-associated neurocognitive disorder, HIV myelopathy, opportunistic infections, cytomegalovirus infection, parasitic infection, and neoplasms. Pathologically, there may be diffuse CNS involvement, focal pathologic changes, and obstructive hydrocephalus.

Demyelinating Disorders

1. Multiple sclerosis (MS) is a relatively chronic inflammatory demyelinating disorder with scarring (sclerosis) and loss of axons. Although the pathogenesis is unknown, the demyelination is thought to result from an immunogenetic-viral cause in genetically susceptible individuals.

2. Guillain-Barré syndrome is a demyelinating disorder caused by a humoral and cell-mediated immunologic reaction directed at the peripheral nerves.

Peripheral Nervous System and Neuromuscular Junction Disorders

1. With disorders of the roots of spinal cord nerves, the roots may be compressed, inflamed, or torn. Clinical manifestations include local pain or paresthesias in the sensory root distribution. Treatment may involve surgery, antibiotics, steroids, radiation therapy, and chemotherapy.

2. Plexus injuries involve the plexus distal to the spinal roots. Paralysis can occur with complete plexus involvement.

3. When peripheral nerves are affected, axon and myelin degeneration may be present. These syndromes are classified as sensorimotor, sensory, or motor and are characterized by varying degrees of sensory disturbance, paresis, and paralysis. Secondary atrophy may be present.

4. Myasthenia gravis is a disorder of voluntary muscles characterized by muscle weakness and fatigability. It is considered an autoimmune disease and is associated with an increased incidence of other autoimmune diseases.

5. Myasthenia gravis results from a defect in nerve impulse transmission at the postsynaptic membrane of the neuromuscular junction. IgG antibody is secreted against the "self" AChR receptors and blocks the binding of acetylcholine. The antibody action destroys the receptor sites, causing decreased transmission of the nerve impulse across the neuromuscular junction.

Tumors of the Central Nervous System

1. Two main types of tumors occur within the cranium: primary and metastatic. Primary tumors are classified as intracerebral tumors (astrocytomas, oligodendrogliomas, and ependymomas) or extracerebral tumors (meningioma or nerve sheath tumors). Metastatic tumors can be found inside or outside the brain substance.

2. CNS tumors cause local and generalized manifestations. The effects are varied, and local manifestations include seizures, visual disturbances, loss of equilibrium, and cranial nerve dysfunction.

3. Spinal cord tumors are classified as intramedullary tumors (within the neural tissues) or extramedullary tumors (outside the spinal cord). Metastatic spinal cord tumors are usually carcinomas, lymphomas, or myelomas.

4. Extramedullary spinal cord tumors produce dysfunction by compression of adjacent tissue, not by direct invasion. Intramedullary spinal cord tumors produce dysfunction by both invasion and compression.

KEY TERMS

REFERENCES

1. Centers for Disease Control and Prevention, National Center for Injury Prevention and Control: *Traumatic brain injury in the United States: fact sheet.* Updated January 12, 2015. Available at: www.cdc.gov/traumaticbraininjury/get_the_facts.html#risk.

2. Perry EC 3rd et al: Neurotraumatology, *Handb Clin Neurol* 121:1751-1772, 2014.

3. Edwards P et al: Final results of MRC CRASH, a randomised placebo-controlled trial of intravenous corticosteroid in adults with head injury—outcomes at 6 months, *Lancet* 365(9475):1957-1959, 2005.

4. Zakaria Z et al: Extradural haematoma—to evacuate or not? Revisiting treatment guidelines, *Clin Neurol Neurosurg* 115(8):1201-1205, 2013.

5. Johnson VE et al: Axonal pathology in traumatic brain injury, *Exp Neurol* 246:35-43, 2013.

6. Jagoda AS: Mild traumatic brain injury: key decisions in acute management, *Psychiatr Clin North Am* 33(4):797-806, 2010.

7. Sauerlaud S, Maegele MA: CRASH landing in severe head injury, *Lancet* 364:729-782, 2004.

8. National Institute for Health and Care Excellence: *Triage, assessment, investigation and early management of head injury in children, young people and adults,* January 2014. Available at: www.nice.org.uk/guidance/CG176.

9. Kabadi SV, Faden AI: Neuroprotective strategies for traumatic brain injury: improving clinical translation, *Int J Mol Sci* 15(1):1216-1236, 2014.

10. Wang X et al: Nutritional support for patients sustaining traumatic brain injury: a systematic review and meta-analysis of prospective studies, *PLoS One* 8(3):e58838, 2013.

11. American College of Emergency Physicians: *Updated mild traumatic brain injury guideline for adults.* Available at: www.cdc.gov/concussion/pdf/TBI_Clinicians_Factsheet-a.pdf. Accessed July 13, 2015.

12. Brain Trauma Foundation: Guidelines for the acute medical management of severe traumatic brain injury in infants, children, and adolescents—second edition, *Pediatr Crit Care Med* 13(1):S1-S82, 2012. Available at: www.braintrauma.org/pdf/guidelines_pediatric2.pdf.

13. Ontario Neurotrauma Foundation: *Guidelines for diagnosing and managing pediatric concussion,* ed 1, Toronto, 2014, Author. Available at: http://onf.org/documents/guidelines-for-pediatric-concussion.

14. Harmon KG et al: American Medical Society for Sports Medicine position statement: concussion in sport, *Br J Sports Med* 47(1):15-26, 2013. Review erratum in *Br J Sports Med* 47(3):184, 2013.

15. Szaflarski JP et al: Post-traumatic epilepsy: current and emerging treatment options, *Neuropsychiatr Dis Treat* 10:1469-1477, 2014.

16. Lucke-Wold BP et al: Linking traumatic brain injury to chronic traumatic encephalopathy: identification of potential mechanisms leading to neurofibrillary tangle development, *J Neurotrauma* 31(13):1129-1138, 2014.

17. Rabinowitz AR, Levin HS: Cognitive sequelae of traumatic brain injury, *Psychiatr Clin North Am* 37(1):1-11, 2014.

18. National Spinal Cord Injury Statistical Center: *Spinal cord injury facts and figures at a glance.* Available at: https://www.nscisc.uab.edu/PublicDocuments/fact_figures_docs/Facts%202013.pdf. Accessed July 13, 2015.

19. Oyinbo CA: Secondary injury mechanisms in traumatic spinal cord injury: a nugget of this multiply cascade, *Acta Neurobiol Exp (Wars)* 71(2):281-299, 2011.

20. Milligan J et al: Autonomic dysreflexia: recognizing a common serious condition in patients with spinal cord injury, *Can Fam Physician* 58(8):831-835, 2012.

21. Priestley JV et al: Limiting spinal cord injury by pharmacological intervention, *Handb Clin Neurol* 109:463-484, 2012.

22. Hansebout RR, Hansebout CR: Local cooling for traumatic spinal cord injury: outcomes in 20 patients and review of the literature, *J Neurosurg Spine* 20(5):550-561, 2014.

23. Rabchevsky AG et al: Pharmacological interventions for spinal cord injury: where do we stand? How might we step forward? *Pharmacol Ther* 132(1):15-29, 2011.

24. Department of Health and Human Services, Centers for Disease Control and Prevention, National Center for Health Statistics: Summary health statistics for U.S. adults: National Health Interview Survey 2010, *Vital Health Stat* 10(252):161, 2012. Available at: www.cdc.gov/nchs/data/series/sr_10/sr10_252.pdf.

25. Hoy D et al: The global burden of low back pain: estimates from the Global Burden of Disease 2010 study, *Ann Rheum Dis* 73(6):968-974, 2014.

26. Golob AL, Wipf JE: Low back pain, *Med Clin North Am* 98(3):405-428, 2014.

27. Ito K, Creemers L: Mechanisms of intervertebral disk degeneration/injury and pain: a review, *Global Spine J* 3(3):145-152, 2013.

28. Chou R et al: Diagnosis and treatment of low back pain: a joint clinical practice guideline from the American College of Physicians and the American Pain Society, *Ann Intern Med* 147(7):478-491, 2007.

29. Koes BW et al: An updated overview of clinical guidelines for the management of non-specific low back pain in primary care, *Eur Spine J* 19(12):2075-2094, 2010.

30. Deyo RA et al: Opioids for low back pain, *Br Med J* 350:g6380, 2015.

31. Kreiner DS et al: North American Spine Society: An evidence-based clinical guideline for the diagnosis and treatment of lumbar disc herniation with radiculopathy. *Spine J* 14(1):180-191, 2014.

32. Jacobs WC et al: Evidence for surgery in degenerative lumbar spine disorders, *Best Pract Res Clin Rheumatol* 27(5):673-684, 2013.

33. Bruggeman AJ, Decker RC: Surgical treatment and outcomes of lumbar radiculopathy, *Phys Med Rehabil Clin North Am* 22(1):161-177, 2011.

34. Go AS et al: Heart disease and stroke statistics—2014 update: a report from the American Heart Association, *Circulation* 131(4):e29-e322, 2014. Available at http://

circ.ahajournals.org/content/129/3/e28.full.pdf +html.

35. Seppa N: Southern blacks face excess risk of stroke, *Sci News* 167:126, 2005.

36. Bradley WG et al: *Neurology in clinical practice,* ed 5, pp 1165-1169, Philadelphia, 2008, Butterworth-Heinemann.

37. Gupta HV et al: Transient ischemic attacks: predictability of future ischemic stroke or transient ischemic attack events, *Ther Clin Risk Manag* 10:27-35, 2014.

38. Wardlaw JM et al: Lacunar stroke is associated with diffuse blood-brain barrier dysfunction, *Ann Neurol* 65(2):194-202, 2009.

39. Klijn CJ, Kappelle LJ: Haemodynamic stroke: clinical features, prognosis, and management, *Lancet Neurol* 9(10):1008-1017, 2010.

40. Jickling GC et al: Hemorrhagic transformation after ischemic stroke in animals and humans, *J Cereb Blood Flow Metab* 34(2):185-199, 2014.

41. Pare JR, Kahn JH: Basic neuroanatomy and stroke syndromes, *Emerg Med Clin North Am* 30(3):601-615, 2012.

42. Kelley RE, Martin-Schild S: Ischemic stroke: emergencies and management, *Neurol Clin* 30(1):187-210, ix, 2012.

43. Maldonado NJ, Kazmi SO, Suarez JI: Update in the management of acute ischemic stroke. *Crit Care Clin* 30(4):673-697, 2014.

44. Jauch EC et al: Guidelines for the early management of patients with acute ischemic stroke: a guideline for healthcare professionals from the American Heart Association/American Stroke Association, *Stroke* 44(3):870-947, 2013. Also available at: http://stroke.ahajournals.org/content/early/2013/01/31/STR.0b013e318284056a.full.

45. Gomes JA, Manno E: New developments in the treatment of intracerebral hemorrhage, *Neurol Clin* 31(3):721-735, 2013.

46. Francis SE et al: A combination of genetic, molecular and haemodynamic risk factors contributes to the formation, enlargement and rupture of brain aneurysms, *J Clin Neurosci* 20(7):912-918, 2013.

47. Connolly ES Jr et al: Guidelines for the management of aneurysmal subarachnoid hemorrhage: a guideline for healthcare professionals from the American Heart Association/American Stroke Association, *Stroke* 43:1711-1737, 2012.

48. Novakovic RL et al: The diagnosis and management of brain arteriovenous malformations, *Neurol Clin* 31(3):749-763, 2013.

49. Gross BA, Du R: Diagnosis and treatment of vascular malformations of the brain, *Curr Treat Options Neurol* 16(1):279, 2014.

50. Budohoski KP et al: Clinical relevance of cerebral autoregulation following subarachnoid haemorrhage, *Nat Rev Neurol* 9(3):152-163, 2013.

51. Ciurea AV et al: Subarachnoid hemorrhage and cerebral vasospasm—literature review, *J Med Life* 6(2):120-125, 2013.

52. Cavanaugh SJ, Gordon VL: Grading scales used in the management of aneurismal subarachnoid

hemorrhage: a critical review, *J Neurosci Nurs* 34:288-295, 2002.

53. Guo LM et al: Risk factors related to aneurysmal rebleeding, *World Neurosurg* 76(3-4):292-298; discussion 253-254, 2011.

54. International Headache Society: *HIS classification ICHD-II 1. Migraine.* Available at: http://ihs-classification.org/en/02_klassifikation/02_teil1/01.00.00_migraine.html. Accessed July 13, 2015.

55. Migraine Research Foundation: *Migraine fact sheet.* Available at: www.migraineresearchfoundation.org/fact-sheet.html. Accessed July 13, 2015.

56. Sacco S et al: Migraine in women: the role of hormones and their impact on vascular diseases, *J Headache Pain* 13(3):177-189, 2012.

57. Ferrari et al: Migraine pathophysiology: lessons from mouse models and human genetics, *Lancet Neurol* 14(1):65-80, 2015.

58. Akerman S, Goadsby PJ: Pathophysiology of migraine. In Aminoff MJ, Daroff RB, editors: *Encyclopedia of the neurological sciences*, ed 2, pp 67-71, London, 2014 Academic Press.

59. Edvinsson L et al: Basic mechanisms of migraine and its acute treatment, *Pharmacol Ther* 136(3):319-333, 2012.

60. Pietrobon D, Moskowitz MA: Pathophysiology of migraine, *Annu Rev Physiol* 75:365-391, 2013.

61. Cutrer FM, Smith JH: Human studies in the pathophysiology of migraine: genetics and functional neuroimaging, *Headache* 53(2):401-412, 2013.

62. Reddy DS: The pathophysiological and pharmacological basis of current drug treatment of migraine headache, *Expert Rev Clin Pharmacol* 6(3):271-288, 2013.

63. Armstrong C: American Academy of Neurology, American Headache Society. AAN/AHS update recommendations for migraine prevention in adults, *Am Fam Physician* 87(8):584-585, 2013. Also available at http://www.aafp.org/afp/2013/0415/p584.html

64. U.S. Food and Drug Administration: *FDA news release: FDA allows marketing of first medical device to prevent migraine headaches*, March 11 2014. Available at: www.fda.gov/newsevents/newsroom/pressannouncements/ucm388765.htm.

65. De Simone R et al: Intracranial pressure in unresponsive chronic migraine, *J Neurol* 261(7):1365-1373, 2014.

66. Benoliel R, Eliav E: Primary headache disorders, *Dent Clin North Am* 57(3):513-539, 2013.

67. Iacovelli E et al: Neuroimaging in cluster headache and other trigeminal autonomic cephalalgias, *J Headache Pain* 13(1):11-20, 2012.

68. Weaver-Agostoni J: Cluster headache, *Am Fam Physician* 88(2):122-128, 2013.

69. Freitag F: Managing and treating tension-type headache, *Med Clin North Am* 97(2):281-292, 2013.

70. Thigpen MC et al Bacterial meningitis in the United States, 1998-2007, *N Engl J Med* 364(21):2016-2025, 2011.

71. Coureuil M et al: Pathogenesis of meningococcemia, *Cold Spring Harb Perspect Med* 3(6), 2013. pii: a012393, 2013.

72. Heckenberg SG et al: Bacterial meningitis, *Handb Clin Neurol* 121:1361-1375, 2014.

73. Putz K et al: Meningitis, *Prim Care* 40(3):707-726, 2013.

74. Centers for Disease Control and Prevention: *Vaccines and vaccination; meningococcal vaccination.* Updated April 1, 2014. Available at: http://www.cdc.gov/meningococcal/vaccine-info.html.

75. Campsall PA et al: Severe meningococcal infection: a review of epidemiology, diagnosis, and management, *Crit Care Clin* 29(3):393-409, 2013.

76. Yan J et al: Meta-analysis of prevention and treatment of toxoplasmic encephalitis in HIV-infected patients, *Acta Trop* 127(3):236-244, 2013.

77. Brouwer MC et al: Clinical characteristics and outcome of brain abscess: systematic review and meta-analysis, *Neurology* 82(9):806-813, 2014.

78. Alvis Miranda H et al: Brain abscess: current management, *J Neurosci Rural Pract* 4(Suppl 1):S67-S81, 2013.

79. Muzumdar D et al: Brain abscess: an overview, *Int J Surg* 9(2):136-144, 2011.

80. Rust RS: Human arboviral encephalitis, *Semin Pediatr Neurol* 19(3):130-151, 2012.

81. Roos KL: Encephalitis, *Handb Clin Neurol* 121:1377-1381, 2014.

82. Sen S et al: Recent developments regarding human immunodeficiency virus infection and stroke, *Cerebrovasc Dis* 33(3):209-218, 2012.

83. Spudich S: HIV and neurocognitive dysfunction, *Curr HIV/AIDS Rep* 10(3):235-243, 2013.

84. Centner CM et al: Manifestations of HIV infection in the peripheral nervous system, *Lancet Neurol* 12(3):295-309, 2013.

85. Alkali NH et al: NeuroAIDS in sub-Saharan Africa: a clinical review, *Ann Afr Med* 12(1):1-10, 2013.

86. Chang CC et al: HIV and co-infections, *Immunol Rev* 254(1):114-142, 2013.

87. Malfitano A et al: Human immunodeficiency virus-associated malignancies: a therapeutic update, *Curr HIV Res* 10(2):123-132, 2012.

88. O'Gorman C et al: Environmental risk factors for multiple sclerosis: a review with a focus on molecular mechanisms, *Int J Mol Sci* 13(9):11718-11752, 2012.

89. Klaver R et al: Grey matter damage in multiple sclerosis: a pathology perspective, *Prion* 7(1):66-75, 2013.

90. Kakalacheva K et al: Viral triggers of multiple sclerosis, *Biochim Biophys Acta* 1812(2):132-140, 2011.

91. Courtney AM: Multiple sclerosis, *Med Clin North Am* 93(2):451-476, 2009:ix-x.

92. Milo R, Miller A: Revised diagnostic criteria of multiple sclerosis, *Autoimmun Rev* 13(4-5):518-524, 2014.

93. Wingerchuk DM, Carter JL: Multiple sclerosis: current and emerging disease-modifying therapies and treatment strategies, *Mayo Clin Proc* 89(2):225-240, 2014.

94. Hewer S et al: Vitamin D and multiple sclerosis, *J Clin Neurosci* 20(5):634-641, 2013.

95. National Institutes of Health, Northwestern University: *Stem cell therapy for patients with multiple sclerosis failing alternate approved therapy—a randomized study.* In Clinical Trials.gov. [Verified March 2015.] Available from http://clinicaltrials.gov/ct2/show/NCT00273364.

96. Winer JB: An update in Guillain-Barré syndrome, *Autoimmune Dis* 2014:793024, 2014.

97. Meyer A, Levy Y: Chapter 33: geoepidemiology of myasthenia gravis, *Autoimmun Rev* 9(5):A383-A386, 2010.

98. Mehndiratta MM et al: Acetylcholinesterase inhibitor treatment for myasthenia gravis, *Cochrane Database Syst Rev* 2:CD006986, 2011.

99. Zieliński M: Management of myasthenic patients with thymoma, *Thorac Surg Clin* 21(1):47-57, 2011:vi.

100. American Cancer Society: *Cancer facts & figures 2015*, Atlanta, 2015, Author. Available at: http://www.cancer.org/acs/groups/content/@editorial/documents/document/acspc-044552.pdf. Accessed July, 2015.

101. Hardell L, Carlberg M: Using the Hill viewpoints from 1965 for evaluating strengths of evidence of the risk for brain tumors associated with use of mobile and cordless phones, *Rev Environ Health* 28(2-3):97-106, 2013.

102. Hardell L et al: Case-control study of the association between malignant brain tumours diagnosed between 2007 and 2009 and mobile and cordless phone use, *Int J Oncol* 43(6):1833-1845, 2013.

103. Grier JT, Batchelor T: Low grade gliomas in adults, *Oncologist* 11:681-693, 2006.

104. Venur VA et al: Current medical treatment of glioblastoma, *Cancer Treat Res* 163:103-115, 2015.

105. Oh MC et al: Prognosis by tumor location in adults with spinal ependymomas, *J Neurosurg Spine* 18(3):226-235, 2013.

106. Ashpole NM et al: Growth hormone, insulin-like growth factor-1 and the aging brain, *Exp Gerontol* 68:76-81, 2015.

107. Ferner RE, Gutmann DH: Neurofibromatosis type 1 (NF1): diagnosis and management, *Handb Clin Neurol* 115:939-955, 2013.

108. Lloyd SK, Evans DG: Neurofibromatosis type 2 (NF2): diagnosis and management, *Handb Clin Neurol* 115:957-967, 2013.

109. DeBella K et al: Use of the National Institutes of Health criteria for diagnosis of neurofibromatosis 1 in children, *Pediatrics* 105(3 Pt 1):608-614, 2000.

110. Walbert T, Gilbert MR: The role of chemotherapy in the treatment of patients with brain metastases from solid tumors, *Int J Clin Oncol* 14(4):299-306, 2009.

111. Gállego Pérez-Larraya J, Hildebrand J: Brain metastases, *Handb Clin Neurol* 121:1143-1157, 2014.

112. Tredway TL: Minimally invasive approaches for the treatment of intramedullary spinal tumors, *Neurosurg Clin North Am* 25(2):327-336, 2014.

17

Alterations of Neurologic Function in Children

Lynne M. Kerr, Sue E. Huether, and Vinodh Narayanan*

Neurologic disorders in children can occur from infancy through adolescence and include congenital malformations, genetic defects in metabolism, brain injuries, infection, tumors, and other disorders that affect neurologic function.

DEVELOPMENT OF THE NERVOUS SYSTEM IN CHILDREN

The nervous system develops from the embryonic ectoderm through a complex, sequential process that can be arbitrarily divided into stages. These include (1) formation of the neural tube (3 to 4 weeks' gestation), (2) development of the forebrain from the neural tube (2 to 3 months' gestation), (3) neuronal proliferation and migration (3 to 5 months' gestation), (4) formation of network connections and synapses (5 months' gestation to many years postnatally), and (5) myelination (birth to many years postnatally). Many different events happen simultaneously and critical periods must pass uninterrupted if the vulnerable fetus is to develop normally. Genetic and environmental factors (e.g., nutrition, hormones, oxygen levels, toxins, alcohol, drugs, maternal infections, maternal disease) can have a significant effect on neural development[1,2] (see *Health Alert:* Alcohol-Related Neurodevelopmental Disorder [ARND]).

The growth and development of the brain occur rapidly from the third month of gestation through the first year of life, reflecting the proliferation of neurons and glial cells. Although basically all of the neurons that an individual will ever have are present at birth,

development of skills, such as walking, talking, and thinking, depends on these cells making correct connections with other cells and on myelination of the axons making those connections. The head is the fastest growing body part during infancy. One half of postnatal brain growth is achieved by the first year and is 90% complete by age 6 years. The cortex thickens with maturation, and the sulci deepen as a result of rapid expansion of the surface area of the brain. Cerebral blood flow and oxygen consumption during these years are about twice those of the adult brain.

The bones of the infant's skull are separated at the suture lines, forming two **fontanelles**, or "soft spots": one diamond-shaped anterior fontanelle and one triangular-shaped posterior fontanelle. The sutures allow for expansion of the rapidly growing brain. The posterior fontanelle may be open until 2 to 3 months of age; the anterior fontanelle normally does not fully close until 18 months of age (Figure 17-1). Head growth almost always reflects brain growth. Monitoring the fontanelles and careful measurement and plotting of the head circumference on standardized growth charts are essential elements of the pediatric examination. A common cause of accelerating head growth and macrocephaly is hydrocephalus, a condition in which the cerebrospinal fluid (CSF) compartment (ventricles) is enlarged. Increased intracranial pressure, with distention or bulging of the fontanelles, and separation of the sutures are key signs of hydrocephalus. Microcephaly (head circumference below the 2nd percentile for age) can be the result of prenatal infection, toxin exposure, or malnutrition, or have a primary genetic etiology (see p. 427).

Because of the immaturity of much of the human forebrain at birth, neurologic examination of the infant detects mostly reflex responses that require an intact spinal cord and brainstem. Some of

*Vinodh Narayanan contributed to the previous edition.

HEALTH ALERT

Alcohol-Related Neurodevelopmental Disorder (ARND)

ARND is a type of alcohol spectrum disorder with long-lasting neurobehavioral and cognitive deficiencies as a result of fetal alcohol exposure. It is among the most common causes of mental deficits that persist throughout adulthood. ARND is 100% preventable and there is no known amount of alcohol that is safe to consume while pregnant. Rates of alcohol consumption by women during pregnancy range from 5% to 15%.[1-3] Alcohol crosses the placenta and the blood-brain barrier and exerts teratogenic effects on the developing brain throughout fetal development. Alcohol exposure during the first trimester can lead to fetal brain volume reduction and can be related to apoptosis, neuro-degeneration, and suppression of neurogenesis.[4] Fetal alcohol exposure during the second trimester is associated with dilation of the lateral ventricles, a reflection of decreased brain growth.[5] Regions shown to be particularly susceptible to third-trimester binge drinking–induced neurodegeneration include the cerebellum; hippocampus; olfactory bulb; corpus callosum; occipital, cingulate, and parietal cortices; caudate nucleus; nucleus accumbens; and anterior thalamic nuclei.[6] MRI imaging reveals delayed white matter development during childhood and adolescence in ARND and may underlie persistent or worsening behavioral and cognitive deficits during this critical period of development.[7] Screening, education, and prevention programs promote alcohol-free pregnancies.[8-10]

References

1. Centers for Disease Control and Prevention (CDC): *MMWR Morb Mortal Wkly Rep* 61(28):534-538, 2012.
2. May PA et al: *Drug Alcohol Depend* 133(2):502-512, 2013.
3. Zelner I, Koren G: *J Popul Ther Clin Pharmacol* 20(2):e201-e206, 2013.
4. Roussotte FF et al: *Hum Brain Mapping* 33(4):920-937, 2012.
5. Sudheendran N et al: *J Biomed Opt* 18(2):20506, 2013.
6. Yang Y et al: *Cereb Cortex* 22(5):1170-1179, 2012.
7. Treit S et al: *J Neurosci* 33(24):10098-10109, 2013.
8. Barry KL et al: *Reducing alcohol-exposed pregnancies: a report of the National Task Force on Fetal Alcohol Syndrome and Fetal Alcohol Effect*, Atlanta, Ga, 2009, Centers for Disease Control and Prevention. Available at: www.cdc.gov/ncbddd/fasd/pastactivities-taskforce.html.
9. Mengel MB et al: *J Am Board Fam Med* 19(5):494-505, 2006.
10. Waterman EH et al: *Obstet Gynecol Surv* 68(5):367-378, 2013.

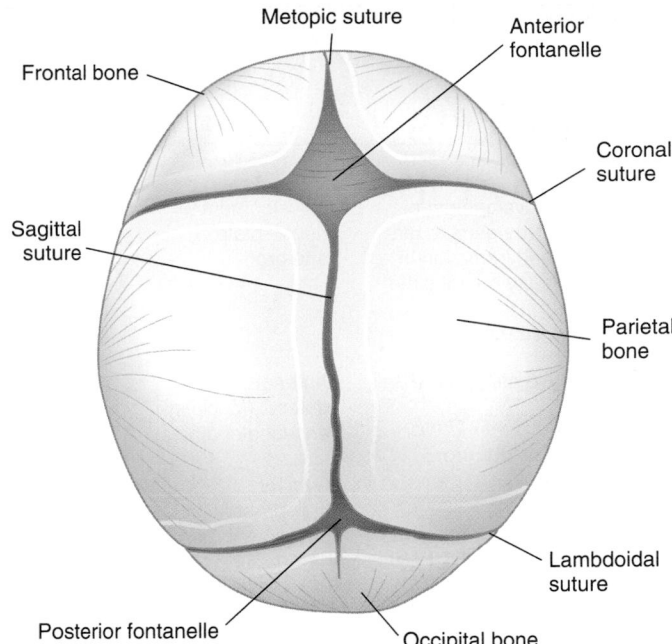

FIGURE 17-1 Cranial Sutures and Fontanelles in Infancy. Fibrous union of suture lines and interlocking of serrated edges (occurs by 6 months; solid union requires approximately 12 years). (Head growth charts are available from the Centers for Disease Control and Prevention at www.cdc.gov/nchs/data/series/sr_11/sr11_246.pdf.)

TABLE 17-1	Reflexes of Infancy	
Reflex	**Age of Appearance of Reflex**	**Age at which Reflex Should No Longer Be Obtainable**
Moro	Birth	3 months
Stepping	Birth	6 weeks
Sucking	Birth	4 months awake 7 months asleep
Rooting	Birth	4 months awake 7 months asleep
Palmar grasp	Birth	6 months
Plantar grasp	Birth	10 months
Tonic neck	2 months	5 months
Neck righting	4 to 6 months	24 months
Landau	3 months	24 months
Parachute reaction	9 months	Persists indefinitely

these reflex patterns are inhibited as cerebral cortical function matures, and these patterns disappear at predictable times during infancy (Table 17-1).

Absence of expected reflex responses at the appropriate age indicates general depression of central or peripheral motor functions. Asymmetric responses may indicate lesions in the motor cortex or peripheral nerves, or may occur with fractures of bones after traumatic delivery or postnatal injury. As the infant matures, the neonatal reflexes disappear in a predictable order as voluntary motor functions supersede them. Abnormal persistence of these reflexes is seen in infants with developmental delays or with central motor lesions.

> **✔ QUICK CHECK 17-1**
> 1. When does development of neuronal myelination occur?
> 2. What is a major function of the fontanelles?
> 3. Why do many of the reflexes of infancy disappear by 1 year of age?

STRUCTURAL MALFORMATIONS

Central nervous system (CNS) malformations are responsible for 75% of fetal deaths and 40% of deaths during the first year of life. CNS malformations account for 33% of all apparent congenital malformations, and 90% of CNS malformations are defects of neural tube closure.

Defects of Neural Tube Closure

Neural tube defects (NTDs) are caused by an arrest of the normal development of the brain and spinal cord during the first month of embryonic development. They occur in about 3000 pregnancies in the United States each year, although there are significant regional prevalence variations.[3] Fetal death often occurs in the more severe forms, thereby reducing the actual prevalence of neural defects at birth.[4] Defects of neural tube closure are divided into two categories: (1) anterior midline defects (ventral induction) and (2) posterior defects

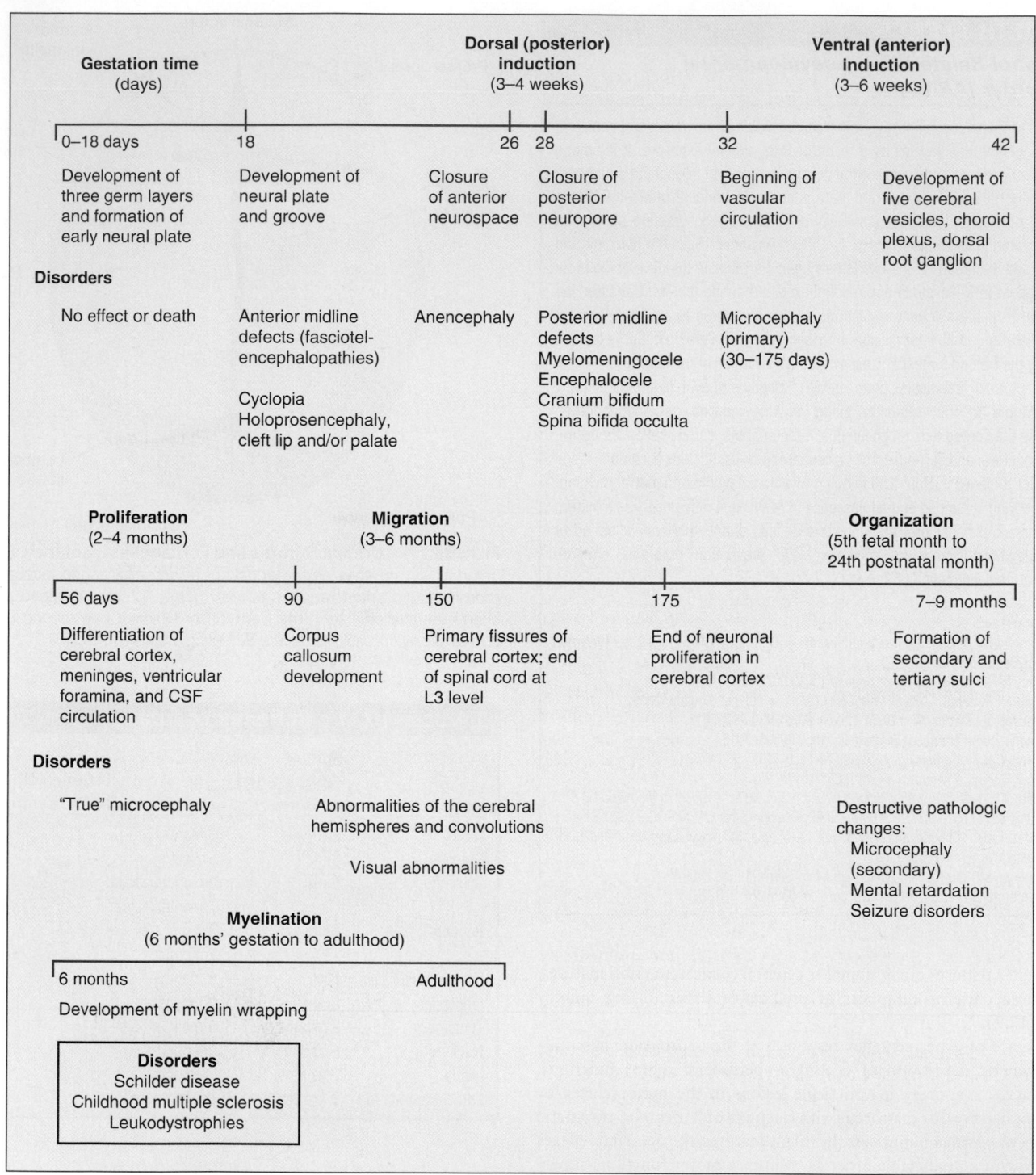

FIGURE 17-2 Disorders Associated with Specific Stages of Embryonic Development. *CSF,* Cerebrospinal fluid.

(dorsal induction). Anterior midline defects may cause brain and face abnormalities with the most extreme form being cyclopia, in which the child has a single midline orbit and eye with a protruding noselike proboscis above the orbit. Spina bifida (split spine) is the most common neural tube defect and includes anencephaly (*an,* "without"; *enkephalos,* "brain"), encephalocele, meningocele, and myelomeningocele. Vertebrae fail to close in spina bifida. Myelomeningocele is a form of spina bifida with incomplete development of the spine and

protrusion of both the spinal cord and the meninges through the skin. Meningocele is a form of spina bifida in which there is protrusion of the meninges but the spinal cord remains in the spinal canal. Disorders of embryonic neural development are summarized in Figure 17-2.

The cause of neural tube defects is believed to be multifactorial (a combination of genes and environment). No single gene has been found to cause neural tube defects but there can be associated mutations in folate-responsive/folate-dependent pathways.[5] Folic acid deficiency during preconception and early stages of pregnancy increases the risk for neural tube defects, and supplementation (400 mcg of folic acid per day) ensures adequate folate status.[6] Other risk factors include a previous NTD pregnancy, maternal diabetes or obesity, use of anticonvulsant drugs (particularly valproic acid), and maternal hyperthermia.[7,8]

Anencephaly is an anomaly in which the soft, bony component of the skull and part of the brain are missing. This is a relatively common disorder, with an incidence of approximately 1 per 4859 total live births in the United States each year.[9] These infants are stillborn or die within a few days after birth. The pathologic mechanism is unknown. Diagnosis is often made prenatally by using ultrasound or evaluating maternal serum alpha fetoprotein (AFP).

Encephalocele refers to a herniation or protrusion of the brain and meninges through a defect in the skull, resulting in a saclike structure. The incidence is approximately 1.0 in 10,000 live births in the United States each year.[10]

Meningocele is a saclike cyst of meninges filled with spinal fluid and is a mild form of spina bifida (Figure 17-3). It develops during the first 4 weeks of pregnancy when the neural tube fails to close completely. The cystic dilation of meninges protrudes through the vertebral defect but does not involve the spinal cord or nerve roots and may produce no neurologic deficit or symptoms. Meningoceles occur with equal frequency in the cervical, thoracic, and lumbar spine areas.

Myelomeningocele (meningomyelocele; spina bifida cystica) is a hernial protrusion of a saclike cyst (containing meninges, spinal fluid, and a portion of the spinal cord with its nerves) through a defect in the posterior arch of a vertebra. Eighty percent of myelomeningoceles are located in the lumbar and lumbosacral regions, the last regions of the neural tube to close. Myelomeningocele is one of the most common developmental anomalies of the nervous system, with an incidence rate ranging from 0.5 to 1.0 per 1000 pregnancies.[11]

Meningocele and myelomeningoceles are evident at birth as a pronounced skin defect on the infant's back (see Figure 17-3). The bony prominences of the unfused neural arches can be palpated at the lateral border of the defect. The defect usually is covered by a transparent membrane that may have neural tissue attached to its inner surface. This membrane may be intact at birth or may leak cerebrospinal fluid (CSF), thereby increasing the risks of infection and neuronal damage.

The spinal cord and nerve roots are malformed below the level of the lesion, resulting in loss of motor, sensory, reflex, and autonomic functions. A brief neurologic examination concentrating on motor function in the legs, reflexes, and sphincter tone is usually sufficient to determine the level above which spinal cord and nerve root function is preserved (Table 17-2). This is useful to predict if the child will ambulate, require bladder catheterization, or be at high risk for developing scoliosis (see Chapter 40).

Hydrocephalus occurs in 85% of infants with myelomeningocele.[12] Seizures also occur in 30% of those with myelodysplasia. Visual and perceptual problems, including ocular palsies, astigmatism, and visuoperceptual deficits, are common. Motor and sensory functions below the level of the lesions are altered. Often these problems worsen as the child grows and the cord ascends within the vertebral canal, pulling primary scar tissue and tethering the cord.[13] Several musculoskeletal deformities are related to this diagnosis, as are spinal deformities.

Myelomeningoceles are almost always associated with the Chiari II malformation (Arnold-Chiari malformation).[12] This is a complex malformation of the brainstem and cerebellum in which the cerebellar tonsils are displaced downward into the cervical spinal canal; the upper

A Normal

B Spina bifida

C Meningocele

D Myelomeningocele

E Myelomeningocele with an intact sac

FIGURE 17-3 Normal Spine, Spina Bifida, Meningocele, and Myelomeningocele. (From Hockenberry MJ, Wilson D: *Wong's nursing care of infants and children*, ed 10, St Louis, 2015, Mosby.)

TABLE 17-2 Functional Alterations in Myelodysplasia Related to Level of Lesion

Level of Lesion	Functional Implications
Thoracic	Flaccid paralysis of lower extremities; variable weakness in abdominal trunk musculature; high thoracic level may mean respiratory compromise; absence of bowel and bladder control
High lumbar	Voluntary hip flexion and adduction; flaccid paralysis of knees, ankles, and feet; may walk with extensive braces and crutches; absence of bowel and bladder control
Mid lumbar	Strong hip flexion and adduction; fair knee extension; flaccid paralysis of ankles and feet; absence of bowel and bladder control
Low lumbar	Strong hip flexion, extension, and adduction and knee extension; weak ankle and toe mobility; may have limited bowel and bladder function
Sacral	Normal function of lower extremities; normal bowel and bladder function

Modified from Sandler AD: *Pediatr Clin North Am* 57(4):879-892, 2010.

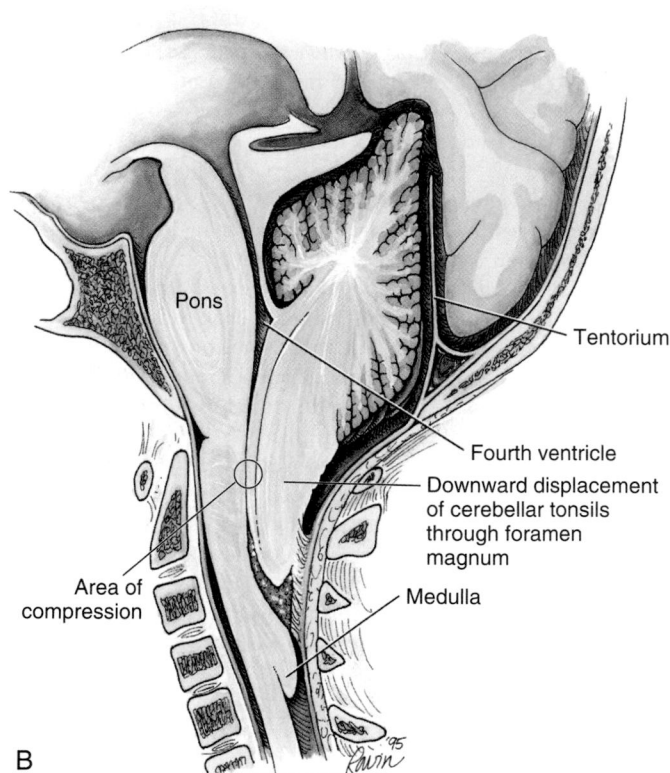

FIGURE 17-4 Normal Brain and Arnold-Chiari II Malformation.
A, Diagram of normal brain. **B,** Diagram of Arnold-Chiari II malformation with downward displacement of cerebellar tonsils and medulla through foramen magnum causing compression and obstruction to flow of CSF. (**B** modified from Barrow Neurological Institute of St Joseph's Hospital and Medical Center. Reprinted with permission.)

medulla and lower pons are elongated and thin; and the medulla is also displaced downward and sometimes has a "kink" (Figure 17-4). The Chiari II malformation is associated with hydrocephalus from pressure that blocks the flow of cerebrospinal fluid; syringomyelia, an abnormality causing cysts at multiple levels within the spinal cord; and cognitive and motor deficits.[14]

Other types of Chiari malformations are not associated with spina bifida. Type I Chiari malformation does not involve the brainstem and may be asymptomatic. In type III, the brainstem or cerebellum extends into a high cervical myelomeningocele. Type IV is characterized by lack of cerebellar development.

Most cases of meningocele and myelomeningocele are diagnosed prenatally by a combination of maternal serologic testing (alpha fetoprotein) and prenatal ultrasound. In these cases, the fetus is usually delivered by elective cesarean section to minimize trauma during labor. Surgical repair is critical and can be performed by in utero fetal surgery or during the first 72 hours of life.[15,16]

It is possible for a defect to occur without any visible exposure of meninges or neural tissue and the term spina bifida occulta is then used. The defect is common and occurs to some degree in 10% to 25% of infants. Spina bifida occulta usually causes no neurologic dysfunction because the spinal cord and spinal nerves are normal. Tethered cord syndrome may develop after surgical correction for myelomeningocele. The cord becomes abnormally attached or tethered as a result of scar tissue as the cord transcends the vertebral canal with growth.[17]

Craniosynostosis

Skull malformations range from minor, insignificant defects to major defects that are incompatible with life. Craniosynostosis (craniostenosis) is the premature closure of one or more of the cranial sutures (sagittal, coronal, lambdoid, metopic) during the first 18 to 20 months of the infant's life. The incidence of craniosynostosis is 1 per 1800 to 2200 live births.[18] Males are affected twice as often as females. Fusion of a cranial suture prevents growth of the skull perpendicular to the suture line, resulting in an asymmetric shape of the skull. The general term *plagiocephaly,* meaning "misshapen skull," is used to describe deformities that result from craniosynostosis or from asymmetric head posture (positional). When a single coronal suture fuses prematurely, the head is flattened on that side in front. When the sagittal suture fuses prematurely, the head is elongated in the anteroposterior direction (scaphocephaly).[19] Single suture craniosynostosis is usually only a cosmetic issue. Rarely, when multiple sutures fuse prematurely, brain growth may be restricted, and surgical repair may prevent neurologic dysfunction (Figure 17-5). Syndromic craniosynostosis involves deformities in other systems (i.e., the heart, limbs, and central nervous system).

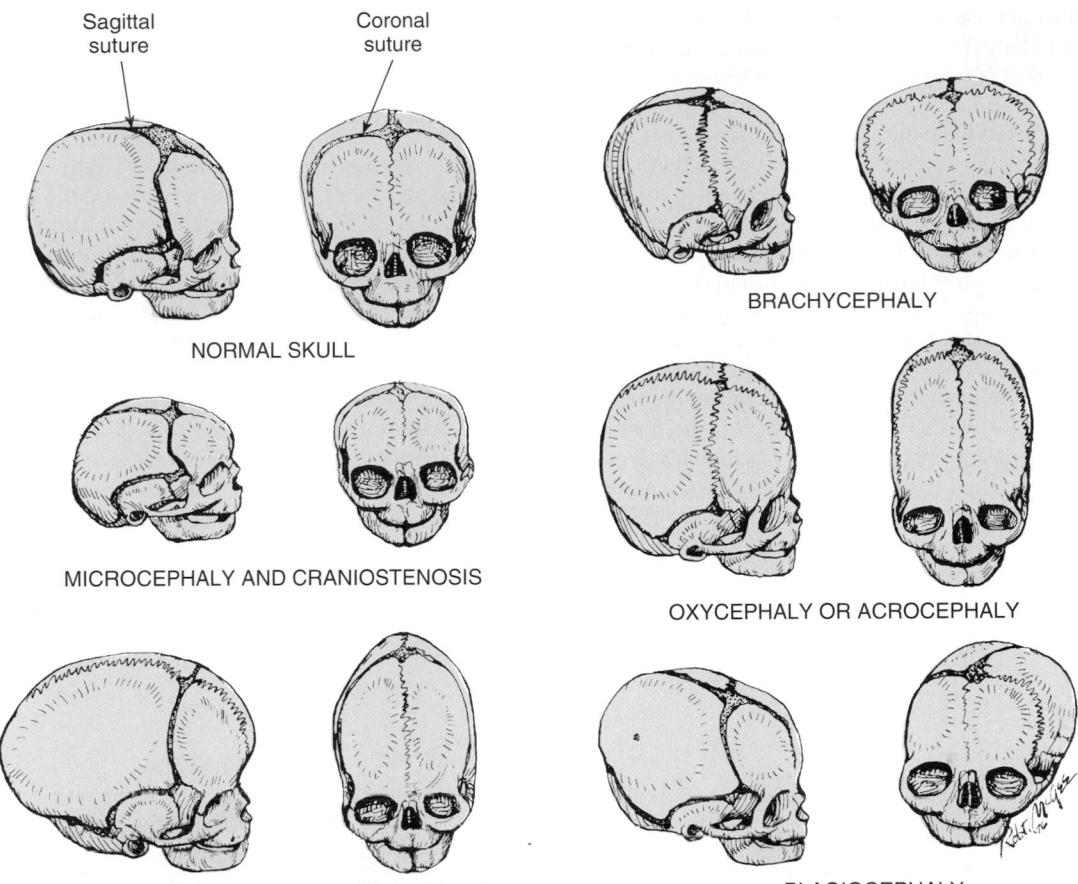

Sagittal suture
Coronal suture

NORMAL SKULL

BRACHYCEPHALY

MICROCEPHALY AND CRANIOSTENOSIS

OXYCEPHALY OR ACROCEPHALY

SCAPHOCEPHALY OR DOLICHOCEPHALY

PLAGIOCEPHALY

FIGURE 17-5 Normal and Abnormal Head Configurations. *Normal skull:* Bones separated by membranous seams until sutures gradually close. *Microcephaly and craniostenosis:* Microcephaly is head circumference more than 2 standard deviations below the mean for age, gender, race, and gestation and reflects a small brain; craniosynostosis is premature closure of sutures. *Scaphocephaly or dolichocephaly* (frequency 56%): Premature closure of sagittal suture, resulting in restricted lateral growth. *Brachycephaly:* Premature closure of coronal suture, resulting in excessive lateral growth. *Oxycephaly or acrocephaly* (frequency 5.8% to 12%): Premature closure of all coronal and sagittal sutures, resulting in accelerated upward growth and small head circumference. *Plagiocephaly* (frequency 13%): Unilateral premature closure of coronal suture, resulting in asymmetric growth. (From Hockenberry MJ, Wilson D: *Wong's nursing care of infants and children,* ed 10, St Louis, 2015, Mosby.)

Malformations of Brain Development

Reduced proliferation or accelerated apoptosis causes congenital microcephaly (microencephaly—small brain) and increased proliferation causes megalencephaly (abnormally large brain).

Microcephaly is a defect in brain growth as a whole (see Figure 17-5). Cranial size is significantly below average for the infant's age, gender, race, and gestation. The small size of the skull reflects a small brain (microencephaly), which is caused by reduced proliferation or accelerated apoptosis (Table 17-3). *True (primary) microcephaly* is usually caused by an autosomal recessive genetic or chromosomal defect. *Secondary (acquired) microcephaly* is associated with various causes including infection, trauma, metabolic disorders, maternal anorexia experienced during the third trimester of pregnancy, and the presence of other genetic syndromes. Children with microcephaly are usually developmentally delayed.

Cortical dysplasias are a heterogeneous group of disorders caused by defects in brain development. These disorders may range from a small area of abnormal tissue (e.g., heterotopia, which are pieces of gray matter that did not migrate to their normal position in the cortex

TABLE 17-3	**Causes of Microcephaly**	
Defects in Brain Development	**Intrauterine Infections**	**Perinatal and Postnatal Disorders**
Hereditary (recessive) microcephaly	Congenital rubella	Intrauterine or neonatal anoxia
Down syndrome and other trisomy syndromes	Cytomegalovirus infection	Severe malnutrition in early infancy
Fetal ionizing radiation exposure	Congenital toxoplasmosis	Neonatal herpesvirus infection
Maternal phenylketonuria		
Cornelia de Lange syndrome		
Rubinstein-Taybi syndrome		
Smith-Lemli-Opitz syndrome		
Fetal alcohol syndrome		
Angelman syndrome		
Seckel syndrome		

of the brain; and focal cortical dysplasias, where brain organization in one small area is abnormal) to an entire brain that is smooth without the normal configuration of gyri and sulci of a developed brain (lissencephaly). The malformation occurs during brain formation. There is a specific genetic defect for some of these disorders; others are multifactorial or acquired (e.g., intrauterine trauma or infection). Cortical dysplasias increase the risk for seizures that are difficult to control, and cause developmental delay and motor dysfunction. Genetic testing assesses risk in other family members and guides therapy.[20]

Congenital hydrocephalus is present at birth and characterized by increased cerebrospinal fluid (CSF) pressure. It may be caused by blockage within the ventricular system where the CSF flows, an imbalance in the production of CSF, or a reduced reabsorption of CSF.[21] The increased pressure within the ventricular system dilates the ventricles and pushes and compresses the brain tissue against the skull cavity (Figure 17-6) When hydrocephalus develops before fusion of the cranial sutures, the skull can expand to accommodate this additional space-occupying volume and preserve neuronal function. The overall incidence of hydrocephalus is approximately 1 to 3 per 1000 live births.[22] The incidence of hydrocephalus that is not associated with myelomeningocele is approximately 0.5 to 1 per 1000 live births.[22] (Types of hydrocephalus are discussed in Chapter 15.)

Congenital hydrocephalus may cause fetal death in utero, or the increased head circumference may require cesarean delivery of the infant. Symptoms depend directly on the cause and rate of hydrocephalus development. When there is separation of the cranial sutures, a resonant note sounds when the skull is tapped, a manifestation termed Macewen sign or "cracked pot" sign. The eyes may assume a staring expression, with sclera visible above the cornea, called *sunsetting*. Cognitive impairment in children with hydrocephalus is often related to associated brain malformations, or episodes of shunt failure or infection. Approximately 30% to 40% of children with uncomplicated congenital hydrocephalus complete schooling and are employed when treated successfully with shunting or endoscopic third ventriculostomy and choroid plexus cauterization.[23-25]

The Dandy-Walker malformation (DWM) is a congenital defect of the cerebellum characterized by a large posterior fossa cyst that communicates with the fourth ventricle and an atrophic, upwardly rotated cerebellar vermis.[26] DWM is commonly associated with hydrocephalus caused by compression of the aqueduct of Sylvius. Other causes of obstructions within the ventricular system that can result in hydrocephalus include brain tumors, cysts, trauma, arteriovenous malformations, blood clots, infections, and the Chiari malformations (see p. 425).

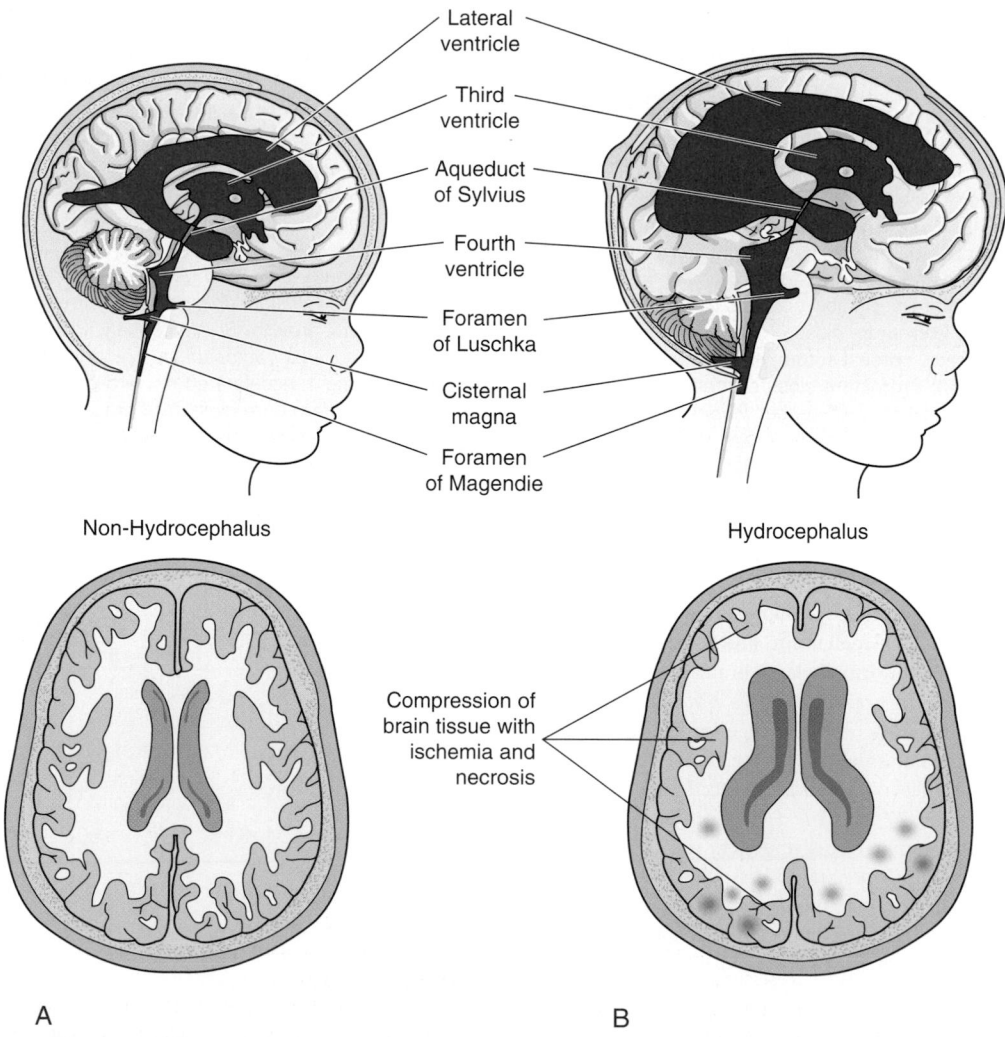

Lateral
ventricle

Third
ventricle

Aqueduct
of Sylvius

Fourth
ventricle

Foramen
of Luschka

Cisternal
magna

Foramen
of Magendie

Non-Hydrocephalus

Hydrocephalus

Compression of
brain tissue with
ischemia and
necrosis

A

B

FIGURE 17-6 Hydrocephalus. A block in the flow of cerebrospinal fluid (CSF). **A,** Patent cerebrospinal fluid circulation. **B,** Enlarged lateral and third ventricles caused by obstruction of circulation (e.g., stenosis of aqueduct of Sylvius).

ALTERATIONS IN FUNCTION: ENCEPHALOPATHIES

Encephalopathy, meaning brain pathology, is a general category that includes a number of syndromes and diseases (see Chapter 16). These disorders may be acute or chronic, as well as static or progressive.

Static Encephalopathies

Static or nonprogressive encephalopathy describes a neurologic condition caused by a fixed lesion without active and ongoing disease. Causes include brain malformations (disorders of neuronal migration) or brain injury that may occur during gestation or birth, or at any time during childhood. The degree of neurologic impairment is directly related to the extent of the injury or malformation. Anoxia, trauma, and infections are the most common factors that cause injury to the nervous system in the perinatal period. Infections, metabolic disturbances (acquired or genetic), trauma, toxins, and vascular disease may injure the nervous system in the postnatal period.[27]

Cerebral palsy is a disorder of movement, muscle tone, or posture that is caused by injury or abnormal development in the immature brain, before, during, or after birth up to 1 year of age. Cerebral palsy is one of the most common crippling disorders of childhood, affecting nearly 500,000 children in the United States alone. Although the exact incidence is unknown, studies suggest that the prevalence is approximately 1 in 323 children in the United States.[28]

Risk factors include prenatal or perinatal cerebral hypoxia, hemorrhage, infection, genetic abnormalities, or low birth weight. It can be classified on the basis of neurologic signs and motor symptoms, with the major types involving spasticity, dystonia, ataxia, or a combination of these symptoms (mixed). Diplegia, hemiplegia, or tetraplegia may be present.

Pyramidal/spastic cerebral palsy results from damage to corticospinal pathways (upper motor neurons) and is associated with increased muscle tone, persistent primitive reflexes, hyperactive deep tendon reflexes, clonus, rigidity of the extremities, scoliosis, and contractures. This accounts for approximately 70% to 80% of cerebral palsy cases. Extrapyramidal/nonspastic cerebral palsy is caused by damage to cells in the basal ganglia, thalamus, or cerebellum and includes two subtypes: dystonic and ataxic. Dystonic cerebral palsy is associated with extreme difficulty in fine motor coordination and purposeful movements. Movements are stiff, uncontrolled, and abrupt, resulting from injury to the basal ganglia or extrapyramidal tracts. This form of cerebral palsy accounts for approximately 10% to 20% of cases. Ataxic cerebral palsy is caused by damage to the cerebellum with alterations in coordination and movement. There is a broad based gait in an attempt to maintain balance and tremor is common with intentional movements. This form of cerebral palsy accounts for approximately 5% to 10% of cases. A child may have symptoms of each of these cerebral palsy types, which leads to a mixed disorder accounting for approximately 13% of cases.[29]

Children with cerebral palsy often have associated neurologic disorders, such as seizures (about 50%), and intellectual impairment ranging from mild to severe (about 67%). Other complications include visual impairment, communication disorders, respiratory problems, bowel and bladder problems, and orthopedic disabilities.[30]

Inherited Metabolic Disorders of the Central Nervous System

A large number of inherited metabolic disorders have been identified, typically leading to diffuse brain dysfunction. Early diagnosis and treatment is vital if these infants are to survive without severe neurologic problems. Newborn metabolic screening for 28 metabolic conditions (in most states) has led to most of these children being identified before symptoms develop. Table 17-4 lists some of these inherited metabolic disorders. Inborn errors of metabolism are present at birth and most cause disturbances of the nervous system, although they may not manifest until childhood or even adulthood. Defects in amino acid and lipid metabolism are among the most common.

Defects in Amino Acid Metabolism

Biochemical defects in amino acid metabolism include (1) those in which the transport of an amino acid is impaired, (2) those involving an enzyme or cofactor deficiency, and (3) those encompassing certain chemical components, such as branched-chain or sulfur-containing amino acids. Most of these disorders are caused by genetic defects resulting in lack of a normal protein and absence of enzymatic activity.

TABLE 17-4	Inherited Metabolic Disorders of the Central Nervous System
Age of Onset	**Disorder**
Neonatal period	Pyridoxine dependency, galactosemia, urea cycle defects, maple syrup urine disease and its variant, phenylketonuria (PKU), Menkes kinky hair syndrome
Early infancy	Tay-Sachs disease and its variants, infantile Gaucher disease, infantile Niemann-Pick disease, Krabbe disease (leukodystrophy), Farber lipogranulomatosis, Pelizaeus-Merzbacher disease and other sudanophilic leukodystrophies, spongy degeneration of CNS (Canavan disease), Alexander disease, Alpers disease, Leigh disease (subacute necrotizing encephalomyelopathy), congenital lactic acidosis, Zellweger encephalopathy, Lowe disease (oculocerebrorenal disease)
Late infancy and early childhood	Disorders of amino acid metabolism, metachromatic leukodystrophy, adrenoleukodystrophy, late infantile GM_1 gangliosidosis, late infantile Gaucher and Niemann-Pick diseases, neuroaxonal dystrophy, mucopolysaccharidosis, mucolipidosis, fucosidosis, mannosidosis, aspartylglycosaminuria, neuronal ceroid lipofuscinoses (Jansky-Bielschowsky disease, Batten disease, Vogt-Spielmeyer disease, neuronal ceroid lipofuscinosis), Cockayne syndrome, ataxia telangiectasia (AT)
Later childhood and adolescence	Progressive cerebellar ataxias of childhood and adolescence, hepatolenticular degeneration (Wilson disease), Hallervorden-Spatz disease, Lesch-Nyhan syndrome, Aicardi-Goutieres syndrome, progressive myoclonus epilepsies, homocystinuria, Fabry disease

Data from Volpe JJ: *Neurology of the newborn*, ed 5, Philadelphia, 2008, Saunders. For information regarding screening and parent education, see Medical Home Portal at www.medicalhomeportal.org/.

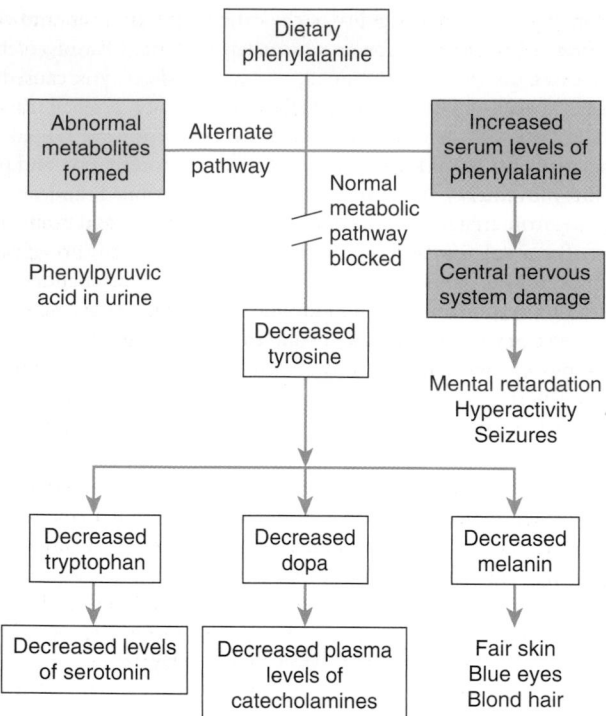

FIGURE 17-7 Metabolic Error and Consequences in Phenylketonuria. (From Hockenberry MJ, Wilson D: *Wong's nursing care of infants and children*, ed 10, St Louis, 2015, Mosby.)

TABLE 17-5	Common Poisons	
Pharmacologic Agents	**Heavy Metals**	**Miscellaneous Agents**
Acetaminophen	Lead	Botulinum toxin
Amphetamines	Acute	Alcohols
Anticonvulsants	Chronic	Ethyl
Antidepressants	Mercury	Isopropyl
Antihistamines	Thallium	Methyl
Atropine	Arsenic	Pesticides
Barbiturates	Iron supplements	Organophosphates
Methadone		Chlorinated hydrocarbons
Phencyclidine		Mushrooms
Salicylates		Venoms
Tranquilizers		Snakebite
		Tick paralysis
		Ethylene glycol
		Furniture polish
		Paint solvents

Data from Shannon MW et al: *Haddad and Winchester's clinical management of poisoning and drug overdose*, ed 4, Philadelphia, 2007, Saunders; Swaiman KF et al: *Pediatric neurology: principles and practice*, ed 5, vol 2, St Louis, 2012, Mosby.

Phenylketonuria. Phenylketonuria (PKU) is an example of an inborn error of metabolism characterized by phenylalanine hydroxylase deficiency and the inability of the body to convert the essential amino acid phenylalanine to tyrosine (Figure 17-7). PKU is an autosomal recessive inborn error of metabolism characterized by mutations of the phenylalanine hydroxylase *(PAH)* gene. PKU has an incidence of 1 per 15,000 live births in the United States.[31,32]

Most natural food proteins contain about 15% phenylalanine, an essential amino acid. Phenylalanine hydroxylase controls the conversion of this essential amino acid to tyrosine in the liver. The body uses tyrosine in the biosynthesis of proteins, melanin, thyroxine, and the catecholamines in the brain and adrenal medulla. Phenylalanine hydroxylase deficiency causes an accumulation of phenylalanine in the serum. Elevated phenylalanine levels result in developmental abnormalities of the cerebral cortical layers, defective myelination, and cystic degeneration of the gray and white matter. Unfortunately, brain damage occurs before the metabolites can be detected in the urine, and damage continues as long as phenylalanine levels remain high. Nonselective newborn screening is used to detect PKU in the United States and in more than 30 other countries. Treatment, consisting of reduction of dietary phenylalanine (PKU diet), is effective and allows for normal development. Mutations in the *PAH* gene are by far the most common cause of PKU, although there are other types of PKU as well. In one such variation, there is impaired synthesis of cofactors (e.g., tetrahydrobiopterin [BH₄]), which contributes to elevated levels of phenylalanine. Individuals with impaired synthesis of BH₄ have a positive response when sapropterin, a synthetic form of tetrahydrobiopterin, is included in their treatment.[33]

Storage Diseases

Disorders of lipid metabolism are termed lysosomal storage diseases because each disorder in this group can be traced to a missing lysosomal enzyme. Lysosomal storage disorders include more than 50 known genetic disorders. The incidence of lysosomal storage disorders is approximately 1 in 7500 live births.[34] These disorders cause an excessive accumulation of a particular cell product, occurring in the brain, liver, spleen, bone, and lung, and thus involving several organ systems. Generally, these disorders are not included in newborn screening. Some of these disorders may be treated with enzyme replacement therapy.[35] Perhaps the best known of the lysosomal storage disorders is Tay-Sachs disease (GM₂ gangliosidosis), an autosomal recessive disorder (*HexA* gene on chromosome 15) caused by deficiency of the lysosomal enzyme hexosaminidase A (HexA), an enzyme that degrades GM₂ gangliosides (fatty acids) within nerve cell lysosomes. Approximately 80% of individuals diagnosed are of Jewish ancestry, although sporadic cases appear in the non-Jewish population. Onset of this disease usually occurs when the infant is 4 to 6 months old. Symptoms of Tay-Sachs include an exaggerated startle response to loud noise, seizures, developmental regression, dementia, and blindness. Death from this disease is almost universal and occurs by 5 years of age. Screening for carriers of the gene defect concomitant with counseling to prevent disease transmission is possible.[36]

> ✔ **QUICK CHECK 17-3**
> 1. List three types of cerebral palsy.
> 2. Why does failure to metabolize phenylalanine produce such widespread and devastating effects on development?

Acute Encephalopathies
Intoxications of the Central Nervous System

Drug-induced encephalopathies must always be considered a possibility in the child with unexplained neurologic changes. Such encephalopathies may result from accidental ingestion, therapeutic overdose, intentional overdose, or ingestion of environmental toxins (the most commonly ingested poisons are listed in Table 17-5). Approximately 1.4 million children were exposed to poisons and approximately

185 children died in the United States in 2012 as a result of poisoning.[37,38]

Lead poisoning results in high blood levels of lead. If lead poisoning is untreated, lead encephalopathy results and is responsible for serious and irreversible neurologic damage. Those at greatest risk are children ages 2 to 3 years and children prone to the practice of pica—the habitual, purposeful, and compulsive ingestion of non–food substances, such as clay, soil, and paint chips or paint dust. Lead intoxication also may occur from chronic exposure to lead in cosmetics, inhalation of gasoline vapors, and ingestion of airborne lead.[39]

An estimated 535,000 children 1 to 5 years of age in the United States (2.2% of children 1 month to 5 years of age) have excessive amounts of lead in their blood.[40] The incidence in black children is greater than that in white children. Most lead exposures are preventable.[41] The American Academy of Pediatrics has published recommendations for the treatment of lead poisoning depending on blood lead levels.[42] Fetal neurotoxicity occurs with maternal lead exposure, particularly during the first trimester.[43]

Infections of the Central Nervous System

Meningitis is an infection of the meninges and subarachnoid space of the brain and spinal cord, whereas the word encephalitis reflects inflammation within the brain. In many infections of the meninges, encephalitis also is present and the term *meningoencephalitis* is used. The origin of such inflammation and acute encephalopathy can be caused by bacteria, viruses, or other microorganisms. Aseptic meningitis has no evidence of bacterial infection but may be associated with viral infection, systemic disease, or drugs.

Bacterial Meningitis

Acute bacterial meningitis is one of the most serious infections to which infants and children are susceptible. In the United States approximately 4100 cases of bacterial meningitis occurred each year between 2003 and 2007, including 500 deaths.[44] Approximately half of these cases occurred in children younger than 18 years of age. The introduction of conjugate vaccines against *Haemophilus influenzae* type B, *Streptococcus pneumoniae*, and *Neisseria meningitidis* (meningococcus) has decreased the incidence of bacterial meningitis.[45] Vaccines for serogroup B *N. meningitidis* are not yet available but clinical trials are in progress.[46]

Group B *Streptococcus* causes lethal meningitis and sepsis in neonates and is transmitted to the child from the mother's birth canal. *S. pneumoniae* is the most common microorganism in children 1 to 23 months of age. Staphylococcal or streptococcal meningitis can occur in children of any age but shows a predilection for children who have had neurosurgery, skull fracture, or a complication of systemic bacterial infection. Infections that originate in the middle ear, sinuses, or mastoid cells also may lead to *S. pneumoniae* infection in children. Children with sickle cell disease or who have had a splenectomy are particularly at high risk for infection.[47]

Escherichia coli and group B beta-hemolytic streptococci are the most common causes of meningitis in the newborn period. The second most common microorganism causing bacterial meningitis, particularly in children younger than 4 years, is *Neisseria meningitidis* (meningococcus) and it has the potential to occur in epidemics. Approximately 2% to 5% of healthy children are carriers of *N. meningitidis*. As the incidence of *N. meningitidis* infection increases in adolescence and with crowded environments, such as in dormitories and among military personnel, it is recommended that all individuals 11 to 18 years of age receive two immunizations against this pathogen.[48]

Pathogens enter the nervous system by direct extension from a contiguous source (e.g., paranasal sinuses or mastoid cells) or, more commonly, by hematogenous spread (e.g., infective endocarditis, pneumonia, neurosurgical procedures, severe burns). Pathogens then cross the blood-brain barrier, enter the cerebrospinal fluid, and multiply. Bacterial toxins increase cerebrovascular permeability, causing alterations in blood flow and edema. Increased ICP may be increased further by obstruction to the CSF circulation. Herniation of the brainstem causes death.

Acute bacterial meningitis often is preceded by an upper respiratory tract or a gastrointestinal infection. Inflammation leads to the general symptoms of fever, headache, vomiting, and irritability and the CNS symptoms of photophobia, nuchal and spinal rigidity, decreased level of consciousness, and seizures. Irritation of the meninges and spinal roots causes pain and resistance to neck flexion (nuchal rigidity), a positive Kernig sign (resistance to knee extension in the supine position with the hips and knees flexed against the body), and a positive Brudzinski sign (flexion of the knees and hips when the neck is flexed forward rapidly). With severe meningeal irritation the child may demonstrate opisthotonic posturing (rigid arching of the back with the head extended). Infants may have bulging fontanelles. Meningococcal meningitis can produce a characteristic petechial rash.

Viral meningitis may result from a direct infection of a virus or it may be secondary to disease, such as measles, mumps, herpes, or leukemia. The hallmark of viral meningitis, or aseptic meningitis, is a mononuclear response in the CSF and the presence of normal glucose levels as well. The clinical manifestations are similar to those in bacterial meningitis, although usually milder.

Viral encephalitis in children is similar to viral encephalitis in adults (see Chapter 16, Figure 16-13 and Table 16-8) and can be difficult to distinguish from viral meningitis. Viruses can directly invade the brain, causing inflammation; or postinfectious encephalitis can develop as a result of an autoimmune response.[49] Encephalopathy resulting from human immunodeficiency virus (HIV) is discussed in Chapter 8 and Chapter 16.

CEREBROVASCULAR DISEASE IN CHILDREN

Perinatal Stroke

Perinatal arterial ischemic stroke is estimated at 1 in 4000 live births and is a leading cause of perinatal brain injury, cerebral palsy, and lifelong disability. Although a cause for perinatal stroke is usually not found, clotting abnormalities may make the child prone to further vascular events.

Childhood Stroke

Childhood stroke occurs in 1.3 to 1.6 per 100,000 children per year and may be divided into two categories: ischemic and hemorrhagic.[50,51]

Ischemic (occlusive) stroke is rare in children and may result from embolism, sinovenous thrombosis, or congenital or iatrogenic narrowing of vessels leading to decreased flow of blood and oxygen to areas of the brain. Children with arterial ischemic stroke do not have the typical adult risk factors of atherosclerosis and hypertension. Risk factors include cardiac diseases, hematologic and vascular disorders, and infection. Approximately 40% of children with acute ischemic stroke have no identifiable risk factors.[52] Sickle cell disease, cerebral arteriopathies, and cardiac anomalies are the common disorders associated with arterial ischemic stroke.[53]

Hemorrhagic stroke is most commonly caused by bleeding from congenital cerebral arteriovenous malformations and is rare in children younger than 19 years. Intraventricular hemorrhage associated with premature birth is related to immature blood vessels and unstable blood pressure. There is a high risk of developing posthemorrhagic hydrocephalus.[54]

Moyamoya disease is a rare, chronic, progressive vascular stenosis of the circle of Willis. There is obstruction of arterial flow to the brain and the development of basal arterial collateral vessels that vascularize hypoperfused brain distal to the occluded vessels.[55] Moyamoya means a "puff of smoke" in Japanese. The disease is idiopathic or associated with other disorders (moyamoya syndrome).

Clinical presentation varies according to the vessels involved, the cause of the disease, and the age of the individual. Symptoms include hemiplegia, weakness, seizures, headaches, high fever, nuchal rigidity, hemianopia, sensory changes, facial palsy, and temporary aphasia. Obtaining a thorough history of evolving symptoms and risk factors is important for diagnosis. Laboratory studies may be indicated. Neuroimaging studies assist in determining the cause of the disease. Surgery is an option for treatment and anticoagulants and antithrombotics may be used in selected cases.

Epilepsy and Seizure Disorders in Children

The incidence of epilepsy varies greatly with age, geographic location, and study design. The incidence is highest younger than age 2 years and older than age 65 years. Approximately 150,000 persons in the United States are newly diagnosed each year.[56]

Seizures are the abnormal discharge of electrical activity within the brain. When a sufficient number of neurons become overexcited, they discharge abnormally, which sometimes results in clinical manifestations (seizures) with alterations in motor function, sensation, autonomic function, behavior, and consciousness. The manifestations depend on the site and spread of abnormal electrical activity. If a child has more than one unprovoked seizure, that child is said to have **epilepsy**, although there are a few exceptions—one example being febrile seizures. Seizures may result from diseases that are primarily neurologic (CNS) or are systemic and affect CNS function secondarily (such as diabetes). Seizures can be caused by structural abnormalities of the brain, hypoxia, intracranial hemorrhage, CNS infection, traumatic injury, electrolyte imbalance, or inborn metabolic disturbances. Febrile seizures occur in about 2% to 5% of children between ages 6 months and 5 years; they are benign and the most common type of childhood seizure. Seizures are sometimes clearly familial. Often the cause of epilepsy is unknown and presumed to have a genetic basis. Table 17-6 summarizes the major types of seizures (also see Chapter 15 and Table 15-14).

CHILDHOOD TUMORS

Brain Tumors

Brain tumors are the most common solid tumor and second most common primary neoplasm in children. Overall, brain tumors account for nearly 20% of all childhood cancers, with an annual incidence of 5.42 per 100,000 for primary malignant tumors and nonmalignant tumors for ages 0 to 19 years in the United States; approximately 43,620 brain tumors are expected to be diagnosed in 2015.[57] Five-year survival for childhood brain tumors is about 73%, varying significantly by tumor type, although there is often significant morbidity.

Primary brain tumors arise from brain tissue and do not metastasize outside the brain. The cause of brain tumors is unknown, although genetic, environmental, and immune factors have been investigated. Exposure to radiation therapy has been the only environmental factor consistently related to the development of brain tumors.[58]

Brain tumors can arise from any CNS cell, and tumors are classified by cell type. The types and characteristics of childhood brain tumors are summarized in Table 17-7. Medulloblastoma, ependymoma, astrocytoma, brainstem glioma, craniopharyngioma, and optic nerve glioma constitute approximately 75% to 80% of all pediatric brain tumors. Germ cell tumors are rare. Two thirds of all pediatric brain tumors in children are located in the posterior fossa (Figure 17-8) Treatment strategies and prognoses are listed in Table 17-8.

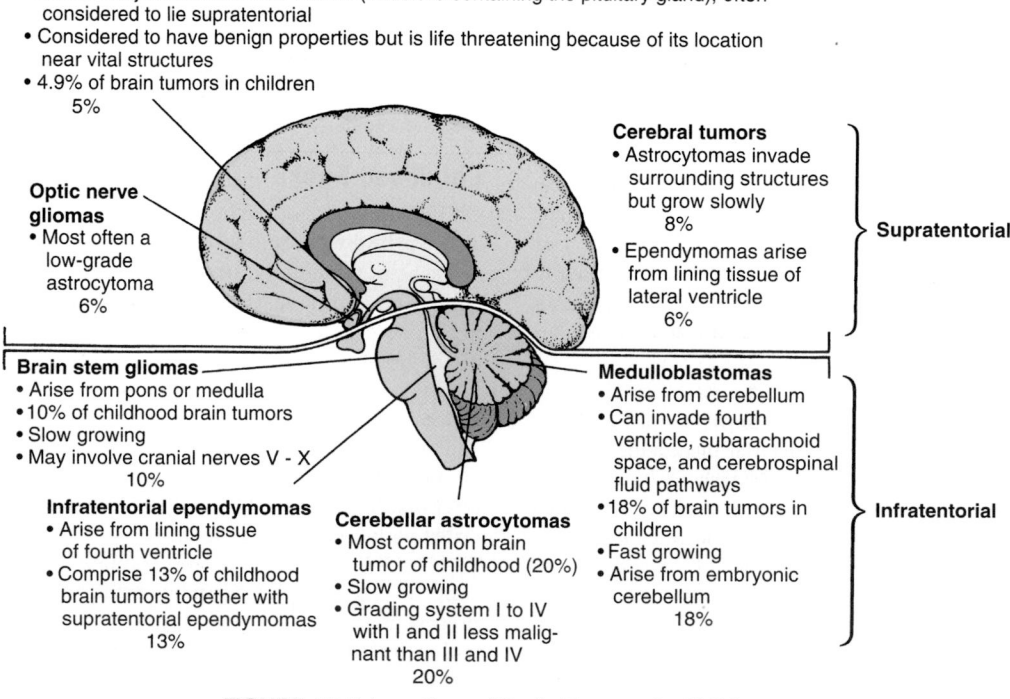

Craniopharyngiomas
- Located adjacent to the sella turcica (structure containing the pituitary gland), often considered to lie supratentorial
- Considered to have benign properties but is life threatening because of its location near vital structures
- 4.9% of brain tumors in children
  5%

Optic nerve gliomas
- Most often a low-grade astrocytoma
  6%

Cerebral tumors
- Astrocytomas invade surrounding structures but grow slowly
  8%
- Ependymomas arise from lining tissue of lateral ventricle
  6%

} **Supratentorial**

Brain stem gliomas
- Arise from pons or medulla
- 10% of childhood brain tumors
- Slow growing
- May involve cranial nerves V - X
  10%

Infratentorial ependymomas
- Arise from lining tissue of fourth ventricle
- Comprise 13% of childhood brain tumors together with supratentorial ependymomas
  13%

Cerebellar astrocytomas
- Most common brain tumor of childhood (20%)
- Slow growing
- Grading system I to IV with I and II less malignant than III and IV
  20%

Medulloblastomas
- Arise from cerebellum
- Can invade fourth ventricle, subarachnoid space, and cerebrospinal fluid pathways
- 18% of brain tumors in children
- Fast growing
- Arise from embryonic cerebellum
  18%

} **Infratentorial**

FIGURE 17-8 Location of Brain Tumors in Children.

TABLE 17-6   Major Types of Seizure Disorders Found in Children

Disorder	Manifestations
Generalized Seizure	First clinical manifestations indicate that seizure activity starts in or involves both cerebral hemispheres; consciousness may be impaired; bilateral manifestations; may be preceded by an aura
Tonic-clonic	Musculature stiffens, then intense jerking as trunk and extremities undergo rhythmic contraction and relaxation
Atonic	Sudden, momentary loss of muscle tone; drop attacks
Myoclonic	Sudden, brief contractures of a muscle or group of muscles
Absence seizure	Brief loss of consciousness with minimal or no loss of muscle tone; may experience 20 or more episodes a day lasting approximately 5 to 10 sec each; may have minor movement, such as lip smacking, twitching of eyelids
Partial (Focal) Seizure	Seizure activity that begins and usually is limited to one part of left or right hemisphere; an aura is common
Simple	Seizure activity that occurs without loss of consciousness
Complex	Seizure activity that occurs with impairment of consciousness
Epilepsy Syndromes	Seizure disorders that display a group of signs and symptoms that occur collectively and characterize or indicate a particular condition
Infantile spasms (West syndrome)	Form of epilepsy with episodes of sudden flexion or extension involving neck, trunk, and extremities; clinical manifestations range from subtle head nods to violent body contractions (jackknife seizures); onset between 3 and 12 months of age; may be idiopathic, genetic, result of metabolic disease, or in response to CNS insult; spasms occur in clusters of 5 to 150 times per day; EEG shows large-amplitude, chaotic, and disorganized pattern called "hypsarrhythmia"
Lennox-Gastaut syndrome	Epileptic syndrome with onset in early childhood, 1 to 5 years of age; includes various generalized seizures—tonic-clonic, atonic (drop attacks), akinetic, absence, and myoclonic; EEG has characteristic "slow spike and wave" pattern; results in mental retardation and delayed psychomotor developments
Juvenile myoclonic epilepsy	Onset in adolescence; multifocal myoclonus; seizures often occur early in morning, aggravated by lack of sleep or after excessive alcohol intake; occasional generalized convulsions; require long-term medication treatment
Benign rolandic epilepsy	Epileptic syndrome typically occurring in the preadolescent age (6 to 12 years); strong association with sleep (seizures typically occur few hours after sleep onset or just before waking in morning); complex partial seizures with orofacial signs (drooling, distortion of facial muscles); characteristic EEG with centrotemporal (Rolandic fissure) spikes
Status Epilepticus	Continuing or recurring seizure activity in which recovery from seizure activity is incomplete; unrelenting seizure activity can last 30 min or more; medical emergency that requires immediate intervention

TABLE 17-7   Brain Tumors in Children

Type	Characteristics
Astrocytoma	Arises from astrocytes, often in cerebellum or lateral hemisphere
	Slow growing, solid or cystic
	Often very large before diagnosed
	Varies in degree of malignancy
Optic nerve glioma	Arises from optic chiasm or optic nerve (association with neurofibromatosis type 1)
	Slow-growing, low-grade astrocytoma
Medulloblastoma (infiltrating glioma)	Often located in cerebellum, extending into fourth ventricle and spinal fluid pathway
	Rapidly growing malignant tumor
	Can extend outside CNS
Brainstem glioma	Arises from pons
	Numerous cell types
	Compresses cranial nerves V through X
Ependymoma	Arises from ependymal cells lining ventricles
	Circumscribed, solid, nodular tumors
Craniopharyngioma	Arises near pituitary gland, optic chiasm, and hypothalamus
	Cystic and solid tumors that affect vision, pituitary, and hypothalamic functions
Germ cell tumor	Arises from germ cells and are most common in pineal and suprasellar region, usually occurring during adolescence

TABLE 17-8   Treatment Strategies for Childhood Brain Tumors

Tumor Type	Treatment and Prognosis
Cerebellar astrocytoma	Surgery; possibly curative
	Radiation and chemotherapy not proved successful but may delay recurrence
	90% to 100% 5-yr survival rate if pilocytic type; if tumor recurs, it does so very slowly
Medulloblastoma	Surgery, primarily as partial resection to relieve increased intracranial pressure and "debulk" tumor
	Type of treatment is age and tumor type dependent
	Radiation as primary treatment; may include spinal radiation
	Chemotherapy showing some promise in conjunction with craniospinal radiation
	65% to 85% 5-yr survival rate depending on stage/type
Brainstem glioma	Surgery, resection occasionally possible
	Radiation, primarily palliative treatment
	Chemotherapy not yet proven beneficial, but new protocols being studied
	20% to 40% 5-yr survival rate
Ependymoma	Tumor possibly indolent for many years
	Surgery rarely curative; risk of resecting an infratentorial tumor too great
	Radiation for palliation (current controversy over whether local or craniospinal radiation is best)
	Chemotherapy used for recurrent disease but with disappointing results
	20% to 80% 5-yr survival rate dependent on total resection
Craniopharyngioma	Surgery possibly successful when complete resection is performed (partial resection usually requires further treatment)
	Radiation after partial surgical resection
	Chemotherapy not commonly used
	80% to 95% 5-yr survival rate
Optic nerve glioma	In setting of visual impairment, or progression (increase in size), chemotherapy is usual initial treatment
	Surgery for hydrocephalus or other complications; rarely for diagnosis
	Radiation therapy for those tumors that progress or recur in spite of chemotherapy
Cerebral astrocytoma	Surgery used if resection is possible, but high rate of recurrence
	Radiation useful for all grades of astrocytoma
	Chemotherapy beneficial in higher grade tumors but further study required 75% 5-yr survival rate with lower grade tumors
Germ cell tumor	Chemotherapy and/or radiotherapy

Data from Cage TA et al: *J Neurosurg Pediatr* 11(6):673-681, 2013; Gerber NU et al: *Cancer Treat Rev* 40(3):356-365, 2014; Grimm SA, Chamberlain MC: *Curr Neurol Neurosci Rep* 13(5):346, 2013; Mufti ST, Jamal A: *Asian J Neurosurg* 7(4):197-202, 2012; Omuro A, DeAngelis LM: *J Am Med Assoc* 310(17):1842-1850, 2013; Shapey J et al: *J Clin Neurosci* 18(12):1585-1591, 2011.

Signs and symptoms of brain tumors in children vary from generalized and vague to localized and related specifically to an anatomic area. Signs of increased intracranial pressure may occur, including headache, vomiting, lethargy, and irritability. If a young child complains of repeated and worsening headache, a thorough investigation should take place because headache is an uncommon complaint in young children. Headache caused by increased intracranial pressure usually is worse in the morning and gradually improves during the day when the child is upright and venous drainage is enhanced. The frequency of headache and other symptoms increases as the tumor grows. Irritability or possible apathy and increased somnolence also may result. Like headache, vomiting occurs more commonly in the morning. Often it is *not* preceded by nausea and may become projectile, differing from a gastrointestinal disturbance in that the child may be ready to eat immediately after vomiting. Other signs and symptoms include increased head circumference with bulging fontanelles in the child younger than 2 years, cranial nerve palsies, and papilledema (Box 17-1).

Localized findings relate to the degree of disturbance in physiologic functioning in the area where the tumor is located. Children with infratentorial tumors exhibit localized signs of impaired coordination and balance, including ataxia, gait difficulties, truncal ataxia, and loss of balance. Medulloblastoma occurs as an invasive malignant tumor that develops in the vermis of the cerebellum and may extend into the fourth ventricle. Ependymoma develops in the fourth ventricle and arises from the ependymal cells that line the ventricular system. Because both tumors are located in the posterior fossa region along the midline, presenting signs and symptoms are similar and are usually related to hydrocephalus and increased intracranial pressure. In contrast, cerebellar astrocytomas are located on the surface of the right or left cerebellar hemisphere and cause unilateral symptoms (occurring on the same side as the tumor), such as head tilt, limb ataxia, and nystagmus.

Brainstem gliomas often cause a combination of cranial nerve involvement (facial weakness, limitation of horizontal eye movement), cerebellar signs of ataxia, and corticospinal tract dysfunction. Increased intracranial pressure generally does not occur.

The area of the sella turcica, the structure containing the pituitary gland, is the site of several childhood brain tumors; most common of this group is the craniopharyngioma. This tumor originates from the pituitary gland or hypothalamus. Usually slow growing, it may be quite large by the time of diagnosis. Symptoms include headache, seizures, diabetes insipidus, early onset of puberty, and growth delay. Other tumors located in this region of the brain include optic gliomas. Optic nerve gliomas are associated with neurofibromatosis type 1, a neurocutaneous condition characterized by café-au-lait macules on the skin and benign tumors of the skin. Tumors that involve the optic tract may cause complete unilateral blindness and hemianopia of the other eye.

BOX 17-1   Clinical Manifestations of Brain Tumors

Headache
Recurrent and progressive
In frontal or occipital area
Worse on arising; pain lessens during the day
Intensified by lowering head and straining, such as when defecating, coughing, sneezing

Vomiting
With or without nausea or feeding
Progressively more projectile
More severe in morning
Relieved by moving and changing position

Neuromuscular Changes
Uncoordination or clumsiness
Loss of balance (use of wide-based stance, falling, tripping, banging into object)
Poor fine motor control
Weakness
Hyporeflexia or hyperreflexia
Positive Babinski sign
Spasticity
Paralysis

Behavioral Changes
Irritability
Decreased appetite

Failure to thrive
Fatigue (frequent naps)
Lethargy
Coma
Bizarre behavior (staring, automatic movements)

Cranial Nerve Neuropathy
Cranial nerve involvement varies according to tumor location
Most common signs:
   Head tilt
   Visual defects (nystagmus, diplopia, strabismus, episodic "graying out" of vision, and visual field defects)

Vital Sign Disturbances
Decreased pulse and respiratory rates
Increased blood pressure
Decreased pulse pressure
Hypothermia or hyperthermia

Other Signs
Seizures
Cranial enlargement*
Tense, bulging fontanelle at rest*
Separating suture*
Nuchal rigidity
Papilledema (edema of optic nerve)

From Hockenberry MN: *Wong's essentials of pediatric nursing*, ed 7, St Louis, 2007, Mosby.
*Present only in infants and young children.

Optic atrophy is another common finding. Supratentorial tumors of the cerebral hemispheres are more common in neonates and adolescents.[59]

Embryonal Tumors
Neuroblastoma

Neuroblastoma is an embryonal tumor originating outside the CNS in the developing sympathetic nervous system (sympathetic ganglia and the adrenal medulla). Because neuroblastoma involves a defect of embryonic tissue and is the most common cancer in infants less than 1 year of age, 75% of neuroblastomas are found before the child is 5 years old and is rare after 10 years of age. Occasionally, these tumors have been diagnosed at birth with metastasis apparent in the placenta. It is seen more commonly in white children (9.6 per million) than in black children (7 per million). Although it accounts for only about 6% of pediatric malignancies, neuroblastoma causes about 15% of cancer deaths in children.[60]

Neuroblastoma is the most common and immature form of the sympathetic nervous system tumors. Areas of necrosis and calcification often are present in the tumor. More than with any other cancer, neuroblastoma has been associated with spontaneous remission, commonly in infants. Prognosis is worse for children older than 2 years of age with disseminated disease.[61]

Although familial tendency has been noted in individual cases, a nonfamilial or sporadic pattern is found in most children with neuroblastoma. Familial cases of neuroblastoma are considered to have an autosomal dominant pattern of inheritance (mechanisms of inheritance are discussed in Chapter 2).

The most common location of neuroblastoma is in the retroperitoneal region (65% of cases), most often the adrenal medulla. The tumor is evident as an abdominal mass and may cause anorexia, bowel and bladder alteration, and sometimes spinal cord compression. The second most common location of neuroblastoma is the mediastinum (15% of cases), where the tumor may cause dyspnea or infection related to airway obstruction. Less commonly, neuroblastoma may arise from the cervical sympathetic ganglion (3% to 4% of cases). Cervical neuroblastoma often causes Horner syndrome, which consists of miosis (pupil contraction), ptosis (drooping eyelid), enophthalmos (backward displacement of the eyeball), and anhidrosis (sweat deficiency). Neuroblastoma rarely presents with a cerebellar neurologic syndrome called opsoclonus-myoclonus syndrome.[62] Children develop conjugate chaotic eye movements, jerky movements of the limbs, and ataxia.

A number of systemic signs and symptoms are characteristic of neuroblastoma, including weight loss, irritability, fatigue, and fever. Intractable diarrhea occurs in 7% to 9% of children and is caused by tumor secretion of a hormone called *vasoactive intestinal polypeptide (VIP)*.

More than 90% of children with neuroblastoma have increased amounts of catecholamines and associated metabolites in their urine. High levels of urinary catecholamines and serum ferritin are associated with a poor prognosis.

Retinoblastoma

Retinoblastoma is a rare congenital eye tumor of young children that originates in the retina of one or both eyes (Figure 17-9). Two forms of retinoblastoma are exhibited: inherited and acquired. The inherited form of the disease generally is diagnosed during the first year of life. The acquired disease most commonly is diagnosed in children 2 to 3 years of age and involves unilateral disease.[63]

Approximately 40% of retinoblastomas are inherited as an autosomal dominant trait with incomplete penetrance (see Figure 2-22). The remaining 60% are acquired. In the early 1970s, Knudson proposed the "two-hit" hypothesis to explain the occurrence of both hereditary and acquired forms of the disease.[64] This hypothesis predicts that two separate transforming events or "hits" must occur in a normal retinoblast cell to cause the cancer. Further, it proposes that in the inherited form, the first hit or mutation occurs in the germ cell (inherited from either parent), and the mutation is contained in every cell of the child's

FIGURE 17-9 Retinoblastoma. The tumor occupies a large portion of the inside of the eye globe. (From Damjanov I: *Pathology for the health professions,* ed 3, St Louis, 2006, Saunders. Courtesy Dr. Walter Richardson and Dr. Jamsheed Khan, Kansas City, Kan.)

body. Only a second, random mutation in a retinoblast cell is needed to transform that cell into cancer. Multiple tumors are observed in the inherited form because these second mutations are likely to occur in several of the approximately 1 to 2 million retinoblast cells. In contrast, the acquired form of retinoblastoma requires two independent hits or mutations to occur in the same somatic cell (after the egg is fertilized) for the transformation to cancer. This is much less likely to happen. Figure 17-10 illustrates the two-mutation model for these two patterns of mutation.

The primary sign of retinoblastoma is leukocoria, a white pupillary reflex (white reflex) also called *cat's eye reflex,* which is caused by the mass behind the lens (see Figure 17-9). This easy to identify sign can be missed. Other signs and symptoms include strabismus; a red, painful eye; and limited vision.

Because retinoblastoma is a treatable tumor, dual priorities are saving the child's life and restoring useful vision. The prognosis for most children with retinoblastoma is excellent, with a greater than 90% long-term survival.

> ✔ **QUICK CHECK 17-4**
> 1. Why are the principal symptoms of brain tumors in children related to brainstem function?

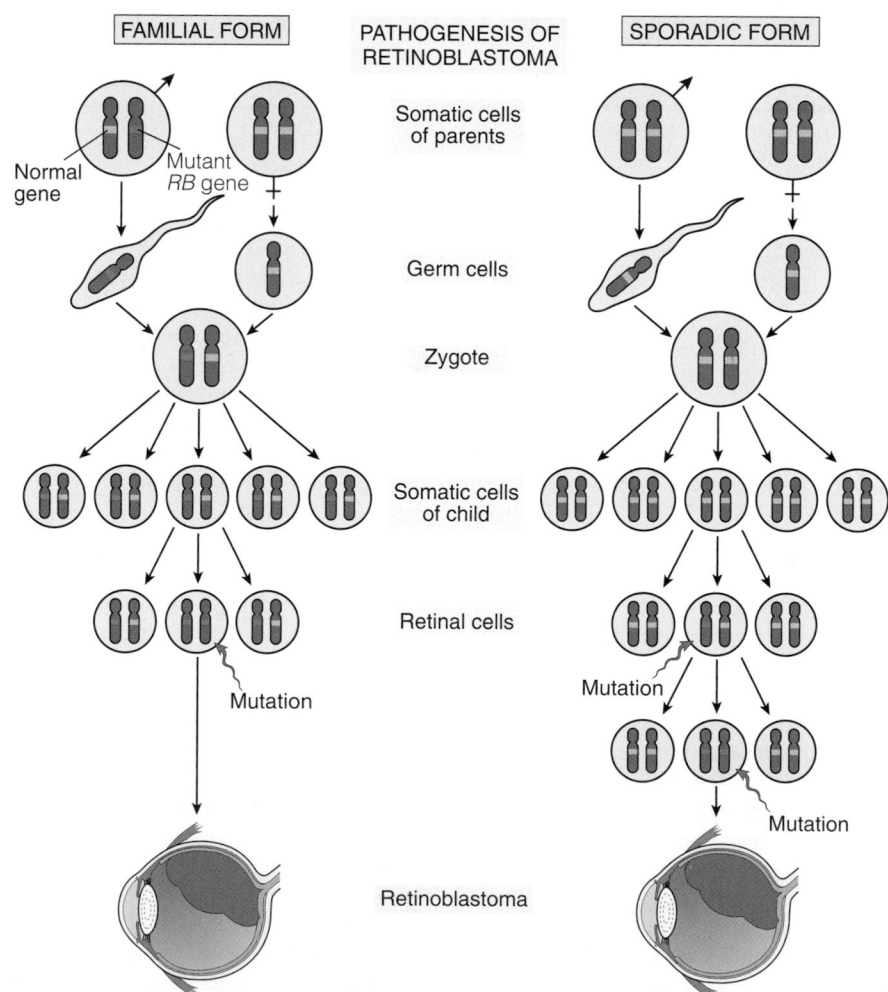

FIGURE 17-10 The Two-Mutation Model of Retinoblastoma Development. In inherited retinoblastoma, the first mutation is transmitted through the germline of an affected parent. The second mutation occurs somatically in a retinal cell, leading to development of the tumor. In sporadic retinoblastoma, development of a tumor requires two somatic mutations.

DID YOU UNDERSTAND?

Development of the Nervous System in Children

1. Growth and development of the brain occur most rapidly during fetal development and during the first year of life.
2. The bones of the skull are joined by sutures, and the wide, membranous junctions of the sutures (known as *fontanelles*) allow for brain growth and close by 18 months of age.
3. At birth neurologic function is primarily at the subcortical level with transition in reflexes as motor development progresses during the first year.

Structural Malformations

1. Spina bifida (failure of vertebral closure) is the most common disorder of neural tube closure and includes anencephaly (absence of part of the skull and brain), encephalocele (herniation of the meninges and brain through a skull defect), meningocele (a saclike meningeal cyst that protrudes through a vertebral defect), and myelomeningocele.
2. Premature closure of the cranial sutures causes craniosynostosis and prevents normal skull expansion, resulting in compression of growing brain tissue.
3. Microcephaly is lack of brain growth with retarded mental and motor development.
4. Congenital hydrocephalus results from overproduction, impaired absorption, or blockage of circulation of cerebrospinal fluid. Dandy-Walker deformity is caused by cystic dilation of the fourth ventricle and aqueductal compression.

Alterations in Function: Encephalopathies

1. Static encephalopathies are nonprogressive disorders of the brain that can occur during gestation, birth, or childhood and can be caused by endogenous or exogenous factors.
2. Cerebral palsy can be caused by prenatal cerebral hypoxia or perinatal trauma, with symptoms of motor dysfunction (including increased muscle tone, increased reflexes, and loss of fine motor coordination), mental retardation, seizure disorders, or developmental disabilities.
3. Inherited metabolic disorders that damage the nervous system include defects in amino acid metabolism (phenylketonuria) and lipid metabolism (Tay-Sachs disease) and result in abnormal behavior, seizures, and deficient psychomotor development.
4. Seizure disorders are abnormal discharges of electrical activity within the brain. They are associated with numerous nervous system disorders and more often are a generalized rather than a partial type of seizure.
5. Generalized forms of seizures include tonic-clonic, myoclonic, atonic, akinetic, and infantile spasms.

6. Partial seizures suggest more localized brain dysfunction.
7. Febrile seizures usually are limited to children ages 6 months to 6 years, with a pattern of one seizure per febrile illness.
8. Accidental poisonings from a variety of toxins can cause serious neurologic damage.
9. Bacterial meningitis is commonly caused by *Neisseria meningitidis* or *Streptococcus pneumoniae* and may result from respiratory tract or gastrointestinal infections; symptoms include fever, headaches, photophobia, seizures, rigidity, and stupor.
10. Viral meningitis may result from direct infection or be secondary to a systemic viral infection (e.g., measles, mumps, herpes, or leukemia).

Cerebrovascular Disease in Children

1. Ischemic (occlusive) cerebrovascular disease is rare in children but can occur from embolism, sickle cell disease, cerebral arteriopathies, and cardiac anomalies.
2. Hemorrhagic stroke can occur in association with immature blood vessel associated with prematurity or cerebral arteriovenous malformations.
3. Moyamoya is a rare, progressive vascular stenosis of the circle of Willis that obstructs arterial blood flow to the brain.

Childhood Brain Tumors

1. Brain tumors are the most common tumors of the nervous system and the second most common type of childhood cancer.
2. Tumors in children most often are located below the tentorial plate (infratentorial tumors).
3. Fast-growing tumors produce symptoms early in the disease, whereas slow-growing tumors may become very large before symptoms appear.
4. Symptoms of brain tumors may be generalized or localized. The most common general symptoms are the result of increased intracranial pressure and include headache, irritability, vomiting, somnolence, and bulging of fontanelles.
5. Localized signs of infratentorial tumors in the cerebellum include impaired coordination and balance. Cranial nerve signs occur with tumors in or near the brainstem.
6. Supratentorial tumors may be located near the cortex or deep in the brain. Symptoms depend on the specific location of the tumor.
7. Neuroblastoma is an embryonal tumor of the sympathetic nervous system and can be located anywhere there is sympathetic nervous tissue. Symptoms are related to tumor location and size of metastasis.
8. Retinoblastoma is a congenital eye tumor that has two forms: inherited and acquired.

KEY TERMS

Acute bacterial meningitis, 431
Anencephaly, 425
Aseptic meningitis, 431
Ataxic cerebral palsy, 429
Brainstem glioma, 434
Cerebellar astrocytoma, 434
Cerebral palsy, 429
Congenital hydrocephalus, 428
Cortical dysphasia, 427
Craniopharyngioma, 434

Craniosynostosis, 426
Cyclopia, 424
Dandy-Walker malformation (DWM), 428
Dystonic cerebral palsy, 429
Encephalitis, 431
Encephalocele, 425
Encephalopathy, 429
Ependymoma, 434
Epilepsy, 432

Extrapyramidal/nonspastic cerebral palsy, 429
Fontanelle, 422
Hemorrhagic stroke, 431
Ischemic (occlusive) stroke, 431
Lead poisoning, 431
Lysosomal storage disease, 430
Macewen sign ("cracked pot" sign), 428

Medulloblastoma, 434
Meningitis, 431
Meningocele, 425
Microcephaly, 427
Moyamoya disease, 432
Myelomeningocele, 425
Neural tube defect (NTD), 423
Neuroblastoma, 435
Optic glioma, 434
Phenylketonuria (PKU), 430

REFERENCES

1. Beard JL: Why iron deficiency is important in infant development, *J Nutr* 138(12):2534-2536, 2008.

2. Todorich B et al: Oligodendrocytes and myelination: the role of iron, *Glia* 57(5):467-478, 2009.

3. National Center on Birth Defects and Developmental Disabilities: *Folic acid: reducing folic acid-preventable neural tube defects.* Updated April 2, 2012. Available at: www.cdc.gov/ncbddd/AboutUs/birthdefects-folicacid.html.

4. Kaufman B: Neural tube defects, *Pediatr Clin North Am* 51(2):389-419, 2004.

5. Copp AJ et al: Neural tube defects: recent advances, unsolved questions, and controversies, *Lancet Neurol* 12(8):799-810, 2013.

6. Khodr ZG et al: Preconceptional folic acid-containing supplement use in the national birth defects prevention study, *Birth Defects Res A Clin Mol Teratol* 100(6):472-482, 2014.

7. Centers for Disease Control and Prevention (CDCP): CDC grand rounds: additional opportunities to prevent neural tube defects with folic acid fortification, *MMWR Morb Mortal Wkly Rep* 59(31):980-984, 2010.

8. Meador KJ: Comment: valproate dose effects differ across congenital malformations, *Neurology* 81(11):1002, 2013.

9. Centers for Disease Control and Prevention (CDCP): *Facts about anecephaly.* Updated March 26, 2013. Available at: www.cdc.gov/ncbddd/birthdefects/Anencephaly.html.

10. Centers for Disease Control and Prevention (CDCP): *Facts about encephalocele.* Updated February 25, 2011. Available at: www.cdc.gov/ncbddd/birthdefects/Encephalocele.html.

11. Behrman R et al: *Nelson's textbook of pediatrics,* ed 17, Philadelphia, 2004, Saunders.

12. Tamburrini G et al: Myelomeningocele: the management of the associated hydrocephalus, *Childs Nerv Syst* 29(9):1569-1579, 2013.

13. Adzick NS: Fetal myelomeningocele: natural history, pathophysiology, and in-utero intervention, *Semin Fetal Neonatal Med* 15(1):9-14, 2009.

14. Salman MS: Posterior fossa decompression and the cerebellum in Chiari type II malformation: a preliminary MRI study, *Childs Nerv Syst* 27(3):457-462, 2011.

15. Adzick NS: MOMS investigators: a randomized trial of prenatal versus postnatal repair of myelomeningocele, *N Engl J Med* 364(11):993-1004, 2011.

16. Adzick NS: Fetal surgery for spina bifida: past, present, future, *Semin Pediatr Surg* 22(1):10-17, 2013.

17. Moldenhauer JS: In utero repair of spina bifida, *Am J Perinatol* 31(7):595-604, 2014.

18. Hukki J et al: Single suture craniosynostosis: diagnosis and imaging, *Front Oral Biol* 12:79-90, 2008.

19. Ciurea AV et al: Actual concepts in scaphocephaly: (an experience of 98 cases), *J Med Life* 4(4):424-431, 2011.

20. Barkovich JA et al: A developmental and genetic classification for malformations of cortical development: update 2012, *Brain* 135(Pt 5):1348-1369, 2012.

21. McAllister JP Jr: Pathophysiology of congenital and neonatal hydrocephalus, *Semin Fetal Neonatal Med* 17(5):285-294, 2012.

22. Garton HJ, Piatt JH Jr: Hydrocephalus, *Pediatr Clin North Am* 51:305-325, 2004.

23. Constantini S et al: Neuroendoscopy in the youngest age group, *World Neurosurg* 79(2 Suppl):S23.e1-e11, 2013.

24. Vinchon M et al: Adult outcome of pediatric hydrocephalus, *Childs Nerv Syst* 28(6):847-854, 2012.

25. Warf BC: Congenital idiopathic hydrocephalus of infancy: the results of treatment by endoscopic third ventriculostomy with or without choroid plexus cauterization and suggestions for how it works, *Childs Nerv Syst* 29(6):935-940, 2013.

26. Gandolfi Colleoni G et al: Prenatal diagnosis and outcome of fetal posterior fossa fluid collections, *Ultrasound Obstet Gynecol* 39(6):625-631, 2012.

27. Marret S et al: Pathophysiology of cerebral palsy, *Handb Clin Neurol* 111:169-176, 2013.

28. Centers for Disease Control and Prevention (CDCP): *Cerebral palsy (CP).* Updated January 12, 2015. Available at: http://www.cdc.gov/ncbddd/cp/data.html.

29. Krigger KW: Cerebral palsy: an overview, *Am Fam Physician* 73(1):91-100, 2006.

30. Pruitt DW, Tsai T: Common medical comorbidities associated with cerebral palsy, *Phys Med Rehabil Clin North Am* 20(3):453-467, 2009.

31. Blau N et al: Phenylketonuria, *Lancet* 376(9750):1417-1427, 2010.

32. Blau N et al: Molecular genetics and diagnosis of phenylketonuria: state of the art, *Expert Rev Mol Diagn* 14(6):655-671, 2014.

33. Burton BK et al: Safety of extended treatment with sapropterin dihydrochloride in patients with phenylketonuria: results of a phase 3b study, *Mol Genet Metab* 103(4):315-322, 2011.

34. Hodges BL, Cheng SH: Cell and gene-based therapies for the lysosomal storage diseases, *Curr Gene Ther* 6(2):227-241, 2006.

35. Parenti G et al: New strategies for the treatment of lysosomal storage diseases (review). *Int J Mol Med* 31(1):11-20, 2013.

36. Patterson MC: Gangliosidoses, *Handb Clin Neurol* 113:1707-1708, 2013.

37. Bronstein AC et al: 2009 Annual Report of the American Association of Poison Control Centers' National Poison Data System (NPDS): 27th Annual Report, *Clin Toxicol* 48:979-1178, 2010. Available at: www.aapcc.org/dnn/Portals/0/correctedannualreport.pdf.

38. Mowry JB et al: 2012 annual report of the American Association of Poison Control Centers' National Poison Data System (NPDS): 30th annual report, *Clin Toxicol* 51(10):949-1229, 2013.

39. Advisory Committee on Childhood Lead Poisoning Prevention: Interpreting and managing blood lead levels <10 µg/dL in children and reducing childhood exposures to lead: recommendations of CDC's Advisory Committee on Childhood Lead Poisoning Prevention, *MMWR Recommend Rep* 56(RR-8):1-14, 2007. Available at: www.cdc.gov/mmwr/preview/mmwrhtml/rr5608a1.htm.

40. Centers for Disease Control and Prevention: Blood lead levels in children aged 1–5 years—United States, 1999–2010, *MMWR Morb Mortal Wkly Rep* 62(13):245-248, 2013.

41. Centers for Disease Control and Prevention: *Lead: prevention tips.* Updated June 19, 2014. Available at http://www.cdc.gov/nceh/lead/tips.htm.

42. American Academy of Pediatrics: Lead exposure in children: prevention, detection, and management, *Pediatrics* 116(4):1036-1046, 2005.

43. Liu J et al: Lead exposure at each stage of pregnancy and neurobehavioral development of neonates, *Neurotoxicology* 44:1-7, 2014.

44. Thigpen MC et al: Bacterial meningitis in the United States, 1998-2007, *N Engl J Med* 364:2016-2025, 2011.

45. Kim KS: Acute bacterial meningitis in infants and children, *Lancet Infect Dis* 10(1):32-42, 2010.

46. Gossger N et al: Immunogenicity and tolerability of recombinant serogroup B meningococcal vaccine administered with or without routine infant vaccinations according to different immunization schedules: a randomized controlled trial, *J Am Med Assoc* 307(6):573-582, 2012.

47. Ramakrishnan M et al: Increased risk of invasive bacterial infections in African people with sickle-cell disease: a systematic review and meta-analysis, *Lancet Infect Dis* 10(5):329-337, 2010.

48. Centers for Disease Control and Prevention (CDCP): *Vaccines and preventable diseases: meningococcal: who needs to be vaccinated?* Page updated April 1, 2014. Available at www.cdc.gov/vaccines/vpd-vac/mening/who-vaccinate.htm.

49. Weingarten L et al: Encephalitis, *Pediatr Emerg Care* 29(2):235-241, 2013.

50. Kirton A, deVeber G: Paediatric stroke: pressing issues and promising directions, *Lancet Neurol* 14(1):92-102, 2015.

51. Mallick AA, O'Callaghan FJ: The epidemiology of childhood stroke, *Eur J Paediatr Neurol* 14(3):197-205, 2010.

52. Lopez-Vicente M et al: Diagnosis and management of pediatric arterial ischemic stroke, *J Stroke Cerebrovasc Dis* 19(3):175-183, 2010.

53. Numis AL, Fox CK: Arterial ischemic stroke in children: risk factors and etiologies, *Curr Neurol Neurosci Rep* 14(1):422, 2014.

54. Tsitouras V, Sgouros S: Infantile posthemorrhagic hydrocephalus, *Childs Nerv Syst* 27(10):1595-1608, 2011.

55. Kronenburg A et al: Recent advances in moyamoya disease: pathophysiology and treatment, *Curr Neurol Neurosci Rep* 14(1):423, 2014.

56. Epilepsy Foundation: *About epilepsy: incidence and prevalence.* Accessed April 15, 2015. Available at: http://www.epilepsy.com/learn/epilepsy-statistics.

57. Central Brain Tumor Registry of the United States: *2014 CBTRUS fact sheet.* Available at: http://www.cbtrus.org/factsheet/factsheet.html.

58. American Cancer Society: *What are the risk factors for brain and spinal cord tumors in children?* Last revised 8/24/14. Available at: www.cancer.org/cancer/braincnstumorsinchildren/detailedguide/brain-and-spinal-cord-tumors-in-children-risk-factors.

59. Jacques G, Cormac O: Central nervous system tumors, *Handb Clin Neurol* 112:931-958, 2013.

60. American Cancer Society: *What are the key statistics about neuroblastoma?* Last revised 3/10/2015. Available at http://www.cancer.org/cancer/neuroblastoma/detailedguide/neuroblastoma-key-statistics.

61. National Cancer Institute: *General information about neuroblastoma.* Updated December 15, 2014. Available at: www.cancer.gov/cancertopics/pdq/treatment/neuroblastoma/HealthProfessional/page1.

62. Singhi P et al: Clinical profile and outcome of children with opsoclonus-myoclonus syndrome, *J Child Neurol* 29(1):58-61, 2014.

63. Rodriguez-Galindo C et al: Retinoblastoma, *Pediatr Clin North Am* 62(1):201-223, 2015.

64. Knudson AG Jr: Mutation and cancer: a statistical study of retinoblastoma, *Proc Natl Acad Sci U S A* 68(4):820-823, 1971.

18

Mechanisms of Hormonal Regulation

Valentina L. Brashers and Sue E. Huether

℮ EVOLVE WEBSITE

CHAPTER OUTLINE

The endocrine system is composed of various glands located throughout the body (Figure 18-1). These glands can synthesize and release special chemical messengers called hormones. The endocrine system has five general functions: (1) differentiation of the reproductive and central nervous systems in the developing fetus; (2) stimulation of sequential growth and development during childhood and adolescence; (3) coordination of the male and female reproductive systems, which makes sexual reproduction possible; (4) maintenance of an optimal internal environment throughout life; and (5) initiation of corrective and adaptive responses when emergency demands occur. The endocrine, nervous, and immune systems work together to regulate responses to the internal and external environments. Hormones convey specific regulatory information among cells and organs and are integrated with the nervous system to maintain communication and control. The mechanisms of communication and control occur within a cell *(autocrine)*, between local cells *(paracrine)*, and between cells located remotely from each other *(endocrine)*. Changes in the structure and function of the endocrine glands occur with aging and are summarized in the *Geriatric Considerations* box.

MECHANISMS OF HORMONAL REGULATION

Endocrine glands respond to specific signals by synthesizing and releasing hormones into the circulation, which then trigger intracellular responses. All hormones share certain general characteristics:

1. Hormones have specific rates and rhythms of secretion. Three basic patterns of secretion are (a) diurnal patterns, (b) pulsatile and cyclic patterns, and (c) patterns that depend on levels of circulating substrates (e.g., calcium, sodium, potassium, or the hormones themselves).
2. Hormones operate within feedback systems, either negative or positive, to maintain an optimal internal environment.

3. Hormones affect only target cells with specific receptors for the hormone and then act on these cells to initiate specific cell functions or activities.
4. Steroid hormones are either excreted directly by the kidneys or metabolized by the liver, which inactivates them and renders the hormone more water soluble for renal excretion. Peptide hormones are catabolized by circulating enzymes and eliminated in the feces or urine.

Hormones may be classified according to structure, gland of origin, effects, or chemical composition. (Table 18-1 categorizes known hormones based on structure.) The secretion and mechanisms of action of hormones represent an extremely complex system of integrated responses. The endocrine and nervous systems work together to regulate responses to the internal and external environments.

Regulation of Hormone Release

Hormones are released either to respond to an altered cellular environment or to maintain the level of another hormone or substance. One or more of the following mechanisms regulates hormone release: (1) chemical factors (such as blood glucose or calcium levels), (2) endocrine factors (a hormone from one endocrine gland controlling another endocrine gland), and (3) neural control. For example, insulin is secreted by the chemical stimulation of increased plasma glucose levels, cortisol from the adrenal cortex is an endocrine factor that regulates and stimulates insulin secretion, and direct stimulation of the insulin-secreting cells of the pancreas by the autonomic nervous system is a form of neural control.

Feedback systems provide precise monitoring and control of the cellular environment. Both negative and positive feedback systems are important for maintaining hormone levels within physiologic ranges. Negative feedback is the most common and occurs when a changing chemical, neural, or endocrine response to a stimulus decreases the

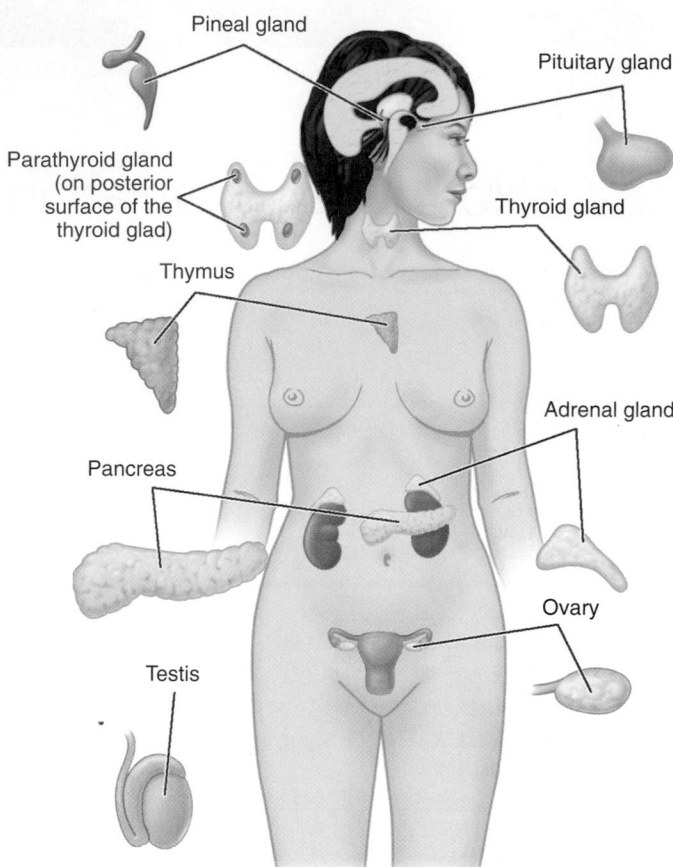

FIGURE 18-1 Major Endocrine Glands. (From Applegate E: *The anatomy and physiology learning system*, ed 4, St Louis, 2011, Saunders.)

TABLE 18-1 **Structural Categories of Hormones**

Structural Category	Examples
Water Soluble	
Peptides	Growth hormone
	Insulin
	Leptin
	Parathyroid hormone
	Prolactin
Glycoproteins	Follicle-stimulating hormone
	Luteinizing hormone
	Thyroid-stimulating hormone
Polypeptides	Adrenocorticotropic hormone
	Antidiuretic hormone
	Calcitonin
	Endorphins
	Glucagon
	Hypothalamic hormones
	Lipotropins
	Melanocyte-stimulating hormone
	Oxytocin
	Somatostatin
	Thymosin
	Thyrotropin-releasing hormone
Amines	Epinephrine
	Norepinephrine
Lipid Soluble	
Thyroxine (an amine but lipid soluble)	Both thyroxine (T_4) and triiodothyronine (T_3)
Steroids (cholesterol is a precursor for all steroids)	Estrogens
	Glucocorticoids (cortisol)
	Mineralocorticoids (aldosterone)
	Progestins (progesterone)
	Testosterone
Derivatives of arachidonic acid (autocrine or paracrine action)	Leukotrienes
	Prostacyclins
	Prostaglandins
	Thromboxanes

synthesis and secretion of a hormone. **Positive feedback** occurs when a neural, chemical, or endocrine response increases the synthesis and secretion of a hormone. For example, Figure 18-2, *A*, illustrates negative feedback within the hypothalamus-pituitary axis and the thyroid gland. Decreased serum levels of the thyroid hormones thyroxine (T_4) and triiodothyronine (T_3) stimulate secretion of **thyrotropin-releasing hormone (TRH)** from the hypothalamus, which stimulates the secretion of **thyroid-stimulating hormone (TSH)**. Secretion of TSH stimulates the synthesis and secretion of T_3 and T_4. Increasing levels of T_4 and T_3 then generate negative feedback on the pituitary and hypothalamus to inhibit TSH and TRH synthesis and decrease the synthesis and production of thyroid hormones. The lack of negative feedback inhibition on hormonal release often results in pathologic excessive hormone production (see Chapter 19).

An example of positive feedback is found in the female reproductive cycle. The cyclic rise of estradiol levels provides positive feedback on the anterior pituitary and hypothalamus, causing a subsequent increase in gonadotropin-releasing hormone and follicle-stimulating hormone. These changes result in ovulation (see Chapter 32).

Hormone Transport

Once hormones are released into the circulatory system, they are distributed throughout the body. The protein (peptide) hormones (see Table 18-1) are water soluble and generally circulate in free (unbound) forms. Water-soluble hormones generally have a half-life of seconds to minutes because they are catabolized by circulating enzymes. For example, insulin has a half-life of 3 to 5 minutes and is catabolized by

insulinases. Lipid-soluble hormones (see Table 18-1), such as cortisol and adrenal androgens, are transported bound to a water-soluble carrier or transport protein and can remain in the blood for hours to days. Only free hormones (those not bound to a carrier protein) can signal a target cell. Because there is an equilibrium between the concentrations of free hormones and hormones bound to plasma proteins, a significant change in the concentration of binding proteins can affect the concentration of free hormones in the plasma (Table 18-2). (Mechanisms of hormone binding are discussed in Chapter 1.)

Mechanisms of Hormone Action

Although a hormone is distributed throughout the body, only those cells with appropriate receptors, termed **target cells**, for that hormone are affected. *Hormone receptors* of the target cell have two main functions: (1) to recognize and bind specifically and with high affinity to their particular hormones and (2) to initiate a signal to appropriate intracellular effectors.

The sensitivity of the target cell to a particular hormone is related to the total number of receptors per cell or the affinity (binding) for

FIGURE 18-2 Feedback Loops. A, Endocrine feedback loops involving the hypothalamus-pituitary gland and end organs; in this example, the thyroid gland is illustrated (endocrine regulation). **B,** General model for control and negative feedback to hypothalamic-pituitary target organ systems. Negative-feedback regulation is possible at three levels: target organ (ultra-short feedback), anterior pituitary (short feedback), and hypothalamus (long feedback). *TRH,* Thyroid-releasing hormone; *TSH,* thyroid-stimulating hormone; *T₃,* triiodothyronine; *T₄,* tetraiodothyronine (thyroxine).

TABLE 18-2 Binding Proteins, Their Hormones, and Variables That Affect Their Circulating Levels

Binding Protein	Hormone	Factors That Increase Binding Protein Levels	Factors That Decrease Binding Protein Levels
Corticosteroid-binding globulin	Cortisol Progesterone	Estrogen	Liver disease
Sex hormone–binding globulin	Dihydrotestosterone Testosterone Estradiol	— Hypothyroidism Liver disease	Androgens
Thyroid-binding globulin	Thyroxine (T₄) Triiodothyronine (T₃)	Estrogen Hyperthyroidism	Testosterone Glucocorticoids Liver disease
Albumin	All lipid-soluble hormones	Estrogen	Liver disease Malnutrition Renal disease

the receptors to the hormone: the more receptors or the higher the affinity of the receptors, the more sensitive the cell to the stimulating effects of the hormone. Low concentrations of hormone increase the number or affinity of receptors per cell; this is called **up-regulation.** High concentrations of hormone decrease the number or affinity of receptors; this is called **down-regulation** (Figure 18-3). Thus the cell can adjust its sensitivity to the concentration of the signaling hormone. The receptors on the plasma membrane are continuously synthesized and degraded, so that changes in receptor concentration or affinity may occur within hours. The regulation of hormone receptors is of particular importance in type 2 diabetes, in which there is a decrease in insulin receptor sensitivity and hyperglycemia (see Chapter 19). Various physiochemical conditions can affect both the receptor number and the affinity of the hormone for its receptor. Some of these physiochemical conditions are the fluidity and structure of the plasma membrane, pH, temperature, ion concentration, diet, and the presence of other chemicals (e.g., drugs).

Hormones affect target cells directly or permissively. **Direct effects** are the obvious changes in cell function that result specifically from stimulation by a particular hormone. **Permissive effects** are less obvious hormone-induced changes that facilitate the maximal response or functioning of a cell. For example, insulin via insulin receptors has

Up-Regulation

Down-Regulation

FIGURE 18-3 Regulation of Target Cell Sensitivity. A, Low hormone level and up-regulation, or an increase in the number of receptors. B, High hormone level and down-regulation, or a decrease in the number of receptors.

BOX 18-1   Methods of Hormone Measurement

Radioimmunoassay (RIA)

In this immunologic technique, known amounts of antibody and radiolabeled hormone are placed in an assay tube with the unlabeled hormone. The radio-labeled hormone competes chemically with the nonlabeled hormone molecules for binding sites on the antibodies. When increasing amounts of unlabeled hormones are added to the assay, the limited binding sites of the antibody can bind less of the radiolabeled hormone. Therefore, the higher the concentration of unlabeled hormone, the fewer the number of radioactive *counts*, or labeled hormone, that bind with the fixed concentration of antibody. A quantitative value is established by use of standard reference curves.

Enzyme-Linked Immunosorbent Assay (ELISA)

This assay is used to determine circulating hormone levels. The method is similar to that of radioimmunoassay (RIA) but is less expensive and easier to conduct. Instead of radiolabeled hormones, an enzyme-labeled hormone is used. The enzyme activity in either the bound or the unbound fraction is determined and related to the concentration of the unlabeled hormone.

Bioassay

This assay uses graded doses of hormone in a reference preparation and then compares the results with an unknown sample. Bioassays are used more commonly in investigative endocrinology than in clinical laboratories.

---

a direct effect on skeletal muscle cells, causing increased glucose transport into these cells. Insulin also has a permissive effect on mammary cells, facilitating the response of these cells to the direct effects of prolactin.

Some hormones have biphasic effects that are dependent on the concentration or secretion pattern of the hormone. For example, in primary hyperparathyroidism, continuous hypersecretion of parathyroid hormone (PTH) leads to bone destruction by osteoclasts. Conversely, bone formation is stimulated when recombinant PTH is given in low doses at intermittent intervals, as a treatment for osteoporosis with high risk for fracture[1] (see Chapter 39). Methods of hormone measurement are summarized in Box 18-1.

Hormone Receptors

Hormone receptors may be located in the plasma membrane or in the intracellular compartment of the target cell (Figure 18-4). Water-soluble (peptide) hormones, which include the protein hormones and the catecholamines, have a high molecular weight and cannot diffuse across the cell membrane. They interact or bind with receptors located in or on the cell membrane. Fat-soluble steroids, vitamin D, retinoic acid, and thyroid hormones diffuse freely across the plasma and nuclear membranes and bind with cytosolic or nuclear receptors. The hormone-receptor complex binds to a specific region in the deoxyribonucleic acid (DNA) and stimulates the expression of a specific gene. Some fat-soluble hormones (e.g., estrogen [see Chapter 32]) may also bind with plasma membrane receptors and can have rapid cellular effects.[2-4]

First and Second Messengers

All water-soluble hormones and some steroid hormones have hormone-specific receptors located in the plasma membranes of cells. Hormone binding with the plasma membrane receptor initiates a complex cascade of intracellular effects. In this cascade, the hormone is termed the first messenger. The hormone-receptor interaction

FIGURE 18-4 Hormone Binding at Target Cell.

initiates a signal that generates a small molecule inside the cell, called the second messenger. Second messengers include cyclic adenosine monophosphate (cAMP), cyclic guanosine monophosphate (cGMP), calcium, inositol triphosphate (IP_3), and the tyrosine kinase system (Table 18-3). The second messenger conveys the signal from the receptor to the cytoplasm and nucleus of the cell and mediates the effect of the hormone on the target cell (e.g., membrane permeability alterations, protein synthesis, inhibition of specific metabolic pathways, enzyme activation, or cellular growth).

When first messengers from the anterior pituitary gland, adrenocorticotropic hormone (ACTH) and thyroid-stimulating hormone

TABLE 18-3 Second Messengers Identified for Specific Hormones

Second Messenger	Associated Hormones
Cyclic AMP	Adrenocorticotropic hormone (ACTH)
	Luteinizing hormone (LH)
	Human chorionic gonadotropin (hCG)
	Follicle-stimulating hormone (FSH)
	Thyroid-stimulating hormone (TSH)
	Antidiuretic hormone (ADH)
	Thyrotropin-releasing hormone (TRH)
	Parathyroid hormone (PTH)
	Glucagon
Cyclic GMP	Atrial natriuretic peptide
Calcium and IP₃	Angiotensin II
	Gonadotropin-releasing hormone (GnRH)
	Antidiuretic hormone (ADH)
	Luteinizing hormone–releasing hormone (LHRH)
Tyrosine kinases	Insulin
	Growth hormone
	Leptin
	Prolactin

AMP, Adenosine monophosphate; *GMP,* guanosine monophosphate; *IP₃,* inositol triphosphate.

FIGURE 18-5 Mechanism of First and Second Messenger Action. The hormone acts as a "first messenger," delivering its message via the bloodstream to a membrane receptor in the target cell much like a key fits into a lock. The "second messenger" causes the cell to respond and perform its specialized function. (From Patton KT, Thibodeau GA: *Structure & function of the body,* ed 15, St Louis, 2016, Mosby.)

(TSH), bind to a cell membrane receptor, intracellular levels of cAMP increase. Second-messenger cAMP activates protein kinases, leading to phosphorylation of cellular proteins. This either activates or deactivates intracellular enzymes, thus directing the actions or products of specific cells (Figure 18-5).

cGMP functions as a second messenger following receptor binding of first messengers (e.g., atrial natriuretic peptide and nitric oxide). These hormones play crucial roles in cardiovascular and pulmonary

health and disease. Drugs such as phosphodiesterase inhibitors that target cGMP are being explored for treatment of various diseases.[5,6]

Hormone-receptor binding of first-messenger angiotensin II and antidiuretic hormone (ADH) results in generation of the second messenger, inositol triphosphate. Inositol triphosphate triggers a release of intracellular calcium, another second messenger. Increased intracellular calcium levels can lead to the formation of the calcium-calmodulin complex, which mediates the effects of calcium on intracellular activities that are crucial for cell metabolism and growth. For example, calmodulin-dependent protein kinases control intracellular contractile components (myosin and actin, which cause muscle contraction), alter plasma membrane permeability to calcium, and regulate the intracellular enzyme activity that promotes hormone secretion.

Some hormone first messengers, such as insulin, growth hormone, and prolactin, bind to surface receptors that directly activate second messengers of the tyrosine kinase family. These tyrosine kinases include the Janus family of tyrosine kinases (JAK) and signal transducers and activators of transcription (STAT). They regulate a wide range of intracellular processes that contribute to cellular metabolism and growth, and are being targeted in emerging treatments for diabetes and cancer.[7-9]

Lipid-Soluble (Steroid) Hormone-Receptor Binding

With the exception of thyroid hormones, the lipid-soluble hormones are synthesized from cholesterol (giving rise to the term "steroid"). These include androgens, estrogens, progestins, glucocorticoids, mineralocorticoids, vitamin D, and retinoid. Because these are relatively small, lipophilic, hydrophobic molecules, lipid-soluble hormones can cross the lipid plasma membrane by simple diffusion (see Chapter 1). Receptors for lipid-soluble hormones are in the cytosol and nucleus and direct gene expression (Figure 18-6). Modulation of gene expression can take hours to days. Studies also reveal that receptors for lipid-soluble hormones are in the plasma membrane and are associated with rapid responses (seconds to minutes) as shown in Figure 18-6.[10,11]

> ✔ **QUICK CHECK 18-1**
> 1. What are hormones? By what mechanisms do they function?
> 2. What is meant by negative-feedback regulation of hormone release?
> 3. How do first messengers differ from second messengers?
> 4. Where are the receptors located for lipid-soluble hormones?

STRUCTURE AND FUNCTION OF THE ENDOCRINE GLANDS

Hypothalamic-Pituitary System

The hypothalamic-pituitary axis (HPA) forms the structural and functional basis for central integration of the neurologic and endocrine systems, creating what is called the neuroendocrine system. The HPA produces several hormones that affect a number of diverse body functions (Figure 18-7), including thyroid, adrenal, and reproductive functions.

The hypothalamus is located at the base of the brain. It is connected to the pituitary gland by the pituitary stalk (Figure 18-8). The hypothalamus is connected to the anterior pituitary through hypophysial portal blood vessels (Figure 18-9) and to the posterior pituitary via a nerve tract referred to as the *hypothalamohypophysial tract* (Figure 18-10). These connections are vital to the functioning of the hypothalamic-pituitary system. The hypothalamus contains special neurosecretory cells that are like other neurons in that they have similar electrical properties, organelles, membranes, and synapses.

FIGURE 18-6 Steroid Hormone Mechanism. Lipid-soluble steroid hormone molecules detach from the carrier protein **(1)** and pass through the plasma membrane **(2)**. Hormone molecules then diffuse into the nucleus, where they bind to a receptor to form a hormone-receptor complex **(3)**. This complex then binds to a specific site on a deoxyribonucleic acid *(DNA)* molecule **(4)**, triggering transcription of the genetic information encoded there **(5)**. The resulting messenger ribonucleic acid *(mRNA)* molecule moves to the cytosol, where it associates with a ribosome, initiating synthesis of a new protein **(6)**. This new protein—usually an enzyme or channel protein—produces specific effects on the target cell **(7)**. The classic genomic action is typically slow *(red arrows)*. Steroids also may exact rapid effects *(green arrows)* by binding to receptors on the plasma membrane **(A)** and activating an intercellular second messenger **(B)**. (From Patton KT, Thibodeau GA: *Anatomy & physiology*, ed 9, St Louis, 2016, Mosby.)

TABLE 18-4 Hypothalamic Hormones (Hypophysiotropic Hormones)

Hormone	Target Tissue	Action
Thyrotropin-releasing hormone (TRH)	Anterior pituitary	Stimulates release of thyroid-stimulating hormone (TSH); modulates prolactin secretion
Gonadotropin-releasing hormone (GnRH)	Anterior pituitary	Stimulates release of follicle-stimulating hormone (FSH) and luteinizing hormone (LH)
Somatostatin	Anterior pituitary	Inhibits release of growth hormone (GH) and TSH
Growth hormone–releasing hormone (GHRH)	Anterior pituitary	Stimulates release of GH
Corticotropin-releasing hormone (CRH)	Anterior pituitary	Stimulates release of adrenocorticotropic hormone (ACTH) and β-endorphin
Substance P	Anterior pituitary	Inhibits synthesis and release of ACTH; stimulates secretion of GH, FSH, LH, and prolactin
Prolactin-inhibiting factor (PIF, dopamine)	Anterior pituitary	Inhibits synthesis and secretion of prolactin
Prolactin-releasing factor (PRF)	Anterior pituitary	Stimulates secretion of prolactin

Hypothalamic neurosecretory cells, however, can synthesize and secrete the hypothalamic-releasing hormones that regulate the release of hormones from the anterior pituitary. In addition, these cells synthesize the hormones antidiuretic hormone (ADH) and oxytocin that are released from the posterior pituitary gland. These hormones are summarized in Table 18-4.

The **pituitary gland** is located in the sella turcica (a saddle-shaped depression of the sphenoid bone at the base of the skull). It weighs approximately 0.5 g, except during pregnancy when its weight increases by about 30%. It is composed of two distinctly different lobes: (1) the anterior pituitary, or adenohypophysis, and (2) the posterior pituitary,

or neurohypophysis (see Figure 18-7). These two lobes differ in their embryonic origins, cell types, and functional relationship to the hypothalamus.

The Anterior Pituitary

The **anterior pituitary** (adenohypophysis) accounts for 75% of the total weight of the pituitary gland. It is composed of three regions: (1) the pars distalis, (2) the pars tuberalis, and (3) the pars intermedia. The **pars distalis** is the major component of the anterior pituitary and is the source of the anterior pituitary hormones. The **pars tuberalis** is a thin layer of cells on the anterior and lateral portions of the

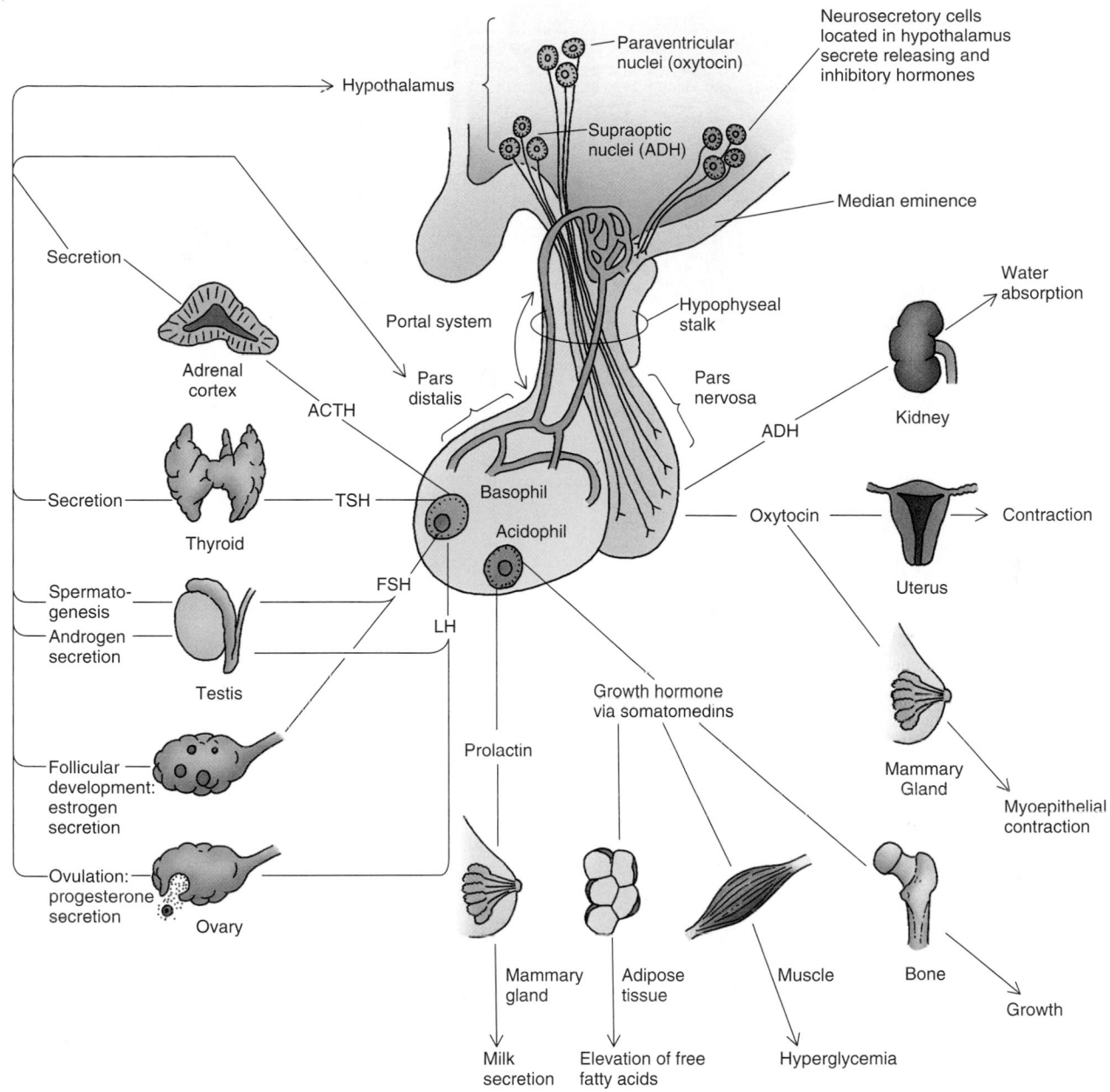

FIGURE 18-7 Pituitary Gland and Its Target Organs. *ACTH*, adrenocorticotropic hormone; *ADH*, antidiuretic hormone; *FSH*, follicle-stimulating hormone; *LH*, luteinizing hormone; *TSH*, thyroid-stimulating hormone. (From Gartner LP, Hiatt JL: *Color textbook of histology*, 3rd ed. Philadelphia, 2007, Saunders.)

pituitary stalk. The **pars intermedia** lies between the two and secretes melanocyte-stimulating hormone in the fetus. In the adult, the distinct pars intermedia disappears and the individual cells are distributed diffusely throughout the pars distalis and pars nervosa (neural lobe) of the posterior pituitary.

The anterior pituitary is composed of two main cell types: (1) the **chromophobes**, which appear to be nonsecretory, and (2) the **chromophils**, which are considered the secretory cells of the adenohypophysis. The chromophils are subdivided into seven secretory cell types, and each cell type secretes a specific hormone or hormones. In general, the anterior pituitary hormones are regulated by (1) secretion of hypothalamic peptide hormones or releasing factors, (2) feedback

effects of the hormones secreted by target glands, and (3) direct effects of other mediating neurotransmitters. (These are summarized in Figure 18-2.)

The anterior pituitary secretes **tropic hormones** that affect the physiologic function of specific target organs (see Figure 18-7 and Table 18-5). **Melanocyte-stimulating hormone (MSH)** promotes the pituitary secretion of melanin, which darkens skin color. The glycoprotein hormones **follicle-stimulating hormone (FSH)** and **luteinizing hormone (LH)** influence reproductive function and are discussed in Chapter 32. **Adrenocorticotropic hormone (ACTH)** regulates the release of cortisol from the adrenal cortex. **Thyroid-stimulating hormone (TSH)** regulates the activity of the thyroid gland. The roles

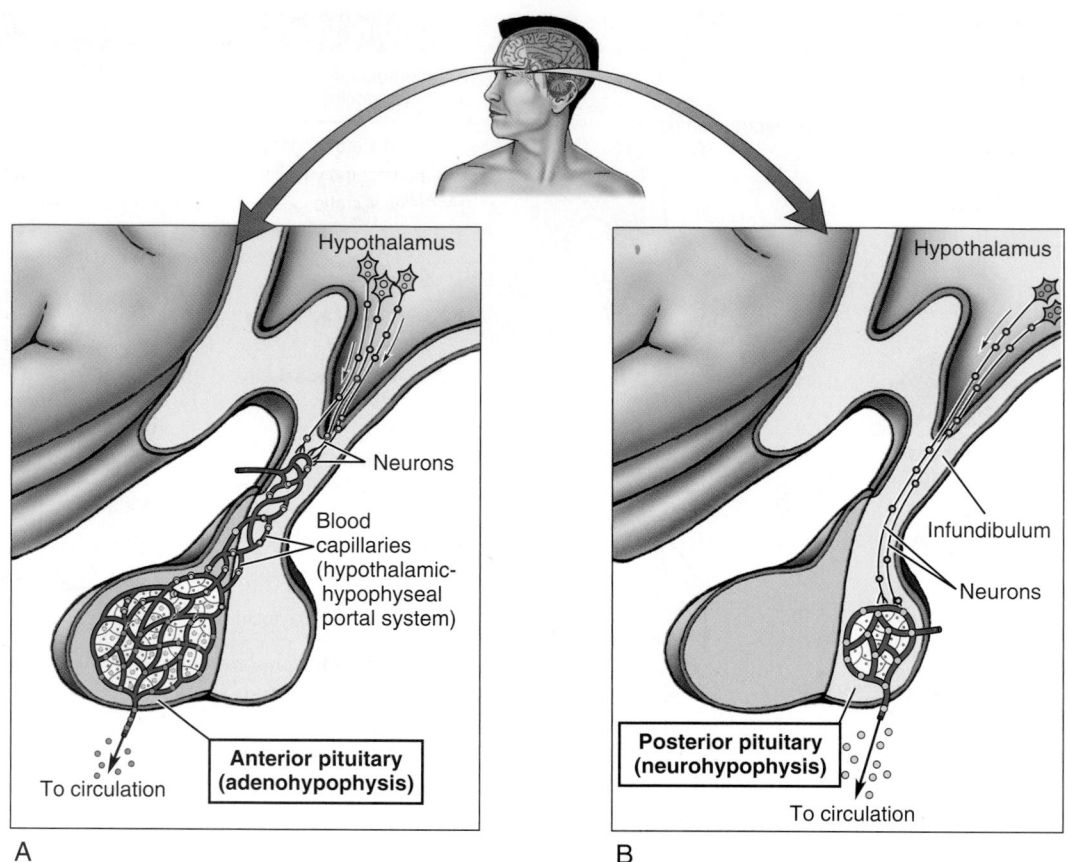

FIGURE 18-8 Pituitary gland. The pituitary gland sits within the sella turcicia of the sphenoid bone of the skull. **A,** Relationship of the hypothalamus to the anterior pituitary gland. **B,** Relationship of the hypothalamus to the posterior pituitary gland. (From Herlihy B: *The human body in health and illness*, ed 5, St Louis, 2015, Saunders.)

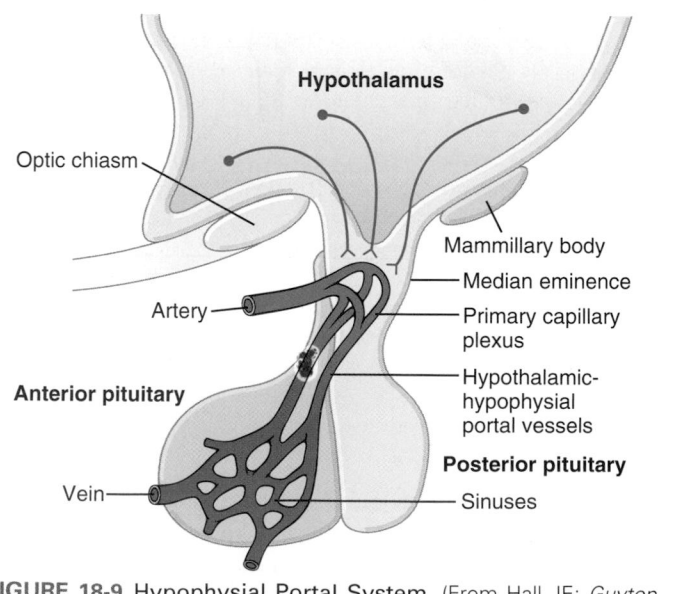

FIGURE 18-9 Hypophysial Portal System. (From Hall JE: *Guyton and Hall textbook of medical physiology*, ed 13, Philadelphia, 2016, Saunders.)

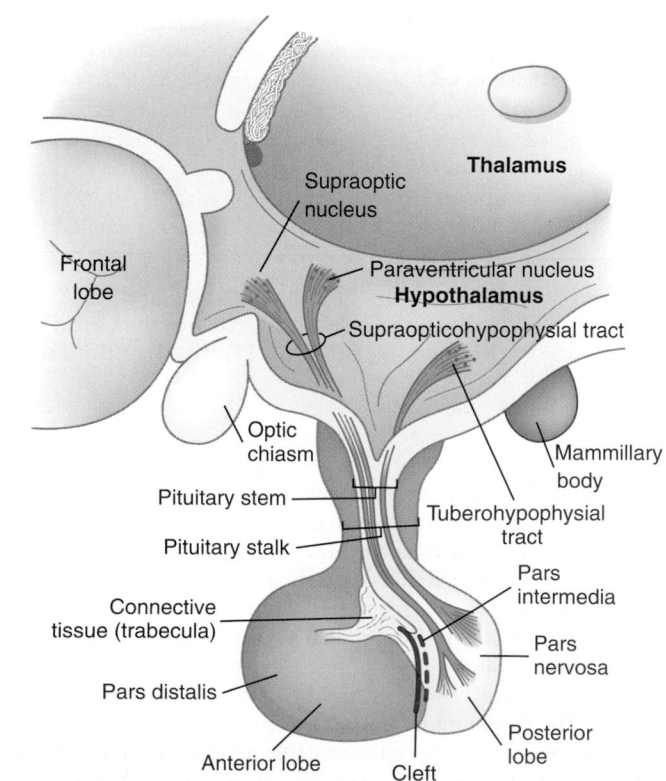

FIGURE 18-10 Nerve Tracts from Hypothalamus to Posterior Lobe of Pituitary Gland. Nerve tracts from hypothalamus to posterior lobe of pituitary gland.

TABLE 18-5 Tropic Hormones of the Anterior Pituitary and Their Functions

Hormone	Secretory Cell Type	Target Organs	Functions
Adrenocorticotropic hormone (ACTH)	Corticotropic	Adrenal gland (cortex)	Increased steroidogenesis (cortisol and androgenic hormones); synthesis of adrenal proteins contributing to maintenance of adrenal gland
Melanocyte-stimulating hormone (MSH)	Melanotropic	Anterior pituitary	Promotes secretion of melanin and lipotropin by anterior pituitary; makes skin darker
Somatotropic Hormones			
Growth hormone (GH)	Somatotropic	Muscle, bone, liver	Regulates metabolic processes related to growth and adaptation to physical and emotional stressors, muscle growth, increased protein synthesis, increased liver glycogenolysis, increased fat mobilization
		Liver	Induces formation of somatomedins, or insulin-like growth factors (IGFs) that have actions similar to insulin
Prolactin	Lactotropic	Breast	Milk production
Glycoprotein Hormones			
Thyroid-stimulating hormone (TSH)	Thyrotropic	Thyroid gland	Increased production and secretion of thyroid hormone
			Increased iodide uptake; promotes hypertrophy and hyperplasia of thymocytes
Luteinizing hormone (LH)	Gonadotropic	In women: granulosa cells; In men: Leydig cells	Ovulation, progesterone production Testicular growth, testosterone production
Follicle-stimulating hormone (FSH)	Gonadotropic	In women: granulosa cells In men: Sertoli cells	Follicle maturation, estrogen production Spermatogenesis
β-Lipotropin	Corticotropic	Adipose cells	Fat breakdown and release of fatty acids
β-Endorphins	Corticotropic	Adipose cells; brain opioid receptors	Analgesia; may regulate body temperature, food and water intake

of ACTH and TSH are discussed later in this chapter. Growth hormone (GH) and prolactin are called the somatotropic hormones and have diverse effects on body tissues. GH secretion is controlled by two hormones from the hypothalamus: growth hormone–releasing hormone (GHRH), which increases GH secretion; and somatostatin, which inhibits GH secretion. GH is essential to normal tissue growth and maturation and also impacts aging, sleep, nutritional status, stress, and reproductive hormones. Many of the anabolic functions of GH are mediated, at least in part, by the insulin-like growth factors (IGFs), which are also known as the somatomedins.[12]

There are two primary forms of IGF: IGF-1 and IGF-2, of which IGF-1 is the most biologically active. They both circulate bound to a group of IGF-binding proteins (IGFBPs) modulating their availability. IGF-1 binds to IGF-1 receptors mediating the anabolic effects of GH. IGF-1 also binds to insulin receptors, providing an insulin-like effect on skeletal muscle. IGF-2 has important effects on fetal growth, but suppresses GH in the adult. Because of the anabolic effects of GH and IGF-1, they can be used to treat growth disorders, increase muscle mass, and potentially slow the aging process; but their use has also been linked to increased rates of cancer[13,14] (see *Health Alert*: Growth Hormone [GH] and Insulin-like Growth Factor [IGF] in Aging).

Prolactin primarily functions to induce milk production during pregnancy and lactation. It has immune stimulatory effects and modulates immune and inflammatory responses with both physiologic and pathologic reactions.[15] Its synthesis is stimulated by vasoactive intestinal polypeptide, serotonin, and growth factors. Release of prolactin is inhibited by dopamine.

The Posterior Pituitary

The embryonic posterior pituitary (neurohypophysis) is derived from the hypothalamus and is comprised of three parts: (1) the median eminence, located at the base of the hypothalamus; (2) the pituitary stalk; and (3) the infundibular process, also known as the pars nervosa

HEALTH ALERT

Growth Hormone (GH) and Insulin-like Growth Factor (IGF) in Aging

Aging is a multifactorial process that is influenced by genetic and environmental factors. The aging process is associated with many hormonal and metabolic changes. The amounts of GH and IGF decline with aging, a process that has been called the "somatopause." Clinical findings related to somatotropic hormone changes with aging include increased visceral fat, decreased lean body mass, decreased bone density, and changes in reproductive and cognitive function. The underlying mechanisms of aging and its relationship to GH and IGF are complex. For example, not only do these hormones promote bone and muscle growth, but also a recent study suggests that the brain IGF-1 receptor may be a significant factor in determining overall life span and ability to respond to physiologic stress. GH and IGF effects on inflammation and immunity also are important in the aging process. Unfortunately, there remains much confusion and controversy over the role of these hormones. Although most studies suggest that it is a deficiency of these hormones that leads to an acceleration of the aging process, there are several studies suggesting that lower lifetime levels of these hormones may confer longevity by providing protection from cancer and other age-related diseases. As these hormones are used to treat a wider range of disorders and for different age groups, more information about their safety is emerging. Despite the initial enthusiasm for the use of therapeutic doses of recombinant human growth hormone (rhGH) as a way to slow the aging process, studies have not been consistently positive and the relationship between GH and IGF supplementation and increased cancer risk is being explored.

Data from Anisimov VN, Bartke A: Crit *Rev Oncol Hematol* 87(3):201-223, 2013; Junnila RK et al: *Nat Rev Endocrinol* 9(6):366-376, 2013; Nass R: *Endocrinol Metab Clin North Am* 42(2):187-199, 2013; Ashpole NM et al: *Exp Gerontol* 68:76-81, 2015; Sattler FR: *Best Pract Res Clin Endocrinol Metab* 27(4):541-555, 2013.

or neural lobe. The median eminence is composed largely of the nerve endings of axons from the ventral hypothalamus. It often is designated as part of the posterior pituitary but contains at least 10 biologically active hypothalamic-releasing hormones, as well as the neurotransmitters dopamine, norepinephrine, serotonin, acetylcholine, and histamine. The pituitary stalk contains the axons of neurons that originate in the supraoptic and paraventricular nuclei of the hypothalamus and connects the pituitary gland to the brain. Axons originating in the hypothalamus terminate in the pars nervosa, which secretes the hormones of the posterior pituitary (see Figure 18-10).

The posterior pituitary secretes two polypeptide hormones: (1) antidiuretic hormone (ADH), also called arginine vasopressin, and (2) oxytocin. These hormones differ by only two amino acids. They are synthesized—along with their binding proteins, the neurophysins—in the supraoptic and paraventricular nuclei of the hypothalamus (see Figure 18-10). They are packaged in secretory vesicles and are moved down the axons of the pituitary stalk to the pars nervosa for storage. The posterior pituitary thus can be seen as a storage and releasing site for hormones synthesized in the hypothalamus. The release of ADH and oxytocin is mediated by cholinergic and adrenergic neurotransmitters. The major stimulus to both ADH and oxytocin release is glutamate, whereas the major inhibitory input is through gamma-aminobutyric acid (GABA).[16] Before release into the circulatory system, ADH and oxytocin are split from the neurophysins and are secreted in unbound form.

Antidiuretic hormone. The major homeostatic function of the posterior pituitary is the control of plasma osmolality as regulated by ADH (see Chapter 5). At physiologic levels, ADH increases the permeability of the distal renal tubules and collecting ducts (see Chapter 29). This increased permeability leads to increased water reabsorption into the blood, thus concentrating the urine and reducing serum osmolality. Hypercalcemia, prostaglandin E, and hypokalemia can inhibit this water reabsorption.

The secretion of ADH is regulated primarily by the osmoreceptors of the hypothalamus, located near or in the supraoptic nuclei. As plasma osmolality increases these osmoreceptors are stimulated, the rate of ADH secretion increases, more water is reabsorbed by the kidney, and the plasma is diluted back to its set-point osmolality. ADH has no direct effect on electrolyte levels, but by increasing water reabsorption, serum electrolyte concentrations may decrease because of a dilutional effect.

ADH secretion also is increased by changes in intravascular volume, as monitored by baroreceptors in the left atrium, in the carotid arteries, and in the aortic arches. A volume loss of 7% to 25% acts on these receptors to stimulate ADH secretion. Stress, trauma, pain, exercise, nausea, nicotine, exposure to heat, and drugs such as morphine also increase ADH secretion. ADH secretion decreases with decreased plasma osmolality, increased intravascular volume, hypertension, alcohol ingestion, and an increase in estrogen, progesterone, or angiotensin II levels.

Physiologic levels of ADH do not significantly impact vessel tone. However, ADH was originally named *vasopressin* because, in extremely high levels, it causes vasoconstriction and a resulting increase in arterial blood pressure. For example, high doses of ADH (given as the drug vasopressin) may be administered to achieve hemostasis during hemorrhage and to raise blood pressure in shock states.[17,18]

Oxytocin. Oxytocin is responsible for contraction of the uterus and milk ejection in lactating women and may affect sperm motility in men. In both genders, oxytocin has an antidiuretic effect similar to that of ADH. In women, oxytocin is secreted in response to suckling and mechanical distention of the female reproductive tract. Oxytocin binds to its receptors on myoepithelial cells in the mammary tissues

and causes contraction of those cells, which increases intramammary pressure and milk expression ("let-down" reflex). Oxytocin also acts on the uterus to stimulate contractions. Oxytocin functions near the end of labor to enhance the effectiveness of contractions, promote delivery of the placenta, and stimulate postpartum uterine contractions, thereby preventing excessive bleeding. The function of this hormone is discussed in detail in Chapter 32.

> ✔**QUICK CHECK 18-2**
> 1. What is the relationship between the hypothalamus and the pituitary?
> 2. What is the action of antidiuretic hormone (ADH)?

Pineal Gland

The pineal gland is located near the center of the brain and is composed of photoreceptive cells that secrete melatonin. It is innervated by noradrenergic sympathetic nerve terminals controlled by pathways within the hypothalamus. Melatonin release is stimulated by exposure to dark and inhibited by light exposure. It is synthesized from tryptophan, which is first converted to serotonin and then to melatonin. Melatonin regulates circadian rhythms and reproductive systems, including the secretion of the gonadotropin-releasing hormones and the onset of puberty. It also plays an important role in immune regulation and is postulated to impact the aging process. Further effects of melatonin include increasing nitric oxide release from blood vessels, removing toxic oxygen free radicals, and decreasing insulin secretion.[19] Melatonin has been used therapeutically in humans to help with sleep disturbances, jet lag, psychological and inflammatory disorders. Its utility for numerous other disorders is being explored.[20]

Thyroid and Parathyroid Glands

The thyroid gland, located in the neck just below the larynx, produces hormones that control the rates of metabolic processes throughout the body. The four parathyroid glands are near the posterior side of the thyroid and function to control serum calcium levels (Figure 18-11).

Thyroid Gland

Two lobes of the thyroid gland lie on either side of the trachea, inferior to the thyroid cartilage and joined by a small band of tissue termed the isthmus. The pyramidal lobe is superior to the isthmus (see Figure 18-11). The normal thyroid gland is not visible on inspection,

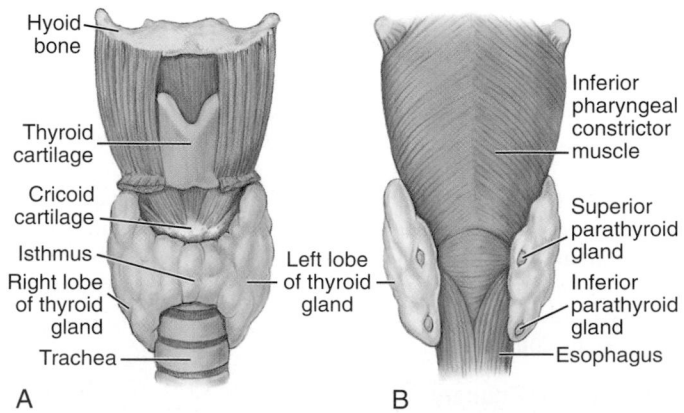

FIGURE 18-11 Thyroid and Parathyroid Glands. **A,** Anterior view. **B,** Posterior view. (From Fehrenbach MJ, et al: *Illustrated anatomy of the head and neck,* ed 4, St Louis, 2012, Saunders.)

but it may be palpated on swallowing, which causes it to be displaced upward.

The thyroid gland consists of follicles that contain follicular cells surrounding a viscous substance called *colloid* (Figure 18-12). The follicular cells synthesize and secrete the thyroid hormones. Neurons terminate on blood vessels within the thyroid gland and on the follicular cells themselves, so neurotransmitters (acetylcholine, catecholamines) may directly affect the secretory activity of follicular cells and thyroid blood flow. Approximately, a 2-month supply of thyroid hormone is stored in the gland.

Also found in the thyroid are parafollicular cells, or C cells (see Figure 18-12). C cells secrete various polypeptides, including calcitonin. At high levels, calcitonin, also called *thyrocalcitonin*, lowers serum calcium levels by inhibiting bone-resorbing osteoclasts (Table 18-6). However, in humans the metabolic consequences of calcitonin deficiency or excess do not appear to be significant. (Bone resorption is explained in Chapter 38.) Calcitonin can be used therapeutically to treat a number of bone disorders, including osteogenesis imperfecta, osteoporosis, and Paget bone disease, among others. Parafollicular cells can give rise to medullary thyroid carcinoma.

Regulation of thyroid hormone secretion. Thyroid hormone (TH) is regulated through a negative-feedback loop involving the hypothalamus, the anterior pituitary, and the thyroid gland (see Figure 18-2). This loop is initiated by thyrotropin-releasing hormone (TRH),

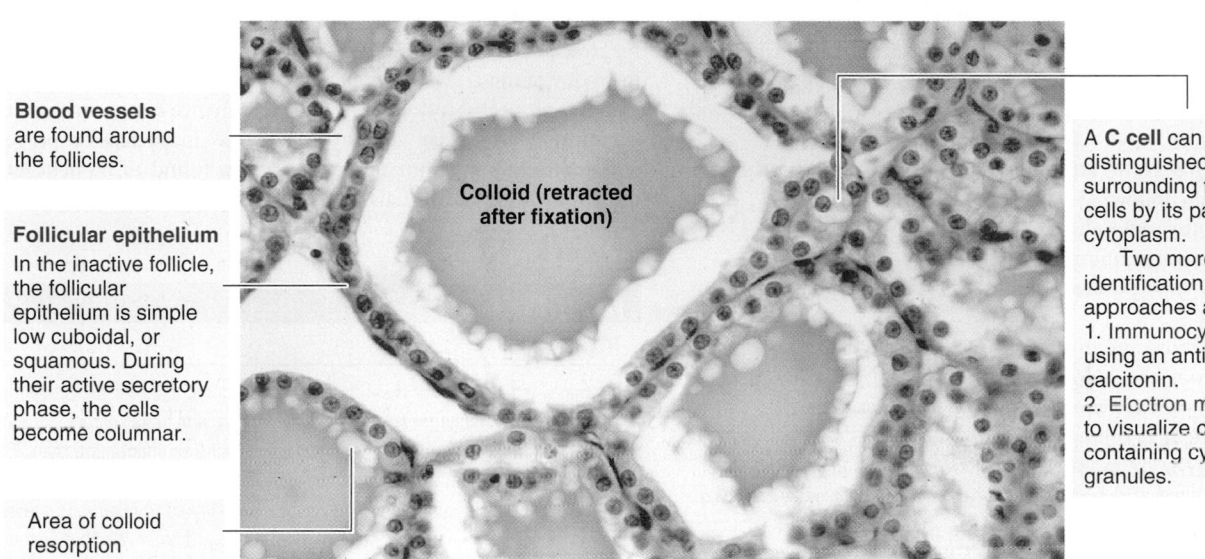

Blood vessels are found around the follicles.

Follicular epithelium In the inactive follicle, the follicular epithelium is simple low cuboidal, or squamous. During their active secretory phase, the cells become columnar.

Area of colloid resorption

Colloid (retracted after fixation)

A **C cell** can be distinguished from surrounding follicular cells by its pale cytoplasm.
Two more effective identification approaches are:
1. Immunocytochemistry, using an antibody to calcitonin.
2. Electron microscopy, to visualize calcitonin-containing cytoplasmic granules.

FIGURE 18-12 Thyroid Follicle Cells.

TABLE 18-6 Thyroid Gland Hormones and Their Regulation and Functions

Hormone	Regulation	Functions

Thyroxine (T_4) and triiodothyronine (T_3)	T_4 and T_3 levels are controlled by TSH; released in response to metabolic demand
	Influences on amount secreted:
	  Gender
	  Pregnancy
	  Gonadal- and adrenocortical-increased steroids = ↑ levels
	  Exposure to extreme cold = ↑ levels
	  Nutritional state
	  Chemicals
	  GHIH = ↓ levels
	  Dopamine = ↓ levels
	  Catecholamines = ↑ levels
		Regulates protein, fat, and carbohydrate catabolism in all cells
		Regulates metabolic rate of all cells
		Regulates body heat production
		Insulin antagonist
		Maintains growth hormone secretion, skeletal maturation
		Affects CNS development
		Necessary for muscle tone and vigor
		Maintains cardiac rate, force, and output
		Maintains secretion of GI tract
		Affects respiratory rate and oxygen utilization
		Maintains calcium mobilization
		Affects RBC production
		Stimulates lipid turnover, free fatty acid release, and cholesterol synthesis

Calcitonin	Elevated serum calcium level—major stimulant for calcitonin
	Other stimulants:
	  Gastrin
	  Calcium-rich foods (regardless of serum Ca^{++} levels)
	  Pregnancy
	Lowered serum calcium level—suppresses calcitonin release
		Lowers serum calcium level by opposing bone-resorbing effects of PTH, prostaglandins, and calciferols by inhibiting osteoclastic activity
		Lowers serum phosphate levels
		Decreases calcium and phosphorous absorption in GI tract

From Monohan FD et al: *Phipps' medical-surgical nursing: health and illness perspective*, ed 8, St Louis, 2007, Mosby.
CNS, Central nervous system; *GHIH,* growth hormone–inhibiting hormone; *GI,* gastrointestinal; *PTH,* parathyroid hormone; *RBC,* red blood cell; *TSH,* thyroid-stimulating hormone.

which is synthesized and stored within the hypothalamus. TRH is released into the hypothalamic-pituitary portal system and circulates to the anterior pituitary, where it stimulates the release of thyroid-stimulating hormone (TSH). TRH levels increase with exposure to cold or stress and from decreased levels of thyroxine (T_4).

TSH is a glycoprotein synthesized and stored within the anterior pituitary. When TSH is secreted by the anterior pituitary, it circulates to bind with receptors on the plasma membrane of the thyroid follicular cells. The primary effect of TSH on the thyroid gland is to cause an immediate release of stored TH and an increase in TH synthesis. TSH also increases growth of the thyroid gland by stimulating thymocyte hyperplasia and hypertrophy. As TH levels rise, there is a negative-feedback effect on the HPA to inhibit TRH and TSH release, which then results in decreased TH synthesis and secretion. TH synthesis is also controlled by serum iodide levels and by circulating selenium-dependent enzymes, called deiodinases, which inactivate the precursor molecule thyroxine.[21] Thyroid gland hormones and their regulation and function are summarized in Table 18-6.

Synthesis of thyroid hormone. Thyroid hormone synthesis is summarized in the following steps:
1. Uniodinated thyroglobulin (a large glycoprotein) is produced by the endoplasmic reticulum of the thyroid follicular cells.
2. Tyrosine is incorporated into the thyroglobulin as it is synthesized.
3. Iodide (the inorganic form of iodine) is actively transferred (pumped) from the blood into the colloid by carrier proteins located in the outer membrane of the follicular cells. This active transport system is called the iodide trap and is very efficient at accumulating the trace amounts of iodide from the blood.
4. Iodide is oxidized and quickly attaches to tyrosine within the thyroglobulin molecule.
5. Coupling of iodinated tyrosine forms thyroid hormones. Triiodothyronine (T_3) is formed from coupling of monoiodotyrosine (one iodine atom and tyrosine) and diiodotyrosine (two iodine atoms and tyrosine). Tetraiodothyronine (T_4), commonly known as thyroxine, is formed from coupling of two diiodotyrosines.
6. Thyroid hormones are stored attached to thyroglobulin within the colloid until they are released into the circulation.

The thyroid gland normally produces 90% T_4 and 10% T_3. Once released into the circulation, T_3 and T_4 are primarily transported bound to thyroxine-binding globulin, though some TH is transported by thyroxine-binding prealbumin (transthyretin), albumin, or lipoproteins. The bound form serves as a reservoir while the unbound form is active. In the body tissues, most of the T_4 is converted to T_3, which acts on the target cell.[22]

Actions of thyroid hormone. TH has a significant effect on the growth, maturation, and function of cells and tissues throughout the body. TH is essential for normal growth and neurologic development in the fetus and infant and affects metabolic, neurologic, cardiovascular, and respiratory functioning across the lifespan. In addition, TH is required for the metabolism and function of blood cells as well as normal muscle functioning and the integrity of skin, nails, and hair. Similar to some steroid hormones, TH binds to intracellular receptor complexes and then influences the genetic expression of specific proteins. TH also affects cell metabolism by altering protein, fat, and glucose metabolism and, as a result, increasing heat production and oxygen consumption. Additionally, TH has permissive effects throughout the body by optimizing the actions of other hormones and neurotransmitters (see Table 18-6). Use of TH and its analogs is being explored for the therapy of many metabolic disorders such as obesity and type 2 diabetes mellitus.[23]

Parathyroid Glands

Normally two pairs of small parathyroid glands are present behind the upper and lower poles of the thyroid gland (see Figure 18-11). However, their number may range from two to six.

The parathyroid glands produce **parathyroid hormone (PTH)**, which is the single most important factor in the regulation of serum calcium concentration. The overall effect of PTH secretion is to increase serum calcium concentration and decrease the level of serum phosphate. A decrease in serum-ionized calcium level stimulates PTH secretion. PTH acts directly on the bone to release calcium by stimulating osteoclast activity. PTH also acts on the kidney to increase calcium reabsorption while phosphate reabsorption is decreased. The resultant increase in serum calcium concentration inhibits PTH secretion. Paradoxically, when PTH is administered intermittently and at a low dose, it stimulates bone formation. This observation led to the use of PTH for treatment of osteoporosis. **1,25-Dihydroxy-vitamin D₃** (the active form of vitamin D) works as a cofactor with PTH to promote calcium and phosphate absorption in the gut and enhance bone mineralization. Vitamin D also plays an important role in metabolic processes and controlling inflammation. It has been found to be deficient in the majority of individuals in the United States (see *Health Alert: Vitamin D*).

HEALTH ALERT
Vitamin D

Vitamin D is essential for bone health and is widely used for the prevention and treatment of postmenopausal osteoporosis and renal osteodystrophy. More recently, vitamin D deficiency has been found to affect more than 75% of all Americans, and more than 90% of Americans with pigmented skin. Inadequate serum levels of vitamin D have been linked to infections, cancer, heart disease, dementia, diabetes, chronic pain syndromes, and autoimmune disorders. Controversies continue as to whether these associations indicate a direct cause and effect between low levels of vitamin D and the pathophysiology of these diseases, and whether vitamin D supplementation reduces risk or improves outcomes. However, many health organizations recommend increased intake of vitamin D–containing foods (seafood, vitamin D–fortified juices, and milk products), increased exposure to sunlight, and supplementation with vitamin D. The Institute of Medicine currently recommends 400 to 600 units of vitamin D per day for adults with a goal of achieving a serum level of 35 to 50 ng/mL.

Data from Balvers MG et al: *J Nutr Sci* 4:e23, 2015; Guessous I: *Biomed Res Int* 2015;2015:563403, 2015; Mozos I, Marginean O: *Biomed Res Int* 2015:109275, 2015; Berridge MJ: *Biochem Biophys Res Commun* 460(1):53-71, 2015; Schöttker B, Brenner H: *Nutrients* 7(5):3264-3278, 2015.

Phosphate and magnesium concentrations also affect PTH secretion. An increase in serum phosphate level decreases serum calcium level by causing calcium-phosphate precipitation into soft tissue and bone, which indirectly stimulates PTH secretion. Hypomagnesemia in persons with normal calcium levels acts as a mild stimulant to PTH secretion; however, in persons with hypocalcemia, hypomagnesemia decreases PTH secretion.[24]

✔QUICK CHECK 18-3
1. How does the anterior pituitary regulate the thyroid gland?
2. What form of thyroid hormone is biologically active?
3. What two organs are the sites of action of parathyroid hormone (PTH)?

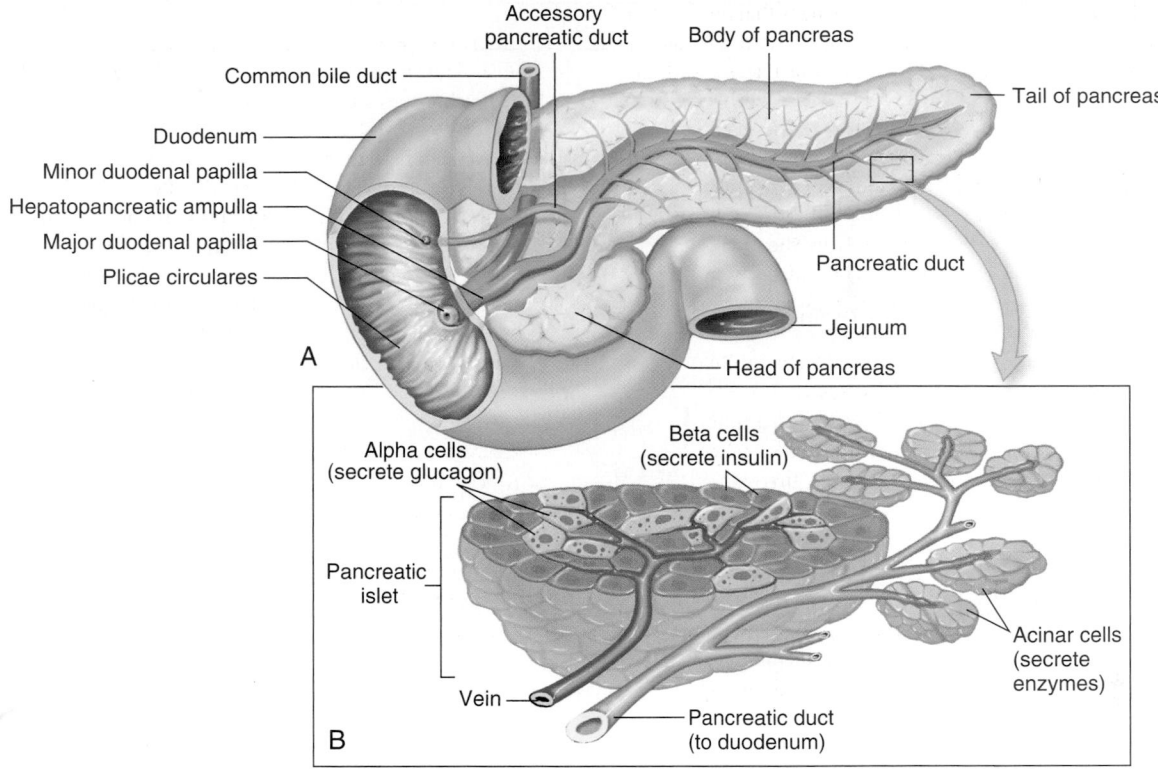

FIGURE 18-13 The Pancreas. A, Pancreas dissected to show main and accessory ducts. The main duct may join the common bile duct, as shown here, to enter the duodenum by a single opening at the major duodenal papilla, or the two ducts may have separate openings. The accessory pancreatic duct is usually present and has a separate opening into the duodenum. **B,** Exocrine glandular cells (around small pancreatic ducts) and endocrine glandular cells of the pancreatic islets (adjacent to blood capillaries). Exocrine pancreatic cells secrete pancreatic juice, alpha endocrine cells secrete glucagon, and beta cells secrete insulin. (From Patton KT, Thibodeau GA: *Structure & function of the body,* ed 15, St Louis, 2016, Mosby.)

Endocrine Pancreas

The pancreas is both an endocrine gland that produces hormones and an exocrine gland that produces digestive enzymes. (The exocrine function of the pancreas is discussed in Chapter 35.) The pancreas is located behind the stomach, between the spleen and the duodenum, and houses the islets of Langerhans. The islets of Langerhans have four types of hormone-secreting cells: alpha cells, which secrete glucagon; beta cells, which secrete insulin and amylin; delta cells, which secrete gastrin and somatostatin; and F (or PP) cells, which secrete pancreatic polypeptide. These hormones regulate carbohydrate, fat, and protein metabolism. (The pancreas is illustrated in Figure 18-13.) Nerves from both the sympathetic and the parasympathetic divisions of the autonomic nervous system innervate the pancreatic islets.

Insulin

The beta cells of the pancreas synthesize insulin from the precursor proinsulin, which is formed from a larger precursor molecule, preproinsulin. Proinsulin is composed of A peptide and B peptide connected by a C peptide and two disulfide bonds. C peptide is cleaved by proteolytic enzymes, leaving the bonded A and B peptides as the insulin molecule. Insulin circulates freely in the plasma and is not bound to a carrier. C peptide level can be measured in the blood and used as an indirect measurement of serum insulin synthesis.

Secretion of insulin is regulated by chemical, hormonal, and neural control. Insulin secretion is pulsatile, increasing when the beta cells are stimulated by the parasympathetic nervous system usually before eating a meal. Other factors stimulating insulin secretion include increased blood levels of glucose, amino acids (leucine, arginine, and lysine), and gastrointestinal hormones (glucagon, gastrin, cholecystokinin, secretin). Insulin secretion diminishes in response to low blood levels of glucose (hypoglycemia), high levels of insulin (through negative feedback to the beta cells), and sympathetic stimulation of the beta cells in the islets. Prostaglandins also inhibit insulin secretion.

At the target cell, insulin signaling is initiated when insulin binds and activates its cell surface receptor. These receptors are found on cells throughout the body. Insulin promotes cellular glucose uptake through glucose transporters (GLUT). An intracellular cascade of phosphorylation events, protein-protein interactions, and second-messenger generation then occurs, resulting in diverse metabolic events throughout the body[25] (see details in Figure 18-14).

The sensitivity of the insulin receptor is a key component in maintaining normal cellular function. Insulin sensitivity is affected by age, weight, abdominal fat, and physical activity. Insulin resistance has been implicated in numerous diseases, including hypertension, heart disease, and type 2 diabetes mellitus. Adipocytes release a number of hormones and cytokines that are altered in obesity and have an important impact on insulin sensitivity. The most effective measures shown to improve insulin sensitivity in humans are weight loss and exercise.[26]

Insulin is an anabolic hormone that promotes glucose uptake primarily in liver, muscle, and adipose tissue. It also increases the synthesis of proteins, carbohydrates, lipids, and nucleic acids. It functions mainly in the liver, muscle, and adipose tissue. Table 18-7 summarizes the

FIGURE 18-14 Insulin Action on Cells. Binding of insulin to its receptor causes autophosphorylation of the receptor, which then itself acts as a tyrosine kinase that phosphorylates insulin receptor substrates 1-4 (*IRS-1-4.* Numerous target enzymes, such as protein kinase B and MAP kinase, are activated and these enzymes have a multitude of effects on cell function. The glucose transporter *(GLUT4)* is recruited to the plasma membrane, where it facilitates glucose entry into the cell. The transport of amino acids, potassium, magnesium, and phosphate into the cell is also facilitated. The synthesis of various enzymes is induced or suppressed, and cell growth is regulated by signal molecules that modulate gene expression. (Redrawn from Levy MN et al, editors: *Berne & Levy principles of physiology,* ed 4, St Louis, 2006, Mosby.)

TABLE 18-7 Insulin Actions

| | SITES OF INSULIN ACTION | | |
Actions	Liver Cells	Muscle Cells	Adipose Cells
Glucose uptake	Increased	Increased	Increased
Glucose use	—	—	Increased glycerol phosphate
Glycogenesis	Increased	Increased	—
Glycogenolysis	Decreased	Decreased	—
Glycolysis	Increased	Increased	Increased
Gluconeogenesis	Increased	—	—
Other	Increased fatty acid synthesis	Increased amino acid uptake	Increased fat esterification
	Decreased ketogenesis	Increased protein synthesis	Decreased lipolysis
	Decreased urea cycle activity	Decreased proteolysis	Increased fat storage

actions of insulin. The net effect of insulin in these tissues is to stimulate protein and fat synthesis and decrease blood glucose level. The brain, red blood cells, kidney, and lens of the eye do not require insulin for glucose transport. Insulin also facilitates the intracellular transport of potassium (K^+), phosphate, and magnesium.

Amylin

Amylin (or islet amyloid polypeptide) is a peptide hormone co-secreted with insulin by beta cells in response to nutrient stimuli. It regulates blood glucose concentration by delaying gastric emptying and suppressing glucagon secretion after meals. Amylin also has a satiety effect, which reduces food intake. Through these mechanisms, amylin has an antihyperglycemic effect.[27]

Glucagon

Glucagon is produced by the alpha cells of the pancreas and by cells lining the gastrointestinal tract. Glucagon acts primarily in the liver and increases blood glucose concentration by stimulating glycogenolysis and gluconeogenesis in muscle and lipolysis in adipose tissue. Amino acids, such as alanine, glycine, and asparagine, stimulate glucagon secretion. Glucagon release is inhibited by high glucose levels and stimulated by low glucose levels and sympathetic stimulation; thus it is antagonistic to insulin.[28]

Pancreatic Somatostatin

Somatostatin is produced by delta cells of the pancreas in response to food intake and is essential in carbohydrate, fat, and protein metabolism. It is different from hypothalamic somatostatin, which inhibits the release of growth hormone and TSH. Pancreatic somatostatin is involved in regulating alpha-cell and beta-cell function within the islets by inhibiting secretion of insulin, glucagon, and pancreatic polypeptide.[29]

Gastrin, Ghrelin, and Pancreatic Polypeptide

Pancreatic gastrin stimulates the secretion of gastric acid. It is postulated that fetal pancreatic gastrin secretion is necessary for adequate islet cell development. Ghrelin stimulates GH secretion, controls appetite, and plays a role in obesity and the regulation of insulin sensitivity. Pancreatic polypeptide is released by F cells in response to hypoglycemia and protein-rich meals. It inhibits gallbladder contraction and exocrine pancreas secretion and is frequently increased in individuals with pancreatic tumors or diabetes mellitus.[30]

Adrenal Glands

The adrenal glands are paired, pyramid-shaped organs behind the peritoneum and close to the upper pole of each kidney. Each gland is surrounded by a capsule, embedded in fat, and well supplied with blood from the aorta and phrenic and renal arteries. Venous return from the left adrenal gland is to the renal vein and from the right adrenal gland is to the inferior vena cava.

Each adrenal gland consists of two separate portions—an outer cortex and an inner medulla. These two portions have different embryonic origins, structures, and hormonal functions. The adrenal cortex and medulla function like two separate but interrelated glands (Figure 18-15).

Adrenal Cortex

The adrenal cortex accounts for 80% of the weight of the adult gland. The cortex is histologically subdivided into the following three zones[31]:

1. The zona glomerulosa, the outer layer, constitutes about 15% of the cortex and primarily produces the mineralocorticoid aldosterone.
2. The zona fasciculata, the middle layer, constitutes 78% of the cortex and secretes the glucocorticoids cortisol, cortisone, and corticosterone.
3. The zona reticularis, the inner layer, constitutes 7% of the cortex and secretes mineralocorticoids (aldosterone), adrenal androgens and estrogens, and glucocorticoids.

The cells of the adrenal cortex are stimulated by adrenocorticotropic hormone (ACTH) from the pituitary gland. All hormones of the adrenal cortex are synthesized from cholesterol. The best known

FIGURE 18-15 Structure of the Adrenal Gland Showing Cell Layers (Zonae) of the Cortex. A, Adrenal glands. Each gland consists of cortex and medulla. The cortex has three layers: zona glomerulosa, zona fasciculata, and zona reticularis. **B,** A portion of the medulla is visible at the lower right in the photomicrograph (× 35) and at the bottom of the drawing. (**A** from Damjanov I: *Pathophysiology,* Philadelphia, 2008, Saunders; **B** from Kierszenbaum A: *Histology and cell biology,* St Louis, 2002, Mosby.)

pathway of steroidogenesis involves the conversion of cholesterol to pregnenolone, which is then converted to the major corticosteroids.

Glucocorticoids

Functions of the glucocorticoids. The glucocorticoids are steroid hormones that have metabolic, neurologic, anti-inflammatory, and growth-suppressing effects. These functions (Figure 18-16) have direct effects on carbohydrate metabolism. These hormones increase blood glucose concentration by promoting gluconeogenesis in the liver and by decreasing uptake of glucose into muscle cells, adipose cells, and lymphatic cells. In extrahepatic tissues, the glucocorticoids stimulate protein catabolism and inhibit amino acid uptake and protein synthesis. The ultimate effect on the body is protein catabolism.

The glucocorticoids act at several sites to suppress immune and inflammatory reactions. One major immunosuppressant effect is the glucocorticoid-mediated decrease in the proliferation of T lymphocytes, primarily T-helper lymphocytes. There is a greater effect on T-helper 1 (Th1) cytokine production (including antiviral interferons) than there is on T-helper 2 (Th2) cytokine production and therefore greater depression of cellular immunity than humoral immunity (see Chapter 7). Glucocorticoids affect innate immunity through several pathways, including decreasing the activity of pattern receptors on the surface of macrophages (see Chapter 6). Anti-inflammatory effects of glucocorticoids also include decreased function of natural killer cells, suppression of inflammatory cytokines, and stabilization of lysosomal membranes, which decreases the release of proteolytic enzymes. The pro-inflammatory effects of glucocorticoids are not clearly understood.[31] Psychological and physiologic stress increases glucocorticoid production, which provides a pathway for the well-described decrease in immunity seen in both acute and chronic stress conditions (see Chapter 9). Use of glucocorticoids for the treatment of disease also leads to suppression of innate and adaptive immunity and the challenging complications of infection and poor wound healing (see Chapter 8).

Other effects of glucocorticoids include inhibition of bone formation, inhibition of ADH secretion, and stimulation of gastric acid secretion. Glucocorticoids appear to potentiate the effects of catecholamines, including sensitizing the arterioles to the vasoconstrictive effects of norepinephrine. Thyroid hormone and growth hormone effects on adipose tissue are also potentiated by glucocorticoids. A metabolite of cortisol may act like a barbiturate and depress nerve cell function in the brain, accounting for the noted effects on mood, such as anxiety and depression, associated with steroid level fluctuation in disease or stress.

Pathologically high levels of glucocorticoids increase the number of circulating erythrocytes (leading to polycythemia), increase the appetite, promote fat deposition in the face and cervical areas, increase uric acid excretion, decrease serum calcium levels (possibly by inhibiting gastrointestinal absorption of calcium), suppress the secretion and synthesis of ACTH, and interfere with the action of growth hormone so that somatic growth is inhibited (see Chapter 19).

Cortisol. The most potent naturally occurring glucocorticoid is cortisol. It is the main secretory product of the adrenal cortex and is needed to maintain life and protect the body from stress (see Figure 9-2). The liver is primarily responsible for the deactivation of cortisol.

Cortisol secretion is regulated primarily by the hypothalamus and the anterior pituitary gland (Figure 18-17). Corticotropin-releasing hormone (CRH) is produced by several nuclei in the hypothalamus and stored in the median eminence. Once released, CRH travels through the portal vessels to stimulate the production of ACTH, β-lipotropin, γ-lipotropin, endorphins, and enkephalins by the anterior pituitary. ACTH is the main regulator of cortisol secretion and adrenocortical growth.

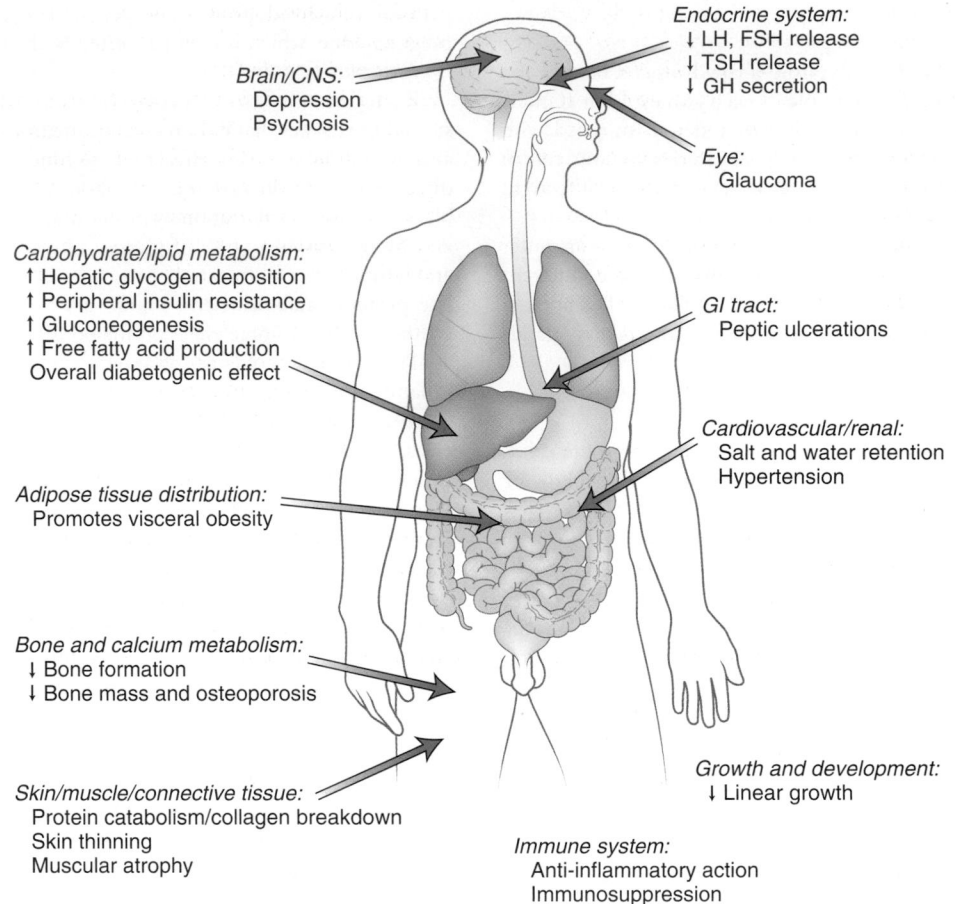

FIGURE 18-16 Effects of Glucocorticoids on the Body. (From Stewart PM, Krone NP: The adrenal cortex. In Melmed S et al, editors: *Williams textbook of endocrinology,* ed 12, Philadelphia, 2011, Saunders.)

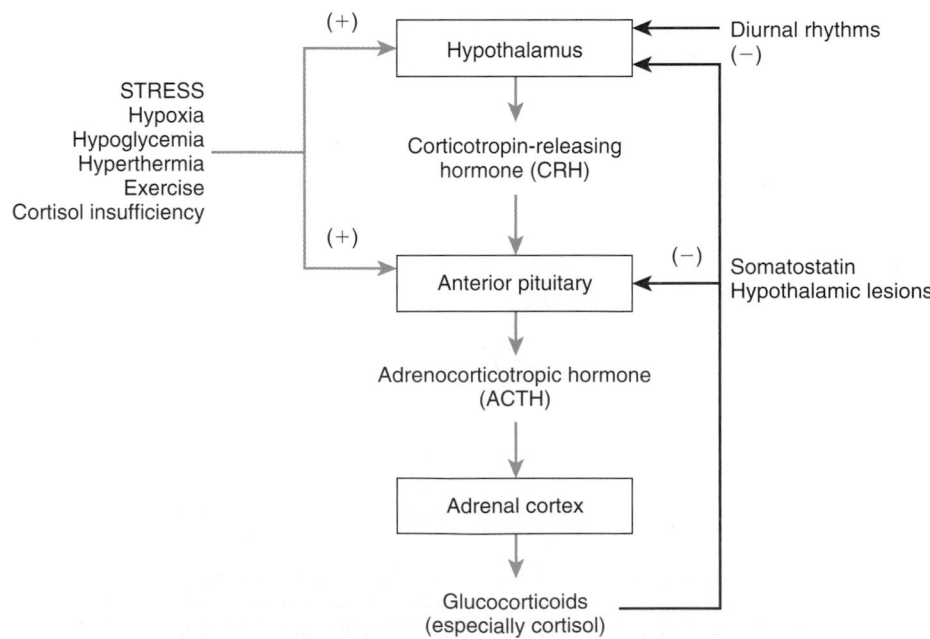

FIGURE 18-17 Feedback Control of Glucocorticoid Synthesis and Secretion.

ACTH is synthesized as part of a precursor called proopiomelano-cortin (POMC). Three factors appear to be primarily involved in regulating the secretion of ACTH: (1) negative-feedback effects of high circulating levels of cortisol and synthetic glucocorticoids suppress both CRH and ACTH, whereas low cortisol levels stimulate their secretion; (2) diurnal rhythms affect ACTH and cortisol levels (in persons with regular sleep-wake patterns, ACTH peaks 3 to 5 hours after sleep begins and declines throughout the day, and cortisol levels follow a similar pattern); and (3) psychological and physiologic (e.g., hypoxia, hypoglycemia, hyperthermia, exercise) stress increases ACTH secretion, leading to increased cortisol levels. (Neurologic mechanisms regulating sleep are discussed in Chapter 14.) A form of immunoreactive ACTH (irACTH) is produced by the cells of the immune system and may account, in part, for integration of the immune and endocrine systems.

Once ACTH is secreted, it binds to specific plasma membrane receptors on the cells of the adrenal cortex and on other extra-adrenal tissues. Because both adrenal and extra-adrenal tissues have ACTH receptors, a number of effects result from stimulation by ACTH. In addition to increasing adrenocortical secretion of cortisol, ACTH maintains the size and synthetic functions of the adrenal cortex through activation of crucial enzymes and storage of cholesterol for metabolism into steroid hormones. Extra-adrenal effects of ACTH include stimulation of melanocytes and activation of tissue lipase.

Once ACTH stimulates the cells of the adrenal cortex, cortisol synthesis and secretion immediately occur. In the healthy person, the secretory patterns of ACTH and cortisol are nearly identical. After secretion, some cortisol circulates in bound form attached to albumin but primarily it is bound to the plasma protein transcortin. A smaller amount circulates in the free form and diffuses into cells with specific intracellular receptors for cortisol. ACTH is rapidly inactivated in the circulation, and the liver and kidneys remove the deactivated hormone.

Mineralocorticoids: aldosterone. Mineralocorticoid steroids directly affect ion transport by epithelial cells, causing sodium retention and potassium and hydrogen loss. **Aldosterone** is the most potent naturally occurring mineralocorticoid and conserves sodium by increasing the activity of the sodium pump of epithelial cells. (The sodium pump is described in Chapter 1.)

The initial stages of aldosterone synthesis occur in the zona fasciculata and zona reticularis. The final conversion of corticosterone to aldosterone is confined to the zona glomerulosa. Aldosterone synthesis and secretion is regulated primarily by the renin-angiotensin system (described in Chapter 29). The renin-angiotensin system is activated by sodium and water depletion, increased potassium levels, and a diminished effective blood volume (Figure 18-18). Angiotensin II is

FIGURE 18-18 The Feedback Mechanisms Regulating Aldosterone Secretion. *ACTH,* Adrenocorticotropic hormone; *cAMP,* cyclic adenosine monophosphate.

the primary stimulant of aldosterone synthesis and secretion; however, sodium and potassium levels also may directly affect aldosterone secretion. ACTH may transiently stimulate aldosterone synthesis but does not appear to be a major regulator of secretion.

When sodium and potassium levels are within normal limits, approximately 50 to 250 mg of aldosterone is secreted daily. Of the secreted aldosterone, 50% to 75% binds to plasma proteins. The large proportion of unbound aldosterone contributes to its rapid metabolic turnover in the liver, its low plasma concentration, and its short half-life (about 15 minutes). Aldosterone is degraded in the liver and is excreted by the kidney.

Aldosterone maintains extracellular volume by acting on distal nephron epithelial cells to increase reabsorption of sodium and excretion of potassium and hydrogen. This renal effect takes 90 minutes to 6 hours. Fluid and electrolyte regulation is addressed in more detail in Chapter 5. Other effects of aldosterone include enhancement of cardiac muscle contraction, stimulation of ectopic ventricular activity through secondary cardiac pacemakers in the ventricles, stiffening of blood vessels with increased vascular resistance, and decrease in fibrinolysis. Pathologically elevated levels of aldosterone have been implicated in the myocardial changes associated with heart failure, resistant hypertension, insulin resistance, and systemic inflammation.[32]

Adrenal estrogens and androgens. The healthy adrenal cortex secretes minimal amounts of estrogen and androgens. ACTH appears to be the major regulator. Some of the weakly androgenic substances secreted by the cortex (dehydroepiandrosterone [DHEA], androstenedione) are converted by peripheral tissues to stronger androgens, such as testosterone, thus accounting for some androgenic effects initiated by the adrenal cortex. Peripheral conversion of adrenal androgens to estrogens is enhanced in aging or obese persons as well as in those with liver disease or hyperthyroidism.[33] The biologic effects and metabolism of the adrenal sex steroids do not vary from those produced by the gonads (see Chapter 32).

Adrenal Medulla

The chromaffin cells (pheochromocytes) of the adrenal medulla secrete and store the catecholamines epinephrine (adrenaline) and norepinephrine (noradrenaline). Both are synthesized from the amino acid phenylalanine (Figure 18-19). The adrenal medulla, together with the sympathetic division of the autonomic nervous system, is embryonically derived from neural crest cells. Only 30% of circulating epinephrine comes from the adrenal medulla; the other 70% is released from nerve terminals. The medulla is only a minor source of norepinephrine. The adrenal medulla functions as a sympathetic ganglion without postganglionic processes. Sympathetic cholinergic preganglion fibers terminate on the chromaffin cells and secrete catecholamines directly into the bloodstream. The catecholamines acting in the blood are therefore hormones and not neurotransmitters.

Physiologic stress to the body (e.g., traumatic injury, hypoxia, hypoglycemia, and many others) triggers release of adrenal catecholamines through acetylcholine (from the preganglionic sympathetic fibers), which depolarizes the chromaffin cells (see Chapter 9). Depolarization causes exocytosis of the storage granules from the chromaffin cells with release of epinephrine and norepinephrine into the bloodstream. Secretion of adrenal catecholamines also is increased by ACTH and the glucocorticoids.[34]

Once released, the catecholamines remain in the plasma for only seconds to minutes. The catecholamines exert their biologic effects after binding to plasma membrane receptors (α_1, α_2, β_1, β_2,

FIGURE 18-19 Synthesis of Catecholamines.

and β_3) in target cells. This binding activates the adenylyl cyclase system. Catecholamines are rapidly removed from the plasma by being absorbed by neurons for storage in new cytoplasmic granules, or they may be metabolically inactivated and excreted in the urine. The catecholamines directly inhibit their own secretion by decreasing the formation of the enzyme tyrosine hydroxylase (the rate-limiting step).

Catecholamines have diverse effects on the entire body. Their release and the body's response have been characterized as the "fight or flight" response (stress response) (see Figures 9-2 and 9-3 and Tables 9-3 and 9-4). Metabolic effects of catecholamines promote hyperglycemia through a variety of mechanisms including interference with the usual glucose regulatory feedback mechanisms.

✔ **QUICK CHECK 18-4**

1. What are the islets of Langerhans? Where are they located?
2. Compare and contrast the actions of alpha, beta, delta, and F cells.
3. What is the most potent naturally occurring glucocorticoid, and how is its secretion related to that of adrenocorticotropic hormone (ACTH)?
4. How does aldosterone influence fluid and electrolyte balance?
5. What are catecholamines?

GERIATRIC CONSIDERATIONS

Aging & Its Effects on Specific Endocrine Glands

General Endocrine Changes with Aging

Aging has many effects on the neuroendocrine system. There are complex changes within the hypothalamic/pituitary axis; and altered biologic activity of hormones, altered circulating levels of hormones, altered secretory response of the endocrine glands, altered metabolism of hormones, and loss of circadian control of hormone secretion are among the findings.

Pituitary

Posterior: Decrease in size; reduced antidiuretic hormone (ADH) secretion.

Anterior: Increased fibrosis and moderate increase in size of gland; decline in growth hormone release.

Thyroid

Glandular atrophy, fibrosis, nodularity, and increased inflammatory infiltrates; decreased T_4 secretion and turnover, decline in T_3 (especially in men), diminished thyroid-stimulating hormone (TSH) secretion; reduced response of plasma TSH concentration to thyroid-releasing hormone (TRH) administration (especially in men).

Growth Hormone and Insulin-like Growth Factors

The amounts of GH and IGF decline with aging, which contributes to decreases in muscle size and function, reduced fat and bone mass, and changes in reproductive and cognitive function. Increased visceral fat, decreased lean body mass, and decreased bone density are common in older adults.

Pancreas

It is common for older individuals to have glucose intolerance or diabetes, and these disorders frequently are undiagnosed in aging adults. Mechanisms include decreased insulin receptor activity and decreased beta-cell secretion of insulin.

Adrenal

Decreased DHEA levels lead to decreased synthesis of androgen-derived estrogen and testosterone; decreased metabolic clearance of glucocorticoids and cortisol causes decreased cortisol secretion; there also are decreased levels of aldosterone. Circadian patterns of ACTH and cortisol secretion may change with aging.

Gonads

Postmenopausal women have decreased estrogen and progesterone, increased follicle-stimulating hormone, and relative increases in androgen levels; these changes have numerous physiologic and pathophysiologic consequences (see Chapter 32); in men there is a gradual decrease in serum testosterone levels, leading to decreased sexual activity, decreased muscle strength, and decreased bone mineralization.

■ DID YOU UNDERSTAND?

Mechanisms of Hormonal Regulation

1. The endocrine system has diverse functions, including sexual differentiation, growth and development, and continuous maintenance of the body's internal environment and responses to stress.
2. Hormones are chemical messengers synthesized by endocrine glands and when released have intracrine, autocrine, paracrine and endocrine effects.
3. Hormones have specific negative- and positive-feedback mechanisms. Most hormone levels are regulated by negative feedback, in which hormone secretion raises the level of a specific hormone, ultimately causing secretion to subside, maintaining the hormone within a normal physiologic range.
4. Endocrine feedback is described in terms of short, long, and ultra-short feedback loops.
5. Water-soluble hormones circulate throughout the body in unbound form, whereas lipid-soluble hormones (e.g., steroid and thyroid hormones) circulate throughout the body bound to carrier proteins.
6. Hormones affect only target cells with appropriate receptors and then act on these cells to initiate specific cell functions or activities.
7. Hormones have two general types of effects on cells: (1) direct effects, or obvious changes in cell function, and (2) permissive effects, or less obvious changes that facilitate cell function.
8. Receptors for hormones may be located on the plasma membrane or in the intracellular compartment of a target cell.
9. Water-soluble hormones act as first messengers, binding to receptors in the cell's plasma membrane. The signals initiated by hormone-receptor binding are then transmitted into the cell by the action of second messengers (i.e., cAMP, cGMP, or tyrosine kinase) and mediate the action of the hormone on the target cell (i.e., protein synthesis or cellular growth).
10. Lipid-soluble hormones (including steroid and thyroid hormones) cross the plasma membrane by diffusion. These hormones diffuse directly into the cell nucleus and bind to nuclear receptors. Rapid responses of steroid hormones may be mediated by plasma membrane receptors.

Structure and Function of the Endocrine Glands

1. The pituitary gland, consisting of anterior and posterior portions, is connected to the central nervous system through the hypothalamus.
2. The hypothalamus regulates anterior pituitary function by secreting releasing or inhibiting hormones and factors into the portal circulation.
3. Hypothalamic hormones include prolactin-releasing factor (PRF), which stimulates secretion of prolactin; prolactin-inhibiting factor (PIF, dopamine), which inhibits prolactin secretion; thyrotropin-releasing hormone (TRH), which affects release of thyroid hormones; growth hormone–releasing hormone (GHRH), which stimulates the release of growth hormone (GH); somatostatin, which inhibits the release of GH; gonadotropin-releasing hormone (GnRH), which facilitates the release of follicle-stimulating hormone (FSH) and luteinizing hormone (LH); corticotropin-releasing hormone (CRH), which facilitates the release of adrenocorticotropic hormone (ACTH) and endorphins; and substance P, which inhibits ACTH release and stimulates the release of a variety of other hormones.

4. Hormones of the anterior pituitary are regulated by (1) secretion of hypothalamic-releasing hormones or factors, (2) negative feedback from hormones secreted by target organs, and (3) mediating effects of neurotransmitters.

5. Hormones of the anterior pituitary include ACTH, melanocyte-stimulating hormone (MSH), somatotropic hormones (growth hormone [GH], prolactin), and glycoprotein hormones—follicle-stimulating hormone (FSH), luteinizing hormone (LH), and thyroid-stimulating hormone (TSH).

6. The posterior pituitary secretes antidiuretic hormone (ADH), which also is called vasopressin, and oxytocin.

7. ADH controls serum osmolality, increases permeability of the renal tubules to water, and causes vasoconstriction when administered pharmacologically in high doses. ADH also may regulate some central nervous system functions.

8. Oxytocin causes uterine contraction and lactation in women and may have a role in sperm motility in men. In both men and women, oxytocin has an antidiuretic effect similar to that of ADH.

9. Melatonin is secreted by the pineal gland and regulates circadian rhythms and reproduction.

10. The two-lobed thyroid gland contains follicles, which secrete some of the thyroid hormones, and C cells, which secrete calcitonin and somatostatin.

11. Regulation of thyroid hormone (TH) levels is complex and involves the hypothalamus, anterior pituitary, thyroid gland, and numerous biochemical variables.

12. Thyroid hormone (TH) secretion is regulated by thyroid-releasing hormone (TRH) through a negative-feedback loop that involves the anterior pituitary and hypothalamus.

13. Thyroid-stimulating hormone (TSH), which is synthesized and stored in the anterior pituitary, stimulates secretion of TH by activating intracellular processes, including uptake of iodine necessary for the synthesis of TH in the thyroid gland.

14. Once secreted, TH acts on the thyroid gland, the anterior pituitary, and the median eminence to regulate further TH production.

15. Synthesis of TH depends on the glycoprotein thyroglobulin (TG), which contains a precursor of TH, tyrosine. Tyrosine then combines with iodine to form precursor molecules of the thyroid hormones thyroxine (T_4) and triiodothyronine (T_3). These hormones are then stored within thyroid colloid until released into the circulation.

16. When released into the circulation, T_3 and T_4 are bound by carrier proteins in the plasma, which store these hormones and provide a buffer for rapid changes in hormone levels. The free form is the active form.

17. Thyroid hormones alter protein synthesis and have a wide range of metabolic effects on proteins, carbohydrates, lipids, vitamins, and other hormones and neurotransmitters. TH also affects heat production and cardiac function.

18. The paired parathyroid glands normally are located behind the upper and lower poles of the thyroid. These glands secrete parathyroid hormone (PTH), an important regulator of serum calcium and phosphate levels.

19. PTH secretion increases levels of ionized calcium and decreases levels of phosphate in the plasma.

20. In bone, PTH causes bone breakdown and resorption. At low doses it can promote bone formation. In the kidney, PTH increases reabsorption of calcium and decreases reabsorption of phosphorus and bicarbonate.

21. The endocrine pancreas contains the islets of Langerhans, which secrete hormones responsible for much of the carbohydrate metabolism in the body.

22. The islets of Langerhans consist of alpha cells, beta cells, delta cells, and F cells, which release hormones that regulate protein, fat, and carbohydrate metabolism.

23. Alpha cells produce glucagon, which is secreted inversely to blood glucose concentrations.

24. Delta cells secrete somatostatin, which inhibits glucagon and insulin secretion.

25. Beta cells secrete preproinsulin, which is ultimately converted to insulin, and amylin, which suppresses glucagon secretion and has a satiety effect.

26. F cells secrete pancreatic polypeptide, which inhibits gallbladder contraction and exocrine pancreatic secretion.

27. Insulin is a hormone that regulates blood glucose concentrations and overall body metabolism of fat, protein, and carbohydrates.

28. The paired adrenal glands are situated above the kidneys. Each gland consists of an adrenal medulla, which secretes catecholamines, and an adrenal cortex, which secretes steroid hormones.

29. The steroid hormones secreted by the adrenal cortex are synthesized from cholesterol. These hormones include glucocorticoids, mineralocorticoids, and adrenal androgens and estrogens.

30. Glucocorticoids directly affect carbohydrate metabolism by increasing blood glucose concentration through gluconeogenesis in the liver and by decreasing use of glucose. Glucocorticoids also inhibit immune and inflammatory responses, suppress growth, and promote protein catabolism.

31. The most potent naturally occurring glucocorticoid is cortisol, which is necessary for the maintenance of life and for protection from stress. Secretion of cortisol is regulated by the hypothalamus and anterior pituitary.

32. Cortisol secretion is related to secretion of adrenocorticotropic hormone (ACTH), which is stimulated by corticotropin-releasing hormone (CRH). ACTH binds with receptors of the adrenal cortex, which activates intracellular mechanisms (specifically cyclic AMP) and leads to cortisol release.

33. Mineralocorticoids are steroid hormones that directly affect ion transport by renal tubular epithelial cells, causing sodium retention and potassium and hydrogen loss.

34. Aldosterone is the most potent of the naturally occurring mineralocorticoids. Its primary role is renal reabsorption of sodium and excretion of potassium and hydrogen.

35. Aldosterone secretion is regulated primarily by the renin-angiotensin system and by the serum sodium concentration.

36. Aldosterone acts by binding to a site on the cell nucleus and altering protein production within the cell. Its principal site of action is the kidney, where it causes sodium reabsorption and potassium and hydrogen excretion.

37. Androgens and estrogens secreted by the adrenal cortex act in the same way as those secreted by the gonads.

38. The adrenal medulla secretes the catecholamines epinephrine and norepinephrine. Epinephrine is 10 times more potent than norepinephrine in exerting metabolic effects. Their release is stimulated by sympathetic nervous system stimulation, ACTH, and glucocorticoids.

39. Catecholamines bind with various target cells and are taken up by neurons or excreted in the urine. They cause a range of metabolic effects characterized as the "fight or flight" response and include hyperglycemia and immunosuppression.

40. The endocrine system acts together with the nervous system to respond to stressors.

41. The response to stressors involves (1) activation of the sympathetic division of the autonomic nervous system and (2) activation of the endocrine system.

42. Other hormones that are secreted in response to stress include growth hormone (GH), prolactin, testosterone, antidiuretic hormone (ADH), and insulin.

43. The adrenal glands and the sympathetic neurons that innervate these glands form the sympathoadrenal axis.

KEY TERMS

Adrenal cortex, 453
Adrenal gland, 453
Adrenal medulla, 456
Adrenocorticotropic hormone (ACTH), 445
Alpha cell, 451
Amylin, 452
Anterior pituitary, 444
Antidiuretic hormone (ADH), 448
Beta cell, 451
C cell, 449
Calcitonin, 449
Chromophil, 445
Chromophobe, 445
Corticotropin-releasing hormone (CRH), 453
Cortisol, 453
Delta cell, 451

1,25-Dihydroxy-vitamin D$_3$, 450
Direct effect, 441
Down-regulation, 441
F (or PP) cell, 451
First messenger, 442
Follicle, 449
Follicle-stimulating hormone (FSH), 445
Gastrin, 452
Ghrelin, 452
Glucagon, 452
Glucocorticoid, 453
Growth hormone (GH), 447
Hormone, 439
Hormone receptor, 442
Hypothalamus, 443
Insulin, 451
Islet of Langerhans, 451
Isthmus, 448
Luteinizing hormone (LH), 445

Median eminence, 448
Melanocyte-stimulating hormone (MSH), 445
Melatonin, 448
Mineralocorticoid, 455
Negative feedback, 439
Oxytocin, 448
Pancreas, 451
Pancreatic polypeptide, 452
Parathyroid hormone (PTH), 450
Pars distalis, 444
Pars intermedia, 445
Pars nervosa, 448
Pars tuberalis, 444
Permissive effect, 441
Pituitary gland, 444
Pituitary stalk, 448
Positive feedback, 440
Posterior pituitary, 447

Prolactin, 447
Second messenger, 442
Somatostatin, 452
Target cell, 440
Thyroid gland, 448
Thyroid hormone (TH), 449
Thyroid-stimulating hormone (TSH), 440
Thyrotropin-releasing hormone (TRH), 440
Thyroxine-binding globulin (TBG), 450
Tropic hormone, 445
Up-regulation, 441
Zona fasciculata, 453
Zona glomerulosa, 453
Zona reticularis, 453

REFERENCES

1. Fujita T et al: Once-weekly injection of low-dose teriparatide (28.2 µg) reduced the risk of vertebral fracture in patients with primary osteoporosis, *Calcif Tissue Int* 94(2):170-175, 2014.
2. Bellavance MA, Rivest S: The HPA-immune axis and the immunomodulatory actions of glucocorticoids in the brain, *Front Immunol* 31(5):136, 2014.
3. Levin ER: Extranuclear steroid receptors are essential for steroid hormoneactions, *Annu Rev Med* 66:271-280, 2015.
4. Spiegel A et al: Mechanisms of action of hormones that act at the cell surface. In Melmed S et al, editors: *Williams textbook of endocrinology*, ed 12, Philadelphia, 2011, Saunders.
5. Das A et al: PDE5 inhibitors as therapeutics for heart disease, diabetes and cancer, *Pharmacol Ther* 147:12-21, 2015.
6. Bubb KJ et al: Inhibition of phosphodiesterase 2 augments cGMP and cAMP signaling to ameliorate pulmonary hypertension, *Circulation* 130(6): 496-507, 2014.
7. Salisbury TB, Tomblin JK: Insulin/Insulin-like growth factors in cancer: new roles for the aryl hydrocarbon receptor, tumor resistance mechanisms, and new blocking strategies, *Front Endocrinol (Lausanne)* 2(6):12, 2015.
8. Miklossy G et al: Therapeutic modulators of STAT signaling for human diseases, *Nat Rev Drug Discov* 12(8):611-629, 2013.
9. Prada PO, Saad MJ: Tyrosine kinase inhibitors as novel drugs for the treatment of diabetes, *Expert Opin Investig Drugs* 22(6):751-763, 2013.
10. Wang C, Liu Y, Cao JM: G protein-coupled receptors: extranuclear mediators for the non-genomic actions of steroids, *Int J Mol Sci* 15(9):15412-15425, 2014.
11. Lazar MA: Mechanism of action of hormones that act on nuclear receptors. In Melmed S et al:

Williams textbook of endocrinology, ed 12, Philadelphia, 2011, Saunders.
12. Annunziata M et al: The IGF system, *Acta Diabetol* 48(1):1-9, 2011.
13. Baxter RC: IGF binding proteins in cancer: mechanistic and clinical insights, *Nat Rev Cancer* 14(5):329-341, 2014.
14. Reed ML et al: Adult growth hormone deficiency—benefits, side effects, and risks of growth hormone replacement, *Front Endocrinol* 4(64):1-14, 2013.
15. Suarez AL et al: Prolactin in inflammatory response, *Adv Exp Med Biol* 846:243-264, 2015.
16. Robinson AG, Verbalis J: Posterior pituitary. In Medmud S et al, editors: *Williams textbook of endocrinology*, ed 12, Philadelphia, 2011, Saunders.
17. Oba Y, Lone NA: Mortality benefit of vasopressor and inotropic agents in septic shock: a Bayesian network meta-analysis of randomized controlled trials, *J Crit Care* 29(5):706-710, 2014.
18. Russell JA: Bench-to-bedside review: vasopressin in the management of septic shock, *Crit Care* 15(4): 226-245, 2011.
19. Lochner A et al: Cardioprotective effect of melatonin against ischaemia/reperfusion damage, *Front Biosci (Elite Ed)* 1(5):305-315, 2013.
20. Anderson G, Maes M. Local melatonin regulates inflammation resolution: a common factor in neurodegenerative, psychiatric and systemic inflammatory disorders, *CNS Neurol Disord Drug Targets* 13(5):817-827, 2014.
21. Verloop H et al: Genetics in endocrinology: genetic variation in deiodinases: a systematic review of potential clinical effects in humans, *Eur J Endocrinol* 171(3):R123-R135, 2014.
22. Salvatore D et al: Thyroid physiology and diagnostic evaluation of patients with thyroid disorders. In Melmed S et al, editors: *Williams textbook of endocrinology*, ed 12, Philadelphia, 2011, Saunders.

23. Shoemaker TJ et al: Thyroid hormone analogues for the treatment of metabolic disorders: new potential for unmet clinical needs? *Endocr Pract* 18(6):954-964, 2012.
24. Castiglioni S et al: Magnesium and osteoporosis: current state of knowledge and future research directions, *Nutrients* 5(8):3022-3033, 2013.
25. Buse JB et al: Type II diabetes mellitus. In Melmed S et al: *Williams textbook of endocrinology*, ed 12, Philadelphia, 2011, Saunders.
26. Conn VS et al: Insulin sensitivity following exercise interventions: systematic review and meta-analysis of outcomes among healthy adults, *J Prim Care Commun Health* 5(3):211-222, 2014.
27. Yang F: Amylin in vasodilation, energy expenditure and inflammation, *Front Biosci (Landmark Ed)* 19:936-944, 2014.
28. Gylfe E, Gilon P: Glucose regulation of glucagon secretion, *Diabetes Res Clin Pract* 103(1):1-10, 2014.
29. Vella A et al: Gastrointestinal hormones and gut endocrine tumors. In Melmed S et al, editors: *Williams textbook of endocrinology*, ed 12, Philadelphia, 2011, Saunders.
30. Stores RD, Cone JK: Neuroendocrine control of energy stores. In Melmed S et al, editors: *Williams textbook of endocrinology*, ed 12, Philadelphia, 2011, Saunders.
31. Stewart PM, Krone NP: The adrenal cortex. In Melmed S et al, editors: *Williams textbook of endocrinology*, ed 12, Philadelphia, 2011, Saunders.
32. Bollag WB: Regulation of aldosterone synthesis and secretion, *Compr Physiol* 4(3):1017-1055, 2014.
33. Lamberts SW: Endocrinology of aging. In Melmed S et al, editors: *Williams textbook of endocrinology*, ed 12, Philadelphia, 2011, Saunders.
34. Young WF: Endocrine hypertension. In Melmed S et al, editors: *Williams textbook of endocrinology*, ed 12, hiladelphia, 2011, Saunders.

19

Alterations of Hormonal Regulation

Valentina L. Brashers, Robert E. Jones, and Sue E. Huether

ⓔ EVOLVE WEBSITE

http://evolve.elsevier.com/Huether/
Student Review Questions
Audio Key Points

Case Studies
Animations
Quick Check Answers

CHAPTER OUTLINE

Functions of the endocrine system involve complex interactions between hormones and most body systems that maintain dynamic steady states and influence tissue growth and reproductive capabilities. Endocrine system dysfunction is usually caused by hypersecretion or hyposecretion of the various hormones, leading to abnormal hormone concentrations in the blood. Dysfunction also may result from abnormal cell receptor function or from altered intracellular response to the hormone-receptor complex.

MECHANISMS OF HORMONAL ALTERATIONS

Significantly elevated or significantly depressed hormone levels may result from various causes (Table 19-1). Dysfunction of an endocrine gland may involve its failure to produce adequate amounts of biologically free or active hormone (hyposecretion), or a gland may synthesize or release too much hormone (hypersecretion). Feedback systems that recognize the need for a particular hormone may fail to function properly or may respond to inappropriate signals. Once hormones are released into the circulation, they may be degraded at an altered rate or be inactivated before reaching the target cell by antibodies that function as circulating hormone inhibitors (e.g., thyroid disease). Other causes of decreased hormone delivery to the target cell include an inadequate blood supply to the gland or target tissues or an insufficient amount of the appropriate carrier proteins in the serum. Ectopic sources of hormones (hormones produced by nonendocrine tissues) may cause abnormally elevated hormone levels without the benefit of the normal feedback system for hormone control (e.g., hormone-

producing tumors); in this case, the ectopic hormone production is said to be autonomous.

Target cells may not respond appropriately to hormonal stimulation for a number of reasons. The following are the two general types of target cell insensitivity to hormones:

1. *Cell surface receptor–associated disorders.* These disorders have been identified primarily in water-soluble hormones, such as insulin. They may involve a decrease in the number of receptors, leading to decreased or defective hormone-receptor binding; impairment of receptor function, resulting in insensitivity to the hormone; presence of antibodies against specific receptors that either reduce available binding sites or mimic hormone action, suppressing or exaggerating, respectively, the target cell response; or unusual expression of receptor function, as occurs in some tumor cells.

2. *Intracellular disorders.* These disorders involve acquired defects in postreceptor signaling cascades or inadequate synthesis of a second messenger, such as cyclic adenosine monophosphate (cAMP), needed to transduce the hormonal signal into intracellular events. The target cell for water-soluble hormones may have a faulty response to hormone-receptor binding and thus fail to generate the required second messenger, or the cell may respond abnormally to the second messenger if levels of intracellular enzymes or proteins are altered. (Second messengers for various hormones are listed in Table 18-3.) As a result, the target cell fails to express the usual hormonal effect (e.g., pseudohypoparathyroidism, see p. 487).

Pathogenic mechanisms affecting target cell response for lipid-soluble hormones are recognized less often than those affecting

TABLE 19-1 **Mechanisms of Hormone Alterations**	
Inappropriate Amounts of Hormone Delivered to Target Cell	**Inappropriate Response by Target Cell**
Inadequate Hormone Synthesis	**Cell Surface Receptor–Associated Disorders**
1. Inadequate quantity of hormone precursors 2. Secretory cell unable to convert precursors to active hormone	1. Decrease in the number of receptors 2. Impaired receptor function (altered affinity for hormones) 3. Presence of antibodies against specific receptors 4. Unusual expression of receptor function
Failure of Feedback Systems 1. Do not recognize positive feedback, leading to inadequate hormone synthesis 2. Do not recognize negative feedback, leading to excessive hormone synthesis	
Inactive Hormones	**Intracellular Disorders**
1. Inadequate biologically free hormone 2. Hormone degraded at an altered rate 3. Circulating inhibitors	1. Acquired defects in postreceptor signaling cascades 2. Inadequate synthesis of a second messenger 3. Intracellular enzymes or proteins are altered 4. Alterations in nuclear co-regulators 5. Altered protein synthesis
Dysfunctional Delivery System 1. Inadequate blood supply 2. Inadequate carrier proteins 3. Ectopic production of hormones	

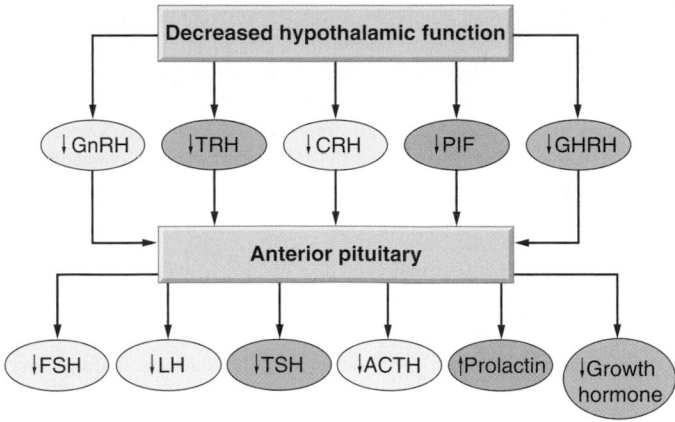

FIGURE 19-1 Loss of Hypothalamic Hormones. *ACTH,* Adrenocorticotropic hormone; *CRH,* corticotropin-releasing hormone; *FSH,* follicle-stimulating hormone; *GHRH,* growth hormone–releasing hormone; *GnRH,* gonadotropin-releasing hormone; *LH,* luteinizing hormone; *PIF,* prolactin inhibitory factor (probably dopamine); *TRH,* thyrotropin-releasing hormone; *TSH,* thyroid-stimulating hormone.

water-soluble hormones. When they do occur, the mechanisms are similar to those for water-soluble hormones, including changes in the number and binding affinity of intracellular receptors or altered generation of new messenger ribonucleic acid (mRNA) and substrates for new protein synthesis. In other cases, hormone responsiveness may be linked to alterations in nuclear co-regulators, which are proteins (such as cAMP response element–binding protein that facilitate or inhibit the transcription of the target gene.[1]

ALTERATIONS OF THE HYPOTHALAMIC-PITUITARY SYSTEM

Perhaps the most common cause of apparent hypothalamic dysfunction is interruption of the pituitary stalk caused by destructive lesions, rupture after head injury, surgical transection, or tumor. In these cases, interruption of the physical connections between the hypothalamus and the pituitary gland causes apparent pituitary disease. For example, without hypothalamic hormones (Figure 19-1), women cease to menstruate and men experience hypogonadism and impaired spermatogenesis. Adrenocorticotropic hormone (ACTH) response to low serum cortisol levels is decreased because of the absence of corticotropin-releasing hormone (CRH). Hypothalamic hypothyroidism is caused by the absence of thyrotropin-releasing hormone (TRH). Low levels of growth hormone–releasing hormone (GHRH) result in growth hormone (GH) deficiency and growth failure in children. Hyperpro-

lactinemia is caused by an absence of the usual inhibitory control of prolactin secretion (dopamine).

Diseases of the Posterior Pituitary

Diseases of the posterior pituitary cause abnormal secretion of antidiuretic hormone (ADH, arginine vasopressin). An excess amount of this hormone results in water retention and a hypoosmolar state, whereas deficiencies in the amount or response to ADH result in serum hyperosmolarity (see Chapter 5). These complex pathophysiologic states not only have significant clinical effects on the modulation of body fluids and electrolytes but also affect cognitive and emotional responses to stress.

Syndrome of Inappropriate Antidiuretic Hormone Secretion

The syndrome of inappropriate ADH secretion (SIADH) is characterized by high levels of ADH in the absence of normal physiologic stimuli for its release. A common cause of SIADH is the ectopic production of ADH by tumors, such as small cell carcinoma of the duodenum, stomach, and pancreas; cancers of the bladder, prostate, and endometrium; lymphomas; and sarcomas. Pulmonary disorders associated with SIADH include bronchogenic carcinoma, pneumonia (e.g., tuberculosis), asthma, cystic fibrosis, and respiratory failure requiring mechanical ventilation. Central nervous system disorders that may cause SIADH include encephalitis, meningitis, intracranial hemorrhage, tumors, and trauma.

Another important cause of SIADH is surgery. Any surgery can result in increased ADH secretion for as long as 5 to 7 days after surgery. The precise mechanism is uncertain but is likely related to fluid and volume changes following surgery, the amount and type of intravenous fluids given, and the use of narcotic analgesics. Transient SIADH also may follow pituitary surgery because stored ADH is released in an unregulated fashion.[2]

Medications are an important cause of SIADH, especially in the elderly. These include hypoglycemic medications (e.g., chlorpropamide), narcotics, general anesthetics, antidepressants, antipsychotics, chemotherapeutic agents, nonsteroidal anti-inflammatory drugs, and synthetic ADH analogs.[3]

PATHOPHYSIOLOGY   The cardinal features of SIADH are the result of enhanced renal water retention. ADH increases renal collecting duct permeability to water by inducing the insertion of aquaporin-2, a water channel protein, into the tubular luminal membrane, which increases water reabsorption by the kidneys.[4] (Renal function is discussed in Chapter 29.) This results in an expansion of extracellular fluid volume that leads to dilutional hyponatremia (low serum sodium concentration), hypoosmolarity, and urine that is inappropriately concentrated with respect to serum osmolarity because water is reabsorbed that normally would be excreted.

CLINICAL MANIFESTATIONS The symptoms of SIADH result from hyponatremia (see Chapter 5) and are determined by its severity and rapidity of onset. Thirst, impaired taste, anorexia, dyspnea on exertion, fatigue, and dulled sensorium occur when the serum sodium level decreases rapidly from 140 to 130 mEq/L. Peripheral edema is absent. Gastrointestinal symptoms, including vomiting and abdominal cramps, occur with a drop in sodium concentration from 130 to 120 mEq/L. There is weight gain from water retention, even with nausea and vomiting. Even if hyponatremia develops slowly, serum sodium levels below 110 to 115 mEq/L cause confusion, lethargy, muscle twitching, and convulsions; severe and sometimes irreversible neurologic damage may occur. Symptoms usually resolve with correction of hyponatremia (see Chapter 5).

EVALUATION AND TREATMENT A diagnosis of SIADH requires the following manifestations: (1) serum hypoosmolality and hyponatremia, (2) urine hyperosmolality (i.e., urine osmolality is greater than expected for the concomitant serum osmolality), (3) urine sodium excretion that matches sodium intake (i.e., sodium excretion is normal in spite of excessive water reabsorption), (4) normal adrenal and thyroid function, and (5) absence of conditions that can alter volume status (e.g., congestive heart failure, hypovolemia from any cause, or renal insufficiency).

The treatment of SIADH involves the correction of any underlying causal problems and fluid restriction with careful monitoring of sodium status and neurologic symptoms. In severe SIADH, emergency correction of severe hyponatremia by careful administration of hypertonic saline may be required. Resolution usually occurs within 3 days, with a 2- to 3-kg weight loss and correction of hyponatremia and salt wasting. If hyponatremia is corrected too rapidly, a severe neurologic syndrome called central pontine myelinolysis can ensue. Demeclocycline, which causes the renal tubules to develop resistance to ADH, may be used to treat resistant or chronic SIADH. Vasopressin (ADH) receptor antagonists, known as vaptans, have recently been shown to be effective in treating SIADH.[5]

Diabetes Insipidus

Diabetes insipidus (DI) is an insufficiency of ADH activity, leading to polyuria (frequent urination) and polydipsia (frequent drinking). The two forms of DI are as follows:
1. *Neurogenic or central DI.* Caused by the insufficient secretion of ADH, it occurs when any organic lesion of the hypothalamus, pituitary stalk, or posterior pituitary interferes with ADH synthesis, transport, or release. Causative lesions include primary brain tumors, hypophysectomy, aneurysms, thrombosis, infections, and immunologic disorders. Central DI is a well-recognized complication of traumatic brain injury. It can also be caused by hereditary disorders that affect ADH genes or result in structural changes in the pituitary gland.
2. *Nephrogenic DI.* Caused by inadequate response of the renal tubules to ADH, nephrogenic DI is usually acquired or may be genetic. Acquired nephrogenic DI is generally related to disorders and drugs that damage the renal tubules or inhibit the generation of cAMP in

the tubules. These disorders include pyelonephritis, amyloidosis, destructive uropathies, and polycystic kidney disease, all of which lead to irreversible diabetes insipidus. Drugs that may induce a reversible form of nephrogenic diabetes insipidus include lithium carbonate, colchicines, amphotericin B, loop diuretics, general anesthetics (such as methoxyflurane), and demeclocycline. Several genetic causes of nephrogenic DI have been identified. One of the best described is a mutation in the gene that codes for aquaporin-2, which is one of the four water transport channels in the renal tubule.[6]

There is a rare form of DI associated with pregnancy. In gestational DI, the level of the vasopressin-degrading enzyme vasopressinase is increased. Clinical manifestations are usually mild and do not require treatment.[4,7]

Dipsogenic or *primary polydipsia* may be confused with diabetes insipidus. It is caused by the chronic ingestion of extremely large quantities of fluid that wash out the renal medullary concentration gradient, which results in a partial resistance to ADH. This condition resolves with decreased fluid ingestion. Psychogenic causes of polydipsia must be differentiated from true DI because administering an ADH analog to an individual with psychogenic DI will result in severe hypoosmolality.

PATHOPHYSIOLOGY Individuals with diabetes insipidus have a partial to total inability to concentrate urine. Insufficient ADH activity causes excretion of large volumes of dilute urine, leading to increased plasma osmolality. In conscious individuals, the thirst mechanism is stimulated and induces polydipsia—usually a craving for cold drinks. Dehydration develops rapidly without ongoing fluid replacement. If the individual with DI cannot conserve as much water as is lost in the urine, serum hypernatremia and hyperosmolality occur. Concentrations of other serum electrolytes generally are not affected.

CLINICAL MANIFESTATIONS The clinical manifestations of diabetes insipidus include polyuria, nocturia, continuous thirst, and polydipsia. The urine output is varied but can increase from the normal output of 1 to 2 L/day to as much as 8 to 12 L/day and can be higher than daily fluid intake. Individuals with long-standing diabetes insipidus develop a large bladder capacity and hydronephrosis (see Chapter 30). Neurogenic diabetes insipidus usually has an abrupt onset and many individuals can specifically recall the date of onset of their symptoms. Nephrogenic DI usually has a more gradual onset. Table 19-2 compares the signs and symptoms of DI and SIADH.

EVALUATION AND TREATMENT Diabetes insipidus must be distinguished from other polyuric states, including diabetes mellitus, osmotically induced diuresis, and psychogenic polydipsia. The criteria for the diagnosis of DI include low urine specific gravity, low urine osmolality, hypernatremia, high serum osmolality, and continued diuresis despite a serum sodium concentration of 145 mEq/L or greater. The diagnosis of DI is generally confirmed through water deprivation testing. Psychogenic polydipsia can be differentiated from nephrogenic DI based on plasma ADH levels. ADH levels are low in psychogenic polydipsia and normal or high in nephrogenic DI.

Treatment of neurogenic DI is based on the extent of the ADH deficiency and on the patient's age, endocrine and cardiovascular status, and lifestyle. Some individuals require ADH replacement, but fluid replacement using oral or intravenous routes is usually adequate. ADH replacement therapy for symptomatic central or neurogenic diabetes insipidus includes intravascular or, more commonly, oral or intranasal administration of the synthetic vasopressin analog DDAVP (desmopressin).[8] Management of nephrogenic DI requires treatment

TABLE 19-2 Signs and Symptoms of Diabetes Insipidus (DI) and Syndrome of Inappropriate Antidiuretic Hormone (SIADH) Secretion

Signs and Symptoms	DI	SIADH
Urine output	High	Low (no hypovolemia)
Urine osmolality	Low (<100-200 mOsm/L)	High (>800 mOsm/L)
Urine specific gravity	Low (<1.010)	High (>1.020)
Serum sodium	Hypernatremia (>145 mEq/L)	Hyponatremia (<135 mEq/L)
Serum osmolality	Hyperosmolar (>300 mOsm/L)	Hypoosmolar (<285 mOsm/L)
Symptoms	Polyuria, thirst, high urine output, signs of dehydration	Water retention, low urine output, nausea, vomiting, mental changes

of any reversible underlying disorders, discontinuation of etiologic medications, and correction of associated electrolyte disorders. Surprisingly, thiazide diuretics may improve renal tubular salt and water retention in individuals with moderate nephrogenic DI. New treatments aimed at reversing aquaporin-2 dysfunction are being developed.[6] Drugs that potentiate the action of otherwise insufficient amounts of endogenous ADH, such as chlorpropamide, carbamazepine, and clofibrate, may be used in individuals with incomplete ADH deficiency.

Diseases of the Anterior Pituitary
Hypopituitarism

Hypopituitarism can be characterized by the absence of one or more anterior pituitary hormones or the complete failure of all anterior pituitary hormone functions. Hypopituitarism results from either an inadequate supply of hypothalamic-releasing hormones, because of damage to the pituitary stalk, or an inability of the gland to produce hormones. The most common causes of hypopituitarism are pituitary infarction or space-occupying lesions, such as pituitary adenomas or aneurysms. Pituitary infarction may occur in women during the postpartum period (Sheehan syndrome) because of blood loss and hypovolemic shock.[9] Traumatic brain injury is increasingly recognized as an important cause of hypopituitarism and can have a significant impact on acute and long-term recovery.[10] Other causes of hypopituitarism include removal or destruction of the gland, infections (e.g., meningitis, syphilis, tuberculosis), autoimmune hypophysitis, certain drugs (e.g., bexarotene, carbamazepine, ipilimumab), or mutation of the prophet of pituitary transcription factor *(PROP-1)* gene involved in early embryonic pituitary development.[11]

PATHOPHYSIOLOGY The pituitary gland is highly vascular and relies heavily upon portal blood flow from the hypothalamus. It is, therefore, vulnerable to ischemia and infarction. Infarction results in tissue necrosis and edema with swelling of the gland. Expansion of the pituitary within the fixed compartment of the sella turcica further impedes blood supply to the pituitary. Over time, fibrosis of pituitary tissue occurs and the symptoms of hypopituitarism develop. Adenomas and aneurysms may compress otherwise normal secreting pituitary cells and lead to compromised hormonal output.

CLINICAL MANIFESTATIONS The signs and symptoms of hypofunction of the anterior pituitary are variable and depend on which hormones are affected. In panhypopituitarism, all hormones are deficient and the individual suffers from multiple complications including cortisol deficiency from lack of ACTH, thyroid deficiency from lack of thyroid-stimulating hormone (TSH), and loss of secondary sex characteristics because of the lack of follicle-stimulating hormone (FSH) and luteinizing hormone (LH). Low levels of growth hormone (GH) and insulin-like growth factor 1 (IGF-1) affect growth in children and can cause physiologic and psychologic symptoms in adults. Finally, postpartum women cannot lactate because of decreased or absent prolactin.

ACTH deficiency with associated loss of cortisol is a potentially life-threatening disorder. ACTH deficiency usually is encountered with generalized pituitary hypofunction; it rarely occurs as an isolated event. Within 2 weeks of the complete absence of ACTH, symptoms of cortisol insufficiency develop, including nausea, vomiting, anorexia, fatigue, and weakness. Hypoglycemia results from increased insulin sensitivity, decreased glycogen reserves, and decreased gluconeogenesis associated with hypocortisolism. ACTH deficiency also limits maximal aldosterone secretion, although the renin-angiotensin system can stimulate some aldosterone secretion. The glomerular filtration rate decreases, causing decreased urine output.

TSH deficiency is rarely seen in isolation but often occurs with other pituitary hormone deficiencies. Symptoms develop 4 to 8 weeks after hypothyrotropinemia occurs and include cold intolerance, skin dryness, mild myxedema, lethargy, and decreased metabolic rate. The symptoms usually are less severe than those of primary hypothyroidism.

The onset of FSH and LH deficiencies in women of reproductive age is associated with amenorrhea and atrophy of the vagina, uterus, and breasts. In postpubertal males, the testicles atrophy and facial hair growth is diminished. Both men and women experience decreased body hair and diminished libido.

GH deficiency occurs in both children and adults. Several genetic defects have been identified in the growth hormone axis in children, including a recessive mutation in the GH gene, resulting in a failure of growth hormone secretion. Mutations also may involve the GH receptor, IGF-1 biosynthesis, IGF-1 receptors, or defects in GH signal transduction.[12] In adults, GH deficiency is most often caused by structural or functional abnormalities of the pituitary. In both children and adults, acute GH and IGF-1 deficiency has been implicated in significant metabolic perturbations seen with critical illness.

GH deficiency in children is manifested by growth failure and a condition known as hypopituitary dwarfism (Figure 19-2); however, not all children with short stature have growth hormone deficiency. Symptoms of chronic adult GH deficiency syndrome include increased body fat, decreased strength and lean body mass, osteoporosis, reduced sweating, dry skin, and psychologic problems, including depression, social withdrawal, fatigue, loss of motivation, and a diminished feeling of well-being. Without adequate GH replacement, increased mortality can occur as a result of myocardial infarction and stroke associated with dyslipidemias and atherosclerosis.[13]

EVALUATION AND TREATMENT The diagnostic evaluation of suspected pituitary disease is often challenging and must be carefully interpreted together with the individual's signs and symptoms. Simultaneous measurements of the levels of tropic hormones from the pituitary and target endocrine glands are crucial, and the more complicated dynamic testing of insulin, TRH, and gonadotropin-releasing hormone (GnRH) may be indicated. Imaging of the pituitary

FIGURE 19-2 Hypopituitary Dwarfism and Pituitary Giantism. A pituitary giant and dwarf contrasted with normal-size men. Excessive secretion of growth hormone by the anterior lobe of the pituitary gland during the early years of life produces giants of this type, whereas deficient secretion of this substance produces well-formed dwarfs. (From Patton KT, Thibodeau GA: *Anatomy & physiology*, ed 8, St Louis, 2013, Mosby.)

(magnetic resonance imaging [MRI] or computed tomography [CT] scans) is critical to assess for anatomic lesions, such as tumors.

Management of hypopituitarism requires correction of the underlying disorder as quickly as possible. Replacement of target gland hormones that are deficient because of lack of tropic anterior pituitary hormones is essential (such as cortisol, thyroid hormone, growth hormone, and gender-specific steroid hormones).[14] In cases of circulatory collapse, immediate therapy with glucocorticoids and intravenous fluids is critical.

Hyperpituitarism: Primary Adenoma

Pituitary adenomas usually are benign, slow-growing tumors that arise from cells of the anterior pituitary. The cause of pituitary adenomas is not known and most occur sporadically. Altered gene expression is commonly detected and familial pituitary adenomas occur as part of syndromes affecting other organs, such as multiple endocrine neoplasia.[15] Most are microscopic (microadenomas) and are found only on postmortem examinations or incidentally discovered on MRI examinations. The majority of pituitary microadenomas are hormonally silent and do not pose significant hazards to the individual. Larger adenomas (macroadenomas) are associated with morbidity and mortality attributable to alterations in hormone secretion or to invasion or impingement of surrounding structures.

PATHOPHYSIOLOGY Local expansion of the adenoma may impinge on the optic chiasma and cause various visual disturbances, depending on the portion of the nerve compressed. If the tumor is locally aggressive, invasion of the cavernous sinuses may occur, resulting in

compromise of the oculomotor, trochlear, abducens, and trigeminal nerves with attending symptoms (see Table 13-6 for review of cranial nerves). Extension to the hypothalamus disturbs control of wakefulness, thirst, appetite, and temperature.

Hormonal effects of adenomas include hypersecretion from the adenoma itself and hyposecretion from surrounding pituitary cells. The adenomatous tissue secretes the hormone of the cell type from which it arose, without regard to the needs of the body and without benefit of regulatory feedback mechanisms (autonomous function). Because of the pressure exerted by the tumor in the unexpandable bony sella turcica, hyposecretion from those cells that are most sensitive to pressure is common (GH-, FSH-, and LH-secreting cells).[16]

CLINICAL MANIFESTATIONS The clinical manifestations of pituitary adenomas are related to tumor growth and hormone hypersecretion or hyposecretion. Increased tumor size causes headache, fatigue, neck pain or stiffness, and seizures. Visual changes include visual field impairments (often beginning in one eye and progressing to the other) and temporary blindness. If the tumor infiltrates other cranial nerves, neuromuscular function is affected.

Pituitary adenomas are most often associated with increased secretion of growth hormone and prolactin (see Hypersecretion of Growth Hormone: Acromegaly and Prolactinoma sections in this chapter). Gonadotropic hyposecretion results in menstrual irregularity in women, decreased libido, and receding secondary sex characteristics in both men and women. If the tumor exerts sufficient pressure, thyroid and adrenal hypofunction may occur because of lack of TSH and ACTH, resulting in the symptoms of hypothyroidism and hypocortisolism, respectively.

EVALUATION AND TREATMENT Diagnosis of pituitary adenoma involves physical and laboratory evaluations, including pertinent hormone assays and radiographic examination of the skull (MRI [preferred] or contrast-enhanced CT). The goal of treatment is to protect the individual from the effects of tumor growth and to control hormone hypersecretion while minimizing damage to appropriately secreting portions of the pituitary. Depending on tumor size and type, individuals may be treated by administration of specific medications to suppress tumor growth, transsphenoidal tumor resection, or radiation therapy including stereotactic treatments.[16]

✔ **QUICK CHECK 19-1**

1. What is the mechanism of receptor-associated hormonal disorder?
2. Why do individuals with the syndrome of inappropriate antidiuretic hormone (SIADH) secrete concentrated urine?
3. Why may individuals with a pituitary adenoma develop visual disturbances?

Hypersecretion of Growth Hormone: Acromegaly

Acromegaly results from continuous exposure to high levels of growth hormone (GH) and insulin-like growth factor 1 (IGF-1); it almost always is caused by a GH-secreting pituitary adenoma (it rarely results from the ectopic production of GHRH).[17]

Acromegaly usually occurs in adults in the 40- to 59-year-old age group, although it is often present for years before diagnosis. It is a slowly progressive disease and, if untreated, is associated with a decreased life expectancy. Deaths from acromegaly are caused by heart disease secondary to hypertension and coronary artery disease, stroke, diabetes mellitus, or malignancy (colon or lung cancers).

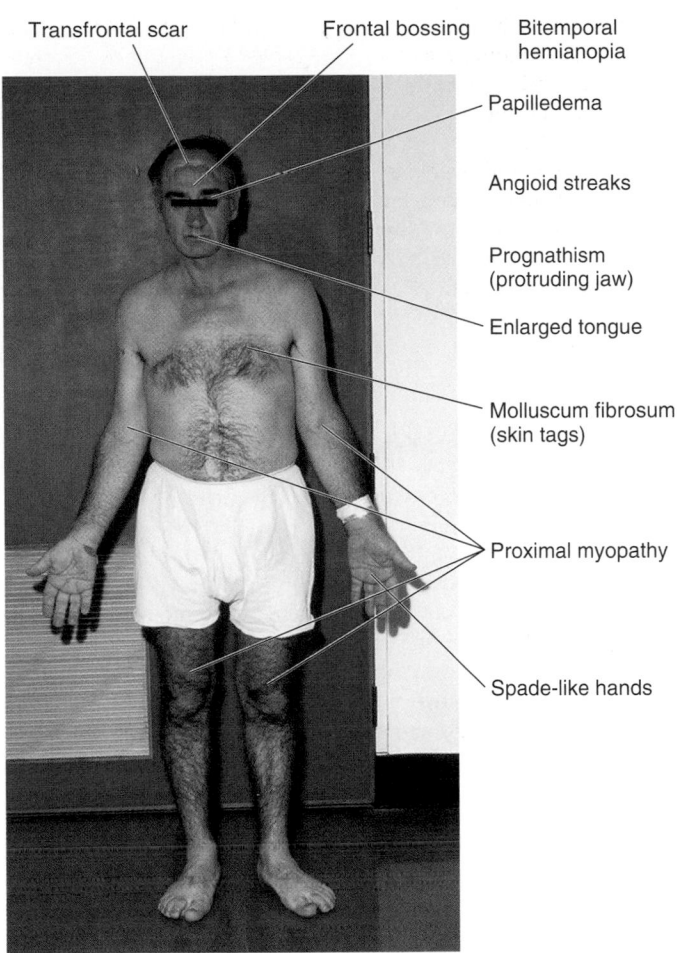

Transfrontal scar   Frontal bossing   Bitemporal
                                                hemianopia

                                                Papilledema

                                                Angioid streaks

                                                Prognathism
                                                (protruding jaw)

                                                Enlarged tongue

                                                Molluscum fibrosum
                                                (skin tags)

                                                Proximal myopathy

                                                Spade-like hands

FIGURE 19-3 Acromegaly. (From Talley NJ, O'Connor S: *Clinical examination*, ed 7, Australia, 2014, Churchill Livingstone.)

PATHOPHYSIOLOGY With a GH-secreting adenoma, the usual GH baseline secretion pattern and sleep-related GH peaks are lost, and a totally unpredictable secretory pattern ensues. However, GH levels in acromegalics are never completely suppressed. Only slight elevations of GH and IGF-1 can stimulate growth. In children and adolescents whose epiphyseal plates have not yet closed, the effect of increased GH levels is termed **giantism** (see Figure 19-2). Skeletal growth is excessive, with some individuals becoming 8 or 9 feet tall. In the adult, epiphyseal closure has occurred, and increased amounts of GH and IGF-1 cause connective tissue proliferation and increased cytoplasmic matrix, as well as bony proliferation that results in the characteristic appearance of acromegaly (Figure 19-3).

GH also has significant effects on glucose, lipid, and protein metabolism. Hyperglycemia results from adipocyte inflammation and GH inhibition of peripheral glucose uptake and increased hepatic glucose production, followed by compensatory hyperinsulinism and, finally, insulin resistance.[18] Diabetes mellitus occurs when the pancreas cannot secrete enough insulin to offset the effects of GH. Excessive levels of GH and IGF-1 also affect the cardiovascular system. Although the associated pathophysiologic mechanism is not clearly understood at present, hypertension and left ventricular heart failure are seen in one third to one half of individuals with acromegaly. Cardiomyopathy associated with progressive and unrestrained myocardial growth is a significant factor.[19] GH also acts on the renal tubules to increase phosphate reabsorption, leading to mild hyperphosphatemia. Because the

adenoma becomes increasingly a space-occupying lesion, hypopituitarism may occur because of compression of surrounding hormone-secreting cells. Hyperprolactinemia can occur in 30% to 40% of individuals with acromegaly.[17]

CLINICAL MANIFESTATIONS With connective tissue proliferation, individuals with acromegaly have an enlarged tongue, interstitial edema, enlarged and overactive sebaceous and sweat glands (leading to increased body odor), and coarse skin and body hair. Bony proliferation involves periosteal vertebral growth and enlargement of the bones of the face, hands, and feet (see Figure 19-3). The lower jaw and forehead also protrude. Skeletal abnormalities are irreversible.

Increased IGF-1 levels cause ribs to elongate at the bone-cartilage junction, leading to a barrel-chested appearance, and increased proliferation of cartilage in joints, which causes backache and arthralgias. With bony and soft tissue overgrowth, nerve entrapment occurs, leading to peripheral nerve damage manifested by weakness, muscular atrophy, footdrop, and sensory changes in the hands.

Symptoms of diabetes mellitus, such as polyuria and polydipsia, may occur because of decreased insulin sensitivity. Acromegaly-associated hypertension is usually asymptomatic until heart failure symptoms develop. Increased tumor size results in central nervous system symptoms of headache, seizure activity, visual disturbances, and papilledema. If compression hypopituitarism occurs, gonadotropin secretion may be affected, causing amenorrhea in women and sexual dysfunction in men. Approximately 20% of growth hormone–secreting tumors also secrete prolactin, resulting in hypogonadism. Cardiovascular, metabolic, and symptoms of tumor compression often improve with treatment.

EVALUATION AND TREATMENT Diagnosis is confirmed by clinical features of the disease, MRI scans, and elevated levels of IGF-1.[20] GH level is typically elevated and not suppressed with oral glucose tolerance testing. The goals of treatment are to normalize or reduce GH secretion and relieve or prevent complications related to tumor expansion. The treatment of choice in acromegaly is transsphenoidal surgical removal of the GH-secreting adenoma. Radiation therapy may be effective when rapid control of GH levels is not essential, when the individual is not a good surgical candidate, or when hyperfunction persists after subtotal resection. Somatostatin analogs, such as octreotide, octreotide LAR, and lanreotide, normalize IGF-1 levels and lower growth hormone levels. Pegvisomant can be used to supplement somatostatin analogs and is an effective drug that induces tissue insensitivity to GH by blocking the GH receptor.[17] Dopaminergic agonists, such as cabergoline, also may be helpful, especially if the tumor also secretes prolactin.

Prolactinoma

Pituitary tumors that secrete prolactin, **prolactinomas**, are the most common hormonally active pituitary tumors. Other conditions or medications can elevate prolactin levels in the absence of a pituitary pathologic condition. For example, renal failure, polycystic ovarian disease, primary hypothyroidism, breast stimulation, or even the stress of venipuncture can increase prolactin levels. Prolactin is under tonic inhibitory hypothalamic control through the secretion of dopamine. Thus medications that block the effects of dopamine can increase prolactin level and stimulate proliferation of prolactin-secreting cells (lactotrophs). These include antipsychotics (risperidone, chlorpromazine), metoclopramide, tricyclic antidepressants, and methyldopa. Estrogens increase prolactin concentration by stimulating hyperplasia of prolactin-secreting cells. Any process that interferes with the delivery of dopamine from the hypothalamus to the lactotrophs (pituitary stalk tumor, pituitary stalk transection, or compressive pituitary tumor) also results in hyperprolactinemia. Because thyrotropin-releasing hormone (TRH) stimulates prolactin secretion, in addition to enhancing TSH release, prolactin concentration may be elevated in individuals with primary hypothyroidism.

PATHOPHYSIOLOGY The hallmark of a prolactinoma is sustained increases in the levels of serum prolactin. The physiologic actions of prolactin include breast development during pregnancy, postpartum milk production, and suppression of ovarian function in nursing women. Pathologic elevation of prolactin levels in women results in amenorrhea, nonpuerperal milk production (galactorrhea), hirsutism, and osteopenia or osteoporosis resulting from estrogen deficiency. Hyperprolactinemia in men causes hypogonadism and erectile dysfunction.

Because the adenoma becomes an increasingly space-occupying lesion, hypopituitarism may occur because of the compression of surrounding hormone-secreting cells. Central nervous system symptoms may develop because of growth and pressure of the adenoma within the sella turcica. These complications are especially common with what are called macro (>1 cm in diameter) or giant (>4 cm in diameter) prolactinomas and are often more difficult to treat.[21]

CLINICAL MANIFESTATIONS Women with hyperprolactinemia generally present with galactorrhea (nonpuerperal milk production) and menstrual disturbances including amenorrhea. In susceptible women, hirsutism develops because of estrogen deficiency. If not detected until after many years, this estrogen deficiency also may result in osteopenia or osteoporosis. Men often present late with symptoms related to the increasing size of the adenoma (i.e., headache or visual impairment).

EVALUATION AND TREATMENT The diagnostic evaluation of hyperprolactinemia includes a careful history to exclude medications that may cause elevations in prolactin concentration. Symptoms of hypothyroidism should be elicited, and screening with a serum TSH level is mandatory. MRI scanning of the pituitary is indicated to determine the size and location of an adenoma. If serum prolactin level is less than 50 ng/ml, a careful search for a nonpituitary cause should be pursued.

Dopaminergic agonists (cabergoline) are the treatment of choice for prolactinomas. Restoration of fertility in previously anovulatory women is common. In individuals resistant or intolerant to these medications, transsphenoidal surgery and radiotherapy are options.[22] New chemotherapeutic and targeted molecular therapies are being explored in selected cases.[23]

ALTERATIONS OF THYROID FUNCTION

Disorders of thyroid function develop as a result of primary dysfunction or disease of the thyroid gland or, secondarily, as a result of pituitary or hypothalamic alterations. Primary thyroid disorders result in alterations of thyroid hormone (TH) levels with secondary feedback effects on pituitary thyroid-stimulating hormone (TSH). For example, when there are primary elevations in TH level, TSH level will secondarily decrease because of negative feedback. When TH level is decreased because of a condition affecting the thyroid gland, TSH level will be elevated. Thyroid disease also can present with minimal or no symptoms but with abnormal laboratory values, known as *subclinical thyroid disease*. Central (secondary) thyroid disorders are related to disorders of pituitary gland TSH production. When there is excessive TSH production, TH level is elevated secondary to the primary

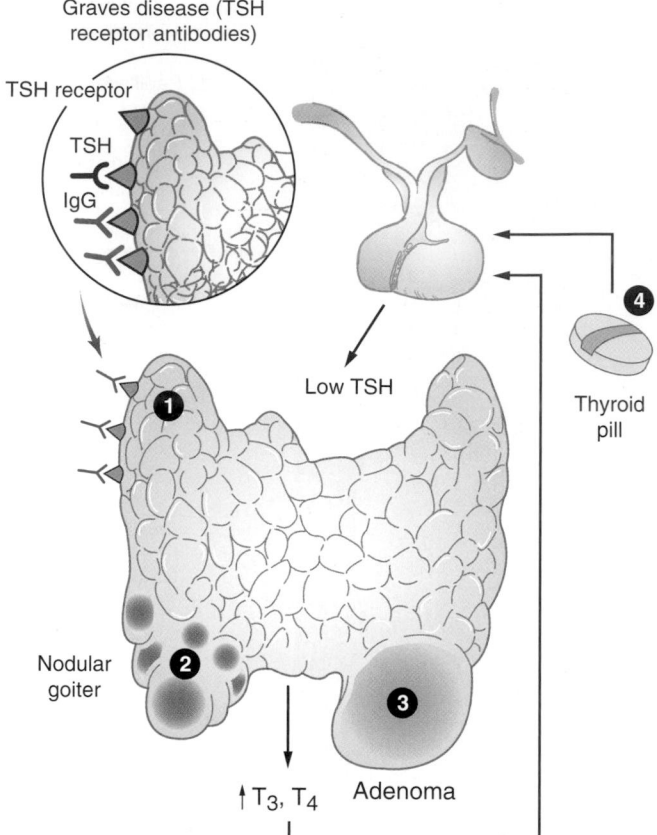

FIGURE 19-4 Common Causes of Hyperthyroidism. Hyperthyroidism may have several causes, among them: **1**, Graves disease; **2**, toxic multinodular goiter; **3**, follicular adenoma; **4**, thyroid medication. (Adapted from Damjanov I: *Pathology for the health professions,* ed 4, St Louis, 2012, Saunders.)

elevation of TSH concentration. The reverse is true with inadequate TSH production.

Thyrotoxicosis/Hyperthyroidism

PATHOPHYSIOLOGY Thyrotoxicosis is a condition that results from any cause of increased TH levels Hyperthyroidism is a form of thyrotoxicosis in which excess amounts of TH are secreted from the thyroid gland (Figure 19-4). The terms *thyrotoxicosis* and *hyperthyroidism* are often used interchangeably. Common diseases that cause primary hyperthyroidism include Graves disease, toxic multinodular goiter, and solitary toxic adenoma. *Central (secondary) hyperthyroidism* is less common and is caused by TSH-secreting pituitary adenomas. Thyrotoxicosis not associated with hyperthyroidism includes ectopic thyroid tissue, and ingestion of excessive TH. Each condition is associated with a specific pathophysiology and manifestations; however, all forms of thyrotoxicosis share some common characteristics.

CLINICAL MANIFESTATIONS The clinical features of thyrotoxicosis are attributable to the metabolic effects of increased circulating levels of thyroid hormones. This usually results in an increased metabolic rate with heat intolerance and increased tissue sensitivity to stimulation by the sympathetic nervous system. The major manifestations are summarized in Figure 19-5. Enlargement of the thyroid gland (goiter) is common in hyperthyroid conditions caused by stimulation of TSH receptors.

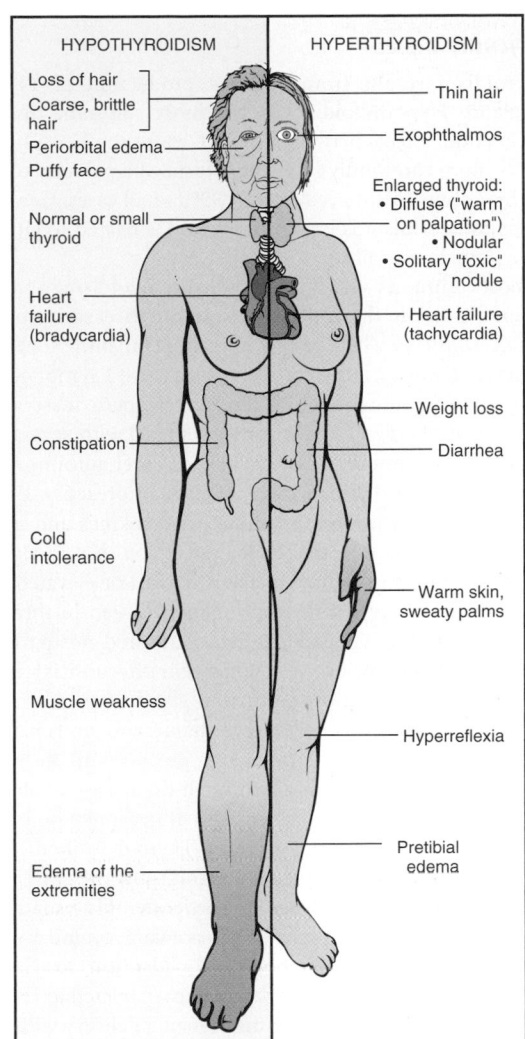

FIGURE 19-5 Clinical Manifestations of Hyperthyroidism and Hypothyroidism. (From Damjanov I: *Pathology for the health professions*, ed 4, St Louis, 2012, Saunders.)

FIGURE 19-6 Evaluation of Hyperthyroidism. Radioactive iodine is used in the differential diagnosis of hyperthyroidism.

FIGURE 19-7 Thyrotoxicosis (Graves Disease). **A,** Exophthalmos (large and protruding eyeballs often in association with a large goiter). **B,** Pretibial myxedema associated with Graves disease; note lumpy and swollen appearance from accumulation of connective tissue and pinkish purple discoloration. (**A** from Belchetz P, Hammond P: *Mosby's color atlas and text of diabetes and endocrinology*, Edinburgh, 2003, Mosby; **B** from Habif T: *Clinical dermatology*, ed 5, St Louis, 2009, Mosby.)

Elevated serum thyroxine (T₄) and triiodothyronine (T₃) levels and suppressed serum TSH levels are diagnostic for primary hyperthyroidism. By contrast, central (secondary) hyperthyroidism caused by TSH-secreting pituitary tumors is characterized by normal to increased TSH levels despite elevated thyroid hormone concentrations. Radioactive iodine is used to test for increased uptake in primary hyperthyroidism (Figure 19-6). Treatment is directed at controlling excessive TH production, secretion, or action and employs antithyroid drug therapy, radioactive iodine therapy (absorbed only by thyroid tissue, causing death of cells), and surgery.[24] A major complication of all forms of treatment for hyperthyroidism is excessive ablation of the gland leading to hypothyroidism.

Graves Disease

Graves disease is the underlying cause of 50% to 80% of cases of hyperthyroidism with a prevalence of approximately 0.5% in the U.S. population. It occurs more commonly in women. Although the exact cause of Graves disease is not known, genetic factors interacting with environmental triggers play an important role in the pathogenesis. Graves disease is classified as an autoimmune disease and results from a form of type II hypersensitivity (see Chapter 8) in which there is stimulation of the thyroid by autoantibodies directed against the TSH receptor. These autoantibodies, called thyroid-stimulating immunoglobulins (TSIs), override the normal regulatory mechanisms. The TSI stimulation of TSH receptors in the gland results in hyperplasia of the gland (goiter) and increased synthesis of TH, especially of triiodo-L-thyronine (T₃). Increased levels of TH result in the classic signs and symptoms of hyperthyroidism illustrated in Figure 19-6. TSH production by the pituitary is inhibited through the usual negative feedback loop.[24]

TSI also contributes to the two major distinguishing clinical manifestations of Graves disease (ophthalmopathy and dermopathy [pretibial myxedema]). Two categories of ophthalmopathy associated with Graves disease (Figure 19-7) are (1) functional abnormalities resulting from hyperactivity of the sympathetic division of the autonomic nervous system (lag of the globe on upward gaze and of the upper lid on downward gaze) and (2) infiltrative changes involving the orbital contents with enlargement of the ocular muscles. These changes affect more than half of individuals with Graves disease. Orbital connective tissue accumulation, inflammation, and edema of the orbital contents result in exophthalmos (protrusion of the eyeball), periorbital edema, and extraocular muscle weakness, leading to diplopia (double vision).[25] The individual may experience irritation, pain, lacrimation, photophobia, blurred vision, decreased visual acuity, papilledema, visual field impairment, exposure keratosis, and corneal ulceration.

A small number of individuals with Graves disease and very high levels of TSI experience pretibial myxedema (Graves dermopathy), characterized by subcutaneous swelling on the anterior portions of the legs and by indurated and erythematous skin. Graves dermopathy is associated with thyrotropin receptor antigens on fibroblasts and recruited T lymphocytes that stimulate excessive amounts of hyaluronic acid production in the dermis and subcutaneous tissue.[26] These manifestations occasionally appear on the hands, giving the appearance of clubbing of the fingers (thyroid acropachy).

Hyperthyroidism resulting from nodular thyroid disease. The thyroid gland normally enlarges in response to the increased demand for TH that occurs in puberty, pregnancy, and iodine-deficient states as well as in individuals with immunologic, viral, or genetic disorders. When the condition resulting in increased TH resolves, TSH secretion normally subsides and the thyroid gland returns to its original size.

Irreversible changes can occur in some follicular cells so these cells function autonomously and produce excessive amounts of TH. On the other hand, some follicular cells may cease to function. The balance between the amount of TH produced by hyperfunctioning nodules and that produced by the remainder of the gland determines whether an individual develops hyperthyroidism. Toxic multinodular goiter occurs when there are several hyperfunctioning nodules leading to hyperthyroidism. Unlike Graves disease, there is absence of an autoimmune stimulus. If only one nodule is hyperfunctioning, it is termed toxic adenoma. The classic clinical manifestations of hyperthyroidism (see Figure 19-5) usually develop slowly, and exophthalmos and pretibial myxedema do not occur. Nodules may be palpable on physical examination and there is increased uptake of radioactive iodine. The incidence of malignancy in toxic nodular goiter is estimated to be as high as 9%, so most individuals should undergo a fine needle aspiration biopsy of suspicious nodules before treatment. Treatment consists of a combination of radioactive iodine, surgery, and antithyroid medications.[27]

Thyrotoxic crisis. Thyrotoxic crisis (thyroid storm) is a rare but dangerous worsening of the thyrotoxic state in which death can occur within 48 hours without treatment. The condition may develop spontaneously, but it usually occurs in individuals who have undiagnosed or partially treated Graves disease and are subjected to excessive stress, such as infection, pulmonary or cardiovascular disorders, trauma, seizures, surgery (especially thyroid surgery), obstetric complications, emotional distress, or dialysis. The symptoms of thyroid crisis are caused by the increased action of thyroxine (T_4) and triiodothyronine (T_3) exceeding metabolic demands.[28]

The systemic symptoms of thyrotoxic crisis include hyperthermia; tachycardia, especially atrial tachydysrhythmias; high-output heart failure; agitation or delirium; and nausea, vomiting, or diarrhea contributing to fluid volume depletion. Treatment includes (1) the use of drugs that block TH synthesis (i.e., propylthiouracil or methimazole), (2) the use of beta-blockers for control of cardiovascular symptoms, the administration of (3) steroids or (4) iodine (e.g., saturated solution of potassium iodide [SSKI]), and (5) supportive care.

Hypothyroidism

Hypothyroidism results from deficient production of TH by the thyroid gland. Hypothyroidism is the most common disorder of thyroid function, affects between 1% and 2% of the U.S. population, and occurs more commonly in women. It may be primary or central. Primary hypothyroidism accounts for 99% of all cases. Central (secondary) hypothyroidism is less common and is related to either pituitary or hypothalamic failure.

The most common cause of primary hypothyroidism in the United States is autoimmune thyroiditis (Hashimoto disease, chronic lymphocytic thyroiditis), which results in gradual inflammatory destruction of thyroid tissue by infiltration of autoreactive T lymphocytes and circulating thyroid autoantibodies (antithyroid peroxidase and antithyroglobulin antibodies). This disorder is linked with several genetic risk factors and is commonly associated with other autoimmune conditions. Infiltration of thyroid autoantibodies, autoreactive T lymphocytes, natural killer cells, and inflammatory cytokines and induction of apoptosis are involved in the tissue destruction seen in Hashimoto thyroiditis.[29] Radioactive iodine uptake is normal or elevated.

Spontaneous recovery of thyroid function is seen in three conditions: subacute thyroiditis, painless thyroiditis, and postpartum thyroiditis. Subacute thyroiditis (de Quervain thyroiditis) is a rare nonbacterial inflammation of the thyroid gland often preceded by a viral infection. It is accompanied by fever, tenderness, and enlargement of the thyroid gland. The inflammatory process initially results in elevated levels of thyroid hormone through the release of stored thyroglobulin, which then is associated with transient hypothyroidism before the gland recovers normal activity. Thyroid antibodies are not present in the blood. Symptoms may last for 2 to 4 months, and nonsteroidal anti-inflammatory drugs or corticosteroids usually resolve symptoms. Painless (silent) thyroiditis has a course similar to that of subacute thyroiditis but is pathologically identical to Hashimoto disease. Postpartum thyroiditis is pathologically related to Hashimoto disease and generally occurs up to 6 months after delivery with a course similar to that seen in subacute thyroiditis. Thus a hyperthyroid phase (with a low thyroid radioiodine uptake) precedes the hypothyroid phase in typical cases of subacute, painless, or postpartum thyroiditis. Spontaneous recovery occurs in 95% of these conditions.

Congenital Hypothyroidism

Hypothyroidism in infants occurs when thyroid tissue is absent (thyroid dysgenesis) or with hereditary defects in TH synthesis. Thyroid dysgenesis occurs more often in female infants, with permanent abnormalities in 1 of every 4000 live births. Because TH is essential for embryonic growth, particularly of brain tissue, the infant will be cognitively disabled if there is no thyroxine during fetal life.[30] The fetus is dependent on maternal thyroxine for the first 20 weeks of gestation.[31] Hypothyroidism may not be evident at birth. Symptoms may include high birth weight, hypothermia, delay in passing meconium, and neonatal jaundice. Cord blood can be examined in the first days of life for measurement of T_4 and TSH levels. The probability of normal growth and intellectual function is high if treatment with levothyroxine is started before the child is 3 or 4 months old. The earlier thyroid hormone replacement is initiated, the better the child's outcome.[32]

Without early screening, hypothyroidism may not be evident until after 4 months of age. Symptoms include difficulty eating, hoarse cry, and protruding tongue caused by myxedema of oral tissues and vocal cords; hypotonic muscles of the abdomen with constipation, abdominal protrusion, and umbilical hernia; subnormal temperature; lethargy; excessive sleeping; slow pulse rate; and cold, mottled skin. Skeletal

FIGURE 19-8 Mechanisms of Primary and Secondary Hypothyroidism.

FIGURE 19-9 Myxedema. Note edema around eyes and facial puffiness. The hair is dry. (From Bolognia JL et al: *Dermatology*, ed 3, St Louis, 2012, Mosby.)

growth is stunted because of impaired protein synthesis, poor absorption of nutrients, and lack of bone mineralization. The child will be dwarfed with short limbs, if not treated. Dentition is often delayed. Cognitive disability varies with the severity of hypothyroidism and the length of delay before treatment is initiated.

PATHOPHYSIOLOGY   In *primary hypothyroidism*, loss of thyroid function leads to decreased production of TH and increased secretion of TSH and TRH (Figure 19-8). The most common causes of primary hypothyroidism in adults include autoimmune thyroiditis (Hashimoto disease), iatrogenic loss of thyroid tissue after surgical or radioactive treatment for hyperthyroidism or after head and neck radiation therapy, medications (e.g., lithium and amiodarone), and endemic iodine deficiency. Infants and children may present with hypothyroidism because of congenital defects. *Central (secondary) hypothyroidism* is caused by the pituitary's failure to synthesize adequate amounts of TSH or a lack of TRH. Pituitary tumors that compress surrounding pituitary cells or the consequences of their treatment are the most common causes of central hypothyroidism. Other causes include traumatic brain injury, subarachnoid hemorrhage, or pituitary infarction. Hypothalamic dysfunction results in low levels of TH, TSH, and TRH.[33] Subclinical hypothyroidism is a mild thyroid failure estimated to occur in 4% to 8% of U.S. adults. It is defined as an elevation in TSH levels with normal levels of circulating TH.[34]

CLINICAL MANIFESTATIONS   Hypothyroidism generally affects all body systems and occurs insidiously over months or years. The decrease in TH level lowers energy metabolism and heat production. The individual develops a low basal metabolic rate, cold intolerance, lethargy, and slightly lowered basal body temperature (see Figure 19-5). The decrease in the level of TH can lead to excessive TSH production, which stimulates thyroid tissue and causes goiter.

The characteristic sign of severe or long-standing hypothyroidism is myxedema, which results from the altered composition of the dermis and other tissues. The connective tissue fibers are separated by large amounts of protein and mucopolysaccharide. This complex binds water, producing nonpitting, boggy edema, especially around the eyes, hands, and feet and in the supraclavicular fossae (Figure 19-9). The tongue and laryngeal and pharyngeal mucous membranes thicken, producing thick, slurred speech and hoarseness. Myxedema coma, a

medical emergency, is a diminished level of consciousness associated with severe hypothyroidism. Signs and symptoms include hypothermia without shivering, hypoventilation, hypotension, hypoglycemia, and lactic acidosis. Older individuals with comorbid conditions, such as pulmonary or urinary infections, congestive heart failure, or cerebrovascular accident, and with moderate or untreated hypothyroidism are particularly at risk for developing myxedema coma. It also may occur after overuse of narcotics or sedatives or after an acute illness in hypothyroid individuals. Symptoms of hypothyroidism in older adults should not be attributed to normal aging changes.[28]

EVALUATION AND TREATMENT   The diagnosis of primary hypothyroidism is made by documentation of the clinical symptoms of hypothyroidism, and measurement of increased levels of TSH and decreased levels of TH (total T_3 and both total and free T_4). When hypothyroidism is caused by pituitary deficiencies, serum TSH levels and basal metabolic rate (BMR) decrease. Hormone replacement therapy with the hormone levothyroxine is the treatment of choice. The restoration of normal TH levels should be timed appropriately; a regimen of hormonal therapy depends on the individual's age, the duration and severity of the hypothyroidism, and the presence of other disorders, particularly cardiovascular disorders.[35] Pregnant women need to be evaluated for thyroid function.[36]

Thyroid Carcinoma

Thyroid carcinoma is the most common endocrine malignancy, accounting for 62,450 estimated new cases and 1950 estimated cancer deaths in 2015 in the United States, less than 4% of all neoplasms.[37] Exposure to ionizing radiation, especially during childhood, is the most consistent causal factor. Papillary and follicular thyroid carcinomas are the most frequent and medullary and anaplastic thyroid carcinomas are less common. Most tumors are well differentiated.

Most individuals with thyroid carcinoma have normal T_3 and T_4 levels and are therefore euthyroid. The cancer is typically discovered as a small thyroid nodule or metastatic tumor in the lungs, brain, or bone. Changes in voice and swallowing and difficulty breathing are related to tumor growth impinging on the trachea or esophagus. Ultrasonographic characteristics may be suggestive of malignancy, but are neither sensitive nor specific.[38] The diagnosis of thyroid cancer is generally made by fine needle aspiration of a thyroid nodule.

Treatment may include partial or total thyroidectomy, TSH suppression therapy (levothyroxine), radioactive iodine therapy (in iodine-concentrating tumors), postoperative radiation therapy, and chemotherapy (especially in anaplastic carcinoma). New insights into the molecular pathogenesis of thyroid carcinoma are leading to new therapies.[39]

> ✔ **QUICK CHECK 19-2**
> 1. Compare the clinical manifestations of hyperthyroidism and hypothyroidism.
> 2. What is Graves disease?
> 3. What is myxedema?
> 4. What is the most common cause of thyroid carcinoma?

ALTERATIONS OF PARATHYROID FUNCTION

Hyperparathyroidism

Hyperparathyroidism is characterized by greater than normal secretion of parathyroid hormone (PTH) and hypercalcemia. Hyperparathyroidism is classified as primary, secondary, or tertiary.[40]

PATHOPHYSIOLOGY **Primary hyperparathyroidism** is characterized by inappropriate excess secretion of PTH by one or more of the parathyroid glands. It is one of the most common endocrine disorders. Approximately 80% to 85% of cases are caused by parathyroid adenomas, another 10% to 15% result from parathyroid hyperplasia, and approximately 1% of cases are caused by parathyroid carcinoma. In addition, primary hyperparathyroidism may be caused by a variety of genetic causes, especially the genes that cause multiple endocrine neoplasia.[41]

In primary hyperparathyroidism, PTH secretion is increased and is not under the usual feedback control mechanisms. The calcium level in the blood increases because of increased bone resorption and gastrointestinal absorption of calcium, but fails to inhibit PTH secretion by the parathyroid gland.

Secondary hyperparathyroidism is a compensatory response of the parathyroid glands to chronic hypocalcemia, which can be associated with decreased renal activation of vitamin D (renal failure) (see Chapter 30). Secretion of PTH is elevated, but PTH cannot achieve normal calcium levels because of insufficient levels of activated vitamin D. Other causes of secondary hyperparathyroidism include dietary deficiency in vitamin D or calcium; decreased intestinal absorption of vitamin D or calcium; and ingestion of drugs, such as phenytoin, phenobarbital, and laxatives, which either accelerate the metabolism of vitamin D or decrease intestinal absorption of calcium.

Tertiary hyperparathyroidism is excessive secretion of PTH and hypercalcemia that occurs after long-standing secondary hyperparathyroidism. The etiology is unknown but represents autonomous secretion of PTH from persistent parathyroid stimulation even after withdrawal of calcium and calcitriol therapy.[42] Treatment is surgical removal of one of the parathyroid glands.

CLINICAL MANIFESTATIONS Hypercalcemia and hypophosphatemia are the hallmarks of primary hyperparathyroidism and may be discovered incidentally. Hypercalcemia and hypophosphatemia may be asymptomatic or affected individuals may present with symptoms related to the muscular, nervous, and gastrointestinal systems, including fatigue, headache, depression, anorexia, and nausea and vomiting. Excessive osteoclastic and osteocytic activity resulting in bone resorption may cause pathologic fractures, kyphosis of the dorsal spine, and compression fractures of the vertebral bodies. (Bone resorption is discussed in Chapter 39.)

The increased renal filtration load of calcium leads to hypercalciuria. Hypercalcemia also affects proximal renal tubular function, causing metabolic acidosis and production of an abnormally alkaline urine.[43] PTH hypersecretion enhances renal phosphate excretion and results in hypophosphatemia and hyperphosphaturia (see Chapter 5). The combination of these three variables—hypercalciuria, alkaline urine, and hyperphosphaturia—predisposes the individual to the formation of calcium stones, particularly in the renal pelvis or renal collecting ducts. These may be associated with infections. Both kidney stones and renal infection can lead to impaired renal function. Hypercalcemia also impairs the concentrating ability of the renal tubule by decreasing its response to ADH. Chronic hypercalcemia of hyperparathyroidism is associated with mild insulin resistance, necessitating increased insulin secretion to maintain normal glucose levels.

Secondary hyperparathyroidism caused by renal disease presents clinically not only with bone resorption but also with the symptoms of hypocalcemia and hyperphosphatemia. Hypocalcemia can cause many significant clinical problems (see Chapter 5) and hyperphosphatemia can cause deleterious effects on the cardiovascular system.

EVALUATION AND TREATMENT The concurrent findings of increased ionized calcium concentration despite elevated PTH concentration are suggestive of primary hyperparathyroidism. PTH levels also may be inappropriately within the normal range because hypercalcemia should completely suppress PTH production. Imaging procedures are used to localize adenomas before surgery. Observation of asymptomatic individuals with mild hypercalcemia is recommended; these individuals are advised to avoid dehydration and limit dietary calcium intake. Definitive treatment of severe primary hyperparathyroidism involves surgical removal of the solitary adenoma or, in the case of hyperplasia, complete removal of three and partial removal of the fourth hyperplastic parathyroid glands. In those individuals who fail surgery, other treatments such as bisphosphonates and calcimimetics (e.g., cinacalcet, a new class of calcium-lowering drugs) may be considered.

If serum calcium concentration is low but PTH level is elevated, secondary hyperparathyroidism is likely. Evaluation for renal function may indicate chronic renal disease. Treatment for secondary hyperparathyroidism in chronic renal disease requires calcium replacement, dietary phosphate restriction and phosphate binders, and vitamin D replacement. Treatment also may include calcimimetics, which work to increase parathyroid calcium receptor sensitivity, thus lowering PTH levels.[44,45]

Hypoparathyroidism

Hypoparathyroidism (abnormally low PTH levels) is most commonly caused by damage to the parathyroid glands during thyroid surgery. This occurs because of the anatomic proximity of the parathyroid glands to the thyroid (see Figure 18-11). Hypoparathyroidism also is associated with genetic syndromes, including familial hypoparathyroidism and DiGeorge syndrome (see Chapter 8). Hypomagnesemia also can cause a decrease in both PTH secretion and PTH function. An idiopathic or autoimmune form of hypoparathyroidism also is recognized.[46] There is an inherited condition associated with hypocalcemia but with normal to elevated levels of PTH called pseudohypoparathyroidism; it is caused by a postreceptor defect in PTH action.

PATHOPHYSIOLOGY A lack of circulating PTH causes depressed serum calcium levels and increased serum phosphate levels. In the absence of PTH, resorption of calcium from bone and regulation of calcium reabsorption from the renal tubules are impaired. Phosphate reabsorption by the renal tubules is therefore increased, causing decreased renal phosphate excretion and hyperphosphatemia.

Hypomagnesemia inhibits PTH secretion. When serum magnesium levels return to normal, however, PTH secretion returns to normal, as does the responsiveness of peripheral tissues to PTH. Hypomagnesemia may be related to chronic alcoholism, malnutrition, malabsorption, increased renal clearance of magnesium caused by the use of aminoglycoside antibiotics or certain chemotherapeutic agents, or prolonged magnesium-deficient parenteral nutritional therapy.

CLINICAL MANIFESTATIONS Symptoms associated with hypoparathyroidism are primarily those of hypocalcemia (see Table 5-7). Hypocalcemia causes a lowered threshold for nerve and muscle excitation so that a nerve impulse may be initiated by a slight stimulus anywhere along the length of a nerve or muscle fiber. This creates tetany, a condition characterized by muscle spasms, hyperreflexia, clonic-tonic convulsions, laryngeal spasms, and, in severe cases, death by asphyxiation. Chvostek and Trousseau signs may be used to evaluate for neuromuscular irritability. Chvostek sign is elicited by tapping the cheek, resulting in twitching of the upper lip. Trousseau sign is elicited by sustained inflation of a sphygmomanometer placed on the upper arm to a level above the systolic blood pressure with resultant painful carpal spasm. Other symptoms of hypocalcemia include dry skin, loss of body and scalp hair, hypoplasia of developing teeth, horizontal ridges on the nails, cataracts, basal ganglia calcifications (which may be associated with a parkinsonian syndrome), and bone deformities, including brachydactyly and bowing of the long bones.

Phosphate retention caused by increased renal reabsorption of phosphate is also associated with hypoparathyroidism (see Table 5-7). Hyperphosphatemia results from PTH deficiency and, in turn, hyperphosphatemia further lowers calcium concentration by inhibiting the activation of vitamin D, thereby lowering the gastrointestinal absorption of calcium.

EVALUATION AND TREATMENT A low serum calcium concentration and a high phosphorous level in the absence of renal failure, intestinal disorders, or nutritional deficiencies suggest hypoparathyroidism. PTH levels are low in hypoparathyroidism and measurement of serum magnesium level and urinary calcium excretion also can help in diagnosis. Treatment is directed toward alleviation of the hypocalcemia. In acute states, this involves parenteral administration of calcium, which corrects serum calcium concentration within minutes. Maintenance of serum calcium level is achieved with pharmacologic doses of cholecalciferol (vitamin D_3) and oral calcium.[47] Hypoplastic dentition, cataracts, bone deformities, and basal ganglia calcifications do not respond to the correction of hypocalcemia, but the other symptoms of hypocalcemia are reversible.

✔**QUICK CHECK 19-3**
1. How does excessive parathyroid hormone (PTH) affect bones?
2. What are the results of a lack of circulating PTH?

DYSFUNCTION OF THE ENDOCRINE PANCREAS: DIABETES MELLITUS

Diabetes mellitus is a group of metabolic diseases characterized by hyperglycemia resulting from defects in insulin secretion, insulin action, or both. In the United States in 2012, 29.1 million people had diabetes and another 8.1 million were estimated to be undiagnosed.[48] The American Diabetes Association (ADA) classifies four categories of diabetes mellitus[49] (Table 19-3), as follows:

1. Type 1 (beta-cell destruction, usually leading to absolute insulin deficiency)
2. Type 2 (ranging from predominantly insulin resistance with relative insulin deficiency to predominantly an insulin secretory defect with insulin resistance)
3. Other specific types
4. Gestational diabetes

The diagnosis of diabetes mellitus is based on glycosylated hemoglobin (HbA$_{1C}$) levels; fasting plasma glucose (FPG) levels; 2-hour plasma glucose levels during oral glucose tolerance testing (OGTT) using a 75-g oral glucose load; or random glucose levels in an individual with symptoms (Box 19-1).[49] Glycosylated hemoglobin refers to the permanent attachment of glucose to hemoglobin molecules and reflects the average plasma glucose exposure over the life of a red blood cell (approximately 120 days). It provides a more accurate measure for monitoring long-term control of blood glucose levels. This test is critically dependent upon the method of measurement and must be related to established standards.

The ADA classification "categories at increased risk for diabetes" (or prediabetes) describes nondiabetic elevations of HbA$_{1C}$, FPG, or 2-hour plasma glucose value during OGTT (see Box 19-1).[49] The Centers for Disease Control and Prevention (CDC) estimates that 37% of U.S. adults aged 20 years or older have prediabetes (51% of those aged 65 years or older).[48] This classification includes impaired glucose tolerance (IGT), which results from diminished insulin secretion, and

---

Box 19-1 Diagnostic Criteria for Diabetes Mellitus

1. HbA$_{1C}$ (as measured in a DCCT-referenced assay) ≥6.5%*
   OR
2. FPG ≥126 mg/dl (7.0 mmol/L); fasting is defined as no caloric intake for at least 8 hr*
   OR
3. 2-hr plasma glucose ≥200 mg/dl (11.1 mmol/L) during OGTT*
   OR
4. In an individual with classic symptoms of hyperglycemia or hyperglycemic crisis, a random plasma glucose ≥200 mg/dl (11.1 mmol/L)

Categories of Increased Risk for Diabetes
1. FPG 100 to 125 mg/dl
2. 2-hr PG 140 to 199 mg/dl during OGTT
3. HbA$_{1C}$ 5.7% to 6.4%

Data from American Diabetes Association: *Diabetes Care* 38: S1-S93, 2015. Available at: http://professional.diabetes.org/admin/UserFiles/0%20-%20Sean/Documents/January%20Supplement%20Combined_Final.pdf.
DCCT, Diabetes Control and Complications Trial; *FPG*, fasting plasma glucose; *HbA$_{1C}$*, hemoglobin A$_{1C}$ or glycosylated hemoglobin; *OGTT*, oral glucose tolerance testing; *PG*, plasma glucose.
*In the absence of unequivocal hyperglycemia, criteria 1 through 3 should be confirmed by repeat testing.

TABLE 19-3	Epidemiology and Etiology of Diabetes Mellitus in the United States	
	Type 1 Diabetes: Primary Beta-Cell Defect or Failure	**Type 2 Diabetes: Insulin Resistance with Inadequate Insulin Secretion**
Incidence		
Frequency	5-10% of all cases of diabetes mellitus Prevalence rate is 0.17%	Accounts for most cases (≈90-95%) Prevalence rate for adults is 9.3%
Change in incidences	No documented increase in incidence in United States	Incidence in adults more than tripled from 1980 to 2011 with no increase from 2006 to 2011.
Characteristics		
Age at onset	Peak onset at age 11-13 yr (slightly earlier for girls than for boys); rare in children younger than 1 yr and adults older than 30 yr	Risk of developing diabetes increases after age 40 yr
Gender	Similar in males and females	Similar in males and females
Racial distribution	Rates for whites 1.5-2 times higher than for nonwhites	Risk is highest for blacks and Native Americans
Obesity	Generally normal or underweight	Frequent contributing factor to precipitate type 2 diabetes among those susceptible
Etiology		
Common theory	*Autoimmune:* genetic and environmental factors, resulting in gradual process of autoimmune destruction in genetically susceptible individuals *Nonautoimmune:* Unknown	Genetic susceptibility (polygenic) combined with environmental determinants; defects in beta-cell function combined with insulin resistance Associated with long-duration obesity
Presence of antibody	Autoantibodies to insulin and to glutamic acid decarboxylase (GAD_{65})	Autoantibodies not present
Insulin resistance	Insulin resistance at diagnosis is unusual, but may occur as individual ages and gains weight	Insulin resistance is virtually universal and multifactorial in origin
Insulin secretion	Severe insulin deficiency or no insulin secretion at all	Typically increased at time of diagnosis, but progressively declines over course of illness

Data from American Diabetes Association: *National diabetes statistics report 2014.* Available at: http://www.cdc.gov/diabetes/data/; Centers for Disease Control: *National diabetes statistics report 2014.* Available at http://www.cdc.gov/diabetes/pubs/statsreport14/national-diabetes-report-web.pdf.

impaired fasting glucose (IFG), which is caused by enhanced hepatic glucose output. Individuals with IGT and IFG are at increased risk of cardiovascular disease and premature death and carry a 15% to 50%, 5-year risk of developing diabetes, particularly type 2 diabetes.[49] Thus, prevention of diabetes with lifestyle interventions is essential.[49]

Types of Diabetes Mellitus
Type 1 Diabetes Mellitus

Type 1 diabetes mellitus is the most common pediatric chronic disease and affects 0.17% of U.S. children, and the incidence is increasing.[48] Between 10% and 13% of individuals with newly diagnosed type 1 diabetes have a first-degree relative (parent or sibling) with type 1 diabetes. There is a 50% concordance rate in twins. Diagnosis is rare during the first 9 months of life and peaks at 12 years of age. Two distinct types of type 1 diabetes have been identified: idiopathic and autoimmune.

PATHOPHYSIOLOGY   Idiopathic type 1 diabetes is far less common than autoimmune diabetes, has a strong genetic component, and occurs mostly in people of Asian or African descent. Affected individuals have varying degrees of insulin deficiency.[48]

Autoimmune type 1 diabetes mellitus is a slowly progressive autoimmune T-cell–mediated disease that destroys beta cells of the pancreas. There is a deficient immune tolerance linked to abnormalities in immune cells and changes in beta-cell antigens.[50] Destruction of beta cells is related to genetic susceptibility and environmental factors. The strongest genetic association is with histocompatibility leukocyte antigen (HLA) class II alleles *HLA-DQ* and *HLA-DR*. The *HLA-DR* marker is associated with other autoimmune disorders, such as celiac,

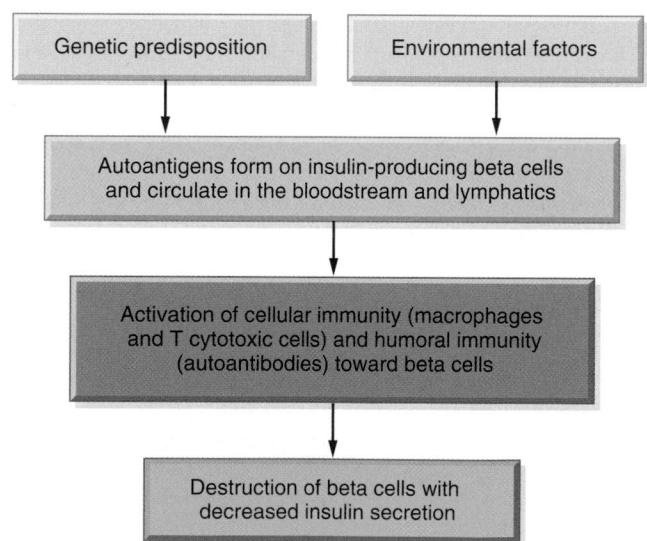

FIGURE 19-10 Pathophysiology of Type 1 Diabetes Mellitus.

Graves, Hashimoto, and Addison diseases. Environmental factors that have been implicated include exposure to certain drugs, foods, and viruses. These gene-environment interactions result in the formation of autoantigens that are expressed on the surface of pancreatic beta cells and circulate in the bloodstream and lymphatics (Figure 19-10). Cellular immunity (T-cytotoxic cells and macrophages) and humoral immunity (autoantibodies) are stimulated, resulting in beta-cell destruction and apoptosis. The destruction of beta cells results from lymphocyte and macrophage infiltration of the islets, resulting in release of inflammatory cytokines, activation of T-helper and T-cytotoxic lymphocytes, and death of islet beta cells. Beta-cell destruction also is mediated by the production of autoantibodies against islet cells, insulin, glutamic acid decarboxylase (GAD), and other cytoplasmic proteins.[50] Insulin synthesis declines and hyperglycemia develops over time.

For insulin synthesis to decline enough such that hyperglycemia occurs, 80% to 90% of the insulin-secreting beta cells of the islet of Langerhans must be destroyed. Insulin normally suppresses secretion of glucagon and, thus, hypoinsulinemia leads to a marked increase in glucagon secretion. Glucagon, a hormone produced by the alpha cells of the islets, acts in the liver to increase blood glucose level by stimulating glycogenolysis and gluconeogenesis. In addition to the decline in insulin secretion, there is decreased secretion of amylin, another beta-cell hormone. One of the critical actions of amylin is to suppress glucagon release from the alpha cells. Thus both alpha-cell and beta-cell functions are abnormal and both a lack of insulin and a relative excess of glucagon contribute to hyperglycemia in type 1 diabetes.

CLINICAL MANIFESTATIONS Historically, type 1 diabetes mellitus was thought to have an abrupt onset. It is now known, however, that the natural history involves a long preclinical period with gradual destruction of beta cells, eventually leading to insulin deficiency and hyperglycemia. In general, this latent period is longer in adults with onset of type 1 diabetes and often results in misclassification of those affected as having type 2 diabetes.

Type 1 diabetes mellitus affects the metabolism of fat, protein, and carbohydrates. Glucose accumulates in the blood and appears in the urine as the renal threshold for glucose is exceeded, producing an osmotic diuresis and symptoms of polyuria and thirst (Table 19-4). Wide fluctuations in blood glucose levels occur. In addition, protein and fat breakdown occurs because of the lack of insulin, resulting in weight loss. Increased metabolism of fats and proteins leads to high levels of circulating ketones, causing a condition known as diabetic ketoacidosis (DKA) (see p. 477).

Currently half of individuals with type 1 diabetes are obese and there are increasing numbers of individuals who have both type 1 diabetes and the clinical manifestations of metabolic syndrome, including obesity, dyslipidemia, and hypertension (see Box 19-1).[51] These individuals are at high risk for chronic complications of diabetes, including heart disease and stroke.

EVALUATION AND TREATMENT The criteria for diagnosis of type 1 diabetes are the same as those for type 2 diabetes.[49] (see Box 19-1). Many children are first diagnosed when they present with the signs and symptoms of DKA. In DKA, acetone (a volatile form of ketones) is exhaled by hyperventilation and gives the breath a sweet or "fruity" odor. Occasionally, diabetic coma is the initial symptom of the disease. The diagnosis of diabetes is not difficult when the symptoms of polydipsia, polyuria, polyphagia, weight loss, and hyperglycemia are present in fasting and postprandial states. C-peptide, a component of proinsulin released during insulin production, can be measured in the serum as a surrogate for insulin levels and is indicative of residual beta-cell mass and function. The zinc transporter 8 autoantibody (ZnT8Ab) test has been approved for diagnosis of type 1 diabetes.[52] Other important aspects of evaluation include looking for evidence of the chronic complications of type 1 diabetes, including renal, nervous system, cardiac, peripheral vascular, retinal, and bony tissue damage.

Currently, treatment regimens are designed to achieve optimal glucose level control (as measured by the HbA_{1C} value) without causing episodes of significant hypoglycemia.[49] Management requires individual planning according to type of disease, age, and activity level, but all individuals require some combination of insulin therapy, meal planning, and exercise regimen. There are several different types of insulin preparations available and there are new technologies for more physiologic insulin delivery systems.[53] Many different kinds of therapies are being tested to prevent the autoimmune destruction of beta cells, including immunosuppression with antirejection drugs (see *Health Alert: Immunotherapy for the Prevention and Treatment of Type 1 Diabetes*). Finally, islet cell, stem cell, and whole pancreas transplantation has been successful in selected individuals.[50,54]

TABLE 19-4 Clinical Manifestations and Mechanisms for Type 1 Diabetes Mellitus

Manifestation	Rationale
Polydipsia	Because of elevated blood glucose levels, water is osmotically attracted from body cells, resulting in intracellular dehydration and stimulation of thirst in hypothalamus
Polyuria	Hyperglycemia acts as an osmotic diuretic; amount of glucose filtered by glomeruli of kidney exceeds that which can be reabsorbed by renal tubules; glycosuria results, accompanied by large amounts of water lost in urine
Polyphagia	Depletion of cellular stores of carbohydrates, fats, and protein results in cellular starvation and a corresponding increase in hunger
Weight loss	Weight loss occurs because of fluid loss in osmotic diuresis and loss of body tissue as fats and proteins are used for energy
Fatigue	Metabolic changes result in poor use of food products, contributing to lethargy and fatigue
Recurrent infections (e.g., boils, carbuncles, and bladder infection)	Growth of microorganisms is stimulated by increased glucose levels and diabetes is associated with some immunocompromised individuals
Prolonged wound healing	Impaired blood supply hinders healing
Genital pruritus	Hyperglycemia and glycosuria favor fungal growth; candidal infections, resulting in pruritus, are a common presenting symptom in women
Visual changes	Blurred vision occurs as water balance in eye fluctuates because of elevated blood glucose levels; diabetic retinopathy may ensue
Paresthesias	Paresthesias are common manifestations of diabetic neuropathies
Cardiovascular symptoms (e.g., chest pain, extremity pain, and neurologic deficits)	Diabetes contributes to formation of atherosclerotic plaques that involve coronary, peripheral, and cerebrovascular circulations and alterations in microvessels

FIGURE 19-11 Pathophysiology of Type 2 Diabetes Mellitus.

HEALTH ALERT

Immunotherapy for the Prevention and Treatment of Type 1 Diabetes

Many different kinds of immunologic approaches are being tested to prevent the autoimmune destruction of beta cells in type 1 diabetes. These treatments are aimed at preserving insulin synthesis early in the course of disease. Some of these interventions create generalized immunosuppression, including mycophenolate mofetil, monoclonal antibodies to B cells (rituximab), mono-clonal antibodies to T cells (otelixizumab, teplizumab), interleukin-1 blockade, and cyclosporine. Studies document their effectiveness in stabilizing beta-cell function but, unfortunately, they also cause many side effects. More focused immunologic therapies are "antigen specific," which means they suppress only the parts of the immune response that are attacking the beta cells. One approach that has shown promising (but mixed) results has been the use of vaccines to induce T-regulatory cells that suppress the immune attack on specific antigens. Vaccines that have currently been tested include dendritic cells, insulin, glutamic acid decarboxylase 65 (GAD-Alum), and heatshock proteins (DiaPep277). Another ambitious new approach to preserving beta-cell function is through the introduction of stem cells, which decrease autoimmune responses and may engraft and become insulin-producing beta cells. Clinical trials are needed to evaluate long term remission.

Data from Atkinson MA et al: *Lancet* 383(9911):69-82, 2014; Canivell S, Gomis R: *Autoimmun Rev* 13(4-5):403-407, 2014; Creusot RJ et al: *Diabetes* 63(1):20-30, 2014; Gupta S et al: *Clin Immunol* 151(2):146-154, 2014; Vetere A et al: *Nat Rev Drug Discov* 13(4):278-289, 2014.

Type 2 Diabetes Mellitus

Type 2 diabetes mellitus (non–insulin-dependent diabetes mellitus) affects 9.3% of adults in the United States.[48] Prevalence is highest among American Indians and Alaska Natives (16%) and lowest among non-Hispanic whites (7.6%). There also is an increased preva-lence of type 2 diabetes in children, especially in obese children (see Table 19-3).

A genetic-environmental interaction appears to be responsible for type 2 diabetes.[55] The most well-recognized risk factors are age, obesity, hypertension, physical inactivity, and family history. More than 60 genes have been identified that are associated with type 2 diabetes, including those that code for beta-cell mass, beta-cell function (ability to sense blood glucose levels, insulin synthesis, and insulin secretion), proinsulin and insulin molecular structures, insulin receptors, hepatic

Box 19-2   Criteria for the Diagnosis of Metabolic Syndrome

Three of the following five traits:
1. Increased waist circumference (>40 inches in men; >35 inches in women)—may be adjusted for ethnic groups
2. Plasma triglycerides ≥150 mg/dl
3. Plasma high-density lipoprotein (HDL) cholesterol <40 mg/dl (men) or <50 mg/dl (women)
4. Blood pressure ≥130/85 mm Hg
5. Fasting plasma glucose ≥100 mg/dl*

From Grundy SM et al: *Circulation* 112(17):2735-52, 2005.
*Criterion decreased from 110 to 100 mg/dl based on 2010 diagnostic category for persons at risk for diabetes mellitus (see Box 19-1).

synthesis of glucose, glucagon synthesis, and cellular responsiveness to insulin stimulation.[56] These genetic abnormalities combined with environmental influences, such as obesity, result in the basic patho-physiologic mechanisms of type 2 diabetes, which are insulin resistance and decreased insulin secretion by beta cells (Figure 19-11).

There is increasing evidence that diet, including diet during preg-nancy, influences the long-term risk of type 2 diabetes in children and adults.[57] Metabolic syndrome is a constellation of disorders (central obesity, dyslipidemia, prehypertension, and an elevated fasting blood glucose level) that together confer a high risk of developing type 2 diabetes and associated cardiovascular complications (Box 19-2). The metabolic syndrome often develops during childhood and is prevalent among overweight children and adolescents. Metabolic syndrome is characterized by many of the same genetic and environmental risks as type 2 diabetes and individuals should be screened on a regular basis (see Box 19-2).[58] Early recognition and treatment, including vigorous lifestyle changes, are critical to reducing cardiovascular events and improving clinical outcomes for individuals with prediabetes and metabolic syndrome.[59]

PATHOPHYSIOLOGY   Many organs contribute to insulin resistance, chronic hyperglycemia, and the consequences of type 2 diabetes (Figure 19-12). Insulin resistance is defined as a suboptimal response of insulin-sensitive tissues (especially liver, muscle, and adipose tissue) to insulin and is associated with obesity. Several mechanisms are involved in abnormalities of the insulin signaling pathway and

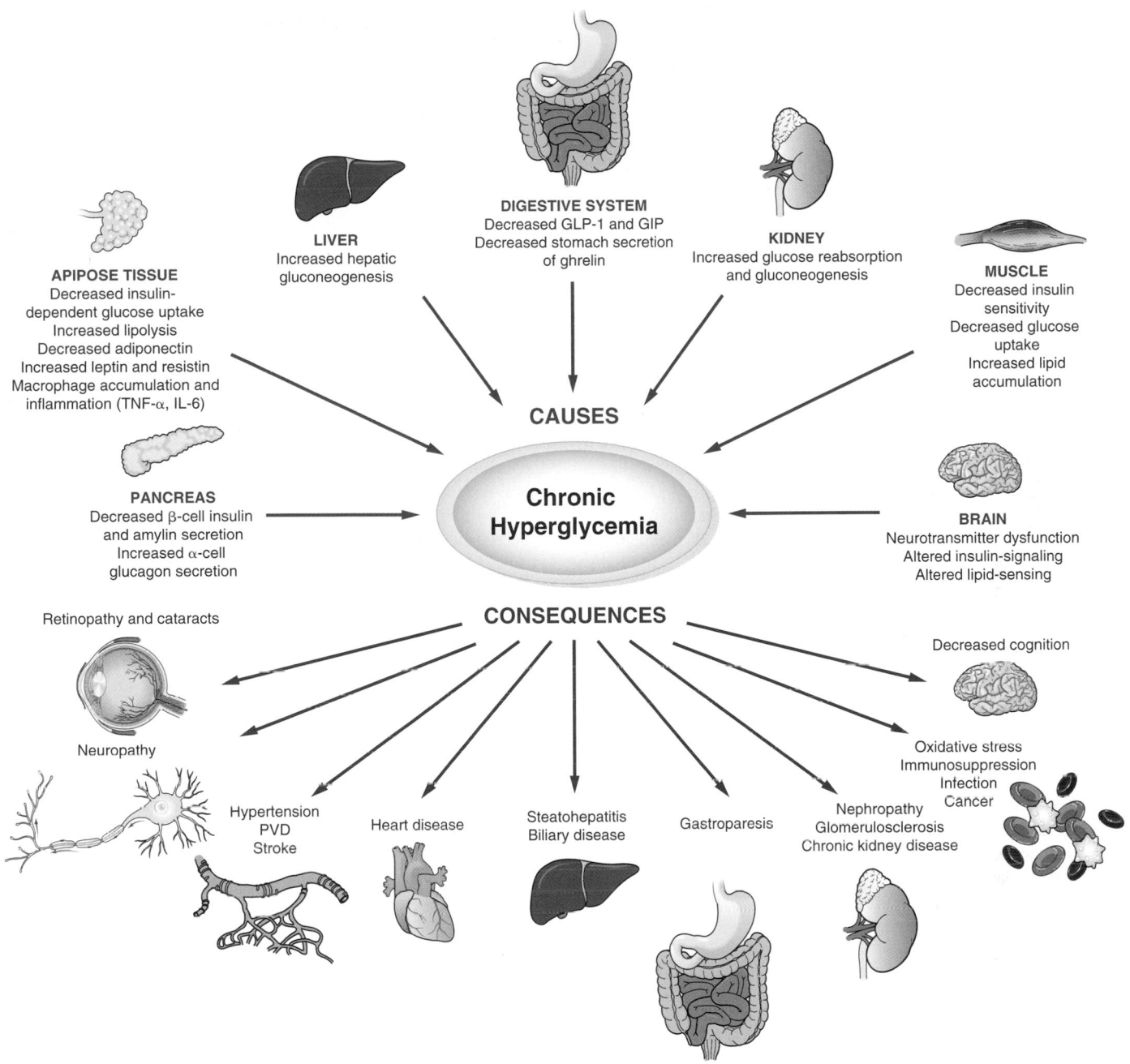

FIGURE 19-12 Multiorgan Causes and Common Consequences of Chronic Hyperglycemia in Type 2 Diabetes. *GLP-1,* Glucagon-like peptide 1; *GIP,* gastric inhibitory polypeptide; *IL,* interleukin; *PVD,* peripheral vascular disease; *TNF,* tumor necrosis factor.

contribute to insulin resistance. These include an abnormality of the insulin molecule, high amounts of insulin antagonists, down-regulation of the insulin receptor, and alteration of glucose transporter (GLUT) proteins.

Obesity is one of the most important contributors to insulin resistance and diabetes and acts through several important mechanisms:
1. Adipokines (leptin and adiponectin) are hormones produced in adipose tissue. Obesity results in increased serum levels of leptin and decreased levels of adiponectin. These changes are associated with inflammation and decreased insulin sensitivity.[60]
2. Elevated levels of serum free fatty acids (FFAs) and intracellular deposits of triglycerides and cholesterol are also found in obese

individuals. These changes interfere with intracellular insulin signaling, decrease tissue responses to insulin, alter incretin actions, and promote inflammation.
3. Inflammatory cytokines are released from intra-abdominal adipocytes or adipocyte-associated mononuclear cells and induce insulin resistance and are cytotoxic to beta cells.[61]
4. Obesity is correlated with hyperinsulinemia and decreased insulin receptor density.

Compensatory hyperinsulinemia prevents the clinical appearance of diabetes for many years. Eventually, however, beta-cell dysfunction develops and leads to a relative deficiency of insulin activity.[55] The islet dysfunction is caused by a combination of a decrease in beta-cell mass and a reduction in normal beta-cell function.[62] A progressive decrease in the weight and number of beta cells occurs and many of the remaining cells develop "exhaustion" from increased demand for insulin biosynthesis.

Glucagon concentration is increased in type 2 diabetes because pancreatic alpha cells become less responsive to glucose inhibition, resulting in an increase in glucagon secretion. These abnormally high levels of glucagon increase blood glucose level by stimulating glycogenolysis and gluconeogenesis. As was discussed under type 1 diabetes, type 2 diabetes also is associated with a deficiency in amylin, further increasing glucagon levels.

Amylin (islet amyloid polypeptide) is another beta-cell hormone that is decreased in both type 1 and type 2 diabetes. Amylin increases satiety and suppresses glucagon release from the alpha cells. It also contributes to islet cell destruction through the deposition of abnormal (misfolded) amyloid polypeptide in the pancreas.[63] Pramlintide, a synthetic analog of amylin, is used for treatment in type 2 diabetes.

Hormones released from the gastrointestinal (GI) tract play a role in insulin resistance, beta-cell function, and diabetes. Ghrelin is a peptide produced in the stomach and pancreatic islets that regulates food intake, energy balance, and hormonal secretion.[64] Decreased levels of circulating ghrelin have been associated with insulin resistance and increased fasting insulin levels. The incretins are a class of peptides that are released from the GI tract in response to food intake and function to increase the secretion of insulin and have many other positive effects on metabolism. The most studied incretin is called glucagon-like peptide 1 (GLP-1), and studies have demonstrated that beta-cell responsiveness to GLP-1 is reduced both in prediabetes and in type 2 diabetes[65] (see *Health Alert:* Incretin Hormones for Type 2 Diabetes Mellitus Therapy).

HEALTH ALERT

Incretin Hormones for Type 2 Diabetes Mellitus Therapy

The incretin hormones are secreted from endocrine intestinal cells in the presence of carbohydrates, proteins, and fats and have many functions including suppressing appetite. The major incretin hormone is glucagon-like peptide-1 (GLP-1). It controls postprandial glucose levels by promoting glucose-dependent insulin secretion, stimulating insulin gene expression, inhibiting glucagon synthesis, and delaying gastric emptying. GLP-1 also reduces beta-cell apoptosis and induces pancreatic acinar cells to differentiate into new beta cells, thus enhancing beta-cell mass and replenishing intracellular stores of insulin. Incretins are inactivated by the enzyme dipeptidyl peptidase IV (DPP-IV). The many positive effects on glucose metabolism without hypoglycemia have led to the use of incretin hormones and incretin enhancers for the treatment of type 2 diabetes. There are two classes of incretin-related therapies: GLP-1 receptor agonists (GLP-1 RAs) and dipeptidyl peptidase IV (DPP-IV) inhibitors. In addition to improving glucose control, many people taking these medications experience weight loss and improvements in measurements of blood pressure, serum lipids, and myocardial function. There also is increasing interest in the use of incretin therapy to reduce the risk of diabetes in individuals with prediabetes.

Data from Angeli FS, Shannon RP: *J Endocrinol* 221(1):T17-T30, 2014; Haluzik M: *J Endocrinol* 221(1):E1-E2, 2014; Lee YS, Jun HS: *Metabolism* 63(1):9-19, 2014; Neumiller JJ: *Med Clin North Am* 99(1):107-129, 2015; Teitelman G: *Endocrinology* 155(4):1175-1177, 2014; Tenzer-Iglesias P: *J Fam Pract* 63(2 suppl):S21-S26, 2014; van Bloemendaal L et al: *J Endocrinol* 221(1):T1-T16, 2014.

The kidneys also influence the pathophysiology of type 2 diabetes. Renal reabsorption of glucose through the sodium-glucose cotransporter 2 (SGLT2) is an important controller of serum glucose levels and new medications aimed at blocking it have resulted in decreased measurements for blood glucose level, weight, and blood pressure.[66]

CLINICAL MANIFESTATIONS The clinical manifestations of type 2 diabetes are nonspecific. The affected individual is often overweight, dyslipidemic, hyperinsulinemic, and hypertensive. The individual with type 2 diabetes may show some classic symptoms of diabetes, such as polyuria and polydipsia, but more often will have nonspecific symptoms such as fatigue, pruritus, recurrent infections, visual changes, or symptoms of neuropathy (paresthesias or weakness). In those whose diabetes has progressed without treatment, symptoms related to coronary artery, peripheral artery, and cerebrovascular disease may develop.

EVALUATION AND TREATMENT The diagnostic criteria for type 2 diabetes are the same as those for type 1 (see Box 19-1).[49] Prevention of type 2 diabetes, especially in those individuals with prediabetes, hinges on diet and exercise, although there is increasing support for the use of some diabetes medications in high-risk individuals.[49]

As with type 1 diabetes, the goal of treatment for individuals with type 2 diabetes is the restoration of near-euglycemia (a normal blood glucose level) and correction of related metabolic disorders. The first approach to treatment of the individual with type 2 diabetes is maintaining an appropriate diet and exercise program.[67] Diet should match activity levels and include more complex carbohydrates (rather than simple sugars), foods low in fats, adequate protein, and fiber. Weight loss results in improved glucose tolerance. Bariatric surgery improves glycemic control, decreases risk of cardiovascular disease, and promotes weight loss in those morbidly obese. For individuals who require further intervention, oral hypoglycemic agents are indicated.[49] Currently, metformin is considered the primary pharmacologic choice for the treatment of type 2 diabetes and a second oral agent, a GLP-1 receptor agonist, or basal insulin is added if the A1C target is not maintained over 3 months. An increasing number of persons are being treated with incretins[49] (see *Health Alert:* Incretin Hormones for Type 2 Diabetes Mellitus Therapy). A combination of drugs may be required. Insulin therapy may be needed in the later stage of type 2 diabetes because of loss of beta-cell function, which is progressive over time.

Other Specific Types of Diabetes Mellitus and Gestational Diabetes Mellitus

As listed in Table 19-3, the American Diabetes Association classification of diabetes mellitus not only includes the most common forms of diabetes (type 1 and type 2) but also encompasses "other specific types of diabetes mellitus" and "gestational diabetes mellitus." Other specific types of diabetes include genetic defects in beta-cell function, genetic defects in insulin action, diseases of the exocrine pancreas, endocrinopathies, drug- or chemical-induced beta-cell dysfunction, infections, and other uncommon autoimmune and inherited disorders that are associated with diabetes.[49] The best-described of these other specific types of diabetes is termed maturity-onset diabetes of youth (MODY). MODY includes six specific autosomal dominant mutations that affect critical enzymes involved in beta-cell function or insulin action. It is estimated that only 1% of cases of diabetes are monogenic and, therefore, are classified as MODY.[68] Diagnosis and management are similar to those techniques used for type 2 diabetes.

Gestational diabetes mellitus (GDM) has been defined as any degree of glucose intolerance with onset or first recognition during pregnancy. However, this definition meant that many women with previously undiagnosed type 1 or type 2 diabetes were diagnosed with

GDM, and many of them had progressive disease after delivery. Therefore the ADA recently recommended that high-risk women found to have diabetes at their initial prenatal visit receive a diagnosis of type 1 or type 2 diabetes, not gestational diabetes.[49] GDM complicates approximately 7% of all pregnancies. Screening for GDM is recommended in asymptomatic, pregnant women after 24 weeks of gestation.[69] An OGTT is used to confirm the diagnosis.[49] Careful glucose control prenatally, during pregnancy, and after delivery is essential to the short- and long-term health of both mother and baby. Women who have GDM have a greatly increased subsequent diabetes risk, making consistent follow-up important.[49]

Acute Complications of Diabetes Mellitus

The major acute complications of diabetes mellitus are hypoglycemia, diabetic ketoacidosis, and hyperosmolar hyperglycemic nonketotic syndrome (see comparison in Table 19-5). The Somogyi effect (low blood glucose level during night that may lead to morning rise in blood glucose level) and dawn phenomenon (early morning rise in blood glucose level related to release of growth hormone, cortisol, and catecholamines without preceding hypoglycemia) also may be seen.

Hypoglycemia in diabetes is sometimes called *insulin shock* or *insulin reaction*. Individuals with type 2 diabetes are at less risk for hypoglycemia than those with type 1 diabetes because they retain relatively intact glucose counterregulatory mechanisms. However, hypoglycemia does occur in type 2 diabetes when treatment involves insulin

secretogogues (e.g., sulfonylureas) or exogenous insulin. Symptoms include pallor, tremor, anxiety, tachycardia, palpitations, diaphoresis, headache, dizziness, irritability, fatigue, poor judgment, confusion, visual disturbances, hunger, seizures, and coma. Treatment requires immediate replacement of glucose either orally or intravenously. Glucagon for home use can be prescribed for individuals who are at high risk.[49] Prevention is achieved with individualized management of medications and diet, monitoring of blood glucose levels, and education.

Diabetic ketoacidosis (DKA) is a serious complication related to a deficiency of insulin and an increase in the levels of insulin counter-regulatory hormones (catecholamines, cortisol, glucagon, growth hormone) (Figure 19-13). DKA occurs in approximately 30% of children with type 1 diabetes, and 5% of children with type 2 diabetes.[70] DKA is much more common in type 1 diabetes because insulin is more deficient (see Table 19-5). It is characterized by hyperglycemia, acidosis, and ketonuria. Insulin normally stimulates lipogenesis and inhibits lipolysis, thus preventing fat catabolism. With insulin deficiency, lipolysis is enhanced and there is an increase in the amount of nonesterified fatty acids delivered to the liver. The consequence is increased gluconeogenesis contributing to hyperglycemia and production of ketone bodies (acetoacetate, hydroxybutyrate, and acetone) by the mitochondria of the liver at a rate that exceeds peripheral use. Accumulation of ketone bodies causes a drop in pH, resulting in metabolic acidosis. Symptoms of diabetic ketoacidosis include Kussmaul respirations

TABLE 19-5 Common Acute Complications of Diabetes Mellitus

Hypoglycemia in Persons with DM	Diabetic Ketoacidosis	Hyperglycemic Nonketotic Syndromes
Synonyms		
Insulin shock, insulin reaction	Diabetic coma syndrome	Hyperosmolar hyperglycemia nonketotic coma
Persons at Risk		
Individuals taking insulin Individuals with rapidly fluctuating blood glucose levels Individuals with type 2 diabetes taking sulfonylurea agents	Individuals with type 1 diabetes Individuals with nondiagnosed diabetes	Older adults or very young individuals with type 2 diabetes, nondiabetic persons with predisposing factors, such as pancreatitis; individuals with undiagnosed diabetes
Predisposing Factors		
Excessive insulin or sulfonylurea agent intake, lack of sufficient food intake, excessive physical exercise, abrupt decline in insulin needs (e.g., renal failure, immediately postpartum), simultaneous use of insulin-potentiating agents or beta-blocking agents that mask symptoms	Stressful situation such as infection, accident, trauma, emotional stress; omission of insulin; medications that antagonize insulin	Infection, medications that antagonize insulin, comorbid condition
Typical Onset		
Rapid	Slow	Slowest
Presenting Symptoms		
Adrenergic reaction: pallor, sweating, tachycardia, palpitations, hunger, restlessness, anxiety, tremors Neurogenic reaction: fatigue, irritability, headache, loss of concentration, visual disturbances, dizziness, hunger, confusion, transient sensory or motor defects, convulsions, coma, death	Malaise, dry mouth, headache, polyuria, polydipsia, weight loss, nausea, vomiting, pruritus, abdominal pain, lethargy, shortness of breath, Kussmaul respirations, fruity or acetone odor to breath	Polyuria, polydipsia, hypovolemia, dehydration (parched lips, poor skin turgor), hypotension, tachycardia, hypoperfusion, weight loss, weakness, nausea, vomiting, abdominal pain, hypothermia, stupor, coma, seizures
Laboratory Analysis		
Serum glucose <30 mg/dl in newborn (first 2-3 days) and <55-60 mg/dl in adults	Glucose levels >250 mg/dl, reduction in bicarbonate concentration, increased anion gap, increased plasma levels of β-hydroxybutyrate, acetoacetate, and acetone	Glucose levels >600 mg/dl, lack of ketosis, serum osmolarity >320 mOsm/L, elevated blood urea nitrogen and creatinine levels

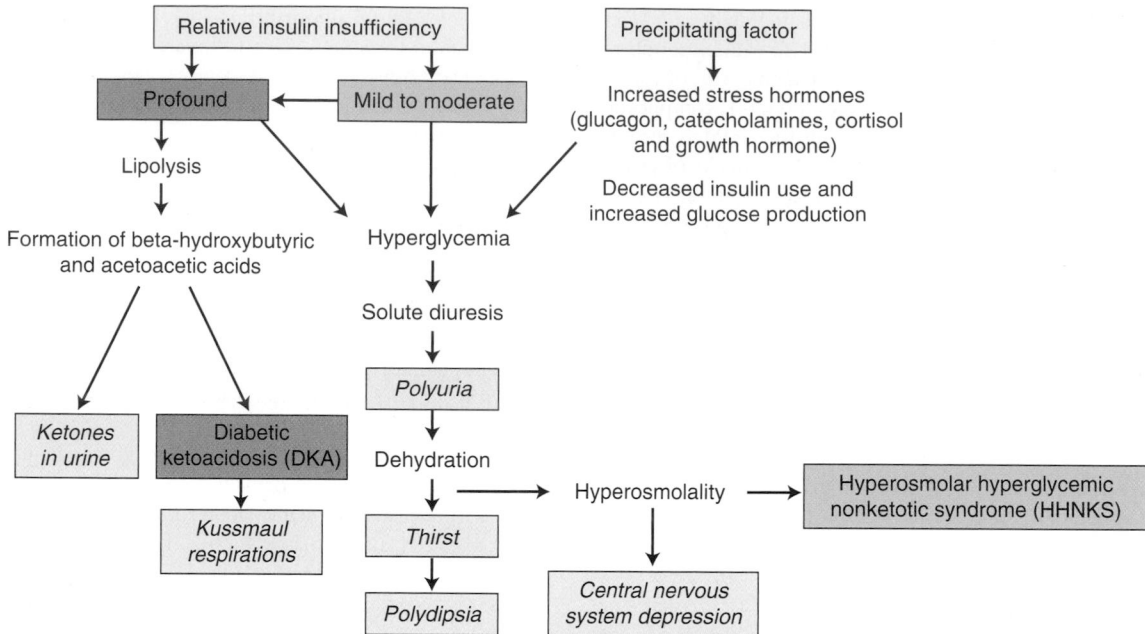

FIGURE 19-13 Pathophysiology of DKA and HHNKS in Diabetes Mellitus.

(hyperventilation in an attempt to compensate for the acidosis), postural dizziness, central nervous system depression, ketonuria, anorexia, nausea, abdominal pain, thirst, and polyuria. DKA is managed with a combination of fluids, insulin, and electrolyte replacement.

Hyperosmolar hyperglycemic nonketotic syndrome (HHNKS) is an uncommon but significant complication of type 2 diabetes mellitus with a high overall mortality. It occurs more often in elderly individuals who have other comorbidities, including infections or cardiovascular or renal disease. HHNKS differs from DKA in the degree of insulin deficiency (which is more profound in DKA) and the degree of fluid deficiency (which is more marked in HHNKS). The clinical features of HHNKS include a very high serum glucose concentration and osmolarity and a near-normal serum bicarbonate level and pH. Glucose levels are considerably higher in HHNKS than in DKA because of volume depletion. Because the amount of insulin required to inhibit fat breakdown is less than that needed for effective glucose transport, insulin levels are sufficient to prevent excessive lipolysis and ketosis (see Figure 19-13). Clinical manifestations include severe dehydration; loss of electrolytes, including potassium; and neurologic changes, such as stupor. Management includes fluid, insulin, and electrolyte replacement.

Chronic Complications of Diabetes Mellitus

A number of serious complications are associated with any type of poorly controlled diabetes mellitus. Most complications are associated with insulin resistance or deficit, chronic hyperglycemia (also known as glucose toxicity), accumulation of advanced glycation end products, and activation of metabolic pathways that cause tissue damage and the chronic complications of diabetes mellitus. These complications include microvascular (damage to capillaries; retinopathies, nephropathies, and neuropathies) and macrovascular (damage to larger vessels; coronary artery, peripheral vascular, and cerebral vascular) disease (Table 19-6). Strict control of blood glucose level reduces some complications, particularly nonfatal myocardial infarction, but increases 5-year mortality. Strict control is not recommended for high-risk individuals with type 2 diabetes mellitus (DM), but the individual risk/benefit profile should be considered.[71,72]

Microvascular Disease

Diabetic microvascular complications (disease in capillaries) are a leading cause of blindness, end-stage kidney failure, and various neuropathies. Occlusion of capillaries is characteristic of diabetic microvascular disease. The frequency and severity of lesions appear to be proportional to the duration of the disease (more or less than 10 years) and the status of glycemic control. Hypoxia and ischemia accompany microvascular disease, especially in the eye, kidney, and nerves. Many individuals with type 2 diabetes will present with microvascular complications because of the long duration of asymptomatic hyperglycemia that generally precedes diagnosis. This underscores the need to screen for diabetes.

Diabetic retinopathy. Diabetic retinopathy is a leading cause of blindness worldwide and in U.S. adults less than 60 years of age.[73] Compared with that in type 1 diabetes, retinopathy seems to develop more rapidly in individuals with type 2 diabetes because of the likelihood of long-standing hyperglycemia before diagnosis. Most individuals with diabetes will eventually develop retinopathy and they are also more likely to develop cataracts and glaucoma (see Chapter 14).

Diabetic retinopathy results from relative hypoxemia, damage to retinal blood vessels, red blood cell (RBC) aggregation, and hypertension (Figure 19-14). The three stages of retinopathy that lead to loss of vision are *nonproliferative* (stage I), characterized by an increase in retinal capillary permeability, vein dilation, microaneurysm formation, and superficial (flame-shaped) and deep (blot) hemorrhages; *preproliferative* (stage II), a progression of retinal ischemia with areas of poor perfusion that culminate in infarcts; and *proliferative* (stage III), the result of neovascularization (angiogenesis) and fibrous tissue formation within the retina or optic disc. Traction of the new vessels on the vitreous humor may cause retinal detachment or hemorrhage into the vitreous humor with severe blurring or loss of vision. Macular edema is the leading cause of blurred vision among persons with diabetes. Blurring of vision also can be a consequence of hyperglycemia and sorbitol accumulation in the lens. Dehydration of the lens, aqueous humor, and vitreous humor also reduces visual acuity.

Diabetic nephropathy. Diabetes is the most common cause of chronic kidney disease and end stage kidney disease. Approximately

TABLE 19-6 Chronic Complications of Diabetes Mellitus

Complications	Pathologic Mechanisms	Associated Symptoms
Microvascular		
Retinopathy		
Nonproliferative	Microaneurysms, capillary dilation, soft and hard exudates, dot and flame hemorrhages, arteriovenous shunts	May have no visual changes
Proliferative	Formation of new blood vessels, vitreal hemorrhage, scarring, retinal detachment	Loss of visual acuity
Maculopathy	Macular edema	Loss of central vision
Hyperglycemic lens edema	Shunting of glucose to polyol pathway: hyperosmolar fluid in lens	Blurring of vision
Cataract formation	Chronic hyperglycemia	Decreasing visual acuity
Nephropathy	Glomerular basement membrane thickening, mesangial expansion, glomerulosclerosis, focal tubular atrophy; hyperperfusion and hyperfiltration	Microalbuminuria and hypertension slowly progressing to end-stage kidney failure
Neuropathy	Oxidative stress, poor perfusion and ischemia, loss of nerve growth factor	Nerve dysfunction and degeneration
Peripheral neuropathy	Same as above	Distal symmetric sensorimotor polyneuropathy with glove and stocking loss of sensation (pain, vibration, temperature, proprioception); loss of motor nerve function with clawed toes and small muscle wasting in hands and flexor muscles; Charcot joints (loss of sensation results in joint and ligament degeneration, particularly of foot)
		Acute painful neuropathy with burning pain in legs and feet
Autonomic neuropathy	Same as above	Heart rate variability and postural hypotension
		Gastroparesis (delayed gastric emptying) and diarrhea
		Loss of bladder tone, urinary retention, and risk for bladder infection
		Erectile dysfunction and impotence in men
Skin and foot lesions	Loss of sensation, poor perfusion, suppressed immunity, and increased risk of infection	High risk for pressure ulcers and delayed wound healing; abscess formation; development of necrosis and gangrene, particularly of toes and foot; infection and osteomyelitis
Macrovascular		
Cardiovascular	Endothelial dysfunction, hyperlipidemia, accelerated atherosclerosis, coagulopathies	Hypertension, coronary artery disease, cardiomyopathy, and heart failure
Cerebrovascular	Same as above	Increased risk for ischemic and thrombotic stroke
Peripheral vascular	Same as above	Claudication, nonhealing ulcers, gangrene
Infection	Impaired immunity, decreased perfusion, recurrent trauma, delayed wound healing, urinary retention	Wound infections, urinary tract infections, increased risk for sepsis

50% of individuals with diabetes mellitus develop diabetic kidney disease.[74]

Hyperglycemia, advanced glycation end products (AGEs), activation of metabolic pathways, and inflammation all contribute to kidney tissue injury; yet the exact process responsible for destruction of kidneys in diabetes is unknown. Renal glomerular changes occur early in diabetes mellitus, occasionally preceding the overt manifestation of the disease. The glomeruli are injured by hyperglycemia with high renal blood flow (hyperfiltration), by increases in proximal tubular reabsorption, and by intraglomerular hypertension exacerbated by systemic hypertension. There is progressive glomerulosclerosis and decreased glomerular blood flow and glomerular filtration. Alterations in glomerular membrane permeability occur with loss of negative charge and albuminuria. Ultimately, there can be tubular and interstitial fibrosis contributing to loss of function.[75]

Microalbuminuria is the first manifestation of diabetic kidney dysfunction. Before proteinuria, no clinical signs or symptoms of progressive glomerulosclerosis are likely to be evident. Later, hypoproteinemia, reduction in plasma oncotic pressure, fluid overload, anasarca (generalized body edema), and hypertension may occur. As renal function continues to deteriorate, individuals with type 1 diabetes may experience hypoglycemia (because of loss of renal insulin metabolism), which necessitates a decrease in insulin therapy. As the glomerular filtration rate drops below 10 ml/min, uremic signs, such as nausea, lethargy, acidosis, anemia, and uncontrolled hypertension, occur (see Chapter 30 for a discussion of renal failure). Proteinuria is strongly correlated with morbidity and mortality from cardiovascular disease.[76] Early diagnosis and control of hypertension and hyperglycemia decreases the severity of nephropathy and delays the onset of end-stage kidney disease.[77]

Diabetic neuropathies. Diabetic neuropathy is the most common cause of neuropathy in the Western world and is the most common complication of diabetes. The underlying pathologic mechanism includes both metabolic and vascular factors related to chronic hyperglycemia with ischemia and demyelination contributing to neural changes and delayed conduction. Both somatic and peripheral nerve cells show diffuse or focal damage, resulting in polyneuropathy. Sensory neuropathies include distal symmetric polyneuropathy, focal neuropathy (wristdrop, footdrop), and diabetic amyotrophy (muscle atrophy; weakness; and pain in the muscles of the hip,

FIGURE 19-14 Diabetic Retinopathy. Neovascularization is present at the optic nerve (1) and along vascular pathways (2). Retinal veins are engorged (3) and a preretinal boat-shaped hemorrhage (4) is present below the fovea. A more diffuse mild vitreous hemorrhage (5) is present below the preretinal hemorrhage. A few small, hard exudates are visible in the fovea (6). (From Palay DA, Krachmer JH: *Primary care ophthalmology,* ed 2, St Louis, 2006, Mosby.)

thigh, and buttocks). Loss of pain, temperature, and vibration sensation is more common than motor involvement and often involves the extremities first in the hands and feet. Motor neuropathies can affect muscle groups, particularly of the feet, contributing to deformity and unstable balance. Peripheral neuropathy can cause Charcot arthropathy, a progressive deterioration of weight-bearing joints, typically in the foot and ankle. Distal neuropathies combined with vascular complications, infection, or injury can lead to amputation[78] (Figure 19-15).

Autonomic neuropathies include delayed gastric emptying, diabetic diarrhea, altered bladder function (e.g., decreased sensation of bladder fullness, urge or overflow incontinence), impotence, orthostatic hypotension, and heart rate variability with both tachycardia and bradycardia.[79] Neuropathy may occur during periods of "good" glucose control and may be the initial clinical manifestation of type 2 diabetes. Chronic hyperglycemia also can cause cognitive dysfunction with alterations in learning and memory.[80]

Macrovascular Disease

Macrovascular disease (lesions in large- and medium-sized arteries) increases morbidity and mortality and increases risk for hypertension, accelerated atherosclerosis, cardiovascular disease, stroke, and peripheral vascular disease, particularly among individuals with type 2 diabetes mellitus. (Atherosclerosis is discussed in Chapter 24.) Children with poorly controlled diabetes have higher risk for macrovascular complications within 1 to 2 decades[81] (Figure 19-16). The process tends to be more severe and accelerated in the presence of other risk factors, including obesity, hyperlipidemia, and smoking.[82]

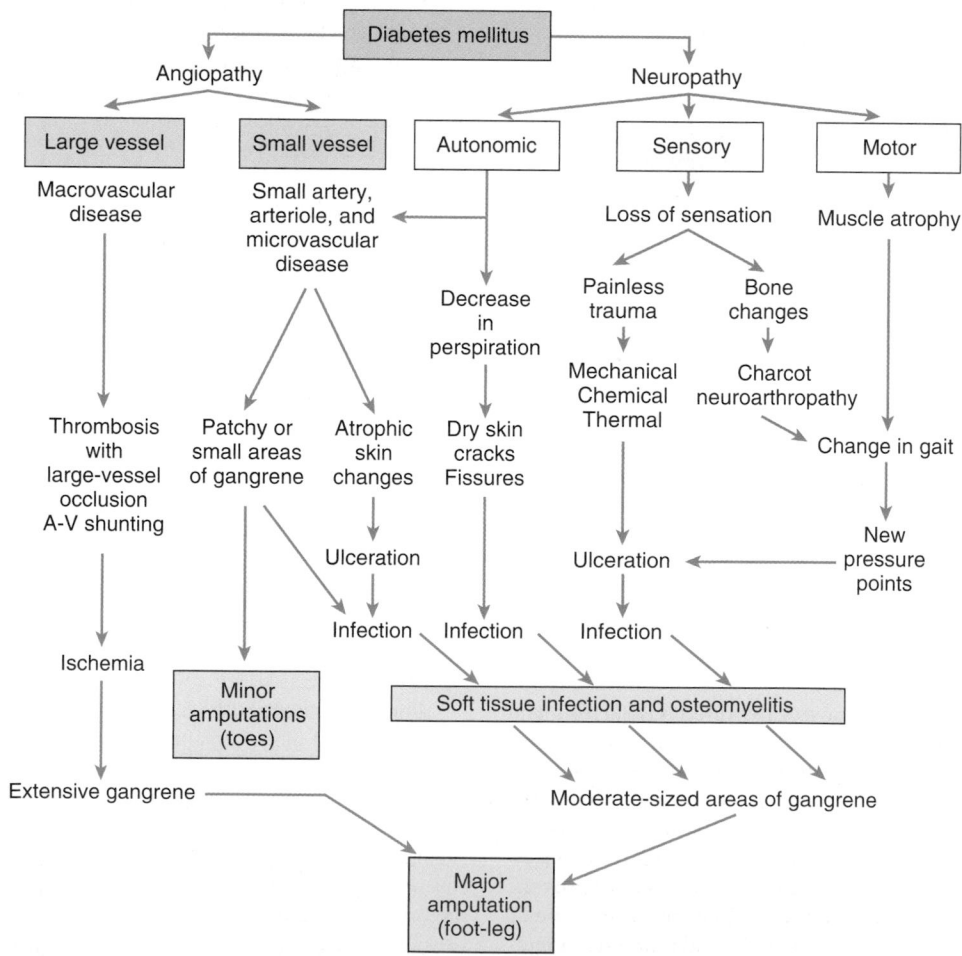

FIGURE 19-15 How Foot Lesions of Diabetes Lead to Amputation. (From Levin ME et al: *The diabetic foot,* ed 5, St Louis, 1993, Mosby.)

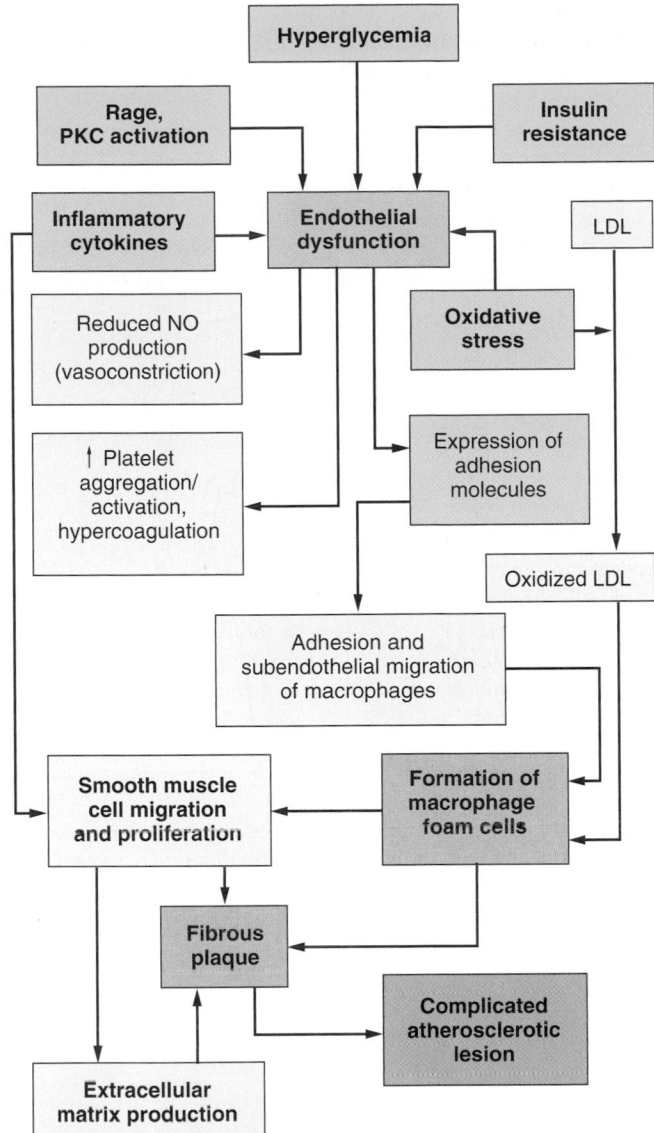

FIGURE 19-16 Diabetes Mellitus and Atherosclerosis. Diabetes with its associated hyperglycemia, relative hypoinsulinemia, oxidative stress, and proinflammatory state contributes to atherogenesis by causing arterial endothelial dysfunction (impaired vasodilation and adhesion of inflammatory cells), dyslipidemia, and smooth muscle proliferation. *LDL,* Low-density lipoprotein; *NO,* nitric oxide; *PKC,* protein kinase C; *Rage,* receptor advanced glycation end product. (Data from Zeadin MG, Petlura CI, Werstuck GH: *Can J Diabetes* 37(5):345-350, 2013; Plutzky K, Zafrir B, Brown JD: *Vascular Biology of Atherosclerosis in Patients with Diabetes, Diabetes in Cardiovascular Disease: A Companion to Braunwald's Heart Disease,* 10, 111-126, Saunders Philadelphia, 2015.)

Cardiovascular disease. Cardiovascular disease is the ultimate cause of death in up to 68% of people with diabetes, with higher risk for women.[83] Hypertension often coexists with diabetes mellitus, is more prevalent than in the nondiabetic population, and can have many causes. In type 1 diabetes hypertension is associated with the development of microalbuminuria. In type 2 diabetes hypertension is associated with metabolic syndrome (see p. 475). Hypertension increases the risk for coronary artery disease and stroke. Coronary artery disease (CAD) is the most common cause of morbidity and mortality in individuals with diabetes mellitus. Mechanisms of disease include vessel injury related to insulin resistance and hyperglycemia oxidative stress,

accelerated atherosclerosis associated with high levels of triglycerides, high levels of small low-density lipoproteins (LDLs), and low levels of high-density lipoproteins (HDLs); platelet activation and prothrombosis; and endothelial cell dysfunction.[84] In general, the prevalence of CAD increases with the duration but not the severity of diabetes and the onset can be silent.

The incidence of *congestive heart failure* is higher in individuals with diabetes, even without myocardial infarction. This may be related to cardiomyopathy and the presence of increased amounts of collagen in the ventricular wall and ventricular hypertrophy. There is reduced mechanical compliance of the heart during filling with diastolic and, eventually, systolic failure.[85] (Heart disease is described in Chapter 24.) Guidelines have been developed to reduce the risk and improve treatment of cardiovascular and coronary artery disease in individuals with diabetes.[49,86,87]

Stroke. Stroke is twice as common in those with diabetes (particularly type 2 diabetes) as in the nondiabetic population.[88] The survival rate for individuals with diabetes after a massive stroke is typically shorter than that for nondiabetic individuals. Hypertension, hyperglycemia, hyperlipidemia, and thrombosis are definite risk factors.

Peripheral vascular disease. Diabetes mellitus increases the incidence of peripheral vascular disease (PVD), with claudication (pain from reduced blood flow during exercise), ulcers, gangrene, and amputation.[82] Age, duration of diabetes, genetics, and additional risk factors (smoking, hyperlipidemia, hypertension) influence the development and management of PVD. Peripheral vascular disease in those with diabetes is more diffuse and often involves arteries below the knee. Occlusions of the small arteries and arterioles cause most of the gangrenous changes of the lower extremities and occur in patchy areas of the feet and toes. The lesions begin as ulcers and progress to osteomyelitis or gangrene requiring amputation. Peripheral neuropathies and increased risk for infection advance the disease[78] (see Figure 19-15). Significant morbidity and mortality are associated with major amputation.

Infection

The individual with diabetes is at an increased risk for infection throughout the body for several reasons[89]:

1. *The senses.* Impaired vision caused by retinal changes and impaired touch caused by neuropathy lead to loss of protection with injury and repeated trauma, open wounds, and soft tissue or osseous infection, particularly in the legs and feet.
2. *Hypoxia.* Once skin integrity is compromised, susceptibility to infection increases as a result of hypoxia. In addition, the glycosylated hemoglobin in the RBCs impedes the release of oxygen to tissues.
3. *Pathogens.* Some pathogens proliferate rapidly because of increased glucose in body fluids, which provides an excellent source of energy.
4. *Blood supply.* Decreased blood supply results from vascular changes and reduces the supply of white blood cells to the affected area.
5. *Suppressed immune response.* Chronic hyperglycemia impairs both innate and adaptive immune responses, including abnormal chemotaxis and vasoactive responses, and defective phagocytosis. Clinical signs of infection may be absent.

> ✔ **QUICK CHECK 19-4**
> 1. What are the major differences between type 1 and type 2 diabetes in relation to insulin?
> 2. How does obesity contribute to the development of type 2 diabetes?
> 3. What are three metabolic alterations related to hyperglycemia that contribute to diabetic complications?
> 4. What is the single most important factor in the management of diabetes mellitus?

ALTERATIONS OF ADRENAL FUNCTION

Disorders of the Adrenal Cortex

Disorders of the adrenal cortex are related either to hyperfunction or to hypofunction. Hyperfunction that causes increased secretion of cortisol (hypercortisolism) leads to Cushing disease or Cushing syndrome. Hyperfunction that causes increased secretion of adrenal androgens or estrogens leads to virilization or feminization. Hyperfunction that causes increased levels of aldosterone leads to hyperaldosteronism, which may be primary or secondary. These syndromes often have overlapping features. Hypofunction of the adrenal cortex leads to Addison disease.

Hypercortical Function (Cushing Syndrome, Cushing Disease)

Cushing syndrome refers to the clinical manifestations resulting from chronic exposure to excess cortisol regardless of cause. Cushing disease refers to excess endogenous secretion of ACTH. It is more common in women but men may have more severe symptoms.[90] ACTH-dependent hypercortisolism results from overproduction of pituitary ACTH by a pituitary adenoma (which can occur at any age) or by an ectopic secreting nonpituitary tumor, such as a small cell carcinoma of the lung (more common in older adults). ACTH-independent hypercortisolism is caused by cortisol secretion from a rare benign or malignant tumor of one or both adrenal glands (more common in children). A Cushing-like syndrome may develop as a side effect of long-term pharmacologic administration of glucocorticoids.[91]

PATHOPHYSIOLOGY Whatever the cause, two observations consistently apply to individuals with hypercortisolism: (1) the normal diurnal or circadian secretion patterns of ACTH and cortisol are lost, and (2) there is no increase in ACTH and cortisol secretion in response to a stressor.[92] With ACTH-dependent hypercortisolism, the excess ACTH stimulates excess production of cortisol and there is loss of feedback control of ACTH secretion. In individuals with ACTH-dependent hypercortisolism, secretion of both cortisol and adrenal androgens is increased, and cortisol-releasing hormone is inhibited. ACTH-independent secreting tumors of the adrenal cortex, however, generally secrete only cortisol. When the secretion of cortisol by the tumor exceeds normal cortisol levels, symptoms of hypercortisolism develop.

CLINICAL MANIFESTATIONS Weight gain is the most common feature and results from the accumulation of adipose tissue in the trunk, facial, and cervical areas. These characteristic patterns of fat deposition have been respectively described as "truncal obesity," "moon face," and "buffalo hump" (Figures 19-17 and 19-18).

Glucose intolerance occurs because of cortisol-induced insulin resistance and increased gluconeogenesis and glycogen storage by the liver. Overt diabetes mellitus develops in approximately 20% of individuals with hypercortisolism. Polyuria is a manifestation of hyperglycemia and resultant glycosuria.

Protein wasting is caused by the catabolic effects of cortisol on peripheral tissues. Muscle wasting leads to muscle weakness. In bone, loss of the protein matrix leads to osteoporosis, with pathologic fractures, vertebral compression fractures, bone and back pain, kyphosis, and reduced height. Cortisol interferes with the action of GH in long bones; thus children who present with short stature may be experiencing growth retardation related to Cushing syndrome rather than GH deficiency. Bone disease may contribute to hypercalciuria and resulting renal stones.

In the skin, loss of collagen leads to thin, weakened integumentary tissues through which capillaries are more visible and are easily

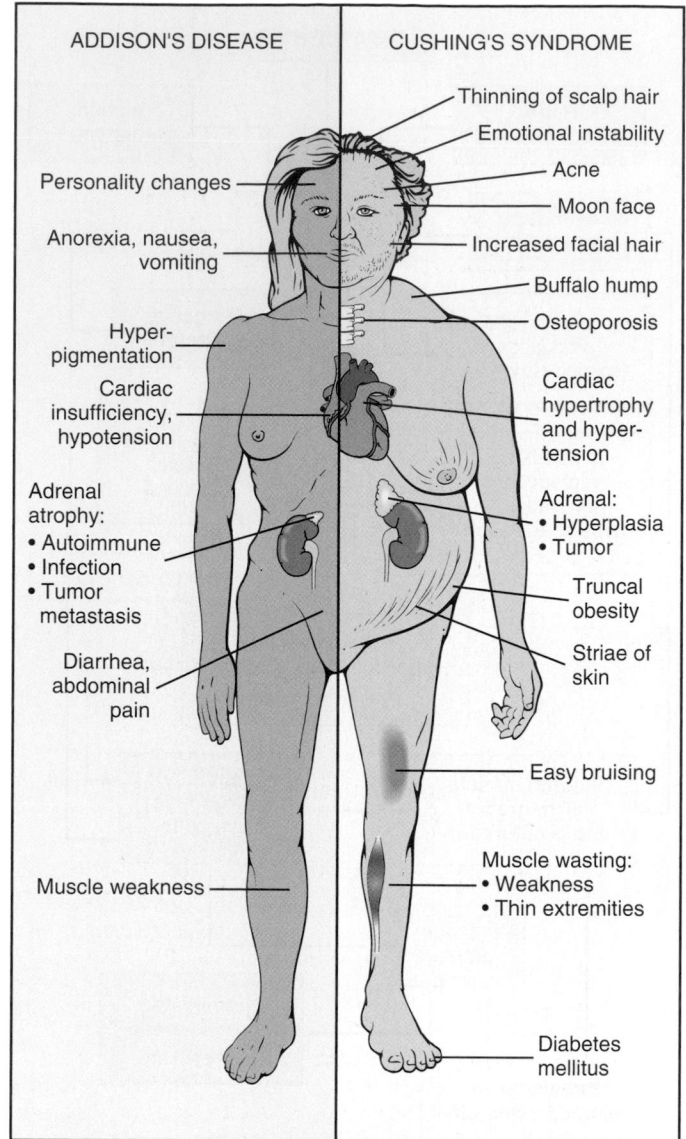

FIGURE 19-17 Symptoms of Addison and Cushing Diseases. (From Goodman CC, Kelly Snyder TE: *Differential diagnosis for physical therapists,* ed 5, Philadelphia, 2013, Saunders.)

stretched by adipose deposits. Together, these changes account for the characteristic purple striae seen in the trunk area. Loss of collagenous support around small vessels makes them susceptible to rupture, leading to easy bruising, even with minor trauma. Thin, atrophied skin is also easily damaged, leading to skin breaks and ulcerations. Bronze or brownish hyperpigmentation of the skin, mucous membranes, and hair occurs when there are very high levels of ACTH.

With elevated cortisol levels, vascular sensitivity to catecholamines increases significantly, leading to vasoconstriction and hypertension. Mineralocorticoid effects promote hypokalemia and sodium and water retention with transient weight gain. Suppression of the immune system and increased susceptibility to infections also occur. Approximately 50% of individuals with Cushing syndrome experience irritability and depression, disturbed sleep, difficulty concentrating, memory loss, and, rarely, schizophrenia-like psychosis.[93] Females with ACTH-dependent hypercortisolism may experience symptoms of increased adrenal androgen levels (virilism), with increased hair growth (especially facial hair), acne, and oligomenorrhea. Rarely, unless an adrenal

FIGURE 19-18 Cushing Syndrome. A, Patient before onset of Cushing syndrome. **B,** Patient 4 months later. Moon facies is clearly demonstrated. (From Zitelli BJ et al: *Zitelli and Davis' atlas of pediatric physical diagnosis,* ed 6, London, 2012, Saunders.)

carcinoma is involved, do androgen levels become high enough to cause changes of the voice, recession of the hairline, and hypertrophy of the clitoris.

EVALUATION AND TREATMENT   Routine laboratory examinations may reveal hyperglycemia, glycosuria, hypokalemia, and metabolic alkalosis. A variety of laboratory tests are used to confirm the diagnosis of hypercortisolism and to determine the underlying disorder. These include urinary free cortisol level higher than 50 mcg in 24 hours, abnormal dexamethasone suppressibility of either urinary or serum cortisol, and simultaneous measurement of ACTH and cortisol levels. Late evening salivary cortisol levels are used as a screening test and to document alterations in the diurnal variation of cortisol level.[94] Tumors are diagnosed using imaging procedures.

Treatment is specific for the cause of hypercorticoadrenalism and includes surgery, medication, and radiation. Differentiation between pituitary ectopic and adrenal causes is essential for effective treatment. Without treatment, approximately 50% of individuals with Cushing syndrome die within 5 years of onset as a result of overwhelming infection, suicide, complications from generalized arteriosclerosis, and hypertensive disease.

Congenital Adrenal Hyperplasia

Congenital adrenal hyperplasia results from an inherited deficiency of an enzyme that is critical in cortisol biosynthesis. Because cortisol is not produced efficiently, the concentration of ACTH increases and causes adrenal hyperplasia, which results in the overproduction of mineralocorticoids or androgens, or both. The most common form is a 21-hydroxylase deficiency, which involves both mineralocorticoid and cortisol synthesis. Affected female children are virilized and may have genital ambiguity. Infants of both genders exhibit salt wasting. Prenatal diagnosis is available and treatment guidelines have been developed. Disease management requires lifelong treatment with glucocorticoids and mineralocorticoids.[95,96]

Hyperaldosteronism

Hyperaldosteronism is characterized by excessive adrenal secretion of aldosterone. Both primary and secondary forms of hyperaldosteronism can occur.

Primary hyperaldosteronism (Conn syndrome, primary aldosteronism) is caused by excessive secretion of aldosterone from an abnormality of the adrenal cortex, usually a single benign aldosterone-producing adrenal adenoma. Bilateral adrenal nodular hyperplasia and adrenal carcinomas account for the remainder of cases. The incidence is estimated to be about 10% of all hypertensive individuals; however, approximately 33% of people with resistant hypertension will have evidence of primary hyperaldosteronism.[97]

Secondary hyperaldosteronism results from an extra-adrenal stimulus of aldosterone secretion, most often by angiotensin II through a renin-dependent mechanism. Examples include decreased circulating blood volume (e.g., in dehydration, shock, or hypoalbuminemia) and decreased delivery of blood to the kidneys (e.g., renal artery stenosis, heart failure, or hepatic cirrhosis). Here, the activation of the renin-angiotensin system and subsequent aldosterone secretion may be seen as compensatory, although in some instances (e.g., congestive heart failure) the increased circulating volume further worsens the condition. Other causes of secondary hyperaldosteronism are Bartter syndrome, a renal tubular defect causing hypokalemia, and renin-secreting tumors of the kidney.

PATHOPHYSIOLOGY   In *primary hyperaldosteronism,* pathophysiologic alterations are caused by excessive aldosterone secretion and the fluid and electrolyte imbalances that ensue. Hyperaldosteronism promotes (1) increased renal sodium and water reabsorption with corresponding hypervolemia (see Chapter 5) and hypertension and (2) renal excretion of hydrogen and potassium (see Chapter 5). The extracellular fluid volume overload, hypertension, and suppression of renin secretion are characteristic of primary disorders. Edema may not occur with primary aldosteronism because hypervolemia-induced atrial natriuretic factor release results in loss of sodium and water.[98] Hypokalemic alkalosis, changes in myocardial conduction, and skeletal muscle weakness may be seen, particularly with severe potassium depletion.

In *secondary hyperaldosteronism,* the effect of increased extracellular volume on renin secretion may vary. If renin secretion is being stimulated by variables other than pressure-initiated cellular changes at the juxtaglomerular apparatus (see Chapter 29), increased circulating blood volume may not decrease renin secretion through feedback mechanisms. This process occurs, for instance, in states of increased estrogen levels.

CLINICAL MANIFESTATIONS   Hypertension, hypokalemia, and neuromuscular manifestations are the hallmarks of primary hyperaldosteronism. Hypertension is resistant to treatment and can lead to the development of left ventricular dilation and hypertrophy, vascular disease, and kidney disease.[99]

EVALUATION AND TREATMENT Various clinical and laboratory evaluations are useful in assessing hyperaldosteronism and include the following:

1. Measurement of blood pressure—hypertension is usually present.
2. Serum and urinary electrolyte levels: serum sodium level is normal or elevated and serum potassium level is depressed, but urinary potassium level is elevated; metabolic alkalosis may be present.
3. Plasma aldosterone-to-renin ratio increases.
4. Aldosterone suppression testing is performed using either salt loading or fludrocortisone acetate (Florinef) if the aldosterone-to-renin ratio is increased.
5. Imaging techniques may be used to localize an aldosterone-secreting adenoma.

Treatment includes management of hypertension and hypokalemia, as well as correction of any underlying causal abnormalities. If an aldosterone-secreting adenoma is present, it must be surgically removed. Medical management with aldosterone receptor antagonists, such as spironolactone or eplerenone (a drug without the side effects of spironolactone), is a viable option in selected cases.

Hypersecretion of Adrenal Androgens and Estrogens

Hypersecretion of adrenal androgens and estrogens may be caused by adrenal tumors, either adenomas or carcinomas; Cushing syndrome; or defects in steroid synthesis. The clinical syndrome that is manifested depends on the hormone secreted, the gender of the individual, and the age at which the hypersecretion is initiated. Hypersecretion of estrogens causes feminization, the development of female secondary sex characteristics. Hypersecretion of androgens causes virilization, the development of male secondary sex characteristics (Figure 19-19).

The effects of an estrogen-secreting tumor are most evident in males and result in gynecomastia (98% of cases), testicular atrophy, and decreased libido. In female children, such tumors may lead to early development of secondary sex characteristics. The changes caused by an androgen-secreting tumor are more easily observed in females and include excessive face and body hair growth (hirsutism), clitoral enlargement, deepening of the voice, amenorrhea, acne, and breast atrophy. In children, virilizing tumors promote precocious sexual development and bone aging. Treatment of androgen-secreting tumors usually involves surgical excision.

Adrenocortical Hypofunction

Hypocortisolism (low levels of cortisol secretion) develops either because of inadequate stimulation of the adrenal glands by ACTH or because of a primary inability of the adrenals to produce and secrete the adrenocortical hormones. Sometimes there is partial dysfunction of the adrenal cortex, so only synthesis of cortisol and aldosterone or the adrenal androgens is affected. Hypofunction of the adrenal cortex may affect glucocorticoid or mineralocorticoid secretion, or both.

Addison disease. Primary adrenal insufficiency is termed Addison disease. It is relatively rare, occurring most often in adults aged 30 to 60 years, although it may appear at any time. Addison disease is caused by autoimmune mechanisms that destroy adrenal cortical cells and is more common in women. Chronic infections, such as tuberculosis, account for the majority of cases of primary adrenal insufficiency in underdeveloped countries.

PATHOPHYSIOLOGY Addison disease is characterized by inadequate corticosteroid and mineralocorticoid synthesis and elevated levels of

FIGURE 19-19 Virilization. Virilization of a young girl by an androgen-secreting tumor of the adrenal cortex. Masculine features include lack of breast development, increased muscle bulk, and hirsutism (excessive hair). (From Thibodeau GA, Patton KT: *The human body in health & disease,* ed 4, St Louis, 2010, Mosby.)

serum ACTH (loss of negative feedback). Before clinical manifestations of hypocortisolism are evident, more than 90% of total adrenocortical tissue must be destroyed.

Idiopathic Addison disease (organ-specific autoimmune adrenalitis) causes adrenal atrophy and hypofunction and is an organ-specific autoimmune disease. It may occur in childhood (type 1) or adulthood (type 2). 21-Hydroxylase autoantibodies and autoreactive T cells specific to adrenal cortical cells are present in 50% to 70% of individuals with idiopathic Addison disease, and this percentage increases in younger persons and in those with other autoimmune diseases. This deficiency allows the proliferation of immunocytes directed against specific antigens within the adrenocortical cells.[100]

The adrenal glands in idiopathic Addison disease are smaller than normal and may be misshapen. Idiopathic Addison disease is often associated with other autoimmune diseases, especially Hashimoto thyroiditis, pernicious anemia, and idiopathic hypoparathyroidism. In these cases, Addison disease may be inherited as an autosomal recessive trait. (Mechanisms of inheritance are described in Chapter 2.)

CLINICAL MANIFESTATIONS The symptoms of Addison disease are primarily a result of hypocortisolism and hypoaldosteronism and are often nonspecific. With mild to moderate hypocortisolism, symptoms begin with weakness and easy fatigability. Skin changes, including hyperpigmentation and vitiligo, may occur. As the condition progresses, anorexia, nausea, vomiting, and diarrhea may develop. Of greatest concern is the development of hypotension that can progress to complete vascular collapse and shock. This is known as *adrenal crisis,* or addisonian crisis, and develops with undiagnosed disease or acute withdrawal of glucocorticoid therapy.

EVALUATION AND TREATMENT   Serum and urine levels of cortisol are depressed with primary hypocortisolism and ACTH levels are increased. Because of dehydration, blood urea nitrogen levels may increase. Serum glucose level is low. Eosinophil and lymphocyte counts often are elevated. Hyperkalemia is seen in Addison disease and may cause mild alkalosis (see Chapter 5). The ACTH stimulation test may be used to evaluate serum cortisol levels.

The treatment of Addison disease involves lifetime glucocorticoid and possibly mineralocorticoid replacement therapy, together with dietary modifications and correction of any underlying disorders.[101] With acute stressors (e.g., infection, surgery, or trauma), additional cortisol must be administered to approximate the amount of cortisol that might be expected if normal adrenal function were present (approximately 100 to 300 mg/day). The individual's diet should include at least 150 mEq of sodium per day, and sodium intake should be increased if the individual experiences excessive sweating or diarrhea.

Secondary hypocortisolism. Secondary hypocortisolism commonly results from prolonged administration of exogenous glucocorticoids; they suppress ACTH secretion and cause adrenal atrophy, resulting in inadequate corticosteroidogenesis once the exogenous glucocorticoids are withdrawn. Decreased ACTH secretion also can result from pituitary infarction, pituitary tumors that compress ACTH-secreting cells, or hypophysectomy. In all instances of low ACTH levels, adrenal atrophy occurs and endogenous adrenal steroidogenesis is depressed. Clinical manifestations of secondary hypocortisolism are similar to those of Addison disease, although hyperpigmentation usually does not occur. The renin-angiotensin system usually is normal, so aldosterone and potassium levels also tend to be normal.

Tumors of the Adrenal Medulla

Hyperfunction of the adrenal medulla is caused by pheochromocytomas (chromaffin cell tumors) or sympathetic paragangliomas of the adrenal medulla. They are rare, and about 10% are malignant and metastasize to the lungs, liver, bones, or paraaortic lymph nodes. The tumors are usually sporadic although up to 40% of them can be inherited.[102]

PATHOPHYSIOLOGY   Pheochromocytomas and sympathetic paragangliomas cause excessive production of norepinephrine, although large tumors secrete epinephrine and norepinephrine because of autonomous secretion of the tumor. Approximately 5% of people with these tumors have no symptoms, apparently because the tumor is nonfunctioning. Such tumors can, however, release catecholamines, especially in response to a stressor, such as surgery.

CLINICAL MANIFESTATIONS   The clinical manifestations of a pheochromocytoma and sympathetic paragangliomas are related to the chronic effects of catecholamine secretion and include persistent hypertension, headache, pallor, diaphoresis, tachycardia, and palpitations. Hypertension results from increased peripheral vascular resistance and may be sustained or paroxysmal. An acute episode of hypertension related to hypersecretion of catecholamines may follow specific events, such as exercise, excessive ingestion of tyrosine-containing foods (aged cheese, red wine, beer, yogurt), ingestion of caffeine-containing foods, external pressure on the tumor, and induction of anesthesia. Hypertension unresponsive to drug therapy is often the first indication of a pheochromocytoma. Headaches appear because of sudden changes in catecholamine levels in the blood, affecting cerebral blood flow. Hypermetabolism and sweating are related to chronic activation of sympathetic receptors in adipocytes, hepatocytes, and other tissues. Glucose intolerance may occur because of catecholamine-induced inhibition of insulin release by the pancreas. These tumors tend to be extremely vascular and can rupture, causing massive and potentially fatal hemorrhage.

EVALUATION AND TREATMENT   Symptoms of pheochromocytoma can be insidious or intermittent and difficult to diagnose. A diagnosis is made when increased catecholamine production is found in the blood or urine. The site of the tumor is then determined using abdominal imaging techniques. Because of the possibility of metastasis, whole-body scanning may be done.

Management of catecholamine excess is essential to prevent hypertensive emergencies and requires the use of α- and β-adrenergic blockers. The usual treatment of pheochromocytoma is laparoscopic surgical excision of the tumor, although open resection is still completed for large tumors or when metastasis is suspected. Medical therapy is continued to stabilize blood pressure before, during, or after surgery.[103] Malignant pheochromocytoma is rarely curable and is usually managed by a combination of surgical debulking of the tumor combined with chemotherapy.[104]

✔ QUICK CHECK 19-5
1. What are the symptoms of hyperaldosteronism?
2. What major diseases are classified as hypocortisolism?
3. What are pheochromocytomas?

■ DID YOU UNDERSTAND?

Mechanisms of Hormonal Alterations
1. Abnormalities in endocrine function may be caused by elevated or depressed hormone levels that result from (1) faulty feedback systems, (2) dysfunction of the gland, (3) altered metabolism of hormones, (4) dysfunction of carrier proteins, or (5) production of hormones from nonendocrine tissues.
2. Target cells may fail to respond to hormones because of (1) cell surface receptor–associated disorders, (2) intracellular disorders, or (3) circulating inhibitors.

Alterations of the Hypothalamic-Pituitary System
1. Dysfunction in the action of hypothalamic hormones is most commonly related to interruption of the connection between the hypothalamus and pituitary—the pituitary stalk.
2. Disorders of the posterior pituitary include syndrome of inappropriate ADH secretion (SIADH) and diabetes insipidus. SIADH is characterized by abnormally high ADH secretion; diabetes insipidus is characterized by abnormally low ADH secretion.

3. In SIADH, high ADH levels interfere with renal free water clearance, leading to hyponatremia and hypoosmolality, and are associated with brain injury, surgical procedures with certain forms of cancer related to ectopic secretion of ADH by tumor cells, and medications.

4. Diabetes insipidus may be neurogenic (caused by insufficient amounts of ADH) or nephrogenic (caused by an inadequate response to ADH). Its principal clinical features are polyuria and polydipsia.

5. Hypopituitarism can be primary (dysfunction of the pituitary) or secondary (dysfunction of the hypothalamus). Primary hypopituitarism can result from a pituitary tumor, trauma, infections, stroke, or surgical removal.

6. Hypopituitarism can affect any or all of the pituitary hormones and symptoms may range from mild to life-threatening.

7. Hyperpituitarism is caused by pituitary adenomas. These are usually benign, slow-growing tumors that arise from cells of the anterior pituitary.

8. Expansion of a pituitary adenoma causes both neurologic and secretory effects. Pressure from the expanding tumor causes hyposecretion of cells, dysfunction of the optic chiasma (leading to visual disturbances), and dysfunction of the hypothalamus and some cranial nerves.

9. Growth hormone deficiency causes increased body fat, decreased muscle mass, and psychologic problems in adults; and hypopituitary dwarfism in children.

10. Hypersecretion of growth hormone (GH) in adults causes acromegaly, in which GH secretion becomes high and unpredictable. Pituitary adenoma is the most common cause of acromegaly. Excessive GH secretion in children with open epiphyseal plates causes giantism.

11. Prolonged, abnormally high levels of GH lead to proliferation of body and connective tissue and slowly developing renal, thyroid, and reproductive dysfunction.

12. Prolactinomas result in galactorrhea, hirsutism, amenorrhea, hypogonadism, and osteopenia.

Alterations of Thyroid Function

1. Thyrotoxicosis is a general condition in which elevated thyroid hormone (TH) levels cause greater than normal physiologic responses. The condition can be caused by a variety of specific diseases, each of which has its own pathophysiology and course of treatment.

2. In general, hyperthyroidism has a range of endocrine, reproductive, gastrointestinal, integumentary, and ocular manifestations. These are caused by increased circulating levels of TH and by stimulation of the sympathetic division of the autonomic nervous system.

3. Graves disease, the most common form of hyperthyroidism, is caused by an autoimmune mechanism that overrides normal mechanisms for control of TH secretion and is characterized by thyrotoxicosis, ophthalmopathy, and circulating thyroid-stimulating immunoglobulins.

4. Toxic nodular goiter and toxic multinodular goiter occur when TH-regulating mechanisms and abnormal hypertrophy of the thyroid gland cause hyperthyroidism. Toxic multinodular goiter is caused by independently functioning follicular cell adenomas.

5. Thyrotoxic crisis is a severe form of hyperthyroidism that is often associated with physiologic or psychologic stress. Without treatment, death occurs quickly.

6. Primary hypothyroidism is caused by deficient production of TH by the thyroid gland. Secondary hypothyroidism is caused by hypothalamic or pituitary dysfunction. Symptoms depend on the degree of TH deficiency. Common manifestations include decreased energy metabolism, decreased heat production, and myxedema.

7. Primary hypothyroidism is characterized by an increased level of TSH, which stimulates goiter formation.

8. Autoimmune thyroiditis (Hashimoto disease) is associated with humoral (antibodies) and cellular autoimmune destruction of the thyroid gland and gradual loss of thyroid function. Autoimmune thyroiditis occurs in those individuals with genetic susceptibility to an autoimmune mechanism that causes thyroid damage and eventual hypothyroidism.

9. Subacute thyroiditis is a self-limiting nonbacterial inflammation of the thyroid gland that damages follicular cells, causing leakage of T_3 and T_4. Hyperthyroidism then is followed by transient hypothyroidism, which is corrected by cellular repair and a return to normal levels in the thyroid.

10. Myxedema is a sign of hypothyroidism caused by alterations in connective tissue with water-binding proteins that lead to edema and thickened mucous membranes.

11. Myxedema coma is a severe form of hypothyroidism that may be life-threatening without emergency medical treatment.

12. Congenital hypothyroidism is the absence of thyroid tissue during fetal development or defects in hormone synthesis.

13. Thyroid carcinoma is a relatively rare cancer associated with exposure to ionizing radiation, especially in childhood.

Alterations of Parathyroid Function

1. Hyperparathyroidism, which may be primary or secondary, is characterized by greater than normal secretion of parathyroid hormone (PTH).

2. Primary hyperparathyroidism is caused by an interruption of the normal mechanisms that regulate calcium and PTH levels. Manifestations include chronic hypercalcemia, increased bone resorption, and hypercalciuria.

3. Secondary hyperparathyroidism is a compensatory response to hypocalcemia and often occurs with chronic renal failure and vitamin D deficiency.

4. Tertiary hyperparathyroidism is persistent secretion of PTH after treatment of secondary hyperparathyroidism.

5. Hypoparathyroidism, defined by abnormally low PTH levels, is caused by thyroid surgery, autoimmunity, or genetic mechanisms.

6. The lack of circulating PTH in hypoparathyroidism causes hypocalcemia, hyperphosphatemia, decreased bone resorption, and hypocalciuria.

Dysfunction of the Endocrine Pancreas: Diabetes Mellitus

1. Diabetes mellitus is a group of disorders characterized by glucose intolerance, chronic hyperglycemia, and disturbances of carbohydrate, protein, and fat metabolism.

2. A diagnosis of diabetes mellitus is based on elevated plasma glucose concentrations and measurement of glycosylated hemoglobin. Classic signs and symptoms are often present as well.

3. The two most common types of diabetes mellitus are type 1 and type 2.

4. Type 1 diabetes mellitus is characterized by loss of beta cells, presence of islet cell antibody, lack of insulin, excess of glucagon, and altered metabolism of fat, protein, and carbohydrates.

5. Type 1 diabetes mellitus is caused by a gradual process of autoimmune destruction of beta cells in genetically susceptible individuals.

6. In type 1 diabetes mellitus, hyperglycemia causes polyuria and polydipsia resulting from osmotic diuresis.

7. Ketoacidosis is caused by increased levels of circulating ketones without the inhibiting effects of insulin. Increased levels of circulating fatty acids and weight loss are both manifestations of type 1 uncontrolled diabetes mellitus.

8. Type 2 diabetes mellitus is caused by genetic susceptibility that is triggered by environmental factors. The most compelling environmental risk factor is obesity.

9. In the obese, many factors, including metabolic syndrome, altered adipokines, increased fatty acids, inflammation, and hyperinsulinemia, contribute to the development of insulin resistance and hyperglycemia.

10. Some insulin production continues in type 2 diabetes mellitus, but the weight and number of beta cells decrease. There are decreased levels of insulin, amylin, ghrelin, and incretins and glucagon concentration is increased. All contribute to chronic hyperglycemia.

11. A rare monogenetic form of diabetes is called maturity-onset diabetes of youth (MODY).

12. Gestational diabetes is glucose intolerance during pregnancy.

13. Acute complications of diabetes mellitus include hypoglycemia, diabetic ketoacidosis, and hyperosmolar hyperglycemic nonketotic syndrome.

14. Hypoglycemia in diabetes is a complication related to insulin treatment.

15. Diabetic ketoacidosis (DKA) develops when there is an absolute or relative deficiency of insulin and an increase in the insulin counterregulatory hormones of catecholamines—cortisol, glucagon, and growth hormone. DKA presents with hyperglycemia, acidosis, and ketonuria.

16. Hyperosmolar hyperglycemic nonketotic syndrome is pathophysiologically similar to diabetic ketoacidosis, although levels of free fatty acids are lower in hyperosmolar nonacidotic diabetes and lack of ketosis indicates some level of insulin action. Severe dehydration and electrolyte imbalance are present.

17. Chronic complications of diabetes mellitus include microvascular disease (e.g., neuropathy, retinopathy, nephropathy), macrovascular disease (e.g., coronary artery disease, stroke, peripheral vascular disease), and infection.

18. Microvascular disease is characterized by thickening of the capillary basement membrane, disruption of the microcirculation, and decreased tissue perfusion.

19. Macrovascular disease associated with diabetes mellitus is most often related to the proliferation of atherosclerotic plaques in the arterial wall and coagulation defects.

20. The incidence of coronary heart disease, peripheral vascular disease, and stroke is greater in those with diabetes than in nondiabetic individuals.

21. Individuals with diabetes are at risk for a variety of infections. Infection may be related to sensory impairment and resulting injury, hypoxia, increased proliferation of pathogens in elevated concentrations of glucose, decreased blood supply associated with vascular damage, and impaired immune protection.

Alterations of Adrenal Function

1. Disorders of the adrenal cortex are related to hyperfunction or hypofunction. No known disorders are associated with hypofunction of the adrenal medulla, but medullary hyperfunction causes clinically defined syndromes.

2. Cortical hyperfunction, or hypercortisolism, causes Cushing syndrome, which does not involve the pituitary gland, and Cushing disease, which is hypercortisolism with pituitary involvement. Congenital adrenal hyperplasia is a genetic disorder with deficient steroidogenesis and excess androgen synthesis.

3. Hypercortisolism is usually caused by Cushing disease (pituitary-dependent) and very rarely can be caused by ectopic production of ACTH. Complications include obesity, diabetes, protein wasting, immune suppression, and mental status changes.

4. Excessive aldosterone secretion causes hyperaldosteronism, which may be primary or secondary. Primary hyperaldosteronism is caused by an abnormality of the adrenal cortex. Secondary hyperaldosteronism involves an extra-adrenal stimulus, often angiotensin.

5. Hyperaldosteronism promotes increased sodium reabsorption (with corresponding hypervolemia), increased extracellular volume (which is variable), hypokalemia related to renal reabsorption of sodium, and excretion of potassium.

6. Hypersecretion of adrenal androgens and estrogens can be a result of adrenal tumors, either adenomas or carcinomas. Hypersecretion of estrogens causes feminization, the development of female secondary sexual characteristics. Hypersecretion of androgens causes virilization, the development of male secondary sexual characteristics.

7. Hypofunction of the adrenal cortex can affect glucocorticoid or mineralocorticoid secretion, or both. Hypofunction can be caused by a deficiency of ACTH or by a primary deficiency in the gland itself.

8. Hypocortisolism, or low levels of cortisol, is caused by inadequate adrenal stimulation by ACTH or by primary cortisol hyposecretion. Primary adrenal insufficiency is termed Addison disease.

9. Addison disease is characterized by elevated ACTH levels with inadequate corticosteroid synthesis and output.

10. Manifestations of Addison disease are related to hypocortisolism and hypoaldosteronism. Symptoms include weakness, fatigability, hypoglycemia and related metabolic problems, lowered response to stressors, hyperpigmentation, vitiligo, and manifestations of hypovolemia and hyperkalemia.

11. Hyperfunction of the adrenal medulla is usually caused by a pheochromocytoma, a catecholamine-producing tumor. Symptoms of catecholamine excess are related to their sympathetic nervous system effects and include hypertension, palpitations, tachycardia, glucose intolerance, excessive sweating, and constipation.

■ KEY TERMS

Acromegaly, 464

Addison disease (primary adrenal insufficiency), 484

Amylin, 473

Autoimmune thyroiditis (Hashimoto disease, chronic lymphocyte thyroiditis), 468

Beta-cell dysfunction, 475

Central (secondary) thyroid disorders, 466

Congenital adrenal hyperplasia, 483

Cushing disease, 482

Cushing-like syndrome, 482

Cushing syndrome, 482

Dawn phenomenon, 477

Diabetes insipidus (DI), 462

Diabetes mellitus, 471

Diabetic ketoacidosis (DKA), 477

Diabetic neuropathy, 479

Diabetic retinopathy, 478

Feminization, 484

Gestational diabetes mellitus (GDM), 476

Ghrelin, 476

Giantism, 465

Glucagon, 473

REFERENCES

1. Sanchez M et al: Coordinate regulation of estrogen receptor beta degradation by Mdm2 and CREB-binding protein in response to growth signals, *Oncogene* 32(1):117-126, 2013.
2. Janneck M et al: Hyponatremia after transsphenoidal surgery, *Minerva Endocrinol* 39(1):27-31, 2014.
3. Ramos-Levi AM et al: Drug-induced hyponatremia: an updated review, *Minerva Endocrinol* 39(1):1-12, 2014.
4. Kortenoeven ML, Fenton RA: Renal aquaporins and water balance disorders, *Biochim Biophys Acta* 1840(5):1533-1549, 2014.
5. Peri A, Giuliani C: Management of euvolemic hyponatremia attributed to SIADH in the hospital setting, *Minerva Endocrinol* 39(1):33-41, 2014.
6. Bockenhauer D, Bichet DG: Pathophysiology, diagnosis and management of nephrogenic diabetes insipidus, *Nat Rev Nephrol* 11(10):576-588, 2015.
7. Wallia A et al: Acute diabetes insipidus mediated by vasopressinase after placental abruption, *J Clin Endocrinol Metab* 98(3):881-886, 2013.
8. Oiso Y et al: Clinical review: treatment of neurohypophyseal diabetes insipidus, *J Clin Endocrinol Metab* 98(10):3958-3967, 2013.
9. Kilicli F et al: Sheehan's syndrome, *Gynecol Endocrinol* 29(4):292-295, 2013.
10. Tanriverdi F, Kelestimur F: Pituitary dysfunction following traumatic brain injury: clinical perspectives, *Neuropsychiatr Dis Treat* 11:1835-1843, 2015.
11. Andrikoula M et al: PROP-1 gene mutations in a 63-year-old woman presenting with osteoporosis and hyperlipidaemia, *Hormones* 12(1):128-134, 2013.
12. Audi L et al: Growth hormone deficiency: an update, *Minerva Endocrinol* 38(1):1-16, 2013.
13. Kargi AY, Merriam GR: Diagnosis and treatment of growth hormone deficiency in adults, *Nat Rev Endocrinol* 9(6):335-345, 2013.
14. Erfurth EM et al: Pituitary disease mortality: is it fiction? *Pituitary* 16(3):402-412, 2013.
15. Gadelha MR et al: Genetics of pituitary adenomas, *Front Horm Res* 41:111-140, 2013.
16. Samarasinghe S et al: Neurology of the pituitary, *Handb Clin Neurol* 120:685-701, 2014.
17. Andersen M: Management of endocrine disease: GH excess: diagnosis and medical therapy, *Eur J Endocrinol* 170(1):R31-R41, 2014.
18. Olarescu NC et al: Inflammatory adipokines contribute to insulin resistance in active acromegaly and respond differently to different treatment modalities, *Eur J Endocrinol* 170(1):39-48, 2014.
19. Arcopinto M et al: The GH/IGF-1 axis in chronic heart failure, *Endocrinol Metab Immune Disord Drug Targets* 13(1):76-91, 2013.

20. Capatina C, Wass JA: 60 YEARS OF NEUROENDOCRINOLOGY, Acromegaly, *J Endocrinol* 226(2):T141-T160, 2015.
21. Glezer A, Bronstein MD: Prolactinomas, *Endocrinol Metab Clin North Am* 44(1):71-78, 2015.
22. Vale FL et al: Medically treated prolactin-secreting pituitary adenomas: when should we operate? *Br J Neurosurg* 27(1):56-62, 2013.
23. Raverot G et al: Management of endocrine disease: clinicopathological classification and molecular markers of pituitary tumours for personalized therapeutic strategies, *Eur J Endocrinol* 170(4):R121-R132, 2014.
24. Menconi F et al: Diagnosis and classification of Graves' disease, *Autoimmun Rev* 13(4-5):398-402, 2014.
25. Barrio-Barrio J et al: Graves' Ophthalmopathy: VISA versus EUGOGO Classification, Assessment, and Management, *J Ophthalmol* 2015:249125, 2015.
26. Dhali TK, Chahar M: Thyroid dermopathy—a diagnostic clue of hidden hyperthyroidism, *Dermatoendocrinol* 6(1):e981078, 2015.
27. Sturniolo G et al: Toxic multinodular goitre. Personal case histories and literature review, *G Chir* 34(9-10):257-259, 2013.
28. Klubo-Gwiezdzinska J, Wartofsky L: Thyroid emergencies, *Med Clin North Am* 96(2):385-403, 2012.
29. Pyzik A et al: Immune disorders in Hashimoto's thyroiditis: what do we know so far? *J Immunol Res* 2015:979167, 2015.
30. Agrawal P et al: Congenital hypothyroidism, *Indian J Endocrinol Metab* 19(2):221-227, 2015.
31. Puig-Domingo M, Vila L: The implications of iodine and its supplementation during pregnancy in fetal brain development, *Curr Clin Pharmacol* 8(2):97-109, 2013.
32. Büyükgebiz A: Newborn screening for congenital hypothyroidism, *J Clin Res Pediatr Endocrinol* 5(Suppl 1):8-12, 2013.
33. Persani L: Clinical review: central hypothyroidism: pathogenic, diagnostic, and therapeutic challenges, *J Clin Endocrinol Metab* 97(9):3068-3078, 2012.
34. Khandelwal D, Tandon N: Overt and subclinical hypothyroidism: who to treat and how, *Drugs* 72(1):17-33, 2012.
35. Suh S, Kim DK: Subclinical Hypothyroidism and Cardiovascular Disease, *Endocrinol Metab (Seoul)* 30(3):246-251, 2015.
36. Hirsch D et al: Pregnancy outcomes in women with severe hypothyroidism, *Eur J Endocrinol* 169(3):313-320, 2013.
37. American Cancer Society: *Cancer facts & figures 2015.* Available at: http://www.cancer.org/acs/groups/content/@editorial/documents/document/acspc-044552.pdf.
38. Brito JP et al: The accuracy of thyroid nodule ultrasound to predict thyroid cancer: systematic

review and meta-analysis, *J Clin Endocrinol Metab* 99(4):1253-1263, 2014.
39. Perri F et al: Targeted therapy: a new hope for thyroid carcinomas, *Crit Rev Oncol Hematol* 94(1):55-63, 2015.
40. Baloch ZW, LiVolsi VA: Pathology of the parathyroid glands in hyperparathyroidism, *Semin Diagn Pathol* 30(3):165-177, 2013.
41. Pasquali D et al: Multiple endocrine neoplasia, the old and the new: a mini review, *G Chir* 33(11-12):370-373, 2012.
42. Jamal SA, Miller PD: Secondary and tertiary hyperparathyroidism, *J Clin Densitom* 16(1):64-68, 2013.
43. Riccardi D, Brown EM: Physiology and pathophysiology of the calcium-sensing receptor in the kidney, *Am J Physiol Renal Physiol* 298(3):F485-F499, 2010.
44. Cunningham J et al: Secondary hyperparathyroidism: pathogenesis, disease progression, and therapeutic options, *Clin J Am Soc Nephrol* 6(4):913-921, 2011.
45. Pyram R et al: Primary hyperparathyroidism: skeletal and non-skeletal effects, diagnosis and management, *Maturitas* 70(3):246-255, 2011.
46. Betterle C et al: Diagnosis and classification of autoimmune parathyroid disease, *Autoimmun Rev* 13(4-5):417-422, 2014.
47. Michels TC, Kelly KM: Parathyroid disorders, *Am Fam Physician* 88(4):249-257, 2013.
48. Centers for Disease Control and Prevention: *National diabetes statistics report, 2014.* Available at: www.cdc.gov/diabeteS/pubs/statsreport14/national-diabetes-report-web.pdf.
49. American Diabetes Association: Standards of medical care in diabetes—2015, *Diabetes Care* 38:S1-S93, 2015. Available at: http://professional.diabetes.org/admin/UserFiles/0%20-%20Sean/Documents/January%20Supplement%20Combined_Final.pdf.
50. Atkinson MA et al: Type 1 diabetes, *Lancet* 383(9911):69-82, 2014.
51. Chillaron JJ et al: Type 1 diabetes, metabolic syndrome and cardiovascular risk, *Metab Clin Exp* 63(2):181-187, 2014.
52. U.S. Food and Drug Administration: *FDA allows marketing of first ZnT8Ab autoantibody test to help diagnose type 1 diabetes, August 20, 2014.* Available at: http://www.fda.gov/NewsEvents/Newsroom/PressAnnouncements/ucm410830.htm.
53. Malik FS, Taplin CE: Insulin therapy in children and adolescents with type 1 diabetes, *Paediatric Drugs* 16(2):141-150, 2014.
54. Cogger K, Nostro MC: Recent advances in cell replacement therapies for the treatment of type 1 diabetes, *Endocrinology* 156(1):8-15, 2015.
55. Kahn SE et al: Pathophysiology and treatment of type 2 diabetes: perspectives on the past, present, and future, *Lancet* 383(9922):1068-1083, 2014.

56. Pal A, McCarthy MI: The genetics of type 2 diabetes and its clinical relevance, *Clin Genet* 83(4):297-306, 2013.

57. Bruce KD: Maternal and in utero determinants of type 2 diabetes risk in the young, *Curr Diab Rep* 14(1):446, 2014.

58. Taylor JY et al: An overview of the genomics of metabolic syndrome, *J Nurs Scholar* 45(1):52-59, 2013.

59. Naci H, Ioannidis JP: Comparative effectiveness of exercise and drug interventions on mortality outcomes: metaepidemiological study, *Br Med J* 347:f5577, 2013.

60. Blüher M, Mantzoros CS: From leptin to other adipokines in health and disease: facts and expectations at the beginning of the 21st century, *Metabolism* 64(1):131-145, 2015.

61. Winer DA et al: B lymphocytes in obesity-related adipose tissue inflammation and insulin resistance, *Cell Mol Life Sci* 71(6):1033-1043, 2014.

62. Vetere A et al: Targeting the pancreatic β-cell to treat diabetes, *Nat Rev Drug Discov* 13(4):278-289, 2014.

63. Gingell JJ et al: Activity of pramlintide, rat and human amylin but not Abeta1-42 at human amylin receptors, *Endocrinology* 155(1):21-26, 2014.

64. Gahete MD et al: Ghrelin gene products, receptors, and GOAT enzyme: biological and pathophysiological insight, *J Endocrinol* 220(1): R1-R24, 2014.

65. Lee YS, Jun HS: Anti-diabetic actions of glucagon-like peptide-1 on pancreatic beta-cells, *Metabolism* 63(1):9-19, 2014.

66. White JR Jr: Sodium glucose cotransporter 2 inhibitors, *Med Clin North Am* 99(1):131-143, 2015.

67. Tenzer-Iglesias P: Type 2 diabetes mellitus in women, *J Fam Pract* 63(2 Suppl):S21-26, 2014.

68. McDonald TJ, Ellard S: Maturity onset diabetes of the young: identification and diagnosis, *Ann Clin Biochem* 50(Pt 5):403-415, 2013.

69. Moyer VA, U.S. Preventive Services Task Force: Screening for gestational diabetes mellitus: U.S. Preventive Services Task Force recommendation statement, *Ann Intern Med* 160(6):414-420, 2014.

70. Dabelea D et al: Trends in the prevalence of ketoacidosis at diabetes diagnosis: the SEARCH for diabetes in youth study, *Pediatrics* 133(4): e938-e945, 2014.

71. ACCORD Study Group et al: Long-term effects of intensive glucose lowering on cardiovascular outcomes, *N Engl J Med* 364(9):818-828, 2011.

72. Giorgino F et al: Cardiovascular disease and glycemic control in type 2 diabetes: now that the dust is settling from large clinical trials, *Ann N Y Acad Sci* 1281:36-50, 2013.

73. Tarr JM et al: Pathophysiology of diabetic retinopathy, *ISRN Ophthalmol* 2013:343560, 2013.

74. Tuttle KR et al: Diabetic kidney disease: a report from an ADA consensus conference, *Am J Kidney Dis* 64(4):510-533, 2014.

75. Blantz RC, Singh P: Glomerular and tubular function in the diabetic kidney, *Adv Chronic Kidney Dis* 21(3):297-303, 2014.

76. Parving HH et al: Microalbuminuria: a parameter that has changed diabetes care, *Diabetes Res Clin Pract* 107(1):1-8, 2015.

77. Marshall SM: Natural history and clinical characteristics of CKD in type 1 and type 2 diabetes mellitus, *Adv Chronic Kidney Dis* 21(3): 267-272, 2014.

78. DiPreta JA: Outpatient assessment and management of the diabetic foot, *Med Clin North Am* 98(2):353-373, 2014.

79. Vinik AI, Erbas T: Diabetic autonomic neuropathy, *Handb Clin Neurol* 117:279-294, 2013.

80. Mayeda ER et al: Diabetes and cognition, *Clin Geriatr Med* 31(1):101-115, ix, 2015.

81. Prendergast C, Gidding SS: Cardiovascular risk in children and adolescent with type 2 diabetes mellitus, *Curr Diab Rep* 14(2):454, 2014.

82. Gibbons GW, Shaw PM: Diabetic vascular disease: characteristics of vascular disease unique to the diabetic patient, *Semin Vasc Surg* 25(2):89-92, 2012.

83. Norhammar A, Schenck-Gustafsson K: Type 2 diabetes and cardiovascular disease in women, *Diabetologia* 56(1):1-9, 2013.

84. Paneni F et al: Diabetes and vascular disease: pathophysiology, clinical consequences, and medical therapy: part I, *Eur Heart J* 34(31): 2436-2443, 2013.

85. Pappachan JM et al: Diabetic cardiomyopathy: pathophysiology, diagnostic evaluation and management, *World J Diabetes* 4(5):177-189, 2013.

86. Nathan DM: Diabetes: Advances in Diagnosis and Treatment, *JAMA* 314(10):1052-1062, 2015.

87. Task Force on diabetes, pre-diabetes, and cardiovascular diseases of the European Society of Cardiology (ESC) and developed in collaboration with the European Association for the Study of Diabetes (EASD): ESC Guidelines on diabetes, pre-diabetes, and cardiovascular diseases developed in collaboration with the EASD—summary, *Diab Vasc Dis Res* 11(3):133-173, 2014.

88. Sander D, Kearney MT: Reducing the risk of stroke in type 2 diabetes: pathophysiology and therapeutic perspectives, *J Neurol* 256(10): 1603-1619, 2009.

89. Gupta S et al: Infections in diabetes mellitus and hyperglycemia, *Infect Dis Clin North Am* 21(3):617-638, 2007.

90. Zilio M et al: Diagnosis and complications of Cushing's disease: gender-related differences, *Clin Endocrinol (Oxf)* 80(3):403-410, 2014.

91. Castinetti F et al: Cushing's disease, *Orphanet J Rare Dis* 7:41, 2012.

92. Bansal V et al: Pitfalls in the diagnosis and management of Cushing's syndrome, *Neurosurg Focus* 38(2):E4, 2015.

93. Starkman MN: Neuropsychiatric findings in Cushing syndrome and exogenous glucocorticoid administration, *Endocrinol Metab Clin North Am* 42(3):477-488, 2013.

94. Elias P et al: A. Late-night salivary cortisol has a better performance than urinary free cortisol in the diagnosis of Cushing's syndrome, *J Clin Endocrinol Metab* 99(6):2014-2051, 2014.

95. Han TS et al: Treatment and health outcomes in adults with congenital adrenal hyperplasia, *Nat Rev Endocrinol* 10(2):115-124, 2014.

96. Speiser PW et al: Congenital adrenal hyperplasia due to steroid 21-hydroxylase deficiency: an Endocrine Society clinical practice guideline, *J Clin Endocrinol Metab* 95(9):4133-4160, 2010.

97. Chao CT et al: Diagnosis and management of primary aldosteronism: an updated review, *Ann Med* 45(4):375-383, 2013.

98. Magill SB: Pathophysiology, diagnosis, and treatment of mineralocorticoid disorders, *Compr Physiol* 4(3):1083-1119, 2014.

99. Harvey AM: Hyperaldosteronism: diagnosis, lateralization, and treatment, *Surg Clin North Am* 94(3):643-656, 2014.

100. Brandão Neto RA, de Carvalho JF: Diagnosis and classification of Addison's disease (autoimmune adrenalitis), *Autoimmun Rev* 13(4-5):408-411, 2014.

101. Husebye ES et al: Consensus statement on the diagnosis, treatment and follow-up of patients with primary adrenal insufficiency, *J Intern Med* 275(2):104-115, 2014.

102. Rana HQ et al: Genetic testing in the clinical care of patients with pheochromocytoma and paraganglioma, *Curr Opin Endocrinol Diabetes Obes* 21(3):166-176, 2014.

103. Tsirlin A et al: Pheochromocytoma: a review, *Maturitas* 77(3):229-238, 2014.

104. Lenders J et al: Pheochromocytoma and paraganglioma: an Endocrine Society clinical practice guideline, *J Clin Endocrinol Metab* 99:1915-1942, 2014.

20

Structure and Function of the Hematologic System

Neal S. Rote and Kathryn L. McCance

All the body's tissues and organs require oxygen and nutrients to survive. These essential needs are provided by the blood that flows through miles of vessels throughout the human body. The red blood cells provide the oxygen, and the fluid portion of the blood carries the nutrients. The blood also cleans discarded waste from the tissues and transports cells (white blood cells) and other ingredients that are necessary for protecting the entire body from injury and infection.

COMPONENTS OF THE HEMATOLOGIC SYSTEM

Composition of Blood

Blood consists of various cells that circulate suspended in a solution of protein and inorganic materials (plasma), which is approximately 91% water and 9% dissolved substances (solutes). The blood volume amounts to about 6 quarts (5.5 L) in adults. The continuous movement of blood guarantees that critical components are available to all parts of the body to carry out their chief functions: (1) delivery of substances needed for cellular metabolism in the tissues, (2) removal of the wastes of cellular metabolism, (3) defense against invading microorganisms and injury, and (4) maintenance of acid-base balance.

Plasma and Plasma Proteins

In adults, plasma accounts for 50% to 55% of blood volume (Figure 20-1). Plasma is a complex aqueous liquid containing a variety of organic and inorganic elements (Table 20-1). The concentration of these elements varies depending on diet, metabolic demand, hormones, and vitamins. Plasma differs from serum in that serum is

plasma that has been allowed to clot in the laboratory in order to remove fibrinogen and other clotting factors that may interfere with some diagnostic tests.

The plasma contains a large number of proteins (plasma proteins). These vary in structure and function and can be classified into two major groups—albumin and globulins. Most plasma proteins are produced by the liver. The major exception is antibody, which is produced by plasma cells in the lymph nodes and other lymphoid tissues (see Chapter 7).

Albumin (about 60% of total plasma protein) serves as a carrier molecule for both normal components of blood and drugs. Its most essential role is regulation of the passage of water and solutes through the capillaries. Albumin molecules are large and do not diffuse freely through the vascular endothelium, and thus they maintain the critical colloidal osmotic pressure (or oncotic pressure) that regulates the passage of fluids and electrolytes into the surrounding tissues (see Chapters 1 and 5). Water and solute particles tend to diffuse out of the arterial portions of the capillaries because blood pressure is greater in arterial than in venous blood vessels. Water and solutes move from tissues into the venous portions of the capillaries where the pressures are reversed, oncotic pressure being greater than intravascular pressure or hydrostatic pressure. In the case of decreased production (e.g., cirrhosis, other diffuse liver diseases, protein malnutrition) or excessive loss of albumin (e.g., certain kidney diseases), the reduced oncotic pressure leads to excessive movement of fluid and solutes into the tissue and decreased blood volume.

The remaining plasma proteins, or globulins, are often classified by their properties in an electric field (serum electrophoresis). Under

FIGURE 20-1 Composition of Whole Blood. Approximate values for the components of blood in a normal adult. (From Patton KT, Thibodeau GA: *Structure & function of the body*, ed 15, St Louis, 2016, Mosby.)

the normal conditions used to perform serum electrophoresis, albumin is the most rapidly moving protein. The globulins are classified by their movement relative to albumin: alpha globulins (those moving most closely to albumin), beta globulins, and gamma globulins (those with the least movement). The alpha and beta globulins may be subdivided into subregions (alpha-1, alpha-2, beta-1, or beta-2 globulins). Fibrinogen is a major plasma protein (about 4% of total plasma protein) that would move between the beta and gamma regions but is removed during the formation of serum. The gamma-globulin region consists primarily of antibodies (see Chapter 7).

Plasma proteins can also be classified by function: clotting, defense, transport, or regulation. The clotting factors promote coagulation and stop bleeding from damaged blood vessels. Fibrinogen is the most plentiful of the clotting factors and is the precursor of the fibrin clot (see Figure 20-18). Proteins involved in defense, or protection, against infection include antibodies and complement proteins (see Chapters 6 and 7). Transport proteins specifically bind and carry a variety of inorganic and organic molecules, including iron (transferrin), copper (ceruloplasmin), lipids and steroid hormones (lipoproteins) (see Chapters 1 and 23), and vitamins (e.g., retinol-binding protein). Regulatory proteins include a variety of enzymatic inhibitors (e.g., α_1-antitrypsin) that protect the tissues from damage, precursor molecules (e.g., kininogen) that are converted into active biologic molecules when needed, and protein hormones (e.g., cytokines) that communicate between cells.

Plasma also contains several inorganic ions that regulate cell function, osmotic pressure, and blood pH. These include electrolytes, sodium, potassium, calcium, chloride, and phosphate. (Electrolytes are described in Chapters 1 and 4.)

Cellular Components of the Blood

The cellular elements of the blood are broadly classified as red blood cells (i.e., erythrocytes), white blood cells (i.e., leukocytes), and platelets. The components of the blood are listed in Table 20-2. Pathways of blood differentiation or maturation are shown in Figure 20-2.

Erythrocytes. Erythrocytes (red blood cells) are the most abundant cells of the blood, occupying approximately 48% of the blood volume in men and about 42% in women. Erythrocytes are primarily responsible for tissue oxygenation. Hemoglobin (Hb) carries the gases, and electrolytes regulate gas diffusion through the cell's plasma membrane. The mature erythrocyte lacks a nucleus and cytoplasmic organelles (e.g., mitochondria), so it cannot synthesize protein or carry out oxidative reactions. Because it cannot undergo mitotic division, the erythrocyte has a limited life span (approximately 80 to 120 days).

The erythrocyte's size and shape are ideally suited to its function as a gas carrier. It is a small disk with two unique properties: (1) a *biconcave* shape and (2) the capacity to be *reversibly deformed*. The flattened, biconcave shape provides a surface area/volume ratio that is optimal for gas diffusion into and out of the cell and for deformity. During its life span, the erythrocyte, which is 6 to 8 μm in diameter, repeatedly circulates through splenic sinusoids (Figure 20-3) and capillaries that are only 2 μm in diameter. Reversible deformity enables the erythrocyte to assume a more compact torpedo-like shape, squeeze through the microcirculation, and return to normal.

TABLE 20-1   Organic and Inorganic Components of Arterial Plasma

Constituent	Amount/Concentration	Major Functions
Water	91% of plasma weight	Medium for carrying all other constituents
Electrolytes	Total >1% of plasma	Maintain H_2O in extracellular compartment; act as buffers; function in membrane excitability
Na^+	142 mEq/L (142 mM)	
K^+	4 mEq/L (4 mM)	
Ca^{++}	5 mEq/L (2.5 mM)	
Mg^{++}	3 mEq/L (1.5 mM)	
Cl^-	103 mEq/L (103 mM)	
HCO_3^-	27 mEq/L (27 mM)	
Phosphate (mostly HPO_4^-)	2 mEq/L (1 mM)	
S_4^-	1 mEq/L (0.5 mM)	
Proteins	7.3 g/dl (2.5 mM)	Provide colloid osmotic pressure of plasma; act as buffers; see text for other functions
Albumins	4.5 g/dl	
Globulins	2.5 g/dl	
Fibrinogen	0.3 g/dl	
Transferrin	250 mg/dl	
Ferritin	15-300 mg/L	
Gases		
CO_2 content	22-20 mmol/L of plasma	By-product of oxygenation, most CO_2 content is from HCO_3^- and acts as buffer
O_2	PaO_2 80 torr or greater (arterial); PvO_2 30-40 torr (venous)	Oxygenation
N_2	0.9 ml/dl	By-product of protein catabolism
Nutrients		Provide nutrition and substances for tissue repair
Glucose and other carbohydrates	100 mg/dl (5.6 mM)	
Total amino acids	40 mg/dl (2 mM)	
Total lipids	500 mg/dl (7.5 mM)	
Cholesterol	150-250 mg/dl (4-7 mM)	
Individual vitamins	0.0001-2.5 mg/dl	
Individual trace elements	0.001-0.3 mg/dl	
Iron	50-150 mg/dl	
Waste Products		
Urea (BUN)	7-18 mg/dl (5.7 mM)	End product of protein catabolism
Creatinine (from creatine)	1 mg/dl (0.09 mM)	End product from energy metabolism
Uric acid (from nucleic acids)	5 mg/dl (0.3 mM)	End product from protein metabolism
Bilirubin (from heme)	0.2-1.2 mg/dl (0.003-0.018 mM)	End product of red blood cell destruction
Individual hormones	0.000001-0.5 mg/dl	Functions specific to target tissue

Data from Vander AJ et al: *Human physiology: the mechanisms of body function,* New York, 2001, McGraw-Hill.

Leukocytes. Leukocytes (white blood cells) defend the body against organisms that cause infection and also remove debris, including dead or injured host cells of all kinds (Figure 20-4). The leukocytes act primarily in the tissues but are transported in the circulation. The average adult has approximately 5000 to 10,000 leukocytes/mm³ of blood.

Leukocytes are classified according to structure as either granulocytes or agranulocytes and according to function as either phagocytes or immunocytes. The granulocytes, which include neutrophils, basophils, and eosinophils, are all phagocytes. (Phagocytic action is described in Chapter 6.) Of the agranulocytes, the monocytes and macrophages are phagocytes, whereas the lymphocytes are immunocytes (cells that create immunity; see Chapter 7).

Granulocytes. The granulocytes have many membrane-bound granules in their cytoplasm. These granules contain enzymes capable of killing microorganisms and catabolizing debris ingested during phagocytosis. The granules also contain powerful biochemical mediators with inflammatory and immune functions. These mediators, along with the digestive enzymes, are released from granulocytes in response to specific stimuli and affect other cells in the circulation. Granulocytes are capable of amoeboid movement, by which they migrate through vessel walls (diapedesis) and then to sites where their action is needed.

The neutrophil (polymorphonuclear neutrophil [PMN]) is the most numerous and best understood of the granulocytes (Figure 20-5). Neutrophils constitute 60% to 70% of the total leukocyte count in adults.

Neutrophils are the chief phagocytes of early inflammation. Soon after bacterial invasion or tissue injury, neutrophils migrate out of the capillaries and into the damaged tissue, where they ingest and destroy contaminating microorganisms and debris. Neutrophils are sensitive to the environment in damaged tissue (e.g., low pH, enzymes released

TABLE 20-2   Cellular Components of the Blood

Cell	Structural Characteristics	Normal Amounts of Circulating Blood	Function	Life Span
Erythrocyte (red blood cell)	Nonnucleated cytoplasmic disk containing hemoglobin	4.2-6.2 million/mm^3	Gas transport to and from tissue cells and lungs	80-120 days
Reticulocyte	60,000/mm^3	Immature erythrocyte		
Absolute reticulocyte count	0.5-2.0% of erythrocytes			
Leukocyte (white blood cell)	Nucleated cell	5000-10,000/mm^3	Body defense mechanisms	See below
Lymphocyte	Mononuclear immunocyte	20-25% of leukocyte count (leukocyte differential)	Humoral and cell-mediated immunity (see Chapter 7)	Days or years depending on type
Natural killer cell	Large granular lymphocyte	5-10% circulatory pool (some in spleen)	Defense against some tumors and viruses (see Chapters 6 and 7)	Unknown
Monocyte and macrophage	Large mononuclear phagocyte	2-8% of leukocyte differential	Phagocytosis; mononuclear phagocyte system	Months or years
Eosinophil	Segmented polymorphonuclear granulocyte	2-4% of leukocyte differential	Control of inflammation, phagocytosis, defense against parasites, allergic reactions	Unknown
Neutrophil	Segmented polymorphonuclear granulocyte	60-70% of leukocyte differential	Phagocytosis, particularly during early phase of inflammation	4 days
Basophil	Segmented polymorphonuclear granulocyte	0.5-1% of leukocyte differential	Mast cell–like functions, associated with allergic reactions and mechanical irritation	Unknown
Platelet	Irregularly shaped cytoplasmic fragment (not a cell)	150,000-400,000/mm^3	Hemostasis after vascular injury; normal coagulation and clot formation/retraction	8-11 days

from damaged cells) and die in 1 or 2 days. The breakdown of dead neutrophils releases digestive enzymes from their cytoplasmic granules. These enzymes dissolve cellular debris and prepare the site for healing.

Eosinophils, which have large, coarse granules, constitute only 2% to 4% of the normal leukocyte count in adults. Using a spectrum of pattern-recognition receptors, eosinophils are capable of amoeboid movement and phagocytosis. Unlike neutrophils, eosinophils ingest antigen-antibody complexes and are induced by immunoglobulin E (IgE)–mediated hypersensitivity reactions to attack parasites (see Chapters 7 and 8). Eosinophil secondary granules contain toxic chemicals (e.g., major basic protein, eosinophil cationic protein, eosinophil peroxidase, eosinophil-derived neurotoxin) that are highly destructive to parasites and viruses.[1] Eosinophil granules also contain a variety of enzymes (e.g., histaminase) that help to control inflammatory processes. Eosinophils also release leukotrienes, prostaglandins, platelet-activating factor (PAF), and a variety of cytokines (e.g., interleukin-1 [IL-1], IL-6, tumor necrosis factor-alpha [TNF-α], granulocyte-macrophage colony-stimulating factor [GM-CSF]) and chemokines (e.g., IL-8) that augment the inflammatory response. During type I hypersensitivity, allergic reactions and asthma are characterized by high eosinophil counts, which may be involved in a dual role of regulation of inflammation and contribute to the destructive inflammatory processes observed in the lungs of persons with asthma.

Basophils, which make up less than 1% of leukocytes, are structurally similar to the mast cells (see Figure 20-5). Basophils contain cytoplasmic granules with histamine, chemotactic factors, proteolytic enzymes (e.g., elastase, lysophospholipase), and an anticoagulant (heparin). Stimulation of basophils also induces synthesis of vasoactive lipid molecules (e.g., leukotrienes) and cytokines, including interleukin-6 (IL-6), which affects differentiation of Th1 cells and Th2 cells. Basophils also are a particularly rich source of the cytokine IL-4, which preferentially guides B-cell differentiation toward plasma cells that secrete IgE (see Chapter 7).

Agranulocytes. The agranulocytes—monocytes, macrophages, and lymphocytes—contain relatively fewer granules than granulocytes. Monocytes and macrophages make up the mononuclear phagocyte system (MPS) (see p. 497, and Chapter 6). Both monocytes and macrophages participate in the immune and inflammatory response, being powerful phagocytes. They also ingest dead or defective host cells, particularly blood cells.

Monocytes are immature macrophages (see Figure 20-5). Monocytes are formed and released by the bone marrow into the bloodstream. As they mature, monocytes migrate into a variety of tissues (e.g., liver, spleen, lymph nodes, peritoneum, gastrointestinal tract) and fully mature into tissue macrophages. Other monocytes may mature into macrophages and migrate out of the vessels in response to infection or inflammation.

Lymphocytes constitute approximately 20% to 25% of the total leukocyte count and are the primary cells of the immune response (see Figure 20-5 and Chapter 7). Most lymphocytes transiently circulate in the blood and eventually reside in lymphoid tissues as mature T cells, B cells, or plasma cells. (Lymphocyte function and dysfunction are described in detail in Unit 2.)

Natural killer (NK) cells, which resemble lymphocytes, kill some types of tumor cells (in vitro) and some virus-infected cells without prior exposure (see Chapters 6 and 7). They develop in the bone marrow and circulate in the blood.

Platelets. Platelets (thrombocytes) are not true cells but irregularly-shaped anuclear cytoplasmic fragments that are essential for blood coagulation and control of bleeding. They are formed by fragmentation of very large (40 to 100 μm in diameter) cells known as megakaryocytes and contain cytoplasmic granules (discussed later in this chapter) capable of releasing potent mediators when stimulated by injury to a blood vessel (Figure 20-6).

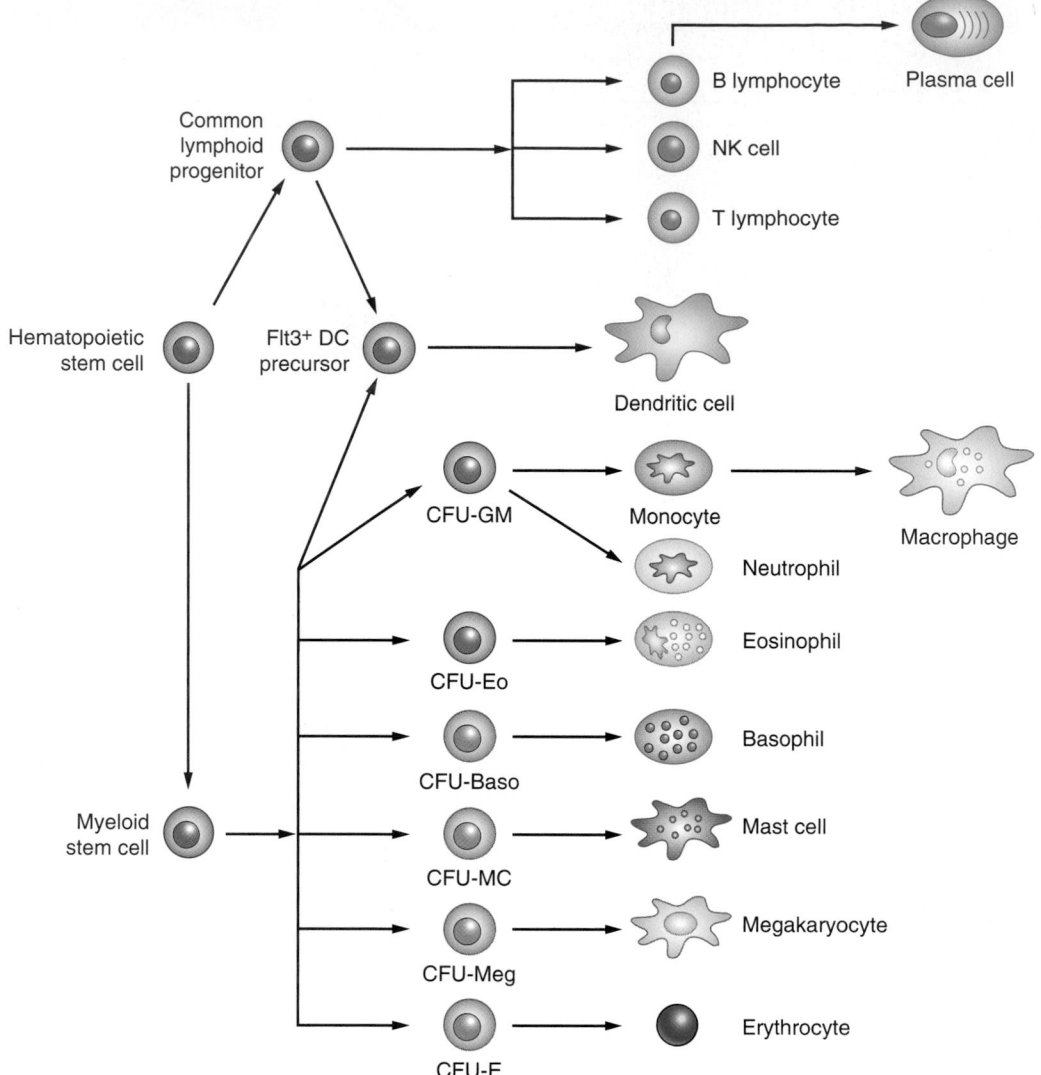

FIGURE 20-2 Differentiation of Hematopoietic Cells. Curved arrows indicate proliferation and expansion of pre-hematopoietic stem cell populations. *CFU,* Colony-forming unit; *NK,* natural killer. (Mast cells are discussed in Chapter 6.)

The normal platelet concentration is approximately 150,000 to 400,000 platelets/mm³ of circulating blood, although the normal ranges may vary slightly from laboratory to laboratory. An additional one third of the body's available platelets are in a reserve pool in the spleen. A platelet circulates for approximately 8 to 11 days, ages, and is removed by macrophages, mostly in the spleen.

QUICK CHECK 20-1
1. What are the unique properties of the erythrocyte's shape?
2. Why are plasma proteins important to blood volume?
3. Which leukocytes are granulocytes?
4. Compare and contrast granulocytes, agranulocytes, phagocytes, and immunocytes.

Lymphoid Organs

The lymphoid system is closely integrated with the circulatory system. The lymphoid organs, some of which stare merely aggregations of lymphoid tissue, are classified as primary or secondary. The **primary**

lymphoid organs are the thymus and the bone marrow. The **secondary lymphoid organs** consist of the spleen, lymph nodes, tonsils, and Peyer patches of the small intestine. All of the lymphoid organs link the hematologic and immune systems in that they are sites of residence, proliferation, differentiation, or function of lymphocytes and mononuclear phagocytes (monocytes and macrophages). (The liver, which also has hematologic functions, is primarily a digestive organ and is described in Chapter 35.)

Spleen

The **spleen** is the largest of the lymphoid organs. It serves as a site of fetal hematopoiesis, filters and cleanses the blood by mononuclear phagocytes, initiates an immune responses to blood-borne microorganisms, and serves as a reservoir for blood.

The spleen is a concave, encapsulated organ that weighs about 150 g and is about the size of a fist. Strands of connective tissue (trabeculae) extend throughout the spleen from the splenic capsule, dividing it into compartments that contain masses of lymphoid tissue called *splenic pulp.* The spleen is interlaced with many blood vessels, some of which can distend to store blood.

FIGURE 20-3 Red Cells in the Spleen. Scanning electron micrograph of spleen, demonstrating erythrocytes (numbered *1* through *6*) squeezing through the fenestrated wall in transit from the splenic cord to the sinus. The view shows the endothelial lining of the sinus wall, to which platelets *(P)* adhere, along with "hairy" white cells, probably macrophages. The arrow shows a protrusion on a red blood cell (×5000). (From Weiss L: *Blood* 43:665, 1974; reprinted with permission.)

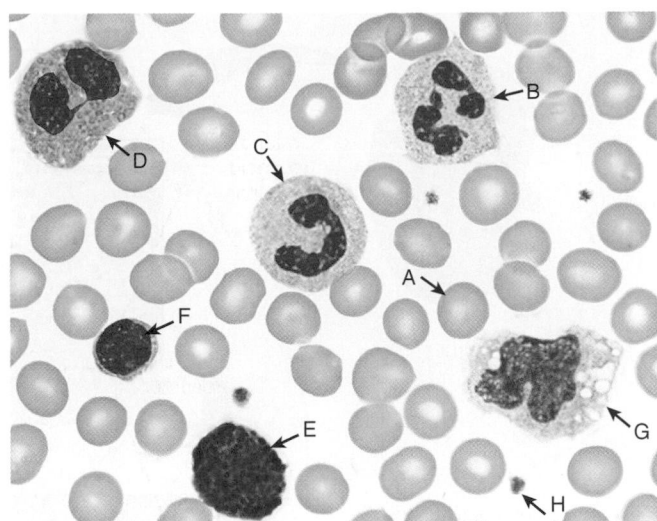

FIGURE 20-5 Leukocytes. Normal cells in peripheral blood: **A,** Erythrocyte (red blood cell); **B,** Neutrophil (segmented); **C,** Neutrophil (banded); **D,** Eosinophil; **E,** Basophil; **F,** Lymphocyte; **G,** Monocyte; **H,** Platelet. (From Keohane E, Smith L, Walenga J: *Rodak's hemotology,* ed 5, St. Louis, 2016, Saunders).

FIGURE 20-4 Blood Cells. Leukocytes are spherical and have irregular surfaces with numerous extending pili. Leukocytes are the cotton candy–like cells *(yellow)*. Erythrocytes are flattened spheres with a depressed center *(red)*. (Copyright Dennis Kunkel Microscopy, Inc.)

FIGURE 20-6 Colored Micrograph of Platelets. The platelet on the left is moderately activated, with a generally round shape and the beginning of formation of pseudopodia (foot-like extensions from the membrane). The platelet on the right is fully activated, with extensive pseudopodia. (Copyright Dennis Kunkel Microscopy, Inc.)

Arterial blood that enters the spleen first encounters the white splenic pulp, which consists of masses of lymphoid tissue containing macrophages and lymphocytes, primarily T lymphocytes in proximity to the arterioles (Figure 20-7). Cellular clumps (lymphoid follicles) are formed in the white pulp around the splenic arterioles. The lymphoid follicles consist primarily of B lymphocytes and are the chief sites of immune function within the spleen. Here blood-borne antigens encounter lymphocytes, initiating the immune response and the conversion of lymphoid follicles into germinal centers (see Chapter 7).

Some of the blood continues through the microcirculation and enters highly distensible storage areas, called *venous sinuses,* in the red pulp of the spleen. The venous sinuses (and the red pulp) can store more than 300 ml of blood. Sudden reductions in blood pressure cause the sympathetic nervous system to stimulate constriction of the sinuses and expel as much as 200 ml of blood into the venous circulation, helping to restore blood volume or pressure in the circulation and increasing the hematocrit by as much as 4%.

The endothelial lining of the venous sinuses is discontinuous (having gaps between endothelial cells) and therefore extremely permeable so that blood cells are allowed to exit the circulation.[2] The red pulp contains a system of loosely interconnected resident macrophages that provide the principal site of splenic filtration. Because of the slow circulation in the sinuses, the macrophages easily phagocytose old, damaged, or dead blood cells of all kinds (but chiefly erythrocytes),

FIGURE 20-7 Diagram of the Spleen. (From Gartner LP, Hiatt JL: *Color textbook of histology,* ed 3, Philadelphia, 2007, Elsevier.)

microorganisms, macromolecules, and particles of debris. Hemoglobin from phagocytosed erythrocytes is catabolized, and heme (iron) is stored in the cytoplasm of the macrophages or released back into the blood. Blood that filters through the red pulp then moves through the venous sinuses and into the portal circulation.

The spleen is not absolutely necessary for life or for adequate hematologic function. However, splenic absence from any cause (atrophy, traumatic injury, or removal because of disease) has several secondary effects on the body. For example, leukocytosis (high levels of circulating leukocytes) often occurs after splenectomy, suggesting that the spleen exerts some control over the rate of proliferation of leukocyte stem cells in the bone marrow or their release into the bloodstream. Circulating levels of iron also may decrease, reflecting the spleen's role in the iron cycle. The immune response to encapsulated bacteria (e.g., *Streptococcus pneumoniae* [pneumococcus], *Neisseria meningiti-*

dis [meningococcus], *Haemophilus influenzae*), which is primarily an IgM response, may be severely diminished resulting in increased susceptibility to disseminated infections. Loss of the spleen results in an increase in morphologically defective blood cells in the circulation, confirming the spleen's role in removing old or damaged cells.

Lymph Nodes

Structurally, **lymph nodes** are part of the lymphatic system. Lymphatic vessels collect interstitial fluid from the tissues and transport it, as lymph, through vessels of increasing size to the thoracic duct, which drains into the superior vena cava, returning the lymph to the circulation. Lymph nodes are distributed throughout the body and provide filtration of the lymph during its journey through the lymphatics. Each lymph node is enclosed in a fibrous capsule, branches of which (trabeculae) extend inward to partition the node into several

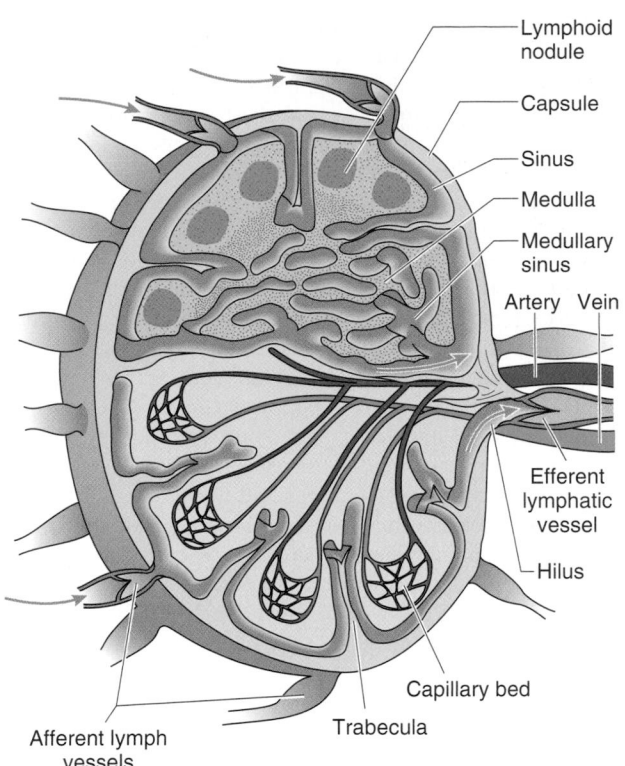

FIGURE 20-8 Cross Section of Lymph Node. Several afferent valved lymphatics bring lymph to node. A single efferent lymphatic leaves the node at the hilus. *Note that the artery and vein also enter and leave at the hilus. Arrows show direction of lymph flow.* (Adapted from Gartner LP, Hiatt JL: *Color textbook of histology,* 3rd ed. Philadelphia, 2007, Saunders.)

compartments (Figure 20-8). Reticular fibers of connective tissue divide the compartments into a meshwork throughout the lymph node. The node consists of outer (cortex) and inner (paracortex) cortical areas and an inner medulla. Lymph enters through multiple small afferent lymphatic vessels into the subcapsular sinus, just beneath the capsule, and drains into the cortical sinuses to the medullary sinuses, from which the lymph is collected and leaves the node by way of the efferent lymphatic vessel. Blood flows into the lymph nodes through the lymphatic artery, which ends in groups of postcapillary venules distributed throughout the outer cortex. The blood is drained through the lymphatic vein.

Functionally, lymph nodes are part of the hematologic and immune systems and are the primary site for the first encounter between antigen and lymphocytes. Lymphocytes enter the lymph node from the blood through the postcapillary venules by means of diapedesis across the endothelial lining. B lymphocytes tend to migrate preferentially to the cortex and medulla of the nodes, whereas T lymphocytes predominantly migrate to the paracortex. Macrophages reside in the lymph node; help filter the lymph of debris, foreign substances, and microorganisms; and provide antigen-processing functions. The dendritic cells encounter and process antigens and microorganisms in other tissues, enter the lymph node through the afferent lymph vessels, and migrate throughout the nodes (see Chapter 6). The reticular network provides adhesive surfaces for trapping large numbers of phagocytes and lymphocytes and facilitates their organization into follicles or primary nodules. The presence of antigen, either removed from the lymph by macrophages or presented on the surface of dendritic cells, results in the production of secondary nodules containing germinal

centers. In the germinal centers lymphocytes, particularly B cells, respond to antigenic stimulation by undergoing proliferation and further differentiation into memory cells and plasma cells (see Chapter 7). Plasma cells migrate to the medullary cords. The B-lymphocyte proliferation in response to a great deal of antigen (e.g., during infection) may result in lymph node enlargement and tenderness (reactive lymph node).

The Mononuclear Phagocyte System

The mononuclear phagocyte system (MPS) consists of monocytes that differentiate without dividing and reside in the tissues for months or perhaps years.[3] Table 20-3 lists the various names given to macrophages localized in specific tissues.

Cells of the MPS ingest and destroy (by phagocytosis) unwanted materials, such as foreign protein particles, circulating immune complexes, microorganisms, debris from dead or injured cells, defective or injured erythrocytes, and dead neutrophils. Recently, the osteoclast was classified as a true member of the MPS. Osteoclasts are multinucleated cells that originate from the monocyte cell lineage (see Figure 20-2) and are specialized for the function of lacunar bone resorption; however, they are also known to have phagocytic abilities.

> ### ✓ QUICK CHECK 20-2
> 1. Why is the spleen considered a hematologic organ? Why can humans live without it?
> 2. Why are lymph nodes considered part of the hematologic system?
> 3. What is the MPS?

DEVELOPMENT OF BLOOD CELLS

Hematopoiesis

The typical human requires about 100 billion new blood cells per day. Blood cell production, termed hematopoiesis, is constantly ongoing, occurring in the liver and spleen of the fetus and only in bone marrow *(medullary hematopoiesis)* after birth. This process involves the biochemical stimulation of populations of relatively undifferentiated cells to undergo mitotic division (i.e., proliferation) and maturation (i.e., differentiation) into mature hematologic cells. Although proliferation and differentiation are usually sequential, certain blood cells proliferate

TABLE 20-3	Mononuclear Phagocyte System (Formerly Called the Reticuloendothelial System)
Name of Cell	**Location**
Monocytes/macrophages	Bone marrow and peripheral blood
Kupffer cells (inflammatory macrophages)	Liver
Alveolar macrophages	Lung
Histiocytes	Connective tissue
Macrophages	Bone marrow
Fixed and free macrophages	Spleen and lymph nodes
Pleural and peritoneal macrophages	Serous cavities
Microglial cells	Nervous system
Mesangial cells	Kidney
Osteoclasts	Bone
Langerhans cells	Skin
Dendritic cells	Lymphoid tissue

and differentiate simultaneously. Erythrocytes and neutrophils generally differentiate fully before entering the blood, but monocytes and lymphocytes continue to mature in the blood and in secondary lymphatic organs.

Hematopoiesis continues throughout life, increasing in response to a need to replenish destroyed circulating cells (e.g., during hemorrhage, hemolytic anemia [peripheral destruction of erythrocytes], consumptive thrombocytopenia) or in response to infection.[4] In general, long-term stimuli, such as chronic diseases, cause a greater increase in hematopoiesis than acute conditions, such as hemorrhage.

Various abnormalities in medullary hematopoiesis have been identified and are discussed in Chapter 21. Extramedullary hematopoiesis—blood cell production in tissues other than bone marrow—of apparently normal blood cells has been reported in the spleen, liver, and, less frequently, lymph nodes, adrenal glands, cartilage, adipose tissue, intrathoracic areas, and kidneys. Extramedullary hematopoiesis, however, is usually a sign of disease, occurring in pernicious anemia, sickle cell anemia, thalassemia, hemolytic disease of the newborn (erythroblastosis fetalis), hereditary spherocytosis, and certain leukemias.

Bone Marrow

Bone marrow is confined to the cavities of bone and is the primary residence of hematopoietic stem cells. It consists of blood vessels, nerves, mononuclear phagocytes, stromal cells, and blood cells in various stages of differentiation. Adults have two kinds of bone marrow: red, or active (hematopoietic), marrow (also called myeloid tissue); and yellow, or inactive, marrow. The large quantities of fat in inactive marrow make it yellow. Not all bones contain active marrow. In adults, active marrow is found primarily in the flat bones of the pelvis (34%), vertebrae (28%), cranium and mandible (13%), sternum and ribs (10%), and in the extreme proximal portions of the humerus and femur (4% to 8%). Inactive marrow predominates in cavities of other bones. (Bones are discussed further in Chapter 38.)

Hematopoietic marrow is vascularized by the primary arteries of the bones, which terminate in a capillary network forming large venous sinuses. Hematopoietic marrow and fat fill the spaces surrounding the network of venous sinuses. Newly produced blood cells traverse narrow openings between endothelial cells in the venous sinus walls and thus enter the circulation. Normally, cells do not enter the circulation until they have differentiated (e.g., developed appropriate surface receptors to interact with the endothelium and enter the circulation), but premature release occurs in certain diseases.

The hematologic compartment of the bone marrow consists of cellular microenvironments or niches that control differentiation of hematopoietic progenitor cells. The cellular composition of niches includes osteoclasts, osteoblasts, sinusoidal endothelial cells, fibroblasts, megakaryocytes, macrophages, and nerve cells. Osteoblasts are derived from fibroblasts and are responsible for construction of bone. Osteoclasts are multinucleate cells of monocytic origin that remodel bone by resorption. Both cells produce cytokines that affect proliferation of hematopoietic cells.[5] At least two populations of stem cells are found in bone marrow niches. Mesenchymal stem cells (MSCs) are stromal cells that can differentiate into a variety of cells, including osteoblasts, adipocytes, and chondrocytes (produce cartilage). Hematopoietic stem cells (HSCs) are progenitors of all hematologic cells. Both populations of stem cells undergo self-renewal in the bone marrow, so that additional MSCs and HSCs are produced to replace those undergoing differentiation.[6]

Two distinct types of niches have been identified—the osteoblastic (also called endosteal) niche and the vascular niche[7] (Figure 20-9). The osteoblastic niche is centralized around osteoblasts, which line the

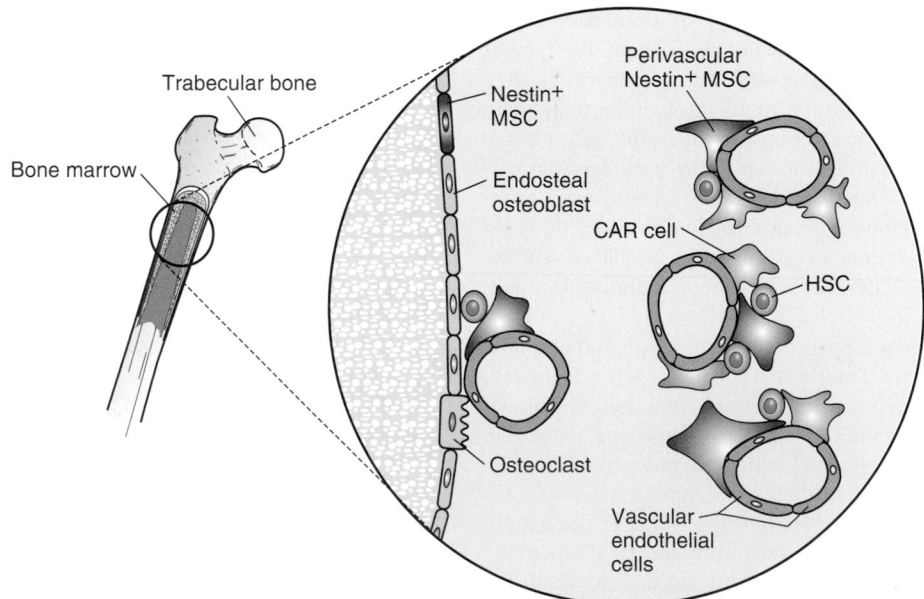

FIGURE 20-9 Bone Marrow Stem Cell Niches. Stem cell niches are microenvironments where stem cells undergo hematopoiesis into all forms of blood cells. Stem cell niches retain and maintain adult resting hematopoietic stem cells *(HSCs)* and are activated after cell injury to promote cell renewal or differentiation to form new tissues. The fate of individual HSCs is determined by interactions (intercellular adherence, cytokines, chemokines) with specialized cells within the niches. Within osteoblastic niches the HSC interacts primarily with the osteoblasts and specialized mesenchymal stem cells *(MSCs)* that include nestin-expressing *(Nestin⁺)* MSCs and CXCL12-abundant reticular *(CAR)* cells. Within the vascular niches, the HSC interacts with vascular endothelial cells, Nestin⁺ MSC, and a more abundant population of CAR cells.

surface of bone, whereas the vascular niche is organized around sinusoidal endothelial cells. In both niches, HSCs are affected by direct cell-to-cell signaling and soluble mediators produced by cells within each niche. Each niche also contains two specialized cells derived from MSCs: CXCL12-abundant reticular (CAR) cells and nestin-expressing cells.[8]

CAR cells resemble reticular cells with long cellular processes and closely interact with HSCs to provide important intercellular signaling through HSC regulatory molecules, including chemokine ligand 12 (CXCL12), stem cell factor (SCF, also called steel factor), vascular cell adhesion molecule 1 (VCAM-1), and angiopoietin 1 (ANG1). CXCL12 is a chemokine that reacts with a chemokine receptor on HSCs. SCF is expressed as a cell surface transmembrane protein or a soluble protein and reacts with the HSC KIT receptor (named stem cell growth factor receptor, proto-oncogene c-Kit, or CD117). VCAM-1 mediates intercellular adhesion through its receptor, integrin $\alpha_4\beta_1$. ANG1 is secreted and reacts with a tyrosine kinase receptor. Nestin-expressing cells express large amounts of the intermediate filament protein, nestin, and particularly SCF and VCAM-1. Although both MSC-derived cells are present in the osteoblastic niche and vascular niche, the CAR cell is the predominant cell in the vascular niche.

Each bone marrow niche affects HSCs differently. In the osteoblastic niche, HSCs are in direct contact with osteoblasts, CAR cells, and nestin-expressing cells. The effect is retention of HSCs in the bone marrow in a quiescent (dormant) state. HSCs that traffic to the vascular niche directly contact endothelial cells, as well as nestin-expressing cells and larger numbers of perivascular CAR cells. The cumulative signaling events induce HSC proliferation and hematopoietic differentiation.

Cellular Differentiation

All humans originate from a single cell (the fertilized egg) that has the capacity to proliferate and eventually differentiate into the huge diversity of cells of the human body. After fertilization, the egg divides over a 5-day period to form a hollow ball (blastocyst) that implants on the uterus. Until about 3 days after fertilization, each cell (blastomere) is undifferentiated and retains the capacity to differentiate into any cell type. In the 5-day blastocyst, the outer layer of cells has undergone differentiation and commitment to become the placenta. Cells of the inner cell mass, however, continue to have unlimited differentiation potential (currently referred to as being *pluripotent*) and can grow into different kinds of tissue—blood, nerves, heart, bone, and so forth. After implantation, cells of the inner cell mass begin differentiation into other cell types. Differentiation is a multistep process and results in intermediate groups of stem cells with more limited, but still impressive, abilities to differentiate into many different types of cells.

Within the bone marrow niches each type of blood cell originates from hematopoietic stem cells that proliferate and differentiate under control of a variety of cytokines and growth factors[9] (see Figure 20-2). As with all stem cells, the hematopoietic stem cells are self-renewing (they have the ability to proliferate without further differentiation) so that a relatively constant population of stem cells is available. Some hematopoietic stem cells will continue differentiation into hematopoietic progenitor cells. Progenitor cells retain proliferative capacity but are committed to possible further differentiation into particular types of hematologic cells: lymphoid (lymphocytes, NK cells), granulocyte/monocyte (granulocytes, monocytes, macrophages), and megakaryocyte/erythroid (platelets, erythrocytes) progenitor cells.

Several cytokines participate in hematopoiesis, particularly colony-stimulating factors (CSFs or hematopoietic growth factors), which stimulate the proliferation of progenitor cells and their progeny and initiate the maturation events necessary to produce fully mature cells. Multiple cell types in hematopoietic organs, including endothelial cells, fibroblasts, and lymphocytes, produce the necessary CSFs.

Hematopoiesis in the bone marrow occurs in two separate pools—the stem cell pool and the bone marrow pool—with eventual release of mature cells into the peripheral circulation (Figure 20-10). The stem cell pool contains pluripotent stem cells and partially committed

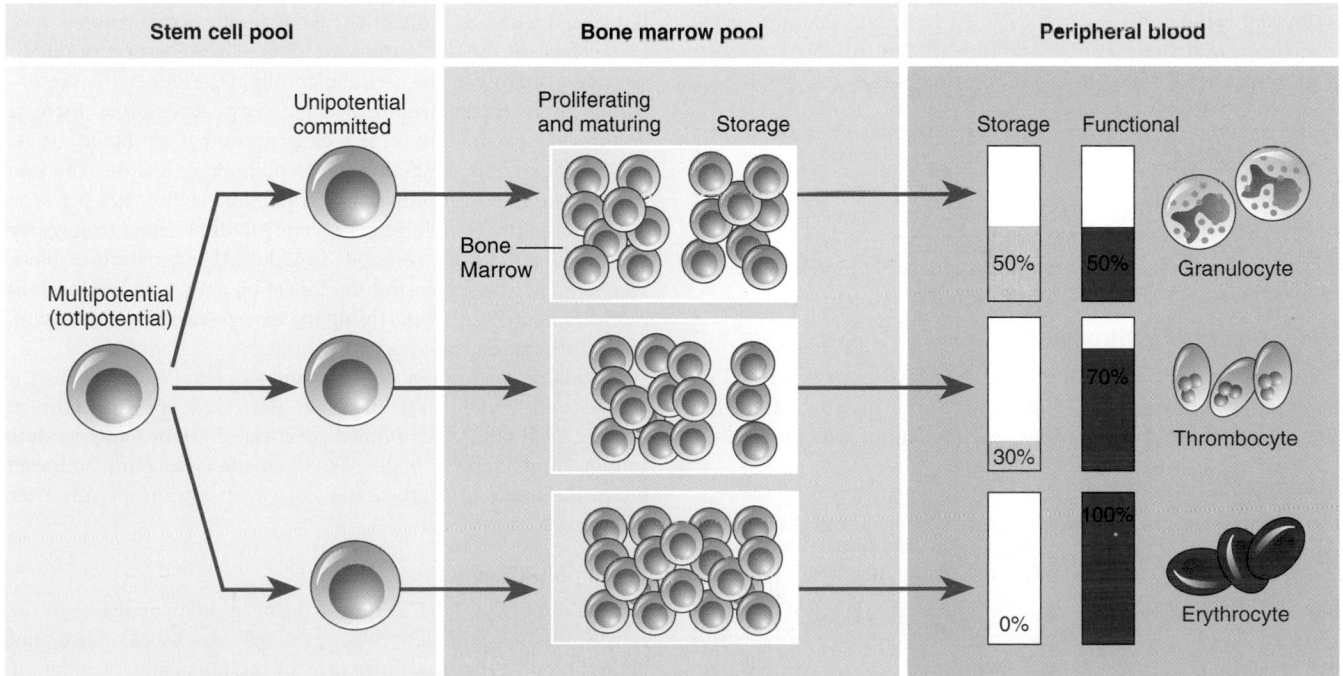

FIGURE 20-10 Hematopoiesis. Hematopoiesis from the stem cell pool; activity mainly in the bone marrow and in the peripheral blood.

FIGURE 20-11 Role of Erythropoietin in Regulation of Erythropoiesis. **(1)** Decreased arterial oxygen levels result in **(2)** decreased tissue oxygen (hypoxia) that **(3)** stimulates the kidney to increase **(4)** production of erythropoietin. Erythropoietin is carried to the bone marrow **(5)** and binds to erythropoietin receptors on proerythroblasts, resulting in increased red cell production and maturation and expansion of the erythron **(6)**. The increased release of red cells into the circulation frequently corrects the hypoxia in the tissues **(7)**. **(8)** Perception of normal oxygen levels by the kidney causes **(9)** diminished production of erythropoietin (negative feedback) and return to normal levels of erythrocyte production. *EPO,* Erythropoietin; *O₂,* oxygen in the blood and tissue; *RBCs,* red blood cells.

progenitor cells. The bone marrow pool contains cells that are proliferating and maturing in preparation for release into the circulation and mature cells that are stored for later release into the peripheral blood. The peripheral blood also contains two pools of cells—those circulating and those stored around the walls of the blood vessels (often called the **marginating storage pool**). The marginating storage pool primarily consists of neutrophils that adhere to the endothelium in vessels where the blood flow is relatively slow. These cells can rapidly move into tissues and mucous membranes when needed.

Under certain conditions, the levels of circulating hematologic cells need to be rapidly replenished. Medullary hematopoiesis can be accelerated by any or all of three mechanisms: (1) conversion of yellow bone marrow, which does not produce blood cells, to red marrow, which does, by the actions of **erythropoietin** (a hormone that stimulates erythrocyte production); (2) faster differentiation of daughter cells; and, presumably, (3) faster proliferation of stem cells.

 QUICK CHECK 20-3

1. Why is the stem cell system important to hematopoiesis?
2. Why are some stem cells called pluripotent?
3. What role do stromal cells play in hematopoiesis?

Development of Erythrocytes

For almost 100 years it was thought that erythrocytes developed in the spleen. It was not until the 1950s that the bone marrow was identified as the site of **erythropoiesis**, or development of red blood cells.

Erythropoiesis

In the confines of the bone marrow erythroid progenitor cells proliferate and differentiate into large, nucleated **proerythroblasts**, which are committed into producing cells of the erythroid series. The proerythroblast differentiates through several intermediate forms of **erythroblast** (sometimes called **normoblast**) while progressively eliminating most intracellular structures (including the nucleus), synthesizing hemoglobin, and becoming more compact, eventually assuming the shape and characteristics of an erythrocyte.

The last immature form is the **reticulocyte**, which contains a mesh-like (reticular) network of ribosomal RNA that is visible microscopically after staining with certain dyes. Reticulocytes remain in the marrow approximately 1 day and are released into the venous sinuses. They continue to mature in the bloodstream and may travel to the spleen for several days of additional maturation. The normal reticulocyte count is 1% of the total red blood cell count. Approximately 1% of the body's circulating erythrocyte mass normally is generated every 24 hours. Therefore, the reticulocyte count is a useful clinical index of erythropoietic activity and indicates whether new red cells are being produced.

Most steps of erythropoiesis are primarily under the control of a feedback loop involving the glycoprotein erythropoietin. In healthy humans, the total volume of circulating erythrocytes remains surprisingly constant. In conditions of tissue hypoxia, erythropoietin is secreted primarily by the peritubular cells of the kidney (Figure 20-11). Rising levels of erythropoietin causes a compensatory increase in erythrocyte production if the oxygen content of blood decreases because of anemia, high altitude, or pulmonary disease. The normal steady-state rate of production (2.5 million erythrocytes per second) can increase (to 17 million per second) under anemic or low-oxygen states. Thus, the body responds to reduced oxygenation of blood in two ways: (1) by increasing the intake of oxygen through increased respiration and (2) by increasing the oxygen-carrying capacity of the blood through increased erythropoiesis.

Recombinant human erythropoietin (r-HuEPO) is used in individuals with anemia secondary to decreased erythropoietin from chronic renal failure. An immediate effect of erythropoietin administration is an increase in the blood reticulocyte count, followed by increasing levels of erythrocytes. The most significant side effect is increased blood pressure.

Hemoglobin Synthesis

Hemoglobin (Hb), the oxygen-carrying protein of the erythrocyte, constitutes approximately 90% of the cell's dry weight. Hemoglobin-packed blood cells take up oxygen in the lungs and exchange it for carbon dioxide in the tissues. Hemoglobin increases the oxygen-carrying capacity of blood by 100-fold. Each hemoglobin molecule is

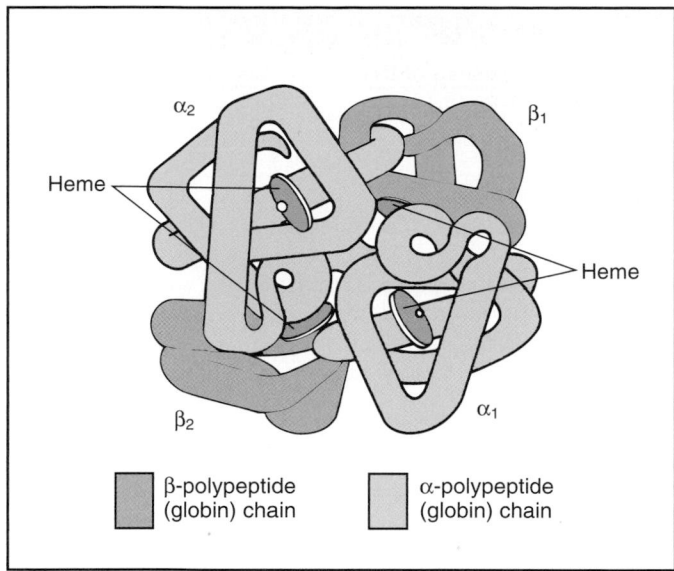

FIGURE 20-12 Molecular Structure of Hemoglobin. Molecule is a spherical tetramer weighing approximately 64,500 daltons. It contains a pair of α-polypeptide chains and a pair of β-polypeptide chains and several heme groups.

FIGURE 20-13 Hemoglobin (Hb) Binding to Nitric Oxide. In the lungs, hemoglobin *(Hb)* binds to nitric oxide *(NO)* as *S*-nitrosothiol *(SNO)*. In tissue, this SNO is released, and free, circulating NO is bound to a different site for exhalation. *Fe,* Iron; *N,* nitrogen.

composed of two pairs of polypeptide chains (the **globins**) and four colorful complexes of iron plus protoporphyrin (the **hemes**), which is responsible for the blood's ruby-red color (Figure 20-12).

Several variants of hemoglobin exist, but they differ only slightly in primary structure based on the use of different polypeptide chains: alpha, beta, gamma, delta, epsilon, or zeta (α, β, γ, δ, ϵ, or ζ).[10] Hemoglobin A, the most common type in adults, is composed of two α- and two β-polypeptide chains ($\alpha_2\beta_2$). A normal variant, fetal hemoglobin (hemoglobin F), is a complex of two α- and two γ-polypeptide chains ($\alpha_2\gamma_2$) that binds oxygen with a much greater affinity than adult hemoglobin.

Heme is a large, flat, iron-protoporphyrin disk that is synthesized in the mitochondria and can carry one molecule of oxygen (O_2).[11] Thus, an individual hemoglobin molecule with its four hemes can carry four oxygen molecules. If all four oxygen-binding sites are occupied by oxygen, the molecule is said to be saturated. Through a series of biochemical reactions, **protoporphyrin**, a complex four-ringed molecule, is produced and bound with ferrous iron. It is crucial that the iron be correctly charged; reduced ferrous iron (Fe^{2+}) can bind oxygen, whereas ferric iron (Fe^{3+}) cannot. Binding of oxygen to ferrous iron temporarily oxidizes Fe^{2+} to Fe^{3+} (**oxyhemoglobin**), but after the release of oxygen the body reduces the iron to Fe^{2+} and reactivates the hemoglobin (**deoxyhemoglobin** [reduced hemoglobin]). Without reactivation, the Fe^{3+}-containing hemoglobin (**methemoglobin**) cannot bind oxygen. An excess of ferric iron occurs with certain drugs and chemicals, such as nitrates and sulfonamides.

Several other molecules can competitively bind to deoxyhemoglobin. Carbon monoxide (CO) directly competes with oxygen for binding to ferrous ion with an affinity that is about 200-fold greater than that of oxygen. Thus, even a small amount of CO can dramatically decrease the ability of hemoglobin to bind and transport oxygen. Hemoglobin also binds carbon dioxide (CO_2), but at a binding site separate from where oxygen binds. In the lungs, CO_2 is released, allowing hemoglobin to bind oxygen.

Erythrocytes may play a role in the maintenance of vascular relaxation. Nitric oxide (NO) produced by blood vessels is a major mediator of relaxation and dilation of the vessel walls. In the lungs, hemoglobin can concurrently bind oxygen to the ferrous ion and NO to cysteine residues in the globins (Figure 20-13). As hemoglobin transfers its oxygen to tissue, it may also shed small amounts of nitric oxide, contributing to dilation of the blood vessels and helping transfer of the oxygen into tissues.

Nutritional Requirements for Erythropoiesis

Normal development of erythrocytes and synthesis of hemoglobin depend on an optimal biochemical state and adequate supplies of the necessary building blocks, including protein, vitamins, and minerals (Table 20-4). If these components are lacking for a prolonged time, erythrocyte production slows and anemia (insufficient numbers of functional erythrocytes) may result (see Chapter 21).

Erythropoiesis cannot proceed in the absence of vitamins, especially B_{12}, folate (folic acid), B_6, riboflavin, pantothenic acid, niacin, ascorbic acid, and vitamin E. Dietary vitamin B_{12} is a large molecule that requires a protein secreted by parietal cells into the stomach (intrinsic factor [IF]) for transport across the ileum. Vitamin B_{12} is stored in the liver and used as needed in erythropoiesis. Decreased B_{12} absorption may lead to pernicious anemia. Folate is necessary for DNA and RNA synthesis. Folate absorption occurs principally in the upper small intestine and is stored in the liver. Folate deficiency is more common than vitamin B_{12} deficiency and occurs more rapidly. Folate supplements are prescribed for pregnant women because pregnancy increases the demand for folate. Supplements can protect against neural tube defects and may prevent anemia.

Normal Destruction of Senescent Erythrocytes

Mature erythrocytes have cytoplasmic enzymes capable of glycolysis (anaerobic glucose metabolism) and production of small quantities of adenosine triphosphate (ATP). ATP provides the energy needed to maintain cell function and keep its plasma membrane pliable[12] (see Figure 1-1). Metabolic processes diminish as the erythrocyte ages, so less ATP is available to maintain plasma membrane function. The aged or senescent red cell becomes increasingly fragile and loses its

TABLE 20-4 **Nutritional Requirements for Erythropoiesis**

Nutrient	Role in Erythropoiesis	Consequence of Deficiency (See Chapter 21)
Protein (amino acids)	Structural component of plasma membrane	Decreased strength, elasticity, and flexibility of membrane; hemolytic anemia
	Synthesis of hemoglobin	Decreased erythropoiesis and life span of erythrocytes
Intrinsic factor	Gastrointestinal absorption of vitamin B_{12}	Pernicious anemia
Cobalamin (vitamin B_{12})	Synthesis of DNA, maturation of erythrocytes, facilitator of folate metabolism	Macrocytic (megaloblastic) anemia
Folate (folic acid)	Synthesis of DNA and RNA, maturation of erythrocytes	Macrocytic (megaloblastic) anemia
Vitamin B_6 (pyridoxine)	Heme synthesis, possibly increases folate metabolism	Hypochromic-microcytic anemia
Vitamin B_2 (riboflavin)	Oxidative reactions	Normochromic-normocytic anemia
Vitamin C (ascorbic acid)	Iron metabolism, acts as reducing agent to maintain iron in its ferrous (Fe^{++}) form	Normochromic-normocytic anemia
Pantothenic acid	Heme synthesis	Unknown in humans*
Niacin	None, but needed for respiration in mature erythrocytes	Unknown in humans
Vitamin E	Synthesis of heme; possible protection against oxidative damage in mature erythrocytes	Hemolytic anemia with increased cell membrane fragility; shortens life span of erythrocytes in individual with cystic fibrosis
Iron	Hemoglobin synthesis	Iron deficiency anemia
Copper	Structural component of plasma membrane	Hypochromic-microcytic anemia

Data from Lee GR et al: *Wintrobe's clinical hematology*, ed 9, Philadelphia, 1993, Lee & Febiger; Harmening DM: *Clinical hematology and fundamentals of hemostasis*, ed 3, Philadelphia, 1997, FA Davis.
DNA, Deoxyribonucleic acid; *RNA*, ribonucleic acid.
*Although pantothenic acid is important for optimal synthesis of heme, experimentally induced deficiency failed to produce anemia or other hematopoietic disturbances.

FIGURE 20-14 Metabolism of Bilirubin Released by Heme Breakdown. *MPS*, Mononuclear phagocyte system.

reversible deformability, becoming susceptible to rupture while passing through narrowed regions of the microcirculation.

Additionally, the plasma membrane of senescent red cells undergoes phospholipid rearrangement with enrichment of surface phosphatidylserine that is recognized by receptors on macrophages (primarily in the spleen), which selectively remove and sequester the red cells. If the spleen is dysfunctional or absent, macrophages in the liver (Kupffer cells) assume control. During digestion of hemoglobin in the macrophage, porphyrin reduces to bilirubin, which is transported to the liver, conjugated, and finally excreted in the bile as glucuronide (Figure 20-14). Bacteria in the intestinal lumen transform conjugated bilirubin into urobilinogen. Although a small portion is reabsorbed, most urobilinogen is excreted in feces. Conditions causing accelerated erythrocyte destruction increase the load of bilirubin for

hepatic clearance, leading to increased serum levels of unconjugated bilirubin and increased urinary excretion of urobilinogen. Gallstones (cholelithiasis) can result from a chronically elevated rate of bilirubin excretion.

Iron cycle. Approximately 67% of total body iron is bound to heme in erythrocytes (hemoglobin) and muscle cells (myoglobin), and approximately 30% is stored in mononuclear phagocytes (i.e., macrophages) and hepatic parenchymal cells as either ferritin or hemosiderin.[13] The remaining 3% (less than 1 mg) is lost daily in urine, sweat, bile, sloughing of epithelial cells from the skin and intestinal mucosa, and minor bleeding. Approximately 25 mg of iron is required daily for erythropoiesis; only 1 to 2 mg of iron is dietary and the remainder is obtained from continual recycling of iron from erythrocytes.

The methemoglobin released from the breakdown of senescent or damaged erythrocytes is dissociated by the enzyme heme oxygenase, and the iron is released into the bloodstream where it is free to bind again to transferrin or be stored in the macrophage's cytoplasm as ferritin or hemosiderin (Figure 20-15). A minute amount of iron is stored in muscle cells by the heme-containing protein myoglobin. Unavailable stores of iron are present in cytochromes, catalases, and peroxidase enzymes.

The protein ferritin is the major intracellular iron storage protein. Apoferritin, which is ferritin without attached iron, can store thousands of atoms of iron. Several apoferritin complexes combine to form the micelle ferritin. Large aggregates of micelles (if a large amount of iron is present) produce large iron storage complexes, known as hemosiderin. Under a light microscope, hemosiderin is visible as an iron-based pigment in cell inclusions. The iron within deposits of hemosiderin is poorly available to supply iron when needed. The most common cause of hemosiderin deposition is simple bruising. Hemosiderin in small amounts within iron-rich tissues (i.e., spleen, liver, bone marrow) is considered normal. Large aggregates or its presence in tissue, such as the lungs or subcutaneous tissue, suggest a pathologic condition.

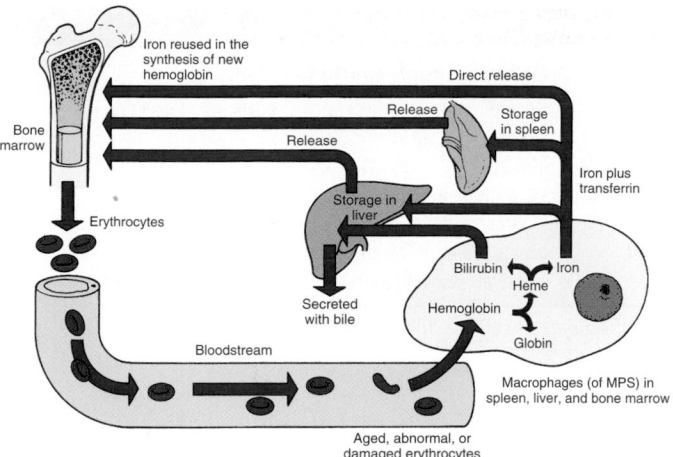

FIGURE 20-15 Iron Cycle. Iron released from gastrointestinal epithelial cells circulates in the bloodstream associated with its plasma carrier, transferrin. It is delivered to erythroblasts in bone marrow, where most of it is incorporated into hemoglobin. Mature erythrocytes circulate for approximately 120 days, after which they become senescent and are removed by the mononuclear phagocyte system (MPS). Macrophages of MPS (mostly in spleen) break down ingested erythrocytes and return iron to the bloodstream directly or after storing it as ferritin or hemosiderin.

Iron from either dietary sources, release of iron stores, or erythrocyte catabolism is transported in the blood bound to apotransferrin, thus becoming transferrin. Apotransferrin is a glycoprotein synthesized primarily by hepatocytes in the liver but also produced in small quantities by tissue macrophages, submaxillary and mammary glands, and ovaries or testes (see Figure 20-15). Transferrin is transported to the bone marrow, where it binds to transferrin receptors on erythroblasts. Transferrin receptors are on the plasma membrane of all nucleated cells, but at particularly high levels on erythroid precursors and rapidly proliferating cells (e.g., lymphocytes), and are thought to be the only route of cellular entry for transferrin-attached iron. Transferrin is recycled (transferrin cycle) by intracellular dissociation of the iron and secretion of the resultant apotransferrin to the bloodstream.

The iron is transported to the erythroblast's mitochondria (the site of hemoglobin production), where the enzyme heme synthetase inserts ferrous iron into protoporphyrin to form heme. Heme then is bound to globin to form hemoglobin. Iron not used in erythropoiesis is stored temporarily as ferritin or hemosiderin and later excreted.

The body's iron homeostasis is primarily controlled by the hormone **hepcidin.** Hepcidin is a 25 amino acid peptide synthesized in the liver and released into the plasma, where it is bound with high affinity to α_2-macroglobulin and with relatively lower affinity to albumin.[14] Hepatocellular hepcidin production is regulated physiologically by the levels of iron in the body, rate of erythropoiesis, and percentage of oxygen saturation. Hepatocytes (liver cells) sense levels of circulating iron by means of receptors for transferrin. Excess iron is stored in hepatocytes and macrophages, and hepatocytes sense these levels by means of receptors for bone morphogenetic protein (BMP), most likely BMP-6, which is a growth factor produced to a large extent by bone marrow sinusoid endothelial cells. Hepcidin production also can be induced by inflammation via IL-6.

Hepcidin regulates iron levels through its binding capacity to ferroportin, which is a transmembrane iron exporter found in the plasma membrane of cells that transport or store iron, including macrophages,

hepatocytes, and enterocytes (intestinal cells).[15] The body's total iron balance is maintained through controlled absorption rather than excretion. Dietary iron (primarily as Fe^{2+}) is transported directly across the membranes of enterocytes in the duodenum and proximal jejunum. (Transport mechanisms are described in Chapter 1.) Hepcidin induces internalization and degradation of ferroportin, thus leading to increased intracellular iron stores, decreased dietary iron absorption, and decreased levels of circulating iron. Decreased production of hepcidin leads to release of stored iron and increased dietary absorption. Thus, if the body's iron stores are low or the demand for erythropoiesis increases, dietary iron is transported rapidly through the epithelial cell and into the plasma. If body stores are high and erythropoiesis is not increased, iron transport is stopped, although iron can cross the epithelial cells' plasma membrane passively and is stored as ferritin.

✔ QUICK CHECK 20-4
1. Why is the reticulocyte count important?
2. Why is iron important to erythropoiesis?
3. What happens to aging erythrocytes?

Development of Leukocytes

Leukocytes consist of lymphocytes, granulocytes, and monocytes. Most leukocytes arise from hematopoietic stem cells in the bone marrow that differentiate into common lymphoid progenitors and common myeloid progenitors (their pathways of differentiation are shown in Figure 20-2). Lymphoid progenitor cells develop into lymphocytes, which are released into the bloodstream to undergo further maturation in the primary and secondary lymphoid organs (see Chapter 7). Common myeloid progenitors further differentiate into progenitors for erythrocytes, megakaryocytes, and mast cells, and into granulocyte/monocyte progenitors. The granulocyte/monocyte progenitors further differentiate into monocyte progenitors and granulocyte progenitors, which develop into monocytes/macrophages and granulocytes (neutrophils, basophils, eosinophils), respectively. Development from hematopoietic stem cell to common granulocyte/monocyte progenitor primarily is under the control of stem cell factor, IL-3, and GM-CSF, whereas further differentiation into granulocytic and monocytic progenitors is controlled by G-CSF and M-CSF, respectively. The ultimate granulocytic phenotype is determined in the bone marrow by relative local concentrations of early and late-acting cytokines, including GM-CSF, G-CSF, IL-3, IL-5, stem cell factor, and others. Granulocytes are released into the blood within 14 days of development. The bone marrow selectively retains immature granulocytes as a reserve pool that can be rapidly mobilized in response to the body's needs.

Monocytic progenitors differentiate into monocytes within 24 hours and are released into the circulation. Monocytes mature into various forms of macrophages, a process that is usually complete within 1 or 2 days after release.

Most leukocytes exist in the body from days to years, depending on type. Maintenance of optimal levels of granulocytes and monocytes in the blood depends on the availability of pluripotent stem cells in the marrow, induction of these into committed stem cells, timely release of new cells from the marrow, and mobilization of the granulocyte reserve pool. Leukocyte production increases in response to infection, to the presence of steroids, and to reduction or depletion of reserves in the marrow. It also is associated with strenuous exercise, convulsive seizures, heat, intense radiation, paroxysmal tachycardias (outbursts of rapid heart rate), pain, nausea and vomiting, and anxiety.

TABLE 20-5 **Types of Bleeding: Sources, Vessel Size, and Sealing Requirements**

Types and Sources of Bleeding	Involved Vessel	Size	Sealing Requirements
Pinpoint petechial hemorrhage (blood leakage from small vessels)	Capillary	Smallest	Generally direct-sealing
	Venule		Mostly fused platelets
	Arteriole		Mostly fused platelets
Ecchymosis (large, soft tissue bleeding)	Vein		Vascular contraction, fused platelets, perivascular and intravascular hemostatic factor activation (see Figure 20-16)
Rapidly expanding "blowout" hemorrhage	Artery	Largest	Greater vascular contraction, more fused platelets, greater perivascular and intravascular hemostatic factor activation

Modified from Harmening DM, editor: *Clinical hematology and fundamentals of hemostasis,* ed 3, Philadelphia, 1997, FA Davis.

Development of Platelets

Platelets (thrombocytes) are derived from stem cells and progenitor cells that differentiate into megakaryocytes. During thrombopoiesis, the megakaryocyte progenitor is programmed to undergo an endomitotic cell cycle (endomitosis) during which DNA replication occurs, but anaphase and cytokinesis are blocked[16] (see Figures 20-2 and 20-6, and Chapter 1). Thus, the megakaryocyte nucleus enlarges and becomes extremely polyploidy (up to 100-fold or more of the normal amount of DNA) without cellular division. Concurrently, the numbers of cytoplasmic organelles (e.g., internal membranes, granules) increase, and the cell develops cellular surface elongations and branches that progressively fragment into platelets. A single large (up to 100 μm) megakaryocyte may produce thousands of smaller platelets (2 to 3 μm). Like erythrocytes, platelets released from the bone marrow lack nuclei.

About two thirds of platelets enter the circulation, and the remainder resides in the splenic pool. Platelets circulate in the bloodstream for about 10 days before beginning to lose their ability to carry out biochemical reactions. Senescent platelets are sequestered and destroyed in the spleen by mononuclear cell phagocytosis. Thrombopoietin (TPO), a hormone growth factor, is the main regulator of the circulating platelet numbers. TPO is primarily produced by the liver and induces platelet production in the bone marrow.[17] Platelets express receptors for TPO and, when circulating platelet levels are normal, TPO is adsorbed onto the platelet surface and prevented from accessing the bone marrow and initiating further platelet production.[18] When platelet levels are low, however, the amount of TPO exceeds the number of available platelet TPO receptors, and free TPO can enter the bone marrow. During inflammation IL-6 induces increased production of TPO, which increases production of newly formed platelets, which are more thrombogenic.

MECHANISMS OF HEMOSTASIS

Hemostasis means arrest of bleeding. As a result of hemostasis, damaged blood vessels may maintain a relatively steady state of blood volume, pressure, and flow. Three equally important components of hemostasis are platelets, clotting factors, and the vasculature (endothelial cells and subendothelial matrix). The following list is the general sequence of events in hemostasis: (1) vascular injury leads to a transient arteriolar vasoconstriction to limit blood flow to the affected site; (2) damage to the endothelial cell lining of the vessel exposes prothrombogenic subendothelial connective tissue matrix leading to platelet adherence and activation and formation of a *hemostatic plug* to prevent further bleeding (primary hemostasis); (3) tissue factor, produced by the endothelium, collaborates with secreted platelet factors and activated platelets to activate the clotting (coagulation) system to form fibrin clots and further prevent bleeding (secondary hemostasis); and (4) the fibrin/platelet clot contracts to form a more permanent plug, and regulatory pathways are activated (fibrinolysis) to limit the size of the plug and begin the healing process. The relative importance of the hemostatic mechanisms clearly varies with vessel size. Damage to large vessels cannot easily be controlled by hemostasis but requires vascular contraction and dramatically decreased blood flow into the damaged vessels (Table 20-5).

Function of Platelets and Blood Vessels

Platelets normally circulate freely, suspended in plasma, in an unactivated state. Endothelial cells lining the vessels produce nitric oxide (NO) and the prostaglandin derivative prostacyclin I_2 (PGI2), which help maintain blood flow and pressure and platelets in an inactive state. NO and PGI_2 are highly synergistic; PGI_2 production varies a great deal in response to stimuli, whereas NO is released continually to regulate vascular tone. Endothelium also produces adenosine diphosphatase, which degrades ADP (a potent activator of platelets).

The endothelial cell surface contains antithrombotic molecules, such as glycosaminoglycans (e.g., heparan sulfate), thrombomodulin, and plasminogen activators. These limit platelet activation and fibrin deposition. Although thrombomodulin and plasminogen activators help control hemostasis in normal vessels, their effects are magnified during vascular damage and clot formation; therefore, further information is provided on these molecules in the following text describing control of hemostatic mechanisms.

When a vessel is damaged, platelet activation may be initiated. The role of platelet activation is to (1) contribute to regulation of blood flow into a damaged site through induction of vasoconstriction (vasospasm), (2) initiate platelet-to-platelet interactions resulting in formation of a platelet plug to stop further bleeding, (3) activate the coagulation (or clotting) cascade to stabilize the platelet plug, and (4) initiate repair processes including clot retraction and clot dissolution. The normal platelet count ranges from 150,000 to 400,000/mm³, and a count below 150,000/mm³ is defined as thrombocytopenia. However, the thrombocytopenia is usually asymptomatic unless the count drops below 100,000/mm³, at which time the number of platelets may be inadequate and abnormal bleeding may occur in response to trauma. Spontaneous major bleeding episodes do not generally occur unless the platelet count falls below 20,000/mm³. However, these values are not absolute and their clinical significance will vary among individuals.

Platelet activation proceeds through a process of (1) increased adhesion to the damaged vascular wall; (2) platelet degranulation, which stimulates changes in platelet shape; (3) aggregation as platelet–vascular wall and platelet-platelet adherence increases; and (4) activation of the clotting system and development of an immobilizing meshwork of platelets and fibrin (Figure 20-16, and see *Health Alert:* Sticky Platelets, Genetic Variations, and Cardiovascular Complications).

FIGURE 20-16 Platelet Activation. **A,** After endothelial denudation, platelets and leukocytes adhere to the subendothelium in a monolayer fashion. **B,** Higher-power view showing leukocytes and platelets adherent to the subendothelium. **C,** High magnification of a thrombus showing a mixture of red cells and platelets incorporated into the fibrin meshwork. (**A** and **B** from Libby P et al: *Braunwald's heart disease: a textbook of cardiovascular medicine,* ed 8, Philadelphia, 2007, Saunders; as reproduced from Faggiotto A, Ross R: *Arteriosclerosis* 4[4]:341-356, 1984; **C** from Damjanov I, Linder J, editors: *Anderson's pathology,* ed 10, St Louis, 1996, Mosby.)

HEALTH ALERT

Sticky Platelets, Genetic Variations, and Cardiovascular Complications

Investigators report that a genetic trait induces some people to make sticky platelets. People with platelets that tend to stick together have an increased risk of suffering complications from heart procedures. After individuals received angioplasty, in which a balloon-tipped catheter opens a blocked artery, investigators compared complications in the group with more sticky, or reactive, platelets with those with less reactive platelets. Of 112 participants, 3 months after the procedure, 15 individuals with sticky platelets experienced chest pain or a heart attack; 4 individuals with less reactive platelets experienced such complications. In addition, 10 people with sticky platelets needed another angioplasty, compared with only 2 from the less reactive platelet group.

In another study, investigators analyzed the receptor glycoprotein GP11b/111a for weaknesses that might direct attempts to prevent clotting, heart attack, and stroke. Blood samples from 1340 people revealed that 72% had inherited from both parents a gene for a version of GP11b/111a called *P1^{A1}*, whereas 28% had inherited 1 or 2 copies of a gene encoding a version called *P1^{A2}*. The blood from the group with two copies of *P1^{A1}* clotted less readily than did the blood of the other group. The degree of clotting also depended on fibrinogen levels in the blood. In individuals with unusually high fibrinogen levels, the presence of *P1^{A1}* glycoprotein seemed to increase clotting more than the presence of *P1^{A2}*. Thus, testing for platelet stickiness and GP11b/111a status could determine which people need anticlotting drugs and also the duration of treatment.

Data from Furlan M: *Swiss Med Wkly* 132(15-16):181-189, 2002; Kubisz P et al: *Semin Thromb Hemost* 39(6):674-683, 2013; Lohse J et al: *Hämostaseologie* 30(suppl 1):S126-S132, 2010.

This process can begin in several ways. If the vessel lining remains intact in an area of inflammation, the endothelial cells may become activated by cytokines and express new proteins on their surface. Several of these, particularly P-selectin, bind specifically yet weakly with receptors on the surface of inactive platelets (e.g., GPIb) (Figure 20-17). As inflammation progresses, the platelets adhere more avidly through additional receptors that bind through a fibrinogen bridge with the endothelial cell surface. The principal fibrinogen receptor on platelets is the integrin αIIbβ3 (also known as GPIIb/IIIa).

During vessel damage, the endothelial layer is frequently compromised, resulting in exposure of the underlying matrix that contains collagen, fibronectin, and other components. The matrix also contains von Willebrand factor (vWF), and the exposed collagen can bind additional vWF from the circulation (see Figure 20-17). Platelets adhere strongly to collagen through the receptor GPα/IIα (as well as other receptors not shown); GPVI and integrin $α_2β_1$) and to vWF through the receptor complex of platelet receptor GPIb and clotting factors IX and V. Progressively the platelets undergo further aggregation through platelet-to-platelet adhesion involving further fibrinogen bridging between receptors (particularly GPIIb/IIIa) on adjacent platelets.

As a result of interactions with the endothelium or the subendothelial matrix, as well as exposure to inflammatory mediators produced by the endothelium and other cells, the platelets are activated. Activation causes reorganization of the platelet cytoskeleton, leading to dynamic changes in platelet shape from smooth spheres to those with spiny projections and degranulation (also called the platelet-release reaction) and resulting in the release of various potent biochemicals.

Platelets contain three types of granules—lysosomes, dense bodies, and alpha granules. The contents of the dense bodies and alpha granules are particularly important in hemostasis. Dense bodies are generally proinflammatory (e.g., adenosine diphosphate [ADP], calcium, and serotonin). ADP recruits and activates other platelets through specific receptors. ADP also induces the platelet plasma membrane to undergo several important changes, including becoming ruffled and sticky; undergoing cellular spreading to make tight contacts between neighboring platelets, causing the platelet plug to seal the injured endothelium; and undergoing externalization of the phospholipid phosphatidylserine, which provides a matrix for activation of clotting factors. Serotonin is a vasoactive amine with histamine-like properties to increase vasodilation and vascular permeability (see Chapter 6). Calcium is necessary for many of the intracellular signaling mechanisms that control platelet activation.

Alpha granules contain a mixture of clotting factors (fibrinogen, factor V), growth and angiogenic factors (e.g., platelet-derived growth factor [PDGF], vascular endothelial growth factor [VEGF], basic fibroblast growth factor), and angiogenesis inhibitors (e.g., platelet factor 4, thrombospondin, inhibitors of metalloproteinases). Platelet factor 4 also is a heparin-binding protein. Depending upon the particular stimulus platelets may selectively release promoters or inhibitors of angiogenesis. Many of these mediators also either promote or inhibit

I. Subendothelial exposure

- Occurs after endothelial sloughing
- Platelets begin to fill endothelial gaps
- Promoted by thromboxane A₂ (TXA₂)
- Inhibited by prostacyclin I₂ (PGI₂)
- Platelet function depends on many factors, especially calcium

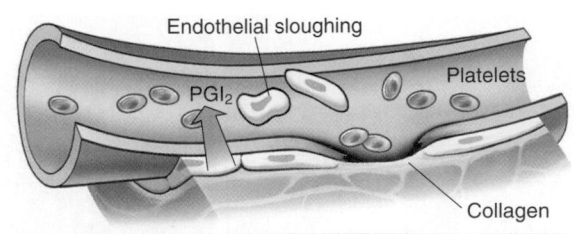

II. Adhesion

- Adhesion is initiated by loss of endothelial cells (or rupture or erosion of atherosclerotic plaque), which exposes adhesive glycoproteins such as collagen and von Willebrand factor (vWF) in the subendothelium. vWF and, perhaps, other adhesive glycoproteins in the plasma deposit on the damaged area. Platelets adhere to the subendothelium through receptors that bind to the adhesive glycoproteins (GPIb, GPIa/IIa, GPIIb/IIIa).

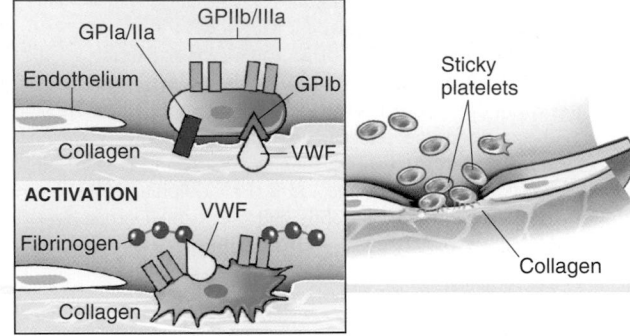

III. Activation

- After platelets adhere they undergo an activation process that leads to a conformational change in GPIIb/IIIa receptors, resulting in their ability to bind adhesive proteins, including fibrinogen and von Willebrand factor
- Changes in platelet shape
- Formation of pseudopods
- Activation of arachidonic pathway

IV. Aggregation

- Induced by release of TXA₂
- Adhesive glycoproteins bind simultaneously to GPIIb/IIIa on two different platelets
- Stabilization of the platelet plug (blood clot) occurs by activation of coagulation factors, thrombin, and fibrin
- Heparin neutralizing factor enhances clot formation

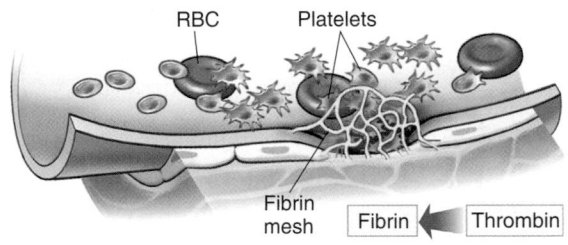

V. Platelet plug formation

- RBCs and platelets enmeshed in fibrin

VI. Clot retraction and clot dissolution

- Clot retraction, using large number of platelets, joins the edges of the injured vessel
- Clot dissolution is regulated by thrombin and plasminogen activators

FIGURE 20-17 Blood Vessel Damage, Blood Clot, and Clot Dissolution.

platelet activity and the eventual process of clot formation (see Figure 20-17). PDGF stimulates smooth muscle cells and promotes tissue repair. Heparin-binding proteins enhance clot formation at the site of injury.

Platelets also begin producing the prostaglandin derivative **thromboxane A₂ (TXA₂)**, which counters the effects of prostacyclin I₂ (PGI₂), produced by endothelial cells (see Figure 20-17). TXA₂ causes vasoconstriction and promotes the degranulation of platelets, whereas PGI₂ promotes vasodilation and inhibits platelet degranulation. In platelets, an isoform of **cyclooxygenase (COX-1)** converts arachidonic acid to

TXA₂. Aspirin, particularly at low doses, specifically and irreversibly inhibits COX-1, decreasing production of TXA₂ and decreasing platelet activation. Daily intake of low doses of aspirin leads to more than 95% inhibition of TXA2 in just a few days.

If blood vessel injury is minor, hemostasis is achieved temporarily by formation of the platelet plug, which usually forms within 3 to 5 minutes of injury. Platelet plugs seal the many minute ruptures that occur daily in the microcirculation, particularly in capillaries. With too few platelets, numerous small hemorrhagic areas called *purpuras* develop under the skin and throughout the tissues (see Chapter 21).

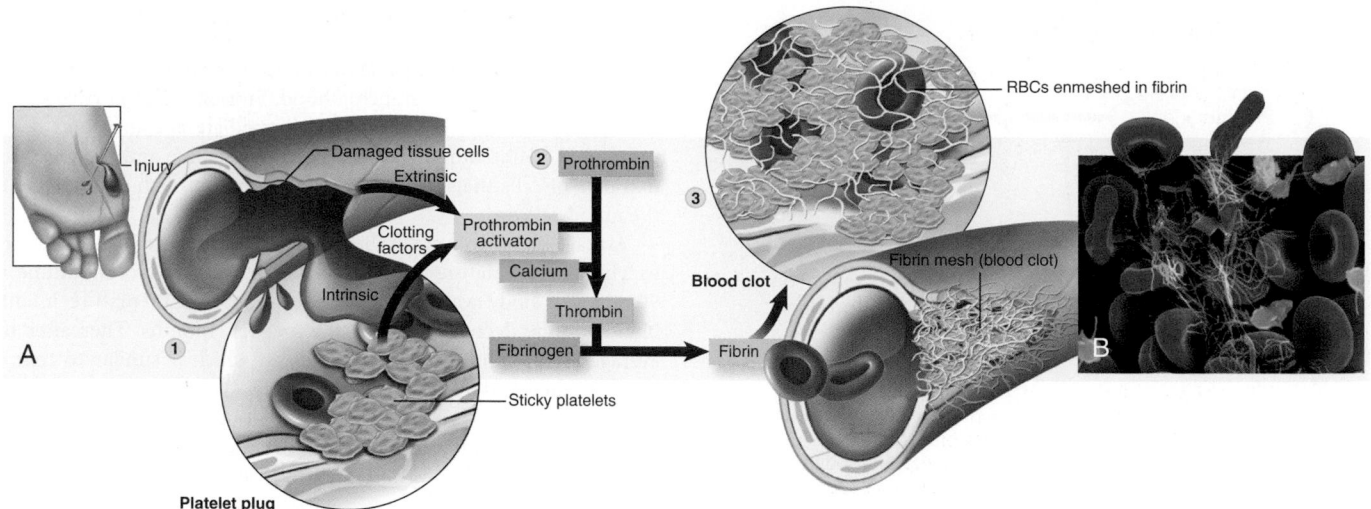

FIGURE 20-18 Blood Clotting Mechanism. A, The complex clotting mechanism can be summarized into three basic steps: **(1)** release of clotting factors from both injured tissue cells and sticky platelets at the injury site (which form temporary platelet plug); **(2)** series of chemical reactions that eventually result in the formation of thrombin; and **(3)** formation of fibrin and trapping of blood cells to form a clot. **B,** An electron micrograph showing entrapped RBCs in a fibrin clot. **(A** from Patton KT, Thibodeau GA: *Structure & function of the body,* ed 14, St Louis, 2012, Mosby; **B** copyright Dennis Kunkel Microscopy, Inc.)

Function of Clotting Factors

A blood clot is a meshwork of protein strands that stabilizes the platelet plug and traps other cells, such as erythrocytes, phagocytes, and microorganisms (Figure 20-18). The strands are made of fibrin, which is produced by the clotting (coagulation) system. The clotting system was described in Chapter 6 and consists of a family of proteins that circulate in the blood in inactive forms. Initiation of the system results in sequential activation (cascade) of multiple members of the system until a fibrin clot is created.

The clotting system is usually presented as two pathways of initiation (intrinsic and extrinsic pathways) that join in a common pathway. The intrinsic pathway is activated when Hageman factor (factor XII) in plasma contacts negatively charged subendothelial substances exposed by vascular injury. The extrinsic pathway is activated when tissue thromboplastin, a substance released by damaged endothelial cells, reacts with clotting factors, particularly factor VII. Both pathways lead to the common pathway and activation of factor X, which proceeds to clot formation.

The extrinsic pathway is clearly predominant; individuals with deficiencies in intrinsic pathway components (i.e., factor XI, factor XII), surprisingly, do not have prolonged bleeding because these factors do not seem to be important for clotting. As with the complement cascade, the clotting system is complex with a large number of alternative activators and inhibitors, and the relative importance of particular factors may differ between in vivo hemostasis and in vitro testing of clotting or may depend on the particular mechanism by which the pathway is activated. There also is interaction between components of the intrinsic and extrinsic pathways so that an activated member of one pathway may activate a member of the other pathway (e.g., factor VIIa of the extrinsic pathway can directly activate factor IX of the intrinsic pathway).

Activated platelets are important participants in clotting. The phosphatidylserine-rich surface produced during platelet activation provides a matrix on which several important complexes of clotting factors are formed. These include the intrinsic pathway's *tenase complex* (factor X and activated factors VIII and IX) that activates factor X and

the *prothrombinase complex* (prothrombin and activated factors X and V) that activates prothrombin into thrombin. Thrombin then converts fibrinogen into fibrin, which polymerizes into a fibrin clot. Thrombin has broad activity in the inflammatory response. In addition to producing fibrin, thrombin is an activator of other coagulation proteins (e.g., factors V, VIII, XI, XIII), platelets (e.g., aggregation, degranulation), endothelial cells (e.g., up-regulation of adhesion molecules for leukocytes, increased NO, PGI_2, PDGF), and monocytes (e.g., cytokine secretion, increased receptors for endothelial cells).

Under normal conditions, spontaneous activation of hemostasis is prevented by factors residing on the endothelial cell surface. These include thrombin inhibitors (e.g., antithrombin III), tissue factor inhibitors (e.g., tissue factor pathway inhibitor), and mechanisms for degrading activated clotting factors (e.g., protein C). Antithrombin III (AT-III) is a circulating inhibitor of plasma serine proteases. AT-III is produced by the liver and binds to heparin sulfate found naturally on the surface of endothelial cells, or with heparin administered clinically to prevent thrombosis. Heparin induces a change in AT-III that greatly enhances its capacity to inhibit thrombin and other activated clotting factors. Tissue factor pathway inhibitor (TFPI) is produced by endothelial cells and platelets; complexes to, and reversibly inhibits, factor Xa in the prothrombinase complex; and also inhibits other activated clotting factors.

Thrombomodulin is a thrombin-binding protein on the surface of endothelial cells. Protein C in the circulation binds to thrombomodulin in a thrombin-dependent manner and is converted to activated protein C.[19] Activated protein C, in association with a cofactor (protein S), degrades factors Va and VIIIa. Deficiencies of AT-III, protein C, or protein S are important causes of hypercoagulation (increased clotting). Expression of thrombomodulin and the endothelial cell protein C receptor is down-regulated by cytokines and other products of inflammation (e.g., IL-1α, tumor necrosis factor-alpha [TNF-α], endotoxin), thereby enhancing clot formation.

Retraction and Lysis of Blood Clots

After a clot is formed, it retracts, or "solidifies." Fibrin strands shorten, becoming denser and stronger, which approximates the edges of the

FIGURE 20-19 The Fibrinolytic System. Fibrinolysis is initiated by the binding of plasminogen to fibrin. Although tissue plasminogen activator *(t-PA)* initiates intravascular fibrinolysis, urokinase plasminogen activator *(u-PA)* is the major activator of fibrinolysis in tissue (extravascular). Plasmin digests the fibrin into smaller soluble pieces (fibrin degradation products). *u-PAR,* Urokinase-like plasminogen activator receptor.

injured vessel wall and seals the site of injury. Retraction is facilitated by the large numbers of platelets trapped within the fibrin meshwork. The platelets contract and "pull" the fibrin threads closer together while releasing a factor that stabilizes the fibrin. Contraction expels serum from the fibrin meshwork (see Figure 20-18). This process usually begins within a few minutes after a clot has formed, and most of the serum is expelled within 20 to 60 minutes.

Lysis (breakdown) of blood clots is carried out by the **fibrinolytic system** (Figure 20-19). Another plasma protein, plasminogen, is converted to **plasmin** by several products of coagulation and inflammation, especially by the enzymatic action of **tissue plasminogen activator (t-PA)**. Endothelial cells express t-PA, which is activated maximally after binding to fibrin. Another activator of plasminogen is **urokinase-like plasminogen activator (u-PA)**. The u-PA binds to a specific cellular u-PA receptor (u-PAR), causing activation of plasminogen. This urokinase is the major activator of fibrinolysis in the *extravascular* or tissue compartment, whereas t-PA is largely involved in *intravascular* fibrinolysis. Several cancers appear to use membrane-bound u-PA to digest intercellular matrix and greatly facilitate tumor invasion and metastasis. Both t-PA and u-PA have been used clinically to treat diseases associated with a blood clot (e.g., pulmonary embolism, myocardial infarction, stroke).[20]

Plasmin is an enzyme that dissolves clots (**fibrinolysis**) by degrading fibrin and fibrinogen into **fibrin degradation products (FDPs)**. A major FDP is D-dimer. **D-dimer** is two D domains from adjacent fibrin monomers that are cross-linked by factor XIIIa and released as a result of enzymatic cleavage by plasmin. Measurement of levels of circulating D-dimer has been used for diagnosis of deep venous thrombosis (DVT) or pulmonary embolism (PE).[21] Blood tests for evaluating the hematologic system are listed in Table 20-6.

✔**QUICK CHECK 20-5**

1. What specific cells are involved in development of leukocytes?
2. Why are platelets necessary to stop bleeding?
3. Briefly describe the steps of platelet adhesion and aggregation.
4. How does plasminogen initiate fibrinolysis?

PEDIATRICS & HEMATOLOGIC VALUE CHANGES

Blood cell counts tend to rise above adult levels at birth and then decline gradually throughout childhood. Table 20-7 lists normal ranges during infancy and childhood. The immediate rise in values is the result of accelerated hematopoiesis during fetal life and the increased numbers of cells that result from the trauma of birth and cutting of the umbilical cord.

Average blood volume in the full-term neonate is 85 ml/kg of body weight. The premature infant has a slightly larger blood volume of 90 ml/kg of body weight. In both full-term and premature infants, blood volume decreases during the first few months. Thereafter the average blood volume is 75 to 77 ml/kg, which is similar to that of older children and adults.

The hypoxic intrauterine environment stimulates erythropoietin production in the fetus and accelerates fetal erythropoiesis, producing polycythemia (excessive proliferation of erythrocyte precursors) in the newborn. After birth, the oxygen from the lungs saturates arterial blood, and more oxygen is delivered to the tissues. In response to the change from a placental to a pulmonary oxygen supply during the first few days of life, levels of erythropoietin and the rate of blood cell formation decrease. The active rate of fetal erythropoiesis is reflected by the large numbers of immature erythrocytes (reticulocytes) in the peripheral blood of full-term neonates. After birth, the number of reticulocytes decreases by 50% every 12 hours, so it is rare to find an elevated reticulocyte count after the first week of life. During this period of rapid growth, the rate of erythrocyte destruction is greater than that in later childhood and adulthood. In full-term infants, the normal erythrocyte life span is 60 to 80 days; in premature infants, it may be as short as 20 to 30 days; and in children and adolescents, it is the same as that in adults—120 days.

The postnatal fall in hemoglobin and hematocrit values is more marked in premature infants than it is in full-term infants. In preschool and school-aged children, hemoglobin, hematocrit, and red blood cell counts gradually rise. Metabolic processes within the erythrocytes of neonates differ significantly from those found in erythrocytes of normal adults. The relatively young population of erythrocytes in newborns consumes greater quantities of glucose than do erythrocytes in adults.

The lymphocytes of children tend to have more cytoplasm and less compact nuclear chromatin than do the lymphocytes of adults. A possible explanation is that children tend to have more frequent viral infections, which are associated with atypical lymphocytes. Minor infections, in which the child fails to exhibit clinical manifestations of illness, and the administration of immunizations also may account for the lymphocyte changes.

At birth the lymphocyte count is high, and it continues to rise during the first year of life. Then it steadily declines until the lower value seen in adults is reached. It is unknown whether these developmental variations are physiologic or a response to frequent viral infection and immunizations in children.

The neutrophil count, like the lymphocyte count, is high at birth and rises during the first days of life. After 2 weeks, the neutrophil count falls to within or below the normal adult range. Although the exact age can vary by approximately 7 years of age, the neutrophil count is the same as that of an adult.

The eosinophil count is higher in the first year of life and higher in children than in teenagers or adults. Monocyte counts also are high in the first year of life but then decrease to adult levels. Platelet counts in full-term neonates are comparable with those in adults and remain so throughout infancy and childhood.

TABLE 20-6   Common Blood Tests for Hematologic Disorders

Cell Type and Test	Property Evaluated by Test	Possible Hematologic Cause of Abnormal Findings
Erythrocyte		
Red cell count	Number (in millions) of erythrocytes/μL of blood	Altered erythropoiesis, anemias, hemorrhage, Hodgkin disease, leukemia
Mean corpuscle volume (MCV)	Size of erythrocytes	Anemias, thalassemias
Mean corpuscle hemoglobin (MCH)	Amount of hemoglobin in each erythrocyte (by weight)	Anemias, hemoglobinopathy
Mean corpuscular hemoglobin concentration (MCHC)	Concentration of hemoglobin in each erythrocyte (percentage of erythrocyte occupied by hemoglobin)	Anemias, hereditary spherocytosis
Hemoglobin determination	Amount of hemoglobin (by weight)/dl of blood	Anemias
Hematocrit determination	Percentage of a given volume of blood that is occupied by erythrocytes	Hemorrhage, polycythemia, erythrocytosis, anemias, leukemia
Reticulocyte count	Number of reticulocytes/μL of blood (also expressed as percentage of reticulocytes in total red blood cell count)	Hyperactive or hypoactive bone marrow function
Erythrocyte osmotic fragility test	Cellular shape (biconcavity), structure of plasma membrane	Anemias, hemolytic disease caused by ABO or Rh incompatibility, Hodgkin disease, polycythemia vera, thalassemia major
Hemoglobin electrophoresis	Relative percentage of different types of hemoglobin in erythrocytes	Sickle cell disease, sickle cell trait, hemoglobin C disease, hemoglobin C trait, thalassemias
Sickle cell test	Presence of hemoglobin S in erythrocytes	Sickle cell trait, sickle cell anemia
Glucose-6-phosphate dehydrogenase (G6PD) deficiency test	Deficiency of G6PD in erythrocytes	Hemolytic anemia
Hemoglobin Metabolism		
Serum ferritin determination	Depletion of body iron (potential deficiency of heme synthesis)	Iron deficiency anemias
Total iron-binding capacity (TIBC)	Amount of iron in serum plus amount of transferrin available in serum ($\mu\gamma/\delta\gamma$)	Hemorrhage, iron deficiency anemia, hemochromatosis, hemosiderosis, iron overload, anemias, thalassemia
Transferrin saturation	Percentage of transferrin that is saturated with iron	Acute hemorrhage, hemochromatosis, hemosiderosis, sideroblastic anemia, iron deficiency anemia, iron overload, thalassemia
Porphyrin analysis (protoporphyrin analysis)	Concentration of protoporphyrin in erythrocytes (mcg/dl), an indicator of iron-deficient erythropoiesis	Megaloblastic anemia, congenital erythropoietic porphyria
Direct antiglobulin test (DAT)	Antibody binding to erythrocytes	Hemolytic disease of newborn, autoimmune hemolytic anemia, drug-induced hemolytic anemia, transfusion reaction
Antibody screen test (indirect Coombs test)	Detection of antibodies to erythrocyte antigens (other than ABO antigens)	Same as for DAT
Leukocytes: Differential White Cell Count (Absolute Number of a Type of Leukocyte/μL of Blood)		
Neutrophil count	Neutrophils/μL	Myeloproliferative disorders, hematopoietic disorders, hemolysis, infection
Lymphocyte count	Lymphocytes/μL	Infectious lymphocytosis, infectious mononucleosis, hematopoietic disorders, anemias, leukemia, lymphosarcoma, Hodgkin disease
Plasma cell count	Plasma cells/μL	Infectious mononucleosis, lymphocytosis, plasma cell leukemia
Monocyte count	Monocytes/μL	Hodgkin disease, infectious mononucleosis, monocytic leukemia, non-Hodgkin lymphoma, polycythemia vera
Eosinophil count	Eosinophils/μL	Hematopoietic disorders, parasitic infections, allergic reactions
Basophil count	Basophils/μL	Chronic myelogenous leukemia, hemolytic anemias, Hodgkin disease, polycythemia vera
Platelets and Clotting Factors		
Platelet count	Number of circulating platelets (in thousands)/μL of blood	Anemias, multiple myeloma, myelofibrosis, polycythemia vera, leukemia, disseminated intravascular coagulation (DIC), hemolytic disease of the newborn, transfusion reaction, lymphoproliferative disorders
Bleeding time	Duration of bleeding following a standardized superficial puncture wound of skin, integrity of platelet plug, measured in minutes following puncture	Leukemia, anemias, DIC, fibrinolytic activity, purpuras, hemorrhagic disease of the newborn, infectious mononucleosis, multiple myeloma, clotting factor deficiencies, thrombasthenia, thrombocytopenia, von Willebrand disease

Continued

TABLE 20-6 Common Blood Tests for Hematologic Disorders—cont'd

Cell Type and Test	Property Evaluated by Test	Possible Hematologic Cause of Abnormal Findings
Clot retraction test	Platelet number and function, fibrinogen quantity and use, measured in hours required for expression of serum from a clot incubated in a test tube	Acute leukemia, aplastic anemia, factor XIII deficiency, increased fibrinolytic activity, Hodgkin disease, hyperfibrinogenemia or hypofibrinogenemia, idiopathic thrombocytopenic purpura, multiple myeloma, polycythemia vera, secondary thrombocytopenia, thrombasthenia
Platelet adhesion studies	Ability of platelets to adhere to foreign surfaces	Anemia, macroglobulinemia, Bernard-Soulier syndrome, multiple myeloma, myeloid metaplasia, plasma cell dyscrasias, thrombasthenia, thrombocytopathy, von Willebrand disease
Platelet aggregation tests	Ability of platelets to adhere to one another	Afibrinogenemia, Bernard-Soulier syndrome, thrombasthenia, hemorrhagic thrombocythemia, myeloid metaplasia, plasma cell dyscrasias, platelet release defects, polycythemia vera, preleukemia, sideroblastic anemia, von Willebrand disease, Waldenström macroglobulinemia, hypercoagulability
Whole blood clotting time (Lee-White coagulation time)	Overall ability of blood to clot, as measured in minutes in a test tube	Afibrinogenemia, clotting factor deficiencies, excessive fibrinolysis, hemorrhagic disease of the newborn, hypofibrinogenemia, hypoprothrombinemia, leukemia
Circulating anticoagulants (immunoglobulin G [IgG] antibodies that inhibit coagulation)	Presence of antibodies that neutralize clotting factors and inhibit coagulation, as indicated by prolonged clotting time, prothrombin time, or partial thromboplastin time	Afibrinogenemia, presence of fibrin-fibrinogen degradation products, macroglobulinemia, multiple myeloma, DIC, plasma cell dyscrasias
Partial thromboplastin time (PTT)	Effectiveness of clotting factors (except factors VII and VIII), effectiveness of intrinsic pathway of coagulation cascade, as measured by a test tube (in seconds)	Presence of circulating anticoagulants, DIC, clotting factor deficiencies, excessive fibrinolysis, hemorrhagic disease of the newborn, hypofibrinogenemia and afibrinogenemia, prothrombin deficiency, von Willebrand disease, acute hemorrhage
Prothrombin time	Effectiveness of activity of prothrombin, fibrinogen, and factors V, VII, and X; effectiveness of vitamin K–dependent coagulation factors of extrinsic and common pathways of coagulation cascade as measured in a test tube (in seconds)	Hypofibrinogenemia, dysfibrinogenemia, and afibrinogenemia; presence of circulating anticoagulants; DIC; deficiency of factors V, VII, or X; presence of fibrin degradation products, increased fibrinolytic activity, hemolytic jaundice, hemorrhagic disease of the newborn; acute leukemia, polycythemia vera, prothrombin deficiency, multiple myeloma
Thrombin time	Quantity and activity of fibrinogen as measured in a test tube (in seconds)	Hypofibrinogenemia, dysfibrinogenemia, and afibrinogenemia; presence of circulating anticoagulants; hemorrhagic disease of the newborn, polycythemia vera; increase in fibrinogen-fibrin degradation products; increased fibrinolytic activity
Fibrinogen assay	Amount of fibrinogen available for fibrin formation	Acute leukemia, congenital hypofibrinogenemia or afibrinogenemia, DIC, increased fibrinolytic activity, severe hemorrhage
Fibrin-fibrinogen degradation products (fibrin-fibrinogen split products)	Fibrinogenic activity as measured by levels of fibrin-fibrinogen degradation products (in µL/ml of blood)	Transfusion reactions, DIC, internal hemorrhage in the newborn, deep vein thrombosis, pulmonary embolism

Data from Bick RL et al: *Hematology: clinical and laboratory practice*, St Louis, 1993, Mosby; Byrne CJ et al: *Laboratory tests: implications for nursing care*, Menlo Park, Calif, 1986, Addison-Wesley.

TABLE 20-7 Mean Hematologic Differential Counts from Birth to Adulthood

Hematologic Differential	Newborn (Cord Blood)	2 Weeks of Age	3 Months of Age	6 Months to 6 Years of Age	7-12 Years of Age	Adult
Hemoglobin (g/dl)	16.8	16.5	12.0	12.0	13.0	13.0
Hematocrit (%)	55	50	36	37	38	40
Reticulocytes (%)	5.0	1.0	1.0	1.0	1.0	1.0
Leukocytes (WBC/mm^3)	18,000	12,000	12,000	10,000	8,000	8,000
Neutrophils (%)	61	40	30	45	55	55
Lymphocytes (%)	31	48	63	48	38	35
Eosinophils (%)	2	3	2	2	2	2
Monocytes (%)	6	9	5	5	5	5
Platelets (10^3/mm^3)	290	252	150-400	150-400	150-400	150-400

AGING & HEMATOLOGIC VALUE CHANGES

Blood composition changes little with age, although some components may be altered by iron deficiency. Total serum iron level, total iron-binding capacity, and intestinal iron absorption are all decreased somewhat in elderly persons. The erythrocyte life span is normal, although the erythrocytes are replenished more slowly after bleeding. Hemoglobin levels may be low, and the plasma membranes of erythrocytes become increasingly fragile, with portions being lost, presumably because of physical trauma inflicted during circulation.

Lymphocyte function decreases with age (see Chapters 7 and 8), causing changes in cellular immunity and some decline in T-cell function. The humoral immune system is less able to respond to antigenic challenge.

No changes in platelet numbers or structure have been observed in elderly persons, yet platelet adhesiveness probably increases. Although fibrinogen levels and levels of factors V, VII, and IX tend to be increased, no major hypercoagulability has been confirmed.

DID YOU UNDERSTAND?

Components of the Hematologic System

1. Blood consists of a variety of components—about 92% water and 8% solutes. In adults, the total blood volume is approximately 5.5 L.
2. Plasma, a complex aqueous liquid, contains two major groups of plasma proteins: albumins and globulins.
3. The cellular elements of blood are the red blood cells (erythrocytes), white blood cells (leukocytes), and platelets.
4. Erythrocytes are the most abundant cells of the blood, occupying approximately 48% of the blood volume in men and approximately 42% in women. Erythrocytes are responsible for tissue oxygenation.
5. Leukocytes are fewer in number than erythrocytes and constitute approximately 5000 to 10,000 cells/mm³ of blood. Leukocytes defend the body against infection and remove dead or injured host cells.
6. Leukocytes are classified as either granulocytes (neutrophils, basophils, eosinophils) or agranulocytes (monocytes/macrophages, lymphocytes).
7. Platelets are anuclear disk-shaped cytoplasmic fragments. Platelets are essential for blood coagulation and control of bleeding.
8. The lymphoid organs are sites of residence, proliferation, differentiation, or function of lymphocytes and mononuclear phagocytes.
9. The spleen is the largest lymphoid organ and functions as the site of fetal hematopoiesis, filters and cleanses the blood, and acts as a reservoir for lymphocytes and other blood cells.
10. The lymph nodes are the site of development or activity of large numbers of lymphocytes, monocytes, and macrophages.
11. The mononuclear phagocyte system (MPS) is composed of monocytes in bone marrow and peripheral blood and macrophages in tissue.
12. The MPS is the main line of defense against bacteria in the bloodstream and cleanses the blood by removing old, injured, or dead blood cells; antigen-antibody complexes; and macromolecules.

Development of Blood Cells

1. Hematopoiesis, or blood cell production, occurs in the liver and spleen of the fetus and in the bone marrow after birth.
2. Hematopoiesis involves two stages: proliferation and differentiation, or maturation. Each type of blood cell has parent cells called *stem cells*.
3. Hematopoiesis continues throughout life to replace blood cells that grow old and die, are killed by disease, or are lost through bleeding.
4. Bone marrow consists of red (hematopoietic) marrow (blood vessels, mononuclear phagocytes, stem cells, blood cells in various stages of differentiation, stromal cells) and yellow marrow (fatty tissue).
5. The bone marrow contains multiple populations of stem cells; mesenchymal stem cells develop into fibroblasts, osteoclasts, and adipocytes; and hematopoietic stem cells develop into blood cells.
6. Regulation of hematopoiesis occurs in bone marrow niches in which hematopoietic stem cells differentiate and are controlled by multiple cytokines and chemokines and through direct contact with osteoblasts (osteoblastic niche) or vascular endothelial cells (vascular niche), as well as several other specialized cells, including CAR cells and nestin-expressing cells.
7. Specific hematopoietic growth factors (e.g., colony-stimulating factors) are necessary for the adequate production of myeloid, erythroid, lymphoid, and megakaryocytic lineages.
8. Hemoglobin, the oxygen-carrying protein of the erythrocyte, enables the blood to transport 100 times more oxygen than could be transported dissolved in plasma alone.
9. Erythropoiesis depends on the presence of vitamins (especially vitamin B_{12}, folate vitamin, vitamin B_6, riboflavin, pantothenic acid, niacin, ascorbic acid, and vitamin E).
10. Regulation of erythropoiesis is mediated by erythropoietin, which is secreted by the kidneys in response to tissue hypoxia and causes a compensatory increase in erythrocyte production if the oxygen content of the blood decreases because of anemia, high altitude, or pulmonary disease.
11. The iron cycle reutilizes iron released from old or damaged erythrocytes. Iron binds to transferrin in the blood, is transported to macrophages of the MPS, and is stored in the cytoplasm as ferritin.
12. Iron homeostasis is controlled by hepcidin, a small hormone produced by hepatocytes, which regulates ferroportin, the principal transporter of iron from stores in hepatocytes and macrophages and from intestinal cells that absorb dietary iron.
13. Maintenance of optimal levels of granulocytes and monocytes in the blood depends on the availability of pluripotential stem cells in the marrow, induction of these into committed stem cells, and timely release of new cells from the marrow.
14. Granulocytes and monocytes in the blood develop from common myeloid progenitor cells in the bone marrow under the direction of several growth factors, including stem cell factor, IL-3, and GM-CSF.
15. Specific humoral colony-stimulating factors (CSFs) are necessary for the adequate growth of myeloid, erythroid, lymphoid, and megakaryocytic lineages.
16. Platelets develop from megakaryocytes by a process called *endomitosis*, which is controlled by thrombopoietin. During endomitosis the megakaryocytes undergo mitosis but not cell

division and the cytoplasm and plasma membrane fragment into platelets.

Mechanisms of Hemostasis

1. Hemostasis, or arrest of bleeding, involves (1) vasoconstriction (vasospasm), (2) formation of a platelet plug, (3) activation of the clotting cascade, (4) formation of a blood clot, and (5) clot retraction and clot dissolution.
2. The normal vascular endothelium prevents spontaneous clotting by producing factors such as nitric oxide (NO) and prostacyclin I_2 (PGI_2) that relax the vessels and prevent platelet activation.
3. Lysis of blood clots is the function of the fibrinolytic system. Plasmin, a proteolytic enzyme, splits fibrin and fibrinogen into fibrin degradation products that dissolve the clot.

Pediatrics & Hematologic Value Changes

1. Blood cell counts tend to rise above adult levels at birth and then decline gradually throughout childhood.
2. The lymphocytes of children tend to have more cytoplasm and less compact nuclear chromatin than do the lymphocytes of adults.

Aging & Hematologic Value Changes

1. Blood composition changes little with age. Erythrocyte replenishment may be delayed after bleeding, presumably because of iron deficiency.
2. Lymphocyte function appears to decrease with age. Particularly affected is a decrease in cellular immunity.
3. Platelet adhesiveness probably increases with age.

KEY TERMS

Agranulocyte, 492
Albumin, 490
Antithrombin III (AT-III), 507
Apoferritin, 502
Apotransferrin, 503
Basophil, 493
Blood clot, 507
Bone marrow (myeloid tissue), 498
Clotting (coagulation) system, 507
Clotting factor, 491
Collagen, 505
Colony-stimulating factor (CSF, hematopoietic growth factor), 499
Cyclooxygenase (COX-1), 506
D-Dimer, 508
Deoxyhemoglobin, 501
Endomitosis, 504
Eosinophil, 493
Erythroblast (normoblast), 500
Erythrocyte, 491
Erythropoiesis, 500

Erythropoietin, 500
Extramedullary hematopoiesis, 498
Fibrin degradation product (FDP), 508
Fibrinolysis, 508
Fibrinolytic system, 508
Globin, 501
Globulin, 490
Granulocyte, 492
Hematopoiesis, 497
Hematopoietic stem cell, 498
Heme, 501
Hemoglobin (Hb), 500
Hemosiderin, 502
Hemostasis, 504
Immunocyte, 492
Integrin $\alpha_{IIb}\beta_3$ (GPIIb/IIIa), 505
Leukocyte, 492
Lipoprotein, 491
Lymph node, 496
Lymphocyte, 493
Macrophage, 493
Marginating storage pool, 500

Megakaryocytes, 493
Mesenchymal stem cells (MSCs), 498
Methemoglobin, 501
Monocyte, 493
Mononuclear phagocyte system (MPS), 497
Myoglobin, 502
Natural killer (NK) cells, 493
Neutrophil (polymorphonuclear neutrophil [PMN]), 492
Niche, 498
Nitric oxide (NO), 504
Osteoblastic niche, 498
Oxyhemoglobin, 501
Phagocyte, 492
Plasma, 490
Plasma protein, 490
Plasmin, 508
Platelet (thrombocyte), 493
Platelet-release reaction, 505
Primary lymphoid organs, 494
Proerythroblast, 500
Prostacyclin I_2 (PGI_2), 504

Protein C, 507
Protein S, 507
Protoporphyrin, 501
Reticulocyte, 500
Secondary lymphoid organs, 494
Serum, 490
Spleen, 494
Stromal cell, 498
Thrombomodulin, 507
Thrombopoietin (TPO), 504
Thromboxane A_2 (TXA_2), 506
Tissue factor pathway inhibitor (TFPI), 507
Tissue plasminogen activator (t-PA), 508
Tissue thromboplastin, 507
Transferrin, 503
Urokinase-like plasminogen activator (u-PA), 508
Vascular niche, 499
von Willebrand factor (vWF), 505

REFERENCES

1. Kita H: Eosinophils: multifunctional and distinctive properties, *Int Arch Allergy Immunol* 161(Suppl 2): 3-9, 2013.
2. Amon TI, Cyster JG: Blood, sphintosine-1-phosphate and lymphocyte migration dynamics in the spleen, *Curr Top Microbiol Immunol* 378(2014): 107-128, 2014.
3. Jenkins SJ, Hume DA: Homeostasis in the mononuclear phagocyte system, *Trends Immunol* 35(8):358-367, 2014.
4. Glatman Zaretsky A et al: Infection-induced changes in hematopoiesis, *J Immunol* 192(1):27-33, 2014.
5. Blin-Wakkach C et al: Roles of osteoclasts in the control of medullary hematopoietic niches, *Arch Biochem Biophys* 561:29-37, 2014.
6. *Stem cell information*, Bethesda, Md, 2010, National Institutes of Health, U.S. Department of Health and Human Services [cited, July 26, 2014]. Available at: http://stemcells.nih.gov/info.
7. He N et al: Bone marrow vascular niche: home for hematopoietic stem cells, *Bone Marrow Res*

2014:128436, 2014. Available at: http://dx.doi.org/10.1155/2014/128436.
8. Morrison SJ, Scadden DT: The bone marrow niche for haematopoietic stem cells, *Nature* 505(7483): 327-334, 2014.
9. Endele M et al: Instruction of hematopoietic lineage choice by cytokine signaling, *Exp Cell Res* 329(2):207-213, 2014.
10. Thom CS et al: Hemoglobin variants: biochemical properties and clinical correlates, *Cold Spring Harb Perspect Med* 3(3):a011858, 2013.
11. Chiabrando D et al: Heme in pathophysiology: a matter of scavenging, metabolism and trafficking across cell membranes, *Front Pharmacol* 5:61, 2014.
12. Simmonds MJ et al: Blood rheology and aging, *J Geriatr Cardiol* 10(3):291-301, 2013.
13. Winter WE et al: The molecular biology of human iron metabolism, *Lab Med* 45(2):92-102, 2014.
14. Loréal O et al: Iron, hepcidin, and the metal connection, *Front Pharmacol* 5:128, 2014.
15. Ganz T: Systemic iron homeostasis, *Physiol Rev* 93(4):1721-1741, 2013.

16. Machlus KR et al: Interpreting the development dance of the megakaryocyte: a review of the cellular and molecular processes mediating platelet formation, *Br J Haematol* 165(2):227-236, 2014.
17. Hitchcock IS, Kaushansky K: Thrombopoietin from beginning to end, *Br J Haematol* 165(2):259-268, 2014.
18. Kuter DJ: Milestones in understanding platelet production: a historical overview, *Br J Haematol* 165(2):248-258, 2014.
19. Spronk HM et al: New insights into modulation of thrombin formation, *Curr Atheroscler Rep* 15(11): 363, 2013.
20. Robertson I et al: Fibrinolytic agents for peripheral arterial occlusion, *Cochrane Database Syst Rev* 12:CD001099, 2013.
21. Wells P, Anderson D: The diagnosis and treatment of venous thromboembolism, *Hematology Am Soc Hematol Educ Program* 2013(1):457-463, 2013.

21

Alterations of Hematologic Function

Anna Schwartz, Kathryn L. McCance, and Neal S. Rote

ⓔ EVOLVE WEBSITE

http://evolve.elsevier.com/Huether/
Student Review Questions
Audio Key Points

Case Studies
Animations
Quick Check Answers

CHAPTER OUTLINE

Alterations of erythrocyte function involve either insufficient or excessive numbers of erythrocytes in the circulation or normal numbers of cells with abnormal components. Anemias are conditions in which there are too few erythrocytes or an insufficient volume of erythrocytes in the blood. Polycythemias are conditions in which erythrocyte numbers or volume is excessive. All of these conditions have many causes and are pathophysiologic manifestations of a variety of disease states.

Many disorders involving leukocytes range from increased numbers of leukocytes (i.e., leukocytosis) in response to infections to proliferative disorders (such as leukemia). Many hematologic disorders are malignancies, and many nonhematologic malignancies metastasize to bone marrow, affecting leukocyte production. Thus a large portion of this chapter is devoted to malignant disease.

The primary role of clotting (hemostasis) is to stop bleeding through an interaction of endothelium lining the vessels, platelets, and clotting factors. A large number of disease states may be associated with a clinically significant increase or decrease in clotting resulting from alterations in any of the three main components of the clotting process.

ALTERATIONS OF ERYTHROCYTE FUNCTION

Classification of Anemias

Anemia is a reduction in the total number of erythrocytes in the circulating blood or a decrease in the quality or quantity of hemoglobin. Anemias commonly result from (1) impaired erythrocyte production, (2) blood loss (acute or chronic), (3) increased erythrocyte destruction, or (4) a combination of these three factors. Anemias are classified by their causes (e.g., anemia of chronic disease) or by the changes that affect the size, shape, or substance of the erythrocyte. The most common classification of anemias is based on the changes that affect the cell's size and hemoglobin content (Table 21-1). Terms used to identify anemias reflect these characteristics. Terms that end with *-cytic* refer to cell size, and those that end with *-chromic* refer to hemoglobin content. Additional terms describing erythrocytes found in some anemias are anisocytosis (assuming various sizes) and poikilocytosis (assuming various shapes).

CLINICAL MANIFESTATIONS The main alteration of anemia is a reduced oxygen-carrying capacity of the blood resulting in tissue hypoxia. Symptoms of anemia vary, depending on the body's ability to compensate for the reduced oxygen-carrying capacity. Anemia that is mild and starts gradually is usually easier to compensate and may cause problems for the individual only during physical exertion. As red cell reduction continues, symptoms become more pronounced and alterations in specific organs and compensation effects are more apparent. Compensation generally involves the cardiovascular, respiratory, and hematologic systems (Figure 21-1).

A reduction in the number of blood cells in the blood causes a reduction in the consistency and volume of blood. Initial compensation for cellular loss is movement of interstitial fluid into the blood, causing an increase in plasma volume. This movement maintains an adequate blood volume, but the viscosity (thickness) of the blood

TABLE 21-1 Morphologic Classification of Anemias

Structure of Erythrocytes	Name and Mechanism of Anemia	Primary Cause
Macrocytic-normochromic anemia: large, abnormally shaped erythrocytes, normal hemoglobin concentrations	Pernicious anemia: lack of vitamin B_{12}; abnormal DNA and RNA synthesis in erythroblast; premature cell death	Congenital or acquired deficiency of intrinsic factor (IF); genetic disorder of DNA synthesis
	Folate deficiency anemia: lack of folate; premature cell death	Dietary folate deficiency
Microcytic-hypochromic anemia: small, abnormally shaped erythrocytes and reduced hemoglobin concentration	Iron deficiency anemia: lack of iron for hemoglobin; insufficient hemoglobin	Chronic blood loss, dietary iron deficiency, disruption of iron metabolism or iron cycle
	Sideroblastic anemia: dysfunctional iron uptake by erythroblasts and defective porphyrin and heme synthesis	Congenital dysfunction of iron metabolism in erythroblasts, acquired dysfunction of iron metabolism as result of drugs or toxins
	Thalassemia: impaired synthesis of α- or β-chain of hemoglobin A; phagocytosis of abnormal erythroblasts in marrow	Congenital genetic defect of globin synthesis
Normocytic-normochromic anemia: normal size, normal hemoglobin concentration	Aplastic anemia: insufficient erythropoiesis	Depressed stem cell proliferation
	Posthemorrhagic anemia: blood loss	Increased erythropoiesis; iron depletion
	Hemolytic anemia: premature destruction (lysis) of mature erythrocytes in circulation	Increased fragility of erythrocytes
	Sickle cell anemia: abnormal hemoglobin synthesis, abnormal cell shape with susceptibility to damage, lysis, and phagocytosis	Congenital dysfunction of hemoglobin synthesis
	Anemia of chronic inflammation; abnormally increased demand for new erythrocytes	Chronic infection or inflammation; malignancy

DNA, Deoxyribonucleic acid; *RNA,* ribonucleic acid.

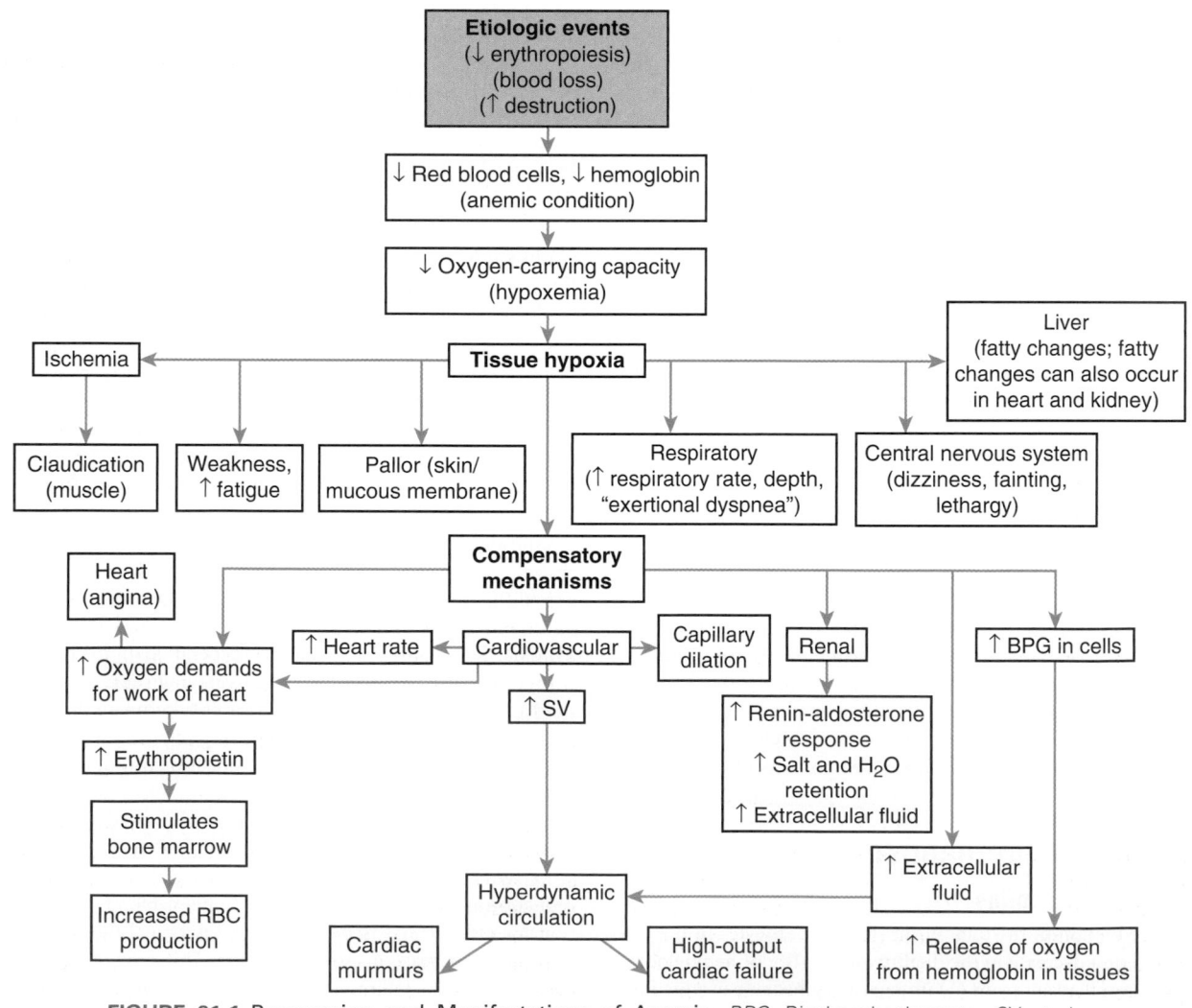

FIGURE 21-1 Progression and Manifestations of Anemia. *BPG,* Bisphosphoglycerate; *SV,* stroke volume.

decreases. The "thinner" blood flows faster and more turbulently than normal blood, causing a hyperdynamic circulatory state. This hyperdynamic state creates cardiovascular changes—increased stroke volume and heart rate. These changes may lead to cardiac dilation and heart valve insufficiency if the underlying anemic condition is not corrected.

Hypoxemia, reduced oxygen level in the blood, further contributes to cardiovascular dysfunction by causing dilation of arterioles, capillaries, and venules, thus increasing flow through them. Increased peripheral blood flow and venous return further contributes to an increase in heart rate and stroke volume in a continuing effort to meet normal oxygen demand and prevent cardiopulmonary congestion. These compensatory mechanisms may lead to heart failure.

Tissue hypoxia creates additional demands and effects on the pulmonary and hematologic systems. The rate and depth of breathing increase in an effort to increase oxygen availability accompanied by an increase in the release of oxygen from hemoglobin. All of these compensatory mechanisms may cause individuals to experience shortness of breath (dyspnea), a rapid and pounding heartbeat, dizziness, and fatigue. In mild chronic cases, these symptoms may be present only when there is an increased demand for oxygen (e.g., during physical exertion), but in severe cases, symptoms may be experienced even at rest.

Manifestations of anemia may be seen in other parts of the body. The skin, mucous membranes, lips, nail beds, and conjunctivae become either pale because of reduced hemoglobin concentration or yellowish (jaundiced) because of accumulation of end products of red cell destruction (hemolysis) if that is the cause of the anemia. Tissue hypoxia of the skin results in impaired healing and loss of elasticity, as well as thinning and early graying of the hair. Nervous system manifestations may occur where the cause of anemia is a deficiency of vitamin B_{12}. Myelin degeneration occurs, causing a loss of nerve fibers in the spinal cord, resulting in paresthesias (numbness), gait disturbances, extreme weakness, spasticity, and reflex abnormalities. Decreased oxygen supply to the gastrointestinal (GI) tract often produces abdominal pain, nausea, vomiting, and anorexia. Low-grade fever (<101° F [38.3° C]) occurs in some anemic individuals and may result from the release of leukocyte pyrogens from ischemic tissues.

When the anemia is severe or acute in onset (e.g., hemorrhage), the initial compensatory mechanism is peripheral blood vessel constriction, diverting blood flow to essential vital organs. Decreased blood flow detected by the kidneys activates the renin-angiotensin response, causing salt and water retention in an attempt to increase blood volume. These situations are considered to be emergencies and require immediate intervention to correct the underlying problem that caused the acute blood loss; therefore, long-term compensatory mechanisms do not develop.

Therapeutic interventions for slowly developing anemic conditions require treatment of the underlying condition and palliation of associated symptoms.[1] Therapies include transfusion, dietary correction, and administration of supplemental vitamins or iron.

Macrocytic-Normochromic Anemias

The macrocytic (megaloblastic) anemias are characterized by unusually large stem cells (megaloblasts) in the marrow that mature into erythrocytes that are unusually large in size (macrocytic), thickness, and volume.[2] The hemoglobin content is normal, thus allowing them to be classified as normochromic. These anemias are the result of ineffective erythrocyte deoxyribonucleic acid (DNA) synthesis, commonly caused by deficiencies of vitamin B_{12} (cobalamin) or folate (folic acid). These defective erythrocytes die prematurely, which decreases

their numbers in the circulation, causing anemia. Premature death of damaged erythrocytes, eryptosis, is a common mechanism of cellular loss in individuals with anemia secondary to deficiencies of iron, infections (e.g., malaria, mycoplasma), chronic diseases (e.g., diabetes, renal disease), genetic diseases (e.g., beta-thalassemia, glucose-6-phosphate dehydrogenase [G6PD] deficiency, sickle cell trait), and myelodysplastic syndrome.[3]

Defective DNA synthesis in megaloblastic anemias causes red cell growth and development to proceed at unequal rates. DNA synthesis and cell division are blocked or delayed. However, ribonucleic acid (RNA) replication and protein (hemoglobin) synthesis proceed normally. Asynchronous development leads to an overproduction of hemoglobin during prolonged cellular division, creating a larger than normal erythrocyte with a disproportionately small nucleus. With each cell division, the disproportion between RNA and DNA becomes more apparent.

Pernicious Anemia

Pernicious anemia (PA), the most common type of macrocytic anemia, is caused by vitamin B_{12} deficiency, which is often associated with the end stage of type A chronic atrophic (autoimmune) gastritis (Figure 21-2, C).[4] Pernicious means highly injurious or destructive and reflects the fact that this condition was once fatal. It most commonly affects individuals older than age 30 who are of Northern European descent; however, it has now been recognized in all populations and ethnic groups.

PATHOPHYSIOLOGY The underlying alteration in PA is the absence of intrinsic factor (IF), a transporter required for gastric absorption of dietary vitamin B_{12}, a vitamin essential for nuclear maturation and DNA synthesis in red blood cells. Deficiency of IF may be congenital or, more often, an autoimmune process directed against gastric parietal cells. Congenital IF deficiency is a genetic disorder with an autosomal recessive inheritance pattern.[5] The autoimmune form of the disease also has a genetic component. Family clusters have been identified; 20% to 30% of individuals related to persons with PA also have PA. These relatives, particularly first-degree female relatives, also demonstrate a higher frequency of the presence of gastric autoantibodies. PA also is frequently a component of autoimmune polyendocrinopathy, which is a cluster of autoimmune diseases of endocrine organs (e.g., chronic autoimmune thyroiditis [Hashimoto thyroiditis], type 1 diabetes mellitus, Addison disease, primary hypoparathyroidism, Graves disease, and myasthenia gravis) that frequently present as comorbidities. Autoimmune thyroiditis and type 1 diabetes mellitus, in particular, are associated with PA.

Most cases of PA result from an autoimmune gastritis (type A chronic gastritis) in which gastric atrophy results from destruction of parietal and zymogenic (relating to an enzyme) cells. Individuals with PA commonly have autoantibodies against the gastric H^+-K^+ ATPase, which is the major protein constituent of parietal cell membranes. Gastric mucosal atrophy, in which gastric parietal cells are destroyed, results in a deficiency of all secretions of the stomach—hydrochloric acid, pepsin, and IF. A direct correlation exists between the severity of the gastric lesion and the degree of malabsorption of vitamin B_{12}.[6,7] Additionally, autoantibodies against IF prevent the formation of the B_{12}-IF complex. Thus, PA is secondary to autoimmune destruction of parietal cells, diminishing the production of IF and the presence of autoantibodies that neutralize the capacity of remaining IF to transport vitamin B_{12}.

Initiation of the autoimmune process may be secondary to a past infection with *Helicobacter pylori*.[8] Although active infection with *H. pylori* is rare in individuals with PA, more than half of these individuals

FIGURE 21-2 Appearance of Red Blood Cells in Various Disorders. A, Normal blood smear. **B,** Hypochromic-microcytic anemia (iron deficiency). **C,** Macrocytic anemia (pernicious anemia). **D,** Macrocytic anemia in pregnancy. **E,** Hereditary elliptocytosis. **F,** Myelofibrosis (teardrop). **G,** Hemolytic anemia associated with prosthetic heart valve. **H,** Microangiopathic anemia. **I,** Stomatocytes. **J,** Spherocytes (hereditary spherocytosis). **K,** Sideroblastic anemia; note the double population of red blood cells. **L,** Sickle cell anemia. **M,** Target cells (after splenectomy). **N,** Basophil stippling in case of unexplained anemia. **O,** Howell-Jolly bodies (after splenectomy). (From Wintrobe MM et al: *Clinical hematology,* ed 8, Philadelphia, 1981, Lea & Febiger.)

CLINICAL MANIFESTATIONS Pernicious anemia develops slowly (over 20 to 30 years), so by the time an individual seeks treatment, it is usually severe. Early symptoms are often ignored because they are nonspecific and vague and include infections, mood swings, and gastrointestinal, cardiac, or kidney ailments. When the hemoglobin level has decreased to 7 to 8 g/dl, the individual experiences classic symptoms of pernicious anemia: weakness, fatigue, paresthesias of feet and fingers, difficulty walking, loss of appetite, abdominal pain, weight loss, and a sore tongue that is smooth and beefy red. The skin may become "lemon yellow" (sallow), caused by a combination of pallor and jaundice. Hepatomegaly, indicating right-sided heart failure, may be present in the elderly along with splenomegaly, which is nonpalpable.

Neurologic manifestations result from nerve demyelination that may produce neuronal death. The posterior and lateral columns of the spinal cord also may be affected, causing a loss of position and vibration sense, ataxia, and spasticity. These complications pose a serious threat because they are not reversible, even with appropriate treatment. The cerebrum also may be involved with manifestations of affective disorders, most commonly of the depressive types. Low levels of vitamin B_{12} have been associated with neurocognitive disorders. An increased prevalence of serum vitamin B_{12} deficiency has been reported among individuals with Alzheimer disease.

EVALUATION AND TREATMENT Evaluation is based on blood tests, bone marrow aspiration, serologic studies, gastric biopsy, and clinical manifestations. The Schilling test (no longer offered in most laboratories) indirectly evaluated vitamin B_{12} absorption by administering radioactive B_{12} and measuring excretion in the urine. Low urinary excretion was significant for PA. The Schilling test has been replaced with serologic studies that measure methylmalonic acid and homocysteine levels, which are elevated early in PA; and this test is more sensitive. The presence of circulating antibodies against parietal cells and intrinsic factor also is useful in diagnosis.[9] Autoimmune gastritis is a chronic progressive inflammatory disorder resulting in replacement of the parietal cell mass by atropic and metaplastic mucosa.[7] The interactions are very complex because of autoantibodies against intrinsic factor that impair the absorption of vitamin B_{12} (cobalamin). The resulting cobalamin deficiency manifests with neurologic and systemic symptoms of PA. The complexity increases with the underappreciated overlap with *Helicobacter pylori* infection. The risk of gastric cancer has not been adequately studied.[7] Gastric biopsy reveals total achlorhydria (absence of hydrochloric acid), which is diagnostic for PA because it occurs only in the presence of this gastric lesion.

Replacement of vitamin B_{12} (cobalamin) is the treatment of choice. Initial injections of vitamin B_{12} are administered weekly until the deficiency is corrected, followed by monthly injections for the remainder of the individual's life. The effectiveness of cobalamin replacement therapy is determined by a rising reticulocyte count. Blood counts return to normal within 5 to 6 weeks. PA cannot be cured so maintenance therapy is lifelong. Conventional wisdom and practice assumed that oral preparations were ineffective because there was no IF to facilitate absorption of vitamin B_{12}. However, recent experience has shown that higher doses of orally administered vitamin B_{12} will be absorbed across the small bowel and that this treatment is beneficial.

Untreated PA is fatal, usually because of heart failure. With replacement therapy of vitamin B_{12}, mortality has decreased significantly. Death from PA is now rare and relapses are often the result of noncompliance with therapy.

Folate Deficiency Anemias

Folate (folic acid) is an essential vitamin required for RNA and DNA synthesis within the maturing erythrocyte. Folates are coenzymes

possess circulating antibodies against this microorganism, suggesting a history of infection. The current opinion is that in genetically prone individuals, antigens expressed by *H. pylori* mimic the parietal cell H^+-K^+ ATPase, resulting in production of an antibody that binds and damages the parietal cell (see Chapter 8 for a discussion of antigenic mimicry and autoimmune disease).

Environmental factors that may contribute to chronic gastritis include excessive alcohol or hot tea ingestion and smoking. Complete or partial removal of the stomach (gastrectomy) causes IF deficiency. Drugs known as proton pump inhibitors (PPIs) are used to decrease gastric acidity and may decrease vitamin B_{12} absorption, but it is not thought that they actually cause PA. Although PA is a benign disorder, people with type A chronic gastritis also are at risk for developing gastric adenocarcinoma and gastric carcinoid type I. The incidence rate of carcinoma in these individuals is 2% to 3%.

required for the synthesis of thymine and purines (adenine and guanine) and the conversion of homocysteine to methionine. Deficient production of thymine, in particular, affects cells undergoing rapid division (e.g., bone marrow cells undergoing erythropoiesis). Humans are totally dependent on dietary intake to meet the daily requirement of 50 to 200 mg/day. Increased amounts are required for lactating and pregnant females. Folate is absorbed from the upper small intestine and does not require any other element (i.e., IF) to facilitate absorption. After absorption, folate circulates through the liver, where it is stored. Folate deficiency occurs more often than B_{12} deficiency, particularly in alcoholics and individuals with chronic malnourishment. It is estimated that at least 10% of North Americans are folate deficient but the incidence has been decreasing in the United States since the fortification of foods with folate and the increased use of folate supplements.

Clinical manifestations are similar to the malnourished appearance of individuals with PA. Specific manifestations include cheilosis (scales and fissures of the mouth), stomatitis (inflammation of the mouth), and painful ulcerations of the buccal mucosa and tongue characteristic of *burning mouth syndrome*. Burning mouth syndrome may be secondary to a large number of disorders (e.g., extremely dry mouth, infection, autoimmune disease, nutritional deficiencies, and other conditions). Dysphagia, flatulence, and watery diarrhea also may be present, as well as histologic changes in the GI tract suggestive of sprue (chronic absorption disorder). Undiagnosed inflammatory bowel disease (e.g., Crohn disease, ulcerative colitis) may be the underlying cause of folate malabsorption in some individuals, and folate deficiency may suppress proliferation of the intestinal mucosa, leading to an increase of gastrointestinal damage. Neurologic manifestations, if present, may be caused by thiamine deficiency, which often accompanies folate deficiency.

Evaluation of folate deficiency is based on blood tests, measurement of serum folate levels, and clinical manifestations. Treatment requires administration of oral folate preparations until adequate blood levels are obtained and manifestations are reduced or eliminated. Long-term therapy is not necessary if the appropriate dietary adjustments are made to maintain adequate intake. After administration of folate, the manifestations of anemia disappear within 1 to 2 weeks.

Microcytic-Hypochromic Anemias

The microcytic-hypochromic anemias are characterized by abnormally small erythrocytes that contain abnormally reduced amounts of hemoglobin (see Figure 21-2, *B*). Hypochromia occurs even in cells of normal size.

Microcytic-hypochromic anemia can result from (1) disorders of iron metabolism, (2) disorders of porphyrin and heme synthesis, or (3) disorders of globin synthesis. Specific conditions include iron deficiency anemia, sideroblastic anemia, and thalassemia.

Iron Deficiency Anemia

Iron deficiency anemia (IDA) is the most common type of anemia throughout the world, occurring in both developing and developed countries.[2,10] Certain populations are at high risk for developing hypoferremia and IDA and include individuals living in poverty, women of childbearing age, and children. Iron deficiency in children is associated with numerous adverse health-related manifestations, especially cognitive impairment, which may be irreversible (see Chapter 22, *Health Alert: A Significant Number of Children Develop and Suffer from Severe Iron Deficiency Anemia*, p. 555). Children in developing countries often are affected by chronic parasite infestations that result in blood and iron loss greater than dietary intake.[11] Treatment of helminth infections results in improvement in appetite, growth, and in

the anemia. Iron deficiency anemia also occurs in individuals with lead poisoning and treatment is associated with a decrease in lead levels. An increased prevalence of iron deficiency has been observed in overweight children.

Females in the United States have a higher incidence than males for both hypoferremia and IDA, with the peak incidence occurring in the reproductive years and decreasing at menopause. Males have a higher incidence during childhood and adolescence.

PATHOPHYSIOLOGY IDA can arise from one of two different etiologies or a combination of both—inadequate dietary intake or chronic blood loss. In both instances there is no intrinsic dysfunction in iron metabolism; however, both etiologies deplete iron stores and reduce hemoglobin synthesis. A second category is a metabolic or functional iron deficiency in which various metabolic disorders lead to either insufficient iron delivery to bone marrow or impaired iron use (or absorption) within the marrow. Paradoxically, iron stores may be sufficient but delivery is inadequate to maintain heme synthesis, thus producing a functional or relative iron deficiency.

In developed countries, pregnancy and a continuous loss of blood are the most common causes of IDA. A blood loss of 2 to 4 ml/day (1 to 2 mg of iron) is enough to cause IDA. Menorrhagia (excessive menstrual bleeding) causes primary IDA in females. Males may experience bleeding as a result of ulcers, hiatal hernia, esophageal varices, cirrhosis, hemorrhoids, ulcerative colitis, or cancer. Other causes of blood loss for both genders include: (1) use of medications that cause GI bleeding (such as aspirin or nonsteroidal anti-inflammatory drugs [NSAIDs]); (2) surgical procedures that decrease stomach acidity, intestinal transit time, and absorption (e.g., gastric bypass); (3) insufficient dietary intake of iron; and (4) eating disorders such as pica—the craving and eating of nonnutritional substances, such as dirt, chalk, and paper. *H. pylori* infections also have been found to cause IDA of unknown origin, although *H. pylori* impairs iron uptake.

Iron in the form of hemoglobin is in constant demand by the body. An important attribute of iron is that it can be recycled; therefore, the body maintains a balance between iron that is in use as hemoglobin and iron that is stored and available for future hemoglobin synthesis (see Figure 21-2, *B*). Blood loss disrupts this balance by creating a need for more iron, thus depleting the iron stores more rapidly to replace the iron lost from bleeding. Iron contributes to immune function by regulating immune effector mechanisms (such as cytokine activities). The precise benefits or detriments of iron deficiency and immunity are controversial.

IDA develops slowly through three overlapping stages. In stage I, the body's iron stores for red cell production and hemoglobin synthesis are depleted. Red cell production proceeds normally with the hemoglobin content of red cells also remaining normal. In stage II, insufficient amounts of iron are transported to the marrow, and iron-deficient red cell production begins. Stage III begins when the hemoglobin-deficient red cells enter the circulation to replace normal, aged erythrocytes that have been destroyed. The manifestations of IDA appear in stage III when there is an insufficient iron supply and diminished hemoglobin synthesis.

CLINICAL MANIFESTATIONS The onset of symptoms is gradual, and individuals usually do not seek medical attention until hemoglobin levels drop to 7 or 8 g/dl. Early symptoms are nonspecific and include fatigue, weakness, shortness of breath, and pale earlobes, palms, and conjunctivae (Figure 21-3).

As the condition progresses and becomes more severe, structural and functional changes occur in epithelial tissue. The fingernails

FIGURE 21-3 Pallor and Iron Deficiency. Pallor of the skin, mucous membranes, and palmar creases in an individual with a hemoglobin level of 9 g/dl. Palmar creases become as pale as the surrounding skin when the hemoglobin level approaches 7 g/dl. (From Hoffbrand AV et al: *Color atlas of clinical hematology,* ed 4, London, 2009, Mosby.)

FIGURE 21-4 Koilonychia. The nails are concave, ridged, and brittle. (Courtesy Dr. S.M. Knowles. From Hoffbrand AV et al: *Color atlas of clinical hematology,* ed 4, London, 2009, Mosby.)

FIGURE 21-5 Glossitis. Tongue of individual with iron deficiency anemia has bald, fissured appearance *(arrow)* caused by loss of papillae and flattening. (From Hoffbrand AV et al: *Color atlas of clinical hematology,* ed 4, London, 2009, Mosby.)

become brittle and "spoon shaped" or concave (koilonychia) (Figure 21-4). Tongue papillae atrophy and cause soreness along with redness and burning (Figure 21-5). These changes can be reversed within 1 to 2 weeks of iron replacement therapy. The corners of the mouth become dry and sore (angular stomatitis), and an individual may experience difficulty with swallowing because of a "web" that develops from mucus and inflammatory cells at the opening of the esophagus. These lesions have the potential to become cancerous.

Nonheme iron is a component of many enzymes in the body, and lack of iron may alter other physiologic processes and contribute to the clinical manifestations. Individuals with IDA exhibit gastritis, neuromuscular changes, irritability, headache, numbness, tingling, and vasomotor disturbances. Gait disturbances are rare. In the elderly,

mental confusion, memory loss, and disorientation may be wrongly perceived as "normal" events associated with aging.

EVALUATION AND TREATMENT Evaluation is based on clinical manifestations and laboratory tests. Iron stores are measured directly, by bone marrow biopsy, or indirectly, by tests that measure serum ferritin level, transferrin saturation, or total iron-binding capacity. A sensitive indicator of heme synthesis is the amount of free erythrocyte protoporphyrin (FEP) within erythrocytes. A test that determines the concentration of soluble fragment transferrin receptor differentiates primary IDA from IDA that is associated with chronic disease.

The first step in treatment of IDA is to find and eliminate, or rule out, sources of blood loss. If this is not done, replacement therapy is ineffective. Iron replacement therapy is required and very effective. Initial doses are 150 to 200 mg/day and are continued until the serum ferritin level reaches 50 mg/L, indicating that adequate replacement has occurred. A rapid decrease in fatigue, lethargy, and other associated symptoms is generally seen within the first month of therapy. Replacement therapy usually continues for 6 to 12 months after the bleeding has stopped but may continue for as long as 24 months. Menstruating females may need daily oral iron replacement therapy (325 mg/day) until menopause.

Sideroblastic Anemia

Sideroblastic anemias (SAs) are a heterogeneous group of inherited and acquired disorders characterized by anemia of varying severity and the presence of ringed sideroblasts in the bone marrow (see Figure 21-2, *K*). Ringed sideroblasts are erythroblasts that contain iron-laden mitochondria arranged in a circle around one third or more of the nucleus. More simply, these are red cells that contain iron granules that have not been synthesized into hemoglobin but instead are arranged in a circle around the nucleus. Individuals with SA also have increased tissue levels of iron.

PATHOPHYSIOLOGY Sideroblastic anemias have various causes but all share the commonality of altered heme synthesis in the erythroid cells in bone marrow. Acquired sideroblastic anemias (ASAs), which are the most common, occur as a primary disorder with no known cause (idiopathic) or are associated with other myeloproliferative or myeloplastic disorders, for example, myeloma, polycythemia vera, and leukemias. Another form, described as reversible sideroblastic anemias (reversible SAs), is secondary to various conditions such as alcoholism, drug reactions, copper deficiency, and hypothermia. Reversible SA, associated with alcoholism, results from nutritional deficiencies of folate. Some drugs also cause reversible SA and include antituberculous agents (isoniazid [INH], pyrazinamide, cycloserine, and chloramphenicol) that interfere with B_{12} metabolism or directly injure the mitochondria. Copper deficiency also causes reversible SA by interfering with conversion of ferric iron to ferrous iron. This is extremely rare and is associated with gastrectomy and prolonged parenteral nutrition without copper supplements. Hypothermia causes decreased heme synthesis and incorporation into hemoglobin.

Hereditary (congenital) sideroblastic anemias are rare and occur almost exclusively in males, supporting a recessive X-linked transmission; however, autosomal transmission affecting females has been reported. Other genetic, chromosomal, or enzyme dysfunctions also have been associated with hereditary SA, for example, mutations in TRNT1 (tRNA nucleotidyl transferase) that lead to metabolic defects in both mitochondria and cytosol.[12] In all instances, SA anemia is present in infancy or childhood but may remain undetected until midlife when other conditions, such as diabetes or cardiac failure from iron overload, cause its manifestation.

The leading known cause of primary ASA, myelodysplastic syndrome (MDS), is a group of disorders of hematopoietic stem cells with all three stem cell lines (erythrocytic, granulocytic, and megakaryocytic) demonstrating abnormal growth or cell characteristics.[13] Pure SA, or cellular features limited to the erythrocytic line, requires blood transfusions that may, over time, produce iron overload. With adequate chelation therapy, individuals are able to survive and thrive for many years. MDS, characterized by abnormalities of multiple cell lineages, may include alterations of neutrophils and platelets. Bleeding from thrombocytopenia and platelet dysfunction is prevalent. Of those who survive, 40% develop acute (myeloblastic) leukemia.

CLINICAL MANIFESTATIONS   The anemias of SA are generally moderate to severe, with hemoglobin levels varying from 4 to 10 g/dl. In addition to the cardiovascular and respiratory manifestations common to all anemias, individuals with SA may show signs of iron overload (hemochromatosis) and mild to moderate enlargement of the liver (hepatomegaly) and spleen (splenomegaly). However, liver function remains normal or only mildly affected. Occasionally, the skin may become abnormally colored (bronze-tinted). Neurologic and skin alterations associated with other anemias are absent. Hemosiderosis of cardiac tissue may result in heart rhythm disturbances, which is a significant but uncommon complication and generally occurs late in the course of the disease. Growth and development impairment may occur in infants and young children who are severely affected.

EVALUATION AND TREATMENT   Initially, SA may be mistaken for deficiency of stem cells in the marrow (hypoplastic anemia) or iron deficiency anemia. The diagnosis of SA is established by bone marrow biopsy, which documents the presence of sideroblasts and confirms the diagnosis. The severity of the anemia is quite variable.

Initial treatment of SA is directed toward identification of a causative agent (i.e., drugs or toxins).[14] Treatment is supportive, with transfusions being the primary intervention. Following removal of the agent, oral pyridoxine (100 mg/day) may be administered on a trial basis. Acquired SA related to alcohol abuse and pyridoxine antagonists often demonstrates a complete response to pyridoxine. SA caused by other etiologies does not demonstrate the same improvement.

Individuals with hereditary SA are initially treated with pyridoxine therapy (50 to 200 mg/day), which is effective in approximately one third of individuals. An optimal response is reticulocytosis with blood hemoglobin levels and low free erythrocyte protoporphyrin levels also returning to normal within 1 to 2 months. Structural abnormalities of cells (microcytosis), however, do not disappear. Hemoglobin levels also may increase in response to therapy but stabilize at less than normal levels. A therapeutic response to pyridoxine may be maintained with lifelong administration of a reduced dosage. Nonresponse to pyridoxine requires blood transfusions for symptom relief and to promote growth and development.

Evidence of iron overload requires iron depletion therapy to prevent or minimize organ damage. Phlebotomy, or removal of blood from the circulation, is used in individuals with mild to moderate anemia without other complications (e.g., heart disease). After iron removal, maintenance phlebotomies are continued. Severely anemic individuals who may require transfusions become extremely iron overloaded, which mandates use of deferoxamine, an iron-chelating agent, to reduce excess iron levels.

Individuals with acquired SA are less likely to respond to pyridoxine, but SA rarely incapacitates them. When SA is secondary to an identifiable cause, treatment or removal of the cause is essential. In the absence of blood cell abnormalities and iron overload, progression

takes place over years. Transfusion and chelation therapy is the same as for hereditary SA when indicated.

Recent advances in treatment for SAs include prolonged administration of erythropoietin and stem cell transplant. Treatment with recombinant human erythropoietin improves anemia in 30% of those with myelodysplastic syndrome.[15] Individuals with the subset of MDS identified as refractory anemia have the overall best response rate. Congenital SA has been treated successfully with stem cell transplants; however, this treatment is in the early stages of use and long-term efficacy has not yet been established. Death from SA is rare and often secondary to complications, such as infection, bone marrow failure, liver failure, or cardiac failure or arrhythmias, or both.

Normocytic-Normochromic Anemias

Normocytic-normochromic anemias (NNAs) are characterized by erythrocytes that are relatively normal in size and hemoglobin content but insufficient in number.[16] These types of anemia do not share any common etiology, pathologic mechanism, or morphologic characteristics. They are less common than the macrocytic-normochromic and the microcytic-hypochromic anemias. The five distinct anemias are aplastic (damage to bone marrow erythropoiesis); posthemorrhagic (acute blood loss); acquired hemolytic (immune destruction of erythrocytes); hereditary hemolytic, such as sickle cell (see Figure 21-2, L) (destruction by eryptosis); and anemia of chronic inflammation (multiple causes). The diversity of the NNAs is summarized in Table 21-2. (Sickle cell anemia is discussed in Chapter 22.)

> ✔ QUICK CHECK 21-1
> 1. How do cell size and content determine classification of anemia?
> 2. Why is iron important to hemoglobin synthesis, and why is iron deficiency related to anemia?
> 3. Discuss the pathophysiology of iron deficiency anemia.
> 4. How is anemia diagnosed?

MYELOPROLIFERATIVE RED CELL DISORDERS

Hematologic dysfunction results from an overproduction of cells, as well as a deficiency. One or more hematopoietic lines may be overproduced in the marrow in response to exogenous (e.g., exposure to radiation, drugs) or endogenous (e.g., physiologic compensatory response, immune disorder) signals. Excessive red cell production is classified as polycythemia (Table 21-3). Polycythemia exists in two forms: relative and absolute. Relative polycythemia results from hemoconcentration of the blood associated with dehydration that may be caused by decreased water intake, diarrhea, excessive vomiting, or increased use of diuretics. Its development is usually of minor consequence and resolves with fluid administration or treatment of underlying conditions.

Absolute polycythemia consists of two forms: primary and secondary. Secondary polycythemia, the most common of the two, is a physiologic response resulting from erythropoietin secretion caused by hypoxia. This hypoxia is noted in individuals living at higher altitudes (>10,000 ft), smokers with increased blood levels of CO, and individuals with chronic obstructive pulmonary disease or coronary heart failure, or both. Abnormal types of hemoglobin (e.g., San Diego, Chesapeake), which have a greater affinity for oxygen, also cause secondary polycythemia, as does inappropriate secretion of erythropoietin by certain tumors (e.g., renal cell carcinoma, hepatoma, and cerebellar hemangioblastomas).

TABLE 21-2 Normocytic-Normochromic Anemias

Anemia	Pathophysiology	Clinical Manifestations	Evaluation and Treatment
Aplastic	Rare; may result from infiltrative disorders of bone marrow, autoimmune diseases, renal failure, splenic dysfunction, vitamin B_{12} or folate deficiency, parvovirus infection, or exposure to radiation, drugs, and toxins; also may be congenital Common stem cell population may be altered so it cannot proliferate or differentiate, or stem cell environment is altered to inhibit erythropoiesis Outcome ranges from death to minimal manifestations	Classic cardiovascular and respiratory manifestations with thrombocytopenia, hemorrhage into tissues, leukopenia, and infection	Bone marrow biopsy determines whether anemia is caused by pure red cell aplasia or hypoplasia Treat underlying disorder or prevent further exposure to causative agent Blood transfusions, marrow transplant, and pharmacologic stimulation of bone marrow function
Posthemorrhagic	Caused by sudden blood loss with normal iron stores	Often obscured by cardiovascular manifestations of acute hemorrhage Severe shock, lactic acidosis, and death can occur if blood loss exceeds 40-50% of plasma volume	Restoration of blood volume by intravenous administration of saline, dextran, albumin, or plasma Transfusion of whole blood also required occasionally
Hemolytic	Acquired: caused by infection, systemic disease, drugs or toxins, liver disease, kidney disease, abnormal immune responses Hereditary: caused by abnormalities of RBC membrane or cytoplasmic contents; present at birth Hemolysis: in blood vessels or lymphoid tissues that filter blood (e.g., spleen, liver) Erythrocytes: rigid, slowing their passage and making them vulnerable to phagocytosis Types: warm antibody disease (mediated by IgG antibody specific for erythrocyte antigens), cold antibody disease (mediated by IgM), and drug induced	Splenomegaly, jaundice, aplastic hemolytic, or megaloblastic crises can develop with viral infection With severe disease, bones become deformed and pathologic fractures occur Cardiovascular and respiratory manifestations correspond with severity of anemia	Blood and bone marrow studies Erythroid hyperplasia is found in marrow and blood smears Treatment of acquired disease involves removing cause or treating underlying disorder Other forms of treatment are transfusions, splenectomy, and steroids or folate
Anemia of chronic inflammation	Associated with chronic infections (e.g., AIDS), chronic inflammatory diseases (e.g., rheumatoid arthritis, SLE), and malignancies Causes are decreased erythrocyte life span, failure of mechanisms of compensatory erythropoiesis, or disturbance of iron cycle	Manifestations fewer and milder than most other anemias General disability caused by chronic disease limits physical activity so hemoglobin levels adequate; if they drop, signs of iron deficiency anemia develop	Blood tests show iron deficiency in marrow despite normal or increased iron stores elsewhere No treatment is needed unless anemia becomes symptomatic Erythropoietin may be used

AIDS, Acquired immunodeficiency syndrome; *RBC*, red blood cell; *SLE*, systemic lupus erythematosus.

TABLE 21-3 Disorders Classified as Polycythemia

Type of Polycythemia	Mechanism of Increased Erythropoiesis	Cause of Associated Disorder
Primary polycythemia (polycythemia vera)	Excessive proliferation of erythroid precursors in marrow; JAK2 mutation, increased sensitivity of stem cell to erythropoietin	Possible mutation in erythropoietin receptor
Secondary polycythemia	Physiologic increase in erythropoietin secretion by kidneys in response to underlying systemic disorder	Tissue hypoxia caused by cardiopulmonary disorders (chronic obstructive pulmonary disease, congestive heart failure), decreased barometric pressure, cardiovascular malformations causing mixing of arterial and venous blood, methemoglobinemia, carboxyhemoglobinemia, smoking, obesity
	"Nonphysiologic"* increase in erythropoietin secretion	Renal disorders, cerebellar hemangioblastomas, hepatoma (liver tumor), ovarian carcinoma, uterine leiomyoma, pheochromocytoma, adrenocortical hypersecretion
Familial polycythemia	Genetically induced increase in erythroid precursors of marrow Abnormal Hb with increased oxygen affinity Decreased 2,3-DPG Increased sensitivity of stem cells to erythropoietin Increased erythropoietin secretion	Genetic defect

2,3-DPG, 2,3-Diphosphoglycerate; *Hb*, hemoglobin.
*Nonphysiologic means that there is no obvious physiologic explanation for hypersecretion of erythropoietin.

Polycythemia Vera

Polycythemia vera (PV) (also known as **primary polycythemia**) is a stem cell disorder with hyperplastic and neoplastic bone marrow alterations. PV is characterized by an abnormal uncontrolled proliferation of red blood cells (frequently with increased levels of white blood cells [leukocytosis] and platelets [thrombocytosis]). The increase in red cells (polycythemia) is responsible for most of the clinical symptoms including an increase in blood volume and viscosity. PV is one of several disorders collectively known as *myeloproliferative neoplasms (MPNs)* (Box 21-1). These disorders include certain leukemias, essential thrombocytosis, and chronic bone marrow fibrosis. The disorders all result from abnormal regulation of the hematopoietic stem cells. Specifically, the common pathogenic feature is the presence of a mutation in the **Janus kinase 2 gene** (*JAK2 gene*) resulting in an overproduction of blood cells. Normally, the *JAC2* gene makes a protein that helps the body produce blood cells (see Pathophysiology). Because of numerous characteristics (e.g., overproduction of different blood cells, marrow hypercellularity, or fibrosis) shared by these disorders and a lack of specific molecular markers, the diagnosis can be quite challenging. The common features include (1) increased proliferative drive in the bone marrow, (2) hematopoiesis of neoplastic stem cells to secondary hematopoietic organs, (3) marrow fibrosis and peripheral deficiencies in blood cells *(cytopenias)*, and (4) variable transformation to acute leukemia.

PV is quite rare with an estimated incidence of 2.3 per 100,000 individuals; peak incidence is between the ages of 60 and 80 years with a median incidence of 55 to 60. However, PV has been observed in individuals younger than the age of 40. Males are twice as likely as females to develop PV. It is more common in whites of Eastern European Jewish ancestry than in blacks. PV is rarely seen in children or in multiple members of a single family; however, an autosomal dominant form exists that causes increased secretion of erythropoietin.

PATHOPHYSIOLOGY Erythrocytosis is the essential component of PV. Proliferation of erythroid progenitors occurs in the bone marrow independent of the hormone erythropoietin, but the cells express a normal erythropoietin receptor. More than 95% of individuals with PV have an acquired mutation in the tyrosine kinase, Janus kinase 2 (JAK2).[17] Normal JAK2 increases the activity of the erythropoietin receptor and is self-regulatory so that JAK2 activity diminishes over time. The mutation associated with PV negates the self-regulatory activity of JAK2 so that the erythropoietin receptor is constantly active regardless of the level of erythropoietin. Overall, the mutated tyrosine kinases bypass normal controls, causing growth factor–independent proliferation and survival of marrow progenitors or precursor cells. The cause of the mutation is unknown.

CLINICAL MANIFESTATIONS PV is uncommon and occurs insidiously. Clinical manifestations of PV are a result of the increased red cell mass and hematocrit. Usually there is an increase in blood volume. Together all of these factors cause abnormal blood flow that increases blood viscosity, creating a hypercoagulable state that results in clogging and occlusion of blood vessels. Tissue injury (ischemia) and death (infarction) is the outcome of blood vessel blockage. These outcomes are directly correlated with hematocrit levels. Increases in numbers of thrombocytes, as well as production of dysfunctional platelets, also contribute to this hypercoagulable condition.

Circulatory alterations caused by the thick, sticky blood give rise to other manifestations, such as plethora (ruddy, red color of the face, hands, feet, ears, and mucous membranes) and engorgement of retinal

BOX 21-1 World Health Organization (WHO) Classification of Myeloid Malignancies

1. Acute myeloid leukemia (AML) and related neoplasms[a]
2. Myeloproliferative neoplasms (MPN)
   2.1. Chronic myeloid leukemia, *BCR-ABL1* positive (CML)
   2.2. *BCR-ABL1*-negative MPN
      2.2.1. Polycythemia vera
      2.2.2. Primary myelofibrosis (PMF)
      2.2.3. Prefibrotic PMF
      2.2.4. Essential thrombocythemia (ET)
   2.3. Other MPN
      2.3.1. Chronic neutrophilic leukemia (CNL)
      2.3.2. Chronic eosinophilic leukemia, not otherwise specified (CEL-NOS)
      2.3.3. Mastocytosis
      2.3.4. Myeloproliferative neoplasm, unclassified (MPN-U)
3. Myelodysplastic syndromes (MDS)
   3.1. Refractory cytopenia[b] with unilineage dysplasia (RCUD)
      3.1.1. Refractory anemia (ring sideroblasts <15% of erythroid precursors)
      3.1.2. Refractory neutropenia
   3.2. Refractory anemia with ring sideroblasts (RARS; dysplasia limited to erythroid lineage and ring sideroblasts ≥15% of bone marrow erythroid precursors)
   3.3. Refractory cytopenia with multilineage dysphasia (RCMD; ring sideroblast count does not matter)
   3.4. Refractory anemia with excess blasts (RAEB)
      3.4.1. RAEB-1 (2-4% circulating *or* 5-9% marrow blasts)
      3.4.2. RAEB-2 (5-19% circulating *or* 10-19% marrow blasts *or* Auer rods present)
   3.5. MDS associated with isolated del(5q)
   3.6. MDS, unclassified
4. MDS/MPN
   4.1. Chronic myelomonocytic leukemia (CMML)
   4.2. Atypical chronic myeloid leukemia, *BCR-AB1* negative
   4.3. Juvenile myelomonocytic leukemia (JMML)
   4.4. MDS/MPN, unclassified
      4.4.1. *Provisional entry: Refractory anemia with ring sideroblastic associated with marked thrombocytosis (RARS-T)*
5. Myeloid and lymphoid neoplasms with eosinophilia and abnormalities of *PDGFRA,*[c] *PDGFRB,*[c] *FGFRI*[c]
   5.1. Myeloid and lymphoid neoplasms with *PDGFRA* rearrangement
   5.2. Myeloid neoplasms with *PDGFRB* rearrangement
   5.3. Myeloid and lymphoid neoplasms with *FGFRI* abnormalities

From Tefferi A, Barbui T: *Am J Hematol* 90(2):162-173, 2015.
[a]Acute myeloid leukemia-related precursor neoplasms include "therapy-related myelodysplastic syndrome" and "myeloid sarcoma."
[b]Either mono- or bi-cytopenia: hemoglobin <10 g/dl, absolute neutrophil count <1.8 × 10^9/L, or platelet count <100 × 10^9/L. However, higher blood counts do not exclude the diagnosis in the presence of unequivocal histologic/cytogenic evidence for myelodysplastic syndrome.
[c]Genetic rearrangements involving platelet-derived growth factor receptor α/β (*PDFRA/PDFRB*) or fibroblast growth factor receptor 1 (*FGFR1*).

and cerebral veins. Other symptoms may include headache, drowsiness, delirium, mania, psychotic depression, chorea, and visual disturbances. Individuals frequently have an enlarged spleen with abdominal pain and discomfort. Death from cerebral thrombosis is approximately five times greater in individuals with PV.[18,19]

Cardiovascular function, despite the vascular alterations, remains relatively normal. Cardiac workload and output remain constant; however, increased blood volume does increase blood pressure. Coronary blood flow may be affected, precipitating angina, although cardiovascular infarctions are uncommon. Other cardiovascular manifestations include Raynaud phenomenon and thromboangiitis obliterans.

A unique feature of PV, and helpful in diagnosis, is the development of intense, painful itching that appears to be intensified by heat or exposure to water (aquagenic pruritus) so that individuals avoid exposure to water, particularly warm water when bathing or showering. The intensity of itching is related to the concentration of mast cells in the skin and is generally not responsive to antihistamines or topical lotions.

EVALUATION AND TREATMENT PV is frequently suspected because of clinical features, such as a thrombotic event, splenomegaly, or aquagenic pruritus. Blood and laboratory findings, characterized by an absolute increase in red blood cells and in total blood volume, confirm the diagnosis. Hematocrit levels may range from 18 to 24 g/dl and red blood cell counts may range from 7×10^{12} to $7 \times 10^{13}/\mu L$. Erythrocytes appear normal, but anisocytosis may be present. There also may be moderate increases in white blood cells and platelets. A bone marrow examination may be done but is not very valuable unless performed in association with cytogenetic and molecular studies for relevant mutations in JAK2.[20] The presence of a JAK2 mutation confirms the diagnosis.[21] Treatment of PV consists of reducing red cell proliferation and blood volume, controlling symptoms, and preventing clogging and clotting of the blood vessels. In low-risk individuals (e.g., those younger than age 60 or with no history of thrombosis and without risk factors for cardiovascular disease), the recommended therapy is phlebotomy (300 to 500 ml at a time to reduce erythrocytosis and blood volume) and low-dose aspirin. Frequent phlebotomies also reduce iron levels, a condition that impedes erythropoiesis.

Hydroxyurea, a nonalkylating myelosuppressive, is the drug of choice for myelosuppression because of a reduced incidence to cause leukemia and thrombosis. Radioactive phosphorus (^{32}P) also is used as an effective and easily tolerated intervention to suppress erythropoiesis. Its effects may last up to 18 months. Side effects of ^{32}P include suppression of hematopoiesis resulting in anemia, leukopenia, and thrombocytopenia. Acute leukemia is also a side effect, although most often it occurs only after 7 or more years of treatment, making its use in elderly persons more common. Interferon-alpha has been used when other forms of treatment have failed.

Survival for 10 to 15 years is common. However, without proper treatment, 50% of individuals with PV die within 18 months of the onset of initial symptoms because of thrombosis or hemorrhage. A significant potential outcome of PV is the conversion to acute myeloid leukemia (AML), occurring spontaneously in 10% of individuals and generally being resistant to conventional therapy. Conversion to AML is most likely related to treatment methods associated with cytotoxic myelosuppressive agents. Although PV is a chronic disorder, appropriate therapy results in remissions and prevention of significant pathologic outcomes.

Iron Overload

Iron overload can be primary, as in hereditary hemochromatosis (HH), or secondary. The secondary causes of iron overload include anemias with inefficient erythropoiesis (e.g., sideroblastic anemia, aplastic anemia), dietary iron overload, or conditions that require repeated blood transfusions or iron dextran injections. Iron absorption is regulated by erythropoietin, tissue oxygenation, and iron stores (see Chapter 20).

Hereditary Hemochromatosis

Hemochromatosis is caused by excessive iron absorption. Hereditary hemochromatosis (HH) is a common inherited, autosomal recessive disorder of iron metabolism[22] and is characterized by increased gastrointestinal iron absorption with subsequent tissue iron deposition. Excess iron is deposited first in the liver and pancreas, followed by the heart, joints, and endocrine glands. Excess iron causes tissue damage that can lead to diseases such as cirrhosis, diabetes, heart failure, arthropathies, and impotence. HH affects more males than females.

HH is caused by two genetic base-pair alterations, C282Y and H63D. These are mutations in the *HFE* gene on chromosome 6. Homozygosity of C282Y is the most common genotype and accounts for 82% to 90% of HH cases. The remaining cases appear to be caused by environmental factors or other genotypes. *HFE* mutations are common in the United States with 1 in 10 white persons heterozygous for *HFE* C282Y mutation and 4.4 in 1000 homozygous for the C282Y mutation. C282Y homozygosity is much lower among Hispanics (0.27 in 1000), Asian Americans (<0.001 per 1000), Pacific islanders (0.12 per 1000), and black persons (0.14 per 1000).

PATHOPHYSIOLOGY In HH, regulation of intestinal absorption of dietary iron is abnormal, causing iron accumulation. The *HFE* gene governs intestinal absorption of dietary iron by regulating the liver-derived protein hepcidin. Hepcidin lowers plasma iron level, and a deficiency in hepcidin, caused by genetic mutations, causes iron overload. The gene mutations in HH reduce hepcidin synthesis, thus reducing the level of circulating plasma hepcidin. The decreased hepcidin-ferroportin (iron transporter) interaction eventually leads to more iron outward flow (efflux) from cells in the small intestinal mucosa, causing a rise in iron concentration and a systemic overload. The iron overload leads to excess iron tissue deposits that can eventually result in liver fibrosis, cirrhosis, hepatocellular carcinoma, diabetes, hypothyroidism, arthritis, cardiomyopathies, and skin hyperpigmentation.

With HH there appears to be a long latent period with individual variation in biochemical expression modified by environmental factors, such as blood loss from menstruation or donation, alcohol intake, and diet. Cirrhosis is a late-stage development of HH that can shorten life expectancy. Cirrhosis also is a risk factor for hepatocellular carcinoma that occurs between 40 and 60 years of age. Cirrhosis prevention is a major goal of HH screening and treatment.

CLINICAL MANIFESTATIONS Clinical manifestations of HH include symptoms such as fatigue, malaise, abdominal pain, arthralgias, and impotence; and clinical findings of hepatomegaly, abnormal liver enzymes, bronzed skin, diabetes, and cardiomegaly. Many individuals are diagnosed as a result of serum iron studies as part of a health screening panel. Most affected individuals (>75%) are asymptomatic and have a low frequency (<25%) of cirrhosis, diabetes, or skin pigmentation.

EVALUATION AND TREATMENT Laboratory findings in individuals with HH show elevations in serum iron levels, transferrin saturation, and ferritin levels. Documentation of iron overload relies on quantitative phlebotomy with calculation of the amount of iron removed or liver biopsy with determination of quantitative hepatic iron. With the advent of genetic testing, individuals who are C282Y homozygous or compound heterozygous, less than 40 years old, and have normal liver functions, no further workup is necessary.

Treatment of HH is simple and consists of phlebotomy of 550 ml of whole blood, which is equivalent to 200 to 250 mg of iron. Frequency of phlebotomy depends on ferritin levels and should continue until the ferritin level is between 20 and 50 ng/ml. Initially, phlebotomy may be needed weekly but once therapeutic ferritin levels are reached, phlebotomy may only be needed every 2 to 3 months. Blood banks now accept blood donations from persons with documented HH. Iron chelating agents are sometimes used in addition to phlebotomy, but this is not the mainstay of treatment. Individuals with HH should be instructed to refrain from taking iron and vitamin C supplements and consuming raw shellfish; in addition, alcohol should be used in moderation. Family screening is recommended and necessary for all first-degree relatives of a person with HH.

ALTERATIONS OF LEUKOCYTE FUNCTION

Leukocyte function is affected if too many or too few white cells are present in the blood or if the cells that are present are structurally or functionally defective. Phagocytic cells (granulocytes, monocytes, macrophages) may lose their ability to act as effective phagocytes, and the lymphocytes may lose their ability to respond to antigens. (Disruptions of inflammatory and immune processes caused by leukocyte disorders are described in Chapter 6.) Other leukocyte alterations include infectious mononucleosis and cancers of the blood—leukemia and multiple myeloma.

Quantitative Alterations of Leukocytes

Quantitative alterations are increases or decreases in numbers and functions of leukocytes in the blood. Leukocytosis is present when the count is higher than normal; leukopenia is present when the count is lower than normal. Leukocytosis and leukopenia may affect a specific type of white blood cell and may result from a variety of physiologic conditions and alterations.

Leukocytosis occurs as a normal protective response to physiologic stressors, such as invading microorganisms, strenuous exercise, emotional changes, temperature changes, anesthesia, surgery, pregnancy, and some drugs, hormones, and toxins. It also is caused by pathologic conditions, such as malignancies and hematologic disorders. Unlike leukocytosis, leukopenia is never normal and is defined as an absolute blood cell count less than 4000 cells/μL. Leukopenia is associated with a decrease in neutrophils, which increases risk for infection. When the neutrophil count falls to less than 1000/μL, the risk of infection increases drastically. With counts below 500/μL, the possibility for life-threatening infections is high. Leukopenia may be caused by radiation, anaphylactic shock, autoimmune disease (e.g., systemic lupus erythematosus), immune deficiencies (see Chapter 8), and certain chemotherapeutic agents.

Granulocyte and Monocyte Alterations

Increased numbers of circulating granulocytes (neutrophils, eosinophils, basophils) and monocytes are chiefly a physiologic response to infection. Increased numbers also occur as a result of myeloproliferative disorders that increase stem cell proliferation in the bone marrow.[23]

Decreased numbers occur when infectious processes deplete the supply of circulating granulocytes and monocytes, drawing them out of the circulation and into infected tissues faster than they can be replaced. Decreases also can be caused by disorders that suppress marrow function, such as severe congenital neutropenia, or immune-related neutropenia.[24]

Granulocytosis—an increase in granulocytes (neutrophils, eosinophils, or basophils)—begins when stored blood cells are released. Neutrophilia is another term that may be used to describe granulocytosis because neutrophils are the most numerous of the granulocytes (Table 21-4). Neutrophilia is seen in the early stages of infection or inflammation and is established when the absolute count exceeds 7500/μL. Release and depletion of stored neutrophils stimulates granulopoiesis

to replenish neutrophil reserves. Specific conditions associated with neutrophilia and other white blood cells are identified in Table 21-4.

When the demand for circulating mature neutrophils exceeds the supply, immature neutrophils (and other leukocytes) are released from the bone marrow. Premature release of the immature cells is responsible for the phenomenon known as a shift-to-the-left, or leukemoid reaction. This refers to the microscopic detection of disproportionate numbers of immature leukocytes in peripheral blood smears. To understand this phenomenon, visualize cellular differentiation, maturation, and release (see Figure 19-7) as progressing from left to right instead of vertically. The early release of immature white cells prevents the completion of the sequence and shifts the distribution of leukocytes in the blood toward those on the left side of the diagram. This phenomenon is also seen in the blood smear of individuals with leukemia, hence the term *leukemoid reaction*. As infection or inflammation diminishes, and granulopoiesis replenishes circulating granulocytes, a shift-to-the-right, or return to normal, occurs.

Neutropenia is a condition associated with a reduction in circulating neutrophils and exists clinically when the neutrophil count is less than 2000/μL. Reduction in neutrophils occurs in severe prolonged infections when production of granulocytes cannot keep up with demand.[23,24]

Other causes of neutropenia, in the absence of infection, may be (1) decreased neutrophil production or ineffective granulopoiesis, (2) reduced neutrophil survival, and (3) abnormal neutrophil distribution and sequestration. Neutropenia also is classified as primary or secondary and primary disorders are further identified as congenital or acquired. Primary acquired neutropenia is associated with multiple conditions, for example, hypoplastic anemia or aplastic anemia, leukemia (acute myelogenous leukemia [AML]/chronic lymphocytic leukemia [CLL]), lymphomas (Hodgkin, non-Hodgkin), and myelodysplastic syndrome (MDS). The megaloblastic anemias (vitamin B_{12} and folate deficiency) as well as starvation and anorexia nervosa cause neutropenia because of an inadequate supply of vitamins and nutrients for protein production.

Congenital defects in neutrophil production include cyclic neutropenia, neutropenia with congenital immunodeficiencies, and multiple syndromes, such as Kostmann, Shwachman-Diamond, Diamond-Blackfan, and Barth syndromes. Reduced neutrophil survival and abnormal distribution and sequestration are usually secondary to other disorders. Neutropenia occurs in a variety of immunologic disorders, particularly systemic lupus erythematosus, rheumatoid arthritis, Felty and Sjögren syndromes, splenomegaly, and drug-related causes.

Severe neutropenia, granulocytopenia (less than 500/μL), or agranulocytosis (complete absence of granulocytes in blood) is usually secondary to arrested hematopoiesis in the bone marrow or massive cell destruction in the circulation. Chemotherapeutic agents used to treat hematologic and other malignancies cause bone marrow suppression. Several other drugs cause agranulocytosis, which occurs rarely but carries a high mortality of 10% to 50%. Clinical manifestations of agranulocytosis include severe infection (particularly of the respiratory system) leading to septicemia, general malaise, fever, tachycardia, and ulcers in the mouth and colon. If this condition remains untreated, sepsis caused by agranulocytosis results in death within 3 to 6 days. Other conditions associated with neutropenia are identified in Table 21-4.

Eosinophilia is an absolute increase (>450/μL) in the total number of circulating eosinophils. Allergic disorders (type 1) associated with asthma, hay fever, parasitic infections, and drug reactions often cause eosinophilia. Hypersensitivity reactions trigger the release of eosinophilic chemotaxic factor of anaphylaxis (ECF-A), and histamine

TABLE 21-4 Other Conditions Associated with Neutrophils, Eosinophils, Basophils, Monocytes, and Lymphocytes

Condition	Cause	Example
Neutrophil		
Neutrophilia (granulocytosis)	Inflammation or tissue necrosis	Surgery, burns, MI, pneumonitis, rheumatic fever, rheumatoid arthritis
	Infection	Bacterial: gram-positive (staphylococci, streptococci, pneumococci), gram-negative (*Escherichia coli*, *Pseudomonas* species)
	Physiologic	Exercise, extreme heat or cold, third-trimester pregnancy, emotional distress
	Hematologic	Acute hemorrhage, hemolysis, myeloproliferative disorder, chronic granulocytic leukemia
	Drugs or chemicals	Epinephrine, steroids, heparin, histamine, endotoxin
	Metabolic	Diabetes (acidosis), eclampsia, gout, thyroid storm
	Neoplasm	Liver, GI tract, bone marrow
Neutropenia	Decreased marrow production	Radiation, chemotherapy, leukemia, aplastic anemia, abnormal granulopoiesis
	Increased destruction	Splenomegaly, hemodialysis, autoimmune disease
	Prolonged infection	Gram-negative (typhoid), viral (influenza, hepatitis B, measles, mumps, rubella), severe infections, protozoal infections (malaria)
Eosinophil		
Eosinophilia	Allergy	Asthma, hay fever, drug sensitivity
	Infection	Parasites (trichinosis, hookworm), chronic (fungal, leprosy, TB)
	Malignancy	CML, lung, stomach, ovary, Hodgkin disease
	Dermatosis	Pemphigus, exfoliative dermatitis (drug-induced)
	Drugs	Digitalis, heparin, streptomycin, tryptophan (eosinophilia-myalgia syndrome), penicillins, propranolol
Eosinopenia	Stress response	Trauma, shock, burns, surgery, mental distress
	Drugs	Steroids (Cushing syndrome)
Basophil		
Basophilia	Inflammation	Infection (measles, chickenpox), hypersensitivity reaction (immediate)
	Hematologic	Myeloproliferative disorders (CML, polycythemia vera, Hodgkin lymphoma, hemolytic anemia)
	Endocrine	Myxedema, antithyroid therapy
Basopenia	Physiologic	Pregnancy, ovulation, stress
	Endocrine	Graves disease
Monocyte		
Monocytosis	Infection	Bacterial (subacute bacterial endocarditis, TB), recovery phase of infection
	Hematologic	Myeloproliferative disorders, Hodgkin disease, agranulocytosis
	Physiologic	Normal newborn
Monocytopenia	Rare	
Lymphocyte		
Lymphocytosis	Physiologic	4 months to 4 years
	Acute infection	Infectious mononucleosis, CMV infection, pertussis, hepatitis, mycoplasma pneumonia, typhoid
	Chronic infection	Congenital syphilis, tertiary syphilis
	Endocrine	Thyrotoxicosis, adrenal insufficiency
	Malignancy	ALL, CLL, lymphosarcoma cell leukemia
Lymphocytopenia	Immunodeficiency syndrome	AIDS, agammaglobulinemia
	Lymphocyte destruction	Steroids (Cushing syndrome), radiation, chemotherapy
		Hodgkin lymphoma
		CHF, renal failure, TB, SLE, aplastic anemia

AIDS, Acquired immunodeficiency syndrome; *ALL,* acute lymphocytic leukemia; *CHF,* congestive (left) heart failure; *CLL,* chronic lymphocytic leukemia; *CML,* chronic myelogenous leukemia; *CMV,* cytomegalovirus; *GI,* gastrointestinal; *MI,* myocardial infarction; *SLE,* systemic lupus erythematosus; *TB,* tuberculosis.

from mast cells attracts eosinophils to the area. Mast cells release interleukin-5 (IL-5), which stimulates the bone marrow to produce more eosinophils into the blood. Areas with abundant mast cells, such as the respiratory and GI tracts, are commonly affected. Eosinophilia also may occur in dermatologic disorders, eosinophilia-myalgia syndrome, and parasitic invasion. Other conditions that cause eosinophilia are detailed in Table 21-4.

Eosinopenia, a decrease in the number of circulating eosinophils, generally is caused by migration of eosinophils into inflammatory sites. It may be seen in Cushing syndrome and as a result of stress caused by surgery, shock, trauma, burns, or mental distress. Other conditions that cause eosinopenia are detailed in Table 21-4.

Basophilia, an increase in the number of circulating basophils, is rare and generally is a response to inflammation and immediate hypersensitivity reactions. Basophils contain histamine that is released during an allergic reaction. Increased numbers of basophils are seen in myeloproliferative disorders, such as chronic myeloid leukemia and myeloid metaplasia. Other conditions that are associated with basophilia are listed in Table 21-4.

Basopenia (also known as *basophilic leukopenia*) is a decrease in circulating numbers of basophils. It is seen in hyperthyroidism, acute infection, ovulation and pregnancy, and long-term therapy with steroids. Other conditions associated with basopenia are listed in Table 21-4.

Monocytosis is an increase in numbers of circulating monocytes (generally greater than 800/μL). It is often transient and not related to a dysfunction of monocyte production. If present, it is usually associated with neutropenia during bacterial infections, particularly in the late stages or recovery stage, when monocytes are needed to phagocytize surviving microorganisms and debris. Increased monocytes also may indicate marrow recovery from agranulocytosis. Monocytosis is often seen in chronic infections such as tuberculosis (TB), brucellosis, listeriosis, and subacute bacterial endocarditis (SBE). Monocytosis has been found to correlate with the extent of myocardial damage following myocardial infarctions. Other conditions associated with monocytosis are identified in Table 21-4. Monocytopenia, a decrease in the number of circulating monocytes, is rare but has been identified with hairy cell leukemia and prednisone therapy.

Lymphocyte Alterations

Quantitative alterations of lymphocytes occur when lymphocytes are activated by antigenic stimuli, usually microorganisms (see Chapter 7). Lymphocytosis is an increase in the number (absolute lymphocytosis) or proportion of lymphocytes in the blood. It is rare in acute bacterial infections and is seen most commonly in acute viral infections, particularly those caused by the Epstein-Barr virus (EBV)—a causative agent in infectious mononucleosis. Other specific disorders associated with lymphocytosis are listed in Table 21-4.

Lymphocytopenia is a decrease in the number of circulating lymphocytes in the blood. It may be attributed to (1) abnormalities of lymphocyte production associated with neoplasias and immune deficiencies and (2) destruction by drugs, viruses, or radiation. It is also known to occur without any detectable cause. Conditions associated with lymphocytopenia are identified in Table 21-4. The lymphocytopenia associated with heart failure and other acute illnesses may be caused by elevated cortisol levels. Lymphocytopenia is a major problem in acquired immunodeficiency syndrome (AIDS). AIDS-related lymphocytopenia is caused by human immunodeficiency virus (HIV), which destroys T-helper lymphocytes. (For a detailed discussion of AIDS, see Chapter 8.)

Infectious Mononucleosis

Infectious mononucleosis (IM) is a benign, acute, self-limiting, lymphoproliferative clinical syndrome characterized by acute infection of B lymphocytes (B cells). The most common cause is Epstein-Barr virus (EBV).[25] EBV is a ubiquitous lymphotropic, herpesvirus and accounts for approximately 85% of IM cases. Other viruses that cause symptoms resembling IM include cytomegalovirus (CMV), adenovirus, HIV, hepatitis A, influenza A and B, and rubella, as well as the bacteria *Toxoplasma gondii*, *Corynebacterium diphtheriae*, and *Coxiella burnetii*. The classic symptoms are pharyngitis, lymphadenopathy, and fever. In individuals with immunodeficiency, the proliferation of infected B cells may be uncontrolled and can lead to the development of B-cell lymphomas.[26] Individuals who are coinfected with malaria or HIV are at increased risk of developing EBV-associated lymphomas, including Burkitt lymphoma (BL). EBV also is etiologically linked to subgroups

of Hodgkin lymphoma (HL). Approximately 50% to 85% of children are infected with EBV by age 4, and more than 90% of adults have indications of subclinical EBV infections. These early infections are usually asymptomatic and provide immunity to EBV; thus early EBV infections rarely develop into IM. IM may arise when the initial infection occurs during adolescence or later, but still only results in IM in 35% to 50% of these individuals. Symptomatic IM usually affects young adults between ages 15 and 35 years, with the peak incidences occurring between 15 and 24 years; males have a later peak (18 to 24 years) than females. The overall incidence rate for this age group is 6 to 8 cases per 1000 persons per year. Children from low socioeconomic environments are particularly susceptible to infections with EBV. IM is uncommon in individuals older than age 40; however, if it does occur, it is commonly caused by CMV.

Transmission of EBV is usually through saliva from close personal contact (e.g., kissing, hence the term *kissing disease*). The virus also may be secreted in other mucosal secretions of the genital, rectal, and respiratory tracts, as well as blood. Transmission through sneezing or coughing has not been documented. The infection begins with widespread invasion of the B lymphocytes, which have receptors for EBV. The virus initially infects the oropharynx, nasopharynx, and salivary epithelial cells with later spread into lymphoid tissues and B cells.

In the immunocompetent individual, unaffected B cells produce antibodies (IgG, IgA, IgM) against the virus. At the same time, there is a massive proliferation of cytotoxic T cells (CD8) that are directed against EBV-infected cells (see Chapter 7). The immune response against EBV-infected cells is largely responsible for the cellular proliferation in the lymphoid tissue (lymph nodes, spleen, tonsils, and, occasionally, liver). Sore throat and fever are caused by inflammation at the site of initial viral entry (the mouth and throat).

CLINICAL MANIFESTATIONS The incubation period for IM is approximately 30 to 50 days. Early flulike symptoms, such as headache, malaise, joint pain, and fatigue, may appear during the first 3 to 5 days, although some individuals are without symptoms. At the time of diagnosis, the individual commonly presents with the classic group of symptoms: fever, sore throat (pharyngitis), cervical lymph node enlargement, and fatigue. The pharyngitis is usually diffuse with a whitish or grayish green, thick exudate. It can be painful, causing the individual to seek treatment. Characteristics with progression may include a generalized lymphadenopathy, enlarged spleen, and appearance in the blood of atypical activated T lymphocytes (mononucleosis cells). IM is usually self-limiting, and recovery occurs in a few weeks. Fatigue, however, may last for 1 to 2 months after resolution of the infection.

Severe clinical complications are rare. With progression of IM, general lymph node enlargement may develop with enlargement of the spleen and liver. Splenomegaly is clinically evident 50% of the time and is demonstrated radiologically 100% of the time. Difficulty in detecting splenomegaly with physical examination contributes to the underestimation of actual enlargement. Splenic rupture is rare (only 0.1% to 0.5% of all cases) and can occur spontaneously as a result of mild trauma, arising primarily in men younger than 25 years of age and between days 4 and 21 after the onset of symptoms. It is the most common cause of death related to IM. Other causes of fatalities are hepatic failure, extensive bacterial infection, or viral myocarditis. Other organ systems are rarely involved, but such involvement may be present with characteristic manifestations, such as fulminant hepatitis with jaundice and anemia, encephalitis, meningitis, Guillain-Barré syndrome, and Bell palsy. Eye manifestations may include eyelid and periorbital edema, dry eyes, keratitis, uveitis, and conjunctivitis. Reye syndrome has been known to develop in children with EBV infection.

Pulmonary and respiratory failure has been documented, but is more likely to occur in immunocompromised individuals. Approximately 3% to 10% of adults older than 40 years of age have never been infected with EBV and are susceptible to IM later in life. In these individuals, the classic symptoms are not generally present, making diagnosis more difficult.

EVALUATION AND TREATMENT The blood of affected individuals contains an increased number of white blood cells with many atypical forms. The diagnosis of IM depends on the following specific findings: (1) an increase in the number of lymphocytes, commonly based on Hoagland criteria of at least 50% lymphocytes and at least 10% atypical lymphocytes in the blood; (2) a positive heterophile antibody reaction (Monospot test, see following text); and (3) a rising titer of specific antibodies for EBV antigens. Heterophilic antibodies are a heterogeneous group of IgM antibodies that are agglutinins against nonhuman red blood cells (e.g., horse, sheep) and are detected by qualitative (Monospot) or quantitative (heterophile antibody test) methods. Use of the Monospot test is limited because other infections (e.g., CMV, adenovirus) and toxoplasmosis also produce heterophilic antibodies. Thus 5% to 15% of Monospot tests yield false-positive results. Heterophilic antibodies in the blood increase as the condition progresses, although some individuals and children younger than 4 years of age do not produce them. Diagnosis of EBV infection specifically may be increased with newer viral-specific tests that identify EBV-specific antibodies.

Treatment is supportive and consists of rest and alleviation of symptoms with analgesics and antipyretics. Aspirin is avoided with children because of its association with Reye syndrome. Streptococcal pharyngitis, which occurs in 20% to 30% of cases, is treated with penicillin or erythromycin, not ampicillin—ampicillin is known to cause a rash. Bed rest with avoidance of strenuous activity and contact sports is indicated. Steroids are used when severe complications, such as impending airway obstruction, or other organ involvement (central nervous system [CNS] manifestations, thrombocytopenic purpura, myocarditis, pericarditis) is evident. Acyclovir has been used in immunocompromised individuals but is not considered standard therapy. In the rare event of splenic rupture, the treatment has been removal of the spleen and continues to be the choice in hemodynamically unstable individuals. Current research, however, is suggesting that it may be better to repair the spleen to avoid overwhelming postsplenectomy infection (OPSI).

QUICK CHECK 21-2

1. What condition is manifested chiefly by an increase in the numbers of circulating granulocytes and monocytes?
2. What is the cause of infectious mononucleosis (IM)?
3. What are the classic symptoms of IM?

Leukemias

Leukemia is a clonal malignant disorder of the bone marrow and usually, but not always, of the blood. The common pathologic feature of all forms of leukemia is an uncontrolled proliferation of malignant leukocytes, causing an overcrowding of bone marrow and decreased production and function of normal hematopoietic cells. Chromosomal abnormalities and translocations are common in the majority of leukemias. When genes become mutated, they create genomic aberrations that block cell maturation and activate pro–growth signaling pathways that prevent apoptotic cell death.

The classification of leukemia is based on (1) the predominant cell of origin (either myeloid or lymphoid) and (2) the rate of progression, which usually reflects the degree at which cell differentiation was arrested when the cell became malignant (acute or chronic) (Figure 21-6). Acute leukemia is characterized by undifferentiated or immature cells, usually a blast cell. The onset of disease is abrupt and rapid. Without treatment, disease progression results in a short survival time. In chronic leukemia, the predominant cell is more differentiated but does not function normally, with a relatively slow progression. There are four types of leukemia: acute lymphocytic (ALL), acute myelogenous (AML), chronic lymphocytic (CLL), and chronic myelogenous (CML).[27-29] Further classification of acute leukemias is based on characteristics that may provide significant therapeutic prognostic information, such as structure, number of cells, genetics, identification of surface markers, and histochemical staining (see Figure 21-6).

Leukemia occurs with varying frequencies at different ages and is more common in adults than in children. It is estimated that more than 52,380 cases of leukemia were newly diagnosed in 2014, with males having a slightly higher incidence than females (Table 21-5). Leukemia accounts for about 34% of all childhood cancers; ALL accounts for almost 78% of all new cases of leukemia in children. CLL and AML are the most common types in adults. CML is found mostly in adults.

Over the past 2 decades, the rates of induced remission and survival in most forms of leukemia have increased. Current survival rates range from 24% for AML to 81% for CLL, and as high as 91% for children and adolescents younger than 15 years of age with ALL.[30]

PATHOPHYSIOLOGY Although the exact cause of leukemia is unknown, several risk factors and related genetic aberrations are associated with the onset of malignancy. The leukemias are clonal disorders driven by genetically abnormal stem-like cancer cells (SLCCs).[31] Abnormal immature white blood cells, called blasts, fill the bone marrow and spill into the blood. The leukemia blasts literally "crowd out" the marrow and cause cellular proliferation of the other cell lines to cease. Normal granulocytic-monocytic, lymphocytic, erythrocytic, and megakaryocytic progenitor cells cease to function, resulting in pancytopenia (a reduction in all cellular components of the blood). Almost 90% of ALLs have chromosomal changes that correlate with immunophenotyping and sometimes confer prognostic significance. Several genetic translocations (mitotic errors) are observed in leukemic cells. One of these translocations, the Philadelphia chromosome, is observed in 95% of those with CML and 30% of adults with ALL (Figure 21-7). The Philadelphia chromosome results from a reciprocal translocation between the long arms of chromosomes 9 and 22. A unique protein (bcr-abl protein) is encoded from two genes (BCR from chromosome 22 and ABL from chromosome 9) artificially linked at the junction of translocation. The bcr-abl protein affects a variety of cell cycle control genes, leading to an increased rate of cellular division, inhibition of DNA repair, and other dysregulations of cell growth. Over time the original tumor becomes genetically unstable and diverse.

Risk factors for the onset of leukemia include environmental factors as well as other diseases. Increased risk for ALL has been linked to exposure to x-rays before birth, being exposed to ionizing radiation (postnatally), past treatment with chemotherapy, and certain genetic conditions including Down syndrome, neurofibromatosis type 1(NF1), Schwachman syndrome, Bloom syndrome, and ataxia telangiectasia. There is growing concern about the effect of low-dose radiation on subsequent risk of leukemia.[32] There is a statistically significant tendency for leukemia to reappear in families. A unique characteristic of ALL, unlike other forms, is that ALL develops at different rates in different geographic locations, although the reason for this is unclear. Individuals in developed countries and in higher socioeconomic categories have an increased incidence of ALL. Acute leukemia also may

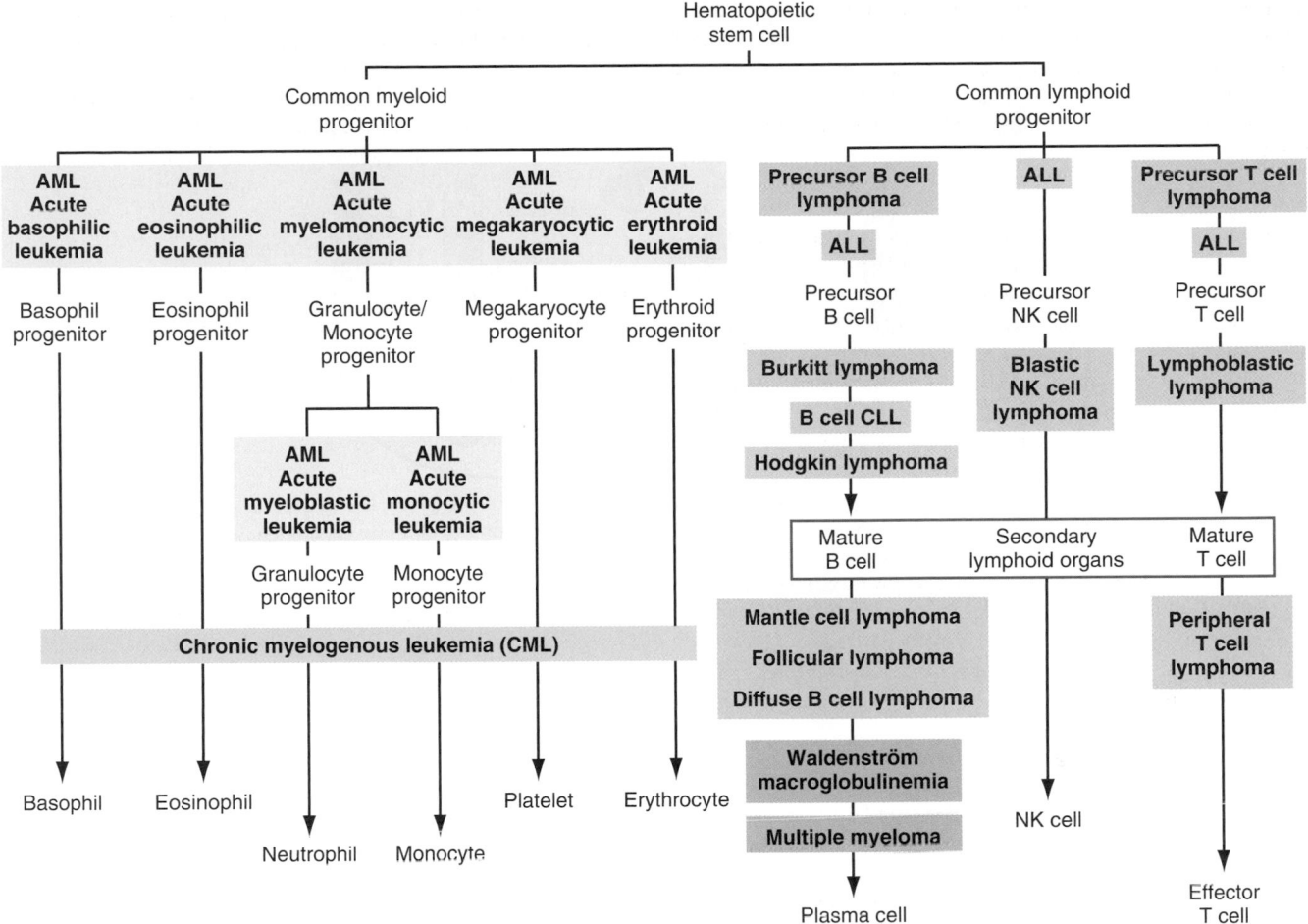

FIGURE 21-6 Origins of Leukemias and Lymphomas. Differentiation pathways of blood-forming cells and reported sites from which specific leukemias and lymphomas originate. Tumors of similar types are given the same background coloring. *ALL*, Acute lymphocytic leukemia; *AML*, acute myelogenous leukemia; *CLL*, chronic lymphocytic leukemia; *CML*, chronic myelogenous leukemia; *NK*, natural killer.

TABLE 21-5 Estimated New Cases and Deaths from Leukemia in the United States—2014

Types of Leukemia	TOTAL NEW CASES (Proportion of New Cases)	NEW CASES BY GENDER		DEATHS BY GENDER	
		Male	Female	Male	Female
All types	52,380 (100%)	30,100	22,280	14,040	10,050
Acute lymphocytic leukemia	6020 (12%)	3140	2880	810	630
Chronic lymphocytic leukemia	15,720 (30%)	9100	6620	2800	1800
Acute myelogenous leukemia	18,860 (36%)	11,530	7330	6010	4450
Chronic myelogenous leukemia	5980 (11%)	3130	2850	550	260
Other	5800 (11%)	3200	2600	3870	2910

Data from American Cancer Society: *Cancer facts and figures—2015*, Atlanta, 2015, The Society.

develop secondary to certain acquired disorders, including CML, CLL, polycythemia vera, myelofibrosis, Hodgkin lymphoma, multiple myeloma, ovarian cancer, and sideroblastic anemia.

Potential risk factors for AML include smoking, previous chemotherapy, and exposure to ionizing radiation. AML is the most frequently reported secondary cancer after high doses of chemotherapy for Hodgkin lymphoma, non-Hodgkin lymphoma, multiple myeloma, ovarian cancer, and breast cancer.

Acute leukemias. Acute leukemias include two types: acute lymphocytic leukemia (ALL) and acute myelogenous leukemia (AML).[32]

ALL is an aggressive, fast growing leukemia with too many lymphoblasts or immature white blood cells found in blood and bone marrow. It also is called *acute lymphoblastic leukemia*. AML is an aggressive fast growing leukemia with too many myeloblasts or immature white blood cells that are not lymphoblasts found in the bone marrow and blood. It also is called *acute myeloblastic leukemia, acute myeloid leukemia,* and *acute nonlymphocytic leukemia (ANLL)*. Acute leukemias are seen in both genders and in all ages with the incidence increasing dramatically in individuals older than 50 years. North American and Scandinavian countries have the highest mortality; Eastern European countries, Asia

FIGURE 21-7 Philadelphia Chromosome. A piece of chromosome 9 and a piece of chromosome 22 break off and trade places. The *bcr-abl* gene is formed on chromosome 22 where the piece of chromosome 9 attaches. The changed chromosome 22 is called Philadelphia chromosome. (Adapted from National Cancer Institute: *Childhood acute lymphoblastic leukemia treatment,* Bethesda, Md, 2014, National Institutes of Health.)

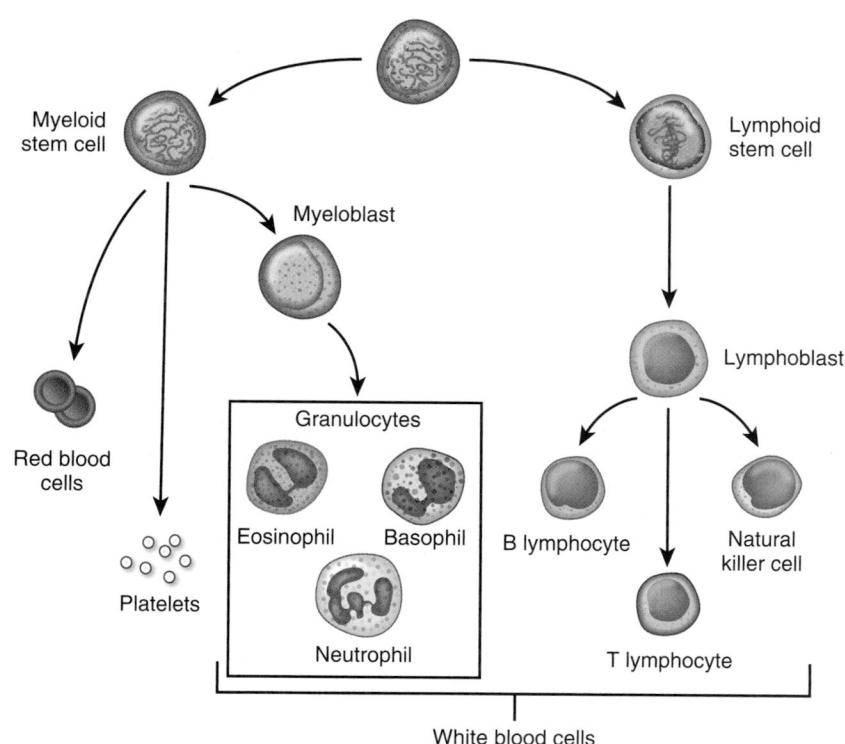

FIGURE 21-8 Leukemia Arises from Stem-like Cells. A blood stem cell undergoes multiple steps to finally become a red blood cell, platelet, or white blood cell. (Modified from National Cancer Institute: *Adult acute lymphoblastic leukemia treatment (PDQ®),* Bethesda, Md, 2014, Author. Available at: www.cancer.gov/cancertopics/pdq/treatment/adultALL/HealthProfessional. Accessed January 9, 2015.)

(except Japan), and Central America have the lowest mortality. Japan's higher mortality is the result of the atomic bombs dropped in World War II. Blacks have consistently shown a lower mortality than whites. More than 6020 new cases of ALL and 18,860 new cases of AML are estimated in 2014, with more than 1440 deaths from ALL and 10,460 deaths from AML.[33] As mentioned earlier, risk factors for ALL include being exposed to x-rays before birth, exposure to ionizing radiation (postnatal), and past treatment with chemotherapy.

PATHOPHYSIOLOGY ALL presumably progresses from malignant transformation of B- or C-cell progenitor cells (like a stem cell) (Figure 21-8). Most cases of ALL occur in children and often in the first decade.

TABLE 21-6 Clinical Manifestations and Related Pathophysiology in Leukemia

Clinical Manifestations	Laboratory Abnormalities	Cause	Comments
Anemia	Relative *proportion* of erythroblasts to total count (decreased in anemia) is key	Decreased stem cell input or ineffective erythropoiesis, or both	In acute leukemia, anemia is usually present from beginning, often first symptom noticed, and severe; mild form without symptoms is common in CML and CLL; hemorrhage common in acute forms, occasional in CML, but rare in CLL
Bleeding (purpura, petechiae, ecchymosis, hemorrhage)	Decreased and possibly abnormal platelets	Reduction in megakaryocytes leading to thrombocytopenia	Bleeding more common in acute than in chronic leukemia
Infection	Increased multisegmented neutrophils	Opportunistic organisms; decreased protection resulting from granulocytopenia or immune deficiency secondary to chemotherapy, corticosteroids, and disease process	Major sites of infection: oral cavity, throat, lower colon, urinary tract, lungs, and skin; prevention of infection focuses on restoring host defenses, decreasing invasive procedures, and reducing colonization of organisms
Weight loss	Decreased 24-hr urinary creatinine excretion; hypoalbuminemia	Condition can be attributed to pain, depression, chemotherapy, radiation therapy, loss of appetite, and alterations in taste	Severe weight loss may be related to excess production of TNF-α
Bone pain	Often no radiographic evidence of bone problems	Result of bone infiltration by leukemic cells or intramedullary infection	If combination drug regimens are ineffective, radiation therapy is used
Liver, spleen, and lymph node enlargement	Biopsy abnormal for liver and spleen	Leukemic cell infiltration	Lymph nodes also undergo leukemia proliferation in CLL
Elevated uric acid level	Normal excretion of uric acid is 300-500 mg/day; leukemic individual can excrete 50 times more	Increased catabolism of protein and nucleic acid; urate precipitation increased from dehydration caused by anorexia or fever and drug therapy	Hyperuricemia is present in both acute leukemia and CML; treatment focuses on increasing urine pH or decreasing acid production with drug allopurinol

CLL, Chronic lymphocytic leukemia; *CMA,* chronic myelocytic leukemia; *RBC,* red blood cell.

Although adults account for about 20% of all cases, their mortality rate is significantly higher. The significant difference between the incidence of ALL in adults and children may be because of differences in the biology of the disease. Approximately 75% of ALL cases in children originate from transformed precursor B cells, whereas adult ALL is a mixture of cancers of precursor B-cell or precursor T-cell origin. Precursor B-cell ALL can be further divided into different phenotypes depending on their progression through the B-cell maturation process. The T-cell lineage ALL is distinguished by T-cell–associated markers.

B-cell ALL is strongly associated with aneuploidy of various types, with more than 50 chromosomes. T-cell ALL generally has fewer cytogenetic abnormalities, and the majority have genetic deletions. Several other translocations are commonly observed in ALL, including the Philadelphia chromosome (discussed earlier) and translocations involving the *ETV6* (formerly *TEL*) and *MLL* genes.

AML is the most common adult leukemia; the mean age of diagnosis is 67 years of age. AML results from an abnormal proliferation of myeloid precursor cells, a decreased rate of apoptosis, and an arrest in cellular differentiation. Therefore the bone marrow and peripheral blood are characterized by leukocytosis and a predominance of blast cells. As these immature blast cells increase, they replace normal myelocytic cells, megakaryocytes, and erythrocytes. This displacement can lead to complications of bleeding, anemia, and infection. Several hereditary conditions are known to increase the risk for AML (e.g., Down syndrome, Fanconi aplastic anemia, Bloom syndrome, and others). More than 150 structural chromosomal abnormalities and several duplications or deletions within genes have been identified in

AML. Although ALL and AML are clinically very similar they are genetically and immunologically distinct.[34]

CLINICAL MANIFESTATIONS Within days to a few weeks of the first symptoms is an abrupt stormy onset, which is more prevalent in ALL. The clinical manifestations of all varieties of acute leukemia are generally similar. Mechanisms associated with common manifestations are summarized in Table 21-6. Signs and symptoms related to bone marrow depression include fatigue caused by anemia, bleeding resulting from thrombocytopenia, and fever caused by infection. Bleeding may occur in the skin, gums, mucous membranes, and GI tract. Visible signs include petechiae and ecchymosis, as well as discoloration of the skin, gingival bleeding, hematuria, and midcycle or heavy menstrual bleeding.

Infection sites include the mouth, throat, respiratory tract, lower colon, urinary tract, and skin and may be caused by gram-negative bacilli (*Escherichia coli*), *Pseudomonas aeruginosa*, and *Klebsiella pneumoniae*. Fever is an early sign often accompanied by chills.

Anorexia is accompanied by weight loss, diminished sensitivity to sour and sweet tastes, wasting of muscle, and difficulty swallowing. Liver, spleen, and lymph node enlargement occurs more commonly in ALL than in AML. Liver and spleen enlargement commonly occur together. The leukemic individual often experiences abdominal pain and tenderness. Pain in the bones and joints is thought to result from leukemia infiltration with secondary stretching of the periosteum.

Neurologic manifestations are common and may be caused by either leukemic infiltration or cerebral bleeding. Headache, vomiting, papilledema, facial palsy, blurred vision, auditory disturbances, and meningeal irritation can occur if leukemic cells infiltrate the cerebral or spinal meninges.

EVALUATION AND TREATMENT Because leukemia often is confused with other conditions, early detection may be difficult. Persistent symptoms need intensive medical investigation. The diagnosis is made through blood tests and examination of bone marrow.

Chemotherapy, used in various combinations, is the treatment of choice for leukemia. Supportive measures include blood transfusions, antibiotics, antifungals, and antivirals. Allopurinol is used to prevent uric acid production and elevation that occurs because of cellular death caused by treatment. Stem cell transplantation is now considered standard therapy for selected individuals with leukemia.

Advances in the treatment of AML have substantially improved the complete remission (CR) rates.[35] Attainment of complete remission requires fairly aggressive treatment. With appropriate induction therapy, approximately 60% to 70% of adults with AML will attain CR status. More than 25% of adults with AML (about 45% of those who attain CR) are expected to survive 3 or more years and may be cured.[35] Since the 1970s, 5-year survival rates for those with ALL have increased from 38% to 66% for adults and from 53% to 91% for children. Factors influencing increased survival rate include the use of combined and multimodality treatment methods; improved supportive services, such as blood banking and nutritional support; and antimicrobial treatment. The presence of the Philadelphia chromosome (observed in about 5% of children with ALL, in 30% of adults with ALL, and occasionally in AML) is a poor prognostic indicator.

Myelosuppression is both a consequence of leukemia and a treatment for the disease. Hematologic support with blood products and granulocyte colony-stimulating factor (G-CSF) or granulocyte-macrophage colony-stimulating factor (GM-CSF) has effectively shortened the time of neutropenia and improved survival by reducing the risk for infection.

Chronic leukemias. The two main types of chronic leukemia are (1) **chronic myelogenous leukemia (CML)** and (2) **chronic lymphocytic leukemia (CLL)**. CML is also called *chronic granulocytic leukemia* and *chronic myeloid leukemia*. Several forms of CML can occur, depending on the lineage of the malignant cells (e.g., chronic neutrophilic leukemia [CNL], chronic eosinophilic leukemia [CEL]). CML is a slowly progressing disease with too many blood cells (not lymphocytes) made in the bone marrow. CLL is a slow-growing cancer in which too many immature lymphocytes (white blood cells) are found mostly in the blood and bone marrow. Cancer cells also may be found in lymphoid tissues. In later stages of the disease, cancer cells are sometimes found in the lymph nodes and the disease is called **small lymphocytic lymphoma (SLL; also known as CLL/SLL)**. SLL cancer cells are found mostly in the lymph nodes; CLL/SLL also is classified as a non-Hodgkin lymphoma. In adults, CLL is the most common leukemia in the Western world.[34] Individuals with chronic leukemia have a longer life expectancy, usually extending several years from the time of diagnosis.

The chronic leukemias account for the majority of cases in adults (see Table 21-5). The incidences of CLL and CML increase significantly in individuals more than 40 years of age, with prevalence in the sixth through eighth decades. CML is one of a group of diseases called **myeloproliferative disorders**—acquired abnormalities in signaling pathways that lead to growth factor–independent proliferation—which also include polycythemia vera, primary thrombocytosis, and idiopathic myelofibrosis (invasion of bone marrow by fibrous tissue).

PATHOPHYSIOLOGY Chronic myelogenous leukemia (CML) is characterized from other myeloproliferative disorders by the presence of a

FIGURE 21-9 Pathogenesis of Chronic Myeloid Leukemia. The breakage and joining of *BCR* and *ABL* creates the chimeric fusion gene *BCR-ABL*. *BCR-ABL* genetically encodes an active BCR-ABL intracellular tyrosine kinase (an enzyme that controls intracellular "on-off" switches). The ABL kinase in turn induces signaling through the same pro-growth and pro-survival pathways that are activated by normal hematologic growth factors. Altogether the activation of many downstream pathways drives growth factor–independent proliferation and survival of bone marrow progenitors. (From Kumar V et al: *Robbins & Cotran pathologic basis of disease,* ed 9, St Louis, 2015, Elsevier.)

chimeric (genetically distinct cells) *BCR-ABL* fusion gene derived from parts of the *BCR* gene on chromosome 22 and parts of the *ABL* gene on chromosome 9 (Figure 21-9).[34] In the majority of cases (i.e., over 90%), *BCR-ABL* is created by a reciprocal translocation of chromosomes (9;22) called the *Philadelphia chromosome* (see Figure 21-7). In the rest of the cases, the *BCR-ABL* fusion gene is made from complex genetic rearrangements and the cell of origin is a hematopoietic stem cell.[34] The *BCR-ABL* gene causes abnormal cell signaling resulting in pro–growth and pro–survival pathways of the leukemic cells. Much is still unknown about these cell-signaling abnormalities and why the *BCR-ABL* fusion gene preferentially drives proliferation of granulocytic and megakaryocytic blood cells. The only known cause of CML is exposure to ionizing radiation.

Chronic lymphocytic leukemia (CLL) involves transformation and progressive accumulation of monoclonal B lymphocytes; rarely (less than 5%) are CLL malignancies of T-cell origin. CLL is derived from a transformation of a partially mature B cell that has not yet encountered antigen. Investigations from the past 2 decades have classified CLL and predicted the outcome based on the immunoglobulin heavy chain variable region (IGHV) gene mutational status. Recent studies are addressing five epigenetic biomarkers to classify CLL, which could result in the use of more targeted therapies for specific subgroups.[36] Additionally, investigators report novel recurrent mutations in CLL, including *SF3B1* and *TP53* mutations, that are independent of *IGHV* mutational status, demanding the need for urgent standardization of detection methods.[37] The notch 1 (*NOTCH1*) gene also has been found recurrently mutated in a subset of individuals, not independent of *IGHV*, and these individuals had a shorter survival.[38] Chromosomal translocations (breakpoints) are rare in CLL. The cause of CLL is unknown.

CLINICAL MANIFESTATIONS   Chronic leukemia advances slowly and insidiously. Approximately 70% of individuals with CLL are asymptomatic at the time of diagnosis. When symptoms do appear, the most common finding is lymphadenopathy. The most significant effect of CLL is suppression of humoral immunity and increased infection with encapsulated bacteria. Frequently, the level of neutrophils is depressed, which adds to the risk of infection. Invasion of most organ cells is uncommon but infiltration does occur in lymph nodes, liver, spleen, and salivary glands. Central nervous system (CNS) involvement is rare. Approximately 10% of individuals develop a more aggressive malignancy, usually a diffuse large B-cell lymphoma. In these individuals, extreme fatigue, weight loss, night sweats, low-grade fever, elevated levels of the enzyme lactic dehydrogenase, hypercalcemia, anemia, and thrombocytopenia are common.

Individuals with CML may progress through three phases of the disease: a chronic phase lasting 2 to 5 years during which symptoms may not be apparent, an accelerated phase of 6 to 18 months during which the primary symptoms develop, and a terminal blast phase ("blast crisis") with a survival of only 3 to 6 months. The accelerated phase is characterized by excessive proliferation and accumulation of malignant cells. Splenomegaly is prominent and becomes painful, but lymphadenopathy generally is not present. Liver enlargement also occurs, but liver function is rarely altered. Hyperuricemia is common and produces gouty arthritis. Infections, fever, and weight loss also are seen often. The terminal blast phase is characterized by rapid and progressive leukocytosis with an increase in basophils. In the later stages of the terminal phase, which then resembles AML, blast cells or promyelocytes predominate, and the individual experiences a "blast crisis."

The acute effects of CML resemble those of acute leukemia but with more prominent and painful splenomegaly. Liver function rarely is altered despite enlargement, and lymphadenopathy generally is found only in the acute phase of the disease. Hyperuricemia invariably is present and produces gouty arthritis. Infections, fever, and weight loss are common findings in individuals with CML.

EVALUATION AND TREATMENT   Diagnosis of chronic leukemia depends on laboratory analyses of peripheral blood and bone marrow. Diagnosis of CLL is based on detection of a monoclonal B-cell lymphocytosis in the blood. The cells must have the characteristic immunophenotype (CD5+, and CD23-positive B cells) at levels in excess of 5000 cells/μL over a sustained period of time (usually 4 weeks). Confusion with other diseases may be avoided by determination of cell surface markers. CLL lymphocytes co-express the B-cell antigens CD19 and CD20 along with the T-cell antigen CD5.[39] This co-expression only occurs in one other disease entity, mantle cell lymphoma.[39] Bone marrow may contain more than 30% lymphocytes and be normocellular or hypercellular. As assays have become more sensitive for detecting monoclonal B-CLL-like cells in peripheral blood, researchers have detected a monoclonal B-cell lymphocytosis (MBL) in 3% of adults older than 40 years and in 6% of adults older than 60 years.[40] Such early detection and diagnosis may falsely suggest improved survival for

the group and may unnecessarily worry or result in therapy for some individuals who would have remained undiagnosed in their lifetime, a circumstance known in the literature as overdiagnosis or pseudodisease.[39,41]

Treatment of CLL ranges from periodic observation with treatment of infection, hemorrhage, or immunologic complications to a variety of options including steroids, alkylating agents, purine analog drugs, combination chemotherapy, monoclonal antibodies, and transplant options.[39] For individuals with progressing CLL, treatment with conventional doses of chemotherapy is not curative; selected individuals treated with allogeneic stem cell transplantation have achieved prolonged disease-free survival.[39] Antileukemic therapy is frequently unnecessary in uncomplicated early disease.[39] From older clinical trials (1970s through the 1990s), the median survival for all individuals ranges from 8 to 12 years.[39] However, a large variation in survival exists, ranging from several months to a normal life expectancy. Treatment must be individualized based on the clinical behavior of the disease.[39] Ongoing clinical trials are testing the concept of T cells directed at specific antigen targets with engineered chimeric antigen receptors.[39] Complications of pancytopenia, including hemorrhage and infection, are a major cause of death for these individuals.

The development and introduction of the tyrosine kinase inhibitor imatinib mesylate (Gleevec) as a treatment modality have changed current management of CML. Imatinib mesylate is highly specific for CML and suppression of BCR-ABL kinase activity and produces a complete cytogenetic response in more than 80% of newly diagnosed persons. Although the *BCR-ABL* inhibitors markedly decrease the number of *BCR-ABL*–positive cells in the marrow and other places, they do not extinguish the CML stem cell, which persists at low levels.[34]

✔ QUICK CHECK 21-3

1. How are leukemias classified?
2. What is the pathogenesis of ALL?
3. What is the significance of the Philadelphia chromosome, and how is it related to leukemia?

ALTERATIONS OF LYMPHOID FUNCTION

Lymphadenopathy

Lymphadenopathy is characterized by enlarged lymph nodes (Figure 21-10). Lymph node enlargement occurs because of an increase in the size and number of its germinal centers caused by proliferation of lymphocytes and monocytes (immature phagocytes) or invasion by malignant cells. Normally, lymph nodes are not palpable or are barely palpable. Enlarged lymph nodes are characterized by being palpable and often also may be tender or painful to touch, although not in all situations.

Localized lymphadenopathy usually indicates drainage of an area associated with an inflammatory process or infection (reactive lymph node). *Generalized lymphadenopathy* occurs less often and is generally seen in the presence of malignant or nonmalignant disease, particularly in adults. Palpable nodes, however, do not always indicate serious disease and may indicate a minor trauma or infection. The location and size of the enlarged nodes are important factors in diagnosing the cause of the lymphadenopathy, as are the individual's age, gender, and geographic location. Generalized lymphadenopathy occurs with non-Hodgkin lymphomas, chronic lymphocytic leukemia, histiocytosis, and disorders that produce lymphocytosis. In general, lymphadenopathy results from four types of conditions: (1) neoplastic disease, (2) immunologic or inflammatory conditions, (3) endocrine disorders, or

FIGURE 21-10 Lymphadenopathy. Individual with lymphocyte leukemia with extreme but symmetric lymphadenopathy. (Courtesy Dr. A.R. Kagan, Los Angeles. From del Regato JA et al: *Cancer: diagnosis, treatment, and prognosis,* ed 6, St Louis, 1985, Mosby.)

(4) lipid storage diseases. Diseases of unknown cause, including autoimmune diseases and reactions to drugs, also may lead to generalized lymphadenopathy.

Malignant Lymphomas

Lymphomas consist of a diverse group of neoplasms that develop from the proliferation of malignant lymphocytes in the lymphoid system (immune system). European and American pathologists have proposed a new classification for lymphoid malignancies—the Revised European American Lymphoma (REAL) classification. The World Health Organization (WHO) modification of the REAL classification recognizes three major categories of lymphoid malignancies based on morphology and cell lineage: (1) B-cell neoplasms; (2) T-cell/natural killer (NK)–cell neoplasms; and (3) Hodgkin lymphoma (Box 21-2); two *basic* categories of lymphomas are Hodgkin lymphoma and non-Hodgkin lymphoma. Non-Hodgkin lymphoma can be further divided into cancers that have an *indolent* or slow-growing course and those with an *aggressive* or fast-growing course. These different subtypes progress and respond to treatment differently. Both Hodgkin lymphoma and non-Hodgkin lymphoma occur in children and adults and the overall treatment and prognosis depend on the stage and type of lymphoma.

Lymphoma is the most common blood cancer in the United States. Incidence rates of lymphoma differ with respect to age, gender, geographic location, and socioeconomic class. The estimated new cases of lymphoma include 9190 cases of Hodgkin lymphoma and 70,800 cases of non-Hodgkin lymphoma. It was estimated in 2014 that 18,990 will

die from non-Hodgkin lymphoma and 1180 from Hodgkin lymphoma. Since the early 1970s, the incidence of non-Hodgkin lymphoma has nearly doubled. The exact reason for this increase remains a mystery; however, a modest portion of the increase had been attributed to lymphomas developing in association with immune deficiencies, including AIDS and organ transplants. Conversely, the incidence of Hodgkin lymphoma has declined over the same time period, especially among older adults.

In general, lymphomas are the result of genetic mutations or viral infection. Malignant transformation produces a cell with uncontrolled and excessive growth that accumulates in the lymph nodes and other sites, producing tumor masses.

BOX 21-2 Updated REAL/WHO Classification

B-Cell Neoplasms

1. Precursor B cell: precursor B-acute lymphoblastic leukemia/lymphoblastic lymphoma (LBL)
2. Peripheral B-cell neoplasms
   a. B-cell CLL/small lymphocytic lymphoma
   b. B-cell prolymphocytic leukemia
   c. Lymphoplasmacytic lymphoma/immunocytoma
   d. Mantle cell lymphoma
   e. Follicular lymphoma
   f. Extranodal marginal zone B-cell lymphoma of mucosa-associated lymphatic tissue (MALT) type
   g. Nodal marginal zone B-cell lymphoma (± monocytoid B cell)
   h. Splenic marginal zone lymphoma (± villous lymphocytes)
   i. Hairy cell leukemia
   j. Plasmacytoma/plasma cell myeloma
   k. Diffuse large B-cell lymphoma
   l. Burkitt lymphoma

T-Cell and Putative NK-Cell Neoplasms

1. Precursor T-cell neoplasm: precursor T-cell acute lymphoblastic leukemia/LBL
2. Peripheral T-cell and NK-cell neoplasms
   a. T-cell CLL/prolymphocytic leukemia
   b. T-cell granular lymphocytic leukemia
   c. Mycosis fungoides/Sézary syndrome
   d. Peripheral T-cell lymphoma, not otherwise characterized
   e. Hepatosplenic gamma/delta T-cell lymphoma
   f. Subcutaneous panniculitis-like T-cell lymphoma
   g. Angioimmunoblastic T-cell lymphoma
   h. Extranodal T-/NK-cell lymphoma, nasal type
   i. Enteropathy-type intestinal T-cell lymphoma
   j. Adult T-cell lymphoma/leukemia (human T-lymphotrophic virus type 1 [HTLV-1])
   k. Anaplastic large cell lymphoma, primary systemic type
   l. Anaplastic large cell lymphoma, primary cutaneous type
   m. Aggressive NK-cell leukemia

Hodgkin Lymphoma

1. Nodular lymphocyte-predominant Hodgkin lymphoma
2. Classic Hodgkin lymphoma
   a. Nodular sclerosis Hodgkin lymphoma
   b. Lymphocyte-rich classic Hodgkin lymphoma
   c. Mixed cellularity Hodgkin lymphoma
   d. Lymphocyte-depleted Hodgkin lymphoma

FIGURE 21-11 Lymph Nodes. Diagnostic Reed-Sternberg cell *(arrow)*. A large multinucleated or multilobed cell with inclusion body–like nucleoli surrounded by a halo of clear nucleoplasm. (From Damjanov I, Linder J, editors, *Anderson's pathology,* ed 10, St Louis, 1996, Mosby.)

FIGURE 21-12 Hodgkin Lymphoma and Enlarged Cervical Lymph Node. Typical enlarged cervical lymph node in the neck *(arrow)* of a 35-year-old woman with Hodgkin lymphoma. (From del Regato JA et al: *Cancer: diagnosis, treatment, and prognosis,* ed 6, St Louis, 1985, Mosby.)

Hodgkin Lymphoma

Hodgkin lymphoma (HL) is a malignant lymphoma that progresses from one group of lymph nodes to another, including the development of systemic symptoms, and the presence of B cells called Reed-Sternberg (RS) cells.[42,43] (see Pathophysiology). In about 70% of cases, RS cells are infected with EBV. The incidence of HL is approximately 3.1/100,000 males and 2.4/100,000 females and peaks at two different times—during the second and third decades of life and later during the sixth and seventh decades. The incidence is greater in whites than in blacks, with Denmark, the Netherlands, and the United States having the highest incidence and Japan and Australia having the lowest.

PATHOPHYSIOLOGY   It is widely accepted that the Reed-Sternberg (RS) cell represents the malignant transformed lymphocyte (Figure 21-11). The RS cells are often large and binucleate with occasional mononuclear variants. The RS cells are necessary for the diagnosis of HL; however, they are not specific to HL. In rare instances, cells resembling RS cells can be found in benign illnesses, as well as in other forms of cancer, including non-Hodgkin lymphomas and solid tissue cancers and in infectious mononucleosis.

The triggering mechanism for the malignant transformation of cells remains unknown. Classic HL appears to be derived from a B cell in the germinal center that has not undergone successful immunoglobulin gene rearrangement (see Chapter 7) and would normally be induced to undergo apoptosis. Survival of this cell may be linked to infection with Epstein-Barr virus (EBV). Laboratory and epidemiologic studies have linked HL with EBV infections, and EBV DNA, RNA, and proteins are frequently observed in HL cells.[44] The EBV epigenome poses a variety of viral-encoded and host-cell factors that control epigenetic regulation by expanding tissue growth, evading immune detection, and driving host-cell carcinogenesis. The RS cells secrete and release cytokines (e.g., interleukin-10 [IL-10], transforming growth factor-beta [TGF-β]) that result in the accumulation of inflammatory cells, which produces the local and systemic effects. HL is subcategorized into two main types: classic Hodgkin and nodular lymphocyte–predominant Hodgkin. Classic HL is subclassified into four types (see Box 21-2) based on the morphology of RS cells and the characteristics of the inflammatory cell infiltrate in the tumor. Lymphocyte-predominant

disease presents with earlier-stage disease, longer survival, and fewer treatment failures than classic HL.[45] However, despite a more favorable prognosis, lymphocyte-predominant HL has a tendency to histologically transform into diffuse large B-cell lymphoma by 10 years in approximately 10% of people.[46]

CLINICAL MANIFESTATIONS   Many clinical features of HL can be explained by the complex action of cytokines and other growth factors that are secreted and released by the malignant cells. These substances induce infiltration and proliferation of inflammatory cells, resulting in an enlarged, painless lymph node in the neck (often the first sign of HL) (Figure 21-12). The discovery of an asymptomatic mediastinal mass on routine chest x-ray is not uncommon. The cervical, axillary, inguinal, and retroperitoneal lymph nodes are commonly affected in HL (Figure 21-13). Local symptoms caused by pressure and obstruction of the lymph nodes are the result of the lymphadenopathy.

About one third of individuals will have some common systemic symptoms, such as intermittent fever, without other symptoms of infection, drenching night sweats, itchy skin (pruritus), and fatigue. These constitutional symptoms accompanied by weight loss are associated with a poor prognosis.

Although HL rarely arises in the lung, mediastinal and hilar node adenopathy can cause secondary involvement of the trachea, bronchi, pleura, or lungs. Retroperitoneal nodes can involve vertebral bodies and nerves and also can cause displacement of ureters. Spinal cord involvement is more common in the dorsal and lumbar regions than in the cervical region. Skin lesions, although uncommon, include psoriasis and eczematoid lesions, causing itching and scratching.

As a result of direct invasion from mediastinal lymph nodes, pericardial involvement can cause pericardial friction rub, pericardial effusion, and engorgement of neck veins. The GI tract and urinary tract are rarely involved. Anemia is often found in individuals with HL accompanied by a low serum iron level and reduced iron-binding capacity. Other laboratory findings include elevated sedimentation rate, leukocytosis, and eosinophilia. Leukopenia occurs in advanced stages of HL.

Splenic involvement in HL depends on histologic type. In mixed cellularity and lymphocytic deletion types of HL, the spleen is involved

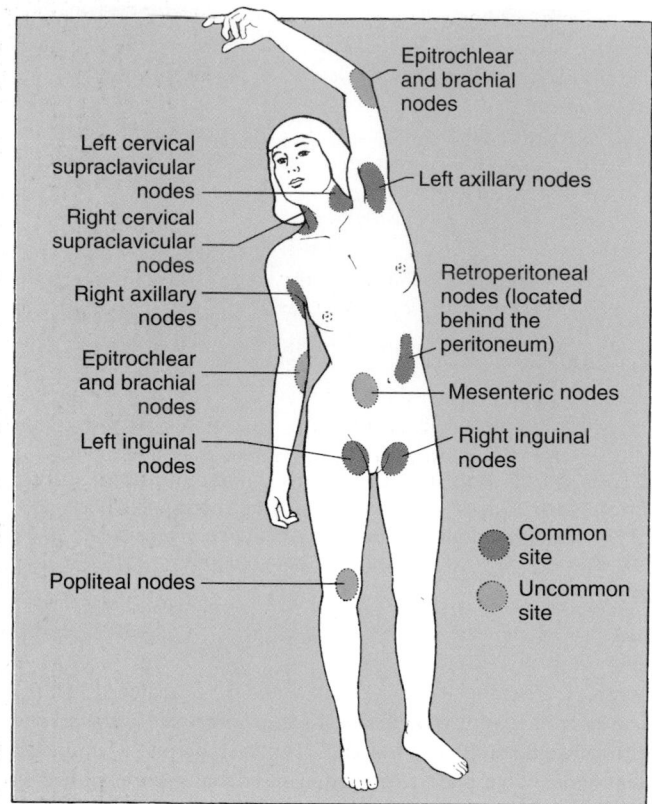

FIGURE 21-13 Common and Uncommon Involved Lymph Node Sites for Hodgkin Lymphoma.

TABLE 21-7 Definitions of Stages of Hodgkin Disease

Stage	Criteria
I	Involvement of a single lymph node region (I) or localized involvement of a single extralymphatic organ or site (I$_E$)*
II	Involvement of two or more lymph node regions on same side of diaphragm (II) or localized involvement of a single associated extralymphatic organ or site and its regional lymph node(s), with or without involvement of other lymph node regions on same side of diaphragm (II$_E$)
III	Involvement of lymph node regions on both sides of diaphragm (III), which may also be accompanied by localized involvement of an associated extralymphatic organ or site (III$_E$), by involvement of the spleen (III$_S$), or by both (III$_{E+S}$).
IV	Disseminated (multifocal) involvement of one or more extralymphatic organs, with or without associated lymph node involvement, or isolated extralymphatic organ involvement with distant (nonregional) nodal involvement

A: No systemic symptoms present

B: Unexplained fevers >38° C (100.4° F), drenching night sweats, or weight loss >10% of body weight

From National Comprehensive Cancer Network: Hodgkin lymphoma. In *NCCN practice guidelines, Version 2.2014: Hodgkin lymphoma* (originally adapted from Carbono PP et al: *Cancer Res* 31[11]:1860-1861, 1971).

*NOTE: The number of lymph node regions involved may be indicated by a subscript (e.g., II$_3$).

in 60% of cases. With lymphocyte and nodular sclerosis types, 34% of cases involve the spleen.

EVALUATION AND TREATMENT Because of the variability in symptoms, early definitive detection may be challenging. Asymptomatic lymphadenopathy can progress undetected for several years. Diagnosis is made from physical examination and history, complete blood count, blood chemistry studies including sedimentation rate, lymph node biopsy, pathology review for Reed-Sternberg cells, and immunophenotyping for disease markers.[47] Clinical staging for individuals with HL includes personal history; physical examination; laboratory studies, including sedimentation rate; and thoracic and abdominal/pelvic CT scans[47] (Table 21-7). Positron emission tomography (PET) scans, usually combined with CT scans, have replaced gallium scans and lymphangiography for clinical staging.[48] Staging laparotomy is no longer recommended; it should be considered only when the results will allow substantial reduction in treatment. It should not be done in individuals who require chemotherapy. If the laparotomy is required for treatment decisions, the risks of potential morbidity should be considered.[48] Prognostic indicators include clinical stage, histologic type, tumor cell concentration and tumor burden, constitutional symptoms, and age of the individual.

The effectiveness of treatment is related to the age, gender, and general health of the individual; signs and symptoms; stage of the disease; blood test results; type of Hodgkin lymphoma; and classification of the disease as recurrent or progressive. Adult Hodgkin lymphoma can usually be cured with early diagnosis and treatment.[47] Three types of treatment are used: chemotherapy, radiation therapy, and surgery. Treatment for pregnant women includes watchful waiting and steroid therapy. Newer treatments undergoing testing include chemotherapy and radiation therapy with stem cell transplant and monoclonal antibody therapy.[47] Treatment with chemotherapy or radiation therapy, or both, may increase the risk of second cancers, cardiovascular disease, and other health problems for many months or years after treatment.

Non-Hodgkin Lymphomas

The NHLs are a heterogeneous group of proliferative lymphoid tissue neoplasms with differing clinical patterns of behavior and responses to treatment. The previously used generic classification of non-Hodgkin lymphoma (NHL) has been reclassified in the WHO/REAL scheme into (1) B-cell neoplasms, a group that consists of a variety of lymphomas including myelomas that originate from B cells at various stages of differentiation; and (2) T-cell and NK-cell neoplasms, a group that includes lymphomas that originate from either T or NK cells. These cancers are differentiated from HL by lack of RS cells and other cellular changes not characteristic of HL.

More than 70,800 new cases of NHL and 18,990 deaths are predicted for 2014.[33] The median age of diagnosis is 67 years and the highest incidences of NHL are in North America, Europe, Oceania, and several African countries.[49] The occurrence of NHL is higher in men than in women. For unknown reasons, incidence increased in many high-income countries between the 1950s and 1990s and no further increase has been observed during the last decade.[49] Part of the increased incidence has been attributed to diagnostic improvements as well as AIDS-related cancers following the HIV epidemic.[49] Conversely, the mortality has risen at a slower rate. It is thought that newer treatment modalities are improving survival rates.

PATHOPHYSIOLOGY NHL is best described as a progressive clonal expansion of B cells, T cells, or NK cells. B cells account for 85% to

TABLE 21-8 Clinical Differences Between Non-Hodgkin Lymphoma and Hodgkin Lymphoma

Characteristics	Non-Hodgkin Lymphoma	Hodgkin Lymphoma
Nodal involvement	Multiple peripheral nodes	Localized to single axial group of nodes (i.e., cervical, mediastinal, paraaortic)
	Mesenteric nodes and Waldeyer ring commonly involved	Mesenteric nodes and Waldeyer ring rarely involved
Spread	Noncontiguous	Orderly spread by contiguity
B symptoms*	Uncommon	Common
Extranodal involvement	Common	Rare
Extent of disease	Rarely localized	Often localized

*Fever, weight loss, night sweats.

90% of NHLs, with most of the remainder being T cells and rarely NK cells. Oncogenes may be activated by chromosomal translocations or the tumor-suppressor loci may be inactivated by deletion or mutation of chromosomes. Certain subtypes may have altered genomes by oncogenic viruses. The various subtypes of NHL may be identified by specific diagnostic markers related to various cytogenetic lesions. The most common type of chromosomal alteration in NHL is translocation, which disrupts the genes encoded at the breakpoints. Unlike Hodgkin lymphoma, NHL spreads in a less predictable way and spreads widely early.[34] Diffuse large B-cell lymphoma (DLBCL) is the most common form of NHL.

Risk factors for adult NHL include being older, male, or white and having one of the following: afflicted by certain inherited immune disorders, an autoimmune disease, or HIV/AIDS; exposure to a variety of mutagenic chemicals or certain pesticides; infection with certain cancer-related viruses (e.g., Epstein-Barr virus, HIV, HTLV-1); consumption of a diet high in meats and fat; and use of immunosuppression drugs after an organ transplant. Gastric infection with *Helicobacter pylori* increases the risk for gastric lymphomas. NHL is a disease of middle age, usually found in persons more than 50 years old.

CLINICAL MANIFESTATIONS Clinical manifestations of NHL usually begin as localized or generalized lymphadenopathy, similar to HL. Differences in clinical features are noted in Table 21-8. The cervical, axillary, inguinal, and femoral lymph node chains are the most commonly affected sites. Generally, the swelling is painless and the nodes have enlarged and transformed over a period of months or years. Other sites of involvement are the nasopharynx, GI tract, bone, thyroid, testes, and soft tissue. Some individuals have retroperitoneal and abdominal masses with symptoms of abdominal fullness, back pain, ascites (fluid in the peritoneal cavity), skin rash or itchy skin, fatigue, fever of unknown origin, drenching night sweats, and leg swelling.

Lymphomas are classified as low, intermediate, or high grade. A low-grade lymphoma, which also may be termed *indolent,* has a slow progression. Individuals with low-grade lymphoma commonly present with a painless, peripheral adenopathy. Spontaneous regression of these nodes may occur, mimicking the presence of an infection. Night sweats with an elevated temperature (more than 38° C [100.4° F]) and weight loss, as well as extranodular involvement, are not commonly present in the early stages but are common in advanced or end-stage disease. *Cytopenia,* or reduction in the number of blood cells, reflective of bone marrow involvement is often observed. Hepatomegaly is common; however, splenomegaly is present in approximately 40% of individuals. Fatigue and weakness are more prevalent with advanced stages.

Intermediate and high-grade lymphomas, which are more aggressive, have a more varied clinical presentation. A high-grade lymphoma also may be termed *aggressive.*

EVALUATION AND TREATMENT The primary means for diagnosis of NHL is physical examination and history, blood tests, urine tests, flow cytometry, and bone marrow aspirate and biopsy. A common finding in NHL is noncontiguous lymph node involvement, which is not common in HL.

Treatment for NHL is quite diverse and depends on type (B cell or T cell), tumor stage, histologic status (low, intermediate, or high grade), symptoms, age, and presence of comorbidities.[50] Depending on the type (B cell or T cell) of the tumor, stage of disease, and aggressiveness of the tumor, treatment is usually initiated at the time of diagnosis. However, because treatment is not curative for some low-grade indolent lymphomas that are widely disseminated, observation without treatment may be the most appropriate choice. These indolent tumors are often not symptomatic for the individual and this approach improves quality of life. In some cases the disease may be so slow growing that treatment is not needed for an extended period of time.

Standard treatment for NHL includes radiation therapy, chemotherapy, target therapy (monoclonal antibody therapy, proteasome inhibitor therapy), plasmapheresis (if the blood becomes thick), biologic therapy (e.g., interferon), and watchful waiting. Several factors affect prognosis, including the stage of the cancer, the type of NHL, the blood levels of lactate dehydrogenase, the amount of β_2-microglobulin in the blood (for Waldenström macroglobulinemia), the age and general health of the patient, and the properties of the lymphoma (i.e., whether it was recently diagnosed or is a recurrence). Indolent NHL types can have a median survival as long as 20 years but are not curable in advanced stages.[51] Those with the aggressive type of NHL have a more limited survival but a significant number of individuals can achieve a cure with an intensive combination of chemotherapy. With modern treatments for NHL, the overall survival at 5 years for nonaggressive NHL is >60%, and for aggressive types >50%. High-grade NHL is seen with increasing frequency in persons with AIDS and has an extremely poor prognosis. New research suggests that a novel therapeutic approach may hold promise for individuals with chemotherapy-refractory advanced large B-cell lymphoma and indolent B-cell malignancies using engineered T cells that express an anti-CD19 chimeric antigen receptor.[52]

Burkitt lymphoma. Burkitt lymphoma is a B-cell tumor with unique clinical and epidemiologic features. Although more common in Africa, Burkitt lymphoma is not confined to the African continent and is documented in the United States, Latin America, and other countries. Classification of Burkitt lymphoma includes (1) African (endemic) Burkitt lymphoma, (2) sporadic (nonendemic) Burkitt lymphoma, and (3) a subset of aggressive lymphomas in individuals infected with HIV. Burkitt lymphomas, in these classifications, are histologically identical but differ in some genetic, virologic, and clinical characteristics.[34] Burkitt lymphoma is a fast-growing tumor that often appears as a large tumor mass in the jaw and sometimes the abdomen (Figure 21-14). It is now understood that Burkitt lymphoma is heterogeneous and pathologic confirmation is sometimes challenging.

PATHOPHYSIOLOGY Basically, all endemic Burkitt lymphomas are latently infected with EBV, which also is present in about 25% of HIV-associated tumors and 15% to 20% of sporadic cases.[34] It is suspected

FIGURE 21-14 Burkitt Lymphoma. Burkitt lymphoma involving the jaw in a young African boy. (Courtesy I. Magrath, MD, Bethesda, Md. From Zitelli BJ et al: *Zitelli and Davis' atlas of pediatric physical diagnosis,* ed 6, Philadelphia, 2012, Saunders.)

FIGURE 21-15 Burkitt Lymphoma Cells. The 8,14 chromosomal translocation and associated oncogenes in Burkitt lymphoma.

that suppression of the immune system by other illnesses (e.g., HIV infection, chronic malaria) increases the individual's susceptibility to EBV. B cells are particularly sensitive because of specific surface receptors for EBV. As a result, the B cell undergoes chromosomal translocations that result in overexpression of the *c-MYC* proto-oncogene and loss of control of cell growth (Figure 21-15). The most common translocation (75% of individuals) is between chromosomes 8 (containing the *c-MYC* gene) and 14 (containing the immunoglobulin heavy chain genes). When the t(8;14) translocation occurs, the *MYC* gene becomes regulated by the B-cell immunoglobulin gene *(IG)* on chromosome 14 and overproduction of MYC protein forces proliferation and blocks cellular differentiation. MYC is a transcriptional regulator that increases genes responsible for aerobic glycolysis (Warburg effect). When glucose and glutamine are available, the Warburg metabolism enables cells to synthesize nutrients that are needed for growth and cell division.

Therefore, investigators believe that Burkitt lymphoma is the fastest growing tumor.[34] Other translocations have been reported between chromosome 8 and chromosomes 2 or 22, which contain genes for immunoglobulin light chains.

CLINICAL MANIFESTATIONS The endemic and sporadic Burkitt lymphomas (the most common type in the United States and without obvious infectious cofactors) are found mostly in children or young adults. Most tumors manifest at extranodal locations. Endemic Burkitt lymphoma usually presents as a mass of the mandible and an unusual tendency for involvement of the abdominal viscera, including the kidneys, ovaries, and adrenal glands. Sporadic Burkitt lymphoma usually appears as a mass involving the ileocecum and peritoneum. More advanced disease may involve other organs—eyes, ovaries, kidneys, glandular tissue (breast, thyroid, tonsil)—and presents with type B symptoms (night sweats, fever, weight loss).

EVALUATION AND TREATMENT The distribution of tumors and biopsies of enlarged lymph nodes or the bone marrow containing malignant B cells are usually indicative of Burkitt lymphoma. It is one of the most aggressive and quickly growing malignancies. Burkitt lymphoma, however, responds successfully to intensive chemotherapy in most children and adults. The outcome is more cautious in older adults.

Lymphoblastic lymphoma. Lymphoblastic lymphoma (LL) is a relatively rare variant of NHL overall (2% to 4%) but accounts for almost one third of cases of NHL in children and adolescents, with a male predominance. The vast majority of LL (90%) is of T-cell origin; the remainder arises from B cells. LL is similar to acute lymphoblastic leukemia and may be considered a variant of that disease.

PATHOPHYSIOLOGY The disease arises from a clone of relatively immature T cells that becomes malignant in the thymus. As with most lymphoid tumors, LL is frequently associated with translocations, primarily of the chromosomes that encode for the T-cell receptor (chromosomes 7 and 14). These aberrations result in increased expression of a variety of transcription factors and loss of growth control.

CLINICAL MANIFESTATIONS The first sign of LL is usually a painless lymphadenopathy in the neck. Peripheral lymph nodes in the chest become involved in about 70% of individuals. Involved nodes are located mostly above the diaphragm. LL is a very aggressive tumor that presents as stage IV in most people. T-cell LL is associated with a unique mediastinal mass (up to 75%) because of the apparent origin of the tumor in the thymus. The mass results in dyspnea and chest pain and may cause compression of bronchi or the superior vena cava. The tumor may infiltrate the bone marrow in about half of those affected, and suppression of bone marrow hematopoiesis leads to increased susceptibility to infections. Other organs, including the liver, kidney, spleen, and brain, also may be affected. Many individuals express type B symptoms: fever, night sweats, and significant weight loss.

EVALUATION AND TREATMENT The most common therapeutic approach is combined chemotherapy (intensive therapy). Bulky tumor masses are sometimes treated with radiation therapy. In early stages of the disease, the response rate is high with increased survival; the 5-year survival in children is 80% to 90% and 45% to 55% in adults. Although LL is easily treated, there is a high relapse rate: 40% to 60% of adults.

Multiple myeloma. Multiple myeloma (MM) is a plasma cell (a white blood cell neoplasm called myeloma cells) cancer characterized by the slow proliferation of malignant cells, with tumor cell masses in the bone marrow usually resulting in destruction of the bone

FIGURE 21-16 Multiple Myeloma, Bone Marrow Aspirate. Normal marrow cells are largely replaced by plasma cells, including atypical forms with multiple nuclei *(arrow)*, and cytoplasmic droplets containing immunoglobulin. (From Kumar V et al: *Robbins and Cotran pathologic basis of disease,* ed 9, Philadelphia, 2015, Saunders.)

(Figure 21-16).[53] Myeloma cells reside in the bone marrow and are usually not found in the peripheral blood. As the number of myeloma cells increases, fewer red blood cells, white blood cells, and platelets are produced. Myeloma may spread to other tissues, especially in very advanced stages of the disease. The reported incidence of MM has doubled in the past 2 decades, possibly as a result of more sensitive testing used for diagnosis. The annual incidence rate in the United States is 6.1/100,000, with 24,050 new cases estimated for 2014. Multiple myeloma occurs in all races, but the incidence in blacks is about twice that of whites. It rarely occurs before the age of 40 years—the peak age of incidence is between 65 and 70 years. It is slightly more common in men (7.7 estimated new cases per 100,000 persons) than in women (4.9 new cases per 100,000 persons). Other risk factors include exposure to radiation or certain chemicals and a history of monoclonal gammopathy of undetermined significance (MGUS, see Clinical Manifestations) or plasmacytoma.

PATHOPHYSIOLOGY   MM is a plasma cell neoplasia that causes lytic bone lesions (bony disease; radiologically appears as punched-out defects), hypercalcemia, renal failure, anemia, and immune abnormalities.[34,54] Multiple mutations in different pathways alter the intrinsic biology of the plasma cell, generating the features of myeloma.[55] MM tumors are highly heterogeneous.[56] Investigators observed frequent mutations in *KRAS, NRAS, BRAF, FAM46C, TP53,* and *DIS3* and many mutations were found in the same pathway.[56] Defining driver mutations and heterogeneity is essential for treatment decisions. Many myelomas are aneuploidy and, in most individuals with myeloma, chromosomal translocations are the most common. The primary translocation involves the immunoglobulin heavy chain on chromosome 14 (IgH locus) that relocates to loci containing genes of the cell cycle (cyclins) on chromosomes 11(q13), 12(p13), and 6(p21); oncogenes on chromosomes 16(q23), 8(q24), and 20; and fibroblast growth factor receptor on chromosome 4(p16).[57] Other reported chromosomal abnormalities include deletion of chromosome 13 and deletion of chromosome 17 on which tumor-suppressor gene *TP53* is localized.[57] Development of further secondary genetic alterations causes progression to an aggressive MM. Investigators are studying various epigenetic alterations and interactions with extracellular matrix proteins. For example, myeloma cells interact and secrete peptides that adhere to stromal cells, inducing cytokines that possibly promote

inflammation. Myeloma cells are prone to the accumulation of misfolded protein, such as unpaired Ig chains. Misfolded proteins activate apoptosis.

Malignant plasma cells arise from one clone of B cells that produce abnormally large amounts of one class of immunoglobulin (usually IgG, occasionally IgA, and rarely IgM, IgD, or IgE). The malignant transformation may begin early in B-cell development, possibly before encountering antigen in the secondary lymphoid organs. The myeloma cells return either to the bone marrow or to other soft tissue sites. Their return is aided by cell adhesion molecules that help them target favorable sites that promote continued expansion and maturation. Cytokines, particularly interleukin-6 (IL-6), have been identified as essential factors that promote the growth and survival of multiple myeloma cells. (Lymphocytes and cytokines are described in Chapter 5.)

Myeloma cells in the bone marrow produce several cytokines themselves (e.g., IL-6, IL-1, IL-11, TNF-α). IL-6 in particular acts as an osteoclast-activating factor and stimulates osteoclasts to reabsorb bone. This process results in bone lesions and hypercalcemia (high calcium levels in the blood) attributable to the release of calcium from the breakdown of bone.

The antibody produced by the transformed plasma cell is frequently defective, containing truncations, deletions, and other abnormalities, and is often referred to as a *paraprotein* (abnormal protein in the blood). Because of the large number of malignant plasma cells, the abnormal antibody, called the **M protein**, becomes the most prominent protein in the blood (see Figure 21-18, p. 539). Suppression of normal plasma cells by the myeloma results in diminished or absent normal antibodies. The excessive amount of M protein also may contribute to many of the clinical manifestations of the disease. Frequently, the myeloma produces free immunoglobulin light chain (Bence Jones protein) that is present in the blood and urine and contributes to damage of renal tubular cells.

CLINICAL MANIFESTATIONS   The common presentation of MM is characterized by elevated levels of calcium in the blood (hypercalcemia), renal failure, anemia, and bone lesions. The hypercalcemia and bone lesions result from infiltration of the bone by malignant plasma cells and stimulation of osteoclasts to reabsorb bone. This process results in the release of calcium (hypercalcemia) and the development of "lytic lesions" (round, "punched out" regions of bone) (Figure 21-17). Destruction of bone tissue causes pain, the most common presenting symptom, and pathologic fractures. The bones most commonly involved, in decreasing order of frequency, are the vertebrae, ribs, skull, pelvis, femur, clavicle, and scapula. Spinal cord compression, because of the weakened vertebrae, occurs in about 10% of individuals. A condition called **amyloidosis** may occur, in which antibody proteins increase and stick together in peripheral nerves and organs, such as the kidney and heart. Signs and symptoms of amyloidosis include fatigue, purple spots on the skin, enlarged tongue, diarrhea, edema, and numbness or tingling in the legs and feet.

Proteinuria is observed in 90% of individuals. Renal failure may be either acute or chronic and is usually secondary to the hypercalcemia. Bence Jones protein may lead to damage of the proximal tubules. Anemia is usually normocytic and normochromic and results from inhibited erythropoiesis caused by tumor cell infiltration of the bone marrow.

The high concentration of paraprotein in the blood may lead to hyperviscosity syndrome. The increased viscosity interferes with blood circulation to various sites (brain, kidneys, extremities). Hyperviscosity syndrome is observed in up to 20% of persons. Additional neurologic symptoms (e.g., confusion, headaches, blurred vision) may occur secondary to hypercalcemia or hyperviscosity.

FIGURE 21-17 Multiple (Plasma Cell) Myeloma. **A,** Roentgenogram of femur showing extensive bone destruction caused by tumor. Note absence of reactive bone formation. **B,** Gross specimen from same individual; myelomatous sections appear as dark granular sections. (From Kissane JM, editor: *Anderson's pathology,* ed 9, St Louis, 1990, Mosby.)

Suppression of the humoral (antibody-mediated) immune response results in repeated infections, primarily pneumonias and pyelonephritis. The most commonly involved microorganisms are encapsulated bacteria that are particularly sensitive to the effects of antibody; pneumonia caused by *Streptococcus pneumoniae, Staphylococcus aureus,* or *Klebsiella pneumonia;* or pyelonephritis caused by *Escherichia coli* or other gram-negative organisms. Cell-mediated (T-cell) function is relatively normal. Overwhelming infection is the leading cause of death from MM.

MM is a progressive disorder and is often preceded by a condition known as monoclonal gammopathy of undetermined significance (MGUS). MGUS is diagnosed by the presence of an M protein in the blood or urine without additional evidence of MM.[58] MGUS is present in approximately 1% of the general population and in 3% of individuals older than 70 years. Although MGUS is considered nonpathologic and requires no treatment, about 2% of individuals with MGUS progress to malignant plasma cell disorders. Progression of MM following MGUS advances to asymptomatic MM and finally symptomatic MM. Asymptomatic MM also may be referred to as smoldering myeloma and indolent myeloma.[58] Smoldering myeloma is usually characterized by the presence of an M protein and clonal bone marrow plasma cells, but with no indication of end-organ damage.

EVALUATION AND TREATMENT   Diagnosis of MM is made by symptoms and radiographic and laboratory studies; a definitive diagnosis requires a bone marrow biopsy. The International Myeloma Working Group's new criteria[58] for the diagnosis of multiple myeloma include biomarkers (monoclonal components in serum and urine; quantification of IgG, IgA, and IgM immunoglobulins; and characterization of the heavy and light chains by immunofixation) and the presence of hypercalcemia, renal failure, anemia, and bone lesions (CRAB). Other criteria include evaluation of bone marrow plasma cell infiltration by bone marrow biopsy and radiologic evaluation of lytic bone lesions. Biomarkers based on quantitation of plasma cells (serum-free light chains) may help stratify risk for people with asymptomatic multiple myeloma and identification, staging, prognosis, and monitoring of those with smoldering multiple myeloma who are at an "ultra-high" risk of developing aggressive multiple myeloma.

New techniques use microRNAs extracted from serum to measure immunoglobulins (IgG, IgM, IgA). Typically, one class of immunoglobulin (the M protein produced by the myeloma cell) is greatly increased, whereas the others are suppressed. Serum electrophoretic analysis shows increased levels of M protein (Figure 21-18). Because the M protein is monoclonal, each molecule has the same electric charge and migrates at about the same site on electrophoresis, resulting in a highly concentrated protein (M spike) (see Figure 21-18). Bence Jones protein may be observed in the urine or serum by immunoelectrophoresis or in the serum using available enzyme-linked immunosorbent assays (ELISAs). Usually an intact antibody paraprotein coexists with Bence Jones protein. However, variants of MM include individuals in which free light chain only is produced and a rare variant that produces only free heavy chain; about 1% of cases are nonsecretory so that neither M protein nor Bence Jones protein is produced. Measurement of another protein, free β2-microglobulin, is used as an indicator of prognosis or effectiveness of therapy.

Although combinations of chemotherapy, radiation therapy, plasmapheresis (exchange), and stem cell transplant have been used for treatment, the prognosis for persons with MM remains poor. However, with the new high-sensitivity biomarkers that are associated with inevitable development of clinical symptoms, early diagnosis and treatment may be possible before individuals develop more advanced disease and organ damage. Conventional combinations of chemotherapeutic agents have included melphalan and prednisone (MP); MP with vincristine, carmustine, and cyclophosphamide; vincristine, doxorubicin, and dexamethasone; and thalidomide and dexamethasone. The drug thalidomide disrupts the stromal marrow–MM cell interaction by modulating cell surface adhesion molecules and inhibiting angiogenesis. In addition, it increases apoptosis and G_1 growth arrest (i.e., the cell cycle gap 1; see Chapter 1) of MM cells. Hematopoietic stem cell transplantation has prolonged life but has not yet proven to be curative.[34] Controversy exists concerning whether tandem stem cell transplant offers the best outcome. Biphosphonate therapy is the primary treatment for bone lesions. Individuals with multiple bone lesions, if untreated, rarely survive more than 6 to 12 months. Individuals with inactive (indolent) myeloma, however, can survive for many years. With chemotherapy and aggressive management of complications, the prognosis can improve significantly, with a median survival of 24 to 30 months and a 10-year survival rate of 3%. Promising new therapies include the use of proteasome inhibitors because proteasome degrades misfolded and unwanted proteins. The rates of new myeloma cases are increasing 0.7% each year and the death rates have decreased an average of 1.3% each year from 2002 to 2011. The 5-year survival for all stages of MM is 45.1%.

> ✔ **QUICK CHECK 21-4**
> 1. What are the risk factors for adult NHL?
> 2. Define what is meant by the following statement: Multiple myeloma is heterogeneous.
> 3. What are the main pathologic features of multiple myeloma?

ALTERATIONS OF SPLENIC FUNCTION

The complexities of splenic function are not totally understood and its mysteries are still being studied. The normal functions of the spleen

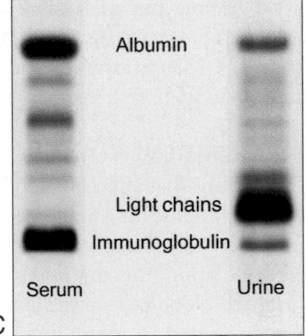

FIGURE 21-18 M Protein. Serum protein electrophoresis *(PEL)* is used to screen for M proteins in multiple myeloma. **A,** In normal serum the proteins separate into several regions between albumin *(Alb)* and a broad band in the gamma (γ) region, where most antibodies (gamma globulins) are found. Immunofixation *(IFE)* can identify the location of IgG *(G)*, IgA *(A)*, IgM *(M)*, and kappa *(κ)* and lambda *(λ)* light chains. **B,** Serum from an individual with multiple myeloma contains a sharp M protein *(M spike)*. The M protein is monoclonal and contains only one heavy chain and one light chain. In this instance the IFE identifies the M protein as an IgG containing a lambda light chain. **C,** Serum and urine protein electrophoretic patterns in an individual with multiple myeloma. Serum demonstrates an M protein *(Immunoglobulin)* in the gamma region, and the urine has a large amount of the smaller-sized light chains with only a small amount of the intact immunoglobulin. (**A** and **B** from Abeloff M et al: *Abeloff's clinical oncology*, ed 4, Philadelphia, 2008, Churchill Livingstone. **C** from McPherson R, Pincus M: *Henry's clinical diagnosis and management by laboratory methods*, ed 22, Edinburgh, 2012, Saunders.)

that may impact disease states include (1) phagocytosis of blood cells and particulate matter (e.g., bacteria), (2) antibody production, (3) hematopoiesis, and (4) sequestration of formed blood elements. The spleen is part of the mononuclear phagocyte system and is involved in all systemic inflammations, hematopoietic disorders, and many metabolic disorders.

In the past, splenomegaly (enlargement of the spleen) has been associated with various disease states. It is now recognized that splenomegaly is not necessarily pathologic; an enlarged spleen may be present in certain individuals without any evidence of disease. Splenomegaly may be, however, one of the first physical signs of underlying conditions, and its presence should not be ignored. In conditions where splenomegaly is present, the normal functions of the spleen may become overactive, producing a syndrome known as hypersplenism. Hypersplenism is characterized by anemia, leukopenia, and thrombocytopenia alone or in combination. Some individuals may seek treatment for problems even though they have not met all the aforementioned clinical criteria; therefore, the relevance and significance of hypersplenism are still uncertain.

PATHOPHYSIOLOGY Specific conditions causing splenomegaly and resulting hypersplenism are many and are related to other categories of disease (Box 21-3). Different pathologic processes that produce splenomegaly are described briefly next.

BOX 21-3 Diseases Related to Classification of Splenomegaly

Inflammation or Infection
Acute: viral (hepatitis, infectious mononucleosis, cytomegalovirus), bacterial (salmonella, gram negative), parasitic (typhoid)
Subacute or chronic: bacterial (subacute bacterial endocarditis, tuberculosis), parasitic (malaria), fungal (histoplasmosis), Felty syndrome, systemic lupus erythematosus, rheumatoid arthritis, thrombocytopenia

Congestive
Cirrhosis, heart failure, portal vein obstruction (portal hypertension), splenic vein obstruction

Infiltrative
Gaucher disease, amyloidosis, diabetic lipemia

Tumors or Cysts
Malignant: polycythemia rubra vera, chronic or acute leukemias, Hodgkin lymphoma, metastatic solid tumors

Nonmalignant: Hamartoma
Cysts: true cysts (lymphangiomas, hemangiomas, epithelial, endothelial); false cysts (hemorrhagic, serous, inflammatory)

Acute inflammatory or infectious processes cause splenomegaly because of an increased demand for defensive activities. Acutely enlarged spleens secondary to infection may become so filled with erythrocytes that their natural rubbery resilience is lost and they become fragile and vulnerable to blunt trauma. Splenic rupture is a complication associated with infectious mononucleosis; rupture occurs mostly in males between days 4 and 21 of acute illness.

Congestive splenomegaly is accompanied by ascites, portal hypertension, and esophageal varices and is most commonly seen in those with hepatic cirrhosis. Splenic hyperplasia develops in disorders that increase splenic workload and is associated most commonly with various types of anemia (hemolytic) and chronic myeloproliferative disorders (i.e., polycythemia vera).

Infiltrative splenomegaly is caused by engorgement by the macrophages with indigestible materials associated with various "storage diseases." Tumors and cysts cause actual growth of the spleen. Metastatic tumors in the spleen are rare and may result from primary tumors of the skin, lung, breast, and cervix.

CLINICAL MANIFESTATIONS Overactivity of the spleen results in hematologic alterations that affect all blood components. Sequestering of red blood cells, granulocytes, and platelets results in a reduction of all circulating blood cells. The spleen may sequester up to 50% of the red blood cell population, thereby upsetting the normal physiologic concentration of red blood cells in the circulation. The rate of splenic pooling is directly related to spleen size and the degree of increased blood flow through it. Sequestering exposes the red blood cells to splenic conditions that accelerate destruction, further contributing to the decreased red blood cell concentration. Anemia is the result of these combined activities. Anemia may be further potentiated by an increase in blood volume, which produces a dilutional effect on the already reduced concentration of red blood cells. The dilutional effect, as well as the removal and destruction of red blood cells, depends primarily on the degree of splenomegaly.

White blood cells and platelets also are affected by sequestering, although not to the same degree as the red blood cell. Again, the size of the spleen is the determining factor in the number of cells sequestered.

EVALUATION AND TREATMENT Treatment for hypersplenism is splenectomy; however, it may not always be indicated. A splenectomy is considered necessary to alleviate the destructive effects on red blood cells. Clinical indicators should determine the need for splenectomy, not necessarily specific conditions. Splenectomy for splenic rupture is no longer considered mandatory because of the possibility of overwhelming sepsis after removal. Repair and preservation are now considered before the decision to remove the spleen. Splenectomy also may be performed as treatment for hairy cell leukemia, Felty syndrome,

agnogenic myeloid metaplasia, thalassemia major, Gaucher disease, hemodialysis, splenomegaly, splenic venous thrombosis, and thrombotic thrombocytopenia purpura (TTP).

Individuals are able to lead normal lives after splenectomy but blood cell abnormalities often exist after removal of the spleen (i.e., red blood cells become thinner, broader, and wrinkled; white blood cell counts initially increase and then plateau; platelet counts rise after surgery and then stabilize). A major postoperative complication following splenectomy is overwhelming postsplenectomy infection (OPSI). Unless treated in time, OPSI may rapidly progress to septic shock and possibly disseminated intravascular coagulation (DIC, see p. 545).

> ✓ **QUICK CHECK 21-5**
> 1. Contrast the principal features of Hodgkin lymphoma with those of non-Hodgkin lymphoma.
> 2. What is Burkitt lymphoma?
> 3. Identify the major causes of splenomegaly. How does it differ from hypersplenism?

HEMORRHAGIC DISORDERS AND ALTERATIONS OF PLATELETS AND COAGULATION

The arrest of bleeding, or hemostasis, is dependent on adequate numbers of platelets, normal levels of coagulation factors, and absence of defects in vessels walls. The spectrum of abnormal bleeding varies widely from massive bleeds, such as rupture of large vessels like the aorta, to small bleeds in skin or mucosal membranes. Diminished or excessive levels of coagulation factors can lead to defective hemostasis or spontaneous and unnecessary clotting. (Hemostasis is discussed in Chapter 20.) Diminished hemostasis results in either internal or external hemorrhage. A classification of hemorrhagic disorders is included in Table 21-9.

Purpuric disorders occur when there is a deficiency of normal platelets necessary to plug damaged vessels or prevent leakage from the tiny tears that occur daily in capillaries. More serious internal bleeding occurs from events that simply overwhelm hemostatic mechanisms, such as rupture of large blood vessels, trauma, and diseases associated with massive hemorrhage including abdominal aneurysm. Between these smaller bleeds and massive bleeds are deficiencies of coagulation factors found with the hemophilias (see Chapter 22). Disorders that result in spontaneous clotting can develop from genetic disorders of the clotting system components or from acquired diseases that activate clotting. These disorders are known collectively as thromboembolic disease. Additionally, any disorder of the blood that predisposes to clotting of blood or thrombosis is called hypercoagulability (thrombophilia).

TABLE 21-9	**Classification of Hemorrhagic Disorders**	
Type of Defect	**Example**	**Manifestation**
Defects of primary hemostasis	Platelet defects or von Willebrand disease	Usually present with small bleeds in skin or mucosal membrane; bleeds are usually petechiae (<3-mm minute hemorrhages) or purpuras (>3-mm red-purple discolorations); common in capillaries; also includes epistaxis (nose bleeds), GI bleeds, or excessive menstruation
Defects of secondary hemostasis	Coagulation factor defects	Bleeds into soft tissue, muscle, or joints; intracranial bleeds may occur
Generalized defects of small vessels	Palpable purpura and ecchymoses	Extravasated blood creates a palpable mass (or palpable purpura), ecchymoses (simply called a *bruise*), or a larger palpable lesion (or hematoma); systemic disorders disrupt small blood vessels, called vasculitis

Disorders of Platelets

Quantitative or qualitative abnormalities of platelets can interrupt normal blood coagulation and prevent hemostasis.[59] The quantitative abnormalities are thrombocytopenia, a decrease in the number of circulating platelets, and thrombocythemia, an increase in the number of platelets. Qualitative disorders affect the structure or function of individual platelets and can coexist with the quantitative disorders. Qualitative disorders usually prevent platelet adherence and aggregation, preventing formation of a platelet plug.

Thrombocytopenia

Thrombocytopenia is defined as a platelet count less than 150,000 platelets/µL of blood, although most individuals do not consider the decrease significant unless it falls below 100,000 platelets/µL of blood.[60] The risk for hemorrhage associated with minor trauma does not appreciably increase until the count falls below 50,000 platelets/µL. Spontaneous bleeding without trauma can occur with counts ranging from 10,000 platelets/µL to 15,000 platelets/µL, resulting in skin manifestations (i.e., petechiae, ecchymoses, and larger purpuric spots) or frank bleeding from mucous membranes. Severe spontaneous bleeding may result if the count is less than 10,000 platelets/µL and can be fatal if it occurs in the gastrointestinal tract, respiratory tract, or central nervous system.

Before the diagnosis of thrombocytopenia is made, pseudothrombocytopenia must be ruled out. This phenomenon occurs in approximately 1 in 1000 to 1 in 10,000 laboratory samples and results from an error in platelet counting when a blood sample is analyzed by an automated cell counter. Platelets in the blood sample may become nonspecifically agglutinated by immunoglobulins in the presence of ethylenediaminetetraacetic acid (EDTA), a preservative in banked blood. The agglutinated platelets are not counted, thus giving an apparent, but false, thrombocytopenia. Thrombocytopenia also may be falsely diagnosed because of a dilutional effect observed after massive transfusion of platelet-poor packed cells to treat a hemorrhage. This occurs when more than 10 units of blood have been transfused within a 24-hour period. The hemorrhage that necessitated the transfusion also accelerates the loss of platelets, contributing to the pseudothrombocytopenic state. Splenic sequestering of platelets in hypersplenism (congestive) also induces an apparent thrombocytopenia as does hypothermia (less than 25° C [77° F]), which is reversed when temperatures return to normal, suggesting an increased platelet sequestration in response to chilling.

PATHOPHYSIOLOGY Thrombocytopenia results from decreased platelet production, increased consumption, or both. The condition may also be either congenital or acquired and may be either primary or secondary to other acquired or congenital conditions.[61,62] Thrombocytopenia secondary to congenital conditions occurs in a large number of different diseases, although each is relatively rare.[63] These include thrombocytopenia–absent radius (TAR) syndrome, Wiskott-Aldrich syndrome (see Chapter 8), various forms of *MYH9* gene mutation (e.g., May-Hegglin anomaly), X-linked thrombocytopenia, and many other examples.

Acquired thrombocytopenia is more common and may occur as a result of decreased platelet production secondary to viral infections (e.g., EBV, rubella, CMV, HIV), drugs (e.g., thiazides, estrogens, quinine-containing drugs, chemotherapeutic agents, ethanol), nutritional deficiencies (vitamin B_{12} or folic acid in particular), chronic renal failure, bone marrow hypoplasia (e.g., aplastic anemia), radiation therapy, or bone marrow infiltration by cancer. Most common forms of thrombocytopenia are the result of increased platelet consumption.

Examples include heparin-induced thrombocytopenia, idiopathic (immune) thrombocytopenia purpura, thrombotic thrombocytopenia purpura, and disseminated intravascular coagulation (discussed later in this chapter).

Heparin-induced thrombocytopenia. Heparin is the most common cause of drug-induced thrombocytopenia.[64] Approximately 1% of individuals treated with unfractionated heparin develop heparin-induced thrombocytopenia (HIT). The incidence is lower (about 0.1%) with the use of low-molecular-weight heparin. HIT is an immune-mediated, adverse drug reaction caused by IgG antibodies against the heparin–platelet factor 4 complex leading to platelet activation through platelet Fc γIIa receptors.[65] The release of additional platelet factor 4 from activated platelets and activation of thrombin lead to increased platelet consumption and a decrease in platelet counts beginning 5 to 10 days after administration of heparin.

CLINICAL MANIFESTATIONS The hallmark of HIT is thrombocytopenia. A decrease of approximately 50% in the platelet count is observed in more than 95% of individuals. However, 30% or more of those with thrombocytopenia are also at risk for venous or arterial thrombosis because a *prothrombotic state* is caused by antibody binding to platelets, inducing activation, aggregation, and consumption (thus the term *thrombocytopenia* in the syndrome name) of platelets. Venous thrombosis is more common and results in deep venous thrombosis and pulmonary emboli. Arterial thrombosis affects the lower extremities, causing limb ischemia. Arterial thrombosis may lead to cerebrovascular accidents and myocardial infarctions. Other major arteries also may be affected (e.g., renal, mesenteric, upper limb). Although platelet counts are low, bleeding is uncommon.

EVALUATION AND TREATMENT Diagnosis is primarily based on clinical observations. The individual presents with dropping platelet counts after 5 days or longer of heparin treatment. On average, platelet counts may reach 60,000/µL. Because most individuals are postsurgery and the onset of symptoms, including thrombosis, may be delayed until after release from the hospital, other possible causes of thrombocytopenia (e.g., infection, other drug reactions) must be considered. Tests are available to measure anti-heparin–platelet factor 4 antibodies. The sensitivity of this test is extremely high (>90%), but the specificity is less because of false-positive reactions (e.g., those receiving dialysis). Treatment is the withdrawal of heparin and use of alternative anticoagulants.

Immune thrombocytopenia purpura. The most common cause of thrombocytopenia secondary to increased platelet destruction is immune thrombocytopenic purpura (ITP). ITP, formerly known as *idiopathic thrombocytopenic purpura*, however, is widely recognized now as an immune process, hence the change from idiopathic to immune.[66] Although results and estimates are conflicting, the incidence of ITP is estimated to range from 9.5 to 20 per 100,000 in the general population and tends to increase with age. In individuals younger than 60 years, females have a higher incidence than males.[67] ITP may be acute or chronic. The acute form is frequently observed in children and typically lasts 1 to 2 months with a complete remission. In some instances it may last for up to 6 months, and some children (7% to 28%) may progress to the chronic condition (see Chapter 22). Acute ITP is usually secondary to infections (particularly viral) or other conditions that lead to large amounts of antigen in the blood, such as drug allergies or systemic lupus erythematosus (SLE). Under these conditions, the antigen usually forms immune complexes with circulating antibody, and it is thought that the immune complexes bind to Fc receptors on platelets, leading to their destruction in the spleen. The acute form of ITP usually resolves as the source of antigen is resolved (infection) or removed (drugs). Recently, *Helicobacter pylori* has been implicated in various autoimmune disorders, including pernicious anemia and immune thrombocytopenic purpura.[68-70] Similar to other autoimmune diseases, the epidemiology and gene-environment interactions and potential triggers for ITP need much study.

Chronic ITP is caused by autoantibody-mediated destruction against platelet-specific antigens. This form is more commonly observed in adults, being most prevalent in women between 20 and 40 years old, although it can be found in all ages. The chronic form tends to get progressively worse. It can occur from a variety of predisposing conditions or exposures (secondary) or have no known risk factors (primary). The autoantibodies are generally of the IgG class and are against one or more of several platelet glycoproteins (e.g., GPIIb/IIIa, GPIIb/IX, GPIa/IIa). The antibodies bind directly to the platelet antigens, after which the antibody-coated platelets are recognized and removed from the circulation by macrophages in the spleen. Autoreactive T cells also play a large role in the crosstalk between antigen-presenting cells and autoantibody-producing B cells and may play a role in ITP.[71]

CLINICAL MANIFESTATIONS Initial manifestations range from minor bleeding problems (development of petechiae and purpura) over the course of several days to major hemorrhage from mucosal sites (epistaxis, hematuria, menorrhagia, bleeding gums). Rarely will an individual present with intracranial bleeding or other sites of internal bleeding.

During pregnancy, a woman with ITP may have a newborn that is also thrombocytopenic. If the fetal platelets express the same antigen as the mother, the maternal antibody will coat the platelets, potentially resulting in thrombocytopenia in utero. A variant of neonatal thrombocytopenia (*neonatal alloimmune thrombocytopenia*) occurs when the mother does not have ITP but makes IgG antibodies against an antigen inherited from the father found on fetal platelets but not on maternal platelets.[72]

EVALUATION AND TREATMENT Diagnosis of ITP is based on a history of bleeding and associated symptoms (weight loss, fever, headache). Physical examination includes notations on the type, location, and severity of bleeding. In addition, evidence of infections (bacterial, HIV and other viral), medication history, family history, and evidence of thrombosis are assessed. Other diagnostic tests include complete blood count (CBC) and peripheral blood smear. Unlike some other forms of thrombocytopenia, there is usually no evidence of splenectomy. Testing for antiplatelet antibodies is usually not helpful. Although most cases of ITP are associated with elevated levels of IgG on platelets, other forms of thrombocytopenia also have a high incidence of platelet-associated antibodies; thus, the specificity is low (50% to 65%).[73] In addition, some cases of ITP will not present with elevated platelet-associated antibodies; the sensitivity is 75% to 94%; therefore, a negative test does not rule out ITP.

The acute form of ITP usually resolves without major clinical consequences but the chronic form, like many autoimmune diseases, is variable with multiple remissions and exacerbations. Treatment is palliative, not curative, and focuses on prevention of platelet destruction. Initial therapy for ITP is glucocorticoids (e.g., prednisone), which suppress the immune response and prevent sequestering and further destruction of platelets. If steroid therapy is ineffective, other reagents have been used. Treatment with intravenous immunoglobulin (IVIg) is used to prevent major bleeding. The response rate is 80%, but the effects are transient, lasting only days to a few weeks. Anti-Rh₀(D) (RhoGAM) has been used with limited success to treat individuals who are Rh-positive. Newer drug therapies are now available.

If platelet counts do not increase appropriately, splenectomy is considered to remove the site of platelet destruction. However, splenectomy is not without risks, and approximately 10% to 20% of individuals who undergo a splenectomy suffer a relapse and require further treatment. In that situation, it is believed that the liver has become the site for platelet destruction. If splenectomy is unsuccessful and life-threatening thrombocytopenia persists, more aggressive immunosuppressive medications (e.g., azathioprine, cyclophosphamide) are usually recommended. Because of potential complications, these medications are reserved for individuals who are severely thrombocytopenic and refractory to other therapies.

Thrombotic thrombocytopenia purpura. Thrombotic thrombocytopenia purpura (TTP) is a multisystem disorder characterized by thrombotic microangiopathy (TMA) (small or microvessel disease) in which platelets aggregate and cause occlusion of arterioles and capillaries within the microcirculation.[74,75] Aggregation may lead to increased platelet consumption and organ ischemia. TTP is relatively uncommon, occurring in about 5 per million individuals per year. The incidence is increasing and does appear to be an actual increase and not just the result of improved recognition. One suspected etiologic factor for TMA, thrombotic thrombocytopenic purpura, and hemolytic-uremic syndrome is drug-induced, and a recent report found definite evidence from three drugs: quinine, cyclosporine, and tacrolimus.[76]

There are two types of TTP: familial and acquired idiopathic. The familial type is the more rare type and is usually chronic, relapsing, and typically seen in children. When recognized and treated early, the child experiences predictable recurring episodes approximately every 3 weeks that are responsive to treatment. Acquired TTP is more common and more acute and severe. It occurs mostly in females in their thirties and is rarely observed in infants and the elderly.

The microthrombi formation is found throughout the entire vascular system, causing damage to multiple organs. The most susceptible organs for damage include the kidney, brain, and heart. Also affected are the pancreas, spleen, and adrenal glands. The thrombi are composed of platelets with minimal fibrin and red cells, differentiating them from thrombi secondary to intravascular coagulation (see p. 545). Most cases of TTP are related to a dysfunction of the plasma metalloprotease ADAMTS13. This enzyme is responsible for digesting large precursor molecules of von Willebrand factor (vWF) produced by endothelial cells into smaller molecules. Defects in ADAMTS13 result in expression of large-molecular-weight vWF on the endothelial cell surface and the formation of large aggregates of platelets, which can break off and form occlusions in smaller vessels. People with TTP (about 80%) have less than 5% of normal plasma ADAMTS13 levels. Most individuals with familial TTP are homozygous for mutations in ADAMTS13. Acquired TTP of unexplained origin is associated in most people with an IgG autoantibody against ADAMTS13 that is able to neutralize the enzyme's activity and accelerate its clearance from the plasma.

CLINICAL MANIFESTATIONS Chronic relapsing TTP is a rare familial form of TTP observed in children and usually recognized and successfully treated. The acquired acute idiopathic TTP is much more common and more severe.[77] TTP is clinically related to and must be distinguished from other thrombotic microangiopathic conditions, including hemolytic uremic syndrome (HUS), malignant hypertension, preeclampsia, and pregnancy-induced HELLP (*h*emolysis, *el*evated *l*iver enzymes, *l*ow *p*latelet count) syndrome. Early diagnosis and treatment is essential because TTP may prove fatal within 90 days.

Acute idiopathic TTP is characterized by a "pentad" of symptoms, including extreme thrombocytopenia (less than 20,000 platelets/μL), intravascular hemolytic anemia, ischemic signs and symptoms most often involving the CNS (about 65% present with memory disturbances, behavioral irregularities, headaches, or coma), kidney failure (present in about 65%), and fever (present in about 33%).

EVALUATION AND TREATMENT A routine blood smear usually shows fragmented red cells *(schizocytes)* produced by shear forces when red cells are in contact with the fibrin mesh in clots that form in the vessels. As a result of tissue injury, serum levels of lactate dehydrogenase (LDH) may be very high, and low-density lipoprotein (LDL) levels may be elevated. Tests for antibody on red cells are negative, excluding immune hemolytic anemia.

Plasma exchange with fresh frozen plasma, which replenishes functional ADAMTS13, is the treatment of choice, achieving a 70% to 85% response rate. Additionally, steroids (glucocorticoids) are administered. In the absence of major organ damage, this approach may lead to complete recovery with no long-term complications. The anti-CD20 monoclonal antibody rituximab has shown some success in people who are refractory to plasma exchange.[20] Relapses do occur at a rate of 13% to 36%, and recurrences have been reported, sometimes delayed until 9 years after treatment. Individuals who do not respond to conventional treatment may be candidates for splenectomy; however, postoperative hemorrhage remains a dangerous complication. Immunosuppression therapy has been successful in some individuals.

Thrombocythemia

Thrombocythemia (also called thrombocytosis) is defined as a platelet count greater than 400,000/μL of blood.[78] Thrombocythemia may be primary or secondary (reactive) and is usually asymptomatic until the count exceeds 1 million/μL. Then intravascular clot formation (thrombosis), hemorrhage, or other abnormalities can occur.

PATHOPHYSIOLOGY Essential (primary) thrombocythemia (ET) is a myeloproliferative neoplasm characterized by an increase in platelet production (or thrombocytosis) and often an increase in red blood cell production (or erythrocytosis).[79] Other disease features include leukocytosis, splenomegaly, thrombosis, bleeding, microcirculatory symptoms, itching (or pruritus), and risk of leukemic or bone marrow fibrotic transformation.[79] Myeloproliferative neoplasms (MPNs) are one of five categories of myeloid malignancies according to the WHO classification for hematologic tumors (see p. 532). ET is characterized by stem cell–derived clonal bone marrow proliferation (myeloproliferation) with a unique "gain-of function" mutation that induces overactivity in cell signaling from Janus kinase 2 (JAK2). JAK2, a tyrosine kinase, is an essential player downstream of cytokine receptors, such as the thrombopoietin (TPO, affects platelet proliferation) and erythropoietin (EPO, affects erythrocyte proliferation) receptors, and a gain-of-function mutation contributes to the development of MPN. More simply, both erythropoietin and thrombopoietin convey their signals and consequent proliferation through JAK2. The alteration is a valine-to-phenylalanine (V617F) mutation that causes constant activation of *JAK2*, leading to an increased responsiveness or production of platelets and other cells in the bone marrow. Along with increased platelets, there may be a concomitant increase in the number of red cells, indicating a myeloproliferative disorder; however, the increase in red cells is not to the extent seen in polycythemia vera (see p. 521). Red blood cells (RBCs) in ET tend to aggregate and adhere to the endothelium and contribute to the blockage of flow in the microvasculature and altered interactions between platelets and the vascular endothelium.[80] The *JAK2* (V617F) mutation is present in 50% to 60% of persons with ET. Other mutually exclusive mutations found include calreticulin (CALR) or leukemia virus oncogene (MPL) mutation. The

overall incidence of ET is 0.8 per 100,000 in the United Kingdom, 2.53 per 100,000 in the United States, and 0.59 per 100,000 in Denmark. It is more common in middle-age individuals, with the majority of cases occurring between ages 50 and 60 years. There is no known gender preference. There also is a rare hereditary type of ET called *familial essential thrombocythemia (FET)* that is inherited in an autosomal dominant pattern.

Secondary thrombocythemia may occur after splenectomy because platelets that normally would be stored in the spleen remain in circulating blood. The increase in platelets may be gradual, with thrombocythemia not occurring for up to 3 weeks after splenectomy. Reactive thrombocythemia may occur during some inflammatory conditions, such as rheumatoid arthritis and cancers. In these conditions, excessive production of some cytokines (e.g., IL-6, IL-11) may induce increased production of thrombopoietin in the liver, resulting in increased megakaryocyte proliferation. Reactive thrombocythemia also may occur during a variety of physiologic conditions, such as after exercise.

CLINICAL MANIFESTATIONS Clinical manifestations vary among individuals. Those with ET are at risk for large-vessel arterial or venous thrombosis, although the most common complication is microvasculature thrombosis leading to ischemia in the fingers, toes, or cerebrovascular regions.[80] The primary presenting symptoms of microvasculature thrombosis are erythromyalgia, headache, and paresthesias. Erythromyalgia is characterized by unilateral or bilateral warm, congested, red hands and feet with painful burning sensations, particularly in the forefoot sole and one or more toes. The lower extremities are affected more often and only one side may be involved. The pain is initiated by standing, exercise, or warmth and relieved by elevation and cooling. In extreme situations, acrocyanosis and gangrene may result.

Arterial thrombosis is more common than venous thrombosis and may involve the coronary and renal arteries. Deep venous thrombosis of the lower extremities and pulmonary embolism are the major sites for venous involvement. Other common venous sites include intraabdominal venous thrombosis (portal and hepatic). People older than 60 years of age or those with prior history of thrombotic events have as much as a 25% chance of developing a cerebral, cardiac, or peripheral arterial thrombus and, less often, developing a pulmonary embolism or deep vein thrombosis.[81,82] Conversion to acute leukemia is found in less than 10%.[83] Symptoms related to microvascular thrombosis in the CNS include headache, dizziness with paresthesias, transient ischemic attacks (TIAs), strokes, visual disturbances, and seizures. Major thrombotic events, not directly related to the platelet count, occur in about 20% to 30% of individuals with ET. Prior history of thrombotic events, advanced age, and duration of thrombocytosis are predictors of future thrombotic complications. Individuals older than age 60 are at greatest risk.

Although thrombosis is the more common symptom, hemorrhage can also occur. Sites for bleeding include the GI tract, skin, mucous membranes, urinary tract, gums, teeth sockets after extraction, joints, eyes, and brain. GI bleeding may be mistaken for a duodenal ulcer. Hemorrhage is not severe and generally occurs in the presence of very high platelet counts; transfusions are required only occasionally. Bleeding and clotting may occur simultaneously, and individuals will not necessarily be "bleeders" or "clotters."

EVALUATION AND TREATMENT Initial diagnosis is not difficult; as many as two thirds of cases are diagnosed from a routine complete blood cell count (CBC). Secondary thrombocytosis also may occur as a moderate rise in the platelet count that resolves with treatment or resolution of the underlying condition. The World Health Organization

(WHO) criteria for the diagnosis of ET require the following four criteria be met: (1) sustained platelet count of at least $450 \times 10^9/L$; (2) bone marrow biopsy showing proliferation of enlarged mature megakaryocytes and no increase of granulocyte or erythrocyte precursors; (3) failure to meet the criteria of polycythemia vera, myelofibrosis, CML, or other myelodysplastic syndrome; and (4) presence of JAK2 617F or another clonal marker or evidence of reactive thrombocytosis.[84] Because ET can be mistaken for CML, careful differentiation is necessary because treatment varies significantly.

Treatment of ET is directed toward preventing thrombosis or hemorrhage.[85] Reducing the platelet count remains a significant treatment issue. Hydroxyurea (HU), a nonalkylating myelosuppressive agent, has been the drug of choice to suppress platelet production; however, long-term use may cause progression to other myeloplastic disorders, particularly acute myeloid leukemia or myelofibrosis.[85] Another drug used to treat ET is interferon (IFN). IFN has a response rate of 80% but may not be effective for everyone because of side effects. Anagrelide is now the drug of choice. Anagrelide interferes with platelet maturation rather than production, thus not interfering with red and white cell growth and development. Low-dose aspirin may be effective to alleviate erthromyalgia and transient neurologic manifestations. ET is not necessarily considered life-threatening but, in those older than age 60 and who have had previous incidences of thrombosis, complications are more common and have a higher risk of mortality.

Alterations of Platelet Function

Qualitative alterations in platelet function are characterized by an increased bleeding time in the presence of a normal platelet count. Associated clinical manifestations include spontaneous petechiae and purpura, and bleeding from the GI tract, genitourinary tract, pulmonary mucosa, and gums. Congenital alterations in platelet function (thrombocytopathies) are quite rare and may be categorized into several types of disorders: (1) platelet–vessel wall adhesion (e.g., defect in GPIb-IX-V expression [Bernard-Soulier syndrome]), (2) platelet-platelet interactions (e.g., deficiency in $\alpha IIb\beta 3$ expression [Glanzmann thrombasthenia]), (3) platelet granules and secretion (e.g., receptor defects [ADP, collagen]), (4) arachidonic acid pathways (defects of prostaglandins and release granules), and (5) membrane phospholipid regulation or coagulation protein-platelet interactions (e.g., Scott syndrome).[86]

Acquired disorders of platelet function are more common than the congenital disorders and may be categorized into three principal causes: (1) drugs, (2) systemic inflammatory conditions, and (3) hematologic alterations.

Multiple drugs are known to interfere with platelet function in several ways: inhibition of platelet membrane receptors, inhibition of prostaglandin pathways, and inhibition of phosphodiesterase activity. Aspirin is the most commonly used drug that affects platelets. It irreversibly inhibits cyclooxygenase function for several days after administration. Nonsteroidal anti-inflammatory drugs also affect cyclooxygenase, although in a reversible fashion.

Systemic disorders that affect platelet function are chronic renal disease, liver disease, cardiopulmonary bypass surgery, and severe deficiencies of iron or folate and antiplatelet antibodies associated with autoimmune disorders. Hematologic disorders associated with platelet dysfunction include chronic myeloproliferative disorders, multiple myeloma, leukemias, and myelodysplastic syndromes and dysproteinemias.

Disorders of Coagulation

Disorders of coagulation are usually caused by defects or deficiencies of one or more of the clotting factors. (Normal function of the clotting factors is described in Chapter 20.) Qualitative or quantitative abnormalities interfere with or prevent the enzymatic reactions that transform clotting factors, circulating as plasma proteins, into a stable fibrin clot (see Figure 20-17). Some clotting factor defects are inherited and involve one a single factor, such as the hemophilias and von Willebrand disease, caused by deficiencies of specific clotting factors. Other coagulation defects are acquired and tend to result from deficient synthesis of clotting factors by the liver. Causes include liver disease and dietary deficiency of vitamin K.

Other coagulation disorders are attributed to pathologic conditions that trigger coagulation inappropriately, engaging the clotting factors and causing detrimental clotting within blood vessels. For example, any cardiovascular abnormality that alters normal blood flow by acceleration, deceleration, or obstruction can create conditions in which coagulation proceeds within the vessels. An example of this is thromboembolic disease, in which blood clots obstruct blood vessels. Coagulation is also stimulated by the presence of *tissue factor* that is released by damaged or dead tissues. Vasculitis, or inflammation of the blood vessels, along with vessel damage activates platelets, which in turn activates the coagulation cascade. In extensive or prolonged vasculitis, blood clot formation can suppress mechanisms that normally control clot formation and dissolution, leading to clogging of the vessels. In each of these acquired conditions, normal hemostatic function proves detrimental to the body by consuming coagulation factors excessively or by overwhelming normal control of clot formation and breakdown (fibrinolysis) (see Figure 20-19).

Impaired Hemostasis

Impaired hemostasis, or the inability to promote coagulation and the development of a stable fibrin clot, is commonly associated with liver dysfunction, which may be caused by either specific liver disorders or lack of vitamin K.

Vitamin K deficiency. Vitamin K, a fat-soluble vitamin, is required for the synthesis and regulation of prothrombin; the procoagulant factors (VII, IX, X); and the anticoagulant factors within the liver (proteins C and S).[87] Unknown is the contribution of vitamin K to the overall supply by the intestinal flora. The primary source of vitamin K is found in green leafy vegetables. The most common cause of vitamin deficiency is parenteral nutrition in combination with antibiotics that destroy normal gut flora. Rarely is the deficiency caused by a lack of dietary intake; however, bulimia can suppress vitamin K–dependent activity. Parenteral administration of vitamin K is the treatment of choice and usually results in correction of the deficiency within 8 to 12 hours. Fresh frozen plasma also may be administered but is usually reserved for individuals with life-threatening hemorrhages or those who require emergency surgery.

Liver disease. Individuals who have liver disease (for example, acute or chronic hepatocellular diseases, cirrhosis, vitamin K deficiency, or liver surgery) present with a broad range of hemostatic derangements that may be characterized by defects in the clotting or fibrinolytic systems and by platelet function. The hepatic parenchyma cells produce most of the factors involved in hemostasis; therefore, damage to the liver frequently results in diminished production of factors involved in clotting. Factor VII level is the first to decline after liver damage because of its rapid turnover. Factor IX levels are less affected and do not decline until the liver destruction is well advanced. The liver also is a major site for production of plasminogen and α_2-antiplasmin of the fibrinolytic system, as well as thrombopoietin and the metalloprotease ADAMTS13. Diminished thrombopoietin may lead to thrombocytopenia from decreased platelet production. Decreased production of ADAMTS13 results in increased levels of large precursor molecules of vWF, which leads to the formation of large aggregates of platelets.

With severe liver disease, such as cirrhosis, most clotting factors are significantly depressed. Levels of clotting system regulators, such as antithrombin, protein C, protein S, and fibrinogen, also are diminished. The fibrolytic system is commonly active because of plasmin inhibitor and unaffected other activators. Thrombocytopenia occurs in affected individuals because of diminished thrombopoietin and ADAMTS13, as well as increased sequestration (pooling) of platelets in the spleen, which is frequently enlarged in cirrhosis and is associated with portal hypertension. Thus, these individuals may appear to have a condition similar to DIC (see Consumptive Thrombohemorrhagic Disorders).

Treatment of hemostasis alterations in liver disease must be comprehensive to cover all aspects of dysfunctions. Fresh frozen plasma (FFP) administration is the treatment of choice; however, not all individuals tolerate the volume needed to adequately replace all deficient factors. Alternative modalities include the addition of exchange transfusions and platelet concentration to plasma administration.

Consumptive Thrombohemorrhagic Disorders

Consumptive thrombohemorrhagic disorders are a heterogeneous group of conditions that demonstrate the entire spectrum of hemorrhagic and thrombotic pathologic findings. Symptoms range from the subtle to the devastating and generally are considered to be intermediary disease processes that complicate a vast number of primary disease states. These disorders are also characterized by confusion and controversy related to their diagnosis, treatment, and management. No one definition can cover all possible varieties of these disorders; however, DIC is most commonly used in the clinical setting to describe a pathologic condition that is associated with hemorrhage and thrombosis.

Disseminated intravascular coagulation. Disseminated intravascular coagulation (DIC) is an acquired clinical syndrome characterized by widespread activation of coagulation resulting in formation of fibrin clots in medium and small vessels or microvasculature throughout the body.[88] Widespread clotting may lead to blockage of blood flow to organs, resulting in multiple organ failure. The magnitude of clotting may result in consumption of platelets and clotting factors, leading to tendency to bleed despite widespread clots.

The clinical course of DIC is largely determined by the stimulus intensity, host response, and comorbidities and ranges from an acute, severe, life-threatening process that is characterized by massive hemorrhage and thrombosis to a chronic, low-grade condition. The chronic condition is characterized by subacute hemorrhage and diffuse microcirculatory thrombosis. DIC may be localized to one specific organ or generalized, involving multiple organs.

The diagnosis of DIC has been confusing and difficult because of the complexity and wide variations in clinical manifestations. Minimally acceptable diagnostic criteria have been established and include a systemic thrombohemorrhagic disorder with laboratory evidence of (1) clotting activation, (2) fibrinolytic activation, (3) coagulation inhibitor consumption, and (4) biochemical evidence of end-organ damage or failure.

DIC is secondary to a wide variety of well-defined clinical conditions, specifically those capable of activating the clotting cascade. Sepsis is the most common condition associated with DIC. Gram-negative microorganisms, as well as some gram-positive microorganisms, fungi, protozoa (malaria), and viruses (influenza, herpes), are capable of precipitating DIC by causing damage to the vascular endothelium. Gram-negative endotoxins are the primary cause of endothelial damage; DIC may occur in up to 50% of individuals with gram-negative sepsis. DIC occurs in approximately 10% to 20% of individuals with metastatic cancer or acute leukemia. The adenocarcinomas most frequently associated with DIC include the lung, pancreas,

colon, and stomach.[34] Direct tissue damage (e.g., massive trauma, extensive surgery, severe burns) also results in release of tissue factor (TF), an initiator of DIC, by the endothelium. Severe trauma, especially to the brain, can induce DIC. DIC occurs in about two thirds of individuals with a systemic inflammatory response to trauma. Some complications of pregnancy also are associated with DIC; incidences range from 50% for women with placental abruptions to less than 10% for severe preeclampsia. Other causes of DIC have been identified, most notably blood transfusion. Transfused blood dilutes the clotting factors, as well as circulating naturally occurring antithrombins. In hemolytic transfusion reactions, the endothelium is damaged by complement-mediated reactions.

PATHOPHYSIOLOGY The coagulation system is designed to function at local areas of vascular damage, resulting in cessation of bleeding and activation of repair to the vessels. The function of clotting is to prevent excessive blood loss and the function of fibrinolysis is to ensure easy circulation within the vasculature (see Chapter 20). DIC results from abnormally widespread and ongoing activation of clotting—*coagulopathy*—in small and midsize vessels that alters the microcirculation, leading to ischemic necrosis in various organs, particularly the kidney and lung. Concomitantly, DIC can be caused by the imbalance between the coagulant system and the fibrinolytic system (which generates plasmin) to maintain normal circulation. DIC can cause widespread deposition of fibrin in the microcirculation that leads to ischemia, microvascular thrombotic obstruction, and organ failure (Figure 21-19).

Seemingly paradoxical, DIC involves both widespread clotting and bleeding because of simultaneous procoagulant activation, fibrinolytic

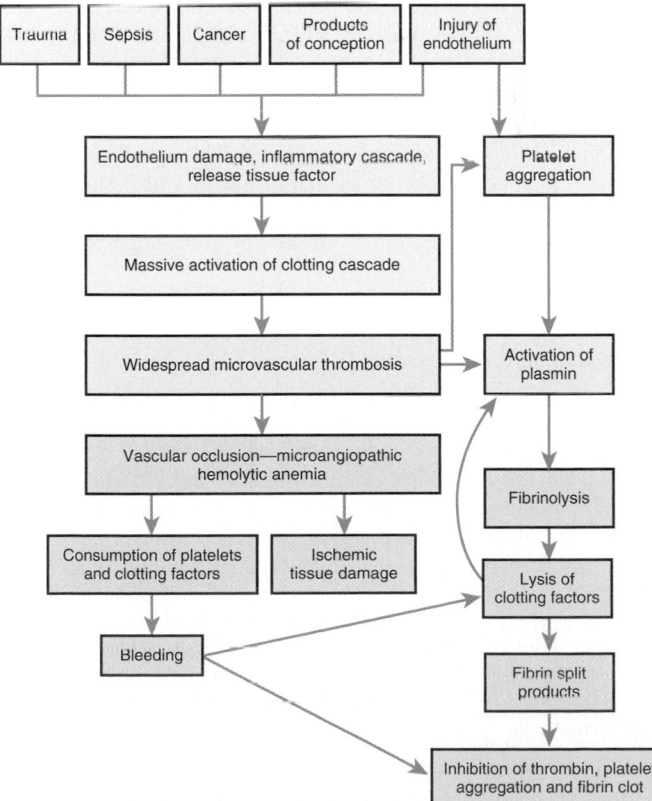

Disseminated Intravascular Coagulation (DIC)

FIGURE 21-19 Pathophysiology of Disseminated Intravascular Coagulation. See text.

BOX 21-4   Conditions Associated with DIC

Malignancy: acute myelocytic leukemia, metastatic solid tumors (pancreas, prostate)

Infections: bacterial (gram-negative endotoxin, gram-positive mucopolysaccharides), viral (hepatitis, CMV, dengue, HIV), fungal, parasitic, rickettsial

Pregnancy complications: eclampsia/preeclampsia, placental abruption, amniotic fluid embolism, dead fetus syndrome

Severe trauma: head injury, burns, crush injuries, tissue necrosis, severe hypo- or hyperthermia

Liver disease: obstructive jaundice, acute liver failure, fatty liver of pregnancy

Intravascular hemolysis: transfusion reactions, drug-induced hemolysis, viper snake bites, graft versus host disease

Medical devices: aortic balloon, prosthetic devices

Hypoxia and low blood flow states: arterial hypotension secondary to shock, cardiopulmonary arrest

Vascular disorders: Giant hemangiomas (Kasabach-Merritt syndrome), aortic aneurysms

---

activation, and consumption of platelets and coagulation factors, which results directly in serious bleeding (see Figure 21-19).

DIC is not a disease but is secondary to a variety of conditions (Box 21-4) because of activation of the clotting cascade. The common pathway for DIC appears to be excessive and widespread exposure to TF. This may occur by several mechanisms: (1) damage to the vascular endothelium results in exposure to TF; (2) when stimulated by inflammatory cytokines, endothelial cells and monocytes express surface TF; (3) endotoxin triggers the release of many cytokines that can both promote and cause progression of DIC; (4) sepsis is associated with many cytokines, interleukins, and platelet activating factor (PAF) that promote DIC as well as activate endothelial cells that stimulate thrombi development; and (5) TF may be released directly into the bloodstream from circulating white blood cells.

TF binds clotting factor VII, which leads to conversion of prothrombin to thrombin and formation of fibrin clots (see Figure 20-19). This pathway appears to be the primary route by which DIC is initiated; in animal models of DIC, inhibition of TF or factor VIIa completely prevents the generation of thrombi by gram-negative bacterial endotoxin.

Not only is the clotting system extensively activated in DIC, but also the activities of the predominant natural anticoagulants (tissue factor pathway inhibitor, antithrombin III, protein C) are greatly diminished. During DIC, the activation of clotting is prolonged and is a result of certain conditions (for example, bacteremia or endotoxemia); thrombin generation is increased and is insufficiently balanced by impaired anticoagulant systems, such as antithrombin and protein C.[89] The overall result is fibrin generation and deposition in the vascular system. In early DIC, plasmin (naturally occurring clot busting or fibrinolytic agent) produced from endothelial cells causes fibrinolysis to maintain circulation. Bleeding can occur with excess fibrinolytic activity. However, fibrinolysis becomes blunted by high levels of plasminogen activator inhibitor-1 (PAI-1), a fibrinolytic inhibitor.[89] Over time the activity of plasmin is diminished by PAI-1. Although some fibrinolytic activity remains, the level is inadequate to control the systemic deposition of fibrin. The slow breakdown of fibrin by plasmin produces fibrin split products (FSPs) (also known as fibrin degradation products [FDPs]). These products are powerful anticoagulants that are normally removed from blood by fibronectin and macrophages. FSPs, along with thrombin, induce further cytokine release from monocytes,

contributing to endothelial damage and TF release. During DIC, the presence of FSPs is prolonged possibly because of diminished production of fibronectin. *Fibronectin* is a glycoprotein with adhesive properties that mediates removal of particulate matter, such as fibrin clumps. Low levels of fibronectin suggest a poor prognosis.

Although thrombosis is generalized and widespread, individuals with DIC are paradoxically at risk for hemorrhage. Hemorrhage is secondary to the abnormally high consumption of clotting factors and platelets, as well as the anticoagulant properties of FSPs, which interfere with fibrin mesh formation or polymerization. Both thrombin and FSPs have a high affinity for platelets and cause platelet activation and aggregation—an event that occurs early in the development of DIC—which facilitates microcirculatory coagulation and obstruction in the initial phase. However, platelet consumption exceeds production, resulting in a thrombocytopenia that increases bleeding.

Activation of clotting also leads to activation of other inflammatory pathways, including the kallikrein-kinin and complement systems (see Chapter 6). Factor XIIa, generated in DIC, converts prekallikrein to kallikrein, ultimately resulting in conversion to circulating kinins. Activation of these systems contributes to increased vascular permeability, hypotension, and shock. Activated complement components also induce platelet destruction, which initially contributes to the thrombosis and later to the thrombocytopenia.

The deposition of fibrin clots in the circulation interferes with blood flow, causing widespread organ hypoperfusion. This condition may lead to ischemia, infarction, and necrosis, further potentiating and complicating the existing DIC process by causing further release of TF and eventually organ failure. Manifestations of multisystem organ dysfunction and failure ultimately result.

In addition to initiation of clotting by tissue factor, DIC may be precipitated by direct proteolytic activation of factor X. This has been described as "thrombin mimicry" and is the result of proteases directly converting fibrinogen to fibrin. These proteases may come from snake venom, some tumor cells, or the pancreas and liver, where they are respectively released during episodes of pancreatitis and various stages of liver disease. Direct proteolytic activity appears to be independent of any type of damage to the endothelium or tissue.

Whatever initiates the process of DIC, the cycle of thrombosis and hemorrhage persists until the underlying cause of the DIC is removed or appropriate therapeutic interventions are used.

CLINICAL MANIFESTATIONS   Clinical signs and symptoms of DIC present a wide spectrum of possibilities, depending on the underlying disease process that initiates DIC and whether the DIC is acute or chronic in nature (Box 21-5). Most symptoms are the result of either bleeding or thrombosis. Acute DIC presents with rapid development of hemorrhaging (oozing) from venipuncture sites, arterial lines, or surgical wounds or development of ecchymotic lesions (purpura, petechiae) and hematomas. Other sites of bleeding include the eyes (sclera, conjunctiva), the nose, and the gums. Most individuals with DIC demonstrate bleeding at three or more unrelated sites, and any combination may be observed. Shock of variable intensity, out of proportion to the amount of blood loss, also may be observed. Hemorrhaging into closed compartments of the body also can occur and may precede the development of shock.

Manifestations of thrombosis are not always as evident, even though it is often the first pathologic alteration to occur. The initial observations may be bleeding and sometimes very extensive hemorrhage. Several organ systems are susceptible to microvascular thrombosis associated with dysfunction: cardiovascular, pulmonary, central nervous, renal, and hepatic systems. Acute and accurate clinical interpretations are critical to preventing progression of DIC that may lead

BOX 21-5 Clinical Manifestations Associated with DIC

Integumentary System
Widespread hemorrhage and vascular lesions
Oozing from puncture sites, incisions, mucous membranes
Acrocyanosis (irregular-shaped cyanotic patches)
Gangrene

Central Nervous System
Subarachnoid hemorrhage
Altered state of consciousness (slight confusion to convulsions and coma)

Gastrointestinal System
Occult bleeding to massive gastrointestinal bleeding
Abdominal distention
Malaise
Weakness

Pulmonary System
Pulmonary infarctions
ARDS
Cyanosis
Tachypnea
Hypoxemia

Renal System
Hematuria
Oliguria
Renal failure

to multisystem organ dysfunction and failure. (Multiple organ dysfunction and failure are discussed further in Chapter 24.) Indicators of multisystem dysfunction include changes in level of consciousness or behavior, confusion, seizure activity, oliguria, hematuria, hypoxia, hypotension, hemoptysis, chest pain, and tachycardia. Symmetric cyanosis of fingers and toes (blue finger/toe syndrome), nose, and breast may be observed and indicates macrovascular thrombosis. This may lead to infarction and gangrene that may require amputation. Jaundice also is observed and most likely results from red cell destruction rather than liver dysfunction.

Individuals with chronic or low-grade DIC do not present with the overt manifestations of hemorrhaging and thrombosis but instead have subacute bleeding and diffuse thrombosis; these individuals are described as having *compensated DIC,* or *non-overt DIC.* The major characteristic of this state is an increased turnover and decreased survival time of the components of hemostasis: platelets and clotting factors. Occasionally, diffuse or localized thrombosis develops, but this is infrequent.

EVALUATION AND TREATMENT No single laboratory test can be used to effectively diagnose DIC. Diagnosis is based primarily on clinical symptoms and confirmed by a combination of laboratory tests. The person must present with a clinical condition that is known to be associated with DIC. The most commonly used combination of laboratory tests usually confirms thrombocytopenia or a rapidly decreasing platelet count on repeated testing, prolongation of clotting times, the presence of fibrin split products, and decreased levels of coagulation inhibitors. Platelet counts below 100,000/μL or a progressive decrease in platelet counts is very sensitive for DIC, although

not greatly specific. These changes usually indicate consumption of platelets.

The standard coagulation tests (e.g., prothrombin time [PT], activated partial thromboplastin time [aPTT]) also have a high degree of sensitivity, but they are not highly specific for DIC. As a result of consumption of circulating clotting factors, these tests are usually abnormal, ranging from shortened to prolonged times. However, conditions other than DIC may prolong clotting times.

Detection of fibrin split products is more specific for DIC. Detection of D-dimers is a widely used test for DIC. A D-dimer is a molecule produced by plasmin degradation of cross-linked fibrin in clots. D-Dimers in the blood can be quantified using ELISA tests that include commercially available and highly specific monoclonal antibody against the D-dimer. Agglutination tests for other fibrin split products are available. Levels of fibrin split products are elevated in the plasma in 95% to 100% of cases; however, they are less specific and only document the presence of plasmin and its action on fibrin. ELISAs for markers of thrombin activity are sometimes used.

Levels of coagulation inhibitors (e.g., antithrombin III [AT-III], protein C) can be measured by assays that rely on function or by ELISAs that quantify the amount of the specific inhibitor. AT-III levels can provide key information for diagnosing and monitoring therapy of DIC. Initial levels of functional AT-III are low in DIC because thrombin is irreversibly complexed with activated clotting factors and AT-III.

Treatment of DIC is directed toward (1) eliminating the underlying pathologic condition, (2) controlling ongoing thrombosis, and (3) maintaining organ function. Elimination of the underlying pathologic condition is the initial intervention in the treatment phase in order to remove the trigger for activation of clotting. Once the stimulus is gone, production of coagulation factors in the liver leads to restoration of normal plasma levels within 24 to 48 hours.

Control of thrombosis is more difficult to attain. Heparin has been used for this; however, its use is controversial because its mechanism of action is binding to and activating AT-III, which is deficient in many types of DIC. Currently, heparin is only indicated in certain types of situations related to DIC. For instance, heparin seems to be effective in DIC caused by a retained dead fetus or associated with acute promyelocytic leukemia. Organ function is compromised by microthrombi, and there is a risk of losing an extremity because of vascular occlusion; thus heparin is also indicated in these conditions. Heparin's usefulness, however, for DIC that is precipitated by septic shock has not been established and so is contraindicated in that instance; heparin is also contraindicated when there is evidence of postoperative bleeding, peptic ulcer, or central nervous system bleeding.

Replacement of deficient coagulation factors, platelets, and other coagulation elements is gaining recognition as an effective treatment modality. Their use is not without controversy, however, because a major concern with replacement therapy is the possible risk of adding components that will increase the rate of thrombosis. Clinical judgment is the key factor in determining whether replacement is to be used as a treatment modality.

Several clinical trials are evaluating replacement of anticoagulants (i.e., AT-III, protein C). Replacement of AT-III appears to be effective in DIC caused by sepsis. Low levels of AT-III correlate with sepsis-initiated DIC, which makes a case for its use. AT-III inactivates thrombin, factor Xa, factor IXa, and other activated components of the clotting system. Heparin augments AT-III, but the effectiveness of the combination of heparin with AT-III replacement has not been established. Antifibrinolytic drugs also are used in treatment but are limited to instances of life-threatening bleeding that have not been controlled by blood component replacement therapy.

FIGURE 21-20 Thrombus. Thrombus arising in valve pocket at upper end of superficial femoral vein *(arrow)*. Postmortem clot on the right is shown for comparison. (From McLachlin J, Paterson JC: *Surg Gynecol Obstet* 93[1]:1-8, 1951.)

Maintenance of organ function is achieved by fluid replacement to sustain adequate circulating blood volume and maintain optimal tissue and organ perfusion. Fluids may be required to restore blood pressure, cardiac output, and urine output to normal parameters.

Thromboembolic Disorders

Certain conditions within the blood vessels predispose an individual to develop clots spontaneously. A stationary clot attached to the vessel wall is called a **thrombus** (Figure 21-20). A thrombus is composed of fibrin and blood cells and can develop in either the arterial or the venous system. **Arterial thrombi** form under conditions of high blood flow and are composed mostly of platelet aggregates held together by fibrin strands. **Venous thrombi** form under conditions of low flow and are composed mostly of red cells with larger amounts of fibrin and few platelets.

A thrombus eventually reduces or obstructs blood flow to tissues or organs, such as the heart, brain, or lungs, depriving them of essential nutrients critical to survival. A thrombus also has the potential of detaching from the vessel wall and circulating within the bloodstream (referred to as an **embolus**). The embolus may become lodged in smaller blood vessels, blocking blood flow into the local tissue or organ and leading to ischemia. Whether episodes of thromboembolism are life-threatening depends on the site of vessel occlusion.

Therapy consists of removal or dissolution of the clot and supportive measures. Anticoagulant therapy is effective in treating or preventing venous thrombosis; it is not as useful in treating or preventing arterial thrombosis. Parenteral heparin is the major anticoagulant used to treat thromboembolism. Oral coumarin drugs also are widely used, including a newer direct factor Xa inhibitor (rivaroxaban). More aggressive therapy may be indicated for such conditions as pulmonary embolism, coronary thrombosis, or thrombophlebitis. Streptokinase, tissue plasminogen activator (t-PA), and urokinase activate the fibrinolytic system and are administered to accelerate the lysis of known thrombi. These drugs are known as fibrinolytic or thrombolytic

therapy and are prescribed with a high degree of caution because they can cause hemorrhagic complications.

The risk for developing spontaneous thrombi is related to several factors, referred to as the **Virchow triad**: (1) injury to the blood vessel endothelium, (2) abnormalities of blood flow, and (3) hypercoagulability of the blood. The role of estrogens as a cause of thrombi has received much attention.

Endothelial injury to blood vessels can result from atherosclerosis (plaque deposits on arterial walls) (see Chapter 24). Atherosclerosis initiates platelet adhesion and aggregation, promoting the development of atherosclerotic plaques that enlarge, causing further damage and occlusion. Other causes of vessel endothelial injury may be related to hemodynamic alterations associated with hypertension and turbulent blood flow. Injury also is caused by radiation injury, exogenous chemical agents (e.g., toxins from cigarette smoke), endogenous agents (e.g., cholesterol), bacterial toxins or endotoxins, or immunologic mechanisms.

Sites of turbulent blood flow in the arteries and stasis of blood flow in the veins are at risk for thrombus formation. In areas of turbulence, platelets and endothelial cells may be activated, leading to thrombosis. In sites of stasis, platelets may remain in contact with the endothelium for prolonged lengths of time, and clotting factors that would normally be diluted with fresh flowing blood are not diluted and may become activated. The most common clinical conditions that predispose to venous stasis and subsequent thromboembolic phenomena are major surgery (e.g., orthopedic surgery), acute myocardial infarction, congestive heart failure, limb paralysis, spinal injury, malignancy, advanced age, the postpartum period, and bed rest longer than 1 week. Turbulence and stasis occur with ulcerated atherosclerotic plaques (myocardial infarction), hyperviscosity (polycythemia), and conditions with deformed red cells (sickle cell anemia).

Hypercoagulability, or **thrombophilia,** is the condition in which an individual is at risk for thrombosis, but by itself it is a rare cause of thrombosis. Hypercoagulability is differentiated according to whether it results from primary (hereditary) or secondary (acquired) causes.

Hereditary thrombophilias. Thrombophilias can result from both inherited conditions and, more commonly, acquired conditions.[90] Several inherited conditions increase the risk of developing thrombosis and most are autosomal dominant. Thus individuals who are homozygous for the mutation are at greatest risk for thrombosis. These include mutations in platelet receptors, coagulation proteins, fibrinolytic proteins, and other factors. The particular mutations that have been most strongly linked as risk factors for venous thrombosis or for arterial thrombosis leading to coronary artery disease or stroke include those that affect fibrinogen, prothrombin (G20210A variant), factor V (factor V Leiden) of the coagulation system, PAI-1 of the fibrinolytic system, the platelet receptor GPIIIa, and methylenetetrahydrofolate reductase (MTHFR), as well as mutations that result in excessive levels of homocysteine (hyperhomocysteinemia). Other inherited thrombophilias are risk factors mostly for venous thrombosis and include deficiencies in protein C, protein S, and AT-III.[90,91] Factor V Leiden results from a single nucleotide mutation that confers partial resistance to inactivation by activated protein C, resulting in prolonged high levels of activated factor V (factor Va) and overproduction of thrombin. Although this mutation increases the risk for thrombosis, most individuals with factor V Leiden do not have clinically relevant thrombotic events. It is the most common hereditary thrombophilia and is primarily observed in individuals of European ancestry. It is observed in about 5% of whites in the United States and in about 30% of individuals presenting with deep venous thrombosis (DVT) or pulmonary embolism.

Other hereditary thrombophilias are less common. Prothrombin mutation, which leads to high levels of circulating prothrombin, is observed in about 2% to 5% of individuals of European ancestry. It is, however, found in 5% to 10% of individuals presenting with thrombosis.

THFR mutation leads to alterations in the metabolism of the amino acid homocysteine into methionine and abnormally elevated levels of that amino acid in the blood (hyperhomocysteinemia). Acquired hyperhomocysteinemia may result from deficiencies in vitamins B_6 or B_{12}, endocrine diseases (e.g., diabetes mellitus, hypothyroidism), pernicious anemia, inflammatory bowel disease, renal failure, and therapy with some drugs. Individuals with homocysteine levels greater than the 95th percentile are 2.5 times more likely to experience an episode of DVT.

More than 100 different known mutations lead to defects of proteins C, protein S, and AT-III and increase the risk of venous thrombosis. Mutations may lead to either quantitative (low levels of protein) or qualitative (production of defective protein) changes.

Tests to diagnose inherited thrombophilias include prothrombin time; partial thromboplastin time; and levels of protein C, protein S, and AT-III. More elaborate tests to detect precise mutations in factor V, prothrombin, or MTHFR may be indicated.

Acquired hypercoagulability. Deficiencies in proteins S and C and AT-III may be acquired and contribute to a hypercoagulable state.[92] Conditions associated with an acquired protein deficiency include DIC, liver disease, infection, DVT, acute respiratory distress syndrome, L-asparaginase therapy, HUS, and TTP. The postoperative state also predisposes an individual to protein C or S deficiency; however, its role in contributing to DVT remains unclear.

Acquired hypercoagulable states include *antiphospholipid syndrome (APS)*.[93] APS is an autoimmune syndrome characterized by autoantibodies against plasma membrane phospholipids and phospholipid-binding proteins. As with most autoimmune diseases, the predominantly affected individual is female and of reproductive age. Those with APS are at risk for both arterial and venous thrombosis and a variety of obstetric complications, including pregnancy loss and preeclampsia/eclampsia. In severe cases the individual may die from recurrent major thrombus formation.[94] The pathophysiology is related to autoantibodies directly reacting with platelets or endothelial cells (increasing the risk for thrombosis) or the placental surface (resulting in damage to the placenta). The predominant diagnostic tests measure prolongation of laboratory blood coagulation tests related to an antibody inhibitor (lupus anticoagulant) and specific ELISAs for antibodies against phospholipids (e.g., anticardiolipin antibody) or proteins that bind to phospholipids (e.g., β_2-glycoprotein I). Highly effective therapy (i.e., unfractionated or low-molecular-weight heparin with low-dose aspirin) is available to prevent the obstetric complications.[95]

✔ **QUICK CHECK 21-6**

1. Identify three pathologic causes of DIC, and describe the manifestations associated with DIC.
2. Compare and contrast thrombocytopenia with thrombocytosis.
3. Why does vitamin K deficiency predispose an individual to a coagulation disorder?
4. Compare and contrast a thrombus with an embolus.

■ DID YOU UNDERSTAND?

Alterations of Erythrocyte Function

1. Anemia is defined as a reduction in the number or volume of circulating red cells or a decrease in the quality or quantity of hemoglobin.
2. The most common classification of anemias is based on changes in the cell size—represented by the cell suffix -*cytic*—and changes in the cell's hemoglobin content—represented by the suffix -*chromic*.
3. Clinical manifestations of anemia can be found in all organs and tissues throughout the body. Decreased oxygen delivery to tissues causes fatigue, dyspnea, syncope, angina, compensatory tachycardia, and organ dysfunction.
4. Macrocytic (megaloblastic) anemias are characterized by unusually large stem cells in the marrow that mature into very large erythrocytes. Macrocytic anemias are caused most commonly by deficiency of vitamin B_{12}. Pernicious anemia, the most common type of macrocytic anemia, can be fatal unless vitamin B_{12} replacement is given (lifelong replacement is required).
5. Microcytic-hypochromic anemias are characterized by abnormally small red cells with insufficient hemoglobin content. The most common cause is iron deficiency.
6. Iron deficiency anemia is the most common type of anemia worldwide and usually develops slowly, with a gradual, insidious onset of symptoms, including fatigue, weakness, dyspnea, alteration of various epithelial tissues, and vague neuromuscular complaints.
7. Iron deficiency anemia is usually a result of a chronic blood loss or decreased iron intake. Once the source of blood loss is identified and corrected, iron replacement therapy can be initiated.
8. Sideroblastic anemias are a heterogeneous group of inherited and acquired disorders. Sideroblastic anemias have various causes but share altered heme synthesis.
9. Normocytic-normochromic anemias are characterized by insufficient numbers of normal erythrocytes. Included in this category are aplastic, posthemorrhagic, acquired hemolytic, hereditary hemolytic, and anemia of chronic inflammation.

Myeloproliferative Red Cell Disorders

1. Polycythemia vera is a stem cell disorder with hyperplastic and neoplastic bone marrow alterations. It is characterized by excessive proliferation of erythrocyte precursors (frequently with increased white blood cells and platelets) in the bone marrow. Polycythemia is responsible for most of the clinical symptoms, including increased blood volume and viscosity. Frequent phlebotomies reduce iron levels and hydroxyurea is the drug of choice for myelosuppression. Use of radioactive phosphorus has been helpful in decreasing the excessive red cell pool.
2. Polycythemia vera may spontaneously convert to acute myelogenous leukemia.

Alterations of Leukocyte Function

1. Quantitative alterations of leukocytes (too many or too few) can be caused by bone marrow dysfunction or premature destruction of cells in the circulation. Many quantitative changes in leukocytes occur in response to invasion by microorganisms.
2. Leukocytosis is a condition in which the leukocyte count is higher than normal and is usually a response to physiologic stressors and invasion of microorganisms.
3. Leukopenia is present when the leukocyte count is lower than normal and is caused by pathologic conditions, such as malignancies and hematologic disorders.

4. Granulocytosis (particularly as a result of an increase in neutrophils, eosinophils, or basophils) occurs in response to infection and inflammation.

5. Eosinophilia results most commonly from allergic disorders, parasitic invasion, and ingestion or inhalation of toxic foreign particles.

6. Basophilia is rare and generally is a response to inflammation and immediate hypersensitivity reactions. Basopenia is a decrease in circulating numbers of basophils.

7. Monocytosis is an increase in numbers of circulating monocytes and is often transient. It occurs during the late or recuperative phase of infection. Monocytopenia is a decrease in circulating monocytes.

8. Granulocytopenia, a significant decrease in the number of neutrophils, can be a life-threatening condition if sepsis occurs; it is often caused by chemotherapeutic agents, severe infection, and radiation.

9. Lymphocytopenia is a decrease in the number of circulating lymphocytes in the blood. It is associated with neoplasias, immune deficiencies, and destruction by drugs, viruses, or radiation.

10. Infectious mononucleosis (IM) is an acute infection of B lymphocytes most commonly (85% of IM cases) associated with the Epstein-Barr virus (EBV). The classic symptoms are pharyngitis, lymphadenopathy, and fever. The proliferation of infected B cells may be uncontrolled and lead to B-cell lymphomas.

11. Transmission of EBV is usually through saliva from close personal contact. IM is self-limiting and treatment consists of rest and symptomatic treatment.

12. The common pathologic feature of all forms of leukemia is an uncontrolled proliferation of leukocytes, overcrowding the bone marrow and resulting in decreased production and function of the other blood cell lines.

13. The classification of leukemias is based on the cell type involved—myeloid or lymphoid—and the rate of progression—acute or chronic. There are four major types of leukemia: acute lymphocytic leukemia (ALL), acute myelogenous leukemia (AML), chronic lymphocytic leukemia (CLL), and chronic myelogenous leukemia (CML).

14. Although the exact cause of leukemia is unknown, several risk factors and related genetic aberrations are associated with the onset of malignancy. The leukemias are clonal disorders driven by genetically abnormal stem-like cancer cells.

15. Abnormal immature white blood cells, called blasts, fill the bone marrow and spill into the blood. The blasts overcrowd the marrow and cause cellular proliferation of the other cell lines to cease.

16. The major clinical manifestations of leukemia include fatigue caused by anemia, bleeding caused by thrombocytopenia, fever secondary to infection, anorexia, and weight loss.

17. Treatment varies depending on the type of leukemia and includes observation, steroids, chemotherapy, monoclonal antibodies, and transplant options.

18. Chronic leukemias progress differently than acute leukemias (which can be abrupt and stormy onset), advancing slowly and insidiously.

Alterations of Lymphoid Function

1. Lymphadenopathy is enlarged lymph nodes.

2. Lymphomas consist of a diverse group of neoplasms that develop from the proliferation of malignant lymphocytes in the lymphoid system. The WHO classification, based on structure and cell lineage, recognizes three major categories of lymphomas: B-cell neoplasms, T-cell/natural killer–cell (NK-cell) neoplasms, and Hodgkin lymphoma. Two *basic* categories of lymphomas are Hodgkin lymphoma and non-Hodgkin lymphoma.

3. In general, lymphomas are the result of genetic mutations or viral infection. Malignant transformation produces a cell with uncontrolled and excessive growth that accumulates in the lymph nodes and other sites, producing tumor masses.

4. Hodgkin lymphoma is characterized by the abnormal cell called the Reed-Sternberg cell.

5. The pathogenesis of Hodgkin lymphoma may be linked to infection with Epstein-Barr virus (EBV).

6. An enlarged, painless mass or swelling, most commonly in the neck, is an initial sign of Hodgkin lymphoma; however, asymptomatic lymphadenopathy can progress undetected for years.

7. Treatment of Hodgkin lymphoma includes chemotherapy, radiation therapy, and surgery. Treatment with chemotherapy or radiation therapy, or both, may increase the risk of second cancers, cardiovascular disease, and other health problems months or years after treatment.

8. The non-Hodgkin lymphomas (NHLs) are a heterogeneous group of proliferative lymphoid tissue neoplasms. Clonal expansion of B cells accounts for the majority of NHLs. Oncogenes may be activated by chromosomal translocation (most common alteration) or by deletion of tumor-suppressor genes. Certain subtypes may have altered genomes by oncogenic viruses.

9. Generally, with non-Hodgkin lymphoma, the swelling of lymph nodes is painless and the nodes enlarge and transform over a period of months or years.

10. Standard treatment for NHL includes radiation therapy, chemotherapy, target therapy (monoclonal antibody therapy, proteasome inhibitor therapy), plasmapheresis, biologic therapy, and watchful waiting.

11. Burkitt lymphoma is a B-cell tumor and involves the jaw and facial bones and sometimes the abdomen. Although more common in Africa, it is documented in the United States, Latin America, and other countries. Burkitt lymphoma is heterogeneous and may involve infection with EBV and suppression of the immune system by other illnesses.

12. Treatment for Burkitt lymphoma is intensive chemotherapy.

13. Multiple myeloma (MM) is a neoplasm of plasma cells in the bone marrow and usually not found in the blood. It is characterized by multiple malignant tumor masses of plasma cells scattered throughout the skeletal system (lytic bone lesions) and sometimes found in soft tissue.

14. MM tumors are highly heterogeneous and involve mutations in different signaling pathways. Chromosomal translocations are common. The exact cause of multiple myeloma is unknown, but risk factors include radiation, certain chemicals, and a history of monoclonal gammopathy of undetermined significance (MGUS).

15. The common presentation of MM is characterized by elevated levels of calcium in the blood, renal failure, anemia, and bone (lytic) lesions.

16. Treatment includes chemotherapy, radiation therapy, plasmapheresis, and stem cell transplant.

Alterations of Splenic Function

1. Splenomegaly (enlargement of the spleen) may be considered normal in certain individuals but its presence is associated with various diseases.

2. Splenomegaly results from (1) acute inflammatory or infectious processes, (2) congestive disorders, (3) infiltrative processes, and (4) tumors or cysts.

3. Hypersplenism (overactivity of the spleen) results from spleno-megaly. Hypersplenism results in sequestering of the blood cells, causing increased destruction of red blood cells, leukopenia, and thrombocytopenia.

Hemorrhagic Disorders and Alterations of Platelets and Coagulation

1. The arrest of bleeding is called hemostasis.
2. Thrombocytopenia is characterized by a platelet count below 150,000/μL of blood; the most significant count is less than 100,000 platelets/μL, and a count less than 50,000/μL increases the potential for hemorrhage associated with minor trauma.
3. Thrombocytopenia exists in primary or secondary forms and is associated with autoimmune diseases, viral infections, drugs, nutritional deficiencies, chronic renal failure, cancer, radiation therapy, bone marrow hypoplasia, and DIC.
4. Immune thrombocytopenic purpura (ITP) is the most common cause of thrombocytopenia secondary to increased platelet destruction.
5. Thrombocythemia is characterized by a platelet count more than 400,000 platelets/μL of blood and is symptomatic when the count exceeds 1 million/μL, at which time the risk for intravascular clotting (thrombosis) is high.
6. Thrombocythemia is a myeloproliferative neoplasm characterized by an increase in platelet production in the bone marrow. It also can include an increase in red blood cell production.
7. Qualitative alterations in normal platelet function prevent platelet plug formation and may result in prolonged bleeding times. Acquired disorders of platelet function are more common than congenital disorders.
8. Disorders of coagulation are usually caused by defects or deficiencies of one or more clotting factors. Coagulation is stimulated by the presence of tissue factor that is released by damaged or dead tissues.
9. Coagulation is impaired when there is a deficiency of vitamin K because of insufficient production of prothrombin and synthesis of clotting factors VII, IX, and X, often associated with liver diseases.
10. Disseminated intravascular coagulation (DIC) is an acquired clinical syndrome characterized by widespread activation of coagulation, resulting in formation of fibrin clots in medium and small vessels or microvasculature throughout the body. Widespread clotting may lead to blockage of blood flow to organs, resulting in multiple organ failure. The magnitude of clotting may result in consumption of platelets and clotting factors, leading to a tendency to bleed despite widespread clots.
11. DIC is secondary to a wide variety of clinical conditions with sepsis as the most common condition associated with DIC.
12. For a diagnosis of DIC, the person must present with a clinical condition that is known to be associated with DIC. The most commonly used combination of laboratory tests usually confirms thrombocytopenia, or a rapidly decreasing platelet count on repeated testing, prolongation of clotting times, the presence of fibrin split products, and decreased levels of coagulation inhibitors may indicate the presence of DIC.
13. Treatment of DIC is directed toward (1) eliminating the underlying pathologic condition, (2) controlling ongoing thrombosis, and (3) maintaining organ function.
14. Thromboembolic disease results from a fixed (thrombus) or moving (embolus) clot that blocks flow within a vessel, denying nutrients to tissues distal to the occlusion; death can result when clots obstruct blood flow to the heart, brain, or lungs.
15. Hypercoagulability, or thrombophilia, is a condition in which an individual is at risk for thrombosis.
16. The term *Virchow triad* refers to three factors that can cause thrombus formation: (1) loss of integrity of the vessel wall, (2) abnormalities of blood flow, and (3) alterations in the blood constituents.

KEY TERMS

REFERENCES

1. Sun CC et al: Targeting the hepcidin-ferroportion axis to develop new treatment strategies for anemia of chronic disease and anemia of inflammation, *Am J Hematol* 87:392-400, 2012.
2. Muñoz M et al: Disorders of iron metabolism. Part II: iron deficiency and iron overload, *J Clin Pathol* 64(4):287-296, 2011.
3. Lang E et al: Killing me softly—suicidal erythrocyte death, *Int J Biochem Cell Biol* 44(8):1236-1243, 2012.
4. den Elzen WP et al: Subnormal vitamin B$_{12}$ concentrations and anaemia in older people: a systematic review, *BMC Geriatr* 10:42, 2010.
5. Banka S et al: Pernicious anemia—genetic insights, *Autoimmun Rev* 10(8):455-459, 2011.
6. Annibale B et al: Diagnosis and management of pernicious anemia, *Curr Gastroenterol Rep* 13(6):518-524, 2011.
7. Neumann WL et al: Autoimmune atropic gastritis-pathogenesis, pathology and management, *Nat Rev Gastroenterol Hepatol* 10:529-541, 2013.
8. Toh BH et al: Cutting edge issues in autoimmune gastritis, *Clin Rev Allerg Immunol* 42(3):269-278, 2012.
9. Vojdani A: Antibodies as predictors of complex autoimmune diseases, *Int J Immunopathol Pharmacol* 21(2):267-278, 2008.
10. Guidi GC, Lechi Santonastaso C: Advancements in anemias related to chronic conditions, *Clin Chem Lab Med* 48(9):1217-1226, 2010.
11. West AR, Oates PS: Mechanisms of heme iron absorption: current questions and controversies, *World J Gastroenterol* 14(26):4101-4110, 2008.
12. Chakraborty PK et al: Mutations in TRNT1 cause congenital sideroblastic anemia with immunodeficiency, fevers, and developmental delay (SIFD), *Blood* 124(18):2867-2871, 2014.
13. Garcia-Manero G: Myelodysplastic syndromes: 2012 update on diagnosis, risk-stratification, and management, *Am J Hematol* 87(7):693-701, 2012.
14. Malcovati L, Nimer SD: Myelodysplastic syndromes: diagnosis and staging, *Cancer Contr* 15(Suppl):4-13, 2008.
15. Moyo V et al: Erythropoiesis-stimulating agents in the treatment of anemia in myelodysplastic syndromes: a meta-analysis, *Ann Hematol* 87(7):527-536, 2008.
16. Scheinberg P, Chen J: Aplastic anemia: what have we learned from animal models and from the clinic, *Semin Hematol* 50(2):156-164, 2013.
17. Finazzi G, Barbui T: Evidence and expertise in the management of polycythemia vera and essential thrombocythemia, *Leukemia* 22(8):1494-1502, 2008.
18. Tefferi A: Polycythemia vera and essential thrombocythemia: 2013 update on diagnosis, risk stratification and management, *Am J Hematol* 88(6):507-516, 2013.

19. Tefferi A, Barbui T: Personalized management of essential thrombocythemia—application of recent evidence to clinical practice, *Leukemia* 27:1617-1620, 2013.
20. Scully M et al: A phase 2 study of the safety and efficacy of rituximab with plasma exchange in acute acquired thrombotic thrombocytopenic purpura, *Blood* 118(7):1746-1753, 2011.
21. *Thrombocytopenia & thrombocytosis*, Bethesda, Md, 2008, National Institutes of Health, U.S. Department of Health and Human Services. Available at: www.nhlbi.nih.gov/health/dci/Diseases/thrm/thrm_all.html. Accessed September 1, 2012.
22. Crownover BK, Covery CH: Hereditory hemochromatosis, *Am Fam Physician* 87(3):183-190, 2013.
23. Greenberg PL: Myelodysplastic syndromes, *J Natl Compr Canc Netw* 9(1):30-56, 2011.
24. Weinzierl EP, Arber DA: The differential diagnosis and bone marrow evaluation of new-onset pancytopenia, *Am J Clin Pathol* 139:9-29, 2013.
25. Thorley-Lawson DA et al: The pathogenesis of Epstein-Barr virus persistent infection, *Curr Opin Virol* 3(3):227-232, 2013.
26. Thorley-Lawson DA, Gross A: Persistence of the Epstein-Barr virus and the origins of associated lymphomas, *N Engl J Med* 350(13):1328-1337, 2004.
27. Konopleva MY, Jordan CT: Leukemia stem cells and microenvironment: biology and therapeutic targeting, *J Clin Oncol* 29(5):591-599, 2011.
28. Pollyea DA et al: Targeting acute myeloid leukemia stem cells: a review and principles for the development of clinical trials, *Haematologica* 99:1277-1284, 2014.
29. Visco C et al: Autoimmune cytopenias in chronic lymphocutic leukemia, *Am J Hematol* 89(11):1055-1062, 2014.
30. *SEER cancer statistics review 1975-2008*, Bethesda, Md, 2011, National Institutes of Health, U.S. Department of Health and Human Services.
31. Radivoyevitch T et al: Etiology and treatment of hematological neoplasms: stochastic mathematical models, *Adv Exp Med Biol* 844:317-346, 2014.
32. Wakeford R: The risk of childhood leukaemia following exposure to ionizing radiation—a review, *Radiol Prot* 33(1):1-25, 2013.
33. American Cancer Society: *Cancer facts & figures 2015*, Atlanta, Ga, 2015, Author.
34. Kumar V et al: *Robbins & Cotran pathologic basis of disease*, ed 9, St Louis, 2015, Elsevier.
35. National Cancer Institute: *Adult acute myeloid leukemia treatment (PDQ®)*, Bethesda, Md, National Cancer Institute. Date last modified January 9, 2015. Available at: www.cancer.gov/

cancertopics/pdq/treatment/adultAML/healthprofessional. Accessed February 23, 2015.
36. Queiros AC et al: A B-cell epigenetic signature defines three biologic subgroups of chronic lymphocytic leukemia with clinical impact, *Leukemia* 252:1-8, 2014.
37. Baliakas P et al: Recurrent mutations refine prognosis in chronic lymphocytic leukemia, *Leukemia* 29(8):329-336, 2015.
38. Villamor N et al: NOTCH1 mutations identify a genetic subgroup of chronic lymphocytic leukemia patients with high risk of transformation and poor outcome, *Leukemia* 27:1100-1106, 2013.
39. National Cancer Institute: *Chronic lymphocytic leukemia treatment (PDQ®)*, Bethesda, Md, 2014, National Cancer Institute, National Institutes of Health. Date last modified December 30, 2004. Available at: http://cancer.gov/cancertopics/pdq/treatment/CLL/Patient. Accessed January 12, 2015.
40. Rawstron AC et al: Monoclonal B-cell lymphocytosis and chronic lymphocytic leukemia, *N Engl J Med* 359(6):575-583, 2008.
41. Fazi C et al: General population low-count CLL-like MBL persists over time without clinical progression, although carrying the same cytogenetic abnormalities of CLL, *Blood* 118(25):6618-6625, 2011.
42. Kreso A, Dick JE: Evolution of the cancer stem cell model, *Cell Stem Cell* 14(3):275-291, 2014.
43. Scott DW, Gascoyne RD: The tumor microenvironment in B cell lymphomas, *Nat Rev Cancer* 14(8):517-534, 2014.
44. Mohamed G et al: Epstein-Barr virus, the germinal centre and the development of Hodgkin's lymphoma, *J Gen Virol* 95(Pt 9):1861-1869, 2014.
45. Nogová L et al: Lymphocyte-predominant and classic Hodgkin's lymphoma: a comprehensive analysis from the German Hodgkin Study Group, *J Clin Oncol* 26(3):434-439, 2008.
46. Al-Mansour M et al: Transformation to aggressive lymphoma in nodular lymphocyte-predominant Hodgkin's lymphoma, *J Clin Oncol* 28(5):793-799, 2010.
47. National Cancer Institute: *Adult Hodgkin lymphoma treatment (PDQ®)*, Bethesda, Md, National Cancer Institute. Date last modified February 25, 2015. Available at: http://cancer.gov/cancertopics/pdq/treatment/adulthodgkins/HealthProfessional. Accessed March 2, 2015.
48. National Cancer Institute: *Adult Hodgkin lymphoma treatment (PDQ®)*, Bethesda, Md, National Cancer Institute. Date last modified January 9, 2015. Available at: http://cancer.gov/cancertopics/pdq/treatment/adulthodgkins/Patient. Accessed February 23, 2015.
49. Boffetta P: Epidemiology of adult non-Hodgkin lymphoma, *Ann Oncol* 22(4):1v27-1v31, 2011.

50. National Cancer Institute: *Adult non-Hodgkin lymphoma treatment (PDQ®)*, Bethesda, Md, National Cancer Institute. Date last modified April 25, 2014. Available at: http://cancer.gov/cancertopics/pdq/treatment/adult-non-hodgkins/Patient. Accessed January 26, 2015.

51. National Cancer Institute: *Adult non-Hodgkin lymphoma treatment (PDQ®)*, Bethesda, Md, National Cancer Institute. Date last modified February 13, 2015. Available at: www.cancer.gov/cancertopics/pdq/treatment/adult-non-hodgkins/HealthProfessional. Accessed March 4, 2015.

52. Kochendorfer JN et al: Chemotherapy-refractory diffuse large B-cell lymphoma and indolent B-cell malignancies can be effectively treated with autologous T cells expressing an anti-CD19 chimeric antigen receptor, *J Clin Oncol* 33(6):540-549 2015.

53. Howlader N et al, editors: *SEER cancer statistics review, 1975-2011*, Bethesda, Md, 2013, National Cancer Institute. Available at: http://seer.cancer.gov/csr/1975_2011/.

54. Rajkumar SV et al: International Myeloma Working Group updated criteria for the diagnosis of multiple myeloma, *Lancet Oncol* 15(12):e528-e548, 2014.

55. Morgan GJ et al: The genetic architecture of multiple myeloma, *Nat Rev Cancer* 12:335-348, 2012.

56. Lohr JG et al: Widespread genetic heterogeneity in multiple myeloma: implications for targeted therapy, *Cancer Cell* 25(1):91-101, 2014.

57. Hattori Y et al: A myeloma cell line established from a patient refractory to thalidomide therapy revealed high-risk cytogenetic abnormalities and produced vascular endothelial growth factor, *Blood Cancer J* 3:e115, 2013.

58. Rajkumar SV et al: Haematological cancer: redefining myeloma, *Nat Rev Clin Oncol* 9(9):494-496, 2012.

59. Ioannou A et al: Platelets, complement and tissue inflammation, *Autoimmunity* 46(1):105, 2013.

60. *Thrombocytopenia*, Bethesda, Md, 2008, National Institutes of Health, U.S. Department of Health and Human Services. Available at: www.nhlbi.nih.gov/health/dci/Diseases/thcp/thcp_all.html. Accessed September 1, 2012.

61. Backmair FM et al: Dietary manipulation of platelet function, *Pharmacol Ther* 144(2):97-113, 2014.

62. Paniccia R et al: Assessment of platelet function: laboratory and point-of-care methods, *World J Transl Med* 3(2):69-83, 2014.

63. Nurden AT, Nurden P: Congential platelet disorders and understanding of platelet function, *Br J Haematol* 165(2):165-178, 2014.

64. Bartholomew JR: Heparin-induced thrombocytopenia. In Lichtin A, Bartholomew J, editors: *The coagulation consult: a case-based guide*, New York, 2014, Springer.

65. Selleng K et al: Heparin-induced thrombocytopenia in intensive care patients, *Semin Thromb Hemost* 34(5):425-438, 2008.

66. Lakshmanan S, Cuker A: Contemporary management of primary immune thrombocytopenia (ITP) in adults, *J Thromb Haemost* 10(10):1988-1998, 2012.

67. Rodeghiero F, Ruggeri M: Treatment of immune thrombocytopenia in adults: the role of thrombopoietin-receptor agonists, *Semin Hematol* 52(1):16-24, 2015.

68. Kuwana M: *Helicobacter pylori*-associated immune thrombocytopenia: clinical features and pathogenic mechanisms, *World J Gastroenterol* 20(3):714-723, 2014.

69. Stasi R, Provan D: *Helicobacter pylori* and chronic ITP. *Hematology Am Soc Hematol Educ Program* 2008:206-211, 2008.

70. Veneri D et al: Analysis of B- and T-cell clonality and HLA class II alleles in patients with idiopathic thrombocytopenic purpura: correlation with *Helicobacter pylori* infection and response to eradication treatment, *Platelets* 16:307-311, 2005.

71. Xie J et al: Changes in follicular helper T cells in idiopathic thrombocytopenic purpura patients, *Int J Biol Sci* 11(2):220-229, 2015.

72. Kuhne T, Imback P: Management of children and adolescents with primary immune thrombocytopenia: controversies and solutions, *Vox Sang* 104(1):55-66, 2013.

73. Bennett CM et al: Targeted ITP strategies: do they elucidate the biology of ITP and related disorders? *Pediatr Blood Cancer* 47(Suppl 5):706-709, 2006.

74. Kashiwagi H, Tomiyama Y: Pathophysiology and management of primary immune thrombocytopenia, *Int J Hematol* 98:24-33, 2013.

75. Lo E, Deane S: Diagnosis and classification of immune-mediated thrombocytopenia, *Autoimmun Rev* 13(3-5):577-583, 2014.

76. Al-Nouri ZL, et al: Drug-induced thrombotic microangiopathy: a systematic review of published reports, *Blood* 125(4):616-618, 2015.

77. Zoller B et al: Autoimmune disease and venous thromboembolism: a review of the literature, *Am J Cardiovasc Dis* 2(3):171-183, 2012.

78. Rodeghiero F, Ruggeri M: ITP and international guidelines: what do we know, what do we need? *La Presse Medicale* 43(4):e61-e67, 2014.

79. Tefferi A, Barbui T: Polycythemia vera and essential thrombocytemia: 2015 update on diagnosis, risk-stratification and management, *Am J of Hematol* 90(2):162-173, 2015.

80. Landolfi R, Fi Gennaro L: Thrombosis in myeloproliferative and myelodysplastic syndromes, *Hematology* 17(Suppl 1):S174-S176, 2012.

81. Harrison C et al: JAK inhibition with ruxolitinib versus best available therapy for myelofibrosis, *N Engl J Med* 366 (9):787-798, 2012.

82. Passamonti F et al: A prognostic model to predict survival in 867 World Health Organization-defined essential thrombocythemia at diagnosis: as study by the international Working Group on Myelofibrosis Research and Treatment, *Blood* 120(6):1197-1201, 2012.

83. Wolanskyj AP et al: Essential thrombocythemia beyond the first decade: life expectancy, long-term complication rates, and prognostic factors, *Mayo Clin Proc* 81(2):159-166, 2006.

84. Tefferi A et al: The 2008 World Health Organization classification system for myeloproliferative neoplasms: order out of chaos, *Cancer* 115(17):3842-3847, 2009.

85. Barbui T et al: Front-line therapy in polycythemia vera and essential thrombocythemia, *Blood Rec* 26(5):205-211, 2012.

86. Salles II et al: Inherited traits affecting platelet function, *Blood Rev* 22(3):155-172, 2008.

87. Lisman T et al: Hemostasis and thrombosis in patients with liver disease: the ups and downs, *J Hepatol* 53(2):362-371, 2010.

88. Wada H et al: Diagnosis and treatment of disseminated intravascular coagulation (DIC) according to four DIC guidelines, *J Intensive Care* 2(1):15, 2014.

89. Venugopal A: Disseminated intravascular coagulation, *Indian J Anaesth* 58(5):603-608, 2014.

90. Nakashima MO, Rogers HJ: Hypercoagulable states: an algorithmic approach to laboratory testing and update on monitoring of direct oral anticoagulants, *Blood Res* 49(2):85-94, 2014.

91. Bruce A, Massicotte MP: Thrombophilia screening: whom to test, *Blood* 120(7):1353-1355, 2012.

92. Baglin T: Inherited and acquired risk factors for venous thromoembolism, *Semin Respir Crit Care Med* 33(2):127-137, 2012.

93. Giannakopoulos B, Krilis SA: The pathogenesis of the antiphospholipid syndrome, *N Engl J Med* 368:1033-1044, 2013.

94. Aksu K et al: Inflammation-induced thrombosis: mechanisms, disease associations and management, *Curr Pharm Des* 18(11):1478-1493, 2012.

95. Heilmann L et al: Pregnancy outcome in women with antiphospholipid antibodies: report on a retrospective study, *Semin Thromb Hemost* 34(8):794-802, 2008.

Alterations of Hematologic Function in Children

Joan Shea, Nancy E. Kline, Anna E. Roche, and Kathryn L. McCance

ⓔ EVOLVE WEBSITE

http://evolve.elsevier.com/Huether/
Student Review Questions
Audio Key Points

Case Studies
Animations
Quick Check Answers

Among the diseases that affect erythrocytes in children are acquired disorders, such as iron deficiency anemia and hemolytic disease of the newborn, and inherited disorders, such as glucose-6-phosphate dehydrogenase deficiency, sickle cell disease, and the thalassemias.

Childhood disorders that involve the coagulation process and platelets include inherited hemorrhagic diseases, such as the hemophilias, and antibody-mediated hemorrhagic diseases, including immune thrombocytopenic purpura. Finally, leukocyte disorders, such as leukemia and the lymphomas (both Hodgkin lymphoma and non-Hodgkin lymphoma), are discussed in this chapter.

DISORDERS OF ERYTHROCYTES

Anemia is the most common blood disorder in children. Like the anemias of adulthood, the anemias of childhood are caused by ineffective erythropoiesis or premature destruction of erythrocytes. The most common cause of insufficient erythropoiesis is iron deficiency, which may result from insufficient dietary intake or chronic loss of iron caused by bleeding. The hemolytic anemias of childhood may be divided into (1) disorders that result from premature destruction caused by intrinsic abnormalities of the erythrocytes and (2) disorders that result from damaging extraerythrocytic factors. The hemolytic anemias are either inherited or acquired.

The most dramatic form of acquired congenital hemolytic anemia is hemolytic disease of the fetus and newborn (HDFN), also termed erythroblastosis fetalis. HDFN is an alloimmunity (isoimmunity) disease in which maternal blood and fetal blood are incompatible, causing the mother's immune system to produce antibodies against fetal erythrocytes. Fetal erythrocytes attacked by (i.e., bound to) maternal antibodies are recognized as foreign or defective by the fetal mononuclear phagocyte system and are removed from the circulation by phagocytosis, usually in the fetal spleen. (For a complete examination

of HDFN, see the discussion that follows.) Other acquired hemolytic anemias—some of which begin in utero—include those caused by infections or the presence of toxic chemicals.

The inherited forms of hemolytic anemia result from intrinsic defects of the child's erythrocytes, any of which can lead to erythrocyte removal by the mononuclear phagocyte system. Structural defects include abnormal cellular size or shape and abnormalities of plasma membrane structure (spherocytosis). Intracellular defects include enzyme deficiencies, the most common of which is glucose-6-phosphate dehydrogenase (G6PD) deficiency, and defects of hemoglobin synthesis, which manifest as sickle cell disease or thalassemia, depending on which component of hemoglobin is defective. These and other causes of childhood anemia are listed in Table 22-1.

Acquired Disorders
Iron Deficiency Anemia

Iron is *critical* to the developing child, especially for normal brain development, and without it the damage from the periods of iron deficiency anemia (IDA) in children is irreversible. IDA is the most common nutritional disorder worldwide with the highest incidence occurring between 6 months and 2 years of age. IDA is common in the United States with prevalence higher in toddlers, adolescent girls, and women of childbearing age; IDA causes clinical manifestations mostly related to inadequate hemoglobin synthesis.[1]

IDA can result from (1) dietary lack of iron, (2) problems with iron absorption, (3) blood loss, and (4) increased requirement for iron. Inadequate intake of iron is the most common cause of IDA during the first few years of life. Blood loss is the most common cause during childhood and adolescence, and for adults in the Western world. Chronic IDA from occult (hidden) blood loss may be caused by a gastrointestinal lesion, parasitic infestation, or hemorrhagic disease. A reasonable hypothesis for infants and young children who develop IDA

TABLE 22-1 Anemias of Childhood

Cause	Anemic Condition
Deficient Erythropoiesis or Hemoglobin Synthesis	
Decreased stem cell population in marrow (congenital or acquired pure red cell aplasia)	Normocytic-normochromic anemia
Decreased erythropoiesis despite normal stem cell population in marrow (infection, inflammation, cancer, chronic renal disease, congenital dyserythropoiesis)	Normocytic-normochromic anemia
Deficiency of a factor or nutrient needed for erythropoiesis	
Cobalamin (vitamin B_{12}), folate	Megaloblastic anemia
Iron	Microcytic-hypochromic anemia
Increased or Premature Hemolysis	
Alloimmune disease (maternal-fetal Rh, ABO, or minor blood group incompatibility)	Autoimmune hemolytic anemia
Autoimmune disease (idiopathic autoimmune hemolytic anemia, symptomatic systemic lupus erythematosus, lymphoma, drug-induced autoimmune processes)	Autoimmune hemolytic anemia
Inherited defects of plasma membrane structure (spherocytosis, elliptocytosis, stomatocytosis) or cellular size or both (pyknocytosis)	Hemolytic anemia
Infection (bacterial sepsis, congenital syphilis, malaria, cytomegalovirus infection, rubella, toxoplasmosis, disseminated herpes)	Hemolytic anemia
Intrinsic and inherited enzymatic defects (deficiencies) of glucose-6-phosphate dehydrogenase (G6PD), pyruvate kinase, 5′-nucleotidase, glucose phosphate isomerase	Hemolytic anemia
Inherited defects of hemoglobin synthesis	Sickle cell anemia
	Thalassemia
Disseminated intravascular coagulation (see Chapter 21)	Hemolytic anemia
Galactosemia	Hemolytic anemia
Prolonged or recurrent respiratory or metabolic acidosis	Hemolytic anemia
Blood vessel disorders (cavernous hemangiomas, large vessel thrombus, renal artery stenosis, severe coarctation of aorta)	Hemolytic anemia

is that it occurs because of chronic intestinal blood loss induced by exposure to a heat-labile protein in cow's milk. Such exposure causes an inflammatory gastrointestinal reaction that damages the mucosa and results in diffuse microhemorrhage. Growing evidence indicates that cellular components of both innate and adaptive immunity play significant roles during the pathogenesis of cow's milk allergy.[2] Dietary lack of iron is not common in developed countries, where iron is in the readily absorbed form from heme found in meat. IDA was recently found in Israel, mainly in children 1.5 to 3 years old, and was associated with low red meat intake.[3] In developing countries, food may be less available and the iron found in plants is in the poorly absorbable inorganic form.[1] Infants are at increased risk for IDA because of very small amounts of iron in milk. Bioavailability of iron from breast milk is higher than that from cow's milk. Impaired absorption is found in chronic diarrhea, fat malabsorption, and sprue (*Health Alert:* A Significant Number of Children Develop and Suffer from Severe Iron Deficiency Anemia).

Children in developing countries are often affected by chronic parasite infestations that result in blood and iron loss greater than dietary intake. Treatment of helminth (parasitic worm) infections results in improvement in both appetite and growth as well as reduction of anemia. The association between iron deficiency anemia and lead poisoning is controversial. Newer areas of investigation include iron deficiency in overweight children and the association of *Helicobacter pylori* infection with IDA.[4]

PATHOPHYSIOLOGY No matter the cause, a deficiency of iron produces a hypochromic-microcytic anemia.[1] Progressive depletion of blood and low serum levels of ferritin and transferrin saturation eventually lead to a lowering of hemoglobin and hematocrit levels. In the early stages, an adaptive increase in red blood cell activity in the bone marrow may prevent the development of anemia. When the iron stores

HEALTH ALERT

A Significant Number of Children Develop and Suffer from Severe Iron Deficiency Anemia

A recent study in the United States found children aged 36 months to 15 years are particularly vulnerable to iron deficiency anemia (IDA), especially those consuming excessive quantities of whole cow's milk. The prevalence of IDA in infancy has not changed in the past four decades and remains about 7%. Several children who were not anemic at 12 months of age went on to develop IDA as their iron stores became depleted. These children had typical signs of anemia although their parents were not aware of the abnormalities. Chronic severe IDA in the first years of life increases the risk of irreversible cognition problems as well as affective and motor development. The American Academy of Pediatrics (AAP) recommends screening for IDA with hemoglobin concentration and clinical assessment at about 1 year of age, and the Centers for Disease Control and Prevention (CDC) recommends that all children aged 2 through 5 years be assessed annually for risk factors for IDA and screened appropriately. IDA is a preventable disease.

Data from Paoletti G et al: *Pediatrics* 53(4):1352-1358, 2014.

are depleted, with accompanying important laboratory indicators, anemia develops.

CLINICAL MANIFESTATIONS The symptoms of mild anemia—listlessness and fatigue—usually are not present or are undetectable in infants and young children, who are unable to describe these symptoms. Therefore parents generally do not note any change in the child's behavior or appearance until moderate anemia has developed. General irritability, decreased activity tolerance, weakness, and lack of interest in play are nonspecific indications of anemia. When hemoglobin levels fall below 5 g/dl, pallor, anorexia, tachycardia, and systolic murmurs may occur.

Other symptoms and signs of chronic IDA include splenomegaly, widened skull sutures, decreased physical growth, developmental delays, *pica* (a behavior in which nonfood substances are eaten, such as clay), and altered neurologic and intellectual functions, especially those involving attention span, alertness, and learning ability.

EVALUATION AND TREATMENT   The diagnosis of IDA is confirmed by laboratory tests. These tests include measurement of hemoglobin, hematocrit, serum iron, and ferritin levels and determination of the total iron binding capacity. Most essential is obtaining a thorough history of present illness and dietary history in addition to performing a complete physical examination. Evaluation and treatment of iron deficiency anemia in children is similar to that used for adults with IDA (see Chapter 21). Oral administration of a simple ferrous salt is usually satisfactory and additional vitamin C helps promote absorption.[5] Iron in a liquid form should be administered through a straw because it can stain teeth. Dietary modification is required to prevent recurrences of iron deficiency anemia. Intake of iron-rich foods is increased and the intake of cow's milk may be restricted.

Hemolytic Disease of the Fetus and Newborn

The most common cause of hemolytic anemia in newborns is alloimmune disease. Hemolytic disease of the fetus and newborn (HDFN) (erythroblastosis fetalis) can occur only if antigens on fetal erythrocytes differ from antigens on maternal erythrocytes. Maternal-fetal incompatibility exists if mother and fetus differ in ABO blood type or if the fetus is Rh-positive and the mother is Rh-negative. Some minor blood antigens also may be involved (see Chapter 7).

ABO incompatibility occurs in about 20% to 25% of all pregnancies, but only 1 in 10 cases of ABO incompatibility results in HDFN. Rh incompatibility occurs in less than 10% of pregnancies and rarely causes HDFN in the first incompatible fetus. Even after five or more pregnancies, only 5% of women have babies with hemolytic disease. Usually erythrocytes from the first incompatible fetus cause the mother's immune system to produce antibodies that affect the fetuses of subsequent incompatible pregnancies. Only one in three cases of HDFN is caused by Rh incompatibility; most cases are caused by ABO incompatibility.

PATHOPHYSIOLOGY   HDFN will result (1) if the mother's blood contains preformed antibodies against fetal erythrocytes or produces them on exposure to fetal erythrocytes, (2) if sufficient amounts of antibody (usually immunoglobulin G [IgG]) cross the placenta and enter fetal blood, and (3) if immunoglobulin G (IgG) binds with sufficient numbers of fetal erythrocytes to cause widespread antibody-mediated hemolysis or splenic removal. (Antibody-mediated cellular destruction is described in Chapter 8.)

Maternal antibodies may be formed against type B erythrocytes if the mother is type A or against type A erythrocytes if the mother is type B. Usually, however, the mother is type O and the fetus is A or B. ABO incompatibility can cause HDFN even if fetal erythrocytes do not escape into the maternal circulation during pregnancy. This occurs because the blood of most adults already contains anti-A or anti-B antibodies, which are produced on exposure to certain foods or infection by gram-negative bacteria. (Anti-O antibodies do not exist because type O erythrocytes are not antigenic.) Therefore IgG against type A or B erythrocytes is usually preformed in maternal blood and can enter the fetal circulation throughout the first incompatible pregnancy.

Anti-Rh antibodies, on the other hand, are formed only in response to the presence of incompatible (Rh-positive) erythrocytes from the fetus in the blood of an Rh-negative mother. Sources of exposure include fetal blood that is mixed with the mother's blood at the time of delivery, transfused blood, and, rarely, previous sensitization of the mother by her own mother's incompatible blood (Figure 22-1).

The first Rh-incompatible pregnancy generally presents no difficulties because few fetal erythrocytes cross the placental barrier during gestation. When the placenta detaches at birth, however, a large number of fetal erythrocytes usually enter the mother's bloodstream. If the mother is Rh-negative and the fetus is Rh-positive, the mother produces anti-Rh antibodies. Anti-Rh antibodies persist in the bloodstream for a long time, and if the next offspring is Rh-positive, the mother's anti-Rh antibodies can enter the bloodstream of the fetus and destroy the erythrocytes. Antibodies against Rh antigen D are of the IgG class and easily cross the placenta.

IgG-coated fetal erythrocytes usually are destroyed in the spleen. As hemolysis proceeds, the fetus becomes anemic. Erythropoiesis accelerates, particularly in the liver and spleen, and immature nucleated cells (erythroblasts) are released into the bloodstream (hence the name *erythroblastosis fetalis*). The degree of anemia depends on the length of time the antibody has been in the fetal circulation, the concentration of the antibody, and the ability of the fetus to compensate for increased hemolysis. Unconjugated (indirect) bilirubin, which is formed during breakdown of hemoglobin, is transported across the placental barrier into the maternal circulation and is excreted by the mother. Hyperbilirubinemia occurs in the neonate after birth because excretion of lipid-soluble unconjugated bilirubin through the placenta is no longer possible.

The pathophysiologic effects of HDFN are more severe in Rh incompatibility than in ABO incompatibility. ABO incompatibility may resolve after birth without life-threatening complications. Maternal-fetal incompatibility in which a mother with type O blood has a child with type A or B blood usually is so mild that it does not require treatment.

Rh incompatibility is more likely than ABO incompatibility to cause severe or even life-threatening anemia, death in utero, or damage to the central nervous system. Severe anemia alone can cause death as a result of cardiovascular complications. Extensive hemolysis also results in increased levels of unconjugated bilirubin in the neonate's circulation. If bilirubin levels exceed the liver's ability to conjugate and excrete bilirubin, some of it is deposited in the brain, causing cellular damage and, eventually, death if the neonate does not receive exchange transfusions.

Fetuses that do not survive anemia in utero usually are stillborn, with gross edema in the entire body, a condition called hydrops fetalis. Death can occur as early as 17 weeks' gestation and results in spontaneous abortion.

CLINICAL MANIFESTATIONS   Neonates with mild HDFN may appear healthy or slightly pale, with slight enlargement of the liver or spleen. Pronounced pallor, splenomegaly, and hepatomegaly indicate severe anemia, which predisposes the neonate to cardiovascular failure and shock. Life-threatening Rh incompatibility is rare today, largely because of the routine use of Rh immunoglobulin.

Because the maternal antibodies remain in the neonate's circulatory system after birth, erythrocyte destruction can continue. This causes hyperbilirubinemia and icterus neonatorum (neonatal jaundice) shortly after birth. Without replacement transfusions, in which the child receives Rh-negative erythrocytes, the bilirubin is deposited in the brain, a condition termed kernicterus. Kernicterus produces cerebral damage and usually causes death (icterus gravis neonatorum). Infants who do not die may have intellectual disabilities, cerebral palsy, or high-frequency deafness.

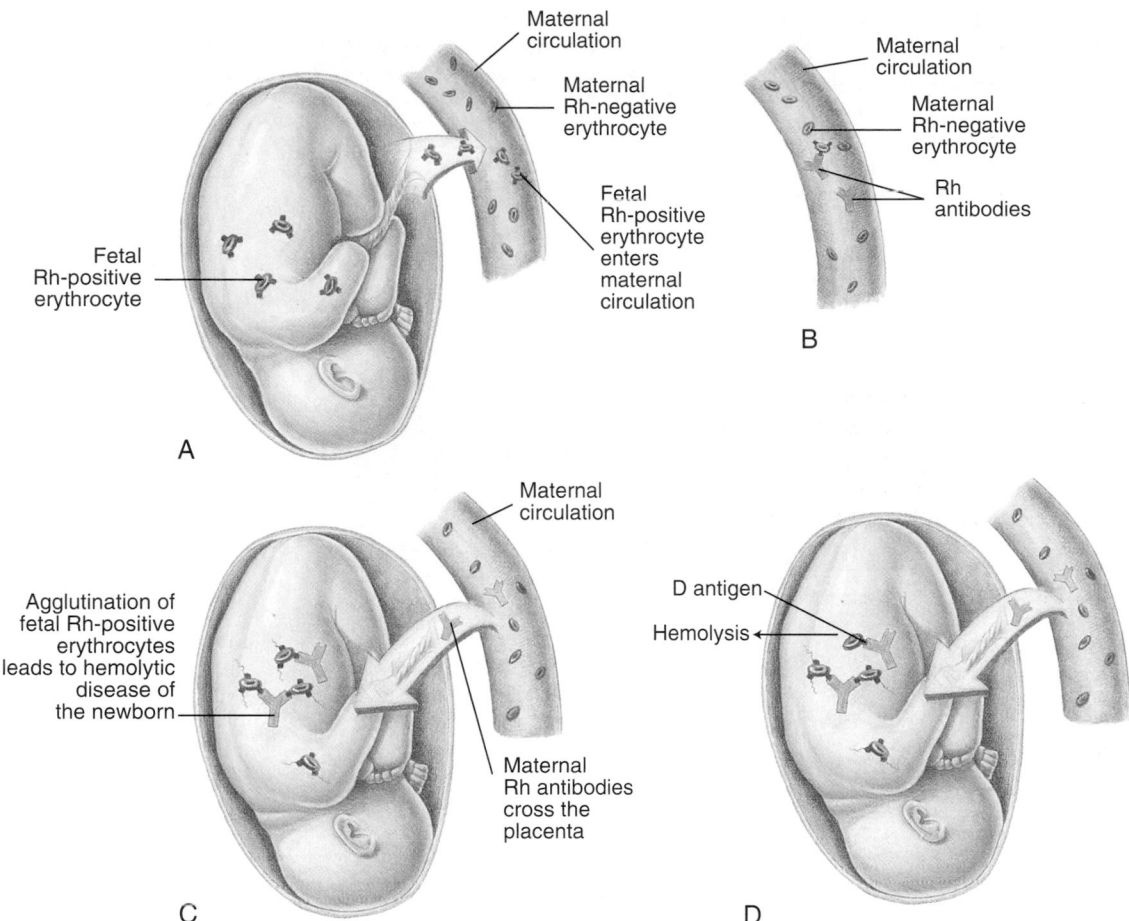

FIGURE 22-1 Hemolytic Disease of the Fetus and Newborn (HDFN). A, Before or during delivery, Rh-positive erythrocytes from the fetus enter the blood of an Rh-negative woman through a tear in the placenta. **B,** The mother is sensitized to the Rh antigen and produces Rh antibodies. Because this usually happens after delivery, there is no effect on the fetus in the first pregnancy. **C,** During a subsequent pregnancy with an Rh-positive fetus, Rh-positive erythrocytes cross the placenta, enter the maternal circulation, and **(D)** stimulate the mother to produce antibodies against the Rh antigen. (Modified from Seeley RR et al: *Anatomy and physiology,* ed 3, St Louis, 1995, Mosby.)

EVALUATION AND TREATMENT   Routine evaluation of fetuses at risk for HDFN (i.e., fetuses resulting from Rh- or ABO-incompatible matings) includes the Coombs test. The indirect Coombs test measures antibody in the mother's circulation and indicates whether the fetus is at risk for HDFN. The direct Coombs test measures antibody already bound to the surfaces of fetal erythrocytes and is used primarily to confirm the diagnosis of antibody-mediated HDFN. With a prior history of fetal hemolytic disease, diagnostic tests are done to determine risk with the current pregnancy. These tests include maternal antibody titers, fetal blood sampling, amniotic fluid spectrophotometry, and ultrasound fetal assessment.

The key to treatment of HDFN resulting from Rh incompatibility lies in prevention (immunoprophylaxis).[6,7] One of the success stories of immunology has been the result obtained with Rh immune globulin (RhoGAM), a preparation of antibody against Rh antigen D (anti-D Ig). If an Rh-negative woman is given Rh immune globulin within 72 hours of exposure to Rh-positive erythrocytes, she will not produce antibody against the D antigen, and the next Rh-positive baby she conceives will be protected. Updated recommendations also state that if anti-D Ig is not given within 72 hours, every effort should still be made to administer the anti-D Ig within 10 days. The newer updates

on the use of anti-D Ig as prophylaxis to prevent sensitization to the D antigen *during* pregnancy or at *delivery* for the prevention of HDFN can be found at the National Guideline Clearinghouse at www.guideline.gov/content.aspx?id=34964#Section 420. The British Committee for Standards in Haematology (BCSH) also established guidelines for the use of anti-D immunoglobulin for rhesus D prophylaxis.[7]

Inherited Disorders
Sickle Cell Disease

Sickle cell disease is a group of disorders characterized by the production of abnormal **hemoglobin S (Hb S)** within the erythrocytes. Hb S is formed by a genetic mutation in which one amino acid (valine) replaces another (glutamic acid) (Figure 22-2). Hb S, the so-called sickle hemoglobin, reacts to deoxygenation and dehydration by solidifying and stretching the erythrocyte into an elongated sickle shape, producing hemolytic anemia (Figure 22-3).

Sickle cell disease is an inherited, autosomal recessive disorder expressed as sickle cell anemia, sickle cell–thalassemia disease, or sickle cell–hemoglobin C disease, depending on mode of inheritance (Table 22-2). (See Chapter 2 for a discussion of genetic inheritance of disease.) Sickle cell anemia, a homozygous form, is the most severe.

Sickle cell anemia is determined by the substitution of normal hemoglobin (Hb A) by hemoglobin S (Hb S) caused by a point mutation (replacement of the nucleotide triplet CTC coding glutamic acid at the mRNA level [GAG] by the CAC triplet [GUG] coding for valine) that modifies the physicochemical properties of the β-globin chain of hemoglobin. All hemoglobin is abnormal in homozygous individuals for the mutant gene, and red blood cells show a sickling deformity and hemolytic anemia in the presence or absence of normal oxygen tension. Heterozygous individuals contain a mixture of Hb A and Hb S, and sickling and anemia are observed when the tension of oxygen decreases.

Irreversibly sickled red blood cells are trapped within the splenic sinusoids and are destroyed by adjacent macrophages. Hemolysis may also occur in the macrophage-sheathed capillaries of the red pulp.

FIGURE 22-2 Sickle Cell Hemoglobin. A, Sickle cell hemoglobin is produced by a recessive allele of the gene encoding the β-chain of the protein hemoglobin. It represents a single amino acid change—from glutamic acid to valine at the sixth position of the chain. In this model of a hemoglobin molecule, the position of the mutation can be seen near the end of the upper arm. **B,** Color-enhanced electron micrograph shows normal erythrocytes and sickled blood cell. **C,** Brief summary of sickle cell. (**A** from Raven PH, Johnson GB: *Biology,* ed 3, St Louis, 1992, Mosby; **B** copyright Dennis Kunkel Microscopy, Inc; **C** from Kierszenbaum A, Tres L: *Histology and cell biology: an introduction to pathology,* ed 3, St Louis, 2012, Mosby.)

Sickle cell–thalassemia and sickle cell–Hb C disease are heterozygous forms in which the child simultaneously inherits another type of abnormal hemoglobin from one parent. Sickle cell trait, in which the child inherits Hb S from one parent and normal hemoglobin (Hb A) from the other, is a heterozygous carrier state that rarely has clinical manifestations. All forms of sickle cell disease are lifelong conditions.

Sickle cell disease tends to occur in persons with origins in equatorial countries, particularly central Africa, the Near East, the Mediterranean area, and parts of India. In the United States, sickle cell disease is most common in blacks, with a reported incidence ranging from 1:400 to 1:500 live births. In the general population, the risk of two black parents having a child with sickle cell anemia is 0.7%. Sickle

TABLE 22-2 Inheritance of Sickle Cell Disease

Hemoglobin Inherited from First Parent	Hemoglobin Inherited from Second Parent	Form of Sickle Cell Disease in Child
Hb S (an abnormal hemoglobin)	Hb S	Sickle cell anemia: homozygous inheritance in which child's hemoglobin is mostly Hb S, with remainder Hb F (fetal hemoglobin)
Hb S	Defective or insufficient α- or β-chains of Hb A (alpha- or beta-thalassemia)	Sickle cell–thalassemia disease (heterozygous inheritance of Hb S and alpha- or beta-thalassemia)
Hb S	Hb C or D (both abnormal hemoglobins)	Sickle cell–hemoglobin C (or D) disease (heterozygous inheritance of hemoglobin S and either C or D)
Hb S	Normal hemoglobins (mostly Hb A)	Sickle cell trait, carrier state (heterozygous inheritance of Hb S and normal hemoglobin)

FIGURE 22-3 Normal and Sickle-Shaped Blood Cells. Scanning electron micrograph of normal and sickle-shaped red blood cells. The irregularly shaped cells are the sickle cells; the circular cells are the normal blood cells. (From Raven PH, Johnson GB: *Biology,* ed 3, St Louis, 1992, Mosby.)

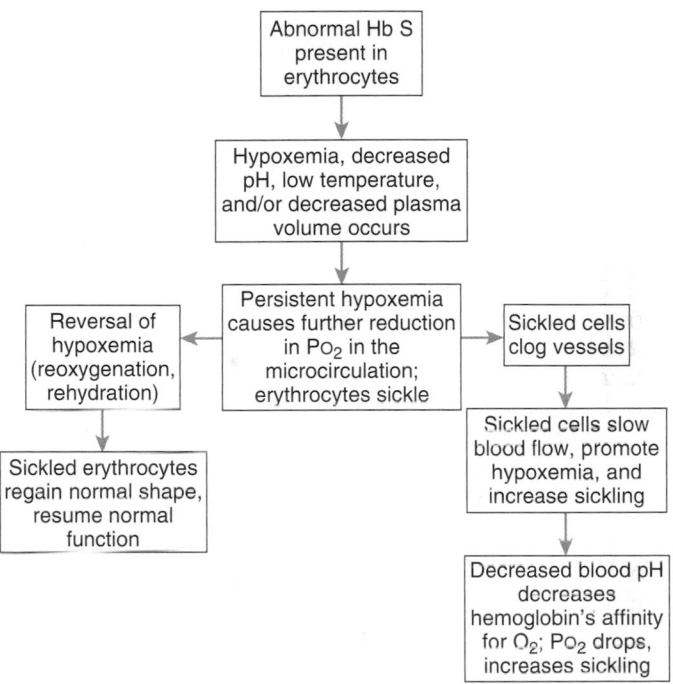

FIGURE 22-4 Sickling of Erythrocytes.

cell–hemoglobin C disease is less common (1 in 800 births), and sickle cell thalassemia occurs in 1 in 1700 births.

Sickle cell trait occurs in 7% to 13% of African Americans, whereas its incidence among East Africans may be as high as 45%. The sickle cell trait may provide protection against lethal forms of malaria, a genetic advantage to carriers who reside in endemic regions for malaria (Mediterranean and African zones) but no advantage to carriers living in the United States.

PATHOPHYSIOLOGY Hemoglobin S is soluble and usually causes no problem when properly oxygenated. When oxygen tension decreases, the single amino acid substitution in the β-globin chain of Hb S polymerizes, forming abnormal fluid polymers. As these polymers realign, they cause the red cell to deform into the sickle shape. Sickling depends on the degree of oxygenation, pH, and dehydration of the individual. A decrease in oxygenation (hypoxemia) and pH, as well as dehydration, increases sickling. Deoxygenation is probably the most important variable in determining the occurrence of sickling.[8] Sickle-trait cells sickle at oxygen tensions of about 15 mm Hg, whereas those from an individual with sickle cell disease begin to sickle at about 40 mm Hg. Sickled erythrocytes tend to plug the blood vessels, increasing the viscosity of the blood, which slows circulation and causes vascular occlusion, pain, and organ infarction. Viscosity increases the time of exposure to less oxygenation, promoting further sickling. Sickled cells undergo hemolysis in the spleen or become sequestered there, causing blood pooling and infarction of splenic vessels. The

anemia that follows triggers erythropoiesis in the marrow and, in extreme cases, in the liver (Figure 22-4).

Sickling usually is not permanent; most sickled erythrocytes regain a normal shape after reoxygenation and rehydration. Irreversible sickling is caused by irreversible plasma membrane damage caused by sickling. In persons with sickle cell anemia, in which the erythrocytes contain a high percentage of Hb S (75% to 95%), up to 30% of the erythrocytes can become irreversibly sickled. Occasionally, irreversible sickling occurs in sickle cell disease but not in the carrier state (sickle cell trait). Sickling also can be triggered by increased plasma osmolality, decreased plasma volume, and low environmental temperature.

CLINICAL MANIFESTATIONS There is much variation in the clinical manifestations of sickle cell disease. Some individuals have mild symptoms and others suffer from repeated vasoocclusive crises.[1] When sickling occurs, the general manifestations of hemolytic anemia—pallor, fatigue, jaundice, and irritability—sometimes are accompanied by acute manifestations called *crises.* Extensive sickling can precipitate the following four types of crises:

1. **Vasoocclusive crisis (thrombotic crisis).** This begins with sickling in the microcirculation. As blood flow is obstructed by sickled cells,

vasospasm occurs and a "logjam" effect blocks all blood flow through the vessel. Unless the process is reversed, thrombosis and infarction of local tissue follow. Vasoocclusive crisis is extremely painful and may last for days or even weeks, with an average duration of 4 to 6 days. The frequency of this type of crisis is variable and unpredictable. Vasoocclusion in vessels to the brain can result in stroke. Chronic vasoocclusion in vessels to the kidneys results in end-stage renal disease.

2. **Sequestration crisis.** Large amounts of blood become acutely pooled in the liver and spleen. This type of crisis is seen only in the young child. Because the spleen can hold as much as one fifth of the body's blood supply at one time, up to 50% mortality has been reported, with death being caused by cardiovascular collapse.

3. **Aplastic crisis.** Profound anemia is caused by diminished erythropoiesis despite an increased need for new erythrocytes. In sickle cell anemia, erythrocyte survival is only 10 to 20 days. Normally a compensatory increase in erythropoiesis (five to eight times normal) replaces the cells lost through premature hemolysis. If this compensatory response is compromised, aplastic crisis develops in a very short time.

4. **Hyperhemolytic crisis.** Although unusual, this may occur in association with certain drugs or infections.

The clinical manifestations of sickle cell disease usually do not appear until the infant is at least 6 months old, at which time the postnatal decrease in concentrations of Hb F causes concentrations of Hb S to rise (Figure 22-5). Infection is the most common cause of death related to sickle cell disease. Sepsis and meningitis develop in as many as 10% of children with sickle cell anemia during the first 5 years of life. Survival time is unpredictable and has improved over the past decades.

Sickle cell–Hb C disease is usually milder than sickle cell anemia. The main clinical problems are related to vasoocclusive crises and are thought to result from higher hematocrit values and viscosity. In older children, sickle cell retinopathy, renal necrosis, and aseptic necrosis of the femoral heads occur along with obstructive crises.

Sickle cell–thalassemia has the mildest clinical manifestations of all the sickle cell diseases. The normal hemoglobins, particularly Hb F, inhibit sickling. In addition, the erythrocytes tend to be small (microcytic) and to contain relatively little hemoglobin (hypochromic), making them less likely to occlude the microcirculation, even when in a sickled state.

EVALUATION AND TREATMENT   The sickle cell trait does not affect life expectancy or interfere with daily activities. However, on rare occasions, severe hypoxia caused by shock, vigorous exercising at high altitudes, flying at high altitudes in unpressurized aircraft, or undergoing anesthesia is associated with vasoocclusive episodes in persons with sickle cell trait. These cells form an ivy shape instead of a sickle shape.

The parents' hematologic history and clinical manifestations may suggest that a child has sickle cell disease, but hematologic tests are necessary for diagnosis. If the sickle solubility test confirms the

FIGURE 22-5 Differences Between Effects of (A) Normal and (B) Sickled RBCs on Blood Circulation and Selected Consequences in a Child. C, Tissue Effects of Sickle Cell Anemia. *CVA,* Cerebrovascular accident. (**A** and **B** adapted from Hockenberry MJ et al, editors: *Wong's nursing care of infants and children,* ed 10, St Louis, 2015, Mosby.)

FIGURE 22-6 Prepregnancy Sickle Cell Test. This technique has potential for detection of other inherited diseases. **1,** Fertilization produces several embryos. **2,** The embryos are tested for the presence of the gene. **3,** The embryos without the gene are implanted. **4,** Amniocentesis confirms whether the fetus (or fetuses) has the sickle cell gene. **5,** Woman has a normal child.

presence of Hb S in peripheral blood, hemoglobin electrophoresis provides information about the amount of Hb S in erythrocytes. Prenatal diagnosis can be made after chorionic villus sampling as early as 8 to 10 weeks' gestation or by amniotic fluid analysis at 15 weeks' gestation (Figure 22-6). Newborn screening for sickle cell disease should be performed according to state law.

The main treatment for sickle cell disease is hydroxyurea; it inhibits DNA synthesis, causes an increase in hemoglobin F concentration, and results in an anti-inflammatory effect (decreases leukocyte production). These outcomes are thought to decrease crises. Treatment of sickle cell disease consists of supportive care aimed at preventing consequences of anemia and avoiding crises, including adequate hydration and pain management. Debate about transfusion therapy exists because of iron overload that can cause liver damage and fibrosis, delayed physical and sexual development, and heart disease; in addition, transfusion therapy requires chelation therapy to remove excess iron.[9] Genetic counseling and psychologic support are important for the child and family.

Thalassemias

The alpha- and beta-thalassemias are inherited autosomal recessive disorders that cause an impaired rate of synthesis of one of the two chains—α or β—of adult hemoglobin (Hb A). The disorder was named **thalassemia**, which is derived from the Greek word for sea, because it was discovered initially in persons with origins near the Mediterranean Sea. Beta-thalassemia, in which synthesis of the β-globin chain is slowed or defective, is prevalent among Greeks, Italians, and some Arabs and Sephardic Jews. Alpha-thalassemia, in which the α-chain is affected, is most common among Chinese, Vietnamese, Cambodians, and Laotians. Both alpha- and beta-thalassemias are common among blacks.

Both alpha- and beta-thalassemias are referred to as major or minor, depending on how many of the genes that control α- or β-chain synthesis are defective and whether the defects are inherited homozygously (thalassemia major) or heterozygously (thalassemia minor). Pathophysiologic effects range from mild microcytosis to death in utero, depending on the number of defective genes and mode of inheritance. The anemic manifestation of thalassemia is microcytic-hypochromic hemolytic anemia.

PATHOPHYSIOLOGY The beta-thalassemias are caused by mutations that decrease the synthesis of β-globin chains, leading to anemia, tissue hypoxia, and red cell hemolysis. β-Chain production is depressed—moderately in the heterozygous form, **beta-thalassemia minor**, and severely in the homozygous form, **beta-thalassemia major** (also called **Cooley anemia**). This results in erythrocytes having a reduced amount of hemoglobin and accumulation of free α-chains (Figure 22-7). The free α-chains are unstable and easily precipitate in the cell. Most erythroblasts that contain precipitates are destroyed by mononuclear phagocytes in the marrow, resulting in ineffective erythropoiesis and anemia. Some of the precipitate-carrying cells do mature and enter the bloodstream, but they are destroyed prematurely in the spleen, resulting in mild hemolytic anemia.

There are four forms of alpha-thalassemia: (1) **alpha trait** (the carrier state), in which a single α-chain–forming gene is defective; (2) **alpha-thalassemia minor**, in which two genes are defective; (3) **hemoglobin H disease**, in which three genes are defective; and (4) **alpha-thalassemia major**, a fatal condition in which all four α-forming genes are defective. Death is inevitable because α-chains are absent and oxygen cannot be released to the tissues.

CLINICAL MANIFESTATIONS Beta-thalassemia occurs more commonly than does alpha-thalassemia. Occasionally, synthesis of γ- or δ-polypeptide chains is defective, resulting in gamma- or delta-thalassemia. (Hemoglobin chains are described in Chapter 20.)

Beta-thalassemia minor causes mild to moderate microcytic-hypochromic anemia, mild splenomegaly, bronze coloring of the skin, and hyperplasia of the bone marrow. The degree of reticulocytosis depends on the severity of the anemia and results in skeletal changes. Hemolysis of immature (and therefore fragile) erythrocytes may cause a slight elevation in serum iron and indirect bilirubin levels. Persons with beta-thalassemia minor are usually asymptomatic.

Persons with beta-thalassemia major may become quite ill. Anemia is severe and results in a significant cardiovascular burden with high-output congestive heart failure. In the past, death resulted from cardiac failure. Today, blood transfusions can increase life span by one to two decades, and death usually is caused by hemochromatosis (from transfusions). Liver enlargement occurs as a result of progressive hemosiderosis, whereas enlargement of the spleen is caused by extramedullary

FIGURE 22-7 Pathogenesis of Beta-thalassemia Major. The aggregates of unpaired α-globin chains are a hallmark of the disease. Blood transfusions can diminish the anemia but they add to the systemic iron overload. (From Kumar V et al: *Robbins & Cotran pathologic basis of disease,* ed 9, Philadelphia, 2015, Saunders.)

hemopoiesis and increased destruction of red blood cells. Growth and maturation are retarded, and a characteristic chipmunk deformity develops on the face, caused by expansion of bones to accommodate hyperplastic marrow.

Persons who inherit the mildest form of alpha-thalassemia (the alpha trait) usually are symptom free or have mild microcytosis. Alpha-thalassemia minor has clinical manifestations that are virtually identical to those of beta-thalassemia minor: mild microcytic-hypochromic reticulocytosis, bone marrow hyperplasia, increased serum iron concentrations, and moderate splenomegaly.

Signs and symptoms of alpha-thalassemia major are similar to those of beta-thalassemia major, but milder. Moderate microcytic-hypochromic anemia, enlargement of the liver and spleen, and bone marrow hyperplasia are evident.

Alpha-thalassemia major causes **hydrops fetalis,** the most severe form of alpha-thalassemia, caused by deletion of all four α-globin genes. The infant suffers from severe tissue anoxia and may develop fulminant intrauterine congestive heart failure. Signs of fetal distress became evident by the third trimester of pregnancy. In the past, severe tissue anoxia led to death in utero; now many such infants are saved by intrauterine transfusions.

Both alpha- and beta-thalassemia major are life-threatening. Children with thalassemia major generally are weak, fail to thrive, show poor development, and experience cardiovascular compromise with high-output failure secondary to anemia. Untreated, they will die by 5 to 6 years of age.

EVALUATION AND TREATMENT Evaluation of thalassemia is based on familial disease history, clinical manifestations, and blood tests. Peripheral blood smears that show microcytosis and hemoglobin electrophoresis that demonstrates diminished amounts of α- or β-chains are used to make the diagnosis. Analysis of fetal DNA from withdrawn amniotic fluid is used as a screening test to detect hydrops fetalis (alpha-thalassemia major). Newborn screening for thalassemia should be done according to state law.

Persons who are silent carriers or have thalassemia minor generally have few if any symptoms and require no specific treatment. However, therapies to support and prolong life are necessary for thalassemia major and include chronic blood transfusion therapy and management of resultant iron overload (see Figure 22-7). Allogeneic hematopoietic stem cell transplantation (HSCT) is the only cure. For both symptom-free carriers and those with the disease, prenatal diagnosis and genetic counseling may be the most important therapeutic measures that can be offered.

DISORDERS OF COAGULATION AND PLATELETS

Inherited Hemorrhagic Disease

Hemophilias

Hemophilia A is defined as factor VIII deficiency and is the most common hereditary disease associated with life-threatening bleeding. It is caused by a mutation in factor VIII, an essential cofactor for factor IX in the coagulation cascade. Factor IX deficiency is most often called hemophilia B (Christmas disease, after the first person identified and not the holiday) but is *clinically* indistinguishable from factor VIII deficiency because factors VIII and IX function together to activate factor X. Both hemophilia A and hemophilia B are inherited as X-linked recessive traits, thus affecting mainly males and homozygous females.[1] Excessive bleeding rarely occurs in heterozygous females. New mutations, not family history, are the cause of about 30% of cases. The incidence of hemophilia A is approximately 1 in 5000 male births, whereas hemophilia B is five times less common, with an incidence of approximately 1 in 30,000 male births. The incidence worldwide of hemophilia is not well known, but it is estimated to be at more than 400,000 people.[10] Races are affected equally for both disorders.

Only hemophilias A and B will be discussed in this chapter. Of note is a third, less common hemophilia, termed hemophilia C, which results from a deficiency of factor XI. Table 22-3 lists the coagulation factors and deficiencies associated with clinical bleeding.

TABLE 22-3 The Coagulation Factors and Associated Disorders

Clotting Factors	Synonym	Disorder
I	Fibrinogen	Congenital deficiency (afibrinogenemia) and dysfunction (dysfibrinogenemia)
II	Prothrombin	Congenital deficiency or dysfunction
V	Labile factor or proaccelerin	Congenital deficiency (parahemophilia)
VII	Stable factor or proconvertin	Congenital deficiency
VIII	Antihemophilic factor (AHF)	Congenital deficiency is hemophilia A (classic hemophilia)
IX	Christmas factor	Congenital deficiency is hemophilia B
X	Stuart-Prower factor	Congenital deficiency
XI	Plasma thromboplastin antecedent	Congenital deficiency, sometimes referred to as hemophilia C
XII	Hageman factor	Congenital deficiency is *not* associated with clinical symptoms
XIII	Fibrin-stabilizing factor	Congenital deficiency

PATHOPHYSIOLOGY Hemophilia may be inherited or caused by a spontaneous mutation of the factor gene. The genetic instructions for both factor VIII and factor IX lie on the long arm of the X chromosome. Deficiencies of factor VIII and factor IX are clinically manifested almost exclusively in males. Because a male's DNA contains only one X chromosome, hemophilia affects mostly males. Women have two X chromosomes, and if one X chromosome has a defective gene, the other X chromosome has the information needed to create clotting factors. A female can have hemophilia because of X-inactivation or lyonization (see Chapter 2). It is possible for one X chromosome to not express itself. If the X chromosome with the hemophilia gene is the active chromosome, the woman will have lower levels of clotting factors. Fifty percent of carriers have low clotting factor levels. There is a known family history of hemophilia A and B in about two thirds of cases; the remaining third are new genetic mutations, either in the individual with hemophilia or in his unaffected carrier mother.

Numerous gene mutations and deletions have been identified at the molecular level in factor VIII and IX deficiency. The molecular defect that leads to hemophilia is identical among members of a given family; however, the deletion mutation has been unique in each family studied.[11]

CLINICAL MANIFESTATIONS The clinical manifestations and severity of hemophilia depend largely on the level of factor VIII and IX activity. The severity designation of an individual's hemophilia will determine the characteristics of the resulting disorder and will direct treatment strategies.[12] Joint bleeding is the most characteristic type of bleeding in hemophilia. Bleeding into muscles, usually from trauma, also occurs with both hemophilia A and hemophilia B. Oral bleeding is common in the setting of dental surgery. Spontaneous painless hematuria, which is relatively common in hemophilia, generally does not result in significant blood loss but requires evaluation. Hematuria accompanied by pain requires prompt evaluation and treatment.

Intracranial bleeds, bleeding of internal organs, and bleeding into the tissues of the neck, chest, or abdomen are all life-threatening. Delayed or suboptimal treatment of these bleeds may lead to permanent brain injury, loss of organ function, or death.

EVALUATION AND TREATMENT Because hemophilia is most often an inherited disease, a positive family history may expedite a diagnosis of hemophilia. When a suspected carrier mother is pregnant, genetic testing in utero through amniocentesis or chorionic villus sampling (CVS) may reveal a hemophilia diagnosis before childbirth. In the absence of a positive family history, when a bleeding disorder is suspected, personal bleed history, laboratory testing, family history, and physical assessment contribute to a thorough evaluation and accurate diagnosis. In general, those with hemophilia A or B will have a prolonged partial thromboplastin time (PTT) and the prothrombin time (PT) will be normal. Measurement of factor VIII (hemophilia A) and factor IX (hemophilia B) levels is necessary for diagnosis.

The majority of children with hemophilia A (factor VIII deficiency) can be treated with recombinant factor VIII, and the majority of children with hemophilia B (factor IX deficiency) can be treated with recombinant factor IX. Recombinant factor is reconstituted in a small volume of diluent, administered by slow intravenous push, and raises the factor level almost immediately.

Antibody-Mediated Hemorrhagic Disease

The antibody-mediated hemorrhagic diseases are a group of disorders caused by the immune response. Antibody-mediated destruction of platelets or antibody-mediated inflammatory reactions to allergens damage blood vessels and cause seepage into tissues. The thrombocytopenic purpuras may be intrinsic or idiopathic, or they may be transient phenomena transmitted from mother to fetus. The inflammatory, or "allergic," purpuras, although rare, occur in response to allergens in the blood. All of these disorders first appear during infancy or childhood.

Immune Thrombocytopenic Purpura

Acute **immune thrombocytopenic purpura (ITP; autoimmune [primary] thrombocytopenic purpura)** is the most common disorder of platelet consumption. Autoantibodies bind to the plasma membranes of platelets, causing platelet sequestration and destruction by mononuclear phagocytes in the spleen and other lymphoid tissues at a rate that exceeds the ability of the bone marrow to produce them. The destruction of platelets is triggered by drugs, infections, lymphomas, or an unknown cause.

PATHOPHYSIOLOGY The autoantibodies that produce the destruction are often of the IgG class and are usually against the platelet membrane glycoproteins (IIb-IIIa or Ib-IX). In approximately 70% of cases of ITP, there is an antecedent viral disease (e.g., cytomegalovirus [CMV], Epstein-Barr virus [EBV], parvovirus, or respiratory tract infection) that precedes the eruption of petechiae or purpura by 1 to 3 weeks.

CLINICAL MANIFESTATIONS Bruising and a generalized petechial rash often occur with acute onset. Petechiae can develop into ecchymoses. Asymmetric bruising is typical and is found most often on the legs and trunk. Hemorrhagic bullae of the gums, lips, and other mucous membranes may be prominent, and epistaxis (nose bleeding) may be severe and difficult to control. Otherwise, the child appears well. The principal changes are found in the spleen, bone marrow, and blood.[1] The acute phase lasts 1 to 2 weeks, but thrombocytopenia often persists. Although the incidence is less than 1%, intracranial hemorrhage is the most serious complication of ITP. In some cases, the onset is more gradual, and clinical manifestations consist of moderate bruising and a few petechiae.

EVALUATION AND TREATMENT Laboratory examination reveals an isolated low platelet count, and the few platelets observed on a smear are large, reflecting increased bone marrow production. The Ivy bleeding time is prolonged. Bone marrow aspiration is not recommended for children with typical features of ITP. The primary treatment for children with ITP is observation regardless of platelet count. When bleeding is present, primary treatment is with an infusion of intravenous immune globulin (IVIG) or a short course of corticosteroids.

Even without treatment, the prognosis for children with ITP is excellent: 75% recover completely within 3 months. After the initial acute phase, spontaneous clinical manifestations subside. By 6 months after onset, 80% of affected children have regained normal platelet counts.[13] ITP that persists longer than 12 months in children is considered chronic and immunosuppressive therapies are utilized.[14,15]

> ✔ **QUICK CHECK 22-2**
> 1. List the major disorders of coagulation and platelets found in children.
> 2. How do gene deletions differ from point mutations?
> 3. Why are persons with hemophilia at risk for developing degenerative joint changes?
> 4. What is the major abnormality in immune thrombocytopenic purpura (ITP)?

NEOPLASTIC DISORDERS

Leukemia

Leukemia is cancer of the blood-forming tissues, such as the bone marrow, that most often produces abnormal white blood cells called **leukemic cells**. Once in the blood, leukemic cells can spread to other organs, such as the lymph nodes, spleen, and brain. Leukemia is the most common malignancy in children and teens.

Among children and teens, about 75% of leukemias are ALL; the remaining cases are AML. ALL is most common in early childhood, peaking between 2 and 4 years of age.[17] AML is slightly more common during the first 2 years of life and during the teenage years, and occurs about equally among boys and girls of all races. ALL is more common in boys than girls and among Hispanic and white children than among black and Asian-American children.[17]

The cause of most childhood cancer is unknown. About 5% of all childhood cancers are caused by inherited mutations. Genetic mutations can occur during fetal development. Other genetic conditions associated with leukemia include Down syndrome, neurofibromatosis, Shwachman syndrome, Bloom syndrome, and ataxia-telangiectasia. Many studies have shown that exposure to ionizing radiation (prenatal exposure to x-rays and postnatal exposure to high doses) can lead to the development of childhood leukemia and possibly other cancers.[18] There is recent concern for performing computed tomography (CT) scans in children because increased use combined with wide variability in radiation doses has resulted in many children receiving a high dose of radiation.[19] Studies of other possible environmental risk factors, including parental exposure to cancer-causing chemicals, prenatal exposure to pesticides, childhood exposure to common infectious agents, and living near a nuclear power plant, have so far produced inconsistent results. Higher risks of cancer have not been seen in children of individuals treated for sporadic cancer (cancer not caused by an inherited mutation).[20,21]

PATHOGENESIS Acute lymphoblastic leukemia (ALL) is composed of immature B (pre-B) or T (pre-T) cells called **lymphoblasts**. The bone marrow is dense with lymphoblasts, considered hypercellular, that replace the normal marrow and disrupt normal function. Many of the chromosomal abnormalities documented in ALL cause dysregulation of the expression and function of transcription factors required for normal B-cell and T-cell development.[1] The mutations can include both gain of function and loss of function that are required for normal development.

Acute myeloid leukemia (AML) is caused by acquired oncogenic mutations that impair differentiation, resulting in the accumulation of immature myeloid blasts in the marrow and other organs. Epigenetic alterations are frequent in AML and have a central role. The bone marrow crowding by blasts produces marrow failure and complications, including anemia, thrombocytopenia, and neutropenia. AML is very heterogeneous because myeloid cell differentiation is very complex. To be called *acute,* the bone marrow usually must include greater than 20% leukemic blasts.

CLINICAL MANIFESTATIONS The onset of leukemia may be abrupt or insidious, but the most common symptoms reflect the consequences of bone marrow failure: decreased levels of both red blood cells and platelets and changes in white blood cells. Pallor, fatigue, petechiae, purpura, bleeding, and fever generally are present. Approximately 45% of children have a hemoglobin level below 7 g/dl. If acute blood loss occurs, characteristic symptoms of tachycardia, air hunger, restlessness, and thirst may be present. Epistaxis often occurs in children with severe thrombocytopenia.

Fever is usually present as a result of (1) infection associated with the decrease in functional neutrophils and (2) hypermetabolism associated with the ongoing rapid growth and destruction of leukemic cells. White blood cell counts greater than 200,000/mm³ can cause leukostasis, an intravascular clumping of cells that results in infarction and hemorrhage, usually in the brain and lung.

Renal failure as a result of hyperuremia (high uric acid levels) can be associated with ALL, particularly at diagnosis or during active treatment. Extramedullary invasion with leukemic cells can occur in nearly all body tissue. The central nervous system (CNS) is a common site of infiltration of extramedullary leukemias, although less than 10% of children with ALL have CNS involvement at diagnosis. The most common symptoms of CNS involvement relate to increased intracranial pressure, causing early morning headaches, nausea, vomiting, irritability, and lethargy.

Gonadal involvement can occur and leukemic infiltration into bones and joints is common. Reports of bone or joint pain actually lead to the diagnosis of leukemia in some children. In most children, bone pain is characterized as migratory, vague, and without areas of swelling or inflammation. However, if joint pain is the primary symptom and some swelling is associated with the pain, misdiagnoses of rheumatoid arthritis and rheumatic fever have occurred.

Other organs reported to be sites of leukemic invasion include the kidneys, heart, lungs, thymus, eyes, skin, and gastrointestinal tract. Children with leukemia can show symptoms only 1 week before diagnosis.

EVALUATION AND TREATMENT The diagnosis of leukemia is made from blood tests and examination of peripheral blood smears. A bone marrow aspiration is usually performed in order to further characterize the leukemia. The blast cell is the hallmark of acute leukemia (Figure 22-8). Healthy children have less than 5% blast cells in the bone marrow and none in the peripheral blood. In ALL, the bone marrow often is replaced by 80% to 100% blast cells, with a reduction in normal developing red blood cells and granulocytes. Occasionally, the marrow appears hypocellular, making the diagnosis difficult to differentiate from aplastic anemia. When this occurs, bone marrow biopsy or biopsy of extramedullary sites is necessary to confirm the diagnosis.

FIGURE 22-8 Monoblasts from Acute Monoblastic Leukemia. Monoblasts in a marrow smear from an individual with acute monoblastic leukemia. The monoblasts are larger than myeloblasts and usually have abundant cytoplasm, often with delicate scattered azurophilic granules (an element that stains well with blue aniline dyes). (From Damjanov I, Linder J, editors: *Anderson's pathology,* ed 10, St Louis, 1996, Mosby.)

Remarkable success has occurred with treatment of ALL in children. Chemotherapy is the treatment of choice for acute leukemia. Radiation has special considerations for use. In ALL, identification of various risk groups has led to the development of different intensities of drug protocols. Thus treatment is tailored specifically for a particular risk group.

Chronic myelogenous leukemia accounts for less than 5% of childhood leukemias. In the past, it was treated with high-dose chemotherapy followed by allogeneic stem cell transplant, resulting in significant treatment-related mortality. However, targeted medications, known as tyrosine kinase inhibitors (TKIs), have revolutionized the treatment of CML. Several TKIs are now approved for use in children; treatment requires continued adherence to an oral regimen and the health impact of long-term TKI therapy is not yet known.[22]

Lymphomas

Lymphoma (Hodgkin lymphoma and non-Hodgkin lymphoma [NHL]) develops from the proliferation of malignant lymphocytes (immune cells) in the lymphoid system (see Chapters 12 and 21). The four most common types of leukemia are (1) acute lymphoblastic leukemia (ALL), (2) acute myeloid leukemia (AML), (3) chronic lymphocytic leukemia (CLL), and (4) chronic myeloid leukemia (CML) (see Chapter 21). Most childhood leukemias are ALL. Chronic leukemias are rare in children.[16]

Lymphomas are malignant proliferations that arise from discrete tissue masses.[1] Lymphoid neoplasms involve some recognizable stage of lymphocyte B- or T-cell differentiation. With time and better understanding, it is clear that some lymphomas occasionally have leukemic presentations and evolution to "leukemia" is not unusual during the progression of incurable "lymphomas." The terms, therefore, merely reflect the usual tissue distribution.[1] Much controversy has surrounded the classifications of lymphoma and a consensus has been reached with the current World Health Organization (WHO) classification scheme found at www.cancer.gov/cancertopics/pdq/treatment/adult-non-hodgkins/HealthProfessional/page3. Non-Hodgkin lymphoma (NHL) and Hodgkin lymphoma constitute approximately 11% of all cases of childhood cancer. Approximately 1800 children younger than 20 years of age are diagnosed with lymphoma in the United States each year.[23] NHL (including Burkitt lymphoma) occurs more often than Hodgkin lymphoma (for newborns to children age 14 years, 5% to 6% versus 4%; and for ages 15 to 19 years, 8% versus 15% of all pediatric malignancies). Either group of diseases is rare before the age of 5 years, and the relative incidence increases throughout childhood. Boys are more likely to be diagnosed with a malignant lymphoma than are girls. At particular risk are children with inherited or acquired immunodeficiency syndromes, who have increased rates of lymphoreticular cancers that range between 100 and 10,000 times the rate of normal children.

Non-Hodgkin lymphoma. Non-Hodgkin lymphomas (NHLs) are neoplasms of immune cells. NHLs are a large and diverse group of tumors; some tumors have a slow-growing (indolent) course, whereas others have a fast-growing (aggressive) course. Almost without exception, childhood NHL becomes evident as a diffuse disease and can be further subdivided into four major types: (1) B-cell non-Hodgkin lymphoma (Burkitt and Burkitt-like lymphoma and Burkitt leukemia); (2) diffuse large B-cell lymphoma; (3) lymphoblastic lymphoma; and (4) anaplastic large cell lymphoma.[24] The common types of NHL in children are different than those in adults. The most common types of NHL in children are Burkitt lymphoma (40%), lymphoblastic lymphoma (25% to 30%), and large cell lymphoma (10%).

PATHOGENESIS Burkitt lymphoma will be discussed as an example of pathogenesis of NHL in children. All forms of Burkitt lymphoma are associated with translocations of the *MYC* gene on chromosome 8 that lead to increased MYC protein levels.[1] MYC is a transcriptional regulator that increases the expression of genes required for aerobic glycolysis, called the Warburg effect (see Chapter 10). Most Burkitt lymphomas are latently infected with the Epstein-Barr virus (EBV).[1] EBV is also present in about 25% of HIV-associated tumors and 15% to 20% of sporadic cases.[1] There is increased evidence of NHL in children with congenital immunodeficiency syndromes, such as Wiskott-Aldrich syndrome, ataxia-telangiectasia, and Bloom syndrome.

CLINICAL MANIFESTATIONS NHL has been found to arise from any lymphoid tissue. Signs and symptoms therefore are specific for the site involved. Associated signs of NHL include swelling of the lymph nodes in the neck, underarm, stomach, or groin; trouble swallowing; painless lump or swelling in a testicle; weight loss for unknown reason; night sweats; and possibly trouble breathing. Involvement of facial bones, particularly the jaw, is common in African Burkitt lymphoma.

EVALUATION AND TREATMENT Diagnosis is made by physical exam and health history, followed by biopsy of disease sites, usually the involved lymph nodes, tonsils, bone marrow, spleen, liver, bowel, or skin. Burkitt lymphoma is very aggressive and responds well to treatment. With intensive chemotherapy most children and young adults can be cured.

Hodgkin Lymphoma

Hodgkin lymphoma (HL) is a group of lymphoid neoplasms that, unlike NHL, arises in a single chain of lymph nodes and spreads first in a contiguous way to lymphoid tissue. NHL frequently arises at extranodal sites and spreads in a noncontiguous or unpredictable way. HL is characterized by the presence of *Reed-Sternberg* cells, which are large cells derived from the germinal center of B cells (Figure 22-9). The World Health Organization (WHO) has identified five types of HL: (1) nodular sclerosis, (2) mixed cellularity, (3) lymphocyte rich, (4) lymphocyte depletion, and (5) lymphocyte predominance. The first four types are considered the *classic* types of HL with similar expression of Reed-Sternberg cells. In the lymphocyte predominance type, the Reed-Sternberg cell is distinctive but different than the others. HL is a common type of cancer in young adults and adolescents but rare in childhood. The average age at diagnosis is 32 years of age.

PATHOGENESIS The Reed-Sternberg cells fail to express most of the B-cell normal genes, including the immunoglobulin (Ig) genes. The causes of the genetic rearrangements or reprogramming are not fully known but are thought to be the result of widespread epigenetic changes. Activation of the transcription factor NF-κB, which controls transcription of DNA, is a very common event in classic HL.[1] NF-κB may be activated by EBV infection. EBV-infected B cells, resembling Reed-Sternberg cells, are found in lymph nodes in individuals with infectious mononucleosis, suggesting that the EBV proteins may have a role in changes of the B cells into Reed-Sternberg cells.[1] NF-κB is involved in many biologic processes, including inflammation, immunity, cell growth, differentiation, and apoptosis. The cytoplasm is abundant with Reed-Sternberg cells and tissue is reactive with many inflammatory type cells and immune cells. These reactive cells cross-talk with Reed-Sternberg cells and support the growth and survival of the tumor cells.

CLINICAL MANIFESTATIONS Painless lymphadenopathy in the lower cervical chain, with or without fever, is the most common symptom in children. Other lymph nodes and organs also may be involved (Figure 22-10). Mediastinal involvement can cause pressure on the trachea or bronchi, leading to airway obstruction. Extranodal primary sites in Hodgkin lymphoma are rare. Initial symptoms consist of anorexia, malaise, and lassitude. Intermittent fever is present in 30% of children, and weight loss also may accompany these symptoms. Hodgkin lymphoma has a well-defined staging system that considers the extent and location of disease and the presence of fever, weight loss, or night sweats at diagnosis.

EVALUATION AND TREATMENT Treatment for Hodgkin lymphoma includes chemotherapy and radiation therapy. Long-term survivors treated with radiotherapy had a much higher incidence of

FIGURE 22-9 Diagnostic Reed-Sternberg Cell. A large multinucleated or multilobated cell with inclusion body–like nucleoli *(arrow)* surrounded by a halo of clear nucleoplasm. (From Damjanov I, Linder J: *Pathology: a color atlas,* St Louis, 2000, Mosby.)

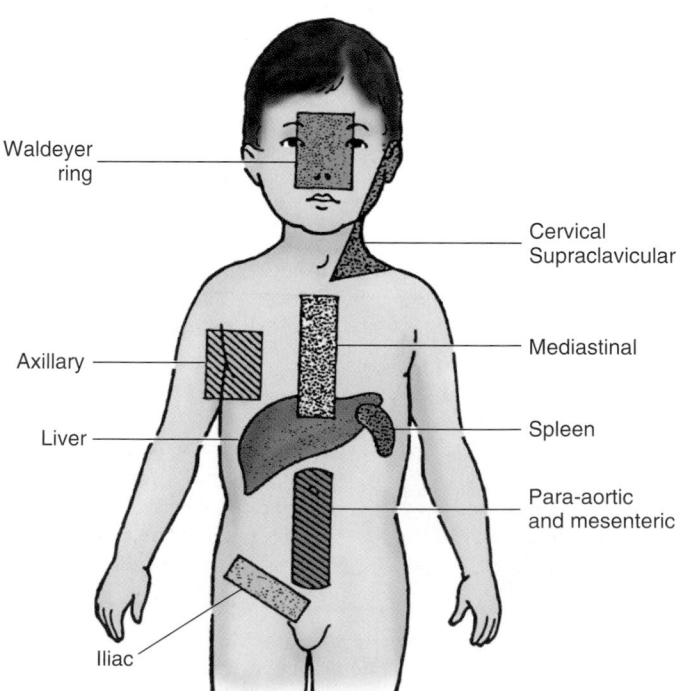

FIGURE 22-10 Main Areas of Lymphadenopathy and Organ Involvement in Hodgkin Lymphoma. (From Hockenberry MJ et al, editors: *Wong's nursing care of infants and children,* ed 10, St Louis, 2015, Mosby.)

secondary cancers, including lung cancer, melanoma, and breast cancer. Individuals previously treated with chemotherapy alkylating agents also had a high incidence of secondary tumors. These results have changed the treatment protocols to minimize the use of radiotherapy and use less toxic chemotherapy. A promising target therapy is anti-CD30.

> ✔ **QUICK CHECK 22-3**
> 1. List the childhood leukemias in order of rate of incidence.
> 2. Why do children with leukemia experience bone or joint pain?
> 3. What are the common types of non-Hodgkin lymphoma (NHL) in children?

▌ DID YOU UNDERSTAND?

Disorders of Erythrocytes

1. Anemia is the most common blood disorder in children. Like the anemias of adulthood, the anemias of childhood are caused by ineffective erythropoiesis or premature destruction of erythrocytes.

2. Iron deficiency anemia (IDA) is the most common nutritional disorder worldwide. IDA has the highest incidence occurring between 6 months and 2 years of age. Iron is critical for the developing child and without it damage from the periods of IDA is irreversible.

3. No matter the cause of IDA it produces a hypochromic-microcytic anemia eventually lowering hemoglobin and hematocrit.

4. Hemolytic disease of the fetus and newborn (HDFN) results from incompatibility between the maternal and the fetal blood, which may involve differences in Rh factors or blood type (ABO). Maternal antibodies (anti-Rh antibodies) formed in response to the presence of fetal incompatible (Rh-positive) erythrocytes in the blood of an Rh-negative mother. The maternal antibodies then enter the fetal circulation and cause hemolysis of fetal erythrocytes. However, ABO incompatibility can cause HDFN even if fetal erythrocytes do not escape into the maternal circulation during pregnancy.

5. The key to treatment of HDFN resulting from Rh incompatibilities lies in prevention or immunoprophylaxis.

6. Sickle cell disease is a group of disorders characterized by the production of abnormal **hemoglobin S (Hb S)** within the erythrocytes.

7. Sickle cell disease is an inherited, autosomal recessive disorder expressed as sickle cell anemia, sickle cell–thalassemia disease, or sickle cell–hemoglobin C disease, depending on mode of inheritance. **Sickle cell anemia**, a homozygous form, is the most severe.

8. **Sickle cell–thalassemia** and **sickle cell–Hb C disease** are heterozygous forms in which the child simultaneously inherits another type of abnormal hemoglobin from one parent. **Sickle cell trait**, in which the child inherits Hb S from one parent and normal hemoglobin (Hb A) from the other, is a heterozygous carrier state that rarely has clinical manifestations. All forms of sickle cell disease are lifelong conditions.

9. Sickle cell disease causes a change in the shape of red blood cells, resulting in deoxygenation or dehydration. It is most common among blacks and those of Mediterranean descent.

10. The alpha- and beta-thalassemias are inherited autosomal recessive disorders that cause an impaired rate of synthesis of one of the two chains—α or β—of adult hemoglobin (Hb A).

Disorders of Coagulation and Platelets

1. Hemophilia A is defined as factor VIII deficiency and is the most common hereditary disease associated with life-threatening bleeding. It is caused by a mutation in factor VIII, an essential cofactor for factor IX in the coagulation cascade. Factor IX deficiency is most often called **hemophilia B**.

2. Hemophilia may be inherited or caused by a spontaneous mutation of the factor gene.

3. The antibody-mediated hemorrhagic diseases are a group of disorders caused by the immune response. Antibody-mediated destruction of platelets or antibody-mediated inflammatory reactions to allergens damage blood vessels and cause seepage into tissues.

4. ITP, the most common of the childhood thrombocytopenic purpuras, is a disorder of platelet consumption in which antiplatelet antibodies bind to the plasma membranes of platelets. This results in platelet sequestration and destruction by mononuclear phagocytes at a rate that exceeds the ability of the bone marrow to produce them.

Neoplastic Disorders

1. Leukemia is cancer of the blood-forming tissues, such as the bone marrow, that most often produces abnormal white blood cells called leukemic cells.

2. Among children and teens, about 75% of leukemias are ALL, the remaining cases are AML. Chronic leukemias are rare in children.

3. The cause of childhood leukemia is unknown. About 5% of all childhood cancers are caused by inherited mutations. Genetic mutations can occur during fetal development.

4. Studies have shown exposure to ionizing radiation can lead to the development of childhood leukemia and possible other cancers.

5. ALL causes dysregulation of the expression and function of transcription factors required for normal B-cell and T-cell development.

6. Epigenetic alterations are frequent in AML and have a central role.

7. The onset of leukemia may be abrupt or insidious and the most common symptoms reflect the consequences of bone marrow failure. These changes can include decreased levels of red blood cells and platelets and changes in white blood cells.

8. Lymphomas are malignant proliferations that arise from discrete tissue masses. Lymphoid neoplasms involve some recognizable stage of lymphocyte B- or T-cell differentiation.

9. With time and better understanding it is now clear that some lymphomas occasionally have leukemic presentations.

10. The lymphomas of childhood are Hodgkin lymphoma (HL) and non-Hodgkin lymphoma (NHL).

11. NHL are neoplasms of immune cells. The most common types of NHL in children are Burkitt lymphoma (40%), lymphoblastic lymphoma (25% to 30%), and large cell lymphoma (10%).

12. Most Burkitt lymphomas are latently infected with the Epstein-Barr virus (EBV). There is increased evidence of NHL in children with congenital immunodeficiency syndromes.

13. Unlike NHL, HL arises in a single chain of lymph nodes and spreads first in a contiguous way to lymphoid tissue.

14. HL is characterized by the presence of Reed-Sternberg cells, which are large cells derived from the germinal center of B cells.

KEY TERMS

REFERENCES

1. Kumar V et al: *Robbins & Cotran pathologic basis of disease*, ed 9, Philadelphia, 2015, Elsevier Saunders.
2. Jo J et al: Role of cellular immunity in cow's milk allergy: pathogenesis, tolerance induction, and beyond, *Mediators Inflamm* 2014:249784, 2014.
3. Moshe G et al: Anemia and iron deficiency in children: association with red meat and poultry consumption, *J Pediatr Gastroenrol Nutr* 57(6): 722-727, 2013.
4. Gheibi SH et al: Refractory iron deficiency anemia and *Helicobacter pylori* infection in pediatrics: a review, *Iran J Ped Hematol Oncol* 5(1):50-64, 2015.
5. Shah M et al: Effect of orange and apple juice on iron absorption in children, *Arch Pediatr Adolesc Med* 157:1232-1236, 2003.
6. Crowther CA et al: Anti-D administration in pregnancy for preventing Rhesus alloimmunization, *Cochrane Database Syst Rev* 2:CD000020, 2013.
7. Qureshi H et al: BCSH guideline for the use of anti-D immunoglobulin for the prevention of haemolytic disease of the fetus and newborn, *Transfus Med* 24(1):8-20, 2014.
8. Kyung P: Sickle cell disease and other hemoglobinopathies, *Int Anesthesiol Clin* 42(3): 77-93, 2004.
9. Yawn BP et al: Management of sickle cell disease summary of the 2014 evidence-based report by

Expert Panel Members, *J Am Med Assoc* 312(10): 1033-1048, 2014.
10. National Hemophilia Foundation: *Information resource center National Hemophilia Foundation*, New York City, New York, 2015, Author.
11. Mariani G, Bernardi F: Factor II deficiency, *Semin Thromb Hemost* 35(4):400-406, 2009.
12. Blanchette VS et al, editors: *Handbook of pediatric thrombosis and hemostasis*, pp 59-78, Basel, 2013, Karger.
13. Gupta V et al: Immune thrombocytopenic purpura, *Indian J Pediatr* 75(7):723-728, 2008.
14. Neunert C et al: The American Society of Hematology 2011 evidence-based practice guideline for immune thrombocytopenia, *Blood* 117: 4190-4207, 2011.
15. Provan D et al: International consensus report on the investigation and management of primary immune thrombocytopenia, *Blood* 115:168-186, 2010.
16. American Cancer Society: *What you need to know about leukemia*, Bethesda, Md, 2015, National Cancer Institute.
17. American Cancer Society: *What are the key statistics for childhood leukemia?* Atlanta, Ga, 2015, Author.
18. National Cancer Institute: *PDQ® childhood acute lymphoblastic leukemia treatment*, Bethesda, Md, 2015, Author. Date last modified April 8, 2015.

Available at: http://cancer.gov/cancertopics/pdq/ treatment/childALL/HealthProfessional. Accessed May 10, 2015.
19. Miglioretti DL et al: The use of computed tomography in pediatrics and the associated radiation exposure and estimated cancer risk, *J Am Med Assoc Pediatr* 167(8):700-707, 2013.
20. Hudson MM: Reproductive outcomes for survivors of childhood cancer, *Obstet Gynecol* 116(5): 1171-1183, 2010.
21. National Cancer Institute: *Cancer in children and adolescents*, Bethesda, Md, 2014, Author. Accessed May 11, 2015.
22. National Cancer Institute: *PDQ® childhood acute myeloid leukemia/other myeloid malignancies treatment*, Bethesda, Md, 2015, Author. Date last modified April 9, 2015. Available at: http://cancer .gov/cancertopics/pdq/treatment/childAML/ HealthProfessional. Accessed May 12, 2015.
23. American Cancer Society: *What are the key statistics for non-Hodgkin lymphoma in children?* Atlanta, Ga, 2014, Author. Accessed May 12, 2015.
24. National Cancer Institute: *PDQ® childhood non-Hodgkin lymphoma treatment*, Bethesda, Md, 2015, Author. Last modified March 16, 2015. Available at: http://cancer.gov/cancertopics/pdq/ treatment/child-non-hodgkins/Patient. Accessed May 11, 2015.

23

Structure and Function of the Cardiovascular and Lymphatic Systems

Susanna G. Cunningham, Valentina L. Brashers, and Kathryn L. McCance

CHAPTER OUTLINE

The functions of the circulatory system include delivery of oxygen, nutrients, hormones, immune system components, and other substances to body tissues and removal of the waste products of metabolism. Delivery and removal are achieved by an extensive array of tubes—the blood and lymphatic vessels—connected to a pump, the heart. The heart continuously pumps blood through the blood vessels in collaboration with other systems, particularly the nervous and endocrine systems, which regulate the heart and blood vessels. Immune system components, nutrients, and oxygen are supplied by the immune, digestive, and respiratory systems; gaseous wastes of metabolism are expired through the lungs; and other wastes are removed by the kidneys and digestive tract.

The vascular endothelium also is a key component of the circulatory system and is sometimes considered a separate endocrine organ. This endothelium is a multifunctional tissue whose health is essential to normal vascular, immune, and hemostatic system function. Endothelial dysfunction is a critical factor in the development of vascular and other diseases.[1]

THE CIRCULATORY SYSTEM

The heart is composed of two conjoined pumps moving blood through two separate circulatory systems in sequence: one pump supplies blood to the lungs, whereas the second pump delivers blood to the rest of the body. Structures on the right side, or **right heart**, pump blood through the lungs. This system is termed the **pulmonary circulation** and is described in Chapter 26. The left side, or **left heart**, sends blood throughout the **systemic circulation**, which supplies all of the body except the lungs (Figure 23-1). These two systems are serially connected; thus the output of one becomes the input of the other.

Arteries carry blood from the heart to all parts of the body, where they branch into arterioles and even smaller vessels, ultimately becoming a fine meshwork of capillaries. Capillaries allow the closest contact and exchange between the blood and the interstitial space, or interstitium—the environment in which cells live. Venules and then veins next carry blood from the capillaries back to the heart. Some of the plasma or liquid part of the blood passes through the walls of the capillaries into the interstitial space. This fluid, lymph, is returned to the cardiovascular system by vessels of the lymphatic system. The lymphatic system is a critical component of the immune system as described in Chapters 6 and 7.

THE HEART

Adult hearts weigh between 200 and 350 grams and are about fist-sized. The heart lies obliquely (diagonally) in the **mediastinum**, the area above the diaphragm and between the lungs. Heart structures can be categorized by function:

1. *Structural support of heart tissues and circulation of pulmonary and systemic blood through the heart.* This category includes the heart wall and fibrous skeleton enclosing and supporting the heart and dividing it into four chambers: the valves directing flow through the chambers and the great vessels conducting blood to and from the heart.

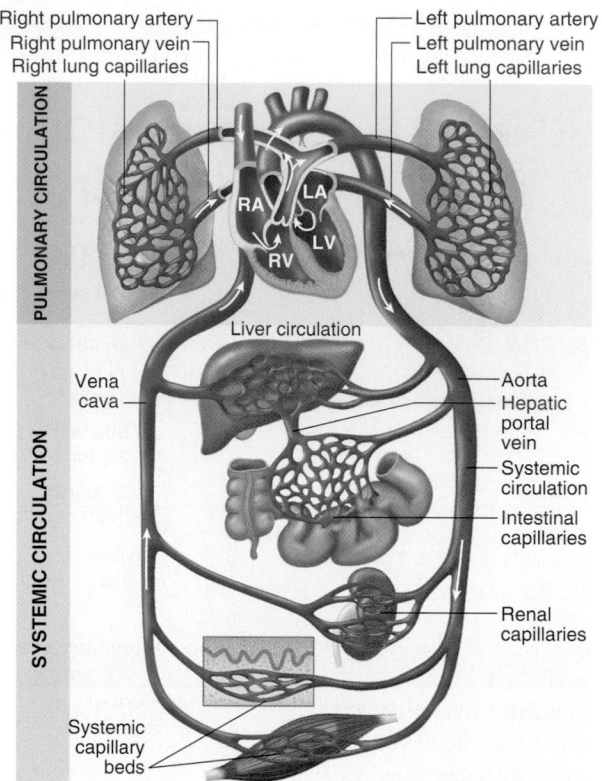

FIGURE 23-1 Diagram of the Pulmonary and Systemic Circulatory Systems. The right heart pumps unoxygenated blood *(blue)* through the pulmonary circulation, where oxygen enters the blood and carbon dioxide is exhaled, and the left heart pumps oxygenated *(red)* blood to and from all the other organ systems in the body. (From Patton KT, Thibodeau GA, Douglas MM: *Essentials of anatomy & physiology,* St Louis, 2012, Elsevier.)

2. *Maintenance of heart cells.* This category includes all the vessels of the coronary circulation—the arteries and veins that serve the metabolic needs of all the heart cells—and the heart's lymphatic vessels.
3. *Stimulation and control of heart action.* Among these structures are the nerves and specialized muscle cells that direct the rhythmic contraction and relaxation of the heart muscles, propelling blood throughout the pulmonary and systemic circulatory systems.

Structures That Direct Circulation Through the Heart
The Heart Wall

The three layers of the heart wall—the epicardium, myocardium, and endocardium—are enclosed in a double-walled membranous sac, the **pericardium** (Figure 23-2). The **pericardial sac** has three main functions: it prevents displacement of the heart during gravitational acceleration or deceleration, serves as a physical barrier to protect the heart against infection and inflammation coming from the lungs and pleural space, and contains pain receptors and mechanoreceptors that can cause reflex changes in blood pressure and heart rate. The two layers of the pericardium, the parietal and the visceral pericardia (see Figure 23-2), are separated by a fluid-containing space called the **pericardial cavity.** The **pericardial fluid** (about 20 ml) is secreted by cells of the mesothelial layer of the pericardium and lubricates the membranes that line the pericardial cavity, enabling them to slide smoothly over one another with minimal friction as the heart beats. The amount and

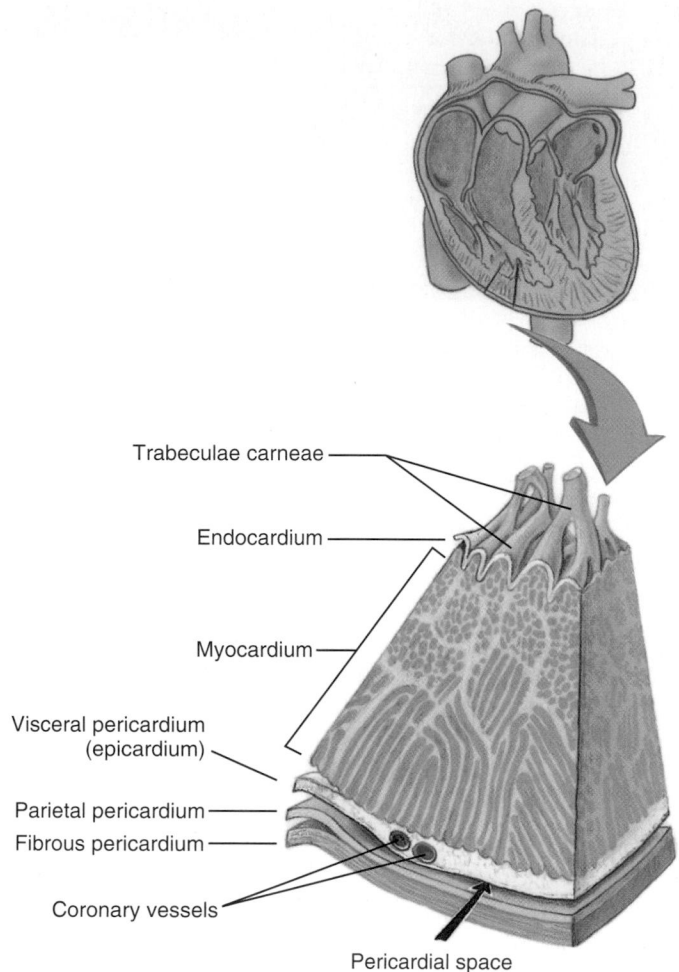

FIGURE 23-2 Wall of the Heart. This section of the heart wall shows the fibrous pericardium, the parietal and visceral layers of the serous pericardium (with the pericardial space between them), the myocardium, and the endocardium. Note the fatty connective tissue between the visceral layer of the serous pericardium (epicardium) and the myocardium. Note also that the endocardium covers tubular projections of myocardial muscle tissue called *trabeculae.* (Revised from Applegate E: *The anatomy and physiology learning system,* ed 4, St Louis, 2011, Saunders.)

character of the pericardial fluid are altered if the pericardium is inflamed (see Chapter 24).

The smoothness of the outer layer of the heart, the epicardium, also minimizes the friction between the heart wall and the pericardial sac. The thickest layer of the heart wall, the **myocardium,** is composed of cardiac muscle and is anchored to the heart's fibrous skeleton. The heart muscle cells, **cardiomyocytes,** provide the contractile force needed for blood to flow through the heart and into the pulmonary and systemic circulations. About 0.5% to 1% of the cardiomyocytes are replaced annually; thus over a lifetime about half of these muscle cells are replaced.[2] There is great interest in finding therapies that will increase the rate of cardiomyocyte replacement for persons who have suffered a myocardial infarction or have heart failure from another cause (see *Health Alert:* Myocardial Regeneration).

The internal lining of the myocardium, the **endocardium,** is composed of connective tissue and squamous cells (see Figure 23-2). This lining is continuous with the endothelium that lines all the arteries, veins, and capillaries of the body, creating a continuous, closed circulatory system.

HEALTH ALERT

Myocardial Regeneration

Myocardial infarction causes the loss of some of the muscle cells needed to maintain cardiac output, thus increasing the risk of heart failure in survivors. Given that heart failure is a growing problem with a poor prognosis in both the United States and internationally, finding an effective therapy is a critical need.

To replace the approximately 1 billion cardiomyocytes that are estimated to be lost with a myocardial infarction, researchers have identified four possible approaches: (1) accelerating the rate of heart cell division, (2) inserting new cells into the heart, (3) stimulating the heart muscle precursor cells already in the heart, and (4) reprogramming other cells so that they will become cardiomyocyte precursor cells. To stimulate adult heart cells to enter the cell cycle and thus accelerate cell division, various signaling molecules, such as neuregulin and fibroblast growth factor 1, have been used with some success. Currently, the most promising cell types that have been injected into the heart include cells from the bone marrow, cardiac-derived cells taken from myocardial biopsies, and human pluripotent stem cells. Although there are cardiac progenitor or precursor cells in the heart, their rate of division is not adequate to replace lost tissue after an infarction. Some of the methods being investigated to stimulate these cardiomyocytes or other progenitor cells in the heart include treatment with peptides that act as paracrines and some types of modified RNAs (ribonucleic acids) for vascular endothelial growth factor (VEGF). Reprogramming from one cell type into a pluripotent stem cell has been attempted with fibroblasts with some success. Each of these four approaches to replacing cardiomyocytes after injury comes with its own set of risks and challenges. Associated risks include increasing the chances for tumor development, damage to other organs, and myocardial scarring.

Data from Gerbin KA, Murray CE: *Cardiovasc Pathol* 2015 Feb 19 [Epub ahead of print]; Laflamme AM, Murry CE: *Nat Biotechnol* 23(7):845-856, 2005; Lin Z, Pu WT: *Sci Transl Med* 6(239):239rv1, 2014; Ounzain S, Pedrazzini T: *Trends Cardiovasc Med* 2015 Feb 7 [Epub ahead of print].

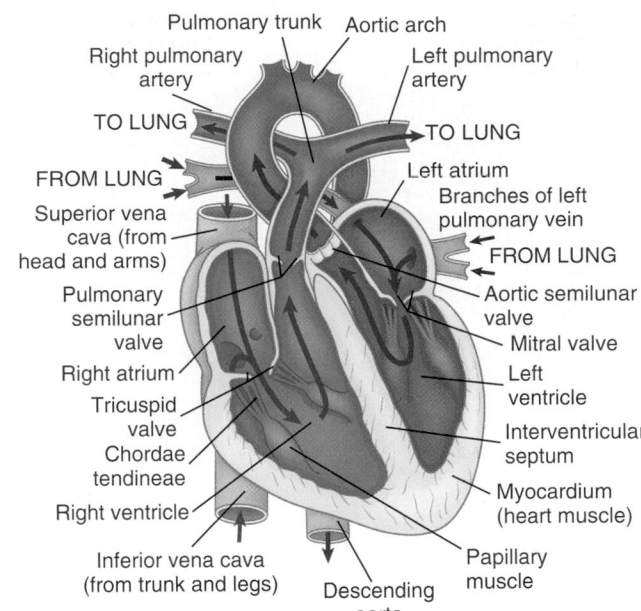

FIGURE 23-3 Structures That Direct Blood Flow Through the Heart. The blue and red arrows indicate the pathways of unoxygenated and oxygenated blood flow through chambers, valves, and major vessels.

Chambers of the Heart

The heart has four chambers: the left atrium, the right atrium, the right ventricle, and the left ventricle. These chambers form two pumps in series: the right heart is a low-pressure system pumping blood through the lungs and the left heart is a high-pressure system pumping blood to the rest of the body (Figure 23-3). The atria are smaller than the ventricles and have thinner walls. The ventricles have a thicker myocardial layer and constitute much of the bulk of the heart. The ventricles are formed by a continuum of muscle fibers originating from the fibrous skeleton at the base of the heart.

The wall thickness of each cardiac chamber depends on the amount of pressure or resistance it must overcome to eject blood. The two atria have the thinnest walls because they are low-pressure chambers that serve as storage units and channels for blood that is emptied into the ventricles. Normally, there is little resistance to flow from the atria to the ventricles. The ventricles, on the other hand, must propel the blood all the way through the pulmonary or systemic vessels. The mean pulmonary artery pressure, the force the right ventricle must overcome, is only 15 mm Hg, whereas the mean arterial pressure the left ventricle must pump against is about 92 mm Hg. Because the pressure is markedly higher in the systemic circulation, the wall of the left ventricle is about three times thicker than that of the right ventricle.

The right ventricle is shaped like a crescent or triangle, enabling a bellows-like action that efficiently ejects large volumes of blood through the pulmonary semilunar valve into the low-pressure pulmonary system. The larger left ventricle is bullet shaped, which allows it to generate enough pressure to eject blood through a relatively larger aortic semilunar valve into the high-pressure systemic circulation.

The septal membrane separates the right and left sides of the heart and prevents blood from crossing between the two circulatory systems. The atria are separated by the interatrial septum, and the ventricles by the interventricular septum. Because the fetus does not depend on the lungs for oxygenation, there is an opening before birth between the right and left atria called the foramen ovale that facilitates circulation. This opening closes functionally at the time of birth as the higher pressure in the left atrium pushes a flap, the septum primum, over the hole. In 75% to 80% of infants these septa are permanently fused within the first year of life[3,4] (see Chapter 25).

Fibrous Skeleton of the Heart

Four rings of dense fibrous connective tissue provide a firm anchorage for the attachments of the atrial and ventricular musculature, as well as the valvular tissue (Figure 23-4). The fibrous rings are adjacent and form a central, fibrous supporting structure collectively termed the *annuli fibrosi cordis.*

Valves of the Heart

Four heart valves and the pressure gradients they maintain ensure that blood only flows one way through the heart. When the ventricles are relaxed, the two atrioventricular valves open and blood flows from the relatively higher pressure in the atria to the lower pressure in the ventricles. As the ventricles contract ventricular pressure increases and causes these valves to close and prevent backflow into the atria. The semilunar valves of the heart open when intraventricular pressure exceeds aortic and pulmonary pressures, and blood flows out of the ventricles and into the pulmonary and systemic circulations. After ventricular contraction and ejection, intraventricular pressure falls and the pulmonic and aortic semilunar valves close when the pressure in

FIGURE 23-4 Transverse section of the heart showing the atrioventricular (AV) (mitral and tricuspid) and semilunar (aortic and pulmonary) valves. Superior view with the atria and vessels removed. *Arrows* indicate direction of blood flow. **(A)** When the heart is filling with blood the AV valves are open and the semilunar valves are closed. **(B)** When blood is leaving the heart the semilunar valves are open and the AV valves are closed. (From Naish J: *Medical sciences,* ed 2, London, 2015, Saunders.)

the vessels is greater than the pressure in the ventricles, thus preventing backflow into the right and left ventricles, respectively. The actions of the heart valves are shown in Figures 23-3 and 23-4.

The atrioventricular (tricuspid and mitral) valve openings are composed of tissue flaps called *leaflets* or *cusps,* which are attached at the upper margin to a ring in the heart's fibrous skeleton and by the **chordae tendineae** at the lower end to the papillary muscles (see Figure 23-3). The **papillary muscles,** extensions of the myocardium, help hold the cusps together and downward at the onset of ventricular contraction, thus preventing their backward expulsion or **prolapse** into the atria.

The atrioventricular valve in the right heart is called the **tricuspid valve** because it has three cusps. The left atrioventricular valve is a bicuspid (two-cusp) valve called the **mitral valve.** The tricuspid and mitral valves function as a unit because the atria, fibrous rings, valvular tissue, chordae tendineae, papillary muscles, and ventricular walls are connected. Collectively, these six structures are known as the **mitral and tricuspid complex.** Damage to any one of the six components of this complex can alter function significantly and contribute to heart failure.

Blood leaves the right ventricle through the pulmonic semilunar valve, and it leaves the left ventricle through the aortic semilunar valve (see Figures 23-3 and 23-4). Both the pulmonic and aortic semilunar valves have three cup-shaped cusps that arise from the fibrous skeleton.

The Great Vessels

Blood moves in and out of the heart through several large veins and arteries (see Figure 23-3). The right heart receives venous blood from the systemic circulation through the **superior** and **inferior venae cavae,** which join and then enter the right atrium. Blood leaving the right ventricle enters the pulmonary circulation through the **pulmonary artery,** which divides into right and left branches to transport unoxygenated blood from the right heart to the lungs. The pulmonary

arteries branch further into the pulmonary capillary beds, where oxygen and carbon dioxide exchange occurs.

Four **pulmonary veins,** two from the right lung and two from the left lung, carry oxygenated blood from the lungs to the left side of the heart. The oxygenated blood moves through the left atrium and ventricle, out into the **aorta** that subsequently branches into the systemic arteries that supply the body.

Blood Flow during the Cardiac Cycle

The pumping action of the heart consists of contraction and relaxation of the heart muscle, or myocardium. Each ventricular contraction and the relaxation that follows it constitute one **cardiac cycle.** (Blood flow through the heart during a single cardiac cycle is illustrated in Figure 23-5.) During the period of relaxation, termed **diastole,** blood fills the ventricles. The ventricular contraction that follows, termed **systole,** propels the blood out of the ventricles and into the pulmonary and systemic circulations. Contraction of the left ventricle occurs slightly earlier than contraction of the right ventricle.

The five phases of the cardiac cycle are said to begin with the opening of the mitral and tricuspid valves and atrial contraction (Figures 23-6 and 23-7). Closing of the mitral and tricuspid valves as passive ventricular filling begins marks the end of one cardiac cycle.

Normal Intracardiac Pressures

Normal intracardiac pressures are shown in Table 23-1.

✔ **QUICK CHECK 23-1**

1. Why are the two separate circulatory systems said to be "serially connected"?
2. What are the functions of the pericardial sac?
3. Why is the thickness of the myocardium different in the right and left ventricles?
4. Trace the flow of blood through the heart during one cardiac cycle.

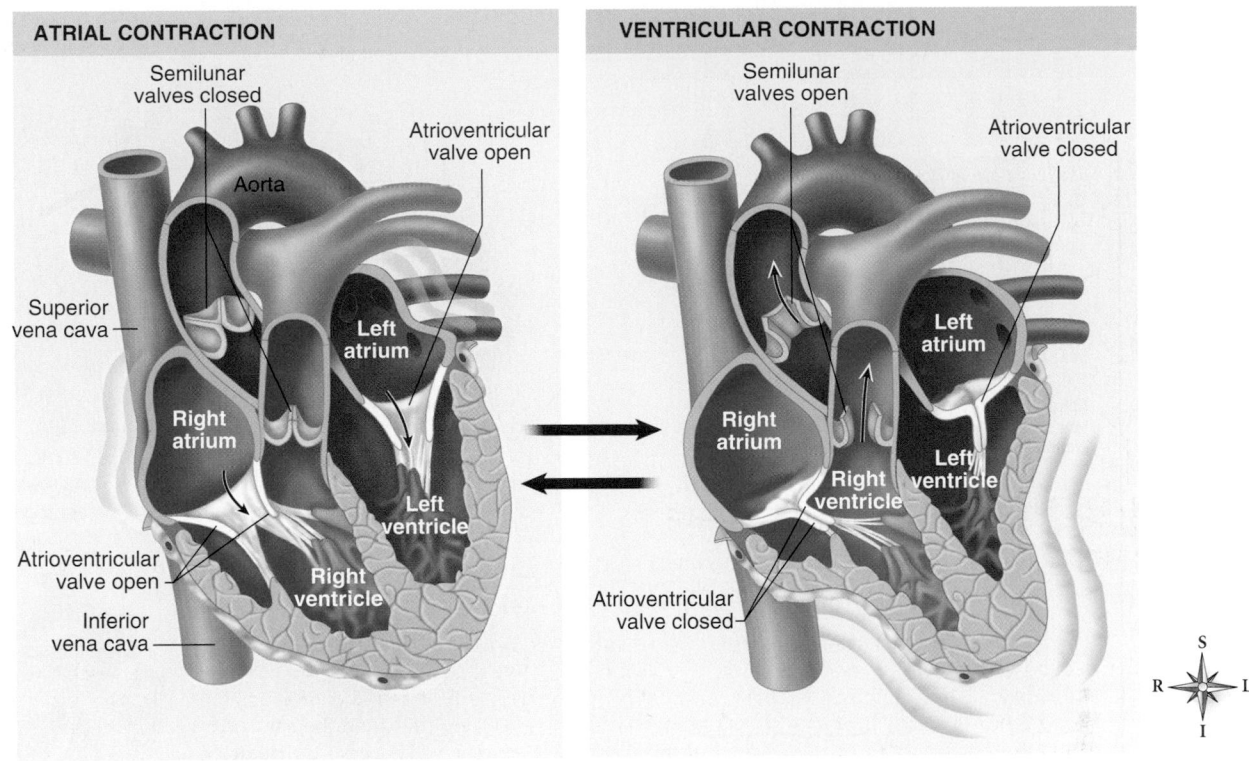

FIGURE 23-5 **Blood Flow Through the Heart during a Single Cardiac Cycle.** A, During diastole, blood flows into atria, atrioventricular valves are pushed open, and blood begins to fill ventricles. Atrial systole squeezes blood remaining in the atria into the ventricles. B, During ventricular systole, the ventricles contract, pushing blood out through semilunar valves into the pulmonary artery (right ventricle) and the aorta (left ventricle). (From Patton KT, Thibodeau GA: *Structure & function of the body,* ed 15, St Louis, 2016, Elsevier.)

TABLE 23-1	Normal Intracardiac Pressures	
	Mean (mm Hg)	Range (mm Hg)
Right atrium	4	0-8
Right ventricle		
Systolic	24	15-28
End-diastolic	4	0-8
Left atrium	7	4-12
Left ventricle		
Systolic	130	90-140
End-diastolic	7	4-12

Structures That Support Cardiac Metabolism: The Coronary Vessels

The myocardium and other heart structures are supplied with oxygen and nutrients by the coronary circulation, which is part of the systemic circulation. The coronary arteries originate at the upper edge of the aortic semilunar valve cusps (Figure 23-8B) and receive blood through openings in the aorta called the coronary ostia. The cardiac veins empty into the right atrium through another ostium, the opening of a large vein called the coronary sinus (Figure 23-8C). (Regulation of the coronary circulation, which is similar to regulation of flow through systemic and pulmonary vessels, is described in a later section.)

Coronary Arteries

The major coronary arteries, the right coronary artery (RCA) and the left coronary artery (LCA) (see Figure 23-8A), traverse the epicardium, myocardium, and endocardium and branch to become arterioles and then capillaries. Their main branches are outlined in Box 23-1. The coronary arteries are smaller in women than in men because women's hearts weigh proportionately less than men's hearts.

Collateral Arteries

Collateral arteries are anastomoses or connections between branches of the same coronary artery or connections of branches of the right coronary artery with branches of the left. The epicardium contains more collateral vessels than the endocardium. New collateral vessels are formed through two processes: arteriogenesis (new artery growth branching from preexisting arteries) and angiogenesis (growth of new capillaries within a tissue).[5] This collateral growth is stimulated by shear stress, that results from increased blood flow speed within and just beyond areas of stenosis, as well as the production of growth factors and cytokines, including monocyte chemoattractant protein-1 (MCP-1) and vascular endothelial growth factor (VEGF).[6] The collateral circulation assists in supplying blood and oxygen to myocardium that has become ischemic following gradual narrowing, or stenosis, of one or more major coronary arteries (coronary artery disease). Unfortunately, diabetes, which predisposes to coronary artery disease, also impedes collateral formation because of increased production of antiangiogenic factors, such as endostatin and angiostatin. Current research is focused on identifying whether some factors that

FIGURE 23-6 Composite Chart of Heart Function. This chart is a composite of several diagrams of heart function (cardiac pumping cycle, blood pressure, blood flow, volume, heart sounds, venous pulse, and electrocardiogram [ECG]), all on the same timescale.

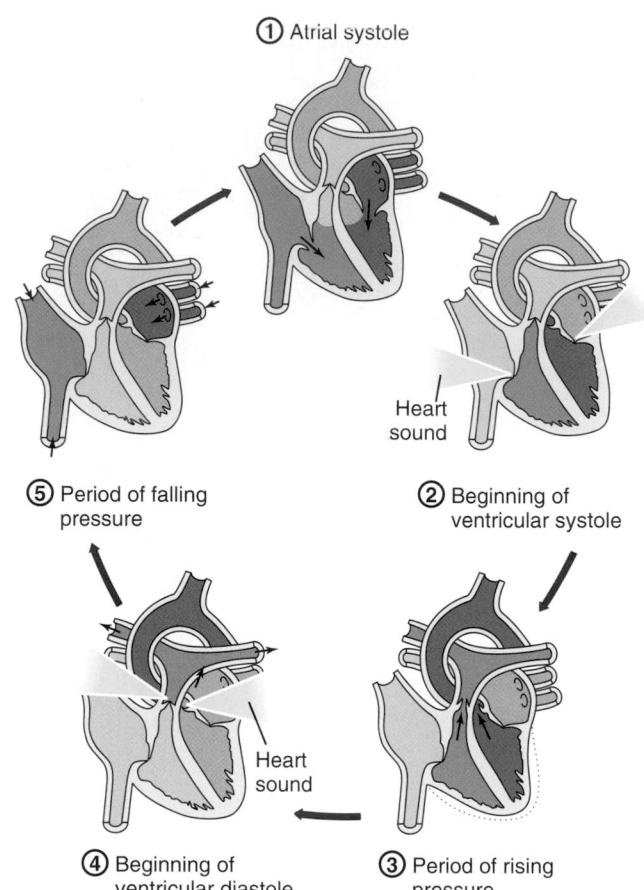

FIGURE 23-7 The Five Phases of the Cardiac Cycle. 1, Atrial systole: Atria contract, pushing blood through the open tricuspid and mitral valves into the ventricles. Semilunar valves are closed. **2,** Beginning of ventricular systole. Ventricles contract, increasing pressure within the ventricles. The tricuspid and mitral valves close, causing the first heart sound. **3,** Period of rising pressure: Semilunar valves open when pressure in the ventricle exceeds that in the arteries. Blood spurts into the aorta and pulmonary arteries. **4,** Beginning of ventricular diastole: Pressure in the relaxing ventricles drops below that in the arteries. Semilunar valves snap shut, causing the second heart sound. **5,** Period of falling pressure: Blood flows from veins into the relaxed atria. Tricuspid and mitral valves open when pressure in the ventricles falls below that in the atria. (Adapted from Solomon E: *Introduction to human anatomy and physiology,* ed 4, St Louis, 2016, Saunders.)

oxygen delivered to it, and coronary blood flow is directly correlated with myocardial oxygen consumption.[7] Any alteration of the cardiac muscles dramatically affects blood flow in the capillaries.

Coronary Veins and Lymphatic Vessels

After passing through the capillary network, blood from the coronary arteries drains into the cardiac veins located alongside the arteries. Most of the venous drainage of the heart occurs through veins in the visceral pericardium. The veins then feed into the great cardiac vein (see Figure 23-8C) and coronary sinus on the posterior surface of the heart, between the atria and ventricles, in the coronary sulcus.

The myocardium has an extensive system of lymphatic capillaries and collecting vessels within the layers of the myocardium and the valves. With cardiac contraction, the lymphatic vessels drain fluid to lymph nodes in the anterior mediastinum that empty into the superior vena cava. The lymphatics are important for protecting the myocardium against infection and injury.

stimulate collateral growth might be useful treatments for myocardial ischemia; so far none have been demonstrated to be effective.[6]

Coronary Capillaries

The heart requires an extensive capillary network to function. Blood travels from the arteries to the arterioles and then into the capillaries, where oxygen and other nutrients enter the myocardium while waste products enter the blood. At rest, the heart extracts 50% to 80% of the

FIGURE 23-8 Coronary Circulation. A, Arteries. **B,** Coronary artery openings from the aorta. **C,** Veins. Both **A** and **C** are anterior views of the heart. Vessels near the anterior surface are more darkly colored than vessels of the posterior surface seen through the heart. **B,** Placement of the coronary artery opening behind the leaflets of the aortic valve allows the coronary arteries to fill during ventricular relaxation. (**A** and **C** from Patton KT, Thibodeau GA: *Anatomy & physiology,* ed 7, St Louis, 2010, Mosby. **B,** Patton KT, Thibodeau GA: *The human body in health & disease,* ed 6, St Louis, 2014, Mosby.)

BOX 23-1 Main Branches of the Coronary Arteries

Left coronary artery. Arises from single ostium behind left cusp of aortic semi-lunar valve; ranges from a few millimeters to a few centimeters long; passes between left arterial appendage and pulmonary artery and generally divides into two branches: the left anterior descending artery and the circumflex artery; other branches are distributed diagonally across the free wall of the left ventricle.

Left anterior descending artery (or anterior interventricular artery). Delivers blood to portions of left and right ventricles and much of interventricular septum; travels down the anterior surface of the interventricular septum toward apex of the heart.

Circumflex artery. Travels in a groove *(coronary sulcus)* that separates left atrium from left ventricle and extends to left border of heart; supplies blood to left atrium and lateral wall of left ventricle; often branches to posterior surfaces of left atrium and left ventricle.

Right coronary artery. Originates from an ostium behind the right aortic cusp, travels from behind the pulmonary artery, and extends around the right heart to the heart's posterior surface, where it branches to atrium and ventricle; three major branches are conus (supplies blood to upper right ventricle), right marginal branch (supplies right ventricle to the apex), and posterior descending branch (lies in posterior interventricular sulcus and supplies smaller branches to both ventricles).

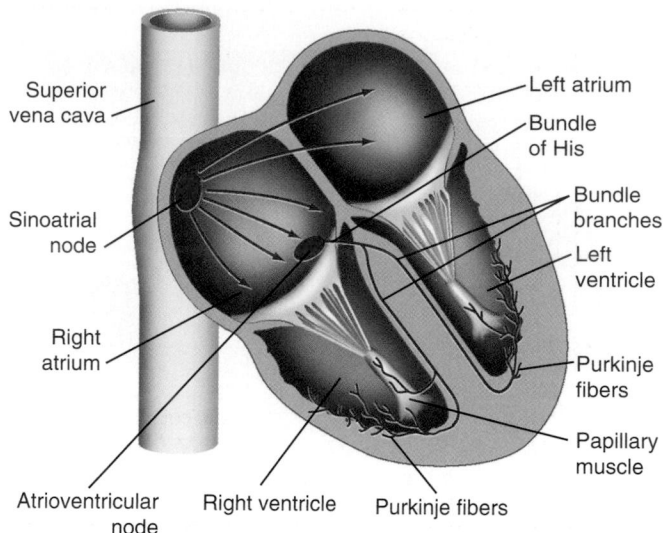

FIGURE 23-9 The Cardiac Conduction System. Specialized cardiac muscle cells in the heart wall rapidly conduct an electrical impulse throughout the myocardium. The signal is initiated by the sinoatrial (SA) node (pacemaker) and spreads through the atrial myocardium to the atrioventricular (AV) node. The AV node then initiates a signal that is conducted through the ventricular myocardium by way of the atrioventricular bundle (of His) and Purkinje fibers. (From Koeppen BM, editor: *Berne & Levy physiology*, ed 6, St Louis, 2010, Mosby.)

Structures That Control Heart Action

Life depends on continuous repetition of the cardiac cycle (systole and diastole), which requires the transmission of electrical impulses, termed **cardiac action potentials**, through the myocardium.[7] (Action potentials are described in Chapters 1 and 5.) The muscle fibers of the myocardium are electrically coupled so that action potentials pass from cell to cell rapidly and efficiently.

The myocardium contains its own pacemakers and **conduction system**—specialized cells that enable it to generate and transmit action potentials without input from the nervous system (Figure 23-9). The pacemaker cells are concentrated at two sites, or nodes, in the myocardium. The cardiac cycle is stimulated by these nodes of specialized cells. Although the heart is innervated by the autonomic nervous system (both sympathetic and parasympathetic fibers), neural impulses are not needed to maintain the cardiac cycle. Thus the heart will beat in the absence of any innervation, one of the many factors that allow heart transplantation to be successful.

Heart action is also influenced by substances delivered to the myocardium in coronary blood. Nutrients and oxygen are needed for cellular survival and normal function. Hormones and biochemical substances, including medications, can affect the strength and duration of myocardial contraction and the degree and duration of myocardial relaxation. Normal or appropriate function depends on the supply of these substances, which is why coronary artery disease can seriously disrupt heart function.

The Conduction System

Normally, electrical impulses arise in the **sinoatrial (SA) node (sinus node)**, the usual pacemaker of the heart. The SA node is located at the junction of the right atrium and superior vena cava, just superior to the tricuspid valve. The SA node is heavily innervated by both sympathetic and parasympathetic nerve fibers.[8] In the resting adult the SA node generates about 60 to 100 action potentials per minute depending on age and physical condition. Each action potential travels rapidly from cell to cell and through the atrial myocardium, carrying the action potential onward to the **atrioventricular node (AV node)**, as well as causing both atria to contract, beginning systole.[8]

The AV node, located in the right atrial wall superior to the tricuspid valve and anterior to the ostium of the coronary sinus, conducts the action potentials onward to the ventricles. It is innervated by nerves from the autonomic parasympathetic ganglia that serve as receptors for the vagus nerve and cause slowing of impulse conduction through the AV node.

Conducting fibers from the AV node converge to form the **bundle of His (atrioventricular bundle)**, within the posterior border of the interventricular septum. The bundle of His then gives rise to the right and left bundle branches. The **right bundle branch (RBB)** is thin and travels without much branching to the right ventricular apex. Because of its thinness and relative lack of branches, the RBB is susceptible to interruption of impulse conduction by damage to the endocardium. The **left bundle branch (LBB)** in some hearts divides into two branches, or fascicles. The left anterior bundle branch (LABB) passes the left anterior papillary muscle and the base of the left ventricle and crosses the aortic outflow tract. Damage to the aortic valve or the left ventricle can interrupt this branch. The left posterior bundle branch (LPBB) travels posteriorly, crossing the left ventricular inflow tract to the base of the left posterior papillary muscle. This branch spreads diffusely through the posterior inferior left ventricular wall. Blood flow through this portion of the left ventricle is relatively nonturbulent, so the LBB is somewhat protected from injury caused by wear and tear.

The **Purkinje fibers** are the terminal branches of the RBB and LBB. They extend from the ventricular apexes to the fibrous rings and penetrate the heart wall to the outer myocardium. The first areas of the ventricles to be excited are portions of the interventricular septum. The septum is activated from both the RBB and the LBB. The extensive network of Purkinje fibers promotes the rapid spread of the impulse to the ventricular apexes. The basal and posterior portions of the ventricles are the last to be activated.

> ✔ **QUICK CHECK 23-2**
> 1. Draw a diagram of the conduction system of the heart.
> 2. Why are the left and right coronary vessels considered the major coronary vessels?

Propagation of cardiac action potentials. Electrical activation of the muscle cells, termed **depolarization**, is caused by the movement of ions, including sodium, potassium, calcium, and chloride, across cardiac cell membranes. Deactivation, called **repolarization**, occurs the same way. (Movement of ions across cell membranes is described in Chapter 1; electrical activation of muscle cells is described in Chapter 38.)

Movement of ions into and out of the cell creates an electrical (voltage) difference across the cell membrane, called the *membrane potential*. The resting membrane potential of myocardial cells is between −80 and −90 millivolts (mV), whereas that of the SA node is between −50 and −60 mV and that of the AV node is between −60 and −70 mV.[8] During depolarization, the inside of the cell becomes less negatively charged. In cardiac cells, as in other excitable cells, when the resting membrane potential (in millivolts) becomes more negative with depolarization and reaches the threshold potential for cardiac cells, a cardiac action potential is fired. Table 23-2 summarizes the intracellular and extracellular ionic concentrations of cardiac muscle. Drugs that alter the movement of these ions (e.g., calcium) have

TABLE 23-2 Intercellular and Extracellular Ion Concentrations in the Myocardium

	Intracellular Concentration (mM)*	Extracellular Concentration (mM)
Sodium (Na$^+$)	15	145
Potassium (K$^+$)	150	4
Chloride (Cl$^-$)	5	120
Calcium (Ca^{++})	10^{-7}	2

*mM, Millimolar (millimoles per kilogram).

profound effects on the action potential and can alter heart rate. The various phases of the cardiac action potential are related to changes in the permeability of the cell membrane to sodium, potassium, chloride, and calcium. Threshold is the point at which the cell membrane's selective permeability to these ions is temporarily disrupted, leading to an "all or nothing" depolarization. If the resting membrane potential becomes more negative because of a decrease in extracellular potassium concentration (hypokalemia), it is termed *hyperpolarization*.

A **refractory period**, during which no new cardiac action potential can be initiated by a stimulus, follows depolarization. This effective or absolute refractory period corresponds to the time needed for the reopening of channels that permit sodium and calcium influx into the cells. A relative refractory period occurs near the end of repolarization, following the effective refractory period. During this time, the membrane can be depolarized again but only by a greater-than-normal stimulus. Abnormal refractory periods as a result of disease can cause abnormal heart rhythms or dysrhythmias, including ventricular fibrillation and cardiac arrest (see Chapter 24).

The electrocardiogram. An electrocardiogram originates from myocardial cell electrical activity as recorded by skin electrodes and is the summation of all the cardiac action potentials (Figure 23-10). The **P wave** represents atrial depolarization. The **PR interval** is a measure of time from the onset of atrial activation to the onset of ventricular activation (normally 0.12 to 0.20 second). The PR interval represents the time necessary for electrical activity to travel from the sinus node through the atrium, AV node, and His-Purkinje system to activate ventricular myocardial cells. The **QRS complex** represents the sum of all ventricular muscle cell depolarization. The configuration and amplitude of the QRS complex may vary considerably among individuals. The duration is normally between 0.06 and 0.10 second. During the **ST interval**, the entire ventricular myocardium is depolarized. The **QT interval** is sometimes called the "electrical systole" of the ventricles. It lasts about 0.4 second but varies inversely with the heart rate. The **T wave** represents ventricular repolarization.

Automaticity. Automaticity, or the property of generating spontaneous depolarization to threshold, enables the SA and AV nodes to generate cardiac action potentials without any external stimulus. Cells capable of spontaneous depolarization are called **automatic cells**. The automatic cells of the cardiac conduction system can stimulate the heart to beat even when it is transplanted and thus has no innervation.

FIGURE 23-10 Electrocardiogram (ECG) and Cardiac Electrical Activity. **A,** Normal ECG. Depolarization and repolarization. **B,** ECG intervals among P, QRS, and T waves. **C,** Schematic representation of ECG and its relationship to cardiac electrical activity. *AV,* Atrioventricular; *LA,* left atrium; *LBB,* left bundle branch; *LV,* left ventricle; *RA,* right atrium; *RBB,* right bundle branch; *RV,* right ventricle.

Spontaneous depolarization is possible in automatic cells because the membrane potential of these special cells does not actually "rest" during return to the resting membrane potential. Instead, it slowly depolarizes toward threshold during the diastolic phase of the cardiac cycle. Because threshold is approached during diastole, return to the resting membrane potential in automatic cells is called **diastolic depolarization**. The electrical impulse normally begins in the SA node because its cells depolarize more rapidly than other automatic cells.

Rhythmicity. **Rhythmicity** is the regular generation of an action potential by the heart's conduction system. The SA node sets the pace because normally it has the fastest rate. The SA node depolarizes spontaneously 60 to 100 times per minute. If the SA node is damaged, the AV node can become the heart's pacemaker at a rate of about 40 to 60 spontaneous depolarizations per minute. Eventually, however, conduction cells in the atria usually take over from the AV node. Purkinje fibers are capable of spontaneous depolarization but at an even slower rate than the AV node.

> ✔ **QUICK CHECK 23-3**
> 1. What are the pathways of conduction through the heart?
> 2. What does each of the electrocardiogram waves (P, Q, R, S, T) represent?
> 3. Define automaticity and rhythmicity.

Cardiac Innervation

Although the heart's nodes and conduction system are able to generate action potentials independently, the autonomic nervous system influences both the rate of impulse generation (firing), depolarization, and repolarization of the myocardium; and the strength of atrial and ventricular contraction. Autonomic neural transmission produces changes in the heart and circulatory system faster than metabolic or humoral agents. Speed is important, for example, in stimulating the heart to increase its pumping action during times of stress and fear—the so-called fight or flight response—or with increased physical activity. Although increased delivery of oxygen, glucose, hormones, and other blood-borne factors sustains increased cardiac activity, the rapid initiation of increased activity depends on the sympathetic and parasympathetic fibers of the autonomic nervous system.

Sympathetic and parasympathetic nerves. Sympathetic and parasympathetic nerve fibers innervate all parts of the atria and ventricles and the SA and AV nodes. In general, sympathetic stimulation increases electrical conductivity and the strength of myocardial contraction, and vagal parasympathetic nerve activity does the opposite, slowing the conduction of action potentials through the heart and reducing the strength of contraction. Thus the sympathetic and parasympathetic nerves affect the speed of the cardiac cycle (**heart rate**, or beats per minute) and the sympathetic nerves also influence the diameter of the coronary vessels (Figure 23-11). Sympathetic nervous activity enhances myocardial performance. Stimulation of the SA node by the sympathetic nervous system rapidly increases heart rate. Furthermore, neurally released norepinephrine or circulating catecholamines interact with β-adrenergic receptors on the cardiac cell membranes. The overall effect is an increased influx of Ca^{++}, which increases the contractile strength of the heart and increases the speed of electrical impulses through the heart muscle and the nodes.[8] Finally, increased sympathetic discharge dilates the coronary vessels by causing the release of vasodilating metabolites resulting from increased myocardial contraction.[7]

The parasympathetic nervous system affects the heart through the vagus nerve, which releases acetylcholine. Acetylcholine causes decreased heart rate and slows conduction through the AV node.

FIGURE 23-11 Autonomic Innervation of Cardiovascular System. Inhibition (−); activation (+).

Myocardial Cells

Cardiomyocytes are composed of long, narrow fibers that contain bundles of longitudinally arranged myofibrils; a nucleus (cardiac muscle); mitochondria; an internal membrane system (the sarcoplasmic reticulum); cytoplasm (sarcoplasm); and a plasma membrane (the sarcolemma), which encloses the cell. Cardiac and skeletal muscle cells also have an "external" membrane system made up of transverse tubules (T tubules) formed by inward pouching of the sarcolemma. The sarcoplasmic reticulum forms a network of channels that surrounds the muscle fiber.

Because the myofibrils in both cardiac and skeletal fibers consist of alternating light and dark bands of protein, the fibers appear striped, or striated. The dark and light bands of the myofibrils create repeating longitudinal units, called *sarcomeres,* which are between 1.6 and 2.2 μm long (Figures 23-12 and 23-13). Length of these sarcomeres determines the limits of myocardial stretch at the end of diastole and subsequently the force of contraction during systole. Alterations in sarcomere size are seen in both physiologic and pathologic myocardial hypertrophy (see *Health Alert:* Regression of Myocardial Hypertrophy).

Differences between cardiac and skeletal muscle reflect heart function. Cardiac cells are arranged in branching networks throughout the myocardium, whereas skeletal muscle cells tend to be arranged in parallel units throughout the length of the muscle. Cardiac fibers have only one nucleus, whereas skeletal muscle cells have many nuclei. Other differences enable cardiac fibers to:

1. *Transmit action potentials quickly from cell to cell.* Electrical impulses are transmitted rapidly from cardiac fiber to cardiac fiber because the network of fibers connects at **intercalated disks**, which are thickened portions of the sarcolemma. The intercalated disks contain three junctions: desmosomes or macula adherens; fascia adherens, which mechanically attach one cell to another; and gap junctions, also known as tight junctions, which allow the electrical impulse to spread from cell to cell through a low-resistance pathway

Regression of Myocardial Hypertrophy

Hypertrophy, or enlargement, of the heart may occur through growth in either the length or the width of the sarcomeres in both normal and disease conditions. When normal stimuli, such as physical activity or pregnancy, cause hypertrophy, myocardial contractility is increased; and when the stimulus is removed, regression of the hypertrophy occurs. Conversely, disease-related hypertrophy caused by conditions such as hypertension or myocardial infarction results in reduced contractility and often heart failure. It has long been thought that this pathologic hypertrophy was not reversible but new research has shown that reversal may be possible.

When patients with hypertrophic heart failure awaiting a heart transplant were treated by the placement of a left ventricular assist device, regression of the ventricular hypertrophy was observed, occasionally to the point that heart transplant was not required. Research on the mechanisms involved in regression has shown that gene activation, several signaling pathways, angiogenesis, and autophagy are all involved. The hope is that identification of these mechanisms will lead to new and more effective pharmaceutical treatments for heart failure that currently is associated with a poor long-term prognosis.

From Hariharan N et al: *PLoS One* 8(1):e51632, 2013; Hou J, Kang YJ: *Pharmacol Ther* 135(3):337-354, 2012; Narula N et al: *Heart Fail Clin* 10(1 Suppl):S63-S74, 2014.

(see Chapter 1). Changes in the function of these junctional elements may cause an increased risk of arrhythmias.[8]

2. *Maintain high levels of energy synthesis.* Unlike skeletal muscle, the heart cannot rest and is in constant need of energy, which is supplied by molecules such as adenosine triphosphate (ATP). Therefore, the cytoplasm surrounding the bundles of myofibrils in each cardiomyocyte contains a large number of mitochondria (25% to 33% of cell volume). Cardiac muscle cells have more mitochondria than do skeletal muscle cells to provide the necessary respiratory enzymes for aerobic metabolism and supply quantities of ATP sufficient for the constant action of the myocardium.[9]

3. *Gain access to more ions, particularly sodium and potassium, in the extracellular environment.* Cardiac fibers contain more T tubules than do skeletal muscle fibers (see Figure 23-12). This increased closeness to the T tubules gives each myofibril in the myocardium faster access to molecules needed for the transmission of action potentials, a process that involves transport of sodium and potassium through the walls of the T tubules. Because the T tubule system is continuous with the extracellular space and the interstitial fluid, it facilitates the rapid transmission of the electrical impulses from the surface of the sarcolemma to the myofibrils inside the fiber. This rapid transmission activates all the myofibrils of one fiber simultaneously. The sarcoplasmic reticulum is located around the myofibrils. As an action potential is transmitted through the T tubules, it induces the sarcoplasmic reticulum to release its stored calcium, thus activating the contractile proteins actin and myosin.

Actin, myosin, and the troponin-tropomyosin complex. Within each myocardial sarcomere are myosin molecules that resemble golf clubs with two large, ovoid heads at one end of the shaft (Figure 23-14, *B*). The two heads contain an actin binding site and a site of ATPase activity. Thick filaments of **myosin** overlapping with thinner actin molecules form the central dark band of the sarcomere called the **anisotropic** or **A band** (see Figures 23-13 and 23-14). A thick filament has about 200 myosin molecules bundled together with their outward-facing heads named *cross-bridges* because they can form

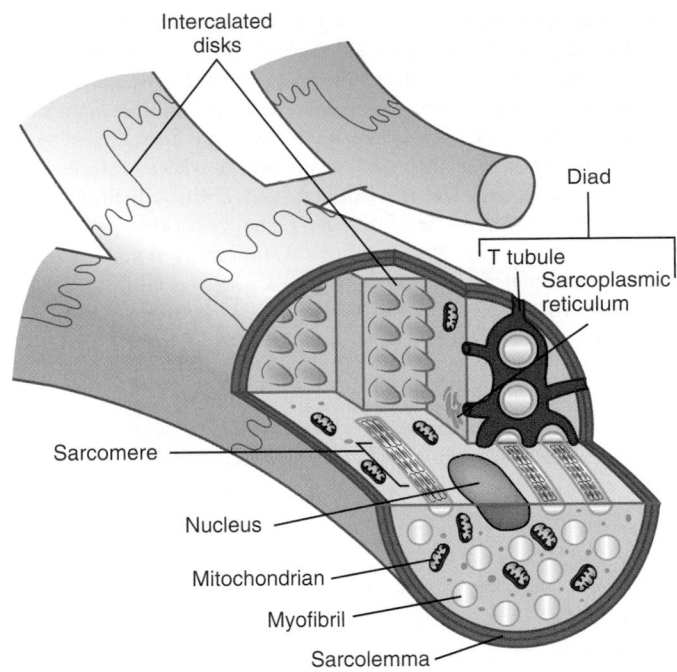

FIGURE 23-12 Cardiac Muscle Fiber. Unlike other types of muscle fibers, cardiac muscle fibers are typically branched with junctions, called *intercalated disks*, between adjacent myocytes. Like skeletal muscle cells, cardiac muscle cells contain sarcoplasmic reticula and T tubules, although these structures are not as highly organized as in skeletal muscle fibers.

FIGURE 23-13 Structure of a Sarcomere. The sarcomere is the basic contractile unit of a muscle cell. The Z disk is the anchor for the contractile elements actin and myosin. Actin attaches directly to the Z disk, whereas myosin is attached to it by elastic titin filaments. The myosin filaments are connected to each other by M-protein at the M line. The A, H, and I bands refer to parts of the sarcomere as they were originally seen by light microscopy.

force-generating bridges by binding with exposed actin molecules, resulting in contraction (Figure 23-14, *A*). **Actin** molecules are part of the thin filaments (see Figures 23-13 and 23-14). The light bands, called **isotropic** or **I bands**, of the sarcomere contain only actin molecules and no myosin (see Figure 23-13). Thin filaments of actin extend from each side of the **Z line**, a dense fibrous structure at the center of each I band. The area from one dark Z line to the next Z line

defines one sarcomere. The center of the sarcomere is the H zone, a less dense region with a central thin, dark **M line**.[9]

A single **tropomyosin** molecule (a relaxing protein) lies alongside seven actin molecules. Troponin, another relaxing protein, associates with the tropomyosin molecule, forming the **troponin-tropomyosin complex** (see Figures 23-14, *A*, and 23-15). The troponin complex itself has three components. **Troponin T** aids in the binding of the troponin complex to actin and tropomyosin; **troponin I** inhibits the ATPase of actomyosin; and **troponin C** contains binding sites for the calcium ions involved in contraction. Troponin T and I molecules are released into the bloodstream during myocardial injury and are measured to evaluate if a myocardial infarction or other damage has occurred. When troponin and tropomyosin cover the myosin binding sites on actin, the cross-bridges release calcium and the myocardium relaxes. The sarcomere also contains a giant elastic protein, **titin**, which attaches myosin to the Z line, acts as a spring, and influences myocardial stiffness.[9] Titin structure impacts myocardial diastolic filling and has been found to play a role in heart failure.[10]

Myocardial metabolism. Cardiomyocytes depend on the constant production of ATP, which is synthesized within the mitochondria mainly from glucose, fatty acids, and lactate. If the myocardium is underperfused because of coronary artery disease, anaerobic metabolism must be used for energy (see Chapter 1). Energy produced by metabolic processes fuels muscle contraction and relaxation, electrical excitation, membrane transport, and synthesis of large molecules. Normally, the amount of ATP produced supplies sufficient energy to pump blood throughout the system.

Cardiac work is expressed as **myocardial oxygen consumption** ($M\dot{V}O_2$), which is closely correlated with total cardiac energy requirements. $M\dot{V}O_2$ is determined by three major factors: (1) amount of wall stress during systole, estimated by measuring the systolic blood pressure; (2) duration of systolic wall tension, measured indirectly by the heart rate; and (3) contractile state of the myocardium, which is not measured clinically.

The coronary arteries deliver oxygen (O_2) to the myocardium. Approximately 70% to 75% of this oxygen is used immediately by cardiac muscle, leaving little O_2 in reserve. Since the O_2 content of the blood and the amount of O_2 extracted from the blood cannot be increased under normal circumstances, any increased energy needs can be met only by increasing coronary blood flow. $M\dot{V}O_2$ increases

F-actin strands   **Troponin**   **Active sites**   **Tropomyosin**

G-actin molecules

A

Myosin

B   **Myosin head**   **Shaft**

FIGURE 23-14 Structure of Myofilaments. **A,** Thin myofilament. **B,** Thick myofilament.

FIGURE 23-15 Cross-Bridge Theory of Muscle Contraction. A, Each myosin cross-bridge in the thick filament moves into a resting position after an adenosine triphosphate (ATP) molecule binds and transfers its energy. **B,** Calcium ions released from the sarcoplasmic reticulum bind to troponin in the thin filament, allowing tropomyosin to shift from its position blocking the active sites of actin molecules. **C,** Each myosin cross-bridge then binds to an active site on a thin filament, displacing the remnants of ATP hydrolysis— adenosine diphosphate (ADP) and inorganic phosphate (Pi). **D,** The release of stored energy from step A provides the force needed for each cross-bridge to move back to its original position, pulling actin along with it. Each cross-bridge will remain bound to actin until another ATP molecule binds to it and pulls it back into its resting position (**A**). (Adapted from Thibodeau GA, Patton KT: *Anatomy & physiology,* ed 4, St Louis, 1999, Mosby.)

with exercise and decreases with hypotension and hypothermia. As myocardial metabolism and consumption of O_2 increase, the local concentration of local vasoactive metabolic factors increases. Some of these, such as adenosine, nitric oxide, and prostaglandins, dilate coronary arterioles, thus increasing coronary blood flow.[11]

Myocardial Contraction and Relaxation

Myocardial contractility is a change in developed tension at a given resting fiber length, which basically is the ability of the heart muscle to shorten. At the molecular level, thin filaments of actin slide over thick filaments of myosin, called the cross-bridge theory of muscle contraction. Anatomically, contraction occurs when the sarcomere shortens, so adjacent Z lines move closer together (see Figure 23-13). The degree of shortening depends on the amount of overlap between the thick and thin filaments.

Calcium and excitation-contraction coupling. Excitation-contraction coupling is the process by which an action potential arriving at the muscle fiber plasma membrane triggers the cycle, leading to cross-bridge formation and contraction. Cycle activation depends on calcium availability, and the amount of force developed is regulated by how much the concentration of calcium ions increases within the cardiomyocytes. Calcium enters the myocardial cell from the interstitial fluid after electrical excitation that increases membrane calcium permeability. Two types of calcium channels (L-type, T-type) are found in cardiac tissues.[9] The L-type, or long-lasting, channels predominate and are the channels blocked by calcium channel–blocking drugs (verapamil, nifedipine, diltiazem).[9] The T-type, or transient, channels are much less abundant in the heart. T-type channels are not blocked by currently available calcium channel–blocking drugs; therefore T-type channel blockers are being investigated.[17] Calcium entering the cell triggers the release of additional calcium from the two storage sites within the sarcomere—the sarcoplasmic reticulum and tubule system. Calcium ions then diffuse toward the myofibrils, where they bind with troponin.

The calcium-troponin complex interaction facilitates the contraction process. In the resting state, troponin I is bound to actin and the tropomyosin molecule covers the sites where the myosin heads bind to actin, thereby preventing interaction between actin and myosin. Calcium binds to troponin C, which ultimately results in tropomyosin moving troponin I, thus uncovering the binding sites on the myosin heads. Myosin and actin can now form cross-bridges, and ATP can be dephosphorylated to adenosine diphosphate (ADP). Under these circumstances, sliding of the thick and thin filaments can occur, and the muscle contracts.[9]

Myocardial relaxation. Relaxation is as vital to optimal cardiac function as contraction; and calcium, troponin, and tropomyosin also facilitate relaxation. After contraction, free calcium ions are actively pumped out of the cell back into the interstitial fluid or taken back into storage by the sarcoplasmic reticulum and tubule system. As the concentration of calcium within the sarcomere decreases, troponin releases its bound calcium. The tropomyosin complex moves and blocks the active sites on the actin molecule, preventing cross-bridge formation with the myosin heads. If the ability of the myocardium to relax is impaired, it can lead to increased diastolic filling pressures and eventually heart failure.[13]

✔ QUICK CHECK 23-4
1. What features distinguish myocardial cells from skeletal cells?
2. Describe the interactions of actin, myosin, and the troponin-tropomyosin complex in controlling heart function.
3. Define excitation-contraction coupling.

Factors Affecting Cardiac Output

Cardiac performance can be evaluated by measuring the cardiac output. Cardiac output is calculated by multiplying heart rate in beats per minute (beats/min) by stroke volume in liters per beat. Normal adult cardiac output is about 5 L/minute at rest given a heart rate of about 70 beats/min and a normal stroke volume of about 70 ml.[7]

With each heartbeat, the ventricles eject much of their blood volume, and the amount ejected per beat is called the ejection fraction. The ejection fraction is estimated by echocardiography, computed tomography (CT) scan, nuclear medicine scan, or cardiac catheterization and is calculated by dividing stroke volume by end-diastolic volume. The end-diastolic volume of the normal ventricle is about 70 to 80 ml/m², and the normal ejection fraction of the resting heart measured with gated myocardial perfusion imaging was 66% ± 8% for women and 58% ± 8% for men.[14]

The ejection fraction is increased by factors that increase contractility, such as increased sympathetic nervous system activity. A decrease in ejection fraction may indicate ventricular failure. The effects of aging on cardiovascular function are summarized in Table 23-3.

The factors that determine cardiac output are (1) preload, (2) afterload, (3) myocardial contractility, and (4) heart rate. Preload, afterload, and contractility all affect stroke volume.

Preload

Preload is the volume and pressure inside the ventricle at the end of diastole (ventricular end-diastolic volume [VEDV] and pressure [VEDP]). Preload is determined by two primary factors: (1) the amount of venous blood returning to the ventricle during diastole and (2) the amount of blood left in the ventricle after systole (end-systolic volume). Venous return is dependent on blood volume and flow through the venous system and the atrioventricular valves. End-systolic volume is dependent on the strength of ventricular contraction and the resistance to ventricular emptying. Clinically, preload is estimated by measuring the central venous pressure (CVP) for the right side of

TABLE 23-3 **Cardiovascular Function in Elderly Persons**		
Determinant	**Resting Cardiac Performance**	**Exercise Cardiac Performance***
Cardiac output	Unchanged	Decreases because of a decrease in maximum heart rate
Heart rate	Slight decrease	Increases less than in younger people
Stroke volume	Slight increase	No change
Ejection fraction	Unchanged	Decreased
Afterload	Increased	Increased
End-diastolic volume	Unchanged	Increased
End-systolic volume	Unchanged	Increased
Contraction	Decreased velocity	Decreased
Myocardial wall stiffness	Increased	Increased
Maximum oxygen consumption	Not applicable	Decreased
Plasma catecholamines	—	Increased

Data from Lakatta EG et al: Aging and cardiovascular disease in the elderly. In Fuster V et al, editors: *Hurst's the heart*, ed 13, Philadelphia, 2011, McGraw-Hill.
*Changes in healthy men and women up to age 80 years as compared to those 20 years of age.

the heart and the pulmonary artery wedge pressure for the left side. Normal values for these two estimates are 1 to 5 mm Hg and 4 to 12 mm Hg, respectively.[15]

Laplace law states that wall tension generated in the wall of the ventricle (or any chamber or vessel) to produce a given intraventricular pressure depends directly on ventricular size or internal radius and inversely on ventricular wall thickness. Ventricular end-diastolic volume, which determines the size of the ventricle and the stretch of the cardiac muscle fibers, therefore affects the tension (or force) for contraction. The Frank-Starling law of the heart indicates that the volume of blood in the heart at the end of diastole, as the volume determines the length of its muscle fibers, is directly related to the force of contraction during the next systole. Muscle fibers have an optimal resting length from which to generate the maximum amount of contractile strength. Within a physiologic range of muscle stretching, increased preload increases stroke volume (and therefore cardiac output and stroke work) (Figure 23-16, curve B). Excessive ventricular filling and preload (increased VEDV) stretches the heart muscle beyond optimal length and stroke volume begins to fall. Factors that

FIGURE 23-16 Frank-Starling Law of the Heart. Relationship between length and tension in heart. End-diastolic volume determines end-diastolic length of ventricular muscle fibers and is proportional to tension generated during systole, as well as to cardiac output, stroke volume, and stroke work. A change in myocardial contractility causes the heart to perform on a different length-tension curve. *A,* Increased contractility; *B,* normal contractility; *C,* heart failure or decreased contractility. (See text for further explanation.)

increase contractility cause the heart to operate on a higher length-tension curve (Figure 23-16, curve *A*). Factors that decrease contractility (Figure 23-16, curve *C*) cause the heart to operate at a lower length-tension curve. Figure 23-17 illustrates the relationship between VEDV and stroke volume, cardiac output, and stroke work.

Increases in preload (VEDV) may not only cause a decline in stroke volume but also result in increases in VEDP. These changes can lead to heart failure (see Chapter 24). Increased VEDP causes pressures to increase or "back up" into the pulmonary or systemic venous circulation, thus increasing the movement of plasma out through vessel walls, causing fluid to accumulate in lung tissues (pulmonary edema; see Chapter 27) or in peripheral tissues (peripheral edema).

Afterload

Left ventricular afterload is the resistance to ejection of blood from the left ventricle. It is the load the muscle must move during contraction. Aortic systolic pressure is an index of afterload. Pressure in the ventricle must exceed aortic pressure before blood can be pumped out during systole. Low aortic pressures (decreased afterload) enable the heart to contract more rapidly and efficiently, whereas high aortic pressures (increased afterload) slow contraction and cause higher workloads against which the heart must function to eject blood. Increased aortic pressure is usually the result of increased systemic vascular resistance (SVR), sometimes referred to as total peripheral resistance (TPR). In individuals with hypertension, increased TPR means that afterload is chronically elevated, resulting in increased ventricular workload and hypertrophy of the myocardium. In some individuals, changes in afterload are the result of aortic valvular disease (see Figure 23-17). SVR is calculated by dividing mean arterial pressure by cardiac output; the normal range is 700 dyne/sec/cm^{-5}.[7,15]

Myocardial Contractility

Stroke volume, or the volume of blood ejected per beat during systole, also depends on the *force* of contraction, myocardial contractility, or the degree of myocardial fiber shortening. Three major factors determine the force of contraction (see Figure 23-17):

1. *Changes in the stretching of the ventricular myocardium caused by changes in VEDV (preload).* As discussed previously, increased

FIGURE 23-17 Factors Affecting Cardiac Performance. Cardiac output, the amount of blood (in liters) ejected by the heart per minute, depends on heart rate (beats per minute) and stroke volume (milliliters of blood ejected during ventricular systole).

venous return to the heart distends the ventricle, thus increasing preload, which increases the stroke volume and, subsequently, cardiac output, up to a certain point. However, an excessive increase in preload leads to decreased stroke volume.

2. *Alterations in the inotropic stimuli of the ventricles.* Hormones, neurotransmitters, or medications that affect contractility are called **inotropic agents**. The most important endogenous positive inotropic agents are epinephrine and norepinephrine released from the sympathetic nervous system. Other positive inotropes include thyroid hormone and dopamine. The most important negative inotropic agent is acetylcholine released from the vagus nerve. Many medications have positive or negative inotropic properties that can have profound effects on cardiac function. In sepsis, a variety of cytokines including tumor necrosis factor-alpha (TNF-α), and interleukin-1β have been shown to impair myocardial contractility.[16]

3. *Adequacy of myocardial oxygen supply.* Oxygen and carbon dioxide levels (tensions) in the coronary blood also influence contractility. With severe hypoxemia (arterial oxygen saturation less than 50%), contractility is decreased. With less severe hypoxemia (saturation more than 50%), contractility is stimulated. Moderate degrees of hypoxemia may increase contractility by enhancing the myocardial response to circulating catecholamines.[17]

Preload, afterload, and contractility all interact with one another to determine stroke volume and cardiac output. Changes in any one of these factors can result in deleterious effects on the others, resulting in heart failure (see Chapter 24).

Heart Rate

As described previously, SA node activity is the primary determinant of the heart rate. The average heart rate in healthy adults is about 70 beats/min. This rate diminishes by 10 to 20 beats/min during sleep and can accelerate to more than 100 beats/min during muscular activity or emotional excitement. In well-conditioned athletes, resting heart rate is normally about 50 to 60 beats/min. In highly trained or elite athletes, the resting heart rate can be below 50 beats/min; these athletes also have a greater stroke volume and lower peripheral resistance in active muscles than they had before training. The control of heart rate includes activity of the central nervous system, autonomic nervous system, neural reflexes, atrial receptors, and hormones (see Figure 23-17).

Cardiovascular control centers in the brain. The **cardiovascular vasomotor control center** is in the medulla and pons areas of the brainstem with additional areas in the hypothalamus, cerebral cortex, and thalamus.[18] The hypothalamic centers regulate cardiovascular responses to changes in temperature, the cerebral cortex centers adjust cardiac reaction to a variety of emotional states, and the brainstem control center regulates heart rate and blood pressure (see Figure 23-11).

The nerve fibers from the cardiovascular control center synapse with autonomic neurons that influence the rate of firing of the SA node. As previously discussed, increased heart rate occurs with sympathetic (adrenergic) stimulation. When the parasympathetic nerves to the heart are stimulated (primarily via the vagus nerve), heart rate slows and the sympathetic nerves to the heart, arterioles, and veins are inhibited.[8] At rest, the heart rate in healthy individuals is primarily under the control of parasympathetic stimulation. Administration of drugs that block parasympathetic function (anticholinergic) or physical interruption of the vagus nerve causes significant tachycardia (abnormally fast heart rate) because this inhibitory parasympathetic influence is lost.

Neural reflexes. Output from the **baroreceptor reflexes** influences short-term regulation of the vascular smooth muscle of resistance arteries, myocardial contractility, and heart rate, all components of blood pressure control. The baroreceptors or pressoreceptors are located in the aortic arch and carotid arteries. If blood pressure decreases, the baroreceptor reflex accelerates heart rate, increases myocardial contractility, and increases vascular smooth muscle contraction in the arterioles, thus raising blood pressure. This reflex is critical to maintaining adequate tissue perfusion. When blood pressure increases, the baroreceptors increase their rate of discharge, sending neural impulses over a branch of the glossopharyngeal nerve (ninth cranial nerve) and through the vagus nerve to the cardiovascular control centers in the medulla. These reflexes increase parasympathetic activity and decrease sympathetic activity, causing the resistance arteries to dilate, decreasing myocardial contractility and heart rate. The role of baroreceptors in influencing blood pressure is discussed in more detail later in this chapter.

Atrial receptors. Mechanoreceptors that influence heart rate exist in both atria.[18] They are located where the veins, venae cavae, and pulmonary veins enter their respective atria. **Bainbridge reflex** is the name for the changes in the heart rate that may occur after intravenous infusions of blood or other fluid. The change in heart rate is thought to be caused by a reflex mediated by these atrial volume receptors that are innervated by the vagus nerve (volume receptors are thought to respond to increased plasma volume). Although this reflex can be elicited in humans, its relevance is uncertain at this time.[19]

Stimulation of these atrial receptors also increases urine volume, presumably because of a neurally mediated reduction in antidiuretic hormone. In addition, peptides of the atrial natriuretic family are released from atrial tissue in response to the increases in blood volume. These peptides have diuretic and natriuretic (salt excretion) properties, resulting in decreased blood volume and pressure. The atrial natriuretic peptides also have been shown to relax vascular smooth muscle and oppose myocardial hypertrophy, leading to measurement of blood levels to evaluate clinical status and raising interest in their use as therapeutic agents.[20]

Hormones and biochemicals. Hormones and other biochemically active substances affect the arteries, arterioles, venules, capillaries, and contractility of the myocardium. Norepinephrine, mainly released as a neurotransmitter from the adrenal medulla, dilates vessels of the liver and skeletal muscle and also causes an increase in myocardial contractility. Some adrenocortical hormones, such as hydrocortisone, potentiate the effects of the catecholamines—norepinephrine and epinephrine.

Thyroid hormones enhance sympathetic activity and increase cardiac output. Growth hormone, working together with insulin-like growth factor-1 (IGF-1), also has been shown to increase myocardial contractility.[21] Decreases in levels of growth hormone or thyroid hormone may result in bradycardia (heart rate below 60 beats/min), reduced cardiac output, and low blood pressure. (Other hormones are discussed in the Regulation of Blood Pressure section.)

> ✔ **QUICK CHECK 23-5**
> 1. Why is the Frank-Starling law of the heart important to the understanding of heart failure?
> 2. Discuss the baroreceptor reflex and explain its influence on blood pressure and heart rate.
> 3. Explain four ways that aging impacts the cardiovascular system.

THE SYSTEMIC CIRCULATION

The arteries and veins of the systemic circulation are illustrated in Figure 23-18. Oxygenated blood leaves the left side of the heart through the aorta and flows into the systemic arteries. These arteries branch into small arterioles, which branch into the smallest vessels, the capillaries, where nutrient and waste product exchange between the blood and tissues occurs. Blood from the capillaries then enters tiny venules that join to form the larger veins, which return venous blood to the right heart. Peripheral vascular system is the term used to describe the part of the systemic circulation that supplies the skin and the extremities, particularly the legs and feet.

Structure of Blood Vessels

Blood vessel walls are composed of three layers: (1) the tunica intima (innermost, or intimal, layer), (2) the tunica media (middle, or medial, layer), and (3) the tunica externa or adventitia (outermost, or

external, layer), which also contains nerves and lymphatic vessels. These layers are illustrated in Figure 23-19. Blood vessel walls vary in thickness depending on the thickness or absence of one or more of these three layers. Cells of the larger vessel walls are nourished by the vasa vasorum, small vessels located in the tunica externa.

Arterial Vessels

An artery is a thick-walled pulsating blood vessel transporting blood away from the heart. In the systemic circulation, arteries carry oxygenated blood. Arterial walls are composed of elastic connective tissue, fibrous connective tissue, and smooth muscle. Elastic arteries, such as the aorta, the branches of the aorta, and the trunk of the pulmonary artery, have a thick tunica media with more elastic fibers than smooth

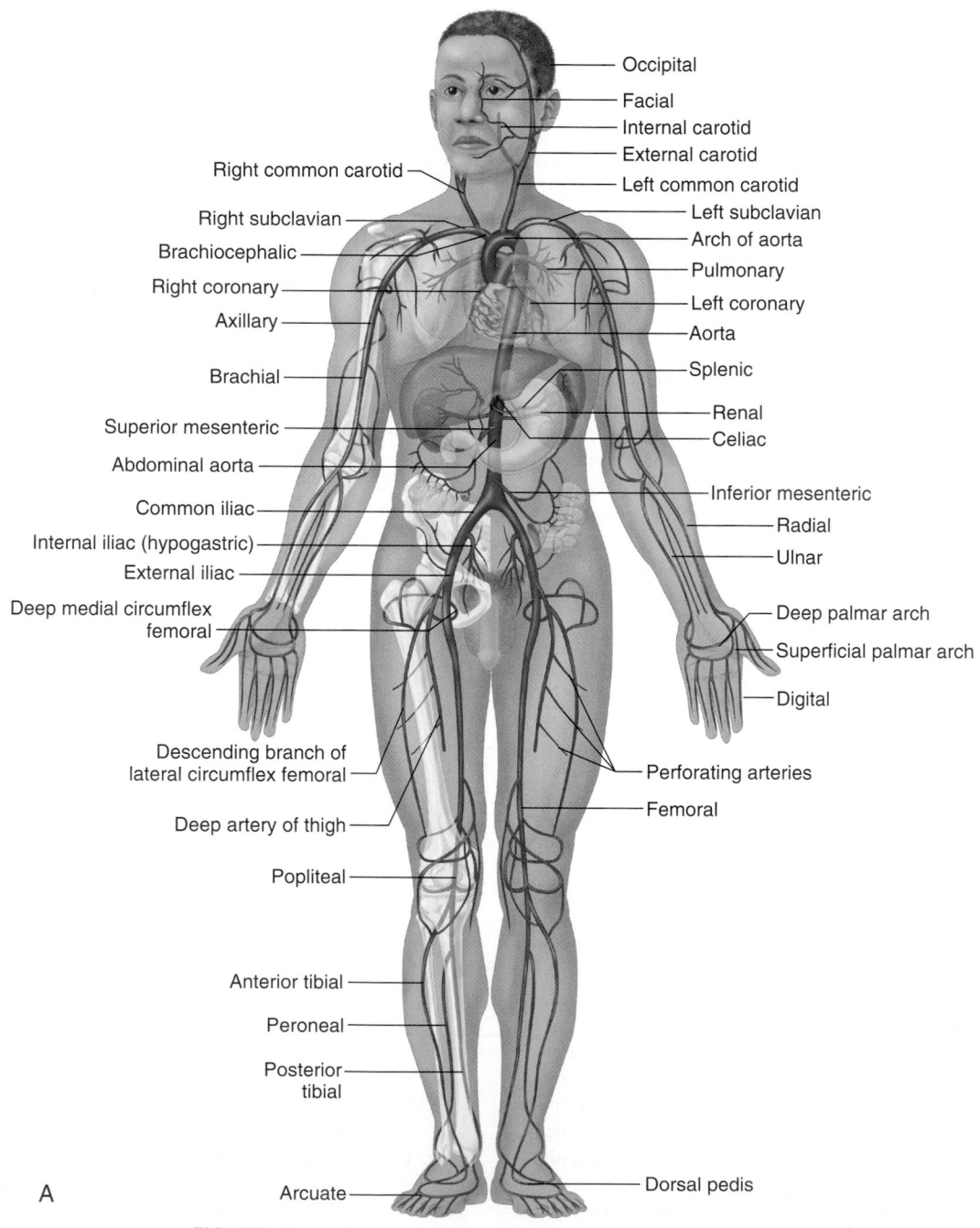

FIGURE 23-18 Circulatory System. **A,** Principal arteries of body.

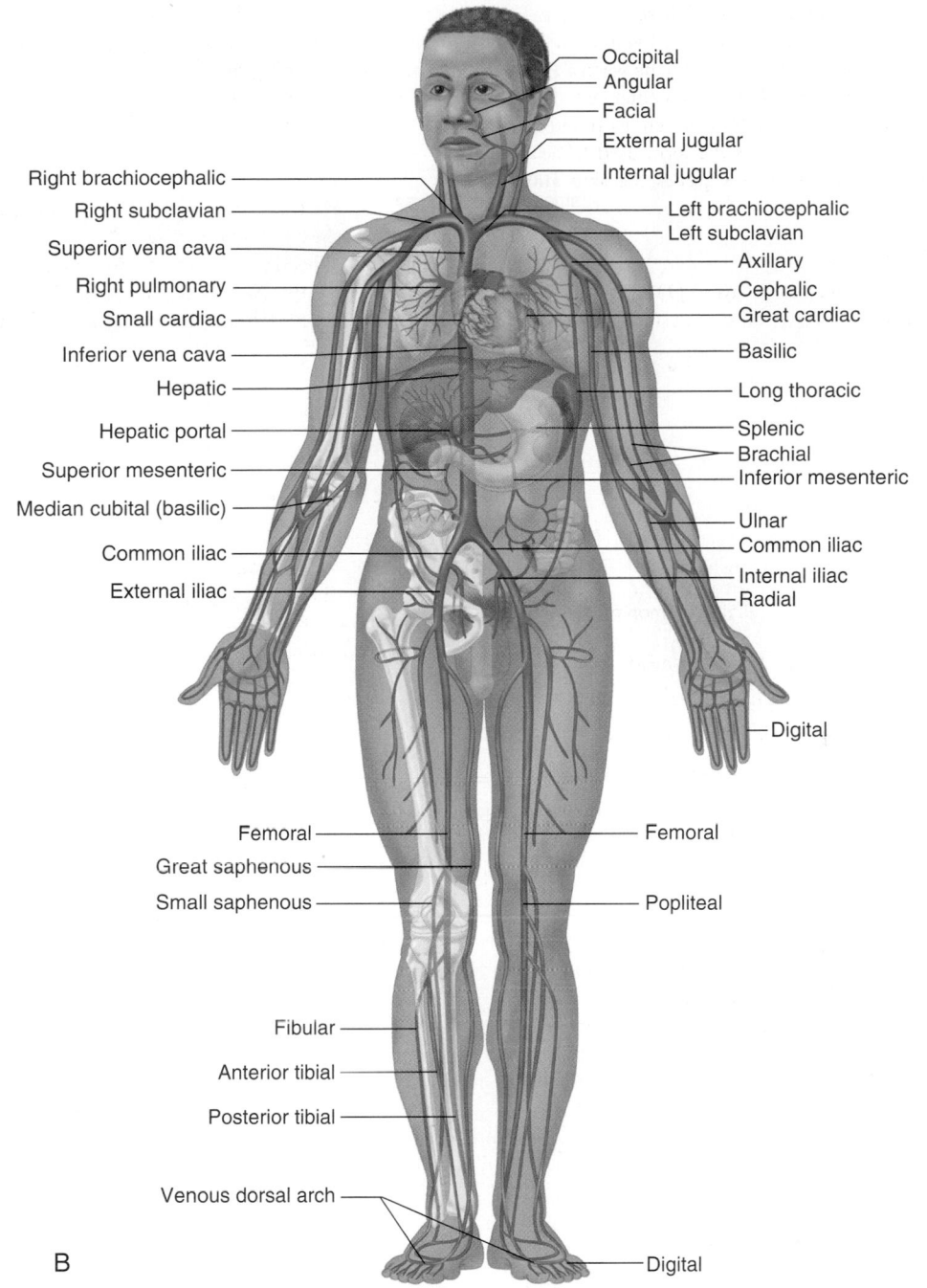

Occipital
Angular
Facial
External jugular
Internal jugular
Right brachiocephalic
Right subclavian
Superior vena cava
Right pulmonary
Small cardiac
Inferior vena cava
Hepatic
Hepatic portal
Superior mesenteric
Median cubital (basilic)
Common iliac
External iliac
Left brachiocephalic
Left subclavian
Axillary
Cephalic
Great cardiac
Basilic
Long thoracic
Splenic
Brachial
Inferior mesenteric
Ulnar
Common iliac
Internal iliac
Radial
Digital
Femoral
Great saphenous
Small saphenous
Femoral
Popliteal
Fibular
Anterior tibial
Posterior tibial
Venous dorsal arch
Digital

B

FIGURE 23-18, cont'd B, Principal veins of body. (From Patton KT, Thibodeau GA, Douglas MM: *Essentials of anatomy & physiology,* St Louis, 2012, Elsevier.)

muscle fibers. Elasticity allows the vessel to absorb energy and stretch as blood is ejected from the heart during systole. During diastole, elasticity promotes recoil of the arteries, maintaining blood pressure within the vessels.

Muscular arteries, medium and small size arteries, are farther from the heart than the elastic arteries. They contain more muscle fibers and fewer elastic fibers than the elastic arteries and they function to distribute blood to arterioles throughout the body. Because their smooth muscle can contract or relax, they play a role in blood flow control and in directing flow to body parts with the highest need at any point in time. Contraction narrows the vessel **lumen** (the internal cavity of the vessel), which diminishes flow through the vessel (**vasoconstriction**).

When the smooth muscle layer relaxes, more blood flows through the vessel lumen (**vasodilation**).

An artery becomes an arteriole where the diameter of its lumen narrows to less than 0.5 mm. **Arterioles** are mainly composed of smooth muscle and regulate the flow of blood into the capillaries by constricting or dilating to either slow or increase the flow of blood into the capillaries (Figure 23-20). The thick smooth muscle layer of the arterioles is a major determinant of the resistance blood encounters as it flows through the systemic circulation.

The capillary network is composed of connective channels called **metarterioles,** and "true" capillaries (see Figure 23-20). Metarterioles have discontinuous smooth muscle cells in their tunica media whereas

FIGURE 23-19 Structure of the Blood Vessels. The tunica externa of the veins is color-coded blue and the arteries red. (From Patton KT, Thibodeau GA: *Structure & function of the body,* ed 15, St Louis, 2016, Elsevier.)

FIGURE 23-20 Microcirculation. Control of local blood flow through a capillary network is regulated by altering the tone of precapillary sphincters surrounding arterioles and metarterioles. In the diagram, the sphincters are relaxed, permitting blood flow to enter the capillary bed. (From Patton KT, Thibodeau GA, Douglas MM: *Essentials of anatomy & physiology,* St Louis, 2012, Elsevier.)

capillaries have no smooth muscle cells. There is a ring of smooth muscle called the precapillary sphincter at the point where capillaries branch from metarterioles. As the sphincters contract and relax, they regulate blood flow through the capillary beds. The precapillary sphincters help to maintain arterial pressure and regulate selective flow to vascular beds.

Capillaries are composed solely of a layer of endothelial cells surrounded by a basement membrane. Their thin walls and unique structure make possible the rapid exchange of water; small (low molecular weight) soluble molecules; some larger molecules, such as albumin; and cells of the innate and adaptive components of the immune system between the blood and the interstitial fluid. In some capillaries, the endothelial cells contain oval windows or pores termed fenestrations covered by a thin diaphragm.

Substances pass between the capillary lumen and the interstitial fluid (1) through junctions between endothelial cells, (2) through fenestrations in endothelial cells, (3) in vesicles moved by active transport across the endothelial cell membrane, or (4) by diffusion through the endothelial cell membrane. A single capillary may be only 0.5 to 1 mm in length and 0.01 mm in diameter, but the capillaries are so numerous their total surface area may be more than 600 m^2 (about 100 football fields).

Endothelium

The vascular endothelium is important to several body functions and is sometimes considered a separate endocrine organ. All tissues depend on a blood supply and the blood supply depends on endothelial cells, which form the lining, or endothelium, of the blood vessel (Figure 23-21). In addition to substance transport, the vascular endothelium has important roles in coagulation, antithrombogenesis, and

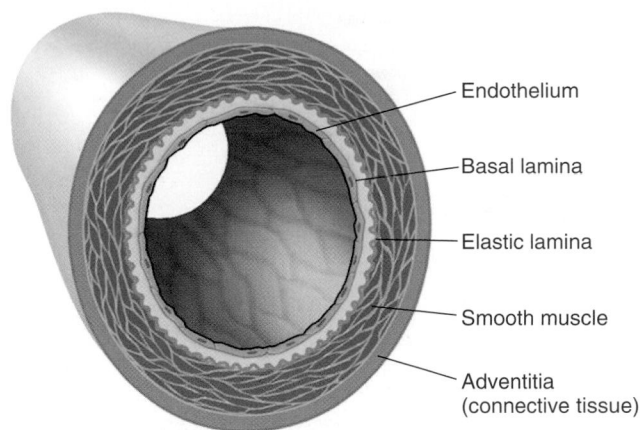

FIGURE 23-21 Vascular Endothelium. The endothelial cells arrange themselves as a single-layer lining that has numerous critical functions (see Table 23-4).

TABLE 23-4	**Functions of the Endothelium**
Function	**Actions Involved**
Filtration and permeability	Facilitates transport of large molecules via vesicular transport movement through intercellular junctions
	Facilitates transport of small molecules via movement of vesicles, through opening of tight junctions, and across cytoplasm
Vasomotion	Stimulates vascular relaxation through production of nitric oxide, prostacyclin, and other vasodilators
	Stimulates vascular constriction through production of endothelin-1 and of angiotensin II by the action of endothelial angiotensin-converting enzyme on angiotensin I
Hemostatic balance	Endothelial surface is normally antithrombotic and maintains a balance between pro- and anticoagulant factors, as well as pro- and antifibrinolytic factors
	Anticoagulant factors include prostacyclin, nitric oxide, antithrombin, thrombomodulin, tissue factor pathway inhibitor, and heparins
	Procoagulant factors include tissue factor (factor VII), factor VIII, factor V, and plasminogen activator inhibitor-1 (PAI-1)
	Profibrinolytic factors are tissue- and urokinase-type plasminogen activating factor and plasminogen activator inhibitor-1 (PAI-1)
	Antifibrinolytic factor is tissue plasminogen activator
Inflammation/ immunity	Expresses chemotactic agents and adhesion molecules that support white blood cells (including monocytes, neutrophils, and lymphocytes) moving into tissues
	Expresses receptors for oxidized lipoproteins, allowing them to enter vascular intima
Angiogenesis/ vessel growth	Releases growth factors such as endothelin-1 and heparins for vascular smooth muscle cells
Lipid metabolism	Expresses receptors for lipoprotein lipase and low-density lipoproteins (LDLs)

From Griendling KK et al: Biology of the vessel wall. In Fuster et al, editors: *Hurst's the heart,* ed 13, Philadelphia, 2011, McGraw-Hill; Rajendran P et al: *Int J Biol Sci* 9(10):1057-1069, 2013.

fibrinolysis; immune system function; tissue and vessel growth and wound healing; and vasomotion, the contraction and relaxation of vessels.[22] Table 23-4 summarizes some of the more important endothelial functions. Endothelial injury and dysfunction are central processes in many of the most common and serious cardiovascular disorders, including hypertension and atherosclerosis (see Chapter 24).

Veins

Compared with arteries, **veins** are thin walled with more fibrous connective tissue and have a larger diameter (see Figure 23-19). Veins also are more numerous than arteries. The smallest venules downstream from the capillaries have an endothelial lining and are surrounded by connective tissue. The largest venules have some smooth muscle fibers in their thin tunica media. The venous tunica externa has less elastic tissue than that in arteries, so veins do not recoil as much or as rapidly after distention. Like arteries, veins receive nourishment from tiny vasa vasorum.

Veins contain valves to facilitate the one-way flow of blood toward the heart (Figure 23-22). These valves are folds of the tunica intima and resemble the semilunar valves of the heart. When a person stands up, contraction of the skeletal muscles of the legs compresses the deep veins of the legs and assists the flow of blood toward the heart. This important mechanism of venous return is called the **muscle pump** (Figure 23-22, *B*).

Factors Affecting Blood Flow

Blood flow, the amount of fluid moved per unit of time, is usually expressed as liters or milliliters per minute (L/min or ml/min). Factors the influence blood flow include pressure, resistance, velocity, turbulent versus laminar flow, and compliance, with the most important of these being pressure and resistance.

Pressure and Resistance

Pressure in a liquid system is the force exerted on the liquid per unit area and is expressed clinically as millimeters of mercury (mm Hg), or torr (1 torr = 1 mm Hg). Blood flow to an organ depends partly on the pressure difference between the arterial and venous vessels supplying that organ. Fluid moves from the arterial "side" of the capillaries where the pressure is higher to the venous side where the pressure is lower.

Resistance is the opposition to blood flow. Most opposition to blood flow results from the diameter and length of the vessels. Changes in blood flow through an organ result from changes in the vascular resistance within the organ because of increases or decreases in vessel diameter and the opening or closing of vascular channels. Resistance in a vessel is inversely related to blood flow—that is, increased resistance leads to decreased blood flow. **Poiseuille law** indicates that resistance is directly related to tube length and blood viscosity and inversely related to the radius of the tube to the fourth power (r^4). Because blood flow is inversely related to resistance, the greater the resistance the lower the blood flow will be. Resistance to flow cannot be measured directly, but it can be calculated if the pressure difference and flow volumes are known. Resistance to blood flow in a single vessel is determined by the radius and length of the blood vessel and by the blood viscosity.

Clinically, the most important factor determining resistance *in a single vessel* is the **radius** or **diameter** of the vessel's lumen. Small changes in the lumen's radius or diameter lead to large changes in vascular resistance. Clinically, vasoconstriction will contribute to an increase in resistance whereas vasodilation will cause a decrease in resistance that may be reflected by a fall in blood pressure. Because

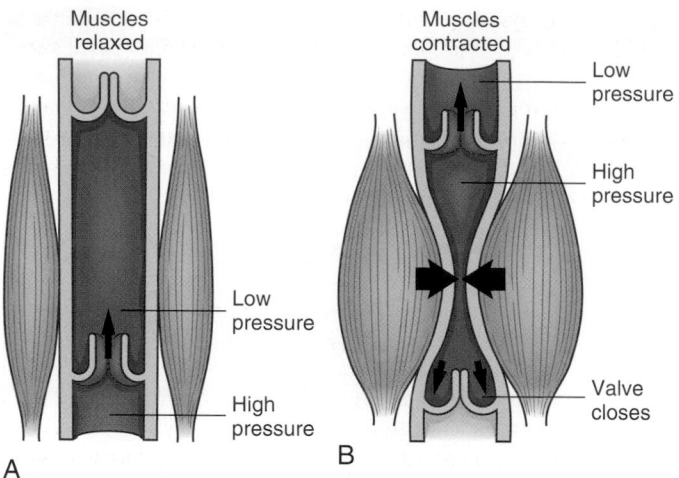

A   B

FIGURE 23-22 Venous Valves and the Muscle Pump. In veins, one-way valves aid circulation by preventing backflow of venous blood when pressure in a local area is low. **A,** Blood is moved toward the heart as valves in the veins are forced open by pressure from volume of blood downstream and the neighboring muscles are relaxed. **B,** When pressure below the valve drops, blood begins to flow backward but fills the "pockets" formed by the valve flaps, pushing the flaps together and thus blocking further backward flow. Contraction in the adjacent muscles and the valves of the systemic veins assist in the return of unoxygenated blood to the right heart.

A

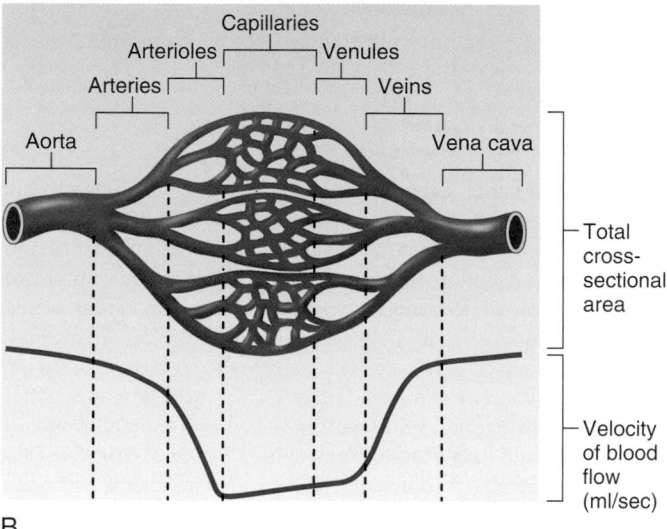

B

FIGURE 23-23 Relationship between Cross-Sectional Area and Velocity of Blood Flow. Blood flows with great speed in the large arteries. However, branching of arterial vessels increases the total cross-sectional area of the arterioles and capillaries, reducing the flow rate. When capillaries merge into venules and venules merge into veins, the total cross-sectional area decreases, causing the flow rate to increase. (From Patton KT, Thibodeau GA: *Anatomy & physiology,* ed 9, St Louis, 2016, Elsevier.)

vessel length is relatively constant whereas lumen size is quite variable, length is not as important as lumen size in determining flow through a single vessel. Because viscosity is relatively constant, blood vessel radius is usually the key factor in determining total peripheral resistance. An exception to this rule is when red blood cell volume, measured as hematocrit, is elevated, which is relatively rare. Conditions with elevated hematocrits include a lack of body water, cyanotic congenital heart disease (see Chapter 25), or polycythemia (see Chapter 21), and can lead to increased cardiac work as a result of increased vascular resistance.

Resistance to flow through a *system of vessels,* or **total resistance,** depends not only on characteristics of individual vessels but also on whether the vessels are arranged in series or in parallel and on the total cross-sectional area of the system. Vessels arranged in parallel provide less resistance than vessels arranged in series. Blood flowing through the distributing arteries, beginning with branches off the aorta and ending at arterioles in the capillary bed, encounters more resistance than blood flowing through the capillary bed itself, where flow is distributed among many short, tiny branches arranged in parallel (see Figure 23-23). The total cross-sectional area of the arteriolar system is greater than that of the arterial system, yet the greater number of arterioles arranged in series leads to great resistance to flow in the arteriolar system. In contrast, the capillary system has a larger number of vessels arranged in parallel than the arteriolar system, and the total cross-sectional area is much greater; thus there is lower resistance overall through the capillary system. The resulting slow velocity of flow in each capillary is optimal for capillary-tissue exchange.

Velocity

Blood velocity or **speed** is the *distance* blood travels in a unit of time, usually centimeters per second (cm/sec). It is directly related to blood flow (*amount* of blood moved per unit of time) and inversely related to the cross-sectional area of the vessel in which the blood is flowing (Figure 23-23). As blood moves from the aorta to the capillaries, the

total cross-sectional area of the vessels increases and the velocity decreases.

Laminar Versus Turbulent Flow

Flow through a tubular system can be either laminar or turbulent. Blood flow through the vessels, except where vessels split or branch, is usually laminar. In **laminar flow,** concentric layers of molecules move "straight ahead" with each layer flowing at a slightly different velocity (Figure 23-24). The cohesive attraction between the fluid and the vessel wall prevents the molecules of blood that are in contact with the wall from moving at all. The next thin layer of blood is able to slide slowly past the stationary layer and so on until, at the center, the blood velocity is greatest. Large vessels have room for a large center layer; therefore they have less resistance to flow and greater flow and velocity than smaller vessels.

Where flow is obstructed, the vessel turns, or blood flows over rough surfaces, the flow becomes **turbulent** with whorls or eddy currents that produce noise, causing a murmur to be heard on auscultation. Resistance increases with turbulence, which frequently occurs in areas with atherosclerotic plaque (see Chapter 24).

Parabolic-shaped velocity profile

A

B

FIGURE 23-24 Laminar and Turbulent Blood Flow. A, Laminar flow. Fluid flows in long, smooth-walled tubes as if it is composed of a large number of concentric layers. **B,** Turbulent flow. Turbulent flow is caused by numerous small currents flowing crosswise or oblique to the long axis of the vessel, resulting in flowing whorls and eddy currents.

Vascular Compliance

Vascular compliance is the increase in volume a vessel can accommodate for a given increase in pressure. Compliance depends on factors related to the nature of a vessel wall, such as the ratio of elastic fibers to muscle fibers in the wall. Elastic arteries are more compliant than muscular arteries. The veins are more compliant than either type of artery, and they can serve as storage areas for the circulatory system.

Compliance determines a vessel's response to pressure changes. For example, a large volume of blood can be accommodated by the venous system with only a small increase in pressure. In the less compliant arterial system, where smaller volumes and higher pressures are normal, even small changes in blood volume can cause significant changes in arterial pressure.

Stiffness is the opposite of compliance. Several conditions and disorders can cause stiffness, with the most common being aging and atherosclerosis (see Chapter 24).

✔ **QUICK CHECK 23-6**
1. What is the function of the arterioles?
2. Identify the functions of the endothelium.
3. Why does the total cross-sectional area in the capillary system lower the resistance to flow?

Regulation of Blood Pressure
Arterial Pressure

Arterial blood pressure is determined by the cardiac output multiplied by the peripheral resistance (Figure 23-25). The systolic blood pressure is the highest arterial blood pressure following ventricular

contraction or systole. The diastolic blood pressure is the lowest arterial blood pressure that occurs during ventricular filling or diastole. The mean arterial pressure (MAP), which is the average pressure in the arteries throughout the cardiac cycle, depends on the elastic properties of the arterial walls and the mean volume of blood in the arterial system. MAP can be approximated from the measured values of the systolic (P_s) and diastolic (P_d) pressures as follows:

$$MAP = P_d + \frac{1}{3}(P_s - P_d)$$

The normal range for MAP is 70 to 110 mm Hg.[23] The difference between the systolic pressure and diastolic pressure ($P_s - P_d$) is called the pulse pressure and typically is between 40 and 50 mm Hg.[7] Pulse pressure is directly related to arterial wall stiffness and stroke volume.

During a wide range of physiologic conditions, including changes in body position, muscular activity, and circulating blood volume, arterial pressure is regulated within a fairly narrow range to maintain tissue perfusion, or blood supply to the capillary beds. The major factors and relationships that regulate arterial blood pressure are summarized in Figure 23-25.

Effects of Cardiac Output

The cardiac output (minute volume) of the heart can be changed by alterations in heart rate, stroke volume (volume of blood ejected during each ventricular contraction), or both. An increase in cardiac output without a decrease in peripheral resistance will cause mean arterial pressure and flow rate to increase. The higher arterial pressure increases blood flow through the arterioles. On the other hand, a decrease in the cardiac output causes a drop in the mean arterial blood pressure and arteriolar flow if peripheral resistance stays constant.

Effects of Total Peripheral Resistance

Total resistance in the systemic circulation, known as either systemic vascular resistance or *total peripheral resistance*, is primarily a function of arteriolar diameter. If cardiac output remains constant, arteriolar constriction raises mean arterial pressure by reducing the flow of blood into the capillaries, whereas arteriolar dilation has the opposite effect. Reflex control of total cardiac output and peripheral resistance includes (1) sympathetic stimulation of heart, arterioles, and veins; and (2) parasympathetic stimulation of the heart (Figure 23-26). The cardiovascular center in the medulla receives input from arterial baroreceptors and chemoreceptors throughout the vascular system and then modifies vagal and sympathetic output to control heart rate and contractility, plus vascular diameter. Vasoconstriction is regulated by an area of the brainstem that maintains a constant (tonic) output of norepinephrine from sympathetic fibers in the peripheral arterioles. This tonic activity is essential for maintenance of blood pressure.

Baroreceptors. As discussed previously, baroreceptors are stretch receptors located predominantly in the aorta and in the carotid sinus (see Figure 23-26, *A*). They respond to changes in smooth muscle fiber length by altering their rate of discharge and supply sensory information to the cardiovascular center in the brainstem. When activated (stretched), the baroreceptors decrease cardiac output by lowering heart rate and stroke volume) and peripheral resistance, and thus lower blood pressure. (Postural changes and the baroreceptor reflex are discussed in Chapter 24.)

Arterial chemoreceptors. Specialized areas within the aortic arch and carotid arteries are sensitive to concentrations of oxygen, carbon dioxide, and hydrogen ions (pH) in the blood (see Figure 23-26, *B*). Although these chemoreceptors are most important for respiratory control, they also transmit impulses to the medullary cardiovascular centers that regulate blood pressure. A decrease in arterial oxygen

FIGURE 23-25 Factors Regulating Blood Pressure.

concentration or an increase in carbon dioxide concentration contributes to an increase in heart rate, stroke volume, and blood pressure, whereas an increase in carbon dioxide concentration causes decreases in these variables. The major chemoreceptive reflex is caused by alterations in arterial oxygen concentration. The effects of altered pH or carbon dioxide levels are minor.[18]

Effect of Hormones

Hormones influence blood pressure regulation through their effects on vascular smooth muscle and blood volume. By constricting or dilating the arterioles in organs, hormones can (1) increase or decrease the flow in response to the body's needs, (2) redistribute blood volume during hemorrhage or shock, and (3) regulate heat loss. The key vasoconstrictor hormones include angiotensin II, vasopressin (or antidiuretic hormone), epinephrine, and norepinephrine. The main vasodilator hormones are the atrial natriuretic hormones. By causing fluid retention or loss, aldosterone, vasopressin, and the natriuretic hormones can influence stroke volume and thus blood pressure.

A variety of other factors, including adipokines and insulin, may be related to the hypertension that occurs with chronic conditions, such as adiposity and diabetes mellitus; but these factors have not been clearly demonstrated to play a role in blood pressure regulation in healthy individuals.[24] Some research has suggested that the risk of cardiovascular disease and hypertension that often co-occurs with diabetes mellitus is more closely related to insulin resistance than to insulin levels.[25] Adrenomedullin (ADM) is a vasodilating peptide present in cardiovascular, pulmonary, renal, and other tissues. Because increases in ADM levels are associated with heart failure and myocardial infarction, ADM levels may be useful for risk categorization in people with these conditions.[26]

Vasoconstrictor hormones. The vasoconstrictor hormones include epinephrine; norepinephrine; angiotensin II, which is part of the renin-angiotensin-aldosterone system; and vasopressin (also known as antidiuretic hormone). Epinephrine, the catecholamine

hormone released from the adrenal medulla, causes vasoconstriction in most vascular beds except the coronary, liver, and skeletal muscle circulations. Norepinephrine mainly acts as a neurotransmitter; however, some also is released from the adrenal medulla. When released into the circulation, it is a more potent vasoconstrictor than epinephrine. Although angiotensin II and vasopressin are vasoconstrictors they are not thought to have a major role in blood pressure control in normal circumstances.

Vasopressin and aldosterone also affect blood pressure by increasing blood volume through their influence on fluid reabsorption in the kidney and by stimulating thirst. Vasopressin causes the reabsorption of water from tubular fluid in the distal tubule and collecting duct of the nephron. Aldosterone, the end product of the renin-angiotensin-aldosterone system, stimulates the reabsorption of sodium, chloride, and water from the same locations in the kidney (Figure 23-27; also see Chapters 5 and 18).

Vasodilator hormones. The natriuretic peptides (NPs) or hormones (see Figure 23-27), including atrial natriuretic peptide (ANP), B-type natriuretic peptide (BNP), C-type natriuretic peptide (CNP), and urodilatin, function as both vasodilators and regulators of sodium and water excretion (natriuresis and diuresis). Increased pressure or diastolic volume in the heart stimulates the release of these peptide hormones. Increased levels of BNP predict increased risk of a poor outcome in heart failure, pulmonary embolism, valvular heart disease, and chronic coronary artery disease.[27]

Effects of Other Mediators

A variety of other mediators have been demonstrated to cause arteriolar vasodilation or vasoconstriction. Some of the vasodilating mediators include nitric oxide (NO), ADM, the endothelins, and prostacyclin. These mediators are being investigated to determine if they or their inhibitors might be useful drugs for the treatment of cardiovascular diseases or if their levels might be useful in determining the prognosis of persons with known disease.

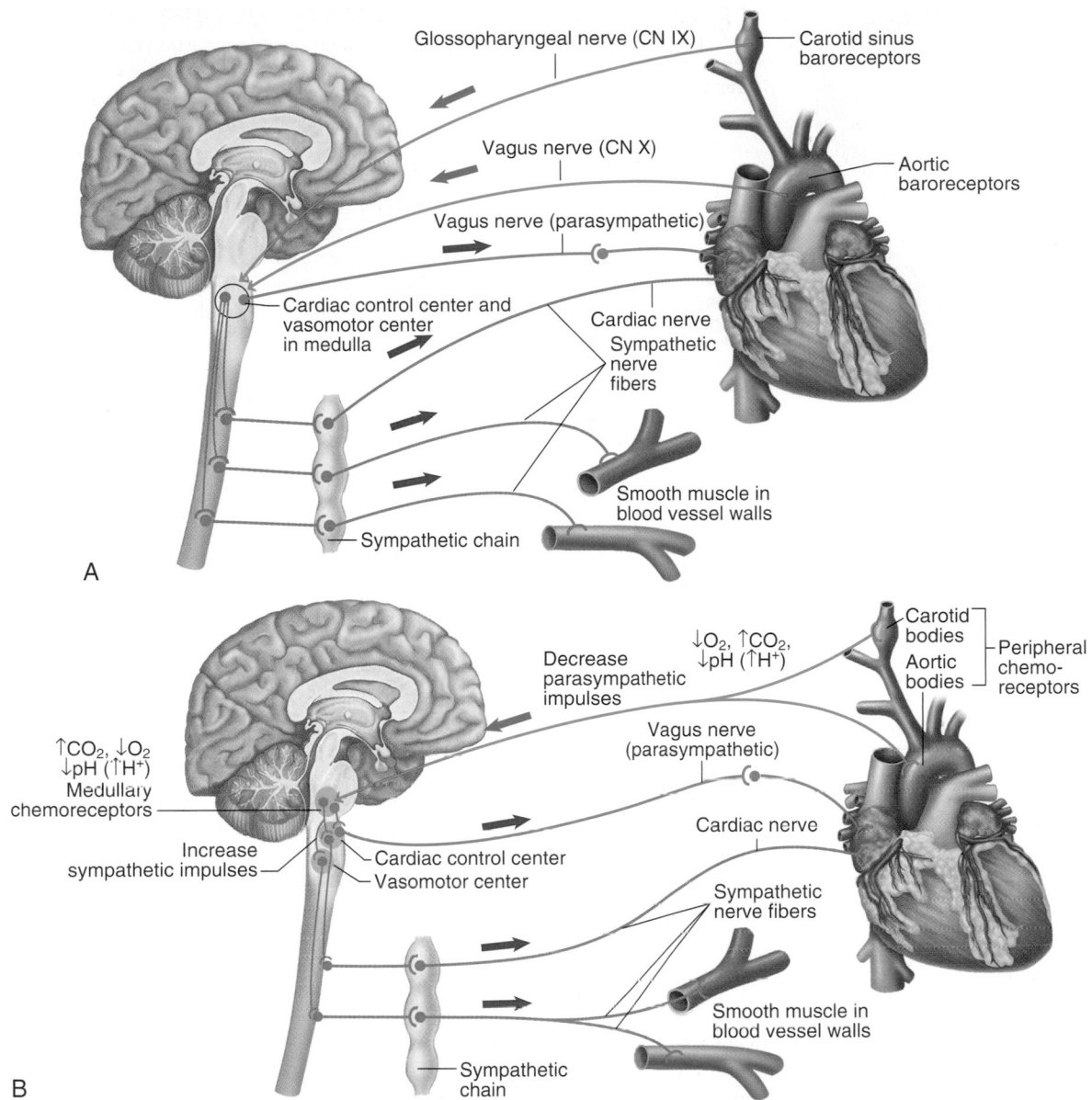

FIGURE 23-26 Baroreceptors and Chemoreceptor Reflex Control of Blood Pressure. A, Baroreceptor reflexes. **B,** Vasomotor chemoreflexes. (Modified from Patton KT, Thibodeau GA: *Anatomy & physiology,* ed 9, St Louis, 2016, Elsevier.)

Nitric oxide (NO), an intercellular and intracellular signaling molecule produced in endothelial cells, has a variety of roles in vascular function including acting as a vasodilator and inhibitor of smooth muscle proliferation. NO also has been called endothelium-derived relaxing factor (EDRF). One way that diabetes may contribute to hypertension is through inhibition of NO production by impeding a family of enzymes—the nitric oxide synthases.[28] Understanding the role of NO in producing vasodilation explains why sublingual nitroglycerin has been a useful treatment for coronary artery spasm.[29]

ADM, a peptide with powerful vasodilatory activity, is present in numerous tissues. It is a member of the calcitonin gene–related peptide family. Although it has been found to have numerous cardiovascular effects, including a role in fetal cardiovascular system development and vasodilation, its exact role in adult human cardiovascular function and disease is unclear. Some research indicates that elevated adrenomedullin levels may be useful disease indicators.[30]

The endothelins are a family of three peptides (ET-1, ET-2, and ET-3) and four receptors produced in cells in the vascular smooth muscle, the endothelium, the kidneys, and other organs. Understanding the physiologic and pathologic roles of these peptides has been complicated by the fact that endothelin binding to the type A receptor causes vasodilation and natriuresis, whereas binding to type B receptor causes the opposite response—vasoconstriction plus sodium and water retention.[31] Inhibitors to endothelin-1 have been approved for the treatment of pulmonary hypertension.[32]

Prostacyclin is a vasodilator that is produced by the actions of cyclooxygenases (COX-1 and COX-2) on arachidonic acid. It also has the additional properties of opposing clot formation (antithrombotic), decreasing platelet activity, and inhibiting the release of growth factors from macrophages and the endothelial cells.[29] Nonsteroidal anti-inflammatory drugs (NSAIDs) that inhibit these cyclooxygenases have been associated with cardiovascular disease risk in healthy people and in those with a known cardiovascular disease.[33,34]

FIGURE 23-27 Three Mechanisms That Influence Total Plasma Volume. The antidiuretic hormone *(ADH)* mechanism and renin-angiotensin-aldosterone system *(RAAS)* tend to increase water, sodium, and chloride retention and thus increase total plasma volume. The atrial natriuretic hormone *(ANH)* mechanism antagonizes these mechanisms by promoting water, sodium, and chloride loss, thus promoting a decrease in total plasma volume. *ACE,* Angiotensin-converting enzyme. (Modified from Patton KT, Thibodeau GA: *Anatomy & physiology,* ed 9, St Louis, 2016, Elsevier.)

Venous Pressure

The main determinants of venous blood pressure are (1) the volume of fluid within the veins and (2) the compliance (distensibility) of the vessel walls. The venous system typically accommodates about 66% of the total blood volume at any time, with venous pressure averaging less than 10 mm Hg. The systemic arteries accommodate about 11% of the total blood volume, with an average arterial pressure (blood pressure) of about 100 mm Hg; the remainder of the blood volume is within the heart, capillaries, and pulmonary circulation.[23]

The sympathetic nervous system controls venous compliance. The walls of the veins are highly innervated by sympathetic fibers that control venous smooth muscle. Rather than constriction that would occur in the arteries, smooth muscle contraction in the veins results in stiffening of the vessel walls. This stiffening reduces venous distensibility and increases venous blood pressure, thus forcing more blood through the veins and into the right heart.

Two other mechanisms that increase venous pressure and venous return to the heart are (1) the skeletal muscle pump and (2) the respiratory pump. During skeletal muscle contraction, the veins within the muscles are partially compressed, causing decreased venous capacity and increased return to the heart (see Figure 23-26). The respiratory pump acts during inspiration, when the veins of the abdomen are partially compressed by the downward movement of the diaphragm. Increased abdominal pressure moves blood toward the heart.

Regulation of the Coronary Circulation

Coronary blood flow is directly proportional to the perfusion pressure and inversely proportional to the vascular resistance of the coronary bed. Coronary perfusion pressure is the difference between pressure in the aorta and pressure in the coronary vessels. Thus, aortic pressure is the driving pressure for the arteries and arterioles that perfuse the myocardium. Vasodilation and vasoconstriction maintain coronary blood flow despite stresses imposed by the constant contraction and relaxation of the heart muscle and despite shifts (within a physiologic range) of coronary perfusion pressure.

Several unique anatomic factors influence coronary blood flow. Because of their anatomic location, the aortic valve cusps can obstruct coronary blood flow by occluding the openings of the coronary arteries during systole. Also during systole, the coronary arteries are compressed by ventricular contraction. The resulting systolic compressive effect is particularly evident in the subendocardial layers of the left ventricular wall and can greatly increase resistance to coronary blood flow with the result that most left ventricular coronary blood flow occurs during diastole. During the period of systolic compression, when flow is slowed or stopped, myoglobin, a protein in heart muscle that binds oxygen, provides the supply of oxygen to the myocardium. Myoglobin's oxygen levels are replenished during diastole.

Autoregulation

Autoregulation (automatic self-regulation) enables organs to regulate blood flow by altering the resistance (diameter) in their arterioles. Autoregulation in the coronary circulation maintains the blood flow at a nearly constant rate at perfusion pressures (mean arterial pressure) between 60 and 140 mm Hg when other influencing factors are held constant.[18] Thus autoregulation helps to ensure constant coronary blood flow despite shifts in the perfusion pressure within the stated range.

Given that blood flow is directly related to pressure and inversely related to resistance, for flow to stay constant as pressure decreases resistance also has to decrease; therefore the mechanisms underlying autoregulation must be related to control of smooth muscle contraction in the arteriolar walls. Although the exact mechanisms underlying autoregulation are unknown, research has indicated that factors influencing calcium release with the myocardium are involved and perhaps also the accumulation of vasodilatory products of metabolism, such as adenosine.[18,35]

Autonomic Regulation

Although the coronary vessels, themselves, contain sympathetic (α- and β-adrenergic) and parasympathetic neural receptors, coronary blood flow during regular activity is regulated locally by the factors that cause autoregulation. During exercise, however, the vasodilating effects of β_2-receptors on the smaller coronary resistance arteries are responsible for about 25% of any increase in blood flow. At the same time, α-adrenergic receptors in larger arteries cause vasoconstriction to direct the blood flow to the inner layers of the myocardium.[18]

> ✔ **QUICK CHECK 23-7**
> 1. Why is capillary flow increased with increased mean arterial pressure?
> 2. Why is angiotensin significant in blood flow?
> 3. Identify the factors regulating blood pressure.
> 4. Define natriuretic peptides and adrenomedullin.

THE LYMPHATIC SYSTEM

The lymphatic system is a one-way network of lymphatic vessels and the lymph nodes (Figures 23-28 and 23-29) that is important

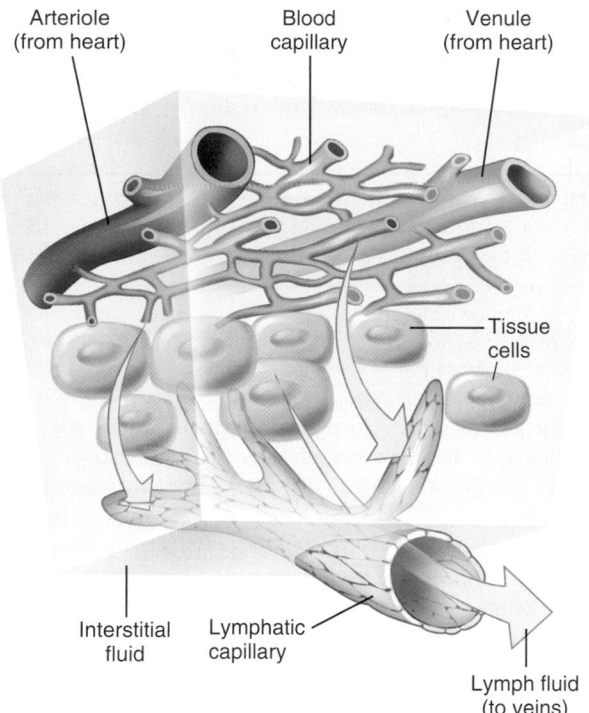

FIGURE 23-28 Role of the Lymphatic System in Fluid Balance.
Fluid from plasma flowing through the capillaries moves into interstitial spaces. Although most of this interstitial fluid is either absorbed by tissue cells or reabsorbed by blood capillaries, some of the fluid tends to accumulate in the interstitial spaces. This lymph then diffuses into the lymphatic vessels that carry it to the lymph nodes and then into the systemic venous blood. Green is used to diagram the lymphatic vessels although the lymphatic vessels, particularly the smaller ones, are almost transparent. (Modified from Thibodeau GA, Patton KT: *Structure & function of the body,* ed 13, St Louis, 2008, Elsevier.)

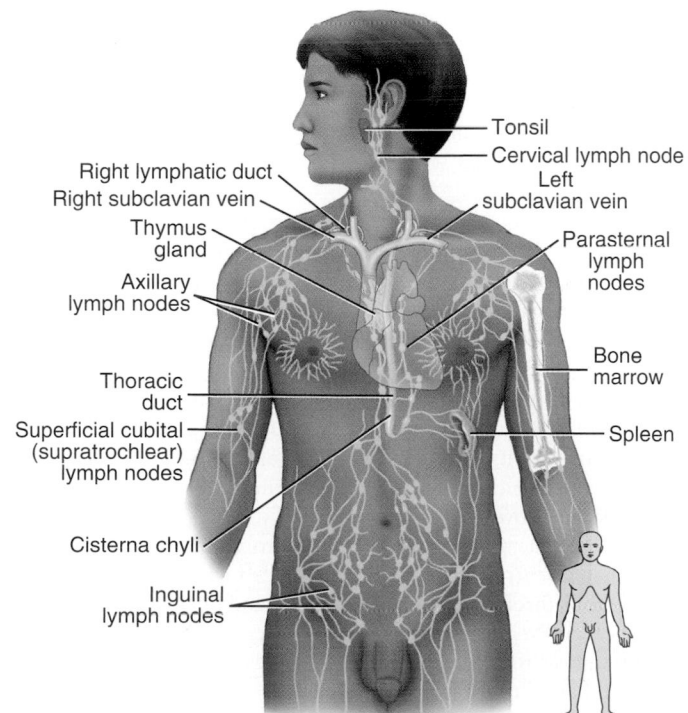

FIGURE 23-29 Principle Organs of the Lymphatic System. (From VanMeter KC, Hubert RJ: *Microbiology for the healthcare professional,* St Louis, 2010, Mosby.)

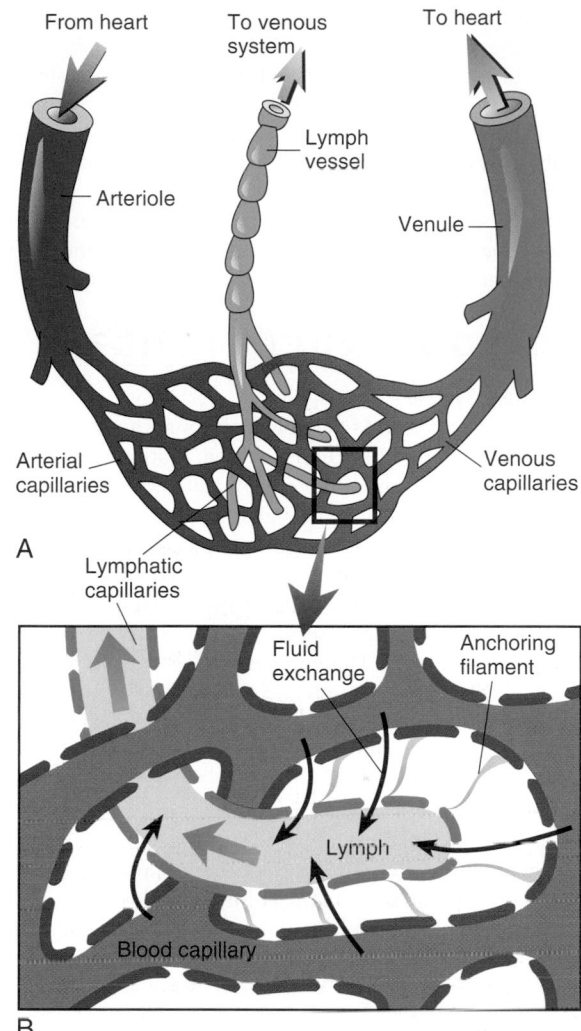

FIGURE 23-30 Lymphatic Capillaries. A, Schematic representation of lymphatic capillaries. **B,** Anatomic components of microcirculation.

for immune function, fluid balance, and transport of lipids, hormones, and cytokines. Every day about 3 liters of fluid filters out of venous capillaries in body tissues and is not reabsorbed. This fluid becomes the lymph that is carried by the lymphatic vessels to the chest, where it enters the venous circulation. The lymphatic vessels run in the same sheaths with the arteries and veins. (Lymph nodes and lymphoid tissues are described in Chapters 6 and 8.) In this pumpless system, a series of valves ensures one-way flow of the excess interstitial fluid (now called lymph) toward the heart. The lymphatic capillaries are closed at the distal ends, as shown in Figure 23-30.

Lymph consists primarily of water and small amounts of dissolved proteins, mostly albumin, that are too large to be reabsorbed into the less permeable blood capillaries. Lymph also carries two types of immune system cells: lymphocytes and antigen-presenting cells. The antigen-presenting cells are carried to the next lymph node in the system while lymphocytes traffic between lymph nodes. Once within the lymphatic system, lymph travels through lymphatic venules and veins that drain into one of two large ducts in the thorax: the right lymphatic duct and the thoracic duct. The right lymphatic duct drains lymph from the right arm and the right side of the head and thorax, whereas the larger thoracic duct receives lymph from the rest of the body (see Figure 23-29). The right lymphatic duct and the thoracic duct drain lymph into the right and left subclavian veins, respectively.

Lymphatic veins are thin walled like the veins of the cardiovascular system. In larger lymphatic veins, endothelial flaps form valves similar to those in blood-carrying veins (see Figure 23-30). The valves allow lymph to flow in only one direction as lymphatic vessels are compressed intermittently by skeletal muscle contraction, pulsatile expansion of the artery in the same sheath, and contraction of the smooth muscles in the walls of the lymphatic vessels.

As lymph is transported toward the heart, it is filtered through thousands of bean-shaped **lymph nodes** clustered along the lymphatic vessels (see Figure 23-29). Lymph enters the nodes through **afferent**

lymphatic vessels, filters through the sinuses in the node, and leaves by way of **efferent lymphatic vessels**. Lymph flows slowly through a node, allowing phagocytosis of foreign substances within the node and delivery of lymphocytes. (Phagocytosis is described in Chapter 7.)

✔ **QUICK CHECK 23-8**
1. Why is the lymphatic system considered a circulatory system?
2. What happens to lymph in lymph nodes?

DID YOU UNDERSTAND?

The Circulatory System

1. The circulatory system is part of the body's transport and communication systems. It delivers oxygen, nutrients, metabolites, hormones, neurochemicals, proteins, and blood cells including lymphocytes and leukocytes throughout the body and carries metabolic wastes to the kidneys, lungs, and liver for excretion.
2. The circulatory system consists of the heart and the blood and lymphatic vessels and is made up of two separate, but conjoined serially connected pump systems: the pulmonary circulation and the systemic circulation. The lymphatic system is a one-way network consisting of lymphatic vessels and lymph nodes.
3. The low-pressure pulmonary circulation is driven by the right side of the heart; its function is to deliver blood to the lungs for oxygenation.
4. The higher pressure systemic circulation is driven by the left side of the heart and functions to provide oxygenated blood, nutrients, and other key substances to body tissues and transport waste products to the lungs, kidneys, and liver for excretion.
5. The lymphatic vessels collect fluids from the interstitium and return the fluids to the circulatory system; lymphatic vessels also deliver antigens, microorganisms, and cells to the lymph nodes.

The Heart

1. The heart consists of four chambers (two atria and two ventricles), four valves (two atrioventricular valves and two semilunar valves), a muscular wall, a fibrous skeleton, a conduction system, nerve fibers, systemic vessels (the coronary circulation), and openings where the great vessels enter the atria and ventricles.
2. The heart wall, which encloses the heart and divides it into chambers, is made up of three layers: the epicardium (outer layer), the myocardium (muscular layer), and the endocardium (inner lining). The heart lies within the pericardium, a double-walled sac.
3. The myocardial layer of the two atria, which receive blood entering the heart, is thinner than the myocardial layer of the ventricles, which have to be stronger to squeeze blood out of the heart.
4. The right and left sides of the heart are separated by portions of the heart wall called the *interatrial septum* and the *interventricular septum.*
5. Deoxygenated (venous) blood from the systemic circulation enters the right atrium through the superior and inferior venae cavae. From the right atrium, the blood passes through the right atrioventricular (tricuspid) valve into the right ventricle. In the ventricle, the blood flows from the inflow tract to the outflow tract and then through the pulmonary semilunar valve (pulmonary valve) into the pulmonary artery, which delivers it to the lungs for oxygenation.
6. Oxygenated blood from the lungs enters the left atrium through the four pulmonary veins (two from the left lung and two from the right lung). From the left atrium, the blood passes through the

left atrioventricular valve (mitral valve) into the left ventricle. In the ventricle, the blood flows from the inflow tract to the outflow tract and then through the aortic semilunar valve (aortic valve) into the aorta, which delivers it to systemic arteries of the entire body.

7. There are four heart valves. The atrioventricular valves ensure one-way flow of blood from the atria to the ventricles. The semilunar valves ensure one-way blood flow from the right ventricle to the pulmonary artery and from the left ventricle to the aorta.
8. Oxygenated blood enters the coronary arteries through openings from the aorta, and deoxygenated blood from the coronary veins enters the right atrium through the coronary sinus.
9. The pumping action of the heart consists of two phases: diastole, during which the myocardium relaxes and the ventricles fill with blood; and systole, during which the myocardium contracts, forcing blood out of the ventricles. A cardiac cycle consists of one systolic contraction and the diastolic relaxation that follows it. Each cardiac cycle represents one heartbeat.
10. The conduction system of the heart generates and transmits electrical impulses (cardiac action potentials) that stimulate systolic contractions. The autonomic nerves (sympathetic and parasympathetic fibers) can adjust heart rate and force of contraction, but they do not originate the heartbeat.
11. The normal electrocardiogram is the sum of all cardiac action potentials. The P wave represents atrial depolarization; the QRS complex is the sum of all ventricular cell depolarizations. The ST interval occurs when the entire ventricular myocardium is depolarized.
12. Cardiac action potentials are generated by the sinoatrial node at a rate of 60 to 100 impulses per minute. The impulses can travel through the conduction system of the heart, stimulating myocardial contraction as they go.
13. Cells of the cardiac conduction system possess the properties of automaticity and rhythmicity. Automatic cells return to threshold and depolarize rhythmically without an outside stimulus. The cells of the sinoatrial node depolarize faster than other automatic cells, making it the natural pacemaker of the heart. If the sinoatrial node is disabled, the next fastest pacemaker, the atrioventricular node, takes over.
14. Each cardiac action potential travels from the sinoatrial node to the atrioventricular node to the bundle of His (atrioventricular bundle), through the bundle branches, and finally to the Purkinje fibers and ventricular myocardium, where the impulse stops. It is prevented from reversing its path by the refractory period of cells that have just been polarized. The refractory period ensures that diastole (relaxation) will occur, thereby completing the cardiac cycle.
15. Adrenergic receptor number, type, and function govern autonomic (sympathetic) regulation of heart rate, contractile force,

and the dilation or constriction of coronary arteries. The presence of specific receptors on the myocardium and coronary vessels determines the effects of the neurotransmitters norepinephrine and epinephrine.

16. Unique features that distinguish myocardial cells from skeletal cells enable myocardial cells to transmit action potentials faster (through intercalated disks), synthesize more ATP (because of a large number of mitochondria), and have readier access to ions in the interstitium (because of an abundance of transverse tubules). These combined differences enable the myocardium to work constantly, which is not required by skeletal muscle.

17. Cross-bridges between actin and myosin enable contraction. Calcium ions interacting with the troponin complex help initiate the contraction process. Subsequently, myocardial relaxation begins as troponin releases calcium ions.

18. Cardiac performance is affected by preload, afterload, myocardial contractility, and heart rate.

19. Preload, or pressure generated in the ventricles at the end of diastole, depends on the amount of blood in the ventricle. Afterload is the resistance to ejection of the blood from the ventricle. Afterload depends on pressure in the aorta.

20. Myocardial stretch determines the force of myocardial contraction; thus the greater the stretch, the stronger the contraction up to a certain point. This relationship is known as the Frank-Starling law of the heart.

21. Contractility is the potential for myocardial fiber shortening during systole. It is determined by the amount of stretch during diastole (i.e., preload) and by sympathetic stimulation of the ventricles.

22. Heart rate is determined by the sinoatrial node and by components of the autonomic nervous system, including cardiovascular control centers in the brain, receptors in the aorta and carotid arteries, and hormones, including catecholamines (epinephrine, norepinephrine).

The Systemic Circulation

1. Blood flows from the left ventricle into the aorta and from the aorta into arteries that eventually branch into arterioles and capillaries, the smallest of the arterial vessels. Oxygen, nutrients, and other substances needed for cellular metabolism pass from the capillaries into the interstitium, where they are taken up by the cells. Capillaries also absorb metabolic waste products from the interstitium.

2. Venules, the smallest veins, receive capillary blood. From the venules, the venous blood flows into larger and larger veins until it reaches the venae cavae, through which it enters the right atrium.

3. Vessel walls have three layers: the tunica intima (inner layer), the tunica media (middle layer), and the tunica externa (the outer layer).

4. Layers of the vessel wall differ in thickness and composition from vessel to vessel, depending on the vessel's size and location within the circulatory system. In general, the tunica media of arteries close to the heart has more elastic fibers because these arteries must be able to distend during systole and recoil during diastole. Distributing arteries farther from the heart contain more smooth muscle fibers because they constrict and dilate to control blood pressure and volume within specific capillary beds.

5. Blood flow into the capillary beds is controlled by the contraction and relaxation of smooth muscle bands (precapillary sphincters) at junctions between metarterioles and capillaries.

6. Endothelial cells line the blood vessels. The endothelium is a life-support tissue; it functions as a filter (altering permeability), changes in vasomotion (constriction and dilation), and is involved in clotting and inflammation.

7. Blood flow through the veins is assisted by the contraction of skeletal muscles (the muscle pump), and backward flow is prevented by one-way valves, which are particularly important in the deep veins of the legs.

8. Blood flow is affected by blood pressure, resistance to flow within the vessels, blood consistency (which affects velocity), anatomic features that may cause turbulent or laminar flow, and compliance (distensibility) of the vessels.

9. Poiseuille law describes the relationship of blood flow, pressure, and resistance as the difference between pressure at the inflow end of the vessel and pressure at the outflow end divided by resistance within the vessel.

10. The greater a vessel's length and the blood's viscosity and the narrower the radius of the vessel's lumen, the greater the resistance within the vessel.

11. Total peripheral resistance, or the resistance to flow within the entire systemic circulatory system, depends on the combined lengths and radii of all the vessels within the system and on whether the vessels are arranged in series (greater resistance) or in parallel (lesser resistance).

12. Blood flow is also influenced by neural stimulation (vasoconstriction or vasodilation) and by autonomic features that cause turbulence within the vascular lumen (e.g., protrusions from the vessel wall, twists and turns, vessel branching).

13. Arterial blood pressure is influenced and regulated by factors that affect cardiac output (heart rate, stroke volume), total resistance within the system, and blood volume.

14. Antidiuretic hormone, the renin-angiotensin-aldosterone system, and natriuretic peptides can all alter blood volume and thus blood pressure.

15. Venous blood pressure is influenced by blood volume within the venous system and compliance of the venous walls.

16. Blood flow through the coronary circulation is governed by the same principles as flow through other vascular beds plus two adaptations dictated by cardiac dynamics. First, blood flows into the coronary arteries during diastole rather than systole, because during systole the cusps of the aortic semilunar valve block the openings of the coronary arteries. Second, systolic contraction inhibits coronary artery flow by compressing the coronary arteries.

17. Autoregulation enables the coronary vessels to maintain optimal perfusion pressure despite systolic compression.

18. Myoglobin in heart muscle stores oxygen for use during the systolic phase of the cardiac cycle.

The Lymphatic System

1. The vessels of the lymphatic system run in the same sheaths as the arteries and veins.

2. Lymph (interstitial fluid) is absorbed by lymphatic venules in the capillary beds and travels through ever larger lymphatic veins until it empties through the right lymphatic duct or thoracic duct into the right or left subclavian veins, respectively.

3. As lymph travels toward the thoracic ducts, it passes through thousands of lymph nodes clustered around the lymphatic veins. The lymph nodes are sites of immune function and are ideally placed to sample antigens and cells carried by the lymph from the periphery of the body into the central circulation.

KEY TERMS

Actin, 580
Adrenomedullin (ADM), 590
Afferent lymphatic vessel, 594
Afterload, 582
Angiogenesis, 573
Anisotropic band (A band), 579
Aorta, 572
Aortic semilunar valve, 571
Arteriogenesis, 573
Arteriole, 584
Artery, 584
Atrioventricular node
    (AV node), 576
Atrioventricular valve, 571
Automatic cell, 577
Automaticity, 577
Autoregulation, 592
Bainbridge reflex, 583
Baroreceptor reflex, 583
Blood flow, 587
Blood velocity, 588
Bundle of His (atrioventricular
    bundle), 576
Capillary, 584
Cardiac action potential, 576
Cardiac cycle, 572
Cardiac output, 581
Cardiac vein, 573
Cardiomyocyte, 570
Cardiovascular vasomotor
    control center, 583
Chordae tendineae, 572
Collateral artery, 573
Conduction system, 576
Coronary artery, 573
Coronary ostium (pl., ostia), 573
Coronary perfusion pressure, 592
Coronary sinus, 573
Cross-bridge theory of muscle
    contraction, 581
Depolarization, 576
Diastole, 572
Diastolic blood pressure, 589

Diastolic depolarization, 578
Efferent lymphatic vessel, 594
Ejection fraction, 581
Elastic artery, 584
Endocardium, 570
Endothelial cell, 586
Endothelium, 586
Epinephrine, 590
Excitation-contraction
    coupling, 581
Fenestration, 586
Frank-Starling law of the
    heart, 582
Great cardiac vein, 574
Heart rate, 578
Inferior vena cava
    (pl., cavae), 572
Inotropic agent, 583
Intercalated disk, 578
Isotropic band (I band), 580
Laminar flow, 588
Laplace law, 582
Left atrium, 571
Left bundle branch (LBB), 576
Left coronary artery (LCA), 573
Left heart, 569
Left ventricle, 571
Lumen, 585
Lymph, 593
Lymph node, 594
Lymphatic vein, 593
Lymphatic venule, 593
M line, 580
Mean arterial pressure
    (MAP), 589
Mediastinum, 569
Metarteriole, 585
Mitral and tricuspid
    complex, 572
Mitral valve (left atrioventricular
    valve, bicuspid valve), 572
Muscle pump, 587
Muscular artery, 585

Myocardial contractility, 581
Myocardial oxygen consumption
    ($M\dot{V}O_2$), 580
Myocardium, 570
Myoglobin, 592
Myosin, 579
Natriuretic peptide (NP), 590
Nitric oxide (NO), 591
P wave, 577
Papillary muscle, 572
Perfusion, 589
Pericardial cavity, 570
Pericardial fluid, 570
Pericardial sac, 570
Pericardium, 570
Peripheral vascular system, 584
Poiseuille law, 587
PR interval, 577
Precapillary sphincter, 586
Preload, 581
Pressure, 587
Prolapse, 572
Pulmonary artery, 572
Pulmonary circulation, 569
Pulmonary vein, 572
Pulmonic semilunar valve, 571
Pulse pressure, 589
Purkinje fiber, 576
QRS complex, 577
QT interval, 577
Radius (diameter), 587
Refractory period, 577
Repolarization, 576
Resistance, 587
Rhythmicity, 578
Right atrium, 571
Right bundle branch (RBB), 576
Right coronary artery
    (RCA), 573
Right heart, 569
Right lymphatic duct, 593
Right ventricle, 571
Semilunar valve, 571

Shear stress, 573
Sinoatrial node (SA node, sinus
    node), 576
Stenosis, 573
ST interval, 577
Stroke volume, 581
Superior vena cava
    (pl., cavae), 572
Systemic circulation, 569
Systemic vascular resistance
    (SVR), 582
Systole, 572
Systolic blood pressure, 589
Systolic compressive
    effect, 592
T wave, 577
Thoracic duct, 593
Titin, 580
Total peripheral resistance
    (TPR), 582
Total resistance, 588
Tricuspid valve, 572
Tropomyosin, 580
Troponin C, 580
Troponin I, 580
Troponin T, 580
Troponin-tropomyosin
    complex, 580
Tunica externa (adventitia), 584
Tunica intima, 584
Tunica media, 584
Turbulent (flow), 588
Vasa vasorum, 584
Vascular compliance, 589
Vasoconstriction, 585
Vasodilation, 585
Vein, 587
Ventricular end-diastolic
    pressure (VEDP), 581
Ventricular end-diastolic volume
    (VEDV), 581
Venule, 584
Z line, 580

REFERENCES

1. Rajendran P et al: The vascular endothelium and human diseases, *Int J Biol Sci* 9(10):1057-1069, 2013.
2. Lin Z, Pu WT: Strategies for cardiac regeneration and repair, *Sci Transl Med* 6(239):239rv1, 2014.
3. Kutty S et al: Patent foramen ovale: the known and the to be known, *J Am Coll Cardiol* 59(19):1665-1671, 2012.
4. Tobis J, Shenoda M: Percutaneous treatment of patent foramen ovale and atrial septal defects, *J Am Coll Cardiol* 60(19):1722-1732, 2012.
5. Faber JE et al: A brief etymology of the collateral circulation, *Arterioscler Thromb Vasc Biol* 34:1854-1859, 2014.
6. Fung E, Helisch A: Macrophages in collateral arteriogenesis, *Front Physiol* 3:353, 2012.
7. Klabunde RE: *Cardiovascular physiology concepts,* ed 2, Baltimore, 2012, Lippincott, Williams & Wilkins.

8. Rubart M, Zipes DP: Genesis of cardiac arrhythmias. In Mann DL et al, editors: *Braunwald's heart disease: a textbook of cardiovascular medicine,* ed 10, pp 33, 629-661, Philadelphia, 2015, Saunders.
9. Opie LH, Bers DM: Mechanisms of cardiac contraction and relaxation. In Mann DL et al, editors: *Braunwald's heart disease: a textbook of cardiovascular medicine,* ed 10, pp 429-453, Philadelphia, 2015, Saunders.
10. Linke WA, Hamdani N: Gigantic business: titin properties and function through thick and thin, *Circ Res* 114:1052-1068, 2014.
11. Deussen A et al: Mechanisms of metabolic coronary flow regulation, *J Mol Cell Cardiol* 52(4):794-801, 2012.
12. Hansen PB: Functional importance of T-type voltage-gated calcium channels in the cardiovascular and renal system: news from the

world of knockout mice, *Am J Physiol Regul Integr Comp Physiol* 308(4):R227-R237, 2015.
13. Sakata Y et al: Left ventricular stiffening as therapeutic target for heart failure with preserved ejection fraction, *Circ J* 77(4):886-892, 2013.
14. Ababneh AA et al: Normal limits for left ventricular ejection fraction and volumes estimated with gated myocardial perfusion imaging in patients with normal exercise test results: influence of tracer, gender, and acquisition camera, *J Nucl Cardiol* 7(6):661-668, 2000.
15. Davidson CJ, Bonow RO: Cardiac catheterization. In Mann DL et al, editors: *Braunwald's heart disease: a textbook of cardiovascular medicine,* ed 10, pp 364-391, Philadelphia, 2015, Saunders.
16. Flynn A et al: Sepsis-induced cardiomyopathy: a review of pathophysiologic mechanisms, *Heart Fail Rev* 15(6):605-611, 2010.

17. Goegel B et al: Impact of acute normobaric hypoxia on regional and global myocardial function: a speckle tracking echocardiography study, *Int J Cardiovasc Imaging* 29(3):561-567, 2013.

18. Hoit BD, Walsh RA: Normal physiology of the cardiovascular system. In Fuster V et al, editors: *Hurst's the heart,* ed 13, Philadelphia, 2011, McGraw-Hill.

19. Crystal GJ, Salem MR: The Bainbridge and the "reverse" Bainbridge reflexes: history, physiology, and clinical relevance, *Anesth Analg* 114(3):520-532, 2012.

20. Volpe M et al: Natriuretic peptides in cardiovascular diseases: current use and perspectives, *Eur Heart J* 35(7):419-425, 2014.

21. Perkel D et al: The potential effects of IGF-1 and GH on patients with chronic heart failure, *J Cardiovasc Pharmacol Ther* 17(1):72-78, 2012.

22. Girard J-P et al: HEVs, lymphatics and homeostatic immune cell trafficking in lymph nodes, *Nat Rev Immunol* 12(11):762-773, 2012.

23. Patton KT, Thibodeau GA: *Anatomy & physiology online package,* ed 9, St Louis, 2016, Elsevier.

24. Kim DH et al: Adiponectin levels and the risk of hypertension: a systematic review and meta-analysis, *Hypertension* 62(1):27-32, 2013.

25. Younk LM et al: The cardiovascular effects of insulin, *Expert Opin Drug Saf* 13(7):955-966, 2014.

26. Yuyun MF et al: Prognostic significance of adrenomedullin in patients with heart failure and with myocardial infarction, *Am J Cardiol* 115(7):986-991, 2015.

27. Bergler-Klein J et al: The role of biomarkers in valvular heart disease: focus on natriuretic peptides, *Can J Cardiol* 30(9):1027-1034, 2014.

28. Lei J et al: Nitric oxide, a protective molecule in the cardiovascular system, *Nitric Oxide* 35:175-185, 2013.

29. Griendling KK et al: Biology of the vessel wall. In Fuster V et al, editors: *Hurst's the heart,* ed 13, Philadelphia, 2011, McGraw-Hill.

30. Nishikimi T et al: Adrenomedullin in cardiovascular disease: a useful biomarker, its pathological roles and therapeutic application, *Curr Protein Pept Sci* 14(4):256-267, 2013.

31. Kohan DE et al: Regulation of blood pressure and salt homeostasis by endothelin, *Physiol Rev* 91(1):1-77, 2011.

32. Nasser SA, El-Mas MM: Endothelin ETA receptor antagonism in cardiovascular disease, *Eur J Pharmacol* 737:210-213, 2014.

33. Schjerning Olsen AM et al: The impact of NSAID treatment on cardiovascular risk—insight from Danish observational data, *Basic Clin Pharmacol Toxicol* 115(2):179-184, 2014.

34. Singh BK et al: Assessment of nonsteroidal anti-inflammatory drug-induced cardiotoxicity, *Expert Opin Drug Metab Toxicol* 10(2):143-156, 2014.

35. Izzard AS, Haegerty AM: Myogenic properties of brain and cardiac vessels and their relation to disease, *Curr Vasc Pharmacol* 12(6):829-835, 2014.

24

Alterations of Cardiovascular Function

Valentina L. Brashers

CHAPTER OUTLINE

Our understanding of the pathophysiology of cardiovascular diseases is evolving rapidly. Neurohumoral, genetic, inflammatory, and metabolic factors are now the focus. This new information is leading to improvements in prevention and treatment.

DISEASES OF THE VEINS

Varicose Veins and Chronic Venous Insufficiency

A **varicose vein** is a vein in which blood has pooled, producing distended, tortuous, and palpable vessels (Figure 24-1). Veins are thin-walled, highly distensible vessels with valves to prevent backflow and pooling of blood (see Figure 23-26). Varicose veins typically involve the saphenous veins of the leg and are caused by (1) trauma to the saphenous veins that damages one or more valves or (2) gradual venous distention caused by the action of gravity on blood in the legs.

If a valve is damaged, a section of the vein is subjected to the pressure of a larger volume of blood under the influence of gravity. Altered connective tissue proteins and proteolytic enzyme activity also play a role in remodeling of the vessel wall.[1] The vein swells as it becomes engorged and surrounding tissue becomes edematous because increased hydrostatic pressure pushes plasma through the stretched

vessel wall. Venous distention can develop over time in individuals who habitually stand for long periods, wear constricting garments, or cross the legs at the knees, which diminishes the action of the muscle pump (see Figure 23-27). Risk factors also include age, female gender, a family history of varicose veins, obesity, pregnancy, deep venous thrombosis, and previous leg injury. Eventually the pressure in the vein damages venous valves, rendering them incompetent and unable to maintain normal venous pressure.

Varicose veins and valvular incompetence can progress to chronic venous insufficiency, especially in obese individuals. **Chronic venous insufficiency (CVI)** is inadequate venous return over a long period. Venous hypertension, circulatory stasis, and tissue hypoxia cause an inflammatory reaction in vessels and tissue leading to fibrosclerotic remodeling of the skin and then to ulceration. Symptoms include edema of the lower extremities and hyperpigmentation of the skin of the feet and ankles. Edema in these areas may extend to the knees. Circulation to the extremities can become so sluggish that the metabolic demands of the cells to obtain oxygen and nutrients and to remove wastes are barely met. Any trauma or pressure can therefore lower the oxygen supply and cause cell death and necrosis (**venous stasis ulcers**) (Figure 24-2). Infection can occur because poor circulation impairs the delivery of the cells and biochemicals necessary for

FIGURE 24-1 Varicose Veins of the Leg *(arrow).* (From Kumar V et al: *Robbins and Cotran pathologic basis of disease,* ed 8, Philadelphia, 2010, Saunders. Courtesy Dr. Magruder C. Donaldson, Brigham and Women's Hospital, Boston, Mass.)

FIGURE 24-2 Venous Stasis Ulcer. (From Rosai J: *Ackerman's surgical pathology,* ed 7, vol 2, St Louis, 1989, Mosby.)

the immune and inflammatory responses. This same sluggish circulation makes infection following reparative surgery a significant risk.

Treatment of varicose veins and CVI begins conservatively, and excellent wound healing results have followed noninvasive treatments such as elevating the legs, wearing compression stockings, and performing physical exercise.[2] Invasive management includes endovenous ablation, sclerotherapy or surgical ligation, conservative vein resection, and vein stripping.[3]

Thrombus Formation in Veins

A **thrombus** is a blood clot that remains attached to a vessel wall (see Figure 21-20). A detached thrombus is a **thromboembolus**. Venous thrombi are more common than arterial thrombi because flow and pressure are lower in the veins than in the arteries. **Deep venous thrombosis (DVT)** occurs primarily in the lower extremity. Three factors (triad of Virchow) promote venous thrombosis: (1) venous stasis (e.g., immobility, age, congestive heart failure), (2) venous

endothelial damage (e.g., trauma, intravenous medications), and (3) hypercoagulable states (e.g., inherited disorders, malignancy, pregnancy, use of oral contraceptives or hormone replacement therapy). Orthopedic trauma or surgery, spinal cord injury, and obstetric/gynecologic conditions can be associated with up to a 100% likelihood of DVT. Numerous genetic abnormalities are associated with an increased risk for venous thrombosis primarily related to states of hypercoagulability. These inherited abnormalities include factor V Leiden mutation, prothrombin mutations, and deficiencies of protein C, protein S, and antithrombin; these abnormalities are commonly found in individuals who develop thrombi in the absence of the usual risk factors.[4]

Accumulation of clotting factors and platelets leads to thrombus formation in the vein, often near a venous valve. Inflammation around the thrombus promotes further platelet aggregation, and the thrombus propagates or grows proximally. This inflammation may cause pain and redness, but because the vein is deep in the leg, it is usually not accompanied by clinical symptoms or signs. If the thrombus creates significant obstruction to venous blood flow, increased pressure in the vein behind the clot may lead to edema of the extremity. Most thrombi will eventually dissolve without treatment; however, untreated DVT is associated with a high risk of embolization of a part of the clot to the lung (pulmonary embolism) (see Chapter 27). Persistent venous obstruction may lead to chronic venous insufficiency and post-thrombotic syndrome with associated pain, edema, and ulceration of the affected limb.[5]

Because DVT is usually asymptomatic and difficult to detect clinically, prevention is important in at-risk individuals and includes early ambulation, pneumatic devices, and prophylactic anticoagulation. If thrombosis does occur, diagnosis is confirmed by a combination of serum D-dimer measurement and Doppler ultrasonography. Management most often consists of anticoagulation therapy using heparin (low-molecular-weight heparin) and warfarin.[6] New oral anticoagulant therapies, such as factor Xa inhibitors and direct thrombin inhibitors, have been shown to have a more favorable benefit-to-risk ratio and are rapidly becoming the treatments of choice.[7] Thrombolytic therapy or placement of an inferior vena cava filter may be indicated in selected individuals.[4,6]

Superior Vena Cava Syndrome

Superior vena cava syndrome (SVCS) is a progressive occlusion of the superior vena cava (SVC) that leads to venous distention in the upper extremities and head. Causes include bronchogenic cancer (75% of cases) followed by lymphomas and metastasis of other cancers.[8] Other less common causes include tuberculosis, mediastinal fibrosis, and cystic fibrosis. Invasive therapies (pacemaker wires, central venous catheters, and pulmonary artery catheters) with associated thrombosis now account for nearly 40% of cases.[9] The SVC is a relatively low-pressure vessel that lies in the closed thoracic compartment; therefore tissue expansion can easily compress the SVC. The right mainstem bronchus abuts the SVC so that cancers occurring in this bronchus may exert pressure on the SVC. Additionally, the SVC is surrounded by lymph nodes and lymph chains that commonly become involved in thoracic cancers and compress the SVC during tumor growth. Because onset of SVCS is most often slow, collateral venous drainage to the azygos vein usually has time to develop.

Clinical manifestations of SVCS are edema and venous distention in the upper extremities and face, including the ocular beds. Affected persons complain of a feeling of fullness in the head or tightness of shirt collars, necklaces, and rings. Cerebral edema may cause headache, visual disturbance, and impaired consciousness. The skin of the face and arms may become purple and taut, and capillary refill time is prolonged. Respiratory distress may be present because of edema of bronchial structures or compression of the bronchus by a carcinoma. In infants, SVCS can lead to hydrocephalus.

Diagnosis is made by chest x-ray, Doppler studies, computed tomography (CT), magnetic resonance imaging (MRI), and ultrasound. Because of its slow onset and the development of collateral venous drainage, SVCS is generally not a vascular emergency, but it is an oncologic emergency. Treatment for malignant disorders can include radiation therapy, surgery, chemotherapy, and the administration of diuretics, steroids, and anticoagulants, as necessary. Treatment for nonmalignant causes may include bypass surgery using various grafts, thrombolysis (both locally and systemically), balloon angioplasty, and placement of intravascular stents.[8]

> ✔ **QUICK CHECK 24-1**
> 1. What is chronic venous insufficiency, and how does it present clinically?
> 2. What are the major risk factors for DVT?
> 3. Name three causes of superior vena cava syndrome.

DISEASES OF THE ARTERIES

Hypertension

Hypertension is consistent elevation of systemic arterial blood pressure. Hypertension (HTN) is the most common primary diagnosis in the United States. One in three Americans has hypertension, and more than two thirds of those older than age 60 are affected.[10] The chance of developing primary hypertension increases with age. Although hypertension is usually considered an adult health problem, it is important to remember that hypertension does occur in children and is being diagnosed with increasing frequency (see Chapter 25). The prevalence of HTN is higher in blacks and in those with diabetes. Hypertension is defined by the Eighth Joint National Committee Report as a sustained systolic blood pressure of 140 mm Hg or greater or a diastolic pressure of 90 mm Hg or greater (Table 24-1).[11] Normal blood pressure is associated with the lowest cardiovascular risk, whereas those who fall into the prehypertension category (which includes between 25% and 37% of the U.S. population) are at risk for developing hypertension and many associated cardiovascular complications unless lifestyle modification and treatment are instituted. All stages of hypertension are associated with increased risk for target organ disease events, such as myocardial infarction, kidney disease, and stroke; thus both stage I and stage II hypertension need effective long-term therapy.

Most cases of hypertension are diagnosed as primary hypertension (also called essential or idiopathic hypertension). From 92% to 95% of hypertensive individuals have primary disease. Secondary hypertension is caused by an underlying disorder such as renal disease. This form of hypertension accounts for only 5% to 8% of cases.

TABLE 24-1 Classification of Blood Pressure for Adults Age 18 Years and Older

Category	Systolic (mm Hg)		Diastolic (mm Hg)
Normal	<120	AND	<80
Prehypertension	120-139	OR	80-89
Stage 1 hypertension	140-159	OR	90-99
Stage 2 hypertension	≥160	OR	≥100

Data from James PA et al: *J Am Med Assoc* 311(5):507-520, 2014.

Factors Associated with Primary Hypertension

A specific cause for primary hypertension has not been identified, and a combination of genetic and environmental factors is thought to be responsible for its development. Genetic predisposition to hypertension is thought to be polygenic and associated with epigenetic changes influenced by diet and lifestyle.[12] Inherited defects are associated with renal sodium excretion, insulin and insulin sensitivity, activity of the sympathetic nervous system (SNS) and the renin-angiotensin-aldosterone system (RAAS), and cell membrane sodium or calcium transport.[13] Factors associated with primary hypertension relate to age, gender, race, and dietary factors (see *Risk Factors:* Primary Hypertension). Many of these factors are also risk factors for other cardiovascular disorders. In fact, obesity, hypertension, dyslipidemia, and glucose intolerance often are found together in a condition called the metabolic syndrome (see Chapter 19).

> ## RISK FACTORS
> ### *Primary Hypertension*
>
> Family history
> Advancing age
> Cigarette smoking
> Obesity
> Heavy alcohol consumption
> Gender (men > women before age 55, women > men after 55)
> Black race
> High dietary sodium intake
> Low dietary intake of potassium, calcium, magnesium
> Glucose intolerance

PATHOPHYSIOLOGY Hypertension results from a sustained increase in peripheral resistance (arteriolar vasoconstriction), an increase in circulating blood volume, or both.

Primary Hypertension

Primary hypertension is the result of an extremely complicated interaction of genetics and the environment mediated by a host of neurohumoral effects. Multiple pathophysiologic mechanisms mediate these effects, including the sympathetic nervous system (SNS), the renin-angiotensin-aldosterone system (RAAS), and natriuretic peptides. Inflammation, endothelial dysfunction, obesity-related hormones, and insulin resistance also contribute to both increased peripheral resistance and increased blood volume. Increased vascular volume is related to a decrease in renal excretion of salt, often referred to as a shift in the pressure-natriuresis relationship (Figure 24-3). This means that for a given blood pressure, individuals with hypertension tend to secrete less salt in their urine.

The sympathetic nervous system has been implicated in both the development and the maintenance of elevated blood pressure and plays a role in hypertensive end-organ damage.[14] Increased SNS activity causes increased heart rate and systemic vasoconstriction, thus raising the blood pressure. Additional mechanisms of SNS-induced hypertension include structural changes in blood vessels (vascular remodeling), renal sodium retention (shift in pressure-natriuresis curve), insulin resistance, increased renin and angiotensin levels, and procoagulant effects.[15]

In hypertensive individuals, overactivity of the RAAS contributes to salt and water retention and increased vascular resistance (see Figure 23-27). High levels of angiotensin II contribute to endothelial

FIGURE 24-3 Factors That Cause a Shift in the Pressure-Natriuresis Relationship. Numerous factors have been implicated in the pathogenesis of sodium retention in individuals with hypertension. These factors cause less renal excretion of salt than would normally occur with increased blood pressure. This is called a shift in the pressure-natriuresis relationship and is thought to be a central process in the pathogenesis of primary hypertension. *RAAS,* Renin-angiotensin-aldosterone system; *SNS,* sympathetic nervous system.

dysfunction, insulin resistance, and platelet aggregation and play an important role in the complications associated with the metabolic syndrome.[16] Further, angiotensin II mediates arteriolar remodeling, which is structural change in the vessel wall that results in permanent increases in peripheral resistance and contributes to atherogenesis[17] (see Figure 23-33). Angiotensin II is associated with end-organ effects of hypertension, including atherosclerosis, renal disease, cardiac hypertrophy, and heart failure.[18,19] Finally, aldosterone not only contributes to sodium retention by the kidney but also has other deleterious effects on the cardiovascular system and contributes to insulin resistance.[20] Medications, such as angiotensin-converting enzyme (ACE) inhibitors and angiotensin receptor blockers (ARBs), oppose the activity of the RAAS and are effective in reducing blood pressure and protecting against target organ damage.[21] A second RAAS also has been described. This system uses ACE2 to create angiotensin 1-7, Ang(1-7), which has cardiovascular, cerebrovascular, and metabolic protective effects.[22] Its discovery may lead to new and more effective medications[23] (see *Health Alert:* The Renin-Angiotensin-Aldosterone System (RAAS) and Cardiovascular Disease).

Populations with high dietary sodium intake have long been shown to have an increased incidence of hypertension.[24] Low dietary potassium, calcium, and magnesium intakes also are risk factors because without their intake, sodium is retained. The natriuretic hormones modulate renal sodium (Na+) excretion and require adequate potassium, calcium, and magnesium to function properly. The natriuretic hormones include atrial natriuretic peptide (ANP), B-type natriuretic peptide (BNP), C-type natriuretic peptide (CNP), and urodilatin. Dysfunction of these hormones, along with alterations in the RAA system and the SNS, causes an increase in vascular tone and a shift in the pressure-natriuresis relationship. When there is inadequate natriuretic function, serum levels of the natriuretic peptides are increased. In hypertension, increased ANP and BNP levels are linked to an increased risk for ventricular hypertrophy, atherosclerosis, and heart failure.[25] Salt retention leads to water retention and increased blood volume, which contributes to an increase in blood pressure. Subtle renal injury

HEALTH ALERT

The Renin-Angiotensin-Aldosterone System (RAAS) and Cardiovascular Disease

The RAAS has multiple effects on the cardiovascular system. There are two primary RAA systems. The best known includes the release of renin, the synthesis of angiotensin II (Ang II) through angiotensin-converting enzyme (ACE), stimulation of the AT1 receptor (AT1R), and secretion of aldosterone. Ang II causes systemic vasoconstriction and renal salt and water retention, and stimulates tissue growth and inflammation. When present in abnormal amounts, Ang II contributes to insulin resistance, remodeling of blood vessels, atherogenesis, and decreased release of endothelial vasodilators and anticoagulants. In the heart, Ang II and aldosterone contribute to hypertensive hypertrophy and fibrosis of heart muscle, decreased contractility, and an increased susceptibility to arrhythmias and heart failure. In the kidney these hormones cause a shift in the pressure-natriuresis curve, inflammation, and glomerular remodeling and are a major contributor to renal failure in individuals with hypertension and diabetes. Drugs that block this RAAS include ACE inhibitors, direct renin inhibitors, Ang II receptor blockers (ARBs), and aldosterone inhibitors. These medications are used widely in managing hypertension, myocardial infarction, and heart failure to lower blood pressure and to protect and improve cardiovascular and renal function. In contrast, the second RAAS serves a counterregulatory system. Activation of a second ACE pathway (ACE2) leads to the synthesis of angiotensin 1-7 from Ang II. Angiotensin 1-7 stimulates Mas receptors in the brain, blood vessels, heart, kidney, gut, pancreas, and inflammatory cells and has vasodilatory, antiproliferative, antifibrotic, and antithrombotic effects. These protective effects lead to lower blood pressure, less vascular inflammation and clotting, and decreased tissue remodeling and damage to target organ tissues. This pathway appears to be especially important in protecting renal tissue and improving insulin sensitivity in those with diabetes and hypertension. Research is underway to develop pharmacologic interventions, such as synthetic Mas agonists, Ang(1-7) formulations, and ACE2 activators that will stimulate these protective RAAS pathways. More recently, additional RAAS pathways have been identified that play a role in proto-oncogene stimulation, hypothalamic function, and central nervous system function.

Data from Clarke C et al: *Future Cardiol* 9(1):23-38, 2013; Dominici FP et al: *Clin Sci* 126(9):613-630, 2014; Farag E et al: *Anesth & Analg* 120(2):275-292, 2015; Fraga-Silva RA et al: *Curr Hypertens Rep* 15(1):31-38, 2013; Henriksen EJ, Prasannarong M: *Mol Cell Endocrinol* 378(1-2):15-22, 2013; McKinney CA et al: *Clin Sci* 126(12):815-827, 2014; Ohishi M et al: *Curr Pharm Des* 19(17):3060-3064, 2013; Regenhardt RW et al: *Clin Sci* 126(3):195-205, 2014; Santos RA et al: *J Endocrinol* 216(2):R1-R17, 2013; Seva Pessoa B et al: *Nat Rev Nephrol* 9(1):26-36, 2013; Wang Y et al: *Atherosclerosis* 226(1):3-8, 2013; Zucker IH et al: *Clin Sci* 126(10):695-706, 2014.

results, with renal vasoconstriction and tissue ischemia. Tissue ischemia causes inflammation of the kidney and contributes to dysfunction of the glomeruli and tubules, which promotes additional sodium retention. Salt restriction combined with adequate intake of dietary potassium, magnesium, and calcium has been linked to improved natriuretic peptide function.[26]

Inflammation plays a role in the pathogenesis of hypertension. One proposed mechanism for initiating hypertension-related inflammation is *peripheral vascular resistance–mediated ischemic cellular injury* and the release of damage-associated molecular patterns (DAMPs) that activate Toll-like receptors on immune cells[27] (see Chapter 5). Activation of innate and adaptive immunity results in damage to endothelial cells.[28] Endothelial injury and tissue ischemia result in the release of vasoactive inflammatory cytokines. Although many of these cytokines (e.g., histamine, prostaglandins) have vasodilatory actions in acute inflammatory injury, chronic inflammation leads to decreased production of vasodilators (such as nitric oxide), vascular remodeling, and smooth muscle contraction. Inflammation also contributes to insulin resistance, decreased natriuresis, and autonomic dysfunction (increased SNS activity).[29-31]

Obesity is recognized as an important risk factor for hypertension in both adults and children and contributes to many of the neurohumoral, metabolic, renal, and cardiovascular processes that cause hypertension.[32] Obesity causes changes in the adipokines (i.e., leptin and adiponectin) and also is associated with increased activity of the SNS and the RAAS.[33] Obesity is linked to inflammation, endothelial dysfunction, and insulin resistance and an increased risk for cardiovascular complications from hypertension[32] (see *Health Alert:* Obesity and Hypertension).

HEALTH ALERT

Obesity and Hypertension

Obesity is a well-known risk factor for hypertension. Obesity and increased caloric intake contribute to adipocyte dysfunction and ectopic fat deposition throughout the cardiovascular system. These dysfunctional adipocytes release inflammatory mediators that contribute to vascular remodeling and endothelial dysfunction with decreased endogenous vasodilator release. Adipocytes secrete adipokines, including leptin and adiponectin. The primary function of leptin is to interact with the hypothalamus to control body weight and fat deposition through appetite inhibition and increased metabolic rate. However, chronically high levels of leptin associated with obesity result in resistance to these weight-reducing functions and have been found to increase sympathetic nervous system activity, decrease renal sodium excretion, promote inflammation, and stimulate myocyte hypertrophy. Adiponectin is a protein that is produced by adipose tissue but is reduced in obesity. Decreased adiponectin is associated with insulin resistance, decreased endothelial-derived nitric oxide (vasodilator) production, and activation of the sympathetic nervous and renin-angiotensin-aldosterone systems. Other less studied adipokines that are altered in obesity-related cardiovascular diseases include resistin, omentin, visfatin, and perivascular adipose tissue–derived relaxing factor. Taken together, these obesity-related changes result in vasoconstriction, salt and water retention, and renal dysfunction that may contribute to the development of hypertension. Obesity-related microvascular dysfunction is linked to the pathogenesis both of hypertension and of hypertension-related target organ damage. Obesity also is linked with insulin resistance, which contributes to vascular dysfunction and the development of sustained hypertension. Weight loss is an essential treatment for obesity-related hypertension and has beneficial effects on these pathogenic pathways. In severe obesity, bariatric surgery has been shown to cause long-standing remission of hypertension in up to 93% of individuals. Further studies aimed at achieving a better understanding of these mechanisms may lead to new treatments for obesity-related hypertension.

Data from Adams ST et al: *Blood Pressure* 22(3):131-137, 2013; Cerezo C et al: *Curr Hypertens Rep* 15(3):196-203, 2013; da Silva AA et al: *Curr Opin Nephrol Hypertens* 22(2):135-140, 2013; Hatzis G et al: *Curr Top Med Chem* 13(2):139-163, 2013; Landsberg L et al: *Obesity* 21(1):8-24, 2013; Stepien M et al: *Angiology* 65(4):333-342, 2014; Van de Voorde J et al: *Metabolism* 62(11):1513-1521, 2013.

Finally, insulin resistance is common in hypertension, even in individuals without clinical diabetes. Insulin resistance is associated with decreased endothelial release of nitric oxide and other vasodilators.[34] It also affects renal function and causes renal salt and water retention. Insulin resistance is associated with overactivity of the sympathetic nervous system and the renin-angiotensin-aldosterone system. It is interesting to note that in many individuals with diabetes treated with drugs that increase insulin sensitivity, blood pressure often declines, even in the absence of antihypertensive drugs. The interactions between obesity, hypertension, insulin resistance, and lipid disorders in the metabolic syndrome result in a high risk of cardiovascular disease.[34]

It is likely that primary hypertension is an interaction between many of these factors leading to sustained increases in blood volume and peripheral resistance. The pathophysiology of primary hypertension is summarized in Figure 24-4.

Secondary Hypertension

Secondary hypertension is caused by an underlying disease process or medication that raises peripheral vascular resistance or cardiac output. Examples include renal vascular or parenchymal disease, adrenocortical tumors, adrenomedullary tumors (pheochromocytoma), and drugs (oral contraceptives, corticosteroids, antihistamines). If the cause is identified and removed before permanent structural changes occur, blood pressure returns to normal.

Complicated Hypertension

As hypertension becomes more severe and chronic, tissue damage can occur in the blood vessels and tissues leading to target organ damage in the heart, kidney, brain, and eyes. Cardiovascular complications of sustained hypertension include left ventricular hypertrophy, angina pectoris, heart failure, coronary artery disease, myocardial infarction, and sudden death. Myocardial hypertrophy in response to hypertension is mediated by several neurohormonal substances, including catecholamines from the SNS and angiotensin II. Hypertrophy is characterized by changes in the myocyte proteins, apoptosis of myocytes, and deposition of collagen in heart muscle, which causes it to become thickened, scarred, and less able to relax during diastole, leading to heart failure with preserved ejection fraction.[35] In addition, the increased size of the heart muscle increases demand for oxygen delivery over time, the contractility of the heart is impaired, and the individual is at increased risk for myocardial infarction and heart failure with reduced ejection fraction. Vascular complications include the formation, dissection, and rupture of aneurysms (outpouchings in vessel walls) and atherosclerosis leading to vessel occlusion.

Renal complications of complicated hypertension include parenchymal damage, nephrosclerosis, renal arteriosclerosis, and renal insufficiency or failure. Microalbuminuria (small amounts of protein in the urine) occurs in 10% to 25% of individuals with primary hypertension and is now recognized as an early sign of impending renal dysfunction and significantly increased risk for cardiovascular events, especially in those who also have diabetes.[36] Complications specific to the retina include retinal vascular sclerosis, exudation, and hemorrhage. Cerebrovascular complications include transient ischemia, stroke, cerebral thrombosis, aneurysm, hemorrhage, and dementia.[37] The pathologic effects of complicated hypertension are summarized in Table 24-2.

Hypertensive crisis (or malignant hypertension) is rapidly progressive hypertension in which diastolic pressure is usually greater than 140 mm Hg. It can occur in those with primary hypertension, but the reason why some people develop this complication and others do not is unknown. Other causes include complications of pregnancy, cocaine or amphetamine use, reaction to certain medications, adrenal tumors, and alcohol withdrawal. High arterial pressure renders the cerebral arterioles incapable of regulating blood flow to the cerebral capillary beds. High hydrostatic pressures in the capillaries cause vascular fluid to exude into the interstitial space. If blood pressure is not reduced, cerebral edema and cerebral dysfunction (encephalopathy) increase until death occurs. Organ damage resulting from malignant

FIGURE 24-4 Pathophysiology of Hypertension. Numerous genetic vulnerabilities have been linked to hypertension and these, in combination with environmental risks, cause neurohumoral dysfunction (sympathetic nervous system *[SNS]*, renin-angiotensin-aldosterone *[RAA]* system, and natriuretic hormones) and promote inflammation and insulin resistance. Insulin resistance and neurohumoral dysfunction contribute to sustained systemic vasoconstriction and increased peripheral resistance. Inflammation contributes to renal dysfunction, which, in combination with the neurohumoral alterations, results in renal salt and water retention and increased blood volume. Increased peripheral resistance and increased blood volume are two primary causes of sustained hypertension.

TABLE 24-2 Pathologic Effects of Sustained, Complicated Primary Hypertension

Site of Injury	Mechanism of Injury	Potential Pathologic Effect
Heart		
Myocardium	Increased workload combined with diminished blood flow through coronary arteries	Left ventricular hypertrophy, myocardial ischemia, heart failure
Coronary arteries	Accelerated atherosclerosis (coronary artery disease)	Myocardial ischemia, myocardial infarction, sudden death
Kidneys	Reduced blood flow, increased arteriolar pressure, RAAS and SNS stimulation, and inflammation	Glomerulosclerosis and decreased glomerular filtration, end-stage renal disease
Brain	Reduced blood flow and oxygen supply; weakened vessel walls, accelerated atherosclerosis	Transient ischemic attacks, cerebral thrombosis, aneurysm, hemorrhage, acute brain infarction
Eyes (retinas)	Retinal vascular sclerosis, increased retinal artery pressures	Hypertensive retinopathy, retinal exudates and hemorrhages
Aorta	Weakened vessel wall	Dissecting aneurysm (see p. 605)
Arteries of lower extremities	Reduced blood flow and high pressures in arterioles, accelerated atherosclerosis	Intermittent claudication, gangrene

hypertension is life-threatening. Besides encephalopathy, hypertensive crisis can cause papilledema, cardiac failure, uremia, retinopathy, and cerebrovascular accident and is considered a medical emergency.[38]

CLINICAL MANIFESTATIONS   The early stages of hypertension have no clinical manifestations other than elevated blood pressure; for this reason, hypertension is called a silent disease. Some hypertensive individuals never have signs, symptoms, or complications, whereas others become very ill, and hypertension can be a cause of death. Still other individuals have anatomic and physiologic damage caused by past hypertensive disease, despite current blood pressure measurements being within normal ranges. If elevated blood pressure is not detected and treated, it becomes established and may begin to accelerate its effects on tissues when the individual is 30 to 50 years of age. This sets the stage for the complications of hypertension that begin to appear during the fourth, fifth, and sixth decades of life.

Most clinical manifestations of hypertensive disease are caused by complications that damage organs and tissues outside the vascular system. Besides elevated blood pressure, the signs and symptoms therefore tend to be specific for the organs or tissues affected. Evidence of heart disease, renal insufficiency, central nervous system dysfunction, impaired vision, impaired mobility, vascular occlusion, or edema can all be caused by sustained hypertension.

EVALUATION AND TREATMENT A single elevated blood pressure reading does not mean that a person has hypertension. Diagnosis requires the measurement of blood pressure on at least two separate occasions, averaging two readings at least 2 minutes apart, with the following conditions: the person is seated, the arm is supported at heart level, the person must be at rest for at least 5 minutes, and the person should not have smoked or ingested any caffeine in the previous 30 minutes.[11] Diagnostic tests for further evaluation of hypertension include 24-hour blood pressure monitoring in selected individuals, complete blood count, urinalysis, biochemical blood profile (measures levels of plasma glucose, sodium, potassium, calcium, magnesium, creatinine, cholesterol, and triglycerides), and an electrocardiogram (ECG). Individuals who have elevated blood pressure are assumed to have primary hypertension unless their history, physical examination, or initial diagnostic screening indicates secondary hypertension. Once the diagnosis is made, a careful evaluation for other cardiovascular risk factors and for end-organ damage should be done.

Treatment of primary hypertension depends on its severity. JNC 8 recommendations begin with lifestyle modification as important for preventing and treating hypertension.[11] Important lifestyle modifications include following an exercise program, making dietary modifications, stopping smoking, and losing weight. Reducing salt intake is an important dietary modification and has been shown to significantly reduce blood pressure in both hypertensive and normotensive individuals.[24,39] Pharmacologic treatment of hypertension reduces the risk of end-organ damage and prevents major diseases, such as myocardial infarction and stroke. Recommendations in the JNC 8 report suggest that treatment should begin with thiazide diuretics alone or in combination with angiotensin II (Ang II) blockers (ACE inhibitors or angiotensin receptor blockers) or calcium channel blockers.[11] Beta-blockers were found to have a higher rate of stroke than Ang II blockers and are no longer recommended as first-line medications. Individuals with heart failure, chronic kidney disease, or a history of myocardial infarction or stroke should begin antihypertensive treatment with an ACE inhibitor or ARB. Some individuals require two or more drugs for blood pressure control. JNC 8 raised the treatment goal for adults 18 to 59 years of age without comorbidities or in those >60 years of age with diabetes or chronic kidney disease to <140/90 mm Hg, and for adults >60 years of age who do not have diabetes or chronic kidney disease to <150/90 mm Hg, which resulted in an overall decrease in the number of individuals requiring treatment compared with previous recommendations.[11,40] In individuals with refractive hypertension, catheter-based renal denervation can result in significant reductions in blood pressure,[41] but many questions remain pertaining to long-term safety, mechanisms of action, and selection of appropriate candidates for the procedure.[42] Careful follow-up to support continued adherence, determine the response, and monitor for potential side effects of these medications is important.

Orthostatic (Postural) Hypotension

The term **orthostatic (postural) hypotension (OH)** refers to a decrease in systolic blood pressure of at least 20 mm Hg or a decrease in diastolic blood pressure of at least 10 mm Hg within 3 minutes of moving to a standing position.[43] *Idiopathic,* or primary, orthostatic hypotension implies no known initial cause. This kind of OH is often called "neurogenic" and is usually the result of primary neurologic disorders or secondary to conditions that affect autonomic function.[44] It affects men more often than women and usually occurs between the ages of 40 and 70 years. Up to 18% of older adults may be affected by primary orthostatic hypotension, and it is a significant risk factor for falls and associated injury, with increased mortality.[45] Recently, OH has been implicated in contributing to depression and dementia.[46]

Normally when an individual stands, the gravitational changes on the circulation are compensated by such mechanisms as baroreceptor-mediated reflex arteriolar and venous constriction and increased heart rate. Other compensatory mechanisms include mechanical factors, such as the closure of valves in the venous system, contraction of the leg muscles, and a decrease in intrathoracic pressure.[46] The normally increased sympathetic activity during upright posture is mediated through a stretch receptor (baroreceptor) reflex that responds to shifts in volume caused by postural changes. This reflex promptly increases heart rate and constricts the systemic arterioles. Thus, arterial blood pressure is maintained. These mechanisms are dysfunctional or inadequate in individuals with orthostatic hypotension; consequently, upon standing, blood pools and normal arterial pressure cannot be maintained.

Orthostatic hypotension may be acute or chronic. Acute orthostatic hypotension is caused when the normal regulatory mechanisms are sluggish as a result of (1) altered body chemistry, (2) drug action (e.g., antihypertensives, antidepressants), (3) prolonged immobility caused by illness, (4) starvation, (5) physical exhaustion, (6) any condition that produces volume depletion (e.g., dehydration, diuresis, potassium or sodium depletion), or (7) any condition that results in venous pooling (e.g., pregnancy, extensive varicosities of the lower extremities). Elderly persons are particularly susceptible to this type of orthostatic hypotension.

Chronic orthostatic hypotension may be (1) secondary to a specific disease or (2) idiopathic or primary. The diseases that cause secondary orthostatic hypotension are endocrine disorders (e.g., adrenal insufficiency, diabetes), metabolic disorders (e.g., porphyria), or diseases of the central or peripheral nervous systems (e.g., Parkinson disease, multiple system atrophy, intracranial tumors, cerebral infarcts, Wernicke encephalopathy, peripheral neuropathies). Cardiovascular autonomic neuropathy is a common cause of orthostatic hypotension in persons with diabetes and is a serious and often overlooked complication. In addition to cardiovascular symptoms, associated impotence and bowel and bladder dysfunction are common.

Orthostatic hypotension is often accompanied by dizziness, blurring or loss of vision, and syncope or fainting caused by insufficient vasomotor compensation and reduction of blood flow through the brain. Although no curative treatment is available for idiopathic orthostatic hypotension, often it can be managed adequately with a combination of nondrug and drug therapies—increasing fluid and salt intake, wearing thigh-high stockings, and taking mineralocorticoids and vasoconstrictors.[44,46]

> ✓ **QUICK CHECK 24-2**
> 1. What are the major risk factors for hypertension?
> 2. Summarize the pathophysiology of primary hypertension.
> 3. What is malignant hypertension?
> 4. What are the causes of orthostatic hypotension?

Aneurysm

An **aneurysm** is a localized dilation or outpouching of a vessel wall or cardiac chamber (Figure 24-5). The law of Laplace (discussed in detail in Chapter 23) can provide an understanding of the hemodynamics of an aneurysm. True aneurysms involve all three layers of the arterial wall and are best described as a weakening of the vessel wall (Figure 24-6, *A*). Most are fusiform and circumferential, whereas *saccular aneurysms* are basically spherical in shape. False aneurysm is an extravascular hematoma that communicates with the intravascular space. A common cause of this type of lesion is a leak between a vascular graft and a natural artery.

Aneurysms most commonly occur in the thoracic or abdominal aorta. The aorta is particularly susceptible to aneurysm formation because of constant stress on the vessel wall and the absence of penetrating vasa vasorum in the media layer. Genetic and environmental risk factors (such as smoking and diet) are implicated in the pathogenesis of aortic aneurysms.[47] Atherosclerosis is the most common cause of arterial aneurysms because plaque formation erodes the vessel wall and contributes to inflammation and release of proteinases that can further weaken the vessel. Hypertension also contributes to aneurysm formation by increasing wall stress. Collagen-vascular disorders (e.g., Marfan syndrome), syphilis, and other infections that affect arterial walls also can cause aneurysms.

Cardiac aneurysms most commonly form after myocardial infarction when intraventricular tension stretches the noncontracting infarcted muscle. The stretching produces infarct expansion, a weak and thin layer of necrotic muscle, and fibrous tissue that bulges with each systole.

Clinical manifestations depend on where the aneurysm is located. Aortic aneurysms often are asymptomatic until they rupture, and then cause severe pain and hypotension. Thoracic aortic aneurysms can cause dysphagia (difficulty swallowing) and dyspnea (breathlessness). An aneurysm that impairs flow to an extremity causes symptoms of ischemia. Cerebral aneurysms, which often occur in the circle of Willis, are associated with signs and symptoms of increased intracranial pressure. Signs and symptoms of stroke occur when cerebral aneurysms leak. (Cerebral aneurysms are described in Chapter 16.) Aneurysms in the heart present with dysrhythmias, heart failure, and embolism of clots to the brain or other vital organs.

FIGURE 24-5 **Aneurysm.** A three-dimensional CT scan shows the aneurysm *(A)* involves the ascending thoracic aorta. *D,* Descending aorta; *LV,* left ventricle.

FIGURE 24-6 Longitudinal Sections Showing Types of Aneurysms. A, The fusiform circumferential and fusiform saccular aneurysms are true aneurysms, caused by weakening of the vessel wall. False and saccular aneurysms involve a break in the vessel wall, usually caused by trauma. **B,** Dissecting aneurysm of thoracic aorta *(arrow).* (**B** from Damjanov I, Linder J, editors: *Anderson's pathology,* ed 10, St Louis, 1996, Mosby.)

Aortic aneurysms can be complicated by the acute aortic syndromes, which include aortic dissection, hemorrhage into the vessel wall, or vessel rupture. Dissection of the layers of the arterial wall occurs when there is a tear in the intima and blood enters the wall of the artery (see Figure 24-6, *B*). Dissections can involve any part of the aorta (ascending, arch, or descending) and can disrupt flow through arterial branches, thus creating a surgical emergency.

The diagnosis of an aneurysm is usually confirmed by ultrasonography, computed tomography, magnetic resonance imaging, or angiography. Medical treatment is indicated for slow-growing aortic aneurysms, particularly in early stages, and includes cessation of smoking, reduction of blood pressure and blood volume, and implementation of β-adrenergic blockade. For those aneurysms that are dilating rapidly or have become large, surgical treatment is indicated and usually includes replacement with a prosthetic graft. Endovascular surgical techniques are commonly used for aneurysm repair and management of acute aortic rupture.[48]

Thrombus Formation

As in venous thrombosis, arterial thrombi tend to develop when intravascular conditions promote activation of coagulation, or when there is stasis of blood flow. These conditions include those in which there is intimal irritation or roughening (such as in surgical procedures), inflammation, traumatic injury, infection, low blood pressures, or obstructions that cause blood stasis and pooling within the vessels. (Mechanisms of coagulation are described in Chapter 20.) Inflammation of the endothelium leads to activation of the clotting cascade, causing platelets to adhere readily. An anatomic change in an artery (such as an aneurysm) can contribute to thrombus formation, particularly if the change results in a pooling of arterial blood. Thrombi also form on heart valves altered by calcification or bacterial vegetation. Valvular thrombi are most commonly associated with inflammation of the endocardium (endocarditis) and rheumatic heart disease. Widespread arterial thrombus formation can occur in shock, particularly shock resulting from septicemia. In septic shock, systemic inflammation activates the intrinsic and extrinsic pathways of coagulation, resulting in microvascular thrombosis throughout the systemic arterial circulation.

Arterial thrombi pose two potential threats to the circulation. First, the thrombus may grow large enough to occlude the artery, causing ischemia in tissue supplied by the artery. Second, the thrombus may dislodge, becoming a thromboembolus that travels through the vascular system until it occludes flow into a distal systemic vascular bed.

Diagnosis of arterial thrombi is usually accomplished through the use of Doppler ultrasonography and angiography. Pharmacologic treatment involves the administration of heparin, warfarin derivatives, thrombin inhibitors, or thrombolytics. A balloon-tipped catheter also can be used to remove or compress an arterial thrombus. Various combinations of drug and catheter therapies are sometimes used concurrently.

Embolism

Embolism is the obstruction of a vessel by an **embolus**—a bolus of matter circulating in the bloodstream. The embolus may consist of a dislodged thrombus; an air bubble; an aggregate of amniotic fluid; an aggregate of fat, bacteria, or cancer cells; or a foreign substance. An embolus travels in the bloodstream until it reaches a vessel through which it cannot pass. No matter how tiny it is, an embolus will eventually lodge in a systemic or pulmonary vessel determined by its source. Pulmonary emboli originate on the venous side (mostly from the deep veins of the legs) of the systemic circulation or in the right heart; arterial emboli most commonly originate in the left heart and are

TABLE 24-3	**Types of Emboli**
Type	**Characteristics**
Arteries	
Arterial thromboembolism	Dislodged thrombus; source is usually from heart; most common sites of obstruction are lower extremities (femoral and popliteal arteries), coronary arteries, and cerebral vasculature
Veins	
Venous thromboembolism	Dislodged thrombus; source is usually from lower extremities; obstructs branches of pulmonary artery
Air embolism	Bolus of air displaces blood in vasculature; source usually room air entering circulation through IV lines; trauma to chest also may allow air from lungs to enter vascular space
Amniotic fluid embolism	Bolus of amniotic fluid; extensive intra-abdominal pressure attending labor and delivery can force amniotic fluid into bloodstream of mother; introduces antigens, cells, and protein aggregates that trigger inflammation, coagulation, and immune responses
Bacterial embolism	Aggregates of bacteria in bloodstream; source is subacute bacterial endocarditis or abscess
Fat embolism	Globules of fat floating in bloodstream associated with trauma to long bones; lungs in particular are affected
Foreign matter	Small particles or fibers introduced during trauma or through an IV or intra-arterial line; coagulation cascade is initiated and thromboemboli form around particles

associated with thrombi after myocardial infarction, valvular disease, left heart failure, endocarditis, and dysrhythmias.

Embolism causes ischemia or infarction in tissues distal to the obstruction, producing organ dysfunction and pain. Infarction and subsequent necrosis of a central organ are life-threatening. For example, occlusion of a coronary artery will cause a myocardial infarction, whereas occlusion of a cerebral artery causes a stroke (see Chapter 16). The types of emboli are summarized in Table 24-3.

> ✓ **QUICK CHECK 24-3**
> 1. How does the law of Laplace function in aneurysms?
> 2. What is a thrombus?
> 3. Why are emboli dangerous?

Peripheral Vascular Disease
Thromboangiitis Obliterans (Buerger Disease)

Thromboangiitis obliterans (Buerger disease) is an inflammatory disease of the peripheral arteries. It is strongly associated with smoking. Thromboangiitis obliterans is an autoimmune condition characterized by the formation of thrombi filled with inflammatory and immune cells.[49] Inflammatory cytokines and toxic oxygen free radicals contribute to accompanying vasospasm.[50] Over time, these thrombi become organized and fibrotic and result in permanent occlusion and obliteration of portions of small- and medium-sized arteries in the feet and sometimes in the hands. Although collateral vessels develop in Buerger disease, they are inadequate to supply the extremities with blood. These collateral vessels have a characteristic corkscrew shape, thought to be a result of dilated vasa vasorum in the affected artery.

The chief symptom of thromboangiitis obliterans is pain and tenderness of the affected part, usually affecting more than one extremity. Clinical manifestations are caused by sluggish blood flow and include rubor (redness of the skin), which is caused by dilated capillaries under the skin, and cyanosis, which is caused by tissue ischemia. Chronic ischemia causes the skin to thin and become shiny and the nails to become thickened and malformed. In advanced disease, profound ischemia of the extremities resulting from vessel obliteration can cause gangrene necessitating amputation. Buerger disease has also been associated with cerebrovascular disease (stroke), mesenteric disease, and rheumatic symptoms (joint pain).

Diagnosis of thromboangiitis obliterans is made by identification of the following common features—age <45 years, smoking history, evidence of peripheral ischemia—and by exclusion of other causes of arterial insufficiency. The most important part of treatment is cessation of cigarette smoking. If the person continues to smoke, the likelihood of recurrence of the disease and gangrene requiring amputation is high. Other measures are aimed at improving circulation to the foot or hand. Vasodilators are prescribed to alleviate vasospasm, and the individual receives instruction in exercises that use gravity to improve blood flow.

Raynaud Phenomenon

Raynaud phenomenon is characterized by attacks of vasospasm in the small arteries and arterioles of the fingers and, less commonly, the toes. Primary Raynaud phenomenon is a common primary vasospastic disorder of unknown origin. Secondary Raynaud phenomenon is associated with systemic diseases, particularly collagen vascular disease (scleroderma), vasculitis, malignancy, pulmonary hypertension, chemotherapy, cocaine use, hypothyroidism, thoracic outlet syndrome, trauma, serum sickness, or long-term exposure to environmental conditions such as cold temperatures or vibrating machinery in the workplace. Blood vessels in affected individuals demonstrate endothelial dysfunction with an imbalance in endothelium-derived vasodilators (e.g., nitric oxide) and vasoconstrictors (e.g., endothelin-1).[51] Platelet activation also may play a role, and autoantibodies have been identified in some individuals. It tends to affect young women and is characterized by vasospastic attacks triggered by brief exposure to cold, vibration, or emotional stress. Genetic predisposition may play a role in its development.

The clinical manifestations of the vasospastic attacks of either disorder are changes in skin color and sensation caused by ischemia. Vasospasm occurs with varying frequency and severity and causes pallor, numbness, and the sensation of coldness in the digits. Attacks tend to be bilateral, and manifestations usually begin at the tips of the digits and progress to the proximal phalanges. Sluggish blood flow resulting from ischemia may cause the skin to appear cyanotic. Rubor, throbbing pain, and paresthesias follow as blood flow returns. Skin color returns to normal after the attack, but frequent, prolonged attacks interfere with cellular metabolism, causing the skin of the fingertips to thicken and the nails to become brittle. In severe, chronic Raynaud phenomenon, ischemia can eventually cause ulceration and gangrene.

Once evident, the clinical manifestations confirm the diagnosis of Raynaud phenomenon; however, nailfold capillaroscopy is a more sensitive method of diagnosis and can improve management and follow-up of individuals with associated collagen-vascular disorders.[52] Treatment for Raynaud phenomenon consists of removing the stimulus or treating the primary disease process. Treatment of Raynaud phenomenon begins with avoidance of stimuli that trigger attacks (e.g., cold temperatures, emotional stress) and cessation of cigarette smoking to eliminate the vasoconstricting effects of nicotine. If attacks of vasospasm become frequent or prolonged, vasodilators, such as calcium channel blockers, nitric oxide agonists, alpha-blockers, prostaglandin analogs, or endothelin antagonists, are administered.[51] Sympathectomy may be indicated in severe cases, but may not be effective. If ischemia leads to ulceration and gangrene, amputation may be necessary.

> ✔ **QUICK CHECK 24-4**
> 1. What is Buerger disease, and why does it occur?
> 2. Compare the physical manifestations of Buerger disease and Raynaud phenomenon.

Atherosclerosis

Arteriosclerosis is a condition characterized by thickening and hardening of the vessel wall. Atherosclerosis is a form of arteriosclerosis that is caused by the accumulation of lipid-laden macrophages within the arterial wall, which leads to the formation of a lesion called a plaque. Atherosclerosis is not a single disease entity but rather a pathologic process that can affect vascular systems throughout the body, resulting in ischemic syndromes that can vary widely in their severity and clinical manifestations. It is the leading cause of coronary artery and cerebrovascular disease. (Atherosclerosis of the coronary arteries is described later in this chapter, and atherosclerosis of the cerebral arteries is described in Chapter 16.)

PATHOPHYSIOLOGY Atherosclerosis begins with injury to the endothelial cells that line artery walls. Pathologically, the lesions progress from endothelial injury and dysfunction to fatty streak to fibrotic plaque to complicated lesion (Figure 24-7). Possible causes of endothelial injury include the common risk factors for atherosclerosis, such as smoking, hypertension, diabetes, increased levels of low-density lipoprotein (LDL), decreased levels of high-density lipoprotein (HDL), and autoimmunity. Other "nontraditional" risk factors include increased serum markers for inflammation and thrombosis (such as high-sensitivity C-reactive protein [hs-CRP], troponin I, adipokines, infection, and air pollution). These risk factors are discussed in more detail in the following section on coronary artery disease (see p. 610).

Injured endothelial cells become inflamed. Inflammation plays a fundamental role in mediating the steps in the initiation and progression of atherogenesis.[53] Inflamed endothelial cells cannot make normal amounts of antithrombic and vasodilating cytokines. Evidence is accumulating that microRNAs (short pieces of RNA that regulate posttranscriptional gene expression) are activated by many of the risk factors for atherosclerosis and impact endothelial cell responses to injury.[54]

The next step in atherogenesis occurs when inflamed endothelial cells express adhesion molecules that bind macrophages and other inflammatory and immune cells (Figure 24-8). Macrophages are activated by binding to damage-associated molecular patterns (DAMPs) released from injured cells, and release numerous inflammatory cytokines (e.g., tumor necrosis factor-alpha [TNF-α], interferons, interleukins, and C-reactive protein) and enzymes that further injure the vessel wall.[53,55] Toxic oxygen free radicals generated by the inflammatory process cause oxidation (i.e., addition of oxygen) of LDL that has accumulated in the vessel intima. Hyperlipidemia, diabetes, smoking, and hypertension contribute to LDL oxidation and its accumulation in the vessel wall.[56] Oxidized LDL causes additional adhesion molecule expression with the recruitment of monocytes that differentiate into macrophages. These macrophages penetrate into the intima, where

**Damaged endothelium:
Chronic endothelial injury**

- Hypertension
- Smoking
- Hyperlipidemia
- Hyperhomocysteinemia
- Hemodynamic factors
- Toxins
- Viruses
- Immune reactions

Endothelium
Tunica intima
Tunic media
Adventitia

Monocyte
Damaged endothelium
Platelets
Macrophage
Lipids

A

Response to injury

Fatty streak

Platelets attach to endothelium
Foamy macrophage ingesting lipids
Migration of smooth muscle into the intima
Lipid accumulation
Fibroblast

B

Fibrous plaque

Collagen cap (fibrous tissue)
Fibroblast
Fissure in plaque
Lipid pool

C

Complicated lesion

Thrombus
Thinning collagen cap
Lipid pool

D

FIGURE 24-7 Progression of Atherosclerosis. A, Damaged endothelium. **B,** Diagram of fatty streak and lipid core formation (see Figure 24-8 for a diagram of oxidized low-density lipoprotein [LDL]). **C,** Diagram of fibrous plaque. Raised plaques are visible: some are yellow; others are white. **D,** Diagram of complicated lesion; thrombus is red; collagen is blue. Plaque is complicated by red thrombus deposition.

FIGURE 24-8 Low-Density Lipoprotein Oxidation. (1) Low-density lipoprotein *(LDL)* enters the arterial intima through an intact endothelium. In hypercholesterolemia, the influx of LDL exceeds the eliminating capacity and an extracellular pool of LDL is formed. This is enhanced by association of LDL with the extracellular matrix. **(2)** Intimal LDL is oxidized through the action of oxygen free radicals formed by enzymatic or nonenzymatic reactions. **(3)** This generates proinflammatory lipids that induce endothelial expression of the adhesion molecule; vascular cell adhesion molecule-1 activates complement and stimulates chemokine secretion. All of these factors cause adhesion and entry of mononuclear leukocytes, particularly monocytes and T lymphocytes. **(4)** Monocytes differentiate into macrophages. Macrophages up-regulate and internalize oxidized LDL and transform into foam cells. Macrophage update of oxidized LDL also leads to presentation of its fragments to antigen-specific T cells. **(5)** This induces an autoimmune reaction that leads to production of proinflammatory cytokines. Such cytokines include interferon-gamma, tumor necrosis factor alpha, and interleukin-1, which act on endothelial cells to stimulate expression of adhesion molecules and procoagulant activity; on macrophages to activate proteases, endocytosis, nitric oxide *(NO)*, and cytokines; and on smooth muscle cells *(SMCs)* to induce NO production and inhibit growth, collagen, and actin expression. (Modified from Crawford MH et al: *Cardiology,* ed 3, London, 2010, Mosby.)

FIGURE 24-9 Histologic features of atheromatous plaque in the coronary artery. A, Overall architecture demonstrating fibrous cap *(F)* and a central necrotic (largely lipid) core *(C)*. The lumen *(L)* has been moderately narrowed. Note that a segment of the wall is plaque free *(arrow)*, so that there is an eccentric lesion. In this section, collagen has been stained blue (Masson's trichrome stain). **B,** Higher power photograph of a section of the plaque shown in **A,** stained for elastin *(black)*, demonstrating that the internal and external elastic membranes are destroyed and the media of the artery is thinned under the most advanced plaque *(arrow)*. **C,** Higher magnification photomicrograph at the junction of the fibrous cap and core, showing scattered inflammatory cells, calcification *(arrowhead)*, and neovascularization *(small arrows)*. (From Kumar V et al: Robbins Basic Pathology, ed 9, St Louis, 2007, Saunders.)

they engulf oxidized LDL. These lipid-laden macrophages are now called **foam cells,** and when they accumulate in significant amounts, they form a lesion called a **fatty streak** (Figures 24-8 and 24-9). These lesions can be found in the walls of arteries of most people, even young children. Once formed, fatty streaks produce more toxic oxygen free radicals, recruit T cells leading to autoimmunity, and secrete additional inflammatory mediators resulting in progressive damage to the vessel wall.[53]

Macrophages also release growth factors that stimulate smooth muscle cell proliferation.[55] Smooth muscle cells in the region of endothelial injury proliferate, produce collagen, and migrate over the fatty streak, forming a fibrous plaque (see Figure 24-9). The fibrous plaque may calcify, protrude into the vessel lumen, and obstruct blood flow to distal tissues (especially during exercise), which may cause symptoms (e.g., angina or intermittent claudication).

Many plaques, however, are "unstable," meaning they are prone to rupture even before they affect blood flow significantly and are clinically silent until they rupture. Plaque rupture occurs because of innate and adaptive immune responses to tissue injury including activation of proteinases (matrix metalloproteinases and cathepsins) and apoptosis of cells within the plaque, and can be accelerated by bleeding within the lesion (plaque hemorrhage).[53] Plaques that have ruptured are called complicated plaques. Once rupture occurs, exposure of underlying tissue results in platelet adhesion, initiation of the clotting cascade, and rapid thrombus formation. The thrombus may suddenly occlude the affected vessel, resulting in ischemia and infarction. Aspirin or other antithrombotic agents are used to prevent this complication of atherosclerotic disease.

CLINICAL MANIFESTATIONS Atherosclerosis presents with symptoms and signs that result from inadequate perfusion of tissues because of obstruction of the vessels that supply them. Partial vessel obstruction may lead to transient ischemic events, often associated with exercise or stress. As the lesion becomes complicated, increasing obstruction with superimposed thrombosis may result in tissue infarction. Obstruction of peripheral arteries can cause significant pain and disability. Coronary artery disease (CAD) caused by atherosclerosis is the major cause of myocardial ischemia and is one of the most important health issues in the United States. Atherosclerotic obstruction of the vessels supplying the brain is the major cause of stroke. Similarly, any part of the body may become ischemic when its blood supply is compromised by atherosclerotic lesions. Often, more than one vessel will become involved with this disease process such that an individual may present with symptoms from several ischemic tissues at the same time, and disease in one area may indicate that the individual is at risk for ischemic complications elsewhere.

EVALUATION AND TREATMENT In evaluating individuals for the presence of atherosclerosis, obtaining a complete health history (including risk factors and symptoms of ischemia) is essential. Physical examination may reveal arterial bruits and evidence of decreased blood flow to tissues. Laboratory data that include measurement of levels of lipids, blood glucose, and hs-CRP are also indicated. Judicious use of x-ray films, electrocardiography, ultrasonography, nuclear scanning, CT, MRI, and angiography may be necessary to identify affected vessels, particularly coronary vessels.[57] New modalities aimed at identifying vulnerable plaques before the rupture are being evaluated.[58]

Current management of atherosclerosis is focused on detection and treatment of preclinical lesions with drugs aimed at stabilizing and reversing plaques before they rupture. Once a lesion obstructs blood flow, the primary goal in the management of atherosclerosis is to restore adequate blood flow to the affected tissues. If an individual has presented with acute ischemia (e.g., myocardial infarction, stroke), interventions are specific to the diseased area (discussed further under those topics). In situations in which the disease process does not require immediate intervention, management focuses on reduction of risk factors and prevention of plaque progression. This includes implementation of an exercise program, cessation of smoking, and control of hypertension and diabetes where appropriate while reducing LDL cholesterol level by diet or medications, or both. Management of atherosclerotic risk factors is discussed further starting on p. 614.

Peripheral Artery Disease

Peripheral artery disease (PAD) refers to atherosclerotic disease of arteries that perfuse the limbs, especially the lower extremities. PAD affects an estimated 8.5 million Americans aged >40 years.[10] The risk factors for PAD are the same as those previously described for atherosclerosis, but it is especially prevalent in elderly individuals with diabetes and has a very strong link with smoking.[59]

Lower extremity ischemia resulting from arterial obstruction in PAD can be gradual or acute. In most individuals, gradually increasing obstruction to arterial blood flow to the legs caused by atherosclerosis in the iliofemoral vessels can result in pain with ambulation called intermittent claudication. If a thrombus forms over the atherosclerotic lesion, complete obstruction of blood flow can occur acutely, causing severe pain, loss of pulses, and skin color changes in the affected extremity.

Although individuals with PAD have an increased mortality, more than two thirds of adults with PAD are asymptomatic even in severe cases.[10] Therefore evaluation for PAD requires a careful history and physical examination that focuses on finding evidence of atherosclerotic disease (e.g., bruits), determining a difference in blood pressure measured at the ankle versus the arm (ankle-brachial index), and measuring blood flow using noninvasive Doppler.[60] Treatment includes risk factor reduction (smoking cessation and treatment of diabetes, hypertension, and dyslipidemia) and antiplatelet therapy. Symptomatic PAD should be managed with vasodilators in combination with antiplatelet or antithrombotic medications (aspirin, cilostazol, ticlopidine, or clopidogrel), and cholesterol-lowering medications.[61] Aerobic exercise is a crucial part of therapy.[10] If acute or refractory symptoms occur, emergent percutaneous or surgical revascularization may be indicated. Newer treatment modalities that are being explored include autologous stem cell therapies and angiogenesis.[62]

Coronary Artery Disease, Myocardial Ischemia, and Acute Coronary Syndromes

Coronary artery disease, myocardial ischemia, and myocardial infarction form a pathophysiologic continuum that impairs the pumping ability of the heart by depriving the heart muscle of blood-borne oxygen and nutrients. The earliest lesions of the continuum are those of coronary artery disease (CAD), which is usually caused by atherosclerosis (see Figure 24-9). CAD can diminish the myocardial blood supply until deprivation impairs myocardial metabolism enough to cause ischemia, a local state in which the cells are temporarily deprived of blood supply. The cells remain alive but cannot function normally. Persistent ischemia or the complete occlusion of a coronary artery causes the acute coronary syndromes including infarction, or irreversible myocardial damage. Infarction constitutes the potentially fatal event known as a *heart attack*.

Development of Coronary Artery Disease

Coronary artery disease affects approximately 6.5% of people in the United States, with an estimated 122,000 deaths caused by myocardial infarction each year.[10] Fortunately, the incidence and mortality statistics for CAD have been decreasing over the past 15 years because of more aggressive recognition, prevention, and treatment. Risk factors for CAD are the same as those for atherosclerosis and can be categorized as conventional (major) versus nontraditional (novel) and as modifiable versus nonmodifiable. The plethora of new information obtained about the conventional risk factors has markedly improved prevention and management of CAD. In addition, nontraditional risk factors have been identified that have provided insight into the pathogenesis of CAD and may lead to more effective interventions in the future.

Conventional or major risk factors for CAD that are nonmodifiable include (1) advanced age, (2) male gender or women after menopause, and (3) family history. Aging and menopause are associated with increased exposure to risk factors and poor endothelial healing. Family history may contribute to CAD through genetics and shared environmental exposures. Many gene polymorphisms have been associated with CAD and its risk factors. Modifiable major risks include (1) dyslipidemia, (2) hypertension, (3) cigarette smoking, (4) diabetes and insulin resistance, (5) obesity, (6) sedentary lifestyle, and (7) atherogenic diet. Fortunately, modification of these factors can dramatically reduce the risk for CAD.[63]

Dyslipidemia. The link between CAD and abnormal levels of lipoproteins is well documented. The term lipoprotein refers to lipids, phospholipids, cholesterol, and triglycerides bound to carrier proteins. Lipids (cholesterol in particular) are required by most cells for the manufacture and repair of plasma membranes. Cholesterol is also a necessary component for the manufacture of such essential substances as bile acids and steroid hormones. Although cholesterol can easily be obtained from dietary fat intake, most body cells also can manufacture cholesterol.

The cycle of lipid metabolism is complex. Dietary fat is packaged into particles known as chylomicrons in the small intestine. Chylomicrons are required for absorption of fat and function by transporting exogenous lipid from the intestine to the liver and peripheral cells. Chylomicrons are the least dense of the lipoproteins and primarily contain triglyceride. Some of the triglyceride may be removed and either stored by adipose tissue or used by muscle as an energy source. The chylomicron remnants, composed mainly of cholesterol, are taken up by the liver. A series of chemical reactions in the liver results in the production of several lipoproteins that vary in density and function. These include very-low-density lipoproteins (VLDLs), primarily triglyceride and protein; low-density lipoproteins (LDLs), mostly cholesterol and protein; and high-density lipoproteins (HDLs), mainly phospholipids and protein.

Dyslipidemia (or dyslipoproteinemia) refers to abnormal concentrations of serum lipoproteins. It has been defined by the Third Report of the National Cholesterol Education Program[64] (Table 24-4), although more recent guidelines place less emphasis on specific serum lipoprotein levels.[65] It is estimated that nearly half of the U.S. population has some form of dyslipidemia, especially among white and Asian populations.[10] These abnormalities are the result of a combination of genetic and dietary factors. Primary or familial dyslipoproteinemias result from genetic defects that cause abnormalities in lipid-metabolizing enzymes and abnormal cellular lipid receptors. Secondary causes of dyslipidemia include the existence of several common systemic disorders, such as diabetes, hypothyroidism, pancreatitis, and renal nephrosis, as well as the use of certain medications, such as some diuretics, glucocorticoids, interferons, and antiretrovirals.

LDL is responsible for the delivery of cholesterol to the tissues, and an increased serum concentration of LDL is a strong indicator of coronary risk. Serum levels of LDL are normally controlled by hepatic receptors that bind LDL and limit liver synthesis of this lipoprotein. High dietary intake of cholesterol and saturated fats, in combination with a genetic predisposition to accumulations of LDL in the serum (e.g., dysfunction of the hepatic LDL receptor), result in high levels of LDL in the bloodstream. LDL migration into the vessel wall, oxidation, and phagocytosis by macrophages are key steps in the pathogenesis of atherosclerosis (see Figure 24-8). LDL also plays a role in endothelial injury, inflammation, and immune responses that have been identified as being important in atherogenesis.[56] The term *LDL* actually describes several types of LDL molecules. Measurement of LDL subfractions allows for a better prediction of coronary risk. For example, LDL-C measurements allow for the detection of the small, dense LDL particles that are the most atherogenic, and apolipoprotein B (structural protein found in both LDL and VLDL) levels are a very strong predictor of future coronary events. New guidelines from the American Heart Association and the American College of Cardiology focus on treating dyslipidemia in the context of other risk factors[65] (see *Health Alert:* New Insights and Guidelines into the Management of Dyslipidemia for the Prevention of Coronary Artery Disease).

Low levels of HDL cholesterol also are a strong indicator of coronary risk. HDL is responsible for "reverse cholesterol transport," which returns excess cholesterol from the tissues to the liver for processing or elimination in the bile. HDL also participates in endothelial repair and decreases thrombosis. It can be fractionated into several particle densities (HDL-2 and HDL-3) that have different effects on vascular function. Exercise, weight loss, fish oil consumption, and moderate alcohol use result in modest increases in HDL level. Despite the wealth of evidence that HDL plays an important role in preventing atherosclerotic coronary disease, studies have suggested that raising overall levels of HDL is not adequate to prevent cardiovascular disease. Niacin and fibrates are drugs that can cause modest increases in HDL levels that are not correlated with an improvement in cardiovascular risk in individuals without documented coronary disease (primary prevention). Drugs that are aimed specifically at increasing HDL levels include recombinant apolipoprotein A-I (ApoA-I) mimetics, thiazolidinediones (used to treat diabetes), and cholesteryl ester transfer protein inhibitors, but they have not been shown to be effective in preventing heart disease. Recent studies suggest that it is not the serum levels of HDL that are key to determining CAD risk, but rather HDL functionality, which is harder to measure.[66,67]

Other lipoproteins associated with increased cardiovascular risk include elevated levels of serum VLDLs (triglycerides) and increased lipoprotein(a) levels. Triglycerides are associated with an increased risk for CAD, especially in combination with other risk factors such as diabetes. Lipoprotein(a) (Lp[a]) is a genetically determined molecular complex between LDL and a serum glycoprotein called apolipoprotein

TABLE 24-4 Criteria for Dyslipidemia*

	Optimal	Near-Optimal	Desirable	Low	Borderline	High	Very High
Total cholesterol			<200		200-239	≥240	
LDL	<100	100-129			130-159	160-189	≥190
Triglycerides			<150		150-199	200-499	≥500
HDL				<40		≥60	

*All units are mg/dl.

Data from Expert Panel on Detection, Evaluation, and Treatment of High Blood Cholesterol in Adults, *JAMA* 285:2486-2497, 2001.

HEALTH ALERT

New Insights and Guidelines into the Management of Dyslipidemia for the Prevention of Coronary Artery Disease

Despite a wealth of evidence that lowering LDL levels decreases the risk for coronary events in individuals with known CAD (secondary prevention), primary prevention of cardiovascular disease through pharmacologic modulation of lipid levels remains controversial. Although many clinical trials and meta-analyses have shown a reduction in primary cardiovascular events with the use of the 3-hydroxy-3-methyl-glutaryl-CoA (HMG-CoA) reductase drugs (statins) in men, other studies have provided mixed results, especially in women. In addition, statin use is linked to several significant complications including muscle soreness, elevation in liver enzymes, and diabetes. There is concern that these complications are being underreported, especially in pharmaceutical company–sponsored research reports. In 2013 the Cochrane Database and the American Heart Association/American College of Cardiology Expert Blood Cholesterol Panel released two comprehensive analyses that documented the effectiveness of statins for primary prevention of coronary events. New guidelines help to weigh the benefits versus risks and guide the intensity of therapy by linking recommendations for statin use with the presence of other risk factors, such as diabetes and age. In contrast, efforts at reducing cardiovascular risk through pharmacologically increased high-density lipoprotein (HDL) levels have failed to demonstrate benefit. New information suggests that the functionality of HDL and its subparticles is more important to reducing risk than is the serum level, and studies are now underway to explore how HDL might be functionality optimized. It is clear from these studies that, despite decades of research, there is still much work needed to fully understand the proper role of medications in the prevention of cardiovascular disease. In the meantime, improved diet and exercise remain the foundation for reducing coronary risk.

Data from Feig JE et al: *Circ Res* 114(1):205-213, 2014; Randolph GJ, Miller NE: *J Clin Invest* 124(3):929-935, 2014; Rosenson RS et al: *Circulation* 128(11):1256-1267, 2013; Stone NJ et al: *Circulation* 2013 Nov 12 [Epub ahead of print]; Taylor F et al: *Cochrane Database Syst Rev* 1:CD004816, 2013.

A and has been shown to be an important risk factor for atherosclerosis, especially in women.

Hypertension. Hypertension is responsible for a twofold to threefold increased risk of atherosclerotic cardiovascular disease. It contributes to endothelial injury, a key step in atherogenesis (see p. 607). It also can cause myocardial hypertrophy, which increases myocardial demand for coronary flow. Overactivity of the SNS and RAAS commonly found in hypertension also contributes to the genesis of CAD.

Cigarette smoking. Both direct and passive (environmental) smoking increase the risk of CAD. Smoking has a direct effect on endothelial cells and the generation of oxygen free radicals that contribute to atherogenesis.[68] Nicotine stimulates the release of catecholamines (epinephrine and norepinephrine), which increase heart rate and peripheral vascular constriction. As a result, blood pressure increases, as do cardiac workload and oxygen demand. Cigarette smoking is associated with an increase in LDL levels and a decrease in HDL levels. The risk of CAD increases with heavy smoking and decreases when smoking is stopped.

Diabetes mellitus. Insulin resistance and diabetes mellitus are extremely important risk factors for CAD. Insulin resistance and diabetes have multiple effects on the cardiovascular system including damage to the endothelium, thickening of the vessel wall, increased inflammation, increased thrombosis, glycation of vascular proteins,

and decreased production of endothelial-derived vasodilators, such as nitric oxide.[69] Diabetes also is associated with dyslipidemia (see Chapter 19). Good diabetic control is linked to reduced risk for CAD.

Obesity/sedentary lifestyle. It is estimated that 65% of the adult population in the United States is overweight or obese, and an estimated 47 million U.S. residents have a combination of obesity, dyslipidemia, hypertension, and insulin resistance, called the **metabolic syndrome**, which is associated with an even higher risk for CAD events.[10] Abdominal obesity has the strongest link with increased CAD risk and is related to inflammation, insulin resistance, decreased HDL level, increased blood pressure, and fewer changes in hormones called adipokines (leptin and adiponectin).[70] A sedentary lifestyle not only increases the risk of obesity but also has an independent effect on increasing CAD risk. Physical activity and weight loss offer substantial reductions in risk factors for CAD.[71] There is emerging evidence that bariatric surgery procedures, such as gastric bypass, can provide sustained improvement in risk factors for cardiovascular disease, such as hypertension, dyslipidemia, and diabetes.[72]

Atherogenic diet. Diet plays a complex role in atherogenic risk. Diets high in salt, fats, trans-fats, and carbohydrates have all been implicated. There are many recommendations regarding diet modification to reduce coronary risk; one of the most effective is called the Mediterranean Diet (see *Health Alert:* Mediterranean Diet).

HEALTH ALERT

Mediterranean Diet

A number of different kinds of studies—observational cohort, secondary prevention trial, and recent randomized intervention trials—show the Mediterranean diet patterns are associated with a reduced cardiovascular disease risk and cardiovascular events. The traditional Mediterranean diet is characterized by a high intake of olive oil, fruits, nuts, vegetables, and cereals; moderate intake of fish and poultry; low intake of dairy products, red meat, processed meats, and sweets; and moderate intake of wine consumed with meals.

A large prospective cohort study showed adherence to the Mediterranean diet was associated with a decrease in incidence of fatal and nonfatal coronary heart disease (CHD) in initially healthy middle-aged individuals. A recent large randomized trial (the Prevención con Dieta Mediterránea Study [PREDIMED]) among individuals at high cardiovascular risk showed that a Mediterranean diet supplemented with extra-virgin olive oil or nuts reduced the incidence of major cardiovascular events, especially stroke. The beneficial effects of the Mediterranean diet are hypothesized to include modulation of all of the following—inflammation and oxidative stress, glucose metabolism, lipid profile, and lipoprotein particle characteristics—and also favorable changes to the vascular endothelium. Additionally, effects may include a favorable interaction between diet and gene polymorphisms related to cardiovascular risk factors and events.

Data from Chiva-Blanch G et al: *Curr Atheroscler Rep* 16(10):446, 2014; deLorgeril M et al: *Circulation* 99:779-785, 1999; Estruch R et al: *N Engl J Med* 368:1279-1290, 2013; Kris-Etherton P et al: *Circulation* 103:1823-1825, 2001; Martinez-Gonzalez MA et al: *Nutr Metab Cardiovasc Dis* 21:237-244, 2011; Willett WC et al: *Am J Clin Nutr* 61(Suppl):1402S-1406S, 1995.

Nontraditional risk factors. Nontraditional, or novel, risk factors for CAD include increased serum markers for inflammation and thrombosis (troponin I, adipokines, infection, and air pollution). The amount of risk conferred by these relatively newly identified factors is still being explored.

FIGURE 24-10 Cycle of Ischemic Events.

Markers of inflammation and thrombosis. Of the numerous markers of inflammation that have been linked to an increase in CAD risk (hs-CRP, fibrinogen, protein C, plasminogen activator inhibitor), the relationship between serum levels of hs-CRP and CAD has been explored in the greatest depth. **High-sensitivity C-reactive protein (hs-CRP)** is a protein mostly synthesized in the liver and is used as an indirect measure of atherosclerotic plaque–related inflammation. An elevated serum level of hs-CRP is strongly correlated with an increased risk for coronary events,[73] but is a nonspecific measure of inflammation and may indicate the presence of other inflammatory conditions. The primary use of hs-CRP is as an aid to decision-making about pharmacologic interventions for individuals with other risk factors for coronary disease.[74] Other markers of inflammation associated with CAD include the erythrocyte sedimentation rate and concentrations of von Willebrand factor, interleukin-6, interleukin-18, tumor necrosis factor, fibrinogen, and CD 40 ligand. Interestingly, the long-term use of some anti-inflammatories, such as ibuprofen, has been linked to increased (rather than decreased) risk for CAD because of their potentiation of clotting in certain tissues.[75]

Troponin I. Troponin I (TnI) is a serum protein whose measurement is used as a sensitive and specific diagnostic test to help identify myocardial injury during acute coronary syndromes. Highly sensitive TnI assays are used in individuals without a history of CAD to assess risk for future CHD events, mortality, and heart failure.

Adipokines. Adipokines are a group of hormones released from adipose cells. Obesity causes increased levels of leptin, which is implicated in hypertension and diabetes, and decreased levels of adiponectin, which is a hormone that functions to protect the vascular endothelium and is anti-inflammatory.[76,77] Other adipokines also have been linked to inflammation in endothelial cells.[78] Weight loss, exercise, and healthy diet improve adipokine levels.

Infection. Infections with various microorganisms, including *Chlamydia pneumoniae, Helicobacter pylori,* and cytomegalovirus, have been linked to an increased risk for CAD, although cause and effect have not been proven. Periodontal disease also has been linked to an increased risk for CAD. One hypothesis is that systemic infection results in increased inflammation of vessels and, therefore, contributes to vascular disease. Unfortunately, the use of antibiotics for the prevention and treatment of CAD has not yielded consistently positive results.

Air pollution. Exposure to air pollution, especially roadway exposures, is strongly correlated with coronary risk. It is postulated that toxins in pollution contribute to macrophage activation, oxidation of LDL, thrombosis, and inflammation of vessel walls.[79]

Myocardial Ischemia

PATHOPHYSIOLOGY The coronary arteries normally supply blood flow sufficient to meet the demands of the myocardium as it labors under varying workloads. Oxygen is extracted from these vessels with maximal efficiency. If demand increases, healthy coronary arteries can dilate to increase the flow of oxygenated blood to the myocardium. Narrowing of a major coronary artery by more than 50% impairs blood flow enough to hamper cellular metabolism when myocardial demand increases.

Myocardial ischemia develops if the flow or oxygen content of coronary blood is insufficient to meet the metabolic demands of myocardial cells (Figure 24-10). Imbalances between coronary blood supply and myocardial demand can result from a number of conditions. The most common cause of decreased coronary blood flow and resultant myocardial ischemia is the formation of atherosclerotic plaques in the coronary circulation. As the plaque increases in size, it may partially occlude the vessel lumina, thus limiting coronary flow and causing ischemia especially during exercise. As discussed earlier in this chapter, some plaques are "unstable," meaning they are prone to ulceration or rupture. When this ulceration or rupture occurs, underlying tissues of the vessel wall are exposed, resulting in platelet adhesion and thrombus formation (see Figures 24-7 and 24-15). Thrombus formation can suddenly stop blood supply to the heart muscle, resulting in acute myocardial ischemia, and if the vessel obstruction cannot be reversed rapidly, ischemia will progress to infarction. Myocardial ischemia also can result from other causes of decreased blood and oxygen delivery to the myocardium, such as coronary spasm, hypotension, dysrhythmias, and decreased oxygen-carrying capacity of the blood (e.g., anemia, hypoxemia). Common causes of increased myocardial demand for blood include tachycardia, exercise, hypertension (hypertrophy), and valvular disease.

Myocardial cells become ischemic within 10 seconds of coronary occlusion, thus hampering pump function and depriving the myocardium of a glucose source necessary for aerobic metabolism. Anaerobic processes take over, and lactic acid accumulates. After several minutes, the heart cells lose the ability to contract and cardiac output decreases. Cardiac cells remain viable for approximately 20 minutes under ischemic conditions. If blood flow is restored, aerobic metabolism resumes, contractility is restored, and cellular repair begins. If perfusion is not restored, then myocardial infarction occurs (see Figure 24-10).

CLINICAL MANIFESTATIONS Individuals with reversible myocardial ischemia present clinically in several ways. Chronic coronary obstruction results in recurrent predictable chest pain called *stable angina*. Abnormal vasospasm of coronary vessels results in unpredictable chest pain called *Prinzmetal angina*. Myocardial ischemia that does not cause detectable symptoms is called *silent ischemia*.

1. **Stable angina pectoris.** Angina is chest pain caused by myocardial ischemia. Stable angina is caused by gradual luminal narrowing and hardening of the arterial walls, with associated inflammation, endothelial cell dysfunction, and a decrease in endogenous vasodilators. These changes are more prevalent in individuals with obesity, diabetes, and dyslipidemia.[80] Affected vessels cannot dilate in response to increased myocardial demand associated with physical exertion or emotional stress. With rest, blood flow is restored and necrosis of myocardial cells does not occur. Angina pectoris is typically experienced as transient substernal chest discomfort, ranging from a sensation of heaviness or pressure to moderately severe pain. Individuals often describe the sensation by clenching a fist over the left sternal border. The discomfort may be mistaken for indigestion. The pain is caused by the buildup of lactic acid or abnormal stretching of the ischemic myocardium that irritates myocardial nerve fibers. These afferent sympathetic fibers enter the spinal cord from levels C3 to T4, accounting for a variety of locations and radiation patterns of anginal pain. Discomfort may radiate to the neck, lower jaw, left arm, and left shoulder, or occasionally to the back or down the right arm. Pallor, diaphoresis, and dyspnea may be associated with the pain. The pain is usually relieved by rest and nitrates. However, myocardial ischemia in women may not present with typical anginal pain. Common symptoms in women include atypical chest pain, palpitations, sense of unease, and severe fatigue. In addition, it is estimated that half of women with stable angina do not have obstructive coronary artery disease, but rather have "microvascular angina" that results from vasoconstriction of small coronary arterioles deep in the myocardium[81] (see *Health Alert: Women and Microvascular Angina*).

2. **Prinzmetal angina.** Prinzmetal angina (also called variant angina) is chest pain attributable to transient ischemia of the myocardium that occurs unpredictably and often at rest. Pain is caused by vasospasm of one or more major coronary arteries with or without associated atherosclerosis. The pain often occurs at night during rapid eye movement sleep and may have a cyclic pattern of occurrence. The angina may result from decreased vagal activity, hyperactivity of the sympathetic nervous system, or decreased nitric oxide activity. Other causes include altered calcium channel function in arterial smooth muscle or impaired production or release of inflammatory mediators, such as serotonin, histamine, endothelin, or thromboxane.[82] Serum markers of inflammation, such as CRP and interleukin-6 (IL-6), are elevated in individuals with this form of angina. Prinzmetal angina is usually a benign condition, but can occasionally cause serious dysrhythmias, especially if treatment is withdrawn; therefore calcium channel blockers or long-acting nitrates, or both, should be continued even if clinical remission is achieved.[83]

3. **Silent ischemia** and **mental stress–induced ischemia.** Myocardial ischemia may not cause detectable symptoms such as angina. Ischemia can be totally asymptomatic and referred to as silent ischemia, or individuals may complain of fatigue, dyspnea, or a feeling of unease. Some individuals only have silent ischemia, and episodes of silent ischemia are common in individuals who also experience angina. One proposed mechanism for the absence of angina in silent myocardial ischemia is the presence of a global or regional abnormality in left ventricular sympathetic afferent innervation. The most common cause of autonomic dysfunction leading to silent ischemia is diabetes mellitus. Other causes include surgical denervation during coronary artery bypass grafting (CABG) or cardiac transplantation, or following ischemic local nerve injury by myocardial infarction. Also of interest is silent ischemia occurring in some individuals during mental stress (Figures 24-11 and 24-12). Chronic stress has been linked to an increase in the number of inflammatory cytokines and a hypercoagulable state that may contribute to acute ischemic events.[84,85] Silent ischemia can be detected by stress radionucleotide imaging. Detection and management of silent ischemia caused by coronary disease is important because it is an indicator of increased risk for serious cardiovascular events.[86]

EVALUATION AND TREATMENT Many individuals with reversible myocardial ischemia will have a normal physical examination between events. Physical examination of those experiencing myocardial ischemia may disclose rapid pulse rate or extra heart sounds (gallops or murmurs), and pulmonary congestion indicating impaired left ventricular function. The presence of xanthelasmas (small fat deposits) around the eyelids or arcus senilis of the eyes (a yellow lipid ring around the cornea) suggests severe dyslipidemia and possible atherosclerosis. The presence of peripheral or carotid artery bruits suggests probable atherosclerotic disease and increases the likelihood that CAD is present.

Electrocardiography is a critical tool for the diagnosis of myocardial ischemia. Ischemic cells distort the electrical impulses that are measured across the myocardium during an electrocardiogram (ECG). Because many individuals have normal ECGs when there is no pain,

---

HEALTH ALERT

Women and Microvascular Angina

More women in the United States die from coronary artery disease (CAD) and stroke than from all cancers combined, and women have a higher rate of CAD-related mortality than men. Women with myocardial ischemia often have either no symptoms or atypical symptoms, such as palpitations, anxiety, weakness, and fatigue. Additionally, many women with angina are found to have cardiac ischemia yet no evidence of obstructive coronary artery disease on cardiac catheterization, a condition sometimes called cardiac syndrome x. Evidence is accumulating that nearly half of women with myocardial ischemia suffer from coronary microvascular disease, a condition often called **microvascular angina (MVA)**. Small intramyocardial arterioles constrict in MVA, causing ischemic pain that is less predictable than with typical epicardial CAD. The pathophysiology is complex and still being elucidated, but there is strong evidence that endothelial dysfunction, decreased endogenous vasodilators, inflammation, changes in adipokines, and platelet activation are contributing factors. Managing MVA can be challenging; for example, women with this condition have less coronary microvascular dilation in response to nitrates than do those without MVA. Aggressive interventions to reduce modifiable risk factors for CAD are an important component of management, especially smoking cessation, exercise, and diabetes management. The combination of nonnitrate vasodilators, such as calcium channel blockers with HMG-CoA reductase inhibitors (statins), also has been shown to be effective in many women, and new drugs, such as ranolazine and ivabradine, have shown promise in the treatment of MVA.

Data from Arthur HM et al: *Can J Cardiol* S28:S42-S49, 2012; Ashley KE, Geraci SA: *South Med J* 106(7):427-433, 2013; Luo C et al: *Circulation* 7(1):43-48, 2014; Recio-Mayoral A et al: *JACC Cardiovas Imaging* 6(6):660-667, 2013; Russo G et al: *Cardiovas Drugs Ther* 27(3):229-234, 2013; Taqueti VR, Ridker PM: *JACC Cardiovas Imaging* 6(6):668-671, 2013; Zhang X et al: *Coron Artery Dis* 25(1):40-44, 2014; Zuchi C et al: *Int J Cardiol* 163(2):132-140, 2013.

FIGURE 24-11 Mental Stress and Angiogram of Coronary Arteries. A, Baseline. **B,** Transient total occlusion of left anterior descending branch of the left coronary artery after mental stress. **C,** After nitrates and nifedipine, artery reopened to same diameter as baseline. (Modified from Stern S, editor: *Silent myocardial ischemia*, St Louis, 1998, Mosby.)

FIGURE 24-12 Pathophysiologic Model of the Effects of Acute Stress as a Trigger of Cardiac Clinical Events. Acting via the central and autonomic nervous systems, stress can produce a cascade of physiologic responses that may lead to myocardial ischemia, especially in persons with coronary artery disease, potentially fatal dysrhythmia, plaque rupture, or coronary thrombosis. *LV,* Left ventricular; *MI,* myocardial infarction; *VF,* ventricular fibrillation; *VT,* ventricular tachycardia. (From Krantz DS et al: Mental stress as a trigger of myocardial ischemia and infarction. In Deedwania PC, Tofler GH, editors: *Triggers and timing of cardiac events,* ed 2, London, 1996, Saunders.)

diagnosis requires that an ECG be performed during an attack of angina or during exercise stress testing. The ST segment and the T wave segments of the ECG respectively correlate with ventricular contraction and relaxation (see Figure 23-10). Transient ST segment depression and T wave inversion are characteristic signs of ischemia that involves only the inner wall of the myocardium (subendocardial ischemia). ST elevation is indicative of ischemia involving the full myocardial wall (transmural ischemia) (Figure 24-13). The ECG tracings correlate with different parts of the myocardium and, therefore, can give some indication of which coronary artery is involved.

Stress radionucleotide imaging is indicated to detect ischemic changes in asymptomatic individuals with multiple risk factors for coronary disease, such as diabetes and dyslipidemia, and for older individuals who plan to start vigorous exercise. Currently, the diagnostic modality of choice for the diagnosis of myocardial ischemia is single photon emission computerized tomography (SPECT), which is effective at identifying ischemia and estimating coronary risk.[87] Stress echocardiography is another technique used to diagnose CAD. Unfortunately

these tests cannot detect the presence of vulnerable plaques that are the cause of the majority of acute coronary syndromes; therefore new diagnostic techniques are being evaluated.[58] Noninvasive tests for evaluating coronary atherosclerotic lesions include measurement of coronary artery calcium concentration by computed tomography (CT), noninvasive coronary angiography using electron beam CT, protein-weighted magnetic resonance imaging, and intravascular ultrasound; however, the sensitivity and specificity of these tests vary widely.[87] Coronary angiography helps determine the anatomic extent of CAD, but the procedure is expensive and carries some risk. It is used primarily to determine whether possible percutaneous coronary intervention (PCI) or coronary artery bypass graft (CABG) surgery is warranted for individuals whose noninvasive studies suggest severe disease.

The primary aims of therapy for myocardial ischemia and stable angina are to increase coronary blood flow and to reduce myocardial oxygen consumption. Recommendations for appropriate diet, exercise, and risk reduction strategies have been widely distributed and the use of lipid-lowering statins has been shown to be effective for both

FIGURE 24-13 Electrocardiogram (ECG) and Ischemia. **A,** Normal ECG. **B,** Electrocardiographic alterations associated with ischemia.

primary and secondary prevention of coronary artery disease.[65,88] Coronary blood flow is improved by reversing vasoconstriction, reducing plaque growth and rupture, and preventing clotting. Myocardial oxygen demand is reduced by manipulation of blood pressure, heart rate, contractility, and left ventricular volume. Several classes of drugs are useful for increasing coronary flow and decreasing myocardial demand, especially nitrates, beta-blockers, and calcium channel blockers.[87,89] Ranolazine represents a relatively new class of antianginal drugs known as sodium ion channel inhibitors and has been found to improve exercise tolerance, lessen anginal symptoms, and reduce the need for nitrates in many individuals with chronic stable angina.[90]

Percutaneous coronary intervention (PCI) is a procedure whereby stenotic (narrowed) coronary vessels are dilated with a catheter. Indications for PCI in stable angina include persistent symptoms despite optimal medical therapy or severe disease that indicates a high risk for infarction.[87] Restenosis of the artery is the major complication of the procedure; however, placement of a coronary stent can reduce this risk. Pharmacologic treatment with antithrombotics, such as aspirin, clopidogrel, or glycoprotein IIb/IIIa receptor antagonists, after stenting also can improve outcomes.

Severe CAD can be surgically treated by a coronary artery bypass graft (CABG), usually using the saphenous vein from the lower leg. In selected individuals, a modified CABG procedure called minimally invasive direct coronary artery bypass (MIDCAB) can be used with much less surgical morbidity and more rapid recovery.

✔ **QUICK CHECK 24-5**

1. Define atherosclerosis, and briefly describe how it develops.
2. Why do hypertension and dyslipidemia increase the likelihood of developing coronary artery disease?
3. Discuss the relationships among myocardial ischemia, angina, and silent ischemia.

Acute Coronary Syndromes

The process of atherosclerotic plaque progression can be gradual. However, when there is sudden coronary obstruction caused by thrombus formation over a ruptured or ulcerated atherosclerotic plaque, the acute coronary syndromes result (Figure 24-14). **Unstable angina** is the result of reversible myocardial ischemia and is a harbinger of impending infarction. **Myocardial infarction (MI)** results when there is prolonged ischemia causing irreversible damage to the heart muscle. MI can be further subdivided into **non-ST elevation MI (non-STEMI)** and **ST elevation MI (STEMI)**. Sudden cardiac death can occur as a result of any of the acute coronary syndromes.

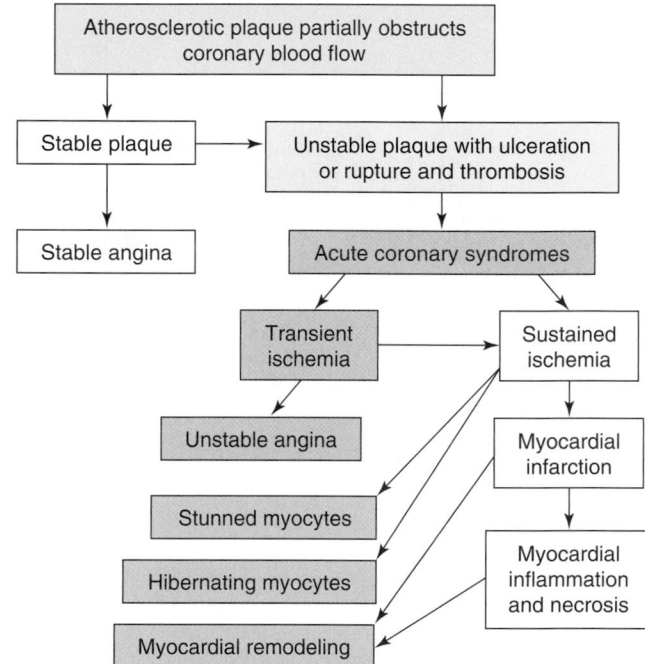

FIGURE 24-14 Pathophysiology of Acute Coronary Syndromes. The atherosclerotic process can lead to stable plaque formation and stable angina or can result in unstable plaques that are prone to rupture and thrombus. Thrombus formation on a ruptured plaque that disperses in less than 20 minutes leads to transient ischemia and unstable angina. If the vessel obstruction is sustained, myocardial infarction with inflammation and necrosis of the myocardium results. In addition, myocardial infarction is associated with other structural and functional changes, including myocyte stunning and hibernation and myocardial remodeling (see Figure 24-34).

An atherosclerotic plaque that is prone to rupture is called "unstable" and has a core that is especially rich in deposited oxidized LDL and a thin fibrous cap (Figure 24-15). These unstable plaques may not extend into the lumen of the vessel and may be clinically silent until they rupture. Plaque disruption (ulceration or rupture) occurs because of the effects of shear forces, inflammation with release of multiple inflammatory mediators, secretion of macrophage-derived degradative enzymes, and apoptosis of cells at the edges of the lesions. Exposure of the plaque substrate activates the clotting cascade. In addition, platelet activation results in the release of coagulants and exposure of platelet glycoprotein IIb/IIIa surface receptors, resulting in further platelet aggregation and adherence. The resulting thrombus can form very quickly (Figure 24-16, *A*). Vessel obstruction is further exacerbated by the release of vasoconstrictors, such as thromboxane A₂ and endothelin. The thrombus may shatter before permanent myocyte damage has occurred (unstable angina) or it may cause prolonged ischemia with infarction of the heart muscle (myocardial infarction) (Figure 24-16, *B*).

Unstable angina. Unstable angina is a form of acute coronary syndrome that results from reversible myocardial ischemia. It is important to recognize this syndrome because it signals that the atherosclerotic plaque has become complicated, and infarction may soon follow. Unstable angina occurs when a fairly small fissuring or superficial erosion of the plaque leads to transient episodes of thrombotic vessel occlusion and vasoconstriction at the site of plaque damage. This thrombus is labile and occludes the vessel for no more than 10 to 20 minutes, with return of perfusion before significant myocardial

necrosis occurs. Unstable angina presents as new-onset angina, angina that is occurring at rest, or angina that is increasing in severity or frequency (Box 24-1). Individuals may experience increased dyspnea, diaphoresis, and anxiety as the angina worsens. Physical examination may reveal evidence of ischemic myocardial dysfunction such as pulmonary congestion. The ECG most commonly shows ST segment depression and T wave inversion during pain that resolve as the pain is relieved. Unstable angina has traditionally been diagnosed by ECG changes without serum cardiac isoenzyme evidence of myocyte necrosis. However, the advent of highly sensitive measurements of myocardial damage (hs-troponin I) that can identify tiny amounts of enzymes released from damaged myocytes has blurred the distinction between unstable angina and myocardial infarction.[91]Therefore, the current guidelines for the management of unstable angina and non-STEMI are identical.[92] Management of unstable angina requires immediate hospitalization with administration of oxygen, aspirin (if not contraindicated), nitrates, and morphine if pain is still present. Additional antithrombotic therapy with clopidogrel or glycoprotein IIb/IIIa platelet receptor antagonists may be indicated. Beta-blockers and ACE inhibitors also may be used. Anticoagulants (such as low-molecular-weight heparin) or direct thrombin inhibitors (e.g., fondaparinux) also can be given. Rapid intervention with PCI also may be indicated.[92]

Myocardial infarction. When coronary blood flow is interrupted for an extended period of time, myocyte necrosis occurs. This results in myocardial infarction (MI). Plaque progression, disruption, and

FIGURE 24-15 Pathogenesis of Unstable Plaques and Thrombus Formation.

BOX 24-1 Three Principal Presentations of Unstable Angina

1. Rest angina—Angina occurring at rest and prolonged, usually >20 minutes
2. New-onset angina—New-onset angina of at least CCS Class III severity
3. Increasing angina—Previously diagnosed angina that has become distinctly more frequent, longer in duration, or lower in threshold (i.e., increased by ≥1 CCS class to at least CCS Class III severity)

From Anderson J et al: *J Am Coll Cardiol* 50:e1-e157, 2007; originally adapted from Braunwald E: *Circulation* 80:410-414, 1989. *CCS,* Canadian Cardiovascular Society.

FIGURE 24-16 Plaque Disruption and Myocardial Infarction. **A,** Plaque disruption. The cap of the lipid-rich plaque has become torn with the formation of a thrombus, mostly inside the plaque. **B,** Myocardial infarction. This infarct is 6 days old. The center is yellow and necrotic with a hemorrhagic red rim. The responsible arterial occlusion is probably in the right coronary artery. The infarct is on the posterior wall. (From Damjanov I, Linder J, editors: *Anderson's pathology,* ed 10, St Louis, 1996, Mosby.)

subsequent clot formation are the same for myocardial infarction as they are for unstable angina (see Figures 24-14, 24-15, and 24-16). In this case, however, the thrombus is less labile and occludes the vessel for a prolonged period, such that myocardial ischemia progresses to myocyte necrosis and death. Pathologically, there are two major types of myocardial infarction: subendocardial infarction and transmural infarction. Clinically, however, myocardial infarction is categorized as non-ST segment elevation myocardial infarction (non-STEMI) or ST segment elevation MI (STEMI).

If the thrombus disintegrates before complete distal tissue necrosis has occurred, the infarction will involve only the myocardium directly beneath the endocardium (subendocardial MI) (Figure 24-17). This infarction will usually present with ST segment depression and T wave

inversion without Q waves; therefore it is termed non-STEMI. It is especially important to recognize this form of acute coronary syndrome because recurrent clot formation on the disrupted atherosclerotic plaque is likely. If the thrombus lodges permanently in the vessel, the infarction will extend through the myocardium all the way from endocardium to epicardium, resulting in severe cardiac dysfunction (transmural MI) (see Figure 24-17). Transmural myocardial infarction will usually result in marked elevations in the ST segments on ECG, and these individuals are categorized as having ST segment elevation MI, or STEMI. Clinically, it is important to identify those individuals with STEMI because they are at highest risk for serious complications and should receive definitive intervention without delay.

PATHOPHYSIOLOGY   After 8 to 10 seconds of decreased blood flow, the affected myocardium becomes cyanotic and cooler. Myocardial oxygen reserves are used quickly (within about 8 seconds) after complete cessation of coronary flow. Glycogen stores decrease as anaerobic metabolism begins. Unfortunately, glycolysis can supply only 65% to 70% of the total myocardial energy requirement and produces much less adenosine triphosphate (ATP) than aerobic processes. Hydrogen ions and lactic acid accumulate. Because myocardial tissues have poor buffering capabilities and myocardial cells are sensitive to low cellular pH, accumulation of these products further compromises the myocardium. Acidosis may make the myocardium more vulnerable to the damaging effects of lysosomal enzymes and may suppress impulse conduction and contractile function, thereby leading to heart failure.

Oxygen deprivation also is accompanied by electrolyte disturbances, specifically the loss of potassium, calcium, and magnesium from cells. Myocardial cells deprived of necessary oxygen and nutrients lose contractility, thereby diminishing the pumping ability of the heart. Ischemia causes the myocardial cells to release catecholamines, predisposing the individual to serious imbalances of sympathetic and parasympathetic function, irregular heartbeats (dysrhythmia), and heart failure. Catecholamines mediate the release of glycogen, glucose, and stored fat from body cells. Therefore plasma concentrations of free fatty acids and glycerol rise within 1 hour after the onset of acute myocardial infarction. Excessive levels of free fatty acids can have a harmful detergent effect on cell membranes. Norepinephrine elevates blood glucose levels through stimulation of liver and skeletal muscle cells and suppresses pancreatic beta-cell activity, which reduces insulin secretion and elevates blood glucose concentration further. Infiltration of inflammatory cells contributes to tissue injury.[93]Angiotensin II is released during myocardial ischemia and contributes to the pathogenesis of myocardial infarction in several ways. First, it results in the systemic effects of peripheral vasoconstriction and fluid retention, which increase myocardial workload. Second, it is a growth factor for vascular smooth muscle cells, myocytes, and cardiac fibroblasts, resulting in structural changes in the myocardium called remodeling. Finally, angiotensin II promotes catecholamine release and causes coronary artery spasm.

Ischemic injury can be exacerbated by reperfusion injury once blood flow is restored. This process involves the release of toxic oxygen free radicals, calcium flux, and pH changes that cause a sustained opening of mitochondrial permeability transition pores (mPTPs) and contribute to resultant cellular death. Many innovative therapies are being explored to reduce reperfusion injury.[93]

Cardiac cells can withstand ischemic conditions for about 20 minutes before irreversible hypoxic injury causes cellular death (apoptosis) and tissue necrosis. This results in the release of intracellular enzymes such as creatine phosphokinase MB (CPK-MB) and myocyte proteins such as the troponins through the damaged cell membranes into the interstitial spaces. The lymphatics absorb the enzymes and

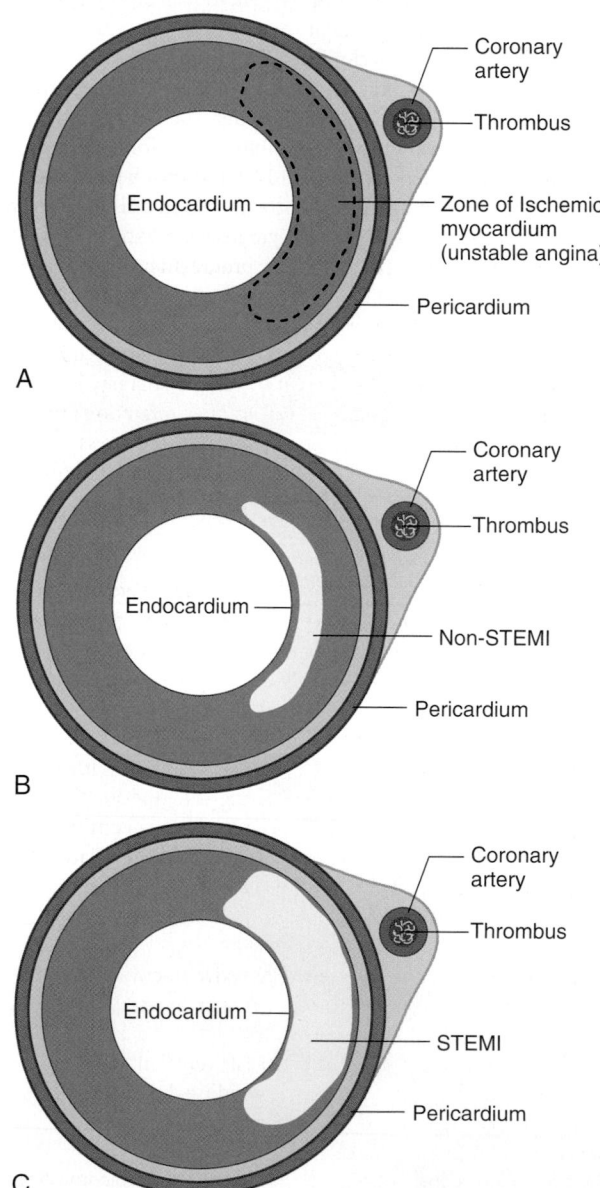

FIGURE 24-17 Unstable Angina, non-STEMI, and STEMI. **A,** Unstable angina. Coronary thrombosis leads to myocardial ischemia. **B,** Non-STEMI. Persistent coronary occlusion leads to infarction of the myocardium closest to the endocardium. **C,** STEMI. Continued coronary occlusion leads to transmural infarction extending from endocardium to pericardium.

FIGURE 24-18 Myocardial Infarction. **A,** Local infarct confined to one region. **B,** Massive large infarct caused by occlusion of three coronary arteries. (From Damjanov I, Linder J, editors: *Anderson's pathology,* ed 10, St Louis, 1996, Mosby.)

transport them into the bloodstream, where they can be detected by serologic tests.

Myocardial infarction results in both structural and functional changes of cardiac tissues (Figure 24-18). Gross tissue changes at the area of infarction may not become apparent for several hours, despite almost immediate onset (within 30 to 60 seconds) of electrocardiographic changes. Cardiac tissue surrounding the area of infarction also undergoes changes. Myocardial stunning is a temporary loss of contractile function that persists for hours to days after perfusion has been restored. This pathophysiologic state can occur both with MI and in individuals who suffer ischemia during cardiovascular procedures or during central nervous system trauma. Stunning is caused by the alterations in electrolyte pumps and calcium homeostasis and by the release of toxic oxygen free radicals; it can contribute to heart failure, shock, and dysrhythmias. Recurrent episodes of transient myocardial ischemia (angina) before MI can result in myocyte adaptation to oxygen deprivation with reduced stunning and preservation of myocardium.[94] This process, termed ischemic preconditioning, is being studied to determine whether it has potential prophylactic or therapeutic uses.[95] Hibernating myocardium describes tissue that is persistently ischemic and undergoes metabolic adaptation to prolong myocyte survival until perfusion can be restored. PCI or surgery aimed at reperfusion of hibernating myocardium can restore significant cardiac function.[96] Myocardial remodeling is a process mediated by angiotensin II, aldosterone, catecholamines, adenosine, and inflammatory cytokines that causes myocyte hypertrophy and loss of contractile function in the areas of the heart distant from the site of infarction. Remodeling can be limited through rapid restoration of coronary flow and the use of renin-angiotensin-aldosterone blockers and beta-blockers after MI.[97]

The severity of functional impairment depends on the size of the lesion and the site of infarction. Functional changes can include (1) decreased cardiac contractility with abnormal wall motion, (2) altered left ventricular compliance, (3) decreased stroke volume, (4) decreased ejection fraction, (5) increased left ventricular end-diastolic pressure, and (6) sinoatrial node malfunction. Life-threatening dysrhythmias and heart failure often follow myocardial infarction.

With infarction, ventricular function is abnormal and the ejection fraction falls, resulting in increases in ventricular end-diastolic volume (VEDV). If the coronary obstruction involves the perfusion to the left ventricle, pulmonary venous congestion ensues; if the right ventricle is ischemic, increases in systemic venous pressures occur.

Myocardial infarction causes a severe inflammatory response that ends with wound repair (see Chapter 6). Damaged cells undergo degradation, fibroblasts proliferate, and scar tissue is synthesized. Many cell types, hormones, and nutrient substrates must be available for optimal healing to proceed. Within 24 hours, leukocytes infiltrate the necrotic area, and proteolytic enzymes from scavenger neutrophils degrade necrotic tissue. The collagen matrix that is deposited is initially weak, mushy, and vulnerable to reinjury. Unfortunately, it is at this time in the recovery period (10 to 14 days after infarction) that individuals feel more like increasing activities and may stress the newly formed scar tissue. After 6 weeks, the necrotic area is completely replaced by scar tissue, which is strong but cannot contract and relax like healthy myocardial tissue.

CLINICAL MANIFESTATIONS   The first symptom of acute myocardial infarction is usually sudden, severe chest pain. The pain is similar to that of angina pectoris but more severe and prolonged. It may be described as heavy and crushing, such as a "truck sitting on my chest." Radiation to the neck, jaw, back, shoulder, or left arm is common. Some individuals, especially those who are elderly or have diabetes, experience no pain, thereby having a "silent" infarction. Infarction often simulates a sensation of unrelenting indigestion. Nausea and vomiting may occur because of reflex stimulation of vomiting centers by pain fibers. Vasovagal reflexes from the area of the infarcted myocardium also may affect the gastrointestinal tract.

Various cardiovascular changes are found on physical examination:

1. The sympathetic nervous system is reflexively activated to compensate, resulting in a temporary increase in heart rate and blood pressure.
2. Abnormal extra heart sounds reflect left ventricular dysfunction.
3. Pulmonary findings of congestion including dullness to percussion and inspiratory crackles at the lung bases can occur if the individual develops heart failure.
4. Peripheral vasoconstriction may cause the skin to become cool and clammy.

The number and severity of postinfarction complications depend on the location and extent of necrosis, the individual's physiologic condition before the infarction, and the availability of swift therapeutic intervention. Sudden cardiac death can occur in individuals with myocardial ischemia even if infarction is absent or minimal, and is a

*See Figure 24-14.

FIGURE 24-19 Three Interacting Factors Related to Sudden Cardiac Death. The three factors are ischemia, left ventricular dysfunction, and electrical instability.

multifactorial problem. Risk factors for sudden death are related to three factors: ischemia, left ventricular dysfunction, and electrical instability. These factors interact with each other (Figure 24-19). Table 24-5 lists the most common complications.

EVALUATION AND TREATMENT The diagnosis of acute myocardial infarction is made on the basis of history, physical examination, ECG results, and serial cardiac troponin elevations (Box 24-2). The cardiac troponins (troponin I and troponin T) are the most specific indicators of MI. A transient rise in these plasma enzyme levels can confirm the occurrence of MI and indicate its severity. Blood is drawn for troponin level determination as soon as possible after the onset of symptoms, and serial serum levels are assessed for several days. If serologic tests show abnormally high levels of troponin, acute myocardial infarction has occurred. Elevation of troponin level may not occur immediately after infarction and laboratory confirmation that an infarction has occurred may be delayed up to 12 hours.

Myocardial infarction can occur in various regions of the heart wall and may be described as anterior, inferior, posterior, lateral, subendocardial, or transmural, depending on the anatomic location and extent of tissue damage from infarction. Twelve-lead ECGs help localize the affected area through identification of changes in ST segments and T waves (Figure 24-20). The infarcted myocardium is surrounded by a zone of hypoxic injury, which may progress to necrosis or return to normal, and adjacent to this zone of hypoxic injury is a zone of reversible ischemia (see Figure 24-20). A characteristic Q wave often develops on ECG some hours later in STEMI.

Cardiac troponin I (cTnI) is the most specific indicator of MI, and measurement of its level should be performed on admission to the

emergency department. cTnI level elevation is detectable 2 to 4 hours after onset of symptoms. Additional measurements within 6 to 9 hours and again at 12 to 24 hours are recommended if clinical suspicion is high and previous samples were negative. Troponin levels also can be used to estimate infarct size and therefore the likelihood of complications. Additional laboratory data may reveal leukocytosis and elevated C-reactive protein (CRP), both of which indicate inflammation. The individual's blood glucose level is usually elevated and the glucose tolerance level may remain abnormal for several weeks.

Acute myocardial infarction requires admission to the hospital, often directly into a coronary care unit. Most guidelines continue to recommend the use of oxygen in acute MI; however, a recent review did not demonstrate a clear benefit of oxygen therapy.[98] The individual should be given an aspirin immediately (ticlopidine if allergic to aspirin). Pain relief is of utmost importance and involves the use of sublingual nitroglycerin and morphine sulfate. Continuous monitoring of cardiac rhythms and enzymatic changes is essential, because the first 24 hours after onset of symptoms is the time of highest risk for sudden death. Non-STEMI is treated in the same way as unstable angina including antithrombotics, anticoagulation or PCI, or both.[92] STEMI is best managed with emergent PCI and antithrombotics.[99] Thrombolytics may be used if PCI is not readily available. Hyperglycemia is treated with insulin. Once the person is stabilized, further management includes ACE inhibitors, beta-blockers, and statins.[99] Individuals who are in shock require aggressive fluid resuscitation, ionotropic drugs, and possible emergent invasive procedures.

Bed rest, followed by gradual return to activities of daily living, reduces the myocardial oxygen demands of the compromised heart.

TABLE 24-5 Complications with Myocardial Infarctions

Type	Characteristics
Dysrhythmias	Disturbances of cardiac rhythm that affect 90% of persons with cardiac infarction
	Caused by ischemia, hypoxia, autonomic nervous system imbalances, lactic acidosis, electrolyte abnormalities, alterations of impulse conduction pathways or conduction abnormalities, drug toxicity, or hemodynamic abnormalities
Left ventricular failure (congestive heart failure)	Characterized by pulmonary congestion, reduced myocardial contractility, and abnormal heart wall motion
	Cardiogenic shock can develop
Inflammation of pericardium (pericarditis)	Includes pericardial friction rubs
	Often noted 2 to 3 days later and associated with anterior chest pain that worsens with respiratory effort
Dressler postinfarction syndrome	Essentially a delayed form of pericarditis that occurs 1 week to several months after acute MI syndrome
	Thought to be immunologic response to necrotic myocardium marked by pain, fever, friction rub, pleural effusion, and arthralgias
Organic brain syndrome	Occurs if blood flow to brain is impaired secondary to MI
Transient ischemic attacks or cerebrovascular accident	Occur if thromboemboli detach from clots that form in cardiac chambers or on cardiac valves
Rupture of heart structures	Caused by necrosis of tissue in or around papillary muscles
	Affects papillary muscles of chordae tendineae cordis
	Predisposing factors include thinning of wall, poor collateral flow, shearing effect of muscular contraction against stiffened necrotic area, marked necrosis at terminal end of blood supply, and aging of myocardium with laceration of myocardial microstructure
Rupture of wall of infarcted ventricle	Can be caused by aneurysm formation when pressure becomes too great
Left ventricular aneurysm	Late (month to years) complication of MI that can contribute to heart failure and thromboemboli
Infarctions around septal structures	Occur in those structures that separate heart chambers and lead to septal rupture
	Associated with audible, harsh cardiac murmurs; increased left ventricular end-diastolic pressure; and decreased systemic blood pressure
Systemic thromboembolism	May disseminate from debris and clots that collect inside dilated aneurysmal sacs or from infarcted endocardium
Pulmonary thromboembolism	Usually from deep venous thrombi of legs
	Reduced incidence associated with early mobilization and prophylactic anticoagulation therapy
Sudden death	Dysrhythmias frequently causative, particularly ventricular fibrillation
	Risk of death increased by age more than 65 years, previous angina pectoris, hypotension or cardiogenic shock, acute systolic hypertension at time of admission, diabetes mellitus, dysrhythmias, and previous MI

BOX 24-2 Universal Definition of Myocardial Infarction

The term *myocardial infarction* should be used when there is evidence of myocardial necrosis in a clinical setting with myocardial ischemia. Under these conditions any one of the following criteria meets the diagnosis for myocardial infarction:

- Detection of rise and/or fall of cardiac biomarkers (preferably troponin) with at least one value above the 99th percentile of the upper reference limit (URL) together with evidence of myocardial ischemia with at least one of the following:
  - Symptoms of ischemia
  - ECG changes indicative of new ischemia (new ST-T changes or new left bundle branch block [LBBB])
  - Development of pathologic Q waves in the ECG
  - Imaging evidence of new loss of viable myocardium or new regional wall motion abnormality
- Sudden, unexpected cardiac death, involving cardiac arrest, often with symptoms suggestive of myocardial ischemia, and accompanied by presumably new ST elevation, or new LBBB, and/or evidence of fresh thrombus by coronary angiography and/or at autopsy; but death occurring before blood samples could be obtained, or at a time before the appearance of cardiac biomarkers in the blood.

- For percutaneous coronary interventions (PCIs) in persons with normal baseline troponin values, elevations of cardiac biomarkers greater than the 99th percentile URL are indicative of periprocedural myocardial necrosis. By convention, increases of biomarkers greater than 3 × 99th percentile URL have been designated as defining PCI-related myocardial infarction. A subtype related to a documented stent thrombosis is recognized.
- For coronary artery bypass grafting (CABG) in persons with normal baseline troponin values, elevations of cardiac biomarkers greater than the 99th percentile URL are indicative of periprocedural myocardial necrosis. By convention, increases of biomarkers greater than 5 × 99th percentile URL plus either new pathologic Q waves or new LBBB, or angiographically documented new graft or native coronary artery occlusion, or imaging evidence of new loss of viable myocardium have been designated as defining CABG-related myocardial infarction.
- Pathologic findings of an acute myocardial infarction.

Data from Thygesen K et al: *J Am Coll Cardiol* 50:2173-2195, 2007.

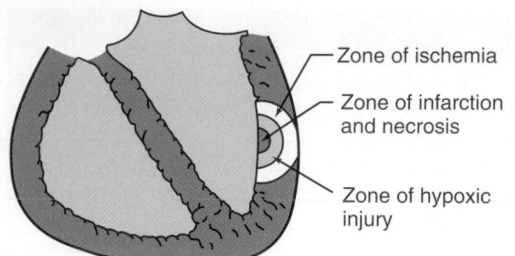

	Normal	Ischemia	Injury	Infarction/necrosis

Zone of ischemia
Zone of infarction and necrosis
Zone of hypoxic injury

FIGURE 24-20 Electrocardiographic Alterations Associated with the Three Zones of Myocardial Infarction.

Individuals not receiving thrombolytic or heparin infusion must receive deep venous thrombosis prophylaxis as long as their activity is significantly limited. Stool softeners are given to eliminate the need for straining, which can precipitate bradycardia and can be followed by increased venous return to the heart, causing possible cardiac overload. Education regarding appropriate diet and caffeine intake, smoking cessation, exercise, and other aspects of risk factor reduction is crucial for secondary prevention of recurrent myocardial ischemia.

> **QUICK CHECK 24-6**
> 1. Describe the coronary artery disease–myocardial ischemia continuum.
> 2. Describe the pathophysiology of myocardial infarction.
> 3. What complications are associated with the period after infarction?

DISORDERS OF THE HEART WALL

Disorders of the Pericardium

Pericardial disease is a localized manifestation of another disorder, such as infection (bacterial, viral, fungal, rickettsial, or parasitic); trauma or surgery; neoplasm; or a metabolic, immunologic, or vascular disorder (uremia, rheumatoid arthritis, systemic lupus erythematosus, periarteritis nodosa). The pericardial response to injury from these diverse causes may consist of acute pericarditis, pericardial effusion, or constrictive pericarditis.

Acute Pericarditis

Acute pericarditis is acute inflammation of the pericardium. The etiology of acute pericarditis is most often idiopathic or caused by viral infection by coxsackie, influenza, hepatitis, measles, mumps, or varicella viruses. It also is the most common cardiovascular complication of human immunodeficiency virus (HIV) infection. Other causes include myocardial infarction, trauma, neoplasm, surgery, uremia, bacterial infection (especially tuberculosis), connective tissue disease (especially systemic lupus erythematosus and rheumatoid arthritis), or radiation therapy.[100] The pericardial membranes become inflamed and roughened, and a pericardial effusion may develop that can be serous, purulent, or fibrinous (Figure 24-21). Possible sequelae of pericarditis include recurrent pericarditis, pericardial constriction, and cardiac tamponade.

Symptoms may follow several days of fever and usually begin with the sudden onset of severe retrosternal chest pain that worsens with respiratory movements and when assuming a recumbent position. The pain may radiate to the back as a result of irritation of the phrenic nerve (innervates the trapezius muscles) as it traverses the pericardium. Individuals with acute pericarditis also report dysphagia, restlessness, irritability, anxiety, weakness, and malaise.

Physical examination often discloses low-grade fever (<38° C [<100.4° F]) and sinus tachycardia. A friction rub—a scratchy, grating

FIGURE 24-21 Acute Pericarditis. Note shaggy coat of fibers covering the surface of heart. (From Damjanov I, Linder J: *Pathology: a color atlas*, St Louis, 2000, Mosby.)

sound—may be heard at the cardiac apex and left sternal border and is highly suggestive of pericarditis. The rub is caused by the roughened pericardial membranes rubbing against each other. Friction rubs are not always present and may be intermittently heard and transient. Hypotension or the presence of a pulsus paradoxus (a decrease in systolic blood pressure of >10 mm Hg with inspiration) is suggestive of cardiac tamponade, which can be life-threatening. Electrocardiographic changes may reflect inflammatory processes through PR segment depression and diffuse ST segment elevation without Q waves, and they may remain abnormal for days or even weeks.[100] Ultrasound, CT scanning, and MRI may be used as diagnostic modalities. Acute pericarditis requires at least two of the following four criteria for diagnosis: (1) chest pain characteristics of pericarditis, (2) pericardial rub, (3) characteristic electrocardiographic (ECG) changes, and (4) new or worsening pericardial effusion.[100]

Treatment for uncomplicated acute pericarditis consists of relieving symptoms and includes administration of anti-inflammatory agents, such as salicylates and nonsteroidal anti-inflammatory drugs, and colchicine. Approximately one third of cases will be complicated by the development of idiopathic recurrent pericarditis.[101] Exploration of the underlying cause is important. If pericardial effusion develops, aspiration of the excessive fluid may be necessary.

Pericardial Effusion

Pericardial effusion is the accumulation of fluid in the pericardial cavity and can occur in all forms of pericarditis. Most are idiopathic (20%) but other causes, such as neoplasm and infection, must be considered.[100] Analysis of the fluid obtained through pericardiocentesis allows for identification of the likely source of the fluid.[102] The fluid may be a transudate, such as the serous effusion that develops with left heart failure, overhydration, or hypoproteinemia. More often, however, the fluid is an exudate, which reflects pericardial inflammation like that seen with acute pericarditis, heart surgery, some chemotherapeutic agents, infections, and autoimmune disorders such as systemic lupus erythematosus. (Types of exudate are described in Chapter 6.) Exudative effusions also are found in up to 12% of individuals with STEMI.[103] If the fluid is serosanguineous, the underlying cause is likely to be tuberculosis, neoplasm, uremia, or radiation. Idiopathic serosanguineous (cause unknown) effusion is possible, however. Effusions of frank blood are generally related to aneurysms, trauma, or coagulation defects (Figure 24-22). If chyle leaks from the thoracic duct, it may enter the pericardium and lead to cholesterol pericarditis.

Pericardial effusion, even in large amounts, is not necessarily clinically significant, except that it indicates an underlying disorder. If an effusion develops gradually, the pericardium can stretch to accommodate large quantities of fluid without compressing the heart. If the fluid accumulates rapidly, however, even a small amount (50 to 100 ml) may create sufficient pressure to cause cardiac compression, a serious condition known as **tamponade**. The danger is that pressure exerted by the pericardial fluid eventually will equal diastolic pressure within the heart chambers, which will interfere with right atrial filling during diastole. This causes increased venous pressure, systemic venous congestion, and signs and symptoms of right heart failure (distention of the jugular veins, edema, hepatomegaly). Decreased atrial filling leads to decreased ventricular filling, decreased stroke volume, and reduced cardiac output. Life-threatening circulatory collapse may occur.

An important clinical finding is pulsus paradoxus, in which arterial blood pressure during expiration exceeds arterial pressure during inspiration by more than 10 mm Hg. Pulsus paradoxus in the setting of a pericardial effusion indicates tamponade and reflects impairment of diastolic filling of the left ventricle plus reduction of blood volume within all four cardiac chambers. The presence of a large pericardial effusion or tamponade magnifies the normally insignificant effect of inspiration on intracardiac flow and volume.

Other clinical manifestations of pericardial effusion are distant or muffled heart sounds, poorly palpable apical pulse, dyspnea on exertion, and dull chest pain. A chest x-ray film may disclose a "water-bottle configuration" of the cardiac silhouette. An echocardiogram can detect an effusion as small as 20 ml and is a reliable and accurate diagnostic test, although CT scans also may be done.[100]

Treatment of pericardial effusion or tamponade generally consists of pericardiocentesis (aspiration of excessive pericardial fluid) and treatment of the underlying condition. Persistent pain may be treated with analgesics, anti-inflammatory medications, or steroids. Surgery may be required if the underlying cause of tamponade is trauma or aneurysm. A pericardial "window" may be surgically created to prevent tamponade.[104]

Constrictive Pericarditis

Constrictive pericarditis, or **restrictive pericarditis (chronic pericarditis)**, was synonymous with tuberculosis years ago, and tuberculosis continues to be an important cause of pericarditis in immunocompromised individuals. Currently in the United States, this form of pericardial disease is more commonly idiopathic or associated with viral infection, radiation exposure, collagen vascular disorders, sarcoidosis, neoplasm, uremia, or cardiac surgery.[100] In constrictive pericarditis, fibrous scarring with occasional calcification of the pericardium causes the visceral and parietal pericardial layers to adhere, obliterating the pericardial cavity. The fibrotic lesions encase the heart in a rigid shell (Figure 24-23). Like tamponade, constrictive pericarditis compresses the heart and eventually reduces cardiac output. Unlike tamponade, however, constrictive pericarditis always develops gradually.

Symptoms tend to be exercise intolerance, dyspnea on exertion, fatigue, and anorexia. Clinical assessment shows edema, distention of

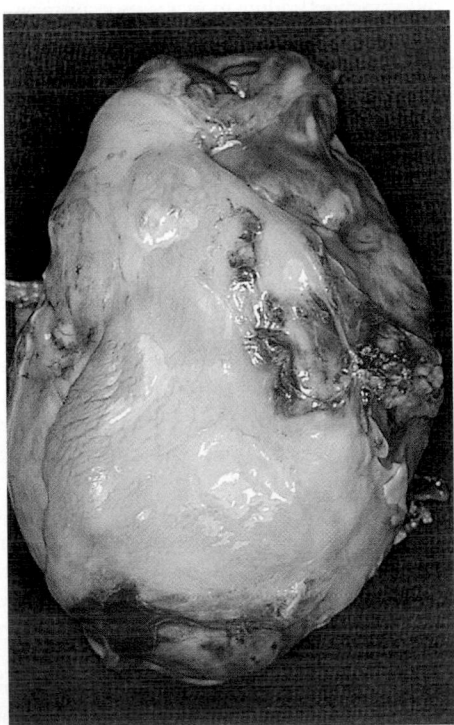

FIGURE 24-23 Constrictive Pericarditis. The fibrotic pericardium encases the heart in a rigid shell. (From Damjanov I, Linder J: *Pathology: a color atlas*, St Louis, 2000, Mosby.)

FIGURE 24-22 Exudate of Blood in the Pericardial Sac from Rupture of Aneurysm. (From Damjanov I, Linder J: *Pathology: a color atlas*, St Louis, 2000, Mosby.)

the jugular vein, hepatic congestion, and systemic hypotension. Restricted ventricular filling may cause a pericardial knock (early diastolic sound).

ECG findings include nonspecific ST and T wave abnormalities and atrial fibrillation. Chest x-ray films often disclose prominent pulmonary vessels and calcification of the pericardium. CT, MRI, and transesophageal echocardiography are used to detect pericardial thickening and constriction and to distinguish constrictive pericarditis from restrictive cardiomyopathy. Pericardial biopsy may be needed to determine the etiology.

Initial treatment for constrictive pericarditis consists of restriction of dietary sodium intake and administration of diuretics to improve cardiac output. Management also may include use of anti-inflammatory drugs and treatment of any underlying disorder. If these modalities are unsuccessful, surgical excision of the restrictive pericardium is indicated (pericardial decortication).[100]

Disorders of the Myocardium: The Cardiomyopathies

The cardiomyopathies are a diverse group of diseases that primarily affect the myocardium itself. They may, however, be secondary to infectious disease, toxin exposure, systemic connective tissue disease, infiltrative and proliferative disorders, or nutritional deficiencies. Many cases are idiopathic; others are caused by ischemia, hypertension, inherited disorders, infections, toxins, or systemic inflammatory disorders. Some are preceded by myocarditis; however, most individuals with acute myocarditis recover without sequelae.[100] The cardiomyopathies are categorized as dilated (formerly, congestive), hypertrophic, or restrictive, depending on their physiologic effects on the heart (Figure 24-24).

Dilated cardiomyopathy is usually the result of ischemic heart disease, valvular disease, diabetes, renal failure, alcohol or drug toxicity, peripartum complications, or infection.[100] There is a strong genetic basis for dilated cardiomyopathy and it can be associated with inherited disorders, such as muscular dystrophy. It is characterized by impaired systolic function leading to increases in intracardiac volume, ventricular dilation, and heart failure with reduced ejection fraction (Figure 24-25) (see p. 632). Individuals complain of dyspnea, fatigue, and pedal edema. Findings on examination include a displaced apical pulse, S_3 gallop, peripheral edema, jugular venous distention, and pulmonary congestion. Diagnosis is confirmed by chest x-ray and echocardiogram, and management is focused on reducing blood volume, increasing contractility, and reversing the underlying disorder if possible.[100] Heart transplant is required in severe cases.

Hypertrophic cardiomyopathy refers to two major categories of thickening of the myocardium: (1) hypertrophic obstructive cardiomyopathy (asymmetric septal hypertrophic cardiomyopathy or subaortic stenosis) and (2) hypertensive or valvular hypertrophic cardiomyopathy. Hypertrophic obstructive cardiomyopathy is the most commonly inherited cardiac disorder. It is characterized by thickening of the septal wall (Figure 24-26), which may cause outflow obstruction to the left ventricle outflow tract.[100] Obstruction of left ventricular outflow can occur when the heart rate is increased and the intravascular volume is decreased. This type of hypertrophic cardiomyopathy is a significant risk factor for serious ventricular dysrhythmias and sudden death.[100,105] There are other conditions that cause hypertrophic changes in the ventricles; hypertensive and valvular hypertrophic cardiomyopathies are the most common.[106] These occur because of increased resistance to ventricular ejection, which is commonly seen in individuals with hypertension or valvular stenosis (usually aortic). In this case, hypertrophy of the myocytes is an attempt to compensate for increased myocardial workload. Long-term dysfunction of the myocytes develops over time, with diastolic dysfunction appearing first

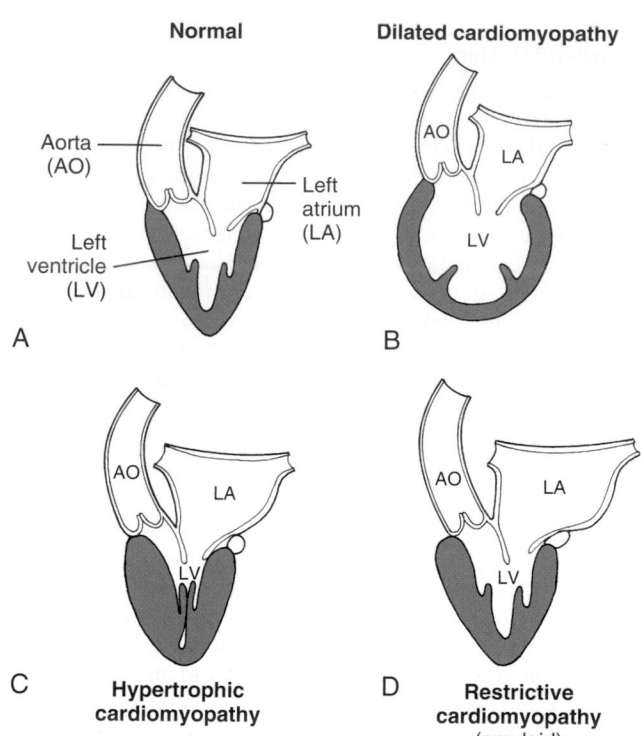

FIGURE 24-24 Diagram Showing Major Distinguishing Pathophysiologic Features of the Three Types of Cardiomyopathy. **A,** The normal heart. **B,** In the dilated type of cardiomyopathy, the heart has a globular shape and the largest circumference of the left ventricle is not at its base but midway between apex and base. **C,** In the hypertrophic type, the wall of the left ventricle is greatly thickened; the left ventricular cavity is small, but the left atrium may be dilated because of poor diastolic relaxation of the ventricle. **D,** In the restrictive (constrictive) type, the left ventricular cavity is normal size, but, again, the left atrium is dilated because of the reduced diastolic compliance of the ventricle. (From Kissane JM, editor: *Anderson's pathology,* ed 9, St Louis, 1990, Mosby.)

FIGURE 24-25 Dilated Cardiomyopathy. The dilated left ventricle has a thin wall *(V).* (From Stevens A et al: *Core pathology,* ed 3, London, 2009, Mosby.)

FIGURE 24-26 Hypertrophic Cardiomyopathy. There is marked left ventricular hypertrophy. This often affects the septum *(S)*. (From Stevens A et al: *Core pathology*, ed 3, London, 2009, Mosby.)

and leading eventually to systolic dysfunction of the ventricle (see Heart Failure, p. 632). Individuals with hypertrophic cardiomyopathy may be asymptomatic or may complain of angina, syncope, dyspnea on exertion, and palpitations. Examination may reveal extra heart sounds and murmurs. Echocardiography and cardiac catheterization can confirm the diagnosis.

Restrictive cardiomyopathy is characterized by restrictive filling and increased diastolic pressure of either or both ventricles with normal or near-normal systolic function and wall thickness. It may occur idiopathically or as a cardiac manifestation of systemic diseases, such as amyloidosis, scleroderma, sarcoidosis, lymphoma, and hemochromatosis, or a number of inherited storage diseases.[100] The myocardium becomes rigid and noncompliant, impeding ventricular filling and raising filling pressures during diastole. The most common clinical manifestation of restrictive cardiomyopathy is right heart failure with systemic venous congestion. Cardiomegaly and dysrhythmias are common. A thorough evaluation for the underlying cause should be initiated (and may include myocardial biopsy). Treatment is aimed at the underlying cause. Death occurs as a result of heart failure or dysrhythmias.

> ✔ **QUICK CHECK 24-7**
> 1. Why does pericarditis develop?
> 2. What are the cardiomyopathies? List the major disorders.
> 3. Briefly describe the pathophysiologic effects of the cardiomyopathies.

Disorders of the Endocardium
Valvular Dysfunction

Disorders of the endocardium (the innermost lining of the heart wall) damage the heart valves, which are composed of endocardial tissue. Endocardial damage can be either congenital or acquired. The acquired forms result from inflammatory, ischemic, traumatic, degenerative, or infectious alterations of valvular structure and function. One of the most common causes of acquired valvular dysfunction is degeneration or inflammation of the endocardium secondary to rheumatic heart disease (Table 24-6). Structural alterations of the heart valves are caused by remodeling changes in the valvular extracellular matrix and lead to stenosis, incompetence, or both.

FIGURE 24-27 Valvular Stenosis and Regurgitation. A, Normal position of the valve leaflets, or cusps, when the valve is open and closed. **B,** Open position of a stenosed valve *(left)* and open position of a closed regurgitant valve *(right)*. **C,** Hemodynamic effect of mitral stenosis. The stenosed valve is unable to open sufficiently during left atrial systole, inhibiting left ventricular filling. **D,** Hemodynamic effect of mitral regurgitation. The mitral valve does not close completely during left ventricular systole, permitting blood to reenter the left atrium.

In **valvular stenosis**, the valve orifice is constricted and narrowed, so blood cannot flow forward and the workload of the cardiac chamber proximal to the diseased valve increases (Figure 24-27). Pressure (intraventricular or atrial) rises in the chamber to overcome resistance to flow through the valve, necessitating greater exertion by the myocardium and producing myocardial hypertrophy.

Although all four heart valves may be affected, in adults those of the left heart (mitral and aortic valves) are far more commonly affected than those of the right heart (tricuspid and pulmonic valves). In **valvular regurgitation** (also called **insufficiency** or **incompetence**), the valve leaflets, or cusps, fail to shut completely, permitting blood flow to continue even when the valve is presumably closed (see Figure 24-27). During systole or diastole, some blood leaks back into the chamber proximal to the diseased valve, which increases the volume of blood the heart must pump and increases the workload of both the atrium and the ventricle. Increased volume leads to chamber dilation, and increased workload leads to hypertrophy, both of which are compensatory mechanisms intended to increase the pumping capability of the heart but that lead to cardiac dysfunction over time. Eventually, myocardial contractility diminishes, ejection fraction drops, and diastolic pressure increases, and the ventricles fail from being overworked. Depending on the severity of the valvular dysfunction and the capacity of the heart to compensate, valvular alterations cause a range of symptoms and some degree of incapacitation (see Table 24-6).

In general, valvular disease is diagnosed by transthoracic echocardiography (TTE), which can be used to assess the severity of valvular obstruction or regurgitation before the onset of symptoms. CT or MRI may be indicated in certain settings. Valvular lesions are staged and appropriate management is determined by using four general categories: (1) at risk, (2) progressive, (3) asymptomatic severe, and (4) symptomatic severe.[107] Management almost always includes careful medical management, valvular repair, or valve replacement followed by long-term anticoagulation therapy and prophylaxis for endocarditis

TABLE 24-6	Clinical Manifestations of Valvular Stenosis and Regurgitation				
Manifestation	Aortic Stenosis	Mitral Stenosis	Aortic Regurgitation	Mitral Regurgitation	Tricuspid Regurgitation
Most common cause	Congenital bicuspid valve, degenerative (calcific) changes with aging, rheumatic heart disease	Rheumatic heart disease	Infective endocarditis; aortic root disease (connective tissue diseases, Marfan syndrome); dilation of aortic root from hypertension and aging	Myxomatous degeneration (mitral valve prolapse)	Congenital
Cardiovascular outcome (untreated)	Left ventricular hypertrophy followed by left heart failure; decreased coronary blood flow with myocardial ischemia	Left atrial hypertrophy and dilation with fibrillation, followed by right ventricular failure	Left ventricular hypertrophy and dilation, followed by left heart failure	Left atrial hypertrophy and dilation, followed by left heart failure	Right heart failure
Pulmonary effects	Pulmonary edema: dyspnea on exertion	Pulmonary edema: dyspnea on exertion, orthopnea, paroxysmal nocturnal dyspnea, predisposition to respiratory tract infections, hemoptysis, pulmonary hypertension	Pulmonary edema with dyspnea on exertion	Pulmonary edema with dyspnea on exertion	Dyspnea
Central nervous system effects	Syncope, especially on exertion	Neural deficits only associated with emboli (e.g., hemiparesis)	Syncope	None	None
Pain	Angina pectoris	Atypical chest pain	Angina pectoris	Atypical chest pain	Palpitations
Heart sounds	Systolic murmur heard best at right parasternal second intercostal space and radiating to neck	Low, rumbling diastolic murmur heard best at apex and radiating to axilla; accentuated first heart sound, opening snap	Diastolic murmur heard best at right parasternal second intercostal space and radiating to neck	Murmur throughout systole heard best at apex and radiating to axilla	Murmur throughout systole heard best at left lower sternal border

With data from Mann DL et al, editors: *Braunwald's heart disease: a textbook of cardiovascular medicine*, ed 10, St Louis, 2014, Elsevier.

as needed. The purpose of valvular intervention is to improve symptoms and prolong survival, as well as to minimize complications such as asymptomatic irreversible ventricular dysfunction, pulmonary hypertension, stroke, and atrial fibrillation (AF).[107]

Stenosis

Aortic stenosis. Aortic stenosis is the most common valvular abnormality, affecting nearly 2% of adults older than 65 years of age.[108] It has three common causes: (1) congenital bicuspid valve, (2) degeneration with aging, and (3) inflammatory damage caused by rheumatic heart disease. Aortic stenosis also is associated with many risk factors for coronary artery disease, including hypertension, smoking, and dyslipidemia. Aortic valve degeneration with aging is associated with chronic inflammation, lipoprotein deposition in the tissue, and leaflet calcification. The orifice of the aortic valve narrows, causing resistance to blood flow from the left ventricle into the aorta (Figure 24-28). Outflow obstruction increases pressure within the left ventricle as it tries to eject blood through the narrowed opening. Left ventricular hypertrophy develops to compensate for the increased workload. Eventually, hypertrophy increases myocardial oxygen demand, which the coronary arteries may not be able to supply. If this occurs, ischemia may cause attacks of angina. In addition, aortic stenosis is frequently accompanied by atherosclerotic coronary disease, further contributing to inadequate coronary perfusion. Untreated aortic stenosis can lead to hypertrophic cardiomyopathy, dysrhythmias, myocardial infarction, and heart failure.[108]

Aortic stenosis usually develops gradually. Classic symptoms include angina, syncope, and dyspnea. Clinical manifestations include

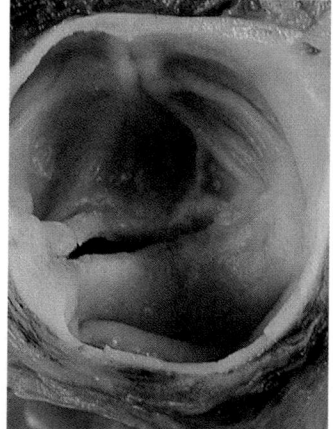

FIGURE 24-28 Aortic Stenosis. Mild stenosis in valve leaflets of a young adult. (From Damjanov I, Linder J: *Pathophysiology: a color atlas*, St Louis, 2000, Mosby.)

decreased stroke volume and narrowed pulse pressure (the difference between systolic and diastolic pressures). Heart rate is often slow, and pulses are delayed. Resistance to flow leads to a crescendo-decrescendo systolic heart murmur heard best at the right parasternal second intercostal space, and may radiate to the neck. Echocardiography can be used to assess the severity of valvular obstruction before the onset of symptoms. Medical management includes vasodilator therapy.

FIGURE 24-29 Mitral Stenosis with Classic "Fish Mouth" Orifice. (From Kumar V et al: *Robins & Cotran pathologic basis of disease,* ed 9, St Louis, 2015, Elsevier.)

Surgical valve replacement with either a mechanical or a bioprosthetic valve is indicated for both symptomatic and asymptomatic individuals with severe stenosis.[107] Percutaneous placement of a prosthetic valve avoids major heart surgery in selected individuals.[107,109] Once individuals become symptomatic from aortic stenosis, the prognosis is poor.

Mitral stenosis. Mitral stenosis impairs the flow of blood from the left atrium to the left ventricle. Mitral stenosis is the most common form of rheumatic heart disease. Autoimmunity in response to group A β-hemolytic streptococcal M protein antigens leads to inflammation and scarring of the valvular leaflets. Scarring causes the leaflets to become fibrous and fused, and the chordae tendineae cordis become shortened (Figure 24-29).

Impedance to blood flow results in incomplete emptying of the left atrium and elevated atrial pressure as the chamber tries to force blood through the stenotic valve. Continued increases in left atrial volume and pressure cause atrial dilation and hypertrophy. The risk of developing atrial fibrillation and dysrhythmia-induced thrombi is high. As mitral stenosis progresses, symptoms of decreased cardiac output occur, especially during exertion. Continued elevation of left atrial pressure and volume causes pressure to rise in the pulmonary circulation. If untreated, chronic mitral stenosis develops into pulmonary hypertension, pulmonary edema, and right ventricular failure.

Blood flow through the stenotic valve results in a rumbling decrescendo diastolic murmur heard best over the cardiac apex and radiating to the left axilla. If the mitral valve is forced open during diastole, it may make a sharp noise called an opening snap. The first heart sound (S_1) is often accentuated and somewhat delayed because of increased left atrial pressure. Other signs and symptoms are generally those of pulmonary congestion and right heart failure. Atrial enlargement and valvular obstruction are demonstrated by chest x-ray films, electrocardiography, and echocardiography. Management includes use of anticoagulation therapy and control of heart rate. Mitral stenosis can often be repaired with percutaneous balloon commissurotomy, but may require valve replacement in advanced cases.[107]

Regurgitation

Aortic regurgitation. Aortic regurgitation results from an inability of the aortic valve leaflets to close properly during diastole because of abnormalities of the leaflets, the aortic root and annulus, or both. It can be primary, caused by congenital bicuspid valve or degeneration in the elderly; or secondary, resulting from chronic hypertension, rheumatic heart disease, bacterial endocarditis, syphilis, connective tissue disorders (e.g., Marfan syndrome and ankylosing

spondylitis), appetite-suppressing medications, trauma, or atherosclerosis.[108] During systole, blood is ejected from the left ventricle into the aorta. During diastole, some of the ejected blood flows back into the left ventricle through the leaking valve. Volume overload occurs in the ventricle because it receives blood both from the left atrium and from the aorta during diastole. The hemodynamic abnormalities depend on the amount of regurgitation. As the end-diastolic volume of the left ventricle increases, myocardial fibers stretch to accommodate the extra fluid. Compensatory dilation permits the left ventricle to increase its stroke volume and maintain cardiac output. Ventricular hypertrophy also occurs as an adaptation to the increased volume and because of increased afterload created by the high stroke volume and resultant systolic hypertension. Over time, ventricular dilation and hypertrophy eventually cannot compensate for aortic incompetence, and heart failure develops.

Clinical manifestations include widened pulse pressure resulting from increased stroke volume and diastolic backflow. Turbulence across the aortic valve during diastole produces a decrescendo murmur in the second, third, or fourth intercostal spaces parasternally and may radiate to the neck. Large stroke volume and rapid runoff of blood from the aorta cause prominent carotid pulsations and bounding peripheral pulses (Corrigan pulse). Other symptoms are usually associated with heart failure that occurs when the ventricle can no longer pump adequately. Dysrhythmias are a common complication of aortic regurgitation. The severity of regurgitation can be estimated by echocardiography, and valve replacement surgery may be delayed for many years through careful use of vasodilators and inotropic agents.[107]

Mitral regurgitation. Mitral regurgitation can be primary because of mitral valve prolapse, rheumatic heart disease, infective endocarditis, MI, connective tissue diseases (Marfan syndrome), and dilated cardiomyopathy. It can also be secondary because of ischemic or nonischemic myocardial disease, which damages the chordae tendineae or the mitral annulus.[107] Mitral regurgitation permits backflow of blood from the left ventricle into the left atrium during ventricular systole, producing a holosystolic (throughout systole) murmur heard best at the apex, which radiates into the back and axilla. Because of increased volume from the left atrium, the left ventricle becomes dilated and hypertrophied to maintain adequate cardiac output. The volume of backflow reentering the left atrium gradually increases, causing atrial dilation and associated atrial fibrillation. As the left atrium enlarges, the valve structures stretch and become deformed, leading to further backflow. As mitral valve regurgitation progresses, left ventricular function may become impaired to the point of failure. Eventually, increased atrial pressure leads to pulmonary hypertension and failure of the right ventricle. Mitral incompetence is usually well tolerated—often for years—until ventricular failure occurs. Most clinical manifestations are caused by heart failure. The severity of regurgitation can be estimated by echocardiography, and transcatheter or surgical repair or valve replacement may become necessary.[110] In acute mitral regurgitation caused by MI, surgical repair must be done emergently.

Tricuspid regurgitation. Tricuspid regurgitation is more common than tricuspid stenosis. Primary tricuspid regurgitation is caused by congenital defects, rheumatic heart disease, endocarditis, or trauma.[108] However, 80% of the cases of tricuspid regurgitation are functional because of annular dilatation and leaflet tethering abnormalities related to dilation of the right ventricle secondary to pulmonary hypertension (see p. 707).[107] Tricuspid valve incompetence leads to volume overload in the right atrium and ventricle, increased systemic venous blood pressure, and right heart failure. Pulmonic valve dysfunction can have the same consequences as tricuspid valve dysfunction.

Mitral Valve Prolapse Syndrome

In **mitral valve prolapse syndrome (MVPS)**, one or both of the cusps of the mitral valve billow upward (prolapse) into the left atrium during systole (Figure 24-30). The most common cause of mitral valve prolapse is myxomatous degeneration of the leaflets in which the cusps are redundant, thickened, and scalloped because of changes in tissue proteoglycans, increased levels of proteinases, and infiltration by myofibroblasts. Mitral regurgitation occurs if the ballooning valve permits blood to leak into the atrium.

Mitral valve prolapse is the most common valve disorder in the United States, with a prevalence of nearly 3% of adults.[108] Because mitral valve prolapse can be associated with other inherited connective tissue disorders (Marfan syndrome, Ehlers-Danlos syndrome, osteogenesis imperfecta), it has been suggested that it results from a genetic or environmental disruption of valvular development during the fifth or sixth week of gestation. There also may be a relationship between symptomatic mitral valve prolapse and hyperthyroidism.

FIGURE 24-30 Mitral Valve Prolapse. A, Prolapsed mitral valve. Prolapse permits the valve leaflets to billow back *(arrow)* into the atrium during left ventricular systole. The billowing causes the leaflets to part slightly, permitting regurgitation into the atrium. **B,** Looking down into the mitral valve, the ballooning *(arrows)* of the leaflets is seen. (From Kumar V et al: *Robins & Cotran pathologic basis of disease*, ed 9, St Louis, 2015, Elsevier. **A** Courtesy William D. Edwards, MD, Mayo Clinic, Rochester, Minn.)

Many cases of mitral valve prolapse are completely asymptomatic. Cardiac auscultation on routine physical examination may disclose a regurgitant murmur or midsystolic click in an otherwise healthy individual, or echocardiography may demonstrate the condition in the absence of auscultatory findings. Symptomatic mitral valve prolapse can cause palpitations related to dysrhythmias, tachycardia, lightheadedness, syncope, fatigue (especially in the morning), lethargy, weakness, dyspnea, chest tightness, hyperventilation, anxiety, depression, panic attacks, and atypical chest pain. Many symptoms are vague and puzzling and are unrelated to the degree of prolapse. Most individuals with mitral valve prolapse have an excellent prognosis, do not develop symptoms, and do not require any restriction in activity or medical management. Occasionally, beta-blockers are needed to alleviate syncope, severe chest pain, or palpitations.

Acute Rheumatic Fever and Rheumatic Heart Disease

Rheumatic fever is a systemic, inflammatory disease caused by a delayed exaggerated immune response to infection by the group A β-hemolytic streptococcus in genetically predisposed individuals. In its acute form, rheumatic fever is a febrile illness characterized by inflammation of the joints, skin, nervous system, and heart.[111] If untreated, rheumatic fever can cause scarring and deformity of cardiac structures, resulting in **rheumatic heart disease (RHD)**.

The incidence of acute rheumatic fever declined in the United States during the 1960s, 1970s, and early 1980s because of medical and socioeconomic improvements. The acute disease occurs most often in children between the ages of 5 and 15 years. Appropriate antibiotic therapy given within the first 9 days of group A β-hemolytic streptococcus infection usually prevents rheumatic fever.[112]

PATHOPHYSIOLOGY Acute rheumatic fever can develop only as a sequel to pharyngeal infection by group A β-hemolytic streptococcus. Streptococcal skin infections do not progress to acute rheumatic fever, although both skin and pharyngeal infections can cause acute glomerulonephritis. This is because the strains of the microorganism that affect the skin do not have the same antigenic molecules in their cell membranes as those that cause pharyngitis and, therefore, do not elicit the same kind of immune response. Acute rheumatic fever is the result of an abnormal humoral and cell-mediated immune response to group A streptococcal cell membrane antigens called M proteins (Figure 24-31).[113,114] This immune response cross-reacts with molecularly similar self-antigens in heart, muscle, brain, and joints, causing an autoimmune response that results in diffuse, proliferative, and exudative inflammatory lesions in these tissues. The inflammation may subside before treatment, leaving behind damage to the heart valves. Repeated attacks of acute rheumatic fever cause chronic proliferative changes in the previously mentioned organs with resultant tissue scarring, granuloma formation, and thrombosis.

Approximately 10% of individuals with rheumatic fever develop rheumatic heart disease (RHD). In developed countries, the peak incidence of the development of RHD occurs in adults between the ages of 25 and 34. Although rheumatic fever can cause carditis in all three layers of the heart wall, the primary lesion usually involves the endocardium. Endocardial inflammation causes swelling of the valve leaflets, with secondary erosion along the lines of leaflet contact. Small, beadlike clumps of vegetation containing platelets and fibrin are deposited on eroded valvular tissue and on the chordae tendineae cordis. These lesions can become progressively adherent. Scarring and shortening of the involved structures occur over time. The valves lose their elasticity, and the leaflets may adhere to each other.

If inflammation penetrates the myocardium, called myocarditis, localized fibrin deposits develop that are surrounded by areas of

FIGURE 24-31 Pathogenesis and Structural Alterations of Acute Rheumatic Heart Disease. Beginning usually with a sore throat, rheumatic fever can develop only as a sequel to pharyngeal infection by group A β-hemolytic streptococcus. Suspected as a hypersensitivity reaction, it is proposed that antibodies directed against the M proteins of certain strains of streptococci cross-react with tissue glycoproteins in the heart, joints, and other tissues. The exact nature of cross-reacting antigens has been difficult to define, but it appears that the streptococcal infection causes an autoimmune response against self-antigens. Inflammatory lesions are found in various sites; the most distinctive within the heart are called Aschoff bodies. The chronic sequelae result from progressive fibrosis because of healing of the inflammatory lesions and the changes induced by valvular deformities. (From Damjanov I: *Pathology for the health professions*, ed 4, Philadelphia, 2012, Saunders.)

necrosis. These fibrinoid necrotic deposits are called Aschoff bodies. Pericardial inflammation is usually characterized by serofibrinous effusion within the pericardial cavity. Cardiomegaly and left heart failure may occur during episodes of untreated acute or recurrent rheumatic fever. Conduction defects and atrial fibrillation often are associated with rheumatic heart disease.

CLINICAL MANIFESTATIONS The common symptoms of acute rheumatic fever are fever, lymphadenopathy, arthralgia, nausea, vomiting, epistaxis (nosebleed), abdominal pain, and tachycardia. The major clinical manifestations of acute rheumatic fever usually occur singly or in combination 1 to 5 weeks after streptococcal infection of the pharynx. They are carditis, acute migratory polyarthritis, chorea, erythema marginatum, and subcutaneous nodules. Criteria for the diagnosis of rheumatic fever (Table 24-7) have not changed since 1992.[111]

EVALUATION AND TREATMENT As described in Table 24-7, supportive evidence for group A β-hemolytic streptococci includes positive throat cultures and measurement of serum antibodies against the hemolytic factor streptolysin O. Cultures may be negative when the rheumatic attack begins, however. Several other antibody tests are sensitive prognosticators of streptococcal infection, including antideoxyribonuclease B (anti-DNase B), antihyaluronidase, and antistreptozyme (ASTZ). Elevated measurements of white blood cell count, erythrocyte sedimentation rate, and C-reactive protein indicate inflammation. All three are usually increased at the time cardiac or joint symptoms begin to appear. Echocardiographic screening for rheumatic heart disease in children with a history of rheumatic fever is controversial because not all detectable abnormalities are clinically relevant.[115]

Therapy for acute rheumatic fever is aimed at eradicating the streptococcal infection and involves a 10-day regimen of oral penicillin or erythromycin administration. Nonsteroidal anti-inflammatory drugs are used as anti-inflammatory agents for both rheumatic carditis and arthritis. Serious carditis may require corticosteroids and diuretics. Because recurrent rheumatic fever occurs in more than half of affected children, continuous prophylactic antibiotic therapy may be necessary for as long as 5 years. Several potential group A streptococcus vaccines are being developed. RHD may require surgical repair of damaged valves.

✓QUICK CHECK 24-8

1. Compare the effect of aortic stenosis with mitral stenosis on the left ventricle and atrium.
2. Describe aortic regurgitation, mitral regurgitation, and tricuspid regurgitation.
3. What are the common symptoms of mitral prolapse?
4. What is the cause of rheumatic heart disease?

Infective Endocarditis

Infective endocarditis is a general term used to describe infection and inflammation of the endocardium—especially the cardiac valves. Bacteria are the most common cause of infective endocarditis, especially streptococci, staphylococci, and enterococci, which account for more than 80% of cases.[116] Other causes include viruses, fungi, rickettsia, and parasites. Infective endocarditis was once a lethal disease, but morbidity and mortality diminished significantly with the advent of antibiotics and improved diagnostic techniques (see *Risk Factors: Infective Endocarditis*).

TABLE 24-7　Jones Criteria (Updated) Used for Diagnosis of Initial Attack of Rheumatic Fever

Criteria	Description
Major Manifestations	
Carditis	Previously undetected murmur, chest pain, pericardial effusion with audible friction rub, extra heart sounds, conduction delays, atrial fibrillation, and prolonged PR interval; valvular diseases (stenosis and regurgitation); recurrent infective endocarditis
Polyarthritis	Migratory polyarthritis (especially large joints of extremities); each joint simultaneously or in succession symptomatic for approximately 2 to 3 days; polyarthritis continued for up to 3 weeks; exudative synovitis (heat, redness, swelling, severe pain)
Chorea	Sudden, aimless, irregular, involuntary movements; more common in females than in males; may occur several months after streptococcal infection; self-limiting, lasting weeks or months; no permanent neural sequelae
Erythema marginatum	Nonpruritic, pink, erythematous macules on trunk that do not occur on face or hands; transitory and may change in appearance within minutes or hours; heat darkens rash; macules may fade in center and be mistaken for ringworm
Subcutaneous nodules	Palpable subcutaneous nodes over bony prominences and along extensor tendons
Minor Manifestations	
Arthralgias	Pain and stiffness in joints without heat, redness, or swelling
Fever	>39° C
Elevated CRP	Indicates inflammation
Prolonged PR interval	Change in ECG consistent with abnormal conduction
Supporting evidence of streptococcal infection	Increased titer of streptococcal antibodies: antistreptolysin O (ASO), positive throat streptococcal infection culture for group A *Streptococcus*

Data from Guidelines for the Diagnosis of Rheumatic Fever: Jones Criteria, 1992 update; Special Writing Group of the Committee on Rheumatic Fever, Endocarditis, and Kawasaki Disease of the Council on Cardiovascular Disease in the Young of the American Heart Association, *JAMA* 268(15):2069-2073, 1992.

RISK FACTORS

Infective Endocarditis

- Acquired valvular heart disease
- Implantation of prosthetic heart valves
- Congenital lesions associated with highly turbulent flow (e.g., ventricular septal defect)
- Previous attack of infective endocarditis
- Intravenous drug use
- Long-term indwelling intravenous catheterization (e.g., for pressure monitoring, feeding, hemodialysis)
- Implantable cardiac pacemakers
- Heart transplant with defective valve

PATHOPHYSIOLOGY　The pathogenesis of infective endocarditis requires at least three critical elements (Figure 24-32):

1. *Endocardial damage.* Trauma, congenital heart disease, valvular heart disease, and the presence of prosthetic valves are the most common risk factors for endocardial damage that leads to infective endocarditis. Turbulent blood flow caused by these abnormalities usually affects the atrial surface of atrioventricular valves or the ventricular surface of semilunar valves. Endocardial damage exposes the endothelial basement membrane, which contains a type of collagen that attracts platelets and thereby stimulates sterile thrombus formation on the membrane. This causes an inflammatory reaction (**nonbacterial thrombotic endocarditis**).
2. *Adherence of blood-borne microorganisms to the damaged endocardial surface.* Bacteria may enter the bloodstream during injection drug use, trauma, dental procedures that involve manipulation of the gingiva, cardiac surgery, genitourinary procedures and indwelling catheters in the presence of infection, or gastrointestinal instrumentation, or they may spread from uncomplicated upper respiratory tract or skin infections. Bacteria adhere to the damaged endocardium using adhesins.[116]

3. *Formation of infective endocardial vegetations* (Figure 24-33). Bacteria infiltrate the sterile thrombi and accelerate fibrin formation by activating the clotting cascade. These vegetative lesions can form anywhere on the endocardium but usually occur on heart valves and surrounding structures. Although endocardial tissue is constantly bathed in antibody-containing blood and is surrounded by scavenging monocytes and polymorphonuclear leukocytes, bacterial colonies are inaccessible to host defenses because they are embedded in the protective fibrin clots. Embolization from these vegetations can lead to abscesses and characteristic skin changes, such as petechiae, splinter hemorrhages, Osler nodes, and Janeway lesions.

CLINICAL MANIFESTATIONS　Fever occurs in 80% of cases.[116] Infective endocarditis causes varying degrees of valvular dysfunction and may be associated with manifestations involving several organ systems (respiratory [lungs], sensory [eyes], genitourinary [kidneys], musculoskeletal [bones, joints], and central nervous systems), making diagnosis exceedingly difficult. Signs and symptoms of infective endocarditis are caused by infection and inflammation, systemic spread of microemboli, and immune complex deposition. The "classic" findings are fever; new or changed cardiac murmur; and petechial lesions of the skin, conjunctiva, and oral mucosa. Characteristic physical findings include Osler nodes (painful erythematous nodules on the pads of the fingers and toes) and Janeway lesions (nonpainful hemorrhagic lesions on the palms and soles). Central nervous system complications are the most frequent and the most severe extracardiac complications and include stroke, abscess, and meningitis.[116,117] Other manifestations include weight loss, back pain, night sweats, and heart failure. Splenic, renal, pulmonary, peripheral arterial, coronary, and ocular emboli may lead to a wide variety of signs and symptoms.

EVALUATION AND TREATMENT　The criteria for the diagnosis of infective endocarditis are called the Duke criteria and include repetitive

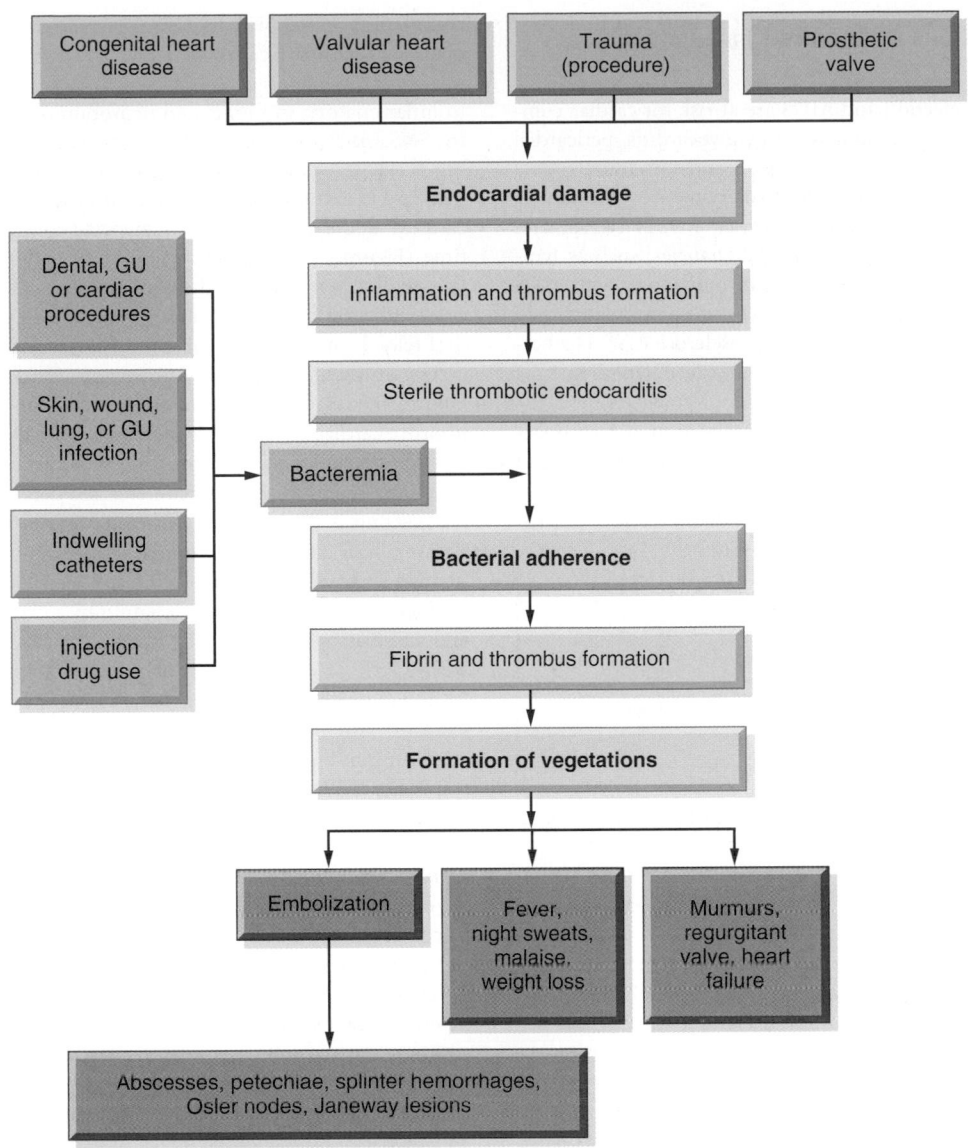

FIGURE 24-32 Pathogenesis of Infective Endocarditis.

FIGURE 24-33 Bacterial Endocarditis of Mitral Valve. The valve is covered with large, irregular vegetations *(arrow)*. (From Damjanov I, Linder J: *Pathology: a color atlas,* St Louis, 2000, Mosby.)

blood cultures positive for bacteria and evidence for endocardial involvement (murmurs or documented regurgitation) along with recognized risk factors, fever, and vascular complications.[116] Serum measures, such as C-reactive protein, also are elevated. Echocardiography should be performed immediately. Antimicrobial therapy is generally given for several weeks, beginning with intravenous and ending with oral administration. In some cases, two different antibiotics are given simultaneously to eliminate the offending microorganism and prevent the development of drug resistance.[107,116] Other drugs may be necessary to treat left heart failure secondary to valvular dysfunction. Surgery that involves excision of infected tissue with or without valve replacement improves outcomes in many persons with infective endocarditis, especially those with severe heart failure or persistent bacteremia despite antibiotic therapy.

Antibiotic prophylaxis to prevent infective endocarditis is indicated for those with prosthetic valves, a history of infective endocarditis, unrepaired cyanotic congenital heart disease, and heart transplant with valvular defect in the setting of gingival procedures or in the presence of documented acute gastrointestinal or genitourinary infection.[107]

Cardiac Complications in Acquired Immunodeficiency Syndrome (AIDS)

Individuals with HIV infection and AIDS are at risk for cardiac complications including dilated cardiomyopathy, myocarditis, pericardial effusion, endocarditis, pulmonary hypertension, and non-antiretroviral drug–related cardiotoxicity. In addition, cardiac involvement may be induced by various bacterial, viral, protozoal, mycobacterial, and fungal pathogens that complicate AIDS. Malignancies, such as lymphoma and Kaposi sarcoma, are seen often in individuals with AIDS and can affect the heart. HIV has been found to cause immune activation that increases the risk for coronary atherosclerosis.[118,119] Furthermore, treatment with antiretroviral therapy can cause hyperlipidemia and atherosclerotic disease.

Left heart failure is the most common complication of HIV infection and is related to left ventricular dilation and dysfunction and sudden death.[120] Pericardial effusion, ventricular dysrhythmias, electrocardiographic changes, and right ventricular dilation and hypertrophy are other less common findings.

> ✔ **QUICK CHECK 24-9**
> 1. What three critical elements are required for the pathogenesis of infective endocarditis?
> 2. Why does infective endocarditis involve several organ systems?
> 3. What effect does AIDS have on the heart?

MANIFESTATIONS OF HEART DISEASE

Heart Failure

Heart failure is when the heart is unable to generate an adequate cardiac output, causing inadequate perfusion of tissues or increased diastolic filling pressure of the left ventricle, or both, so that pulmonary capillary pressures are increased. It affects nearly 10% of individuals older than age 65 and is the most common reason for admission to the hospital in that age group. Ischemic heart disease and hypertension are the most important predisposing risk factors.[10] Other risk factors include age, obesity, diabetes, renal failure, valvular heart disease, cardiomyopathies, myocarditis, congenital heart disease, and excessive alcohol use. Numerous genetic polymorphisms have been linked to an increased risk for heart failure, including genes for cardiomyopathies, myocyte contractility, and neurohumoral receptors. Most causes of heart failure result from dysfunction of the left ventricle (heart failure with reduced ejection fraction and heart failure with preserved ejection fraction). The right ventricle also may be dysfunctional, especially in pulmonary disease (right ventricular failure). Finally, some conditions cause inadequate perfusion despite normal or elevated cardiac output (high-output failure).

Left Heart Failure (Congestive Heart Failure)

Left heart failure, commonly called congestive heart failure, is further categorized as heart failure with reduced ejection fraction or heart failure with preserved ejection fraction. It is possible for these two types of heart failure to occur simultaneously in one individual.

Heart failure with reduced ejection fraction (HFrEF), or systolic heart failure, is defined as an ejection fraction of <40% and an inability of the heart to generate an adequate cardiac output to perfuse vital tissues. Cardiac output depends on the heart rate and stroke volume. Stroke volume is influenced by three major determinants: contractility, preload, and afterload (see Chapter 23).

Contractility is reduced by diseases that disrupt myocyte activity. Myocardial infarction is the most common primary cause of decreased contractility. Other primary causes include myocarditis and cardiomyopathies. Secondary causes of decreased contractility, such as recurrent myocardial ischemia and increased myocardial workload, contribute to inflammatory, immune, and neurohumoral changes (activation of the SNS and RAAS) that mediate a process called ventricular remodeling.[121] Ventricular remodeling results in disruption of the normal myocardial extracellular structure with resultant dilation of the myocardium and causes progressive myocyte contractile dysfunction over time (Figure 24-34). When contractility is decreased, stroke volume falls and left ventricular end-diastolic volume (LVEDV) increases. This causes dilation of the heart and an increase in preload.

Preload, or LVEDV, increases with decreased contractility or an excess of plasma volume (intravenous fluid administration, renal failure, mitral valvular disease). Increases in LVEDV can actually improve cardiac output up to a certain point, but as preload continues to rise, it causes a stretching of the myocardium that eventually can lead to dysfunction of the sarcomeres and decreased contractility. This relationship is described by the Frank-Starling law of the heart (see Figure 23-16). Decreased contractility leads to further increases in preload (Figure 24-35).

Increased afterload is most commonly a result of increased peripheral vascular resistance (PVR), such as that seen with hypertension. Nearly 75% of cases of heart failure have antecedent hypertension.[10] Although much less common, it also can be the result of aortic valvular disease. With increased afterload, there is resistance to ventricular emptying and more workload for the ventricle; and the ventricle responds with hypertrophy, which is a form of myocardial remodeling. This process differs from the physiologic myocyte response to increased workload (exercise) in which the workload is intermittent rather than sustained, resulting in an increase in muscle mass but no distortion of the cardiac architecture. Sustained afterload leads to pathologic hypertrophy mediated by angiotensin II and catecholamines and results in an increase in oxygen demand by the thickened myocardium.[122] A state of relative ischemia develops that further contributes to changes in the myocytes themselves and ventricular remodeling (Figure 24-36). In addition, hypertrophic remodeling results in alteration of the cardiac extracellular matrix and deposition of collagen between the myocytes, which can disrupt the integrity of the muscle, decrease contractility, and increase the likelihood that the ventricle will dilate and fail.[123] These changes in ventricular structure and function are referred to as hypertensive hypertrophic cardiomyopathy (see p. 624).

As cardiac output falls, renal perfusion diminishes with activation of the RAAS, which acts to increase PVR and plasma volume, thus further increasing afterload and preload. In addition, baroreceptors in the central circulation detect the decrease in perfusion and stimulate the SNS to cause yet more vasoconstriction and the hypothalamus to produce antidiuretic hormone. This vicious cycle of decreasing contractility, increasing preload, and increasing afterload causes progressive worsening of left heart failure.

In addition to these hemodynamic interactions, HFrEF is characterized by a complex constellation of neurohumoral, inflammatory, and metabolic processes. Ang II and aldosterone have direct toxicity to the myocardium, contributing to remodeling, myocyte death, and fibrosis. Catecholamines released by the SNS also are toxic to the myocardium and contribute to remodeling.[121] Natriuretic peptides are released in an effort to improve renal salt and water excretion but are inadequate to compensate for these neurohumoral perturbations.[124] Insulin resistance and diabetes not only contribute to heart failure but also are a complication of heart failure with changes in myocyte metabolism. Inflammatory cytokines, such as TNF-α, are released in heart failure, contributing to myocardial damage as well as systemic weight loss (cardiac cachexia). Finally, changes in the metabolic processes

FIGURE 24-34 Pathophysiology of Ventricular Remodeling. Myocardial dysfunction activates the renin-angiotensin-aldosterone and sympathetic nervous systems, releasing neurohormones (angiotensin II, aldosterone, catecholamines, and cytokines). These neurohormones contribute to ventricular remodeling. (Redrawn from Carelock J, Clark AP: *Am J Nurs* 101[12]:27, 2001.)

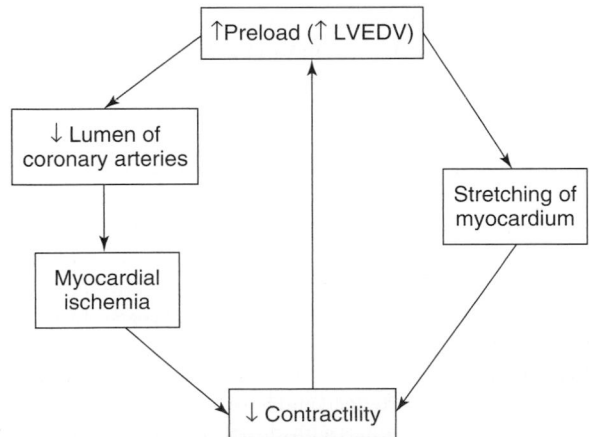

FIGURE 24-35 Effect of Elevated Preload on Myocardial Oxygen Supply and Demand. *LVEDV,* Left ventricular end-diastolic volume.

within the myocardium also are affected with a decreased ability of the heart to produce energy and an increase in release of toxic metabolites.[125] (see *Health Alert:* Metabolic Changes in Heart Failure). These neurohumoral, inflammatory, and metabolic aspects of left HFrEF have led to the routine use of combinations of medications

that inhibit angiotensin, aldosterone, and catecholamines and increase salt excretion in an effort to prevent long-term damage to the myocardium, as well as the exploration of new treatment modalities focused on reducing inflammation and improving myocardial metabolic function.[125,126]

The interaction of these hemodynamic, neurohumoral, inflammatory, and metabolic processes results in a steady decline in myocardial function. Pathologically, the heart muscle exhibits gradual changes in myocyte structure and function, with apoptosis of cells, deposition of fibrin, and remodeling of the myocardium such that contractility and cardiac output decline. A vicious cycle of decreasing contractility, increasing preload, and increasing afterload develops, causing the progressive worsening of symptoms associated with left heart failure (Figure 24-37).

The clinical manifestations of left heart failure are the result of pulmonary vascular congestion and inadequate perfusion of the systemic circulation. Individuals experience dyspnea, orthopnea, cough of frothy sputum, fatigue, decreased urine output, and edema. Physical examination often reveals pulmonary edema (cyanosis, inspiratory crackles, pleural effusions), hypotension or hypertension, an S_3 gallop, and evidence of underlying CAD or hypertension. The diagnosis can be further confirmed with echocardiography showing decreased cardiac output and cardiomegaly. The level of serum B-type natriuretic

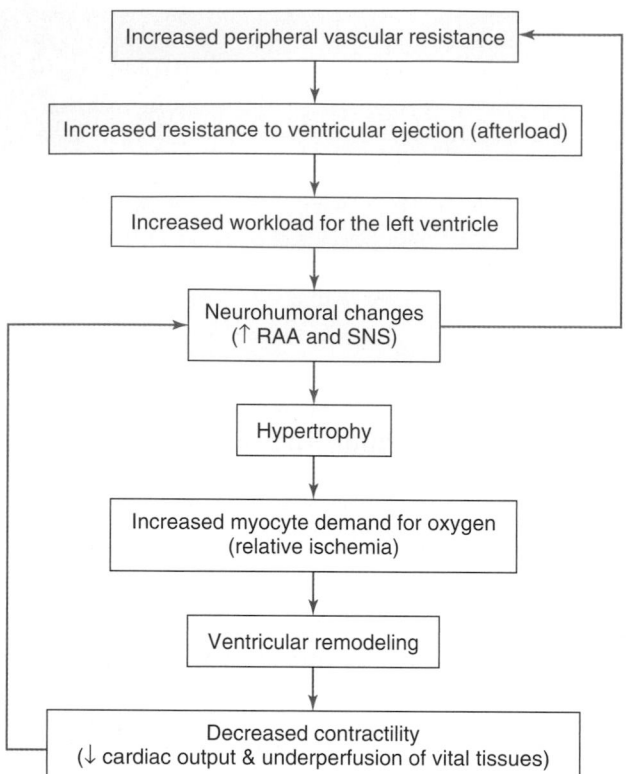

FIGURE 24-36 Role of Increased Afterload in the Pathogenesis of Heart Failure.

FIGURE 24-37 Vicious Cycle of Heart Failure with Reduced Ejection Fraction. Although the initial insult may be one of primary decreased contractility (e.g., myocardial infarction), increased preload (e.g., renal failure), or increased afterload (e.g., hypertension), all three factors play a role in the progression of left heart failure. *LVEDV*, Left ventricular end-diastolic volume.

peptide (BNP) can also help make the diagnosis of heart failure and give some insight into its severity.[127]

Management of HFrEF is aimed at interrupting the worsening cycle of decreasing contractility, increasing preload, and increasing afterload. The acute onset of left heart failure is most often the result of acute myocardial ischemia and must be managed in conjunction with management of the underlying coronary disease (see p. 614). Oxygen, nitrate, and morphine administration improves myocardial oxygenation and helps relieve coronary spasm while lowering preload through systemic venodilation. Inotropic drugs, such as dopamine, dobutamine, and milrinone, increase contractility and can help raise the

HEALTH ALERT
Metabolic Changes in Heart Failure

Although the use of medications that block the renin-angiotensin-aldosterone and sympathetic nervous systems reduces remodeling and improves outcomes in heart failure, morbidity and mortality from this condition are still high. The heart is the largest consumer of energy in the body and relies on the efficient production of adenosine triphosphate (ATP), yet it has very little capacity for energy storage. In the failing heart, increased demand for oxygen and energy is coupled with a decreased ability to utilize fatty acids as an energy source. As a result, several genes are activated that alter the ability of myocytes to use lipids and glucose as fuel sources, the most studied of which are the peroxisome proliferator–activated receptor (PPAR) family of genes. These genes control fatty acid oxidation and are of particular importance in heart failure associated with insulin resistance and diabetes. Energy starvation and high levels of catecholamines associated with heart failure lead to altered fatty acid oxidation and decreased effective ATP generation and utilization. This results in decreased myocardial contractility and structural changes in the myocardium (remodeling). Increasing knowledge of these mechanisms has led to the exploration of potential new therapies for heart failure. For example, although currently available PPAR-γ agonists (thiazolidinediones) are contraindicated in worsening heart failure because of increased fluid retention at the renal tubule, new insulin sensitizers are being explored that may improve myocardial metabolic function. In addition, inhibitors of fatty acid oxidation (e.g., trimetazidine) have been tried in several small studies with some improvement in cardiac function. Other metabolic abnormalities in the failing heart are being discovered, including changes in the pentose phosphate pathway, ketone bodies, uncoupled electron transfer, and lipotoxins. Many new potential drugs are under investigation and mechanical support devices, such as left ventricular assist devices, are promising in reversing these metabolic changes. In the meantime, most researchers agree that exercise and a healthy diet are the most effective approaches to improving myocardial metabolic function.

Data from Carley AN et al: *Circ Res* 114(4):717-729, 2014; Chen YR, Zweier JL: *Circ Res* 114(3):524-537, 2014; Dominic EA et al: *Heart* 100(8):611-618, 2014; Turer AT: *J Mol Cell Cardiol* 55:12-18, 2013; Wang XM et al: *Cardiovasc Drugs Ther* 27(4):297-307, 2013; Weitzel LB et al: *PLoS ONE* 8(4):e60292, 2013.

blood pressure in hypotensive individuals but must be monitored carefully.[128] Diuretics reduce preload. ACE inhibitors, ARBs, and aldosterone blockers reduce both preload and afterload by decreasing aldosterone levels and reducing PVR. Finally, individuals with severe HFrEF failure may benefit from acute coronary bypass or percutaneous coronary intervention (PCI). These people often are supported with the intra-aortic balloon pump (IABP) or left ventricular assist devices (LVADs) until surgery can be performed.

Management of chronic left heart failure is based on current clinical guidelines and clinical severity.[129] The overall goals are to reduce preload and afterload. Salt restriction and diuretics (loop diuretics) are effective in reducing preload. ACE inhibitors (or Ang II receptor blockers) reduce preload and afterload and have been shown to significantly reduce mortality in individuals with chronic left heart failure. Aldosterone blockers, such as spironolactone, also are associated with improved outcomes.[130] Beta-blockers improve symptoms and increase survival but must be used carefully to avoid hypotension. The inotropic drug digoxin may be considered in selected individuals, especially those with refractory heart failure or atrial fibrillation.[129] Although many individuals with left heart failure die suddenly from dysrhythmias, prophylactic administration of antidysrhythmics has not been shown to improve survival. In individuals with sustained ventricular tachycardia, implantable cardioverter-defibrillators should be considered. Cardiac resynchronization therapy is proving to be an important modality in selected individuals.[131] For those individuals with coronary artery disease, coronary bypass surgery or PCI may improve perfusion to ischemic myocardium (hibernating myocardium) and improve cardiac output. Surgical interventions may be performed (including improving ventricular geometry, implanting assist devices) or heart transplantation may need to be considered. Experimental therapies, including natriuretic peptide analogs, gene transfer, and stem cell therapies, are being explored.[132] Gene therapy offers some exciting new hope for severe heart failure (see *Health Alert:* Gene Therapy for Heart Failure).

HEALTH ALERT

Gene Therapy for Heart Failure

The effectiveness and safety of recent gene therapy trials for heart failure have led to an explosion of interest in innovative methods for restoring cardiac function. Multiple components of cardiac contractility have been identified as targets for gene therapy, including calcium channel cycling, β-adrenergic functioning, and cellular proliferation. The most studied of the potential gene targets include sarcoendoplasmic reticulum calcium ATPase (SERCA2a) and S100A1, which affect intracellular myocyte calcium handling. Another exciting target is adenylyl cyclase 6 (AC6), the enzyme catalyzing cAMP formation and β-adrenergic receptor function. Other targets include SDF1/CXCR4 complex, which promotes homing of stem cells to infarcted myocardium; microRNAs; and genes that code for critical neurohumoral factors, including insulin-like growth factor-1 (IGF-1), growth hormone, and B-type natriuretic peptide. Gene delivery vectors fall into one of two categories: nonviral or viral. Nonviral gene delivery vectors are safe and have minimal immunogenicity but do not appear to be efficient at delivering the genes to the tissues. Viral vectors are more efficient at delivering genes to cells but safety concerns persist. Today the viruses most widely used for cardiovascular gene transfer are adenovirus, Sendai virus, and adeno-associated virus (AAV). These viruses exhibit fairly good cardiotropism and various methods are being explored for delivering these gene vectors most efficiently to the myocardium, including antegrade or retrograde coronary infusion, intravenous infusion, direct myocardial injection, and pericardial injection. One recent report documented that intracoronary infusion of AAV with SERCA2a for individuals with severe heart failure significantly improved mortality and heart failure outcomes with positive effects and no reported safety concerns reported at 3 years. It is clear that the future will reveal many new and potentially lifesaving gene therapies for those with intractable heart failure.

Data from Lipskaia L et al: *Curr Vasc Pharmacol* 11(4):465-479, 2013; Naim C et al: *Curr Cardiol Rep* 15(2):333, 2013; Papolos A, Frishman WH: *Cardiol Rev* 21(3):151-154, 2013; Park WJ: *BMB Rep* 46(5):237-243, 2013; Pleger ST et al: *Circ Res* 113(6):792-809, 2013; Siddiqi S, Sussman MA: *Exp Rev Cardiovas Ther* 11(8):949-957, 2013; Watts G: *Br Med J* 346:f2795, 2013.

Heart failure with preserved ejection function (HFpEF), or **diastolic heart failure**, can occur singly or along with HFrEF. Isolated HFpEF is defined as pulmonary congestion despite a normal stroke volume and cardiac output. It is estimated that HFpHF affects more than 25% of adults in the United States.[10] HFpEF is preceded by a condition called preclinical diastolic dysfunction (PDD) in which affected individuals do not have symptoms, but have early changes in ventricular relaxation and a high untreated risk for developing heart failure.[133] HFpHF results from decreased compliance of the left ventricle and abnormal diastolic relaxation such that a normal left ventricular end-diastolic volume (LVEDV) results in an increased left ventricular end-diastolic pressure (LVEDP). This pressure is reflected

TABLE 24-8 Comparison of Heart Failure with Reduced Ejection Fraction (HFrEF) and Heart Failure with Preserved Ejection Fraction (HFpEF)

Characteristic	HFrEF	HFpEF
Gender	Male > female	Female > male
Left ventricular ejection fraction	Decreased	Normal
Left ventricular chamber size	Increased	Decreased
Left ventricular hypertrophy on electrocardiogram	Possible	Probable
Chest radiography	Pulmonary congestion with cardiomegaly	Pulmonary congestion without cardiomegaly
Gallop	S_3	S_4

Adapted from Jessup M, Brozena S: *N Engl J Med* 348(20):2007-2018, 2003.

back into the pulmonary circulation and results in pulmonary edema, pulmonary hypertension, and right ventricular hypertrophy.[134] The amount of LV stiffness and RV hypertrophy are the strongest pathophysiologic predictors of complications from HFpEF.[135] The major causes of diastolic dysfunction include hypertension-induced myocardial hypertrophy and myocardial ischemia–induced ventricular remodeling. Hypertrophy and ischemia cause a decreased ability of the myocytes to actively pump calcium from the cytosol, resulting in impaired relaxation. Other causes include aortic valvular disease, mitral valve disease, pericardial diseases, and cardiomyopathies. Diabetes also increases the risk for diastolic dysfunction. Like HFrEF, HFpEF is characterized by sustained activation of the RAAS and the SNS.

Individuals with diastolic dysfunction present with dyspnea on exertion and fatigue. Evidence of pulmonary edema (inspiratory crackles on auscultation, pleural effusions) is usually not present in resting individuals without tachycardia. Late in diastole, atrial contraction with rapid ejection of blood into the noncompliant ventricle may give rise to an S_4 gallop. Electrocardiography often reveals evidence of left ventricular hypertrophy, and chest x-ray may show pulmonary congestion without cardiomegaly (Table 24-8). There also may be evidence of underlying coronary disease, hypertension, or valvular disease. Diagnosis is based upon three factors: signs and symptoms of heart failure, normal left ventricular (LV) ejection fraction, and evidence of diastolic dysfunction. The diagnosis is confirmed by clinical Doppler echocardiography, which demonstrates poor ventricular filling with normal ejection fractions.[136]

Management is aimed at improving ventricular relaxation and prolonging diastolic filling times to reduce diastolic pressure. No therapy has been shown to improve survival, and calcium channel blockers, beta-blockers, ACE inhibitors, and ARBs have been used with only varying success.[137] Treatment with the 3-hydroxy-3-methyl-glutaryl-coenzyme A (HMG-CoA) reductase inhibitors (statins) has consistently resulted in improvements in LV diastolic function.[137,138] Inotropic drugs are not indicated in isolated HFpEF because contractility and ejection fraction are not affected; however, digoxin may be used to slow the heart rate in individuals with atrial fibrillation. Outcomes for individuals with HFpEF are as poor as those with HFrEF, and there has been no improvement in prognosis despite numerous new treatment trials.[139]

Right Heart Failure

Right heart failure is defined as the inability of the right ventricle to provide adequate blood flow into the pulmonary circulation at a normal central venous pressure. It can result from left heart failure when an increase in left ventricular filling pressure is reflected back into the pulmonary circulation. As pressure in the pulmonary circulation rises, the resistance to right ventricular emptying increases (Figure 24-38). The right ventricle is poorly prepared to compensate for this increased afterload and will dilate and fail. When this happens, pressure will rise in the systemic venous circulation, resulting in peripheral edema and hepatosplenomegaly. Treatment relies on management of the left ventricular dysfunction as just outlined. When right heart failure occurs in the absence of left heart failure, it is typically attributable to diffuse hypoxic pulmonary disease such as chronic obstructive pulmonary disease (COPD), cystic fibrosis, and acute respiratory distress syndrome (ARDS). These disorders result in an increase in right ventricular afterload. The mechanisms for this type of right ventricular failure (cor pulmonale) are discussed in Chapter 27. Finally, myocardial infarction, cardiomyopathies, and pulmonic valvular disease interfere with right ventricular contractility and can lead to right heart failure.

High-Output Failure

High-output failure is the inability of the heart to adequately supply the body with blood-borne nutrients, despite adequate blood volume and normal or elevated myocardial contractility. In high-output failure, the heart increases its output but the body's metabolic needs are still not met. Common causes of high-output failure are anemia, septicemia, hyperthyroidism, and beriberi (Figure 24-39).

Anemia decreases the oxygen-carrying capacity of the blood. Metabolic acidosis occurs as the body's cells switch to anaerobic metabolism (see Chapter 5). In response to metabolic acidosis, heart rate and stroke volume increase in an attempt to improve tissue perfusion. If anemia is severe, however, even maximum cardiac output does not supply the cells with enough oxygen for metabolism.

In septicemia, disturbed metabolism, bacterial toxins, and the inflammatory process cause systemic vasodilation and fever. Faced with a lowered systemic vascular resistance (SVR) and an elevated metabolic rate, cardiac output increases to maintain blood pressure and prevent metabolic acidosis. In overwhelming septicemia, however, the heart may not be able to raise its output enough to compensate for vasodilation. Body tissues show signs of inadequate blood supply despite a high cardiac output.

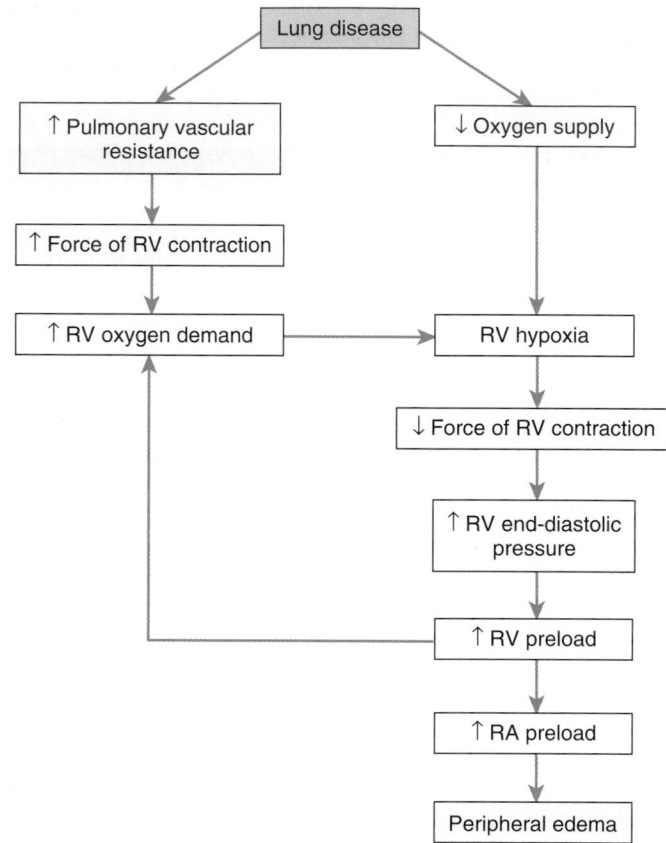

FIGURE 24-38 Right Heart Failure. *RA,* Right atrial; *RV,* right ventricular.

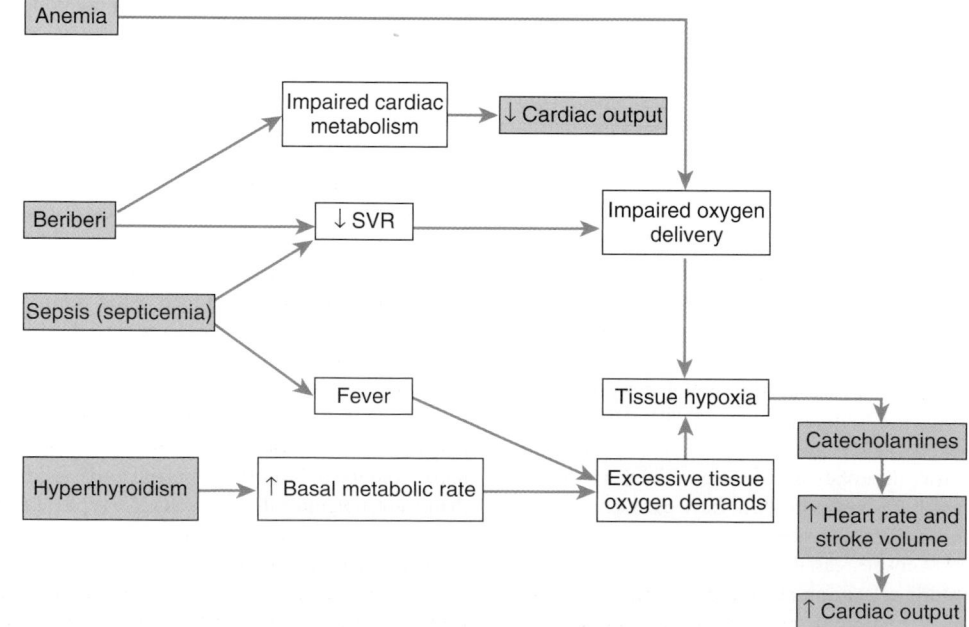

FIGURE 24-39 High-Output Failure. *SVR,* Systemic vascular resistance.

Hyperthyroidism accelerates cellular metabolism through the actions of elevated levels of thyroxine from the thyroid gland. This may occur chronically (thyrotoxicosis) or acutely (thyroid storm). Because the body's increased demand for oxygen threatens to cause metabolic acidosis, cardiac output increases. If blood levels of thyroxine are high and the metabolic response to thyroxine is vigorous, even an abnormally elevated cardiac output may be inadequate.

In the United States, beriberi (thiamine deficiency) usually is caused by malnutrition secondary to chronic alcoholism. Beriberi actually causes a mixed type of heart failure. Thiamine deficiency impairs cellular metabolism in all tissues, including the myocardium. In the heart, impaired cardiac metabolism leads to insufficient contractile strength. In blood vessels, thiamine deficiency leads to peripheral vasodilation, which decreases SVR. Heart failure ensues as decreased SVR triggers increased cardiac output, which the impaired myocardium is unable to deliver. The strain of demands for increased output in the face of impaired metabolism may deplete cardiac reserves until low-output failure begins.

Dysrhythmias

A dysrhythmia, or arrhythmia, is a disturbance of heart rhythm. Normal heart rhythms are generated by the sinoatrial (SA) node and travel through the heart's conduction system, causing the atrial and ventricular myocardium to contract and relax at a regular rate that is appropriate to maintain circulation at various levels of physical activity (see Chapter 23). Dysrhythmias range in severity from occasional "missed" or rapid beats to serious disturbances that impair the pumping ability of the heart, contributing to heart failure and death. Dysrhythmias can be caused either by an abnormal rate of impulse generation (Table 24-9) from the SA node or other pacemaker or by the abnormal conduction of impulses (Table 24-10) through the heart's conduction system, including the myocardial cells themselves.

✔**QUICK CHECK 24-10**
1. Why are changes in LVEDV important for left heart failure?
2. What is ventricular remodeling?
3. What is the vicious cycle of heart failure with preserved ejection fraction?

SHOCK

In shock the cardiovascular system fails to perfuse the tissues adequately, resulting in widespread impairment of cellular metabolism. Because tissue perfusion can be disrupted by any factor that alters heart function, blood volume, or blood pressure, shock has many causes and various clinical manifestations. Ultimately, however, shock progresses to organ failure and death, unless compensatory mechanisms reverse the process or clinical intervention succeeds. Untreated severe shock overwhelms the body's compensatory mechanisms through positive feedback loops that initiate and maintain a downward physiologic spiral.

The term *multiple organ dysfunction syndrome* (MODS) describes the failure of two or more organ systems after severe illness and injury and is a frequent complication of severe shock. The disease process is initiated and perpetuated by uncontrolled inflammatory and stress responses. It is progressive and is associated with significant mortality.

Impairment of Cellular Metabolism

The final common pathway in shock of any type is impairment of cellular metabolism. Figure 24-40 illustrates the pathophysiology of shock at the cellular level.

Impairment of Oxygen Use

In all types of shock, the cell either is not receiving an adequate amount of oxygen or is unable to use oxygen. Without oxygen, the cell shifts from aerobic to anaerobic metabolism. Anaerobic metabolism is a less efficient method of extracting energy from carbon bonds, and the cell begins to use its stores of adenosine triphosphate (ATP) faster than stores can be replaced. Without ATP, the cell cannot maintain an electrochemical gradient across its selectively permeable membrane. Specifically, the cell cannot operate the sodium-potassium pump. Sodium and chloride accumulate inside the cell, and potassium exits the cell. Cells of the nervous system and myocardium are profoundly and immediately affected. The resting potentials of these cells are reduced, and action potentials decrease in amplitude. Various clinical manifestations of impaired central nervous system and myocardial function result.

As sodium moves into the cell, water follows. Throughout the body, the water drawn from the interstitium into the cells is "replaced" by water that is, in turn, drawn out of the vascular space. This decreases circulatory volume. Within the cells, water causes cellular edema that disrupts cellular membranes, releasing lysosomal enzymes that injure the cells internally and then leak into the interstitium. Compensatory mechanisms, including inflammation and activation of the clotting cascade, further impair oxygen use and contribute to the complications of shock, such as acute tubular necrosis (ATN), acute respiratory distress syndrome (ARDS), and disseminated intravascular coagulation (DIC).

In addition to decreasing ATP stores, anaerobic metabolism affects the pH of the cell, and metabolic acidosis develops. A compensatory mechanism enables cardiac and skeletal muscles to use lactic acid as a fuel source, but only for a limited time. The decreasing pH of the cell that is functioning anaerobically has serious consequences. Enzymes necessary for cellular function dissociate under acid conditions. Enzyme dissociation stops cell function, repair, and division. As lactic acid is released systemically, blood pH drops, reducing the oxygen-carrying capacity of the blood (see Chapter 4). Therefore less oxygen is delivered to the cells. Further acidosis triggers the release of more lysosomal enzymes because the low pH disrupts lysosomal membrane integrity.

Impairment of Glucose Use

Impaired glucose use can be caused by either impaired glucose delivery or impaired glucose uptake by the cells (see Figure 24-40). The reasons for inadequate glucose delivery are the same as those enumerated for inadequate oxygen delivery. In addition, in septic and anaphylactic shock, glucose metabolism may be increased or disrupted because of fever or bacteria, and glucose uptake can be prevented by the presence of vasoactive toxins, endotoxins, histamine, and kinins.

Some compensatory mechanisms activated by shock contribute to decreased glucose uptake by the cells. High serum levels of cortisol, thyroid hormone, and catecholamines account for hyperglycemia and insulin resistance, tachycardia, increased SVR, and increased cardiac contractility. Cells shift to glycogenolysis, gluconeogenesis, and lipolysis to generate fuel for survival (see Chapter 1). Except in the liver, kidneys, and muscles, the body's cells have extremely limited stores of glycogen. In fact, total body stores can fuel the metabolism for only about 10 hours. The depletion of fat and glycogen stores is not itself a cause of organ failure, but the energy costs of glycogenolysis and lipolysis are considerable and contribute to cell failure.

The depletion of protein also is a cause of organ failure. When gluconeogenesis causes proteins to be used for fuel, these proteins are no longer available to maintain cellular structure, function, repair, and replication. The breakdown of protein occurs in starvation states,

TABLE 24-9 Disorders of Impulse Formation

Type	Electrocardiogram	Effect	Pathophysiology	Treatment
Sinus bradycardia	P rate 60 or less PR interval normal QRS for each P	Increased preload Decreased mean arterial pressure	Hyperkalemia: slows depolarization Vagal hyperactivity: unknown Digoxin toxicity common Late hypoxia: lack of adenosine triphosphate (ATP)	If hypotensive, treat cause Sympathomimetics, anticholinergics Pacemaker placement
Simple sinus tachycardia	P rate 100-150 PR interval normal QRS for each P	Decreased filling times Decreased mean arterial pressure Increased myocardial demand	Catecholamines: rise in resting potential and calcium influx Fever: unknown Early heart failure: compensatory response to decreased stroke volume Lung disease: hypoxic cell metabolism Hypercalcemia	Oxygen, bed rest Calcium blockers
Premature atrial contractions (PACs) or beats*	Early P waves that may have morphologic changes PR interval normal QRS for each P	Occasional decreased filling time and mean arterial pressure	Electrolyte disturbances (especially hypercalcemia): alter action potentials Hypoxia and elevated preload: cell membrane disturbances	Treat underlying cause Digoxin
Sinus dysrhythmias	Rate varies P-P regularly irregular, short with inspiration, long with exhalation PR interval normal QRS for each P	Variable filling times Variable mean arterial pressure Variable oxygen demand	Unknown Common in young children and young adults	None
Atrial tachycardia (includes premature atrial tachycardia if onset is abrupt)	P rate 151-250 P morphology may differ from sinus P PR interval normal P/QRS ratio variable	Decreased filling time Decreased mean arterial pressure Increased myocardial demand	Same as PACs: leads to increased atrial automaticity, atrial reentry Digoxin toxicity: common Aging	Control ventricular rate Digoxin, calcium channel blockers, vagus stimulation Pacemaker to override atrial conduction Cardioversion
Atrial flutter*	P rate 251-300, morphology may vary from sinus P PR interval usually not observable P/QRS ratio variable	Decreased filling time Decreased mean arterial pressure	Same as atrial tachycardia	Same as atrial tachycardia
Atrial fibrillation*	P rate >300 and usually not observable No PR interval QRS rate variable and rhythm irregular	Same as atrial flutter	Same as atrial tachycardia	Same as atrial tachycardia
Idiojunctional rhythm	P absent or independent QRS normal, rate 41-59, regular	Decreased cardiac output from loss of atrial contribution to ventricular preload	Atrial and sinus bradycardia, standstill, or block	Same as sinus bradycardia
Junctional bradycardia	P absent or independent QRS normal, rate 40 or less	Same as idiojunctional rhythm	Same as idiojunctional rhythm Vagal hyperactivity	Same as sinus bradycardia
Premature junctional contractions (PJCs) or beats	Early beats without P waves QRS morphology normal	Decreased cardiac output from loss of atrial contribution to ventricular preload for that beat	Hyperkalemia (5.4-6 mEq/L) Hypercalcemia, hypoxia, and elevated preload (see PACs)	Same as PAC
Accelerated junctional rhythm	P absent or independent QRS morphology normal, rate 60-99	Decreased cardiac output from loss of atrial contribution to ventricular preload	Same as PJCs	Same as PAC
Junctional tachycardia	P absent or independent QRS morphology normal, rate 100 or more	Decreased cardiac output from loss of atrial contribution to ventricular preload Increased myocardial demand because of tachycardia	Same as PJCs	Same as PAC

TABLE 24-9	Disorders of Impulse Formation—cont'd			
Type	**Electrocardiogram**	**Effect**	**Pathophysiology**	**Treatment**
Idioventricular rhythm[†]	P absent or independent QRS >0.11 and rate 20-39	Same as idiojunctional rhythm	Sinus, atrial, and junctional bradycardia, standstill, or block	Same as sinus bradycardia
Ventricular bradycardia[†]	P absent or independent QRS >0.11 and rate 60-<60	Same as idiojunctional rhythm	Same as idiojunctional rhythm	Same as sinus bradycardia
Agonal rhythm/ electromechanical dissociation[†]	P absent or independent QRS >0.11 and rate 20 or less	Absent or barely present cardiac output and pulse Not compatible with life	Depolarization and contraction not coupled: electrical activity present with little or no mechanical activity Usually caused by profound hypoxia	Vigorous pharmacologic treatment aimed at restoring rate and force Usually ineffective May attempt to use pacemaker
Ventricular standstill or asystole[†]	P absent or independent QRS absent	No cardiac output Not compatible with life	Profound ischemia, hyperkalemia, acidosis	Same as agonal rhythm, plus electrical defibrillation
Premature ventricular contractions (PVCs) or depolarizations*	Early beats with P waves QRS occasionally opposite in deflection from usual QRS	Same as premature junctional contractions	Same as PJCs, aging and induction of anesthesia Impulse originates in cell outside normal conduction system and spreads through intercalated disks	Pharmacologic interventions to change thresholds, refractory periods; reduce myocardial demand, increase supply
Accelerated ventricular rhythm	P absent or independent QRS >0.11 and rate of 41-99	Same as accelerated junctional rhythm	Same as PVCs	Removal of cause Same as PVCs
Ventricular tachycardia[†]	P absent or independent QRS >0.11 and rate 100 or more	Same as junctional tachycardia	Same as PVCs	Same as PVCs, plus electrical cardioversion
Ventricular fibrillation[†]	P absent QRS >300 and usually not observable	Same as ventricular standstill	Same as PVCs Rapid infusion of potassium	Same as PVCs, plus electrical cardioversion

*Most common in adults.
[†]Life-threatening in adults.

TABLE 24-10	Disorders of Impulse Conduction			
Type	**ECG**	**Effect**	**Pathophysiology**	**Treatment**
Sinus block	Occasionally absent P, with loss of QRS for that beat	Occasional decrease in cardiac output Increase in preload for following beat	Local hypoxia, scarring of intra-atrial conduction pathways, electrolyte imbalances Increased atrial preload	Conservative Usually do not progress in severity Pharmacologic treatment includes vagolytics, sympathomimetics, pacing
First-degree block*	PRI >0.2 sec	None	Same as sinus block Hyperkalemia (>7 mEq/L) Hypokalemia (<3.5 mEq/L) Formation of myocardial abscess in endocarditis	Conservative Discovery and correction of cause
Second-degree block, Mobitz I, or Wenckebach*	Progressive prolongation of PRI until one QRS is dropped Pattern of prolongation resumes	Same as sinus block	Hypokalemia (<3.5 mEq/L) Faulty cell metabolism in AV node Severity increases as heart rate increases Supports theory that AV node is fatiguing Digoxin toxicity, beta blockade CAD, MI, hypoxia, increased preload, valvular surgery and disease, diabetes	Same as sinus block
Second-degree block or Mobitz II	Same as sinus block	Same as sinus block	Hypokalemia (<3.5 mEq/L) Faulty cell metabolism below AV node Antidysrhythmics, tricyclic antidepressants CAD, MI, hypoxia, increased preload, valvular surgery and disease, diabetes	More aggressively than Mobitz I, because can progress to type III Pacemaker after pharmacologic treatment

Continued

TABLE 24-10   Disorders of Impulse Conduction—cont'd

Type	ECG	Effect	Pathophysiology	Treatment
Third-degree block[†]	P waves present and independent of QRS No observed relationship between P and QRS Always AV dissociation	Same as idiojunctional rhythm	Hypokalemia (<3.5 mEq/L) Faulty cell metabolism low in bundle of His MI, especially inferior wall, as nodal artery interrupted; results in ischemia of AV node	Pacemaker after pharmacologic treatment Temporary pacing if caused by inferior MI, because ischemia usually resolves
Atrioventricular dissociation	P waves present and independent of QRS, but not always because of block (e.g., ventricular tachycardia) AV dissociation not always third-degree block	Decreased cardiac output from loss of atrial contribution to ventricular preload Variable effect on myocardial demand, depending on ventricular rate	May result from third-degree block or accelerated junctional or ventricular rhythm or be caused by sinus, atrial, and junctional bradycardias	Treat according to cause Pacemaker or reducing rate of AV or ventricular discharge, or increasing rate of sinus or AV node discharge
Ventricular block	QRS >0.11 sec R-S-R″ in V_1, V_2, V_5, V_6	None	Faulty cell metabolism in right and left bundle branches RBBB more common than LBBB because of dual blood supply to left bundle branch CHF, MR, especially anterior MI, because of infarct of fascicles Left anterior hemiblock more common than left posterior hemiblock because posterior fascicles have dual blood supply	Isolated RBBB or LBBB or hemiblock not treated If acute and/or associated with acute anterior MI, treated with permanent pacer and vigorous pharmacologic therapy
Aberrant conduction	QRS >0.11 sec	None, unless ventricular rate abnormalities present	Conduction of impulse through intercalated disks because conduction system transiently blocked as a result of hypoxia, electrolyte imbalances, digoxin toxicity, excessively rapid rate of discharge	Correct underlying cause
Preexcitation syndromes (Wolff-Parkinson-White and Lown-Ganong-Levine)	P present with QRS for each PPRI <0.12 sec and QRS <0.11 sec because of delta wave in PRI	None	Congenital presence of accessory pathways (bundle of Kent and fiber of Mahaim) that conduct very rapidly and bypass AV node, causing early ventricular depolarization in relation to atrial depolarization Prone to tachycardias and atrial fibrillation that can result in very rapid ventricular rates (reason unknown)	Aimed at aligning refractory periods of accessory pathway and AV node to prevent reentry May slow rate with drug therapy May surgically cut pathways

AV, Atrioventricular; *CAD,* coronary artery disease; *CHF,* congestive heart failure; *LBBB,* left bundle branch block; *MI,* myocardial infarction; *MR,* mitral regurgitation; *PRI,* PR interval; *RBBB,* right bundle branch block.
*Most common in adults.
[†]Life-threatening in adults.

hyperdynamic metabolic states, and septic shock. During anaerobic metabolism, protein metabolism liberates alanine, which is converted to pyruvate. In sepsis, pyruvic acid is changed into lactic acid, and a positive feedback loop is formed. As proteins are broken down anaerobically, ammonia and urea are produced. Ammonia is toxic to living cells. Uremia develops, and uric acid further disrupts cellular metabolism. Serum albumin and other plasma proteins are consumed for fuel first. Serum protein consumption decreases capillary osmotic pressure and contributes to the development of interstitial edema, creating another positive feedback loop that decreases circulatory volume. In septic shock, plasma protein breakdown includes metabolism of immunoglobulins, thereby impairing immune system function when it is most needed.

Muscle wasting caused by protein breakdown weakens skeletal and cardiac muscle. Skeletal muscle wasting impairs the muscles that facilitate breathing. Muscle wasting therefore alters the actions of both the heart and the lungs. The delivery of oxygen and glucose to the cells is directly reduced, as is the removal of waste products, forming another positive feedback loop.

A final outcome of impaired cellular metabolism is the buildup of metabolic end products in the cell and interstitial spaces. Waste products are toxic to the cells and further disrupt cellular function and membrane integrity. Once a sufficiently large number of cells from vital organs have damage to cellular membranes, leakage of lysosomal enzymes, and depletion of ATP, shock can be irreversible.

Clinical Manifestations of Shock

The clinical manifestations of shock are variable depending on the type of shock, and observable and measurable signs and symptoms are often conflicting in nature. Subjective complaints in shock are usually

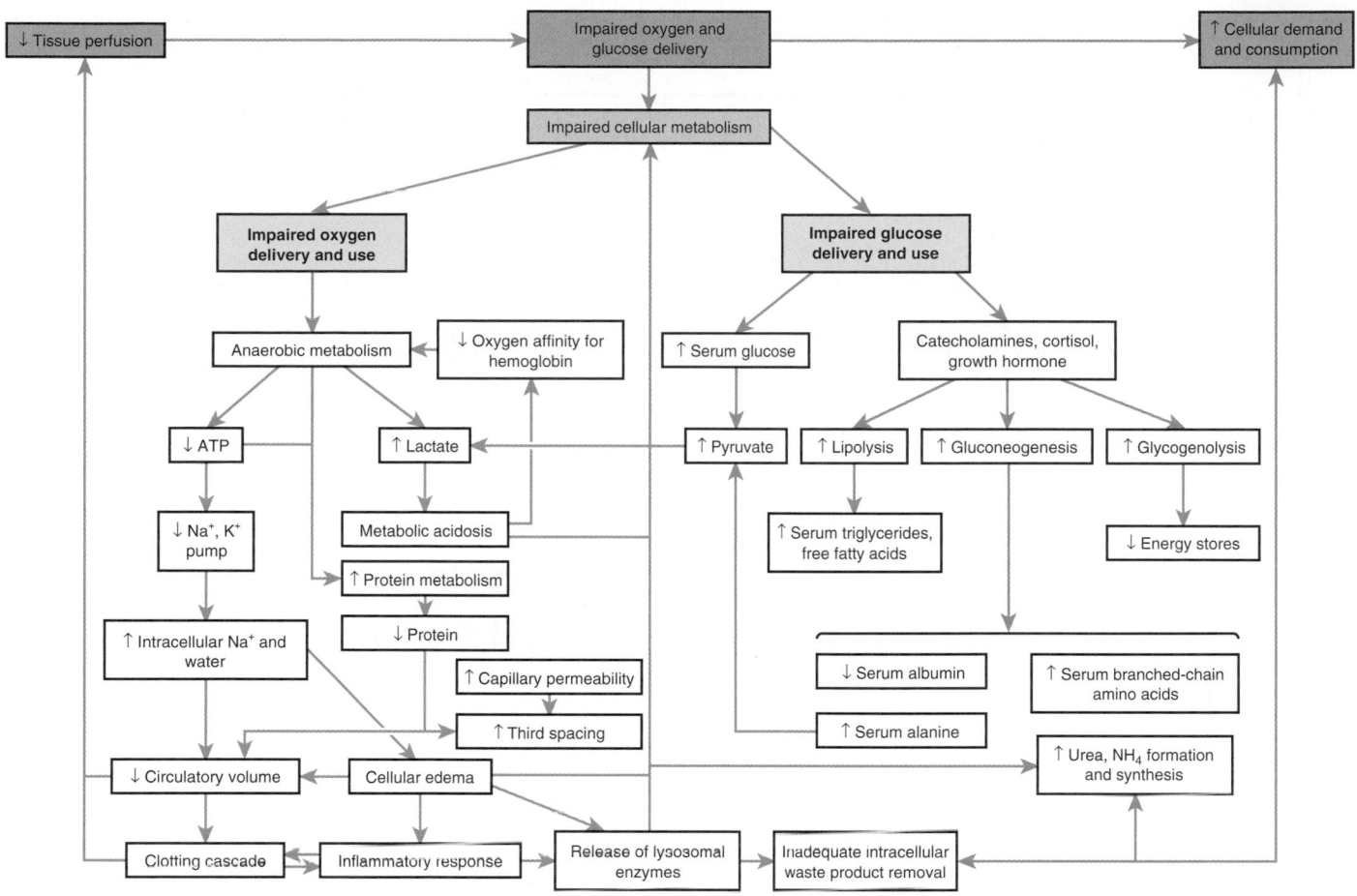

FIGURE 24-40 Impaired Cellular Metabolism in Shock. *ATP,* Adenosine triphosphate.

nonspecific. The individual may report feeling sick, weak, cold, hot, nauseated, dizzy, confused, afraid, thirsty, and short of breath. Hypotension, characterized by a mean arterial pressure below 60 mm Hg, is common to almost all shock states; however, it is a late sign of decreased tissue perfusion. Cardiac output and urinary output are usually variable early in shock states but generally become decreased as the shock syndrome progresses. Respiratory rate is usually increased, and respiratory alkalosis may be an important early indicator of impending shock. Other variable indicators of shock include alterations of heart rate, core body temperature, skin temperature, systemic vascular resistance (SVR), and skin color. Altered sensorium may be another indicator of poor tissue perfusion. Decreased mixed venous oxygen saturation indicates poor tissue oxygenation and an alteration in cellular oxygen extraction and can be used to monitor response to therapy.

Treatment for Shock

The first treatment for shock is to discover and correct or remove the underlying cause. Simultaneously, management should begin directed at improvement in microcirculatory tissue perfusion. General supportive treatment includes administration of intravenous fluids to expand intravascular volume, use of vasopressors and supplemental oxygen, and control of glucose levels. Further treatment depends on the cause and severity of the shock syndrome, which is discussed with each type of shock. Once positive feedback loops are established, intervention in shock is difficult. Prevention and very early treatment offer the best prognosis.

Types of Shock

Shock is classified by cause as cardiogenic (caused by heart failure), hypovolemic (caused by insufficient intravascular fluid volume), neurogenic (caused by neural alterations of vascular smooth muscle tone), anaphylactic (caused by immunologic processes), or septic (caused by infection). As described previously, each of these share similar effects on tissues and cells but can vary in their clinical manifestations and severity.

Cardiogenic Shock

Cardiogenic shock is defined as decreased cardiac output and evidence of tissue hypoxia in the presence of adequate intravascular volume. Most cases of cardiogenic shock follow myocardial infarction, but shock also can follow left heart failure, dysrhythmias, acute valvular dysfunction, ventricular or septal rupture, myocardial or pericardial infections, massive pulmonary embolism, cardiac tamponade, and drug toxicity. Microcirculation changes within the myocardium contribute to decreased contractility and worsening cardiac output.[140] Compensatory neurohumoral responses contribute to the overall pathophysiology (Figure 24-41).

The clinical manifestations of cardiogenic shock are caused by widespread impairment of cellular metabolism. They include impaired mentation, dyspnea and tachypnea, systemic venous and pulmonary edema, dusky skin color, marked hypotension, oliguria, and ileus. Management of cardiogenic shock includes careful fluid and vasopressor administration followed by early angiography, intra-aortic balloon

FIGURE 24-41 Cardiogenic Shock. Shock becomes life-threatening when compensatory mechanisms (in orange boxes) cause increased myocardial oxygen requirements. Renal and hypothalamic adaptive responses (i.e., renin-angiotensin-aldosterone and antidiuretic hormone [ADH]) maintain or increase blood volume. The adrenal gland releases catecholamines (e.g., mostly epinephrine, some norepinephrine), causing vasoconstriction and increases in contractility and heart rate. These adaptive mechanisms, however, increase myocardial demands for oxygen and nutrients. These demands further strain the heart, which can no longer pump an adequate volume, resulting in shock and impaired metabolism. *SVR*, Systemic vascular resistance.

pump counterpulsation, ventricular assist devices, extracorporeal membrane oxygenation, and early revascularization (PCI or bypass surgery).[141] Cardiogenic shock is often unresponsive to treatment, with a mortality of more than 70% reported. New therapies being explored include anti-inflammatory drugs and nitric oxide synthase inhibitors.

Hypovolemic Shock

Hypovolemic shock is caused by loss of whole blood (hemorrhage), plasma (burns), or interstitial fluid (diaphoresis, diabetes mellitus, diabetes insipidus, emesis, diarrhea, or diuresis) in large amounts. Hypovolemic shock begins to develop when intravascular volume has decreased by about 15%.

Hypovolemia is offset initially by compensatory mechanisms (Figure 24-42). Heart rate and SVR increase, boosting both cardiac output and tissue perfusion pressures. Interstitial fluid moves into the vascular compartment. The liver and spleen add to blood volume by disgorging stored red blood cells and plasma. In the kidneys, renin stimulates aldosterone release and the retention of sodium (and hence water), whereas antidiuretic hormone (ADH) from the posterior pituitary gland increases water retention. However, if the initial fluid or blood loss is great or if loss continues, compensation fails, resulting in decreased tissue perfusion. As in cardiogenic shock, oxygen and

nutrient delivery to the cells is impaired and cellular metabolism fails. Anaerobic metabolism and lactate production result in lactic acidosis and serum and cellular electrolyte abnormalities.

The clinical manifestations of hypovolemic shock include high SVR, poor skin turgor, thirst, oliguria, low systemic and pulmonary preloads, rapid heart rate, thready pulse, and mental status deterioration. The differences between the signs and symptoms of hypovolemic shock and those of cardiogenic shock are mainly caused by differences in fluid volume and cardiac muscle health. Management begins with rapid fluid replacement with crystalloids and blood products.[142] For hemorrhagic hypovolemic shock, the administration of pharmacologic doses of ADH can improve blood pressure. Hypothermia and coagulopathies frequently complicate treatment.[142] If adequate tissue perfusion cannot be restored promptly, systemic inflammation and multiple organ dysfunction are likely.

Neurogenic Shock

Neurogenic shock (sometimes called **vasogenic shock**) is the result of widespread and massive vasodilation that results from parasympathetic overstimulation and sympathetic understimulation (Figure 24-43) (see Chapter 23). This type of shock can be caused by any factor that stimulates parasympathetic or inhibits sympathetic stimulation of vascular smooth muscle. Trauma to the spinal cord or medulla and

FIGURE 24-42 Hypovolemic Shock. This type of shock becomes life-threatening when compensatory mechanisms (in orange boxes) are overwhelmed by continued loss of intravascular volume. *ADH,* Antidiuretic hormone; *SVR,* systemic vascular resistance.

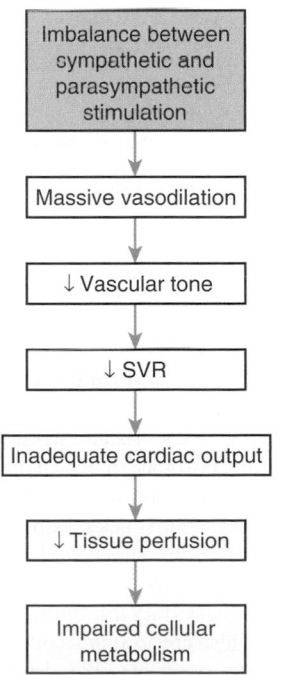

FIGURE 24-43 Neurogenic Shock. *SVR,* Systemic vascular resistance.

conditions that interrupt the supply of oxygen or glucose to the medulla can cause neurogenic shock by interrupting sympathetic activity. Depressive drugs, anesthetic agents, and severe emotional stress and pain are other causes. The loss of vascular tone results in "relative hypovolemia," in which blood volume has not changed but SVR decreases drastically so that the amount of space containing the blood has increased.[143] The pressure in the vessels falls below that which is needed to drive nutrients across capillary membranes to the cells. In addition, neurologic insult may cause bradycardia, which decreases cardiac output and further contributes to hypotension and underperfusion of tissues. As with other types of shock, this leads to impaired cellular metabolism. Management includes the careful use of fluids and vasopressors until blood pressure stabilizes.

Anaphylactic Shock

Anaphylactic shock results from a widespread hypersensitivity reaction known as **anaphylaxis**. The lifetime prevalence of anaphylaxis is 0.5% to 2%.[144] The basic physiologic alteration is the same as that of neurogenic shock: vasodilation and relative hypovolemia, leading to decreased tissue perfusion and impaired cellular metabolism (Figure 24-44). Anaphylactic shock is characterized by other effects that rapidly involve the entire body.

Anaphylactic shock begins with exposure of a sensitized individual to an allergen. Common allergens known to cause these reactions are insect venoms, shellfish, peanuts, latex, and medications such as penicillin. In genetically predisposed individuals, these allergens initiate a vigorous humoral immune response (type I hypersensitivity reaction)

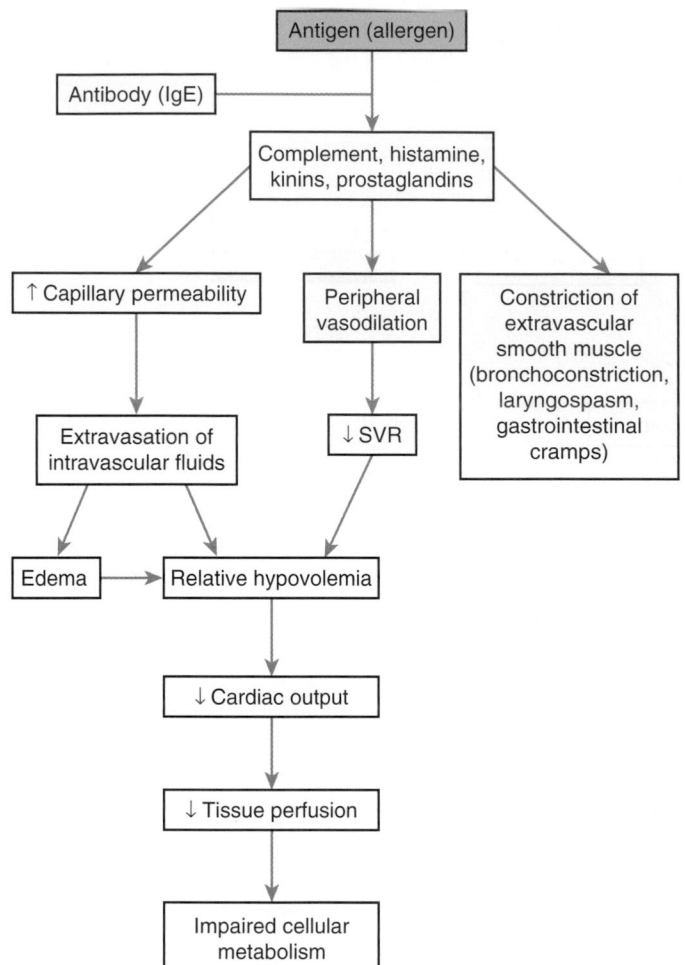

FIGURE 24-44 Anaphylactic Shock. *DIC,* Disseminated intravascular coagulation; *ECF-A,* eosinophil chemotactic factor anaphylaxis; *IgE,* immunoglobulin E; *SVR,* systemic vascular resistance.

TABLE 24-11	Causes and Definitions of Septic Shock
Cause	**Definition**
Infection	Microbial phenomenon characterized by inflammatory response to presence of microorganisms or invasion of normally sterile host tissue by those microorganisms
Bacteremia	Presence of viable bacteria in blood
Systemic inflammatory response syndrome (SIRS)	Systemic inflammatory response to a variety of severe clinical insults manifested by two or more of the following signs: Temperature >38° C or <36° C Heart rate >90 beats/min Respiratory rate >20 breaths/min or arterial blood carbon dioxide level <32 mm Hg White blood cell count >12,000 cells/mm^3, <4000 cells/mm^3, or containing <10% immature forms (bands)
Sepsis	Systemic response to infection characterized by two or more of SIRS criteria
Severe sepsis	Sepsis associated with organ dysfunction
Septic shock	Severe sepsis complicated by persistent hypotension refractory to early fluid therapy
Multiple organ dysfunction syndrome	Presence of altered organ function in an acutely ill individual such that homeostasis cannot be maintained without intervention

Data adapted from American College of Chest Physicians/Society of Critical Care Medicine Consensus Conference: *Crit Care Med* 20(6):864-874, 1992; Levy MM et al: SCCM/ES/CM/ACCP/ATS/SIS International Sepsis Definitions Conference, *Crit Care Med* 31(4):1250-1256, 2003.

✔ QUICK CHECK 24-11
1. Describe the mechanisms operative in shock.
2. Why does myocardial infarction often cause cardiogenic shock?
3. How is hypovolemic shock manifested?
4. Why is anaphylactic shock considered a medical emergency?

that results in the production of large quantities of immunoglobulin E (IgE) antibody (see Chapter 6). Allergen bound to IgE causes degranulation of mast cells. Mast cells release a large number of vasoactive and inflammatory cytokines. This provokes an extensive immune and inflammatory response, including vasodilation and increased vascular permeability, resulting in peripheral pooling and tissue edema. Extravascular effects include constriction of extravascular smooth muscle, often causing laryngospasm and bronchospasm (see Chapter 27) and cramping abdominal pain with diarrhea.

The onset of anaphylactic shock is usually sudden, and progression to death can occur within minutes unless emergency treatment is given. The primary clinical manifestations of anaphylaxis include anxiety, dizziness, difficulty breathing, stridor, wheezing, pruritus with hives (urticaria), swollen lips and tongue, and abdominal cramping. A precipitous fall in blood pressure occurs, followed by impaired mentation. Other signs include decreased SVR, with high or normal cardiac output, and oliguria. The diagnosis can be confirmed by a number of serum markers, such as plasma histamine and tryptase.[145] Treatment begins with removal of the antigen (if possible). Epinephrine is administered intramuscularly to cause vasoconstriction and reverse airway constriction.[146] Fluids are given intravenously to reverse the relative hypovolemia, and antihistamines and corticosteroids are administered to stop the inflammatory reaction. Vasopressors and inhaled β-adrenergic agonist bronchodilators may also be necessary.

Septic Shock

Septic shock begins with an infection that progresses to bacteremia, then systemic inflammatory response syndrome (SIRS) with sepsis, then severe sepsis, then septic shock, and finally multiple organ dysfunction syndrome (MODS). Causes and definitions of each component of septic shock are presented in Table 24-11.[147]

In the United States, severe sepsis and septic shock occur in 2% of persons admitted to the hospital, of which half are treated in the intensive care unit (ICU), accounting for 10% of ICU admissions.[148] Although death rates from septic shock have been declining, it remains a highly lethal condition.[149] Septic shock can be caused by community-acquired or healthcare-associated infections, especially pneumonia, intra-abdominal, and urinary tract infections. Indwelling arterial and central venous catheters also are an important source of infection (see *Health Alert:* Central Line–Associated Bloodstream Infection).[150] Bacteria cause most sepsis, with *Staphylococcus aureus* and *Streptococcus pneumoniae* as the most common gram-positive causes; and *Escherichia coli, Klebsiella* species, and *Pseudomonas aeruginosa* as the most common gram-negative causes.[148] Septic shock also can be caused by fungi and viruses, and in almost one third of cases, the infectious organism is never identified. The source and virulence of the infectious microorganism, as well as the underlying health of the affected individual, significantly affect prognosis. Risk factors for septic shock include the individual's genetic composition, underlying chronic diseases, immune deficiency states, and timeliness of therapeutic interventions for infection.

HEALTH ALERT

Central Line–Associated Bloodstream Infection

Central line–associated bloodstream infection (CLABSI) is an important cause of sepsis and septic shock and occurs in more than 40,000 people each year. Central lines are most commonly placed in the central venous circulation for administering medications, performing hemodialysis, and monitoring hemodynamics. Catheters can be placed in several ways, including surgical and percutaneous access methods, depending on the purpose of the catheter. Risk factors for CLABSI include extremes of age, underlying systemic and immunocompromising conditions, and catheter-related factors, such as number of catheters, site of catheter insertion, and length of time the catheter has been in place. The Centers for Disease Control and Prevention (CDC) has determined that nearly one in four individuals who contracts CLABSI dies from associated complications and the CDC has been active in educating healthcare providers in CLABSI prevention. Prevention consists of appropriate patient selection and guideline-driven placement and management techniques.

Data from Centers for Disease Control and Prevention: *Central line-associated bloodstream infection (CLABSI) event,* January 2014, available at: www.cdc.gov/nhsn/pdfs/pscmanual/4psc_clabscurrent.pdf; Huber K et al: *Am J Infect Control* 42(6 Suppl): S166, 2014; The Joint Commission: *Preventing central line–associated bloodstream infections: a global challenge, a global perspective,* Oak Brook, Ill, 2012, Joint Commission Resources (available at: www.PreventingCLABSIs.pdf).

FIGURE 24-45 Septic Shock. *SIRS,* Systemic inflammatory response syndrome; *TLR,* Toll-like receptor.

Most septic shock begins when bacteria enter the bloodstream to produce bacteremia. These bacteria and their associated toxins initiate an innate immune response. Gram-negative microorganisms release endotoxins, and gram-positive microorganisms release exotoxins, lipoteichoic acids, and peptidoglycans. These pathogen-associated molecular patterns (PAMPs), as well as molecules released from injured cells (damage-associated molecular patters), trigger the septic syndrome by interacting with pattern-associated receptors on macrophages, such as Toll-like receptor 2 (TLR-2) for gram-positive PAMPs and Toll-like receptor 4 (TLR-4) for gram-negative PAMPs (Figure 24-45).[148,151] These microbial molecules also activate complement, coagulation, kinins, and inflammatory cells.

The release of inflammatory mediators triggers intense cellular responses and the subsequent release of secondary mediators, including cytokines, complement fragments, prostaglandins, platelet-activating factor, oxygen free radicals, nitric oxide, and proteolytic enzymes. (see *Risk Factors:* Proinflammatory Mediators Contributing to Septic Shock). Chemotaxis, activation of granulocytes, and reactivation of the phagocytic cells and inflammatory cascades result. This systemic inflammation, especially through the action of nitric oxide, leads to widespread vasodilation with compensatory tachycardia and increased cardiac output in the early stages of septic shock (hyperdynamic phase).[151] Later in the course of disease, inflammatory mediators, such as complement and interleukins, depress myocardial contractility such that cardiac output falls and tissue perfusion decreases. Tissue perfusion and cellular oxygen extraction also are

affected by activation of the clotting cascade through the action of platelet-activating factor and depletion of the endogenous anticoagulant protein C.[148,151] Furthermore, unresponsiveness to or depletion of vasoactive factors such as vasopressin contributes to hypotension and tissue hypoperfusion. The inflammatory response can become overwhelming, leading to the systemic inflammatory response syndrome (SIRS).[152] SIRS can progress to widespread tissue hypoxia, necrosis, and apoptosis, leading to septic shock and MODS. It has been determined that there is a parallel release of anti-inflammatory mediators and impairment of phagocytic and adaptive immune cell function that accompanies SIRS, causing a depression in the immune response to infection that contributes to the overall shock syndrome.[148,152]

Clinical manifestations of septic shock are the result of inflammation, decreased perfusion of vital tissues, and an alteration in oxygen extraction by all cells. In early shock, tachycardia causes cardiac output to remain normal or become elevated, although myocardial contractility is reduced. Temperature instability is present, ranging from hyperthermia to hypothermia. Effects on other organ systems may result in deranged renal function, jaundice, clotting abnormalities with disseminated intravascular coagulation (DIC), deterioration of mental status, and ARDS. Gastrointestinal mucosa changes cause the translocation of bacteria from the gut into the bloodstream. Increased permeability of the gut also can lead to increased inflammation and immune reactions attributable to toxins carried by the intestinal lymphatics.

RISK FACTORS

Proinflammatory Mediators Contributing to Septic Shock

More than 100 inflammatory mediators have been implicated in the pathogenesis of septic shock. The following are some of the most important contributors:

Tumor Necrosis Factor-alpha (TNF-α)
Produced from macrophages, natural killer cells, and mast cells in response to endotoxin and interleukins
Net effect: generates same symptoms of septic shock as those seen with interleukins; thus is redundant

Interleukin-1β (IL-1β)
Released by macrophages and lymphocytes in septic shock in response to bacterial toxins
Net effect: produces fever, vasodilation and hypotension, edema, myocardial depression, and elevated white blood count

Interleukin-6 (IL-6)
Released by macrophages and lymphocytes during infection
Net effect: fever, elevated white blood count

Nitric Oxide (NO)
Released by activated macrophages and neutrophils
Net effect: damages tissues and causes systemic vasodilation and hypotension

Platelet-Activating Factor (PAF)
Released from mononuclear phagocytes, platelets, and some endothelial cells in response to endotoxin
Net effect: contributes to widespread clotting, generates same symptoms of shock as those seen with interleukins and tumor necrosis factor-alpha, and may initiate multiple organ failure

Complement
Activated by bacterial products and antigen/antibody complexes
Net effect: damages tissues and amplifies the inflammatory process by cellular chemotaxis and promotion of phagocytosis

HEALTH ALERT

The Surviving Sepsis Guidelines

Mortality rates for severe sepsis and septic shock have declined because of more rapid recognition of systemic infection and more effective management. Current Surviving Sepsis Guidelines for the management of sepsis were developed based on an in-depth analysis of the pathophysiology, clinical manifestations, and management outcomes reported over the past decade of sepsis care. The Guidelines provide a prioritized list of interventions that seek to quickly restore tissue perfusion, control infection, and support adequate oxygenation and ventilation. Intravenous infusion of fluids along with vasopressors, such as norepinephrine and vasopressin, is implemented quickly. Blood cultures, imaging modalities to determine the source of infection, and administration of appropriate antimicrobials are essential components of care. Respiratory support often includes mechanical ventilation, proper patient positioning, and careful monitoring of outcomes. Sedation is implemented as needed and general supportive care includes glucose management with insulin, stress ulcer prevention, and nutrition. These Surviving Sepsis Guidelines have improved morbidity and mortality outcomes for individuals with septic shock.

Data from Dellinger RP et al: *Crit Care Med* 41:580-637, 2013.

✔ QUICK CHECK 24-12
1. What are some of the important causes of septic shock?
2. What is the systemic inflammatory response syndrome?
3. Why is correction of the underlying problem the most important treatment for all kinds of shock?

dysfunction can progress to organ failure and death (Figure 24-46). Although sepsis and septic shock are the most common causes, any severe injury or disease process that activates a massive systemic inflammatory response in the host can initiate MODS. These triggers include severe trauma, burns, acute pancreatitis, obstetric complications, major surgery, circulatory shock, some drugs, and gangrenous or necrotic tissue.

MODS is a common cause of mortality in intensive care units. Mortality for individuals ranges from 36% to 100% if there is failure of five or more organs, with liver and kidney failure being the most common.[157] People at greatest risk for developing MODS are elderly individuals and persons with significant tissue injury or preexisting disease (Box 24-3).

PATHOPHYSIOLOGY   As a result of the initiating insult (sepsis, injury, or disease), the neuroendocrine system is activated with the release of the stress hormones cortisol, epinephrine, and norepinephrine into the bloodstream (see Chapter 8). Vascular endothelial damage occurs as a direct result of injury or from damage by bacterial toxins and inflammatory mediators, such as nitric oxide, TNF, and IL-1, which are released into the circulation. The vascular endothelium becomes permeable, allowing fluid and protein to leak into the interstitial spaces, contributing to hypotension and hypoperfusion. Leakage of fluid into the lungs causes a condition called acute respiratory distress syndrome (ARDS). When the endothelium is damaged, platelets and tissue thromboplastin are activated, resulting in systemic microvascular coagulation that may lead to DIC (see Chapter 20).[158]

Because of the release of inflammatory mediators, four major plasma enzyme cascades are activated: complement, coagulation, fibrinolytic, and kallikrein/kinin. The overall effect of the activation of these cascades is a hyperinflammatory and hypercoagulant state that

The diagnosis of septic shock rests on the recognition of the systemic manifestations of overwhelming inflammation (SIRS) in individuals with suspected or documented infection. Determining the cause and severity of septic shock can be aided by measurement of levels of serum lactate, troponin,[153] C-reactive protein, and procalcitonin.[154] The management of septic shock has improved outcomes[155] by following the Surviving Sepsis Guidelines (see *Health Alert: The Surviving Sepsis Guidelines*). These guidelines include rapid goal-directed resuscitation with fluids and vasopressors, antibiotic administration, and respiratory support.[155] Control of hyperglycemia with insulin, treatment of complications associated with MODS, careful nutritional support, and prevention of stress ulcers and deep venous thrombosis are also essential. Despite improvements in septic shock–related mortality in recent years, mortality remains high and new treatments are being explored.[156]

Multiple Organ Dysfunction Syndrome

Multiple organ dysfunction syndrome (MODS) is the progressive dysfunction of two or more organ systems resulting from an uncontrolled inflammatory response to a severe illness or injury. The organ

FIGURE 24-46 Pathogenesis of Multiple Organ Dysfunction Syndrome.

maintains the interstitial edema formation, cardiovascular instability, endothelial damage, and clotting abnormalities characteristic of MODS.[159] A massive systemic immune/inflammatory response then develops involving neutrophils, macrophages, and mast cells (Table 24-12). The inflammatory process initiated is the same as that described in septic shock and SIRS (see p. 644) and sets the stage for MODS.

The numerous inflammatory and clotting processes operating in MODS cause maldistribution of blood flow and hypermetabolism. Oxygen delivery to the tissues decreases despite the supranormal systemic blood flow for several reasons:

1. Shunting of blood past selected regional capillary beds is caused when inflammatory mediators override the normal vascular tone.
2. Interstitial edema, resulting from microvascular changes in permeability, contributes to decreased oxygen delivery by creating a relative hypovolemia and by increasing the distance oxygen must travel to reach the cells.
3. Capillary obstruction occurs because of formation of microvascular thrombi and the aggregation of white blood cells.

Hypermetabolism in MODS with accompanying alterations in carbohydrate, fat, and lipid metabolism is initially a compensatory

TABLE 24-12   Cells of Inflammation and Multiple Organ Dysfunction

Cell	Activators	Contribution to Multiple Organ Dysfunction
Neutrophils	Complement, kinins, endotoxin, clotting factors	Release of phagocytic products: toxic oxygen free radicals, superoxide ion, hydrogen peroxide, hydroxyl radicals, proteases, platelet-activating factor (PAF), arachidonic acid metabolites (prostaglandins, thromboxane, leukotrienes)
		Endothelial damage, vasodilation, vasopermeability, microvascular coagulation, selective vasoconstriction, hypotension, shock
Macrophages	Complement, endotoxin, chemotactic factors	Release of same phagocytic products as neutrophils
		Release of monokines: tumor necrosis factor (TNF), interleukin-1 (IL-1)
		TNF produces fever, anorexia, hyperglycemia, weight loss
Mast cells	Direct injury, endotoxin, complement	Release of histamine, PAF, arachidonic acid metabolites Vasodilation, vasopermeability, hypotension, shock

BOX 24-3   Other Common Triggers of MODS

Severe trauma
Major surgery
Burns
Circulatory shock
Acute pancreatitis
Acute renal failure
Acute respiratory distress syndrome
Blood transfusion
Heat stroke
Liver failure
Mesenteric ischemia
Propofol infusion syndrome
Persistent inflammatory foci
Necrotic tissue
Disseminated intravascular coagulation

Data from Abboud B et al: *World J Gastroenterol* 14(35):5361-5370, 2008; Adukauskiené D et al: *Medicina (Kaunas)* 44(7):536-540, 2008; Beger HG, Rau BM: *World J Gastroenterol* 13(38):5043-5051, 2007; Bouchama A, Knochel JP: *N Engl J Med* 346:1978-1988, 2002; Broessner G et al: *Crit Care* 9(5):R498-R501, 2006; Carnovale A et al: *J Pancreas (Online)* 6(5):438-444, 2005; Ciesla DJ et al: *Arch Surg* 140(5):432-440, 2005; Gando S: *Crit Care Med* 38(2):S35-S42, 2010; Kam PCA, Cardone D: *Anesthesia* 62(1):690-701, 2007; Oeckler RA, Hubmayr RD: *Eur Respir J* 30(6):1216-1226, 2007; Shaheem MA, Akhtar AJ: *J Nat Med Assoc* 99(12):1402-1406, 2007; Varghese GM et al: *Emerg Med J* 22:185-187, 2005; Vincent JL et al: *Crit Care Med* 39(5):1050-1055, 2011; Zaccheo MM, Bucher DH: *Crit Care Nurse* 28(3):18-26, 2008.

measure to meet the body's increased demands for energy. The alterations in metabolism affect all aspects of substrate utilization. The net result of hypermetabolism is depletion of oxygen and fuel supplies.

Myocardial depression also accompanies MODS. The cause is unclear but inflammatory cytokines, bacterial products, and ischemia have been implicated. Decreased cardiac output contributes to poor perfusion of tissues and exacerbation of MODS.

Maldistribution of blood flow, coagulation, myocardial depression, ARDS, and the hypermetabolic state combine to create an imbalance in oxygen supply and demand. This imbalance is critical in the pathogenesis of MODS because it results in a pathologic condition known as **supply-dependent oxygen consumption**. Ordinarily, the amount of oxygen consumed by the cells depends only on the demands of the cells, because there is an adequate reserve of oxygen that can be delivered if needed. The reserve, however, has been exhausted in MODS, and the amount of oxygen consumed becomes dependent on the amount the circulation is able to deliver; this amount is inadequate in MODS. Therefore tissue hypoxia with cellular acidosis and impaired cellular function ensue and result in multiple organ failure.

CLINICAL MANIFESTATIONS   There may be a lag time between the inciting event and the onset of symptoms that may last for as long as 24 hours. The individual develops a low-grade fever, tachycardia, dyspnea, altered mental status, and hyperdynamic and hypermetabolic states. ARDS is often an early manifestation of MODS (see Chapter 27) and is characterized by tachypnea, pulmonary edema with crackles and diminished breath sounds, use of accessory muscles, and hypoxemia.

As the syndrome continues, hypermetabolic and hyperdynamic states intensify and signs of liver and kidney failure appear. Liver failure presents with jaundice, abdominal distention, liver tenderness, muscle wasting, and hepatic encephalopathy. All facets of metabolism, substance detoxification, and immune response are impaired; albumin and clotting factor synthesis decreases; protein wastes accumulate; and liver tissue macrophages (Kupffer cells) no longer function effectively. Progressive oliguria, azotemia, and edema mark the development of renal failure. Anuria, hyperkalemia, and metabolic acidosis may occur if renal shutdown is severe.

The gastrointestinal system also shows evidence of dysfunction. The gastrointestinal system is sensitive to ischemic and inflammatory injury. Clinical manifestations of bowel involvement are hemorrhage, ileus, malabsorption, diarrhea or constipation, vomiting, anorexia, and abdominal pain. Stress ulceration of the stomach lining is a common complication of shock and MODS and, although usually painless, can result in massive blood loss and death. Compounding the damage caused by injury to the bowel is the phenomenon of bacterial translocation. When mediators and severe ischemia injure the mucosal epithelium, bacteria and toxins pass from the gut into the portal circulation. The overwhelmed liver is unable to clear these products and they move into the systemic circulation. Thus, whether infection or some other injury was the precipitating cause of MODS, sepsis occurs once the gut barrier is damaged.

Hematologic failure and myocardial failure are usually later manifestations. The signs and symptoms of cardiac failure in the hypermetabolic, hyperdynamic phase of MODS are similar to those of septic shock: tachycardia, bounding pulse, increased cardiac output, decreased systemic vascular resistance, and hypotension. In the terminal stages, hypodynamic circulation with bradycardia, profound hypotension, and ventricular dysrhythmias may develop. Encephalopathy, characterized by mental status changes ranging from confusion to deep coma, may occur at any time. Ischemia and inflammation are responsible for the central nervous system manifestations, which include apprehension, confusion, disorientation, restlessness, agitation, headache, decreased cognitive ability and memory, and decreased level of consciousness. When ischemia is severe, seizures and coma can occur. Death may occur as early as 14 days or after a period of several weeks.

EVALUATION AND TREATMENT Early detection of organ failure is extremely important so that supportive measures can be initiated immediately. Frequent assessment of the clinical status of individuals at known risk is essential. The Acute Physiology and Chronic Health Evaluation (APACHE) II and III systems assess for severity and progression of MODS. Once organ failure develops, monitoring of laboratory values and hemodynamic parameters also can be used to assess the degree of impairment.

There is no specific treatment for MODS and therapeutic management consists of prevention and support. Prevention consists of controlling the initial insult, treating infections quickly, and supporting healing. Management goals include controlling infection, restoring oxygenation and perfusion, and supporting organ function. Sources of infection are removed and antimicrobials are administered. Ventilatory support is initiated to maintain adequate oxygen saturation and fluids are administered to maintain vascular volume. Nutritional support must be provided to meet metabolic demand. Dialysis also may be required.

✔ QUICK CHECK 24-13
1. Why can MODS be initiated by either a septic or a nonseptic insult?
2. Why are inflammation and clotting triggered when the vascular endothelium is injured?
3. Describe the mechanisms that result in decreased oxygen delivery to the tissues in MODS.

▌ DID YOU UNDERSTAND?

Diseases of the Veins and Arteries

1. Varicosities are areas of veins in which blood has pooled, usually in the saphenous veins. Varicosities may be caused by damaged valves as a result of trauma to the valve or by chronic venous distention involving gravity and venous constriction.
2. Chronic venous insufficiency is inadequate venous return over a long period of time that causes pathologic ischemic changes in the vasculature, skin, and supporting tissues.
3. Venous stasis ulcers follow the development of chronic venous insufficiency and probably develop as a result of the borderline metabolic state of the cells in the affected extremities.
4. Deep venous thrombosis results from stasis of blood flow, endothelial damage, or hypercoagulability. The most serious complication of deep venous thrombosis is pulmonary embolism.
5. Superior vena cava syndrome is a progressive occlusion of the superior vena cava that leads to venous distention in the upper extremities and head. Because this syndrome is usually caused by bronchogenic cancer, it is generally considered an oncologic emergency rather than a vascular emergency.
6. Hypertension is the elevation of systemic arterial blood pressure resulting from increases in cardiac output (blood volume), total peripheral resistance, or both.
7. Hypertension can be primary, without a known cause, or secondary, caused by an underlying disease.
8. The risk factors for hypertension include a positive family history; male gender; advancing age; black race; obesity; high sodium intake; low magnesium, potassium, or calcium intake; diabetes mellitus; cigarette smoking; and heavy alcohol consumption.
9. The exact cause of primary hypertension is unknown, although several hypotheses are proposed, including overactivity of the sympathetic nervous system; overactivity of the renin-angiotensin-aldosterone system; sodium and water retention by the kidneys; hormonal inhibition of sodium-potassium transport across cell walls; and complex interactions involving insulin resistance, inflammation, and endothelial function.
10. Clinical manifestations of hypertension result from damage of organs and tissues outside the vascular system. These include retinal changes, heart disease, renal disease, and central nervous system disorders, such as stroke and dementia.
11. Hypertension is managed with both pharmacologic and nonpharmacologic methods that lower the blood volume and the total peripheral resistance.
12. Orthostatic hypotension is a drop in blood pressure that occurs on standing. The compensatory vasoconstriction response to standing is replaced by a marked vasodilation and blood pooling in the muscle vasculature.
13. The clinical manifestations of orthostatic hypotension include fainting and may involve cardiovascular symptoms, as well as impotence and bowel and bladder dysfunction.
14. An aneurysm is a localized dilation of a vessel wall; the aorta is particularly susceptible.
15. A thrombus is a clot that remains attached to a vascular wall. An embolus is a mobile aggregate of a variety of substances that occludes the vasculature. Sources of emboli include clots, air, amniotic fluid, bacteria, fat, and foreign matter. These emboli cause ischemia and necrosis when a vessel is totally blocked.
16. The most common source of arterial thrombotic emboli is the heart as a result of mitral and aortic valvular disease and atrial fibrillation, followed by myxomas. Tissues affected include the lower extremities, the brain, and the heart.
17. Emboli to the central organs cause tissue death in lungs, kidneys, and mesentery.
18. Peripheral vascular diseases include Buerger disease and Raynaud phenomenon, involving arterioles of the extremities.
19. Atherosclerosis is a form of arteriosclerosis and is the leading contributor to coronary artery disease (CAD) and cerebrovascular disease (CVD).
20. Atherosclerosis is an inflammatory disease that begins with endothelial injury.
21. Important steps in atherogenesis include vasoconstriction, adherence of macrophages, release of inflammatory mediators, oxidation of LDL, formation of foam cells and fatty streaks, and development of fibrous plaque.
22. Once a plaque has formed, it can rupture, resulting in clot formation and instability and vasoconstriction, which lead to obstruction of the lumen and inadequate oxygen delivery to tissues.
23. Peripheral artery disease is the result of atherosclerotic plaque formation in the arteries that supply the extremities, and it causes pain and ischemic changes in the nerves, muscles, and skin of the affected limb.
24. Coronary artery disease (CAD) is the result of an atherosclerotic plaque that gradually narrows the coronary arteries or that ruptures and causes sudden thrombus formation.

25. Many risk factors contribute to the onset and escalation of CAD, including traditional risk factors such as dyslipidemia, smoking, hypertension, diabetes mellitus (insulin resistance), and obesity/sedentary lifestyle and nontraditional risk factors such as elevated C-reactive protein levels, hyperhomocysteinemia, and changes in adipokines.

26. Ischemic heart disease is most commonly the result of coronary artery disease and the ensuing decrease in myocardial blood supply.

27. Atherosclerotic plaque progression can be gradual and cause stable angina pectoris, which is predictable chest pain caused by myocardial ischemia in response to increased demand (e.g., exercise) without infarction.

28. Prinzmetal angina results from coronary artery vasospasm.

29. Myocardial ischemia may be asymptomatic, which is called silent ischemia, and is a risk factor for the development of the acute coronary syndromes.

30. Sudden coronary obstruction because of thrombus formation causes the acute coronary syndromes. These include unstable angina, non-ST elevation myocardial infarction (non-STEMI), and ST elevation myocardial infarction (STEMI).

31. Unstable angina results in reversible myocardial ischemia.

32. Myocardial infarction is caused by prolonged, unrelieved ischemia that interrupts blood supply to the myocardium. After about 20 minutes of myocardial ischemia, irreversible hypoxic injury causes cellular death and tissue necrosis.

33. Myocardial infarction is clinically classified as non-STEMI or STEMI based on electrocardiographic findings that suggest the extent of myocardial damage (subendocardial versus transmural).

34. An increase in plasma enzyme levels is used to diagnose the occurrence of myocardial infarction as well as indicate its severity. Elevations of the isoenzymes creatine kinase-myocardial bound (CK-MB), troponins, and lactate dehydrogenase 1 (LDH-1) are most predictive of a myocardial infarction.

35. Treatment of a myocardial infarction includes revascularization (thrombolytics or PCI) and administration of antithrombotics, ACE inhibitors, and beta-blockers. Pain relief and fluid management also are key components of care. Dysrhythmias and cardiac failure are the most common complications of acute myocardial infarction.

Disorders of the Heart Wall

1. Inflammation of the pericardium, or pericarditis, may result from several sources (infection, drug therapy, tumors). Pericarditis presents with symptoms that are physically troublesome, but in and of themselves they are not life-threatening.

2. Fluid may collect within the pericardial sac (pericardial effusion). Cardiac function may be severely impaired if the accumulation of fluid occurs rapidly and involves a large volume.

3. Cardiomyopathies are a diverse group of primary myocardial disorders that are usually the result of remodeling, neurohumoral responses, and hypertension. The cardiomyopathies are categorized as dilated (congestive), restrictive (rigid and noncompliant), and hypertrophic (asymmetric). The size of the cardiac muscle walls and chambers may increase or decrease depending on the type of cardiomyopathy, thereby altering contractile activity.

4. The hemodynamic integrity of the cardiovascular system depends to a great extent on properly functioning cardiac valves. Congenital or acquired disorders that result in stenosis, regurgitation, or both can structurally alter the valves.

5. Characteristic heart sounds, cardiac murmurs, and systemic complaints assist in identification of an abnormal valve. If severely compromised function exists, a prosthetic heart valve may be surgically implanted to replace the faulty one.

6. Mitral valve prolapse (MVP) describes the condition in which the mitral valve leaflets do not position themselves properly during systole. Mitral valve prolapse may be a completely asymptomatic condition or can result in unpredictable symptoms.

7. Rheumatic fever is an inflammatory disease that results from a delayed immune response to a streptococcal infection in genetically predisposed individuals. The disorder usually resolves without sequelae if treated early.

8. Severe or untreated cases of rheumatic fever may progress to rheumatic heart disease, a potentially disabling cardiovascular disorder.

9. Infective endocarditis is a general term for infection and inflammation of the endocardium, especially the cardiac valves. In the mildest cases, valvular function may be slightly impaired by vegetations that collect on the valve leaflets. If left unchecked, severe valve abnormalities, chronic bacteremia, and systemic emboli may occur as vegetations detach from the valve surface and travel through the bloodstream. Antibiotic therapy can limit the extension of this disease.

10. Human immunodeficiency virus (HIV) infection and AIDS are associated with cardiac abnormalities, including myocarditis, endocarditis, pericarditis, and cardiomyopathy.

Manifestations of Heart Disease

1. A dysrhythmia (arrhythmia) is a disturbance of heart rhythm. Dysrhythmias range in severity from occasional missed beats or rapid beats to disturbances that impair myocardial contractility and are life-threatening.

2. Dysrhythmias can occur because of an abnormal rate of impulse generation or an abnormal conduction of impulses.

3. Heart failure (HF) can be divided into heart failure with reduced ejection fraction (systolic) and heart failure with preserved ejection fraction (diastolic).

4. The most common causes of left ventricular failure are myocardial infarction and hypertension.

5. Heart failure with reduced ejection fraction (systolic) is caused by increased preload, decreased contractility, or increased afterload. These processes result in an increased left ventricular end-diastolic volume and an increased left ventricular end-diastolic pressure that cause increased pulmonary venous pressures and pulmonary edema.

6. In addition to the hemodynamic changes of left ventricular failure, there is a neuroendocrine response that tends to exacerbate and perpetuate the condition.

7. The neuroendocrine mediators of heart failure include the sympathetic nervous system and the renin-angiotensin-aldosterone system; thus diuretics, beta-blockers, and angiotensin-converting enzyme (ACE) inhibitors are important components of the pharmacologic therapy.

8. Heart failure with preserved ejection fraction (diastolic heart failure) is a clinical syndrome characterized by the symptoms and signs of heart failure, a preserved ejection fraction, and abnormal diastolic function.

9. Diastolic dysfunction means that the left ventricular end-diastolic pressure is increased, even if volume and cardiac output are normal.

10. Right heart failure can result from left heart failure or pulmonary disease.

Shock

1. Shock is a widespread impairment of cellular metabolism involving positive feedback loops that places the individual on a downward physiologic spiral leading to multiple organ dysfunction syndrome.

2. Types of shock are cardiogenic, hypovolemic, neurogenic, anaphylactic, and septic. Multiple organ dysfunction syndrome can develop from all types of shock.

3. The final common pathway in all types of shock is impaired cellular metabolism—cells switch from aerobic to anaerobic metabolism. Energy stores drop, and cellular mechanisms relative to membrane permeability, action potentials, and lysozyme release fail.

4. Anaerobic metabolism results in activation of the inflammatory response, decreased circulatory volume, and decreasing pH.

5. Impaired cellular metabolism results in cellular inability to use glucose because of impaired glucose delivery or impaired glucose intake, resulting in a shift to glycogenolysis, gluconeogenesis, and lipolysis for fuel generation.

6. Glycogenolysis is effective for about 10 hours. Gluconeogenesis results in the use of proteins necessary for structure, function, repair, and replication that leads to more impaired cellular metabolism.

7. Gluconeogenesis contributes to lactic acid, uric acid, and ammonia buildup, interstitial edema, and impairment of the immune system, as well as general muscle weakness, leading to decreased respiratory function and cardiac output.

8. Cardiogenic shock is decreased cardiac output, tissue hypoxia, and the presence of adequate intravascular volume.

9. Hypovolemic shock is caused by loss of blood or fluid in large amounts. The use of compensatory mechanisms may be vigorous, but tissue perfusion ultimately decreases and results in impaired cellular metabolism.

10. Neurogenic shock results from massive vasodilation, causing a relative hypovolemia even though cardiac output may be high, and leads to impaired cellular metabolism.

11. Anaphylactic shock is caused by physiologic recognition of a foreign substance. The inflammatory response is triggered, and a massive vasodilation with fluid shift into the interstitium follows. The relative hypovolemia leads to impaired cellular metabolism.

12. Septic shock begins with impaired cellular metabolism caused by uncontrolled septicemia. The infecting agent triggers the inflammatory and immune responses. This inflammatory response is accompanied by widespread changes in tissue and cellular function.

13. Multiple organ dysfunction syndrome (MODS) is the progressive failure of two or more organ systems after a severe illness or injury. It can be triggered by chronic inflammation, necrotic tissue, severe trauma, burns, adult respiratory distress syndrome, acute pancreatitis, and other severe injuries.

14. MODS involves the stress response; changes in the vascular endothelium resulting in microvascular coagulation; release of complement, coagulation, and kinin proteins; and numerous inflammatory processes. Consequences of all these mediators are a maldistribution of blood flow, hypermetabolism, hypoxic injury, and myocardial depression.

15. Clinical manifestations of MODS include inflammation, tissue hypoxia, and hypermetabolism. All organs can be affected including the kidney, lung, liver, gastrointestinal tract, and central nervous system.

KEY TERMS

Acute coronary syndrome, 610
Acute pericarditis, 622
Anaphylactic shock, 643
Anaphylaxis, 643
Aneurysm, 604
Aortic regurgitation, 627
Aortic stenosis, 626
Arteriolar remodeling, 601
Arteriosclerosis, 607
Atherosclerosis, 607
Cardiogenic shock, 641
Cardiomyopathy, 624
Chronic orthostatic hypotension, 604
Chronic venous insufficiency (CVI), 598
Chylomicron, 611
Complicated plaque, 610
Constrictive pericarditis (restrictive pericarditis [chronic pericarditis]), 623
Coronary artery disease (CAD), 610
Damage-associated molecular patterns (DAMP), 601
Deep venous thrombosis (DVT), 599

Diastolic heart failure, 635
Dilated cardiomyopathy, 624
Dyslipidemia (dyslipoproteinemia), 611
Dysrhythmia (arrhythmia), 637
Electrocardiogram (ECG), 614
Embolism, 606
Embolus, 606
False aneurysm, 605
Fatty streak, 609
Fibrous plaque, 610
Foam cell, 609
Heart failure, 632
Heart failure with reduced ejection fraction (HFrEF; systolic heart failure), 632
Heart failure with preserved ejection fraction HFpEF; diastolic heart failure), 635
Hibernating myocardium, 619
High-sensitivity C-reactive protein (hs-CRP), 613
High-output failure, 636
Hypertension, 600
Hypertensive crisis (malignant hypertension), 602

Hypertensive hypertrophic cardiomyopathy, 624
Hypertrophic cardiomyopathy, 624
Hypertrophic obstructive cardiomyopathy, 624
Hypovolemic shock, 642
Infarction, 610
Infective endocarditis, 629
Intermittent claudication, 610
Ischemia, 610
Left heart failure, 632
Lipoprotein, 611
Lipoprotein(a) (Lp[a]), 611
Mental stress–induced ischemia, 614
Metabolic syndrome, 612
Microvascular angina (MVA), 614
Mitral regurgitation, 627
Mitral stenosis, 627
Mitral valve prolapse syndrome (MVPS), 628
Multiple organ dysfunction syndrome (MODS), 646
Myocardial infarction (MI), 616

Myocardial remodeling, 619
Myocardial stunning, 619
Neurogenic shock (vasogenic shock), 642
Nonbacterial thrombotic endocarditis, 630
Non-ST elevation MI (non-STEMI), 616
Orthostatic (postural) hypotension (OH), 604
Percutaneous coronary intervention (PCI), 616
Pericardial effusion, 623
Peripheral artery disease (PAD), 610
Plaque, 607
Pressure-natriuresis relationship, 600
Primary hypertension (essential hypertension, idiopathic hypertension), 600
Prinzmetal angina, 614
Raynaud phenomenon, 607
Restrictive cardiomyopathy, 625
Rheumatic fever, 628
Rheumatic heart disease (RHD), 628

REFERENCES

1. Pfisterer L et al: Pathogenesis of varicose veins—lessons from biomechanics, *Vasa* 43(2):88-99, 2014.
2. Poynter E et al: Clinical inquiry what is the best initial treatment for venous stasis ulcers? *J Fam Practice* 62(8):433-434, 2013.
3. Gohel M: Which treatments are cost-effective in the management of varicose veins? *Phlebology* 28(Suppl 1):153-157, 2013.
4. Bates SM et al: Diagnosis of DVT: antithrombotic therapy and prevention of thrombosis, ed 9, American College of Chest Physicians Evidence-Based Clinical Practice Guidelines, *Chest* 143I(2 Suppl):e351S-e418S, 2012.
5. Baldwin MJ et al: Post-thrombotic syndrome: a clinical review, *J Thromb Haemost* 11(5):795-805, 2013.
6. Pollak AW, McBane RD: Succinct review of the new VTE prevention and management guidelines, *Mayo Clin Proc* 89(3):394-408, 2014.
7. Prandoni P: Venous thromboembolism in 2013: the advent of the novel oral anticoagulants, *Nat Rev Cardiol* 11(2):70-72, 2014.
8. Shaheen K, Alraies M: Superior vena cava syndrome, *Clev Clin J Med* 79(6):410-412, 2012.
9. Quinn KL, Smith CA: Nonmalignant superior vena cava syndrome, *J Gen Intern Med* 28(7):970-971, 2013.
10. Go AS et al: Heart disease and stroke statistics—2014 update: a report from the American Heart Association, *Circulation* 129(3):e28-e292, 2014.
11. James PA et al: 2014 evidence-based guideline for the management of high blood pressure in adults. Report from the panel members appointed to the Eighth Joint National Committee (JNC 8), *J Am Med Assoc* 311(5):507-520, 2014.
12. Friso S et al: Epigenetics and arterial hypertension: the challenge of emerging evidence, *Transl Res* 165(1):154-165, 2015.
13. Lind JM, Chiu CL: Genetic discoveries in hypertension: steps on the road to therapeutic translation, *Heart* 99(22):1645-1651, 2013.
14. DiBona GF: Sympathetic nervous system and hypertension, *Hypertension* 61(3):556-560, 2013.
15. Grassi G et al: Sympathetic nervous system: role in hypertension and in chronic kidney disease, *Curr Opin Nephrol Hypertens* 21(1):46-51, 2012.
16. Ohishi M et al: Angiotensin (1-7) and other angiotensin peptides, *Curr Pharm Des* 19(17):3060-3064, 2013.
17. McKinney CA et al: Angiotensin-(1-7) and angiotensin-(1-9): function in cardiac and vascular remodeling, *Clin Sci* 126(12):815-827, 2014.
18. Clarke C et al: Regulation of cardiovascular remodeling by the counter-regulatory axis of the renin-angiotensin system, *Future Cardiol* 9(1):23-38, 2013.
19. Zucker IH et al: The central renin-angiotensin system and sympathetic nerve activity in chronic heart failure, *Clin Sci* 126(10):695-706, 2014.
20. Bender SB et al: Mineralocorticoid receptor-mediated vascular insulin resistance: an early contributor to diabetes-related vascular disease? *Diabetes* 62(2):313-319, 2013.

21. Sevá Pessôa B et al: Key developments in renin-angiotensin-aldosterone system inhibition, *Nat Rev Nephrol* 9(1):26-36, 2013.
22. Santos RA et al: Angiotensin-converting enzyme 2, angiotensin-(1-7) and Mas: new players of the renin-angiotensin system, *J Endocrinol* 216(2):R1-R17, 2013.
23. Fraga-Silva RA et al: Opportunities for targeting the angiotensin-converting enzyme 2/angiotensin-(1-7)/mas receptor pathway in hypertension, *Curr Hypertens Rep* 15(1):31-38, 2013.
24. Bibbins-Domingo K: The Institute of Medicine report sodium intake in populations: assessment of evidence: summary of primary findings and implications for clinicians, *J Am Med Assoc Intern Med* 174(1):136-137, 2014.
25. Rubattu S et al: Atrial natriuretic peptide and regulation of vascular function in hypertension and heart failure: implications for novel therapeutic strategies, *J Hypertens* 31(6):1061-1072, 2013.
26. Koliaki C, Katsilambros N: Dietary sodium, potassium, and alcohol: key players in the pathophysiology, prevention, and treatment of human hypertension, *Nutr Rev* 71(6):402-411, 2013.
27. McCarthy CG et al: Toll-like receptors and damage-associated molecular patterns: novel links between inflammation and hypertension, *Am J Physiol Heart Circ Physiol* 306(2):H184-H196, 2014.
28. Schiffrin EL: Immune mechanisms in hypertension and vascular injury, *Clin Sci* 126(4):267-274, 2014.
29. Aroor AR et al: Maladaptive immune and inflammatory pathways lead to cardiovascular insulin resistance, *Metabolism* 62(11):1543-1552, 2013.
30. Johns EJ, Abdulla MH: Renal nerves in blood pressure regulation, *Curr Opin Nephrol Hypertens* 22(5):504-510, 2013.
31. Santisteban MM et al: Dysfunctional brain-bone marrow communication: a paradigm shift in the pathophysiology of hypertension, *Curr Hypertens Rep* 15(4):377-389, 2013.
32. Landsberg L et al: Obesity-related hypertension: pathogenesis, cardiovascular risk, and treatment—a position paper of the Obesity Society and the American Society of Hypertension, *Obesity* 21(1):8-24, 2013.
33. Van de Voorde J et al: Adipocytokines in relation to cardiovascular disease, *Metabolism* 62(11):1513-1521, 2013.
34. Kovacic JC et al: The relationships between cardiovascular disease and diabetes: focus on pathogenesis, *Endocrinol Metab Clin North Am* 43:41-57, 2014.
35. Ishizu T et al: Left ventricular strain and transmural distribution of structural remodeling in hypertensive heart disease, *Hypertension* 63(3):500-506, 2014.
36. Lioudaki E et al: Microalbuminuria: a neglected cardiovascular risk factor in non-diabetic individuals? *Curr Pharm Des* 19(27):4964-4980, 2013.

37. Kohler S et al: Temporal evolution of cognitive changes in incident hypertension: prospective cohort study across the adult age span, *Hypertension*. 63(2):245-251, 2014.
38. Johnson W et al: Hypertension crisis in the emergency department, *Cardiol Clin* 30(4):533-543, 2012.
39. He FJ et al: Effect of longer term modest salt reduction on blood pressure: Cochrane systematic review and meta-analysis of randomised trials, *Br Med J* 346:f1325, 2013.
40. Navar-Boggan AM et al: Proportion of US adults potentially affected by the 2014 hypertension guideline, *J Am Med Assoc* 311(14):1424-1429, 2014.
41. Krum H et al: Percutaneous renal denervation in patients with treatment-resistant hypertension: final 3-year report of the Symplicity HTN-1 study, *Lancet* 383(9917):622-629, 2014.
42. Bhatt DL et al: A controlled trial of renal denervation for resistant hypertension, *N Engl J Med* 370(15):1393-1401, 2014.
43. Freeman R et al: Consensus statement on the definition of orthostatic hypotension, neurally mediated syncope and the postural tachycardia syndrome, *Clin Auton Res* 21:69-72, 2011.
44. Metzler M et al: Neurogenic orthostatic hypotension: pathophysiology, evaluation, and management, *J Neurol* 260(9):2212-2219, 2013.
45. Xin W et al: Orthostatic hypotension and mortality risk: a meta-analysis of cohort studies, *Heart* 100(5):406-413, 2014.
46. Perlmuter LC et al: A review of the etiology, associated comorbidities, and treatment of orthostatic hypotension, *Am J Ther* 20(3):279-291, 2013.
47. Bjorck M, Wanhainen A: Pathophysiology of AAA: heredity vs environment, *Prog Cardiovasc Dis* 56(1):2-6, 2013.
48. Singh MJ et al: Ruptured abdominal aortic aneurysms: is open surgery an outdated operation? *J Cardiovasc Surg* 55(2):137-149, 2014.
49. Ketha SS, Cooper LT: The role of autoimmunity in thromboangiitis obliterans (Buerger's disease), *Ann N Y Acad Sci* 1285:15-25, 2013.
50. Alamdari DH et al: B. Oxidative and antioxidative pathways might contribute to thromboangiitis obliterans pathophysiology, *Vascular* 22(1):46-50, 2014.
51. Prete M et al: Raynaud's phenomenon: from molecular pathogenesis to therapy, *Autoimmun Rev* 13(6):655-667, 2014.
52. Cutolo M, Smith V: State of the art on nailfold capillaroscopy: a reliable diagnostic tool and putative biomarker in rheumatology? *Rheumatology* 52(11):1933-1940, 2013.
53. Witztum JL, Lichtman AH: The influence of innate and adaptive immune responses on atherosclerosis, *Annu Rev Pathol* 9:73-102, 2014.
54. Madrigal-Matute J et al: MicroRNAs and atherosclerosis, *Curr Atheroscler Rep* 15(5):322, 2013.
55. Jaipersad AS et al: The role of monocytes in angiogenesis and atherosclerosis, *J Am Coll Cardiol* 63(1):1-11, 2014.

56. Arai H: Oxidative modification of lipoproteins, *Subcell Biochem* 77:103-114, 2014.

57. Pattanayak P, Bluemke DA: New era of evidence-based medicine with noninvasive imaging, *Nat Rev Cardiol* 11:74-76, 2014.

58. Bourantas CV et al: Early detection and invasive passivation of future culprit lesions: a future potential or an unrealistic pursuit of chimeras? *Am Heart J* 165(6):869-881.e4, 2013.

59. Lu L et al: Meta-analysis of the association between cigarette smoking and peripheral arterial disease, *Heart* 100(5):414-423, 2014.

60. Wennberg PW: Approach to the patient with peripheral arterial disease, *Circulation* 128(20):2241-2250, 2013.

61. Tattersall MC et al: Contemporary and optimal medical management of peripheral arterial disease, *Surg Clin North Am* 93(4):761-778, vii, 2013.

62. Szabo GV et al: Peripheral blood-derived autologous stem cell therapy for the treatment of patients with late-stage peripheral artery disease—results of the short- and long-term follow-up, *Cytotherapy* 15(10):1245-1252, 2013.

63. Jhamnani S et al: Meta-analysis of the effects of lifestyle modifications on coronary and carotid atherosclerotic burden, *Am J Cardiol* 115(2):268-375, 2015.

64. Expert Panel on Detection: Evaluation and treatment of high blood cholesterol in adults: executive summary of the third report of the National Cholesterol Education Program (NCEP) Expert Panel on Detection, Evaluation, and Treatment of High Blood Cholesterol in Adults (Adult Treatment Panel III), *J Am Med Assoc* 285(19):2486-2497, 2001.

65. Stone NJ et al: 2013 ACC/AHA guideline on the treatment of blood cholesterol to reduce atherosclerotic cardiovascular risk in adults: a report of the American College of Cardiology/American Heart Association Task Force on Practice Guidelines, *J Am Coll Cardiol* 63(25 Pt B):3024-3025, 2014.

66. Feig JE et al: High-density lipoprotein and atherosclerosis regression: evidence from preclinical and clinical studies, *Circ Res* 114(1):205-213, 2014.

67. Rosenson RS et al: Translation of high-density lipoprotein function into clinical practice: current prospects and future challenges, *Circulation* 128(11):1256-1267, 2013.

68. Messner B, Bernhard D: Smoking and cardiovascular disease: mechanisms of endothelial dysfunction and early atherogenesis, *Arterioscler Thromb Vasc Biol* 34(3):509-515, 2014.

69. Bornfeldt KE: 2013 Russell Ross memorial lecture in vascular biology: cellular and molecular mechanisms of diabetes mellitus-accelerated atherosclerosis, *Arterioscler Thromb Basc Biol* 34(4):705-714, 2014.

70. Bastien M et al: Overview of epidemiology and contribution of obesity to cardiovascular disease, *Prog Cardiovasc Dis* 56(4):369-381, 2014.

71. Ades PA, Savage PD: Potential benefits of weight loss in coronary heart disease, *Prog Cardiovasc Dis* 56(4):448-456, 2014.

72. Tschoner A et al: Long-term effects of weight loss after bariatric surgery on functional and structural markers of atherosclerosis, *Obesity* 21(10):1960-1965, 2013.

73. Goff DC et al: 2013 ACC/AHA guideline on the assessment of cardiovascular risk: a report of the American College of Cardiology/American Heart Association Task Force on Practice Guidelines, *J Am Coll Cardiol* 63(25 Pt B):3026, 2014.

74. The Emerging Risk Factors Collaboration: C-reactive protein, fibrinogen, and cardiovascular disease prediction, *N Engl J Med* 367:1310-1320, 2012.

75. Bhala N et al: Coxib and traditional NSAID Trialists' (CNT) Collaboration, vascular and upper gastrointestinal effects of non-steroidal anti-inflammatory drugs: meta-analyses of individual participant data from randomised trials, *Lancet* 382:769, 2013.

76. Van de Voorde J et al: Adipocytokines in relation to cardiovascular disease, *Metabolism* 62(11):1513-1521, 2013.

77. Yanai H, Hirowatari Y: Serum adiponectin levels are significantly associated with favorable metabolic parameters and elevation of atherosclerotic markers, *Int J Cardiol* 167(6):3065-3066, 2013.

78. Ntaios G et al: Adipokines as mediators of endothelial function and atherosclerosis, *Atherosclerosis* 227(2):216-221, 2013.

79. Adar SD et al: Fine particulate air pollution and the progression of carotid intima-medial thickness: a prospective cohort study from the multi-ethnic study of atherosclerosis and air pollution, *PLoS Med* 10(4):e1001430, 2013.

80. Thomsen M, Nordestgaard BG: Myocardial infarction and ischemic heart disease in overweight and obesity with and without metabolic syndrome, *J Am Med Assoc* 174(1):15-22, 2014.

81. Zuchi C et al: Angina pectoris in women: focus on microvascular disease, *Int J Cardiol* 163(2):132-140, 2013.

82. Moukarbel GV, Weinrauch LA: Disruption of coronary vasomotor function: the coronary spasm syndrome, *Cardiovasc Ther* 30(2):e66-e73, 2012.

83. Seo SM et al: Persistent coronary artery spasm documented by follow-up coronary angiography in patients with symptomatic remission of variant angina, *Heart Vessels* 28(3):301-307, 2013.

84. Chen H et al: Relationship of depression, stress and endothelial function in stable angina patients, *Physiol Behav* 118:152-158, 2013.

85. Paine NJ et al: Inflammation and vascular responses to acute mental stress: implications for the triggering of myocardial infarction, *Curr Pharm Des* 18(11):1494-1501, 2012.

86. Conti CR et al: Silent ischemia: clinical relevance, *J Am Coll Cardiol* 59(5):435-441, 2012.

87. Fihn SD et al: ACCF/AHA/ACP/AATS/PCNA/SCAI/STS guideline for the diagnosis and management of patients with stable ischemic heart disease: a report of the American College of Cardiology Foundation/American Heart Association Task Force on Practice Guidelines, and the American College of Physicians, American Association for Thoracic Surgery, Preventive Cardiovascular Nurses Association, Society for Cardiovascular Angiography and Interventions, and Society of Thoracic Surgeons, *Circulation.* 126:e354-e471, 2012.

88. Taylor F et al: Statins for the primary prevention of cardiovascular disease, *Cochrane Database Syst Rev* 1:CD004816, 2013.

89. Wilson JF: In the clinic. Stable ischemic heart disease, *Ann Intern Med* 160(1):ITC1-1-16; quiz ITC1-16, 2014.

90. Banon D et al: The usefulness of ranolazine for the treatment of refractory chronic stable angina pectoris as determined from a systematic review of randomized controlled trials, *Am J Cardiol* 113(6):1075-1082, 2014.

91. Braunwald E, Morrow DA: Unstable angina: is it time for a requiem? *Circulation* 127(24):2452-2457, 2013.

92. Jneid H et al: 2012 ACCF/AHA focused update of the guideline for the management of patients with unstable angina/non-ST-elevation myocardial infarction (updating the 2007 guideline and replacing the 2011 focused update): a report of the American College of Cardiology Foundation/American Heart Association Task Force on Practice Guidelines, *Circulation* 126(7):875-910, 2012.

93. Lin L, Knowlton AA: Innate immunity and cardiomyocytes in ischemic heart disease, *Life Sci* 100(1):1-8, 2014.

94. Reiter R et al: Preinfarction angina reduces infarct size in ST-elevation myocardial infarction treated with percutaneous coronary intervention, *Circ Cardiovasc Interven* 6(1):52-58, 2013.

95. Schevchuck A, Laskey WK: Ischemic conditioning as an adjunct to percutaneous coronary intervention, *Circ Cardiovasc Interven* 6(4):484-492, 2013.

96. Shah BN et al: The hibernating myocardium: current concepts, diagnostic dilemmas, and clinical challenges in the post-STICH era, *Eur Heart J* 34(18):1323-1336, 2013.

97. Ozaki Y et al: Effect of direct renin inhibitor on left ventricular remodeling in patients with primary acute myocardial infarction, *Int Heart J* 55(1):17-21, 2014.

98. Cabello JB et al: Oxygen therapy for acute myocardial infarction, *Cochrane Database Syst Rev* 8:CD007160, 2013.

99. O'Gara PT et al: 2013 ACCF/AHA guideline for the management of ST-elevation myocardial infarction: a report of the American College of Cardiology Foundation/American Heart Association Task Force on Practice Guidelines, *Circulation* 127:e362–e425, 2013. Available at: http://circ.ahajournals.org/content/127/4/e362.full.pdf+html.

100. Shammas NW et al: Pericarditis, myocarditis, and other cardiomyopathies, *Prim Care Clin Office Pract* 40(1):213-236, 2013.

101. Cantarini L et al: Role of autoimmunity and autoinflammation in the pathogenesis of idiopathic recurrent pericarditis, *Clin Rev Allergy Immunol* 44(1):6-13, 2013.

102. Kopcinovic LM, Culej J: Pleural, peritoneal and pericardial effusions—a biochemical approach, *Biochem Med* 24(1):123-237, 2014.

103. Figueras J et al: Predictors of moderate-to-severe pericardial effusion, cardiac tamponade, and electromechanical dissociation in patients with ST-elevation myocardial infarction, *Am J Cardiol* 113(8):1291-1296, 2014.

104. Imazio M, Adler Y: Management of pericardial effusion, *Eur Heart J* 34(16):1186-1197, 2013.

105. Smith KM, Squires J: Hypertrophic cardiomyopathy: an overview, *Crit Care Nurs Clin North Am* 25(2):263-272, 2013.

106. Yilmaz A, Sechtem U: Diagnostic approach and differential diagnosis in patients with hypertrophied left ventricles, *Heart* 100(8):662-671, 2014.

107. Nishimura RA et al: 2014 AHA/ACC guideline for the management of patients with valvular heart disease: executive summary: a report of the American College of Cardiology/American Heart Association Task Force on Practice Guidelines, *J Thorac Cardiovasc Surg* 148(1):e1-e132, 2014.

108. Brinkley DM, Gelfand EV: Valvular heart disease: classic teaching and emerging paradigms, *Am J Med* 126(12):1035-1042, 2013.

109. Holmes DR Jr et al: Clinical outcomes at 1 year following transcatheter aortic valve replacement, *J Am Med Assoc* 313(10):1019-1-28, 2015.

110. O'Gara PT et al: Transcatheter therapies for mitral regurgitation: a professional society overview from the American College of Cardiology, the American Association for Thoracic Surgery, Society for Cardiovascular Angiography and Interventions Foundation, and the Society of Thoracic Surgeons, *J Am Coll Cardiol* 63(8):840-852, 2014.

111. Burke RJ, Chang C: Diagnostic criteria of acute rheumatic fever, *Autoimmun Rev* 13(4-5):503-507, 2014.

112. Spinks A et al: Antibiotics for sore throat, *Cochrane Database Syst Rev* 11:CD000023, 2013.

113. Nitsche-Schmitz DP, Chhatwal GS: Host-pathogen interactions in streptococcal immune sequelae, *Curr Top Microbiol Immunol* 368:155-171, 2013.

114. Nussinovitch U, Shoenfeld Y: The clinical and diagnostic significance of anti-myosin autoantibodies in cardiac disease, *Clin Rev Allergy Immunol* 44(1):98-108, 2013.

115. Roberts K et al: Screening for rheumatic heart disease: current approaches and controversies, *Nat Rev Cardiol* 10(1):49-58, 2013.

116. Hoen B, Duval X: Clinical practice. Infective endocarditis, *N Engl J Med* 368(15):1425-1433, 2013.

117. Ferro JM, Fonseca AC: Infective endocarditis, *Handbook Clin Neurol* 119:75-91, 2014.

118. Fitch KV et al: Noncalcified coronary atherosclerotic plaque and immune activation in

HIV-infected women, *J Infect Dis* 208(11): 1737-1746, 2013.

119. Gupta M et al: Biomarkers and electrocardiographic evidence of myocardial ischemia in patients with human immunodeficiency virus infection, *Am J Cardiol* 111(5):760-764, 2013.

120. Moyers BS et al: Effect of left ventricular dysfunction and viral load on risk of sudden cardiac death in patients with human immunodeficiency virus, *Am J Cardiol* 113(7): 1260-1265, 2014.

121. Zucker IH et al: The central renin-angiotensin system and sympathetic nerve activity in chronic heart failure, *Clin Sci* 126(10):695-706, 2014.

122. Oka T et al: Angiogenesis and cardiac hypertrophy: maintenance of cardiac function and causative roles in heart failure, *Circ Res* 114(3): 565-571, 2014.

123. Li AH et al: Dynamic changes in myocardial matrix and relevance to disease: translational perspectives, *Circ Res* 114(5):916-927, 2014.

124. D'Alessandro R et al: Natriuretic peptides: molecular biology, pathophysiology and clinical implications for the cardiologist, *Future Cardiol* 9(4):519-534, 2013.

125. Turer AT: Using metabolomics to assess myocardial metabolism and energetics in heart failure, *J Mol Cell Cardiol* 55:12-18, 2013.

126. Dominic EA et al: Mitochondrial cytopathies and cardiovascular disease, *Heart* 100(8):611-618, 2014.

127. Reddy P, Samson R: Clinical utility of natriuretic peptides in left ventricular failure, *South Med J* 106(2):182-187, 2013.

128. Charisopoulou D et al: Milrinone in advanced heart failure: dose and therapeutic monitor outside intensive care unit, *Angiology* 65(4): 343-349, 2014.

129. Writing Committee Members et al: 2013 ACCF/AHA guideline for the management of heart failure: a report of the American College of Cardiology Foundation/American Heart Association Task Force on practice guidelines, *Circulation* 128(16):e240-e327, 2013.

130. Vizzardi E et al: Effects of spironolactone on long-term mortality and morbidity in patients with heart failure and mild or no symptoms, *Am J Med Sci* 347(4):271-276, 2014.

131. Kosmala W, Marwick TH: Meta-analysis of effects of optimization of cardiac resynchronization therapy on left ventricular function, exercise capacity, and quality of life in patients with heart failure, *Am J Cardiol* 113(6):988-994, 2014.

132. Braunwald E: The war against heart failure: the Lancet lecture, *Lancet* 385(9970):812-824, 2015.

133. Wan SH et al: Pre-clinical diastolic dysfunction, *J Am Coll Cardiol* 63(5):407-416, 2014.

134. Guazzi M: Pulmonary hypertension in heart failure preserved ejection fraction: prevalence, pathophysiology, and clinical perspectives, *Circ Heart Fail* 7(2):367-377, 2014.

135. Burke Ma et al: Prognostic importance of pathophysiologic markers in patients with heart failure and preserved ejection fraction, *Circ Heart Fail* 7(2):288-299, 2014.

136. Penicka M et al: Diagnosis of heart failure with preserved ejection fraction: role of clinical Doppler echocardiography, *Heart* 100(1):68-76, 2014.

137. Liu G et al: Meta-analysis of the effect of statins on mortality in patients with preserved ejection fraction, *Am J Cardiol* 113(7):1198-1204, 2014.

138. Athyros VG et al: Treating heart failure with preserved ejection fraction: statins could make the difference, *Angiology* 65(4):328-329, 2014.

139. Quiroz R et al: Comparison of characteristics and outcomes of patients with heart failure preserved ejection fraction versus reduced left ventricular ejection fraction in an urban cohort, *Am J Cardiol* 113(4):691-696, 2014.

140. Ashruf JF et al: New insights into the pathophysiology of cardiogenic shock: the role of the microcirculation, *Curr Opin Crit Care* 19(5): 381-386, 2013.

141. Tharmaratnam D et al: Management of cardiogenic shock complicating acute coronary syndromes, *Heart* 99(21):1614-1623, 2013.

142. Gann DS, Drucker WR: Hemorrhagic shock, *J Trauma Acute Care Surg* 75(5):888-895, 2013.

143. Summers RL et al: Characterization of the spectrum of hemodynamic profiles in trauma patients with acute neurogenic shock, *J Crit Care* 28(4):531.e1-5, 2013.

144. Samant SA et al: Anaphylaxis: diagnostic criteria and epidemiology, *Allergy Asthma Proc* 34(2): 115-119, 2013.

145. Sicherer SH, Leung DY: Advances in allergic skin disease, anaphylaxis, and hypersensitivity reactions to foods, drugs, and insects in 2013, *J Allergy Clin Immunol* 133(2):324-334, 2014.

146. Lieberman PL: Recognition and first-line treatment of anaphylaxis, *Am J Med* 127(1 Suppl): S6-S11, 2014.

147. Levy MM et al: 2001 SCCM/ESICM/ACCP/ATS/SIS international sepsis definitions conference, *Crit Care Med* 31:1250-1256, 2003.

148. Angus DC, van der Poll T: Severe sepsis and septic shock, *N Engl J Med* 369(9):840-851, 2013.

149. Stevenson EK et al: Two decades of mortality trends among patients with severe sepsis: a comparative meta-analysis, *Crit Care Med* 42(3): 625-631, 2014.

150. Centers for Disease Control: *Central line-associated bloodstream infection (CLABSI) event.* Available at: www.cdc.gov/nhsn/pdfs/pscmanual/4psc_clabscurrent.pdf. Accessed January 2014.

151. King EG et al: Pathophysiologic mechanisms in septic shock, *Lab Invest* 94(1):4-12, 2014.

152. Bosmann M, Ward PA: The inflammatory response in sepsis, *Trends Immunol* 34(3):129-136, 2013.

153. Landesberg G et al: Troponin elevation in severe sepsis and septic shock: the role of left ventricular diastolic dysfunction and right ventricular dilatation, *Crit Care Med* 42(4):790-800, 2014.

154. Corona A, De Iaco M: Procalcitonin or C-reactive protein: that is the question? *Crit Care Med* 42(4): e310-e311, 2014.

155. Dellinger RP et al: Surviving Sepsis Campaign: international guidelines for management of severe sepsis and septic shock: 2012, *Crit Care Med* 41:580-637, 2013.

156. Huet O, Chin-Dusting JP: Septic shock: desperately seeking treatment, *Clin Sci* 126(1): 31-39, 2014.

157. Sauaia A et al: Temporal trends of postinjury multiple-organ failure: still resource intensive, morbid, and lethal, *J Trauma Acute Care Surg* 76(3):582-592, discussion 592-593, 2014.

158. Levi M et al: Sepsis and thrombosis, *Semin Thromb Hemost* 39(5):559-566, 2013.

159. Bosmann M, Ward PA: The inflammatory response in sepsis, *Trends Immunol* 34(3):129-136, 2013.

25

Alterations of Cardiovascular Function in Children

Nancy Pike and Nancy L. McDaniel

CHAPTER OUTLINE

Cardiovascular disorders in children are classified as congenital or acquired. Congenital heart disease is the most common. The diagnosis and management of congenital heart disease continues to improve with the use of fetal echocardiography and early interventional catheterization or surgical repair. Acquired heart disease in children continues to present challenges to the practitioner. Although guidelines for diagnosing acquired diseases are available, work is still needed in developing standards of treatment and long-term follow-up protocols.

CONGENITAL HEART DISEASE

The incidence of congenital heart disease (CHD) varies from 4 to 8 per 1000 live births and is the major cause of death in the first year of life other than prematurity. Several environmental and genetic risk factors are associated with the incidence of different types of CHD. Among the environmental factors are (1) maternal conditions, such as intrauterine viral infections (especially rubella), diabetes mellitus, phenylketonuria, alcoholism, hypercalcemia, drugs (e.g., thalidomide, phenytoin), and complications of increased age; (2) antepartal bleeding; and (3) prematurity (Table 25-1).[1,2]

Genetic factors also have been implicated in the incidence of CHD, although the mechanism of causation is often unknown (Table 25-2). The incidence of CHD is three to four times higher in siblings of affected children, and chromosomal defects account for about 6% of all cases of CHD. Down syndrome, trisomies 13 and 18, Turner syndrome, and cri du chat syndrome (chromosome 5p deletion syndrome) have been associated with a relatively high incidence of heart defects. Only a small percentage of cases of CHD are clearly linked solely to genetic or environmental factors. There also are multiple hereditary and nonhereditary syndromes that are associated with cardiovascular abnormalities in children.[2] However, the cause of most defects is multifactorial.[1,2]

Congenital heart defects can be categorized according to (1) whether the defect causes cyanosis, (2) whether the defect causes increased or decreased blood flow into the pulmonary circulation, and (3) whether the defect causes obstruction of blood flow from the ventricles (Figure 25-1). The normal movement of blood through the right side of the heart and into the pulmonary system is separate from the blood flow through the left side of the heart into the systemic circulation (Figure 25-2, *A*). Abnormal movement from one side of the heart to the other is termed a shunt. Shunting of blood flow from the left heart into the right heart is called a left-to-right shunt and occurs in conditions such as atrial septal defect and ventricular septal defect (see Figure 25-2, *B*). This increases blood flow into the pulmonary circulation. Because blood continues to flow through the lungs before passing into the systemic circulation, there is no decrease in tissue oxygenation or cyanosis. Thus defects that cause left-to-right shunt are termed acyanotic heart defects. Other types of acyanotic heart defects obstruct blood flow from the ventricles but do not cause shunting. Cyanotic heart defects frequently cause shunting of blood from the right side of the heart directly into the left side of the heart (right-to-left shunt). This type of shunt decreases blood flow through the pulmonary system, causing less than normal oxygen delivery to the tissues and resultant cyanosis (see Chapter 27). Tetralogy of Fallot (TOF) occurs in 5% to 10% of all CHD and is the most common cyanotic heart defect.[2] In this condition, narrowing of the pulmonary outflow tract increases right heart pressures, thus forcing blood through a defect in the ventricular septum into the left heart (see Figure 25-2, *C*). Cyanosis, a bluish discoloration of the skin indicating that tissues are not receiving normal amounts of oxygen, also can be caused by other types of heart defects that result in the mixing of venous and arterial blood that enter the systemic circulation.

Most congenital heart defects are named to describe the underlying defect (for example, valvular abnormalities; abnormal openings in the septa, including persistence of the foramen ovale; continued patency

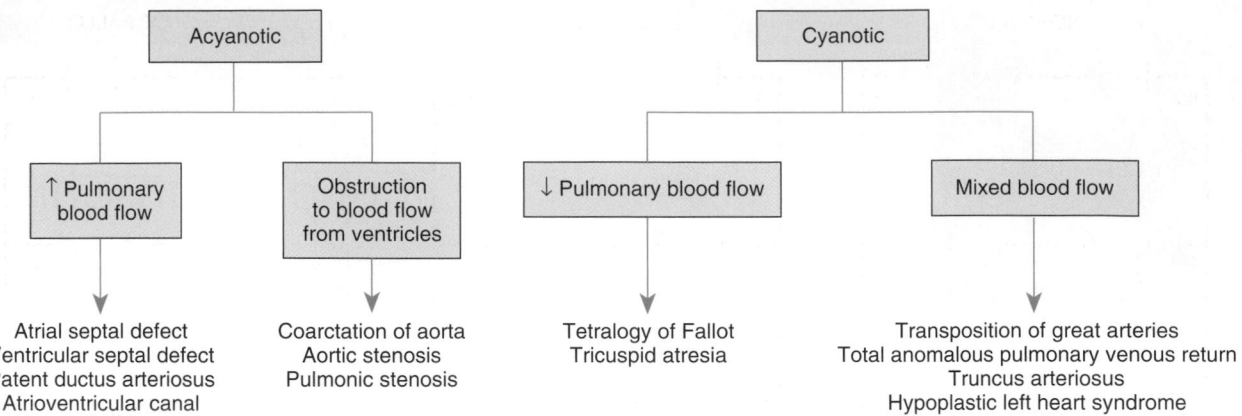

FIGURE 25-1 Comparison of Acyanotic-Cyanotic and Hemodynamic Classification Systems of Congenital Heart Disease. (From Hockenberry MJ, Wilson D: *Wong's nursing care of infants and children,* ed 10, St Louis, 2015, Mosby.)

TABLE 25-1 Maternal Conditions and Environmental Exposures and the Associated Congenital Heart Defects

Cause	Type of Congenital Heart Defect
Infection	
Intrauterine	Patent ductus arteriosus (PDA), pulmonary stenosis (PS), coarctation of the aorta (COA)
Systemic viral	PDA, PS, COA
Rubella	PDA, PS, COA
Coxsackie B5	Endocardial fibroelastosis
Radiation	Specific cardiovascular effect not known
Metabolic Disorders	
Diabetes	Ventricular septal defect (VSD), cardiomegaly, transposition of the great vessels
Phenylketonuria (PKU)	COA, PDA
Hypercalcemia	Supravalvular aortic stenosis (AS), PS; aortic hyperplasia
Drugs	
Thalidomide	No specific lesion
Dextroamphetamine	One case of reported transposition
Alcohol	Tetralogy of Fallot (TOF), atrial septal defect (ASD), VSD
Peripheral Conditions	
Increased maternal age	VSD, TOF (relationship unclear)
Antepartal bleeding	Various defects (relationship unclear)
Prematurity	PDA, VSD
High altitude	PDA, ASD (increased incidence)

TABLE 25-2 Congenital Heart Disease in Selected Fetal Chromosomal Aberrations

Conditions	Incidence of CHD (%)	Common Defects (in Decreasing Order of Frequency)
5p (cri du chat syndrome)	25	VSD, PDA, ASD
Trisomy 13 syndrome	90	VSD, PDA, dextrocardia
Trisomy 18 syndrome	99	VSD, PDA, PS
Trisomy 21 (Down syndrome)	50	AVSD, VSD
Turner syndrome (XO)	35	COA, AS, ASD
Klinefelter variant (XXXXY)	15	PDA, ASD

From Park MK: *Pediatric cardiology for practitioners,* ed 6, St Louis, 2014, Mosby.
AS, Aortic stenosis; *ASD,* atrial septal defect; *AVSD,* atrioventricular septal defect; *COA,* coarctation of the aorta; *PDA,* patent ductus arteriosus; *PS,* pulmonary stenosis; *VSD,* ventricular septal defect.

of the ductus arteriosus; and malformation or abnormal placement of the great vessels). Descriptions of the most common defects follow.

Obstructive Defects
Coarctation of the Aorta

PATHOPHYSIOLOGY Coarctation of the aorta (COA) is an abnormal localized narrowing of the aorta just proximal to the insertion of the ductus arteriosus. Before birth, the ductus arteriosus bypasses this obstruction and allows for blood to flow from the pulmonary artery into the distal aorta. However, once the ductus functionally closes within 15 hours after birth, blood flow to the lower extremities is then restricted by the coarctation. Clinically, there is increased blood pressure proximal to the defect (head and upper extremities, right greater than left) and decreased blood pressure distal to the obstruction (torso and lower extremities) (Figure 25-3).

CLINICAL MANIFESTATIONS The location and severity of the COA determine whether an infant will become symptomatic after the ductus arteriosus closes. If the COA is severe, infants will present with low cardiac output, poor tissue perfusion, acidosis, and hypotension. Physical examination of the infant will reveal weak or absent femoral pulses. Some infants with COA will remain asymptomatic after the closure of the ductus arteriosus. As they age, children with undiagnosed COA will present with unexplained upper extremity hypertension. Children may complain of leg pain or cramping with exercise. Although rare, they also may experience dizziness, headaches, fainting, or epistaxis from hypertension.[1,2]

EVALUATION AND TREATMENT Physical examination and measurement of upper and lower extremity blood pressures will often suggest the diagnosis. Echocardiography, magnetic resonance imaging (MRI), and cardiac catheterization may be needed to confirm the diagnosis.

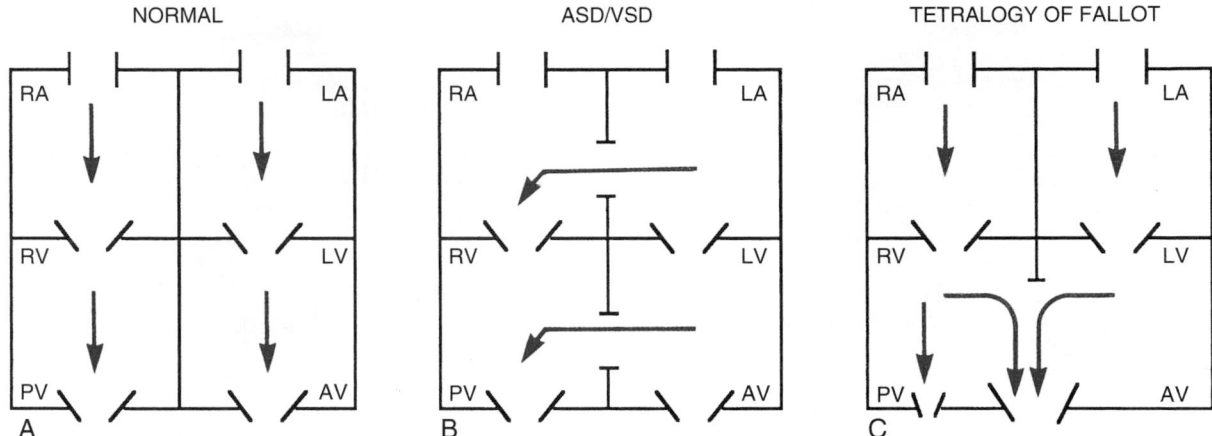

FIGURE 25-2 Shunting of Blood in Congenital Heart Disease. A, Normal. **B,** Acyanotic defect. **C,** Cyanotic defect. *ASD,* Atrial septal defect; *AV,* aortic valve; *LA,* left atrium; *LV,* left ventricle; *PV,* pulmonic valve; *RA,* right atrium; *RV,* right ventricle; *VSD,* ventricular septal defect. (From Hockenberry MJ, Wilson D: *Wong's nursing care of infants and children,* ed 10, St Louis, 2015, Mosby.)

Initial treatment in the symptomatic newborn consists of continuous intravenous infusion of prostaglandin E_1 to maintain the patency of the ductus arteriosus. Once the symptomatic newborn is stabilized, surgical correction is indicated.[3]

Surgical correction consists of either resection of the narrowed portion of the aorta with an end-to-end anastomosis or enlargement of the constricted section using a graft taken from a portion of the left subclavian artery. Because this defect is outside the heart and pericardium, cardiopulmonary bypass usually is not required and a thoracotomy incision is used. However, coarctation repair may be part of a more complex operation, which might require a sternotomy incision and cardiopulmonary bypass. Postoperative hypertension is treated with intravenous medication, often a short-acting beta-blocker, followed by oral medications, such as an angiotensin-converting enzyme inhibitor. Residual hypertension after repair of COA seems to be related to age and time of repair.

Studies have shown percutaneous balloon angioplasty with or without the use of a stent to be an effective, less invasive option for treating native COA or for reducing residual postoperative coarctation in most children.[1,2,4] Balloon angioplasty of COA as an initial intervention can also be considered. However, in infants younger than 6 months of age, most will experience recoarctation in only a short period of time after primary angioplasty. Other complications include aneurysm formation and blood vessel injury from arterial access. Data exist that support balloon angioplasty as an effective therapy in selected infants older than 6 months of age with a decreased risk of aneurysm formation as compared to younger infants.[4]

Aortic Stenosis

PATHOPHYSIOLOGY Aortic stenosis (AS) is a narrowing or stricture of the left ventricular outlet, causing resistance of blood flow from the left ventricle into the aorta (Figure 25-4). The physiologic consequence of severe AS is hypertrophy of the left ventricular wall, which eventually leads to increased end-diastolic pressure, resulting in pulmonary venous and pulmonary arterial hypertension. If severe, there may be decreased cardiac output and pulmonary vascular congestion. Left ventricular hypertrophy impedes coronary artery perfusion and may result in subendocardial ischemia and associated papillary muscle dysfunction that cause mitral insufficiency.

There are three types of AS. Valvular AS occurs as a consequence of malformed or fused cusps, resulting in a unicuspid or bicuspid valve.

Valvular AS is a serious defect because (1) the obstruction tends to be progressive; (2) there may be sudden episodes of myocardial ischemia or low cardiac output that, on rare occasions, can result in sudden death in late childhood or adolescence; and (3) surgical repair will not result in a normal valve. This is one of the rare forms of congenital heart disease in which strenuous physical activity may be curtailed because of the cardiac condition.[1,2]

Subvalvular AS is a stricture caused by a fibrous ring below a normal valve. It can also be caused by a narrowed left ventricular outflow tract in combination with a small aortic valve annulus. Supravalvular AS, a narrowing of the aorta just above the valve, occurs infrequently. It can occur as a single defect (familial supravalvular stenosis syndrome) or as a part of Williams syndrome, which also is characterized by unusual elfin-like facial appearance and mental disability.[5]

CLINICAL MANIFESTATIONS Infants with significant AS demonstrate signs of decreased cardiac output with faint pulses, hypotension, tachycardia, and poor feeding. A loud, harsh systolic ejection murmur is expected. Older children also may have complaints of exercise intolerance and, rarely, chest pain. Children are at risk for bacterial endocarditis, although prophylaxis with antibiotics is no longer routinely recommended (see *Health Alert:* Endocarditis Risk). Aortic stenosis, when severe, also can be complicated by coronary insufficiency, ventricular dysfunction, and, rarely, sudden death.

EVALUATION AND TREATMENT Valvular aortic stenosis (AS) diagnosis is confirmed by echocardiography. Mild to moderate valvular AS does not usually require intervention or restriction of activity. Treatment of severe valvular AS varies, with nonsurgical palliation the initial treatment of choice by many interventional cardiologists. Dilation of the stenotic valve with balloon angioplasty, which is performed in the cardiac catheterization laboratory, still carries a high morbidity and mortality in the critically ill neonate; however, in older infants and children it compares favorably with surgical valvotomy.[4] Balloon angioplasty is, however, associated with the risk of aortic regurgitation (insufficiency). Children undergoing this procedure almost always require surgical intervention at some time to relieve recurrent narrowing or worsening regurgitation.[4]

Surgical treatment for valvular AS depends on the severity of the stenosis, previous interventions, and age of the child. Aortic valve

FIGURE 25-3 Postductal and Preductal Coarctation of the Aorta. **A,** Postductal coarctation occurs distal to ("after") the insertion of the closed ductus arteriosus into the aortic arch. Preductal coarctation occurs proximal to ("before") the insertion of the patent ductus arteriosus. The coarctation consists of a flap of tissue that protrudes from the tunica media of the aortic wall. **B,** Coarctation of the aorta with typical indentation of the aortic wall *(arrow)* opposite the ductal arterial ligament *(asterisk)*. *Ao,* Aorta. (**A** from Hockenberry MJ, Wilson D: *Wong's essentials of pediatric nursing,* ed 9, St Louis, 2013, Mosby; **B** from Damjanov I, Linder J, editors: *Anderson's pathology,* ed 10, St Louis, 1996, Mosby.)

FIGURE 25-4 Aortic Stenosis (AS). Narrowing of the aortic valve causing resistance to blood flow in the left ventricle, decreased cardiac output, left ventricular hypertrophy, and pulmonary congestion. (From Hockenberry MJ et al: *Wong's essentials of pediatric nursing,* ed 9, St Louis, 2013, Mosby.)

HEALTH ALERT

Endocarditis Risk

Children with CHD are at risk for developing endocarditis. Although the risk is low, a transient bacteremia has been noted to follow dental and surgical procedures and instrumentation involving mucosal surfaces. A blood-borne pathogen can inhabit areas of the heart where there is high turbulence (such as an abnormal valve or vessel) or reside on artificial material (such as a valve or homograft). *Streptococcus viridans* (α-hemolytic streptococci) is the most commonly found pathogen following dental or oral procedures. *Enterococcus faecalis* (enterococci) is the most common bacterium found following genitourinary and gastrointestinal tract surgery or instrumentation. The American Heart Association has provided updated guidelines for the prevention of bacterial endocarditis. The type and dose of antibiotic prophylaxis recommended depend on the procedure and the cardiac classification of risk for endocarditis. Good dental hygiene with daily brushing and flossing is critically important along with regular dental check-ups.

Data from the American Heart Association: available at www.americanheart.org.

commissurotomy or valvotomy may be used as an early intervention. Aortic valve replacement may be required if the valve is severely dysplastic. The Ross procedure, which involves moving the native pulmonary valve (autograft) into the aortic position and replacing the pulmonary valve with an allograft (cadaver), and coronary artery reimplantation have become an option. The advantage of the Ross procedure over mechanical valve replacement, especially in a young child, is that there is no requirement for long-term anticoagulation therapy; however, the valve may fail with time. Mechanical valve replacement is usually deferred as long as possible to minimize the number of valve replacements related to growth. Aortic stenosis requires lifelong evaluation and treatment. Multiple surgical or catheterization interventions are expected. Mortality for sick infants and young children is higher than that for older children.

Subvalvular Aortic Stenosis. Surgical correction for subvalvular as involves incising the constricting fibromuscular ring. if the obstruction results from a narrow left ventricular outflow tract and a small aortic valve annulus, a patch may be required to enlarge the entire left ventricular outflow tract and annulus and replace the aortic valve, an approach known as the Konno procedure. an aortic homograft with a valve also may be used (extended aortic root replacement).

Supravalvular Aortic Stenosis. Surgery is usually required for management of moderate-to-severe supravalvular AS. Balloon angioplasty and stent insertion have been successful but carry a higher risk of rupture.[1,2,4] An extended graft with coronary reimplantation may be needed if narrowing is severe.

Pulmonic Stenosis

PATHOPHYSIOLOGY Pulmonic stenosis (PS) is a narrowing or stricture of the pulmonary valve that causes resistance to blood flow from

FIGURE 25-5 Pulmonic Stenosis (PS). A, The pulmonary valve narrows at the entrance of the pulmonary artery. **B,** Balloon angioplasty is used to dilate the valve. A catheter is inserted across the stenotic pulmonic valve into the pulmonary artery, and a balloon at the end of the catheter is inflated while it is positioned across the narrowed valve opening. (**A** from Hockenberry MJ et al: *Wong's essentials of pediatric nursing,* ed 9, St Louis, 2013, Mosby.)

the right ventricle to the pulmonary artery (Figure 25-5). Generally moderate to severe stenosis causes right ventricular hypertrophy. **Pulmonary atresia** is an extreme form of PS with total fusion of the valve leaflets (blood cannot flow to the lungs); the right ventricle may be hypoplastic. In some cases of right ventricular outflow obstruction, the narrowing is below the valve (infundibular or subvalve PS).

CLINICAL MANIFESTATIONS Most infants are asymptomatic if the PS is mild to moderate. Newborns with severe PS or pulmonary atresia will be cyanotic (from a right-to left shunt through an atrial septal defect [ASD]) and may have signs of decreased cardiac output. A harsh systolic murmur is expected with PS. Pulmonary atresia produces a continuous murmur.

EVALUATION AND TREATMENT Echocardiography confirms the diagnosis and determines the severity of the PS. The treatment of choice for infants with moderate to severe pulmonary stenosis is balloon angioplasty (see Figure 25-5, *B*). A catheter with a special balloon device is used to dilate the area of narrowing. Multiple studies have proven the effectiveness and safety of balloon angioplasty in reducing the pressure gradient across the pulmonic valve.[4] In rare cases, surgical valvotomy may be required. Pulmonary blood flood is supported with prostaglandin E_1 infusion to maintain the patency of the ductus arteriosus in cases of pulmonary atresia with right ventricle–dependent coronary circulation in the neonatal period until surgery is performed to supply pulmonary blood flow.[4]

Both balloon dilation and surgical valvotomy leave the pulmonary valve incompetent (insufficient); however, most children are usually able to tolerate pulmonary valve incompetence and are asymptomatic. Long-term problems with restenosis are rare for uncomplicated PS.[1,2,4] However, clinically significant valve incompetence that results in right ventricle dilation and dysfunction may occur, requiring surgical intervention.[1,2,4]

Defects with Increased Pulmonary Blood Flow
Patent Ductus Arteriosus
PATHOPHYSIOLOGY Patent ductus arteriosus (PDA) is failure of the fetal ductus arteriosus (artery connecting the aorta and pulmonary

artery) to functionally close within the first 15 hours after birth. However, several weeks after birth (Figure 25-6) may be needed for attainment of true anatomic closure, in which the ductus loses the ability to reopen. The continued patency of this vessel allows blood to flow from the higher pressure aorta to the lower pressure pulmonary artery, causing a left-to-right shunt.

CLINICAL MANIFESTATIONS Infants may be asymptomatic or show signs of pulmonary overcirculation, such as dyspnea, fatigue, and poor feeding. There is a characteristic machinery-like murmur in both systole and diastole. Aortic flow (run-off) into the lower pressure pulmonary circulation produces low diastolic blood pressure, widened pulse pressure, and bounding pulses. Children are at risk for bacterial endocarditis and may develop pulmonary hypertension in later life from chronic excessive pulmonary blood flow.

EVALUATION AND TREATMENT Diagnosis is confirmed with echocardiography. Administration of indomethacin (a prostaglandin inhibitor) has proved successful in closing a PDA in premature infants and some newborns. Surgical division of the PDA through a left thoracotomy also may be done; in some cases the procedure can be performed with thoracoscopy. Closure with an occlusion device during cardiac catheterization is performed in select children older than 6 months of age. Both surgical and nonsurgical procedures are considered low risk.[2,4]

Atrial Septal Defect
PATHOPHYSIOLOGY An atrial septal defect (ASD) is an opening in the septal wall between the two atria. This opening allows blood to shunt from the left atrium to the right atrium. There are three types of ASDs. An ostium primum ASD is an opening low in the atrial septum and may be associated with abnormalities of the mitral valve. An ostium secundum ASD is an opening in the middle of the atrial septum and is the most common type. A sinus venosus ASD is an opening usually high in the atrial wall near the junction of the superior vena cava and may be associated with partial anomalous pulmonary venous connection.[6] Left-to-right shunting of blood can occur with a large ASD.

FIGURE 25-6 Patent Ductus Arteriosus (PDA). **A,** PDA with left-to-right shunt. **B,** PDA in an adult with pulmonary hypertension. *Ao,* Aorta; *LPA,* left pulmonary artery; *RPA,* right pulmonary artery; *SCV,* subclavian vein. (**A** from Hockenberry MJ, Wilson D: *Wong's essentials of pediatric nursing,* ed 9, St Louis, 2013, Mosby; **B** from Damjanov I, Linder J, editors: *Anderson's pathology,* ed 10, St Louis, 1996, Mosby.)

Another opening in the atrial septal wall that is part of normal fetal communication, which usually closes after birth, is the foramen ovale. When the lungs become functional at birth, the pulmonary pressure decreases and the left atrial pressure exceeds that of the right. The pressure change forces the septum to functionally close the foramen ovale. If it does not close, it is called a patent foramen ovale (PFO). About one out of four adults has a PFO without CHD; however, in children with CHD the foramen ovale often remains open.

CLINICAL MANIFESTATIONS Children with an ASD are usually asymptomatic. Infants with a large ASD may, in rare cases, develop pulmonary overcirculation and slow growth. Some older children and adults will experience shortness of breath with activity as the right ventricle becomes less compliant with age. Pulmonary hypertension and stroke are associated rare complications. A systolic ejection murmur and a widely split second heart sound are the expected findings on physical examination.

EVALUATION AND TREATMENT Diagnosis is confirmed by echocardiography. The ASD may be closed surgically with primary repair

(sutured closed) or with a patch (pericardium or Dacron). Surgical repair involves open-heart surgery with cardiopulmonary bypass. Catheterization device closure offers a less invasive alternative for children with an ASD that meets anatomic and size criteria.[7] All options have low morbidity and mortality. Atrial dysrhythmias persist in about 5% to 10% of individuals in both groups after closure.[7]

Ventricular Septal Defect

PATHOPHYSIOLOGY A ventricular septal defect (VSD) is an opening of the septal wall between the ventricles. VSDs are the most common type of congenital heart defect and account for 15% to 20% of all such defects.[2] VSDs are classified by location. Perimembranous VSDs are located high in the ventricular septal wall underneath the atrioventricular valves, and VSDs located under the aortic valve are subarterial. Muscular VSDs are located low in the septal wall. VSDs also can be located in the inlet or outlet portion of the ventricle. VSDs are similar to ASDs in that blood will shunt from left to right. Left-to-right shunting of blood can occur with a large VSD. Depending on the size and location, many VSDs close spontaneously, most often within the first 2 years of life.

CLINICAL MANIFESTATIONS Depending on the size, location, and degree of shunting and pulmonary vascular resistance, children may have no symptoms or have clinical effects from excessive pulmonary blood flow. In the infant, excessive pulmonary blood flow from left-to-right shunting causes dyspnea and tachypnea symptoms, commonly referred to as heart failure (HF), even though the heart muscle functions well with a VSD. A holosystolic (pansystolic) murmur is expected.

If the degree of shunting is significant and not corrected, the child is at risk for developing pulmonary hypertension. Irreversible pulmonary hypertension can result in Eisenmenger syndrome, a condition in which shunting of blood is reversed because of high pulmonary pressure and resistance (right-to-left shunt with cyanosis).

EVALUATION AND TREATMENT Diagnosis is confirmed by echocardiogram. Cardiac catheterization may be needed to calculate the degree of shunting and to directly measure the pressures in the heart. Smaller VSDs require minimal treatment and may close completely or become small enough that surgical closure is not required. If the infant has severe HF or failure to thrive that is unmanageable with medical therapy, early surgical repair is performed. Surgical repair involves open-heart surgery with cardiopulmonary bypass. The opening is either sutured closed (primary) or covered with a patch (pericardium or Dacron). Nonsurgical device closure is available but only under restricted conditions.[4,8] Endocarditis prophylaxis is only recommended for 6 months after surgical or device closure and indefinitely with a residual VSD after patch closure.[8]

Atrioventricular Canal Defect

PATHOPHYSIOLOGY Atrioventricular canal (AVC) defect, also known as atrioventricular septal defect (AVSD) or by the traditional term endocardial cushion defect (ECD), is the result of incomplete fusion of endocardial cushions (Figure 25-7). AVC defect consists of an ostium primum ASD and inlet VSD with associated abnormalities of the atrioventricular valve tissue. These valve abnormalities range from a cleft in the mitral valve to a common mitral and tricuspid valve. The directions and pathways of flow are determined by pulmonary and systemic resistance, left and right ventricular pressures, and the compliance of each chamber. Flow is generally from left to right. AVC is a common cardiac defect in children with Down syndrome. However, children with this defect can have a normal karyotype.

FIGURE 25-7 Atrioventricular Canal (AVC) Defect. (From Hockenberry MJ, Wilson D: *Wong's essentials of pediatric nursing*, ed 9, St Louis, 2013, Mosby.)

CLINICAL MANIFESTATIONS Infants with this defect often display moderate to severe heart failure attributable to left-to-right shunting and pulmonary overcirculation. Infants with pulmonary hypertension and high pulmonary resistance have less shunting and therefore minimal signs of HF. There may be mild cyanosis that increases with crying. Those with a large left-to-right shunt will have a murmur, and those with minimal shunt may not have a murmur. Children with AVC are at risk for developing irreversible pulmonary hypertension if left surgically untreated.

EVALUATION AND TREATMENT AVC is one of the most frequent diagnoses made with fetal echocardiography. Cardiac catheterization usually is not needed. Initial treatment goals include aggressive medical management of HF and nutritional supplementation. Infants are followed closely for signs or symptoms of failure to thrive. Pulmonary artery banding is occasionally performed in small infants with severe symptoms. However, complete surgical repair is most common and typically performed between 3 and 6 months of age to prevent irreversible pulmonary hypertension. This procedure consists of patch closure of the septal defects and reconstruction of the AV valve tissue (either repair of the mitral valve cleft or fashioning of two AV valves). If the mitral valve defect is severe, valve replacement may be needed. A potential problem following repair is mitral regurgitation, which may later require valve replacement.

Defects with Decreased Pulmonary Blood Flow
Tetralogy of Fallot

PATHOPHYSIOLOGY The classic form of tetralogy of Fallot (TOF) includes four defects: (1) VSD, (2) PS, (3) overriding aorta, and (4) right ventricular hypertrophy (Figure 25-8). The pathophysiology varies widely, depending not only on the degree of PS but also on the pulmonary and systemic vascular resistance to flow. If total resistance to pulmonary flow is greater than systemic resistance, the shunt is from right to left. If systemic resistance is more than pulmonary resistance, the shunt is from left to right. PS decreases blood flow to the lungs and, consequently, the amount of oxygenated blood that returns to the left heart. Physiologic compensation to chronic, severe hypoxia includes production of more red blood cells (polycythemia),

FIGURE 25-8 Tetralogy of Fallot (TOF). **A,** TOF hemodynamics. **B,** Right ventricular *(RV)* hypertrophy and overriding aorta. (**A** from Hockenberry MJ, Wilson D: *Wong's essentials of pediatric nursing*, ed 9, St Louis, 2013, Mosby; **B** from Damjanov I, Linder J, editors: *Anderson's pathology*, ed 10, St Louis, 1996, Mosby.)

development of collateral bronchial vessels, and enlargement of the nail beds (clubbing).

CLINICAL MANIFESTATIONS Some infants may be acutely cyanotic at birth. In others, progression of hypoxia and cyanosis may be more gradual over the first year of life as the pulmonary stenosis worsens. Acute episodes of cyanosis and hypoxia can occur, called *hypercyanotic spells, blue spells,* or *"tet" spells.* These spells (increased right-to-left shunt) may occur during crying or after feeding. Oxygen has little effect in improving hypoxemia but placing the infant in a knee-chest position (Figure 25-9) and administering morphine sulfate subcutaneously or intravenously is most commonly used to treat "tet" spells. If prolonged or frequent, these spells are an indication for emergent evaluation and surgical treatment.

FIGURE 25-9 Infant held in a Knee-Chest Position. (From Hockenberry MJ, Wilson D: *Wong's essentials of pediatric nursing,* ed 9, St Louis, 2013, Mosby.)

Chronic cyanosis may cause clubbing of the fingers and poor growth in children. Squatting or the knee-chest position can help with cyanosis in these children because it increases peripheral resistance in the systemic circulation, which causes an increase in pressures in the left heart and consequent reduction in right-to-left shunting and improvement in pulmonary perfusion. Children with unrepaired TOF are at risk for emboli, stroke, brain abscess, seizures, and loss of consciousness or sudden death following a "tet" spell.

EVALUATION AND TREATMENT   Diagnosis is confirmed with echocardiography. Elective surgical repair is usually performed in the first year of life. Indications for earlier repair include increasing cyanosis or the development of hypercyanotic spells. Complete repair involves closure of the VSD, resection of the infundibular stenosis, and application of a pericardial patch to enlarge the right ventricular outflow tract that can extend across the pulmonary valve annulus (transannular patch).

In very small infants who cannot undergo primary repair, a palliative procedure to increase pulmonary blood flow and increase oxygen saturation may be performed. This systemic artery to pulmonary artery anastomosis is the *Blalock-Taussig* or modified *Blalock-Taussig shunt,* which provides blood flow to the pulmonary arteries.

Tricuspid Atresia

PATHOPHYSIOLOGY   Tricuspid atresia is failure of the tricuspid valve to develop; consequently, there is no communication from right atrium to right ventricle (Figure 25-10). Blood flows through an ASD or a patent foramen ovale (PFO) to the left atrium and through a VSD to the right ventricle. This condition is often associated with PS or transposition of the great arteries. There is complete mixing of unoxygenated and oxygenated blood in the left side of the heart, resulting in systemic desaturation and mild cyanosis. The physiologic process that causes lesion development is variable, depending on the great vessel anatomy and amount of pulmonary stenosis.

CLINICAL MANIFESTATIONS   A murmur is noted, and cyanosis is usually seen in the newborn period. Tachycardia, dyspnea, fatigue, and poor feeding may be noted with excessive pulmonary blood flow. Older

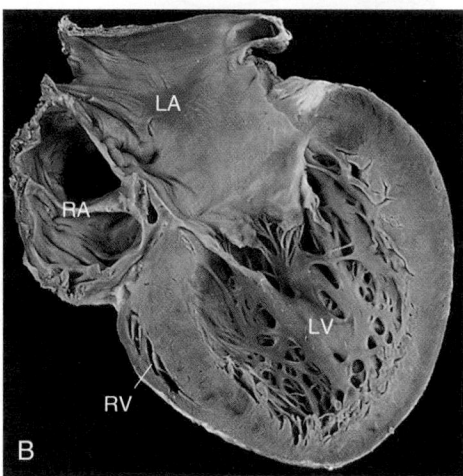

FIGURE 25-10 Tricuspid Atresia. **A,** Tricuspid atresia hemodynamics. **B,** Small right ventricle *(RV)* slit of VSD; left ventricle *(LV)* is enlarged. (**A** from Hockenberry MJ, Wilson D: *Wong's essentials of pediatric nursing,* ed 9, St Louis, 2013, Mosby; **B** from Damjanov I, Linder J, editors: *Anderson's pathology,* ed 10, St Louis, 1996, Mosby.)

children may have signs of chronic hypoxemia with clubbing. Children are at risk for bacterial endocarditis, brain abscess, and stroke.

EVALUATION AND TREATMENT   After diagnosis is confirmed by echocardiography, the neonate with decreased pulmonary blood flow is treated with a continuous infusion of prostaglandin E_1 to maintain the patency of the ductus arteriosus until surgical intervention. If the ASD is restrictive, an atrial septostomy is performed during cardiac catheterization or under echocardiographic guidance.[9] Treatment is accomplished in staged procedures. Once the infant is stabilized, a *Blalock-Taussig shunt* (systemic to pulmonary artery anastomosis) is placed to increase blood flow to the lungs.

Further surgery is undertaken between 4 and 8 months of age, depending on the child's growth and degree of cyanosis. The second-stage procedure is the *bidirectional Glenn shunt* in which the superior vena cava is anastomosed to the pulmonary artery. At that time, the pulmonary artery may be ligated and the Blalock-Taussig shunt is removed. The final separation of the pulmonary circulation from the systemic circulation is the *modified Fontan procedure.* In this stage, the inferior vena cava blood flow is routed to the pulmonary artery using an intra- or extracardiac tube graft or baffle. The procedure is typically

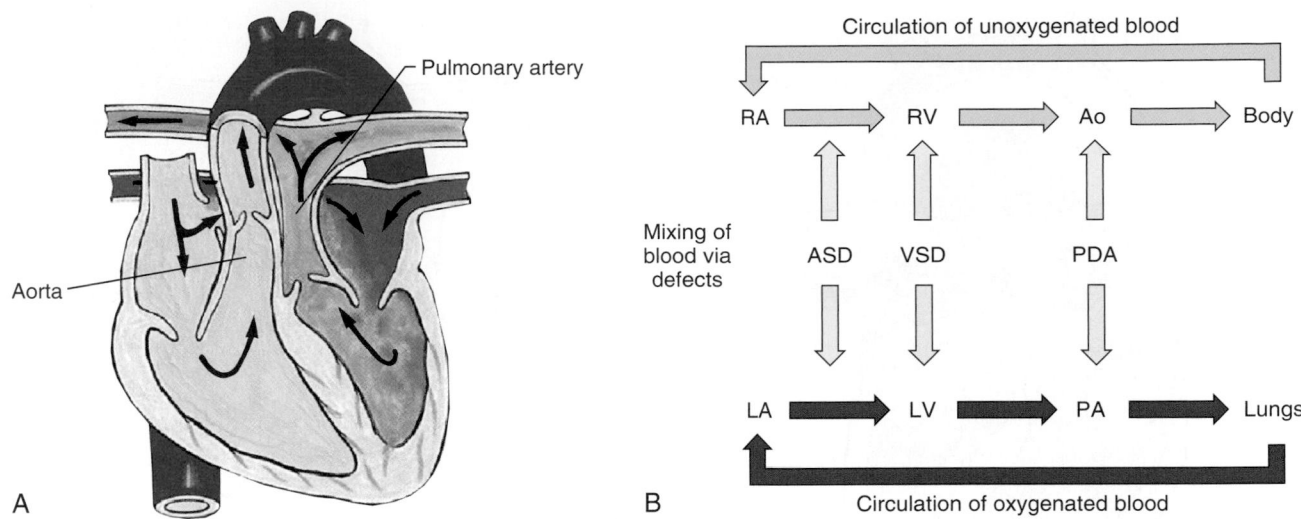

FIGURE 25-11 Hemodynamics in Transposition of the Great Vessels (TGV). **A,** Complete transposition of the great vessels with an intact interventricular septum. The aorta arises from the right ventricle and the pulmonary artery from the left ventricle. **B,** Oxygen saturation in the two, parallel circuits. *Ao,* Aorta; *ASD,* atrial septal defect; *LA,* left atrium; *LV,* left ventricle; *PA,* pulmonary artery; *PDA,* patent ductus arteriosus; *RA,* right atrium; *RV,* right ventricle; *VSD,* ventricular septal defect. (**A** from Hockenberry MJ, Wilson D: *Wong's essentials of pediatric nursing,* ed 9, St Louis, 2013, Mosby.)

performed between 2 and 4 years of age. Surgical outcomes are best in the child with normal ventricular function and low pulmonary vascular resistance (PVR). For children with borderline PVR, a fenestration (opening) can be created in the baffle or graft to relieve high systemic pulmonary venous pressures if needed.

Postoperative complications that increase hospital stay include pleural and pericardial effusions, elevated PVR, and ventricular dysfunction. Exercise tolerance is limited in many children with the Fontan procedure, but general health is considered good.

Mixing Defects
Transposition of the Great Arteries or Transposition of the Great Vessels

PATHOPHYSIOLOGY In transposition of the great arteries (TGA) or transposition of the great vessels (TGV), the pulmonary artery leaves the left ventricle and the aorta exits the right ventricle (Figure 25-11). Associated defects, such as ASD, VSD, or PDA, permit mixing of saturated and desaturated blood, which maintains adequate tissue oxygenation for a limited time.

CLINICAL MANIFESTATIONS Clinical manifestations depend on the type and size of the associated defects. Children with limited communication between cardiac chambers are severely cyanotic, acidotic, and ill at birth. Those with large septal defects or a PDA may be less severely cyanotic but may have symptoms of pulmonary overcirculation. Classically, no murmur is heard unless there is an associated VSD.

EVALUATION AND TREATMENT Diagnosis is suspected by physical examination and confirmed with echocardiography. Administration of intravenous prostaglandin E₁ to maintain the patency of the ductus arteriosus may be initiated to temporarily increase oxygen delivery. Enlargement of the PFO by balloon atrial septostomy may be performed during cardiac catheterization or under echocardiographic guidance to increase mixing and maintain cardiac output.[4,9]

The most preferred type of surgical repair for TGA performed in the first weeks of life is the *arterial switch procedure.* It involves

transecting the great arteries and anastomosing the main pulmonary artery to the native proximal aorta (just above the aortic valve) and anastomosing the ascending aorta to the native proximal pulmonary artery. The coronary arteries are moved with a "button" of tissue from the proximal aorta to the proximal pulmonary artery, creating a new aorta. Reimplantation of the coronary arteries is critical to the infant's survival, and the arteries must be reattached without torsion or kinking to provide the heart with its supply of oxygen. The advantage of the arterial switch procedure is the reestablishment of normal circulation with the left ventricle acting as the systemic pump. Potential complications of the arterial switch include narrowing at the great artery anastomoses, neoaortic valve regurgitation, or coronary artery insufficiency.[?] Long-term results for the arterial switch operation are usually good.

Total Anomalous Pulmonary Venous Connection

PATHOPHYSIOLOGY Total anomalous pulmonary venous connection (TAPVC) is a rare defect characterized by failure of the pulmonary veins to join the left atrium during cardiac development. TAPVC is also called *total anomalous pulmonary venous return (TAPVR)* or *total anomalous pulmonary venous drainage (TAPVD)* (Figure 25-12). The pulmonary venous return is connected to the right side of the circulation rather than to the left atrium. The type of TAPVC is classified according to the pulmonary venous point of attachment:

- *Supracardiac:* Attachment above the diaphragm, usually to the superior vena cava (most common form)
- *Cardiac:* Direct attachment to the heart, usually to the right atrium or coronary sinus
- *Infracardiac:* Attachment below the diaphragm, such as to the inferior vena cava (most severe and least common form)

The right atrium receives all the blood that normally would flow into the left atrium. As a result, the right side of the heart is enlarged and the left side, especially the left atrium, is smaller than normal. An associated ASD or PFO allows systemic venous blood to shunt from the right atrium to the left side of the heart. As a result, the oxygen saturation of the blood in both sides of the heart (and, ultimately, in the systemic arterial circulation) is the same. If the pulmonary blood

FIGURE 25-12 Total Anomalous Pulmonary Venous Connection (TAPVC).

FIGURE 25-13 Truncus Arteriosus (TA). The truncus arteriosus fails to divide into the pulmonary artery and aorta, and the interventricular septum fails to close at the top. Blood from both ventricles mixes in the truncus arteriosus and then enters the pulmonary and systemic circuits. (From Hockenberry MJ, Wilson D: *Wong's essentials of pediatric nursing,* ed 9, St Louis, 2013, Mosby.)

flow is increased, pulmonary venous return is also large, and the amount of saturated blood is relatively high. However, if there is obstruction to pulmonary venous drainage, the infant has severe cyanosis and low cardiac output. Infracardiac TAPVC often is associated with obstruction of pulmonary venous drainage and is a surgical emergency with higher mortality than the unobstructed types.

CLINICAL MANIFESTATIONS Most infants develop cyanosis early in life. The degree of cyanosis is inversely related to the amount of pulmonary blood flow. Children with unobstructed TAPVC may be asymptomatic until PVR decreases during infancy, increasing pulmonary blood flow, with resulting signs of pulmonary overcirculation. Cyanosis becomes worse with pulmonary vein obstruction; once obstruction occurs, the infant's condition usually deteriorates rapidly. Without intervention, cardiac failure will progress to death. Murmur is not a common feature of TAPVC.

EVALUATION AND TREATMENT Diagnosis is suspected with echocardiography but may require confirmative angiography. Corrective repair is usually required in early infancy. The surgical approach varies with the anatomic defect. In general, however, the common pulmonary vein (venous confluence) is sutured to the left atrium, the ASD is closed, and the anomalous pulmonary venous connection or vertical vein may be ligated.

Truncus Arteriosus

PATHOPHYSIOLOGY Truncus arteriosus (TA) is failure of normal septation and division of the embryonic outflow tract into a pulmonary artery and an aorta, resulting in a single vessel that exits the heart. There is always an associated VSD with mixing of the systemic and arterial circulations (Figure 25-13) causing some degree of cyanosis. Blood ejected from the heart flows preferentially to the lower pressure pulmonary arteries, causing increased pulmonary blood flow. The three types are as follows:

- *Type I:* A single pulmonary trunk arises near the base of the truncus and divides into the left and right pulmonary arteries.

- *Type II:* The left and right pulmonary arteries arise separately from the posterior aspect of the truncus.
- *Type III:* The pulmonary arteries arise independently and from the lateral aspect of the truncus.

CLINICAL MANIFESTATIONS Most infants are symptomatic with moderate heart failure and variable cyanosis, poor growth, and activity intolerance. Children are at risk for brain abscess and bacterial endocarditis.

EVALUATION AND TREATMENT Diagnosis is made by echocardiography. Corrective repair is a modification of the Rastelli procedure and is performed in the first few weeks or months of life. It involves closing the VSD so that the truncus arteriosus receives the outflow from the left ventricle, and excising the pulmonary arteries from the aorta and attaching them to the right ventricle by means of a homograft (cadaver) conduit. These children require additional procedures to replace the conduit since its size becomes inadequate in relation to growth or narrows because of calcification over time.

Hypoplastic Left Heart Syndrome

PATHOPHYSIOLOGY Hypoplastic left heart syndrome (HLHS) is underdevelopment of the left side of the heart. Features include small left atrium, small or absent mitral valve, small or absent left ventricle, and small or absent aortic valve. Coarctation also is expected (Figure 25-14). Most blood from the left atrium flows across the PFO to the right atrium, to the right ventricle, and out the pulmonary artery. The descending aorta receives blood from the PDA supplying systemic blood flow and filling the aorta and coronary arteries as well.

CLINICAL MANIFESTATIONS HLHS presents in the early newborn period as mild cyanosis, tachypnea, and low cardiac output if not already detected by fetal echocardiogram. Support of the systemic circulation is accomplished with prostaglandin E_1 infusion. If HLHS is not suspected and the PDA closes, there is progressive deterioration

FIGURE 25-14 Hypoplastic Left Heart Syndrome (HLHS). (From Hockenberry MJ et al: *Wong's essentials of pediatric nursing,* ed 8, St Louis, 2009, Mosby.)

with cyanosis and decreased cardiac output, leading to cardiovascular collapse. If untreated, HLHS is usually fatal in the first months of life.

EVALUATION AND TREATMENT Echocardiography shows all of the features of HLHS. Cardiac catheterization is rarely required. A multistage repair approach is used. The first stage is the *Norwood procedure,* which is anastomosis of the main pulmonary artery to the aorta to create a new aorta, construction of either a modified Blalock-Taussig (systemic to pulmonary artery) or Sano (**right** ventricle to pulmonary artery) shunt to provide pulmonary blood flow, creation of a large ASD, and repair of the coarctation. The second stage is a *bidirectional Glenn shunt* performed at 3 to 6 months of age by connecting the superior vena cava to the pulmonary artery, which minimizes cyanosis and reduces the volume load on the right ventricle. The final stage is a modified Fontan procedure that relieves cyanosis by connecting the inferior vena cava blood to the pulmonary artery using an intra- or extracardiac tube graft or baffle. Few centers perform heart transplantation in the newborn period rather than the staged procedure (Norwood, Glenn, Fontan) because of the scarcity of newborn donor hearts. Disadvantages of neonatal transplantation include shortage of newborn organ donors, risk of rejection, long-term problems with chronic immunosuppression, and infection. For infants who are not candidates for staged procedures or transplantation, the family is then offered palliative care.

Infants successfully treated for HLHS have improved survival rates related to advances in surgical and medical technology. Long-term (10 to 15 years) health problems after the Fontan procedure related to reduced right ventricular function and high central venous pressures have been reported to impact quality of life.[10,11]

TABLE 25-3 Causes of Heart Failure Resulting from Congenital Heart Disease

Age of Onset	Cause
At birth	HLHS
	Volume overload lesions
	Severe tricuspid or pulmonary insufficiency
	Large systemic AV fistula
First week	TGA
	PDA in small premature infants
	HLHS (with more favorable anatomy)
	TAPVR, particularly those with pulmonary venous obstruction
	Others
	Systemic AV fistula
	Critical AS or PS
1-4 weeks	COA with associated anomalies
	Critical AS
	Large left-to-right shunt lesions (VSD, PDA) in premature infants
	All other lesions previously listed
4-6 weeks	Some left-to-right shunt lesions, such as AVSD
6 weeks to 4 months	Large VSD
	Large PDA
	Others, such as anomalous left coronary artery from PA

Modified from Park MK: *Pediatric cardiology for practitioners,* ed 6, St Louis, 2014, Mosby.
AS, Aortic stenosis; *AV,* atrioventricular; *AVSD,* atrioventricular septal defect; *COA,* coarctation of the aorta; *HLHS,* hypoplastic left heart syndrome; *PA,* pulmonary artery; *PDA,* patent ductus arteriosus; *PS,* pulmonary stenosis; *TAPVR,* total anomalous pulmonary venous return; *TGA,* transposition of the great vessels; *VSD,* ventricular septal defect.

Heart Failure

Heart failure (HF) is a common complication of many congenital heart defects. HF occurs when the heart is unable to maintain sufficient cardiac output to meet the metabolic demands of the body. The most common congenital causes of HF in infancy and childhood are listed in Table 25-3. Classic HF in children also can be acquired, usually resulting from cardiomyopathies, dysrhythmias, or electrolyte disturbances. Pulmonary overcirculation from a large left-to-right shunt is often called congestive heart failure but is not usually associated with decreased ventricular function and failure to meet metabolic demands. However, the clinical manifestations are similar, such as failure to thrive, tachypnea, tachycardia, and exercise intolerance.[2]

In general, the pathophysiologic mechanisms of HF in infants and children are similar to those in adults. It is most often a result of decreased left ventricular systolic function and the associated left atrial and pulmonary venous hypertension and pulmonary venous congestion. The same compensatory mechanisms are activated in the face of inadequate cardiac output. Right ventricular failure is rare in childhood.

Left heart failure in infants is manifested as poor feeding and sucking, often leading to failure to thrive. In left heart failure, dyspnea, tachypnea, and diaphoresis may be accompanied by retractions, grunting, and nasal flaring. Wheezing, coughing, and rales are rare in childhood HF.[1,2,12] Common skin changes, such as pallor or mottling, are

BOX 25-1 Clinical Manifestations of Heart Failure

Impaired Myocardial Function
Tachycardia
Sweating (inappropriate)
Decreased urinary output
Fatigue
Weakness
Restlessness
Anorexia
Pale, cool extremities
Weak peripheral pulses
Decreased blood pressure
Gallop rhythm
Cardiomegaly

Pulmonary Congestion
Tachypnea
Dyspnea

Retractions (infants)
Flaring nares
Exercise intolerance
Orthopnea
Cough, hoarseness
Cyanosis
Wheezing
Grunting

Systemic Venous Congestion
Weight gain
Hepatomegaly
Peripheral edema, especially periorbital
Ascites
Neck vein distention

From Hockenberry MJ et al: *Wong's essentials of pediatric nursing*, ed 9, St Louis, 2013, Mosby.

often present (Box 25-1). Signs of systemic venous congestion, such as hepatomegaly, weight gain, ascites, and peripheral edema, can be present but could be suggestive of other medical conditions such as renal or nutritional deficiencies.

A thorough physical examination with emphasis on cardiac and pulmonary findings will often reveal the degree of HF. Plotting a child's growth (height, weight, head circumference) is an important method of assessing a child's health. Infants with HF or pulmonary overcirculation usually have low weight with normal length and head circumference measurements. The failure to thrive is usually the result of increased metabolic expenditure relative to caloric intake. An electrocardiogram (ECG) also should be performed to determine the presence of dysrhythmia or hypertrophy. A chest x-ray is useful in assessing the presence of cardiomegaly and signs of increased pulmonary circulation or pulmonary edema with echocardiogram to assess impaired function and possible etiology. B-type natriuretic peptide (BNP) has emerged as another diagnostic test of HF in children to confirm or exclude a cardiac cause for the symptoms.[2,13]

Treatment is aimed at decreasing cardiac workload and increasing the efficiency of heart function. Severe CHD is typically managed with surgical repair if applicable. Medical management initially consists of diuretics, such as furosemide. Depending on the degree of HF, other diuretics can be used in combination with furosemide to counteract potassium losses. Agents that reduce afterload, such as captopril or enalapril and beta-blockers, are employed to further manage severe HF.[1,2,12] Children with end-stage HF on maximal medical therapy can be supported on a ventricular assist device (VAD) while awaiting cardiac transplantation in severe cases that meet eligibility.[12]

ACQUIRED CARDIOVASCULAR DISORDERS

Acquired heart diseases refer to disease processes or abnormalities that occur after birth. They result from various causes, such as infection, genetic disorders, autoimmune processes in response to infection, environmental factors, or autoimmune diseases. Examples of acquired heart diseases include Kawasaki disease, myocarditis, rheumatic heart disease, cardiomyopathy, and systemic hypertension. This chapter discusses Kawasaki disease and systemic hypertension. Myocarditis, rheumatic heart disease, and cardiomyopathy are discussed in Chapter 24.

Kawasaki Disease

Kawasaki disease (KD), formerly known as mucocutaneous lymph node syndrome, is an acute, usually self-limiting systemic vasculitis that may result in cardiac sequelae without treatment. Although KD occurs throughout the world, the greatest number of cases are seen in Japan.[1,2] This reflects the genetic component of KD, with the case rate being highest among Asians and less among white and black children.

Kawasaki disease is primarily a condition of young children. Eighty percent of cases are seen in children younger than 5 years of age, with the incidence peaking in the toddler age group. Males are affected slightly more than females. The peak incidence is in the winter and spring.[1,2]

The etiology of KD remains unknown. Current etiologic theories center on an immunologic response to an infectious, toxic, or antigenic substance.[2,13]

PATHOPHYSIOLOGY Kawasaki disease progresses pathologically and clinically in the following stages. In the early or acute phase, small capillaries, arterioles, and venules become inflamed, as does the heart itself. In the subacute state, inflammation spreads to larger vessels and aneurysms of the coronary arteries may develop. In the convalescent stage, medium-sized arteries begin the granulation process and may cause coronary artery thickening with increased risk for thrombosis. After the convalescent stage, inflammation wanes with potential scarring of the affected vessels, calcification, and stenosis.

CLINICAL MANIFESTATIONS The clinical course of KD progresses in three stages: acute, subacute, and convalescent. In the acute phase, the child with classic or typical KD has fever, conjunctivitis, oral changes ("strawberry" tongue), rash, erythema of the palms and soles, and lymphadenopathy, and is often irritable. During this phase, myocarditis may develop. The subacute phase begins when the fever ends and continues until the clinical signs have resolved. It is at this time that the child is most at risk for coronary artery aneurysm development. Desquamation of the palms and soles occurs at this time, as well as marked thrombocytosis. The convalescent phase is marked by the elevation of the erythrocyte sedimentation rate and C-reactive protein level, as well as by an increased platelet count. Arthritis or arthralgia of the joints may be present. This phase continues until all laboratory values return to normal—usually about 6 to 8 weeks after onset.[1,2] Atypical or "incomplete" KD can be seen in infants and children who lack the diagnostic criteria (have fewer than four signs) or "classic" physical findings. Recognition can be difficult and often results in delay of treatment with possible cardiovascular sequelae.[2,13]

EVALUATION AND TREATMENT The diagnostic criteria for KD is based on clinical features, which state that the child must exhibit fever for more than 5 days along with four of five criteria (Box 25-2). These children usually have leukocytosis, increased erythrocyte sedimentation rates, thrombocytosis, and elevated liver enzymes. An echocardiogram is obtained at the time of diagnosis as a baseline measurement to assess for coronary aneurysms or inflammation. Serial echocardiograms are obtained after treatment to assess for development of coronary aneurysms or regression of those present early in the course of

BOX 25-2 Diagnostic Criteria for Kawasaki Disease

The child must exhibit five of the following six criteria, including fever:
1. Fever for 5 or more days (often diagnosed with shorter duration of fever if other symptoms are present)
2. Bilateral conjunctival infection without exudation
3. Changes in the oral mucous membranes, such as erythema, dryness, and fissuring of the lips; oropharyngeal reddening; or "strawberry tongue"
4. Changes in the extremities, such as peripheral edema, peripheral erythema, and desquamation of palms and soles, particularly periungual peeling
5. Polymorphous rash, often accentuated in the perineal area
6. Cervical lymphadenopathy (one lymph node >1.5 cm)

Modified from Hockenberry MJ et al: *Wong's essentials of pediatric nursing*, ed 9, St Louis, 2013, Mosby.

TABLE 25-4 Normative Blood Pressure Levels (Systolic/Diastolic [Mean]) by DINAMAP Monitor in Children 5 Years Old and Younger

Age	Mean BP Levels (mm Hg)	90th Percentile	95th Percentile
1-3 days	64/41 (50)	75/49 (50)	78/52 (62)
1 month to 2 years	95/58 (72)	106/68 (83)	110/71 (86)
2-5 years	101/57 (74)	112/66 (82)	115/68 (85)

Data from Park MK: *Pediatric cardiology for practitioners*, ed 6, St Louis, 2014, Mosby; modified from Park MK, Menard SM: *Am J Dis Children* 143:860, 1989.
BP, Blood pressure.

TABLE 25-5 Auscultatory Blood Pressure Values for Boys and Girls Aged 6 to 17 Years (Systolic/Diastolic K5)

Age & Gender	Mean BP Levels	90th Percentile	95th Percentile
6-7 yrs			
Boys	95-96 / 53-55	105-107 / 64-66	108-110 / 67-70
Girls	94-94 / 52-54	103-104 / 63-65	106-107 / 66-68
8-9 yrs			
Boys	97-99 / 56-57	108-109 / 68-68	111-113 / 71-71
Girls	96-98 / 56-56	106-108 / 67-67	109-111 / 70-70
10-11 yrs			
Boys	100-102 / 57-57	111-113 / 68-68	114-116 / 71-71
Girls	100-102 / 57-57	110-112 / 68-68	113-115 / 71-71
12-13 yrs			
Boys	105-108 / 56-56	116-118 / 68-68	119-122 / 71-71
Girls	104-105 / 57-57	113-115 / 68-68	116-118 / 71-71
14-15 yrs			
Boys	110-113 / 57-57	121-124 / 68-69	122-127 / 71-72
Girls	106-107 / 58-58	116-117 / 68-69	119-119 / 72-72
16-17 yrs			
Boys	114-114 / 59-62	125-125 / 71-73	128-128 / 74-77
Girls	107-108 / 59-59	117-118 / 69-70	120-121 / 73-73

From Park MK: *Pediatric cardiology for practitioners*, ed 6, St Louis, 2014, Mosby.
BP, Blood pressure; K5, Korotkoff phase 5.

the disease. Treatment includes oral administration of aspirin and intravenous infusion of gamma globulin (most often only one dose). Aspirin is continued until the manifestations of inflammation are resolved but may be used indefinitely in children with residual coronary artery abnormalities.

Treatment with aspirin and intravenous immunoglobulin during the acute phase has decreased the morbidity of KD and has reduced the incidence of coronary abnormalities from approximately 20% to less than 10% at 6 to 8 weeks after initiation of therapy. Most children recover completely from KD, including regression of aneurysms. The most common cardiovascular sequela is coronary thrombosis.[13]

Systemic Hypertension

Systemic hypertension in children is defined as systolic and diastolic blood pressure levels greater than the 95th percentile for age and gender on at least three occasions (Tables 25-4 and 25-5). The Fourth Task Force on Blood Pressure Control in Children uses height as an additional criterion to the blood pressure guidelines.[1,14]

Hypertension is classified into two categories: primary, or essential, hypertension, in which a specific cause cannot be identified; and secondary hypertension, in which a cause *can* be identified (Box 25-3). Hypertension (HTN) in children differs from adult hypertension in etiology and presentation. Young children, when diagnosed with HTN, are often found to have secondary hypertension caused by some underlying disease, such as renal disease or COA (see Box 25-3). An increased prevalence of primary HTN in older children has been noted. Researchers are now focusing on primary HTN in older children in relation to morbidity and the presence of early atherosclerotic disease. Certain factors influence blood pressure in children. Children who are overweight are often hypertensive (see *Health Alert:* U.S. Childhood Obesity and Its Association with Cardiovascular Disease). Smoking also is associated with an increased risk for HTN.[15-17]

PATHOPHYSIOLOGY In infants and children, a cause of HTN is almost always found. In general, the younger the child with significant hypertension, the more likely a correctable cause can be determined. Therefore a thorough evaluation needs to be performed.[2,15]

The pathophysiology of primary HTN in children is not clearly understood but may result from a complex interaction of a strong predisposing genetic component with disturbances in sympathetic vascular smooth muscle tone, humoral agents (angiotensin, catecholamines), renal sodium excretion, and cardiac output. New studies have shown an increased level of leptin, a hormone produced by adipose tissue, to be associated with hypertension in obese children.[17] Ultimately, these factors impair the ability of the peripheral vascular bed to relax.

CLINICAL MANIFESTATIONS Most children with systemic HTN are asymptomatic. It is necessary that a thorough history and physical examination be obtained. The examination should include an accurate blood pressure measurement obtained in the right arm with the arm supported at the level of the heart; three separate measurements using

---

BOX 25-3 **Conditions Associated with Secondary Hypertension in Children**

Renal

Renal parenchymal disease

Glomerulonephritis, acute and chronic

Pyelonephritis, acute and chronic

Congenital anomalies (polycystic or dysplastic kidneys)

Obstructive uropathies (hydronephrosis)

Hemolytic-uremic syndrome

Collagen disease (periarteritis, lupus)

Renal damage from nephrotoxic medications, trauma, or radiation

Renovascular disease

Renal artery disorders (e.g., stenosis, polyarteritis, thrombosis)

Renal vein thrombosis

Cardiovascular

Coarctation of the aorta

Conditions with large stroke volume (patent ductus arteriosus, aortic insufficiency, systemic arteriovenous fistula, complete heart block) (these conditions cause only systolic hypertension)

Endocrine

Hyperthyroidism (systolic hypertension)

Excessive catecholamine levels

Pheochromocytoma

Neuroblastoma

Adrenal dysfunction

Congenital adrenal hyperplasia

11-β-Hydroxylase deficiency

17-Hydroxylase deficiency

Cushing's syndrome

Hyperaldosteronism

Primary

Conn's syndrome

Idiopathic nodular hyperplasia

Dexamethasone-suppressible hyperaldosteronism

Secondary

Renovascular hypertension

Renin-producing tumor (juxtaglomerular cell tumor)

Hyperparathyroidism (and hypercalcemia)

Neurogenic

Increased intracranial pressure (any cause, especially tumors, infections, trauma)

Poliomyelitis

Guillain-Barré syndrome

Dysautonomia (Riley-Day syndrome)

Drugs and chemicals

Sympathomimetic drugs (nose drops, cough medications, cold preparations, theophylline)

Amphetamines

Corticosteroids

Nonsteroidal anti-inflammatory drugs

Oral contraceptives

Heavy-metal poisoning (mercury, lead)

Cocaine, acute or chronic use

Cyclosporine

Thyroxine

Tacrolimus

Miscellaneous

Hypervolemia and hypernatremia

Stevens-Johnson syndrome

Bronchopulmonary dysplasia (newborns)

From Park MK: *Pediatric cardiology for practitioners,* ed 6, St Louis, 2014, Mosby.

HEALTH ALERT

U.S. Childhood Obesity and Its Association with Cardiovascular Disease

Childhood obesity prevalence remains high in the United States. Approximately 17% (or 12.7 million) of children and adolescents ages 2 to 19 years are obese. This number has not changed significantly since 2003. However, the number of obese children between 2 and 5 years of age has decreased significantly from 13.9% between 2003 and 2004 to 8.4% between 2011 and 2012. Obesity continues to be a major health concern in children and is linked to insulin resistance and diabetes and increased cardiovascular risk, especially atherosclerosis, hypertension, and lipid abnormalities. The mechanisms by which insulin resistance and diabetes cause cardiovascular diseases include endothelial dysfunction, structural changes in arterial walls, abnormal vasoconstriction, and changes in renal function and salt transport. Research into genetics and insulin-regulated transcription factors suggests that obesity, insulin resistance, diabetes, and cardiovascular disease share important molecular etiologies and processes. These findings may lead investigators to important new treatments. For now, helping children develop good exercise and dietary habits has been shown to significantly improve arterial function and reduce cardiovascular risk.

Content and updated references and statistics can be found at www.cdc.gov/obesity/childhood/index.html.

---

an appropriate-size cuff also are needed for an accurate blood pressure reading.[15-17]

EVALUATION AND TREATMENT In children, the history and physical examination should be directed at determining the etiology of HTN, such as COA or renal disease (Table 25-6). A complete blood count, serum chemistry levels (including blood urea nitrogen and creatinine), uric acid level, urinalysis, urine culture, lipid profile, and renal ultrasound are part of the routine evaluation for renal disease (Table 25-7). Blood pressure differential between upper and lower extremities and

TABLE 25-6   Most Common Causes of Chronic Sustained Hypertension

Age Group	Causes
Newborn	Renal artery thrombosis, renal artery stenosis, congenital renal malformation, COA, bronchopulmonary dysplasia
<6 yr	Renal parenchymal disease, COA, renal artery stenosis
6-10 yr	Renal artery stenosis, renal parenchymal disease, primary hypertension
>10 yr	Primary hypertension, renal parenchymal disease

From Park MK: *Pediatric cardiology for practitioners*, ed 6, St Louis, 2014, Mosby.
COA, Coarctation of the aorta.

TABLE 25-7   Routine and Special Laboratory Tests for Hypertension

Laboratory Tests	Significance of Abnormal Results
Urinalysis, urine culture, blood urea nitrogen, and creatinine levels	Renal parenchymal disease
Serum electrolyte levels (hypokalemia)	Hyperaldosteronism, primary or secondary Adrenogenital syndrome Renin-producing tumors
ECG, chest x-ray studies	Cardiac cause of hypertension, also baseline function
Intravenous pyelography (or ultrasonography, radionuclide studies, computed tomography of kidneys)	Renal parenchymal diseases Renovascular hypertension Tumors (neuroblastoma, Wilms tumor)
Plasma renin activity, peripheral	High-renin hypertension Renovascular hypertension Renin-producing tumors Some caused by Cushing syndrome Some caused by essential hypertension Low-renin hypertension Adrenogenital syndrome Primary hyperaldosteronism
24-hr urine collection for 17-ketosteroids and 17-hydroxycorticosteroids	Cushing syndrome Adrenogenital syndrome
24-hr urine collection for catecholamine levels and vanillylmandelic acid	Pheochromocytoma Neuroblastoma
Aldosterone	Hyperaldosteronism, primary or secondary Renovascular hypertension Renin-producing tumors
Renal vein plasma renin activity	Unilateral renal parenchymal disease Renovascular hypertension
Abdominal aortogram	Renovascular hypertension Abdominal COA Unilateral renal parenchymal diseases Pheochromocytoma
Intra-arterial digit subtraction angiography	Renovascular hypertension

COA, Coarctation of the aorta; ECG, electrocardiogram.
From Park MK: *Pediatric cardiology for practitioners*, ed 6, St Louis, 2014, Mosby.

echocardiogram can be used to identify COA. If COA is found, surgical correction or balloon angioplasty with or without a stent is initiated depending on age and severity of the coarctation. If HTN is determined to be essential, or primary, in nature, nonpharmacologic therapy is used initially. Moderate weight loss and exercise can decrease systolic and diastolic pressures in many children. Appropriate diet, regular physical activity, and avoidance of smoking have been shown to be effective in reducing blood pressure.[1] Ambulatory blood pressure monitoring (ABPM) has the potential to become an important tool in the evaluation and management of childhood hypertension.[18]

Medication therapy is controversial in children with primary hypertension; however, when nonpharmacologic therapy fails, the approach is similar to the treatment of hypertension in adults with the use of angiotensin-converting enzyme inhibitors or angiotensin receptor blocker medications.[2,16] The current emphasis on preventive cardiology, especially for children, is significant because many investigators believe signs of atherosclerosis are present during childhood.[1,15-17]

✔ QUICK CHECK 25-2

1. Why are the infant's height and weight important in the assessment of HF?
2. Why is it critical to recognize and treat children during the acute phase of KD?
3. Discuss the causes of obesity in children and the cardiovascular effects.

DID YOU UNDERSTAND?

Congenital Heart Disease

1. Most congenital heart defects have begun to develop by the eighth week of gestation, and some have associated causes, both environmental and genetic.
2. Environmental risk factors associated with the incidence of congenital heart defects typically are maternal conditions. Maternal conditions include viral infections, diabetes, drug intake, and advanced maternal age.
3. Genetic factors associated with congenital heart defects include, but are not limited to, Down syndrome, trisomy 13, trisomy 18, cri du chat syndrome, and Turner syndrome.
4. Classification of congenital heart defects is based on (1) whether they cause blood flow to the lungs to increase, decrease, or remain normal; (2) whether they cause cyanosis; and (3) whether they cause obstruction to flow.
5. Cyanosis, a bluish discoloration of the skin, indicates that the tissues are not receiving normal amounts of oxygenated blood. Cyanosis can be caused by defects that (1) restrict blood flow into the pulmonary circulation; (2) overload the pulmonary circulation, causing pulmonary overcirculation, pulmonary edema, and respiratory difficulty; or (3) cause large amounts of unoxygenated blood to shunt from the pulmonary to the systemic circulation.

6. Congenital defects that maintain or create direct communication between the pulmonary and systemic circulatory systems cause blood to shunt from one system to another, mixing oxygenated and unoxygenated blood and increasing blood volume and, occasionally, pressure on the receiving side of the shunt.

7. The direction of shunting through an abnormal communication depends on differences in pressure and resistance between the two systems. Flow is always from an area of high pressure to an area of low pressure.

8. Obstruction of ventricular outflow is commonly caused by PS (right ventricle) or AS (left ventricle).

9. In less severe obstruction, ventricular outflow remains normal because of compensatory ventricular hypertrophy stimulated by increased afterload and, in postductal COA, development of collateral circulation around the coarctation.

10. Acyanotic congenital defects that increase pulmonary blood flow consist of abnormal openings (ASD, VSD, PDA, or AVC) that permit blood to shunt from left (systemic circulation) to right (pulmonary circulation). Cyanosis does not occur because the left-to-right shunt does not interfere with the flow of oxygenated blood through the systemic circulation.

11. If the abnormal communication between the left and right circuits is large, volume and pressure overload in the pulmonary circulation can lead to left-sided HF.

12. Cyanotic congenital defects in which saturated and desaturated blood mix within the heart or great arteries include TA, TOF, TGA, TAPVC, and HLHS.

13. In cyanotic heart defects that decrease pulmonary blood flow (TOF), myocardial hypertrophy cannot compensate for restricted right ventricular outflow. Flow to the lungs decreases, and cyanosis is caused by an insufficient volume of oxygenated blood and right-to-left shunt.

14. Initial treatment for CHD, depending on the defect, is aimed at controlling the level of HF symptoms or cyanosis. Interventional procedures in the cardiac catheterization laboratory and surgical palliation or repair are performed to establish a source of pulmonary blood flow or restore normal circulation.

15. Heart failure is usually the result of congenital heart defects that increase blood volume in the pulmonary circulation. A clinical manifestation of HF unique to children is failure to thrive.

Acquired Cardiovascular Disorders in Children

1. Two examples of acquired heart disease in children are Kawasaki disease and systemic hypertension.

2. Kawasaki disease is an acute systemic vasculitis that also may result in the development of coronary artery aneurysms and thrombosis if untreated.

3. Systemic hypertension in children differs from HTN in adults in etiology and presentation. When significant hypertension is found in a young child, the examiner should evaluate for the presence of secondary hypertension, most commonly renal disease or COA.

KEY TERMS

Acyanotic heart defect, 655
Aortic stenosis (AS), 657
Atrial septal defect (ASD), 659
Atrioventricular canal (AVC) defect (atrioventricular septal defect [AVSD], endocardial cushion defect [ECD]), 660
Coarctation of the aorta (COA), 656
Congenital heart disease (CHD), 655
Cyanosis, 655
Cyanotic heart defect, 655

Eisenmenger syndrome, 660
Foramen ovale, 660
Heart failure (HF), 665
Hypoplastic left heart syndrome (HLHS), 664
Kawasaki disease (KD), 666
Left-to-right shunt, 655
Muscular VSD, 660
Ostium primum ASD, 659
Ostium secundum ASD, 659
Patent ductus arteriosus (PDA), 659
Patent foramen ovale (PFO), 660

Perimembranous VSD, 660
Pulmonary atresia, 659
Pulmonic stenosis (PS), 658
Right-to-left shunt, 655
Shunt, 655
Sinus venosus ASD, 659
Subvalvular AS, 657
Supravalvular AS, 657
Systemic hypertension, 667
Tetralogy of Fallot (TOF), 661
Total anomalous pulmonary venous connection (TAPVC), 663

Transposition of the great arteries (TGA; transposition of the great vessels [TGV]), 663
Tricuspid atresia, 662
Truncus arteriosus (TA), 664
Valvular AS, 657
Ventricular septal defect (VSD), 660

REFERENCES

1. Allen HD, editor: *Moss and Adams' heart disease in infants, children, and adolescents including the fetus and young adults*, ed 8, Philadelphia, 2012, Lippincott Williams & Wilkins.
2. Park MK: *Pediatric cardiology for practitioners*, ed 6, St Louis, 2014, Mosby. Available at: http://mdconsult/book.
3. Vergales JE et al: Coarctation of the aorta—the current state of surgical and transcatheter therapies, *Curr Cardiol Rev* 9(3):211-219, 2013.
4. Feltes TF et al: Indications for cardiac catheterization and intervention in pediatric heart disease: a scientific statement from the American Heart Association, *Circulation* 123(22):2607-2625, 2011.
5. Rowena N et al: Characterizing associations and dissociations between anxiety, social and cognitive phenotypes of Williams syndrome, *Res Dev Disabil* 35(10):2403-2415, 2014.
6. Wong D et al: *Whaley and Wong's nursing care of infants and children*, ed 9, St Louis, 2013, Mosby.

7. Geva T et al: Atrial septal defects, *Lancet* 383(9932):1921-1932, 2014.
8. Penny DJ, Vick GW: Ventricular septal defect, *Lancet* 377(9771):1103-1112, 2011.
9. Schranz D, Michel-Behnke I: Advances in interventional and hybrid therapy in neonatal congenital heart disease, *Semin Fetal Neonatal Medicine* 18(5):311-321, 2013.
10. Pike NA et al: Clinical profile of the adolescent/adult Fontan survivor, *Congenit Heart Dis* 6(1):9-17, 2011.
11. Pike NA et al: Quality of life, health status and depression in adolescents and adults after the Fontan procedure compared to healthy counterparts, *J Cardiovasc Nurs* 27(6):539-546, 2012.
12. Rossano JW, Shaddy RE: Heart failure in children: etiology and treatment, *J Pediatr* 165(2):228-233, 2014.
13. Eleftheriou D et al: Management of Kawasaki disease, *Arch Dis Child* 99:74-83, 2014.

14. National High Blood Pressure Education Program Working Group on High Blood Pressure in Children and Adolescents: The fourth report on the diagnosis, evaluation and treatment of high blood pressure in children and adolescents, *Pediatrics* 114(suppl 2, 4th rep):555-576, 2004.
15. Gauer R et al: Pediatric hypertension: often missed and mismanaged, *J Fam Pract* 63(3):129-136, 2014.
16. Riley M, Bluhm B: High blood pressure in children and adolescents, *Am Fam Physician* 85(7):693-700, 2012.
17. Flynn JT: The changing face of pediatric hypertension in the era of the childhood obesity epidemic, *Pediatr Nephrol* 28(7):1059-1066, 2012.
18. Flynn JT et al: Update: ambulatory blood pressure monitoring in children and adolescents: a scientific statement from the American Heart Association Atherosclerosis, Hypertension and Obesity in Youth Committee of the Council on Cardiovascular Disease in the Young, *Hypertension* 63(5):1116-1135, 2014.

26

Structure and Function of the Pulmonary System

Valentina L. Brashers

CHAPTER OUTLINE

The primary function of the pulmonary system is the exchange of gases between the environmental air and the blood. The three steps in this process are (1) ventilation, the movement of air into and out of the lungs; (2) diffusion, the movement of gases between air spaces in the lungs and the bloodstream; and (3) perfusion, the movement of blood into and out of the capillary beds of the lungs to body organs and tissues. The first two functions are carried out by the pulmonary system and the third by the cardiovascular system (see Chapter 23). Normally the pulmonary system functions efficiently under a variety of conditions and with little energy expenditure.

STRUCTURES OF THE PULMONARY SYSTEM

The pulmonary system includes two lungs, the upper and lower airways, the blood vessels that serve these structures (Figure 26-1), the diaphragm, and the chest wall or thoracic cage. The lungs are divided into lobes: three in the right lung (upper, middle, lower) and two in the left lung (upper, lower). Each lobe is further divided into segments and lobules. The mediastinum is the space between the lungs and contains the heart, great vessels, and esophagus. A set of conducting airways, or bronchi, delivers air to each section of the lung. The lung tissue that surrounds the airways supports them, preventing distortion or collapse of the airways as gas moves in and out during ventilation. The diaphragm is a dome-shaped muscle that separates the thoracic and abdominal cavities and is involved in ventilation.

The lungs are protected from exogenous contaminants by a series of mechanical barriers (Table 26-1). These defense mechanisms are so effective that, in the healthy individual, contamination of the lung tissue itself, particularly by infectious agents, is rare.

Conducting Airways

The conducting airways allow air into and out of the gas-exchange structures of the lung. The nasopharynx, oropharynx, and related structures are often called the *upper airway* (Figure 26-2). These structures are lined with a ciliated mucosa that warms and humidifies inspired air and removes foreign particles from it. The mouth and oropharynx are used for ventilation when the nose is obstructed or when increased flow is required (e.g., during exercise). Filtering and humidifying are not as efficient with mouth breathing.

The larynx connects the upper and lower airways and consists of the endolarynx and its surrounding triangular-shaped bony and cartilaginous structures. The endolarynx encompasses two pairs of folds: the false vocal cords (supraglottis) and the true vocal cords. The slit-shaped space between the true cords forms the glottis (see Figure 26-2). The vestibule is the space above the false vocal cords. The laryngeal box is formed of three large cartilages (epiglottis, thyroid, cricoid) and three smaller cartilages (arytenoid, corniculate, cuneiform) connected by ligaments. The supporting cartilages prevent collapse of the larynx during inspiration and swallowing. The internal laryngeal muscles control vocal cord length and tension, and the external laryngeal muscles move the larynx as a whole. Both sets of muscles are important to swallowing, ventilation, and vocalization.[1] The internal muscles contract during swallowing to prevent aspiration into the trachea. These muscles also contribute to voice pitch.

The trachea, which is supported by U-shaped cartilage, connects the larynx to the bronchi, the conducting airways of the lungs. The trachea branches into two main airways, or bronchi (sing., bronchus), at the carina (see Figure 26-1). The right and left main bronchi enter the lungs at the hila (sing., hilum), or "roots" of the lungs, along with the pulmonary blood and lymphatic vessels. From the hila the main bronchi branch farther, as shown in Figure 26-3.

The bronchial walls have three layers: an epithelial lining, a smooth muscle layer, and a connective tissue layer. The epithelial lining of the bronchi contains single-celled exocrine glands—the mucus-secreting goblet cells—and ciliated cells. The goblet cells produce a mucous blanket that protects the airway epithelium, and the ciliated epithelial

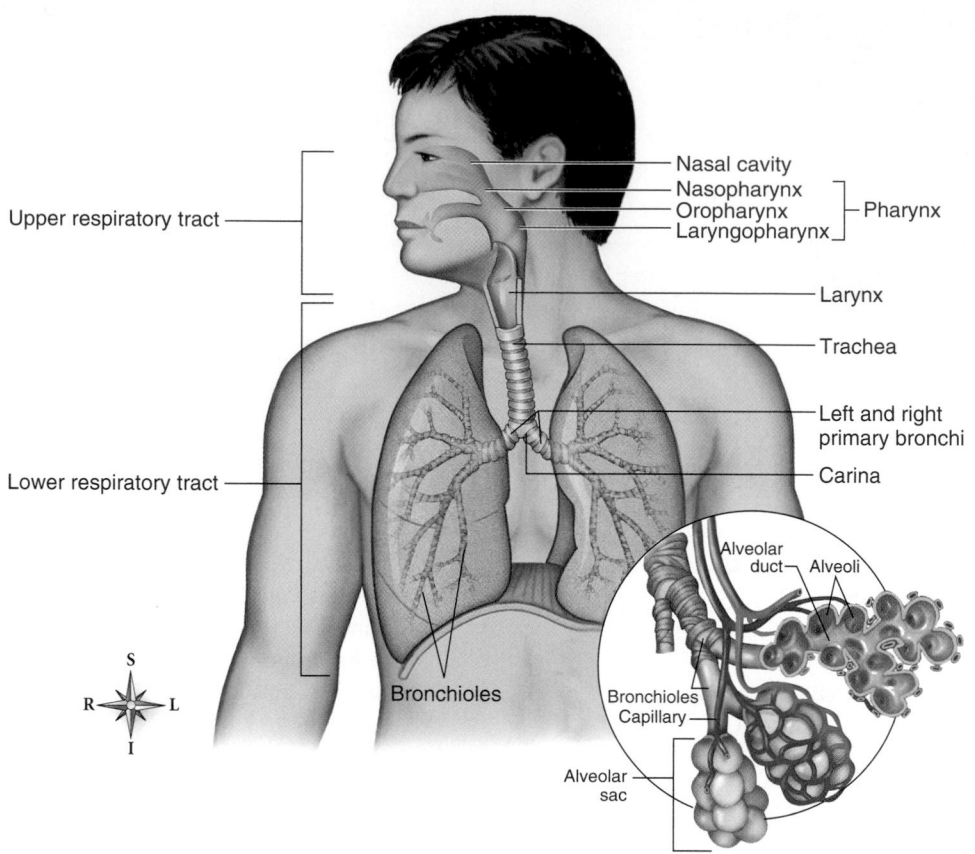

FIGURE 26-1 Structure of the Pulmonary System. The upper and lower respiratory tracts (airways) are illustrated. The enlargement in the circle depicts the acinus, where oxygen and carbon dioxide are exchanged. (From Patton KT, Thibodeau GA: *Structure & function of the body*, ed 15, St Louis, 2016, Mosby.)

TABLE 26-1	Pulmonary Defense Mechanisms
Structure or Substance	**Mechanism of Defense**
Upper respiratory tract mucosa	Maintains constant temperature and humidification of gas entering lungs; traps and removes foreign particles, some bacteria, and noxious gases from inspired air
Nasal hairs and turbinates	Trap and remove foreign particles, some bacteria, and noxious gases from inspired air
Mucous blanket	Protects trachea and bronchi from injury; traps most foreign particles and bacteria that reach lower airways
Cilia	Propel mucous blanket and entrapped particles toward oropharynx, where they can be swallowed or expectorated
Irritant receptors in nares (nostrils)	Stimulation by chemical or mechanical irritants triggers sneeze reflex, which results in rapid removal of irritants from nasal passages
Irritant receptors in trachea and large airways	Stimulation by chemical or mechanical irritants triggers cough reflex, which results in removal of irritants from lower airways
Alveolar macrophages	Ingest and remove bacteria and other foreign material from alveoli by phagocytosis (see Chapters 6 and 7)

cells rhythmically beat this mucous blanket toward the trachea and pharynx where it can be swallowed or expectorated by coughing. The layers of epithelium that line the bronchi become thinner with each successive branching (see Figure 26-3).

Gas-Exchange Airways

The conducting airways terminate in the respiratory bronchioles, alveolar ducts, and alveoli (sing., alveolus). These thin-walled structures together are sometimes called the acinus (see Figures 26-1 and 26-3), and all of them participate in gas exchange.[2]

The alveoli are the primary gas-exchange units of the lung, where oxygen enters the blood and carbon dioxide is removed (Figure 26-4). Tiny passages called *pores of Kohn* permit some air to pass through the septa from alveolus to alveolus, promoting collateral ventilation and even distribution of air among the alveoli. The lungs contain approximately 25 million alveoli at birth and 300 million by adulthood.

Lung epithelial cells provide a protective interface with the environment and are essential for adequate gas exchange, preventing entry of foreign agents, regulating ion and water transport, and maintaining mechanical stability of the alveoli.[3] Two major types of epithelial cells appear in the alveolus. Type I alveolar cells provide structure, and type II alveolar cells secrete surfactant, a lipoprotein that coats the inner surface of the alveolus and lowers alveolar surface tension at end-expiration, thereby preventing lung collapse.[1,2,4,5]

Like the bronchi, alveoli contain cellular components of immunity and inflammation, particularly the mononuclear phagocytes (called

FIGURE 26-2 Structures of the Upper Airway. (Redrawn from Thompson JM et al: *Mosby's clinical nursing*, ed 5, St Louis, 2002, Mosby.)

alveolar macrophages). These cells ingest foreign material that reaches the alveolus and prepare it for removal through the lymphatics. (Phagocytosis and the mononuclear phagocyte system are described in Chapters 6 and 7.)

✔**QUICK CHECK 26-1**
1. List the major components of the pulmonary system.
2. What are conducting airways?
3. Describe an alveolus.
4. Which components of the pulmonary system contribute to the body's defense?

Pulmonary and Bronchial Circulation

The pulmonary circulation facilitates gas exchange, delivers nutrients to lung tissues, acts as a reservoir for the left ventricle, and serves as a filtering system that removes clots, air, and other debris from the circulation.

Although the entire cardiac output from the right ventricle goes into the lungs, the pulmonary circulation has a lower pressure and resistance than the systemic circulation. Pulmonary arteries are exposed to about one fifth the pressure of the systemic circulation. Usually about one third of the pulmonary vessels are filled with blood (perfused) at any given time. More vessels become perfused when right ventricular cardiac output increases. Therefore increased delivery of blood to the lungs does not normally increase mean pulmonary artery pressure.

The pulmonary artery divides and enters the lung at the hila, branching with each main bronchus and with all bronchi at every division. Thus, every bronchus and bronchiole has an accompanying artery or arteriole. The arterioles divide at the terminal bronchioles to form a network of pulmonary capillaries around the acinus. Capillary walls consist of an endothelial layer and a thin basement membrane, which often fuses with the basement membrane of the alveolar septum. Consequently, there is very little separation between blood in the capillary and gas in the alveolus.

The shared alveolar and capillary walls compose the **alveolocapillary membrane** (respiratory membrane) (Figure 26-5). Gas exchange occurs across this membrane. With normal perfusion, approximately 100 ml of blood in the pulmonary capillary bed is spread very thinly

FIGURE 26-3 Structures of the Lower Airway. A, Structures of lower respiratory airway. **B,** Changes in bronchial wall with progressive branching. **C,** Electron micrograph of alveoli: long white arrow identifies type II pneumocyte (secretes surfactant); white arrow identifies pores of Kohn; red arrow identifies alveolar capillary. **D,** Plastic cast of pulmonary capillaries at high magnification. (**A** redrawn from Thompson JM et al: *Mosby's clinical nursing,* ed 5, St Louis, 2002, Mosby; **B** from Wilson SF, Thompson JM: *Respiratory disorders,* St Louis, 1990, Mosby; **C** from Mason RJ et al: *Murray and Nadel's textbook of respiratory medicine,* ed 5, Philadelphia, 2010, Saunders; **D** courtesy A. Churg, MD, and J. Wright, MD, Vancouver, Canada. From Leslie KO, Wick MR: *Practical pulmonary pathology: a diagnostic approach,* ed 2, Philadelphia, 2011, Saunders.)

over 70 to 100 m^2 of alveolar surface area. Any disorder that thickens the membrane impairs gas exchange.

Each pulmonary vein drains several pulmonary capillaries. Unlike the pulmonary arteries, pulmonary veins are dispersed randomly throughout the lung and then leave the lung at the hila and enter the left atrium. They have no valves.

The bronchial circulation is part of the systemic circulation, and it both moistens inspired air and supplies nutrients to the conducting airways, large pulmonary vessels, and membranes (pleurae) that surround the lungs. Not all of its capillaries drain into its own venous system. Some empty into the pulmonary vein and contribute to the normal venous mixture of oxygenated and deoxygenated blood or right-to-left shunt (right-to-left shunts are described in Chapter 27). The bronchial circulation does not participate in gas exchange.[6]

Lung vasculature also includes deep and superficial pulmonary lymphatic capillaries. Fluid and alveolar macrophages migrate from the alveoli to the terminal bronchioles, where they enter the lymphatic system. Both deep and superficial lymphatic vessels leave the lung at the hilum through a series of mediastinal lymph nodes. The lymphatic system plays an important role in both providing immune defense and keeping the lung free of fluid. (The lymphatic system is described in Chapter 23.)

Control of the Pulmonary Circulation

The caliber of pulmonary artery lumina decreases as smooth muscle in the arterial walls contracts. Contraction increases pulmonary artery pressure. Caliber increases as these muscles relax, decreasing blood pressure. Contraction (vasoconstriction) and relaxation (vasodilation)

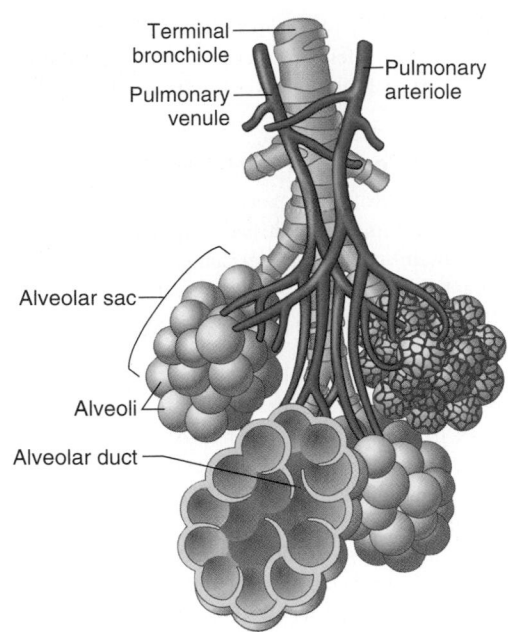

FIGURE 26-4 Alveoli. Bronchioles subdivide to form tiny tubes called *alveolar ducts,* which end in clusters of alveoli called *alveolar sacs.* (From Patton KT, Thibodeau GA: *The human body in health & disease,* ed 6, St Louis, 2014, Mosby.)

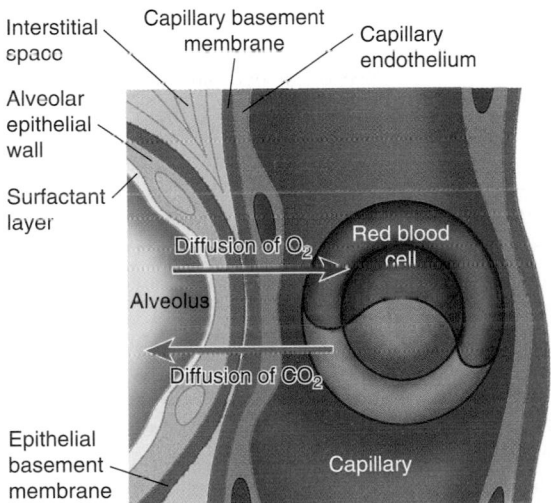

FIGURE 26-5 Cross-Section Through an Alveolus Showing Histology of the Alveolar-Capillary Membrane (Respiratory Membrane). The dense network of capillaries forms an almost continuous sheet of blood in the alveolar walls, providing a very efficient arrangement for gas exchange. (Adapted from Montague SE, Watson R, Herbert R: *Physiology for nursing practice,* ed 3, London, 2005, Elsevier.)

primarily occur in response to local humoral conditions, even though the pulmonary circulation is innervated by the autonomic nervous system (ANS), as is the systemic circulation.

The most important cause of pulmonary artery constriction is a low alveolar Po_2 (P_Ao_2). Vasoconstriction is caused by alveolar and pulmonary venous hypoxia, often termed **hypoxic pulmonary vasoconstriction,** and results from an increase in intracellular calcium levels in vascular smooth muscle cells in response to low oxygen concentration and the presence of charged oxygen molecules called oxygen

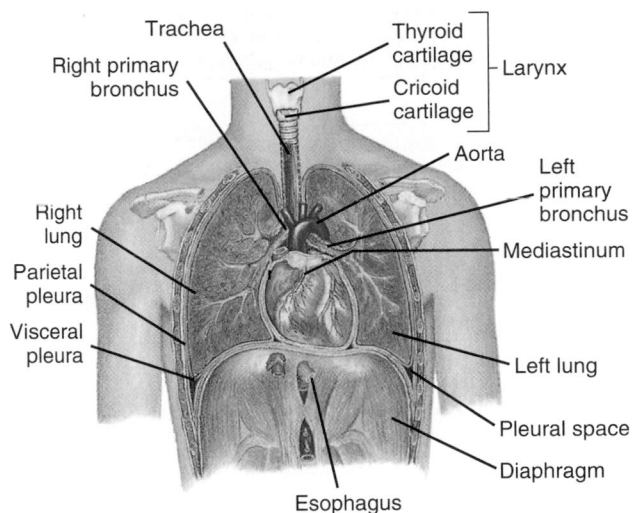

FIGURE 26-6 Thoracic (Chest) Cavity and Related Structures. The thoracic (chest) cavity is divided into three subdivisions (left and right pleural divisions and mediastinum) by a partition formed by a serous membrane called the *pleura.* (From Thibodeau GA, Patton KT: *Anatomy & physiology,* ed 3, St Louis, 1996, Mosby.)

radicals.[7] It can affect only one portion of the lung (i.e., one lobe that is obstructed, decreasing its P_Ao_2) or the entire lung. If only one segment of the lung is involved, the arterioles to that segment constrict, shunting blood to other, well ventilated portions of the lung. This reflex improves the lung's efficiency by better matching ventilation and perfusion. If all segments of the lung are affected, however, vasoconstriction occurs throughout the pulmonary vasculature and pulmonary hypertension (elevated pulmonary artery pressure) can result. The pulmonary vasoconstriction caused by low alveolar Po_2 is reversible if the alveolar Po_2 is corrected. Chronic alveolar hypoxia can result in structural changes in pulmonary arterioles causing permanent pulmonary artery hypertension, which eventually leads to right heart failure (cor pulmonale).[7]

Acidemia also causes pulmonary artery constriction. If the acidemia is corrected, the vasoconstriction is reversed. (Respiratory acidosis and metabolic acidosis are described in Chapter 5.) An elevated $Paco_2$ value without a drop in pH does not cause pulmonary artery constriction. Other biochemical factors that affect the caliber of vessels in pulmonary circulation are histamine, prostaglandins, serotonin, nitric oxide, and bradykinin (see *Geriatric Considerations:* Aging & the Pulmonary System, p. 684).

Chest Wall and Pleura

The chest wall (skin, ribs, intercostal muscles) protects the lungs from injury. The intercostal muscles of the chest wall, along with the diaphragm, accessory muscles, and abdominal muscles, perform the muscular work of breathing. The **thoracic cavity** is contained by the chest wall and encases the lungs (Figure 26-6). A serous membrane called the **pleura** adheres firmly to the lungs and then folds over itself and attaches firmly to the chest wall. The membrane covering the lungs is the *visceral pleura;* that lining the thoracic cavity is the *parietal pleura.* The area between the two pleurae is called the **pleural space,** or **pleural cavity.** Normally, only a thin layer of fluid secreted by the pleura (pleural fluid) fills the pleural space, lubricating the pleural surfaces and allowing the two layers to slide over each other without separating. Pressure in the pleural space is usually negative or subatmospheric (−4 to −10 mm Hg).

FIGURE 26-7 Functional Components of the Respiratory System. The central nervous system responds to neurochemical stimulation of ventilation and sends signals to the chest wall musculature. The response of the respiratory system to these impulses is influenced by several factors that impact the mechanisms of breathing and, therefore, affect the adequacy of ventilation. Gas transport between the alveoli and pulmonary capillary blood depends on a variety of physical and chemical activities. Finally, the control of the pulmonary circulation plays a role in the appropriate distribution of blood flow.

QUICK CHECK 26-2

1. What are the functions of the pulmonary circulation and of the bronchial circulation?
2. What is the most important factor causing pulmonary artery constriction? What other factors are involved?
3. What are the visceral and parietal pleurae?
4. What are the characteristics of the pleural space?

FUNCTION OF THE PULMONARY SYSTEM

The pulmonary system (1) ventilates the alveoli, (2) diffuses gases into and out of the blood, and (3) perfuses the lungs so that the organs and tissues of the body receive blood that is rich in oxygen and deficient in carbon dioxide. Each component of the pulmonary system contributes to one or more of these functions (Figure 26-7).

Ventilation

Ventilation is the mechanical movement of gas or air into and out of the lungs. It is often misnamed *respiration,* which is actually the exchange of oxygen and carbon dioxide during cellular metabolism. "Respiratory rate" is actually the ventilatory rate, or the number of times gas is inspired and expired per minute. The amount of effective ventilation is calculated by multiplying the ventilatory rate (breaths per minute) by the volume or amount of air per breath (liters per breath or tidal volume). This is called the minute volume (or minute ventilation) and is expressed in liters per minute.

Carbon dioxide (CO_2), the gaseous form of carbonic acid (H_2CO_3), is produced by cellular metabolism. The lung eliminates about 10,000 milliequivalents (mEq) of carbonic acid per day in the form of CO_2, which is produced at the rate of approximately 200 ml/min. Carbon dioxide is eliminated to maintain a normal arterial CO_2 pressure ($Paco_2$) of 40 mm Hg and normal acid-base balance (see Chapter 5 for a discussion of acid-base regulation). Adequate ventilation is necessary to maintain normal $Paco_2$ levels. Diseases that limit ventilation result in CO_2 retention. The adequacy of alveolar ventilation *cannot* be accurately determined by observation of ventilatory rate, pattern, or effort. If a healthcare professional needs to determine the adequacy of ventilation, an arterial blood gas analysis must be performed to measure $Paco_2$.

Neurochemical Control of Ventilation

Breathing is usually involuntary, because homeostatic changes in ventilatory rate and volume are adjusted automatically by the nervous system to maintain normal gas exchange. Voluntary breathing is necessary for talking, singing, laughing, and deliberately holding one's breath. The mechanisms that control respiration are complex (Figure 26-8).

The respiratory center in the brainstem controls respiration by transmitting impulses to the respiratory muscles, causing them to contract and relax. The respiratory center is composed of several groups of neurons: the dorsal respiratory group (DRG), the ventral respiratory group (VRG), the pneumotaxic center, and the apneustic center.[1,2,4]

The basic automatic rhythm of respiration is set by the DRG, which receives afferent input from peripheral chemoreceptors in the carotid and aortic bodies; from mechanical, neural, and chemical stimuli; and from receptors in the lungs.[8] The VRG contains both inspiratory and expiratory neurons and is almost inactive during normal, quiet respiration, becoming active when increased ventilatory effort is required. The pneumotaxic center and apneustic center, situated in the pons, do not generate primary rhythm but, rather, act as modifiers of the rhythm established by the medullary centers. The pattern of breathing can be influenced by emotion, pain, and disease.

Lung Receptors

Three types of lung receptors send impulses from the lungs to the DRG:

1. Irritant receptors (C fibers) are found in the epithelium of all conducting airways. They are sensitive to noxious aerosols (vapors), gases, and particulate matter (e.g., inhaled dusts), which cause them to initiate the cough reflex.[9] When stimulated, irritant receptors also cause bronchoconstriction and increased ventilatory rate.
2. Stretch receptors are located in the smooth muscles of airways and are sensitive to increases in the size or volume of the lungs. They decrease ventilatory rate and volume when stimulated, an occurrence sometimes referred to as the Hering-Breuer expiratory reflex. This reflex is active in newborns and assists with ventilation. In adults, this reflex is active only at high tidal volumes (such as with exercise) and may protect against excess lung inflation. Bronchopulmonary C fibers and a subset of stretch-sensitive, acid-sensitive myelinated sensory nerves mediate the cough reflex.[10]
3. J-receptors (juxtapulmonary capillary receptors) are located near the capillaries in the alveolar septa. They are sensitive to increased pulmonary capillary pressure, which stimulates them to initiate rapid, shallow breathing; hypotension; and bradycardia.[5]

The lung is innervated by the autonomic nervous system (ANS). Fibers of the sympathetic division in the lung branch from the upper thoracic and cervical ganglia of the spinal cord. Fibers of the parasympathetic division of the ANS travel in the vagus nerve to the lung. (Structures and function of the ANS are discussed in detail in Chapter 13.) The parasympathetic and sympathetic divisions control airway caliber (interior diameter of the airway lumen) by stimulating bronchial smooth muscle to contract or relax. The parasympathetic receptors cause smooth muscle to contract, whereas sympathetic receptors cause it to relax. Bronchial smooth muscle tone depends on equilibrium—that is, equal stimulation of contraction and relaxation. The parasympathetic division of the ANS is the main controller of airway caliber under normal conditions. Constriction occurs if

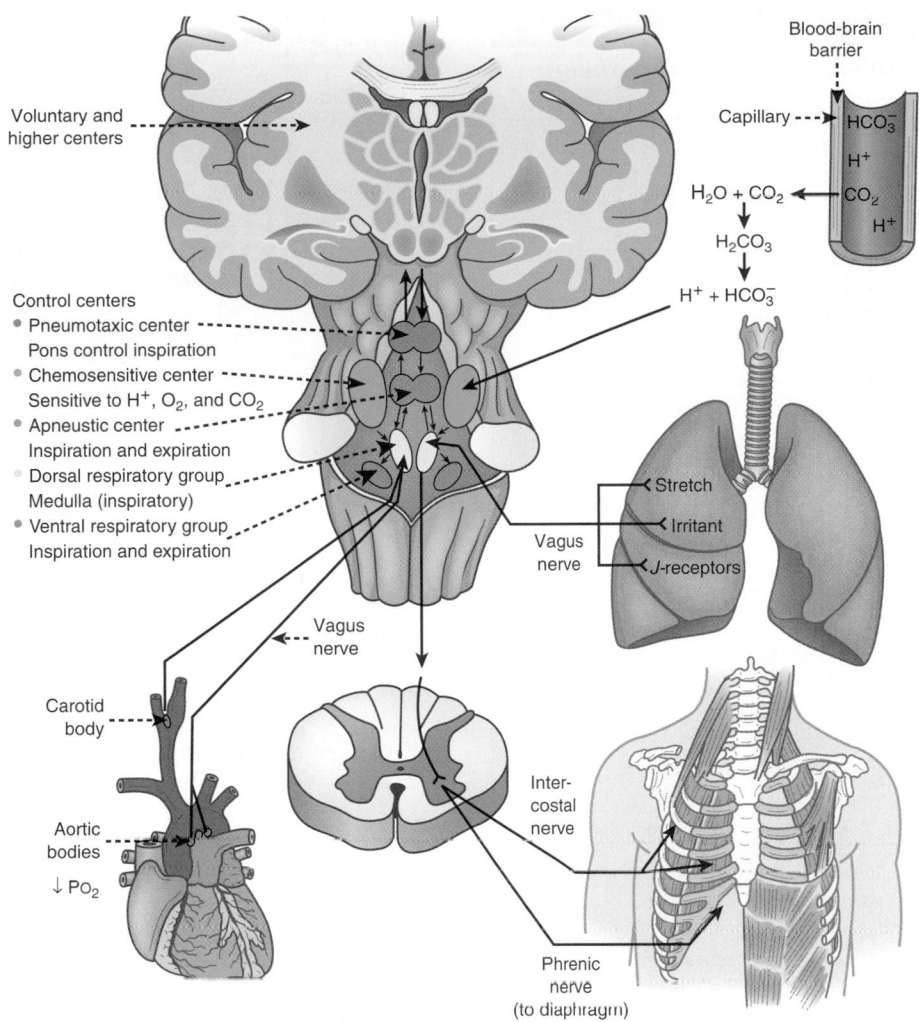

FIGURE 26-8 Neurochemical Respiratory Control System.

the irritant receptors in the airway epithelium are stimulated by irritants in inspired air, by inflammatory mediators (e.g., histamine, serotonin, prostaglandins, leukotrienes), by many drugs, and by humoral substances.

Chemoreceptors

Chemoreceptors monitor the pH, Paco$_2$, and Pao$_2$ (arterial pressure of oxygen) of arterial blood. **Central chemoreceptors** monitor arterial blood indirectly by sensing changes in the pH of cerebrospinal fluid (CSF) (see Figure 26-8).[11] They are located near the respiratory center and are sensitive to hydrogen ion concentration in the CSF. (Chapter 5 describes the relationship between ions and the pH, or acid-base status, of body fluids.) The pH of the CSF reflects arterial pH because carbon dioxide in arterial blood can diffuse across the blood-brain barrier (the capillary wall separating blood from cells of the central nervous system) into the CSF until the partial pressure of carbon dioxide (Pco$_2$) is equal on both sides. Carbon dioxide that has entered the CSF combines with H$_2$O to form carbonic acid, which subsequently dissociates into hydrogen ions that are capable of stimulating the central chemoreceptors. In this way, Paco$_2$ regulates ventilation through its impact on the pH (hydrogen ion content) of the CSF.[1,2,4,11]

If alveolar ventilation is inadequate, Paco$_2$ increases. Carbon dioxide diffuses across the blood-brain barrier until Pco$_2$ values in the blood and the CSF reach equilibrium. As the central chemoreceptors

sense the resulting decrease in pH (increase in hydrogen ion concentration), they stimulate the respiratory center to increase the depth and rate of ventilation. Increased ventilation causes the Pco$_2$ of arterial blood to decrease below that of the CSF, and carbon dioxide diffuses out of the CSF, returning its pH to normal.

The central chemoreceptors are sensitive to very small changes in the pH of CSF (equivalent to a 1 to 2 mm Hg change in Pco$_2$) and can maintain a normal Paco$_2$ under many different conditions, including strenuous exercise.[11] If inadequate ventilation, or hypoventilation, is long term (e.g., in chronic obstructive pulmonary disease), these receptors become insensitive to small changes in Paco$_2$ ("reset") and regulate ventilation poorly (see *Health Alert:* Changes in the Chemical Control of Breathing During Sleep).[12]

The **peripheral chemoreceptors** are somewhat sensitive to changes in Paco$_2$ and pH but are sensitive primarily to oxygen levels in arterial blood (Pao$_2$). As Pao$_2$ and pH decrease, peripheral chemoreceptors, particularly in the carotid bodies, send signals to the respiratory center to increase ventilation. However, the Pao$_2$ must drop well below normal (to approximately 60 mm Hg) before the peripheral chemoreceptors have much influence on ventilation. If Paco$_2$ is elevated as well, ventilation increases much more than it would in response to either abnormality alone. The peripheral chemoreceptors become the major stimulus to ventilation when the central chemoreceptors are reset by chronic hypoventilation.[13]

HEALTH ALERT

Changes in the Chemical Control of Breathing During Sleep

There are multiple sites of central carbon dioxide chemosensitivity in the brainstem, and there are specialized chemosensory sites that function only during certain sleep states. Chemical control of ventilation, related to both hypercapnia and hypoxia, appears to be blunted during sleep. The orexins are neurohormones that control feeding, vigilance, and sleep. It is postulated that changes in orexin activity contribute to the blunting of chemoreceptor sensitivity seen in many states, including obesity and sleep apnea. Congestive heart failure, chronic obstructive pulmonary disease, and hypertension also are associated with abnormal breathing responses during sleep. Changes in the chemical control of breathing during sleep may contribute to morbidity and mortality seen in individuals with these disorders.

Data from; Fung ML: *Respir Physiol Neurobiol* 209:6-12, 2015; Guyenet PG et al: *Brain Res* 1511:126-137, 2013; Mansukhani MP et al: *Exp Physiol* 100(2):130-135, 2015; Nattie E, Li A: *Prog Brain Res* 198:25-46, 2012; Urfy MZ, Suarez JI: *Handb Clin Neurol* 119:241-250, 2014; Wang W et al: *Peptides* 42:48-54, 2013.

✔ QUICK CHECK 26-3

1. What are the functions of the pulmonary system?
2. How do ventilation and respiration differ?
3. Describe three functions of the respiratory center in the brainstem.
4. What are the three types of lung receptors?
5. How do the functions of central and peripheral chemoreceptors differ?

Mechanics of Breathing

The mechanical aspects of inspiration and expiration are known collectively as the mechanics of breathing and involve (1) major and accessory muscles of inspiration and expiration, (2) elastic properties of the lungs and chest wall, and (3) resistance to airflow through the conducting airways. Alterations in any of these properties increase the work of breathing or the metabolic energy needed to achieve adequate ventilation and oxygenation of the blood.

Major and Accessory Muscles

The major muscles of inspiration are the diaphragm and the external intercostal muscles (muscles between the ribs) (Figure 26-9). The diaphragm is a dome-shaped muscle that separates the abdominal and thoracic cavities. When it contracts and flattens downward, it increases the volume of the thoracic cavity, creating a negative pressure that draws gas into the lungs through the upper airways and trachea. Contraction of the external intercostal muscles elevates the anterior portion of the ribs and increases the volume of the thoracic cavity by increasing its front-to-back (anterior-posterior [AP]) diameter. Although the external intercostals may contract during quiet breathing, inspiration at rest is usually assisted by the diaphragm only.

The accessory muscles of inspiration are the sternocleidomastoid and scalene muscles. Like the external intercostals, these muscles enlarge the thorax by increasing its AP diameter. The accessory muscles assist inspiration when the minute volume (volume of air inspired and expired per minute) is high, as during strenuous exercise, or when the work of breathing is increased because of disease. The accessory muscles do not increase the volume of the thorax as efficiently as the diaphragm does.

There are no major muscles of expiration because normal, relaxed expiration is passive and requires no muscular effort. The accessory muscles of expiration, the abdominal and internal intercostal muscles,

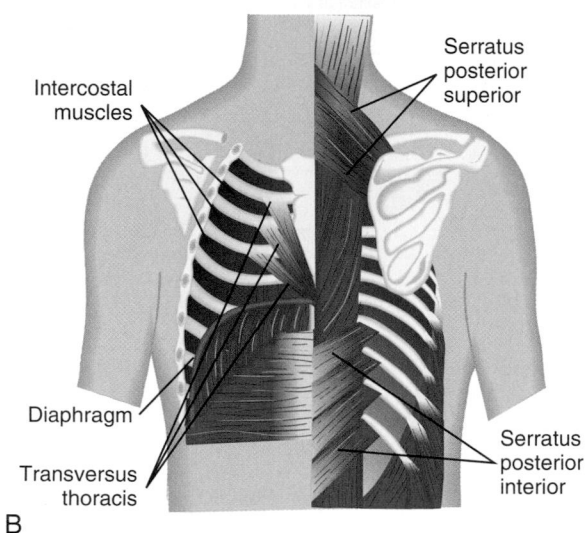

FIGURE 26-9 Muscles of Ventilation. **A,** Anterior view. **B,** Posterior view. (Modified from Thompson JM et al: *Mosby's clinical nursing,* ed 5, St Louis, 2002, Mosby.)

assist expiration when minute volume is high, during coughing, or when airway obstruction is present. When the abdominal muscles contract, intra-abdominal pressure increases, pushing up the diaphragm and decreasing the volume of the thorax. The internal intercostal muscles pull down the anterior ribs, decreasing the AP diameter of the thorax.

Alveolar Surface Tension

Surface tension occurs at any gas-liquid interface and refers to the tendency for liquid molecules that are exposed to air to adhere to one another. This phenomenon can be seen in the way liquids "bead" when splashed on a waterproof surface.

Within a sphere, such as an alveolus, surface tension tends to make expansion difficult. According to the law of Laplace, the pressure (P) required to inflate a sphere is equal to two times the surface tension $(2T)$ divided by the radius (r) of the sphere, or $P = 2T/r$. As the radius of the sphere (or alveolus) decreases, more and more pressure is required to inflate it. If the alveoli were lined only with a water-like fluid, taking breaths would be extremely difficult.

Alveolar ventilation, or distention, is made possible by surfactant, which lowers surface tension by coating the air-liquid interface in the alveoli. Surfactant, a lipoprotein (90% lipids and 10% protein) produced by type II alveolar cells, includes two groups of *surfactant* proteins. One group consists of small hydrophobic molecules that have a detergent-like effect that separates the liquid molecules, thereby decreasing alveolar surface tension.[2,14] The second group of surfactant proteins consists of large hydrophilic molecules called collectins that are capable of inhibiting foreign pathogens (see Chapter 6).[15]

As the radius of an alveolus shrinks, the surface tension of the surfactant-lined sphere decreases, and as the radius expands, the surface tension increases. Thus, normal alveoli are much easier to inflate at low lung volumes (i.e., after expiration) than at high volumes (i.e., after inspiration). The decrease in surface tension caused by surfactant also is responsible for keeping the alveoli free of fluid. If surfactant is not produced in adequate quantities, alveolar surface tension increases, causing alveolar collapse, decreased lung expansion, increased work of breathing, and severe gas-exchange abnormalities.

Elastic Properties of the Lung and Chest Wall

The lung and chest wall have elastic properties that permit expansion during inspiration and return to resting volume during expiration. The elasticity of the lung is caused both by elastin fibers in the alveolar walls and surrounding the small airways and pulmonary capillaries, and by surface tension at the alveolar air-liquid interface.[13] The elasticity of

the chest wall is the result of the configuration of its bones and musculature.

Elastic recoil is the tendency of the lungs to return to the resting state after inspiration. Normal elastic recoil permits passive expiration, eliminating the need for major muscles of expiration. Passive elastic recoil may be insufficient during labored breathing (high minute volume), when the accessory muscles of expiration may be needed. The accessory muscles are used also if disease compromises elastic recoil (e.g., in emphysema) or blocks the conducting airways.

Normal elastic recoil depends on an equilibrium between opposing forces of recoil in the lungs and chest wall. Under normal conditions, the chest wall tends to recoil by expanding outward. The tendency of the chest wall to recoil by expanding is balanced by the tendency of the lungs to recoil or inward collapse around the hila. The opposing forces of the chest wall and lungs create the small negative intrapleural pressure.

Balance between the outward recoil of the chest wall and inward recoil of the lungs occurs at the resting level, the end of expiration, where the functional residual capacity (FRC) is reached. However, muscular effort is needed to overcome lung resistance to expansion. During inspiration, the diaphragm and intercostal muscles contract, air flows into the lungs, and the chest wall expands. During expiration, the muscles relax and the elastic recoil of the lungs causes the thorax to decrease in volume until, once again, balance between the chest wall and lung recoil forces is reached (Figure 26-10).

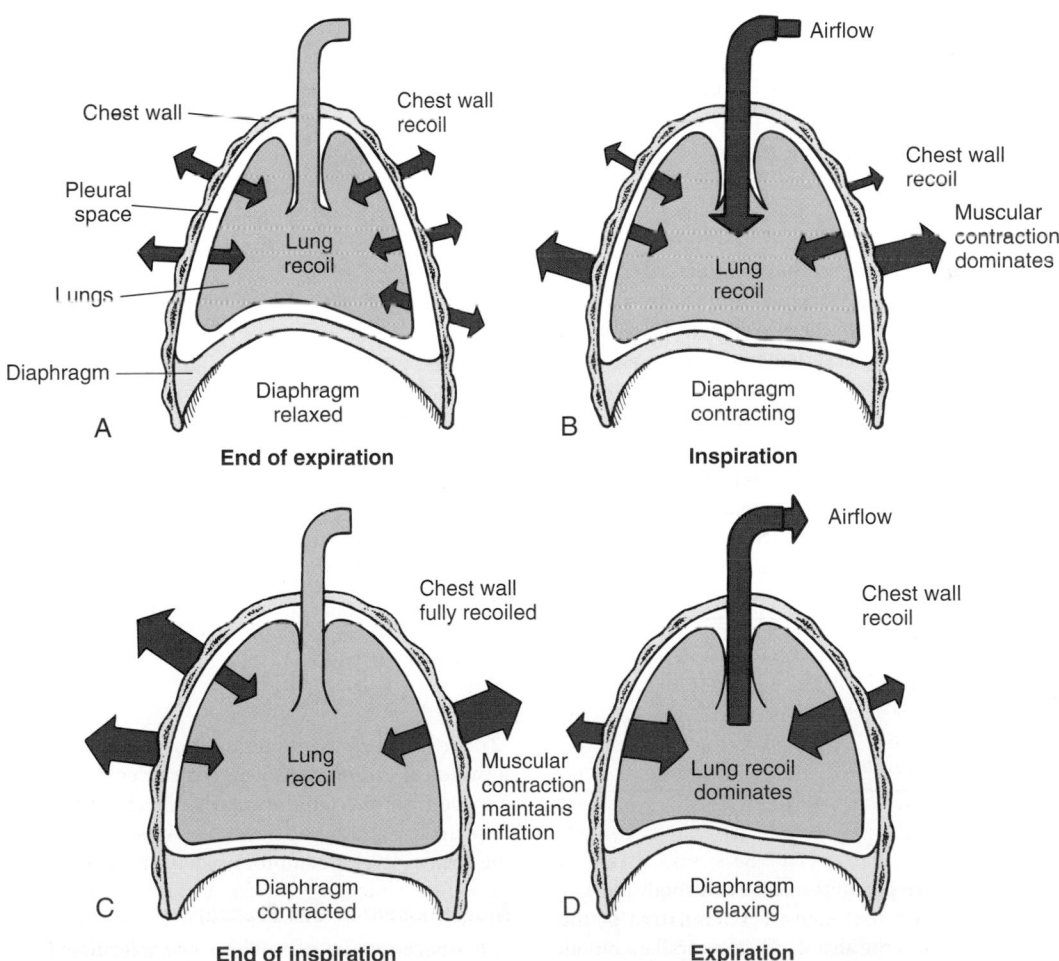

FIGURE 26-10 Interaction of Forces During Inspiration and Expiration. A, Outward recoil of the chest wall equals inward recoil of the lungs at the end of expiration. **B,** During inspiration, contraction of respiratory muscles, assisted by chest wall recoil, overcomes the tendency of lungs to recoil. **C,** At the end of inspiration, respiratory muscle contraction maintains lung expansion. **D,** During expiration, respiratory muscles relax, allowing elastic recoil of the lungs to deflate the lungs.

Compliance is the measure of lung and chest wall distensibility and is defined as volume change per unit of pressure change. It represents the relative ease with which these structures can be stretched and is, therefore, the opposite of elasticity. Compliance is determined by the alveolar surface tension and the elastic recoil of the lung and chest wall.

Increased compliance indicates that the lungs or chest wall is abnormally easy to inflate and has lost some elastic recoil. A decrease in compliance indicates that the lungs or chest wall is abnormally stiff or difficult to inflate. Compliance increases with normal aging and with disorders such as emphysema; it decreases in individuals with acute respiratory distress syndrome, pneumonia, pulmonary edema, and fibrosis. (These disorders are described in Chapter 27.)

Airway Resistance

Airway resistance, which is similar to resistance to blood flow (described in Chapter 23), is determined by the length, radius, and cross-sectional area of the airways and by the density, viscosity, and velocity of the gas (Poiseuille law). Resistance *(R)* is computed by dividing change in pressure *(P)* by rate of flow *(F)*, or $R = P/F$ (Ohm law). Airway resistance is normally very low. One half to two thirds of total airway resistance occurs in the nose. The next highest resistance is in the oropharynx and larynx. There is very little resistance in the conducting airways of the lungs because of their large cross-sectional area. Airway resistance is affected by the diameter of the airways. Bronchodilation, which decreases resistance to airflow, is caused by β_2-adrenergic receptor stimulation. Bronchoconstriction, which increases airway resistance, can be caused by stimulation of parasympathetic receptors in the bronchial smooth muscle and by numerous irritants and inflammatory mediators.[2] Airway resistance can also be increased by edema of the bronchial mucosa and by airway obstructions such as mucus, tumors, or foreign bodies. Pulmonary function tests (PFTs) measure lung volumes and flow rates and can be used to diagnose lung disease.

Work of Breathing

The work of breathing is determined by the muscular effort (and therefore oxygen and energy) required for ventilation. Normally very low, the work of breathing may increase considerably in diseases that disrupt the equilibrium between forces exerted by the lung and chest wall. More muscular effort is required when lung compliance decreases (e.g., in pulmonary edema), chest wall compliance decreases (e.g., in spinal deformity or obesity), or airways are obstructed by bronchospasm or mucous plugging (e.g., in asthma or bronchitis). An increase in the work of breathing can result in a marked increase in oxygen consumption and an inability to maintain adequate ventilation (Figure 26-11).

> ✔ **QUICK CHECK 26-4**
> 1. Describe the work of the diaphragm in ventilation.
> 2. What is surfactant? What is its function?
> 3. How is elastic recoil related to compliance?
> 4. What causes changes in airway resistance?

Gas Transport

Gas transport is the delivery of oxygen to the cells of the body and the removal of carbon dioxide. It has four steps: (1) ventilation of the lungs, (2) diffusion of oxygen from the alveoli into the capillary blood, (3) perfusion of systemic capillaries with oxygenated blood, and (4) diffusion of oxygen from systemic capillaries into the cells. Steps in the transport of carbon dioxide occur in reverse order: (1) diffusion of carbon dioxide from the cells into the systemic capillaries,

FIGURE 26-11 Pulmonary Ventilation and Lung Volumes. The chart in **A** shows a tracing like that produced with a spirometer. The diagram in **B** shows the pulmonary volumes as relative proportions of an inflated balloon. During normal, quiet breathing, about 500 ml of air is moved into and out of the respiratory tract (TV). During forceful breathing (like that during and after heavy exercise), an extra 3300 ml can be inspired (IRV), and an extra 1000 ml or so can be expired (ERV). The largest volume of air that can be moved in and out during ventilation is called the vital capacity (VC). Air that remains in the respiratory tract after a forceful expiration is called the residual volume (RV). (From Patton KT, Thibodeau GA: *The human body in health & disease*, ed 4, St Louis, 2010, Mosby.)

(2) perfusion of the pulmonary capillary bed by venous blood, (3) diffusion of carbon dioxide into the alveoli, and (4) removal of carbon dioxide from the lung by ventilation. If any step in gas transport is impaired by a respiratory or cardiovascular disorder, gas exchange at the cellular level is compromised.

Measurement of Gas Pressure

A gas is composed of millions of molecules moving randomly and colliding with each other and with the wall of the space in which they are contained. These collisions exert pressure. If the same number of gas molecules is contained in a small and a large container, the pressure is greater in the small container because more collisions occur in

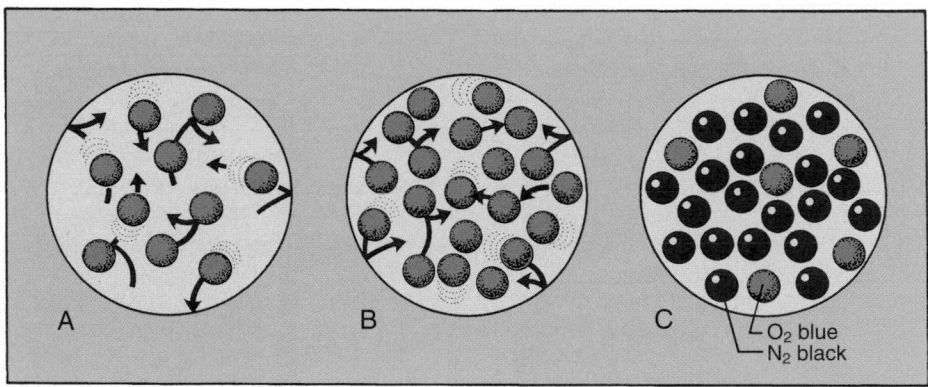

FIGURE 26-12 Relationship Between Number of Gas Molecules and Pressure Exerted by the Gas in an Enclosed Space. **A,** Theoretically, 10 molecules of the same gas exert a total pressure of 10 within the space. **B,** If the number of molecules is increased to 20, total pressure is 20. **C,** If there are different gases in the space, each gas exerts a partial pressure: here the partial pressure of nitrogen (N_2) is 20, that of oxygen (O_2) is 6, and the total pressure is 26.

the smaller space (Figure 26-12). Heat increases the speed of the molecules, which also increases the number of collisions and therefore the pressure.

Barometric pressure (P_B) (atmospheric pressure) is the pressure exerted by gas molecules in air at specific altitudes. At sea level, barometric pressure is 760 mm Hg and is the sum of the pressures exerted by each gas in the air at sea level. The portion of the total pressure exerted by any individual gas is its partial pressure (see Figure 26-12). At sea level the air consists of oxygen (20.9%), nitrogen (78.1%), and a few other trace gases. The **partial pressure** of oxygen is equal to the percentage of oxygen in the air (20.9%) times the total barometric pressure (760 mm Hg at sea level), or 159 mm Hg ($760 \times 0.209 = 158.84$ mm Hg). (Symbols used in the measurement of gas pressures and pulmonary ventilation are defined in Table 26-2.)

The amount of water vapor contained in a gas mixture is determined by the temperature of the gas and is unrelated to barometric pressure. Gas that enters the lungs becomes saturated with water vapor (humidified) as it passes through the upper airway. At body temperature (37° C [98.6° F]), water vapor exerts a pressure of 47 mm Hg regardless of total barometric pressure. The partial pressure of water vapor must be subtracted from the barometric pressure before the partial pressures of other gases in the mixture can be determined. In saturated air at sea level, the partial pressure of oxygen is therefore $(760 - 47) \times 0.209 = 149$ mm Hg. All pressure and volume measurements made in pulmonary function laboratories specify the temperature and humidity of a gas at the time of measurement.

Many pressure measurements are stated as variations from barometric pressure, rather than percentages of it. On such scales, barometric pressure is considered zero, and pressure varies up or down from zero. Physiologic pressure measurements that involve fluids, rather than gases, are measured as variations from barometric pressure. For example, a systolic blood pressure of 120 mm Hg indicates that the systolic pressure is 120 mm Hg higher than the barometric pressure.

Distribution of Ventilation and Perfusion

Effective gas exchange depends on an approximately even distribution of gas (ventilation) and blood (perfusion) in all portions of the lungs.[1] The lungs are suspended from the hila in the thoracic cavity. When an individual is in an upright position (sitting or standing), gravity pulls the lungs down toward the diaphragm and compresses their lower portions or bases. The alveoli in the upper portions, or apices, of the lungs contain a greater residual volume of gas and are larger and less

TABLE 26-2	**Common Pulmonary Abbreviations**
Symbol	**Definition**
V	Volume or amount of gas
Q	Perfusion or blood flow
P	Pressure (usually partial pressure) of a gas
PaO_2	Partial pressure of oxygen in arterial blood
P_AO_2	Partial pressure of oxygen in alveolar gas
$PaCO_2$	Partial pressure of carbon dioxide in arterial blood
PvO_2	Partial pressure of oxygen in mixed venous or pulmonary artery blood
$P(A-a)O_2$	Difference between alveolar and arterial partial pressure of oxygen (A–a gradient)
P_B	Barometric or atmospheric pressure
SaO_2	Saturation of hemoglobin (in arterial blood) with oxygen
SvO_2	Saturation of hemoglobin (in mixed venous blood) with oxygen
V_A	Alveolar ventilation
V_D	Dead-space ventilation
V_E	Minute capacity
V_T	Tidal volume or average breath
$\dot{V}/\dot{Q}$*	Ratio of ventilation to perfusion
FiO_2	Fraction of inspired oxygen
FRC	Functional residual capacity
FVC	Forced vital capacity
FEV_1	Forced expiratory volume in 1 second

*An overhead dot means measurement over time, usually 1 minute.

numerous than those in the lower portions. Because surface tension increases as the alveoli become larger, the larger alveoli in the upper portions of the lung are more difficult to inflate (less compliant) than the smaller alveoli in the lower portions of the lung. Therefore, during ventilation most of the tidal volume is distributed to the bases of the lungs, where compliance is greater.

The heart pumps against gravity to perfuse the pulmonary circulation. As blood is pumped into the lung apices of a sitting or standing individual, some blood pressure is dissipated in overcoming gravity. As a result, blood pressure at the apices is lower than that at the bases. Because greater pressure causes greater perfusion, the bases of the lungs are better perfused than the apices (Figure 26-13). Thus, ventilation and perfusion are greatest in the same lung portions—the lower

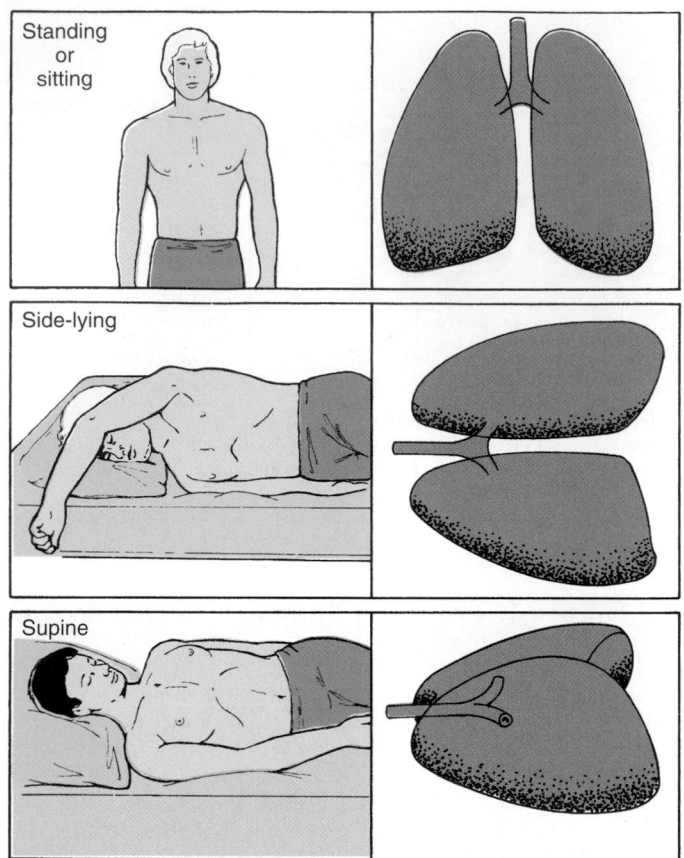

FIGURE 26-13 Pulmonary Blood Flow and Gravity. The greatest volume of pulmonary blood flow normally will occur in the gravity-dependent areas of the lung. Body position has a significant effect on the distribution of pulmonary blood flow. Shaded areas represent gravity dependent pulmonary blood flow.

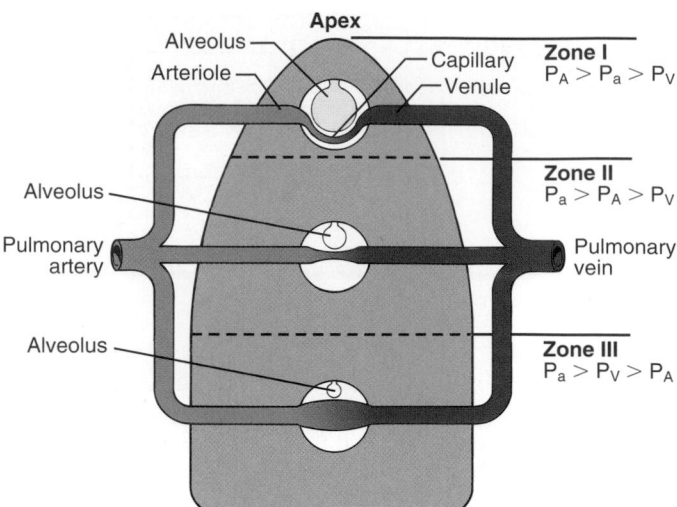

FIGURE 26-14 Gravity and Alveolar Pressure. Effects of gravity and alveolar pressure on pulmonary blood flow in the three lung zones. In zone I, alveolar pressure (P_A) is greater than arterial and venous pressures, and no blood flow occurs. In zone II, arterial pressure (P_a) exceeds alveolar pressure, but alveolar pressure exceeds venous pressure (P_V). Blood flow occurs in this zone, but alveolar pressure compresses the venules (venous ends of the capillaries). In zone III, both arterial and venous pressures are greater than alveolar pressure and blood flow fluctuates depending on the difference between arterial pressure and venous pressure.

Perfusion exceeds ventilation in the bases, and ventilation exceeds perfusion in the apices of the lung. The relationship between ventilation and perfusion is expressed as a ratio called the **ventilation-perfusion ratio ($\dot{V}/\dot{Q}$)**.[1] The normal $\dot{V}/\dot{Q}$ is 0.8. This is the amount by which perfusion exceeds ventilation under normal conditions.

Oxygen Transport

Approximately 1000 ml (1 L) of oxygen is transported to the cells of the body each minute. Oxygen is transported in the blood in two forms: a small amount dissolves in plasma, and the remainder binds to hemoglobin molecules. Without hemoglobin, oxygen would not reach the cells in amounts sufficient to maintain normal metabolic function. (Hemoglobin is discussed in detail in Chapter 20, and cellular metabolism is explored in Chapter 1.)

Diffusion across the alveolocapillary membrane. The alveolocapillary membrane is ideal for oxygen diffusion because it has a large total surface area (70 to 100 m^2) and is very thin (0.5 micrometer [μm]). In addition, the partial pressure of oxygen molecules in alveolar gas ($P_{A_{O_2}}$) is much greater than that in capillary blood, a condition that promotes rapid diffusion down the concentration gradient from the alveolus into the capillary. The partial pressure of oxygen (oxygen tension) in mixed venous or pulmonary artery blood (Pv_{O_2}) is approximately 40 mm Hg as it enters the capillary, and alveolar oxygen tension ($P_{A_{O_2}}$) is approximately 100 mm Hg at sea level. Therefore a pressure gradient of 60 mm Hg facilitates the diffusion of oxygen from the alveolus into the capillary (Figure 26-15).

Blood remains in the pulmonary capillary for about 0.75 second, but only 0.25 second is required for oxygen concentration to equilibrate (equalize) across the alveolocapillary membrane. Therefore oxygen has ample time to diffuse into the blood, even during increased cardiac output, which speeds blood flow and shortens the time the blood remains in the capillary.

Determinants of arterial oxygenation. As oxygen diffuses across the alveolocapillary membrane, it dissolves in the plasma, where it exerts pressure (the partial pressure of oxygen in arterial blood, or

lobes—and depend on body position. If a standing individual assumes a supine or side-lying position, the areas of the lungs that are then most dependent become the best ventilated and perfused.

Distribution of perfusion in the pulmonary circulation also is affected by alveolar pressure (gas pressure in the alveoli). The pulmonary capillary bed differs from the systemic capillary bed in that it is surrounded by gas-containing alveoli. If the gas pressure in the alveoli exceeds the blood pressure in the capillary, the capillary collapses and flow ceases. This is most likely to occur in portions of the lung where blood pressure is lowest and alveolar gas pressure is greatest—that is, at the apex of the lung.

The lungs are divided into three zones on the basis of relationships among all the factors affecting pulmonary blood flow. Alveolar pressure and the forces of gravity, arterial blood pressure, and venous blood pressure affect the distribution of perfusion, as shown in Figure 26-14.

In zone I, alveolar pressure exceeds pulmonary arterial and venous pressures. The capillary bed collapses, and normal blood flow ceases. Normally zone I is a very small part of the lung at the apex. In zone II, alveolar pressure is greater than venous pressure but not arterial pressure. Blood flows through zone II, but it is impeded to a certain extent by alveolar pressure. Zone II is normally above the level of the left atrium. In zone III, both arterial and venous pressures are greater than alveolar pressure and blood flow is not affected by alveolar pressure. Zone III is in the base of the lung. Blood flow through the pulmonary capillary bed increases in regular increments from the apex to the base.

Although both blood flow and ventilation are greater at the base of the lungs than at the apices, they are not perfectly matched in any zone.

FIGURE 26-15 Partial Pressure of Respiratory Gases in Normal Respiration. The numbers shown are average values near sea level. The values of P_{O_2}, P_{CO_2}, and P_{N_2} fluctuate from breath to breath. (Modified from Thompson JM et al: *Mosby's clinical nursing*, ed 5, St Louis, 2002, Mosby.)

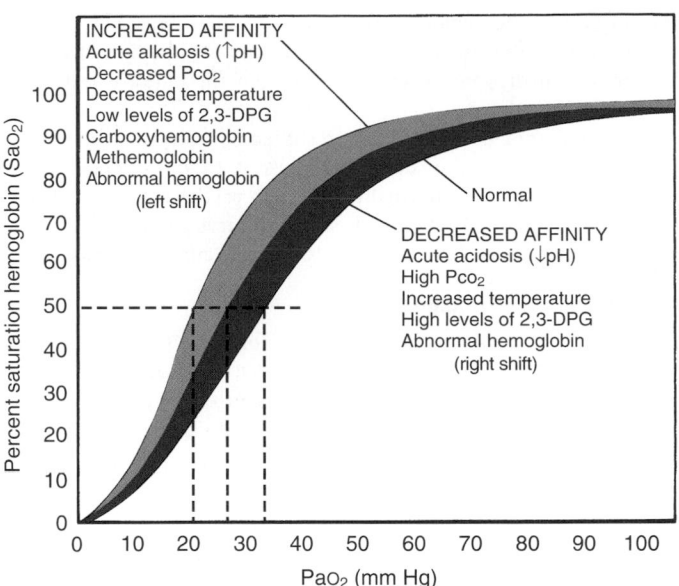

FIGURE 26-16 Oxyhemoglobin Dissociation Curve. The horizontal or flat segment of the curve at the top of the graph is the arterial or association portion, or that part of the curve where oxygen is bound to hemoglobin and occurs in the lungs. This portion of the curve is flat because partial pressure changes of oxygen between 60 and 100 mm Hg do not significantly alter the percentage saturation of hemoglobin with oxygen and allow adequate hemoglobin saturation at a variety of altitudes. If the relationship between SaO_2 and PaO_2 was linear (in a downward sloping straight line) instead of flat between 60 and 100 mm Hg, there would be inadequate saturation of hemoglobin with oxygen. The steep part of the oxyhemoglobin dissociation curve represents the rapid dissociation of oxygen from hemoglobin that occurs in the tissues. During this phase there is rapid diffusion of oxygen from the blood into tissue cells. The P_{50} is the PaO_2 at which hemoglobin is 50% saturated, normally 26.6 mm Hg. A lower than normal P_{50} represents increased affinity of hemoglobin for O_2; a high P_{50} is seen with decreased affinity. Note that variation from the normal is associated with decreased (low P_{50}) or increased (high P_{50}) availability of O_2 to tissues *(dashed lines)*. The shaded area shows the entire oxyhemoglobin dissociation curve under the same circumstances. *2,3-DPG*, 2,3-Diphosphoglycerate. (From Lane EE, Walker JF: *Clinical arterial blood gas analysis*, St Louis, 1987, Mosby.)

PaO_2). As the PaO_2 increases, oxygen moves from the plasma into the red blood cells (erythrocytes) and binds with hemoglobin molecules. Oxygen continues to bind with hemoglobin until the hemoglobin-binding sites are filled or *saturated*. Oxygen then continues to diffuse across the alveolocapillary membrane until the PaO_2 (oxygen dissolved in plasma) and P_{AO_2} (oxygen in the alveolus) equilibrate, eliminating the pressure gradient across the alveolocapillary membrane. At this point, diffusion ceases (see Figure 26-15).

The majority (97%) of the oxygen that enters the blood is bound to hemoglobin. The remaining 3% stays in the plasma and creates the partial pressure of oxygen (PaO_2). The PaO_2 can be measured in the blood by obtaining an arterial blood gas measurement. The **oxygen saturation** (SaO_2) is the percentage of the available hemoglobin that is bound to oxygen and can be measured using a device called an oximeter.

Because hemoglobin transports all but a small fraction of the oxygen carried in arterial blood, changes in hemoglobin concentration affect the oxygen content of the blood. Decreases in hemoglobin concentration below the normal value of 15 g/dl of blood reduce oxygen content, and increases in hemoglobin concentration may increase oxygen content, minimizing the impact of impaired gas exchange. In fact, increased hemoglobin concentration is a major compensatory mechanism in pulmonary diseases that impair gas exchange. For this reason, measurement of hemoglobin concentration is important in assessing individuals with pulmonary disease. If cardiovascular function is normal, the body's initial response to low oxygen content is to accelerate cardiac output. In individuals who also have cardiovascular disease, this compensatory mechanism is ineffective, making increased hemoglobin concentration an even more important compensatory mechanism. (Hemoglobin structure and function are described in Chapter 20.)

Oxyhemoglobin association and dissociation. When hemoglobin molecules bind with oxygen, **oxyhemoglobin** (HbO_2) forms.

Binding occurs in the lungs and is called *oxyhemoglobin association* or *hemoglobin saturation with oxygen* (SaO_2). The reverse process, where oxygen is released from hemoglobin, occurs in the body tissues at the cellular level and is called *hemoglobin desaturation*. When hemoglobin saturation and desaturation are plotted on a graph, the result is a distinctive **S**-shaped curve known as the **oxyhemoglobin dissociation curve** (Figure 26-16).

Several factors can change the relationship between PaO_2 and SaO_2, causing the oxyhemoglobin dissociation curve to shift to the right or left (see Figure 26-16). A shift to the right depicts hemoglobin's decreased affinity for oxygen or an increase in the ease with which oxyhemoglobin dissociates and oxygen moves into the cells. A shift to the left depicts hemoglobin's increased affinity for oxygen, which promotes association in the lungs and inhibits dissociation in the tissues.

The oxyhemoglobin dissociation curve is shifted to the right by acidosis (low pH) and hypercapnia (increased $PaCO_2$). In the tissues, the increased levels of carbon dioxide and hydrogen ions produced by metabolic activity decrease the affinity of hemoglobin for oxygen. The curve is shifted to the left by alkalosis (high pH) and hypocapnia (decreased $PaCO_2$). In the lungs, as carbon dioxide diffuses from the blood into the alveoli, the blood carbon dioxide level is reduced and the affinity of hemoglobin for oxygen is increased. The shift in the oxyhemoglobin dissociation curve caused by changes in carbon dioxide and hydrogen ion concentrations in the blood is called the **Bohr effect**.

The oxyhemoglobin curve is also shifted by changes in body temperature and increased or decreased levels of 2,3-diphosphoglycerate (2,3-DPG), a substance normally present in erythrocytes. Hyperthermia and increased 2,3-DPG levels shift the curve to the right. Hypothermia and decreased 2,3-DPG levels shift the curve to the left.

Carbon Dioxide Transport

Carbon dioxide is carried in the blood in three ways: (1) dissolved in plasma (P_{CO_2}), (2) as bicarbonate (HCO_3^-), and (3) as carbamino compounds. As CO_2 diffuses out of the cells into the blood, it dissolves in the plasma. Approximately 10% of the total CO_2 in venous blood and 5% of the CO_2 in arterial blood are transported dissolved in the plasma ($P_{V_{CO_2}}$ and Pa_{CO_2}, respectively). As CO_2 moves into the blood, it diffuses into the red blood cells. Within the red blood cells, CO_2, with the help of the enzyme carbonic anhydrase, combines with water to form carbonic acid and then quickly dissociates into H^+ and HCO_3^-. As carbonic acid dissociates, the H^+ binds to hemoglobin, where it is buffered, and the HCO_3^- moves out of the red blood cell into the plasma. Approximately 60% of the CO_2 in venous blood and 90% of the CO_2 in arterial blood are carried in the form of bicarbonate. The remainder combines with blood proteins, hemoglobin in particular,

to form carbamino compounds. Approximately 30% of the CO_2 in venous blood and 5% of the CO_2 in arterial blood are carried as carbamino compounds.

CO_2 is 20 times more soluble than O_2 and diffuses quickly from the tissue cells into the blood. The amount of CO_2 able to enter the blood is enhanced by diffusion of oxygen out of the blood and into the cells. Reduced hemoglobin (hemoglobin that is dissociated from oxygen) can carry more CO_2 than can hemoglobin saturated with O_2. Therefore the drop in S_{O_2} at the tissue level increases the ability of hemoglobin to carry CO_2 back to the lung.

The diffusion gradient for CO_2 in the lung is only approximately 6 mm Hg (venous P_{CO_2} = 46 mm Hg; alveolar P_{CO_2} = 40 mm Hg) (see Figure 26-15). Yet CO_2 is so soluble in the alveolocapillary membrane that the CO_2 in the blood quickly diffuses into the alveoli, where it is removed from the lung with each expiration. Diffusion of CO_2 in the lung is so efficient that diffusion defects that cause hypoxemia (low oxygen content of the blood) do not as readily cause hypercapnia (excessive carbon dioxide in the blood).

The diffusion of CO_2 out of the blood is also enhanced by oxygen binding with hemoglobin in the lung. As hemoglobin binds with O_2, the amount of CO_2 carried by the blood decreases. Thus, in the tissue capillaries, O_2 dissociation from hemoglobin facilitates the pickup of CO_2, and the binding of O_2 to hemoglobin in the lungs facilitates the release of CO_2 from the blood. This effect of oxygen on CO_2 transport is called the **Haldane effect**.

GERIATRIC CONSIDERATIONS
Aging & the Pulmonary System

Elasticity/Chest Wall

Chest wall compliance decreases because ribs become ossified and joints are stiffer, which results in increased work of breathing.

Kyphoscoliosis may curve the vertebral column, decreasing lung volumes.

Intercostal muscle strength decreases.

Elastic recoil diminishes, possibly the result of loss of elastic fibers.

Result: Lung compliance increases and ventilatory capacity (VC) declines, residual volume (RV) increases, total lung capacity (TLC) is unchanged, ventilatory reserves decline, and ventilation-perfusion ratios fall.

Gas Exchange

Pulmonary capillary network decreases.

Alveoli dilate, and peripheral airways lose supporting tissues.

Surface area for gas exchange decreases.

pH and P_{CO_2} do not change much, but P_{O_2} declines.

Sensitivity of respiratory centers to hypoxia or hypercapnia decreases.

Ability to initiate an immune response against infection decreases.

NOTE: Maximum Pa_{O_2} at sea level can be estimated by multiplying person's age by 0.3 and subtracting the product from 100.

Exercise

Decreased Pa_{O_2} and diminished ventilatory reserve lead to decreased exercise tolerance.

Early airway closure inhibits expiratory flow.

Changes depend on activity and fitness levels earlier in life.

An active, physically fit individual has fewer changes in function at any age than does a sedentary individual.

Respiratory muscle strength and endurance decrease but can be enhanced by exercise.

Lung Immunity

Alterations in alveolar complement and surfactant and an increase in proinflammatory cytokines increase the risk for pulmonary disease and infection.

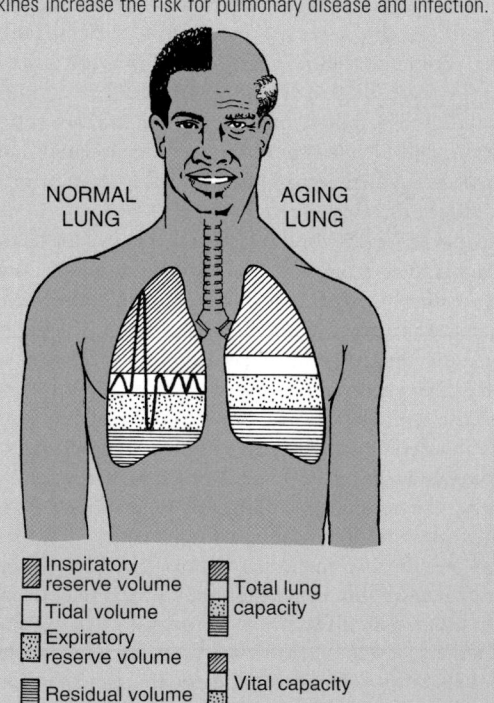

NORMAL LUNG   AGING LUNG

Inspiratory reserve volume
Tidal volume
Expiratory reserve volume
Residual volume
Total lung capacity
Vital capacity

Changes in Lung Volumes with Aging. With aging, note particularly the decreased vital capacity and the increase in residual volume.

Data from Carpagnano GE et al: *Aging Clin Exp Res* 25(3):239-245, 2013; Lalley PM: *Respir Physiol Neurobiol* 187(3):199-210, 2013; Lowery EM et al: *Clin Interv Aging* 8:1489-1496, 2013; Miller MR: *Semin Respir Crit Care Med* 31(5):521-527, 2010; Moliva JI et al: *Age (Dordr)* 36(3):9633, 2014; Weiss CO et al: *J Gerontol A Biol Sci Med Sci* 65(3):287-294, 2010. Ramly E et al: *Surg Clin North Am* 95(1):53-69, 2015.

✔**QUICK CHECK 26-5**
1. What are the eight steps of gas transport?
2. Describe the relationship between ventilation and pulmonary blood flow.
3. What is the alveolocapillary membrane? How does it function in ventilation and perfusion?
4. Describe the process of oxyhemoglobin association and dissociation.
5. What is barometric pressure? How is it related to physiologic pressure measurements?

DID YOU UNDERSTAND?

Structures of the Pulmonary System

1. The pulmonary system consists of the lungs, upper and lower airways, chest wall, and pulmonary and bronchial circulation.
2. Air is inspired and expired through the conducting airways: nasopharynx, oropharynx, trachea, bronchi, and bronchioles.
3. Gas exchange occurs in structures beyond the respiratory bronchioles: in the alveolar ducts and the alveoli. Together these structures compose the acinus.
4. The chief gas-exchange units of the lungs are the alveoli. The membrane that surrounds each alveolus and contains the pulmonary capillaries is called the *alveolocapillary membrane.*
5. The gas-exchange airways are perfused by the pulmonary circulation, a separate division of the circulatory system. The bronchi and other lung structures are perfused by a branch of the systemic circulation called the *bronchial circulation.*
6. The chest wall, which contains and protects the contents of the thoracic cavity, consists of the skin, ribs, and intercostal muscles, which lie between the ribs.
7. The chest wall is lined by a serous membrane called the *parietal pleura;* the lungs are encased in a separate membrane called the *visceral pleura.* The *pleural space* is the area where these two pleurae contact and slide over one another.

Function of the Pulmonary System

1. The pulmonary system enables oxygen to diffuse into the blood and carbon dioxide to diffuse out of the blood.
2. Ventilation is the process by which air flows into and out of the gas-exchange airways.
3. Most of the time, ventilation is involuntary. It is controlled by the sympathetic and parasympathetic divisions of the autonomic nervous system, which adjust airway caliber (by causing bronchial smooth muscle to contract or relax) and control the rate and depth of ventilation.
4. Neuroreceptors in the lungs (lung receptors) monitor the mechanical aspects of ventilation. Irritant receptors sense the need to expel unwanted substances, stretch receptors sense lung volume (lung expansion), and J-receptors sense pulmonary capillary pressure.
5. Chemoreceptors in the circulatory system and brainstem sense the effectiveness of ventilation by monitoring the pH status of cerebrospinal fluid and the oxygen content (Po_2) of arterial blood.
6. Successful ventilation involves the mechanics of breathing: the interaction of forces and counterforces involving the muscles of inspiration and expiration, alveolar surface tension, elastic properties of the lungs and chest wall, and resistance to airflow.
7. The major muscle of inspiration is the diaphragm. When the diaphragm contracts, it moves downward in the thoracic cavity, creating a vacuum that causes air to flow into the lungs.

8. The type II alveolar cells produce surfactant, a lipoprotein that lines the alveoli. Surfactant reduces alveolar surface tension and permits the alveoli to expand as air enters.
9. Compliance is the ease with which the lungs and chest wall expand during inspiration. Lung compliance is ensured by an adequate production of surfactant, whereas chest wall expansion depends on elasticity.
10. Elastic recoil is the tendency of the lungs and chest wall to return to their resting state after inspiration. The elastic recoil forces of the lungs and chest wall are in opposition and pull on each other, creating the normally negative pressure of the pleural space.
11. Gas transport depends on ventilation of the alveoli, diffusion across the alveolocapillary membrane, perfusion of the pulmonary and systemic capillaries, and diffusion between systemic capillaries and tissue cells.
12. Efficient gas exchange depends on an even distribution of ventilation and perfusion within the lungs. Both ventilation and perfusion are greatest in the bases of the lungs because the alveoli in the bases are more compliant (their resting volume is low) and perfusion is greater in the bases as a result of gravity.
13. Almost all the oxygen that diffuses into pulmonary capillary blood is transported by hemoglobin, a protein contained within red blood cells. The remainder of the oxygen is transported dissolved in plasma.
14. Oxygen enters the body by diffusing down the concentration gradient, from high concentrations in the alveoli to lower concentrations in the capillaries. Diffusion ceases when alveolar and capillary oxygen pressures equilibrate.
15. Oxygen is loaded onto hemoglobin by the driving pressure exerted by Pao_2 in the plasma. As pressure decreases at the tissue level, oxygen dissociates from hemoglobin and enters tissue cells by diffusion, again down the concentration gradient.
16. Compared with oxygen, carbon dioxide is more soluble in plasma. Therefore carbon dioxide diffuses readily from tissue cells into plasma and from plasma into the alveoli. Carbon dioxide returns to the lungs dissolved in plasma, as bicarbonate, or in carbamino compounds (e.g., bound to hemoglobin).
17. The pulmonary circulation is innervated by the autonomic nervous system (ANS), but vasodilation and vasoconstriction are controlled mainly by local and humoral factors, particularly arterial oxygenation and acid-base status.

Geriatric Considerations: Aging & the Pulmonary System

1. Aging affects the mechanical aspects of ventilation by decreasing chest wall compliance and elastic recoil of the lungs. Changes in these elastic properties reduce the ventilatory reserve.
2. With aging, the surface area for gas exchange and capillary perfusion may decrease, reducing exercise capacity.
3. Level of fitness and associated systemic disease affect individual lung function.

KEY TERMS

Acinus, 672
Alveolar duct, 672
Alveolar ventilation, 676
Alveolocapillary membrane, 673
Alveolus (pl., alveoli), 672
Bohr effect, 684
Bronchus (pl., bronchi), 671
Carina, 671
Central chemoreceptor, 677
Collectin, 679
Compliance, 680
Elastic recoil, 679

Goblet cell, 671
Haldane effect, 684
Hilum (pl., hila), 671
Hypoxic pulmonary
  vasoconstriction, 675
Irritant receptor, 676
J-receptor, 676
Larynx, 671
Mediastinum, 671
Minute volume (minute
  ventilation), 676
Nasopharynx, 671

Oropharynx, 671
Oxygen saturation (Sao$_2$), 683
Oxyhemoglobin (HbO$_2$), 683
Oxyhemoglobin dissociation
  curve, 683
Partial pressure (of a gas), 681
Peripheral chemoreceptor, 676
Pleura (pl., pleurae), 675
Pleural space (pleural
  cavity), 675
Respiratory bronchiole, 672
Respiratory center, 676

Stretch receptor, 676
Surface tension, 678
Surfactant, 672
Thoracic cavity, 675
Trachea, 671
Ventilation, 676
Ventilation-perfusion ratio
  ($\dot{V}/\dot{Q}$), 682

REFERENCES

1. Lumb A: *Nunn's applied respiratory physiology*, ed 7, St Louis, 2011, Mosby.
2. Barrett KE et al: *Ganong's review of medical physiology*, ed 25, New York, 2015, McGraw-Hill.
3. Guillot L et al: Alveolar epithelial cells: master regulators of lung homeostasis, *Int J Biochem Cell Biol* 45(11):2568-2573, 2013.
4. Clouter M, Thrall R: The respiratory system. In Koeppen BM, Stanton BA, editors: *Berne and Levy physiology*, ed 6, St Louis, 2010, Mosby.
5. West JB, Luks AM: *West's respiratory physiology: the essentials*, ed 10, Philadelphia, 2015, Lippincott, Wolters Kluwer.
6. Osiro S et al: A friend to the airways: review of the emerging clinical importance of the bronchial arterial circulation, *Surg Radiol Anat* 34(9):791-798, 2012.
7. Ariyaratnam P et al: Hypoxic pulmonary vasoconstriction in humans, *BioMed Res Int* 2013:623684, 2013.
8. Urfy MZ, Suarez JI: Breathing and the nervous system, *Handb Clin Neurol* 119:241-250, 2014.
9. Nattie E et al: Distinguished lecture: central chemoreception: then … and now, *J Appl Physiol* 110(1):1-8, 2011.
10. Canning BJ et al: Anatomy and neurophysiology of cough: CHEST guideline and expert panel report, *Chest* 146(6):1633-1648, 2014.
11. Guyenet PG et al: The respiratory chemoreception conundrum: light at the end of the tunnel? *Brain Res* 1511:126-137, 2013.
12. Jacono FJ: Control of ventilation in COPD and lung injury, *Respir Physiol Neurobiol* 189(2): 371-376, 2013.
13. Kacmarek R et al: *Egan's fundamentals of respiratory care,* ed 10, St Louis, 2013, Mosby.
14. Brown LK: Hypoventilation syndromes, *Clin Chest Med* 31(2):249-270, 2010.
15. Jakel A et al: Ligands and receptors of lung surfactant proteins SP-A and SP-D, *Front Biosci (Landmark Ed)* 18:1129-1140, 2013.

27

Alterations of Pulmonary Function

Valentina L. Brashers and Sue E. Huether

EVOLVE WEBSITE

CHAPTER OUTLINE

Pulmonary disease is often classified as acute or chronic, obstructive or restrictive, or infectious or noninfectious. Symptoms of lung disease are common and associated not only with primary lung disorders but also with diseases of other organ systems, particularly the heart.

CLINICAL MANIFESTATIONS OF PULMONARY ALTERATIONS

Signs and Symptoms of Pulmonary Disease

Pulmonary disease is associated with many signs and symptoms, the most common of which are dyspnea and cough. Others include abnormal sputum, hemoptysis, altered breathing patterns, hypoventilation and hyperventilation, cyanosis, clubbing, and chest pain.

Dyspnea

Dyspnea is a subjective experience of breathing discomfort that is comprised of qualitatively distinct sensations that vary in intensity. Dyspnea is an individual experience and derives from interactions among multiple physiologic, psychologic, social, and environmental factors, and it may induce secondary physiologic and behavioral responses.[1] It is often described as breathlessness, air hunger, shortness of breath, labored breathing, and preoccupation with breathing. Dyspnea may be the result of pulmonary disease, or many other conditions such as pain, heart disease, trauma, and psychogenic disorders.[2]

The severity of the experience of dyspnea may not directly correlate with the severity of underlying disease. Either diffuse or focal disturbances of ventilation, gas exchange, or ventilation-perfusion relationships can cause dyspnea, as can increased work of breathing or any disease that damages lung tissue (lung parenchyma). Neurophysiologic mechanisms of dyspnea involve an impaired sense of effort in which the perceived work of breathing is greater than the actual motor response that is generated. Stimulation of many receptors can contribute to the sensation of dyspnea, including afferent receptors in the cortex and medulla and mechanoreceptors in the chest wall, upper airway receptors, and central and peripheral chemoreceptors.[3]

The more severe signs of dyspnea include flaring of the nostrils and use of accessory muscles of respiration. Retraction (pulling back) of the supercostal or intercostal muscles is predominant in children. Dyspnea can be quantified by the use of both ordinal rating scales and visual analog scales and is frequently associated with significant anxiety.

Dyspnea may occur transiently or can become chronic. Dyspnea first presents during exercise and is called *dyspnea on exertion*. Orthopnea is dyspnea that occurs during heart failure when an individual lies flat, which causes the abdominal contents to exert pressure on the diaphragm, and decreases the efficiency of the respiratory muscles. Paroxysmal nocturnal dyspnea (PND) occurs when individuals with pulmonary or cardiac disease awake at night gasping for air and have to sit or stand to relieve the dyspnea. Dyspnea may be unrecognized in mechanically ventilated individuals and is often accompanied by pain and anxiety. A focused assessment and change in ventilator settings may be required.[4]

Cough

Cough is a protective reflex that helps clear the airways by an explosive expiration. Inhaled particles, accumulated mucus, inflammation, or the presence of a foreign body initiates the cough reflex by stimulating the irritant receptors in the airway. There are few such receptors in the most distal bronchi and the alveoli; thus it is possible for significant amounts of secretions to accumulate in the distal respiratory tree without cough being initiated. The cough reflex consists of inspiration, closure of the glottis and vocal cords, contraction of the expiratory muscles, and reopening of the glottis, causing a sudden, forceful expiration that removes the offending matter. The effectiveness of the cough depends on the depth of the inspiration and the degree to which the airways narrow, increasing the velocity of expiratory gas flow. Those with an inability to cough effectively are at greater risk for pneumonia.

Acute cough is cough that resolves within 2 to 3 weeks of the onset of illness or resolves with treatment of the underlying condition. It is most commonly the result of upper respiratory tract infections, allergic rhinitis, acute bronchitis, pneumonia, congestive heart failure, pulmonary embolus, or aspiration. *Chronic cough* is defined as cough that is persistent and in individuals who do not smoke. Chronic cough is commonly caused or triggered by postnasal drainage syndrome, asthma, eosinophilic bronchitis, laryngeal hypersensitivity, and gastroesophageal reflux disease or there may be no identifiable underlying cause.[5] In persons who smoke, chronic bronchitis is the most common cause of chronic cough, although lung cancer must always be considered. Individuals taking angiotensin-converting enzyme inhibitors for cardiovascular disease may develop chronic cough that resolves with discontinuation of the drug.

Abnormal Sputum

Changes in the amount, color, and consistency of sputum provide information about progression of disease and effectiveness of therapy. The gross and microscopic appearances of sputum enable the clinician to identify cellular debris or microorganisms, which aids in diagnosis and choice of therapy.

Hemoptysis

Hemoptysis is the coughing up of blood or bloody secretions. This is sometimes confused with hematemesis, which is the vomiting of blood. Blood produced with coughing is usually bright red, has an alkaline pH, and is mixed with frothy sputum. Blood that is vomited is dark, has an acidic pH, and is mixed with food particles.

Hemoptysis usually indicates infection or inflammation that damages the bronchi (bronchitis, bronchiectasis) or the lung parenchyma (pneumonia, tuberculosis, lung abscess). Other causes include cancer, pulmonary infarction, or pulmonary venous stenosis. The amount and duration of bleeding provide important clues about its source. Bronchoscopy, combined with chest computed tomography (CT), is used to confirm the site of bleeding.

Abnormal Breathing Patterns

Normal breathing (eupnea) is rhythmic and effortless. The resting ventilatory rate is 8 to 16 breaths per minute, and tidal volume ranges from 400 to 800 ml. A short expiratory pause occurs with each breath, and the individual takes an occasional deeper breath, or sighs. Sigh breaths, which help to maintain normal lung function, are usually 1.5 to 2 times the normal tidal volume and occur approximately 10 to 12 times per hour.

The rate, depth, regularity, and effort of breathing undergo characteristic alterations in response to physiologic and pathophysiologic conditions. Patterns of breathing automatically adjust to minimize the work of respiratory muscles. Strenuous exercise or metabolic acidosis induces Kussmaul respiration (hyperpnea), which is characterized by a slightly increased ventilatory rate, very large tidal volumes, and no expiratory pause.

Labored breathing occurs whenever there is an increased work of breathing, especially if the airways are obstructed. In large airway obstruction, a slow ventilatory rate, large tidal volume, increased effort, prolonged inspiration and expiration, and stridor or audible wheezing

(depending on the site of obstruction) are typical. In small airway obstruction, such as that seen in asthma and chronic obstructive pulmonary disease, a rapid ventilatory rate, small tidal volume, increased effort, prolonged expiration, and wheezing are often present. *Restricted breathing* is commonly caused by disorders, such as pulmonary fibrosis, that stiffen the lungs or chest wall and decrease compliance, resulting in small tidal volumes and rapid ventilatory rate (tachypnea).

Shock and severe cerebral hypoxia (insufficient oxygen in the brain) contribute to gasping respirations that consist of irregular, quick inspirations with an expiratory pause. Anxiety can cause sighing respirations, which consist of irregular breathing characterized by frequent, deep sighing inspirations. Cheyne-Stokes respirations are characterized by alternating periods of deep and shallow breathing. Apnea lasting from 15 to 60 seconds is followed by ventilations that increase in volume until a peak is reached; then ventilation (tidal volume) decreases again to apnea. Cheyne-Stokes respirations result from any condition that reduces blood flow to the brainstem, which in turn slows impulses sending information to the respiratory centers of the brainstem. Neurologic impairment above the brainstem is also a contributing factor (see Figure 15-1).

Hypoventilation and Hyperventilation

Hypoventilation is inadequate alveolar ventilation in relation to metabolic demands. Hypoventilation occurs when minute volume (tidal volume × respiratory rate) is reduced. It is caused by alterations in pulmonary mechanics or in the neurologic control of breathing.[6] When alveolar ventilation is normal, carbon dioxide (CO_2) is removed from the lungs at the same rate as it is produced by cellular metabolism and arterial and alveolar P_{CO_2} values remain at normal levels (40 mm Hg). With hypoventilation, CO_2 removal does not keep up with CO_2 production and Pa_{CO_2} increases, causing hypercapnia (Pa_{CO_2} greater than 44 mm Hg) (see Table 26-2 for a definition of gas partial pressures and other pulmonary abbreviations). This results in respiratory acidosis that can affect the function of many tissues throughout the body. Hypoventilation is often overlooked until it is severe because breathing pattern and ventilatory rate may appear to be normal and changes in tidal volume can be difficult to detect clinically. Blood gas analysis (i.e., measurement of the Pa_{CO_2} of arterial blood) reveals the hypoventilation. Pronounced hypoventilation can cause secondary hypoxemia, somnolence, or disorientation.

Hyperventilation is alveolar ventilation exceeding metabolic demands. The lungs remove CO_2 faster than it is produced by cellular metabolism, resulting in decreased Pa_{CO_2}, or hypocapnia (Pa_{CO_2} less than 36 mm Hg). Hypocapnia results in a respiratory alkalosis that also can interfere with tissue function. Like hypoventilation, hyperventilation can be determined by arterial blood gas analysis. Hyperventilation commonly occurs with severe anxiety, acute head injury, pain, and in response to conditions that cause hypoxemia.

Cyanosis

Cyanosis is a bluish discoloration of the skin and mucous membranes caused by increasing amounts of desaturated or reduced hemoglobin (which is bluish) in the blood. It generally develops when 5 g of hemoglobin is desaturated, regardless of hemoglobin concentration.

Peripheral cyanosis (slow blood circulation in fingers and toes) is most often caused by poor circulation resulting from intense peripheral vasoconstriction, like that observed in persons who have Raynaud disease, are in cold environments, or are severely stressed. Peripheral cyanosis is best seen in the nail beds. *Central cyanosis* is caused by decreased arterial oxygenation (low Pa_{O_2}) from pulmonary diseases or pulmonary or cardiac right-to-left shunts. Central cyanosis is best detected in buccal mucous membranes and lips.

Lack of cyanosis does not necessarily indicate that oxygenation is normal. In adults, cyanosis is not evident until severe hypoxemia is present and, therefore, is an insensitive indication of respiratory failure. For example, severe anemia (inadequate hemoglobin concentration) and carbon monoxide poisoning (in which hemoglobin binds to carbon monoxide instead of to oxygen) can cause inadequate oxygenation of tissues without causing cyanosis. Individuals with polycythemia (an abnormal increase in numbers of red blood cells), however, may have cyanosis when oxygenation is adequate. Therefore, cyanosis must be interpreted in relation to the underlying pathophysiologic condition. If cyanosis is suggested, the PaO_2 should be measured.

Clubbing

Clubbing is the selective bulbous enlargement of the end (distal segment) of a digit (finger or toe) (Figure 27-1); its severity can be graded from 1 to 5 based on the extent of nail bed hypertrophy and the amount of changes in the nails themselves. It is usually painless. Clubbing is commonly associated with diseases that disrupt the normal pulmonary circulation and cause chronic hypoxemia, such as bronchiectasis, cystic fibrosis, pulmonary fibrosis, lung abscess, and congenital heart disease, and is rarely reversible. It is proposed that whole megakaryocytes enter the systemic circulation and become impacted in the fingertip circulation. Megakaryocytes and megakaryocyte fragments are activated to release platelet-derived growth factor (PDGF). PDGF promotes growth, vascular permeability, and monocyte and neutrophil chemotaxis and leads to an increased number of vascular smooth muscle cells and fibroblasts, all of which are seen in the pathology of clubbing.[7] It can sometimes be seen in individuals with lung cancer even without hypoxemia because of the effects of inflammatory cytokines and growth factors (hypertrophic osteoarthropathy).[8]

Pain

Pain caused by pulmonary disorders originates in the pleurae, airways, or chest wall.[9] Infection and inflammation of the parietal pleura cause sharp or stabbing pain (pleurodynia) when the pleura stretches during inspiration. The pain is usually localized to a portion of the chest wall, where a unique breath sound called a *pleural friction rub* may be heard over the painful area. Laughing or coughing makes pleural pain worse. Pleural pain is common with pulmonary infarction (tissue death) caused by pulmonary embolism and emanates from the area around the infarction.

Infection and inflammation of the trachea or bronchi (tracheitis or tracheobronchitis, respectively) can cause central chest pain that is pronounced after coughing. It can be difficult to differentiate from cardiac pain. High blood pressure in the pulmonary circulation (pulmonary hypertension) can cause pain during exercise that is often mistaken for cardiac pain (angina pectoris).

Pain in the chest wall is muscle pain or rib pain. Excessive coughing (which makes the muscles sore) and rib fractures or thoracic surgery produce such pain. Inflammation of the costochondral junction (costochondritis) also can cause chest wall pain. Chest wall pain can often be reproduced by pressing on the sternum or ribs.

Conditions Caused by Pulmonary Disease or Injury
Hypercapnia

Hypercapnia, or increased carbon dioxide concentration in the arterial blood (increased $PaCO_2$), is caused by hypoventilation of the alveoli. As discussed in Chapter 26, carbon dioxide is easily diffused from the blood into the alveolar space; thus, minute volume (respiratory rate × tidal volume) determines not only alveolar ventilation but also $PaCO_2$. Hypoventilation is often overlooked because the breathing pattern and ventilatory rate may appear to be normal; therefore it is important to obtain blood gas analysis to determine the severity of hypercapnia and resultant respiratory acidosis (acid-base balance is described in Chapter 5).

There are many causes of hypercapnia. Most are a result of a decreased drive to breathe or an inadequate ability to respond to ventilatory stimulation. Some of these causes include (1) depression of the respiratory center by drugs; (2) diseases of the medulla, including infections of the central nervous system or trauma; (3) abnormalities of the spinal conducting pathways, as in spinal cord disruption or poliomyelitis; (4) diseases of the neuromuscular junction or of the respiratory muscles themselves, as in myasthenia gravis or muscular dystrophy; (5) thoracic cage abnormalities, as in chest injury or congenital deformity; (6) large airway obstruction, as in tumors or sleep apnea; and (7) increased work of breathing or physiologic dead space, as in emphysema.

Hypercapnia and the associated respiratory acidosis result in electrolyte abnormalities that may cause dysrhythmias. Individuals also may present with somnolence and even coma because of changes in intracranial pressure associated with high levels of arterial carbon dioxide, which causes cerebral vasodilation. Alveolar hypoventilation with increased alveolar CO_2 concentration limits the amount of oxygen available for diffusion into the blood, thereby leading to secondary hypoxemia.

Hypoxemia

Hypoxemia, or reduced oxygenation of arterial blood (reduced PaO_2), is caused by respiratory alterations, whereas hypoxia (or ischemia) is reduced oxygenation of cells in tissues. Although hypoxemia can lead to tissue hypoxia, tissue hypoxia can result from other abnormalities unrelated to alterations of pulmonary function, such as low cardiac output or cyanide poisoning.

Hypoxemia results from problems with one or more of the major mechanisms of oxygenation:
1. Oxygen delivery to the alveoli
   a. Oxygen content of the inspired air (FiO_2)
   b. Ventilation of alveoli

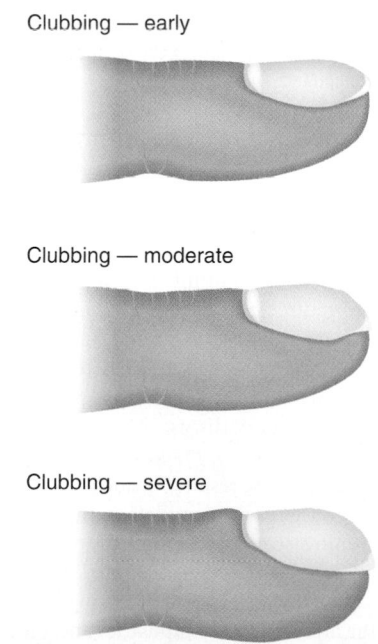

Clubbing — early

Clubbing — moderate

Clubbing — severe

FIGURE 27-1 Clubbing of Fingers Caused by Chronic Hypoxemia. (Modified from Seidel HM et al: *Mosby's guide to physical examination,* ed 7, St Louis, 2011, Mosby.)

2. Diffusion of oxygen from the alveoli into the blood
   a. Balance between alveolar ventilation and perfusion ($\dot{V}/\dot{Q}$ match)
   b. Diffusion of oxygen across the alveolar capillary barrier
3. Perfusion of pulmonary capillaries

The amount of oxygen in the alveoli is called the $P_{A}O_2$ and is dependent on two factors. The first factor is the presence of adequate oxygen content of the inspired air. The amount of oxygen in inspired air is expressed as the percentage or fraction of air that is composed of oxygen, called the Fio_2. The Fio_2 of air at sea level is approximately 21% or 0.21. Anything that decreases the Fio_2 (such as high altitude) decreases the $P_{A}O_2$. A second factor is the amount of alveolar minute volume (tidal volume × respiratory rate). Hypoventilation results in an increase in $P_{A}CO_2$ and a decrease in $P_{A}O_2$ such that there is less oxygen available in the alveoli for diffusion into the blood. This type of hypoxemia can be completely corrected if alveolar ventilation is improved by increases in the rate and depth of breathing. Hypoventilation causes hypoxemia in unconscious persons; in persons with neurologic, muscular, or bone diseases that restrict chest expansion; and in individuals who have chronic obstructive pulmonary disease.

Diffusion of oxygen from the alveoli into the blood is also dependent on two factors. The first is the balance between the amount of air that enters alveoli ($\dot{V}$) and the amount of blood perfusing the capillaries around the alveoli ($\dot{Q}$). An abnormal ventilation-perfusion ratio ($\dot{V}/\dot{Q}$) is the most common cause of hypoxemia (Figure 27-2). The normal $\dot{V}/\dot{Q}$ is 0.8 because perfusion is somewhat greater than ventilation in the lung bases and because some blood is normally shunted to the bronchial circulation. $\dot{V}/\dot{Q}$ mismatch refers to an abnormal distribution of ventilation and perfusion. Hypoxemia can be caused by inadequate ventilation of well-perfused areas of the lung (low $\dot{V}/\dot{Q}$). Mismatching of this type, called shunting, occurs in atelectasis, in asthma as a result of bronchoconstriction, and in pulmonary edema and pneumonia when alveoli are filled with fluid. When blood passes through portions of the pulmonary capillary bed that receive no ventilation, the pulmonary capillaries in that area constrict and a right-to-left shunt occurs, resulting in decreased systemic Pao_2 and

hypoxemia. Hypoxemia also can be caused by poor perfusion of well-ventilated portions of the lung (high $\dot{V}/\dot{Q}$), resulting in wasted ventilation. The most common cause of high $\dot{V}/\dot{Q}$ is a pulmonary embolus that impairs blood flow to a segment of the lung. An area where alveoli are ventilated but not perfused is termed alveolar dead space.

The second factor affecting diffusion of oxygen from the alveoli into the blood is the alveolocapillary membrane. Diffusion of oxygen through the alveolocapillary membrane is impaired if the membrane is thickened or the surface area available for diffusion is decreased. Thickened alveolocapillary membranes, as occur with edema (tissue swelling) and fibrosis (formation of fibrous lesions), increase the time required for oxygen to diffuse from the alveoli into the capillaries. If diffusion is slowed enough, the Po_2 levels of alveolar gas and capillary blood do not have time to equilibrate during the fraction of a second that blood remains in the capillary. Destruction of alveoli, as in emphysema, decreases the alveolocapillary membrane surface area available for diffusion. Hypercapnia is seldom produced by impaired diffusion because carbon dioxide diffuses so easily from capillary to alveolus that the individual with impaired diffusion would die from hypoxemia before hypercapnia could occur.

Hypoxemia can result from blood flow bypassing the lungs. This can occur because of intracardiac defects that cause right-to-left shunting or because of intrapulmonary arteriovenous malformations.

Hypoxemia is most often associated with a compensatory hyperventilation and the resultant respiratory alkalosis (i.e., decreased $Paco_2$ and increased pH). However, in individuals with associated ventilatory difficulties, hypoxemia may be complicated by hypercapnia and respiratory acidosis. Hypoxemia results in widespread tissue dysfunction and, when severe, can lead to organ infarction. In addition, hypoxic pulmonary vasoconstriction can contribute to increased pressures in the pulmonary artery (pulmonary artery hypertension) and lead to right heart failure or *cor pulmonale*. Clinical manifestations of acute hypoxemia may include cyanosis, confusion, tachycardia, edema, and decreased renal output.

✔ QUICK CHECK 27-1
1. List the primary signs and symptoms of pulmonary disease.
2. What abnormal breathing patterns are seen with pulmonary disease?
3. What mechanisms produce hypercapnia?
4. What mechanisms produce hypoxemia?

Acute Respiratory Failure

Respiratory failure is defined as inadequate gas exchange such that $Pao_2 \leq 60$ mm Hg or $Paco_2 \geq 50$ mm Hg, with pH ≤ 7.25.[10] Respiratory failure can result from direct injury to the lungs, airways, or chest wall or indirectly because of disease or injury involving another body system, such as the brain, spinal cord, or heart. It can occur in individuals who have an otherwise normal respiratory system or in those with underlying chronic pulmonary disease. Most pulmonary diseases can cause episodes of acute respiratory failure. If the respiratory failure is primarily hypercapnic, it is the result of inadequate alveolar ventilation and the individual must receive ventilatory support, such as with a bag-valve mask, noninvasive positive pressure ventilation, or intubation and placement on mechanical ventilation. If the respiratory failure is primarily hypoxemic, it is the result of inadequate exchange of oxygen between the alveoli and the capillaries and the individual must receive supplemental oxygen therapy. Many people will have combined hypercapnic and hypoxemic respiratory failure and will require both kinds of support.

FIGURE 27-2 Ventilation-Perfusion ($\dot{V}/\dot{Q}$) Abnormalities.

Respiratory failure is an important potential complication of any major surgical procedure, especially those that involve the central nervous system, thorax, or upper abdomen. The most common postoperative pulmonary problems are atelectasis, pneumonia, pulmonary edema, and pulmonary emboli. People who smoke are at risk, particularly if they have preexisting lung disease. Limited cardiac reserve, neurologic disease, chronic renal failure, chronic hepatic disease, and infection also increase the tendency to develop postoperative respiratory failure.

Prevention of postoperative respiratory failure includes frequent turning and position changes, deep-breathing exercises, and early ambulation to prevent atelectasis and accumulation of secretions. Humidification of inspired air can help loosen secretions. Incentive spirometry gives individuals immediate feedback about tidal volumes, which encourages them to breathe deeply. Supplemental oxygen is given for hypoxemia, and antibiotics are given as appropriate to treat infection. If respiratory failure develops, the individual may require mechanical ventilation or extracorporeal membrane oxygenation.

Disorders of the Chest Wall and Pleura

There are many conditions that can affect the chest wall or pleura, or both, and influence the function of the respiratory system. Chest wall disorders primarily affect tidal volume and, therefore, result in hypercapnia. Pleural diseases impact both ventilation and oxygenation.

Chest Wall Restriction

If the chest wall is deformed, traumatized, immobilized, or heavy from the accumulation of fat, the work of breathing increases and ventilation may be compromised because of a decrease in tidal volume. The degree of ventilatory impairment depends on the severity of the chest wall abnormality. Grossly obese individuals are often dyspneic on exertion or when recumbent. Individuals with severe kyphoscoliosis (lateral bending and rotation of the spinal column, with distortion of the thoracic cage) often present with dyspnea on exertion that can progress to respiratory failure. Obesity and kyphoscoliosis are risk factors for respiratory failure or infections in individuals admitted to the hospital for other problems, particularly those who require surgery. Other musculoskeletal abnormalities that can impair ventilation are ankylosing spondylitis (see Chapter 39) and pectus excavatum (a deformity characterized by depression of the sternum).

Impairment of respiratory muscle function caused by neuromuscular diseases such as poliomyelitis, muscular dystrophy, myasthenia gravis, and Guillain-Barré syndrome (see Chapter 16) also can restrict the chest wall and impair pulmonary function. Muscle weakness can result in hypoventilation, inability to remove secretions, and hypoxemia.

Pain from chest wall injury, surgery, or disease can cause significant hypoventilation, especially in those with underlying lung disease. Trauma to the thorax not only can restrict chest expansion because of pain but also can cause structural and mechanical changes that impair the ability of the chest to expand normally. **Flail chest** results from the fracture of several consecutive ribs in more than one place or fracture of the sternum and several consecutive ribs. These multiple fractures result in instability of a portion of the chest wall, causing paradoxical movement of the chest with breathing. During inspiration the unstable portion of the chest wall moves inward and during expiration it moves outward, impairing movement of gas in and out of the lungs (Figure 27-3).

Chest wall restriction results in a decrease in tidal volume. An increase in respiratory rate can compensate for small decreases in tidal volume, but many individuals will progress to hypercapnic respiratory failure. Diagnosis of chest wall restriction is made by pulmonary

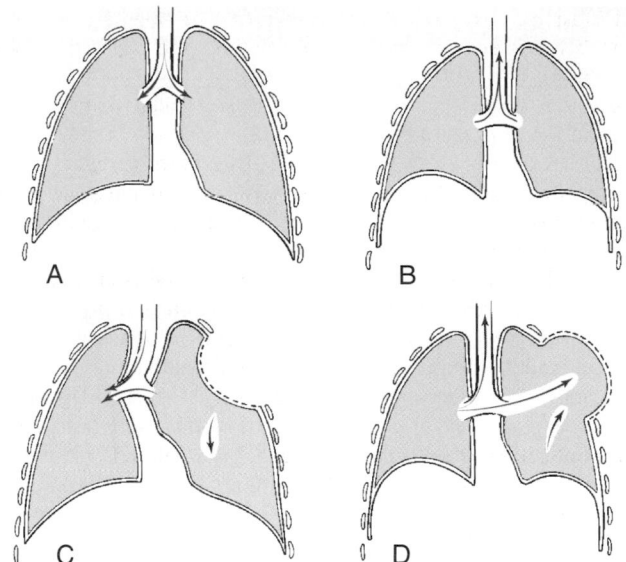

FIGURE 27-3 Flail Chest. Normal respiration: **A,** inspiration; **B,** expiration. Paradoxical motion: **C,** inspiration, area of lung underlying unstable chest wall flattens on inspiration; **D,** expiration, unstable area inflates. Note movement of mediastinum toward opposite lung during inspiration.

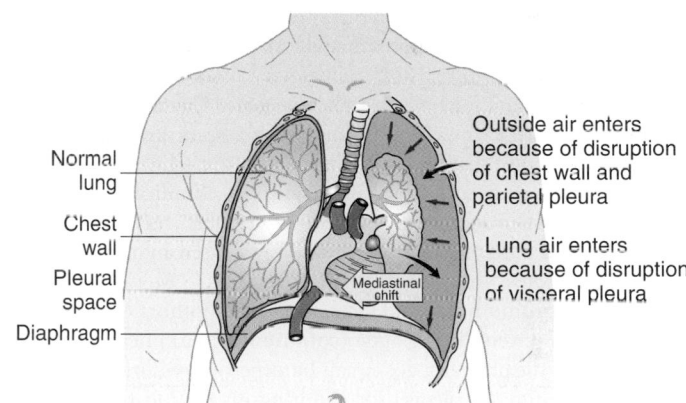

FIGURE 27-4 Pneumothorax. Air in the pleural space causes the lung to collapse around the hilus and may push mediastinal contents (heart and great vessels) toward the other lung.

function testing (reduction in forced vital capacity [FVC]), arterial blood gas measurement (hypercapnia), and radiographs. Treatment is aimed at any reversible underlying cause but is otherwise supportive. In severe cases, mechanical ventilation may be indicated.

Pleural Abnormalities
Pneumothorax

Pneumothorax is the presence of air or gas in the pleural space caused by a rupture in the visceral pleura (which surrounds the lungs) or the parietal pleura and chest wall. As air separates the visceral and parietal pleurae, it destroys the negative pressure of the pleural space and disrupts the equilibrium between elastic recoil forces of the lung and chest wall. The lung then tends to recoil by collapsing toward the hilum (Figure 27-4).

Primary (spontaneous) pneumothorax occurs unexpectedly in healthy individuals (usually men) between 20 and 40 years of age and is caused by the spontaneous rupture of blebs (blister-like formations)

TABLE 27-1 Mechanism of Pleural Effusion*

Type of Fluid/Effusion	Source of Accumulation	Primary or Associated Disorder
Transudate (hydrothorax)	Watery fluid that diffuses out of capillaries beneath pleura (i.e., capillaries in lung or chest wall)	Cardiovascular disease that causes high pulmonary capillary pressures; liver or kidney disease that disrupts plasma protein production, causing hypoproteinemia (decreased oncotic pressure in blood vessels)
Exudate	Fluid rich in cells and proteins (leukocytes, plasma proteins of all kinds; see Chapter 5) that migrates out of capillaries	Infection, inflammation, or malignancy of pleura that stimulates mast cells to release biochemical mediators that increase capillary permeability
Pus (empyema)	Microorganisms and debris of infection (leukocytes, cellular debris) accumulate in pleural space	Pulmonary infections, such as pneumonia; lung abscesses; infected wounds
Blood (hemothorax)	Hemorrhage into pleural space	Traumatic injury, surgery, rupture, or malignancy that damages blood vessels
Chyle (chylothorax)	Chyle (milky fluid containing lymph and fat droplets) that moves from lymphatic vessels into pleural space instead of passing from gastrointestinal tract to thoracic duct	Traumatic injury, infection, or disorder that disrupts lymphatic transport

*The principles of diffusion are described in Chapter 1; mechanisms that increase capillary permeability and cause exudation of cells, proteins, and fluid are discussed in Chapter 5.

on the visceral pleura. Bleb rupture can occur during sleep, rest, or exercise. The ruptured blebs are usually located in the apexes of the lungs. The cause of bleb formation is not known, although more than 80% of these individuals have been found to have emphysema-like changes in their lungs even if they have no history of smoking or no known genetic disorder. Approximately 10% of affected individuals have a significant family history of primary pneumothorax that has been linked to mutations in the folliculin gene.[11] *Secondary pneumothorax* can be caused by chest trauma (such as a rib fracture or stab and bullet wounds that tear the pleura; rupture of a bleb or bulla [larger vesicle], as occurs in emphysema; or mechanical ventilation, particularly if it includes positive end-expiratory pressure [PEEP]). *Iatrogenic pneumothorax* is most commonly caused by transthoracic needle aspiration.

Primary pneumothorax and secondary pneumothorax can present as either open or tension. In open (communicating) pneumothorax, air pressure in the pleural space equals barometric pressure because air that is drawn into the pleural space during inspiration (through the damaged chest wall and parietal pleura or through the lungs and damaged visceral pleura) is forced back out during expiration. In tension pneumothorax, however, the site of pleural rupture acts as a one-way valve, permitting air to enter on inspiration but preventing its escape by closing during expiration. As more and more air enters the pleural space, air pressure in the pneumothorax begins to exceed barometric pressure. Air pressure in the pleural space pushes against the already recoiled lung, causing compression atelectasis, and against the mediastinum, compressing and displacing the heart, great vessels, and trachea (*mediastinal shift*). The pathophysiologic effects of tension pneumothorax are life-threatening (see Figure 27-4).

Clinical manifestations of spontaneous or secondary pneumothorax begin with sudden pleural pain, tachypnea, and dyspnea. Depending on the size of the pneumothorax, physical examination may reveal absent or decreased breath sounds and hyperresonance to percussion on the affected side. Tension pneumothorax may be complicated by severe hypoxemia, tracheal deviation away from the affected lung, and hypotension (low blood pressure). Deterioration occurs rapidly and immediate treatment is required. Diagnosis of pneumothorax is made with chest radiographs, ultrasound, and computed tomography (CT). Pneumothorax is treated by aspiration, usually with insertion of a chest tube that is attached to a water-seal drainage system with suction or a small-bore catheter with a one-way valve.[12] After the pneumothorax is evacuated and the pleural rupture is healed, the chest tube is removed. For individuals with persistent air leaks, other interventions may be needed including thoracoscopic surgical techniques or pleurodesis (instillation of a caustic substance, such as talc, into the pleural space).

Pleural Effusion

Pleural effusion is the presence of fluid in the pleural space. The source of the fluid is usually from blood vessels or lymphatic vessels lying beneath the pleural space, but occasionally an abscess or other lesion may drain into the pleural space. Pleural effusions that enter the pleural space from intact blood vessels can be transudative (watery) or exudative (high concentrations of white blood cells and plasma proteins). Other types of pleural effusion are characterized by the presence of pus (empyema), blood (hemothorax), or chyle (chylothorax). Mechanisms of pleural effusion are summarized in Table 27-1.

Small collections of fluid may not affect lung function and remain undetected. Most will be removed by the lymphatic system once the underlying condition is resolved. In larger effusions, dyspnea, compression atelectasis with impaired ventilation, and pleural pain are common. Mediastinal shift and cardiovascular manifestations occur in a large, rapidly developing effusion. Physical examination shows decreased breath sounds and dullness to percussion on the affected side. A pleural friction rub can be heard over areas of inflamed pleura.

Diagnosis is confirmed by chest x-ray and thoracentesis (needle aspiration), which can determine the type of effusion and provide symptomatic relief. If the effusion is large, drainage usually requires the placement of a chest tube and surgical interventions may be needed to prevent recurrence of the effusion.

Empyema

Empyema (infected pleural effusion) is the presence of pus in the pleural space and develops when the pulmonary lymphatics become blocked, leading to an outpouring of contaminated lymphatic fluid into the pleural space. Empyema occurs most commonly in older adults and children and usually develops as a complication of pneumonia, surgery, trauma, or bronchial obstruction from a tumor. Commonly documented infectious organisms include *Staphylococcus aureus*, *Escherichia coli*, anaerobic bacteria, and *Klebsiella pneumoniae*.

Individuals with empyema present clinically with cyanosis, fever, tachycardia (rapid heart rate), cough, and pleural pain. Breath sounds are decreased directly over the empyema. Diagnosis is made by chest radiographs, thoracentesis, and sputum culture. The treatment for empyema includes the administration of appropriate antimicrobials and drainage of the pleural space with a chest tube. In severe cases, ultrasound-guided pleural drainage, instillation of fibrinolytic agents, or introduction of deoxyribonuclease (DNase) into the pleural space is needed for adequate drainage. Surgical debridement may be required.[13]

> ✔ **QUICK CHECK 27-2**
> 1. How does chest wall restriction affect ventilation?
> 2. How does pneumothorax differ from pleural effusion?
> 3. What causes empyema?

PULMONARY DISORDERS

Restrictive Lung Diseases

Restrictive lung diseases are characterized by decreased compliance of the lung tissue. This means that it takes more effort to expand the lungs during inspiration, which increases the work of breathing. Individuals with lung restriction have dyspnea, an increased respiratory rate, and a decreased tidal volume. Pulmonary function testing reveals a decrease in FVC. Restrictive lung diseases can cause $\dot{V}/\dot{Q}$ mismatch and affect the alveolocapillary membrane, which reduces the diffusion of oxygen from the alveoli into the blood and results in hypoxemia. Some of the most common restrictive lung diseases in adults are aspiration, atelectasis, bronchiectasis, bronchiolitis, pulmonary fibrosis, inhalation disorders, pneumoconiosis, allergic alveolitis, pulmonary edema, and acute respiratory distress syndrome.

Aspiration

Aspiration is the passage of fluid and solid particles into the lung. It tends to occur in individuals whose normal swallowing mechanism and cough reflex are impaired by central or peripheral nervous system abnormalities. Predisposing factors include an altered level of consciousness caused by substance abuse, sedation, or anesthesia; seizure disorders; stroke; neuromuscular disorders that cause dysphagia; and feeding through a nasogastric tube. The right lung, particularly the right lower lobe, is more susceptible to aspiration than the left lung because the branching angle of the right mainstem bronchus is straighter than the branching angle of the left mainstem bronchus.

Aspiration of large food particles or gastric fluid with pH of less than 2.5 has serious consequences. Solid food particles can obstruct a bronchus, resulting in bronchial inflammation and collapse of airways distal to the obstruction. If the aspirated solid is not identified and removed by bronchoscopy, a chronic, local inflammation develops that may lead to recurrent infection and bronchiectasis (permanent dilation of the bronchus).

Aspiration of oral or pharyngeal secretions can lead to aspiration pneumonia. Intubation of the trachea also can cause aspiration and bacterial pneumonia. Aspiration of acidic gastric fluid may cause severe pneumonitis. Bronchial damage includes inflammation, loss of ciliary function, and bronchospasm. In the alveoli, acidic fluid damages the alveolocapillary membrane. This allows plasma and blood cells to move from capillaries into the alveoli, resulting in hemorrhagic pneumonitis. The lung becomes stiff and noncompliant as surfactant production is disrupted, leading to further edema and collapse.

Hypoventilation may develop as this process progresses and systematic complications, such as hypotension, may occur.

Clinical manifestations of aspiration include the sudden onset of choking and intractable cough with or without vomiting, fever, dyspnea, and wheezing. Some individuals have no symptoms acutely; instead they have recurrent lung infections, chronic cough, or persistent wheezing over months and even years.

Preventive measures for individuals at risk are more effective than treatment of known aspiration. The most important preventive measures include use of a semirecumbent position, surveillance of enteral feeding, use of promotility agents, and avoidance of excessive sedation. Nasogastric tubes, which are often used to remove stomach contents, are used to prevent aspiration but also can cause aspiration if fluid and particulate matter are regurgitated as the tube is being placed.

Treatment of aspiration pneumonitis includes use of supplemental oxygen and mechanical ventilation with positive end-expiratory pressure (PEEP) and administration of corticosteroids. Fluids are restricted to decrease blood volume and minimize pulmonary edema. Bacterial pneumonia may develop as a complication of aspiration pneumonitis and must be treated with broad-spectrum antimicrobials.

Atelectasis

Atelectasis is the collapse of lung tissue. There are three types of atelectasis:

1. **Compression atelectasis** is caused by external pressure exerted by tumor, fluid, or air in the pleural space or by abdominal distention pressing on a portion of lung, causing alveoli to collapse.
2. **Absorption atelectasis** results from removal of air from obstructed or hypoventilated alveoli or from inhalation of concentrated oxygen or anesthetic agents.
3. **Surfactant impairment** results from decreased production or inactivation of surfactant, which is necessary to reduce surface tension in the alveoli and thus prevent lung collapse during expiration. Surfactant impairment can occur because of premature birth, acute respiratory distress syndrome, anesthesia induction, or mechanical ventilation.

Atelectasis tends to occur after surgery, especially in those who have been administered general anesthetics.[14] Postoperative individuals are often in pain, breathe shallowly, are reluctant to change position, and produce viscous secretions that tend to pool in dependent portions of the lung, especially following thoracic or upper abdominal surgery. Atelectasis increases shunt, decreases compliance, and may lead to perioperative hypoxemia.

Clinical manifestations of atelectasis are similar to those of pulmonary infection including dyspnea, cough, fever, and leukocytosis. Prevention and treatment of postoperative atelectasis usually include deep-breathing exercises (often with the aid of an incentive spirometer), frequent position changes, and early ambulation. Deep breathing promotes ciliary clearance of secretions, stabilizes the alveoli by redistributing surfactant, and promotes collateral ventilation through the *pores of Kohn*, promoting expansion of collapsed alveoli (Figure 27-5). Postoperative noninvasive positive-pressure ventilation (NIPPV) has been shown to improve oxygenation and ventilation for high-risk individuals (i.e., individuals who are obese or in respiratory distress).

Bronchiectasis

Bronchiectasis is persistent abnormal dilation of the bronchi. There may be a genetic predisposition or a defect in host defense.[15] It usually occurs in conjunction with other respiratory conditions that are associated with chronic bronchial inflammation, such as obstruction of an airway with mucous plugs, atelectasis, aspiration of a foreign body, infection, cystic fibrosis (see Chapter 28), tuberculosis, congenital

FIGURE 27-5 Pores of Kohn. A, Absorption atelectasis caused by lack of collateral ventilation through pores of Kohn. **B,** Restoration of collateral ventilation during deep breathing.

weakness of the bronchial wall, or immunocompromised health status. Chronic inflammation of the bronchi leads to destruction of elastic and muscular components of their walls, obstruction of the bronchial lumen, traction from adjacent fibrosis, and permanent dilation. Bronchiectasis also is associated with a number of systemic disorders, such as rheumatologic disease, inflammatory bowel disease, and immunodeficiency syndromes (e.g., acquired immunodeficiency syndrome [AIDS]). There may be no known cause.

The primary symptom of bronchiectasis is a chronic productive cough that may date back to a childhood illness or infection. The disease is commonly associated with recurrent lower respiratory tract infections and expectoration of voluminous amounts of foul-smelling purulent sputum (measured in cupfuls). Hemoptysis and clubbing of the fingers (from chronic hypoxemia) are common. Pulmonary function studies show decreases in FVC and expiratory flow rates. Hypoxemia eventually leads to cor pulmonale (see p. 708). Diagnosis is usually confirmed by the use of high-resolution computed tomography. Bronchiectasis is treated with sputum culture, antibiotics, anti-inflammatory drugs, bronchodilators, chest physiotherapy, and supplemental oxygen.

Bronchiolitis

Bronchiolitis is a diffuse, inflammatory obstruction of the small airways or bronchioles occurring most commonly in children. In adults it usually occurs with chronic bronchitis but can occur in otherwise healthy individuals in association with an upper or lower respiratory tract viral infection or with inhalation of toxic gases, or be of unknown etiology.[16] Bronchiolitis also is a serious complication of stem cell and lung transplantation and can progress to **bronchiolitis obliterans**, a fibrotic process that occludes airways and causes permanent scarring of the lungs. **Bronchiolitis obliterans organizing pneumonia (BOOP)** is a complication of bronchiolitis obliterans in which the alveoli and bronchioles become filled with plugs of connective tissue.

Clinical manifestations include a rapid ventilatory rate; marked use of accessory muscles; low-grade fever; dry, nonproductive cough; and hyperinflated chest. A decrease in the ventilation-perfusion ratio results in hypoxemia. Diagnosis is made by spirometry and bronchoscopy with biopsy. Bronchiolitis is treated with appropriate antibiotics,

corticosteroids, immunosuppressive agents, and chest physical therapy (humidified air administration, coughing and deep-breathing exercises, postural drainage).

Pulmonary Fibrosis

Pulmonary fibrosis is an excessive amount of fibrous or connective tissue in the lung. Pulmonary fibrosis can be caused by formation of scar tissue after active pulmonary disease (e.g., acute respiratory distress syndrome, tuberculosis), in association with a variety of autoimmune disorders (e.g., rheumatoid arthritis, progressive systemic sclerosis, sarcoidosis), or by inhalation of harmful substances (e.g., coal dust, asbestos). Chronic inflammation leads to fibrosis and causes a marked loss of lung compliance. The lung becomes stiff and difficult to ventilate, and the diffusing capacity of the alveolocapillary membrane may decrease, causing hypoxemia. Diffuse pulmonary fibrosis has a poor prognosis.

Pulmonary fibrosis is known as idiopathic pulmonary fibrosis when there is no specific cause. **Idiopathic pulmonary fibrosis (IPF)** is the most common idiopathic interstitial lung disorder. It is more common in men than in women and most cases occur after age 60. Although IPF is characterized by chronic inflammation, recent studies suggest that it results from multiple injuries at different lung sites with aberrant healing responses to alveolar epithelial cell injury, which probably occurs in response to a combination of environmental insults and genetic predispositions.[17] Fibroproliferation of the interstitial lung tissue around the alveoli causes decreased oxygen diffusion across the alveolocapillary membrane and hypoxemia. As the disease progresses, decreased lung compliance leads to increased work of breathing, decreased tidal volume, and resultant hypoventilation with hypercapnia.

The primary symptom of IPF is increasing dyspnea on exertion. Physical examination reveals diffuse inspiratory crackles. The diagnosis is confirmed by pulmonary function testing (decreased FVC), high-resolution computed tomography, and lung biopsy. Treatment includes oxygen, corticosteroids, and cytotoxic drugs, although success rates are low and toxicities are high. Newer therapies include antifibrotic drugs (*N*-acetylcysteine, pirfenidone), nintedanib (angiogenesis inhibitor), interferon, and anticoagulation therapy.[18] Selected individuals may benefit from lung transplantation.

Inhalation Disorders

Exposure to toxic gases. Inhalation of gaseous irritants can cause significant respiratory dysfunction. Commonly encountered toxic gases include smoke, ammonia, hydrogen chloride, sulfur dioxide, chlorine, phosgene, and nitrogen dioxide. Inhalation injuries in burns can include toxic gases from household or industrial combustants, heat, and smoke particles. Inhaled toxic particles cause damage to the airway epithelium and promote mucus secretion, inflammation, mucosal edema, ciliary damage, pulmonary edema, and surfactant inactivation. The cellular effects of toxic gases and polluted air are described in Chapter 4. Acute toxic inhalation is frequently complicated by acute respiratory distress syndrome (ARDS) and pneumonia. Initial symptoms include burning of the eyes, nose, and throat; coughing; chest tightness; and dyspnea. Hypoxemia is common. Treatment includes administration of supplemental oxygen, mechanical ventilation with PEEP, and support of the cardiovascular system. Corticosteroids are sometimes used, although their effectiveness has not been well documented. Most individuals respond quickly to therapy. Some, however, may improve initially and then deteriorate as a result of bronchiectasis or bronchiolitis.

Prolonged exposure to high concentrations of supplemental oxygen can result in a relatively rare condition known as oxygen toxicity. The basic underlying mechanism of injury is a severe inflammatory response mediated by oxygen free radicals. Damage to alveolocapillary membranes results in disruption of surfactant production, production of interstitial and alveolar edema, and a reduction in lung compliance. In infants this can lead to a condition known as bronchopulmonary dysplasia in which there is severe scarring of the lung. Treatment involves ventilatory support and a reduction of inspired oxygen concentration to less than 60% as soon as tolerated.

Pneumoconiosis. Pneumoconiosis represents any change in the lung caused by inhalation of inorganic dust particles, usually occurring in the workplace. As in all cases of environmentally acquired lung disease, the individual's history of exposure is important in determining the diagnosis. Pneumoconiosis often occurs after years of exposure to the offending dust, with progressive fibrosis of lung tissue.

The dusts of silica, asbestos, and coal are the most common causes of pneumoconiosis. Others include talc, fiberglass, clays, mica, slate, cement, cadmium, beryllium, tungsten, cobalt, aluminum, and iron. Deposition of these materials in the lungs causes the release of proinflammatory cytokines. This leads to chronic inflammation with scarring of the alveolocapillary membrane, resulting in pulmonary fibrosis and progressive pulmonary deterioration. Clinical manifestations with advancement of disease include cough, chronic sputum production, dyspnea, decreased lung volumes, and hypoxemia. In most cases, diagnosis is confirmed by performing chest x-ray or CT and obtaining a complete occupational history. Treatment is usually palliative and focuses on preventing further exposure and improving working conditions, along with pulmonary rehabilitation and management of associated hypoxemia and bronchospasm.

Hypersensitivity pneumonitis. Hypersensitivity pneumonitis (extrinsic allergic alveolitis) is an allergic, inflammatory disease of the lungs caused by inhalation of organic particles or fumes. Many allergens can cause this disorder, including grains, silage, bird droppings or feathers, wood dust (particularly redwood and maple), cork dust, animal pelts, coffee beans, fish meal, mushroom compost, and molds that grow on sugarcane, barley, and straw. The lung inflammation is a hypersensitivity response that occurs after repeated, prolonged exposure to the allergen causing pneumonitis. Lymphocytes and inflammatory cells infiltrate the interstitial lung tissue, releasing a variety of autoimmune and inflammatory cytokines.[19]

Hypersensitivity pneumonitis can be acute, subacute, or chronic. The acute form causes fever, cough, and chills a few hours after exposure. With continued exposure, the disease becomes chronic and pulmonary fibrosis develops. Diagnosis is made by obtaining a history of allergen exposure and by performing serum antibody testing, chest x-ray, bronchoalveolar lavage, CT, and, in some cases, lung biopsy. Treatment consists of removal of the offending agent and administration of corticosteroids.[20]

Pulmonary Edema

Pulmonary edema is excess water in the lung. The normal lung is kept dry by lymphatic drainage and a balance among capillary hydrostatic pressure, capillary oncotic pressure, and capillary permeability. In addition, surfactant lining the alveoli repels water, keeping fluid from entering the alveoli. Predisposing factors for pulmonary edema include heart disease, acute respiratory distress syndrome, and inhalation of toxic gases. The pathogenesis of pulmonary edema is shown in Figure 27-6.

The most common cause of pulmonary edema is left-sided heart disease. When the left ventricle fails, filling pressures on the left side of the heart increase and cause a concomitant increase in pulmonary capillary hydrostatic pressure. When the hydrostatic pressure exceeds the oncotic pressure (which holds fluid in the capillary), fluid moves from the capillary into the interstitial space (the space within the alveolar septum between the alveolus and capillary). When the flow of fluid out of the capillaries exceeds the lymphatic system's ability to remove it, pulmonary edema develops.

Another cause of pulmonary edema is capillary injury that increases capillary permeability, as in cases of adult respiratory distress syndrome or inhalation of toxic gases, such as ammonia. Capillary injury and inflammation causes water and plasma proteins to leak out of the capillary and move into the interstitial space, increasing the interstitial oncotic pressure (which is usually very low). As the interstitial oncotic pressure begins to exceed the capillary oncotic pressure, water moves out of the capillary and into the lung. (Mechanisms of edema are discussed in Chapter 5, Figures 5-1 and 5-2.) Pulmonary edema also can result from obstruction of the lymphatic system by tumors and fibrotic tissue and by increased systemic venous pressure.

Clinical manifestations of pulmonary edema include dyspnea, hypoxemia, and increased work of breathing. Physical examination may disclose inspiratory crackles (rales) and dullness to percussion over the lung bases. In severe edema, pink frothy sputum is expectorated, hypoxemia worsens, and hypoventilation with hypercapnia may develop.

The treatment of pulmonary edema depends on its cause. If the edema is caused by increased hydrostatic pressure resulting from heart failure, therapy is directed toward improving cardiac output with diuretics, vasodilators, and drugs that improve the contraction of the heart muscle. If edema is the result of increased capillary permeability resulting from injury, the treatment is focused on removing the offending agent and implementing supportive therapy to maintain adequate ventilation and circulation. Individuals with either type of pulmonary edema require supplemental oxygen. Mechanical ventilation may be needed if edema significantly impairs ventilation and oxygenation.

Acute Lung Injury/Acute Respiratory Distress Syndrome

Acute lung injury (ALI)/acute respiratory distress syndrome (ARDS) represents a spectrum of acute lung inflammation and diffuse alveolocapillary injury. Both ALI and ARDS are defined as (1) the acute onset of bilateral infiltrates on chest radiograph, (2) a low ratio of

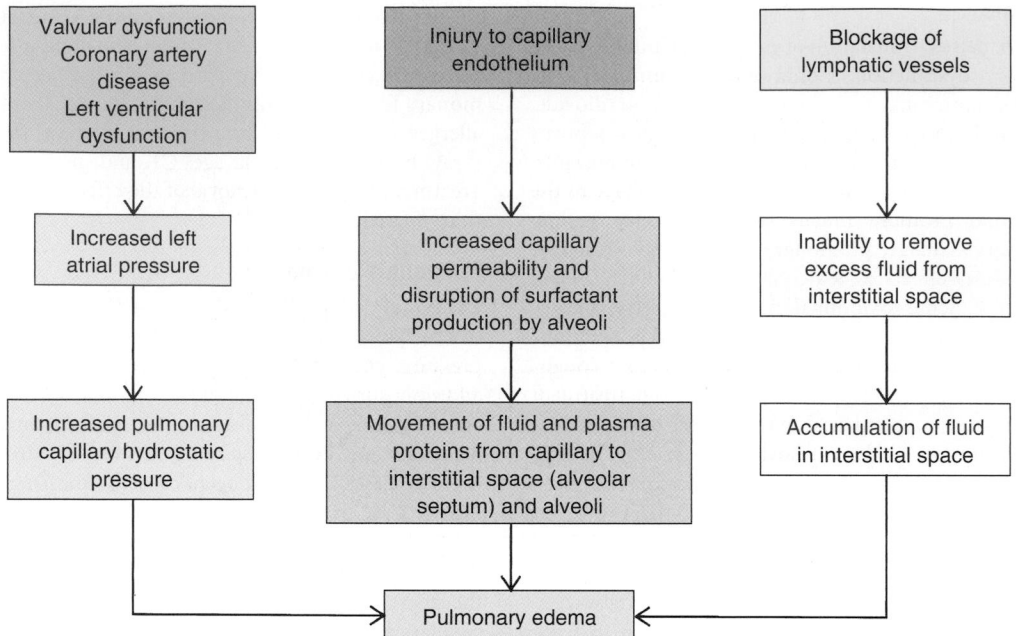

FIGURE 27-6 Pathogenesis of Pulmonary Edema.

partial pressure of arterial oxygen to the fraction of inhaled oxygen under positive airway pressure, and (3) is not derived from hydrostatic pulmonary edema. Biomarkers that can be used to diagnose ARDS are under investigation.[21] In the United States more than 30% of intensive care unit (ICU) admissions are complicated by ARDS. Advances in therapy have decreased overall mortality in people younger than 60 years to approximately 40%, although mortality in older adults and those with severe infections remains much higher. The most common predisposing factors are genetic factors, sepsis, and multiple trauma. There are many other causes, including pneumonia, burns, aspiration, cardiopulmonary bypass surgery, pancreatitis, blood transfusions, drug overdose, inhalation of smoke or noxious gases, fat emboli, high concentrations of supplemental oxygen, radiation therapy, and disseminated intravascular coagulation.

PATHOPHYSIOLOGY   All disorders causing ALI/ARDS cause acute injury to the alveolocapillary membrane, producing massive pulmonary inflammation, increased capillary permeability, severe pulmonary edema, shunting, $\dot{V}/\dot{Q}$ mismatch, and hypoxemia. ARDS can occur directly (from aspiration of highly acidic gastric contents, inhalation of toxic gases) or indirectly (from circulating inflammatory mediators released in response to systemic disorders, such as sepsis and trauma). Lung injury and inflammation damages the alveolocapillary membrane, causing pulmonary edema, often referred to as *noncardiogenic pulmonary edema*. ARDS progresses through three overlapping phases characterized by histologic changes in the lung: exudative (inflammatory), proliferative, and fibrotic[22,23] (Figure 27-7). The three phases are described as follows:

Exudative phase (within 72 hours): activation of neutrophils and other cells (platelets, macrophages, lung epithelial and endothelial cells) that release a cascade of inflammatory cytokines causing damage to the alveolocapillary membrane and greatly increased capillary membrane permeability. Fluids, proteins, and blood cells leak from the capillary bed into the pulmonary interstitium and flood the alveoli (hemorrhagic exudate). Surfactant is inactivated. The resulting pulmonary edema and hemorrhage severely reduce lung

compliance and impair alveolar ventilation. The inflammatory mediators also cause pulmonary vasoconstriction, contributing to ventilation/perfusion mismatch. The inflammatory mediators causing the alveolocapillary damage of ARDS often cause inflammation, endothelial damage, and capillary permeability throughout the body, resulting in systemic inflammatory response syndrome (SIRS). SIRS then leads to multiple organ dysfunction syndrome (MODS) and may cause death (see Chapter 24 and Figure 24-46).

Proliferative phase (within 4 to 21 days): after the initial lung injury, resolution of the pulmonary edema and proliferation of type II pneumocytes, fibroblasts, and myofibroblasts. The intra-alveolar hemorrhagic exudate becomes a cellular granulation tissue appearing as hyaline membranes and there is progressive hypoxemia.

Fibrotic phase (within 14 to 21 days): remodeling and fibrosis of lung tissue. The fibrosis progressively obliterates the alveoli, respiratory bronchioles, and interstitium, leading to a decrease in functional residual capacity (FRC) and continuing $\dot{V}/\dot{Q}$ mismatch with severe right-to-left shunt. The result of this overwhelming inflammatory response by the lungs is acute respiratory failure.

CLINICAL MANIFESTATIONS   The clinical manifestations of ARDS are progressive as follows:

1. Dyspnea and hypoxemia with poor response to oxygen supplementation
2. Hyperventilation and respiratory alkalosis
3. Decreased tissue perfusion, metabolic acidosis, and organ dysfunction
4. Increased work of breathing, decreased tidal volume, and hypoventilation
5. Hypercapnia, respiratory acidosis, and worsening hypoxemia
6. Respiratory failure, decreased cardiac output, hypotension, and death

EVALUATION AND TREATMENT   Diagnosis is based on a history of the lung injury, physical examination, blood gas analysis, and radiologic examination. Measurement of serum biomarkers (i.e., surfactant

FIGURE 27-7 Pathogenesis of Acute Respiratory Distress Syndrome (ARDS). *IL-1,* Interleukin-1; *ROS,* reactive oxygen species; *TGF-β,* transforming growth factor-beta; *TNF,* tumor necrosis factor.

proteins, mucin-associated antigens and interleukins) may aid in the diagnosis and prognosis of ARDS.[24] Treatment is based on early detection, supportive therapy, and prevention of complications. Supportive therapy is focused on maintaining adequate oxygenation and ventilation while preventing infection. This often requires various modes of mechanical ventilation. Pharmacologic therapy continues to be explored. Low-dose corticosteroids may improve survival in selected individuals but needs further investigation.[25]

✔ **QUICK CHECK 27-3**
1. Contrast aspiration and atelectasis.
2. What are some of the causes of pulmonary fibrosis?
3. What symptoms are produced by inhalation of toxic gases?
4. Describe pneumoconiosis, and give two examples.
5. Briefly describe the role of neutrophils in acute respiratory distress syndrome (ARDS).

Obstructive Lung Diseases

Obstructive lung disease is characterized by airway obstruction that is worse with expiration. More force (i.e., use of accessory muscles of expiration) is required to expire a given volume of air and emptying of the lungs is slowed. The unifying symptom of obstructive lung diseases is dyspnea, and the unifying sign is wheezing. Individuals have an increased work of breathing, ventilation-perfusion mismatching, and a decreased forced expiratory volume in 1 second (FEV$_1$). The most common obstructive diseases are asthma, chronic bronchitis, and emphysema. Because many individuals have chronic bronchitis with emphysema, these diseases together are often called chronic obstructive pulmonary disease (COPD).

Asthma

Asthma is a chronic inflammatory disorder of the bronchial mucosa that causes bronchial hyperresponsiveness, constriction of the airways, and variable airflow obstruction that is reversible. Asthma occurs at all ages, with approximately 6.8 million cases among children (see Chapter 28) and 18.7 million cases among adults in the United States. The prevalence is increasing.[26]

Asthma is a familial disorder, and more than 100 genes have been identified that may play a role in the susceptibility, pathogenesis, and treatment response of asthma. Specific gene expressions may impart associated *phenotypes* with specific inflammatory markers (i.e., cells, cytokines, or exhaled nitric oxide) or *endotypes* including clinical characteristics, biomarkers, lung physiology, genetics, histopathology, epidemiology, and treatment response.[27] Other risk factors include age at onset of disease, levels of allergen exposure, urban residence, exposure to indoor and outdoor air pollution, tobacco smoke, recurrent respiratory tract viral infections, gastroesophageal reflux disease, and obesity (which promotes a proinflammatory state).[28-30] Exposure to inhaled irritants can cause inflammation and damage to airways independent of allergen sensitivity. This leads to irritant (or nonallergic) asthma, as well as increases the hyperresponsiveness of the airways to allergens in those with a history of atopy (allergy).[31] Inhaled irritants affect both the epigenetics of asthma and asthma presentation, including age of onset, symptoms, and gender differences.[32]

Exposure to high levels of certain allergens during childhood increases the risk for asthma. Furthermore, decreased exposure to certain infectious organisms appears to create an immunologic imbalance that favors the development of allergy and asthma. This complex relationship has been called the *hygiene hypothesis*.[33] Recently, the relationship between the microbiome and asthma risk is shedding light on these complex interactions[34] (see *Health Alert:* The Microbiome and Asthma).

PATHOPHYSIOLOGY Airway epithelial exposure to antigen initiates both an innate and an adaptive immune response in sensitized individuals[35] (see Chapter 8). Many cells and cellular elements contribute to the persistent inflammation of the bronchial mucosa and hyperresponsiveness of the airways, including dendritic cells (antigen-presenting macrophages), T helper 2 (Th2) lymphocytes, B lymphocytes, mast cells, neutrophils, eosinophils, and basophils. There is both an immediate (early asthmatic response) and a late (delayed) response.

During the *early asthmatic response,* antigen exposure to the bronchial mucosa activates dendritic cells, which present antigen to T-helper cells. T-helper cells differentiate into Th2 cells releasing inflammatory cytokines and interleukins that activate B lymphocytes (plasma cells) and eosinophils. Plasma cells produce antigen-specific IgE, which binds to the surface of mast cells. Subsequent cross-linking of IgE molecules with the antigen causes mast cell degranulation with the

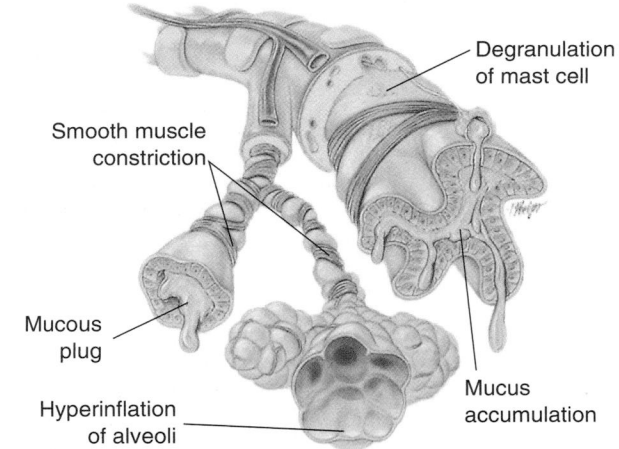

FIGURE 27-8 Bronchial Asthma. Thick mucus, mucosal edema, and smooth muscle spasm cause obstruction of small airways; breathing becomes labored and expiration is difficult. (Modified from Des Jardins T, Burton GG: *Clinical manifestations and assessment of respiratory disease,* ed 3, St Louis, 1995, Mosby.)

release of inflammatory mediators including histamine, bradykinins, leukotrienes and prostaglandins, platelet-activating factor, and interleukins[36] (see Figures 8-11 and 8-12 for additional details). These inflammatory mediators cause vasodilation, increased capillary permeability, mucosal edema, bronchial smooth muscle contraction (bronchospasm), and mucus secretion from mucosal goblet cells with narrowing of the airways and obstruction to airflow. Eosinophils cause direct tissue injury and release of toxic neuropeptides that contribute to increased bronchial hyperresponsiveness[37] (Figures 27-8, 27-9, and 27-10).

The *late asthmatic response* begins 4 to 8 hours after the early response. Chemotactic recruitment of eosinophils, neutrophils, and lymphocytes during the acute response causes a latent release of inflammatory mediators, again inciting bronchospasm, edema, and

FIGURE 27-9 Pathophysiology of Asthma. Allergen or irritant exposure results in a cascade of inflammatory events leading to acute and chronic airway dysfunction. *IgE,* Immunoglobulin E; *IL,* interleukin.

mucus secretion with obstruction to airflow. Synthesis of leukotrienes contributes to prolonged smooth muscle contraction. Eosinophils cause direct tissue injury with fibroblast proliferation and airway scarring. Damage to ciliated epithelial cells contributes to impaired mucociliary function, with the accumulation of mucus and cellular debris forming plugs in the airways. Untreated inflammation can lead to long-term airway damage that is irreversible and is known as *airway remodeling* (subepithelial fibrosis, smooth muscle hypertrophy).[38]

Airway obstruction increases resistance to airflow and decreases flow rates, especially expiratory flow. Impaired expiration causes air trapping, hyperinflation distal to obstructions, and increased work of breathing. Changes in resistance to airflow are not uniform throughout the lungs and the distribution of inspired air is uneven, with more air flowing to the less resistant portions. Continued air trapping increases intrapleural and alveolar gas pressures and causes decreased perfusion of the alveoli. Increased alveolar gas pressure, decreased ventilation, and decreased perfusion lead to variable and uneven ventilation-perfusion relationships within different lung segments. Hyperventilation is triggered by lung receptors responding to increased lung volume and obstruction. The result is early hypoxemia without CO_2 retention. Hypoxemia further increases hyperventilation through stimulation of the respiratory center, causing $Paco_2$ to decrease and pH to increase (respiratory alkalosis). With progressive obstruction of expiratory airflow, air trapping becomes more severe and the lungs and thorax become hyperexpanded, positioning the respiratory muscles at a

mechanical disadvantage. This leads to a decrease in tidal volume with increasing CO_2 retention and respiratory acidosis. Respiratory acidosis signals respiratory failure, especially when left ventricular filling, and thus cardiac output, becomes compromised because of severe hyperinflation.

CLINICAL MANIFESTATIONS   Individuals are asymptomatic between attacks and pulmonary function tests are normal. At the beginning of an attack, the individual experiences chest constriction, expiratory wheezing, dyspnea, nonproductive coughing, prolonged expiration, tachycardia, and tachypnea. Severe attacks involve the accessory muscles of respiration and wheezing is heard during both inspiration and expiration. A **pulsus paradoxus** (decrease in systolic blood pressure during inspiration of more than 10 mm Hg) may be noted. Peak flow measurements should be obtained. Because the severity of blood gas alterations is difficult to evaluate by clinical signs alone, arterial blood gas tensions should be measured if oxygen saturation falls below 90%. Usual findings are hypoxemia with an associated respiratory alkalosis. In the *late asthma response,* symptoms can be even more severe than the initial attack.

If bronchospasm is not reversed by usual treatment measures, the individual is considered to have acute severe bronchospasm or **status asthmaticus**.[39] If status asthmaticus continues, hypoxemia worsens, expiratory flows and volumes decrease further, and effective ventilation decreases. Acidosis develops as the $Paco_2$ level begins to rise. Asthma

FIGURE 27-10 Acute Asthmatic Responses. Inhaled antigen (**1**) binds to mast cells covered with pre-formed IgE. Mast cells degranulate (**2**) and release inflammatory mediators such as histamine, bradykinins, leukotrienes, prostaglandins, platelet-activating factor, and interleukins. Secreted mediators (**3**) induce active bronchospasm (airway smooth muscle constriction), edema from increased capillary permeability, and airway mucus secretion from goblet cells. At the same time, antigen is detected by (**4**) dendritic cells that process and present it to Th2 cells (**5**), which produce interleukin-4 (*IL-4*) and many other interleukins (see text). IL-4 promotes switching of B cells to favor immunoglobulin E (*IgE*) production. Th2 cells also produce IL-5 (**6**), which activates eosinophils. Eosinophil products, such as major basic protein and eosinophilic cationic protein, damage the respiratory epithelium. Many inflammatory cells, including neutrophils (**7**), also contribute to the inflammatory process and airway obstruction. *IgE,* Immunoglobulin E.

becomes life-threatening at this point if treatment does not reverse this process quickly. A silent chest (no audible air movement) and a·Paco$_2$ >70 mm Hg are ominous signs of impending death.

EVALUATION AND TREATMENT The diagnosis of asthma is supported by a history of allergies and recurrent episodes of wheezing, dyspnea, and cough or exercise intolerance. Further evaluation includes spirometry, which may document reversible decreases in FEV$_1$ during an induced attack.

The evaluation of an acute asthma attack requires the rapid assessment of arterial blood gases and expiratory flow rates (using a peak flow meter) and a search for underlying triggers, such as infection. Hypoxemia and respiratory alkalosis are expected early in the course of an acute attack. The development of hypercapnia with respiratory acidosis signals the need for mechanical ventilation. Management of the acute asthma attack requires immediate administration of oxygen and inhaled beta-agonist bronchodilators. In addition, oral corticosteroids should be administered early in the course of management.[40] Careful monitoring of gas exchange and airway obstruction in response to therapy provides information necessary to determine whether hospitalization is necessary. Antibiotics are not indicated for acute asthma unless there is a documented bacterial infection.

Management of asthma begins with avoidance of allergens and irritants. Individuals with asthma tend to underestimate the severity of their asthma and extensive education is important, including use of a peak flow meter and adherence to an action plan. In the mildest form of asthma (intermittent), short-acting beta-agonist inhalers are prescribed. For all categories of persistent asthma, anti-inflammatory medications are essential and inhaled corticosteroids are the mainstay of therapy. In individuals who are not adequately controlled with inhaled corticosteroids, leukotriene antagonists can be considered. In more severe asthma, long-acting beta agonists can be used to control persistent bronchospasm; however, these agonists can actually worsen asthma in some individuals with certain genetic polymorphisms.[40a] Immunotherapy has been shown to be an important tool in reducing asthma exacerbations and can now be given sublingually.[41] Monoclonal antibodies to IgE (omalizumab) have been found to be helpful as adjunctive therapy to inhaled steroids.[42] The National Asthma Education and Prevention Program offers stepwise guidelines for the diagnosis and management of chronic asthma based on clinical severity; they may be reviewed at www.nhlbi.nih.gov/guidelines/asthma/asthgdln.htm. Biomarkers and epigenetic markers are being evaluated to personalize treatment and reduce mortality.[43,44]

Chronic Obstructive Pulmonary Disease

Chronic obstructive pulmonary disease (COPD) is defined as a common preventable and treatable disease characterized by persistent airflow limitation that is usually progressive and associated with an enhanced chronic inflammatory response in the airways and the lung to noxious particles or gases. Exacerbations and comorbidities contribute to the overall severity of disease.[45] COPD is the most common chronic lung disease in the world, and the fourth leading cause of death in the United States and globally. Overall mortality from COPD has increased in the United States over the past 30 years; however, COPD

Enlarged
submucosal
gland

Mucus
accumulation

Mucous
plug

Inflammation
of epithelium

Hyperinflation
of alveoli

FIGURE 27-11 Chronic Bronchitis. Inflammation and thickening of mucous membrane with accumulation of mucus and pus leading to obstruction characterized by productive cough. (Modified from Des Jardins T, Burton GG: *Clinical manifestations and assessment of respiratory disease,* ed 3, St Louis, 1995, Mosby.)

TABLE 27-2 Clinical Manifestations of Chronic Obstructive Lung Disease

Clinical Manifestations	Bronchitis	Emphysema
Productive cough	Classic sign	With infection
Dyspnea	Late in course	Common
Wheezing	Intermittent	Common
History of smoking	Common	Common
Barrel chest	Occasionally	Classic
Prolonged expiration	Always present	Always present
Cyanosis	Common	Uncommon
Chronic hypoventilation	Common	Late in course
Polycythemia	Common	Late in course
Cor pulmonale	Common	Late in course

prevalence in women is higher throughout the life span. Risk factors for COPD include tobacco smoke (cigarette, pipe, cigar, and environmental tobacco smoke), occupational dusts and chemicals (vapors, irritants, and fumes), indoor air pollution from biomass fuel used for cooking and heating (in poorly vented dwellings), outdoor air pollution, and any factor that affects lung growth during gestation and childhood (low birth weight, respiratory tract infections).[46] Genetic and epigenetic susceptibilities have been identified including polymorphisms of genes that code for tumor necrosis factor, surfactant, proteases, and antiproteases and acquired failure of DNA repair.[47] The clinical phenotypes of COPD discussed here are chronic bronchitis and emphysema. An inherited mutation in the α_1-antitrypsin gene results in the development of COPD at an early age, even in individuals who do not smoke.

Chronic Bronchitis

Chronic bronchitis is defined as hypersecretion of mucus and chronic productive cough for at least 3 months of the year (usually the winter months) for at least 2 consecutive years.

PATHOPHYSIOLOGY Inspired irritants result in airway inflammation with infiltration of neutrophils, macrophages, and lymphocytes into the bronchial wall. Continual bronchial inflammation causes bronchial edema, an increase in the size and number of mucous glands and goblet cells in the airway epithelium, smooth muscle hypertrophy with fibrosis, and narrowing of airways. Thick, tenacious mucus is produced and cannot be cleared because of impaired ciliary function (Figure 27-11). The lung's defense mechanisms are, therefore, compromised, increasing susceptibility to pulmonary infection and injury and ineffective repair. Frequent infectious exacerbations from bacterial colonization of damaged airways are complicated by bronchospasm with dyspnea and productive cough.[48,49] The pathogenesis of chronic bronchitis is shown in Figure 27-12.

This process initially affects only the larger bronchi, but eventually all airways are involved. The thick mucus and hypertrophied bronchial smooth muscle constrict the airways and lead to obstruction, particularly during expiration when the airways are narrowed (Figure 27-13). Obstruction eventually leads to ventilation-perfusion mismatch with hypoxemia. The airways collapse early in expiration, trapping gas in

the distal portions of the lung (hyperinflation).[50] Air trapping expands the thorax and positions the respiratory muscles at a mechanical disadvantage. This leads to decreased tidal volume, hypoventilation, and hypercapnia.

CLINICAL MANIFESTATIONS Table 27-2 lists the common clinical manifestations of chronic obstructive lung disease, chronic bronchitis, and emphysema.

EVALUATION AND TREATMENT Diagnosis is based on history of symptoms, physical examination, chest imaging, pulmonary function tests (i.e., a FEV_1/forced vital capacity ratio <0.7), and blood gas analyses. These tests reflect the progressive nature of the disease. Prevention of chronic bronchitis is essential because pathologic changes are not reversible. By the time an individual seeks medical care for symptoms, considerable airway damage is present. If the individual stops smoking, disease progression can be halted.[51] Influenza and pneumococcal vaccinations should be up to date.

Bronchodilators, mucolytics, antioxidants, and anti-inflammatory drugs are prescribed as needed to control cough and reduce dyspnea. Chest physical therapy may be helpful and includes deep breathing and postural drainage. During acute exacerbations (infection and bronchospasm), individuals require treatment with antibiotics and steroids and may need mechanical ventilation.[52] Chronic use of oral steroids may be needed late in the course of the disease but should be considered a last resort. Individuals with severe hypoxemia will require home oxygen therapy. Oxygen is administered with care to individuals with severe hypoxemia and CO_2 retention. Chronic elevation of $Paco_2$ diminishes the sensitivity of central chemoreceptors and they no longer act as the primary stimulus for breathing. Teaching includes nutritional counseling, respiratory hygiene, recognition of the early signs of infection, and techniques that relieve dyspnea, such as pursed-lip breathing. In addition, many comorbidities accompany COPD and require monitoring and therapy, including cardiovascular disorders, metabolic diseases, bone disease, stroke, lung cancer, cachexia, skeletal muscle weakness, anemia, depression, and cognitive decline. Chronic low-grade systemic inflammation may be associated with these conditions.[53]

Emphysema

Emphysema is abnormal permanent enlargement of gas-exchange airways (acini) accompanied by destruction of alveolar walls without obvious fibrosis. Obstruction results from changes in lung tissues, rather than mucus production and inflammation as in chronic

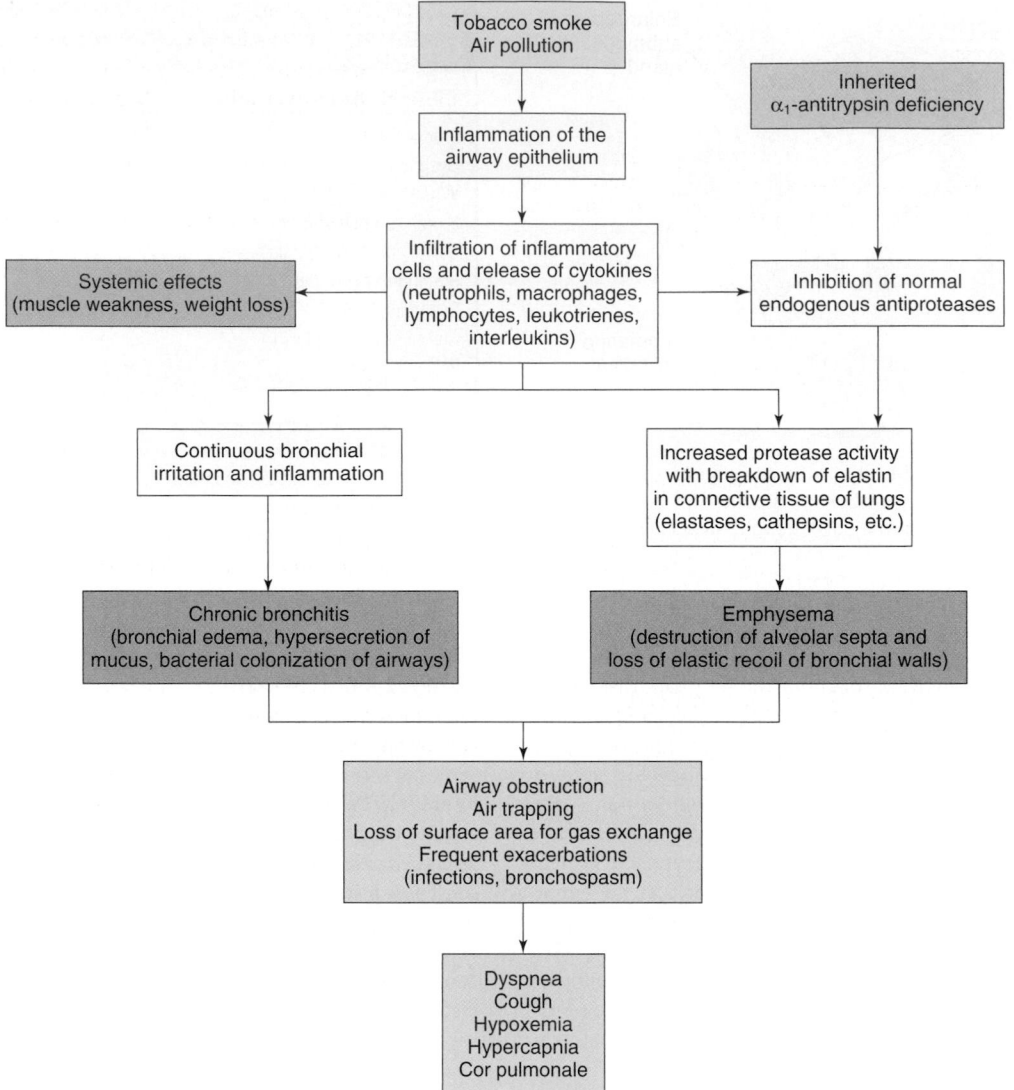

FIGURE 27-12 Pathogenesis of Chronic Bronchitis and Emphysema (Chronic Obstructive Pulmonary Disease [COPD]).

bronchitis. The major mechanism of airflow limitation is loss of elastic recoil.

Primary emphysema, which accounts for 1% to 3% of all cases of emphysema, is commonly linked to an inherited deficiency of the enzyme α_1-antitrypsin. Normally α_1-antitrypsin inhibits the action of many proteolytic enzymes (i.e., elastases released by neutrophils); therefore α_1-antitrypsin deficiency (an autosomal recessive trait) increases the likelihood of developing emphysema because proteolysis in lung tissues is not inhibited.[54] α_1-Antitrypsin deficiency is suggested in individuals who develop emphysema before 40 years of age and in individuals who do not smoke but still develop the disease. The major cause of secondary emphysema is the inhalation of cigarette smoke, although air pollution, occupational exposures, and childhood respiratory tract infections are known to be contributing factors.

PATHOPHYSIOLOGY Emphysema is characterized by destruction of alveoli through the breakdown of elastin within the septa by an imbalance between proteases and antiproteases, oxidative stress, and apoptosis of lung structural cells (see Figure 27-12).[55] Alveolar destruction also produces large air spaces within the lung parenchyma (bullae) and air spaces adjacent to pleurae (blebs) (Figure 27-14). Bullae and blebs

are not effective in gas exchange and result in significant ventilation-perfusion ($\dot{V}/\dot{Q}$) mismatching and hypoxemia. Expiration becomes difficult because loss of elastic recoil reduces the volume of air that can be expired passively and air is trapped in the lungs (see Figure 27-13). **Air trapping** causes hyperexpansion of the chest, placing the muscles of respiration at a mechanical disadvantage. This results in increased workload of breathing, so that late in the course of disease, many individuals will develop hypoventilation and hypercapnia. Persistent inflammation in the airways can result in hyperreactivity of the bronchi with bronchoconstriction, which may be partially reversible with bronchodilators. Destruction of alveolar walls and pulmonary capillaries also causes pulmonary artery hypertension and cor pulmonale (see pp. 707-708). Chronic inflammation also can have significant systemic effects including weight loss, muscle weakness, and increased susceptibility to comorbidities, such as infection.

CLINICAL MANIFESTATIONS The clinical manifestations of emphysema are listed in Table 27-2.

EVALUATION AND TREATMENT Emphysema is usually diagnosed and staged by pulmonary function measures. In COPD, pulmonary

Air movement during INSPIRATION

Air movement during EXPIRATION

Mucous plug

Muscle

Bronchial walls collapse

Alveolar walls

FIGURE 27-13 Mechanisms of Air Trapping in COPD. Mucous plugs and narrowed airways cause air trapping and hyperinflation of alveoli on expiration. During inspiration, the airways are pulled open, allowing gas to flow past the obstruction. During expiration, decreased elastic recoil of the bronchial walls results in collapse of the airways and prevents normal expiratory airflow.

FIGURE 27-14 Bullous Emphysema with Large Apical and Subpleural Bullae (arrows). (From Kumar V et al, editors: *Robbins basic pathology,* ed 8, Philadelphia, 2007, Saunders/Elsevier.)

function tests indicate obstruction to gas flow during expiration with a marked decrease in FEV$_1$. Chronic management of emphysema begins with smoking cessation. Pharmacologic management is based on clinical severity (mild, moderate, severe, or very severe). Inhaled anticholinergic agents and beta agonists should be prescribed. Inhaled corticosteroids are indicated for severe COPD, although long-term therapy with oral steroids should be avoided if possible. Pulmonary rehabilitation, improved nutrition, and breathing techniques can improve symptoms. Progressive pulmonary dysfunction with hypoxemia and hypercapnia may require long-term oxygen therapy and ventilation if indicated.[56] A class of drugs called *phosphodiesterase E4*

(PDE4) inhibitors is proving to be effective in selected individuals with severe COPD.[52] α_1-Antitrypsin augmentation may be indicated for primary emphysema.[57] Selected individuals with severe emphysema can benefit from lung volume reduction surgery.[58]

> ✔ **QUICK CHECK 27-4**
> 1. What mechanisms cause airway obstruction in asthma?
> 2. How does emphysema affect oxygenation and ventilation?
> 3. Define chronic bronchitis.

Respiratory Tract Infections

Respiratory tract infections are the most common cause of short-term disability in the United States. Most of these infections—the common cold, pharyngitis (sore throat), and laryngitis—involve only the upper airways. Although the lungs have direct contact with the atmosphere, they usually remain sterile. Infections of the lower respiratory tract occur most often in the very young and very old or those with impaired immunity.

Acute Bronchitis

Acute bronchitis is acute infection or inflammation of the airways or bronchi and is usually self-limiting. The vast majority of cases of acute bronchitis are caused by viruses. Many of the clinical manifestations are similar to those of pneumonia (i.e., fever, cough, chills, malaise), but physical examination does not reveal signs of pulmonary consolidation and chest radiographs do not show infiltrates. Individuals with viral bronchitis usually have a nonproductive cough that often occurs in paroxysms and is aggravated by cold, dry, or dusty air. In some cases, purulent sputum is produced. Chest pain often develops from the effort of coughing. Treatment consists of rest, aspirin, humidity, and a cough suppressant, such as codeine. Bacterial bronchitis is treated with rest, antipyretics, humidity, and antibiotics.

Pneumonia

Pneumonia is infection of the lower respiratory tract caused by bacteria, viruses, fungi, protozoa, or parasites. It is the sixth leading cause of death in the United States. The incidence and mortality of pneumonia are highest in the elderly. Risk factors for pneumonia include advanced age, compromised immunity, underlying lung disease, alcoholism, altered consciousness, impaired swallowing, smoking, endotracheal intubation, malnutrition, immobilization, underlying cardiac or liver disease, and residence in a nursing home. The causative microorganism influences the clinical presentation of the individual, the treatment plan, and the prognosis.

Pneumonia can be categorized as community-acquired (CAP), health care–associated (HCAP), hospital-acquired (HAP), or ventilator-associated (VAP). CAP is one of the most common reasons for hospitalization in the United States. HCAP is defined as occurring in individuals with recent hospitalization, residence in a nursing home or extended care facility, home infusion therapy, chronic dialysis, or home wound care, although more recent studies suggest nonambulatory status, tube feedings, and the use of gastric acid suppressive agents also should be considered as criteria for HCAP.[59] It is estimated that nearly one third of all hospital admissions for pneumonia are now considered HCAP. HAP is the second most common nosocomial infection (urinary tract infection [UTI] is the most common) but has the greatest mortality (overall 20% to 50% mortality). VAP is a nosocomial infection that occurs in 9% to 27% of individuals who require intubation and mechanical ventilation.[60-62]

BOX 27-1   **Etiologic Microorganisms for Pneumonia in Adults**

CAP	HCAP/HAP/ VAP	Immunocompromised Individuals
Streptococcus pneumoniae	Pseudomonas aeruginosa	Pneumocystis jirovecii
Moraxella catarrhalis	Staphylococcus aureus	Mycobacterium tuberculosis
Haemophilus influenzae		Atypical mycobacteria
Oral anaerobic bacteria	Klebsiella pneumoniae	Fungi
Influenza virus		Respiratory viruses
Respiratory syncytial virus	Escherichia coli	Protozoa
Staphylococcus aureus		Parasites
Chlamydia pneumoniae		
Legionella pneumophila		
Mycoplasma pneumoniae		

CAP, Community-acquired pneumonia; HAP, hospital-acquired pneumonia; HCAP, health care–associated pneumonia; VAP, ventilator-associated pneumonia.

The microorganisms that most commonly cause CAP are different from those infections that cause HCAP, HAP, and VAP (Box 27-1). The most common community-acquired pneumonia is caused by *Streptococcus pneumoniae* (also known as *pneumococcus*), which results in hospitalization in more than half of affected individuals and an overall hospital mortality of about 10%.[63] *Mycoplasma pneumoniae* is a common cause of atypical pneumonia in young people, especially those living in group housing such as dormitories and army barracks. Community-acquired methicillin-resistant *Staphylococcus aureus* (MRSA) is becoming more common.[64,65] Influenza and respiratory syncytial virus are the most common viral causes of viral community-acquired pneumonia in adults.[66] VAP is a frequent complication in the intensive care unit (see *Health Alert*: Ventilator-Associated Pneumonia [VAP]). Immunocompromised individuals (e.g., those with human immunodeficiency virus [HIV] or those undergoing organ transplantation) are especially susceptible to *Pneumocystis jirovecii* (formerly called *P. carinii*), mycobacterial infections, and fungal infections of the respiratory tract. These infections can be difficult to treat and have a high mortality.

PATHOPHYSIOLOGY   Aspiration of oropharyngeal secretions is the most common route of lower respiratory tract infection; thus, the nasopharynx and oropharynx constitute the first line of defense for most infectious agents. Another route of infection is through the inhalation of microorganisms that have been released into the air when an infected individual coughs, sneezes, or talks, or from aerosolized water such as that from contaminated respiratory therapy equipment. This route of infection is most important in viral and mycobacterial pneumonias and in *Legionella* outbreaks. Endotracheal tubes become colonized with bacteria that form biofilms (protected colonies of bacteria that are resistant to host defenses and treatment with antibiotics) and can seed the lung with microorganisms, especially during endotracheal suctioning. Pneumonia also can occur when bacteria are spread to the lung in the blood from bacteremia that can result from infection elsewhere in the body or from intravenous (IV) drug abuse.

In healthy individuals, pathogens that reach the lungs are expelled or controlled by mechanisms of self-defense (see Chapters 6, 7, and 8). If a microorganism evades the upper airway defense mechanisms, such as the cough reflex and mucociliary clearance, the next line of defense

HEALTH ALERT
Ventilator-Associated Pneumonia (VAP)

Ventilator-associated pneumonia (VAP) is a common complication of mechanical ventilation and is the most serious infection in the intensive care unit. VAP is associated with higher mortality, morbidity, and costs. Although there are many risk factors, including age greater than 65 years, presence of comorbidities, use of sedation, supine posture, poor oral hygiene, and immunocompromised status, the principal determinant of VAP development is the presence of the endotracheal (ET) tube. Common etiologic microorganisms include *Staphylococcus aureus* and *Pseudomonas aeruginosa;* multidrug-resistant strains are common. Bacterial colonization of the oropharynx occurs soon after placement of the ET tube with subsequent aspiration and pooling of bacteria near the ET tube cuff. Many bacteria are capable of forming a protective coating, called a biofilm, on the surface of the ET tube that contributes to bacterial replication and makes microorganisms less vulnerable to antibiotics. Injury to the tracheal mucosa and decreased mucociliary clearance contribute to lower airway infection. Analgesic and sedation agents alter cellular function and reduce the immune response. Implementation of certain treatment protocols has shown improved outcomes regarding VAP prevention and mortality reduction, especially the use of a "bundle" of techniques including raising the head of the bed, improving oral hygiene, providing continuous suction of subglottic secretions by antimicrobial-impregnated ET tubes, using checklists, and encouraging effective team communication. Recent studies have suggested that surveillance cultures could improve the prescribing of appropriate antibiotics and that the addition of aerosolized antibiotics may improve treatment outcomes.

Data from Klompas M et al: *J Am Med Assoc Int Med* 174(5):751-761, 2014; Kollef MH et al: *Curr Opin Infect Dis* 26(6):5385-5344, 2013; Luna CM et al: *Curr Opin Infect Dis* 27(2):184-193, 2014; Mietto C et al: *Resp Care* 58(6):990-1007, 2013; Rouze A, Nseir S: *Curr Opin Crit Care* 19(5):440-447, 2013; Smith MA et al: *Ann Pharmacother* 48(1):77-85, 2014. Kallet RH: *Respir Care,* 60(10): 1495-1508, 2015.

is the airway epithelial cell. Airway epithelial cells can recognize some pathogens directly (e.g., *Pseudomonas aeruginosa* and *Staphylococcus aureus*). The most important guardian cell of the lower respiratory tract is the alveolar macrophage; it recognizes pathogens through its pattern-recognition receptors (e.g., Toll-like receptors). Macrophages present infectious antigens to the adaptive immune system, activating T cells and B cells with the induction of both cellular and humoral immunity. Release of tumor necrosis factor-alpha (TNF-α) and interleukin-1 (IL-1) from macrophages and chemokines and chemotactic signals from mast cells and fibroblasts contributes to widespread inflammation in the lung and recruitment of neutrophils from the capillaries of the lungs into the alveoli. The resulting inflammatory mediators and immune complexes can damage bronchial mucous membranes and alveolocapillary membranes, causing the acini and terminal bronchioles to fill with infectious debris and exudate. Some microorganisms release toxins from their cell walls that can cause further lung damage and consolidation of lung tissue. The accumulation of exudate in the acinus leads to dyspnea and to $\dot{V}/\dot{Q}$ mismatching and hypoxemia.

Pneumococcus *(Streptococcus pneumoniae)* is the most common and lethal cause of outpatient and inpatient pneumonias.[67] Pneumococci can infect the lungs through inhalation of aerosolized bacteria or more commonly by aspiration of colonized oropharyngeal secretions. These bacteria have several virulence factors; most importantly, they have capsules that make phagocytosis by alveolar macrophages more difficult and they have the ability to release a variety of toxins,

FIGURE 27-15 Pathophysiologic Course of Pneumococcal Pneumonia.

including pneumolysin, which damages airway and alveolar cells.[68] An intense inflammatory response is initiated with release of TNF-α and IL-1.[67] Neutrophils and inflammatory exudates cause alveolar edema, which leads to the other changes shown in Figure 27-15.

Viral pneumonia is a seasonal and usually mild and self-limiting CAP. It can set the stage for a secondary bacterial infection by damaging ciliated epithelial cells, which normally prevent pathogens from reaching the lower airways. Immunocompromised individuals are at risk for very serious viral infections, such as pneumonia caused by cytomegalovirus. Viral pneumonia also can be a complication of another viral illness, such as chickenpox or measles (spread from the blood). New or atypical forms of viral infection, such as swine influenza A (H1N1) virus, avian influenza A (H5N1) virus, and the coronavirus that causes the severe acute respiratory syndrome (SARS), are affecting previously healthy populations and pose a considerable threat for pandemics.[69]

Viruses destroy the ciliated epithelial cells and invade the goblet cells and bronchial mucous glands. Sloughing of destroyed bronchial epithelium occurs throughout the respiratory tract, preventing mucociliary clearance. Bronchial walls become edematous and infiltrated with leukocytes. In severe cases, the alveoli are involved with decreased compliance and increased work of breathing.

CLINICAL MANIFESTATIONS Most cases of pneumonia are preceded by a viral upper respiratory tract infection. Individuals then develop fever, chills, productive or dry cough, malaise, pleural pain, and sometimes dyspnea and hemoptysis. Physical examination may show signs of pulmonary consolidation, such as dullness to percussion, inspiratory crackles, increased tactile fremitus, egophony, and whispered pectoriloquy. Individuals also may demonstrate symptoms and signs of underlying systemic disease or sepsis.

EVALUATION AND TREATMENT Diagnosis is made on the basis of history and physical examination (tachypnea, tachycardia, crackles, bronchial breath sounds, findings of pleural effusion), white blood cell count, oxygenation and pH, chest x-rays, stains and cultures of respiratory tract secretions, and blood cultures before starting antibiotics. The white blood cell count is usually elevated, although it may be low if the individual is debilitated or immunocompromised. Serum procalcitonin level can be used to help differentiate bacterial from viral infection and guide therapy. Chest radiographs show infiltrates that may involve a single lobe of the lung or may be more diffuse. Once the diagnosis of pneumonia has been made, the pathogen is identified by means of sputum characteristics (Gram stain, color, odor) and cultures or, if sputum is absent, blood cultures. Because many pathogens exist in the normal oropharyngeal flora, the specimen may be contaminated with pathogens from oral secretions. If sputum studies fail to identify the pathogen, the individual is immunocompromised, or the individual's condition worsens, further diagnostic studies may include thoracentesis, bronchoscopy, or lung biopsy. Urine antigen testing offers rapid pathogen identification for Legionella pneumophila, Streptococcus pneumoniae, and Histoplasma capsulatum but requires culture for microbial specificity.[70]

Prevention of pneumonia includes avoidance of aspiration, respiratory isolation of immunocompromised individuals, and vaccination. The first step in the management of pneumonia is establishing adequate ventilation and oxygenation. Adequate hydration and good pulmonary hygiene (e.g., deep breathing, coughing, chest physical therapy) also are important. Antibiotics are given within 4 hours to treat bacterial pneumonia; however, resistant strains of microorganisms are becoming more prevalent and require secondary antibiotics.[71] When a specific microorganism is not identified, empirical antibiotics are chosen based on the likely causative microorganism.[59] Viral pneumonia is usually treated with supportive therapy alone; however, antivirals may be needed in severe cases. Infections with opportunistic microorganisms may be polymicrobial and require multiple drugs, including antifungals.

Tuberculosis

Tuberculosis (TB) is an infection caused by *Mycobacterium tuberculosis,* an acid-fast bacillus that usually affects the lungs but may invade other body systems. TB is a leading cause of death from a curable infectious disease in the world. TB cases increased greatly during the mid-1990s as a result of acquired immunodeficiency syndrome (AIDS) but both have decreased since 2000.[72] Emigration of infected individuals from high-prevalence countries, transmission in crowded institutional settings, homelessness, substance abuse, and lack of access to screening and medical care have contributed to the spread of TB.

PATHOPHYSIOLOGY TB is highly contagious and is transmitted from person to person in airborne droplets. In immunocompetent individuals, the microorganism is usually contained by the inflammatory and immune response systems. This results in latent TB infection (LTBI) and is associated with no clinical evidence of disease.

Once the bacilli are inspired, they lodge in the lung periphery, usually in the upper lobe, and cause localized nonspecific pneumonitis (lung inflammation). Some bacilli migrate through the lymphatics and become lodged in the lymph nodes, where they encounter lymphocytes and initiate the immune response. Inflammation in the lung causes activation of alveolar macrophages and neutrophils. These phagocytes engulf the bacilli and begin the process by which the body's defense mechanisms isolate the bacilli, preventing them from spreading. However, the bacterium is successful as a pathogen because it can survive and multiply within macrophages and resist lysosomal killing, forming a granulomatous lesion called a *tubercle* (see Chapter 6). Infected tissues within the tubercle die, forming cheeselike material called *caseation necrosis.* Collagenous scar tissue then grows around the tubercle, completing isolation of the bacilli. The immune response is complete after about 10 days, preventing further multiplication of the bacilli.

Once the bacilli are isolated in tubercles and immunity develops, tuberculosis may remain dormant for life. If the immune system is impaired, reactivation with progressive disease occurs and may spread through the blood and lymphatics to other organs. Infection with human immunodeficiency virus (HIV) is the single greatest risk factor for reactivation of tuberculosis infection. Cancer, immunosuppressive medications (e.g., corticosteroids), poor nutritional status, and renal failure can also reactivate disease.

CLINICAL MANIFESTATIONS LTBI is asymptomatic. Symptoms of active disease often develop so gradually that they are not noticed until the disease is advanced. Common clinical manifestations include fatigue, weight loss, lethargy, anorexia (loss of appetite), and a low-grade fever that usually occurs in the afternoon. A cough that produces purulent sputum develops slowly and becomes more frequent over several weeks or months. Night sweats and general anxiety are often present. Dyspnea, chest pain, and hemoptysis may occur as the disease progresses. Extrapulmonary TB disease is common in HIV-infected individuals and may cause neurologic deficits, meningitis symptoms, bone pain, and urinary symptoms.

EVALUATION AND TREATMENT Tuberculosis is diagnosed by a positive tuberculin skin test (TST; purified protein derivative [PPD]), sputum culture, immunoassays, and chest radiographs.[73] A positive skin test indicates the need for yearly chest radiographs to detect active

disease. In addition, individuals who have received the TB vaccine with bacille Calmette-Guérin (BCG) will have a positive TST even if they have never had TB. When active pulmonary disease is present, the tubercle bacillus can be cultured from the sputum and may be seen with an acid-fast stain. However, sputum culture can take up to 6 weeks to become positive. Two immunoassays (enzyme-linked immunospot and quantitative blood interferon-gamma assay) are available. These new tests are more sensitive and specific than TST for the diagnosis of latent TB and are not confounded by previous BCG vaccination.[74]

Treatment consists of combination antibiotic therapy to control active disease or prevent reactivation of LTBI. Side effects are common and new drugs are being explored.[75] Two worrisome treatment categories of TB have become more prevalent in recent years. "Multidrug-resistant TB" and "extensively resistant TB" now account for approximately 2% to 5% of cases worldwide. Multiple second-line drugs are required for treatment success.[76] The bacillus Calmette-Guérin (BCG) vaccine is used in countries where TB is endemic but not in the United States, where TST is used for screening. New vaccines are in clinical trials.[77] Treatment of TB HIV coinfection requires monitoring of drug interactions and toxicities.[78]

Abscess Formation and Cavitation

An abscess is a circumscribed area of suppuration and destruction of lung parenchyma. Abscess formation follows consolidation of lung tissue, in which inflammation causes alveoli to fill with fluid, pus, and microorganisms. Aspiration abscess can occur from aspiration of anaerobes, such as those found in individuals who have pneumonia or who are infected with *Klebsiella* or *Staphylococcus.* Aspiration abscess is usually associated with alcohol abuse, seizure disorders, general anesthesia, and swallowing disorders. Necrosis (death and decay) of consolidated tissue may progress proximally until it communicates with a bronchus. Cavitation is the process of the abscess emptying into a bronchus and cavity formation. Abscess communication with a bronchus causes production of copious amounts of often foul-smelling sputum, and occasionally hemoptysis. Other clinical manifestations include fever, cough, chills, and pleural pain. The diagnosis is made by chest radiography. Treatment includes appropriate antibiotics and chest physical therapy (chest percussion and postural drainage). Bronchoscopy may be performed to drain the abscess.

✔ **QUICK CHECK 27-5**
1. Compare pneumococcal and viral pneumonia as to severity of disease.
2. Describe the pathophysiologic features of tuberculosis.
3. How does lung abscess present clinically?

Pulmonary Vascular Disease

Blood flow through the lungs can be disrupted by disorders that occlude the vessels, increase pulmonary vascular resistance, or destroy the vascular bed. Effects of altered pulmonary blood flow may range from insignificant dysfunction to severe and life-threatening changes in ventilation-perfusion ratios. Major disorders include pulmonary embolism, pulmonary hypertension, and cor pulmonale.

Pulmonary Embolism

Pulmonary embolism (PE) is occlusion of a portion of the pulmonary vascular bed by an embolus. PE most commonly results from embolization of a clot from deep venous thrombosis involving the lower leg (see Chapter 24). Other less common emboli include tissue fragments, lipids (fats), a foreign body, an air bubble, or amniotic fluid. Risk factors for PE include conditions and disorders that promote blood clotting as a result of venous stasis (immobilization, heart failure), hypercoagulability (inherited coagulation disorders, malignancy, hormone replacement therapy, oral contraceptives), and injuries to the endothelial cells that line the vessels (trauma, infection, caustic intravenous infusions). Genetic risks include factor V Leiden, antithrombin II, protein S, protein C, and prothrombin gene mutations. No matter its source, a blood clot becomes an embolus when all or part of it detaches from the site of formation and begins to travel in the bloodstream.

PATHOPHYSIOLOGY   The effect of the embolus depends on the extent of pulmonary blood flow obstruction, the size of the affected vessels, the nature of the embolus, and the secondary effects. Pulmonary emboli can result in any of the following:

1. *Embolus with infarction:* an embolus that causes infarction (death) of a portion of lung tissue
2. *Embolus without infarction:* an embolus that does not cause permanent lung injury (perfusion of the affected lung segment is maintained by the bronchial circulation)
3. *Massive occlusion:* an embolus that occludes a major portion of the pulmonary circulation (i.e., main pulmonary artery embolus)
4. *Multiple pulmonary emboli:* multiple emboli may be chronic or recurrent

Significant obstruction of the pulmonary vasculature leads to increased pulmonary artery vasoconstriction, pulmonary hypertension and right ventricular dilation and afterload.[79] The pathogenesis of pulmonary embolism caused by a thrombus is summarized in Figure 27-16.

If the embolus does not cause infarction, the clot is dissolved by the fibrinolytic system and pulmonary function returns to normal. If pulmonary infarction occurs, shrinking and scarring develop in the affected area of the lung.

CLINICAL MANIFESTATIONS   In most cases, the clinical manifestations of PE are nonspecific; therefore, evaluation of risk factors and predisposing factors is an important aspect of diagnosis. Although most emboli originate from clots in the lower extremities, deep vein thrombosis is often asymptomatic, and clinical examination has low sensitivity for the presence of clot, especially in the thigh and pelvis.

An individual with PE usually presents with the sudden onset of pleuritic chest pain, dyspnea, tachypnea, tachycardia, and unexplained anxiety. Occasionally syncope (fainting) or hemoptysis occurs. With large emboli, a pleural friction rub, pleural effusion, fever, and leukocytosis may be noted. Recurrent small emboli may not be detected until progressive incapacitation, precordial pain, anxiety, dyspnea, and right ventricular enlargement are exhibited. Massive occlusion causes severe pulmonary hypertension and shock.

EVALUATION AND TREATMENT   Routine chest radiographs and pulmonary function tests are not definitive for pulmonary embolism in the first 24 hours. Arterial blood gas analyses usually demonstrate hypoxemia and hyperventilation (respiratory alkalosis). The diagnosis is made by measuring elevated levels of d-dimer in the blood (a product of thrombus degradation) in combination with CT scanning or MRI. Measurement of the levels of brain natriuretic peptide and troponin is useful in PE associated with right ventricular dysfunction.[80]

Prevention of PE includes elimination of predisposing factors for individuals at risk. Venous stasis in hospitalized persons is minimized by leg elevation, bed exercises, position changes, early postoperative ambulation, and pneumatic calf compression. Clot formation is also prevented by prophylactic low-dose anticoagulant therapy.

FIGURE 27-16 Pathogenesis of Massive Pulmonary Embolism Caused by a Thrombus (Pulmonary Thromboembolism).

Anticoagulant therapy is the primary treatment for pulmonary embolism. Initial anticoagulant therapy usually includes low-molecular-weight heparins (e.g., enoxaparin) and factor Xa inhibitors. If a massive life-threatening embolism occurs, a fibrinolytic agent, such as streptokinase, is sometimes used, and some individuals will require catheter directed therapies or surgical thrombectomy. A filter in the inferior vena cava can prevent emboli from reaching the lungs. After stabilization, anticoagulation is continued for several months.[81]

Pulmonary Artery Hypertension

Pulmonary artery hypertension (PAH) is defined as a mean pulmonary artery pressure greater than 25 mm Hg at rest. PAH is classified into several groups[82]:

1. No known cause or associated with inheritance, drugs or toxins, connective tissue disease or infection
2. Pulmonary hypertension attributable to left heart disease (see Chapter 24)
3. Pulmonary hypertension caused by chronic lung disease or hypoxia, or both
4. Chronic thromboembolic pulmonary hypertension
5. Pulmonary hypertension caused by other multifactorial mechanisms including blood, metabolic and systemic disorders.

COPD is the most common lung disease associated with PAH, but any condition that causes chronic hypoxemia can result in pulmonary hypertension.

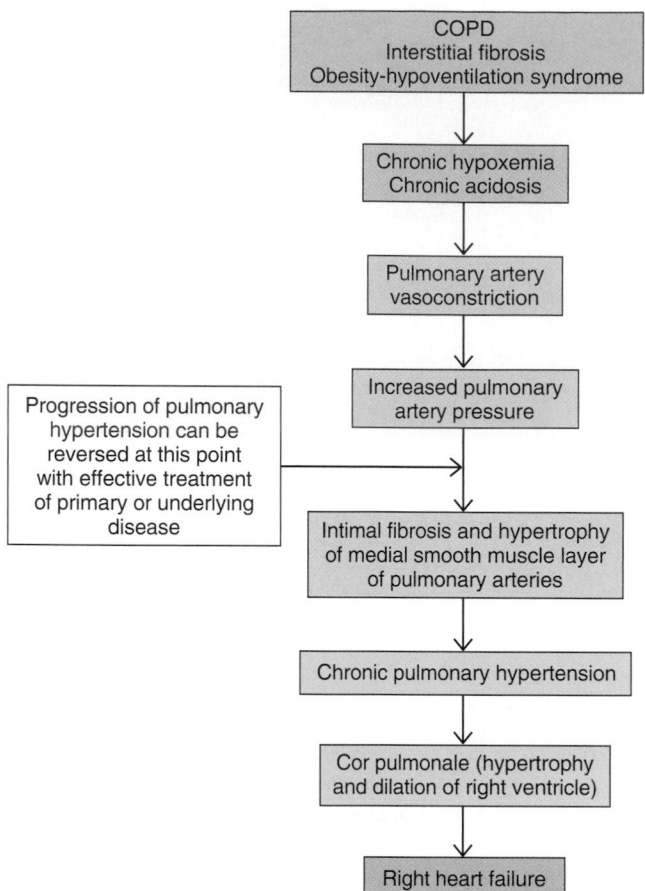

FIGURE 27-17 Pathogenesis of Pulmonary Hypertension and Cor Pulmonale.

PATHOPHYSIOLOGY *Idiopathic pulmonary arterial hypertension (IPAH)* (also called pulmonary hypertension caused by unclear multifactorial mechanisms) is characterized by endothelial dysfunction with overproduction of vasoconstrictors, such as thromboxane and endothelin, and decreased production of vasodilators, such as prostacyclin and nitric oxide. Vascular growth factors are released, causing fibrosis and thickening of vessel walls (called *remodeling*) with luminal narrowing and abnormal vasoconstriction.[83] These changes cause resistance to pulmonary artery blood flow, thus increasing the pressure in the pulmonary arteries and right ventricle. Gas exchange is reduced with restriction in lung volumes. As resistance and pressure increase, the workload of the right ventricle increases and subsequent right ventricular hypertrophy, followed by failure, may occur (cor pulmonale). The pathogenesis of PAH and cor pulmonale resulting from disease of the respiratory system or hypoxia is shown in Figure 27-17.

Pulmonary hypertension associated with lung respiratory disease or hypoxia, or both, is a serious complication of many acute and chronic pulmonary disorders, such as COPD and hypoventilation associated with obesity. These conditions are complicated by hypoxic pulmonary vasoconstriction, which further increases pulmonary artery pressure.

CLINICAL MANIFESTATIONS Pulmonary hypertension may not be detected until it is quite severe. The symptoms are often masked by other forms of pulmonary or cardiovascular disease. The first indication of PAH may be an abnormality seen on a chest radiograph (enlarged right heart border) or an electrocardiogram that shows right ventricular hypertrophy. Manifestations of fatigue, chest discomfort, tachypnea, and dyspnea (particularly with exercise) are common. Examination may reveal peripheral edema, jugular venous distention, a precordial heave, and accentuation of the pulmonary component of the second heart sound.

EVALUATION AND TREATMENT Definitive diagnosis of PAH can be made only with right heart catheterization. Common diagnostic modalities used to determine the cause include chest x-ray, echocardiography, and computed tomography. The diagnosis of IPAH is made when all other causes of pulmonary hypertension have been ruled out.

General therapies for PAH include administration of oxygen, diuretics, and anticoagulants and avoidance of contributing factors, such as air travel, decongestant medications, nonsteroidal anti-inflammatory medications, pregnancy, and tobacco use. Medications used in the treatment of PAH include prostacyclin and its analogs, endothelin antagonists, phosphodiesterase-5 inhibitors, and a soluble guanylate cyclase activator. None of these drugs are curative but there is improved morbidity and mortality.[84] Percutaneous catheter-based therapies are under development.[85] Individuals who do not achieve adequate clinical remission may require lung transplantation.

The most effective treatment for pulmonary hypertension associated with lung respiratory disease or hypoxia, or both, is treatment of the primary disorder. Supplemental oxygen may be indicated to reverse hypoxic vasoconstriction.

Cor Pulmonale

Cor pulmonale is defined as right ventricular enlargement (hypertrophy, dilation, or both) caused by PAH (see Figure 27-17).[86]

PATHOPHYSIOLOGY Cor pulmonale develops as PAH exerts chronic pressure overload in the right ventricle. Pressure overload increases the work of the right ventricle and causes hypertrophy of the normally thin-walled heart muscle. This eventually progresses to dilation and failure of the ventricle.

CLINICAL MANIFESTATIONS The clinical manifestations of cor pulmonale may be obscured by underlying respiratory or cardiac disease and appear only during exercise testing. The heart may appear normal at rest, but with exercise, cardiac output falls. The electrocardiogram may show right ventricular hypertrophy. The pulmonary component of the second heart sound, which represents closure of the pulmonic valve, may be accentuated, and a pulmonic valve murmur also may be present. Tricuspid valve murmur may accompany the development of right ventricular failure. Increased pressures in the systemic venous circulation cause jugular venous distention, hepatosplenomegaly, and peripheral edema.

EVALUATION AND TREATMENT Diagnosis is based on physical examination, imaging, and electrocardiography or echocardiography, or both. The goal of treatment for cor pulmonale is to decrease the workload of the right ventricle by lowering pulmonary artery pressure. Treatment is the same as that for pulmonary hypertension, and its success depends on reversal of the underlying lung disease.

✔ **QUICK CHECK 27-6**

1. What factors influence the impact of an embolus?
2. List three causes of pulmonary hypertension.
3. What is cor pulmonale?

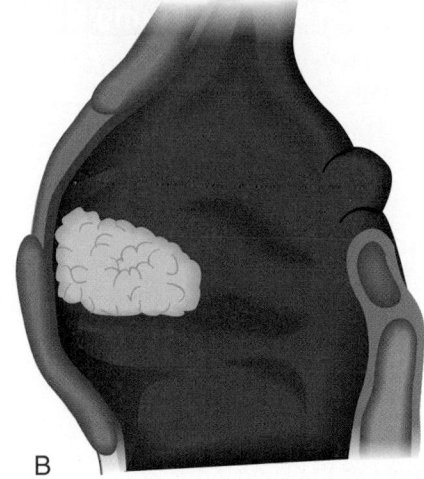

A   R   L   B

FIGURE 27-18 Laryngeal Cancer. A, Mirror view of carcinoma of the right false cord partially hiding the true cord. **B,** Lateral view. (Redrawn from del Regato JA et al: *Ackerman and del Regato's cancer,* ed 2, St Louis, 1985, Mosby.)

Malignancies of the Respiratory Tract
Laryngeal Cancer

Cancer of the larynx (laryngeal cancer) represents less than 1% of all cancers in the United States, with an estimated 13,560 new cases and 3640 deaths in 2015.[87] The primary risk factor for laryngeal cancer is tobacco smoking; risk is further heightened with the combination of smoking and alcohol consumption. The human papillomavirus (HPV 6 and 11) also has been linked to both benign and malignant disease of the larynx.[88] The highest incidence is in men between 50 and 75 years of age.

PATHOPHYSIOLOGY   Carcinoma of the true vocal cords (glottis) is more common than that of the supraglottic structures (epiglottis, aryepiglottic folds, arytenoids, false cords). Tumors of the subglottic area are rare. Squamous cell carcinoma is the most common cell type, although small cell carcinomas also occur (Figure 27-18). Metastasis develops by spread to the draining lymph nodes, and distant metastasis is rare.

CLINICAL MANIFESTATIONS   The presenting symptoms of laryngeal cancer include hoarseness, dyspnea, and cough. Progressive hoarseness can result in voice loss. Dyspnea is rare with supraglottic tumors but can be severe in subglottic tumors. Cough may follow swallowing. Laryngeal pain is likely with supraglottic lesions.

EVALUATION AND TREATMENT   Evaluation of the larynx includes external inspection and palpation of the larynx and the lymph nodes of the neck. Indirect laryngoscopy provides a stereoscopic view of the structure and movement of the larynx. A biopsy also can be obtained during this procedure. Direct laryngoscopy provides more thorough visualization of the tumor. Imaging procedures facilitate the identification of tumor boundaries and the degree of extension to surrounding tissue.

Combined chemotherapy and radiation or surgical resection can result in cure in selected cases; however, sequelae such as swallowing and speech difficulties may result.[89] Total laryngectomy is required when lesions are extensive and involve the cartilage. Swallowing and speech therapy after treatment can significantly improve recovery.

Lung Cancer

The term **lung cancer** refers to tumors that arise from the epithelium of the respiratory tract (bronchogenic carcinomas). Other pulmonary tumors, such as mesotheliomas (associated with asbestos exposure), occur less commonly (Table 27-3). Lung cancer is the second most common cancer in the United States, with an estimated 221,200 new cases and 158,040 deaths in 2015, the most common cause of cancer deaths.[87] Overall 5-year survival remains low at 17%.

The most common cause of lung cancer is tobacco smoking (see Figure 11-5). Smokers with obstructive lung disease (low FEV₁ measurements) are at much greater risk. Other risk factors for lung cancer include radon gas exposure, secondhand (environmental) smoke, occupational exposures to certain workplace toxins, radiation, and air pollution (see Chapter 11 and Figures 11-20 and 11-21). Genetic risks include polymorphisms of the genes responsible for growth factor receptors, angiogenesis, apoptosis, DNA repair, and detoxification of inhaled smoke.[90] Lung cancers are classified by cell type and molecular profiling. The most common types of lung cancer are presented here.

Types of lung cancer. Primary lung cancers arise from cells that line the bronchi within the lungs and are therefore called *bronchogenic carcinomas.* Although there are many types of lung cancer, they can be divided into two major categories: non–small cell lung carcinoma (NSCLC) and neuroendocrine tumors of the lung. The category of non–small cell lung carcinoma accounts for 75% to 85% of all lung cancers and can be subdivided into three types of lung cancer: squamous cell carcinoma, adenocarcinoma, and large cell undifferentiated carcinoma. They are further described by genotyping (i.e., epidermal growth factor receptor [EGFR] gene or anaplastic lymphoma kinase [ALK] gene mutations and rearrangements), which is important for targeted personalized therapy.[91] Neuroendocrine tumors of the lung arise from the bronchial mucosa and include small cell carcinoma, large cell neuroendocrine carcinoma, and typical carcinoid and atypical carcinoid tumors. Small cell carcinoma is the most common of these neuroendocrine tumors, accounting for 15% to 20% of all lung cancers. Characteristics of these tumors, including clinical manifestations, are listed in Table 27-3. Many cancers that arise in other organs of the body metastasize to the lungs; however, these are not considered lung cancers and are categorized by their primary site of origin.

TABLE 27-3   Characteristics of Lung Cancers

Tumor Type	Growth Rate	Metastasis	Means of Diagnosis	Clinical Manifestations and Treatment
Non–Small Cell Carcinoma				
Squamous cell carcinoma	Slow	Late; mostly to hilar lymph nodes	Biopsy, sputum analysis, bronchoscopy, electron microscopy, immunohistochemistry	Cough, hemoptysis, sputum production, airway obstruction, hypercalcemia; treated surgically, chemotherapy and radiation as adjunctive therapy
Adenocarcinoma	Moderate	Early; to lymph nodes, pleura, bone, adrenal glands, and brain	Radiography, fiberoptic bronchoscopy, electron microscopy	Pleural effusion; treated surgically, chemotherapy as adjunctive therapy
Large cell carcinoma	Rapid	Early and widespread	Sputum analysis, bronchoscopy, electron microscopy (by exclusion of other cell types)	Chest wall pain, pleural effusion, cough, sputum production, hemoptysis, airway obstruction resulting in pneumonia; treated surgically
Neuroendocrine Tumors of the Lung				
Small cell carcinoma	Very rapid	Very early; to mediastinum, lymph nodes, brain, bone marrow	Radiography, sputum analysis, bronchoscopy, electron microscopy, immunohistochemistry	Cough, chest pain, dyspnea, hemoptysis, localized wheezing, airway obstruction, signs and symptoms of excessive hormone secretion; treated by chemotherapy and ionizing radiation to thorax and central nervous system
Other Pulmonary Tumors				
Malignant pleural mesothelioma (MPM)	Rapid	Early; to lymph nodes, lungs, heart, bone	Radiography, thoracentesis	Chest pain, chronic cough, signs of pleural effusion

Non–small cell lung cancer. Squamous cell carcinoma accounts for about 30% of bronchogenic carcinomas and is associated with smoking and COPD. These tumors are typically located near the hila and project into bronchi (Figure 27-19, *A*). Because of this central location, symptoms of nonproductive cough or hemoptysis are common. Pneumonia and atelectasis are often associated with squamous cell carcinoma (see Figure 27-19, *A*). Chest pain is a late symptom associated with large tumors. These tumors are often fairly well localized and tend not to metastasize until late in the course of the disease.

Adenocarcinoma (tumor arising from glands) of the lung constitutes 35% to 40% of all bronchogenic carcinomas (Figure 27-19, *B*). Pulmonary adenocarcinoma develops in a stepwise fashion through atypical adenomatous hyperplasia, adenocarcinoma in situ, and minimally invasive adenocarcinoma to invasive carcinoma.[92] These tumors, which are usually smaller than 4 cm, more commonly arise in the peripheral regions of the pulmonary parenchyma. They may be asymptomatic and discovered by routine chest roentgenogram in the early stages, or the individual may present with pleuritic chest pain and shortness of breath from pleural involvement by the tumor.

Included in the category of adenocarcinoma is bronchioloalveolar cell carcinoma. These tumors arise from terminal bronchioles and alveoli and are now being referred to as adenocarcinoma in situ or minimally invasive adenocarcinoma.[93] They are slow-growing tumors with an unpredictable pattern of metastasis through the pulmonary arterial system and mediastinal lymph nodes.

Large cell carcinoma (undifferentiated). Large cell carcinomas constitute approximately 10% of bronchogenic carcinomas. These transformed epithelial cells have lost all evidence of differentiation and are considered an undifferentiated non–small cell carcinoma. Recent studies have confirmed that these tumors arise from squamous, glandular, or neuroendocrine precursor cells, and molecular analyses have made it possible to target some of these aggressive cancers for immunologic therapy.[94] These tumors commonly arise centrally and can grow to distort the trachea and cause widening of the carina.

Neuroendocrine tumors. Small cell (oat cell) carcinomas are the most common type of neuroendocrine lung tumors and have the highest correlation with tobacco smoking. Small cell carcinoma arises from neuroendocrine cells that contain neurosecretory granules. Most of these tumors are central in origin (hilar and mediastinal) (see Figure 27-19, *C*). Cell sizes range from 6 to 8 μm, have a rapid rate of growth, and tend to metastasize early and widely.[95] Small cell carcinomas tend to present at TNM stage IV and have the worst prognosis. They are often associated with ectopic hormone production. Ectopic hormone production is important to the clinician because resulting signs and symptoms called *paraneoplastic syndromes* may be the first manifestation of the underlying cancer. Examples include hyponatremia (antidiuretic hormone), Cushing syndrome (adrenocorticotropic hormone), hypocalcemia (calcitonin), gynecomastia (gonadotropins), carcinoid syndrome (serotonin), and Lambert-Eaton myasthenic syndrome (paneoplastic cerebellar degeneration).

PATHOPHYSIOLOGY Tobacco smoke contains more than 30 carcinogens and is responsible for causing 80% to 90% of lung cancers. These carcinogens, along with inherited genetic predisposition to cancers, result in tumor development. Once lung cancer is initiated by these carcinogen-induced mutations, further tumor development is promoted by growth factors that alter cell growth and differentiation, such as epidermal growth factor, and by production of inflammatory mediators, such as toxic oxygen free radicals. The bronchial mucosa suffers multiple carcinogenic "hits" because of repetitive exposure to tobacco smoke and, eventually, epithelial cell changes begin to be visible on biopsy. These changes progress from metaplasia to carcinoma in situ and finally to invasive carcinoma. Further tumor progression includes invasion of surrounding tissues and finally metastasis to distant sites including the brain, bone marrow, and liver (see Chapter 10 for details of cancer biology).

CLINICAL MANIFESTATIONS Table 27-3 summarizes the characteristic clinical manifestations according to tumor type. Symptoms are

FIGURE 27-19 Lung Cancer. A, Squamous cell carcinoma. This hilar tumor originates from the main bronchus. **B,** Peripheral adenocarcinoma. The tumor shows prominent black pigmentation, suggestive of having evolved in an anthracotic scar. **C,** Small cell carcinoma. The tumor forms confluent nodules. On cross section, the nodules have an encephaloid appearance. (From Damjanov I, Linder J, editors: *Anderson's pathology,* ed 10, St Louis, 1996, Mosby.)

often attributed to side effects of smoking; and when they are severe enough to motivate the individual to seek medical advice, the disease is usually advanced.

EVALUATION AND TREATMENT Screening for lung cancer remains controversial but low-dose spiral CT scans decrease the risk of dying from lung cancer by 20% in heavy smokers.[96] Diagnostic tests for the evaluation of lung cancer include sputum cytologic studies, chest imaging, virtual bronchoscopy, radial probe endobronchial ultrasound, electromagnetic navigational bronchoscopy, and biopsy. Biopsy determines the cell type, and the evaluation of lymph nodes and other organ systems is used to determine the stage of the cancer.[97] The histologic cell type, the genotype, and the stage of the disease are major factors that influence choice of therapy. The current accepted system for the staging of non–small cell cancer is the TNM classification (*T* denotes the extent of the primary tumor, *N* indicates the nodal involvement, *M* describes the extent of metastasis) (see Chapter 10). In contrast, small cell lung cancers are only staged as either limited (confined to the area of origin in the lung) or extensive.

The only proven way of reducing the risk for lung cancer is the cessation of smoking and avoidance of environmental toxins.[98] For all types of early-stage lung carcinoma, the preferred treatment is surgical resection. Once metastasis has occurred, total surgical resection is more difficult and survival rates dramatically decrease. For individuals with non–small cell carcinoma with metastasis at diagnosis, adjunctive radiation and chemotherapy and treatment based on molecular markers may improve outcomes.[99] Treatment modalities, including dose-intensified radiation, radiofrequency ablation, microwave ablation, cryotherapy, and brachytherapy, may be available as primary or palliative treatment for those for whom surgical removal is not an

option. Research is in progress to advance personalized genetic and immunologic approaches to treatment[100,101] (see *Health Alert:* Molecular Targets in Lung Cancer Treatment).

✓ QUICK CHECK 27-7
1. Describe squamous cell carcinoma of the vocal cords.
2. Differentiate the two types of non–small cell lung cancer.
3. What are paraneoplastic syndromes?

DID YOU UNDERSTAND?

Clinical Manifestations of Pulmonary Alterations

1. Dyspnea is the feeling of breathlessness and increased respiratory effort.
2. Coughing is a protective reflex that expels secretions and irritants from the lower airways.
3. Changes in the sputum volume, consistency, or color may indicate underlying pulmonary disease.
4. Hemoptysis is expectoration of bloody mucus.
5. Abnormal breathing patterns are adjustments made by the body to minimize the work of respiratory muscles. They include Kussmaul, obstructed, restricted, gasping, and Cheyne-Stokes respirations as well as sighing.
6. Hypoventilation is decreased alveolar ventilation caused by airway obstruction, chest wall restriction, or altered neurologic control of breathing and results in increased $Paco_2$ (hypercapnia).
7. Hyperventilation is increased alveolar ventilation produced by anxiety, head injury, or severe hypoxemia and causes decreased $Paco_2$ (hypocapnia).
8. Cyanosis is a bluish discoloration of the skin caused by desaturation of hemoglobin, polycythemia, or peripheral vasoconstriction.
9. Clubbing of the fingertips is associated with diseases that interfere with oxygenation of the tissues.
10. Chest pain can result from inflamed pleurae, trachea, bronchi, ribs, or respiratory muscles.
11. Hypoxemia is a reduced Pao_2 caused by (1) decreased oxygen content of inspired gas, (2) hypoventilation, (3) diffusion abnormality, (4) ventilation-perfusion mismatch, or (5) shunting.

Disorders of the Chest Wall and Pleura

1. Chest wall compliance is diminished by obesity and kyphoscoliosis, which compress the lungs, and by neuromuscular diseases that impair chest wall muscle function.
2. Flail chest results from rib or sternal fractures that disrupt the mechanics of breathing.
3. Pneumothorax is the accumulation of air in the pleural space. It can be caused by spontaneous rupture of weakened areas of the pleura or can be secondary to pleural damage caused by disease, trauma, or mechanical ventilation.
4. Tension pneumothorax is a life-threatening condition caused by trapping of air in the pleural space, producing displacement of the great vessels and heart.
5. Pleural effusion is the accumulation of fluid in the pleural space resulting from disorders that promote transudation or exudation from capillaries underlying the pleura or from blockage or injury to lymphatic vessels that drain into the pleural space.
6. Empyema is the presence of pus in the pleural space (infected pleural effusion); it usually occurs because of lymphatic drainage from sites of bacterial pneumonia.

Pulmonary Disorders

1. Pulmonary disorders can be restrictive (limiting lung volumes) or obstructive (limiting airflow) or both.
2. Aspiration of food particles or pharyngeal or gastric secretions can cause obstruction, inflammation, or pneumonitis.
3. Atelectasis is the collapse of alveoli resulting from compression of lung tissue or absorption of gas from obstructed alveoli.
4. Bronchiectasis is abnormal dilation of the bronchi secondary to another pulmonary disorder, usually infection or inflammation.

5. Bronchiolitis is the inflammatory obstruction of small airways. It is most common in children.
6. Pulmonary fibrosis is excessive connective tissue in the lung that diminishes lung compliance; it may be idiopathic or caused by disease and is associated with chronic inflammation.
7. Inhalation of noxious gases or prolonged exposure to high concentrations of oxygen can damage the bronchial mucosa or alveolocapillary membrane and cause inflammation or acute respiratory failure.
8. Pneumoconiosis, which is caused by inhalation of dust particles in the workplace, can cause pulmonary fibrosis, increase susceptibility to lower airway infection, and initiate tumor formation.
9. Hypersensitivity pneumonitis (extrinsic allergic alveolitis) is an allergic or hypersensitivity reaction to many allergens causing lung inflammation.
10. Pulmonary edema is excess water in the lung caused by increased capillary hydrostatic pressure, decreased capillary oncotic pressure, or increased capillary permeability. Causes include left heart failure that increases capillary hydrostatic pressure in the pulmonary circulation, inflammation of alveoli, or lymphatic obstruction.
11. Acute lung injury (ALI)/acute respiratory distress syndrome (ARDS) results from an acute, diffuse injury to the alveolocapillary membrane and decreased surfactant production, which increases membrane permeability and causes edema, atelectasis, and hypoxemia.
12. Obstructive lung disease is characterized by airway obstruction that causes difficult expiration. Obstructive disease can be acute or chronic and includes asthma, chronic bronchitis, and emphysema.
13. Asthma is an inflammatory disease of the airways resulting from a type I hypersensitivity immune response involving the activity of antigen, IgE, mast cells, eosinophils, and other inflammatory cells and mediators.
14. In asthma, airway obstruction is caused by episodic attacks of bronchospasm, bronchial inflammation, mucosal edema, and increased mucus production.
15. Chronic obstructive pulmonary disease (COPD) is the coexistence of chronic bronchitis and emphysema and is an important cause of hypoxemic and hypercapnic respiratory failure.
16. Chronic bronchitis causes airway obstruction resulting from inflammation, bronchial smooth muscle hypertrophy, and production of thick, tenacious mucus.
17. In emphysema, destruction of the alveolar septa and loss of passive elastic recoil lead to alveolar enlargement, airway collapse, obstruction of gas flow, and air trapping during expiration.
18. Acute bronchitis is usually a self-limiting viral infection.
19. Pneumococcal pneumonia (*Streptococcus pneumoniae*) is the most common acute lung infection, resulting in an inflammatory response with four phases: (1) consolidation, (2) red hepatization, (3) gray hepatization, and (4) resolution.
20. Viral pneumonia can be severe, but is more often an acute, self-limiting lung infection usually caused by the influenza virus. Atypical forms and new forms can cause severe acute respiratory syndrome (SARS).
21. Tuberculosis (TB) is a lung infection caused by *Mycobacterium tuberculosis* (tubercle bacillus). In tuberculosis, the inflammatory response proceeds to isolate colonies of bacilli by enclosing them in tubercles and surrounding the tubercles with scar

tissue. TB bacilli escape immune defenses by surviving within macrophages.

22. Pulmonary vascular diseases are caused by embolism or hypertension in the pulmonary circulation.

23. Pulmonary embolism is most often the result of embolism of part of a clot from deep venous thrombosis and causes vascular obstruction, $\dot{V}/\dot{Q}$ mismatch, hypoxemia, and pulmonary hypertension; it may or may not cause infarction.

24. Pulmonary artery hypertension (pulmonary artery pressure >25 mm Hg) can be idiopathic or associated with left heart failure, lung disease, or recurrent pulmonary emboli that increase resistance to blood flow in the pulmonary artery or its branches.

25. Cor pulmonale is right ventricular enlargement or failure caused by pulmonary hypertension.

26. Laryngeal cancer occurs primarily in men and represents 2% to 3% of all cancers. Squamous cell carcinoma of the true vocal cords is most common and presents with a clinical symptom of progressive hoarseness.

27. Lung cancer, the most common cause of cancer death in the United States, is commonly caused by tobacco smoking.

28. Lung cancer (bronchogenic carcinomas) cell types include non–small cell carcinoma (squamous cell, adenocarcinoma, and large cell) and, less commonly, neuroendocrine tumors (small cell carcinoma, large cell neuroendocrine carcinoma, and typical carcinoid and atypical carcinoid tumors). Each type arises in a characteristic site or type of tissue, causes distinctive clinical manifestations, and differs in likelihood of metastasis and prognosis.

KEY TERMS

Abscess, 706
Absorption atelectasis, 693
Acute bronchitis, 703
Acute lung injury (ALI), 695
Acute respiratory distress syndrome (ARDS), 695
Adenocarcinoma, 710
Alveolar dead space, 690
Aspiration, 693
Asthma, 698
Atelectasis, 693
Bronchiectasis, 693
Bronchiolitis, 694
Bronchiolitis obliterans, 694
Bronchiolitis obliterans organizing pneumonia (BOOP), 694
Cavitation, 706
Cheyne-Stokes respiration, 688
Chronic bronchitis, 701

Chronic obstructive pulmonary disease (COPD), 700
Clubbing, 689
Compression atelectasis, 693
Consolidation, 704
Cor pulmonale, 708
Cough, 687
Cyanosis, 688
Dyspnea, 687
Emphysema, 701
Empyema (infected pleural effusion), 692
Extrinsic allergic alveolitis (hypersensitivity pneumonitis), 695
Flail chest, 691
Hemoptysis, 688
Hypercapnia, 689
Hyperventilation, 688
Hypocapnia, 688

Hypoventilation, 688
Hypoxemia, 689
Hypoxia, 689
Idiopathic pulmonary fibrosis (IPF), 694
Kussmaul respiration (hyperpnea), 688
Large cell carcinoma, 710
Laryngeal cancer, 709
Latent TB infection (LTBI), 706
Lung cancer, 709
Open pneumothorax (communicating pneumothorax), 692
Orthopnea, 687
Oxygen toxicity, 695
Paroxysmal nocturnal dyspnea (PND), 687
Pleural effusion, 692
Pneumoconiosis, 695

Pneumonia, 703
Pneumothorax, 691
Pulmonary artery hypertension (PAH), 707
Pulmonary edema, 695
Pulmonary embolism (PE), 706
Pulmonary fibrosis, 694
Pulsus paradoxus, 699
Respiratory failure, 690
Shunting, 690
Small cell (oat cell) carcinoma, 710
Squamous cell carcinoma, 710
Status asthmaticus, 699
Surfactant impairment, 693
Tension pneumothorax, 692
TNM classification, 711
Transudative effusion, 692
Tuberculosis (TB), 706

REFERENCES

1. Hayen A et al: Understanding dyspnea as a complex individual experience, *Maturitas* 76(1):45-50, 2013.
2. Peters SP: When the chief complaint is (or should be) dyspnea in adults, *J Allergy Clin Immunol Pract* 1(2):129-136, 2013.
3. Parshall MB et al: An official American Thoracic Society statement: update on the mechanisms, assessment, and management of dyspnea, *Am J Respir Crit Care Med* 185(4):435-452, 2012.
4. Schmidt M et al: Unrecognized suffering in the ICU: addressing dyspnea in mechanically ventilated patients, *Intensive Care Med* 40(1):1-10, 2014.
5. Gibson PG et al: Mechanisms of cough, *Curr Opin Allergy Clin Immunol* 14(1):55-61, 2014.
6. Guyton AC, Hall JE, editors: *Textbook of medical physiology*, ed 13, Philadelphia, 2015, Saunders.
7. Spicknall KE et al: Clubbing: an update on diagnosis, differential diagnosis, pathophysiology, and clinical relevance, *J Am Acad Dermatol* 52(6):1020-1028, 2005.
8. Nguyen S, Hojjati M: Review of current therapies for secondary hypertrophic pulmonary osteoarthropathy, *Clin Rheumatol* 30(1):7-13, 2011.
9. Brims FJ et al: Respiratory chest pain: diagnosis and treatment, *Med Clin North Am* 94(2):217-232, 2010.

10. Oana S, Mukherji J: Acute and chronic respiratory failure, *Handb Clin Neurol* 119:273-288, 2014.
11. Sundaram S et al: Familial spontaneous pneumothorax and lung cysts due to a Folliculin exon 10 mutation, *Eur Respir J* 33(6):1510-1512, 2009.
12. Repanshek ZD et al: Alternative treatments of pneumothorax, *J Emerg Med* 44(2):457-466, 2013.
13. Psallidas I et al: Management of parapneumonic effusions and empyema, *Semin Respir Crit Care Med* 35(6):715-722, 2014.
14. O'Brien J: Absorption atelectasis: incidence and clinical implications, *AANA J* 81(3):205-208, 2013.
15. McDonnell MJ et al: Non-cystic fibrosis bronchiectasis, *QJM* 106(8):709-715, 2013.
16. Papiris SA et al: Bronchiolitis: adopting a unifying definition and a comprehensive etiological classification, *Exp Rev Respir Med* 7(3):289-306, 2013.
17. Wolters PJ et al: Pathogenesis of idiopathic pulmonary fibrosis, *Annu Rev Pathol* 9:157-179, 2014.
18. Ahluwalia N et al: New therapeutic targets in idiopathic pulmonary fibrosis. Aiming to rein in runaway wound-healing responses, *Am J Respir Crit Care Med* 190(8):867-878, 2014.

19. Grunes D, Beasley MB: Hypersensitivity pneumonitis: a review and update of histologic findings, *J Clin Pathol* 66(10):888-895, 2013.
20. Ohshimo S et al: Hypersensitivity pneumonitis, *Immunol Allergy Clin North Am* 32(4):537-556, 2012.
21. Fujishima S: Pathophysiology and biomarkers of acute respiratory distress syndrome, *J Intensive Care* 2(1):32, 2014.
22. Bakowitz M et al: Acute lung injury and the acute respiratory distress syndrome in the injured patient, *Scand J Trauma Resusc Emerg Med* 20:54, 2012.
23. Matthay MA et al: The acute respiratory distress syndrome, *J Clin Invest* 122(8):2731-2740, 2012.
24. Fujishima S: Pathophysiology and biomarkers of acute respiratory distress syndrome, *J Intensive Care* 2(1):32, 2014.
25. Ruan SY et al: Exploring the heterogeneity of effects of corticosteroids on acute respiratory distress syndrome: a systematic review and meta-analysis, *Crit Care* 18(2):R63, 2014.
26. Centers for Disease Control and Prevention: *FastStats: asthma.* Last update July 14, 2014. Available at www.cdc.gov/nchs/fastats/asthma.htm.
27. Corren J: Asthma phenotypes and endotypes: an evolving paradigm for classification, *Discov Med* 15(83):243-249, 2013.

28. Guarnieri M, Balmes JR: Outdoor air pollution and asthma, *Lancet* 383(9928):1581-1592, 2014.

29. Mackenzie KJ et al: Viral respiratory tract infections and asthma in early life: Cause and effect? *Clin Exp Allergy* 44(1):9-19, 2014.

30. Sutherland ER: Linking obesity and asthma, *Ann N Y Acad Sci* 1311:31-41, 2014.

31. Yoo Y, Perzanowski MS: Allergic sensitization and the environment: latest update, *Curr Allergy Asthma Rep* 14(10):465, 2014.

32. Kabesch M: Epigenetics in asthma and allergy, *Curr Opin Allergy Clin Immunol* 14(1):62-68, 2014.

33. Kramer A et al: Maintaining health by balancing microbial exposure and prevention of infection: the hygiene hypothesis versus the hypothesis of early immune challenge, *J Hosp Infect* 83(Suppl 1): S29-S34, 2013.

34. Beigelman A et al: The relationships between environmental bacterial exposure, airway bacterial colonization, and asthma, *Curr Opin Allergy Clin Immunol* 14(2):137-142, 2014.

35. Holgate ST: Innate and adaptive immune responses in asthma, *Nat Med* 18(5):673-683, 2012.

36. Deckers J et al: Innate immune cells in asthma, *Trends Immunol* 34(11):540-547, 2013.

37. Busse WW: The relationship of airway hyperresponsiveness and airway inflammation: airway hyperresponsiveness in asthma: its measurement and clinical significance, *Chest* 138(Suppl 2):4S-10S, 2010.

38. Bai TR: Evidence for airway remodeling in chronic asthma, *Curr Opin Allergy Clin Immunol* 10(1):82-86, 2010.

39. Shah R, Saltoun CA: Chapter 14: Acute severe asthma (status asthmaticus), *Allergy Asthma Proc* 33(Suppl 1):S47-S50, 2012.

40. Murata A, Ling PM: Asthma diagnosis and management, *Emerg Med Clin North Am* 30(2): 203-222, vii, 2012.

40a. Fajt ML, Wenzel SE: Asthma phenotypes and the use of biologic medications in asthma and allergic disease: the next steps toward personalized care, *J Allergy Clin Immunol* 135(2):299-310, 2015.

41. Penagos M et al: Metaanalysis of the efficacy of sublingual immunotherapy in the treatment of allergic asthma in pediatric patients, 3 to 18 years of age, *Chest* 133(3):599-609, 2008.

42. Normansell R et al: Omalizumab for asthma in adults and children, *Cochrane Database Syst Rev* 1:CD003559, 2014.

43. Apter AJ: Advances in adult asthma diagnosis and treatment in 2013, *J Allergy Clin Immunol* 133(1): 49-56, 2014.

44. Lovinsky-Desir S, Miller RL: Epigenetics, asthma, and allergic diseases: a review of the latest advancements, *Curr Allergy Asthma Rep* 12(3): 211-220, 2012.

45. Vestbo J et al: Global strategy for the diagnosis, management and prevention of chronic obstructive pulmonary disease, GOLD executive summary, *Am J Respir Crit Care Med* 187:347-365, 2013.

46. Diaz-Guzman E, Mannino DM: Epidemiology and prevalence of chronic obstructive pulmonary disease, *Clin Chest Med* 35(1):7-16, 2014.

47. Tzortzaki EG et al: Immune and genetic mechanisms in COPD: possible targets for therapeutic interventions, *Curr Drug Targets* 14(2):141-148, 2013.

48. Kim V, Criner GJ: Chronic bronchitis and chronic obstructive pulmonary disease, *Am J Respir Crit Care Med* 187(3):228-237, 2013.

49. Vijayan VK: Chronic obstructive pulmonary disease, *Indian J Med Res* 137(2):251-269, 2013.

50. Gagnon P et al: Pathogenesis of hyperinflation in chronic obstructive pulmonary disease, *Int J Chron Obstruct Pulmon Dis* 9:187-201, 2014.

51. Csikes NG, Gartman EJ: New developments in the assessment of COPD: early diagnosis is key, *Int J Chron Obstruct Pulmon Dis* 9:277-286, 2014.

52. Kim V, Criner GJ: Chronic bronchitis and chronic obstructive pulmonary disease, *Am J Respir Crit Care Med* 187(3):228-237, 2013.

53. Martinez CH, Han MK: Contribution of the environment and comorbidities to chronic obstructive pulmonary disease phenotypes, *Med Clin North Am* 96(4):713-727, 2012.

54. Stockley RA: Alpha1-antitrypsin review, *Clin Chest Med* 35(1):39-50, 2014.

55. Tuder RM, Petrache I: Pathogenesis of chronic obstructive pulmonary disease, *J Clin Invest* 122(8):2749-2755, 2012.

56. Kent BD et al: Hypoxemia in patients with COPD: cause, effects, and disease progression, *Int J Chron Obstruct Pulmon Dis* 6:199-208, 2011.

57. Stockley RA, Turner AM: α-1-Antitrypsin deficiency: clinical variability, assessment, and treatment, *Trends Mol Med* 20(2):105-115, 2014.

58. Murphy PB et al: Noninvasive ventilation and lung volume reduction, *Clin Chest Med* 35(1): 251-269, 2014.

59. Wunderink RG, Waterer GW: Clinical practice. Community-acquired pneumonia, *N Engl J Med* 370(6):543-551, 2014.

60. Ashraf M, Ostrosky-Zeichner L: Ventilator-associated pneumonia: a review, *Hosp Pract (Minneap)* 40(1):93, 2012.

61. Charles MP et al: Ventilator-associated pneumonia, *Australas Med J* 7(8):334-344, 2014.

62. Lobdell KW et al: Hospital-acquired infections, *Surg Clin North Am* 92(1):65-77, 2012.

63. Remington LT, Sligl WI: Community-acquired pneumonia, *Curr Opin Pulm Med* 20(3):215-224, 2014.

64. Hidron AI et al: Emergence of community-acquired methicillin-resistant *Staphylococcus aureus* strain USA3 00 as a cause of necrotising community-onset pneumonia, *Lancet Infect Dis* 9(6):384-392, 2009.

65. Klevens RM et al: Invasive methicillin-resistant *Staphylococcus aureus* infections in the United States, *J Am Med Assoc* 298:1763-1771, 2007.

66. Lieberman D et al: Respiratory viruses in adults with community-acquired pneumonia, *Chest* 138(4):811-816, 2010.

67. Vernatter J, Pirofski LA: Current concepts in host-microbe interaction leading to pneumococcal pneumonia, *Curr Opin Infect Dis* 26(3):277-283, 2013.

68. Mitchell TJ, Dalziel CE: The biology of pneumolysin, *Subcell Biochem* 80:145-160, 2014.

69. Ramsey CD, Kumar A: Influenza and endemic viral pneumonia, *Crit Care Clin* 29(4):1069-1086, 2013.

70. Couturier MR et al: Urine antigen tests for the diagnosis of respiratory infections: legionellosis, histoplasmosis, pneumococcal pneumonia, *Clin Lab Med* 34(2):219-236, 2014.

71. Yayan J: The comparative development of elevated resistance to macrolides in community-acquired pneumonia caused by *Streptococcus pneumoniae*, *Drug Des Devel Ther* 8:1733-1743, 2014.

72. Murray CJ et al: Global, regional, and national incidence and mortality for HIV, tuberculosis, and malaria during 1990-2013: a systematic analysis for the Global Burden of Disease Study 2013, *Lancet* 384(9947):1005-1070, 2014.

73. Pai M et al: New and improved tuberculosis diagnostics: evidence, policy, practice, and impact, *Curr Opin Pulmon Med* 16(3):271-284, 2010.

74. Moon HW, Hur M: Interferon-gamma release assays for the diagnosis of latent tuberculosis infection: an updated review, *Ann Clin Lab Sci* 43(2):221-229, 2013.

75. Zumla AI et al: New antituberculosis drugs, regimens, and adjunct therapies: needs, advances, and future prospects, *Lancet Infect Dis* 14(4): 327-340, 2014.

76. Günther G: Multidrug-resistant and extensively drug-resistant tuberculosis: a review of current concepts and future challenges, *Clin Med* 14(3): 279-285, 2014.

77. Weiner J 3rd, Kaufmann SH: Recent advances towards tuberculosis control: vaccines and biomarkers, *J Intern Med* 275(5):467-480, 2014.

78. Regazzi M et al: Treatment optimization in patients co-infected with HIV and Mycobacterium tuberculosis infections: focus on drug-drug interactions with rifamycins, *Clin Pharmacokinet* 53(6):489-507, 2014.

79. Konstantinides SV et al: 2014 ESC guidelines on the diagnosis and management of acute pulmonary embolism, *Eur Heart J* 35(43):3033-3069, 3069a-3069k, 2014.

80. Moorjani N, Price S: Massive pulmonary embolism, *Cardiol Clin* 31(4):503-518, vii, 2013.

81. Wells PS et al: Treatment of venous thromboembolism, *J Am Med Assoc* 311(7): 717-728, 2014.

82. National Heart Lung and Blood Institute: *Types of pulmonary hypertension*, August 2, 2011. Available at http://www.nhlbi.nih.gov/health/health-topics/topics/pah/types. Accessed May 2, 2015.

83. Roden AC: Pulmonary pathology: LC22-1 PULMONARY HYPERTENSION, *Pathology* 46(Suppl 2):S37, 2014.

84. Zamanian RT et al: Current clinical management of pulmonary arterial hypertension, *Circ Res* 115(1):131-147, 2014.

85. Rosanio S et al: Pulmonary arterial hypertension in adults: novel drugs and catheter ablationtechniques show promise? Systematic review on pharmacotherapy and interventional strategies, *Biomed Res Int* 2014:743868, 2014.

86. Rich S: Right ventricular adaptation and maladaptation in chronic pulmonary arterial hypertension, *Cardiol Clin* 30(2):257-269, 2012.

87. American Cancer Society: *Cancer facts and figures 2015*, Atlanta, 2015, Author.

88. Grce M, Mravak-Stipetić M: Human papillomavirus-associated diseases, *Clin Dermatol* 32(2):253-258, 2014.

89. Agra IM et al: Diagnosis and treatment of recurrent laryngeal cancer following initial nonsurgical therapy, *Head Neck* 34(5):727-735, 2012.

90. Sakashita S et al: Genes and pathology of non-small cell lung carcinoma, *Semin Oncol* 41(1):28-39, 2014.

91. Hensing T et al: A personalized treatment for lung cancer: molecular pathways, targeted therapies, and genomic characterization, *Adv Exp Med Biol* 799:85-117, 2014.

92. Noguchi M: Stepwise progression of pulmonary adenocarcinoma—clinical and molecular implications, *Cancer Metastasis Rev* 29(1):15-21, 2010.

93. Kerr KM: Clinical relevance of the new IASLC/ERS/ATS adenocarcinoma classification, *J Clin Pathol* 66(10):832-838, 2013.

94. Rossi G et al: Large cell carcinoma of the lung: clinically oriented classification integrating immunohistochemistry and molecular biology, *Virchows Archiv* 464(1):61-68, 2014.

95. Detterbeck FC: Clinical presentation and evaluation of neuroendocrine tumors of the lung, *Thorac Surg Clin* 24(3):267-276, 2014.

96. Nanavaty P et al: Lung cancer screening: advantages, controversies, and applications, *Cancer Control* 21(1):9-14, 2014.

97. Rivera MP et al: Establishing the diagnosis of lung cancer: diagnosis and management of lung cancer, 3rd ed: American College of Chest Physicians evidence-based clinical practice guidelines, *Chest* 143(5 Suppl):e142S-e165S, 2013.

98. Groot P, Munden RF: Lung cancer epidemiology, risk factors, and prevention, *Radiol Clin North Am* 50(5):863-876, 2012.

99. Carnio S et al: Extending survival of stage IV non-small cell lung cancer, *Semin Oncol* 41(1): 69-92, 2014.

100. Declerck S, Vansteenkiste J: Immunotherapy for lung cancer: ongoing clinical trials, *Future Oncol* 10(1):91-105, 2014.

101. Freitas DP et al: Therapy-induced enrichment of putative lung cancer stem-like cells, *Int J Cancer* 134(6):1270-1278, 2014.

28

Alterations of Pulmonary Function in Children

Valentina L. Brashers and Sue E. Huether

CHAPTER OUTLINE

Alterations of respiratory function in children are influenced by physiologic maturation, which is determined by age, genetics, and environmental conditions. Infants, especially premature infants, may present special problems because of incomplete development of the airways, circulation, chest wall, and immune system. A variety of upper and lower airway infections can cause respiratory compromise or play a role in the pathogenesis of more chronic pulmonary disease. Pulmonary dysfunction can be categorized into disorders of either the upper or the lower airways.

DISORDERS OF THE UPPER AIRWAYS

Disorders of the upper airways can cause significant obstruction to airflow. Common causes of upper airway obstruction in children are infections, foreign body aspiration, obstructive sleep apnea, and trauma.

Infections of the Upper Airways

Table 28-1 compares some of the more common upper airway infections.

Croup

Croup illnesses can be divided into two categories: (1) acute laryngotracheobronchitis (croup) and (2) spasmodic croup.[1] Diphtheria can also be considered a croup illness but is now rare because of vaccinations. Croup illnesses are all characterized by infection and obstruction of the upper airways.

Croup is an acute *laryngotracheitis* and almost always occurs in children between 6 months and 5 years of age with a peak incidence at 2 years of age. In 85% of cases, croup is caused by a virus, most commonly parainfluenza. Other causes include respiratory syncytial virus, rhinovirus, adenovirus, rubella virus, or atypical bacteria. The incidence of croup is higher in males and is most common during the winter months. Approximately 15% of affected children have a strong family history of croup.[2] *Spasmodic croup* usually occurs in older children. The etiology is unknown but can be triggered by cold, allergy, or viral infection.[2,3] Spasmodic croup develops acutely, usually without fever, and tends to recur.

PATHOPHYSIOLOGY The pathophysiology of viral croup is caused primarily by subglottic inflammation and edema from the infection. The mucous membranes of the larynx are tightly adherent to the underlying cartilage, whereas those of the subglottic space are looser and thus allow accumulation of mucosal and submucosal edema (Figure 28-1). Furthermore, the cricoid cartilage is structurally the narrowest point of the airway, making edema in this area critical. Spasmodic croup also causes obstruction but with less inflammation and edema. As illustrated in Figure 28-2, increased resistance to airflow leads to increased work of breathing, which generates more negative intrathoracic pressure that, in turn, may exacerbate dynamic collapse of the upper airway.

CLINICAL MANIFESTATIONS Typically, the child experiences rhinorrhea, sore throat, and low-grade fever for a few days, and then develops a harsh (seal-like) barking cough, inspiratory stridor, and hoarse voice. The quality of voice, cough, and stridor may suggest the location of the obstruction (Figure 28-3). Most cases resolve spontaneously within 24 to 48 hours and do not warrant hospital admission. A child with severe croup usually displays deep retractions (Figure 28-4), stridor, agitation, tachycardia, and sometimes pallor or cyanosis.

TABLE 28-1 Comparison of Upper Airway Infections

Condition	Age	Onset	Etiology	Pathophysiology	Symptoms
Acute laryngotracheobronchitis	6 months to 3 yr	Usually gradual	Viral	Inflammation from larynx to bronchi	Harsh cough; stridor; low-grade fever; may have nasal discharge, conjunctivitis
Acute tracheitis	1 to 12 yr	Abrupt or following viral illness	*Staphylococcus aureus*	Inflammation of upper trachea	High fever; toxic appearance; harsh cough; purulent secretions
Acute epiglottitis	2 to 6 yr	Abrupt	*Haemophilus influenzae,* group A streptococci	Inflammation of supraglottic structures	Severe sore throat; dysphagia; high fever; toxic appearance; muffled voice; may drool; dyspnea; sits erect and quietly

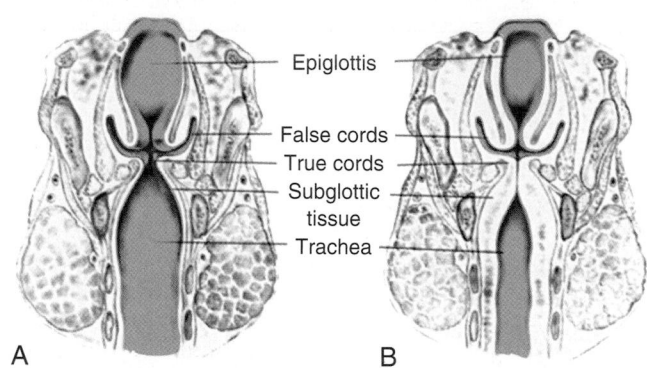

FIGURE 28-1 The Larynx and Subglottic Trachea. A, Normal trachea. **B,** Narrowing and obstruction from edema caused by croup. (From Hockenberry MJ, Wilson D: *Wong's nursing care of infants and children,* ed 10, St Louis, 2015, Mosby.)

Labels: Epiglottis, False cords, True cords, Subglottic tissue, Trachea

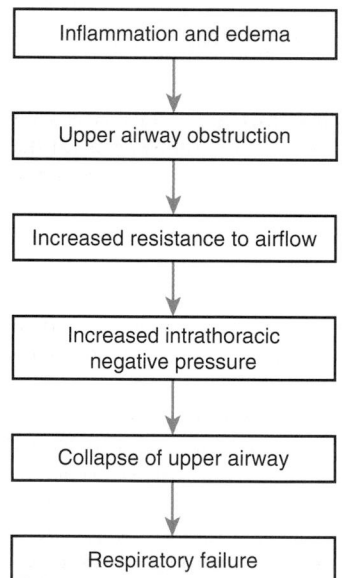

Inflammation and edema
↓
Upper airway obstruction
↓
Increased resistance to airflow
↓
Increased intrathoracic negative pressure
↓
Collapse of upper airway
↓
Respiratory failure

FIGURE 28-2 Upper Airway Obstruction with Croup.

Labels: Snoring zone, Inspiratory stridor zone, Voice quality zone, Cough quality zone, Expiratory stridor zone

FIGURE 28-3 Listening Can Help Locate the Site of Airway Obstruction. A loud, gasping snore suggests enlarged tonsils or adenoids. In inspiratory stridor, the airway is compromised at the level of the supraglottic larynx, vocal cords, subglottic region, or upper trachea. Expiratory stridor results from a narrowing or collapse in the trachea or bronchi. Airway noise during both inspiration and expiration often represents a fixed obstruction of the vocal cords or subglottic space. Hoarseness or a weak cry is a by-product of obstruction at the vocal cords. If a cough is croupy, suspect constriction below the vocal cords. (Redrawn from Eavey RD: *Contemp Ped* 3[6]:79, 1986; original illustration by Paul Singh-Roy.)

Spasmodic croup is characterized by similar hoarseness, barking cough, and stridor. It is of sudden onset and usually occurs at night and without prodromal symptoms. It usually resolves quickly.

EVALUATION AND TREATMENT The degree of symptoms determines the level of treatment. The most common tool for estimating croup severity is the Westley croup score.[4] Most children with croup require no treatment; however, some cases require outpatient treatment. These children usually have only mild stridor or retractions and appear alert, playful, and able to eat. There has been much debate about the most effective outpatient treatments for croup. Humidified air does not improve symptoms in mild to moderate croup.[5]

Glucocorticoids—either injected, oral (dexamethasone), or nebulized (budesonide)—have been shown to improve symptoms.[6] The presence of stridor at rest, moderate or severe retractions of the chest, or agitation suggests more severe disease and does require inpatient observation and treatment. For acute respiratory distress, nebulized epinephrine stimulates α- and β-adrenergic receptors and decreases mucosal edema and airway secretions.[7]

Oxygen should be administered. Heliox (helium-oxygen mixture) also can be used in severe cases although it is not yet considered a

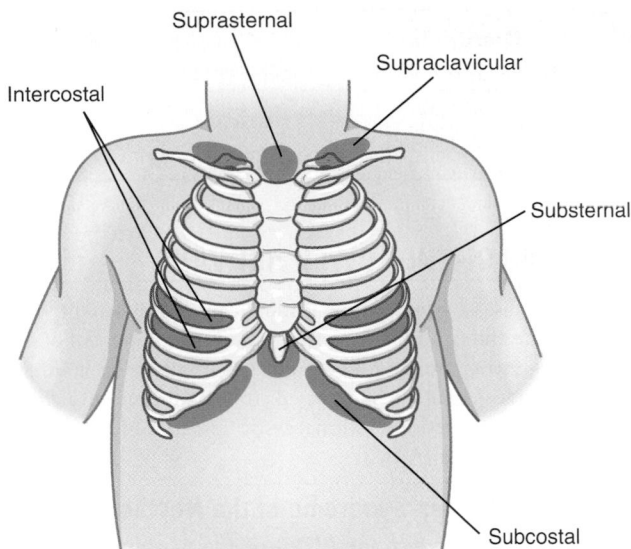

FIGURE 28-4 Areas of Chest Muscle Retraction.

mainstay of routine treatment. This works by improving gas flow and thus decreasing the flow resistance of the narrowed airway.[8] In rare cases, croup and spasmodic croup may require placement of an endotracheal tube.

Bacterial tracheitis. Bacterial tracheitis (pseudomembranous croup) is the most common potentially life-threatening upper airway infection in children. It is most often caused by *Staphylococcus aureus (S. aureus)* (including methicillin-resistant *S. aureus* [MRSA] strains), *Haemophilus influenzae (H. influenzae),* or group A beta-hemolytic *Streptococcus* (GABHS). Treatment of viral croup with corticosteroids has increased the risk for bacterial tracheitis. The presence of airway edema and copious purulent secretions leads to airway obstruction that can be worsened by the formation of a tracheal pseudomembrane and mucosal sloughing. Bacterial tracheitis is treated with immediate administration of antibiotics and endotracheal intubation to prevent total upper airway obstruction.[15]

Acute Epiglottitis

Historically, acute epiglottitis was caused by *Haemophilus influenzae* type B (HiB). Since the advent of *H. influenzae* vaccine, the overall incidence of acute epiglottitis has been reduced; however, up to 25% of epiglottitis cases are still caused by HiB, which is now more common in adults.[9] Current cases in children usually are related to vaccine failure or are caused by other pathogens.

PATHOPHYSIOLOGY The epiglottis arises from the posterior tongue base and covers the laryngeal inlet during swallowing. Bacterial invasion of the mucosa with associated inflammation leads to the rapid development of edema, causing severe, life-threatening obstruction of the upper airway.[9]

CLINICAL MANIFESTATIONS In the classic form of the disease, a child between 2 and 7 years of age suddenly develops high fever, irritability, sore throat, inspiratory stridor, and severe respiratory distress. The child appears anxious and has a voice that sounds muffled ("hot potato" voice). Drooling, absence of cough, preference to sit, and dysphagia (inability to swallow) are common.[10] In addition to appearing ill, the child will generally adopt a position of leaning forward

(tripoding) to try to improve breathing. Death can occur in a few hours. Pneumonia, cervical lymph node inflammation, otitis, and, rarely, meningitis or septic arthritis may occur concomitantly because of bacterial sepsis.

EVALUATION AND TREATMENT Acute epiglottitis is a life-threatening emergency. Efforts should be made to keep the child calm and undisturbed. Examination of the throat should not be attempted because it may trigger laryngospasm and cause respiratory collapse. With severe airway obstruction, the airway may be secured with intubation, and antibiotics are administered promptly. Racemic epinephrine and corticosteroids may be given until definitive management of the airway can be achieved.[11] Resolution with treatment is usually rapid. Postexposure prophylaxis with rifampin is recommended for all household unvaccinated contacts after a child is diagnosed.

Tonsillar Infections

Tonsillar infections (tonsillitis) are occasionally severe enough to cause upper airway obstruction. As with other infections of the upper airway, the incidence of tonsillitis secondary to group A beta-hemolytic *Streptococcus* (GABHS) and methicillin-resistant *Staphylococcus aureus* (MRSA) has risen in the past 15 years. Upper airway obstruction because of tonsillitis is a well-known complication of infectious mononucleosis, especially in a young child. Tonsillitis may be complicated by formation of a tonsillar abscess, which can further contribute to airway obstruction. Peritonsillar abscess is usually unilateral and is most often a complication of acute tonsillitis.[12] The abscess must be drained and the child given antibiotics.[13] The development of significant obstruction in tonsillar infections may require the use of corticosteroids, especially in the case of mononucleosis. The management of severe bacterial tonsillitis requires the use of antibiotics. Some children with recurrent tonsillitis benefit from adenotonsillectomy.[14]

Aspiration of Foreign Bodies

Aspiration of foreign bodies (FBs) into the airways usually occurs in children 1 to 4 years of age. More than 100,000 cases and 100 deaths occur each year.[16] Most objects are expelled by the cough reflex, but some objects may lodge in the larynx, trachea, or bronchi. Large objects (e.g., hard candy, a bite of hot dog, nuts, popcorn, grapes, beans, toy pieces, fragments of popped balloons, or coins) may occlude the airway and become life-threatening. Items of particular concern would be batteries and magnets. The aspiration event commonly is not witnessed or is not recognized when it happens because the coughing, choking, or gagging symptoms may resolve quickly. Foreign bodies lodged in the larynx or upper trachea cause cough, stridor, hoarseness or inability to speak, respiratory distress, and agitation or panic; the presentation is often dramatic and frightening. If the child is acutely hypoxic and unable to move air, immediate action such as sweeping the oral airway or performing abdominal thrusts (formerly called the Heimlich maneuver) may be required to prevent tragedy. Otherwise, bronchoscopic removal should be performed urgently. If an aspirated foreign body is small enough, it will be transferred to a bronchus before becoming lodged. If the foreign body is lodged in the airway for a notable period of time, local irritation, granulation, obstruction, and infection will ensue. Thus children may present with cough or wheezing, atelectasis, pneumonia, lung abscess, or blood-streaked sputum. These children are treated by prompt bronchoscopic removal of the object and administration of antibiotics as necessary.[17]

Obstructive Sleep Apnea

Obstructive sleep apnea syndrome (OSAS) is defined by partial or intermittent complete upper airway obstruction during sleep with disruption of normal ventilation and sleep patterns. Childhood OSAS is common, with an estimated prevalence of 2% to 3% of children 12 to 14 years of age and up to 13% of children between 3 and 6 years of age.[18,19] Prevalence is estimated to be two to four times higher in vulnerable populations (blacks, Hispanics, and preterm infants).[18] In children, unlike adults, OSAS occurs equally among girls and boys. Possible influences early in life may include passive smoke inhalation, socioeconomic status, and snoring together with genetic modifiers that promote airway inflammation.

PATHOPHYSIOLOGY Reduced airway diameter and increased upper airway collapsibility are the common causes of OSAS. Obstruction of the upper airway during sleep results in cyclic episodes of increasing respiratory effort and changes in intrathoracic pressures with oxygen desaturation, hypercapnia, and arousal. The child goes back to sleep and the cycle repeats. Adenotonsillar hypertrophy, obesity, and craniofacial anomalies are associated with decreased airway diameter. Infants are at risk because they have both anatomic and physiologic predispositions toward airway obstruction and gas exchange abnormalities.[20]

Reduced motor tone of the upper airways may be seen in neurologic disorders, such as cerebral palsy, and Down syndrome. Upper airway inflammation and altered neurologic reflexes involving respiratory control of upper airway muscles are significant factors in reducing airway diameter. Allergy and asthma may contribute to inflammation, and children who have a history of a clinically significant episode of respiratory syncytial virus (RSV) bronchiolitis in infancy may exhibit altered neuroimmunomodulatory pathways toward inflammation in the upper airway.[21] In obese children, current research links OSAS with airway inflammation and elevated levels of C-reactive protein, which also contribute to increased risk for cardiovascular and metabolic disease.[22,23] OSAS also may cause pulmonary disease, insulin resistance, and growth failure.[24]

CLINICAL MANIFESTATIONS Common manifestations of OSAS include snoring and labored breathing, sweating, and restlessness during sleep, which may be continuous or intermittent. There may be episodes of increased respiratory effort but no audible airflow, often terminated by snorting, gasping, repositioning, or arousal. Daytime sleepiness/napping is occasionally reported, as well as nocturnal enuresis. There is no correlation between sleep position and OSAS in children, except for those children who are notably obese. Obese children may adopt the prone position to attempt improved ventilation. Cognitive and neurobehavioral impairment, excessive daytime sleepiness, impaired school performance, and poor quality of life are consequences of OSAS.[25]

EVALUATION AND TREATMENT All parents should be asked if their child exhibits snoring, followed by a careful history and physical examination. A variety of screening tools are available. Imaging of the upper airway may be used to rule out adenoidal hypertrophy or upper airway narrowing.[26] The most definitive evaluation is the polysomnographic sleep study, which documents obstructed breathing and physiologic impairment. If obstructive sleep apnea is documented or strongly suspected clinically, children are most often referred for tonsillectomy and adenoidectomy (T & A) on the basis of described symptoms and physical findings, such as enlarged tonsils, adenoidal facies, and mouth breathing. For severely affected children who do not respond to T & A or who have different problems, such as obesity, continuous positive airway pressure (CPAP), anti-inflammatories, dental treatments, high-flow nasal cannula, and weight loss can be considered. Treatment is important to minimize associated morbidities.[27,28]

✔ **QUICK CHECK 28-1**
1. Compare and contrast pathology, clinical presentations, and severity of croup and epiglottitis.
2. What symptoms indicate aspiration of a foreign body?
3. What signs and symptoms suggest obstructive sleep apnea?

DISORDERS OF THE LOWER AIRWAYS

Lower airway disease is one of the leading causes of morbidity in the first year of life and continues to be an important component of other illnesses progressing into childhood. Pulmonary disorders commonly observed include neonatal respiratory distress syndrome, bronchopulmonary dysplasia, infections, asthma, cystic fibrosis, and acute respiratory distress syndrome (ARDS).

Respiratory Distress Syndrome of the Newborn

Respiratory distress syndrome (RDS) of the newborn (previously known as *hyaline membrane disease [HMD]*) is a significant cause of neonatal morbidity and mortality. It occurs almost exclusively in premature infants and the incidence has increased in the United States over the past 2 decades.[29] RDS occurs in 50% to 60% of infants born at 29 weeks' gestation and decreases significantly by 36 weeks. Risk factors are summarized in *Risk Factors*: Respiratory Distress Syndrome of the Newborn. Death rates have declined significantly since the introduction of antenatal steroid therapy and postnatal surfactant therapy.

RISK FACTORS
Respiratory Distress Syndrome of the Newborn

- Premature birth/low birth weight
- Male gender
- Cesarean delivery without labor
- Diabetic mother
- Perinatal asphyxia

PATHOPHYSIOLOGY RDS is caused by surfactant deficiency, which decreases the alveolar surface area available for gas exchange. Surfactant is a lipoprotein with a detergent-like effect that separates the liquid molecules inside the alveoli, thereby decreasing alveolar surface tension. Without surfactant, alveoli collapse at the end of each exhalation. Surfactant normally is not secreted by the alveolar cells until approximately 30 weeks' gestation. In addition to surfactant deficiency, premature infants are born with underdeveloped and small alveoli that are difficult to inflate and have thick walls and inadequate capillary blood supply such that gas exchange is significantly impaired. Furthermore, the infant's chest wall is weak and highly compliant and, thus, the rib cage tends to collapse inward with respiratory effort. The net effect is *atelectasis* (collapsed alveoli), resulting in significant hypoxemia. Atelectasis is difficult for the neonate to overcome because it requires a significant negative inspiratory pressure to open the alveoli with each breath. This increased work of breathing may result in hypercapnia. Hypoxia and hypercapnia cause pulmonary vasoconstriction and increase intrapulmonary resistance and shunting. This results in hypoperfusion of the lung and a decrease in effective pulmonary blood flow. Increased pulmonary vascular resistance may even cause a partial return to fetal circulation, with right-to-left shunting of blood through the ductus arteriosus and foramen ovale. Inadequate perfusion of tissues and hypoxemia contribute to metabolic acidosis.

FIGURE 28-5 Pathogenesis of Respiratory Distress Syndrome (RDS) of the Newborn.

Inadequate alveolar ventilation can be further complicated by increased pulmonary capillary permeability. Many premature infants with RDS will require mechanical ventilation, which damages the alveolar epithelium. Together these conditions result in the leakage of plasma proteins into the alveoli. Fibrin deposits in the air spaces create the appearance of *"hyaline membranes,"* for which the disorder was originally named. The plasma proteins leaked into the air space have the additional adverse effect of inactivating any surfactant that may be present. The pathogenesis of RDS is summarized in Figure 28-5.

CLINICAL MANIFESTATIONS Signs of RDS appear within minutes of birth and include tachypnea (respiratory rate greater than 60 breaths/min), expiratory grunting, intercostal and subcostal retractions, nasal flaring, and cyanosis. Severity tends to increase over the first 2 days of life. Apnea and irregular respirations occur as the infant tires. Severity of hypoxemia and difficulty in providing supplemental oxygenation have resulted in the Vermont Oxford Neonatal Network definition of RDS: a Pao_2 less than 50 mm Hg in room air, central cyanosis in room air, or a need for supplemental oxygen to maintain Pao_2 greater than 50 mm Hg, as well as classic chest film appearance.[30] The typical chest radiograph shows diffuse, fine granular densities within the first 6 hours of life. This "ground glass" appearance is associated with alveolar flooding. Ventilatory support is often required. In most cases the clinical manifestations reach a peak within 3 days, after which there is gradual improvement.

EVALUATION AND TREATMENT Diagnosis is made on the basis of premature birth or other risk factors, chest radiographs, pulse oximetry measurements, and, if needed, analysis of amniotic fluid or tracheal aspirates to estimate lung maturity (lecithin/sphingomyelin ratio [L/S ratio]). Some neonates require immediate resuscitation because of asphyxia or severe respiratory distress. The ultimate treatment for RDS would be prevention of premature birth. For women at risk of preterm birth, antenatal treatment with glucocorticoids induces a significant and rapid acceleration of lung maturation and stimulation of surfactant production in the fetus and significantly reduces the incidence of RDS and death.[31,32]

Current recommendations for infants weighing less than 1000 g include prophylaxis beginning within 15 to 30 minutes of birth by administration of exogenous surfactant (either synthetic or natural) through nebulizer or nasal continuous positive airway pressure (CPAP) ventilation. Repeat doses are given every 12 hours for the first few days. There is usually a dramatic improvement in oxygenation as well as a decreased incidence of RDS death, pneumothorax, and pulmonary interstitial emphysema. For infants weighing more than 1000 g, surfactant replacement is based on clinical need. Surfactant therapy should be considered complementary to antenatal glucocorticoids. The two therapies together appear to have an additive effect on improving lung function.[33]

Supportive care includes oxygen administration and often such measures as mechanical ventilation. Mechanical ventilation can result in a proinflammatory state that may contribute to the development of chronic lung disease, such as bronchopulmonary dysplasia (BPD). Strategies that are lung protective include greater reliance on nasal CPAP, permissive hypercapnia, lower oxygen saturation targets, modulation of tidal volume (V_t) settings, and use of high-frequency oscillation. Further studies are needed to evaluate the effectiveness of inhaled nitric oxide (iNO) in preterm infants.[34] Most infants survive RDS and, in many cases, recovery may be complete within 10 to 14 days. However, the incidence of subsequent chronic lung disease (i.e., bronchopulmonary dysplasia) is significant among very low birth weight infants.[35]

Bronchopulmonary Dysplasia

Bronchopulmonary dysplasia (BPD), also known as *chronic lung disease (CLD) of prematurity,* is the major cause of pulmonary disease in infants. It is associated with premature birth (usually before 28 weeks' gestation), prolonged (at least 28 days) perinatal supplemental oxygen, and positive pressure ventilation. There are approximately 60,000 U.S. infants born weighing less than 1500 g on an annual basis. About 20% to 30% of these infants develop BPD.[36] Risk factors for BPD[37] are summarized in *Risk Factors:* Bronchopulmonary Dysplasia (BPD).

RISK FACTORS

Bronchopulmonary Dysplasia (BPD)

- Premature birth (especially ≤28 weeks)
- Positive-pressure ventilation
- Supplemental oxygen administration
- Antenatal chorioamnionitis
- Postnatal sepsis or pneumonia
- Patent ductus arteriosus
- Nutritional deficiencies
- Early adrenal insufficiency
- Genetic susceptibility

The widespread use of antenatal glucocorticoids and postnatal surfactant has lessened the incidence and severity of RDS, and BPD is occurring primarily in the smallest premature infants (23 to 28 weeks' gestation) who have received mechanical ventilation. The presence of antenatal chorioamnionitis with fetal involvement, postnatal sepsis, a patent ductus arteriosus, and genetic susceptibility confer additional risks of developing BPD.[37] Surprisingly, some of these tiny infants who develop BPD have shown few or no clinical signs of RDS at birth or have initially received only low levels of supplemental oxygen or ventilatory support, sometimes for other reasons such as apnea.

PATHOPHYSIOLOGY Lung immaturity and inflammation contributes to the development of BPD. Before the widespread use of surfactant therapy, BPD was a disease characterized by airway injury, inflammation, and parenchymal fibrosis (*classic BPD*). With the initiation of surfactant therapy, what is called the *new BPD* is most common and is a form of arrested lung development. There is poor formation of the alveolar structure with fewer and larger alveoli and decreased surface area for gas exchange. Persistent inflammation contributes to

---

TABLE 28-2 Comparison of Classic and New Bronchopulmonary Dysplasia (BPD)

Classic BPD	New BPD
Metaplasia of respiratory epithelium	Less severe squamous metaplasia
Smooth muscle hypertrophy	Less smooth muscle hypertrophy
Significant fibrosis	Less fibrosis
Large vascular modifications	Abnormal pulmonary vascular structure
	Small number and increased diameter of alveoli
	Increase in elastic tissue

Adapted from Monte LF et al: *J Pediatr (Rio J)* 81(2):99-110, 2005 (Table 3). Available at: www.scielo.br/scielo.php?pid=s0021 -75572005000300004&script=sci_arttext&tlng=en.

---

pulmonary capillary fibrosis, perfusion mismatch, pulmonary hypertension, and decreased exercise capacity.[38,39] The predominant mediators of *new BPD* are profibrotic and angiogenic cytokines rather than proinflammatory cytokines, which contribute to pulmonary hypertension.[40] Table 28-2 and Figure 28-6 illustrate the pathophysiology of BPD.

CLINICAL MANIFESTATIONS The clinical definition of BPD includes need for supplemental oxygen at 36 weeks' postmenstrual age or gestational age (the time elapsed between the first day of the last normal menstrual period and the day of birth), and for at least 28 days after birth. It also details a graded severity dependent on required respiratory support at term (mild, moderate, and severe, based on oxygen requirements and ventilatory needs). Clinically, the infant exhibits hypoxemia and hypercapnia caused by ventilation-perfusion mismatch and diffusion defects. The work of breathing increases and the ability to feed may be impaired. Intermittent bronchospasm, mucus plugging, and pulmonary hypertension characterize the clinical course. Of the most severely affected infants, dusky spells may occur with agitation, feeding, or gastroesophageal reflux. Infants with mild BPD may demonstrate only mild tachypnea and difficulty handling respiratory tract infections.

EVALUATION AND TREATMENT Infants with severe BPD require prolonged assisted ventilation. Prevention of lung damage with noninvasive respiratory support, such as early nasal CPAP or nasal intermittent positive-pressure ventilation (IPPV), is used in clinical situations when permitted. When compared to mechanical ventilation, use of CPAP has resulted in fewer days of oxygen and ventilator requirement by reducing the amount of lung injury.[41] Diuretics are used to control pulmonary edema. Bronchodilators reduce airway resistance. Inhaled corticosteroids improve the rate of extubation and reduce the time that mechanical ventilation is required.[42] Prophylactic caffeine citrate administration, vitamin A supplementation, and careful fluid and nutritional support are routinely used and have resulted in improved outcomes.[43] Children with BPD will need to be monitored into adulthood for the development of chronic lung disease.

✔ QUICK CHECK 28-2

1. Why are premature infants susceptible to RDS?
2. Describe the pathologic findings of "new BPD."

FIGURE 28-6 Pathophysiology of Bronchopulmonary Dysplasia (BPD).

Respiratory Tract Infections

Respiratory tract infections are common in children and are a frequent cause for emergency department visits and hospitalizations. Clinical presentation, age of the child, and season of the year can often provide clues to the etiologic agent, even when the agent cannot be proved.

Bronchiolitis

Bronchiolitis is a common, viral respiratory tract infection of the small airways that occurs almost exclusively in infants and young toddlers and is a major reason for hospitalization. It has a seasonal, yearly incidence, from approximately November to April, and is the leading cause of hospitalization for infants during the winter season. The most common associated pathogen is respiratory syncytial virus (RSV), but bronchiolitis also may be associated with human metapneumovirus and human bocavirus. Healthy infants usually make a full recovery from RSV bronchiolitis, but infants who were premature (birth weight <2500 g) or who have underlying BPD or heart disease may have a much higher risk for a more severe or even deadly course. Bronchiolitis has been linked to an increased risk for asthma later in childhood.[44] Associations with rhinovirus and low vitamin D levels also are being investigated because they appear to correlate with the increased likelihood that children develop asthma after they have experienced bronchiolitis.[45]

PATHOPHYSIOLOGY Viral infection causes necrosis of the bronchial epithelium and destruction of ciliated epithelial cells. There is infiltration with lymphocytes around the bronchioles and a cell-mediated hypersensitivity to viral antigens with release of lymphokines causing inflammation, as well as activation of eosinophils, neutrophils, and monocytes. The submucosa becomes edematous and cellular debris and fibrin form plugs within the bronchioles. Edema of the bronchiolar wall, accumulation of mucus and cellular debris, and bronchospasm narrow many peripheral airways. Other airways become partially or completely occluded. Atelectasis occurs in some areas of the lung and hyperinflation in others.

The mechanics of breathing are disrupted by bronchiolitis. Airway narrowing causes obstruction of airflow that is worse on expiration. This leads to air trapping, hyperinflation, and increased functional residual capacity (FRC). Airway resistance and hyperinflation result in increased work of breathing and the development of hypercapnia in severe cases.

CLINICAL MANIFESTATIONS Symptoms usually begin with significant rhinorrhea followed by a tight cough over the next several days, along with systemic signs of decreased appetite, lethargy, and fever. Infants typically have tachypnea, variable degrees of respiratory distress, and abnormal auscultatory findings of the chest. Wheezing is most common, but rales or rhonchi also may be present. Chest radiographs often reveal hyperexpanded lungs, patchy or peribronchial infiltrates, and, sometimes, atelectasis of the right upper lobe. Very young infants may present with severe apnea before lower respiratory tract symptoms appear, and these apneas frequently require mechanical ventilation. Many children also may present with conjunctivitis or otitis media.

EVALUATION AND TREATMENT Guidelines from the American Academy of Pediatrics are available for the evaluation, treatment, and prevention of bronchiolitis.[46] Diagnosis of bronchiolitis is made by review of history, signs, and symptoms (e.g., rhinitis, cough, wheezing, chest retractions, tachypnea). Laboratory and radiologic examination are not routinely performed.

Treatment for bronchiolitis is determined by the severity of the disease and the age of the child. Most cases are mild and require no specific treatment and may be monitored as outpatients. When treatment is indicated, it is primarily supportive in nature. Preventive treatment with RSV-specific monoclonal antibody (palivizumab), provided as a monthly injection for 5 months through the RSV season, is recommended for high-risk infants younger than 2 years who meet specific criteria (e.g., hemodynamically significant heart disease and chronic lung disease of prematurity). Other preventive measures include use of hand washing and alcohol-based decontamination, prevention of exposure to tobacco smoke, and promotion of infant breast feeding.

Pneumonia

Pneumonia is infection and inflammation in the terminal airways and alveoli. Community-acquired pneumonia (CAP) is a major cause of morbidity and mortality in children, particularly in developing countries. The most common agents are viruses, followed by bacteria and atypical microorganisms (e.g., mycoplasma) (Table 28-3), and clinical symptoms often do not differentiate viral from bacterial or atypical pneumonia. Risk factors for developing CAP are age younger than 2 years, overcrowded living conditions, winter season, recent antibiotic treatment, daycare attendance, and passive smoke exposure. Nutritional status, age, and underlying disease process influence morbidity and mortality rates related to CAP.

PATHOPHYSIOLOGY Viral pneumonia is two to three times more likely to occur in children than in adults, and incidence generally follows a seasonal pattern. Bacterial coinfections are common. RSV (respiratory syncytial virus) is the most common viral pneumonia in young children. A number of other viruses are important, including parainfluenza, influenza, human rhinovirus, human metapneumovirus, adenoviruses, and *Mycoplasma pneumoniae*.[47] Acquisition of these viruses is by direct contact, droplet transmission, or aerosol exposure. There is initial destruction of the ciliated epithelium of the distal airway with sloughing of cellular material. A mononuclear-predominant inflammatory response occurs, in the interstitium initially, and later may involve the alveoli as well. Early in the course of the disease, it is often difficult to determine whether the pneumonia is viral or bacterial. Viral pneumonia often presents with cough and no fever. Differences in the clinical presentation can help to determine origin, such as degree of elevation of temperature, absolute neutrophil counts, and percentage of bands. Ultimately, diagnosis requires laboratory confirmation using immunofluorescence tests. Development of safe agents to treat and prevent viral pneumonia continues to be a focus of much research.[48]

Bacterial pneumonia beyond the neonatal period is most commonly the result of infection with streptococci and staphylococci microorganisms. Pneumococcal (*Streptococcus pneumoniae*) pneumonia is the most common cause of community-acquired bacterial pneumonia and presents acutely and with variable severity.[49] Childhood immunization with polyvariant pneumococcal conjugate vaccine appears to decrease the incidence of pneumococcal pneumonia in children younger than 2 years of age.[50] Staphylococcal pneumonia and group A streptococcal pneumonia can be particularly fulminant (sudden, severe) and necrotizing (causing cell death) with a high incidence of accompanying empyema, pneumatocele (a lung lesion filled with air), and sepsis. *H. influenzae* pneumonia has become rare because of widespread immunization.

Bacterial pneumonia usually begins with aspiration of nasopharyngeal bacteria. A preceding viral infection sometimes sets the stage for bacterial infection by causing epithelial damage, reduced mucociliary clearance in the trachea and major bronchi, and a reduced immune response. Once in the alveolar region, bacteria encounter local host defenses, such as antibodies, complement, and cytokines, which prepare bacteria for ingestion by alveolar macrophages. Alveolar macrophages recognize bacteria with their surface receptors and phagocytose them. If these mechanisms fail, macrophages release numerous inflammatory cytokines and neutrophils will be recruited into the lung.[51] An intense, cytokine-mediated inflammation will ensue. Vascular engorgement, edema, and a fibrinopurulent exudate occur. Alveolar filling precludes gas exchange and, if extensive, can lead to respiratory failure. If sepsis occurs at the same time, shock and end-organ hypoperfusion will cause metabolic acidosis.

The clinical presentation of bacterial pneumonia, particularly pneumococcal, may include a preceding viral illness followed by fever with chills and rigors, shortness of breath, and an increasingly productive cough. Occasionally, there is blood streaking of the sputum. Respiratory rate and oxygen saturation also are important clinical indicators.

TABLE 28-3	Common Types of Pneumonia in Children			
Type	**Causal Agent**	**Age**	**Onset**	**Signs/Symptoms**
Viral pneumonia	Respiratory syncytial virus (RSV), influenza, adenovirus, others	Infants for RSV, all ages for others	Acute or gradual, winter and early spring	Mild to high fever, cough, rhinorrhea, malaise, rales, rhonchi, wheezing, or apnea; variable radiographic pattern
Pneumococcal pneumonia	Pneumococci (*Streptococcus pneumoniae*)	Usually 1 to 4 yr	Acute, follows an upper respiratory tract infection, winter and early spring	High fever, productive cough, pleuritic pain, increased respiration rate, decreased breath sounds in area of consolidation; lobar infiltrate or "round pneumonia" on radiograph
Staphylococcal pneumonia	*Staphylococcus aureus* (including methicillin-resistant strains)	1 wk to 2 yr	Acute, winter	High fever, cough, respiratory distress; empyema or pneumatoceles common
Streptococcal pneumonia	Group A beta-hemolytic streptococci	All ages	Acute, any season	High fever, chills, respiratory distress, sepsis, or shock
Mycoplasmal and chlamydial pneumonia	*Mycoplasma pneumoniae, Chlamydophila pneumonia*	School-age and adolescents	Gradual	Low-grade fever, cough

Auscultation usually shows such abnormalities as crackles or decreased breath sounds. Other, less specific findings may include malaise, emesis, abdominal pain, and chest pain. Chest films will usually present with a lobar pattern in older children and adolescents but may appear patchier with a bronchopneumonic pattern in younger children.

Atypical pneumonia (*Mycoplasma* pneumoniae, *Chlamydophila pneumoniae*) is the most common cause of community-acquired pneumonia for school-age children and young adults. *Chlamydophila* pneumonia is clinically indistinguishable from and is typically grouped with *Mycoplasma* as "atypical pneumonia." Transmission is from person-to-person with a 2- to 3-week incubation period.

Mycoplasmic microorganisms lack cell walls but have a limiting membrane and a specialized receptor for attaching to ciliated respiratory epithelial cells. Local sloughing of cells occurs. Peribronchial lymphocytic infiltration develops, along with neutrophil recruitment to the airway lumen. The pattern resembles bronchitis or bronchopneumonia. Onset is usually gradual, resembling a typical upper respiratory tract infection but with low-grade fever, cough, and chest pain.[52] *Mycoplasma* can cause a wide spectrum of disease and is more extensive as a cause of complications than previously noted. It also is occurring more frequently in infants and younger children. Most cases are not clinically severe and full recovery should be expected. Complications, when they do occur, can include bronchopneumonia, parapneumonic effusions, and necrotizing pneumonitis.

EVALUATION AND TREATMENT Guidelines have been developed to improve and aid assessment and management of pediatric pneumonia.[53,54] Diagnosis of pneumonia is based on clinical and laboratory findings. The etiologic agent can sometimes be inferred from the age of the child and clinical scenario.[55] Chest x-ray in bacterial pneumonia often will initially produce a patchy infiltration and later reveal a segmental or lobar disease. A viral infection is more likely to be associated with an interstitial pattern. Biomarkers (i.e., procalcitonin) facilitate more rapid diagnosis and guide antibiotic therapy. The highly sensitive C-reactive protein (hs-CRP) is less specific and its level is elevated in both viral and bacterial infections.[56] Several microbiologic tests are available, such as polymerase chain reaction (PCR) and nucleic acid amplification tests (NAATs).

Some pneumonias may be treated on an outpatient basis; however, many children require oxygen supplementation and, occasionally, assisted ventilation. This is particularly true with infants who have a viral interstitial pneumonia, such as RSV. In addition, adequate hydration, proper nutrition, and supportive pulmonary therapy are required to reduce the duration and severity of illness. Many infants are markedly tachypneic and unable to coordinate their breathing with swallowing; they may require enteral feeding. Aspiration is always a risk with infants in respiratory distress.

Appropriate antibiotic administration for bacterial pneumonias is dependent on age and severity assessment. Local patterns of resistance must be considered when choosing appropriate antibiotics. Pneumococcal and mycoplasmal pneumonias present some unique treatment obstacles and may need a multifaceted approach to care including vaccine antigens and immune adjuvant therapies in addition to antibiotics.[57] Children should be vaccinated against influenza and pneumococcus.

> ✔ **QUICK CHECK 28-3**
> 1. Describe the typical presentation of RSV bronchiolitis.
> 2. What clinical features distinguish bacterial pneumonia from atypical pneumonia?

Aspiration Pneumonitis

Aspiration pneumonitis is caused by a foreign substance, such as food, meconium, secretions (saliva or gastric), or environmental compounds, entering the lung and resulting in inflammation of the lung tissue. The aspiration of meconium from amniotic fluid can occur at birth.[58] Neurologically compromised children or children with chronic lung disease may have chronic pulmonary aspiration (CPA), which can cause progressive lung disease, bronchiectasis, and respiratory failure. This is the leading cause of death in children who are neurologically compromised because of failure of protective reflexes and difficulty swallowing.[59] Children undergoing sedation or anesthesia also may aspirate oral secretions contaminated with anaerobic bacteria or acidic stomach contents. The severity of lung injury after an aspiration incident is determined by the volume and pH of the material aspirated and the presence of pathogenic bacteria. Very low pH or extremely high pH will cause a significant inflammatory response. With hydrocarbon ingestions, lung injury is determined by the volatility and viscosity of the aspirated substance. A low-viscosity substance, such as gasoline or lighter fluid, is the most toxic, and high-viscosity hydrocarbons, such as petroleum jelly or mineral oil, are much less likely to cause a pneumonitis. Treatment for aspiration pneumonitis depends on the material aspirated but can include broad-spectrum antibiotics with failure to improve after 48 hours. Children with CPA and a large amount of upper respiratory tract secretions may benefit from salivary gland injection with botulinum toxin A (BTX-A) to suppress secretion.[60]

Bronchiolitis Obliterans

Bronchiolitis obliterans (BO) is fibrotic obstruction of the respiratory bronchioles and alveolar ducts secondary to intense inflammation. It is relatively rare in children. There are two types: proliferative and constrictive (obstructive), with the latter being the more common form. BO most often occurs as a sequela of a severe viral pulmonary infection (e.g., influenza, adenovirus, pertussis [whooping cough], or measles). Other cases may be secondary to parainfluenza, RSV, human immunodeficiency virus (HIV), or *M. pneumoniae* infection or lung transplant. It also may occur after lung, heart-lung, or bone marrow transplantation, or be associated with collagen vascular disease, toxic fume inhalation, chronic hypersensitivity pneumonitis, Crohn disease, and Stevens-Johnson syndrome.[61,62] Although the child may initially improve after the acute insult, the progression of disease is then reflected by increasing tachypnea, dyspnea, cough, sputum production, crackles, wheezing, increased chest anteroposterior diameter (APD), and hypoxemia.

There is no specific treatment for bronchiolitis obliterans and, because it is so rare, there have been no randomized clinical trials. Therapeutic options include inhaled corticosteroids, bronchodilators, antibiotics, and oxygen supplementation. Mechanical ventilation may contribute to the progression of the disease. Some children deteriorate rapidly and die within weeks, whereas others follow a more chronic course. Antiviral agents may assist in blunting the initial viral response but otherwise have limited effect on the illness. Anti-inflammatory agents are showing promise in reducing airway inflammation and improving pulmonary function. For those children having undergone lung transplantation, increased immunosuppressive regimens are sometimes helpful.[63,64]

Asthma

Asthma is a chronic inflammatory disease characterized by bronchial hyperreactivity and reversible airflow obstruction, usually in response to an allergen (see Chapter 27). It is the most prevalent chronic disease in childhood, affecting about 10% of U.S. children between birth and

17 years of age, and prevalence is increasing. Populations most affected include black, American Indian, Alaska Native, and Hispanic children; those living in an urban setting; and those of low socioeconomic status.[65]

Childhood asthma results from a complex interaction between *genetic* susceptibility and *environmental* factors. Many genotypes are associated with susceptibility and phenotypes of asthma, including early-onset mild allergic asthma, asthma with severe exacerbations, later-onset asthma associated with obesity, severe nonatopic asthma, and corticosteroid-dependent asthma. Important risk factors include early exposure to allergens (e.g., air pollution, dust mites, cockroach antigen, cat exposure, and tobacco smoke), respiratory tract infections, preterm birth, and childhood obesity.[66-69] The *hygiene hypothesis* proposes that infants and children exposed to a highly hygienic environment and who receive vaccinations to prevent certain infections lack adequate exposure to common pathogens and therefore do not achieve balanced immune responses as they mature[70] (see Chapter 27).

About 70% to 80% of acute wheezing episodes in children with asthma are associated with viral respiratory tract infection (i.e., respiratory syncytial virus, human rhinoviruses, and parainfluenza viruses). In infants and toddlers less than 2 years old, the most common of these is respiratory syncytial virus (RSV). In older children and adults, the major viral trigger is rhinovirus (the "common cold" virus). Bacterial respiratory tract infections also can trigger asthma.[71] Vitamin D insufficiency may be a risk factor for airway inflammation and wheezing in children because vitamin D suppresses Th2-mediated allergic disease.[72]

PATHOPHYSIOLOGY The pathophysiology of asthma in children is similar to that for adults and is described in Chapter 27. Asthma is initiated by a type I hypersensitivity reaction primarily mediated by Th2 lymphocytes whose cytokines activate mast cells, eosinophilia, leukocytosis, and enhanced B-cell IgE production (see Chapter 8) (see Figures 27-8, 27-9, 27-10). As in adults, inflammation, bronchospasm, and mucus production in the airways lead to ventilation and perfusion mismatch with hypoxemia and expiratory airway obstruction with air trapping and increased work of breathing. In young children, airway obstruction can be more severe because of the smaller diameter of their airways.

CLINICAL MANIFESTATIONS Clinical manifestations of an acute asthma attack include coughing, expiratory wheezing, and shortness of breath. Breath sounds may become faint when air movement is poor. The child may speak in clipped sentences or not at all because of dyspnea. Sometimes hyperinflation (barrel chest) is visible. Respiratory rate and heart rate are elevated. Nasal flaring and use of accessory muscles with retractions in the substernal, subcostal, intercostal, suprasternal, or sternocleidomastoid areas are evident. Infants may appear to be "head bobbing" because of sternocleidomastoid muscle use. Pulsus paradoxus (decrease in systolic blood pressure of more than 10 mm Hg during inspiration) may be present. The child may appear anxious or diaphoretic, important signs of respiratory compromise.

Findings in chronic asthma may include hyperinflation of the thorax or pectus excavatum. Clubbing should not be seen with asthma and, if present, should trigger evaluation for other conditions such as cystic fibrosis. Exercise intolerance may indicate underlying asthma (see *Health Alert*: Exercise-Induced Bronchoconstriction).

EVALUATION AND TREATMENT Asthma is often underdiagnosed and undertreated, especially in preschool-age children because asthma symptoms overlap with other respiratory illnesses, such as bronchitis or upper respiratory tract infections. Diagnosis of asthma is based on

HEALTH ALERT

Exercise-Induced Bronchoconstriction

Exercise-induced bronchoconstriction (EIB) occurs in 90% of children diagnosed with asthma. It is estimated to occur in 10% to 15% of all U.S. children without diagnosed asthma and is surprisingly common among young, elite athletes, who have been found to have EIB prevalence rates of 20% to 40%. A proposed mechanism for EIB is epithelial injury and inflammation, which results from drying of the mucosa and changes in the osmolarity in the airway epithelium leading to degranulation of mast cells. Another contributing factor is the inhalation of particles and toxins at high flow rates; this is of particular importance in urban areas and in swimmers in chlorinated pools. These changes result in increased type I hypersensitivity and airway hyperresponsiveness (AHR) in those with asthma and are associated with an increase in leukotriene release. Eosinophil activation also plays a role in airway hyperreactivity and tissue damage. Finally, it has been found that obese children who have high levels of the inflammatory adipokine leptin are more likely to develop EIB than nonobese children. Symptoms are a poor indicator of the severity of bronchoconstriction, especially in obese children, and spirometry with exercise challenge testing is needed to make the diagnosis. Warm-up exercises and cooling down slowly after exercise, along with the use of facemasks in cold weather, can be helpful. A recent study reported that yoga training can markedly improve EIB in children aged 6 to 17. Although bronchodilators remain the most commonly used medications for EIB, studies suggest that inhaled corticosteroids or leukotriene inhibitors are more effective and safer in children with EIB and asthma.

Data from Baek HS et al: *Ann Allergy Asthma Immunol* 111(2):112-117, 2013; Lazarinis N et al: *Thorax* 69(2):130-136, 2014; Molphy J et al: *J Asthma* 51(1):44-50, 2014; Pasnick SD et al: *Ann Am Thorac Soc* 11(10):1651-1652, 2014; Randolph C: *Curr Allergy Asthma Rep* 13(6):662-671, 2013; Tahan F et al: *Altern Ther Health Med* 20(2):18-23, 2014.

episodes of wheezing as well as a variety of risk factors including parental history of asthma, atopic dermatitis, sensitization to aeroallergens or foods, blood eosinophilia, or wheezing not associated with upper respiratory tract illnesses. The modified Asthma Predictive Index (API) can be used to help with asthma diagnosis and is recommended by the National Institutes of Health (NIH) guidelines.[73] Confirmation of the diagnosis of asthma relies on pulmonary function testing using spirometry, which can be accomplished only after the child is 5 to 6 years of age. For younger children, an empirical trial of asthma medications is commonly initiated.

The goal of asthma therapy is to achieve long-term control by reduction in impairment and risk.[73,74] Child/family education and appropriate allergen avoidance techniques should begin immediately. Care providers need to periodically assess asthma control in children. Key features for assessment include nighttime awakenings, interference with normal activities, use of short-acting beta$_2$ agonists, pulmonary function testing, and exacerbations requiring steroids. Peak flow meters are often used to help guide treatment. Before therapy is augmented, care providers need to assess medication administration techniques, environmental controls, and comorbidities. For reduction in therapy, the asthma needs to be under good control for a minimum of 3 months.[74]

The pharmacologic treatment of asthma in children is essentially the same as that for adults and is initiated in a stepwise sequence based on asthma severity and response to treatment (see Chapter 27). Management of asthma medications in children is often difficult because fluctuation in severity of symptoms is common.

Acute Lung Injury/Acute Respiratory Distress Syndrome

Acute respiratory distress syndrome (ARDS) occurs in all children and is a dramatic, life-threatening condition resulting from a direct *acute lung injury (ALI)*, such as pneumonia, aspiration, near drowning, or smoke inhalation; or from a systemic insult, such as sepsis or multiple trauma, either of which activates an inflammatory response that causes alveolocapillary injury. ARDS accounts for approximately 10% of total patient days and one third of all deaths in pediatric intensive care units. Mortality in pediatric ARDS remains high, at approximately 40%.[75]

PATHOPHYSIOLOGY   The pathophysiology of ARDS in children is the same as that described for adults in Chapter 27 (see Figure 27-7).

CLINICAL MANIFESTATIONS   ARDS develops acutely after ALI, usually within 24 hours, though occasionally it is delayed up to a few days. ARDS is characterized by progressive respiratory distress, severe hypoxemia, decreased pulmonary compliance, and diffuse densities on chest radiograph. Initially, hyperventilation occurs, but CO_2 retention may ultimately occur as well because of inadequate functional air space and respiratory muscle fatigue. The severity of the overall picture is modified by comorbid factors, such as the presence of sepsis or multiorgan failure, and by the presence or absence of complications, such as nosocomial pneumonia. Some children who recover have residual pulmonary abnormalities.

EVALUATION AND TREATMENT   Treatment for ARDS remains supportive in nature, and the goals are to maintain adequate tissue oxygenation, minimize acute lung injury, and avoid iatrogenic pulmonary complications. Most individuals with ARDS require mechanical ventilation and often relatively high levels of positive end-expiratory pressure (PEEP) to promote alveolar ventilation and stabilization, and redistribution of alveolar edema fluid into the interstitium. Lung-protective ventilation strategies may include low tidal volume and permissive hypercapnia, permissive hypoxemia to prevent oxygen toxicity, prone positioning, high-frequency oscillatory ventilation, and airway pressure release ventilation. Use of corticosteroids in children with ARDS is controversial and remains at the discretion of the clinician. Extracorporeal membrane oxygenation (ECMO) can provide cardiac or respiratory support, or both, but does not heal the underlying condition.[76]

Cystic Fibrosis

Cystic fibrosis (CF) is an autosomal recessive inherited disease that results from defective epithelial chloride ion transport. The CF gene is located on chromosome 7. There are more than 1800 known mutations of this gene divided into 6 classes with varying severity of disease expression. Classes 1 through 3 are associated with more severe disease and 4 through 6 with milder pulmonary disease and pancreatic sufficiency. Mortality correlates respectively with the aforementioned classes.[77] CF primarily affects whites (approximately 1 in 3000 whites). There are approximately 1000 new cases of CF diagnosed each year and the median age at diagnosis is 6 months. The projected mean age of survival is the early forties. The estimated carrier frequency is high, 1 in 29 whites in the United States. Carriers are not affected by the mutation.[78,79] The median age of survival in the United States is projected at 37 years for females and 40 years for males; mortality has decreased by 1.8% per year from 2000 to 2010.[80]

PATHOPHYSIOLOGY   CF is a multiorgan disease that affects the lungs, digestive tract (see Chapter 37), and reproductive organs. The *cystic fibrosis transmembrane conductance regulator (CFTCR) gene* mutation results in the abnormal expression of cystic fibrosis transmembrane conductance regulator (CFTCR) protein, which is an activated chloride channel present on the surface of many types of epithelial cells, including those lining airways, bile ducts, pancreas, sweat ducts, and vas deferens. The most important effects are on the lungs, and respiratory failure is almost always the cause of death. The typical features of CF lung disease are mucus plugging, chronic inflammation, and chronic infection of the small airways. The mucus plugging results from both increased production and altered physicochemical properties of the mucus. Mucus-secreting airway cells (goblet cells and submucosal glands) are increased in number and size. CF mucus is dehydrated and viscous because of defective chloride secretion and excess sodium absorption. The periciliary fluid layer is depleted in volume, impairing the mobility of the cilia and thereby allowing mucus to adhere to the airway epithelium, along with bacteria and injurious by-products from neutrophils. Neutrophils are present in great excess in the airways and release damaging oxidants and proteases (i.e., elastase) that cause direct damage to lung structural proteins, induce airway cells to produce interleukin-8 (IL-8) (which attracts more neutrophils and stimulates mucus secretion), and destroy immunoglobulin G (IgG) and complement components important for opsonization and phagocytosis of pathogens[81] (Figure 28-7).

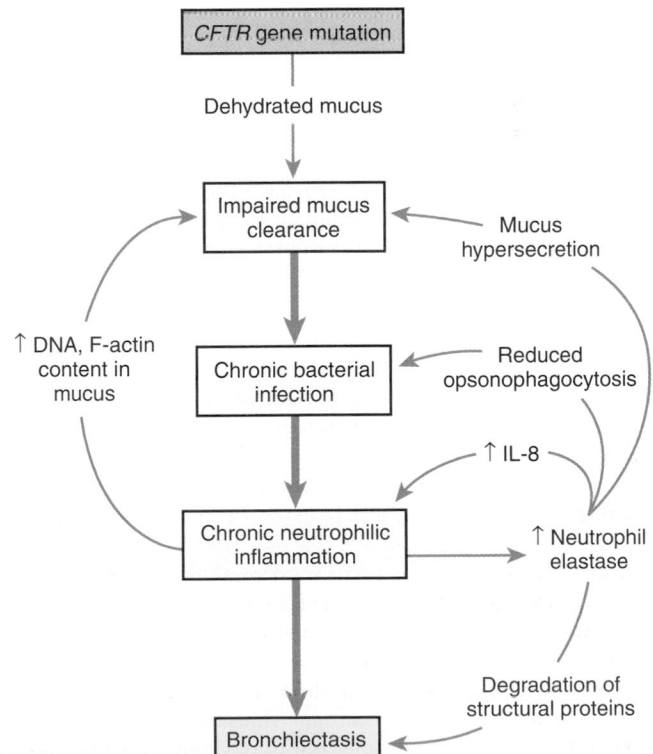

FIGURE 28-7 Pathogenesis of Cystic Fibrosis Lung Disease. *CFTR*, Cystic fibrosis transmembrane conductance regulator, *IL-8*, interleukin-8.

FIGURE 28-8 Pathology of the Lung in End-Stage Cystic Fibrosis. Key features are widespread mucus impaction of airways and bronchiectasis, especially from the upper lobe *(U)*, with hemorrhagic pneumonia in the lower lobe *(L)*. Small cysts *(C)* are present at the apex of the lung. (From Kleinerman J, Vauthy P: *Pathology of the lung in cystic fibrosis,* Atlanta, 1976, Cystic Fibrosis Foundation.)

The CF airway microenvironment favors bacterial colonization. *Staphylococcus aureus* and *Haemophilus influenzae* are common in younger children and *Pseudomonas aeruginosa* ultimately colonizes airways in at least 75% of children with CF.[82] Their biofilm resists beta-lactam antibiotics, and rapid mutation of the biofilm makes these children antibiotic resistant.[83] Persistence of these microorganisms incites chronic local inflammation and airway damage with microabscess formation, bronchiectasis, patchy consolidation and pneumonia, peribronchial fibrosis, and cyst formation (Figure 28-8).[84] Peripheral bullae may develop and pneumothorax may occur. Hemoptysis, sometimes life-threatening, may occur because of the erosion of enlarged bronchial arteries. Over time, pulmonary vascular remodeling occurs because of localized hypoxia and arteriolar vasoconstriction. Pulmonary hypertension and cor pulmonale may develop in the late stages of disease.

CLINICAL MANIFESTATIONS The most common presenting symptoms of CF are respiratory or gastrointestinal (see Chapter 37). Respiratory symptoms include persistent cough or wheeze, excessive sputum production, and recurrent or severe pneumonia. Physical signs that develop over time include barrel chest and digital clubbing. More subtle presentations include chronic sinusitis and nasal polyps. Newborn screening for CF is universal throughout the United States and will increase the numbers of children provided early, presymptomatic diagnosis and treatment[85] (see *Health Alert:* Newborn Screening for Cystic Fibrosis).

HEALTH ALERT
Newborn Screening for Cystic Fibrosis

Newborn screening for cystic fibrosis (CF) is now conducted in all 50 states in the United States and many other countries. The newborn screen for CF is a quantitative measure of immunoreactive trypsinogen (IRT) performed on a dried blood spot on a filter paper card. IRT is a pancreatic enzyme precursor that is persistently elevated in infants with CF. If a child is found to have an elevated IRT concentration, the next step is defined by state newborn screening protocols. Some states repeat the IRT level measurement, whereas others proceed to genetic testing for common mutations in the cystic fibrosis transmembrane conductance regulator (CFTR) gene. If the secondary testing is suggestive of a diagnosis of CF, the child is then referred to a Cystic Fibrosis Center for further evaluation and confirmatory sweat chloride testing. Research suggests that early diagnosis of CF has favorable effects on outcome. Children who are diagnosed with CF in infancy have improved nutritional outcomes compared to children who are diagnosed later in life. Establishing good nutrition in infants with CF has been correlated with improved lung function later in life. It is these improved clinical outcomes that have led the Centers for Disease Control and Prevention to support universal screening for CF.

Data from Grosse SD et al: *MMWR Recomm Rep* 53:1-36, 2004; National Newborn Screening and Global Resource Center: *Newborn national screening status report (updated 11/3/14),* available at http://genes-r-us.uthscsa.edu/sites/genes-r-us/files/nbsdisorders.pdf; O'Sullivan BP, Freedman SD: *Lancet* 373:1891-1904, 2009; Wagener JS et al: *Curr Opin Pediatr* 24(3):329-335, 2014.

EVALUATION AND TREATMENT The standard method of diagnosis (screening) are the immunoreactive trypsinogen (IRT) blood test and the sweat test, which reveal sweat chloride concentration in excess of 60 mEq/L. Alternative or supplemental methods include genotyping for CFTR mutations. Newborn screening for CF is universal in the United States.

Treatment is primarily focused on pulmonary health and nutrition (see Chapter 37). Common pulmonary therapies include techniques to promote mucus clearance, such as chest physical therapy and related mechanical devices; use of bronchodilators; and administration of aerosolized dornase alfa and hypertonic saline, which liquefy mucus.[87,88] Oral, inhaled, or intravenous antibiotics are used to treat exacerbations of pulmonary infection. Different classes of antibiotics are used to treat different pathogens and to overcome antibiotic resistance.[89,90] Recombinant human growth hormone has been shown to improve lung function, height, and weight in children with severe CF.[91] Individuals with end-stage lung disease may consider lung transplantation.[92] Newer approaches to gene therapy are being explored including mutation-specific targets.[86]

SUDDEN INFANT DEATH SYNDROME (SIDS)

Sudden infant death syndrome (SIDS)/sudden unexpected infant death remains a disease of unknown cause and is the most common cause of unexplained infant death in Western countries. It is defined as "sudden death of an infant under 1 year of age which remains unexplained after a thorough case investigation, including performance of a complete autopsy, examination of the death scene, and review of the clinical history."[93]

The incidence of SIDS is low during the first month of life with the peak incidence at 2 to 4 months of age. It is unusual after 6 months of age. The incidence of SIDS in the United States is about 3500 deaths per year.[93] SIDS almost always occurs during nighttime sleep, when infants are least likely to be observed. A seasonal variation has been noted, with higher frequencies during the winter months. This has been related to a higher rate of respiratory tract infections during those months, and such infections are often reported to have preceded the death. The sleeping room also may be overheated or the infant overwrapped.

Clinical risk groups are summarized in *Risk Factors*: Sudden Infant Death Syndrome (SIDS). About 75% of all SIDS victims have no known predisposing clinical risk factor.[94] SIDS rates decreased where

massive public campaigns warned against prone sleeping for infants (e.g., the Back-to-Sleep campaign).[95]

The etiology of SIDS remains unknown but probably involves a combination of predisposing factors, including a vulnerable infant and environmental stressors. There has been long-standing interest in hypotheses involving impaired autonomic regulation and failure of cardiovascular, ventilatory, and arousal responses to hypoxemia or hypercapnia. There also is a potential relationship between SIDS, auditory function, and central chemosensitivity to CO_2.[96,97]

Alternative theories involve airway obstruction events, such as control of tongue movements related to inspiratory activity, increased vagal tone, sudden intrapulmonary shunting because of abnormalities of surfactant or pulmonary vessels, exaggerated inflammation, or exaggerated inflammation in response to bacterial pathogens from the nasopharynx or viral respiratory tract infections.[98] Genetic factors may predispose certain individuals to SIDS. The most important risk factor genes include those involved in the regulation of the immune system, cardiac abnormalities, and brainstem function.[99-102]

Currently, the best strategies for reducing SIDS seem to be avoidance of all the controllable risk factors. Parents of infants with clinical risk should be taught cardiopulmonary resuscitation (CPR) as a precaution. Home monitoring has not been demonstrated to decrease the incidence of SIDS, and more research is needed.[103] Some at-risk infants may warrant cardiorespiratory monitoring after careful consideration of the individual situation.

RISK FACTORS
Sudden Infant Death Syndrome (SIDS)

- Prone and side-lying sleeping positions
- Sleeping on soft bedding
- Overheated sleeping environment
- Lower socioeconomic status
- Mothers younger than 20
- Blacks, Native Americans, Alaska Natives
- Low birth weight or growth restricted infants
- Male infants
- Preterm delivery
- Multiple gestations
- Sibling who died of SIDS
- Smoking during pregnancy
- Exposure to tobacco smoke
- Lack of prenatal care
- Illicit drug use or binge-drinking
- Larger family size

Data from Bergman NJ: *Pediatr Res* 77(1-1):10-19, 2015; Blackwell C et al: *Front Immunol* 6:44, 2015; Hakeem GF et al: *World J Pediatr* 11(1):41-47, 2015; Van Nguyen JM, Abenhaim HA: *Am J Perinatol* 30(9):703-714, 2013.

✔ QUICK CHECK 28-5
1. How are the alveoli and capillaries affected by the inflammation of acute respiratory distress syndrome (ARDS)?
2. What aspects of lung disease in cystic fibrosis are the focus of current therapies?
3. What are the risk factors for SIDS?

▮ DID YOU UNDERSTAND?

Disorders of the Upper Airways

1. Croup is an acute laryngotracheobronchitis, usually caused by parainfluenza virus. This infection causes swelling of the upper trachea. The typical sign is a seal-like barking cough, which appears after a few days of rhinorrhea, sore throat, and low-grade fever.
2. Spasmodic croup is characterized by a similar barking cough but occurs in older children, is of sudden onset at night and without fever, and has unknown etiology.
3. Acute epiglottitis is a potentially life-threatening airway infection whose incidence in children has decreased dramatically since the advent of *H. influenzae* vaccine. Now other pathogens, such as group A beta-hemolytic *Streptococcus*, *Candida* species, *S. aureus*, MRSA, or viral pathogens, are usually the causative agents.
4. Tonsillar infections are usually caused by group A beta-hemolytic *Streptococcus* and can be complicated by tonsillar abscesses.
5. Aspiration of foreign bodies that lodge in the airways may cause cough, hoarseness, stridor or wheezing, and dyspnea. The severity depends on the location of the foreign body within the airway and the degree of obstruction. Blockage of the larynx or trachea can be fatal, whereas bronchial obstruction may not be diagnosed immediately.
6. Obstructive sleep apnea syndrome (OSAS) is defined by partial or intermittent upper airway obstruction during sleep with disruption of normal ventilation and normal sleep patterns.

Disorders of the Lower Airways

1. Respiratory distress syndrome (RDS) of the newborn usually occurs in premature infants who are born before surfactant production and alveolocapillary development are complete. Atelectasis and hypoventilation cause shunting, hypoxemia, and hypercapnia. Prenatal steroids and postnatal surfactant are beneficial preventive therapies.
2. Bronchopulmonary dysplasia (BPD) is the result of tissue injury and repair and disrupted alveolar development in the lungs of infants who required ventilatory support during a time when their lungs were underdeveloped because of their prematurity. Surfactant therapy has improved outcomes. Infants with BPD may require oxygen and additional therapies for many months.
3. Bronchiolitis is a viral lower respiratory tract infection that presents with runny nose, wheezing, cough, and tachypnea in infants and is usually caused by infection with respiratory syncytial virus (RSV). Infants with risk factors of prematurity or underlying lung or heart disease are at high risk and may receive RSV-specific monoclonal antibody to prevent RSV disease.
4. Viral pneumonia and bacterial pneumonia cause varying degrees of illness in children and viral pneumonia is the most common and frequently precedes bacterial pneumonia. Community-acquired bacterial pneumonia is one of the leading causes of hospitalization and is prevented with polyvariant pneumococcal conjugate vaccine.

5. Aspiration pneumonitis is caused by inhalation of a foreign substance, such as food, milk, secretions, or environmental compounds, into the lung, and results in inflammation.
6. Bronchiolitis obliterans is a rare postinflammatory condition in which the bronchioles and some small bronchi are partially or completely obliterated by fibrous tissue, causing pulmonary impairment and disability.
7. Asthma is a chronic inflammatory disease characterized by bronchial hyperreactivity and reversible airflow obstruction, and is usually a type I hypersensitivity response to an antigen. Its origins are multifactorial, including genetic, allergic, and viral-triggered mechanisms.
8. Acute respiratory distress syndrome (ARDS) results from acute lung injury and can occur when there is an insult to the lung that activates an inflammatory response causing alveolar capillary injury, usually within 24 hours. There is progressive respiratory distress with severe hypoxemia and respiratory failure.
9. Cystic fibrosis is an autosomal recessive genetic disease that affects the epithelial lining of many organ systems, especially the respiratory and gastrointestinal systems. Airway secretions are particularly thick and tenacious, and the airways develop chronic bacterial infection with pathogens such as *Pseudomonas aeruginosa* and *Staphylococcus aureus*. Chronic infection, plugged airways, and severe inflammation cause long-term lung damage and ultimately death. However, the prognosis is improving, and most children with CF now survive to adulthood.

Sudden Infant Death Syndrome (SIDS)
1. Sudden infant death syndrome is the leading cause of postnatal death for infants outside of the hospital setting and is associated with low birth weight, prone sleeping position, and other environmental factors. There has been a significant reduction in SIDS since widespread adoption of recommendations for supine positioning of infants during sleep.

KEY TERMS

Acute epiglottitis, 717
Acute respiratory distress syndrome (ARDS), 725
Aspiration pneumonitis, 723
Asthma, 723
Atypical pneumonia (*Mycoplasma pneumoniae, Chlamydophila pneumoniae*), 723
Bacterial pneumonia, 722
Bacterial tracheitis (pseudomembranous croup), 717
Bronchiolitis, 721
Bronchiolitis obliterans (BO), 723
Bronchopulmonary dysplasia (BPD), 720
Croup, 715
Cystic fibrosis (CF), 725
Cystic fibrosis transmembrane conductance regulator (CFTR) protein, 725
Obstructive sleep apnea syndrome (OSAS), 717
Peritonsillar abscess, 717
Pneumonia, 722
Respiratory distress syndrome (RDS) of the newborn, 718
Sudden infant death syndrome (SIDS)/sudden unexpected infant death, 726
Tonsillar abscess, 717
Tonsillar infections, 717
Upper airway obstruction, 715
Viral pneumonia, 722

REFERENCES

1. Choi J, Lee GL: Common pediatric respiratory emergencies, *Emerg Med Clin North Am* 30(2):529-563, x, 2012.
2. Zoorob R et al: Croup: an overview, *Am Fam Physician* 83(9):1067-1073, 2011.
3. Sammer M, Pruthi S: Membranous croup (exudative tracheitis or membranous laryngotracheobronchitis), *Pediatr Radiol* 40:781, 2010.
4. Li SF: The Westley croup score, *Acad Emerg Med* 10(3):289, 2003: author reply 289.
5. Pitluk JD et al: Clinical inquiries. What's best for croup? *J Fam Pract* 60(11):680-681, 2011.
6. Dobrovoljac M, Geelhoed GC: How fast does oral dexamethasone work in mild to moderately severe croup? A randomized double-blinded clinical trial, *Emerg Med Australas* 24(1):79-85, 2012.
7. Bjornson C et al: Nebulized epinephrine for croup in children, *Cochrane Database Syst Rev* 2:CD006619, 2011.
8. Moraa I et al: Heliox for croup in children, *Cochrane Database Syst Rev* 12:CD006822, 2013.
9. Cirilli AR: Emergency evaluation and management of the sore throat, *Emerg Med Clin North Am* 31(2):501-515, 2013.
10. Tibballs J, Watson T: Symptoms and signs differentiating croup and epiglottitis, *J Paediatr Child Health* 47(3):77-82, 2011.
11. Shah RK, Stocks C: Epiglottitis in the United States: national trends, variances, prognosis, and management, *Laryngoscope* 120(6):1256-1262, 2010.
12. Kordeluk S et al: Relation between peritonsillar infection and acute tonsillitis: myth or reality? *Otolaryngol Head Neck Surg* 145(6):940-945, 2011.
13. Powell J, Wilson JA: An evidence-based review of peritonsillar abscess, *Clin Otolaryngol* 37(2):136-145, 2012.
14. Yenigun A: The efficacy of tonsillectomy in chronic tonsillitis patients as demonstrated by the neutrophil-to-lymphocyte ratio, *J Laryngol Otol* 129(4):386-391, 2015.
15. Kuo CY, Parikh SR: Bacterial tracheitis, *Pediatr Rev* 35(11):497-499, 2014.
16. Kim IA et al: The national cost burden of bronchial foreign body aspiration in children, *Laryngoscope* 125(5):1221-1224, 2015.
17. Shlizerman L et al: Foreign body aspiration in children: the effects of delayed diagnosis, *Am J Otolaryngol* 31(5):320-324, 2010.
18. Katz ES, D'Ambrosio CM: Pediatric obstructive sleep apnea syndrome, *Clin Chest Med* 31:221-234, 2010.
19. Snow A et al: Pediatric obstructive sleep apnea: a potential late consequence of respiratory syncytial virus bronchiolitis, *Pediatr Pulmonol* 44:1186-1191, 2009.
20. Katz ES et al: Obstructive sleep apnea in infants, *Am J Respir Crit Care Med* 185(8):805-816, 2012.
21. Tan HL et al: Obstructive sleep apnea in children: a critical update, *Nat Sci Sleep* 5:109-123, 2013.
22. Gozal D et al: C-reactive protein and obstructive sleep apnea syndrome in children, *Front Biosci (Elite Ed)* 4:2410-2422, 2012.
23. Kim J et al: Inflammatory pathways in children with insufficient or disordered sleep, *Respir Physiol Neurobiol* 178(3):465-474, 2011.
24. Alexander NS, Schroeder JW Jr: Pediatric obstructive sleep apnea syndrome, *Pediatr Clin North Am* 60(4):827-840, 2013.
25. Lal C et al: Neurocognitive impairment in obstructive sleep apnea, *Chest* 141(6):1601-1610, 2012.
26. Donnelly LF: Magnetic resonance sleep studies in the evaluation of children with obstructive sleep apnea, *Semin Ultrasound CT MR* 31(2):107-115, 2010.
27. Marcus CL et al: Diagnosis and management of childhood obstructive sleep apnea syndrome, *Pediatrics* 130(3):e714-e755, 2012.
28. Tapia IE, Marcus CL: Newer treatment modalities for pediatric obstructive sleep apnea, *Paediatr Respir Rev* 14(3):199-203, 2013.
29. Shapiro-Mendoza CK, Lackritz EM: Epidemiology of late and moderate preterm birth, *Semin Fetal Neonatal Med* 17(3):120-125, 2012.
30. Sweet D et al: European consensus guidelines on the management of neonatal respiratory distress syndrome, *J Perinatal Med* 35:175-186, 2007.
31. Kamath-Rayne BD et al: Antenatal steroids for treatment of fetal lung immaturity after 34 weeks of gestation: an evaluation of neonatal outcomes, *Obstet Gynecol* 119(5):909-916, 2012.
32. McKinlay CJ et al: Repeat antenatal glucocorticoids for women at risk of preterm birth: a Cochrane Systematic Review, *Am J Obstet Gynecol* 206(3):187-941, 2012.
33. Smolarova S et al: Impact of updated European Consensus Guidelines on the management of neonatal respiratory distress syndrome on clinical outcome of preterm infants, *Adv Exp Med Biol* 835:61-66, 2015.
34. Dani C, Pratesi S: Nitric oxide for the treatment of preterm infants with respiratory distress syndrome, *Expert Opin Pharmacother* 14(1):97-103, 2013.
35. Bhandari A, McGrath-Morrow S: Long-term pulmonary outcomes of patients with bronchopulmonary dysplasia, *Semin Perinatol* 37(2):132-137, 2013.
36. Van Marter LJ: Epidemiology of bronchopulmonary dysplasia, *Semin Fetal Neonatal Med* 14(6):358-366, 2009.

37. Trembath A, Laughon MM: Predictors of bronchopulmonary dysplasia, *Clin Perinatol* 39(3):585-601, 2012.

38. Berkelhamer SK et al: Pulmonary hypertension in bronchopulmonary dysplasia, *Semin Perinatol* 37(2):124-131, 2013.

39. Simpson SJ et al: Lung function following very preterm birth in the era of 'new' bronchopulmonary dysplasia, *Respirology* 20(4):535-540, 2015.

40. Viscardi RM: Perinatal inflammation and lung injury, *Semin Fetal Neonatal Med* 17(1):30-35, 2012.

41. Pfister RH, Soll RF: Initial respiratory support of preterm infants: the role of CPAP, the INSURE method, and noninvasive ventilation, *Clin Perinatol* 39(3):459-481, 2012.

42. Picone S et al: Caffeine citrate: when and for how long. A literature review, *J Matern Fetal Neonatal Med* 25(Suppl 3):11-14, 2012.

43. Lodha A et al: Association of early caffeine administration and neonatal outcomes in very preterm neonates, *JAMA Pediatr* 169(1):33-38, 2015.

44. Teshome G et al: Acute bronchiolitis, *Pediatr Clin North Am* 60(5):1019-1034, 2013.

45. Beigelman A, Bacharier LB: The role of early life viral bronchiolitis in the inception of asthma, *Curr Opin Allergy Clin Immunol* 13(2):211-216, 2013.

46. Ralston SL et al: Clinical practice guideline: the diagnosis, management, and prevention of bronchiolitis, *Pediatrics* 134(5):e1474-e1502, 2014. Available at http://pediatrics.aappublications.org/content/134/5/e1474.full.pdf+html.

47. Jain S et al: Community-acquired pneumonia requiring hospitalization among U.S. children, *N Engl J Med* 372(9):835-845, 2015.

48. Pavia AT: What is the role of respiratory viruses in community-acquired pneumonia? What is the best therapy for influenza and other viral causes of community-acquired pneumonia? *Infect Dis Clin North Am* 27(1):157-175, 2013.

49. Yamad M et al: Rising rates of macrolide-resistant *Mycoplasma pneumoniae* in the central United States, *Pediatr Infect Dis J* 31(4):409-410, 2012.

50. Durando P et al: Improving the protection against *Streptococcus pneumoniae* with the new generation 13-valent pneumococcal conjugate vaccine, *J Prev Med Hyg* 53(2):68-77, 2012.

51. van der Sluijs KF et al: Bench-to-bedside review: bacterial pneumonia with influenza—pathogenesis and clinical implications, *Crit Care* 14(2):219, 2010.

52. Wang K et al: Clinical symptoms and signs for the diagnosis of *Mycoplasma pneumoniae* in children and adolescents with community-acquired pneumonia, *Cochrane Database Syst Rev* 10:CD009175, 2012.

53. Bradley JS et al: The management of community-acquired pneumonia in infants and children older than 3 months of age: clinical practice guidelines by the Pediatric Infectious Diseases Society and the Infectious Diseases Society of America, *Clin Infect Dis* 53:e25-e76, 2011.

54. Schauner S et al: Community-acquired pneumonia in children: a look at the IDSA guidelines, *J Fam Pract* 62(1):9-15, 2013.

55. Patria F et al: Clinical profile of recurrent community-acquired pneumonia in children, *BMC Pulm Med* 13:60, 2013.

56. Krüger S, Welte T: Biomarkers in community-acquired pneumonia, *Expert Rev Respir Med* 6(2):203-214, 2012.

57. Mulholland S et al: Antibiotics for community-acquired lower respiratory tract infections secondary to *Mycoplasma pneumoniae* in children, *Cochrane Database Syst Rev* 9:CD004875, 2012.

58. Swarnam K et al: Advances in the management of meconium aspiration syndrome, *Int J Pediatr* 2012:359571, 2012.

59. Boesch RP et al: Advances in the diagnosis and management of chronic pulmonary aspiration in children, *Eur Respir J* 28:847-861, 2006.

60. Pena A et al: Botulinum toxin A injection of salivary glands in children with drooling and chronic aspiration, *J Vasc Interv Radiol* 20(3):368-373, 2009.

61. Fischer GB et al: Post infectious bronchiolitis obliterans in children, *Paediatr Respir Rev* 11(4):233-239, 2010.

62. Moonnumakal SP, Fan LL: Bronchiolitis obliterans in children, *Curr Opin Pediatr* 20(3):272-278, 2008.

63. Champs NS et al: Post-infectious bronchiolitis obliterans in children, *J Pediatr (Rio J)* 87(3):187-198, 2011.

64. Sacher VY et al: Effects of prophylactic use of sirolimus on bronchiolitis obliterans syndrome development in lung transplant recipients, *Ann Thorac Surg* 97(1):268-274, 2014.

65. Lara J et al: *Trends in asthma prevalence, health care use, and mortality in the United States, 2001–2010,* NCHS Data Brief Number 94, Hyattsville, Md, May 2012, Author. Available at: www.cdc.gov/nchs/data/databriefs/db94.htm. Reviewed January 30, 2014.

66. Been JV et al: Preterm birth and childhood wheezing disorders: a systematic review and meta-analysis, *PLoS Med* 11(1):e1001596, 2014.

67. Blumenthal MN: Genetic, epigenetic, and environmental factors in asthma and allergy, *Ann Allergy Asthma Immunol* 108(2):69-73, 2012.

68. Hakimeh D, Tripodi S: Recent advances in diagnosis and management of childhood asthma and food allergies, *Ital J Pediatr* 39:80, 2013.

69. Papoutsakis C et al: Childhood overweight/obesity and asthma: is there a link? A systematic review of recent epidemiologic evidence, *J Acad Nutr Diet* 113(1):77-105, 2013.

70. Prokopakis E et al: The pathophysiology of the hygiene hypothesis, *Int J Pediatr Otorhinolaryngol* 77(7):1065-1071, 2013.

71. Fuchs O, von Mutius E: Prenatal and childhood infections: implications for the development and treatment of childhood asthma, *Lancet Respir Med* 1(9):743-754, 2013.

72. Keating P et al: Effect of vitamin D on T-helper type 9 polarized human memory cells in chronic persistent asthma, *Ann Allergy Asthma Immunol* 112(2):154-162, 2014.

73. National Heart, Lung, and Blood Institute: *National Asthma Education and Prevention Program Expert Panel Report 3: guidelines for the diagnosis and management of asthma,* 2007. Available at: http://www.nhlbi.nih.gov/guidelines/asthma/asthgdln.htm Accessed May 8, 2015.

74. Agency for Healthcare Quality and Research: *National Guideline Clearing House and the Institute for Clinical Systems Improvement (ICSI): Diagnosis and management of asthma.* Available at http://www.guideline.gov/content.aspx?id=38255#Section420. Accessed May 8, 2015.

75. Willson DF et al: Surfactant for pediatric acute lung injury, *Pediatr Clin North Am* 55(3):545-575, 2008:ix.

76. Cheifetz IM: Advances in monitoring and management of pediatric acute lung injury, *Pediatr Clin North Am* 60(3):621-639, 2013.

77. CFTR.INFO: *Classification of CFTR mutations.* Available at: www.cftr.info/about-cf/role-of-ctfr-in-cf/cftr-mutations/the-six-classes-of-cftr-defects/. Accessed January 30, 2014.

78. Cystic Fibrosis Foundation: *CF genetics: updated 7/18/13.* Available at: www.cff.org/AboutCF/Testing/Genetics/. Accessed January 30, 2014.

79. Cystic Fibrosis Foundation: *Testing cystic fibrosis: updated 12/17/10.* Available at: www.cff.org/AboutCE/Testing/. Accessed January 30, 2014.

80. MacKenzie T et al: Longevity of patients with cystic fibrosis in 2000 to 2010 and beyond: survival analysis of the Cystic Fibrosis Foundation Patient Registry, *Ann Intern Med* 161(4):233-241, 2014.

81. Gifford AM, Chalmers JD: The role of neutrophils in cystic fibrosis, *Curr Opin Hematol* 21(1):16-22, 2014.

82. Lobo J et al: Recent advances in cystic fibrosis, *Clin Chest Med* 33(2):307-328, 2012.

83. López-Causapé C et al: The problems of antibiotic resistance in cystic fibrosis and solutions, *Expert Rev Respir Med* 9(1):73-88, 2015.

84. O'Sullivan BP, Freedman SD: Cystic fibrosis, *Lancet* 373(9678):1891-1904, 2009.

85. Wagener JS et al: Newborn screening for cystic fibrosis, *Curr Opin Pediatr* 24(3):329-335, 2012.

86. Amaral MD: Novel personalized therapies for cystic fibrosis: treating the basic defect in all patients, *J Intern Med* 277(2):155-166, 2015.

87. Dentice R, Elkins M: Timing of dornase alfa inhalation for cystic fibrosis, *Cochrane Database Syst Rev* 6:CD007923, 2013.

88. Elkins M, Dentice R: Timing of hypertonic saline inhalation for cystic fibrosis, *Cochrane Database Syst Rev* 2:CD008816, 2013.

89. Chmiel JF et al: Antibiotic management of lung infections in cystic fibrosis. I. The microbiome, methicillin-resistant Staphylococcus aureus, gram-negative bacteria, and multiple infections, *Ann Am Thorac Soc* 11(7):1120-1129, 2014.

90. Chmiel JF et al: Antibiotic management of lung infections in cystic fibrosis. II. Nontuberculous mycobacteria, anaerobic bacteria, and fungi, *Ann Am Thorac Soc* 11(8):1298-1306, 2014.

91. Thaker V et al: Recombinant growth hormone therapy for cystic fibrosis in children and young adults, *Cochrane Database Syst Rev* 6:CD008901, 2013.

92. Lynch JP 3rd et al: Lung transplantation for cystic fibrosis: results, indications, complications, and controversies, *Semin Respir Crit Care Med* 36(2):299-320, 2015.

93. Centers for Disease Control and Prevention: *Sudden unexpected infant death and sudden infant death syndrome.* Updated May 11, 2015. Available at: www.cdc.gov/sids/index.htm. Accessed May 19, 2015.

94. Bergman NJ: Proposal for mechanisms of protection of supine sleep against sudden infant death syndrome: an integrated mechanism review, *Pediatr Res* 77(1 1):10-19, 2015.

95. Trachtenberg FL et al: Risk factor changes for sudden infant death syndrome after initiation of Back-to-Sleep campaign, *Pediatrics* 129(4):630-638, 2012.

96. Garcia AJ 3rd et al: The physiological determinants of sudden infant death syndrome, *Respir Physiol Neurobiol* 189(2):288-300, 2013.

97. Rubens D, Sarnat HB: Sudden infant death syndrome: an update and new perspectives of etiology, *Handb Clin Neurol* 112:867-874, 2013.

98. Alfelali M, Khandaker G: Infectious causes of sudden infant death syndrome, *Paediatr Respir Rev* 15(4):307-311, 2014.

99. Kinney HC et al: Dentate gyrus abnormalities in sudden unexplained death in infants: morphological marker of underlying brain vulnerability, *Acta Neuropathol* 129(1):65-80, 2015.

100. Klaver EC et al: Cardiac ion channel mutations in the sudden infant death syndrome, *Int J Cardiol* 152(2):162-170, 2011.

101. Salomonis N: Systems-level perspective of sudden infant death syndrome, *Pediatr Res* 76(3):220-229, 2014.

102. Sweeting J, Semsarian C: Cardiac abnormalities and sudden infant death syndrome, *Paediatr Respir Rev* 15(4):301-306, 2014.

103. Strehle EM et al: Can home monitoring reduce mortality in infants at increased risk of sudden infant death syndrome? A systematic review, *Acta Paediatr* 101(1):8-13, 2012.

29

Structure and Function of the Renal and Urologic Systems

Sue E. Huether

The primary function of the kidney is to maintain a stable internal environment for optimal cell and tissue metabolism. The kidneys accomplish these life-sustaining tasks by balancing solute and water transport, excreting metabolic waste products, conserving nutrients, and regulating acids and bases. The kidney also has an endocrine function and secretes the hormones renin, erythropoietin, and 1,25-dihydroxy-vitamin D_3 for regulation of blood pressure, erythrocyte production, and calcium metabolism, respectively. The kidney also can release glucose into the circulation by the processes of glycogenolysis and gluconeogenesis. The formation of urine is achieved through the processes of glomerular filtration, tubular reabsorption, and secretion within the kidney. The bladder stores the urine received from the kidney by way of the ureters. Urine is then released from the bladder through the urethra.

STRUCTURES OF THE RENAL SYSTEM

Structures of the Kidney

The kidneys are paired organs located in the posterior region of the abdominal cavity behind the peritoneum. They lie on either side of the vertebral column with their upper and lower poles extending from the twelfth thoracic vertebra to the third lumbar vertebra (Figure 29-1). The right kidney is slightly lower and is displaced downward by the overlying liver. Each kidney is approximately 11 cm long, 5 to 6 cm wide, and 3 to 4 cm thick. A tightly adhering capsule (the renal capsule) surrounds each kidney, which is embedded in a mass of perirenal fat. The capsule and fatty layer are covered with a double layer of renal fascia composed of fibrous tissue. The cushion of adipose tissue (paranephric fat) and the position of the kidney between the

abdominal organs and muscles of the back protect it from trauma. The hilum is a medial indentation in the kidney and is the location of the entry and exit for the renal blood vessels, nerves, lymphatic vessels, and ureter.

The structures of the kidney are summarized in Figure 29-2. The outer layer of the kidney is called the cortex and contains all of the glomeruli, most of the proximal tubules, and some segments of the distal tubule. The medulla forms the inner part of the kidney and consists of regions call pyramids. Renal columns are an extension of the cortex and extend between the pyramids to the renal pelvis. The pyramids extend into the renal pelvis and contain the loops of Henle and collecting ducts. The minor and major calyces are chambers receiving urine from the collecting ducts and form the entry into the renal pelvis, which is an extension of the upper ureter. The structural unit of the kidney is the lobe. Each lobe is composed of a pyramid and the overlying cortex. There are about 14 to 18 lobes in each kidney.

Nephron

The nephron is the functional unit of the kidney. Each kidney contains approximately 1.2 million nephrons. The nephron is a tubular structure with subunits that include the renal corpuscle, proximal convoluted tubule, loop of Henle, distal convoluted tubule, and collecting duct, all of which contribute to the formation of final urine (Figure 29-3). The different structures of the epithelial cells lining various segments of the tubule facilitate the special functions of secretion and reabsorption (Figure 29-4).

The kidney has three kinds of nephrons: (1) superficial cortical nephrons (85% of all nephrons), which extend partially into the medulla; (2) midcortical nephrons with short or long loops; and

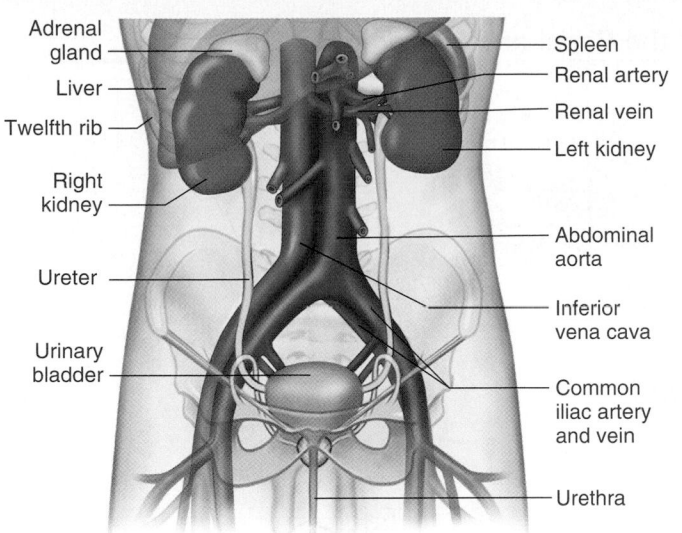

FIGURE 29-1 Organs of the Urinary System. (From Patton KT, Thibodeau GA: *The human body in health & disease,* ed 6, St Louis, 2014, Mosby.)

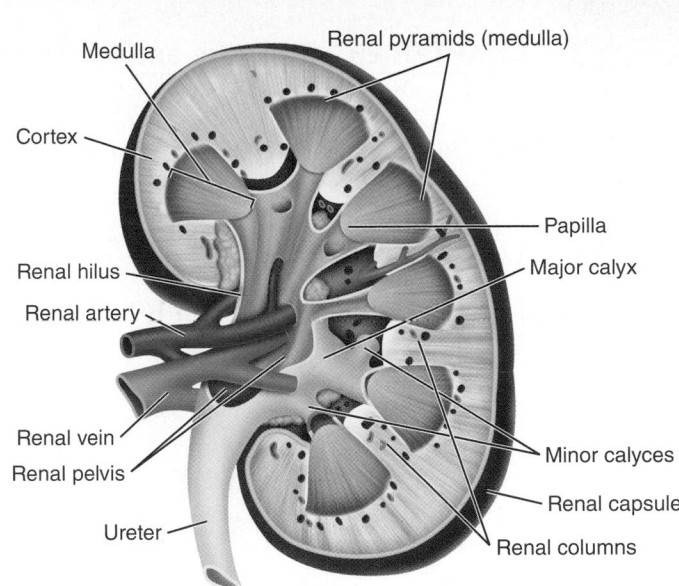

FIGURE 29-2 Internal Structure of the Kidney. (From Solomon E: *Introduction to human anatomy and physiology,* ed 4, St Louis, 2016, Saunders.)

Renal corpuscle
- Bowman capsule
- Glomerulus

Distal convoluted tubule (DCT)

Proximal convoluted tubule (PCT)

Descending limb of Henle (DLH)

Renal tubule

Thick ascending limb of Henle (TAL)

Cortex

Medulla

Collecting duct (CD)

Henle (nephron) loop

Thin ascending limb of Henle (tALH)

Papillary duct

Papilla of renal pyramid

Afferent arteriole

Juxtaglomerular cells

Juxtaglomerular apparatus

Macula densa

Afferent arteriole

Afferent arteriole

Visceral wall

Parietal wall

Juxtaglomerular cells

Proximal tubule

Distal tubule

Bowman capsule

Efferent arteriole

Glomerulus

FIGURE 29-3 Components of the Nephron. (From Patton KT, Thibodeau GA, Douglas MM: *Essentials of anatomy & physiology,* St Louis, 2012, Mosby; Damjanov I: *Pathology for the health professions,* ed 4, St Louis, 2012, Mosby.)

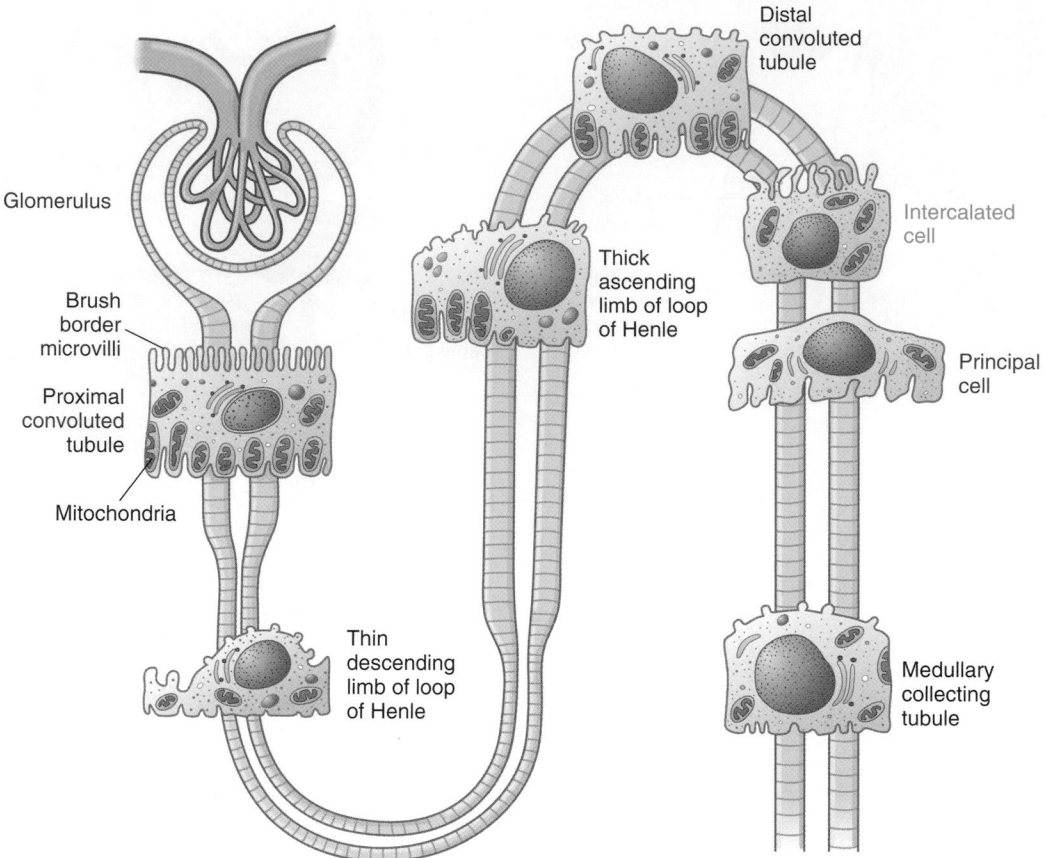

FIGURE 29-4 Epithelial Cells of the Various Segments of Nephron Tubules. The brush border and high number of mitochondria in cells of the proximal tubule promote reabsorption of 50% of the glomerular filtrate. Intercalated cells secrete H^+ (through K^+ exchange) or reabsorb HCO_3^-. Principal cells are influenced by aldosterone and reabsorb Na^+ and water and secrete K^+.

(3) **juxtamedullary nephrons** (about 12% of nephrons), which lie close to and extend deep into the medulla (about 40 mm) and are important for the concentration of urine (Figure 29-5). The **glomerulus** is a tuft of capillaries that loop into **Bowman capsule (Bowman space)**, like fingers pushed into bread dough. **Mesangial cells** (shaped like smooth muscle cells) secrete the **mesangial matrix** (a type of connective tissue) and lie between and support the capillaries (Figure 29-6). Mesangial cells also have phagocytic abilities similar to monocytes, release inflammatory cytokines, and can contract to regulate glomerular capillary blood flow.[1] Together, the glomerulus, Bowman capsule, and mesangial cells are called the **renal corpuscle**.

The **glomerular filtration membrane** filters blood components through its three layers: (1) an inner capillary endothelium, (2) a middle basement membrane, and (3) an outer layer of capillary epithelium. The capillary endothelium is composed of cells in continuous contact with the basement membrane and contains pores. The middle basement membrane is a selectively permeable network of glycoproteins and mucopolysaccharides. The epithelium has specialized cells called **podocytes** from which pedicles (foot projections) radiate and adhere to the basement membrane. The pedicles interlock with the pedicles of adjacent podocytes, forming an elaborate network of intercellular clefts (**filtration slits**, or slit membranes). The endothelium, basement membrane, and podocytes are covered with protein molecules bearing anionic (negative) charges that retard the filtration of anionic proteins and prevent proteinuria. The glomerular filtration membrane separates the blood of the glomerular capillaries from the fluid in Bowman space and allows all components of the blood to be filtered, with the exception of blood cells and plasma proteins with a molecular weight greater than 70,000. The glomerular filtrate passes through the three layers of the glomerular membrane and forms the primary urine.

The glomerulus is supplied by the afferent arteriole and drained by the efferent arteriole. A group of specialized cells known as **juxtaglomerular cells** (renin-releasing cells) are located around the afferent arteriole where it enters the glomerulus (see Figure 29-3). Between the afferent and efferent arterioles is the **macula densa** (sodium-sensing cells) of the distal tubule (see Figure 29-6). Together the juxtaglomerular cells and macula densa cells form the **juxtaglomerular apparatus** (see Figure 29-3). Control of renal blood flow, glomerular filtration, and renin secretion occurs at this site.[2]

The **proximal convoluted tubule** continues from Bowman space and has an initial convoluted segment (pars convoluta) and then a straight segment (pars recta) that descends toward the medulla (see Figure 29-3). The wall of the proximal tubule consists of one layer of cuboidal epithelial cells with a surface layer of microvilli (a brush border) that increases reabsorptive surface area. This is the only surface inside the nephron where the cells are covered with a brush border of microvilli (see Figure 29-4). The proximal convoluted tubule joins the **loop of Henle**, which extends into the medulla. The cells of the thick segment are cuboidal and actively transport several solutes, but not water. The thin ascending segment of the loop of Henle narrows and is composed of thin squamous cells with no active transport function.

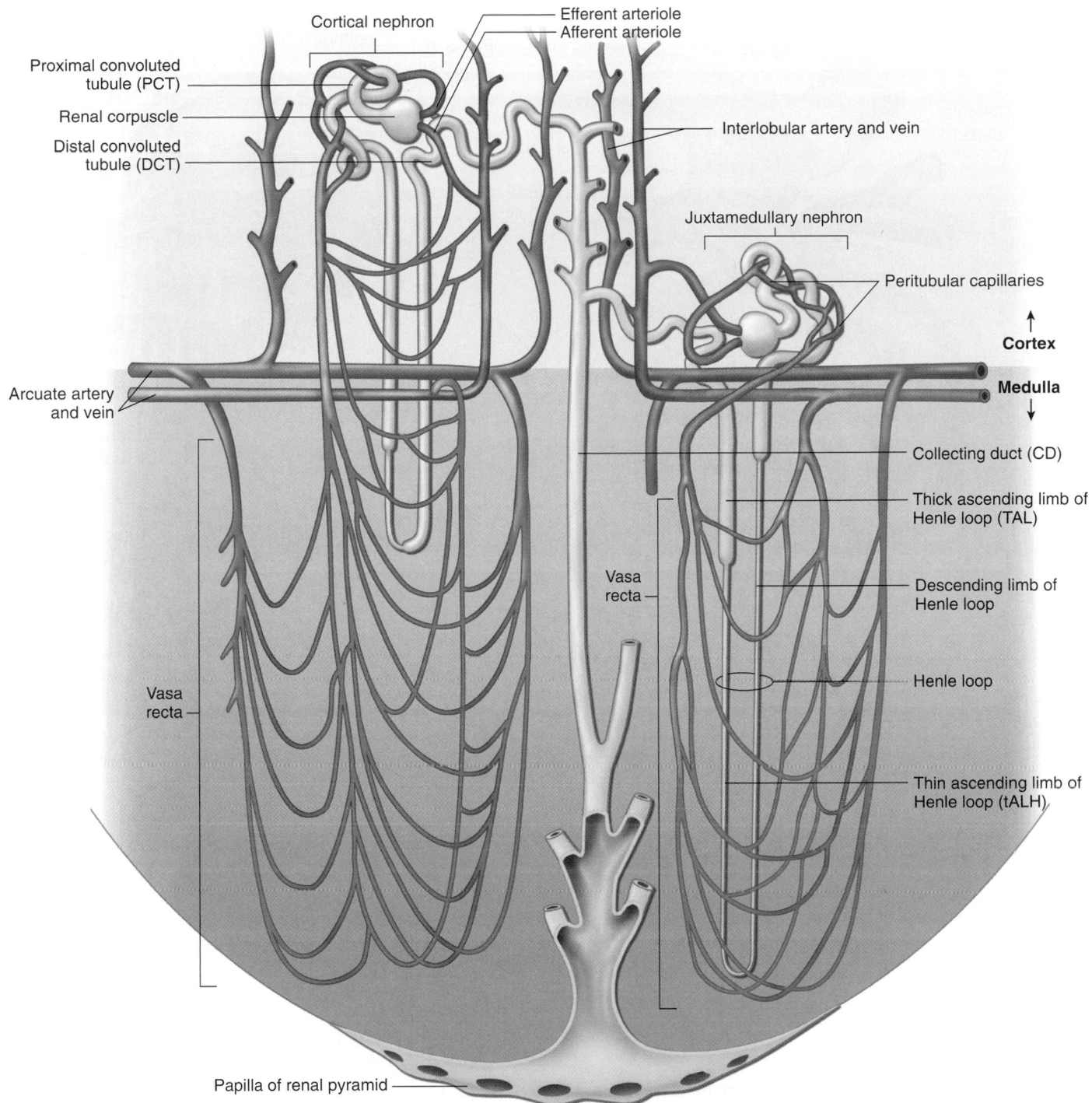

FIGURE 29-5 Nephron Unit with Its Blood Vessels. Blood flows through nephron vessels as follows: interlobular artery, afferent arteriole, glomerulus, efferent arteriole, peritubular capillaries (around the tubules), venules, interlobular vein. (From Patton KT, Thibodeau GA, Douglas MM: *Essentials of anatomy & physiology,* St Louis, 2012, Mosby.)

The **distal tubule** has straight and convoluted segments. It extends from the macula densa to the **collecting duct,** a large tubule that descends down the cortex and through the renal pyramids of the inner and outer medullae, draining urine into the minor calyx. In the distal tubule **principal cells** reabsorb sodium and secrete potassium, and **intercalated cells** secrete hydrogen and reabsorb potassium and bicarbonate.

Blood Vessels of the Kidney

The blood vessels of the kidney closely parallel nephron structure. The major vessels are as follows:

1. **Renal arteries** arise as the fifth branches of the abdominal aorta, divide into anterior and posterior branches at the renal hilum, and then subdivide into lobar arteries supplying blood to the lower, middle, and upper thirds of the kidney.

FIGURE 29-6 Anatomy of the Glomerulus and Juxtaglomerular Apparatus. A, Longitudinal cross section of glomerulus and juxtaglomerular apparatus. **B,** Horizontal cross section of glomerulus. **C,** Enlargement of glomerular capillary filtration membrane.

2. **Interlobar artery** subdivisions travel down renal columns and between pyramids and form afferent glomerular arteries.
3. **Arcuate arteries** consist of branches of interlobar arteries at the cortical-medullary junction; they arch over the base of the pyramids and run parallel to the surface.
4. **Glomerular capillaries** consist of four to eight vessels and are arranged in a fistlike structure; they arise from the **afferent arteriole** and empty into the **efferent arteriole**, which carries blood to the peritubular capillaries. They are the major resistance vessels for regulating intrarenal blood flow (see Autoregulation of Intrarenal Blood Flow, p. 735).
5. **Peritubular capillaries** surround convoluted portions of the proximal and distal tubules and the loop of Henle; they are adapted for cortical and juxtamedullary nephrons.
6. **Vasa recta** is a network of capillaries that forms loops and closely follow the loops of Henle; it is the only blood supply to the medulla (important for formation of concentrated urine).
7. **Renal veins** follow the arterial path in reverse direction and have the same names as the corresponding arteries; they eventually empty into the inferior vena cava. The lymphatic vessels also tend to follow the distribution of the blood vessels.

> ✔ **QUICK CHECK 29-1**
> 1. What is the major structural difference between the cortex and medulla of the kidney?
> 2. What is the function of the nephron?
> 3. Why are proteins not filtered at the glomerulus?

Urinary Structures
Ureters

The urine formed by the nephrons flows from the distal tubules and collecting ducts through the papillary ducts to the **renal papillae** (projections of the ducts) into the calyces, where it is collected in the renal pelvis (see Figures 29-2 and 29-5), and then funneled into the **ureters.** Each adult ureter is approximately 30 cm long and is composed of long, intertwining smooth muscle bundles. The lower ends pass obliquely through the posterior aspect of the bladder wall. The close approximation of smooth muscle cells permits the direct transmission of electrical stimulation from one cell to another. The resulting downward peristaltic contraction from intrinsic pacemaker activity propels urine into the bladder. Contraction of the bladder during **micturition** (urination) compresses the lower end of the ureter, preventing reflux. Peristalsis is maintained even when the ureter is denervated, so ureters can be transplanted.

Sensory innervation for the upper part of the ureter arises from sympathetic inputs from the tenth thoracic nerve roots, with referred pain to the umbilicus. The innervation of lower segments arises from the parasympathetic sacral nerves, with referred pain to the vulva or penis. The ureters have a rich blood supply. The primary arteries come from the kidney, with contributions from the lumbar and superior vesical arteries.

Bladder and Urethra

The bladder is a bag of smooth muscle fibers that forms the detrusor muscle and its smooth lining of uroepithelium. As the bladder fills with urine, it distends and the layers of uroepithelium within the lining slide past each other and become thinner as bladder volume increases. The uroepithelium forms the interface between the urinary space and the underlying vasculature and connective, nervous, and muscle tissue. Uroepithelium also lines the urinary tract from the renal pelvis to the urethra. The uroepithelium maintains an important barrier function to prevent movement of water and solutes between the urine and the blood. It communicates information about urine pressure and composition to surrounding nerve and muscle cells.[3] The trigone is a smooth triangular area between the openings of the two ureters and the urethra (Figure 29-7). The position of the bladder varies with age and sex. The bladder has a profuse blood supply, accounting for the bleeding that readily occurs with trauma, surgery, or inflammation.

The urethra extends from the inferior side of the bladder to the outside of the body. A ring of smooth muscle forms the internal urethral sphincter at the junction of the urethra and bladder. The external urethral sphincter is composed of striated skeletal muscle and is under voluntary control. The entire urethra is lined with mucus-secreting glands. The female urethra is short (3 to 4 cm). The male urethra is long (18 to 20 cm) and has three main segments: prostatic, membranous, and penile. The prostatic urethra is closest to the bladder. It passes through the prostate gland and contains the openings of the ejaculatory ducts. The membranous urethra passes through the floor of the pelvis. The penile segment forms the remainder of the tube. It is surrounded by the corpous spongiosum erectile tissue and contains the openings of the bulbourethral mucous glands.

The innervation of the bladder and internal urethral sphincter is supplied by parasympathetic fibers of the autonomic nervous system. The reflex arc required for micturition is stimulated by mechanoreceptors that respond to stretching of tissue, sensing bladder fullness and sending impulses to the sacral level of the cord. When the bladder accumulates 250 to 300 ml of urine, the bladder contracts and the internal urethral sphincter relaxes through activation of the spinal reflex arc (known as the *micturition reflex*). At this time, a person feels the urge to void. The reflex can be inhibited or facilitated by impulses coming from the brain, resulting in voluntary control of micturition by the relaxation or contraction of the external sphincter.

RENAL BLOOD FLOW

The kidneys are highly vascular organs and usually receive 1000 to 1200 ml of blood per minute, or about 20% to 25% of the cardiac output. With a normal hematocrit of 45%, about 600 to 700 ml of blood flowing through the kidney per minute is plasma. From the renal plasma flow (RPF), 20% (approximately 120 to 140 ml/min) is filtered at the glomerulus and passes into Bowman capsule. The filtration of the plasma per unit of time is known as the glomerular filtration rate (GFR), which is directly related to the perfusion pressure of the glomerular capillaries.

The remaining 80% (about 480 ml/min) of plasma flows through the efferent arterioles to the peritubular capillaries. The ratio of glomerular filtrate to renal plasma flow per minute (125/600 − 0.20) is called the *filtration fraction*. Normally all but 1 to 2 ml/min of the glomerular filtrate is reabsorbed from nephron tubules and returned to the circulation by the peritubular capillaries.

The GFR is directly related to renal blood flow (RBF), which is regulated by intrinsic autoregulatory mechanisms, by neural regulation, and by hormonal regulation. In general, blood flow to any organ is determined by the arteriovenous pressure differences across the vascular bed. If mean arterial pressure decreases or vascular resistance increases, RBF declines and urinary output decreases. Normal urinary output is about 30 ml/hour minimum in adults or 0.5 to 1.0 ml/kg/hr.

Autoregulation of Intrarenal Blood Flow

In the kidney, a local mechanism tends to keep the rate of glomerular perfusion and therefore the GFR fairly constant over a range of arterial pressures between 80 and 180 mm Hg (Figure 29-8). Changes in afferent arteriolar resistance occur in the same direction. Therefore, RBF and GFR are relatively constant, a relationship maintained by an intrinsic autoregulatory myogenic mechanism of contraction when blood vessels are stretched. The purpose of autoregulation of intrarenal blood flow is to keep RBF and GFR constant when there are increases or decreases in systemic blood pressure. Solute and water excretion, and thus blood volume, are regulated despite arterial pressure changes.[4]

A second mechanism of autoregulation is tubuloglomerular feedback. Because the glomerular filtration rate in an individual nephron increases or decreases, the macula densa cells in the distal tubule sense the increasing or decreasing amounts of filtered sodium. When GFR and sodium concentration increase, the macula densa cells stimulate

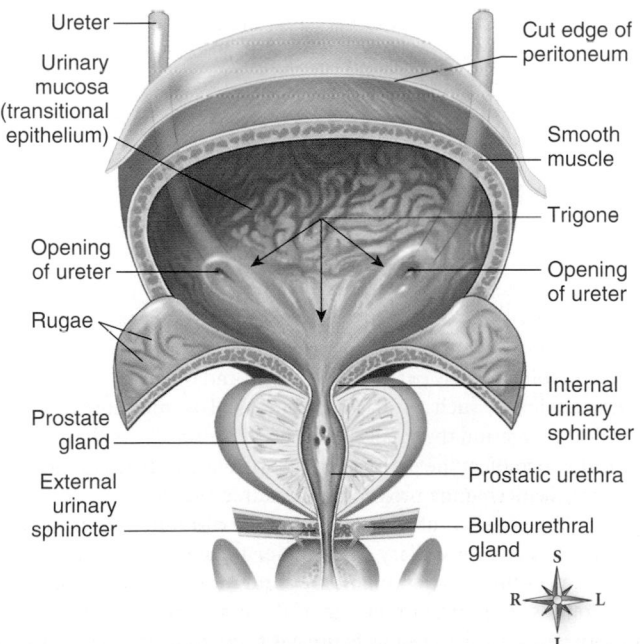

FIGURE 29-7 Structure of the Urinary Bladder. Frontal view of a dissected urinary bladder (male) in a fully distended position. (From Patton KT, Thibodeau GA: *The human body in health & disease*, ed 6, St Louis, 2014, Mosby.)

Ureter —
Urinary mucosa (transitional epithelium) —
Opening of ureter —
Rugae —
Prostate gland —
External urinary sphincter —

— Cut edge of peritoneum
— Smooth muscle
— Trigone
— Opening of ureter
— Internal urinary sphincter
— Prostatic urethra
— Bulbourethral gland

FIGURE 29-8 Renal Autoregulation. Blood flow and glomerular filtration rate are stabilized in the face of changes in perfusion pressure. (From Koeppen BM, Stanton BA: *Berne and Levy physiology* [updated], ed 6, St Louis, 2010, Mosby.)

afferent arteriolar vasoconstriction and decrease GFR. The opposite occurs with decreases in GFR and sodium concentration at the macula densa. This mechanism prevents large fluctuations in body water and salt.[5]

Neural Regulation of Renal Blood Flow

The blood vessels of the kidney are innervated by sympathetic nerve fibers located primarily on afferent arterioles. When systemic arterial pressure decreases, increased renal sympathetic nerve activity is mediated reflexively through the carotid sinus and the baroreceptors of the aortic arch. The sympathetic nerves release catecholamines. This stimulates afferent renal arteriolar vasoconstriction and decreases RBF and GFR, increases renal tubular sodium and water reabsorption, and increases blood pressure. Decreased afferent renal sympathetic nerve activity produces the opposite effects. The integrated response regulates water and sodium balance. Renalase is a hormone released by the kidney and heart that promotes the metabolism of catecholamines and in this way participates in blood pressure regulation.[6] The sympathetic nervous system also participates in hormonal (i.e., angiotensin II) regulation of renal blood flow. There is no significant parasympathetic innervation. The innervation of the kidney arises primarily from the celiac ganglion and greater splanchnic nerve.

Hormones and Other Factors Regulating Renal Blood Flow

Hormones and other mediators can alter the resistance of the renal vasculature by stimulating vasodilation or vasoconstriction. A major hormonal regulator of renal blood flow is the renin-angiotensin-aldosterone system (RAAS), which can increase systemic arterial pressure and change RBF. Renin is an enzyme formed and stored in the cells of the arterioles of the juxtaglomerular apparatus (see Figure 29-3). Renin release is triggered by decreased blood pressure in the afferent arterioles, decreased sodium chloride concentration in the distal convoluted tubule, sympathetic nerve stimulation of β-adrenergic receptors on the juxtaglomerular cells, and the release of prostaglandins.[7] Numerous physiologic effects of the RAAS stabilize systemic blood

pressure and preserve the extracellular fluid volume during hypotension or hypovolemia. Actions include sodium reabsorption, systemic vasoconstriction, sympathetic nerve stimulation, and thirst stimulation with increased fluid intake. The effects of aldosterone combine with those of antidiuretic hormone in regulating blood volume are summarized in Figure 29-9 (also see Figures 5-4 and 18-18).

Natriuretic peptides are synthesized and released from the heart and are natural antagonists to the renin-angiotensin-aldosterone system. Natriuretic peptides cause vasodilation and increase sodium and water excretion and decrease blood pressure (see p. 741). They assist in protecting the heart from volume overload. Urodilatin is renal natriuretic peptide produced by cells in the distal tubule and collecting duct. It increases renal blood flow, causing diuresis.

> ✔ **QUICK CHECK 29-2**
> 1. Where is pain from the ureters referred?
> 2. How do the bladder and urethra function in urine regulation?
> 3. What is autoregulation in the kidney? What other regulatory mechanisms are at work in renal function?

KIDNEY FUNCTION

Nephron Function

The nephron can perform many functions simultaneously (Figure 29-10), as follows:
1. Filters plasma at glomerulus.
2. Reabsorbs and secretes different substances along tubular structures.
3. Forms a filtrate of protein-free fluid (ultrafiltration).
4. Regulates the filtrate to maintain body fluid volume, electrolyte composition, and pH within narrow limits.

Glomerular filtration is the movement of fluid and solutes across the glomerular capillary membrane into the Bowman space. Tubular reabsorption is the movement of fluids and solutes from the tubular lumen to the peritubular capillary plasma. Tubular secretion is the transfer of substances from the plasma of the peritubular capillary to the tubular lumen. The transport mechanisms are both active and passive (processes defined in Chapter 1). Excretion is the elimination of a substance in the final urine (Figure 29-11).

Glomerular Filtration

The fluid filtered by the glomerular capillary filtration membrane and released into the proximal convoluted tubule is protein free but contains electrolytes (such as sodium, chloride, and potassium) and organic molecules (such as creatinine, urea, and glucose) in the same concentrations as found in plasma. Like other capillary membranes, the glomerulus is freely permeable to water and relatively impermeable to large colloids, such as plasma proteins. The molecule's size and electrical charge and the small size of the filtration slits in the glomerular epithelium affect the permeability of substances crossing the glomerulus and entering the proximal convoluted tubule.

Capillary pressures also affect glomerular filtration. The hydrostatic pressure within the capillary is the major force for moving water and solutes across the filtration membrane and into Bowman capsule. Two forces oppose the filtration effects of the glomerular capillary hydrostatic pressure (P_{GC}): (1) the hydrostatic pressure in Bowman space (P_{BC}) and (2) the effective oncotic pressure of the glomerular capillary blood (π_{GC}). Because the fluid in Bowman space normally contains only minute amounts of protein, it does not usually have an oncotic influence on the plasma of the glomerular capillary (Figure 29-12).

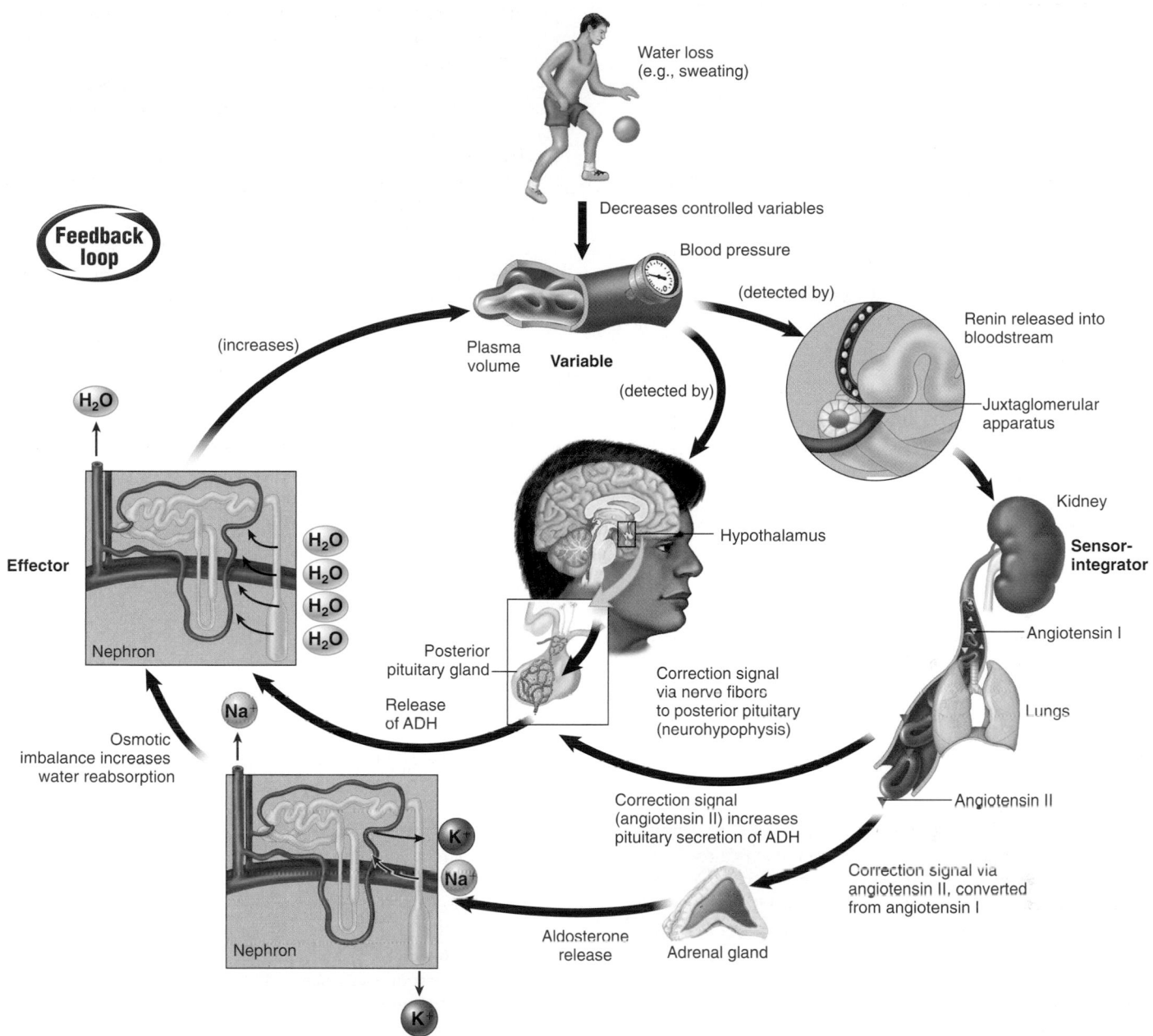

FIGURE 29-9 Cooperative Roles of Antidiuretic Hormone (ADH) and Aldosterone in Regulating Urine and Plasma Volume. The drop in blood pressure that accompanies loss of fluid from the internal environment triggers the hypothalamus to rapidly release ADH from the posterior pituitary gland. ADH increases water reabsorption by the kidney by increasing water permeability of the distal tubules and collecting ducts. The drop in blood pressure also is detected by each nephron's juxtaglomerular apparatus, which responds by secreting renin. Renin triggers the formation of angiotensin II, which stimulates release of aldosterone from the adrenal cortex. Aldosterone then slowly boosts water reabsorption by the kidneys by increasing reabsorption of Na^+. Because angiotensin II also stimulates secretion of ADH, it serves as an additional link between the ADH and aldosterone mechanisms. (From Patton KT, Thibodeau GA: *Anatomy & physiology,* ed 9, St Louis, 2016, Mosby.)

The combined effect of forces favoring and forces opposing filtration determines the filtration pressure. The net filtration pressure (NFP) is the sum of forces favoring and opposing filtration. The estimated values contributing to the forces of net filtration are presented in Table 29-1.

As the protein-free fluid is filtered into Bowman capsule, the plasma oncotic pressure increases and the hydrostatic pressure decreases. The increase in glomerular capillary oncotic pressure is great enough to reduce the net filtration pressure to zero at the efferent end of the capillary and to stop the filtration process effectively. The low hydrostatic pressure and the increased oncotic pressure in the efferent arteriole then are transferred to the peritubular capillaries and facilitate reabsorption of fluid from the proximal convoluted tubules.

Filtration rate. The total volume of fluid filtered by the glomeruli averages 180 L/day, or approximately 120 ml/min, a phenomenal amount considering the size of the kidneys. Because only 1 to 2 L

FIGURE 29-10 Major Functions of Nephron Segments. *ADH*, Antidiuretic hormone. (Modified from Hockenberry MJ et al: *Wong's nursing care of infants and children*, ed 8, St Louis, 2007, Mosby.)

		PRESSURES (mm Hg)	
Forces	**Pressures**	**Beginning of Capillary**	**End of Capillary**
Promoting Filtration			
Glomerular capillary hydrostatic pressure	P_{GC}	47	45
Bowman capsule oncotic pressure	π_{BC}	Negligible effect	Negligible effect
Opposing Filtration			
Bowman capsule hydrostatic pressure	P_{BC}	10	10
Glomerular capillary oncotic pressure	π_{GC}	25	35
Net filtration pressure		12	0

TABLE 29-1 Glomerular Filtration Pressures

of urine is excreted per day, 99% of the filtrate is reabsorbed into the peritubular capillaries and returned to the blood. The factors determining the GFR are directly related to the pressures that favor or oppose filtration (see Figure 29-12 and Table 29-1).

Obstruction to the outflow of urine (caused by strictures, stones, or tumors along the urinary tract) can cause a retrograde increase in hydrostatic pressure at Bowman space and a decrease in GFR. Low levels of plasma protein in the blood can result in a decrease in glomerular capillary oncotic pressure, which increases GFR. Excessive loss of *protein-free fluid* from vomiting, diarrhea, use of diuretics, or excessive sweating can increase glomerular capillary oncotic pressure and decrease the GFR. Renal disease also can cause changes in pressure relationships by altering capillary permeability and the surface area available for filtration (see Chapter 30).

Proximal convoluted tubule. By the end of the proximal tubule, approximately 60% to 70% of filtered sodium and water and about 50% of urea have been actively reabsorbed, along with 90% or more of potassium, glucose, bicarbonate, calcium, phosphate, amino acids, and uric acid. Chloride, water, and urea are reabsorbed passively but linked to the active transport of sodium (a cotransport mechanism). For some molecules, active transport in the renal tubules is limited as the carrier molecules become saturated, a phenomenon known as transport maximum (T_m). For example, when the carrier molecules for glucose reabsorption in the proximal convoluted tubule become saturated (i.e., with the development of hyperglycemia), the excess will be excreted in the urine.

Proximal convoluted tubule. Active reabsorption of sodium is the primary function of the proximal convoluted tubule. Water, most other electrolytes, and organic substances are cotransported with sodium. The osmotic force generated by active sodium transport promotes the passive diffusion of water out of the tubular lumen and into the peritubular capillaries. Passive transport of water is further enhanced by the elevated oncotic pressure of the blood in the peritubular capillaries, which is created by the previous filtration of water at the glomerulus. The reabsorption of water leaves an increased

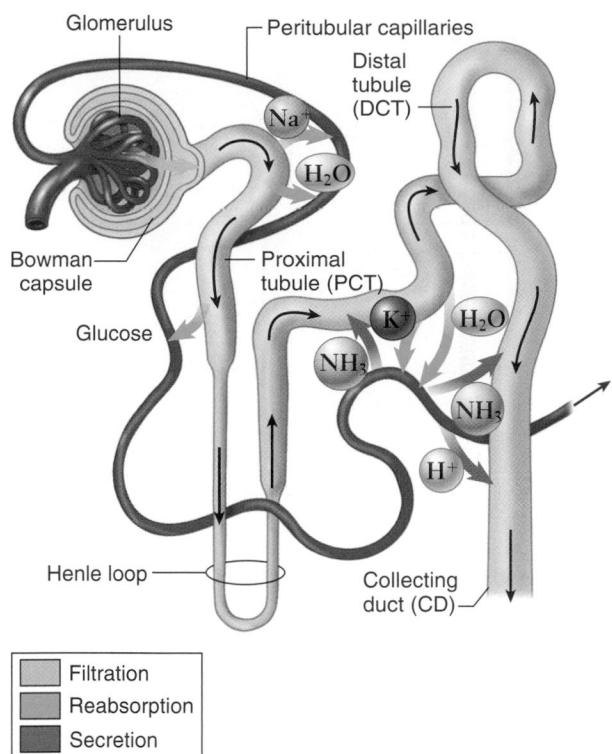

FIGURE 29-11 Urine Formation: Glomerular Filtration, Tubular Reabsorption, and Tubular Secretion. These are the three processes by which the kidneys excrete urine. Water, electrolytes, glucose, and organic molecules are filtered at the glomerulus. Sodium and glucose are reabsorbed into peritubular capillaries by active transport from the proximal convoluted tubules, and water reabsorption follows by osmosis. Sodium is reabsorbed by active transport from distal convoluted tubules; more sodium is conserved when aldosterone is secreted. Osmotic reabsorption of water from the distal tubules occurs when ADH is present. Secretion of ammonia (NH_3), hydrogen, and potassium occurs from peritubular capillaries into distal tubules by active transport. (From Patton KT, Thibodeau GA: *The human body in health & disease*, ed 6, St Louis, 2014, Mosby.)

concentration of urea within the tubular lumen, creating a gradient for its passive diffusion to the peritubular plasma. As the positively charged sodium ions leave the tubular lumen, negatively charged chloride ions passively follow to maintain electroneutrality. Because the inner membrane of the proximal tubular cell has a limited permeability to chloride, chloride reabsorption lags behind sodium.

Hydrogen ions are actively exchanged for sodium ions in the tubular lumen. The hydrogen ions (H^+) then combine with bicarbonate (HCO_3^-).

Bicarbonate is completely filtered at the glomerulus, and approximately 90% is reabsorbed in the proximal tubule. In the tubular lumen, hydrogen and bicarbonate ions form carbonic acid (H_2CO_3), which rapidly breaks down, or dissociates, to carbon dioxide (CO_2) and water (H_2O). These then diffuse into the tubular cell, where carbonic anhydrase again catalyzes the CO_2 and H_2O to form HCO_3^- and H^+. The H^+ is secreted again, and HCO_3^- combines with sodium and is transported to the peritubular capillary blood as $NaHCO_3$ (a sodium bicarbonate buffer). Bicarbonate is thus conserved, and the hydrogen is reabsorbed as water. Therefore, these ions normally do not contribute to the urinary excretion of acid or the addition of acid to the blood.

In addition to the proximal tubular secretion of hydrogen ions, secretory transport mechanisms exist for creatinine, other organic

FIGURE 29-12 Glomerular Filtration Pressures.

BOX 29-1   Substances Transported by Renal Tubules

Reabsorption	Secretion
Albumin	Choline
Ascorbate	Creatinine
Fructose	Histamine
Galactose	Methylguanidine
Glutamate	*para*-Aminohippurate
Glucose	Penicillin and many other drugs
Phosphate	Steroid glucuronides
Sulfate	Thiamine
Xylose	

bases, and endogenous and exogenous organic acids including *para*-aminohippurate (PAH) and penicillin (Box 29-1). These secretory mechanisms eliminate drugs and other exogenous chemical products from the body, often after first conjugating them with sulfate and glucuronic acid in the liver. Many drugs and their metabolites are eliminated from the body in this way. When the renal tubules are damaged, metabolic by-products and drugs may accumulate, causing toxic levels in the body.

Normally, 99% of the glomerular filtrate is reabsorbed. When the GFR spontaneously decreases or increases, the renal tubules, primarily the proximal tubules, automatically adjust their rate of reabsorption of sodium and water to balance the change in GFR. This prevents wide fluctuations in the excretion of sodium and water into the urine and is known as glomerulotubular balance.

Loop of henle and distal convoluted tubule. Urine can be hypotonic, isotonic, or hypertonic. Urine concentration or dilution occurs principally in the loop of Henle, distal tubules, and collecting ducts.

FIGURE 29-13 Countercurrent Mechanism for Concentrating and Diluting Urine. A, Urine dilution; **B,** urine concentration. **1,** Filtrate isotonic to plasma. **2,** Descending thin limb permeable to water. **3,** Ascending thin limb impermeable to water; permeable to ions. **4,** Ascending thick limb actively transports NaCl; impermeable to water and urea. **5,** Distal tubule actively resorbs NaCl; resorbs water in presence of antidiuretic hormone. **6,** Medullary collecting duct actively resorbs NaCl, and slightly permeable to water and urea. (NOTE: Numbers on illustration represent milliosmoles [mOsm]). H_2O, water; *NaCl*, sodium chloride. See text for details. (From Koeppen BM, Stanton BA: *Berne and Levy physiology* [updated], ed 6, St Louis, 2010, Mosby.)

The structural features of the medullary hairpin loops allow the kidney to concentrate urine and conserve water for the body. The transition of the filtrate into the final urine reflects the concentrating ability of the loops. Final adjustments in urine composition are made by the distal tubule and collecting duct according to body needs.

Production of concentrated urine involves a **countercurrent exchange system,** in which fluid flows in opposite directions through the parallel tubes of the loop of Henle. A concentration gradient causes fluid to be exchanged across the parallel pathways. The longer the loop, the greater the concentration gradient; the concentration gradient increases from the cortex to the tip of the medulla. The loops of Henle multiply the concentration gradient, and the vasa recta blood vessels act as a countercurrent exchanger for maintaining the gradient. The process is initiated in the thick ascending limb of the loop of Henle with the active transport of chloride and sodium out of the tubular lumen and into the medullary interstitium (Figure 29-13). Because the lumen of the ascending limb is impermeable to water, water cannot follow the sodium-chloride transport. This causes the ascending tubular fluid to become hypoosmotic and the medullary interstitium to become hyperosmotic. The descending limb of the loop, which receives fluid from the proximal tubule, is highly permeable to water but it is the only place in the nephron that does not actively transport either sodium or chloride. Sodium and chloride may, however, diffuse into the descending tubule from the interstitium. The hyperosmotic medullary interstitium causes water to move out of the descending limb, and the remaining fluid in the descending tubule becomes increasingly concentrated while it flows toward the tip of the medulla. While the tubular fluid rounds the loop and enters the ascending limb, sodium and chloride are removed and water is retained. The fluid then becomes more and more dilute as it encounters the distal tubule.

The slow rate of blood flow and the hairpin structure of the vasa recta blood vessels allow blood to flow through the medullary tissue without disturbing the osmotic gradient. When blood flows into the descending limb of the vasa recta, it encounters the increasing osmotic concentration gradient of the medullary interstitium. Water moves out and sodium and chloride diffuse into the descending vasa recta. The plasma becomes increasingly concentrated as it flows toward the tip of the medulla.

As blood flows away from the tip of the medulla and toward the cortex, the surrounding interstitial fluid becomes comparatively more dilute. Water then moves back into the vasa recta, and sodium and chloride diffuse out and the plasma again becomes more dilute. The net result is a preservation of the medullary osmotic gradient. If blood were to flow rapidly through the vasa recta, as occurs in some renal diseases, the medullary concentration gradient would be washed away and the ability to concentrate urine and conserve water would be lost. The efficiency of water conservation is related to the length of the loops of Henle: the longer the loops, the greater the ability to concentrate the urine.

Urea is the major constituent of urine along with water. The glomerulus freely filters urea, and tubular reabsorption depends on urine flow rate, with less reabsorption at higher flow rates. Approximately 50% of urea is excreted in the urine, and 50% is recycled within the kidney. This recycling contributes to the osmotic gradient within the medulla and is necessary for the concentration and dilution of urine (see Figure 29-13). Because urea is an end product of protein metabolism, individuals with protein deprivation cannot maximally concentrate their urine.[8]

Another function of the loop of Henle is the production of **uromodulin** (also known as **Tamm-Horsfall protein [THP]**), the most abundant protein in human urine. This protein binds to uropathogens to prevent urinary tract infection, protects the uroepithelium from injury, protects against kidney stone formation and is associated with progression of kidney disease.[9]

The convoluted portion of the distal tubule is poorly permeable to water but readily reabsorbs ions and contributes to the dilution of the tubular fluid. The later, straight segment of the distal tubule and the collecting duct are permeable to water as controlled by antidiuretic hormone (ADH) released from the posterior pituitary gland. Sodium is readily reabsorbed by the later segment of the distal tubule and collecting duct under the regulation of the hormone aldosterone (see Chapter 18). Potassium is actively secreted in these segments and is also controlled by aldosterone and other factors related to the concentration of potassium in body fluids (see Chapter 5).

Hydrogen is secreted by the distal tubule and combines with nonbicarbonate buffers (i.e., ammonium and phosphate) for the elimination of acids in the urine (see Figure 5-11). The distal tubule thus contributes to the regulation of acid-base balance by excreting hydrogen ions into the urine and by adding new bicarbonate to the plasma. The mechanism is similar to the conservation of bicarbonate by the proximal tubule, except that the hydrogen ion is excreted in the urine and influences acid-base balance (see Figure 5-11). The specific mechanisms of acid-base balance and acid excretion are described in Chapter 5.

Urine Composition

Urine is normally clear yellow or amber in color. Cloudiness may indicate the presence of bacteria, cells, or high solute concentration. The pH ranges from 4.6 to 8.0, but it is normally acidic, providing protection against bacteria. Specific gravity ranges from 1.001 to 1.035. Normal urine does not contain glucose or blood cells and only occasionally contains traces of protein, usually in association with rigorous exercise.

Hormones and Nephron Function
Antidiuretic Hormone

The distal tubule in the cortex receives the hypoosmotic urine from the ascending limb of the loop of Henle. The concentration of the final urine is controlled by antidiuretic hormone (ADH), which is secreted from the posterior pituitary or neurohypophysis. ADH increases water permeability and reabsorption in the last segment of the distal tubule and along the entire length of the collecting ducts, which pass through the inner and outer zones of the medulla. The water diffuses into the ascending limb of the vasa recta and returns to the systemic circulation. The excreted urine can have a high osmotic concentration, up to 1400 mOsm. The volume is normally reduced to about 1% of the amount filtered at the glomerulus. (The mechanism for the regulation of ADH and plasma osmolality is described in Chapters 5 and 18.)

Aldosterone

Aldosterone is synthesized and secreted by the adrenal cortex under the regulation of the renin-angiotensin-aldosterone system (see Chapter 18, and the previous discussion of the renin-angiotensin-aldosterone system on p. 736). Aldosterone stimulates the epithelial cells of the distal tubule and collecting duct to reabsorb sodium (promoting water reabsorption) and increases the excretion of potassium and hydrogen ion.

Natriuretic Peptides

Natriuretic peptides are a group of peptide hormones, including atrial natriuretic peptide (ANP), secreted from myocardial cells in the atria, and brain natriuretic peptide (BNP), secreted from myocardial cells in the cardiac ventricles.[10] When the heart dilates during volume expansion or heart failure, ANP and BNP inhibit sodium and water absorption by kidney tubules, inhibit secretion of renin and aldosterone, vasodilate the afferent arterioles, and constrict the efferent arterioles. The result is increased urine formation leading to a decrease in blood volume and blood pressure. *C-type natriuretic peptide* is secreted from the vascular endothelium and causes vasodilation in the nephron. *Urodilatin* is secreted by the distal convoluted tubules and collecting ducts and causes vasodilation and natriuretic and diuretic effects.

Diuretics as a Factor in Urine Flow

A diuretic is any agent enhancing the flow of urine. Clinically, diuretics interfere with renal sodium reabsorption and reduce extracellular fluid volume. Diuretics are commonly used to treat hypertension and edema caused by heart failure, cirrhosis, and nephrotic syndrome.

Diuretics are divided into five general categories: (1) osmotic diuretics, (2) carbonic anhydrase inhibitors (inhibitors of urinary acidification), (3) inhibitors of loop sodium or chloride transport, (4) aldosterone antagonists (potassium sparing), and (5) aquaretics. (The physiologic mechanism related to each category is summarized in Table 29-2.)

Renal Hormones

Certain hormones are either activated or synthesized by the kidney. These hormones have significant systemic effects and include urodilatin (see earlier text), the active form of vitamin D, and erythropoietin.

Vitamin D

Vitamin D is a hormone that can be obtained in the diet or synthesized by the action of ultraviolet radiation (sun exposure) on cholesterol in the skin. These forms of vitamin D_3 (cholecalciferol) are inactive and require two hydroxylations to establish a metabolically active form. The first step occurs in the liver and the second in the kidneys.

Vitamin D is necessary for the absorption of calcium and phosphate by the small intestine. The renal hydroxylation step is stimulated by parathyroid hormone (see Chapter 18). A decreased plasma calcium level (less than 10 mg/dl) stimulates the secretion of parathyroid hormone. Parathyroid hormone then stimulates a sequence of events to help restore plasma calcium concentration toward normal levels (9 to 10.5 mg/dl):

1. Calcium mobilization from bone
2. Synthesis of 1,25-dihydroxy-vitamin D_3
3. Absorption of calcium from the intestine
4. Increased renal calcium reabsorption
5. Decreased renal phosphate reabsorption

Serum phosphate concentration fluctuations also influence the renal hydroxylation of vitamin D. Decreased levels stimulate active 1,25-dihydroxy-vitamin D_3 formation, and increased levels inhibit formation. This results in compensatory changes in phosphate absorption from bone and intestine. Individuals with renal disease have a deficiency of 1,25-dihydroxy-vitamin D_3 (1,25-OH$_2$D$_3$) and manifest symptoms of disturbed calcium and phosphate balance (see Chapters 5, 18, and 30).

Erythropoietin

Erythropoietin (Epo) stimulates the bone marrow to produce red blood cells in response to tissue hypoxia and may have tissue protective effects[11] (see *Health Alert:* The Many Effects of Erythropoietin [Epo]). Erythrocyte production is discussed in Chapter 20. The stimulus for Epo release is decreased oxygen delivery in the kidneys. Oxygen-sensing erythropoietin-producing cells are peritubular fibroblasts located in the juxtamedullary cortex.[12] The anemia of chronic renal failure, in which kidney cells have become nonfunctional, can be related to the lack of this hormone (see Chapter 30).

Kidney function changes throughout the life span and major changes are summarized in the boxes: *Pediatric Considerations:* Pediatrics & Renal Function and *Geriatric Considerations:* Aging & Renal Function.

TESTS OF RENAL FUNCTION
Renal Clearance

A number of specific renal functions can be measured by renal clearance. Renal clearance techniques determine how much of a substance can be cleared from the blood by the kidneys per given unit of time. The application of this principle permits an indirect measure of GFR, tubular secretion, tubular reabsorption, and RBF.

TABLE 29-2 Action of Diuretics

Diuretic	Site of Action	Action	Common Side Effects
Osmotic Diuretics			
Mannitol	Proximal tubule	Freely filtered but not reabsorbed; osmotically attract water and diminish sodium reabsorption	Hypokalemia, dehydration
Glycerol			
Urea			
Carbonic Anhydrase Inhibitors			
Acetazolamide	Proximal tubule	Inhibits carbonic anhydrase; blocks hydrogen ion secretion and reabsorption of sodium and bicarbonate	Hypokalemia, systemic acidosis, alkaline urine
Inhibitors of Sodium/Chloride Reabsorption			
Thiazides	Distal convoluted tubules	Inhibit sodium and chloride reabsorption; mildly suppress carbonic anhydrase; reduce calcium excretion	Hypokalemia, metabolic alkalosis
Furosemide	Thick ascending limb of loop of Henle	Inhibit active transport of chloride, sodium, and potassium	Hypokalemia, uric acid retention
Ethacrynic acid			
Torsemide	Cortical vasodilation	Increase rate of urine formation	Hypokalemia, uric acid retention
Bumetanide			
Potassium-Sparing Diuretics			
Spironolactone	Distal tubule/collecting duct	Inhibits aldosterone, blocks sodium reabsorption, and results in potassium retention	Hyperkalemia, nausea, confusion, gynecomastia
Triamterene and amiloride	Distal tubule/collecting duct	Inhibit sodium reabsorption and inhibit potassium excretion	Nausea, vomiting, headache, granulocytopenia, skin rash
Aquaretics			
Vasopressin (V_2) blockers (e.g., conivaptan)	Distal tubule/collecting ducts	Block action of antidiuretic hormone	Dehydration

HEALTH ALERT

The Many Effects of Erythropoietin (Epo)

Receptors for Epo are found in many body cells other than hematopoietic cells (i.e., neurons, immune cells, cancer cell lines, endothelial cells, bone marrow myocardium, skeletal muscle, kidney cells, pancreatic cells, and cells of the reproductive system and gastrointestinal tract). Epo-related tissue protective effects include anti-apoptotic, anti-inflammatory, and angiogenic actions. In acute kidney injury, Epo reduces ischemia, oxidative stress, and inflammation, protecting cells from injury. These same effects, including angiogenesis, limit myocardial infarction size and left ventricular remodeling. Epo also is anti-inflammatory and inhibits inflammation in chronic inflammatory diseases. Epo is neuroprotective in conditions associated with hypoxia, neurodegeneration, and inflammation. Epo is used for the treatment of anemia in chronic kidney disease and anemia related to cancer chemotherapy. Studies are currently evaluating if the angiogenic and growth factor effects of Epo promote tumor growth.

Data from Glaspy J: *Semin Thromb Hemost* 40(3):306-312, 2014; Nguyen AQ et al: *Exp Biol Med (Maywood)* 239(11):1461-1475, 2014; Sanchis-Gomar F et al: *Int J Cardiol* 171(2):116-125, 2014; Zhang Y et al: *Int J Mol Sci* 15(6):10296-10333, 2014.

✔QUICK CHECK 29-3

1. Outline the process of glomerular filtration.
2. What types of absorption/reabsorption take place in the proximal tubule, the loops of Henle, and the distal tubule?
3. What is the countercurrent exchange system? What substances are involved?
4. What hormones are activated or synthesized by the kidney?

Clearance and Renal Blood Flow

A clearance formula also can be used to estimate RPF and RBF using a molecule called *para*-aminohippuric acid (PAH). Some PAH is filtered at the glomerulus and most of the remainder is secreted into the tubules in one circulation through the kidney. If all the PAH were removed from the plasma during a single pass through the kidney, total RPF could be determined. Because the supporting and nonsecreting structures of the kidney receive 10% to 15% of the **effective renal blood flow (ERBF)**, clearance of PAH measures only what is known as the **effective renal plasma flow (ERPF)**, which is 85% to 90% of the true renal plasma flow.

Clearance and Glomerular Filtration Rate

The GFR provides the best estimate of functioning renal tissue and is important for assessing or monitoring kidney damage and drug dosing. Damage to the glomerular membrane or loss of nephrons leads to a corresponding decrease in GFR. The measurement of GFR requires the use of a substance that has a stable plasma concentration; is freely filtered at the glomerulus; is not secreted, reabsorbed, or metabolized by the tubules; and is easy to measure. *Inulin* (a fructose polysaccharide) is one substance that meets the criteria for measurement of GFR.

The accurate determination of inulin clearance requires constant infusion to maintain a stable plasma level. This is time-consuming and inconvenient. Therefore the clearance of creatinine, a natural substance produced by muscle and released into the blood at a relatively constant rate, is commonly used as an estimate clinically. It is freely filtered at the glomerulus, but a small amount is secreted by the renal tubules. Therefore creatinine clearance overestimates the GFR, but within tolerable limits. Creatinine clearance provides a good clinical measure of GFR because only one blood sample is required in addition to an accurately collected 24-hour volume of urine. Cystatin C is a stable protein in serum filtered at the glomerulus and metabolized in the tubules. Serum levels of cystatin C also are a marker for estimating GFR, particularly for mild to moderate impaired renal function.[13] A combined creatinine and cystatin C estimate of GFR was developed in 2012 and considers age, race, and sex.[14]

Formulas are used to estimate GFR.[15] The Cockcroft and Gault creatinine-based formula is commonly used and considers age, body weight, and plasma creatinine (P_{cr}) values: The National Kidney Foundation recommends the Modification of Diet in Renal Disease (MDRD) equation.[16] The Chronic Kidney Disease Epidemiology Collaboration (2009 CKD-EPI) equation has been developed as a more precise estimate of GFR than the MDRD and considers age, sex, and race.[17] In 2012, cystatin C and combined creatinine and cystatin C equations were developed. Calculators for estimates of GFR using these formulas are readily available on the Internet (see example at http://touchcalc.com/ip_epi_gfr/ip_ckd_epi). Normal GFR values are 90 to 120 ml/min.

Plasma Creatinine Concentration

A chronic decline in the GFR over weeks or months is reflected in the plasma creatinine (P_{cr}) concentration (normal value = 0.7 to 1.2 mg/dl). The P_{cr} concentration has a stable value when the GFR is stable, because creatinine has a constant rate of production as a product of muscle metabolism. The amount filtered is approximately equal to the amount excreted. When the GFR declines, the P_{cr} increases proportionately. Thus the GFR and P_{cr} are inversely related. If the GFR were to decrease by 50%, the filtration and excretion of creatinine would be reduced by 50% and creatinine would accumulate in plasma to twice the normal value. Therefore, elevated P_{cr} values represent decreasing GFR. In the new steady state, however, the total amount of creatinine excreted in the urine would remain the same because of the proportionate decrease in GFR and increase in P_{cr}.

The application of this principle is simple and useful for monitoring progressive changes in renal function. The test is most valuable for monitoring the progress of chronic rather than acute renal disease because it takes 7 to 10 days for the plasma creatinine level to stabilize when GFR declines. Serial measures can be obtained over a long time and plotted as a curve of glomerular function. The P_{cr} also becomes elevated during trauma or the breakdown of muscle tissue. In such instances, the value is then not useful for estimating GFR.

Blood Urea Nitrogen

The concentration of urea nitrogen in the blood reflects glomerular filtration and urine-concentrating capacity. Because urea is filtered at the glomerulus, blood urea nitrogen (BUN) levels increase as glomerular filtration drops. Because urea is reabsorbed by the blood through the permeable tubules, the BUN value rises in states of dehydration and with acute and chronic renal failure when passage of fluid through the tubules slows. BUN values also change as a result of altered protein intake and protein catabolism. The normal range for BUN level in the adult is 10 to 20 mg/dl of blood.

Urinalysis

Urinalysis is a noninvasive and relatively inexpensive diagnostic procedure. The best results are obtained from a fresh, cleanly voided specimen because decay permits changes in the composition of urine. Urinalysis includes evaluation of color, turbidity, protein, pH, specific gravity, sediment, and supernatant. Urine tests are listed in Table 29-3 and bladder function tests are listed in Table 29-4.

✔**QUICK CHECK 29-4**
1. Why is creatinine clearance a good estimate of glomerular filtration rate?
2. What is the relationship between plasma creatinine concentration and glomerular filtration rate?

PEDIATRIC CONSIDERATIONS

Pediatrics & Renal Function

Glomerular filtration rate in infants does not reach adult levels until 1 to 2 years of age, and newborns have a decreased ability to efficiently remove excess water and solutes. Their shorter loops of Henle also decrease concentrating ability and produce a more dilute urine than that produced by adults. Risks for metabolic acidosis are increased during the first few months of life while the mechanisms for excreting acid and retaining bicarbonate are maturing. These normal developmental processes result in a narrow safety margin for fluid and electrolyte balance when there is any disturbance such as diarrhea, infection, fever, fasting for diagnostic tests, improper feeding, fluid replacement, or drug administration. Newborns diurese 2 to 3 days after birth, which is reflected by a decrease in total body water and body weight. An increased risk of toxicity accompanies drug administration. Low birth weight infants have a delay in achieving full renal function and may not have full GFR until 8 years of age. They also are at greater risk for low nephron numbers and chronic kidney disease as adults.

Data from Filler G et al: *Pediatr Nephrol* 29(2):183-192, 2014; Hoseini R et al: *Iran J Kidney Dis* 6(3):166-172, 2012; Lankadeva YR et al: *Am J Physiol Renal Physiol* 306(8):F791-F800, 2014; Sulemanji M, Vakili K: *Semin Pediatr Surg* 22(4):195-198, 2013.

GERIATRIC CONSIDERATIONS

Aging & Renal Function

- Structural changes commonly occur in the kidney with aging, including loss of renal mass, arterial sclerosis, an increased number of sclerotic glomeruli, loss of tubules, and interstitial fibrosis. These changes contribute to a slow decline in GFR and a reduction in creatinine clearance in most individuals, but it generally is not significant enough to lead to severe loss of renal function. As the number of nephrons decreases and degenerative changes occur, nephrons are less able to concentrate urine and less able to tolerate dehydration, excessive water loads, or electrolyte imbalances, particularly with physiologic stress. Up to 45% of people older than 70 years of age have chronic kidney disease.
- The presence of comorbid conditions, such as hypertension and diabetes mellitus, accelerates the decline of renal function. Obesity does not accelerate a decline in GFR.
- Response to acid-base changes and reabsorption of glucose may be delayed.
- Drugs eliminated by the kidney can accumulate in the plasma, causing toxic reactions; GFR and drug dosage should be carefully evaluated.
- Decreased thirst sensation and diminished water intake may alter water balance.
- Impairment in renal blood flow, hormonal regulatory systems, and metabolism of medications may alter sodium and water balance.
- Older donor kidneys show decreased regenerative capacity.

Data from Baldea AJ: *Surg Clin North Am* 95(1):71-83, 2009; Bolignano D et al: *Ageing Res Rev* 14:65-80, 2014; Karam Z, Tuazon J: *Clin Geriatr Med* 29(3):555-564, 2013; Presta P et al: *Int Urol Nephrol* 44(2):625-632, 2012; Sands JM: *J Gerontol A Biol Sci Med Sci* 67(12):1352-1357, 2012; Schmitt R, Melk A: *Am J Transplant* 12(11):2892-2900, 2012; Tonelli M, Riella MC: *Nat Rev Nephrol* 10(3):127-128, 2014.

TABLE 29-3 Normal Renal Function Tests

Test	Normal Value	Interpretation
Urine		
Color	Amber-yellow	Drugs and foods may change color
Turbidity	Clear	Purulent matter will make cloudy
pH	4.6-8.0	Bacteria create an alkaline urine
Specific gravity (density of water = 1.000)		Represents concentrating ability or density of urine in relation to density of water (i.e., higher when contains glucose or protein; lower with dilute urine)
Adults	1.010-1.025	
Infants	1.010-1.018	
Blood	Negative	Bleeding along urinary tract
Microscopic Urine		
Bacteria	None	Infection
Red blood cells	Negative	Bleeding along urinary tract
White blood cells	Negative	Urinary tract infection
Crystals	Negative	May have potential for stones
Fat	Negative	Can be associated with nephrosis
Casts	Occasional	A few are normal; may represent renal disease
Urinary Chemistry		
Bilirubin	Negative	Increases may cause dark orange color
Urobilinogen	Less than 4 mg/24 hr	Increases may indicate red blood cell hemolysis
Ketones	Negative	Represents an increase in fat metabolism
Glucose	Negative	Usually signifies hyperglycemia
Sodium	100-260 mEq/24 hr	Can increase or decrease with renal disease
Potassium	25-100 mEq/24 hr	Can increase or decrease with renal disease, potassium intake, aldosteronism, or diuretic use
Protein	Negative-trace	Dysfunction of glomerulus
Normal Serum Values		
BUN	7-18 mg/dl	Elevated with diseased kidneys
Creatinine	Elevated with decreased GFR	
Male	0.6-1.5 mg/dl	
Female	0.6-1.1 mg/dl	
Cystatin C	0.8-2.1 mg/L	Early detection of decreased GFR
Potassium		Elevated in renal failure

TABLE 29-4 Bladder Function Tests

Procedure	Description
Urodynamic Tests	
Cystometry (cystometrogram)	Measurement of bladder pressure determined using a pressure-measuring catheter; fluid volume and pressures are measured as bladder is filled with fluid; simultaneous pressures may be measured in rectum; sensations of bladder fullness are also recorded; coughing or straining can lead to involuntary bladder contractions
	Bladder capacity: male, 350-750 ml; female, 350-550 ml
	Intrabladder pressure with empty bladder: 40 cm H_2O
	Detrusor pressure: <10 cm H_2O
	Residual urine: <30 ml
Uroflowmetry	Measures time it takes to empty a full bladder of urine; flow rates may be faster with urge incontinence or slower with prostatic obstruction
Postvoid residual urine	Measures residual urine in bladder after voiding; urine can be removed with catheter and measured, or ultrasound imaging can be used to measure urine; postvoid residual of more than 200 ml is abnormal and requires further evaluation
Measurement of leak point pressure	Pressure at which bladder fluid will leak from bladder without warning
Pressure flow study	Measures pressure required to empty bladder; pressure flow study identifies bladder outlet obstruction such as that occurring with prostate enlargement
Electromyography	Measures nerve impulses and muscle activity in urethral sphincter by placing sensors on skin near urethra and rectum or by placing sensors on catheter placed in urethra or rectum
Video urodynamics	Imaging of x-rays or ultrasound waves during fluid filling of bladder; shows size and shape of urinary tract
Direct Visualization Diagnostic Procedures	
Cystoscopy	Cystoscope (a type of endoscope) is inserted through urethra and is used to visualize inside of bladder
Ureteroscopy	Ureteroscope is inserted through urethra and bladder and directly into ureter and upper urinary tract to visualize upper urinary tract

DID YOU UNDERSTAND?

Structures of the Renal System

1. The kidneys are paired structures lying bilaterally between the twelfth thoracic and third lumbar vertebrae and behind the peritoneum of the abdominal cavity.
2. The kidney is composed of an outer cortex and an inner medulla.
3. The calyces receive urine from the distal tubules and join to form the renal pelvis, which is continuous with the upper end of the ureter.
4. The nephron is the urine-forming unit of the kidney and is composed of the glomerulus, proximal convoluted tubule, hairpin loops of Henle, distal tubule, and collecting duct.
5. The glomerulus contains loops of capillaries supported by mesangial cells. The capillary walls serve as a filtration membrane for the formation of the primary urine.
6. The proximal tubule is lined with microvilli to increase surface area and enhance reabsorption of water, solutes, and electrolytes.
7. The hairpin loops of Henle transport solutes and water, contributing to the hypertonic state of the medulla, and are important for the concentration and dilution of urine.
8. The distal convoluted tubule adjusts acid-base balance by excreting acid into the urine and forming new bicarbonate ions. It reabsorbs water with the influence of ADH and reabsorbs sodium and excretes potassium with the influence of aldosterone.
9. The ureters extend from the renal pelvis to the posterior wall of the bladder. Urine flows through the ureters and into the bladder by means of peristaltic contraction of the ureteral muscles.
10. The bladder is a bag composed of the detrusor and trigone muscles and innervated by parasympathetic fibers. When accumulation of urine reaches 250 to 300 ml, mechanoreceptors, which respond to stretching of tissue, stimulate the micturition reflex.

Renal Blood Flow

1. Renal blood flows at about 1000 to 1200 ml/min, or 20% to 25% of the cardiac output.
2. Blood flow through the glomerular capillaries is maintained at a constant rate in spite of a wide range of arterial pressures by autoregulation of the glomerular capillaries.
3. The glomerular filtration rate (GFR) is the filtration of plasma per unit of time and is directly related to the perfusion pressure of renal blood flow.
4. Renin is an enzyme secreted from the juxtaglomerular apparatus in response to decreased blood pressure and causes the generation of angiotensin II, a potent vasoconstrictor. The renin-angiotensin-aldosterone system is thus a regulator of renal blood flow.

Kidney Function

1. The major function of the nephron is urine formation, which involves the processes of glomerular filtration, tubular reabsorption, and tubular secretion and excretion.
2. Glomerular filtration is favored by capillary hydrostatic pressure and opposed by oncotic pressure in the capillary and hydrostatic pressure in Bowman capsule. The balance of favoring and opposing filtration forces is known as net filtration pressure (NFP).
3. The GFR is approximately 120 ml/min, and 99% of the filtrate is reabsorbed.
4. The proximal convoluted tubule reabsorbs about 60% to 70% of the filtered sodium and water and 90% of other electrolytes.
5. Because most molecules are reabsorbed by active transport, the carrier mechanism can become saturated at a point known as the transport maximum (T_m). Molecules not reabsorbed are excreted with the urine.
6. The concentration or specific gravity of the final urine is a function of the level of antidiuretic hormone (ADH). This hormone stimulates the distal tubules and collecting ducts to reabsorb water. The countercurrent exchange system of the long loops of Henle and their accompanying capillaries establishes a concentration gradient within the renal medulla to facilitate the reabsorption of water from the collecting duct.
7. The kidney secretes or activates a number of hormones having systemic effects, including vitamin D, erythropoietin, and the natriuretic hormone urodilatin.

Tests of Renal Function

1. Creatinine, a substance produced by muscle, is measured in both plasma and urine to calculate a commonly used clinical measurement of GFR.
2. Plasma creatinine concentration, cystatin C level, and blood urea nitrogen (BUN) level are estimates of glomerular function. BUN value also is an indicator of hydration status.
3. Formulas for estimating GFR can be helpful clinical indicators of renal function.
4. Urinalysis involves evaluation of color, turbidity, protein, pH, specific gravity, sediment, and supernatant. Presence of bacteria, red blood cells, white blood cells, casts, or crystals in the urine sediment may indicate a renal or bladder disorder.

PEDIATRIC CONSIDERATIONS: Pediatrics & Renal Function

1. Compared with adults, infants and children have more dilute urine because of higher blood flow and shorter loops of Henle.
2. Children are more affected than adults by fluid imbalances resulting from diarrhea, infection, or improper feeding because of their limited ability to quickly regulate changes in pH or osmotic pressure.

GERIATRIC CONSIDERATIONS: Aging & Renal Function

1. Older adults have a decreased ability to concentrate urine and are less able to tolerate dehydration or water loads because they have fewer nephrons.
2. Responses to acid-base changes and reabsorption of glucose are delayed in older adults.
3. In older adults, drugs eliminated by the kidney can accumulate in the plasma, causing toxic reactions.

KEY TERMS

Afferent arteriole, 734
Aldosterone, 741
Antidiuretic hormone (ADH), 741
Arcuate artery, 734
Atrial natriuretic peptide (ANP), 741
Autoregulation of intrarenal blood flow, 735
Bladder, 735
Bowman capsule, 732
Bowman space, 732
Calyx (pl., calyces), 730
Collecting duct, 733
Cortex, 730
Cortical nephron, 730
Countercurrent exchange system, 740
Cystatin C, 743
Detrusor muscle, 735

REFERENCES

1. Abboud HE: Mesangial cell biology, *Exp Cell Res* 318(9):979-985, 2012.
2. Friis UG et al: Regulation of renin secretion by renal juxtaglomerular cells, *Pflugers Arch* 465(1):25-37, 2013.
3. Birder LA et al: Is the urothelium intelligent? *Neurourol Urodyn* 29(4):598-602, 2010.
4. Guan Z et al: P2 receptors in renal autoregulation, *Curr Vasc Pharmacol* 12(6):818-828, 2014.
5. Singh P, Thomson SC: Renal homeostasis and tubuloglomerular feedback, *Curr Opin Nephrol Hypertens* 19(1):59-64, 2010.
6. Desir GV et al: Human renalase: a review of its biology, function, and implications for hypertension, *J Am Soc Hypertens* 6(6):417-426, 2012.
7. Castrop H et al: Physiology of kidney renin, *Physiol Rev* 90(2):607-673, 2010.

8. Benabe JE, Martinez-Maldonado M: The impact of malnutrition on kidney function, *Miner Electrolyte Metab* 24(1):20-26, 1998.
9. Iorember FM, Vehaskari VM: Uromodulin: old friend with new roles in health and disease, *Pediatr Nephrol* 29(7):1151-1158, 2014.
10. Januzzi JL Jr: Natriuretic peptides as biomarkers in heart failure, *J Investig Med* 61(6):950-955, 2013.
11. Bartnicki P et al: The influence of the pleiotropic action of erythropoietin and its derivatives on nephroprotection, *Med Sci Monit* 19:599-605, 2013.
12. Bunn HF: Erythropoietin, *Cold Spring Harb Perspect Med* 3(3):aD11619, 2013.
13. Shlipak MG et al: Update on cystatin C: incorporation into clinical practice, *Am J Kidney Dis* 62(3):595-603, 2013.
14. KDIGO 2012 clinical practice guideline for the evaluation and management of chronic kidney

disease, *Kidney Int Supp* 3(1):1-150, 2013. Available at: www.kdigo.org/clinical_practice_guidelines/pdf/CKD/KDIGO_2012_CKD_GL.pdf. Accessed May 11, 2015.
15. Levey AS et al: GFR estimation: from physiology to public health, *Am J Kidney Dis* 63(5):820-834, 2014.
16. Botev R et al: Estimating glomerular filtration rate: Cockcroft-Gault and modification of diet in renal disease formulas compared to renal insulin clearance, *Clin J Am Soc Nephrol* 4(5):899-906, 2009.
17. Levey AS et al: A new equation to estimate glomerular filtration rate, *Ann Intern Med* 150(9):604-612, 2009.

Alterations of Renal and Urinary Tract Function

Sue E. Huether

CHAPTER OUTLINE

Renal and urinary function can be affected by a variety of disorders. The most common type of urinary dysfunction is infection of the bladder. Stones, tumors, or inflammation also can obstruct the urinary tract. Renal function can be impaired by disorders of the kidney itself or by systemic diseases and may ultimately result in acute kidney injury or chronic kidney disease. Because the kidney filters the blood, it is directly linked to every other organ system. Renal failure, whether acute or chronic, is therefore a life-threatening condition.

URINARY TRACT OBSTRUCTION

Urinary tract obstruction is an interference with the flow of urine at any site along the urinary tract (Figure 30-1). An obstruction may be anatomic or functional. The obstruction impedes flow proximal to the blockage, dilates structures distal to the obstruction, increases the risk for infection, and compromises renal function. Anatomic changes in the urinary system caused by obstruction are referred to as **obstructive uropathy**. The severity of an obstructive uropathy is determined by (1) the location of the obstructive lesion, (2) the involvement of ureters and kidneys, (3) the severity (completeness) of the blockage, (4) the duration of the blockage, and (5) the nature of the obstructive lesion.[1,2] Obstructions may be relieved or partially alleviated by correction of the obstruction, although permanent impairments occur if a complete or partial obstruction persists over a period of weeks to months or longer.

Upper Urinary Tract Obstruction

Common causes of upper urinary tract obstruction include stricture or congenital compression of a calyx at the ureteropelvic-ureterovesical junction (e.g., stones [calculi], or vesicoureteral reflux) (see Chapter 31); compression from an aberrant vessel, tumor, or abdominal inflammation and scarring (retroperitoneal fibrosis); or ureteral blockage from stones or a malignancy of the renal pelvis or ureter.

Obstruction of the upper urinary tract causes dilation of the ureter, renal pelvis, calyces, and renal parenchyma proximal to the site of urinary blockage resulting from a "backing up" of urine. The increased pressure is transmitted to the glomerulus, which decreases filtration. Dilation of the ureter is referred to as **hydroureter** (accumulation of urine in the ureter), and dilation of the renal pelvis and calyces proximal to a blockage is referred to as **hydronephrosis** or **ureterohydronephrosis** (dilation of both the ureter and the pelvicaliceal system) (Figure 30-2). Dilation of the upper urinary tract is an early response to obstruction and includes smooth muscle hypertrophy and accumulation of urine above the level of blockage (urinary stasis). Unless the obstruction is relieved, the dilation leads to enlargement and **tubulointerstitial fibrosis** with deposition of excessive amounts of collagen and other proteins. These changes occur in the distal nephrons and affect renal function within approximately 7 days. By 14 days, obstruction has adversely affected both distal and proximal tubular aspects of the nephron units. Within 28 days, the glomeruli of the kidney have been

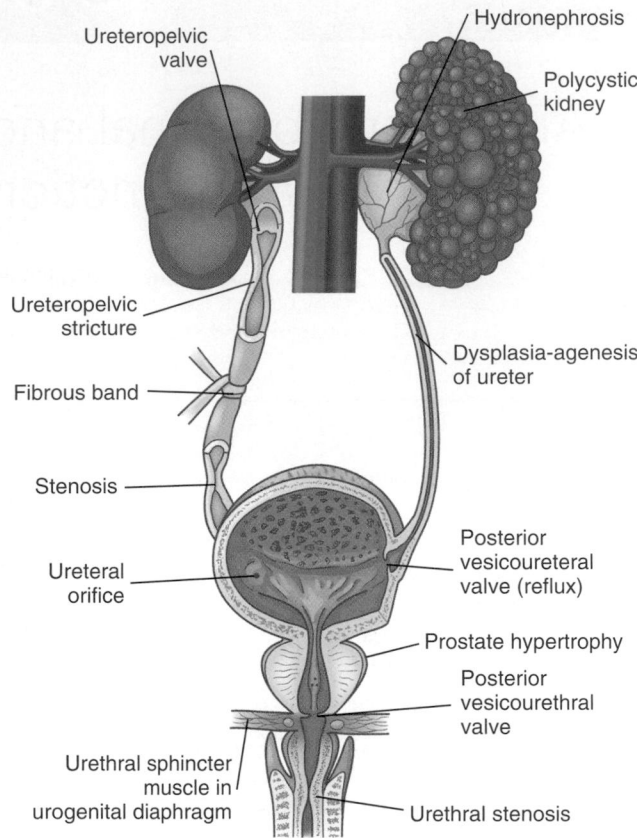

Hydronephrosis

Ureteropelvic valve

Polycystic kidney

Ureteropelvic stricture

Dysplasia-agenesis of ureter

Fibrous band

Stenosis

Ureteral orifice

Posterior vesicoureteral valve (reflux)

Prostate hypertrophy

Posterior vesicourethral valve

Urethral sphincter muscle in urogenital diaphragm

Urethral stenosis

FIGURE 30-1 Major Sites of Urinary Tract Obstruction.

FIGURE 30-2 Hydronephrosis of the kidney. There is marked dilation of the renal pelvis and calyces with thinning of the overlying cortex and medulla due to compression atrophy. (From Kumar V et al: *Robbins and Cotran pathologic basis of disease*, ed 9, Philadelphia, 2015, Saunders.)

damaged and the renal cortex and medulla are reduced in size (thinned). Tubular damage initially decreases the kidney's ability to concentrate urine, causing an increase in urine volume despite a decrease in glomerular filtration rate (GFR). The affected kidney is unable to conserve sodium, bicarbonate, and water or to excrete hydrogen or potassium, leading to metabolic acidosis and dehydration. The magnitude of this damage, and the kidney's ability to recover normal

regulatory function, is affected by the severity and duration of the obstruction. With complete obstruction and compression of the renal vasculature, damage to the renal tubules occurs in a matter of hours, and irreversible damage occurs within 4 weeks. Nevertheless, even in the face of a complete obstruction, the human kidney may recover at least partial function provided the blockage is removed within 56 to 69 days.[3] This recovery requires a period of approximately 4 months. Partial obstruction, in the absence of renal infection, leads to subtler but ultimately permanent impairments including loss of the kidney's ability to concentrate urine, reabsorb bicarbonate, excrete ammonia, or regulate metabolic acid-base balance.

The body is able to partially counteract the negative consequences of unilateral obstruction by a process called **compensatory hypertrophy** and **hyperfunction**.[4] Compensatory response is the result of two growth processes: obligatory growth occurs under the influence of somatomedins, and compensatory growth occurs under the influence of still unidentified hormone(s). These processes cause the unobstructed kidney to increase the size of individual glomeruli and tubules but not the total number of functioning nephrons. The ability of the body to engage in compensatory hypertrophy and hyperfunction diminishes with age, and the process is reversible when relief of obstruction results in recovery of function by the obstructed kidney.

Relief of bilateral, partial urinary tract obstruction or complete obstruction of one kidney is usually followed by a brief period of diuresis (commonly called **postobstructive diuresis**).[5] Postobstructive diuresis is a physiologic response and is typically mild, representing a restoration of fluid and electrolyte imbalance caused by the obstructive uropathy. Occasionally, relief of obstruction will cause rapid excretion of large volumes of water, sodium, or other electrolytes, resulting in a urine output of 10 L/day or more. Rapid postobstructive diuresis causes dehydration and fluid and electrolyte imbalances that must be promptly corrected. Risk factors for severe postobstructive diuresis include chronic, bilateral obstruction; impairment of one or both kidneys' ability to concentrate urine or reabsorb sodium *(acquired nephrogenic diabetes insipidus);* hypertension; edema and weight gain; congestive heart failure; and uremic encephalopathy.

Kidney Stones

Calculi, or **urinary stones**, are masses of crystals, protein, or other substances that are a common cause of urinary tract obstruction in adults. Calculi can be located in the kidneys, ureters, and urinary bladder. The prevalence of stones in the United States is approximately 7% in women and 10% in men and has increased in the past 20 years.[6] The recurrence rate is approximately 30% to 50% within 5 years.[7] Most renal stones are unilateral. The risk of urinary calculi formation is influenced by a number of factors, including age, sex, race, geographic location, seasonal factors, fluid intake, diet, and occupation. Most persons develop their first stone before age 50 years. Geographic location influences the risk of stone formation because of indirect factors, including average temperature, humidity, and rainfall, and their influence on fluid intake and dietary patterns. Persons who regularly consume an adequate volume of water and those who are physically active are at reduced risk when compared with persons who are inactive or consume lower volumes of water.

Urinary calculi can be classified according to the primary minerals (salts) that make up the stones. The most common stone types include calcium oxalate or phosphate (70% to 80%), struvite (magnesium-ammonium-phosphate) (15%), and uric acid (7%). Cystine stones are rare (<1%).[8]

PATHOPHYSIOLOGY Calculus formation is complex and related to (1) supersaturation of one or more salts in the urine, (2) precipitation of the salts from a liquid to a solid state, (3) growth through crystallization or agglomeration (sometimes called *aggregation*), and (4) the presence or absence of stone inhibitors (e.g., uromodulin [Tamm-Horsfall protein]).[9] *Supersaturation* is the presence of a higher concentration of a salt within a fluid (in this case, the urine) than the volume is able to dissolve to maintain equilibrium.

Human urine contains many ions capable of *precipitating* from solution and forming a variety of salts. The salts form crystals that are retained and grow into stones. *Crystallization* is the process by which crystals grow from a small *nidus* or nucleus to larger stones in the presence of supersaturated urine. Although supersaturation is essential for free stone formation, the urine need not remain continuously supersaturated for a calculus to grow once its nidus has precipitated from solution. Intermittent periods of supersaturation after the ingestion of a meal or during times of dehydration from limited oral intake or secondary to continued use of diuretics are sufficient for stone growth in many individuals. In addition, the renal tubules and papillae have many surfaces that may attract a crystalline nidus (Randall plaque) and add biologic material (matrix) forming a stone.[10] *Matrix* is an organic material (i.e., mucoprotein) in which the components of a kidney stone are embedded.

The temperature and pH of the urine also influence the risk of precipitation and calculus formation, and pH is most important. An alkaline urinary pH (pH >7.0) significantly increases the risk of calcium phosphate stone formation, whereas acidic urine (pH <5.0) increases the risk of uric acid stone formation. Cystine and xanthine also precipitate more readily in acidic urine.

Stone or *crystal growth inhibiting substances,* such as potassium citrate, Tamm-Horsfall protein, pyrophosphate, and magnesium, are capable of crystal growth inhibition, thereby reducing the risk of calcium phosphate or calcium oxalate precipitation in the urine and preventing subsequent stone formation.

The size of a stone determines the likelihood that it will pass through the urinary tract and be excreted through micturition.[11] Stones smaller than 5 mm have about a 50% chance of spontaneous (painful) passage, whereas stones that are 1 cm have almost no chance of spontaneous passage.

Retention of *crystal particles* occurs primarily at the papillary collecting ducts. Although most crystals are flushed from the tract through antegrade urine flow, urinary stasis (i.e., from benign prostatic hyperplasia, neurogenic bladder), anatomic abnormalities (strictures), or inflamed epithelium within the urinary tract may prevent prompt flushing of crystals from the system, thus increasing the risk of calculus formation.

Calcium stones account for 70% to 80% of all stones requiring treatment. Calcium oxalate accounts for about 80% of these stones and calcium phosphate about 15%. Most individuals have *idiopathic calcium urolithiasis (ICU)*, a condition whose exact etiology has not yet been defined. Stones can form freely in supersaturated urine or detach from interstitial sites within the tubules (Randall plaque formation) near the tip of the renal papillae. Hypercalciuria, hyperoxaluria, hyperuricosuria, hypocitraturia, mild renal tubular acidosis, or crystal growth inhibitor deficiencies and alkaline urine are associated with calcium stones. Hypercalciuria is attributable to intestinal hyperabsorption of dietary calcium and decreased renal calcium reabsorption. Hyperparathyroidism and bone demineralization associated with prolonged immobilization are also known to cause hypercalciuria. Although oxalate in the diet influences the risk of calcium stones, primary hyperoxaluria is a rare, inherited disorder.

Struvite stones primarily contain magnesium-ammonium-phosphate as well as varying levels of matrix. Matrix forms in an alkaline urine and during infection with a urease-producing bacterial pathogen, such as a *Proteus, Klebsiella,* or *Pseudomonas*. Struvite calculi may grow quite large and branch into a staghorn configuration (**staghorn calculus**) that approximates the pelvicaliceal collecting system.

Uric acid stones occur in persons who excrete excessive uric acid in the urine, such as those with gouty arthritis. Uric acid is primarily a product of biosynthesis of endogenous purines and is secondarily affected by consumption of purines (e.g., meat and beer) in the diet. A consistently acidic urine (pH <5.0) greatly increases this risk. Cystine and xanthine are amino acids that precipitate more readily in acidic urine. *Cystinuria* and *xanthinuria* are both genetic disorders of amino acid metabolism, and excess of these amino acids in urine can cause **cystinuric**, or **xanthine**, stone formation in the presence of a low urine pH of 5.5 or less.

CLINICAL MANIFESTATIONS Renal colic, described as moderate to severe pain often originating in the flank and radiating to the groin, usually indicates obstruction of the renal pelvis or proximal ureter.[12] Colic that radiates to the lateral flank or lower abdomen typically indicates obstruction in the midureter, and bothersome lower urinary tract symptoms (urgency, frequent voiding, urge incontinence) indicate obstruction of the lower ureter or ureterovesical junction. The pain can be severe and incapacitating and may be accompanied by nausea and vomiting. Gross or microscopic hematuria may be present.

EVALUATION AND TREATMENT The evaluation and diagnosis of urinary calculi is based on presenting symptoms and history combined with a focused physical assessment. Imaging studies determine the location of the calculi, the severity of obstruction, and associated obstructive uropathy. The history queries dietary habits, the age of the first stone episode, stone analysis, and presence of complicating factors including hyperparathyroidism or recent gastrointestinal or genitourinary surgery. Urinalysis (including pH) is obtained and a 24-hour urine is completed to identify calcium oxalate, calcium citrate, and other significant constituents. In addition, every effort is made to retrieve and analyze calculi that are passed spontaneously or retrieved through aggressive intervention. To diagnose and manage underlying metabolic disorders, additional tests are completed for those with suspected hyperparathyroidism (elevated serum calcium levels) or cystine or uric acid (high purine diet) stones.

The goals of treatment are to manage acute pain, promote stone passage, reduce the size of stones already formed, and prevent new stone formation. The components of treatment include (1) managing pain, (2) reducing the concentration of stone-forming substances by increasing urine flow rate with high fluid intake, (3) adjusting the pH of the urine (e.g., make it more alkaline with potassium citrate administration), (4) decreasing the amount of stone-forming substances in the urine by decreasing dietary intake or endogenous production or by altering urine pH, and (5) removing stones using percutaneous nephrolithotomy, ureteroscopy, or ultrasonic or laser lithotripsy to fragment stones for excretion in the urine. Prevention of recurrent stones includes increasing fluid intake to generate 2.5 L of urine per day, avoiding intake of colas and other soft drinks acidified with phosphoric acid, avoiding dietary oxalate (e.g., chocolate, beets, nuts, rhubarb, spinach, strawberries, tea, wheat bran), eating less animal protein, limiting sodium intake, and, for calcium stone prevention, maintaining a dietary calcium intake of 1000 to 1200 mg/day. Potassium citrate may be used to raise urinary pH.[13,14]

Lower Urinary Tract Obstruction

Obstructive disorders of the lower urinary tract (LUT) are primarily related to storage of urine in the bladder or emptying of urine through the bladder outlet. The causes of obstruction include both neurogenic

TABLE 30-1	Types of Incontinence
Type	**Description**
Urge incontinence (most common in older adults)	Involuntary loss of urine associated with abrupt and strong desire to void (urgency); often associated with involuntary contractions of detrusor; when associated with neurologic disorder, this is called detrusor hyperreflexia; when no neurologic disorder exists, this is called detrusor instability; may be associated with decreased bladder wall compliance
Stress incontinence (most common in women <60 years and men who have had prostate surgery)	Involuntary loss of urine during coughing, sneezing, laughing, or other physical activity associated with increased abdominal pressure
Overflow incontinence	Involuntary loss of urine with overdistention of bladder; associated with neurologic lesions below S1, polyneuropathies, and urethral obstruction (e.g., enlarged prostate)
Mixed incontinence (most common in older women)	Combination of both stress and urge incontinence
Functional incontinence	Involuntary loss of urine attributable to dementia or immobility

Data from Agency for Health Care Policy and Research, National Guideline Clearing House: *Assessment and diagnosis. In: Guidelines on urinary incontinence.* Updated March 4, 2014. Available at: http://www.guideline.gov/content.aspx?id=47640&search=urinary+incontinence; Khandelwal C, Kistler C: Diagnosis of urinary incontinence, *Am Fam Physician* 87(8):543-550, 2013.

TABLE 30-2	Neurogenic Bladder	
Site of Lesion	**Cause (Symptoms)**	**Diseases**
Lesions above C2 involve pontine micturition center (UMN disorder)	Detrusor hyperreflexia (urgency and urine leakage)	Stroke, traumatic brain injury, multiple sclerosis (MS), hydrocephalus, cerebral palsy, Alzheimer disease, brain tumors
Lesions between C2 and S1 (UMN disorder)	Detrusor hyperreflexia with vesicosphincter dyssynergia (functional bladder outlet obstruction)	Spinal cord injury C2-T12, MS, transverse myelitis, Guillain-Barré syndrome, disk problems
Lesions below S1 (cauda equina syndrome) (LMN disorder)	Acontractile detrusor, with or without urethral sphincter incompetence (stress urinary incontinence)	Myelodysplasia, peripheral polyneuropathies, MS, tabes dorsalis, spinal injury T12-S1, cauda equina syndrome, herpes simplex/zoster

LMN, Lower motor neuron; UMN, upper motor neuron.

and anatomic alterations or, in some instances, a combination of both. Incontinence is a common symptom and types of incontinence are reviewed in Table 30-1.

Neurogenic Bladder

Neurogenic bladder is a general term for bladder dysfunction caused by neurologic disorders (Table 30-2). The types of dysfunction are related to the sites in the nervous system controlling sensory and motor bladder function. Lesions developing in upper motor neurons of the brain and spinal cord result in dyssynergia (loss of coordinated neuromuscular contraction) and overactive or hyperreflexive bladder function. Lesions in the sacral area of the spinal cord or peripheral nerves result in underactive, hypotonic, or atonic (flaccid) bladder function, often with loss of bladder sensation.

Neurologic disorders that develop above the pontine micturition center result in detrusor hyperreflexia (overactivity), also known as an uninhibited or reflex bladder. This is an upper motor neuron disorder in which the bladder empties automatically when it becomes full and the external sphincter functions normally. Because the pontine micturition center remains intact, there is coordination between detrusor muscle contraction and relaxation of the urethral sphincter. Stroke, traumatic brain injury, dementia, and brain tumors are examples of disorders that result in detrusor hyperreflexia. Symptoms include urine leakage and incontinence.

Neurologic lesions that occur below the pontine micturition center but above the sacral micturition center (between C2 and S1) are also upper motor neuron lesions and result in detrusor hyperreflexia with vesicosphincter dyssynergia. There is loss of pontine coordination of detrusor muscle contraction and external sphincter relaxation, so both the bladder and the sphincter are contracting at the same time,

causing a functional obstruction of the bladder outlet.[15] Spinal cord injury, multiple sclerosis, Guillain-Barré syndrome, and vertebral disk problems are causes of this disorder. There is diminished bladder relaxation during storage with small urine volumes and high intravesicular (inside the bladder) pressures. The result is an overactive bladder syndrome with symptoms of frequency, urgency, urge incontinence, and increased risk for urinary tract infection.

Lesions involving the sacral micturition center (below S1; may also be termed *cauda equina syndrome*) or peripheral nerve lesions result in detrusor areflexia (acontractile detrusor), a lower motor neuron disorder. The result is an acontractile detrusor or atonic bladder with retention of urine and distention. If the sensory innervation of the bladder is intact, the full bladder will be sensed but the detrusor may not contract. This is an *underactive bladder syndrome* and may have symptoms of stress and overflow incontinence. Myelodysplasia, multiple sclerosis, tabes dorsalis, and peripheral polyneuropathies are associated with this disorder.

Overactive Bladder Syndrome

Overactive bladder syndrome (OAB) is a syndrome of detrusor overactivity characterized by urgency with involuntary detrusor contractions during the bladder filling phase that may be spontaneous or provoked.[16] There is coordination between the contracting bladder and the external sphincter, but the detrusor is too weak to empty the bladder, resulting in urinary retention with overflow or stress incontinence. Overactive bladder is defined by the International Continence Society as a symptom syndrome of urgency, with or without urge incontinence and usually associated with frequency and nocturia.[17] Overactive bladder syndrome affects millions of adults and children. Adults are often reluctant to discuss this syndrome with their healthcare provider.

Anatomic Obstructions to Urine Flow

Anatomic causes of resistance to urine flow include urethral stricture, prostatic enlargement in men, pelvic organ prolapse in women, and tumor compression. Symptoms of obstruction are more common in men and include (1) frequent daytime voiding (urination more than every 2 hours while awake); (2) nocturia (awakening more than once each night to urinate for adults younger than 65 years of age or more than twice for older adults); (3) poor force of stream; (4) intermittency of urinary stream; (5) bothersome urinary urgency, often combined with hesitancy; and (6) feelings of incomplete bladder emptying despite micturition.

A **urethral stricture** is a narrowing of its lumen and occurs when infection, injury, or surgical manipulation produces a scar that reduces the caliber of the urethra. The vast majority of urethral strictures occur in men; they are rare in women. The severity of obstruction is influenced by its location within the urethra, its length, and the minimum caliber of urethral lumen within the stricture. Specifically, proximal urethral strictures cause more severe obstruction than do strictures of the distal urethra, longer strictures tend to be more obstructive, and the magnitude of blockage is *inversely* proportional to the urethral caliber.[18,19]

Prostate enlargement is caused by acute inflammation, benign prostatic hyperplasia, or prostate cancer (see Chapter 33). Each of these disorders can cause encroachment on the urethra with obstruction to urine flow and the symptoms summarized previously.

Severe **pelvic organ prolapse** (see Chapter 33) in a woman causes bladder outlet obstruction when a cystocele (the downward protrusion/herniation of the bladder into the vagina) descends below the level of the urethral outlet. A cystocele reaching or protruding beyond the vaginal introitus creates the greatest risk for obstruction, particularly if the bladder neck has been surgically repaired without simultaneous repair of the cystocele. In men the bladder may rarely herniate into the scrotum, causing a similar type of obstruction.

Partial obstruction of the bladder outlet or urethra initially causes an increase in the force of detrusor contraction. If the blockage persists, afferent nerves within the bladder wall are adversely affected, leading to urinary urgency and, in some cases, overactive detrusor contractions (a myogenic cause of overactive bladder). When obstruction persists, there is an increased deposition of collagen within the smooth muscle bundles of the detrusor muscle (*trabeculation*), possibly in an attempt to increase the force of its contraction strength. Ultimately, the bladder wall loses its ability to stretch and accommodate urine, a condition called **low bladder wall compliance**, and the detrusor loses its ability to contract efficiently. Low bladder wall compliance chronically elevates intravesicular pressure, greatly increasing the likelihood of hydroureter, hydronephrosis, and impaired renal function.

EVALUATION AND TREATMENT Although the history and physical examination are critical to the evaluation of lower urinary tract disorders, it must be remembered that no symptom or cluster of symptoms has been identified that accurately differentiates the various causes of these disorders. For example, symptoms such as urgency, urge incontinence, frequent urination, and nocturia may develop because of overactive bladder or either increased or decreased bladder outlet resistance. Reduced resistance is associated with the symptom of stress incontinence (incontinence with coughing or sneezing) and symptoms of increased resistance are similar to bladder outlet obstruction, including poor force of urinary stream, hesitancy, and feelings of incomplete bladder emptying.

Various diagnostic tests assist with evaluation. The *postvoid urine* is measured by catheterization within 5 to 15 minutes of urination or through a bladder ultrasound machine that measures bladder height and width to provide an approximation of urine within the vesicle. This measurement may be combined with *uroflowmetry,* a graphic representation of the force of the urinary stream expressed as milliliters voided per second. A *cystometric test* uses a catheter and manometer to evaluate bladder urine volume and pressure in relation to involuntary bladder contraction (the leak point pressure) and the urge to void. Each of these measurements assesses the lower urinary tract's efficiency in evacuating urine through micturition but neither differentiates poor detrusor contraction strength from obstruction as a cause of urinary retention. Instead, *multichannel urodynamic testing* is used to identify obstruction, quantify its severity, and measure detrusor contraction strength (Figure 30-3). *Video-urodynamic recordings* can also demonstrate overactive bladder and detrusor sphincter dyssynergia. An evaluation of renal function, including functional imaging studies and measurement of serum creatinine level, is completed particularly when obstruction is severe and associated with elevated residuals or urinary tract infection.

Because the bladder neck consists of circular smooth muscle with adrenergic innervation, OAB and detrusor sphincter dyssynergia may be managed by α-adrenergic blocking (antimuscarinic) medications. In intractable cases, botulinum toxin A injections or surgery is recommended.[20] Detrusor sphincter dyssynergia may be managed by intermittent catheterization in combination with higher dose antimuscarinic drugs to prevent overactive detrusor contractions and associated dyssynergia while ensuring regular, complete bladder evacuation by catheterization. Alternatively, men with dyssynergia may be managed by condom catheter containment, supplemented by an α-adrenergic-blocking drug or transurethral sphincterotomy (surgical incision of the striated sphincter) to relieve obstruction. Low bladder wall compliance may be managed by antimuscarinic drugs and intermittent catheterization; however, more severe cases may require augmentation enterocystoplasty (enlargement of the low compliant bladder wall using a detubularized piece of small bowel), urinary diversion, or long-term indwelling catheterization. Untreated OAB impairs health and quality of life, causes depression, leads to social isolation, and causes significant economic burden. In the elderly, OAB may cause risk for falls and urinary tract infection.[21]

Prostate enlargement is managed by treating the underlying cause of the prostate enlargement with medication or surgery. Urinary retention may require transient placement of a suprapubic catheter. Urethral stricture is treated with urethral dilation accomplished by using a steel instrument shaped like a catheter (urethral sound) or a series of incrementally increasing catheter-like tubes (filiforms and followers). Long, dense strictures typically require surgical repair to prevent recurrence.

Tumors

Renal Tumors

Renal tumors are estimated at 61,560 (3.7%) of new cancer cases and 14,080 deaths for 2015.[22] There are a number of different types of kidney tumors. **Renal adenomas** (benign tumors) are uncommon but are increasing in number. The tumors are encapsulated and are usually located near the cortex of the kidney. Because the tumors can become malignant, they are usually surgically removed. **Renal cell adenocarcinoma (RCC)** is the most common renal neoplasm (85% of all renal neoplasms) and represents about 2% of cancer deaths. **Renal transitional cell carcinoma (RTCC)** is rare and primarily arises in the renal parenchyma and renal pelvis. Renal cell carcinoma usually occurs in men (two times more often than in women) between 50 and 60 years of age. Risk factors include cigarette smoking, obesity, and uncontrolled hypertension. With surgical resection 5-year survival is about 90% for stage I (encapsulated) cancer.[22]

FIGURE 30-3 Neurogenic Detrusor Overactivity with Detrusor Sphincter Dyssynergia. The arrow indicates narrowing of the striated sphincter consistent with electromyographic activity *(line 6)* noted on the urodynamic tracing. Note the characteristic poor flow pattern *(line 1)* with elevated voiding pressures *(lines 4 and 5)* indicating obstruction. *Line 1,* Urine flow rate; *line 2,* urine volume; *line 3,* abdominal pressure *(Pabd); line 4,* intravesicular (inside bladder) pressure *(Pves); line 5,* detrusor muscle pressure *(Pdet); line 6,* bladder electromyelogram *(EMG).*

PATHOGENESIS Renal cell carcinomas are adenocarcinomas that usually arise from tubular epithelium commonly in the renal cortex. The etiology is unknown. They are classified according to cell type and extent of metastasis. *Clear cell tumors,* the most common, present a better prognosis than granular cell or spindle tumors. Confinement within the renal capsule, together with treatment, is associated with a better survival rate. The tumors usually occur unilaterally (Figure 30-4). About 25% of individuals with RCC present with metastasis.[23]

FIGURE 30-4 Renal Cell Carcinoma. Renal cell carcinomas usually are spheroidal masses composed of yellow tissue mottled with hemorrhage, necrosis, and fibrosis. (From Damjanov I, Linder J, editors: *Anderson's pathology,* ed 10, St Louis, 1996, Mosby.)

CLINICAL MANIFESTATIONS The classic clinical manifestations of renal tumors are hematuria, dull and aching flank pain, palpable flank mass, and weight loss, but all of these symptoms occur in fewer than 10% of cases. Further, they represent an advanced stage of disease, whereas earlier stages are often silent (painless hematuria). The most common sites of distant metastasis are the lung, lymph nodes, liver, bone, thyroid gland, and central nervous system.

EVALUATION AND TREATMENT Diagnosis is based on the clinical symptoms, plain x-ray films of the abdomen, intravenous pyelography, renal angiography, computed tomography (CT) or positron emission tomography using [124]I-girentuximab, and a radiolabeled monoclonal antibody that binds to clear cell cancer cells. The TNM classification is used to stage renal cell carcinoma.[24] Staging systems using molecular tumor markers are rapidly improving.[25] Treatment for localized disease is surgical removal of the affected kidney (radical nephrectomy) or partial nephrectomy for smaller tumors, with combined use of chemotherapeutic agents. Radiofrequency abalation also may be used for early stage tumors when surgery is not an option. Metastatic disease is treated with immunotherapy (i.e., bevacizumab [angiogenesis inhibitor such as sunitinib or sorafenib], T-cell activators, interferon-alpha, and interleukin-2) and target therapies including vascular endothelial growth factor (VEGF) or the mammalian target of rapamycin (mTOR) pathways, or both. Cell-based vaccines are showing promise.[26,27] Survival is related to tumor grade, tumor cell type, and extent of metastasis.

Bladder Tumors

Bladder tumors are the fifth most common malignancy and represent about 1% of all malignant tumors with 70,530 new cases each year and 14,680 deaths.[22] The development of bladder cancer is most common in men older than 60 years. *Transitional cell (urothelial) carcinoma* is the most common bladder malignancy and tumors are usually superficial. More advanced tumors are muscle invasive. Less common forms are squamous cell and adenocarcinoma (cells that produce mucus).

PATHOGENESIS The risk of primary bladder cancer is greater among people who smoke or are exposed to metabolites of aniline dyes, high levels of arsenic in drinking water, heavy consumption of phenacetin, or have uroepithelial Schistosomiasis infection. Bladder cancer results from a genetic alteration in normal bladder epithelium.[28] Metastasis is usually to lymph nodes, liver, bones, or lungs. The TNM classification is used for staging bladder carcinoma.[29] Secondary bladder cancer develops by invasion of cancer from bordering organs, such as cervical carcinoma in women or prostatic carcinoma in men.

CLINICAL MANIFESTATIONS Gross painless hematuria is the archetypal clinical manifestation of bladder cancer. Episodes of hematuria tend to recur, and they are often accompanied by bothersome lower urinary tract symptoms including daytime voiding frequency, nocturia, urgency, and urge urinary incontinence, particularly for carcinoma in situ. Flank pain may occur if tumor growth obstructs one or both ureterovesical junctions.

EVALUATION AND TREATMENT Cystoscopy with tissue biopsy confirms the diagnosis of bladder cancer. Urine cytologic study (pathologic analysis of sloughed cells within the urine) is used for screening-high risk individuals. Use of biologic markers for bladder cancer diagnosis and treatment prognosis are under investigation.[30] Transurethral resection or laser ablation, combined with intravesical chemotherapy or biologic therapy, is effective for superficial tumors. Radical cystectomy with urinary diversion and adjuvant chemotherapy is required for locally invasive tumors.[31]

 QUICK CHECK 30-1
1. List two typical complications of urinary tract obstruction, and briefly describe them.
2. How do kidney stones form?
3. Which population group is at greatest risk for bladder tumors?

URINARY TRACT INFECTION

Causes of Urinary Tract Infection

A **urinary tract infection (UTI)** is an inflammation of the urinary epithelium usually caused by bacteria from gut flora. A UTI can occur anywhere along the urinary tract including the urethra, prostate, bladder, ureter, or kidney. At risk are premature newborns; prepubertal children; sexually active and pregnant women; women treated with antibiotics that disrupt vaginal flora; spermicide users; estrogen-deficient postmenopausal women; individuals with indwelling catheters; and persons with diabetes mellitus, neurogenic bladder, or urinary tract obstruction. Cystitis is more common in women because of the shorter urethra and the closeness of the urethra to the anus (increasing the possibility of bacterial contamination). Up to 50% of women may have a lower UTI at some time in their life.[32] Generally, UTIs are mild and without complications, and they occur in individuals with a normal urinary tract; these infections are termed *uncomplicated UTIs*. A *complicated* UTI develops when there is an abnormality in the urinary system or a health problem that compromises host defenses, such as human immunodeficiency virus (HIV), renal transplant, diabetes, or spinal cord injury. UTI may occur alone or in association with pyelonephritis, prostatitis, or kidney stones.[33] Up to 40% of cases of septic shock are caused by urosepsis.[34] Factors associated with UTI are summarized in Figure 30-5.

Several factors normally combine to protect against UTIs. Most bacteria are washed out of the urethra during micturition. The low pH and high osmolality of urea, the presence of Tamm-Horsfall protein or uromodulin (secreted by renal tubular cells in the distal loop of Henle), and secretions from the uroepithelium provide a bactericidal

Bacterial factors

Capsular antigens resist phagocytosis

Hemolysin damages epithelium

Urease positive bacteria promote infection i.e. *Proteus* and *Kebsiella*

Adhesins: *E. coli* type I and P fimbria bind to uroepithelium

Host factors

Kidney stones

Diabetes mellitus

Immunosuppression

Ureteral reflux

Pregnancy Neurogenic bladder

P blood group antigens

Prostatic hypertrophy

Short urethra in women Indwelling catheters

E. coli contamination from colon

FIGURE 30-5 Mechanisms of Urinary Tract Infection.

effect. The ureterovesical junction closes during bladder contraction, preventing reflux of urine to the ureters and kidneys. Both the longer urethra and the presence of prostatic secretions decrease the risk of infection in men. A UTI occurs when a pathogen circumvents or overwhelms the host's defense mechanisms and rapidly reproduces.

Types of Urinary Tract Infection
Acute Cystitis

Acute cystitis is an inflammation of the bladder and is the most common site of UTI. The morphologic appearance of the bladder through cystoscopy describes different types of cystitis. With mild inflammation, the mucosa is hyperemic (red). More advanced cases may show diffuse hemorrhage (termed *hemorrhagic cystitis*), pus formation, or suppurative exudates (termed *suppurative cystitis*) on the epithelial surface of the bladder. Prolonged infection may lead to sloughing of the bladder mucosa with ulcer formation (termed *ulcerative cystitis*). The most severe infections may cause necrosis of the bladder wall (termed *gangrenous cystitis*).

PATHOPHYSIOLOGY The most common infecting microorganisms are uropathic strains of *Escherichia coli* and the second most common is *Staphylococcus saprophyticus*. Less common microorganisms include *Klebsiella, Proteus, Pseudomonas,* fungi, viruses, parasites, or tubercular bacilli. Schistosomiasis is the most common cause of parasitic invasion of the urinary tract on a global basis; it infects more than 200 million people and has a strong association with bladder cancer.[35]

Bacterial contamination of the normally sterile urine usually occurs by retrograde movement of gram-negative bacilli into the urethra and bladder and then to the ureter and kidney. Uropathic strains of *E. coli* have *type-1 fimbriae* that bind to latex catheters and receptors on the uroepithelium. They resist flushing during normal micturition. These strains also have *P fimbriae* (pyelonephritis-associated fimbriae) that bind to the uroepithelium of individuals with P blood group antigen and readily ascend the urinary tract (see Figure 30-5). Some women may be genetically susceptible to certain strains of *E. coli* attachment.[36] Hematogenous infections are uncommon and often preceded by septicemia. Infection initiates an inflammatory response and the symptoms of cystitis. The inflammatory edema in the bladder wall stimulates discharge of stretch receptors initiating symptoms of bladder fullness with small volumes of urine and producing the urgency and frequency of urination associated with cystitis.

CLINICAL MANIFESTATIONS Many individuals with bacteriuria are asymptomatic, and the elderly have the highest risk. Clinical manifestations of cystitis are related to the inflammatory response and usually include frequency, urgency, dysuria (painful urination), and suprapubic and low back pain. Hematuria, cloudy urine, and flank pain are more serious symptoms. Approximately 10% of individuals with bacteriuria have no symptoms, and 30% of individuals with symptoms are abacteriuric. Elderly persons with cystitis may be asymptomatic or demonstrate confusion or vague abdominal discomfort. The elderly with recurrent UTIs and other concurrent illness have a higher risk of mortality.[37]

EVALUATION AND TREATMENT Infections in symptomatic individuals are diagnosed by urine culture of specific microorganisms with counts of 10,000/ml or more from freshly voided urine. Urine dipstick testing that is positive for leukocyte esterase or nitrite reductase can be used for the diagnosis of uncomplicated UTI. Risk factors, such as urinary tract obstruction, should be identified and treated. Evidence of bacteria from urine culture and antibiotic sensitivity warrants treatment with a microorganism-specific antibiotic. Acute uncomplicated cystitis in nonpregnant women can be diagnosed without an office visit or urine culture. If a urine culture and sensitivity are ordered, the urine specimen must be obtained before the initiation of any antibiotic therapy; 3 to 7 days of treatment is most common.[38] Complicated UTI requires 7 to 14 days of treatment. From 20% to 25% of women have relapsing infection within 7 to 10 days requiring prolonged antibiotic treatment. Follow-up urine cultures should be obtained 1 week after initiation of treatment and at monthly intervals for 3 months. Clinical symptoms are frequently relieved, but bacteriuria may still be present. Repeat cultures should be obtained every 3 to 4 months until 1 year after treatment for evaluation and treatment of recurrent infection[39] (see *Health Alert:* Urinary Tract Infection and Antibiotic Resistance).

Painful Bladder Syndrome/Interstitial Cystitis

Painful bladder syndrome/interstitial cystitis (PBS/IC) is a condition that includes nonbacterial infectious cystitis (viral, mycobacterial, chlamydial, fungal), noninfectious cystitis (radiation, chemical, autoimmune, hypersensitivity), and interstitial cystitis. It occurs most commonly in women ages 20 to 30 years who have symptoms of cystitis, such as frequency, urgency, dysuria, and nocturia, but with negative urine cultures and no other known etiology. Nonbacterial infectious cystitis is most common among those who are immunocompromised. Noninfectious cystitis is associated with radiation or chemotherapy treatment for pelvic and urogenital cancers.

The cause of PBS/IC is unknown. An autoimmune reaction may be responsible for the inflammatory response, which includes mast cell activation, altered uroepithelial permeability, and increased sensory nerve sensitivity. Inflammation and fibrosis of the bladder wall are accompanied by the presence of hemorrhagic ulcers (Hunner ulcers), and bladder volume may decrease as a result of fibrosis. Alteration of

the bladder uroepithelial proteoglycan layer makes it more susceptible to penetration by bacteria. Characteristic symptoms of PBS/IC include bladder fullness, urinary frequency (including nocturia), small urine volume, and chronic pelvic pain with symptoms lasting longer than 9 months. Diagnosis of PBS/IC requires the exclusion of other diagnoses, and extensive evaluations are completed. No single treatment is effective. Oral and intravesical therapies, sacral nerve stimulation, and onabotulinumtoxinA (Botox) are used for symptom relief. Surgery is used in refractory cases.[40,41]

Acute Pyelonephritis

Pyelonephritis is an infection of one or both upper urinary tracts (ureter, renal pelvis, and interstitium). Common causes are summarized in Table 30-3. Urinary obstruction and reflux of urine from the bladder (vesicoureteral reflux) are the most common underlying risk factors. One or both kidneys may be involved. Most cases occur in women.

PATHOPHYSIOLOGY Microorganisms usually associated with acute pyelonephritis include *E. coli*, *Proteus*, or *Pseudomonas*. The latter two microorganisms are more commonly associated with infections after urethral instrumentation or urinary tract surgery. These

TABLE 30-3 Common Causes of Pyelonephritis

Predisposing Factor	Pathologic Mechanisms
Kidney stones	Obstruction and stasis of urine contributing to bacteriuria and hydronephrosis; irritation of epithelial lining with entrapment of bacteria
Vesicoureteral reflux	Chronic reflux of urine up the ureter and into kidney during micturition, contributing to bacterial infection
Pregnancy	Dilation and relaxation of ureter with hydroureter and hydronephrosis; partly caused by obstruction from enlarged uterus and partly from ureteral relaxation caused by higher progesterone levels
Neurogenic bladder	Neurologic impairment interfering with normal bladder contraction with residual urine and ascending infection
Instrumentation	Introduction of organisms into urethra and bladder by catheters and endoscopes introduced into urinary tract for diagnostic purposes
Female sexual trauma	Movement of organisms from urethra into bladder with infection and retrograde spread to kidney

microorganisms also split urea into ammonia, making alkaline urine that increases the risk of stone formation. The infection is probably spread by ascending uropathic microorganisms along the ureters, but dissemination also may occur by way of the bloodstream. The inflammatory process is usually focal and irregular, primarily affecting the pelvis, calyces, and medulla. The infection causes medullary infiltration of white blood cells with renal inflammation, renal edema, and purulent urine. In severe infections, localized abscesses may form in the medulla and extend to the cortex. Primarily affected are the tubules; the glomeruli usually are spared. Necrosis of renal papillae can develop. After the acute phase, healing occurs with fibrosis and atrophy of affected tubules. The number of bacteria decreases until the urine again becomes sterile. Acute pyelonephritis rarely causes renal failure.[42]

CLINICAL MANIFESTATIONS The onset of symptoms is usually acute, with fever, chills, and flank or groin pain. Symptoms characteristic of a UTI, including frequency, dysuria, and costovertebral tenderness, may precede systemic signs and symptoms. Older adults may have nonspecific symptoms, such as low-grade fever and malaise.

EVALUATION AND TREATMENT Differentiating symptoms of cystitis from those of pyelonephritis by clinical assessment alone is difficult. The specific diagnosis is established by urine culture, urinalysis, and clinical signs and symptoms. White blood cell casts indicate pyelonephritis, but they are not always present in the urine. Complicated pyelonephritis requires blood cultures and urinary tract imaging.[43] Uncomplicated acute pyelonephritis responds well to 2 to 3 weeks of microorganism-specific antibiotic therapy. Follow-up urine cultures are obtained at 1 and 4 weeks after treatment if symptoms recur. Antibiotic-resistant microorganisms or reinfection may occur in cases of urinary tract obstruction or reflux. Intravenous pyelography and voiding cystourethrography identify surgically correctable lesions.

Chronic Pyelonephritis

Chronic pyelonephritis is a persistent or recurrent infection of the kidney leading to scarring of one or both kidneys. The specific cause of chronic pyelonephritis is difficult to determine. Recurrent infections from acute pyelonephritis may be associated with chronic pyelonephritis. Generally, chronic pyelonephritis is more likely to occur in individuals who have renal infections associated with some type of obstructive pathologic condition, such as renal stones and vesicoureteral reflux.

PATHOPHYSIOLOGY Chronic urinary tract obstruction prevents elimination of bacteria and starts a process of progressive inflammation, alterations of the renal pelvis and calyces, destruction of the tubules, atrophy or dilation and diffuse scarring, and, finally, impaired urine-concentrating ability, leading to chronic kidney failure. The lesions of chronic pyelonephritis are sometimes termed *chronic interstitial nephritis* because the inflammation and fibrosis are located in the interstitial spaces between the tubules.

CLINICAL MANIFESTATIONS The early symptoms of chronic pyelonephritis are often minimal and may include hypertension, frequency, dysuria, and flank pain. Progression can lead to kidney failure, particularly in the presence of obstructive uropathy or diabetes mellitus.

EVALUATION AND TREATMENT Urinalysis, intravenous pyelography, and ultrasound are used diagnostically. Treatment is related to the underlying cause. Obstruction must be relieved. Antibiotics may be given, with prolonged antibiotic therapy for recurrent infection.

> ✔ **QUICK CHECK 30-2**
> 1. Why is cystitis more common in women?
> 2. What is interstitial cystitis?
> 3. How does pyelonephritis differ from cystitis?

GLOMERULAR DISORDERS

Glomerulonephritis

Acute glomerulonephritis is an inflammation of the glomerulus caused by *primary glomerular injury*, including immunologic responses, ischemia, free radicals, drugs, toxins, vascular disorders, and infection. *Secondary glomerular injury* is a consequence of systemic diseases, including diabetes mellitus, hypertension, bacterial toxins, systemic lupus erythematosus, congestive heart failure, and human immunodeficiency virus (HIV) related kidney disease.

PATHOPHYSIOLOGY Immune mechanisms are a major cause of injury for primary and secondary causes of glomerulonephritis (Figure 30-6). The injury damages the glomerular capillary filtration membrane, including the endothelium, basement membrane, and epithelium (podocytes). The most common types of immune injury are (1) deposition of circulating antigen-antibody immune complexes into the glomerulus (type III hypersensitivity) and (2) reaction of antibodies in situ against planted antigens within the glomerulus (type II hypersensitivity, cytotoxic) (see Chapter 8). Nonimmune glomerular injury is related to ischemia, metabolic disorders (e.g., diabetes mellitus), toxin exposure, drugs, vascular disorders (e.g., vasculitis), and infection with direct injury to glomerular cells. Different causes of injury may result in more than one type of glomerular lesion; thus lesions are not necessarily disease specific (Table 30-4).

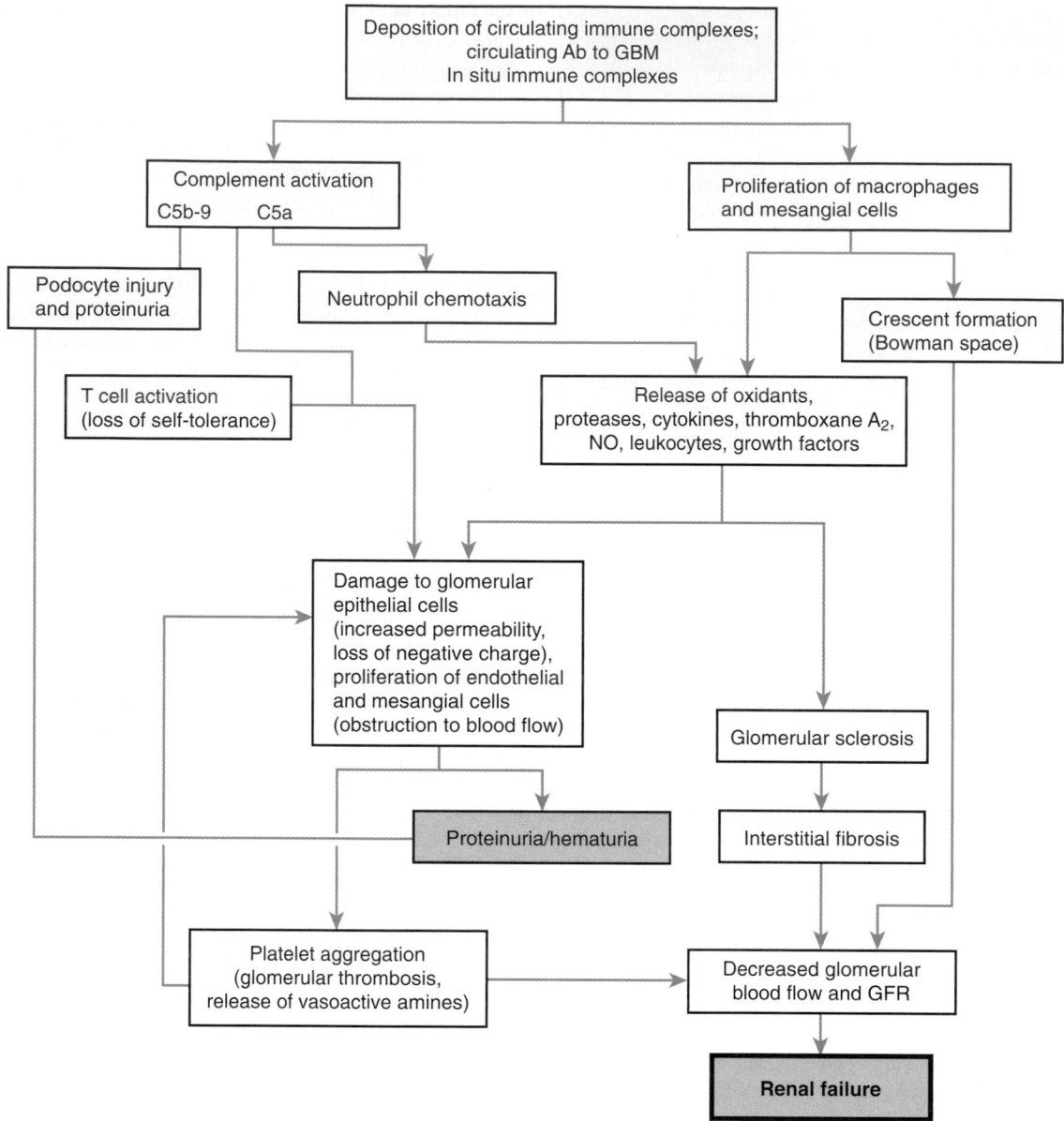

FIGURE 30-6 Mechanisms of Glomerular Injury. *Ab,* Antibody; *GBM,* glomerular basement membrane; *GFR,* glomerular filtration rate; *NO,* nitric oxide.

TABLE 30-4	Types of Glomerular Lesions
Lesion	**Characteristics**
Glomerular Lesions	
Diffuse	Relatively uniform involvement of most or all glomeruli; most common form of glomerulonephritis
Focal	Changes in only some glomeruli, whereas others are normal
Segmental-local	Changes in one part of glomerulus with other parts unaffected
Lesion Characteristics	
Mesangial	Deposits of immunoglobulins in mesangial matrix, mesangial cell proliferation
Membranous	Thickening of glomerular capillary wall with immune deposits
Proliferative	Increase in number of glomerular cells
Sclerotic	Glomerular scarring from previous glomerular injury
Crescentic	Accumulation of proliferating cells within Bowman space, making crescent appearance
Interstitial fibrosis	Scarring between glomerulus and tubules

TABLE 30-5 Immunologic Pathogenesis of Glomerulonephritis

Glomerular Injury	Mechanism
Soluble immune-complex glomerulonephritis (90%)	Formation of antibodies stimulated by presence of endogenous or exogenous antigens; results in circulating soluble antigen-antibody complexes deposited in glomerular capillaries or formation of complexes within the glomerular membrane; glomerular injury occurs with complement activation and release of immunologic substances that lyse cells and increase membrane permeability; severity of glomerular injury related to number of complexes formed; type III hypersensitivity reaction
Anti–glomerular basement membrane glomerulonephritis (5%)	Antibodies are formed and act directly against glomerular basement membrane; immune response causes accumulation of inflammatory cells in Bowman space (in shape of a crescent moon) surrounding and compressing glomerular capillaries; generally associated with rapidly progressive renal failure, such as Goodpasture syndrome; type II hypersensitivity reaction
Alternative complement pathway	Relatively rare, mechanism associated with low levels of complement and membranoproliferative glomerulonephritis; type III hypersensitivity reaction
Cell-mediated immunity	Delayed hypersensitivity response that damages glomerulus; actual cellular mechanism not clearly understood; type IV hypersensitivity reaction

Immune injury is caused by activation of biochemical mediators of inflammation (i.e., complement and cytokines from leukocytes) and begins after the antigen-antibody complexes have deposited or formed in the glomerular capillary wall or mesangium. Complement is deposited with the antibodies, and activation can cause cell lysis or serve as a chemotactic stimulus for attraction of neutrophils, monocytes, and T lymphocytes. These phagocytes, along with activated platelets, further the inflammatory reaction by releasing mediators that injure the glomerular filtration membrane, including epithelial cells, glomerular basement membrane, and endothelial cells (podocytes and filtration slits).[44] The injury increases glomerular membrane permeability and reduces glomerular membrane surface area. The GFR decreases, resulting in increased serum creatinine levels. There also may be swelling and proliferation of mesangial cells and expansion of the extracellular matrix in the Bowman space, contributing to crescent formation (deposition of substances in the Bowman space, forming the shape of a crescent moon). The result is decreased glomerular blood flow, decreased driving hydrostatic pressure, decreased GFR, and hypoxic injury.[45]

Loss of negative electrical charge across the glomerular filtration membrane and increase in filtration pore size enhance movement of proteins into the urine. Proteins are normally repelled because they also have a negative charge. Red blood cells also escape if pore size is large enough. Proteinuria or hematuria, or both, develops. The severity of glomerular damage and decline in glomerular function is related to the size, number, and location (focal or diffuse) of cells injured, duration of exposure, and type of antigen-antibody complexes.

CLINICAL MANIFESTATIONS The onset of glomerulonephritis may be sudden or insidious and significant loss of nephron function can occur before symptoms develop. Acute glomerulonephritis may be silent, mild, moderate, or severe in symptom presentation. Severe or progressive glomerular disease causes oliguria (urine output of 30 ml/hour or less), hypertension, and renal failure. Focal lesions tend to produce less severe clinical symptoms. Salt and water are reabsorbed, contributing to fluid volume expansion, edema, and hypertension.

Two major symptoms distinctive of more severe glomerulonephritis (i.e., associated with rapidly progressive glomerulonephritis) are (1) hematuria with red blood cell casts and (2) proteinuria exceeding 3 to 5 g/day with albumin (macroalbuminuria) as the major protein. Different types of acute glomerulonephritis may be associated with different patterns of urinary sediment and nephrotic or nephritic syndrome (see p. 759).

EVALUATION AND TREATMENT The diagnosis of glomerular disease is confirmed by the progressive development of clinical manifestations and laboratory findings of abnormal urinalysis with proteinuria, red blood cells, white blood cells, and casts. Microscopic evaluation from renal biopsy provides a specific determination of renal injury and type of pathologic condition. Patterns of antigen-antibody complex deposition within the glomerular capillary filtration membrane have been established using light, electron, and immunofluorescent microscopy for different disease processes. The findings with light microscopy provide information about the distribution and extent of immune response injury (Table 30-5). Electron microscopy differentiates morphologic changes within the glomerular capillary wall. Staining with fluorescein identifies different antibodies (i.e., immunoglobulin G [IgG] or immunoglobulin A [IgA]) and their configurations when viewed under ultraviolet (black) light with a microscope.

Reduced GFR during glomerulonephritis is evidenced by elevated plasma urea, cystatin C, and creatinine concentrations, or by reduced creatinine clearance (see Chapter 29). Edema, caused by excessive sodium and water retention, may require the use of diuretics or dialysis.

Management principles for treating glomerulonephritis are related to treating the primary disease, preventing or minimizing immune responses, and correcting accompanying problems, such as edema, hypertension, hypoalbuminemia, and hyperlipidemia. Specific treatment regimens are necessary for particular types of glomerulonephritis. Antibiotic therapy is essential for the management of underlying infections that may be contributing to ongoing antigen-antibody responses. Corticosteroids decrease antibody synthesis and suppress inflammatory responses. Cytotoxic agents (e.g., cyclophosphamide) may be used to suppress the immune response in corticosteroid-resistant cases. Anticoagulants may be useful for controlling fibrin crescent formation in rapidly progressive glomerulonephritis.

Types of Glomerulonephritis

The classification of glomerulonephritis can be described according to cause, pathologic lesions, disease progression (acute, rapidly progressive, chronic), or clinical presentation (nephrotic syndrome, nephritic syndrome, acute or chronic renal failure). In nearly all types of glomerulonephritis, the epithelial or podocyte layer of the glomerular capillary membrane is disturbed with loss of negative charges and changes in membrane permeability; the mesangial matrix may be expanded or the basement membrane thickened. Features of the patterns of glomerular injury are summarized in Table 30-6. Many types

TABLE 30-6   Features of the Common Types of Glomerulonephritis

Type and Cause	Pathophysiology
Associated with Nephritic Syndrome	
Acute postinfectious/infection-related glomerulonephritis (group A β-hemolytic streptococcus or staphylococcus)	Diffuse deposits of immune complexes (IgG and complement) in glomerular capillary wall; infiltration of leukocytes; endocapillary proliferation and mesangial proliferation
Occurs with untreated primary infection in throat or skin	Decreased capillary blood flow and GFR
Crescentic or rapidly progressive glomerulonephritis	Accumulation of immune deposits and inflammatory cells and debris that proliferate into Bowman space and form crescent-shaped lesions
In situ formation of anti–glomerular basement membrane antibodies or immune complex deposition	Decreased capillary blood flow and GFR
Nonspecific response to glomerular injury; can occur in any severe glomerular disease	Can result in renal failure within 3 months
Can be associated with Goodpasture syndrome	Formation of Ab against both pulmonary capillary and GBM
Mesangial proliferative glomerulonephritis	Deposits of immune complexes in mesangium with mesangial proliferation
IgA nephropathy	Decreased glomerular blood flow and GFR
	Abnormal glycosylated IgA-1 and complement bind to mesangial cells causing proliferation
Associated with Nephrotic Syndrome	
Minimal change disease (lipoid nephrosis)	Uniform diffuse thinning of epithelial (podocyte) foot processes; loss of negative charge in basement membrane and increased permeability
Glomerular basement membrane appears normal	
Usually idiopathic	Severe proteinuria and nephrotic syndrome
No immune deposits	
Focal segmented glomerulosclerosis	Similar to minimal change disease
Usually idiopathic	
Membranous nephropathy (autoimmune response to unknown renal antigen)	Thickening of glomerular capillary wall caused by antibody and complement deposition and release of inflammatory cytokines with focal segmental sclerosis and increased permeability, proteinuria, and nephrotic syndrome
Usually idiopathic	
Can be associated with systemic diseases (i.e., hepatitis B virus, systemic lupus erythematous, solid malignant tumors)	
Membranoproliferative glomerulonephritis	Mesangial cell proliferation; thickening of basement membrane; subendothelial deposits of immune complex occlude glomerular capillary blood flow
Usually idiopathic; associated with low complement levels	
	Decreased GFR
IgA nephropathy (Berger disease)	Mesangial deposits of IgA and proliferation of inflammatory cells into Bowman space, with sclerosis and fibrosis of glomerulus and crescent formation
Usually idiopathic; elevated IgA plasma levels	
	Decreased GFR and hematuria; usually focal, some diffuse lesions
Chronic glomerulonephritis	Glomerular fibrosis and scarring, interstitial and tubular fibrosis and vascular sclerosis; original glomerular lesions may not be definable; progression to end-stage kidney disease with uremia
Can be a consequence of any type of glomerulonephritis; more common with crescentic or rapidly progressive glomerulonephritis	

Ab, Antibody; *GBM,* glomerular basement membrane; *GFR,* glomerular filtration rate; *IgA,* immunoglobulin A.

of glomerular injury occur most often in children or young adults, including acute postinfectious glomerulonephritis and minimal change nephropathy (lipoid nephrosis). Details of these diseases are presented in Chapter 31.

Complications of diabetic nephropathy and systemic lupus erythematosus can affect the entire nephron and glomerular injury is significant. Different patterns of injury develop over the course of these diseases. Diabetic nephropathy develops from metabolic and vascular complications (see Chapter 19). Changes in the glomerulus are characterized by progressive thickening and fibrosis of the glomerular basement membrane, and nodular expansion of the mesangial matrix with albuminuria, podocyte loss, tubular epithelial cell atrophy, and progression to chronic renal failure (Figure 30-7). Diabetic nephropathy is the most common cause of chronic kidney disease and end-stage renal failure. Glomerular structure and function can return to normal after pancreatic transplantation and years of normoglycemia.[46] Lupus nephritis is caused by the formation of autoantibodies against double-stranded DNA with glomerular deposition of the immune complexes and alteration in B cell and T cell subsets. There is complement activation and a cascade of inflammatory events resulting in damage to the glomerular membrane with mesangial expansion.[47]

Chronic Glomerulonephritis

Chronic glomerulonephritis encompasses several glomerular diseases with a progressive course leading to chronic kidney failure. There may be no history of kidney disease before the diagnosis. Hypercholesterolemia and proteinuria have been associated with progressive glomerular and tubular injury. The proposed mechanism is related to those observed in glomerulosclerosis and interstitial injury, such as hyperfiltration and inflammatory processes.[48] The primary cause may be difficult to establish because advanced pathologic changes may obscure specific disease characteristics (see Figure 30-7). Diabetes mellitus and lupus erythematosus are examples of secondary causes of chronic glomerular injury.[49] Renal insufficiency usually begins to develop after 10 to 20 years, followed by nephrotic syndrome and an accelerated progression to end-stage renal failure. Symptom patterns vary depending on the underlying cause. The specific pathologic condition is identified by renal biopsy and is best performed in early stages

FIGURE 30-7 Diabetic Glomerulopathy. (Used with permission from Reidy K et al: *J Clin Invest* 124[6]:2333-2340, 2014.)

of chronic kidney disease to identify specific treatment options.[50] Use of steroids and immunosuppressive agents can prolong remissions and preserve renal function. Dialysis or kidney transplantation ultimately may be needed.

Nephrotic and Nephritic Syndromes

Nephrotic syndrome is the excretion of 3.5 g or more of protein in the urine per day and is characteristic of glomerular injury. It occurs when filtration of proteins exceeds tubular reabsorption. *Primary causes of nephrotic syndrome* include minimal change nephropathy (lipoid nephrosis) (see Chapter 31), membranous glomerulonephritis, and focal segmental glomerulosclerosis.[51] *Secondary forms of nephrotic syndrome* occur in systemic diseases, including diabetes mellitus (see Chapter 19), amyloidosis, systemic lupus erythematosus, and Henoch-Schönlein purpura (see Chapter 31). Nephrotic syndrome also is associated with certain drugs (e.g., nonsteroidal anti-inflammatory drugs), infections, malignancies, and vascular disorders. When present as a secondary complication with renal diseases, nephrotic syndrome often signifies a more serious prognosis.[51] Nephrotic syndrome is more common in children than adults (see Chapter 31).

Nephritic syndrome is hematuria and red blood cell casts in the urine. Proteinuria is usually less severe than in nephrotic syndrome. It occurs primarily with infection-related glomerulonephritis and rapidly progressive crescentic glomerulonephritis.

PATHOPHYSIOLOGY In nephrotic syndrome, disturbances in the glomerular basement membrane and podocyte injury lead to increased permeability to protein and loss of electrical negative charge. Loss of plasma proteins, particularly albumin and some immunoglobulins, occurs across the injured glomerular filtration membrane. Loss of plasma proteins decreases plasma oncotic pressure, resulting in edema. The predominant cause of nephrotic syndrome is minimal change nephropathy, which is common in children (see Chapter 31). Hypoal-

buminemia results from urinary loss of albumin combined with a diminished synthesis of replacement albumin by the liver. Albumin is lost in the greatest quantity because of its high plasma concentration and low molecular weight. Decreased dietary intake of protein from anorexia or malnutrition or accompanying liver disease may also contribute to lower levels of plasma albumin. Loss of albumin stimulates lipoprotein synthesis by the liver and hyperlipidemia and can promote progression of glomerular disease. Loss of immunoglobulins may increase susceptibility to infections. Sodium retention is common.[52]

In nephritic syndrome, hematuria (usually microscopic) is present and red blood cell casts are present in the urine in addition to proteinuria, which is not severe. It is caused by increased permeability of the glomerular filtration membrane with pore sizes large enough to allow the passage of red blood cells and protein. Nephritic syndrome is associated with postinfectious glomerulonephritis, rapidly progressive (crescentic) glomerulonephritis, IgA nephropathy, lupus nephritis, and diabetic nephropathy. The pathophysiology is related to immune injury of the glomerulus as previously described. Hypertension and uremia occur in advanced stages of disease.

CLINICAL MANIFESTATIONS Many clinical manifestations of nephrotic and nephritic syndrome are related to loss of serum proteins and associated sodium retention (Table 30-7). They include edema, hypoproteinemia, proteinuria, hyperlipidemia, lipiduria, vitamin D deficiency, and hypothyroidism.[53] Vitamin D deficiency is related to loss of serum transport proteins and decreased vitamin D activation by the kidney. Hypothyroidism can result from urinary loss of thyroid-binding protein and thyroxine. Alterations in coagulation factors can cause hypercoagulability and may lead to thromboembolic events.[54]

EVALUATION AND TREATMENT Nephrotic syndrome is diagnosed when the protein level in a 24-hour urine collection is greater than 3.5 g. Serum albumin level decreases (to less than 3 g/dl), and

TABLE 30-7	**Clinical Manifestations of Nephrotic Syndrome**	
Manifestation	**Contributing Factors**	**Result**
Significant proteinuria	Increased glomerular permeability, decreased proximal tubule reabsorption	Edema, increased susceptibility to infection from loss of immunoglobulins
Hypoalbuminemia	Increased urinary losses of protein	Edema
Edema	Hypoalbuminemia (decreased plasma oncotic pressure, sodium and water retention, increased aldosterone and antidiuretic hormone [ADH] secretion), unresponsiveness to atrial natriuretic peptides	Soft, pitting, generalized edema
Hyperlipidemia	Decreased serum albumin level; increased hepatic synthesis of very-low-density lipoproteins; increased levels of cholesterol, phospholipids, triglycerides	Increased atherogenesis
Lipiduria	Sloughing of tubular cells containing fat (oval fat bodies); free fat from hyperlipidemia	Fat droplets that may float in urine

concentrations of serum cholesterol, phospholipids, and triglycerides increase. Fat bodies may be present in the urine.

Nephrotic syndrome is commonly treated by consuming a moderate protein restriction (i.e., 0.8 g/kg body weight/day), low-fat, salt-restricted diet, and by prescribing diuretics. Diuretics are used to control hypertension and eliminate fluid. Care must be taken to observe for hypovolemia and hypokalemia or potassium toxicity in the presence of renal insufficiency. Spironolactone may be combined with loop diuretics to suppress aldosterone activity to conserve potassium. Heparinoids are used for prophylactic anticoagulation. Glucocorticoids are used to control immune-mediated disease or may be combined with immunosuppressive drugs. Angiotensin-converting enzyme (ACE) inhibitors or angiotensin receptor blockers (ARBs) lower urine protein excretion.[55]

The evaluation and treatment of nephritic syndrome are similar to those described for nephrotic syndrome. The course of glomerulonephritis is usually more severe with nephritic syndrome. High-dose corticosteroids and cyclophosphamide represent the standard therapy for rapidly progressive crescentic glomerulonephritis. The addition of plasma exchange (plasmapheresis) also may be helpful.[56]

> **QUICK CHECK 30-3**
> 1. What is glomerulonephritis? List two types.
> 2. What immune mechanisms are operative in glomerulonephritis?
> 3. Why is edema present in individuals with nephrotic syndrome?

ACUTE KIDNEY INJURY

Classification of Kidney Dysfunction

Kidney injury may be acute and rapidly progressive (within hours), and the process may be reversible. Kidney failure also can be chronic, progressing to end-stage kidney failure over a period of months or years. The terms *renal insufficiency, renal failure, uremia,* and *azotemia* are associated with decreasing renal function but are not specific in relation to the cause of kidney disease. They are often used synonymously, although with some distinctions. Generally, renal insufficiency refers to a decline in renal function to about 25% of normal or a GFR of 25 to 30 ml/minute. Levels of serum creatinine and urea are mildly elevated. The term acute kidney injury is preferred to the term *acute renal failure* because it captures the diverse nature of this syndrome, ranging from minimal or subtle changes in renal function to complete renal failure requiring renal replacement therapy. Renal failure refers to significant loss of renal function. When less than 10% of renal function remains, this is termed end-stage kidney disease

(ESKD). Specific criteria for acute renal dysfunction are discussed in the next section. Uremia (uremic syndrome) is a syndrome of renal failure and includes elevated blood urea and creatinine levels accompanied by fatigue, anorexia, nausea, vomiting, pruritus, and neurologic changes. Uremia represents numerous consequences related to renal failure, including retention of toxic wastes, deficiency states, electrolyte disorders, and immune activation promoting a proinflammatory state. Azotemia is characterized by increased blood urea nitrogen levels (normal is 8 to 20 mg/dl) and frequently increased serum creatinine levels (normal is 0.7 to 1.4 mg/dl). Renal insufficiency or renal failure causes azotemia. Both azotemia and uremia indicate an accumulation of nitrogenous waste products in the blood, a common characteristic that explains the overlap in definitions of terms.

Acute Kidney Injury

Acute kidney injury (AKI) is a sudden decline in kidney function with a decrease in glomerular filtration and urine output with accumulation of nitrogenous waste products in the blood as demonstrated by an elevation in plasma creatinine and blood urea nitrogen levels. Classification criteria have been developed to guide the diagnosis of kidney injury and are described by the acronym RIFLE (R = risk, I = injury, F = failure, L = loss, and E = end-stage kidney disease [ESKD]), representing three levels of renal dysfunction of increasing severity (Table 30-8). A similar set of criteria have been published by the Acute Kidney Injury Network and Kidney Disease Improving Global Outcomes.[57]

PATHOPHYSIOLOGY AKI results from ischemic injury related to extracellular volume depletion and decreased renal blood flow, toxic injury from chemicals, or sepsis-induced injury. The injury initiates an inflammatory response, vascular responses, and cell death. Alterations in renal function may be minimal or severe.[58] Acute kidney injury can be classified as prerenal (renal hypoperfusion), intrarenal (disorders involving renal parenchymal or interstitial tissue), or postrenal (urinary tract obstructive disorders) (Table 30-9 and Figure 30-8).

Prerenal acute kidney injury is the most common reason for AKI and is caused by inadequate kidney perfusion. Poor perfusion can result from hypotension, hypovolemia associated with hemorrhage or fluid loss (e.g., burns), sepsis, inadequate cardiac output (e.g., myocardial infarct [heart attack]), or renal vasoconstriction (e.g., caused by nonsteroidal anti-inflammatory drugs [NSAIDs] or radiocontrast agents) or renal artery stenosis. The GFR declines because of the decrease in filtration pressure. Failure to restore blood volume or blood pressure and oxygen delivery can cause ischemic cell injury and acute tubular necrosis or acute interstitial necrosis, a more severe form of AKI. Reperfusion injury with cell death also can occur[59] (see Figure 4-11). AKI can occur during chronic renal failure if a sudden stress is imposed on already marginally functioning kidneys.

Mechanisms of oliguria in acute kidney injury

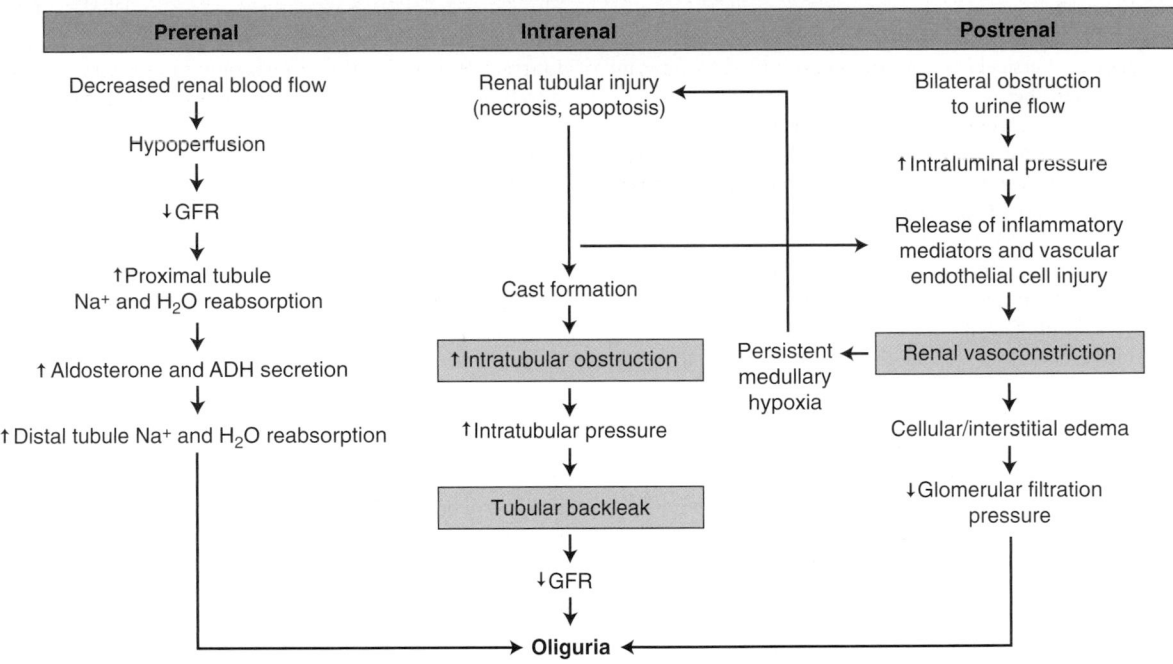

FIGURE 30-8 Acute Kidney Injury and Mechanisms of Oliguria. *ADH*, Antidiuretic hormone; *GFR*, glomerular filtration rate.

TABLE 30-8 RIFLE Criteria for Acute Kidney Dysfunction/Failure

Category	GFR Criteria	Urine Output (UO) Criteria
Risk	Increased creatinine × 1.5 or GFR decrease >25%	UO <0.5 ml/kg/hr × 6 hr
Injury	Increased creatinine × 2 or GFR decrease >50%	UO <0.5 ml/kg/hr × 12 hr
Failure	Increased creatinine × 3 or GFR decrease >75%	UO <0.3 ml/kg/hr × 24 hr or anuria × 12 hr
Loss	Persistent ARF = complete loss of kidney function >4 weeks	
ESKD	End-stage kidney disease (>3 months)	

Adapted from Bellomo R et al: *Curr Opin Crit Care* 8(6):505-508, 2002; Bellomo R et al: *Crit Care* 8(4):R204-R212, 2004.

TABLE 30-9 Classification of Acute Kidney Injury

Area of Dysfunction	Possible Causes
Prerenal	*Hypovolemia*
	Hemorrhagic blood loss (trauma, gastrointestinal bleeding, complications of childbirth)
	Loss of plasma volume (burns, peritonitis)
	Water and electrolyte losses (severe vomiting or diarrhea, intestinal obstruction, uncontrolled diabetes mellitus, inappropriate use of diuretics)
	Hypotension or hypoperfusion
	Septic shock
	Cardiac failure or shock
	Massive pulmonary embolism
	Stenosis or clamping of renal artery
Intrarenal	*Acute tubular necrosis (postischemic or nephrotoxic)*
	Glomerulopathies
	Acute interstitial necrosis (tumors or toxins)
	Vascular damage
	Malignant hypertension, vasculitis
	Coagulation defects
	Renal artery/vein occlusion
	Bilateral acute pyelonephritis
Postrenal	*Obstructive uropathies (usually bilateral)*
	Ureteral destruction (edema, tumors, stones, clots)
	Bladder neck obstruction (enlarged prostate)
	Neurogenic bladder

Intrarenal (intrinsic) acute kidney injury can result from ischemic **acute tubular necrosis (ATN)** related to prerenal AKI, nephrotoxic ATN (e.g., exposure to radiocontrast media), acute glomerulonephritis, vascular disease (malignant hypertension, disseminated intravascular coagulation, and renal vasculitis), allograft rejection, or interstitial disease (drug allergy, infection, tumor growth). ATN caused by ischemia occurs most often after surgery (40% to 50% of cases) but also is associated with sepsis, obstetric complications, and severe hemorrhagic trauma or severe burns. Hypotension associated with hypovolemia produces ischemia and the inflammatory response, generating toxic oxygen free radicals that cause cellular swelling, injury, and necrosis. Intrarenal microcirculatory vasoconstriction occurs in response to injury and inflammation. Ischemic necrosis tends to be patchy and may be distributed along any part of the nephron. Sepsis-related tubular injury can occur in the absence of hypoperfusion and may be related to inflammation and changes in microcirculation and mitochondrial function.[60]

Nephrotoxic ATN can be produced by radiocontrast media and numerous antibiotics, particularly the aminoglycosides (neomycin, gentamicin, tobramycin) because these drugs accumulate in the renal cortex. Other substances, such as excessive myoglobin (oxygen-transporting substance from muscles released with crush injuries), carbon tetrachloride, heavy metals (mercury, arsenic), or methoxyflurane anesthetic, and bacterial toxins may promote renal failure. Dehydration, advanced age, concurrent renal insufficiency, and diabetes mellitus tend to enhance nephrotoxicity. Necrosis caused by nephrotoxins is usually uniform and limited to the proximal tubules.

Postrenal acute kidney injury is rare and usually occurs with urinary tract obstruction that affects the kidneys bilaterally (e.g., bladder outlet obstruction, prostatic hypertrophy, bilateral ureteral obstruction), tumors, or neurogenic bladder. A pattern of several hours of anuria with flank pain followed by polyuria is a characteristic finding. The obstruction causes an increase in intraluminal pressure upstream from the site of obstruction with a gradual decrease in GFR. This type of renal failure can occur after diagnostic catheterization of the ureters, a procedure that may cause edema of the tubular lumen.

Oliguria (<400 ml/24 hours) can occur in AKI, and three mechanisms have been proposed to account for the decrease in urine output.[61] All three mechanisms probably contribute to oliguria in varying combinations and degrees throughout the course of the disease (see Figure 30-8). These mechanisms are as follows:

1. *Alterations in renal blood flow.* Efferent arteriolar vasoconstriction may be produced by intrarenal release of angiotensin II or there may be redistribution of blood flow from the cortex to the medulla. Autoregulation of blood flow may be impaired, resulting in decreased GFR. Changes in glomerular permeability and decreased GFR also may result from ischemia.
2. *Tubular obstruction.* Necrosis of the tubules causes sloughing of cells, cast formation, or ischemic edema that results in tubular obstruction, which in turn causes a retrograde increase in pressure and reduces the GFR. Renal failure can occur within 24 hours.
3. *Tubular backleak.* Glomerular filtration remains normal, but tubular reabsorption of filtrate is accelerated as a result of permeability caused by ischemia and increased tubular pressure from obstruction.

CLINICAL MANIFESTATIONS   The clinical progression of AKI with recovery of renal function occurs in three overlapping phases: initiation phase, maintenance phase, and recovery phase. The *initiation phase* is the phase of reduced perfusion or toxicity in which kidney injury is evolving. Prevention of injury is possible during this phase. The *maintenance* or *oliguric phase* is the period of established kidney injury and dysfunction after the initiating event has been resolved, and

may last from weeks to months. Urine output is lowest during this phase and serum creatinine and blood urea nitrogen (BUN) levels both increase. The *recovery* or *polyuric phase* is the interval when glomerular function returns but the regenerating tubules cannot concentrate the filtrate. Diuresis is common during this phase, with a decline in serum creatinine and urea concentrations and an increase in creatinine clearance.

Oliguria begins within 1 day after a hypotensive event and lasts 1 to 3 weeks, but may regress in several hours or extend for several weeks, depending on the duration of ischemia or the severity of injury or obstruction. Anuria (urine output less than 50 ml/day) is uncommon in ATN, involves both kidneys, and suggests bilateral renal artery occlusion, obstructive uropathy, or acute cortical necrosis. Renal failure can present with nonoliguric renal failure and represents less severe injury, particularly with intrinsic kidney injury associated with nephrotoxins. The urine output may vary in volume, but the BUN and plasma creatinine concentrations increase (plasma creatinine concentration is inversely proportional to the GFR). Other manifestations include hyperkalemia, hyperphosphatemia, and metabolic acidosis from decreased urine excretion. Edema and congestive heart failure can be associated with fluid retention.

As renal function improves, increase in urine volume (diuresis) is progressive. The tubules are still damaged early in the recovery phase but are recovering function. Polyuria can result in excessive loss of sodium, potassium, and water. Fluid and electrolyte balance must be carefully monitored and excessive urinary losses replaced.

Serial measurements of plasma creatinine concentration provide an index of renal function during the *recovery phase*. Return to normal status may take from 3 to 12 months, and some individuals do not have full recovery of a normal GFR or tubular function.

EVALUATION AND TREATMENT   The diagnosis of AKI is related to the cause of the disease. A history of surgery, trauma, or cardiovascular disorders is common, and exposure to nephrotoxins, obstructive uropathies (e.g., an enlarged prostate), or infection must be considered. The diagnostic challenge is to differentiate prerenal AKI from intrarenal AKI, and some evidence is available from urinalysis and measurement of plasma creatinine and BUN levels (Table 30-10). However, more than 50% of glomerular filtration must be lost before there is elevation of serum creatinine level. *Cystatin C*, a serum protein freely filtered at the glomerulus, can serve as a measure of GFR. Biomarkers are being developed to assess the extent of kidney injury before elevation of serum creatinine level.[62] Prevention of AKI is the most important therapeutic approach and involves avoidance of hypotension, hypovolemia, and nephrotoxicity.

The primary goal of therapy is to maintain the individual's life until renal function has recovered. Management principles directly related to physiologic alterations generally include (1) correcting fluid and

TABLE 30-10	**Differentiation of Acute Oliguric Kidney Failure**					
	Urine Volume	Urine Specific Gravity	Urine Osmolality	Urine Sodium Concentration	BUN/Plasma Creatinine Ratio	FE$_{Na}$*
Prerenal failure	<400 ml	1.016-1.020	>500 mOsm	<10 mEq/L	>15:1	<1% (also seen in acute glomerulonephritis)
Intrarenal failure (i.e., acute tubular necrosis)	<400 ml	1.010-1.012	<400 mOsm	>30 mEq/L	<15:1	>1% (also seen in acute urinary tract obstruction and renal parenchymal disease)

*$FE_{Na} = \dfrac{Urine\ Na/plasma\ Na}{Urine\ creatinine/plasma\ creatinine} = 100.$

electrolyte disturbances, particularly hyperkalemia; (2) managing blood pressure; (3) preventing and treating infections; (4) maintaining nutrition; and (5) remembering that certain drugs or their metabolites are not excreted and can be toxic. Renal replacement therapy (hemodialysis or peritoneal dialysis) may be indicated for uncontrollable hyperkalemia, acidosis, or severe fluid overload.[63,64]

CHRONIC KIDNEY DISEASE

Chronic kidney disease (CKD) is the progressive loss of renal function associated with systemic diseases, such as diabetes mellitus (most significant risk factor), hypertension, or systemic lupus erythematosus, or with intrinsic kidney diseases, such as acute kidney injury, chronic glomerulonephritis, chronic pyelonephritis, obstructive uropathies, or vascular disorders. Acute kidney injury can progress to CKD. The National Kidney Foundation defines kidney damage as a glomerular filtration rate (GFR) <60 ml/min/1.73 m² for 3 months or more, irrespective of cause. *Chronic kidney disease* is the preferred terminology and refers to declining glomerular filtration rate (GFR). The terms *renal insufficiency* and *chronic renal failure* are still often used to describe declining renal function, but they do not have the specificity of the stages based on GFR recommended by the National Kidney Foundation (Table 30-11). CKD decreases GFR and tubular functions with changes manifested throughout all organ systems (Table 30-12 and Figure 30-9).[65]

PATHOPHYSIOLOGY The kidneys have a remarkable ability to adapt to loss of nephron mass. Symptomatic changes result from increased levels of creatinine, urea, and potassium. Alterations in salt and water balance usually do not become apparent until renal function declines to less than 25% of normal when adaptive renal reserves have been exhausted.

Different theories have been proposed to account for the adaptation to loss of renal function. The *intact nephron hypothesis* proposes that loss of nephron mass with progressive kidney damage causes the surviving nephrons to sustain normal kidney function. These nephrons are capable of a compensatory hypertrophy and expansion or hyperfunction in their rates of filtration, reabsorption, and secretion and can maintain a constant rate of excretion in the presence of overall declining GFR.[66] The intact nephron hypothesis explains adaptive changes in solute and water regulation that occur with advancing renal failure. Although the urine of an individual with chronic kidney disease may contain abnormal amounts of protein and red and white blood cells or casts, the major end products of excretion are similar to those of normally functioning kidneys until the advanced stages of renal failure, when there is a significant reduction of functioning nephrons.[67]

With severe or repeated injury, epithelial cells have an impaired proliferative response resulting in interstitial capillary loss and fibroblast proliferation. The progressive process of glomerulosclerosis and tubulointerstitial fibrosis contributes to chronic kidney disease and end-stage kidney disease.[68] The *particular location of kidney damage* also influences loss of kidney function. For example, tubular interstitial diseases damage primarily the tubular or medullary parts of the nephron, producing problems such as renal tubular acidosis, salt wasting, and difficulty diluting or concentrating the urine. When the damage is primarily vascular or glomerular, proteinuria, hematuria, and nephrotic syndrome are more prominent. A summary of factors involved in the progression of chronic kidney disease is outlined in Table 30-13 and Figure 30-10.

Two factors that have consistently been recognized to advance renal disease are proteinuria and angiotensin II activity. Glomerular hyperfiltration and increased glomerular capillary permeability and loss of negative charge lead to proteinuria. *Proteinuria* contributes to tubulointerstitial injury by accumulating in the interstitial space of the

TABLE 30-11	**Stages of Chronic Kidney Disease**	
Stage	**Description**	**Signs/Symptoms**
I	Normal kidney function Normal or high GFR (>90 ml/min)	*Usually none* Hypertension common
II	Mild kidney damage, mild reduction in GFR (60-89 ml/min)	*Subtle* Hypertension Increasing creatinine and urea levels
III	Moderate kidney damage GFR 30-59 ml/min	*Mild* As above
IV	Severe kidney damage GFR 15-29 ml/min	*Moderate* As above Erythropoietin deficiency anemia Hyperphosphatemia Increased triglycerides Metabolic acidosis Hyperkalemia Salt/water retention
V	End-stage kidney disease Established kidney failure GFR <15 ml/min	*Severe* As above

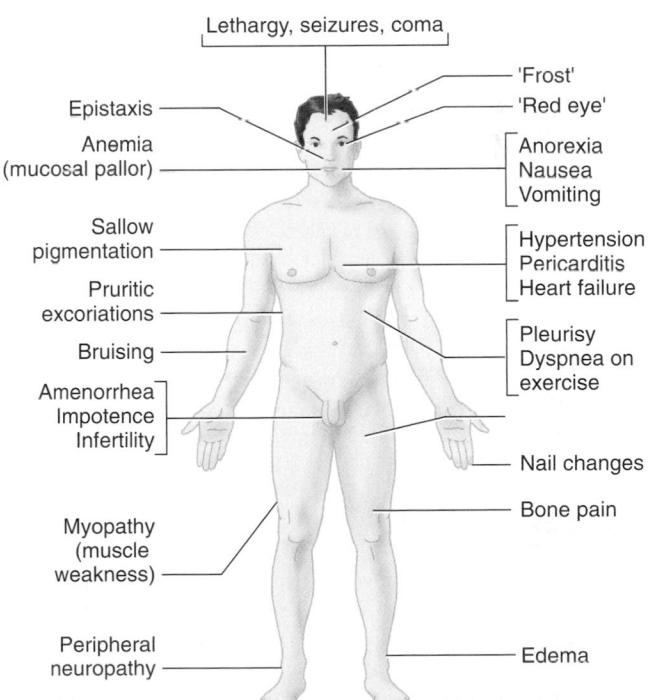

FIGURE 30-9 Common Signs and Symptoms of Kidney Failure (see text for reference site). (From Goldman L, Schafer AI: *Goldman's Cecil medicine*, ed 24, Philadelphia, 2012, Saunders; redrawn from Forbes CD, Jackson WF: *Color atlas and text of clinical medicine*, ed 3, London, 2003, Mosby.)

TABLE 30-12   Systemic Effects of Chronic Kidney Failure

System	Manifestations	Mechanisms	Treatment
Skeletal	Spontaneous fractures and bone pain Deformities of long bones	Osteitis fibrosa: bone inflammation with fibrous degeneration related to hyperparathyroidism Osteomalacia: bone resorption associated with vitamin D and calcium deficiency	Control of hyperphosphatemia to reduce hyperparathyroidism; administration of calcium and aluminum hydroxide antacids, which bind phosphate in the gut, together with a phosphate-restricted diet; vitamin D replacement; avoidance of magnesium antacids because of impaired magnesium excretion
Cardiopulmonary	Pulmonary edema, Kussmaul respirations	Fluid overload associated with pulmonary edema and metabolic acidosis leading to Kussmaul respirations	ACE inhibitors; combination of propranolol, hydralazine, and minoxidil for those with high levels of renin; bilateral nephrectomy with dialysis or transplantation
Cardiovascular	Left ventricular hypertrophy, cardiomyopathy, and ischemic heart disease; hypertension, dysrhythmias, accelerated atherosclerosis; pericarditis with fever, chest pain, and pericardial friction rub	Extracellular volume expansion and hypersecretion of renin associated with hypertension; anemia increases cardiac workload; hyperlipidemia promotes atherosclerosis; toxins precipitate into pericardium	Volume reduction with diuretics that are not potassium sparing (to avoid hyperkalemia); dialysis
Neurologic	Encephalopathy (fatigue, reduced attention span, difficulty with problem solving); peripheral neuropathy (pain and burning in legs and feet, loss of vibration sense and deep tendon reflexes); loss of motor coordination, twitching, fasciculations, stupor, and coma with advanced uremia	Progressive accumulation of uremic toxins associated with end-stage renal disease Stroke or intracerebral hemorrhage associated with chronic dialysis	Dialysis or successful kidney transplantation
Hematologic	Anemia, usually normochromic-normocytic; platelet disorders with prolonged bleeding times	Reduced erythropoietin secretion and reduced red cell production; uremic toxins shorten red blood cell survival and alter platelet function	Dialysis; recombinant human erythropoietin and iron supplementation; conjugated estrogens; DDAVP (1-desamino-8-D-arginine vasopressin); transfusion
Gastrointestinal	Anorexia, nausea, vomiting; mouth ulcers, stomatitis, urine odor of breath (uremic fetor), hiccups, peptic ulcers, gastrointestinal bleeding, and pancreatitis associated with end-stage renal failure	Retention of metabolic acids and other metabolic waste products	Protein-restricted diet for relief of nausea and vomiting
Integumentary	Abnormal pigmentation and pruritus	Retention of urochromes, contributing to sallow yellow color; high plasma calcium levels and neuropathy associated with pruritus	Dialysis with control of serum calcium levels
Immunologic	Increased risk of infection that can cause death; increased risk of carcinoma	Suppression of cell-mediated immunity; reduction in number and function of lymphocytes, diminished phagocytosis	Routine dialysis
Reproductive	Sexual dysfunction: menorrhagia, amenorrhea, infertility, and decreased libido in women; decreased testosterone levels, infertility, and decreased libido in men	Dysfunction of ovaries and testes; presence of neuropathies	No specific treatment

With data from Almeras C, Argilés A: *Semin Dial* 22(4):329-333, 2009; Keane WF: *Kidney Int Suppl* 75:S27-S31, 2000; Thomas R et al: *Prim Care* 35(2):329-344, 2008.

nephron tubules and activating complement proteins and other mediators and cells, such as macrophages, that promote inflammation and progressive fibrosis.[69] *Angiotensin II* (from activation of the renin-angiotensin-aldosterone system [RAAS]) promotes glomerular hypertension and hyperfiltration caused by efferent arteriolar vasoconstriction and also promotes systemic hypertension. The chronically high intraglomerular pressure increases glomerular capillary permeability, contributing to proteinuria. Angiotensin II also may promote the activity of inflammatory cells and growth factors that participate in tubulointerstitial fibrosis and scarring.[70]

CLINICAL MANIFESTATIONS   The clinical manifestations of chronic kidney disease include uremia and azotemia (see p. 760) with many systemic effects.[71] The many systemic manifestations associated with chronic kidney disease are discussed in the following sections and summarized in Table 30-12 and Figure 30-9.

Creatinine and Urea Clearance

Creatinine is constantly released from muscle and excreted primarily by glomerular filtration. In chronic kidney disease (CKD), as glomerular filtration rate (GFR) declines, the plasma creatinine level increases

TABLE 30-13 Factors Representing Progression of Chronic Kidney Failure

Factor	Characteristics
Proteinuria	Glomerular hyperfiltration of protein contributes to tubular interstitial injury by accumulating in interstitial space and promoting inflammation and progressive fibrosis.
Creatinine and urea clearance	In chronic renal failure, the GFR falls and the plasma creatinine concentration increases by a reciprocal amount; because there is no regulatory adjustment for creatinine, plasma levels continue to rise and serve as an index of changing glomerular function. As GFR declines, urea clearance increases. (**NOTE:** Urea is both filtered and reabsorbed and varies with state of hydration.)
Sodium and water balance	In chronic renal failure, sodium load delivered to nephrons exceeds normal, so excretion must increase; thus less is reabsorbed. Obligatory loss occurs, leading to sodium deficits and volume depletion. As GFR is reduced, ability to concentrate and dilute urine diminishes.
Phosphate and calcium balance	Changes in acid-base balance affect phosphate and calcium balance. Major disorders associated with chronic renal failure are reduced renal phosphate excretion, decreased renal synthesis of 1,25-dihydroxy-vitamin D_3, and hypocalcemia. Hypocalcemia leads to secondary hyperparathyroidism, GFR falls, and progressive hyperphosphatemia, hypocalcemia, and dissolution of bone result.
Hematocrit	Because of anemia that accompanies chronic renal failure, lethargy, dizziness, and low hematocrit are common.
Potassium balance	In chronic renal failure, tubular secretion of potassium increases until oliguria develops. Use of potassium-sparing diuretics also may precipitate elevated serum potassium levels. As disease progresses, total body potassium levels can rise to life-threatening levels and dialysis is required.
Acid-base balance	In early renal insufficiency, acid excretion and bicarbonate reabsorption are increased to maintain normal pH. Metabolic acidosis begins when GFR reaches 30% to 40%. Metabolic acidosis and hyperkalemia may be severe enough to require dialysis when end-stage renal failure develops.
Dyslipidemia	Chronic hyperlipidemia may induce glomerular and tubulointerstitial injury, contributing to progression of chronic renal disease.

GFR, Glomerular filtration rate.

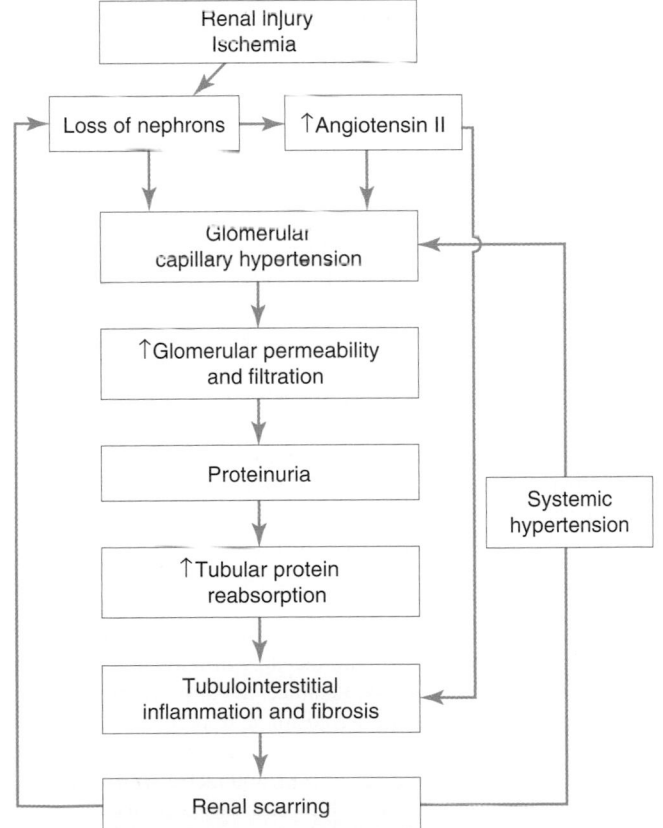

FIGURE 30-10 Mechanisms Related to the Progression of Chronic Kidney Disease.

by a reciprocal amount to maintain a constant rate of excretion. As GFR continues to decline, plasma creatinine concentration increases. The clearance of *urea* follows a similar pattern, but urea is both filtered and reabsorbed and its level varies with the state of hydration; therefore urea concentration is not a good index of GFR. However, as the GFR decreases, plasma urea concentration also increases.

Fluid and Electrolyte Balance

Fluid and electrolyte and acid-base balance is significantly disturbed with chronic kidney disease. When the GFR decreases to 25%, there is an adaptive loss of 20 to 40 mEq of *sodium* per day with osmotic loss of water. Dietary intake must be maintained to prevent sodium deficits and volume depletion. As GFR continues to decline, there also is loss of tubular function to dilute and concentrate the urine and urine specific gravity becomes fixed at about 1.010. Ultimately the kidney loses its ability to regulate sodium and water balance. Both sodium and water are retained, contributing to edema, proteinuria, and hypertension.

In early kidney failure, tubular secretion of *potassium* is maintained and larger amounts of potassium are lost through the bowel. With the onset of oliguria, total body potassium concentration can increase to life-threatening levels and must be controlled by dialysis.

Metabolic acidosis develops when the GFR decreases to less than 20% to 25% of normal. The causes of acidosis are primarily related to decreased hydrogen ion elimination and decreased bicarbonate reabsorption. With end-stage kidney disease, metabolic acidosis may be severe enough to require alkali therapy and dialysis.[72]

Calcium, Phosphate, and Bone

Bone and skeletal changes develop with alterations in calcium and phosphate metabolism. These changes begin when the GFR decreases to 25% or less. *Hypocalcemia* is accelerated by impaired renal synthesis of 1,25-dihydroxy-vitamin D_3 (calcitriol) with decreased intestinal absorption of calcium. Renal phosphate excretion also decreases and the increased serum phosphate binds calcium, further contributing to hypocalcemia. Acidosis also contributes to a negative calcium balance. Decreased serum calcium level stimulates parathyroid hormone secretion with mobilization of calcium from bone. The combined effect of *hyperparathyroidism* related to elevated phosphate levels and *vitamin D deficiency* can result in renal osteodystrophies (i.e., *osteoporosis, osteomalacia,* and *osteitis fibrosa*) with increased risk for fractures.[73]

Protein, Carbohydrate, and Fat Metabolism

Protein, carbohydrate, and fat metabolism are altered in CKD. Proteinuria, metabolic acidosis, inflammation, and a catabolic state contribute to a negative nitrogen balance. Levels of serum proteins diminish, including albumin, complement, and transferrin, and there is loss of muscle mass. Insulin resistance and glucose intolerance are common and may be related to proinflammatory cytokines, and alterations in adipokines (high leptin and low adiponectin levels) that interfere with insulin action.[74]

Dyslipidemia is common among individuals with CKD. There is a high ratio of low-density lipoprotein (LDL) to high-density lipoprotein (HDL), a high level of triglycerides, and an accumulation of LDL particles with accelerated atherosclerosis and vascular calcification. Uremia causes a deficiency in lipoprotein lipase and a decreased level of hepatic triglyceride lipase. Decreased lipolytic activity results in a reduction in HDL level. The concentration of apolipoprotein B is also elevated, thereby accelerating atherogenesis.[75]

Cardiovascular System

Cardiovascular disease is a major cause of morbidity and mortality in CKD. Proinflammatory cytokines, oxidative stress, metabolic derangements, and uremic toxins are significant contributors. *Hypertension* is the result of excess sodium and fluid volume and arteriosclerosis. Endothelial cell dysfunction and calcium deposits lead to a loss of vessel elasticity and vascular calcification. Elevated renin concentration also stimulates the secretion of aldosterone, increasing sodium reabsorption. *Dyslipidemia* promotes atheromatous plaque formation. The resulting vascular disease increases the risk for *ischemic heart disease, left ventricular hypertrophy, congestive heart failure, stroke,* and *peripheral vascular disease* in individuals with uremia. Declining erythropoietin production causes anemia, thereby increasing demands for cardiac output and adding to the cardiac workload. *Pericarditis* can develop from inflammation caused by the presence of uremic toxins. Accumulation of fluid in the pericardial space can compromise ventricular filling and cardiac output.[76] Fluid overload and hypertension can promote congestive heart failure (cardiorenal syndrome).

Pulmonary System

Pulmonary complications are associated with fluid overload, congestive heart failure, and dyspnea. Pulmonary edema develops and metabolic acidosis can cause Kussmaul respirations. Pulmonary hypertension can develop because of left ventricular dysfunction or uremic-associated vascular changes.[77]

Hematologic System

Hematologic alterations include *normochromic-normocytic anemia, impaired platelet function,* and *hypercoagulability.* Inadequate production of erythropoietin decreases red blood cell production and uremia decreases red blood cell life span. Lethargy, dizziness, and low hematocrit values are common findings. Defective platelet aggregation, decreased platelet numbers, and altered vascular endothelium promote an increased bleeding tendency, increased risk for bruising, epistaxis, gastrointestinal bleeding, or cerebrovascular hemorrhage. Alterations in thrombin and other clotting factors contribute to hypercoagulability; thus control of coagulation is essential during dialysis.[78]

Immune System

Immune system dysregulation develops with the uremia of CRF. Chemotaxis, phagocytosis, antibody production, and cell-mediated immune responses are suppressed. Malnutrition, metabolic acidosis, and hyperglycemia may amplify immunosuppression. Release of inflammatory cytokines results in systemic inflammation. Failure of antioxidant systems also promotes inflammation. There are deficient responses to vaccination, increased risk for infection, and virus-associated cancers (e.g., human papillomavirus, hepatitis B and C viruses, Epstein-Barr virus).[71]

Neurologic System

Neurologic symptoms are common and progressive with CKD. Symptoms may include headache, pain, drowsiness, sleep disorders, impaired concentration, memory loss, and impaired judgment (known as uremic encephalopathy). In advanced stages of renal failure, symptoms may progress to seizures and coma. Neuromuscular irritation can cause hiccups, muscle cramps, and muscle twitching. Peripheral neuropathies associated with uremic toxins also can develop with impaired sensations, particularly in the lower limbs. Symptoms improve with hemodialysis.[79]

Gastrointestinal System

Gastrointestinal complications are common in individuals with CKD. Uremic gastroenteritis can cause bleeding ulcer and significant blood loss. Nonspecific symptoms include anorexia, nausea, vomiting, constipation, or diarrhea. Uremic fetor is a form of bad breath caused by the breakdown of urea by salivary enzymes. Malnutrition is common.[80]

Endocrine and Reproductive Systems

Endocrine and reproductive alterations develop with progression of CKD. Both males and females have a decrease in levels of circulating sex steroids. Males often experience a reduction in testosterone levels and may be impotent. Oligospermia and germinal cell dysplasia can result in infertility. Females have reduced estrogen levels, amenorrhea, and difficulty maintaining a pregnancy to term.[81] A decrease in libido and fertility can occur in both genders.[82]

Insulin resistance is common in uremia, and as CKD progresses the ability of the kidney to degrade insulin is reduced and the half-life of insulin is prolonged. Individuals with diabetes mellitus and CRF need to carefully manage their insulin dosages.[83]

CRF also causes alterations in thyroid hormone metabolism, particularly hypothyroidism, known as nonthyroidal illness syndrome. Uremia delays the response of thyroid-stimulating hormone receptors and triiodothyronine (T_3) levels are often low.[84]

Integumentary System

Skin changes are associated with other complications that develop with CKD. Anemia can cause pallor and bleeding into the skin and results in hematomas and ecchymosis. Retained urochromes manifest as a sallow skin color. Hyperparathyroidism and uremic skin residues (known as uremic frost) are associated with inflammation, irritation, and pruritus with scratching, excoriation, and increased risk for infection. Half-and-half nails (half white and half red or brown) are common. Local bullous lesions and nephrogenic systemic fibrosis are less common.[85]

EVALUATION AND TREATMENT   Early screening and evaluation of CKD is based on the risk factors, history, presenting signs and symptoms, and diagnostic testing. Elevated serum creatinine and serum urea nitrogen concentrations are consistent with chronic renal failure.

Markers of kidney damage include measurement of urine protein level, particularly albumin, and examination of urine sediment. Ultrasound, CT scan, or plain x-ray films will show small kidney size. Renal biopsy confirms the diagnosis.

Management involves dietary restriction of protein, sodium, potassium, and phosphate, supplementation with vitamin D or vitamin D receptor activators, maintenance of sodium and fluid balance, restriction of potassium, promotion of adequate caloric intake, management of dyslipidemias, and use of erythropoietin as needed. Angiotensin-converting enzyme (ACE) inhibitors or angiotensin receptor blockers are often used to control systemic hypertension, reduce proteinuria, provide renoprotection, and prevent progressive renal damage.[86,87]

End-stage renal failure related to diabetic nephropathy can be significantly reduced with glycemic control.[83] End-stage renal failure is treated with conservative care, continuous renal replacement therapy, supportive therapy, and renal transplantation.[88,89] Portable and wearable dialysis devices are in clinical trials.[90]

✔ QUICK CHECK 30-4

1. What mechanisms cause prerenal acute renal failure?
2. How does intrarenal acute renal failure differ from postrenal failure?
3. Briefly describe the causes of anemia, cardiovascular disease, and bone and neurologic changes associated with chronic renal failure.

■ DID YOU UNDERSTAND?

Urinary Tract Obstruction

1. Obstruction can occur anywhere in the urinary tract, and it may be anatomic or functional, including renal stones, an enlarged prostate gland, urethral strictures, or neurogenic bladder. The most serious complications are hydronephrosis, hydroureter, ureterohydronephrosis, and infection caused by the accumulation of urine behind the obstruction.

2. Hypertrophy of the opposite kidney compensates for loss of function of the kidney with obstructive disease.

3. Relief of obstruction is usually followed by postobstructive diuresis and may cause fluid and electrolyte imbalance.

4. Persistent obstruction of the bladder outlet leads to residual urine volumes, low bladder wall compliance, and risk for vesicoureteral reflux and infection.

5. Kidney stones are caused by supersaturation of the urine with precipitation of stone-forming substances, changes in urine pH, or urinary tract infection.

6. The most common kidney stone is formed from calcium oxalate and most often causes obstruction by lodging in the ureter.

7. Obstructions of the bladder are a consequence of neurogenic or anatomic alteration of the bladder, or both.

8. A neurogenic bladder is caused by a neural lesion that interrupts innervation of the bladder.

9. Upper motor neuron lesions result in overactive or hyperreflexive bladder function.

10. Lower motor neuron lesions result in underactive, hypotonic, or atonic bladder function.

11. Underactive bladder (UAB) is a condition in which the duration or strength of contraction is inadequate to empty the bladder, resulting in distention and overflow incontinence.

12. Overactive bladder (OAB) syndrome is an uncontrollable or premature contraction of the bladder that results in urgency with or without incontinence, frequency, and nocturia.

13. Detrusor sphincter dyssynergia is failure of the urethrovesical junction smooth muscle to release urine during bladder contraction and causes a functional obstruction.

14. Other causes of lower urinary tract obstruction include prostatic enlargement, urethral stricture, and pelvic organ prolapse in women.

15. Partial obstruction of the bladder can result in overactive bladder contractions with urgency. There is deposition of collagen in the bladder wall over time, resulting in decreased bladder wall compliance and ineffective detrusor muscle contraction.

16. Renal cell carcinoma is the most common renal neoplasm and usually presents with hematuria. The larger neoplasms tend to metastasize to the lung, liver, and bone.

17. Bladder tumors are commonly composed of transitional cells with a papillary appearance and a high rate of recurrence.

Urinary Tract Infection

1. Urinary tract infections (UTIs) are commonly caused by the retrograde movement of bacteria into the urethra and bladder. UTIs are uncomplicated when the urinary system is normal or complicated when there is an abnormality.

2. Cystitis is an inflammation of the bladder commonly caused by bacteria and may be acute or chronic.

3. Painful bladder syndrome/interstitial cystitis includes nonbacterial infectious cystitis (viral, mycobacterial, chlamydial, fungal), noninfectious cystitis (i.e., radiation injury), and interstitial cystitis, which is related to autoimmune injury.

4. Pyelonephritis is an acute or chronic inflammation of the renal pelvis often related to obstructive uropathies and may cause abscess formation and scarring with an alteration in renal function.

Glomerular Disorders

1. Glomerular disorders are a group of related diseases of the glomerulus that can be caused by immune responses, toxins or drugs, vascular disorders, and other systemic diseases.

2. Acute glomerulonephritis commonly results from inflammatory damage to the glomerular filtration membrane as a consequence of immune reactions after a streptococcal infection.

3. Immune mechanisms in glomerulonephritis include the deposition of circulating antigen-antibody complexes often with complement components or the in situ formation of antibodies, or both, specific for the glomerular basement membrane.

4. Diabetic nephropathy is the most common cause of glomerular injury progressing to chronic kidney disease.

5. Chronic glomerulonephritis is related to a variety of diseases that cause deterioration of the glomerulus and a progressive loss of renal function.

6. Nephrotic syndrome is the excretion of at least 3.5 g of protein (primarily albumin) in the urine per day because of glomerular injury with increased capillary permeability and loss of membrane negative charge. Its principal signs are hypoproteinuria, hyperlipidemia, and edema. The liver cannot produce enough protein to adequately compensate for urinary loss.

7. Nephritic syndrome is characterized by hematuria and red blood cell casts with less severe proteinuria.

Acute Kidney Injury

1. Acute kidney injury is a sudden decline in kidney function with a decrease in GFR and urine output and with an elevation in plasma creatinine and blood urea nitrogen levels.
2. Prerenal acute kidney injury is caused by decreased renal perfusion with a decreased GFR, ischemia, and tubular necrosis.
3. Intrarenal acute kidney injury is associated with several systemic diseases but is commonly related to acute tubular necrosis (ATN).

4. Postrenal kidney injury is associated with diseases that obstruct the flow of urine from the kidneys.
5. Oliguria is urine output that is less than 400 ml/24 hours.

Chronic Kidney Disease

1. Chronic kidney disease is the progressive loss of renal function. Plasma creatinine levels gradually become elevated as GFR declines; sodium is lost in the urine; potassium is retained; acidosis develops; calcium and phosphate metabolism are altered; and erythropoietin production is diminished. All organs systems are affected by CRF.

■ KEY TERMS

Acute cystitis, 753
Acute glomerulonephritis, 755
Acute kidney injury (AKI), 760
Acute tubular necrosis (ATN), 761
Anuria, 762
Azotemia, 760
Calcium stone, 749
Calculus (pl., calculi) (urinary stone), 748
Chronic glomerulonephritis, 758
Chronic kidney disease (CKD), 763
Chronic pyelonephritis, 755
Compensatory hypertrophy, 748
Cystinuric (xanthine) stone, 749
Detrusor areflexia, 750
Detrusor hyperreflexia (overactivity), 750

Detrusor hyperreflexia with vesicosphincter dyssynergia, 750
Diabetic nephropathy, 758
Dyssynergia, 750
End-stage kidney disease (ESKD), 760
Hydronephrosis, 747
Hydroureter, 747
Hyperfunction, 748
Intrarenal (intrinsic) acute kidney injury, 761
Low bladder wall compliance, 751
Lupus nephritis, 758
Nephritic syndrome, 759
Nephrotic syndrome, 759
Neurogenic bladder, 750
Nonbacterial infectious cystitis, 754

Noninfectious cystitis, 754
Nonoliguric renal failure, 762
Obstructive uropathy, 747
Oliguria, 762
Overactive bladder syndrome (OAB), 750
Painful bladder syndrome/interstitial cystitis (PBS/IC), 754
Partial obstruction of the bladder outlet or urethra, 751
Pelvic organ prolapse, 751
Postobstructive diuresis, 748
Postrenal acute kidney injury, 762
Prerenal acute kidney injury, 760
Prostate enlargement, 751
Pyelonephritis, 754
Renal adenoma, 751
Renal cell carcinoma (RCC), 751

Renal colic, 749
Renal failure, 760
Renal insufficiency, 760
Renal transitional cell carcinoma (RTCC), 751
Staghorn calculus, 749
Struvite stone, 749
Tubulointerstitial fibrosis, 747
Uremia (uremic syndrome), 760
Ureterohydronephrosis, 747
Urethral stricture, 751
Uric acid stone, 749
Urinary tract infection (UTI), 753

REFERENCES

1. Siddiqui MM, McDougal WS: Urologic assessment of decreasing renal function, *Med Clin North Am* 95(1):161-168, 2011.
2. Tseng TY, Stoller ML: Obstructive uropathy, *Clin Geriatr Med* 25(3):437-443, 2009.
3. Klatt EC: *Robbins and Cotran atlas of pathology*, ed 3, Philadelphia, 2015, Saunders.
4. Maarten TW, Brenner BM: Adaptation to nephron loss and mechanisms of progression chronic kidney disease. In Brenner BM, editor: *Brenner and Rector's the kidney*, ed 9, Philadelphia, 2012, Saunders.
5. Frokiaer J, Zeidel ML: Urinary tract obstruction. In Brenner BM, editor: *Brenner and Rector's the kidney*, ed 8, Philadelphia, 2008, Saunders.
6. Roudakova K, Monga M: The evolving epidemiology of stone disease, *Indian J Urol* 30(1):44-48, 2014.
7. Lotan Y et al: Primary prevention of nephrolithiasis is cost-effective for a national healthcare system, *BJU Int* 110(11 Pt C):E1060-E1067, 2012.
8. Sakhaee K et al: Clinical review. Kidney stones 2012: pathogenesis, diagnosis, and management, *J Clin Endocrinol Metab* 97(6):1847-1860, 2012.
9. Argade S et al: An evaluation of Tamm-Horsfall protein glycans in kidney stone formers using novel techniques, *Urolithiasis* 2015 May 3. [Epub ahead of print.]

10. Daudon M et al: Randall's plaque as the origin of calcium oxalate kidney stones, *Urolithiasis* 43 Suppl 1:5-11, 2015.
11. Matlaga BR, Lingeman JE: Surgical management of upper urinary tract calculi. In Wein A et al, editors: *Campbell-Walsh urology*, ed 10, Philadelphia, 2012, Saunders.
12. Dalziel PJ, Noble VE: Bedside ultrasound and the assessment of renal colic: a review, *Emerg Med J* 30(1):3-8, 2013.
13. Pearle MS et al: Medical management of kidney stones: AUA guideline, *J Urol* 192(2):316-324, 2014.
14. Qaseem A et al: Dietary and pharmacologic management to prevent recurrent nephrolithiasis in adults: a clinical practice guideline from the American College of Physicians, *Ann Intern Med* 161:659-667, 2014.
15. Unger CA et al: Neuroanatomy, neurophysiology, and dysfunction of the female lower urinary tract: a review, *Female Pelvic Med Reconstr Surg* 20(2):65-75 2014.
16. Banakhar MA et al: Pathophysiology of overactive bladder, *Int Urogynecol J* 23(8):975-982, 2012.
17. Abrams P et al: The standardisation of terminology of lower urinary tract function: report from the Standardisation Sub-committee of the International

Continence Society, *Am J Obstet Gynecol* 187(1):116-126, 2002.
18. Hampson LA et al: Male urethral strictures and their management, *Nat Rev Urol* 11(1):43-50, 2014.
19. Osman NI et al: A systematic review of surgical techniques used in the treatment of female urethral stricture, *Eur Urol* 64(6):965-973, 2013.
20. Chibelean C, Nechifor-Boila IA: Botulinum neurotoxin A for overactive bladder treatment: advantages and pitfalls, *Can J Urol* 22(2): 7681-7689, 2015.
21. Coyne KS et al: Comorbidities and personal burden of urgency urinary incontinence: a systematic review, *Int J Clin Pract* 67(10):1015-1033, 2013.
22. American Cancer Society: *Cancer facts & figures—2015*, Atlanta, 2015, Author.
23. Bhatt JR, Finelli A: Landmarks in the diagnosis and treatment of renal cell carcinoma, *Nat Rev Urol* 11(9):517-525, 2014.
24. National Cancer Institute: *Renal cell cancer treatment (PDQ®)*. Updated May 12, 2015. Available at http://www.cancer.gov/types/kidney/patient/kidney-treatment-pdq#section/all.
25. Ridge CA et al: Epidemiology and staging of renal cell carcinoma, *Semin Intervent Radiol* 31(1):3-8, 2014.

26. Bedke J et al: Targeted therapy in renal cell carcinoma: moving from molecular agents to specific immunotherapy, *World J Urol* 32(1):31-38, 2014.

27. Su D et al: Renal cell carcinoma: molecular biology and targeted therapy, *Curr Opin Oncol* 26(3):321-327, 2014.

28. Sapre N et al: Gene-based urinary biomarkers for bladder cancer: an unfulfilled promise? *Urol Oncol* 32(1):48.e9-e17, 2014.

29. National Cancer Institute: *Bladder cancer treatment (PDQ®)*. Updated May 12, 2015. Available at http://www.cancer.gov/types/bladder/patient/bladder-treatment-pdq#section/all.

30. Sonpavde G et al: Future directions and targeted therapies in bladder cancer, *Hematol Oncol Clin North* 29(2):361-376, 2015.

31. Lee RK et al: Urinary diversion after radical cystectomy for bladder cancer: options, patient selection, and outcomes, *BJU Int* 113(1):11-23, 2014.

32. Dielubanza EJ, Schaeffer AJ: Urinary tract infections in women, *Med Clin North Am* 95(1):27-41, 2011.

33. Dielubanza EJ et al: Management of non-catheter-associated complicated urinary tract infection, *Infect Dis Clin North Am* 28(1):121-123, 2014.

34. Nicolle LE: Urinary tract infection, *Crit Care Clin* 29(3):699-715, 2013.

35. Rinaldi G et al: New research tools for urogenital schistosomiasis, *J Infect Dis* 211(6):861-869, 2015.

36. Stapleton AE: Urinary tract infection pathogenesis: host factors, *Infect Dis Clin North Am* 28(1):149-159, 2014.

37. Rowe TA, Juthani-Mehta M: Diagnosis and management of urinary tract infection in older adults, *Infect Dis Clin North Am* 28(1):75-89, 2014.

38. Grigoryan L et al: Diagnosis and management of urinary tract infections in the outpatient setting: a review, *J Am Med Assoc* 312(16):1677-1684, 2014.

39. National Guideline Clearinghouse (NGC): *Guideline synthesis: diagnosis and management of lower urinary tract infection*, Rockville, Md, 2008 Jan (revised 2012 March), National Guideline Clearinghouse, Agency for Healthcare Research and Quality. Available at: www.guideline.gov. Accessed December 2, 2014.

40. Dyer AJ, Twiss CO: Painful bladder syndrome: an update and review of current management strategies, *Curr Urol Rep* 15(2):384, 2014.

41. Hanno PM et al: Diagnosis and treatment of interstitial cystitis/bladder pain syndrome: AUA guideline amendment, *J Urol* 2015 Jan 23. [Epub ahead of print.]

42. Hooton T: Chapter 53: Bacterial urinary tract infections. In Johnson RJ et al, editors: *Comprehensive clinical nephrology*, ed 5, pp 632-643, Philadelphia, 2015, Saunders.

43. Takhar SS, Moran GF: Diagnosis and management of urinary tract infection in the emergency department and outpatient settings, *Infect Dis Clin North Am* 28(1):33-48, 2014.

44. Kościelska-Kasprzak K et al: The complement cascade and renal disease, *Arch Immunol Ther Exp (Warsz)* 62(1):47-57, 2014.

45. Hénique C et al: Update on crescentic glomerulonephritism, *Semin Immunopathol* 36(4):479-490, 2014.

46. Fioretto P et al: Is diabetic nephropathy reversible? *Diabetes Res Clin Pract* 104(3):323-328, 2014.

47. Yap DY, Lai KN: Pathogenesis of renal disease in systemic lupus erythematosus—the role of autoantibodies and lymphocytes subset abnormalities, *Int J Mol Sci* 16(4):7917-7931, 2015.

48. Reidy K et al: Molecular mechanisms of diabetic kidney disease, *J Clin Invest* 124(6):2333-2340, 2014.

49. Sun YM et al: Recent advances in understanding the biochemical and molecular mechanism of diabetic nephropathy, *Biochem Biophys Res Commun* 433(4):359-361, 2013.

50. Haider DG et al: Kidney biopsy in patients with glomerulonephritis: is the earlier the better? *BMC Nephrol* 13:34, 2012.

51. Kodner C: Nephrotic syndrome in adults: diagnosis and management, *Am Fam Physician* 80(10):1129-1134, 2009.

52. Siddall EC, Radhakrishnan J: The pathophysiology of edema formation in the nephrotic syndrome, *Kidney Int* 82(6):635-642, 2012.

53. Yee J: Treatment of nephrotic syndrome: retrospection, *Adv Chronic Kidney Dis* 21(2):115-118, 2014.

54. Gigante A et al: Hypercoagulability and nephrotic syndrome, *Curr Vasc Pharmacol* 12(3):512-517, 2014.

55. Ponticelli C, Glassock RJ: Glomerular diseases: membranous nephropathy—a modern view, *Clin J Am Soc Nephrol* 9(3):609-616, 2014.

56. Moroni G, Ponticelli C: Rapidly progressive crescentic glomerulonephritis: early treatment is a must, *Autoimmun Rev* 13(7):723-729, 2014.

57. Thomas ME et al: The definition of acute kidney injury and its use in practice, *Kidney Int* 87(1):62-73, 2014.

58. Tögel F, Westenfelder C: Recent advances in the understanding of acute kidney injury, *F1000Prime Rep* 6:83, 2014.

59. Chatauret N et al: Ischemia-reperfusion: from cell biology to acute kidney injury, *Prog Urol* 24(Suppl 1):S4-S12, 2014.

60. Gomez H et al: A unified theory of sepsis-induced acute kidney injury: inflammation, microcirculatory dysfunction, bioenergetics, and the tubular cell adaptation to injury, *Shock* 41(1):3-11, 2014.

61. Glodowski SD, Wagener G: New insights into the mechanisms of acute kidney injury in the intensive care unit, *J Clin Anesth* 27(2):175-180, 2015.

62. Obermüller N et al: Current developments in early diagnosis of acute kidney injury, *Int Urol Nephrol* 46(1):1-7, 2014.

63. Chionh CY et al: Use of peritoneal dialysis in AKI: a systematic review, *Clin J Am Soc Nephrol* 8(10):1649-1660, 2013.

64. Macedo E, Mehta RL: Timing of dialysis initiation in acute kidney injury and acute-on-chronic renal failure, *Semin Dial* 26(6):675-681, 2013.

65. Thomas R et al: Chronic kidney disease and its complications, *Prim Care* 35(2):329-344, vii, 2008.

66. Cleper R: Mechanisms of compensatory renal growth, *Pediatr Endocrinol Rev* 10(1):152-163, 2012.

67. Fong D et al: Compensatory responses to nephron deficiency: adaptive or maladaptive? *Nephrology (Carlton)* 19(3):119-128, 2014.

68. Grgic I et al: Targeted proximal tubule injury triggers interstitial fibrosis and glomerulosclerosis, *Kidney Int* 82(2):172-183, 2012.

69. Gorriz JL, Martinez-Castelao A: Proteinuria: detection and role in native renal disease progression, *Transplant Rev (Orlando)* 26(1):3-13, 2012.

70. Navar LG: Intrarenal renin-angiotensin system in regulation of glomerular function, *Curr Opin Nephrol Hypertens* 23(1):38-45, 2014.

71. Betjes MG: Immune cell dysfunction and inflammation in end-stage renal disease, *Nat Rev Nephrol* 9(5):255-265, 2013.

72. Dobre M et al: Current status of bicarbonate in CKD, *J Am Soc Nephrol* 26(3):515-523, 2015.

73. Kazama JJ et al: Chronic kidney disease and bone metabolism, *J Bone Miner Metab* 33(3):245-252, 2015.

74. Liao MT et al: Insulin resistance in patients with chronic kidney disease, *J Biomed Biotechnol* 2012:691369, 2012.

75. Keane WF et al: Lipid abnormalities in patients with chronic kidney disease: implications for the pathophysiology of atherosclerosis, *J Atheroscler Thromb* 20(2):123-133, 2013.

76. Johnson RJ et al: Chapter 82: Cardiovascular disease in chronic kidney disease. In Johnson RJ et al, editors: *Comprehensive clinical nephrology*, pp 949-966, Philadelphia, 2015, Saunders.

77. Kawar B et al: Pulmonary hypertension in renal disease: epidemiology, potential mechanisms and implications, *Am J Nephrol* 37(3):281-290, 2013.

78. Leung N: Hematologic manifestations of kidney disease, *Semin Hematol* 50(3):207-215, 2013.

79. Baumgaertel MW et al: Neurologic complications of acute and chronic renal disease, *Handb Clin Neurol* 119:383-393, 2014.

80. Thomas R et al: Gastrointestinal complications in patients with chronic kidney disease—a 5-year retrospective study from a tertiary referral center, *Ren Fail* 35(1):49-55, 2013.

81. Vellanki K: Pregnancy in chronic kidney disease, *Adv Chronic Kidney Dis* 20(3):223-228, 2013.

82. Holley JL, Schmidt RJ: Changes in fertility and hormone replacement therapy in kidney disease, *Adv Chronic Kidney Dis* 20(3):240-245, 2013.

83. Williams ME, Garg R: Glycemic management in ESRD and earlier stages of CKD, *Am J Kidney Dis* 63(2 Suppl 2):S22-S38, 2014.

84. Mohamedali M et al: Thyroid disorders and chronic kidney disease, *Int J Nephrol* 2014:520281, 2014.

85. Galperin TA et al: Cutaneous manifestations of ESRD, *Clin J Am Soc Nephrol* 9(1):201-218, 2014.

86. Levey AS, Coresh J: Chronic kidney disease, *Lancet* 379(9811):165-180, 2012.

87. Ruggenenti P et al: Mechanisms and treatment of CKD, *J Am Soc Nephrol* 23(12):1917-1928, 2012.

88. Kane PM et al: Palliative care for advanced renal disease: a summary of the evidence and future direction, *Palliat Med* 27(9):817-821, 2013.

89. Legendre C et al: Factors influencing long-term outcome after kidney transplantation, *Transpl Int* 27(1):19-27, 2014.

90. Davenport A: Portable and wearable dialysis devices for the treatment of patients with end-stage kidney failure: wishful thinking or just over the horizon? *Pediatr Nephrol* 2014 Oct 21. [Epub ahead of print.]

31

Alterations of Renal and Urinary Tract Function in Children

Patricia Ring and Sue E. Huether

ⓔ EVOLVE WEBSITE

CHAPTER OUTLINE

The incidence and type of renal and urinary tract disorders experienced by children vary with age and maturation. Newborn disorders may involve congenital malformations. During childhood, the kidney and genitourinary structures continue to develop, so renal dysfunction may be associated with mechanisms and manifestations that differ from those found in adults.

STRUCTURAL ABNORMALITIES

Congenital abnormalities of the kidney and urinary tract occur in about 1% to 2% of newborns.[1] These abnormalities range from minor, nonpathologic, or easily correctable anomalies to those that are incompatible with life. For example, the kidneys may fail to ascend from the pelvis to the abdomen, causing ectopic kidneys—which usually function normally. The kidneys may fuse as they ascend, causing a single, U-shaped horseshoe kidney. Approximately one third of individuals with horseshoe kidneys are asymptomatic, with the most common problems being hydronephrosis, infection, stone formation, and, rarely, renal malignancies.[2] Collectively, structural anomalies of the renal system account for approximately 45% of cases of renal failure in children in developed countries.[3] Many are linked to gene defects.[4] Certain structural anomalies are associated with urinary tract malformations,[4,5] including:

Low-set, malformed ears
Sensorineural deafness
Chromosomal disorders, including trisomy 13 (Patau syndrome) and trisomy 18 (Edward syndrome)
Absent abdominal muscles (prune-belly syndrome)
Anomalies of the spinal cord and lower and upper extremities
Imperforate anus and Hirschsprung disease
Optic nerve coloboma (hole)
Nephroblastoma (Wilms tumor)
Cystic disease of the liver

Hypospadias

Hypospadias is a congenital condition in which the urethral meatus is located on the ventral side or undersurface of the penis. The meatus can be located anywhere on the glans, on the penile shaft, at the base of the penis, at the penoscrotal junction, or in the perineum (Figure 31-1). This is the most common anomaly of the penis; it occurs in about 1 in 300 infant boys.[6] The cause of this condition is multifactorial and includes genetic, endocrine, and environmental factors. Advanced maternal age and low birth weight also have been implicated.[7,8] Chordee (penile torsion) may accompany cases of hypospadias. In chordee, skin tethering and shortening of subcutaneous tissue cause the penis to bend or "bow ventrally" (Figure 31-2). Penile torsion is rotation of the penile shaft to either the right or the left. Partial absence of the foreskin and cryptorchidism (undescended testes; see Chapter 32) are associated with the anomaly.

The goals for corrective surgery on the child with hypospadias are (1) a straight penis when erect to facilitate intercourse as an adult, (2) a uniform urethra of adequate caliber to prevent spraying during urination, (3) a cosmetic appearance satisfactory to the individual, and (4) repair completed in as few procedures as possible. Surgery is most effective, psychologically as well as physically, when performed between 6 and 12 months of age.[9]

FIGURE 31-1 Hypospadias. (Courtesy H. Gil Rushton, MD, Children's National Medical Center, Washington, DC; from Hockenberry MJ, Wilson D: *Wong's nursing care of infants and children*, ed 10, St Louis, 2015, Mosby.)

FIGURE 31-3 Exstrophy of Bladder. (Courtesy H. Gil Rushton, MD, Children's National Medical Center, Washington, DC; from Hockenberry MJ, Wilson D: *Wong's nursing care of infants and children*, ed 10, St Louis, 2015, Mosby.)

Chordee

Urethral meatus

Two halves of the scrotum located lateral to penile shaft

FIGURE 31-2 Hypospadias with Significant Chordee. (From Kliegman RM et al, editors: *Nelson textbook of pediatrics*, ed 19, Philadelphia, 2011, Saunders.)

Epispadias and Exstrophy of the Bladder

Epispadias and exstrophy of the bladder are the same congenital defect expressed to differing degrees. In male epispadias, the urethral opening is on the dorsal surface of the penis. In females, a cleft along the ventral urethra usually extends to the bladder neck. The incidence of epispadias is about 9.25 per 100,000 in-hospital live births.[10] This is seen predominantly in males.

In boys, the urethral opening may be small and situated behind the glans (anterior epispadias), or a fissure may extend the entire length of the penis and into the bladder neck (posterior epispadias). Continence is determined in part by the location of the defect, with urinary incontinence rates of up to 75% in children with distal epispadias.[11] Treatment is surgical reconstruction.

Exstrophy of the bladder is a rare, extensive congenital anomaly of herniation of the bladder through the abdominal wall. The bony part of the pelvis remains open (Figure 31-3), and the posterior portion of the bladder mucosa is exposed through the abdominal opening and appears bright red. The incidence of bladder exstrophy in the United States is about 1.7 per 100,000 live births.[10] Studies vary widely concerning male versus female prevalence.[12]

Exstrophy of the bladder is caused by intrauterine failure of the abdominal wall and the mesoderm of the anterior bladder to fuse. The rectus muscles below the umbilicus are separated, and the pubic rami (bony projections of the pubic bone) are not joined. This causes a waddling gait when the child first learns to walk, but most children quickly learn to compensate. The clitoris in girls is divided into two parts with the urethra between each half. The penis in boys is epispadiac. Urine seeps onto the abdominal wall from the ureters, causing a constant odor of urine and excoriation of the surrounding skin. Because the exposed bladder mucosa becomes hyperemic and edematous, it bleeds easily and is painful.

The unrepaired exstrophic bladder is prone to cancerous changes as soon as 1 year after birth. Ideally, the bladder and pubic defect should be closed before the infant is 72 hours old. Surgical reconstruction is usually performed within the first year either as a complete primary repair or as staged procedures. Staged procedures may include bladder augmentation, bladder neck reconstruction, and epispadias repair.[13] Objectives of management include preservation of renal function, attainment of urinary control, prevention of infection, and improvement of sexual function. Diagnosis is often made by prenatal ultrasound.

Cloacal exstrophy is the most rare and severe form of bladder exstrophy. The intestine and spine may be involved, and reconstruction with restored urine and fecal control is difficult.

Bladder Outlet Obstruction

Congenital causes of bladder outlet obstruction are rare and include urethral valves and polyps. A urethral valve is a thin membrane of tissue that occludes the urethral lumen and obstructs urinary outflow in males. Most valves occur in the posterior urethra, although a few arise from the embryologically distinct anterior urethra. Urethral polyps are rare.[14] The timing and presentation of these conditions depend on the degree of obstruction they cause. Severe obstruction may impair renal embryogenesis and lead to renal failure.[15] Urethral valves or polyps are resected as soon as they are diagnosed.

Ureteropelvic Junction Obstruction

Ureteropelvic junction (UPJ) obstruction is a blockage of the tapered point where the renal pelvis transitions into the ureter. UPJ obstruction is the most common cause of hydronephrosis in neonates. An intrinsic malformation of smooth muscle or urothelial development produces obstruction in the majority of cases. Extrinsic compression abnormalities are less common.[16] **Secondary ureteropelvic junction obstruction** is caused by kinking or secondary scarring in the presence of high-grade vesicoureteral reflux (see p. 775). There is an increased risk of vesicoureteral reflux in children with UPJ obstruction in the obstructed or contralateral kidney, or both; whether this represents a sequela of the embryonic defect leading to the UPJ defect is not known. Diagnosis of a UPJ obstruction can be made by ultrasound. Obstruction of the distal ureter (**ureterovesical junction obstruction**) causes dilation of the entire ureter, renal pelvis, and calyceal system. An **ureterocele** is a cystic dilation of the intravesical ureter. Open or endoscopic surgery to relieve an obstruction occurs if there is decline of renal drainage or function.[17]

Hypoplastic/Dysplastic Kidneys

During embryologic development, the ureteric duct grows into the metanephric tissue, triggering the formation of the kidneys. If this growth does not occur, the kidney is absent—a condition called **renal aplasia**. A **hypoplastic kidney** is small with a decreased number of nephrons. These conditions may be unilateral or bilateral; the occurrence may be incidental or familial. Bilateral hypoplastic kidneys are a common cause of chronic renal failure in children.[18] Segmental hypoplasia—the **Ask-Upmark kidney**—may be congenital or secondary to vesicoureteral reflux. Systemic hypertension is a common presentation.[19]

Renal dysplasia usually results from abnormal differentiation of the renal tissues; for example, primitive glomeruli and tubules, cysts, and nonrenal tissue (such as cartilage) are found in the dysplastic kidney. Dysplasia may be secondary to antenatal obstruction of the urinary tract from ureteroceles, posterior urethral valves, or prune-belly syndrome (congenital absence of abdominal muscles).

Polycystic Kidney Disease

Polycystic kidney disease (PKD) is an autosomal dominant disease (*PDK1* or *PDK2* gene) occurring in 1 of 1000 live births, or an autosomal recessive (*PKHD1* gene) inherited disorder with an incidence of 1 in 20,000 to 1 in 40,000.[20] Affected kidneys have multiple cysts that interfere with renal function. Autosomal dominant PKD (ADPKD) usually presents in late childhood or adulthood with the development of cysts. Defects in the formation of epithelial cells and their cilia result in cyst formation in all parts of the nephron. Cysts in other organs, including the liver, pancreas, and ovaries, may occur. Hypertension, aortic and intracranial aneurysms, and heart valve defects may develop. Autosomal recessive PKD (ARPKD) is often first suspected on a prenatal ultrasound. Epithelial hyperplasia and fluid secretion result in collecting duct cysts. Hepatic disease and hypertension typically accompany PKD. Clinical trials for various potential treatment modalities are ongoing.[21]

Renal Agenesis

Renal agenesis (the absence of one or both kidneys) may be unilateral or bilateral, and may occur randomly or be hereditary. It may be an isolated entity or be associated with anomalies in other organs.

Unilateral renal agenesis occurs in approximately 1 in 1000 live births. Males are more often affected, and it is usually the left kidney that is absent. The single remaining kidney is often completely normal so that the child can expect a normal, healthy life. By the time the child is several years old, the volume of this kidney may approach twice the normal size to compensate for the absence of a second kidney. In some instances, however, the single kidney is abnormally formed and associated with abnormalities of its collecting system. Because the child has a decreased number of nephrons, there is a risk of "hyperfiltration injury," increasing the chance of developing proteinuria, hypertension, and chronic kidney disease.[22] Extrarenal congenital abnormalities of the urogenital, skeletal, cardiac, and other systems may coexist.

Bilateral renal agenesis is a rare disorder incompatible with extrauterine life. Approximately 75% of affected children are males. **Oligohydramnios** (low amount of amniotic fluid) resulting from inadequate fetal urine production leads to underdeveloped lungs and **Potter syndrome** (wide-set eyes, parrot-beak nose, low-set ears, and receding chin). Approximately 40% of affected infants are stillborn. Infants with this condition rarely live more than 24 hours because of pulmonary insufficiency.[23] Renal agenesis can be detected prenatally by ultrasound.

✔ **QUICK CHECK 31-1**
1. Describe hypospadias.
2. Why does bladder exstrophy occur?
3. Contrast dysplastic kidney and hypoplastic kidney.

GLOMERULAR DISORDERS

Common glomerular disorders in children are glomerulonephritis, nephrotic syndrome, immunoglobulin A (IgA) nephropathy, and hemolytic uremic syndrome. Most glomerular diseases are acquired and immunologically mediated (see Chapter 30 and Figure 30-6, and Tables 29-5 and 29-7). The disease can be acute or chronic. The likelihood of developing renal failure depends on the specific condition.

Glomerulonephritis

Glomerulonephritis includes a number of renal disorders in which proliferation and inflammation of the glomeruli are secondary to an immune mechanism (the pathophysiology is described in Chapter 30). Chronic glomerulonephritis accounts for about 14% of the cases of renal failure in children in the United States[3] and is the causative factor for 9% to 35% of end-stage renal disease in children worldwide.[24]

Acute Poststreptococcal Glomerulonephritis

Acute poststreptococcal glomerulonephritis (APGN) is one of the most common immune complex–mediated renal diseases in children. It most commonly occurs after a throat or skin infection with a nephritogenic strain of group A β-hemolytic streptococci, although other bacteria and viruses also may be responsible.[25] Occurrences have been observed after bacterial endocarditis, which may be associated with streptococcal or staphylococcal microorganisms, or after viral diseases, such as varicella-zoster virus and hepatitides B and C. Glomerulonephritis develops with the deposition of antigen-antibody complexes in the glomerulus. The antigen-antibody complex activates complement and the release of inflammatory mediators that damage endothelial and epithelial cells lying on the glomerular basement membrane. Damage to the glomerular basement membrane leads to hematuria and proteinuria.

Symptoms usually begin 1 to 2 weeks after an upper respiratory tract infection (more common during cold weather) and up to 6 weeks after skin infections such as impetigo (more common during warm weather).

The onset of symptoms is abrupt, varying with disease severity. The child typically has gross or microscopic hematuria, proteinuria, edema, and renal insufficiency. Oliguria may be present. Hypertension occurs because of increased vascular volume. Acute hypertension may cause headache, vomiting, somnolence, and other central nervous system manifestations. Cardiovascular symptoms are related to circulatory overload and are compounded by hypertension. These include dyspnea, tachypnea, and an enlarged, tender liver. The most severely affected children develop acute renal failure with oliguria. As many as half of affected children are asymptomatic.

The disease usually runs its course in 1 month, but urine abnormalities may be found for up to 1 year or longer after the onset. Prolonged proteinuria and abnormal glomerular filtration rate (GFR) indicate an unfavorable prognosis. More than 95% of affected children recover completely. Less than 1% of children develop end-stage renal disease.[26] Treatment is supportive and symptom specific.

Immunoglobulin A Nephropathy

Immunoglobulin A (IgA) nephropathy is the most common form of glomerulonephritis worldwide and occurs more often in males. It is characterized by deposition primarily of immunoglobulin A and complement proteins in the mesangium of the glomerulus. Children with the disease have recurrent gross hematuria concurrent with a respiratory tract infection. Most continue to have microscopic hematuria between the attacks of gross hematuria and have a mild proteinuria as well. Treatment is supportive. Some children recover completely, whereas 20% or more will eventually require dialysis and transplantation.[27] IgA nephropathy may recur following transplantation.[28]

Henoch-Schönlein purpura nephritis is a particular form of IgA nephropathy that involves a systemic vasculitis. Symptoms vary widely. In addition to palpable purpura, children may experience abdominal pain, arthralgia, hematuria, and/or proteinuria. Complete recovery may occur, but some children progress to end-stage kidney disease.[29]

Nephrotic Syndrome

Nephrotic syndrome is characterized by severe proteinuria, hypoalbuminemia, hyperlipidemia, and edema. The syndrome is more common in children than in adults. When no identifiable cause is found, the condition is primary (idiopathic) nephrotic syndrome. If it results from a systemic disease or other causes (e.g., drugs, toxins), it is called secondary nephrotic syndrome. Primary nephrotic syndrome is found predominantly in the preschool-age child, with a peak incidence of onset between 2 and 3 years of age. It is rare after 8 years of age. Boys are affected more often than girls. No prevalent racial or geographic distributions are evident. The incidence is approximately 3 per 100,000 children per year.

PATHOPHYSIOLOGY   The most common causes of primary nephrotic syndrome in children are minimal change nephropathy and focal segmental glomerulosclerosis. Minimal change nephropathy (MCN) (lipoid nephrosis) is characterized by fusion of the glomerular podocyte foot processes, which are seen by electron microscopy. The glomeruli appear normal by light microscopy. A systemic immune mechanism is a likely cause of the disease, but the true etiology is unknown. An unidentified circulating permeability factor released by T lymphocytes has been proposed.[30] Loss of the electrical negative charge and increased permeability within the glomerular capillary wall lead to albuminuria. Hypoalbuminemia (causing decreased plasma oncotic pressure) and sodium retention contribute to edema.[31] Hyperlipidemia leads to hyperlipiduria and primarily results from increased hepatic lipid synthesis and decreased plasma lipid catabolism.

In idiopathic focal segmental glomerulosclerosis (FSGS), there is segmental loss of glomerular capillaries with proliferation of the mesangial matrix and adhesion of the capillaries to Bowman capsule.

CLINICAL MANIFESTATIONS   Onset of nephrotic syndrome can be insidious, with periorbital edema as the usual first sign. The edema is most noticeable in the morning and subsides during the day as fluid shifts to the abdomen, genitalia, and lower extremities. Parents may notice diminished, frothy, or foamy urine output; or when edema becomes pronounced with ascites, respiratory difficulty from pleural effusion or labial or scrotal swelling may occur. Edema of the intestinal mucosa may cause diarrhea, anorexia, and poor absorption. Edema often masks the malnutrition caused by malabsorption and protein loss. Pallor, with shiny skin and prominent veins, also is common. Blood pressure is usually normal. The child has an increased susceptibility to infection, especially pneumonia, peritonitis, cellulitis, and septicemia. Irritability, fatigue, and lethargy are common. Congenital nephrotic syndrome (Finnish type) is caused by an autosomal recessive mutation of the NPHS1 gene that encodes an immunoglobulin-like protein, nephrin, at the podocyte slit membrane.[32] Congenital nephrotic syndrome (Finnish type) presents with heavy proteinuria, hypoproteinemia, and edema in the first 3 months of life. These babies do not respond to steroid treatment and require albumin infusion and diuretics.[33]

EVALUATION AND TREATMENT   The diagnosis of nephrotic syndrome is evident from the findings of proteinuria, hyperlipidemia, and edema. Diagnostic testing, including kidney biopsy, may be required to determine whether the cause is an intrinsic renal disease or a consequence of systemic disease. Basic management of nephrotic syndrome includes administering glucocorticosteroids (prednisone); adhering to a low-sodium, well-balanced diet; performing good skin care; and, if edema becomes problematic, prescribing diuretics (furosemide, metolazone). Immunosuppressive agents (i.e., cyclophosphamide) may be used with children who have frequent relapses or who are resistant to steroid therapy. Long-term outcomes depend on the underlying cause of the nephrotic syndrome. Children with minimal change disease tend to do very well, whereas those with other conditions may develop end-stage kidney disease.

Hemolytic Uremic Syndrome

Hemolytic uremic syndrome (HUS) is an acute disorder characterized by hemolytic anemia, thrombocytopenia, and acute renal failure. HUS is the most common cause of acute renal failure in children. The disease occurs most often in infants and children younger than 4 years of age but has been known to occur in adolescents and adults.

PATHOPHYSIOLOGY   HUS has been associated with bacterial and viral agents, as well as endotoxins, especially that from *Escherichia coli* 0157:H7 and more recently *Escherichia coli* 0104:H4 (Shiga toxins).[34] In HUS, the endothelial lining of the glomerular arterioles becomes swollen and occluded with platelets and fibrin clots. Narrowed vessels damage passing erythrocytes. These damaged red blood cells are removed by the spleen, causing acute hemolytic anemia. Fibrinolysis, the process of dissolution of a clot, acts on precipitated fibrin, causing the fibrin split products to appear in serum and urine. Platelet thrombi develop within damaged vessels, and platelet removal produces thrombocytopenia. Varying degrees of vascular occlusion cause altered renal perfusion and renal insufficiency or failure.[35]

CLINICAL MANIFESTATIONS   A prodromal gastrointestinal illness (fever, vomiting, diarrhea) or, less frequently, an upper respiratory tract infection often precedes the onset of HUS by 1 to 2 weeks. After a symptom-free 1- to 5-day period, the sudden onset of pallor, bruising or purpura, irritability, and oliguria heralds the commencement of the disease. Slight fever, anorexia, vomiting, diarrhea (with the stool characteristically watery and blood stained), abdominal pain, mild jaundice, and circulatory overload are accompanying symptoms. Seizures and lethargy indicate central nervous system (CNS) involvement. Renal failure is apparent within the first days of onset. The renal failure causes metabolic acidosis, azotemia, hyperkalemia, and often hypertension.

EVALUATION AND TREATMENT Clinical evaluation includes history of preexisting illness, presenting symptoms, and urine and blood analysis. Management is supportive. When renal failure occurs, dialysis is indicated. Blood transfusions with packed red cells are needed to maintain reasonable hemoglobin levels. Seventy percent of children recover completely. Potential long-term sequelae include renal (hypertension, proteinuria, chronic kidney disease, and end-stage kidney disease) and nonrenal abnormalities (diabetes mellitus, neurologic manifestations). In cases unresponsive to treatment, splenectomy may be indicated.[36]

NEPHROBLASTOMA

Nephroblastoma (Wilms tumor) is a rare embryonal tumor of the kidney arising from undifferentiated mesoderm and represents 5% of childhood cancers in the United States. Approximately 500 children are diagnosed each year in the United States, most younger than 5 years of age.[37] The peak incidence occurs between 2 and 3 years of age. Nephroblastoma is slightly more common in black children than in white children. Maternal preconception toxin exposure (e.g., pesticides) may be associated with increased risk in offspring.[38]

PATHOGENESIS Nephroblastoma has both sporadic and inherited origins. The sporadic form occurs in children with no known genetic predisposition. Inherited cases, which are relatively rare, are transmitted in an autosomal dominant fashion. Syndromic and nonsyndromic causes of nephroblastoma have been linked to mutation of several tumor-suppressor genes (i.e., *WT1* and *WT2* mutations).[39]

Eighteen percent of children who have nephroblastoma also have other congenital anomalies. The anomalies associated with nephroblastoma include aniridia (lack of an iris in the eye), hemihyperplasia (an asymmetry of the body), and genitourinary malformations (i.e., horseshoe kidneys, hypospadias, ureteral duplication, polycystic kidneys).[40] Children with both congenital anomalies and nephroblastoma are more likely to have the inherited bilateral form of the disease.

CLINICAL MANIFESTATIONS Most children with nephroblastoma present with an enlarging asymptomatic abdominal mass before the age of 5 years. Many tumors are actually discovered by the child's parent, who feels or notices an abdominal swelling, usually while dressing or bathing the child. The child appears healthy and thriving. Other presenting complaints include vague abdominal pain, hematuria, anemia, and fever. Hypertension may be present, often as a result of excessive renin secretion by the tumor.[41]

Nephroblastoma may occur in any part of the kidney and varies greatly in size at the time of diagnosis. The tumor generally appears as a solitary mass surrounded by a smooth, fibrous external capsule and also may contain cystic or hemorrhagic areas. A pseudocapsule generally separates the tumor from the renal parenchyma.

TABLE 31-1	Staging of Nephroblastoma Tumor*
Stage	**Tumor Characteristics**
I	Tumor limited to kidney; can be completely resected
II	Tumor ascending beyond kidney but is totally resected
III	Residual nonhematogenous tumor confined to abdomen
IV	Hematogenous metastases to organs such as lungs, liver, bone, or brain
V	Bilateral disease either at diagnosis or later, then staged for each kidney

*Staging system of the National Wilms Tumor Study Group.

EVALUATION AND TREATMENT On physical examination, the tumor feels firm, nontender, and smooth, and is generally confined to one side of the abdomen. If the tumor is palpable past the midline of the abdomen, it may be large or may be arising from a horseshoe or ectopic kidney. Once an abdominal mass is detected, diagnostic imaging demonstrates a solid intrarenal mass.

Diagnosis is based on surgical biopsy. Imaging studies are used to evaluate the presence or absence of metastasis.[42] The most common sites of metastasis are regional lymph nodes and the lungs, and less commonly the liver, brain, and bone.

Several staging systems for nephroblastoma have been developed and serve as guides to treatment. The most widely accepted system was developed by the National Wilms Tumor Study Group (Table 31-1). Primary treatment is usually surgical exploration and resection or chemotherapy and then surgical resection. Radiation therapy may be used for children with higher stages of disease and metastases. Survival is greater than 90% for localized disease and up to 80% for higher stages, although congestive heart failure, renal failure, and hypertension occur more frequently in long-term survivors than in the general population.[43]

> **QUICK CHECK 31-2**
> 1. What is the cause of proteinuria?
> 2. What is Wilms tumor and what cellular components are involved?

BLADDER DISORDERS

Urinary Tract Infections

Urinary tract infections (UTIs) are rare in newborns, and children with congenital renal abnormalities and noncircumcised males are at increased risk.[44] UTIs in children are most common in 7- to 11-year-old girls as a result of perineal bacteria, especially *E. coli*, ascending the urethra. Susceptibility, bacterial virulence, and, perhaps, genetics affect the severity of the disease.[45] An abnormal urinary tract (presence of reflux, obstruction, stasis, or stones) is particularly susceptible to infection. Sexually active female adolescents are at increased risk to have a UTI.

Cystitis, or infection of the bladder, results in mucosal inflammation and congestion. This causes detrusor muscle hyperactivity and a resulting decrease in bladder capacity, resulting in urgency and frequency. It may also cause distortion of the ureterovesical (UV) junction leading to transient reflux of infected urine up the ureters, causing acute or chronic pyelonephritis.

Differentiating whether an infection is in the bladder or in the kidneys is difficult based on symptoms alone. Infants may be asymptomatic or develop fever, lethargy, abdominal pain, vomiting, diarrhea, or asymptomatic jaundice. Children may present with fever of undetermined origin, frequency, urgency, dysuria, enuresis or incontinence in a previously dry child, flank or back pain, and sometimes hematuria. Acute pyelonephritis usually causes chills, high fever, and flank or abdominal pain, along with enlarged kidney(s) caused by inflammatory edema. Chronic pyelonephritis may be asymptomatic.

Diagnosis of UTIs is by urine culture. Dipstick analyses for nitrite, leukocyte esterase, and blood may be used as a screening tool. Any positive or strong suspicion of a UTI, including unexplained jaundice in infants,[46] requires urine culture. Diagnostic imaging may be necessary to rule out obstructions, renal scarring, or functional abnormalities. With treatment, UTI symptoms are usually relieved in 1 to 2 days, and the urine becomes sterile. A 2- to 4-day course of oral antibiotics is effective for uncomplicated UTI.[47] Longer treatment may be required if the child has a history of recurrent UTIs or has congenital abnormalities of the urinary tract. If there is no improvement in 2 days, the child should be reevaluated (see *Health Alert:* Childhood Urinary Tract Infections).

FIGURE 31-4 Normal and Abnormal Configurations of the Ureterovesical Ureter. A refluxing ureterovesical ureter has the same anatomic features as a nonrefluxing ureter, except for the shorter length of the intravesical ureter, which allows reflux of urine during filling of the bladder.

HEALTH ALERT

Childhood Urinary Tract Infections

Childhood urinary tract infections (UTIs) are often seen in primary care settings and can cause significant longer term morbidity if not treated. Children younger than 2 years often have few, nonspecific signs of infection, including fever, irritability, poor feeding, failure to thrive, and diarrhea. Obtaining a proper urine sample and culture is vital because true infections require further examination. Antibiotic prophylaxis may be considered because of the link between vesicoureteral reflux (VUR), recurrent UTIs, and renal scarring and hypertension; however, this is a controversial issue because of the risk of antibiotic resistance. Current recommendations are to *consider* prophylaxis for children younger than 1 year of age with VUR and a history of febrile UTIs, and other children as indicated. Circumcision status is controversial; however, recent studies have shown a decreased rate of UTIs in circumcised boys. The position of the American Academy of Pediatrics is that scientific evidence shows medical benefits of neonatal circumcision, but data are insufficient to support routine neonatal circumcision. Abnormalities in bowel and bladder function must be addressed because they can impact the development of UTIs and affect the resolution of VUR. Surgical management of VUR is considered based on failure of medical management to prevent recurrent infections, VUR grade, and degree of renal scarring.

Data from American Academy of Pediatrics: *Pediatrics* 130(3):585-586, 2012; Arshad M, Seed PC: *Clin Perinatol* 42(1):17-28, vii, 2015; Paintsil E: *Curr Opin Pediatr* 25(1):88-94, 2013; Saperston KN et al: *J Urol* 191(5 Suppl):1608-1613, 2014.

Vesicoureteral Reflux

Vesicoureteral reflux (VUR) is the retrograde flow of urine from the bladder into the kidney or ureters, or both. This allows infected urine from the bladder to reach the kidneys. Vesicoureteral reflux occurs more often in girls by a ratio of 10:1 and is uncommon in blacks. The actual incidence is unknown because VUR is often undiagnosed. An estimated 30% to 40% of children younger than 5 years who develop a UTI have VUR. Siblings of those affected have about a 27% to

51% chance of having reflux, and children with parents who had childhood reflux have almost a 70% chance of reflux.[48] Although reflux is considered abnormal at any age, the shortness of the submucosal tunnel of the ureter during infancy and childhood renders the antireflux mechanism relatively inefficient and delicate. Thus reflux is seen commonly in association with infections during early childhood but rarely in older children and adults.

PATHOPHYSIOLOGY The normal distal ureter enters the bladder through the detrusor muscle and passes through a submucosal tunnel before opening into the bladder lumen via the ureteral orifice. As the bladder fills with urine the ureter is compressed within the bladder wall, preventing reflux. Primary VUR results from a congenital abnormally short submucosal tunnel and ureter that permits reflux by the rising pressure of the filling bladder (Figure 31-4). Urine sweeps up into the ureter and then flows back into the empty bladder. The reflux perpetuates infection by preventing complete emptying of the bladder and providing a reservoir for infection. With bladder filling, the maximal intravesical pressure can be transmitted up the ureter to the renal pelvis and calyces. The combination of reflux and infection is an important cause of pyelonephritis. Renal parenchymal injury, scarring, hypertension, and chronic renal insufficiency can occur many years later, making early diagnosis and treatment important. Secondary reflux develops in association with acquired conditions (e.g., neurogenic bladder dysfunction, ureteral obstruction, voiding disorders, or surgery on the ureterovesical [UV] junction). Reflux may be unilateral or bilateral, and is graded using the International Reflux Grading System[49] (Figure 31-5):

Grade I: reflux into a nondilated distal ureter
Grade II: reflux into the upper collecting system without dilation
Grade III: reflux into a dilated ureter or blunting of calyceal fornices
Grade IV: reflux into a grossly dilated ureter and calyces
Grade V: massive reflux with urethral dilation and tortuosity and effacement of the calyceal details

CLINICAL MANIFESTATIONS Children with reflux may be asymptomatic or have recurrent urinary tract infections, unexplained fevers,

FIGURE 31-5 Grades of Vesicoureteral Reflux. (From Johnson JR, Feehally J, Floege J: *Comprehensive clinical nephrology*, ed 5, Philadelphia, Saunders.)

TABLE 31-2	Classification of Incontinence
Type	**Definition**
Daytime voiding frequency	Decreased: 3 or fewer voids per day Increased: 8 or more voids per day
Dysfunctional voiding	Habitual contraction of urethral sphincter during voiding; observed by uroflow measurements
Enuresis	Incontinence of urine while sleeping
Incontinence, continuous	Continuous leakage, not in discrete portions
Incontinence, stress	Leakage with raised intra-abdominal pressure
Urgency	Sudden, unexpected, immediate need to void
Overactive bladder	Child with urgency; increased voiding frequency and/or incontinence may or may not be present
Underactive bladder	Decreased voiding frequency with use of raised intra-abdominal pressure to void
Urge incontinence	Incontinence in children with urgency

From Nevéus T et al: *J Urol* 176(1):314-324, 2006.

poor growth and development, irritability, and feeding problems. The family history may reveal VUR or urinary tract infections.

EVALUATION AND TREATMENT In addition to the history of recurrent urinary tract infection and other symptoms, a voiding cystourethrogram is the primary diagnostic procedure. Most children with VUR respond to nonoperative management aimed at prevention and treatment of infection. Spontaneous remission of grades I, II, and III reflux may occur in 50% to 80% of children younger than 5 years. Approximately 20% of grades IV and V will resolve.[50] Recurrent infection may require endoscopic, open, laparoscopic, and robotic procedures to stop the refluxing ureter.[51]

URINARY INCONTINENCE

Urinary incontinence refers to the involuntary passage of urine by a child who is beyond the age when voluntary bladder control should have been acquired. Bladder control is accomplished by most children before the age of 5 years, although this is largely influenced by cultural beliefs and parental toilet training practices.

Types of Incontinence

Wetness that occurs during the day is called daytime incontinence. Nighttime wetting is called enuresis. Primary incontinence (enuresis) means the child has never been continent, whereas secondary incontinence (enuresis) means the child has been continent for at least 6 months before wetting recurs. A child may have daytime incontinence, enuresis, or a combination of both. (Types of incontinence and clinical manifestations are defined in Table 31-2.)

The incidence of incontinence (enuresis) is difficult to determine because it is not a problem parents often discuss. Enuresis occurs in as many as 10% of 7-year-old males and resolves at a rate of 15% per year. Daytime incontinence occurs in up to 9% of early school age children.[52]

PATHOGENESIS A combination of factors is likely to be responsible for incontinence or enuresis. Organic causes account for a minority of cases and include UTIs; neurologic disturbances; congenital defects of the meatus, urethra, or bladder neck; and allergies. Disorders that increase the normal output of urine, such as diabetes mellitus and diabetes insipidus, or disorders that impair the concentrating ability of the kidney, such as chronic renal failure or sickle cell disease, should be considered during evaluation. Other conditions that may be associated with incontinence include perinatal anoxia, CNS trauma, seizures, attention-deficit/hyperactivity disorder,[53] developmental delay, imperforate anus, bladder trauma or surgery, obesity,[54] and occult spinal dysraphism. Altered sleep arousal or obstructive sleep apnea[55] may be associated with enuresis. Stressful psychologic situations, such as a new sibling, may cause incontinence or enuresis to develop. Constipation is frequently present in children with urinary incontinence.[56] Incontinence or enuresis in which no structural or neurologic abnormality is identified is common in children.

Genetic factors contribute to some types of incontinence. At least four gene loci associated with enuresis have been identified. Enuresis occurs with high frequency among parents, siblings, and other near relatives of symptomatic children. There is a high concordance rate in monozygotic twins with enuresis.[57]

EVALUATION AND TREATMENT Diagnostic evaluation of childhood incontinence includes a thorough history, voiding diary, physical examination, and urinalysis. Urodynamic flow studies or imaging may be required based on the history and physical findings. Therapeutic management of incontinence or enuresis begins with education. If the child and family understand the probably etiology of the child's condition, they are better able to choose and participate in therapies that are most likely to succeed. Treatment of daytime incontinence includes behavioral therapy, including timed voiding; fluid management; treatment of constipation, urinary tract infections, and other coexisting conditions if present; and medication (anticholinergic or alpha-blocker medications). Enuresis treatment also may include enuresis alarms or other medications (e.g., desmopressin acetate).[58]

> ✔ **QUICK CHECK 31-3**
> 1. How does the cause of urinary tract infections (UTIs) in newborns differ from that in older children?
> 2. How does vesicoureteral reflux occur?
> 3. What organic causes are operative in enuresis?

DID YOU UNDERSTAND?

Structural Abnormalities

1. Congenital renal disorders affect about 10% to 15% of the population. These disorders range in severity from minor conditions that need no treatment to those incompatible with life.
2. Hypospadias is a congenital condition in which the urethral meatus can be located anywhere on the ventral surface of the glans, the penile shaft, the midline of the scrotum, or the perineum.
3. Exstrophy of the bladder is a congenital malformation in which the pubic bones are separated, the lower portion of the abdominal wall and anterior wall of the bladder are missing, and the posterior wall of the bladder is everted through the opening.
4. Urethral valves and polyps are congenital formations of tissue that block the urethra.
5. Ureteropelvic junction obstruction is blockage where the renal pelvis joins the ureter and is often caused by smooth muscle or urothelial malformation or by scarring that leads to hydronephrosis.
6. A dysplastic kidney is the result of abnormal differentiation of renal tissues. A hypoplastic kidney is small with a decreased number of nephrons.
7. Polycystic kidney disease is a cystic genetic disorder resulting in multiple, bilateral renal cysts.
8. Renal agenesis is the failure of a kidney to grow or develop. The condition may be unilateral or bilateral and may occur as an isolated entity or in association with other disorders.

Glomerular Disorders

1. Glomerulonephritis is an inflammation of the glomeruli characterized by hematuria, edema, and hypertension. The cause is unknown but is often immune mediated. Glomerulonephritis may follow infections, especially those of the upper respiratory tract caused by strains of group A β-hemolytic streptococcus. Increases in glomerular capillary permeability lead to hematuria and proteinuria.
2. IgA nephropathy occurs with deposition of IgA in the glomerulus, causing glomerular injury with gross hematuria.
3. *Nephrotic syndrome* is a term used to describe a symptom complex characterized by proteinuria, hypoproteinemia, hyperlipidemia, and edema. Metabolic, biochemical, or physiochemical disturbances in the glomerular basement membrane may lead to increased permeability to protein.
4. Hemolytic uremic syndrome is an acute disorder characterized by hemolytic anemia, acute renal failure, and thrombocytopenia.

Nephroblastoma

1. Nephroblastoma (Wilms tumor) is an embryonal tumor of the kidney that usually presents between birth and 5 years of age. Survival is high following treatment by surgery, a combination of drugs, and, sometimes, radiation therapy.

Bladder Disorders

1. Urinary tract infections can result from general sepsis in the newborn but are caused by bacteria ascending the urethra in older children. The bladder alone is infected in cystitis. The infection ascends to one or both kidneys in pyelonephritis. Urinary tract anomalies may require surgical correction to prevent frequent recurrent infections.
2. Vesicoureteral reflux is the retrograde flow of bladder urine into the kidney or ureter, or both, increasing the risk for pyelonephritis. It can be unilateral or bilateral; primary or secondary.

Urinary Incontinence

1. Urinary incontinence is the involuntary passage of urine. It may occur during the day (incontinence) or at night (enuresis), or both. Maturational delay, UTIs, constipation, and many other factors may contribute.

KEY TERMS

Acute poststreptococcal glomerulonephritis (APGN), 772
Acute pyelonephritis, 775
Ask-Upmark kidney, 772
Chordee (penile torsion), 770
Chronic pyelonephritis, 775
Congenital nephrotic syndrome (Finnish type), 773
Cystitis, 774
Daytime incontinence, 776
Enuresis, 776
Epispadias, 771
Exstrophy of the bladder, 771

Focal segmental glomerulosclerosis (FSGS), 773
Glomerulonephritis, 772
Hemolytic uremic syndrome (HUS), 773
Henoch-Schönlein purpura nephritis, 773
Horseshoe kidney, 770
Hypoplastic kidney, 772
Hypospadias, 770
Immunoglobulin A (IgA) nephropathy, 773
Minimal change nephropathy (MCN) (lipoid nephrosis), 773

Nephroblastoma (Wilms tumor), 774
Oligohydramnios, 772
Polycystic kidney disease (PKD), 772
Potter syndrome, 772
Primary incontinence, 776
Primary (idiopathic) nephrotic syndrome, 773
Renal agenesis, 772
Renal aplasia, 772
Renal dysplasia, 772
Secondary incontinence, 776
Secondary nephrotic syndrome, 773

Secondary ureteropelvic junction (UPJ) obstruction, 772
Ureterocele, 772
Ureteropelvic junction (UPJ) obstruction, 772
Urethral polyp, 771
Urethral valve, 771
Urethrovesical junction obstruction, 772
Urinary incontinence, 776
Urinary tract infection (UTI), 774
Vesicoureteral reflux (VUR), 775

REFERENCES

1. Caiulo VA et al: Ultrasound mass screening for congenital anomalies of the kidney and urinary tract, *Pediatr Nephrol* 27(6):949-953, 2012.
2. Natsis K et al: Horseshoe kidney: a review of anatomy and pathology, *Surg Radiol Anat* 36(6):517-526, 2013.
3. Harambat J et al: Epidemiology of chronic kidney disease in children, *Pediatr Nephrol* 27(3):363-373, 2012.
4. Vivante A et al: Single-gene causes of congenital anomalies of the kidney and urinary tract (CAKUT) in humans, *Pediatr Nephrol* 29(4):695-704, 2014.
5. Yosypiv IV: Congenital anomalies of the kidney and urinary tract: a genetic disorder? *Int J Nephrol* 2012:909083, 2012.
6. Montag S, Palmer LS: Abnormalities of penile curvature: chordee and penile torsion, *ScientificWorldJournal* 11:1470-1478, 2011.

7. Carmichael SL et al: Environmental and genetic contributors to hypospadias: a review of the epidemiologic evidence, *Birth Defects Res A Clin Mol Teratol* 94(7):499-510, 2012.

8. Gill SK et al: National Birth Defects Prevention Study: association between maternal age and birth defects of unknown etiology: United States, 1997-2007, *Birth Defects Res A Clin Mol Teratol* 94(12):1010-1018, 2012.

9. Springer A, Baskin LS: Timing of hypospadias repair in patients with disorders of sex development, *Endocr Dev* 27:197-202, 2014.

10. Lloyd JC et al: Contemporary epidemiological trends in complex congenital genitourinary anomalies, *J Urol* 190(4 Suppl):1590-1595, 2013.

11. Frimberger D: Diagnosis and management of epispadias, *Semin Pediatr Surg* 20(2):85-90, 2011.

12. Siffel C et al: Bladder exstrophy: an epidemiologic study from the International Clearinghouse for Birth Defects Surveillance and Research, and an overview of the literature, *Am J Med Genet C Semin Med Genet* 157C(4):321-332, 2011.

13. Inouye BM et al: Modern management of bladder exstrophy repair, *Curr Urol Rep* 14(4):359-365, 2013.

14. Akbarzadeh A et al: Congenital urethral polyps in children: report of 18 patients and review of literature, *J Pediatr Surg* 49(5):835-839, 2014.

15. Pereira PL et al: Long-term consequences of posterior urethral valves, *J Pediatr Urol* 9(5):590-596, 2013.

16. Alberti C: Congenital ureteropelvic junction obstruction: physiopathology, decoupling of tout court pelvic dilatation-obstruction semantic connection, biomarkers to predict renal damage evolution, *Eur Rev Med Pharmacol Sci* 16(2):213-219, 2012.

17. Pohl HG: Recent advances in the management of ureteroceles in infants and children: why less may be more, *Curr Opin Urol* 21(4):3227, 2011.

18. Cain JE et al: Genetics of renal hypoplasia: insights into the mechanisms controlling nephron endowment, *Pediatr Res* 68(2):91-98, 2010.

19. Prasad S et al: Ask-Upmark kidney: a report of 2 cases, *IJHSR* 3(1):61-64, 2013. Available at: www.ijhsr.org. Downloaded July 21, 2014.

20. Sweeney WE Jr, Avner ED: Pathophysiology of childhood polycystic kidney diseases: new insights into disease-specific therapy, *Pediatr Res* 75(1-2):148-157, 2014.

21. Ong AC et al; ERA-EDTA Working Group for Inherited Kidney Diseases: Autosomal dominant polycystic kidney disease: the changing face of clinical management, *Lancet* 385(9981):1993-2002, 2015.

22. Westland R et al: Clinical implications of the solitary functioning kidney, *Clin J Am Soc Nephrol* 9(5):978-986, 2014.

23. Shastry SM et al: Potter's sequence, *J Clin Neonatol* 1(3):157-159, 2012.

24. Rizvi SA et al: Pediatric kidney transplantation in the developing world: challenges and solutions, *Am J Transplant* 13(9):2441-2449, 2013.

25. Stratta P et al: New trends of an old disease: the acute post infectious glomerulonephritis at the beginning of the new millennium, *J Nephrol* 27(3):229-239, 2014.

26. Nast CC: Infection-related glomerulonephritis: changing demographics and outcomes, *Adv Chronic Kidney Dis* 19(2):68-75, 2012.

27. Wyatt RJ, Julian BA: IgA nephropathy, *N Engl J Med* 368(25):2402-2414, 2013.

28. Floege J, Gröne HJ: Recurrent IgA nephropathy in the renal allograft: not a benign condition, *Nephrol Dial Transplant* 28(5):1070-1073, 2013.

29. Davin JC, Coppo R: Henoch-Schönlein purpura nephritis in children, *Nat Rev Nephrol* 10(10):563-73, 2014.

30. Sinha A, Bagga A: Nephrotic syndrome, *Indian J Pediatr* 79(8):1045-1055, 2012.

31. Cadnapaphornchai MA et al: The nephrotic syndrome: pathogenesis and treatment of edema formation and secondary complications, *Pediatr Nephrol* 29(7):1159-1167, 2014.

32. Avni EF et al: Update on congenital nephrotic syndromes and the contribution of US, *Pediatr Radiol* 41(1):76-81, 2011.

33. Rheault MN: Nephrotic and nephritic syndrome in the newborn, *Clin Perinatol* 41(3):605-618, 2014.

34. Petruzziello-Pellegrini TN, Marsden PA: Shiga toxin-associated hemolytic uremic syndrome: advances in pathogenesis and therapeutics, *Curr Opin Nephrol Hypertens* 21(4):433-440, 2012.

35. Trachtman H: HUS and TTP in children, *Pediatr Clin North Am* 60(6):1513-1526, 2013.

36. Rosales A et al: Need for long-term follow-up in enterohemorrhagic Escherichia coli-associated hemolytic uremic syndrome due to late-emerging sequelae, *Clin Infect Dis* 54(10):1413-1421, 2012.

37. Ward E et al: Childhood and adolescent cancer statistics, 2014, *CA Cancer J Clin* 64(2):83-103, 2014.

38. Chu A et al: Wilms' tumour: a systematic review of risk factors and meta-analysis, *Paediatr Perinat Epidemiol* 24(5):449-469, 2010.

39. National Cancer Institute: *Wilms tumor and other childhood kidney tumors treatment–for health professionals (PDQ®)*. Updated May 14, 2015. Available at http://www.cancer.gov/types/kidney/hp/wilms-treatment-pdq#section/_1.

40. Dumoucel S et al: Malformations, genetic abnormalities, and Wilms tumor, *Pediatr Blood Cancer* 61(1):140-144, 2014.

41. Davidoff AM: Wilms tumor, *Adv Pediatr* 59(1):247-267, 2012.

42. Kembhavi SA et al: Understanding the principles in management of Wilms' tumour: can imaging assist in patient selection? *Clin Radiol* 68(7):646-653, 2013.

43. Termuhlen AM et al: Twenty-five year follow-up of childhood Wilms tumor: a report from the Childhood Cancer Survivor Study, *Pediatr Blood Cancer* 57(7):1210-1216, 2011.

44. Becknell B et al: The diagnosis, evaluation and treatment of acute and recurrent pediatric urinary tract infections, *Expert Rev Anti Infect Ther* 13(1):81-90, 2015.

45. Ragnarsdóttir B, Svanborg C: Susceptibility to acute pyelonephritis or asymptomatic bacteriuria: host-pathogen interaction in urinary tract infections, *Pediatr Nephrol* 7(11):2017-2029, 2012.

46. Mutlu M et al: Urinary tract infections in neonates with jaundice in their first two weeks of life, *World J Pediatr* 10(2):164-167, 2014.

47. Fitzgerald A et al: Antibiotics for treating lower urinary tract infection in children, *Cochrane Database Syst Rev* 8:CD006857, 2012.

48. Hunziker M, Puri P: Familial vesicoureteral reflux and reflux related morbidity in relatives of index patients with high grade vesicoureteral reflux, *J Urol* 188(4 Suppl):1463-1466, 2012.

49. Lebowitz RL et al: International system of radiographic grading of vesicoureteric reflux. International Reflux Study in Children, *Pediatr Radiol* 15(2):105-109, 1985.

50. Tullus K: Vesicoureteric reflux in children, *Lancet* 385(9965):371-379, 2015.

51. Altobelli E et al: Vesicoureteral reflux in pediatric age: where are we today? *Urologia* 81(2):76-87, 2014

52. Buckley BS, Lapitan MC: Prevalence of urinary incontinence in men, women, and children—current evidence: findings of the Fourth International Consultation on Incontinence, *Urology* 76(2):265-270, 2010.

53. Mellon MW et al: Incidence of enuresis and encopresis among children with attention-deficit/hyperactivity disorder in a population-based birth cohort, *Acad Pediatr* 13(4):322-327, 2013.

54. Weintraub Y et al: Enuresis—an unattended comorbidity of childhood obesity, *Int J Obes (Lond)* 37(1):75-78, 2013.

55. Su MS et al: Nocturnal enuresis in children: prevalence, correlates, and relationship with obstructive sleep apnea, *J Pediatr* 159(2):238-242, 2011.

56. Burgers RE et al: Management of functional constipation in children with lower urinary tract symptoms: report from the Standardization Committee of the International Children's Continence Society, *J Urol* 190(1):29-36, 2013.

57. von Gontard A et al: Family history of nocturnal enuresis and urinary incontinence: results from a large epidemiological study, *J Urol* 185(6):2303-2306, 2011.

58. Maternik M et al: The management of childhood urinary incontinence, *Pediatr Nephrol* 30(1):41-50, 2014.

32

Structure and Function of the Reproductive Systems

Afsoon Moktar, George W. Rodway, and Sue E. Huether

EVOLVE WEBSITE

http://evolve.elsevier.com/Huether/
Student Review Questions
Audio Key Points

Case Studies
Animations
Quick Check Answers

CHAPTER OUTLINE

The male and female reproductive systems have several anatomic and physiologic features in common. Most obvious is their major function—reproduction—through which a 23-chromosome female gamete, the ovum, and a 23-chromosome male gamete, the **spermatozoon (sperm cell)**, unite to form a 46-chromosome zygote that is capable of developing into a new individual. The male reproductive system produces sperm that can be transferred to the female reproductive tract. The female reproductive system produces the **ovum** (pl., **ova**), and if the ovum is fertilized it is then called the embryo and developing fetus. These functions are determined not only by anatomic structures but also by complex hormonal and neurologic factors.[1,2]

DEVELOPMENT OF THE REPRODUCTIVE SYSTEMS

The structure and function of both male and female reproductive systems depend on steroid hormones called **sex hormones** and their precursors. Cholesterol is the precursor for steroid hormones, including the sex hormones. Other hormones support reproduction. The actions of both sex and reproductive hormones are summarized in Table 32-1. Sex hormones, like all hormones, act on target tissues by binding with cellular receptors (see Chapter 18). Hormonal effects on the reproductive systems begin during embryonic development and continue in varying degrees throughout life.

Sexual Differentiation in Utero

Initially, in embryonic development, the reproductive structures of male and female embryos are homologous (the same) or undifferenti-

ated. They consist of one pair of primary sex organs, or **gonads**, and two pairs of ducts—the mesonephric ducts (wolffian ducts) and the paramesonephric ducts (müllerian ducts) (Figure 32-1). The müllerian ducts are the precursor of the internal female sex organs (oviducts, uterus, cervix, and upper vagina). Müllerian ducts are initially formed regardless of genotypic sex and require no *SRY* signaling for development. *SRY* signaling is required in males to cause regression of the müllerian ducts, which in turn prevents the development of the female reproductive tract. The wolffian ducts are the precursor of male internal sex organs (secrete testosterone and promote development of the male sex organs).

The first sign of development of reproductive organs (male or female) occurs during the fifth week of gestation. Between 6 and 7 weeks' gestation, the male embryo will differentiate under the influence of testes-determining factor (TDF), a protein expressed by a gene in the sex-determining region on the Y chromosome *(SRY)*. When the *SRY* gene is expressed, male gonadal development prevails. TDF stimulates the male gonads to develop into the two testes, and by 8 weeks' gestation testosterone secretion begins. Müllerian inhibitory hormone (MIF), secreted by Sertoli cells in the testes, promotes degeneration of the müllerian ducts. Without MIF, the müllerian ducts would develop and the wolffian ducts would degenerate with loss of male sex organ development. By 9 months' gestation, the male gonads (testes) have descended into the scrotum. The testes produce sperm after puberty.

Female gonadal development occurs in the absence of *SRY* expression and with the expression of other genes.[3] The presence of *estrogen* and the absence of *testosterone* and MIF cause a loss in the wolffian

TABLE 32-1	**Summary of Female and Male Sex and Reproductive Hormones**	
Hormone (Source)	**Action in Females**	**Action in Males**
Dehydroepiandrosterone (DHEA) (adrenal gland, ovary, other tissues)	Converted to androstenedione and then to estrogens, testosterone, or both	Converted to androstenedione and then to estrogens, testosterone, or both
Estrogens (estrone, estradiol, estriol) function through estrogen receptors alpha and beta (ovary and placenta, small amounts in other tissues)	Stimulates development of female sexual characteristics: maturation of breast, uterus, and vagina; promotes proliferative development of endometrium during menstrual cycle; during pregnancy promotes mammary gland development, fetal adrenal gland function, and uteroplacental blood flow (see Box 32-1)	Growth at puberty, growth plate fusion in bone, prevention of apoptosis of germ cells
Testosterone (adrenal glands from DHEA, ovaries)	Libido, learning, sleep, protein anabolism, growth of muscle and bone; growth of pubic and axillary hair; activation of sebaceous glands, accounting for some cases of acne during puberty	Stimulates spermatogenesis, stimulates development of primary and secondary sexual characteristics, promotes growth of muscle and bone (anabolic effect); growth of pubic and axillary hair; activates sebaceous glands, accounting for some cases of acne during puberty; maintains libido
Gonadotropin-releasing hormone (GnRH) (hypothalamus-neuroendocrine cells)	Stimulates secretion of gonadotropins (FSH and LH) from anterior pituitary	Stimulates secretion of gonadotropins (FSH and LH) from anterior pituitary
Follicle-stimulating hormone (FSH) (anterior pituitary, gonadotroph cells)	Gonadotropin; promotes development of ovarian follicle; stimulates estrogen secretion	Gonadotropin; promotes development of testes and stimulates spermatogenesis by Sertoli cells
Luteinizing hormone (LH) (anterior pituitary, gonadotroph cells)	Gonadotropin; triggers ovulation; promotes development of corpus luteum	Gonadotropin; stimulates testosterone production by Leydig cells of testis
Inhibin (ovary and testes)	Inhibits FSH production in anterior pituitary (perhaps by limiting GnRH)	Inhibits FSH production in anterior pituitary
Human chorionic gonadotropin (hCG) (placenta)	Supports corpus luteum, which secretes estrogen and progesterone during first 7 weeks of pregnancy	
Activin (ovary)	Stimulates secretion of FSH and pituitary response to GnRH and FSH binding in dominant granulosa cells	
Progesterone (ovary and placenta)	Promotes secretory changes in endometrium during luteal phase of menstrual cycle; quiets uterine myometrium (muscle) activity and prevents lactogenesis during pregnancy	
Relaxin (corpus luteum, myometrium and placenta)	Inhibits uterine contractions during pregnancy and softens pelvic joints and cervix to facilitate childbirth	

system, and at 6 to 8 weeks' gestation the two female gonads develop into ovaries, which will produce ova. In females, the mesonephric ducts deteriorate and the upper ends of paramesonephric ducts become the fallopian tubules, whereas the lower ends join to become the uterus, cervix, and upper two thirds of the vagina (see Figure 32-1). The fallopian tubes will carry ova from the ovaries to the uterus during a woman's reproductive years. Lack of testosterone and the presence of estrogen promote the development of external genitalia (lower end of vagina, labia, and clitoris).

Like the internal reproductive structures, the external structures develop from homologous embryonic tissues. During the first 7 to 8 weeks' gestation, both male and female embryos develop an elevated structure called the *genital tubercle* (Figure 32-2). Testosterone is necessary for the genital tubercle to differentiate into external male genitalia; otherwise, female genitalia develop, which may occur even in the absence of ovaries, possibly because of the presence of placental estrogens.

Anterior pituitary development begins between the fourth and fifth weeks of fetal life, and the vascular connection between the hypothalamus and the pituitary is established by the twelfth week. Gonadotropin-releasing hormone (GnRH) is produced in the hypothalamus by 10 weeks' gestation and controls the production of two gonadotropins, luteinizing hormone (LH) and follicle-stimulating hormone (FSH), by the anterior pituitary gland. In the female fetus, high levels of FSH

and LH are excreted. FSH and LH stimulate the production of estrogen and progesterone by the ovary. The production of FSH and LH increases until about 28 weeks' gestation, when the production of estrogen and progesterone by the ovaries and placenta is high enough to result in the decline of gonadotropin production.[4] Production of primitive female gametes (ova) occurs solely during fetal life. From puberty to menopause, one female gamete matures per menstrual cycle. Production of the male gametes (sperm) begins at puberty; after that, millions are produced daily, usually for life.

By the end of pregnancy, a sensitive negative feedback system, which includes the gonadostat (also known as the gonadotropin-releasing hormone pulse generator), is operative in the human fetus. The gonadostat responds to high levels of placental estrogens by releasing low levels of GnRH. Soon after birth, steroid hormone levels drop because of the loss of maternal placental hormones. Hypothalamic pulsatile GnRH is secreted and gonadotropins LH and FSH are released; their levels peak at 3 to 6 months for boys and at 12 to 18 months for girls and then fall steadily. The gonadotropins will be suppressed until the onset of puberty.

Puberty and Reproductive Maturation

Puberty is the onset of sexual maturation and differs from adolescence. Adolescence is the stage of human development between childhood and adulthood and includes social, psychologic, and biologic changes.

FIGURE 32-1 Internal Genitalia Development. Embryonic and fetal development of the internal genitalia. *MIF,* Müllerian inhibitory factor; *SRY,* gene that produces TDF; *TDF,* testosterone development factor; see text for additional details.

In girls, puberty begins at about age 8 to 9 years with thelarche (breast development). In boys, it begins later—at about age 11 years and occurs earlier with increased weight and body mass index.[5] Genetics, environment, ethnicity, general health, and nutrition can influence the timing of puberty. There is an association between obesity and earlier puberty in girls perhaps from higher estrogen levels related to leptin, gonadotropin, and estrogen secretion.[6] Girls who have low body fat and reduced body weight and perform intense exercise may experience delayed maturation.[7]

Reproductive maturation involves the hypothalamic-pituitary-gonadal axis, the central nervous system, and the endocrine system (Figure 32-3). There is a sequential series of hormonal events that promote sexual maturation as puberty approaches. About 1 year before puberty in girls, nocturnal pulses of gonadotropin secretion (i.e., LH and FSH) and an increased response in the pituitary to GnRH occur. This, in turn, stimulates gonadal maturation (**gonadarche**) with estradiol secretion in girls and testosterone secretion in boys. Estradiol causes development of the breasts (**thelarche**), maturation

of the reproductive organs (vagina, uterus, ovaries), and deposition of fat in the female's hips. Estrogen and increased production of growth factors cause rapid skeletal growth in both boys and girls. Testosterone causes growth of the testes, scrotum, and penis. A positive feedback loop is created with gonadotropins stimulating the gonads to produce more sex hormones. The most important hormonal effects occur in the gonads. In males, the testes begin to produce mature sperm that are capable of fertilizing an ovum. Male puberty is complete with the first ejaculation that contains mature sperm. In females, the ovaries begin to release mature ova. Female puberty is complete at the time of the first ovulatory menstrual period; however, this can take up to 1 to 2 years after menarche. **Adrenarche** is the increased production of adrenal **androgens** (dehydroepiandrosterone and androstenedione, which are converted to testosterone and estrogen) before puberty, which occurs in both sexes and is manifested by growth of axillary and pubic hair and activation of sweat and sebaceous glands. Puberty is complete when an individual is capable of reproduction.

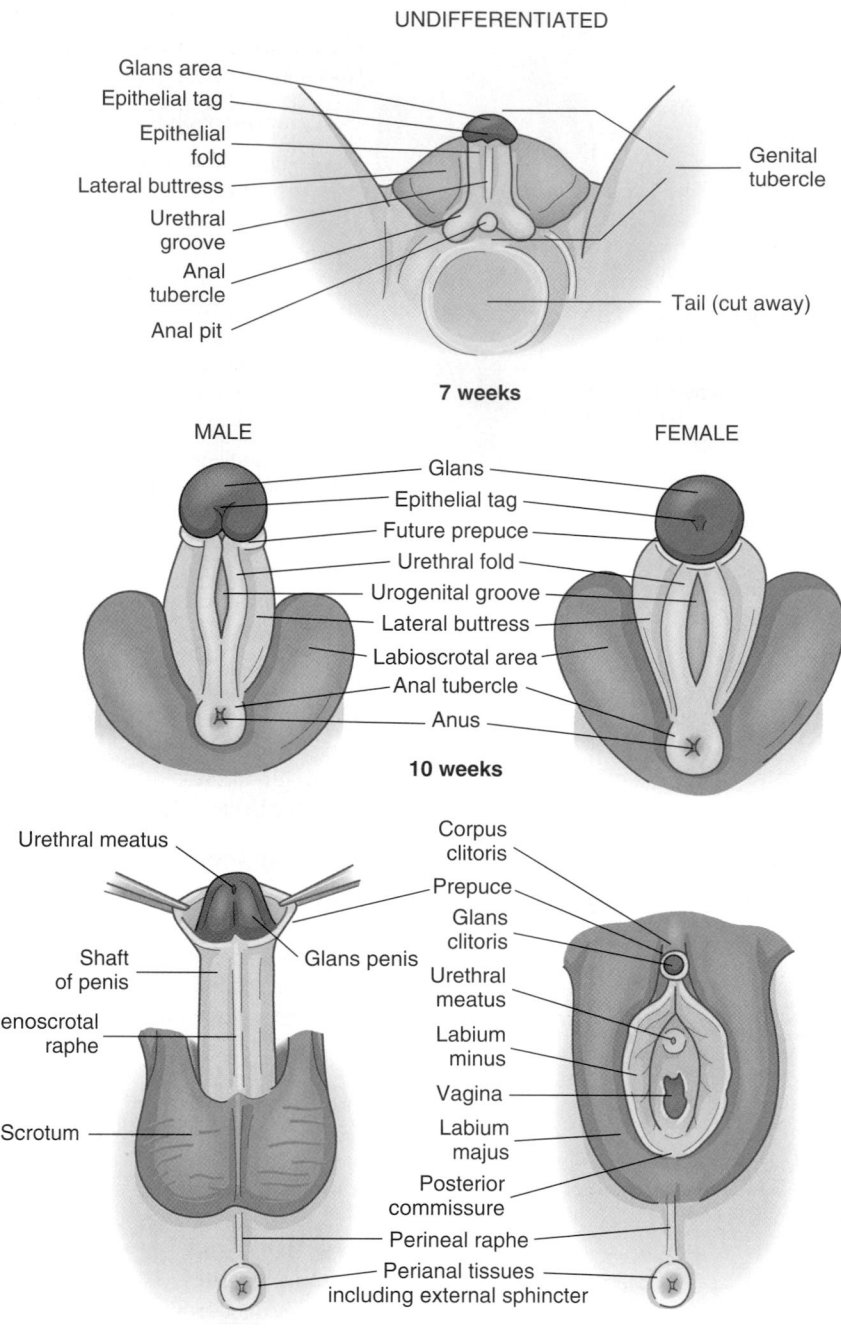

UNDIFFERENTIATED

7 weeks

10 weeks

Near 40 weeks

FIGURE 32-2 External Genitalia Development. Embryonic and fetal development of the external genitalia.

> **QUICK CHECK 32-1**
> 1. When do sex hormones first exhibit an effect on sexual development?
> 2. Why are sex hormones necessary for reproduction?

THE FEMALE REPRODUCTIVE SYSTEM

The function of the female reproductive system is to produce mature ova; if fertilization occurs, the female reproductive system provides protection and nourishment of the fetus until it is expelled at birth.

The most important internal reproductive organs in females are the ovaries, fallopian tubes, uterus, and vagina. The external genitalia protect body openings and play an important role in sexual functioning.

External Genitalia

Figure 32-4 shows the external female genitalia, known collectively as the **vulva**, or pudendum. The major structures are as follows:

Mons pubis: Fatty layer of tissue over pubic symphysis (joint formed by union of the pubic bones). During puberty it becomes covered with pubic hair, and sebaceous and sweat glands become more

FIGURE 32-3 Hormonal Stimulation of the Gonads. The hypothalamic-pituitary-gonadal axis.

active. Estrogen causes fat to be deposited under the skin, gives the mons pubis a moundlike shape, and protects the pubic symphysis during sexual intercourse.

Labia majora (sing., labium majus): Two folds of skin arising at the mons pubis and extending back to the fourchette, forming a cleft. During puberty the amount of fatty tissue increases, pubic hair grows on lateral surfaces, and sebaceous glands on hairless medial surfaces secrete lubricants. This structure is highly sensitive to temperature, touch, pressure, and pain; it is homologous to the male scrotum; and it protects the inner structures of the vulva.

Labia minora (sing., labium minus): Two smaller, thinner, asymmetric folds of skin within the labia majora that form the clitoral hood (prepuce) and frenulum, then split to enclose the vestibule, and converge near the anus to form the fourchette. The labia minora are hairless, pink, and moist; they are well supplied by nerves, blood vessels, and sebaceous glands that secrete bactericidal fluid with a distinctive odor that lubricates and waterproofs vulvar skin. The labia swell with blood during sexual arousal.

Clitoris: Richly innervated erectile organ between the labia minora. It is a small, cylindric structure having a visible glans and a shaft that lies beneath the skin; the clitoris is homologous to the penis. It secretes smegma, which has a unique odor that may be sexually arousing to the male. Like the penis, the clitoris is a major site of

sexual stimulation and orgasm. With sexual arousal, erectile tissue fills with blood, causing the clitoris to enlarge slightly.

Vestibule: An area protected by the labia minora that contains the external opening of the vagina, called the *introitus* or vaginal orifice. A thin, perforated membrane, the *hymen,* may cover the introitus. The vestibule also contains the opening of the urethra, or *urinary meatus* (orifice). These structures are lubricated by two pairs of glands: Skene glands and Bartholin glands. The ducts of the *Skene glands* (also called the *lesser vestibular* or *paraurethral glands*) open on both sides of the urinary meatus. The ducts of the *Bartholin glands (greater vestibular* or *vulvovaginal glands)* open on either side of the introitus. In response to sexual stimulation, Bartholin glands secrete mucus that lubricates the inner labial surfaces, as well as enhances the viability and motility of sperm. Skene glands help lubricate the urinary meatus and the vestibule. Secretions from both sets of glands facilitate coitus. In response to sexual excitement, the highly vascular tissue just beneath the vestibule also fills with blood and becomes engorged.

Perineum: An area with less hair, skin, and subcutaneous tissue lying between the vaginal orifice and anus. Unlike the rest of the vulva, this area has little subcutaneous fat so the skin is close to the underlying muscles. The perineum covers the muscular *perineal body,* a fibrous structure that consists of elastic fibers and connective tissue and serves as the common attachment for the bulbocavernosus, external anal sphincter, and levator ani muscles. The perineum varies in length from 2 to 5 cm or more and has elastic properties. The length of the perineum and the elasticity of the perineal body influence tissue resistance and injury during childbirth.

Internal Genitalia
Vagina

The **vagina** is an elastic, fibromuscular canal that is 9 to 10 cm long in a reproductive-age female. It extends up and back from the introitus to the lower portion of the uterus. As Figure 32-5 shows, the vagina lies between the urethra (and part of the bladder) and the rectum. Mucosal secretions from the upper genital organs, menstrual fluids, and products of conception leave the body through the vagina, which also receives the penis during coitus. During sexual excitement, the vagina lengthens and widens and the anterior third becomes congested with blood.

The vaginal wall is composed of four layers:
1. Mucous membrane lining of squamous epithelial cells that thickens and thins in response to hormones, particularly estrogen. The squamous epithelial membrane is continuous with the membrane that covers the lower part of the uterus. In women of reproductive age, the mucosal layer is arranged in transverse wrinkles, or folds, called **rugae** (sing., **ruga**) that permit stretching during coitus and childbirth
2. Fibrous connective tissue containing numerous blood and lymphatic vessels
3. Smooth muscle
4. Connective tissue and a rich network of blood vessels

The upper part of the vagina surrounds the cervix, the lower end of the uterus (see Figure 32-5). The recessed space around the cervix is called the **fornix** of the vagina. The posterior fornix is "deeper" than the anterior fornix because of the angle at which the cervix meets the vaginal canal. In most women this angle is about 90 degrees. A pouch called the **cul-de-sac** separates the posterior fornix and the rectum.

Its elasticity and relatively sparse nerve supply enhance the vagina's function as the birth canal. During sexual arousal, the vaginal wall becomes engorged with blood, like the labia minora and clitoris. Engorgement pushes some fluid to the surface of the mucosa,

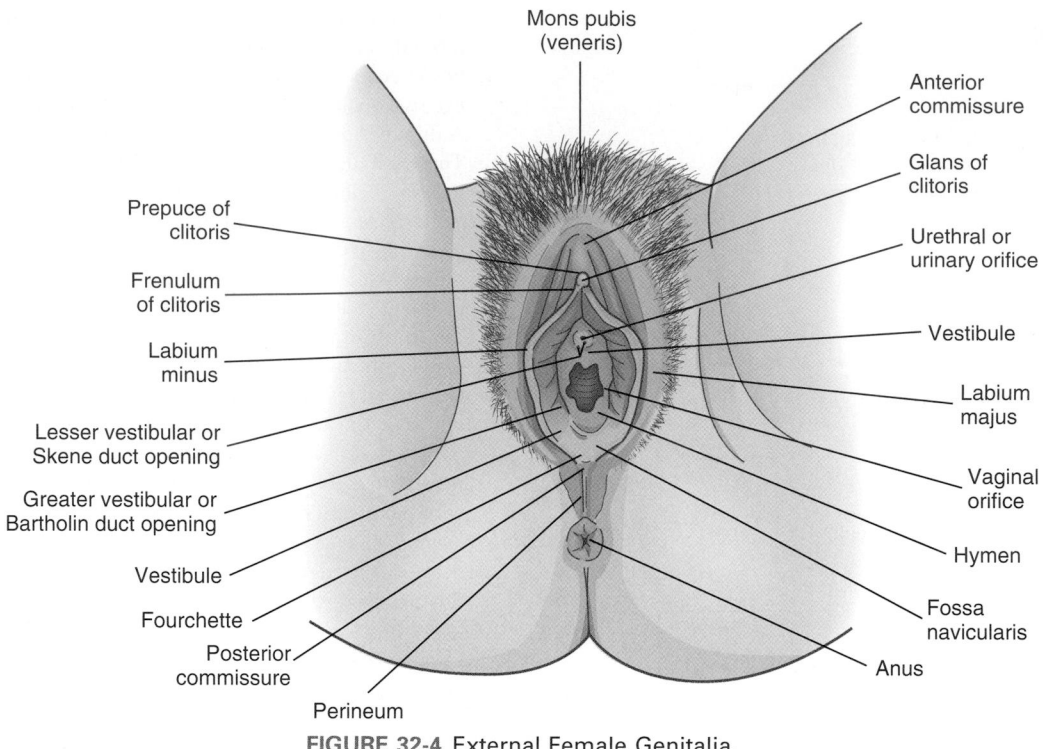

FIGURE 32-4 External Female Genitalia.

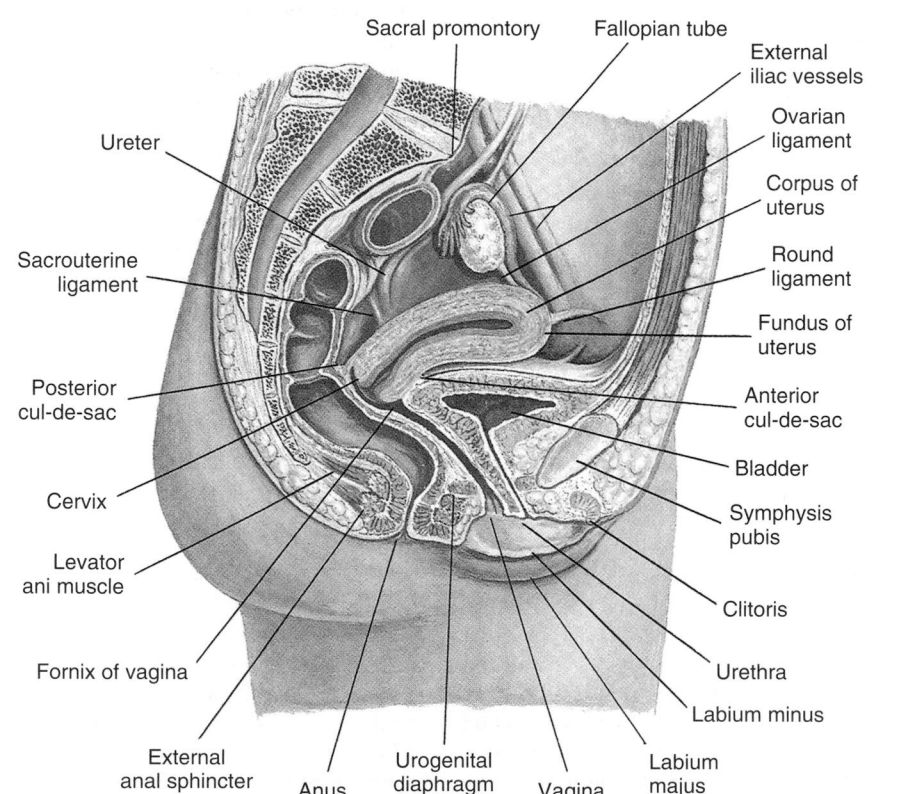

FIGURE 32-5 Internal Female Genitalia and Other Pelvic Organs. (From Ball JW et al: *Seidel's guide to physical examination,* ed 8, St Louis, 2015, Mosby.)

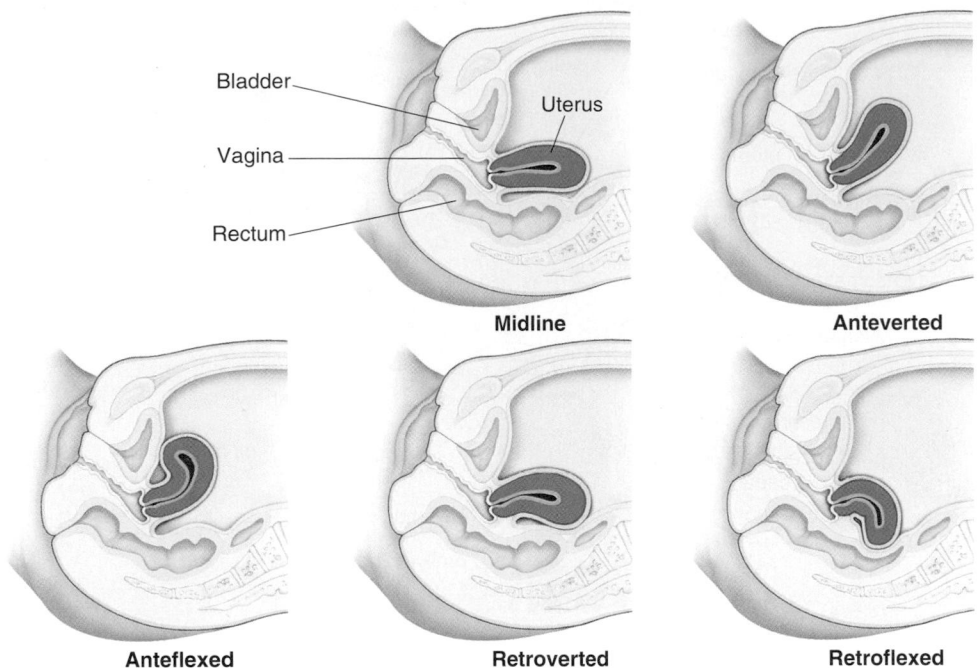

Bladder

Vagina

Rectum

Uterus

Midline

Anteverted

Anteflexed

Retroverted

Retroflexed

FIGURE 32-6 Variations in Uterine Positions.

enhancing lubrication. The vaginal wall does not contain mucus-secreting glands; rather, secretions drain into the vagina from the endocervical glands or from the Bartholin and Skene glands of the vestibule.

Two factors help to maintain the self-cleansing action of the vagina and to defend it from infection, particularly during the reproductive years. They are (1) an acid-base balance that discourages the proliferation of most pathogenic bacteria and (2) the thickness of the vaginal epithelium. Before puberty, vaginal pH is about 7.0 (neutral) and the vaginal epithelium is thin. At puberty, the pH becomes more acidic (4.0 to 5.0) and the squamous epithelial lining thickens. These changes are maintained until menopause (cessation of menstruation), when the pH rises again to more alkaline levels and the epithelium thins. Therefore protection from infection is greatest during the years when a woman is most likely to be sexually active. Both defense factors are greatest when estrogen levels are high and the vagina contains a normal population of *Lactobacillus acidophilus*, a harmless resident bacterium that helps to maintain pH at acidic levels. Any condition that causes vaginal pH to rise—such as douching or use of vaginal sprays or deodorants, the presence of low estrogen levels, or destruction of *L. acidophilus* by antibiotics—lowers vaginal defenses against infection.

Uterus

The **uterus** is a hollow, pear-shaped organ whose lower end opens into the vagina. It anchors and protects a fertilized ovum, provides an optimal environment while the ovum develops, and pushes the fetus out at birth. In addition, the uterus plays an important role in sexual response and conception. During sexual excitement, the opening of the lower uterus (the cervix) dilates slightly. At the same time, the uterus increases in size and moves upward and backward, creating a tenting effect in the midvagina that results in the cervix "sitting" in a pool of semen. During orgasm, rhythmic contractions facilitate movement of sperm through the cervical os while also enhancing physical pleasure.

At puberty, the uterus attains its adult size and proportions and descends from the abdomen to the lower pelvis, between the bladder and the rectum (see Figure 32-5). The uterus of a mature, nonpregnant female is approximately 7 to 9 cm long and 6.5 cm wide, with muscular walls 3.5 cm thick, and enlarges about 1 cm in all dimensions after pregnancy.[8] It is loosely held in position by ligaments, peritoneal tissue folds, and the pressure of adjacent organs, especially the urinary bladder, sigmoid colon, and rectum. In most women, the uterus is tipped forward (anteverted) so that it rests on the urinary bladder; however, it may be tipped backward (retroverted). Various degrees of flexion are normal (Figure 32-6).

The uterus has two major parts: the body, or **corpus**, and the cervix (Figure 32-7). The top of the corpus, above the insertion of the fallopian tubes, is called the **fundus**. The diameter of the uterine cavity is widest at the fundus and narrowest at the **isthmus**, just above the **cervix** (see Figure 32-5). The cervix, or "neck of the uterus," extends from the isthmus to the vagina. The passageway between the upper opening (the internal os) and the lower opening (the external os) of the cervix is called the **endocervical canal** (see Figure 32-7). The entire uterus, like the upper vagina, is innervated exclusively by motor and sensory fibers of the autonomic nervous system.

The uterine wall is composed of three layers (see Figure 32-7). The **perimetrium (parietal peritoneum)** is the outer serous membrane that covers the uterus. The **myometrium** is the thick, muscular middle layer. It is thickest at the fundus, apparently to facilitate birth. The **endometrium**, or uterine lining, is composed of a functional layer (superficial compact layer and spongy middle layer) and a basal layer. The functional layer of the endometrium responds to the sex hormones estrogen and progesterone. Between puberty and menopause, this layer proliferates and is shed monthly. The basal layer, which is attached to the myometrium, regenerates the functional layer after shedding (menstruation).

The endocervical canal does not have an endometrial layer but is lined with columnar epithelial cells. It is continuous with the lining of

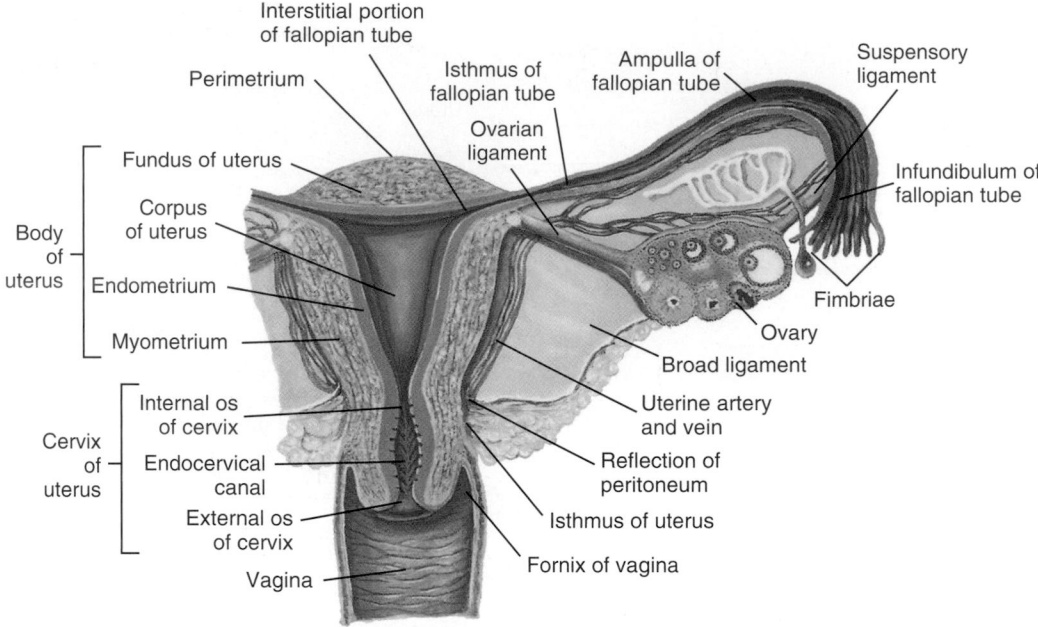

FIGURE 32-7 Cross Section of Uterus, Fallopian Tube, and Ovary. (From Ball JW et al: *Seidel's guide to physical examination,* ed 8, St Louis, 2015, Mosby.)

the outer cervix and vagina, which are lined with squamous epithelial cells. The point where the two types of cells meet is called the *transformation zone,* or **squamous-columnar junction**. The transformation zone is vulnerable to the human papillomavirus, which can lead to cervical dysplasia or carcinoma in situ (see Figure 33-16). Cells of the transformation zone are removed for examination during a Papanicolaou (Pap test) smear.[8]

The cervix acts as a mechanical barrier to infectious microorganisms from the vagina. The external cervical os is a very small opening that contains thick, sticky mucus (the mucous "plug") during the luteal phase of the menstrual cycle and throughout pregnancy. During ovulation, the mucus changes under the influence of estrogen and forms watery strands, or **spinnbarkeit mucus**, to facilitate the transport of sperm into the uterus. In addition, the downward flow of cervical secretions moves microorganisms away from the cervix and uterus. In women of reproductive age, the pH of these secretions is inhospitable to many bacteria. Further, mucosal secretions contain enzymes and antibodies (mostly immunoglobulin A [IgA]) of the secretory immune system. Uterine pathophysiologic disorders include infection, displacement of the uterus within the pelvis, benign growths (fibroids) of the uterine wall, hyperplasia of the endometrium, endometriosis, and cancer (see Chapter 33).

✔ QUICK CHECK 32-2

1. Name three functions of the uterus.
2. Where are the Bartholin glands located? What is their function?
3. What is the name of the cells in which cervical cancer is most likely to grow?

Fallopian Tubes

The two **fallopian tubes** (oviducts, **uterine tubes**) enter the uterus bilaterally just beneath the fundus (see Figure 32-7). They direct the ova from the spaces around the ovaries to the uterus. From the uterus,

the fallopian tubes curve up and over the two ovaries. Each tube is 8 to 12 cm long and about 1 cm in diameter, except at its ovarian end, which resembles the bell of a trumpet and is fringed or fimbriated (**infundibulum**). The fimbriae (fringes) move, creating a current that draws the ovum into the infundibulum. Once the ovum enters the fallopian tube, cilia (hairlike structures) and peristalsis (muscle contractions) keep it moving toward the uterus.

The ampulla, or distal third, of the fallopian tube is the usual site of fertilization (see Figure 32-7). Sperm released into the vagina travel upward through the endocervical canal and uterine cavity and enter the fallopian tubes. If an ovum is present in either tube, fertilization can occur. Whether or not the ovum encounters sperm, it continues to travel through the fallopian tube to the uterus. If fertilized, the ovum (then called a *blastocyst*) implants itself in the endometrial layer of the uterine wall. If not fertilized, the ovum fragments and leaves the uterus with menstrual fluids. Disorders that affect the fallopian tubes (e.g., congenital malformations, infection, and inflammation) block the path of both sperm and the ovum and may cause infertility or ectopic (tubal) pregnancy.

Ovaries

The **ovaries**, the female gonads, are the primary female reproductive organs (Figure 32-8). Their two main functions are secretion of female sex hormones and development and release of female gametes, or ova.

The almond-shaped ovaries are located on both sides of the uterus and are suspended and supported by the mesovarium portions of the broad ligament, ovarian ligaments, and suspensory ligaments (see Figure 32-7). The ovaries are smaller than their male homologs, the testes. In women of reproductive age, each ovary is about 3 to 5 cm long, 2.5 cm wide, and 2 cm thick and weighs 4 to 8 g. Size and weight vary slightly during each phase of the menstrual cycle (see pp. 788-790).

At birth, the cortex of each ovary contains approximately 1 to 2 million ova within primordial (immature) **ovarian follicles**. By puberty, the number ranges between 300,000 and 500,000, and some of the follicles and the ova within them begin to mature. Between

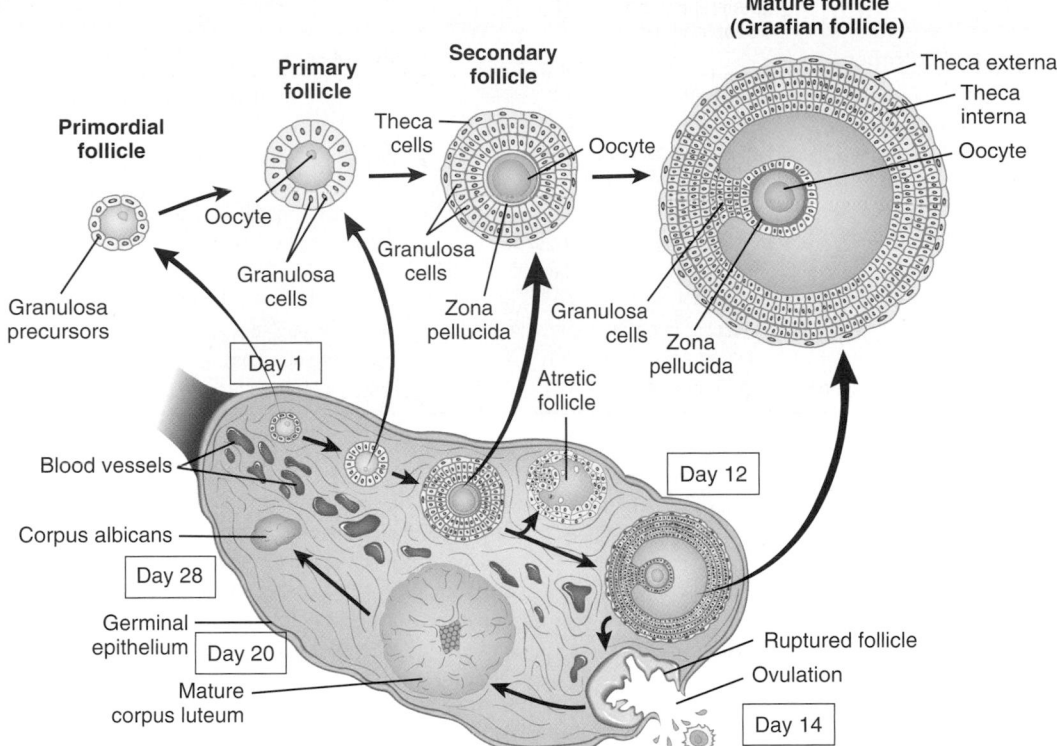

FIGURE 32-8 Cross Section of Ovary and Development of an Ovarian Follicle. Schematic representation (not to scale) of the structure of the ovary, showing the various stages in the development of the follicle and its successor structure, the corpus luteum. (Adapted from Berne RM, Levy MN, editors: *Physiology*, ed 5, St Louis, 2003, Mosby.)

puberty and menopause, the ovarian cortex always contains follicles and ova in various stages of development (primary and secondary follicles). Once every menstrual cycle (about every 28 days), one of the follicles reaches maturation and discharges its ovum through the ovary's outer covering, the germinal epithelium. During the reproductive years, 400 to 500 ovarian follicles mature completely and release an ovum (ovulation). The remaining follicles either fail to develop at all or degenerate without maturing completely and are known as atretic follicles[8] (see Figure 32-8).

After release of the mature ovum (ovulation), the follicle develops into another structure, the corpus luteum (see Figure 32-8). If fertilization occurs, the corpus luteum enlarges and begins to secrete hormones that maintain and support pregnancy. If fertilization does not occur, the corpus luteum secretes these hormones for approximately 14 days and then degenerates, which triggers the maturation of another follicle. The ovarian cycle—the process of follicular maturation, ovulation, corpus luteum development, and corpus luteum degeneration—is continuous from puberty to menopause, except during pregnancy or hormonal contraceptive use. At menopause, this process ceases and the ovaries atrophy to the point that they cannot be felt during a pelvic examination.

Sex hormones are secreted by cells present within the ovarian cortex, including two types of cells in the ovarian follicle—theca cells (produce androgens that migrate to granulosa cells) and granulosa cells (convert androgens to estradiol)—and cells of the corpus luteum (secrete primarily progesterone, estrogen, and inhibin) (see Figure 32-8). These cells all contain receptors for the gonadotropins (LH, FSH) or for the sex hormones, which are discussed in the next section.

Female Sex Hormones

The sex hormones are all steroid hormones and are synthesized from cholesterol (see Chapter 18). Both male and female sex hormones are present in all adults. However, the female body contains low levels of testosterone and other androgens, and the male body contains low levels of estrogen. Individual effects of sex hormones depend on the amount and concentration in the blood.

Estrogens and Androgens

Estrogen is a generic term for any of three similar hormones derived from cholesterol: estradiol, estrone, and estriol. Estradiol (E_2) is the most potent and plentiful of the three and is principally produced (95%) by the ovaries (ovarian follicle and corpus luteum). Limited amounts are secreted by the cortices of the adrenal glands and the placenta during pregnancy. Androgens are converted to estrone in ovarian and adipose tissue; estriol is the peripheral metabolite of estrone and estradiol.

Estrogen has numerous biologic effects, many of which involve interactions with other hormones. It is needed for maturation of reproductive organs, development of secondary sex characteristics, growth, and maintenance of pregnancy, as well as the many nonreproductive effects of estrogen, including closure of long bones after the pubertal growth spurt (in both males and females), maintenance of bone and skin, and systemic organ function (see Table 32-1 and Box 32-1). After menopause, the ovaries dramatically reduce production of estradiol and secretion of estrone is markedly diminished (see Aging and the Female Reproductive System, p. 797). At this time, the majority

TABLE 32-2 Complementary and Opposing Effects of Estrogen and Progesterone

Structure	Effect of Estrogen	Effect of Progesterone
Vaginal mucosa	Proliferation of squamous epithelium; increase in glycogen content of cells; layering (cornification) of cells	Thinning of squamous epithelium; decornification
Cervical mucosa	Production of abundant fluid secretions that favor survival and enhance motility of sperm	Production of thick, sticky secretions that tend to plug cervical os
Fallopian tube	Increase of motility and ciliary action	Decrease of motility and ciliary action
Uterine muscle	Increase of blood flow; increase of contractile proteins; increase of uterine muscle and myometrial excitability to action potential; increase of sensitization to oxytocin	Relaxation of myometrium; decrease of sensitization to oxytocin
Endometrium	Stimulation of growth; increase in number of progesterone receptors	Activation of glands and blood vessels; decrease in number of estrogen receptors
Breasts	Growth of ducts; promotion of prolactin effects	Growth of lobules and alveoli; inhibition of prolactin effects

BOX 32-1 Summary of Nonreproductive Effects of Estrogen

- Estrogens (including estrone, estradiol, estriol) function through estrogen receptors alpha and beta, have different roles in different cells and tissues, and have paracrine or intracrine function.
- Maintains bone density.
- Acts in liver to decrease cholesterol level, increase high-density lipoprotein (HDL) level, and decrease low-density lipoprotein (LDL) level (antiatherosclerotic); promotes fat deposition.
- Maintains nervous system (neurotrophic and neuroprotective); facilitates memory and cognition.
- Increases collagen content, dermal thickness, elasticity, water content, and healing ability of skin.
- Protects against chronic kidney disease in individuals without diabetes.
- Prevents vascular injury and early atheroma formation through endothelial mechanisms.
- Inhibits platelet adhesiveness.
- Can promote inflammation and have variable effects on immunity.
- Estrogen associated with pregnancy or use in contraceptive pills promotes clotting and increased risk of thromboembolism.

follicular phase, the ovary and adrenal glands each contribute approximately 50% of the progesterone production. Conversely, large amounts are cyclically secreted from the ovary while the corpus luteum is active for about 9 to 13 days after ovulation. The complementary and opposing effects of progesterone and estrogen are listed in Table 32-2. Progesterone secreted by the corpus luteum stimulates the thickened endometrium to become more complex in preparation for implantation of a blastocyte. If conception and implantation do occur, the corpus luteum persists and secretes progesterone (and estrogen) until the placenta is well established at approximately 8 to 10 weeks' gestation and undertakes progesterone production.

Progesterone is sometimes called the *hormone of pregnancy*. Progesterone's effects in pregnancy include (1) maintaining the thickened endometrium; (2) relaxing smooth muscle in the myometrium, which prevents premature contractions and helps the uterus to expand; (3) thickening (hypertrophy) the myometrium, which prepares it for the muscular work of labor; (4) promoting growth of lobules and alveoli in the breast in preparation for lactation, but preventing lactation until the fetus is born and then promoting lactation in collaboration with prolactin after birth[10]; (5) preventing additional maturation of ova by suppressing FSH and LH, thereby stopping the menstrual cycle; and (6) providing immune modulation, allowing tolerance against fetal antigens (the mother's immune system does not attack the fetus).[11]

QUICK CHECK 32-3
1. What hormones does the ovary produce?
2. Why is the ovary the most essential female reproductive organ?

of estradiol is derived from intracellular synthesis in peripheral tissues. Estradiol acts locally to meet physiologic needs according to cell type and is then inactivated without systemic effects.[9]

Although **androgens** are primarily male sex hormones produced in the testes, small amounts are produced in the adrenal cortex in both men and women, and in the ovaries in women. Some androgens (dehydroepiandrosterone and its metabolite androstenedione) are precursors of estrogens (estrone, estradiol) (see Table 32-1). At puberty, androgens contribute to the skeletal growth spurt and cause growth of pubic and axillary hair. Androgens also activate sebaceous glands, accounting for some cases of acne during puberty, and play a role in libido.

Progesterone

Luteinizing hormone (LH) from the anterior pituitary stimulates the corpus luteum to secrete progesterone, the second major female sex hormone. With estrogen, progesterone controls the ovarian menstrual cycle. LH surge occurs when there is a peak level of estrogen, about 24 to 36 hours before ovulation. LH promotes luteinization of the granulosa in the dominant follicle, resulting in progesterone production and the development of blood vessels and connective tissue. During the

Menstrual (Ovarian) Cycle

In addition to pregnancy, the obvious manifestation of female reproductive functioning is menstrual bleeding (the menses), which starts with menarche (first menstruation) and ends with menopause (cessation of menstrual flow for 1 year). In the United States, the median age of first menstruation is about 12.14 years in black females, 12.25 years in Latina or Hispanic females, and 12.6 years in white females, with a range from 9 to 13.5 years.[12] Menarche appears to be related to body weight, especially percentage of body fat (ratio of fat to lean tissue), which may trigger a change in the metabolic rate and lead to hormonal changes associated with early menarche (age 11 years or younger).[13] There is an increased sensitivity to leptin (a regulatory hormone of appetite and energy metabolism) during puberty and, in theory, the adolescent consumes more calories to meet the caloric needs of the pubertal growth spurt.[14]

Cycles are anovulatory at first and may vary in length from 10 to 60 days or more. As adolescence proceeds, regular patterns of menstruation and ovulation are established at intervals ranging between 21 and 45 days.[15] Menstruation continues to recur in a recognizable and characteristic pattern during adulthood, with the length of the menstrual cycle varying considerably among women. The commonly accepted cycle average is 28 (25 to 30) days, with rhythmic intervals of 21 to 35 days considered normal (see Figure 32-9). Approximately 2 to 8 years before menopause, cycles begin to lengthen again. Menstrual cyclicity and regular ovulation are dependent on (1) the activity of GnRH; (2) the initial pituitary secretion of the gonadotropin FSH; and (3) the estrogen (estradiol) positive feedback mechanism for preovulatory FSH and LH surge, oocyte maturation, corpus luteum formation, and progesterone production.[16]

Phases of the Menstrual Cycle

The menstrual (ovarian) cycle (Figure 32-9) consists of two phases: the follicular/proliferative phase (postmenstrual) followed by the luteal/secretory phase (premenstrual).

During menstruation (menses), the functional layer of the endometrium disintegrates and is discharged through the vagina. Menstruation is followed by the follicular/proliferative phase. This phase is named for two simultaneous processes: maturation of an ovarian follicle and proliferation of the endometrium (see Figure 32-9). During this phase, GnRH and a balance between activin and inhibin levels from the granulosa cells contribute to the increase of FSH level, which stimulates a number of follicles. The pulsatile secretion of FSH from the anterior pituitary gland rescues a dominant ovarian follicle from apoptosis by days 5 to 7 of the cycle. Together, estrogen and FSH increase the number of FSH receptors in the granulosa cells of the primary follicle, making them more sensitive to FSH. FSH and estrogen combine to induce production of LH receptors on the granulosa cells, thus promoting LH stimulation to combine with FSH stimulation and cause a more rapid secretion of follicular estrogen. As estrogen level increases, FSH level drops because of an increase in inhibin-B secreted by the granulosa cells in the dominant follicle. This drop in FSH concentration decreases the growth of less developed follicles (see Figure 32-8). Estrogen causes cells of the endometrium to proliferate and stimulates production of LH. A surge in the levels of both FSH and LH is required for final follicular growth and ovulation.

Ovulation is the release of an ovum from a mature follicle and marks the beginning of the luteal/secretory phase of the menstrual cycle. The ovarian follicle begins its transformation into a corpus luteum (see Figure 32-8), hence the name *luteal phase*. Pulsatile secretion of LH from the anterior pituitary stimulates the corpus luteum to secrete progesterone, which in turn initiates the secretory phase of endometrial development. Glands and blood vessels in the endometrium branch and curl throughout the functional layer, and the glands

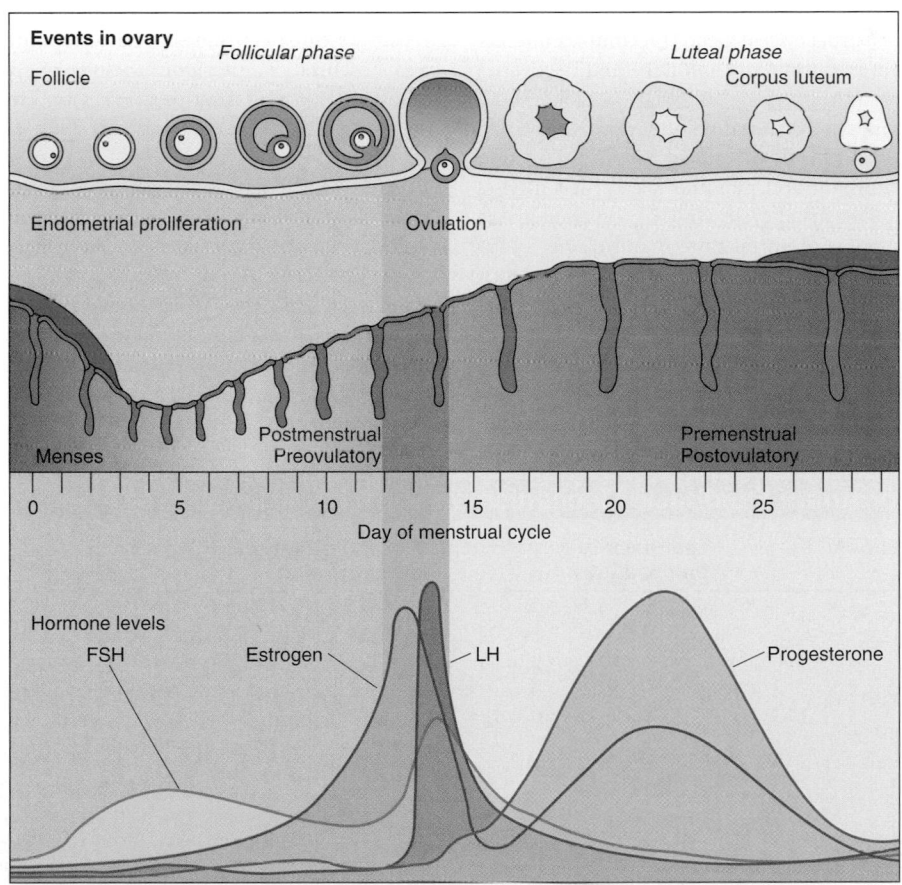

FIGURE 32-9 Female Reproductive Cycle. Correlation of events in follicular development, ovulation, hormonal interrelationships, and the menstrual cycle. Note: levels of estrogen (from ovarian follicle) and luteinizing hormone (LH) (from pituitary) are highest at the time of ovulation; progesterone from corpus luteum is highest during postovulation. FSH, follicle-stimulating hormone (From Gartner LP, Hiatt JL: *Color textbook of histology,* ed 3, Philadelphia, 2007, Saunders.)

begin to secrete a thin, glycogen-containing fluid, hence the name *secretory phase*. If conception occurs, the nutrient-laden endometrium is ready for implantation. Human chorionic gonadotropin (hCG) is secreted 3 days after fertilization by the blastocytes and maintains the corpus luteum once implantation occurs at about day 6 or 7. hCG can be detected in maternal blood and urine 8 to 10 days after ovulation. The production of estrogen and progesterone will continue until the placenta can adequately maintain hormonal production. If conception and implantation do not occur, the corpus luteum degenerates and ceases its production of progesterone and estrogen. Without progesterone or estrogen to maintain it, the endometrium enters the ischemic ("blood-starved") phase and disintegrates, hence the name ischemic/menstrual phase. Then menstruation occurs, marking the beginning of another cycle.

Ovulatory cycles appear to have a minimum length of 24 to 26.5 days: the ovarian follicle requires 10 to 12.5 days to develop, and the luteal phase appears fixed at 14 days (±3 days). Menstrual blood flow usually lasts 3 to 7 days but may last as long as 8 days or stop after 2 days and still be considered within normal limits. Bleeding is consistently scant to heavy and varies from 30 to 80 ml, with most blood loss occurring during the first 3 days of menses. Menstrual discharge consists of blood, mucus, and desquamated endometrial tissue and does not clot under normal circumstances. It is usually dark and produces a characteristic musty odor on oxidation. Environmental factors, such as severe emotional stress, illness, malnutrition, obesity, and seasonal variation, may affect the length of the menstrual cycle.[17-19]

Hormonal Controls

Hormonal control of the menstrual cycle depends on complex interactions among the hypothalamus, the anterior pituitary, and the ovaries (or hypothalamic-pituitary-ovarian [H-P-O] axis)[20] (Table 32-3). Hormonal control is dependent on negative and positive ovarian feedback mechanisms. GnRH controls the gonadotropin production of FSH and LH, and the constant and pulsatile release of GnRH is critical to the timing of the menstrual cycle. GnRH is secreted by the hypothalamus into the hypophysial portal system and travels to the anterior pituitary, where it stimulates the secretion of FSH and LH. FSH and LH are released from the anterior pituitary in pulses that correspond to the secretion of GnRH.

During the early follicular phase, estrogen levels rise steadily and, through negative feedback, suppress FSH production and positively increase the production of LH. During the late follicular phase, the preovulatory rise in progesterone level facilitates a positive feedback loop whereby estrogen levels begin to increase, stimulating a surge of FSH and LH secretion from the anterior pituitary. The midcycle surge of LH and FSH induces ovulation. A nonsteroidal ovarian factor, gonadotropin surge-attenuating factor (GnSAF), may antagonize the effect of estrogen on the pituitary and regulate the surge of LH at midcycle.[21] Rising estrogen and progesterone levels during the luteal phase may inhibit the anterior pituitary and thus reduce LH and FSH secretion. Just before menstruation, FSH and LH levels begin to increase slightly, probably because of declining estrogen and progesterone levels (see Figure 32-9).

A variety of growth factors and autocrine/paracrine peptides influence hormonal control and follicular response. During the early follicular stage, FSH stimulates FSH receptors, LH receptors and release of insulin-like growth factor 1 as well as the production of inhibin and activin in the ovary. Activin from granulosa cells stimulates the secretion of FSH, increases the pituitary response to GnRH, and increases FSH binding in the granulosa cells in the dominant follicle. FSH stimulates inhibin secretion from granulosa cells and it, in turn, suppresses FSH synthesis. Inhibin B is primarily secreted in the follicular phase of the cycle but sharply spikes when ovulation occurs. Inhibin A is secreted in the luteal phase and further suppresses FSH. Inhibin also restrains prolactin and growth hormone release, interferes with GnRH receptors, and promotes breakdown of intracellular gonadotropins. In summary, the balance between activin and inhibin regulates FSH secretion and follistatin inhibits activin and boosts inhibin activity. Inhibin and activin also regulate LH stimulation of androgen synthesis in theca cells.[22] Research continues to advance understanding of the function and structural complexity of these polypeptides and their interaction with GnRH, gonadotropins, and sex hormones.

Ovarian Cycle

By stimulating follicles, gonadotropins initiate their growth and maturation. The most important hormonal event is a rise in FSH level. The decline in luteal phase estrogen, progesterone, and inhibin secretion allows FSH level to rise; concurrently there is a slight increase in LH levels (see Figure 32-9). FSH stimulates granulosa cell growth and initiates estrogen production in these cells. At this time, a group of ovarian follicles is recruited and begins to mature; the exact number depends on the remaining pool of inactive follicles. As the follicles mature,

TABLE 32-3 Hormonal Feedback Mechanism in the Menstrual Cycle

Phase of Cycle and Ovarian Hormone Levels	Feedback to Hypothalamus and Anterior Pituitary	Resultant GnRH, FSH, and LH Levels	Ovarian and Menstrual Events
Early follicular phase: estrogen levels low; minute amount of progesterone secreted	Negative and inhibitory	All low	Ovarian follicle develops; endometrium proliferates
Late follicular (preovulatory) phase: estrogen levels high; progesterone level increases with small surge before ovulation	Positive and stimulatory	All surge; LH dominates	Process of ovulation begins; endometrial proliferation complete
Ovulatory phase: estrogen levels dip; progesterone levels begin to rise	Negative and inhibitory	All fall sharply	Corpus luteum begins to develop; endometrium enters secretory phase
Early luteal phase: estrogen and progesterone levels high; progesterone dominates	Negative and inhibitory	All continue to decline, but gradually	Corpus luteum fully developed; endometrium ready for implantation
Late luteal phase: estrogen and progesterone levels fall sharply	Negative and inhibitory; feedback lessens slightly	All rise slightly	Corpus luteum regresses; endometrium disintegrates; menstruation begins
Menstrual phase: estrogens levels low; minute amount of progesterone secreted	Negative and inhibitory	All low	More ovarian follicles begin to develop; functional layer of endometrium is shed

FSH, Follicle-stimulating hormone; *GnRH,* gonadotropin-releasing hormone; *LH,* luteinizing hormone.

granulosa cells multiply, increasing estradiol secretion. Within a few days of the cycle, one follicle becomes dominant and the others atrophy. The mechanism for follicular recruitment or dominance is unknown. The dominant follicle begins to secrete progressively larger amounts of estrogen (estradiol), which exerts an increase in GnRH receptor concentration and an increase in pituitary sensitivity to GnRH, creating a positive feedback effect that causes a FSH and LH surge. Ovulation occurs 1 to 2 hours before the final progesterone surge, or about 12 to 36 hours after the onset of the FSH and LH surge. Progesterone, proteolytic enzymes, and prostaglandins trigger mechanisms controlling follicular rupture and release of the ovum.[23] The FSH and LH surge also transforms the granulosa cells of the ovulatory follicle into the corpus luteum. The corpus luteum secretes both estrogen and progesterone in amounts that depend, in part, on adequate development of the follicle before ovulation. Progesterone acts both centrally and locally within the ovary to suppress new follicular growth during the early to midluteal phases. If pregnancy does not occur, the corpus luteum persists for 11 to 14 days and then regresses and eventually disappears. An increase in pulse frequency of GnRH from a low level reactivates hormonal control of the menstrual cycle.

Uterine Phases

Uterine phases of the menstrual cycle—the follicular/proliferative phase, the luteal/secretory phase, and menstruation—involve the cyclic changes that occur in the endometrium controlled by estrogen and progesterone. Hormonal effects are influenced by the presence of receptors and numerous growth factors, peptides, and enzymes that act as intermediaries between the sex steroids and the endometrium.[23] During the midfollicular/proliferative phase, increasing levels of estrogen contribute to endometrial repair and proliferation, thus increasing endometrial thickness (luteal phase). Once ovulation occurs and serum progesterone levels increase, the endometrial tissue develops secretory characteristics (secretory phase). If implantation of a fertilized ovum does not take place, endometrial tissue begins to break down approximately 11 days after ovulation (ischemic phase of menstruation; see Figure 32-9). Shedding of tissue (menstrual bleeding) begins about 14 days after ovulation.

Cervical mucus also undergoes cyclic changes. During the proliferative phase, the cervical mucus is thin and watery. Peak estrogen levels occur just before ovulation and maximally stimulate the cervical glands to produce mucus. Cervical mucus becomes abundant and more elastic (spinnbarkeit). Increasing estrogen levels apparently contribute to the development of tiny channels in cervical mucus, providing access for sperm into the interior of the uterus. Changes in the consistency of cervical mucus can be used to identify fertile intervals.[24]

Vaginal Response

The vaginal endothelium also responds to the cyclic hormonal changes of the menstrual cycle. Under the influence of estrogen, cells of the vaginal epithelium grow maximally during the follicular/proliferative phase. After ovulation, layers of keratinized cells overgrow the basal epithelium, a process known as cornification. Near the end of the luteal phase, leukocytes invade vaginal epithelium, removing the outer layers in a process termed decornification.

Body Temperature

Basal body temperature (BBT) undergoes characteristic biphasic changes during menstrual cycles in which ovulation occurs. During the follicular phase, the BBT fluctuates around 98° F (37° C). During the luteal phase, the average temperature increases by 0.4° to 1.0° F (0.2° to 0.5° C). At the end of the luteal phase, 1 to 3 days before the onset of menstruation, BBT declines to follicular-phase levels. The shift in temperature is related to ovulation, corpus luteum formation, and increased serum progesterone levels. Progesterone probably acts on the thermoregulatory center of the hypothalamus to increase body temperature. Changes in BBT are used to document ovulatory cycles but when used alone are not the best method to predict the exact timing of ovulation.[25]

QUICK CHECK 32-4
1. Why does menstruation occur?
2. What event is associated with the luteal/secretory phase of the menstrual cycle?

STRUCTURE AND FUNCTION OF THE BREAST

The breasts are modified sebaceous glands that lie on the ventral surface of the thorax, within the superficial fascia of the chest wall. They extend vertically from the second rib to the sixth or seventh intercostal space and laterally from the side of the sternum to the midaxillary line. Breast tissue also may extend into the axilla; this tissue is known as the *tail of Spence*.

Female Breast

The female breast is composed of 15 to 20 pyramid-shaped lobes that are separated and supported by Cooper ligaments (Figure 32-10). Each lobe contains 20 to 40 lobules (alveoli), which subdivide further into many functional units called acini (sing., acinus). Each acinus is lined with a layer of epithelial cells capable of secreting milk and a layer of subepithelial cells capable of contracting to squeeze milk from the acinus. Biochemical signaling and density within the extracellular matrix is essential for differentiation and function of the acini glandular epithelium. The acini empty into a network of lobular collecting ducts, which empty into interlobular collecting and ejecting ducts. Collagen fiber alignment is required for ductal elongation and organized branching.[26] The ducts reach the skin through openings (pores) in the nipple. The lobes and lobules are surrounded and separated by muscle strands and fatty connective tissue. The amount of fatty connective tissue varies among individuals, depending on weight and genetic and endocrine factors, and contributes to the diversity of breast size and shape and the function of the mammary epithelium. Fat increases in the breast after menopause.[27]

An extensive capillary network surrounds the acini and is supplied by the internal and lateral thoracic arteries and the intercostal arteries. Venous return follows arterial supply, with relatively rapid emptying into the superior vena cava. The breasts receive sensory innervation from branches of the second through sixth intercostal nerves and the cervical plexus. This accounts for the fact that breast pain may be referred to the chest, back, scapula, medial arm, and neck. Lymphatic drainage of the breast occurs largely through axillary nodes, but there may be predominance of superficial mammary routes with resultant asymmetry between a person's breasts[27] (Figure 32-11).

The nipple is a pigmented cylindric structure usually located at the fourth or fifth intercostal space. On its surface lie multiple openings, one from each lobe. It measures 0.5 to 1.3 cm in diameter and is approximately 10 to 12 mm in height when erect. The areola is the pigmented circular area around the nipple. It may be 15 to 60 mm in diameter. A number of sebaceous glands, the glands of Montgomery, are located within the areola and aid in lubrication of the nipple during lactation. The nipple and areola contain smooth muscles, which receive motor innervation from the sympathetic nervous system. Sexual

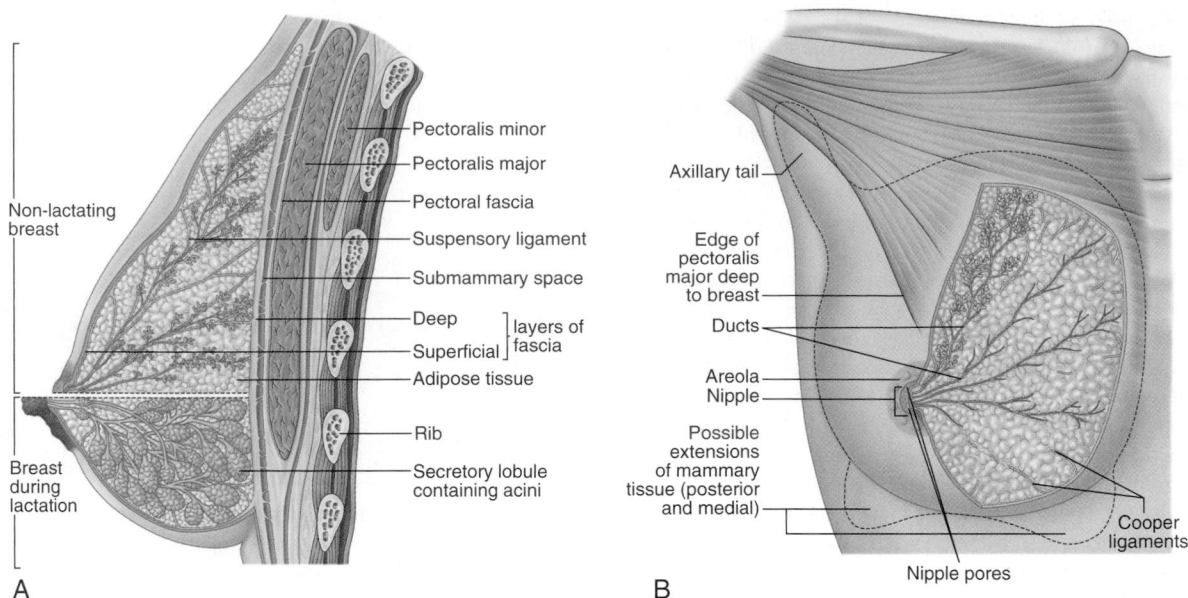

FIGURE 32-10 Schematic Diagram of the Breast. (From Standring S: *Gray's anatomy*, ed 40, London, 2009, Churchill Livingstone.)

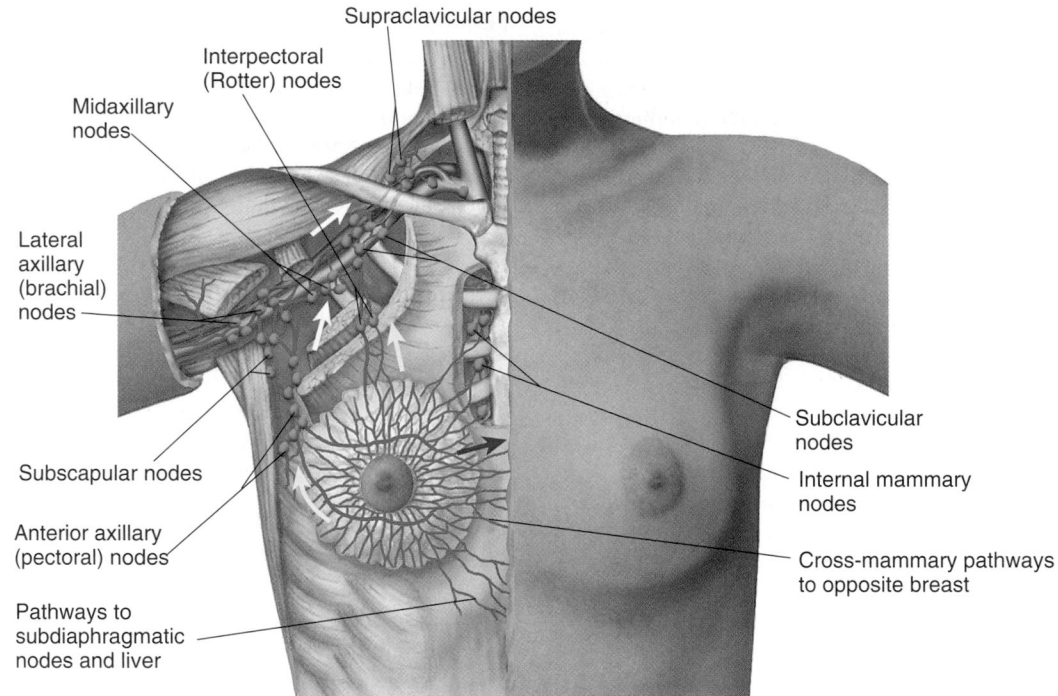

FIGURE 32-11 Lymphatic Drainage of the Female Breast. (From Ball JW et al: *Seidel's guide to physical examination*, ed 8, St Louis, 2015, Mosby.)

stimulation, breast-feeding, and exposure to cold cause the nipple to become erect.

The fetal and early postnatal development of breast tissue does not depend on hormones, although fetal breast tissue does become progressively responsive to hormonal stimulation. During childhood, breast growth is latent and growth of the nipple and areola keeps pace with body surface growth. At the onset of puberty in the female, estrogen secretion stimulates mammary growth. Breast development, or thelarche, is usually the first sign of puberty in the female. Full differentiation and development of breast tissue are mediated by several hormones, including estrogen, progesterone, prolactin, growth hormone, thyroid and parathyroid hormones, insulin, and cortisol.

During the reproductive years, the breast undergoes cyclic changes in response to changes in the levels of estrogen and progesterone associated with the menstrual cycle. Estrogen promotes development of the lobular ducts; progesterone stimulates development of cells lining the acini. Lactation (milk production) occurs after childbirth in response to increased levels of prolactin. Prolactin secretion, in turn, increases by continued breast-feeding. Oxytocin, another hormone released after delivery, controls milk ejection (let down) from acini cells. During the follicular/proliferative phase of the menstrual cycle, high estradiol levels increase the vascularity of breast tissue and stimulate proliferation of ductal and acinar tissue. This effect is sustained into the luteal/secretory phase of the cycle. During this phase, progesterone levels increase and contribute to the breast changes induced by estradiol. Specific effects of progesterone include dilation of the ducts and conversion of the acinar cells into secretory cells. Most women experience some degree of premenstrual breast fullness, tenderness, and increased breast nodularity. Breast volume may increase as much as 10 to 30 ml. Because the length of the menstrual cycle does not allow for complete regression of new cell growth, breast growth continues at a slow rate until approximately 35 years of age. Because of the cyclic changes that occur in breast tissue, breast examination should be conducted at the conclusion of or a few days after the menstrual cycle, when hormonal effects are minimal and breasts are at their smallest.

The function of the female breast is primarily to provide a source of nourishment for the newborn. Physiologically, breast milk is the most appropriate nourishment for newborns. Colostrum, produced in low quantities in the first few days postpartum, is rich in immunologic components, including secretory IgA, lactoferrin, leukocytes, and developmental factors, such as epidermal growth factor. The nutrient composition changes over time to meet the changing digestive capabilities and nutritional requirements of the infant. Secretory IgA and nonspecific antimicrobial factors, such as lysosomes and lactoferrin, protect the infant against infection.[28] During lactation, high prolactin levels interfere with hypothalamic-pituitary hormones that stimulate ovulation. This mechanism suppresses the menstrual cycle and can prevent ovulation.[29] In some parts of the world breast-feeding is the major means of contraception (lactational amenorrhea method).[30,31] However, it is not absolute that ovulation will not occur and this method will not ensure that pregnancy will not occur. Breasts are also a source of pleasurable sexual sensation and in Western cultures have become a sexual symbol.

Male Breast

Until puberty, development of the male breast is similar to that of the female breast. In the absence of sufficiently high levels of estrogen and progesterone, and with antagonistic effects of androgens, the male breast does not develop any further. The normal male breast consists mostly of fat with a small, underdeveloped nipple and a few ductlike structures in the subareolar area. The male breast may appear enlarged in obese men because of accumulation of fatty tissue. During puberty, some males experience benign gynecomastia (benign proliferation of male breast glandular tissue), a condition in which the breasts enlarge temporarily as a result of hormonal fluctuations, and should be differentiated from any underlying systemic disorders.[32]

> **QUICK CHECK 32-5**
> 1. How does breast development differ between adult men and women?
> 2. What happens to estradiol levels in perimenopausal women?

THE MALE REPRODUCTIVE SYSTEM

The external genitalia in men perform the major functions of reproduction. Sperm are produced in the male gonads and the testes, and delivered by the penis. The internal male genitalia consist of conducting tubes and fluid-producing glands, all of which aid in the transport of sperm from the testes to the urethral opening of the penis. The male reproductive and urinary structures are shown in Figure 32-12.

External Genitalia

Testes

The testes are the essential organs of male reproduction. Like the ovaries, the testes have two functions: (1) production of gametes (i.e.,

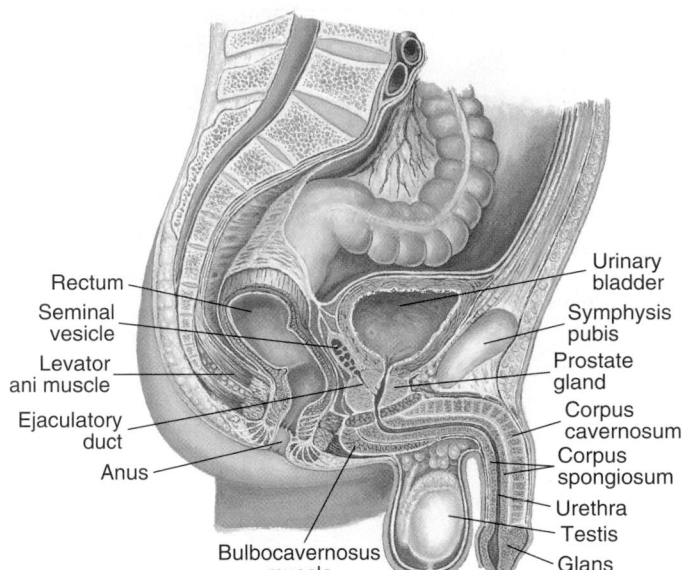

FIGURE 32-12 Structure of the Male Reproductive Organs. (From Ball JW et al: *Seidel's guide to physical examination,* ed 8, St Louis, 2015, Mosby.)

sperm) and (2) production of sex hormones (i.e., androgens and testosterone).

During embryonic and fetal life, the testes develop within the abdomen (see Figure 32-1). About 3 months before birth, the testes start to descend toward the developing scrotum. About 1 month before birth, they enter twin passageways called **inguinal canals**. The inguinal canals are vaginal processes created by outpouchings of the peritoneum (lining of the abdominal cavity). The descent of a testis is shown in Figure 32-13. When descent is complete, the abdominal end of each vaginal process closes and the inguinal canal disappears. Failure of the testes to descend through the inguinal canal is known as cryptorchidism. The scrotal end of each vaginal process becomes the outer covering of the testis, the **tunica vaginalis**.

Figure 32-14 shows a sagittal section of a mature testis. The adult **testis** is oval and varies considerably in length (3 to 6 cm), width (2 to 3.5 cm), depth (3 to 4 cm), and weight (10 to 40 g). The testis is almost entirely surrounded by the tunica vaginalis, which separates the testis from the scrotal wall, and the **tunica albuginea**. Inward extensions of the tunica albuginea separate the testis into about 250 compartments, or lobules, each of which contains several tortuously coiled ducts called **seminiferous tubules**. Sperm are produced in these tubules. (Sperm production, termed *spermatogenesis,* is described on p. 796.) Tissue surrounding these ducts contains **Leydig cells**, which occur in clusters and produce androgens, chiefly testosterone.

The two ends of each seminiferous tubule join and leave the lobule through the **tubulus rectus**, which leads to the central portion of the testis, the **rete testis**. The sperm then move through the **efferent tubules**, or vasa efferentia, to the epididymis, where they mature.

The testes are innervated by adrenergic fibers whose sole function apparently is to regulate blood flow to the Leydig cells. Arterial blood from the internal spermatic and differential arteries flows over the surface of the testes before entering the parenchyma (functional tissues). Surface flow cools the blood to temperatures that promote spermatogenesis, approximately 1° to 7° C (33.8° to 44.6° F) below body core temperature.[33] Additionally, the testes are suspended outside the pelvic cavity to facilitate cooling.

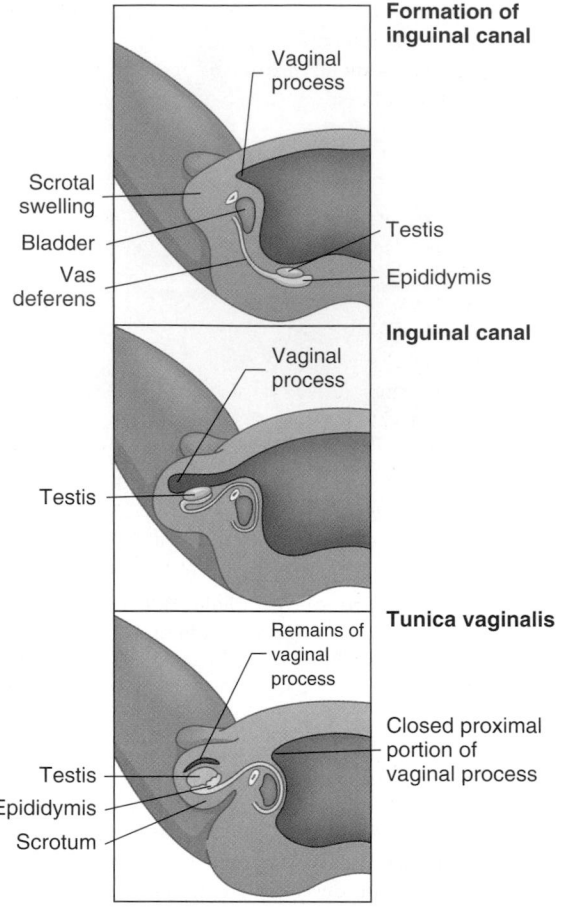

Formation of inguinal canal

- Vaginal process
- Scrotal swelling
- Bladder
- Vas deferens
- Testis
- Epididymis

Inguinal canal

- Vaginal process
- Testis

Tunica vaginalis

- Remains of vaginal process
- Closed proximal portion of vaginal process
- Testis
- Epididymis
- Scrotum

FIGURE 32-13 Descent of a Testis. The testes descend from the abdominal cavity to the scrotum during the last 3 months of fetal development.

Epididymis

The epididymis (pl., epididymides) is a comma-shaped structure that curves over the posterior portion of each testis (see Figure 32-14). It consists of a single, densely packed and markedly coiled duct measuring 5 to 7 cm in length (but about 6 meters in length when uncoiled). The epididymis has structural and physiologic functions. Its structural function is to conduct sperm from the efferent tubules to the vas deferens, whereas physiologic functions include sperm maturation, mobility, and fertility. When sperm enter the head of the epididymis, they are not fully mature or motile, nor can they fertilize an ovum. During the 12 days (or more) sperm take to travel the length of the epididymis, they receive nutrients and testosterone and their capacity for fertilization is enhanced.[34] After traveling the length of the epididymis, sperm are stored in the epididymal tail and vas deferens. The vas deferens is a duct with muscular layers capable of powerful peristalsis that transports sperm toward the urethra. The vas deferens enters the pelvic cavity through the spermatic cord (see Figure 32-14).

Scrotum

The testes, epididymides, and spermatic cord are enclosed and protected by the scrotum, a skin-covered, fibromuscular sac homologous to the female labia majora (see Figure 32-2). The skin of the scrotum is thin and has rugae (wrinkles or folds), which enable it to enlarge or relax away from the body. At puberty the scrotal skin darkens, develops active sebaceous glands, and becomes sparsely covered with hair. Just under the skin lies a layer of connective tissue (fascia) and smooth muscle, the tunica dartos (see Figure 32-14). The tunica dartos also forms a septum that separates the two testes. Exposure to cold temperatures causes the tunica dartos to contract, pulling the testes close to the warm body. In warm temperatures, the tunica dartos relaxes, suspending the testes away from body heat. These mechanisms promote optimal temperatures for spermatogenesis. In addition, scrotal sensitivity to touch, pressure, temperature, and pain protects

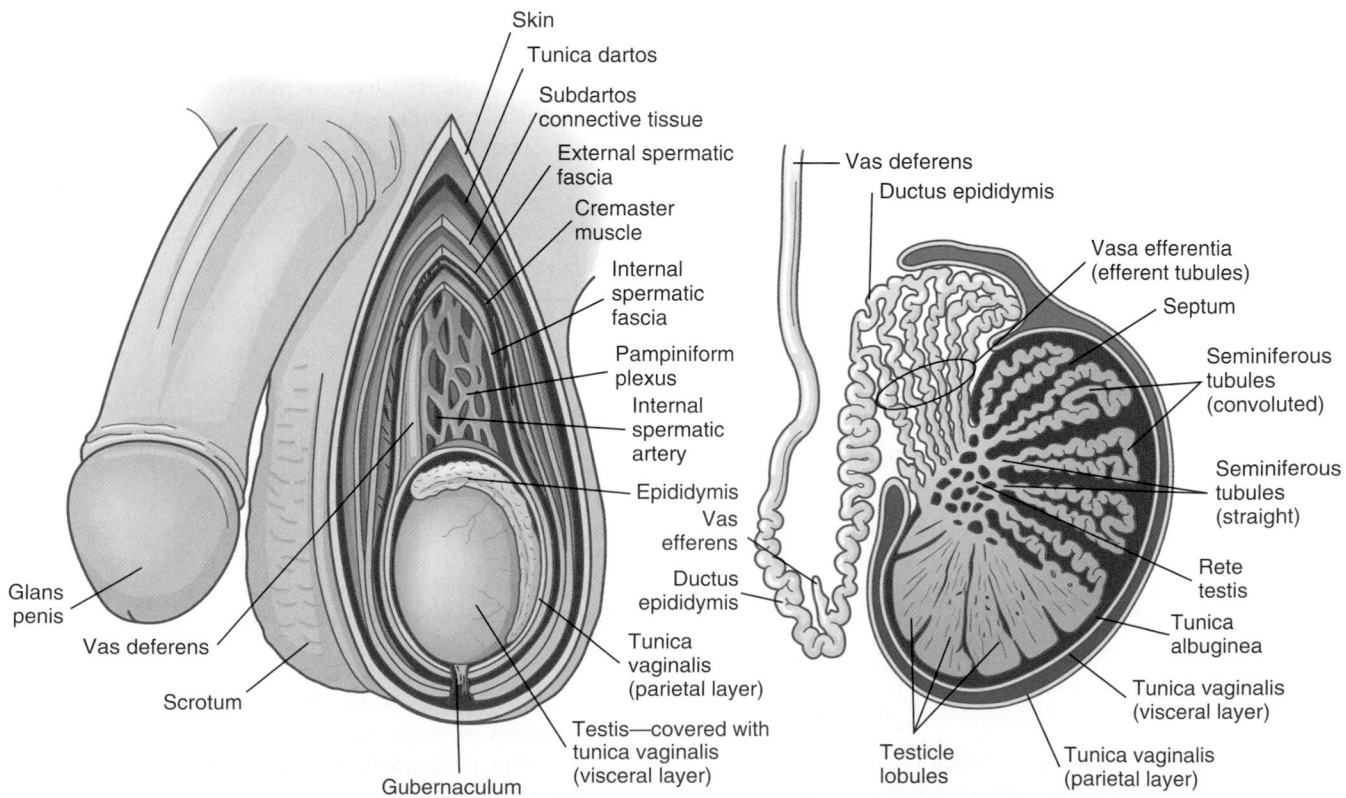

Labels: Skin · Tunica dartos · Subdartos connective tissue · External spermatic fascia · Cremaster muscle · Internal spermatic fascia · Pampiniform plexus · Internal spermatic artery · Epididymis · Vas efferens · Ductus epididymis · Tunica vaginalis (parietal layer) · Testis—covered with tunica vaginalis (visceral layer) · Glans penis · Vas deferens · Scrotum · Gubernaculum · Vas deferens · Ductus epididymis · Vasa efferentia (efferent tubules) · Septum · Seminiferous tubules (convoluted) · Seminiferous tubules (straight) · Rete testis · Tunica albuginea · Tunica vaginalis (visceral layer) · Tunica vaginalis (parietal layer) · Testicle lobules

FIGURE 32-14 The Testes. External and sagittal views showing interior anatomy.

the testes from potential harm. During sexual excitement, the scrotal skin and tunica thicken, the scrotum tightens and lifts, and the spermatic cords shorten, partially elevating the testes toward the body. As excitement plateaus, the engorged testes increase 50% in size, rotate anteriorly, and flatten against the body, signaling impending ejaculation.

Penis

The **penis** has two main functions: delivery of sperm to the female vagina and elimination of urine. (Urine formation and excretion are discussed in Chapter 29.) Embryonically, the penis is homologous to the female clitoris (see Figure 32-2).

Figure 32-15 shows a sagittal section of the adult penis and its anatomic relation to other urogenital structures. Externally, the penis consists of a shaft with a tip (the **glans**) that contains the opening of the urethra (see Figures 32-14 and 32-15). The skin of the glans folds over the tip of the penis, forming the **prepuce**, or **foreskin**. The skin of the penis is continuous with that of the groin, scrotum, and inner thighs. It is hairless, movable, and darker than surrounding skin.

Internally, the penis consists of the urethra and three compartments or sinusoids: two **corpora cavernosa** and the **corpus spongiosum** (see Figure 32-15) separated by Buck fascia. Like the testes, these compartments are enclosed by the fibrous tunica albuginea. The **urethra** passes through the corpus spongiosum and ends at a sagittal slit in the glans.

Penetration of the female vagina is made possible by the **erectile reflex**, a process in which erectile tissues within the corpora cavernosa and corpus spongiosum become engorged with blood. The erectile tissues consist of vascular spaces, or chambers, supplied with blood by arterioles (small arteries). Usually, the arterioles are constricted, so that not much blood flows through the erectile tissues. Sexual stimulation, however, causes the arterioles to dilate and fill with blood, expanding the erectile tissues and causing an erection. Erection apparently is maintained by compression or constriction of veins that drain the corpora cavernosa and corpus spongiosum. When sexual stimulation ceases or orgasm and ejaculation occur, these veins open, blood flows out of the arterioles, and the penis becomes flaccid (soft and pendulous). Erection is under the control of the autonomic nervous system but can be stimulated or inhibited by central nervous system input.

Erections begin in utero and continue throughout life, but ejaculation does not occur until sperm production begins at puberty. Growth of the penis and scrotal contents continues well past puberty, however, and may not be complete until the late teens or early twenties. Penis size, when flaccid, varies considerably; with an erection, difference in penis size diminishes. Sexual excitement causes the corpora cavernosa to increase in length and width and become rigid; the penis becomes erect. Stimulation of the glans, which is endowed with copious sensitive nerve endings, provides maximum erotic sensation. With sexual arousal, skin color deepens, the glans doubles in size, and the urethral meatus dilates. Ejaculation occurs with frequent, strong contractions of the vas deferens, epididymis, seminal vesicles, prostate, urethra, and penis. Erection and ejaculation can occur independently of each other.[35,36]

Internal Genitalia

Figure 32-12 shows the anatomy of the internal genitalia and their relation to other pelvic organs. The internal genitalia consist of ducts and glands, as follows:

Ducts—consist of two vasa deferentia, ejaculatory duct, and urethra; conduct sperm and glandular secretions from the testes to the urethral opening of the penis

Glands—consist of prostate gland, two seminal vesicles, and two Cowper (bulbourethral) glands; secrete fluids that serve as a vehicle for sperm transport and create nutritious alkaline medium that promotes sperm motility and survival

Together the sperm and the glandular fluids compose **semen**.

Sperm leave the epididymides and travel rapidly through the internal ducts (**emission**). Emission occurs just seconds before ejaculation, at the moment when sexual arousal peaks. It always leads to ejaculation.

Emission occurs as smooth muscle in the walls of the epididymides and vasa deferentia begins to contract rhythmically, pushing sperm and epididymal secretions through the vasa deferentia. Each vas deferens is a firm, elastic, fibromuscular tube that begins at the tail of the epididymis, enters the pelvic cavity within the spermatic cord, loops up and over the bladder, and ends in the prostate gland (Figure 32-16). Sperm are conducted by peristaltic contractions of smooth muscle in the walls of the vas deferens.

As sperm leave the ampulla (wide portion) of the vas deferens, the seminal vesicles secrete a nutritive, glucose-rich fluid into the ejaculate (semen). The **seminal vesicles** are glands about 4 to 6 cm long that lie behind the urinary bladder and in front of the rectum. The ducts of the seminal vesicles join the ampulla of the vas deferens to become the **ejaculatory duct**, which contracts rhythmically during emission and ejaculation. As seen in Figures 32-13 and 32-16, the ejaculatory duct joins the urethra, where both pass through the prostate gland. During emission and ejaculation, a sphincter (muscle surrounding a duct) closes, preventing urine from entering the prostatic urethra.

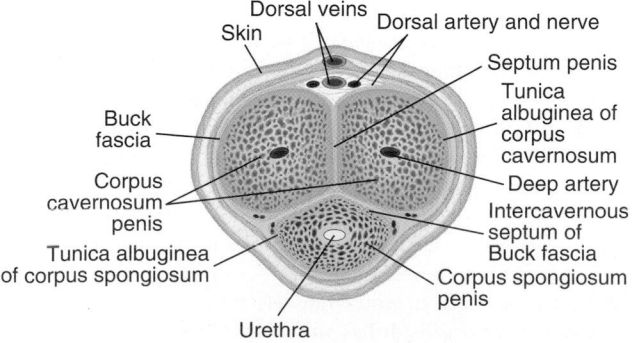

FIGURE 32-15 Cross Section of the Penis. (From Thompson JM et al, editors: *Mosby's clinical nursing*, ed 5, St Louis, 2002, Mosby.)

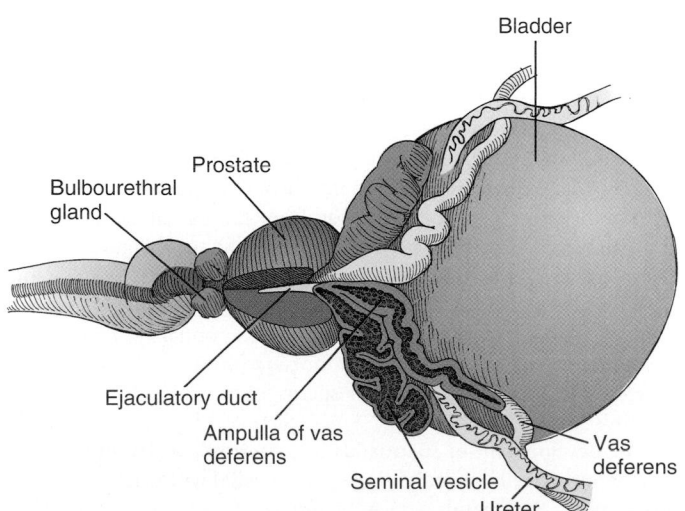

FIGURE 32-16 Prostate Gland, Seminal Vesicles, and Vas Deferens. (From Huguet J: *Hinman's atlas of urosurgical anatomy*, ed 2, pp 249-286, Philadelphia, 2012, Saunders.)

FIGURE 32-17 Seminiferous Tubule and Spermatogenesis. Cross section of a seminiferous tubule showing the different cell types. Interstitial cells that produce testosterone are between the seminiferous tubules. Spermatids in the lumen become sperm by a process called spermiogenesis. The numbers in white represent the number of chromosomes. (From Applegate E: *The anatomy and physiology learning system,* ed 4, St Louis, 2011, Saunders.)

The **prostate gland** is about the size of a walnut, surrounds the urethra, and is composed of glandular alveoli and ducts embedded in fibromuscular tissue. Nerves required for penile erection travel along the posterolateral surface of the prostate. While semen moves through the prostatic portion of the urethra, the prostate gland contracts rhythmically and secretes prostatic fluid (a thin, milky substance with an alkaline pH that helps sperm to survive in the acidic environment of the female reproductive tract) into the mixture. In addition, substances in seminal and prostatic fluids help to mobilize sperm after ejaculation.

Bulbourethral glands (Cowper glands) are the last pair of glands to add fluid to the ejaculate; their ducts secrete mucus into the urethra near the base of the penis. Ejaculation occurs as semen reaches the base of the penis, where muscles rhythmically contract and expel semen. Normally a man ejaculates between 2 and 6 ml of semen, containing 75 million to 400 million sperm. About 98% of the ejaculate consists of glandular fluids; 60% to 70% of the volume originates from the seminal vesicles and 20% from the prostate. Therefore the ejaculate of a man who has undergone a vasectomy (a surgical procedure for permanent male birth control) is reduced by only about 2%.

Spermatogenesis

Spermatogenesis begins at puberty and continues for life. In this respect, spermatogenesis differs markedly from oogenesis (production of primordial ova), which occurs during fetal life only. **Spermatogenesis** takes place within the seminiferous tubules of the testes (see Figures 32-14 and 32-17). The basement membrane of each seminiferous tubule is lined with diploid (46-chromosome) germ cells called **spermatogonia** (sing., **spermatogonium**). These cells undergo continuous mitotic division (division into two identical cells, see Chapter 1.) Some spermatogonia move away from the basement membrane and mature, becoming **primary spermatocytes** (Figure 32-17). These undergo meiosis, cell division that results in two haploid (23-chromosome) cells called **secondary spermatocytes**. (Meiosis is described and illustrated in Chapter 2.) The secondary spermatocytes also undergo meiosis, resulting in four **spermatids**. The spermatids differentiate into spermatozoa, or sperm, each of which contains 23 chromosomes (Figure 32-18).

The development of spermatids into sperm depends on the presence of **Sertoli cells (nondividing support cells)** within the seminiferous tubules. Spermatids attach themselves to the Sertoli cells (see Figure 32-17), where they receive nutrients and hormonal signals necessary to develop into sperm.[37]

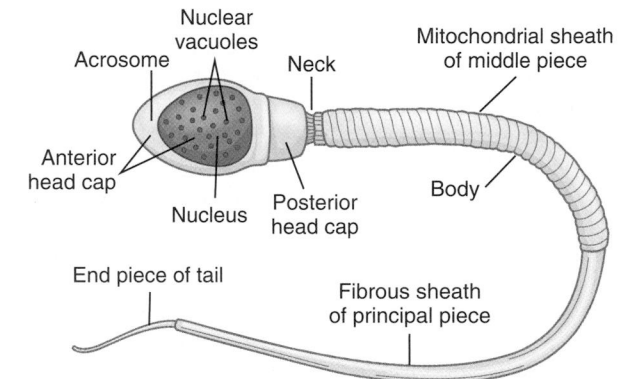

FIGURE 32-18 Mature Sperm Cell (Spermatozoon). Anatomy of mature sperm cell.

The process of spermatogenesis, from mitotic division of a spermatogonium to maturation of the spermatids, takes about 70 to 80 days. Mature sperm migrate from the seminiferous tubules to the epididymides, where their capacity for fertilization continues to develop. Although they are completely mature by the time they are ejaculated, the sperm do not become motile (capable of movement) until they are activated by biochemicals in semen and in the female reproductive tract (known as sperm capacitation).[38]

Male Sex and Reproductive Hormones

The male sex hormones are androgens. Testosterone, the primary male sex hormone, and other androgens are produced mainly by Leydig cells of the testes, but they are also produced by the adrenal glands (see Table 32-1 and discussion about adrenarche under Puberty and Reproductive Maturation, p. 780). In men, sex hormone production is relatively constant and does not occur in a cyclic pattern, as it does in women.

The physiologic actions of androgen are related to the growth and development of male tissues and organs.[39] Androgens are responsible for the fetal differentiation and development of the male urogenital system and have some effects on the fetal brain. After birth, the Leydig cells become quiescent until activated by the gonadotropins during puberty. Then androgens cause the sex organs to grow and secondary sex characteristics to develop.

Testosterone affects nervous and skeletal tissues, bone marrow, skin and hair, and sex organs. It has an anabolic effect on skeletal muscle tissue, thereby contributing to the difference in body weight and composition between men and women. Testosterone also stimulates growth of the musculature and cartilage of the larynx, causing a permanent deepening of the voice. Testosterone directly stimulates the bone marrow and indirectly stimulates renal erythropoietin production to achieve increased hemoglobin and hematocrit levels. Because sebaceous gland activity is stimulated by testosterone, acne may develop. Hair becomes coarser in texture, and facial, axillary, and pubic hair grows in male patterns. Later in life, testosterone causes baldness in genetically susceptible individuals. Testosterone is required for spermatogenesis and for secretion of fluid by the prostate gland, seminal vesicles, and Cowper glands. Testosterone is also associated with libido (sex drive). Other, less-understood effects of testosterone include alterations in fatty acid and cholesterol metabolism.

The regulation of androgen production and spermatogenesis is achieved by a complex feedback system involving the extrahypothalamic central nervous system, the hypothalamus, the anterior pituitary, the testes, and the androgen-sensitive end organs. These relationships are essentially the same in women (see Figure 32-3).

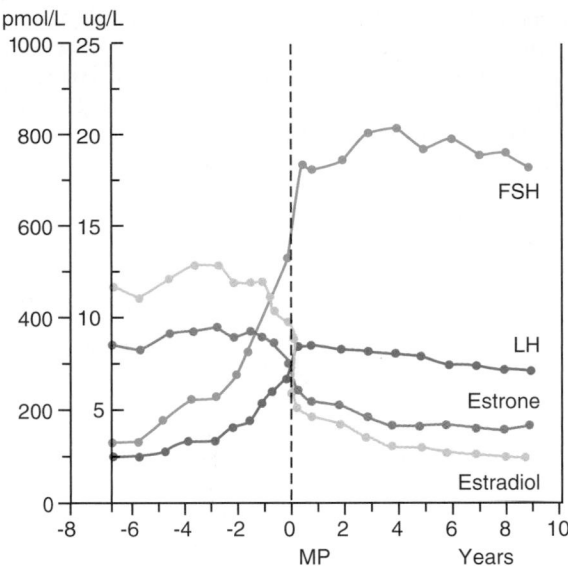

FIGURE 32-19 Perimenopausal Hormone Transition. Mean circulating hormone levels. *FSH,* Follicle-stimulating hormone; *LH,* luteinizing hormone.

> ✔ **QUICK CHECK 32-6**
> 1. Which cells produce testosterone?
> 2. Why do sperm take 12 days to travel the length of the epididymis?
> 3. What is the purpose of prostatic secretion?

AGING & REPRODUCTIVE FUNCTION

Aging and the Female Reproductive System

Menopause is a normal developmental and transitional event that is universally experienced by the average age of about 51 years with a range of 40 to 60 years. Genetics are associated with timing of menopause and menopause can occur 2 years sooner on average for smokers. Findings from studies of body mass index, physical activity, and race are inconsistent in relation to timing of menopause.[40] Changes are caused primarily by declining ovarian function and a resulting decrease in ovarian hormone secretion. The primary changes of menopause are as follows[41]:

Perimenopause: This is the transitional period between reproductive and nonreproductive years and can last 1 to 8 years. About 5 to 10 years before menopause, approximately 90% of women note mild to extreme variability in frequency and quality of menstrual flow. Symptoms usually begin with a shortening of the menstrual cycle, which correlates with a shorter follicular phase, followed by unpredictable or irregular ovulation and a lengthening of the menstrual cycle. The perimenopause varies between women and from cycle to cycle in the same woman.

Menopause: Menopause is defined by the point that marks 12 consecutive months of amenorrhea. This means that it is determined retrospectively after a woman has not had a menstrual period for 1 year. It is characterized by loss of ovarian function, low estrogen and progesterone levels, and high FSH and LH levels (Figure 32-19).[42] Early menopause is the 5 years after menopause onset. Late menopause follows and continues until death.[43]

Ovarian changes: Around 37 to 38 years of age, women experience accelerated follicular loss, which ends when the supply of follicles is depleted at menopause. This accelerated loss is correlated with increased FSH stimulation, declining inhibin production, and slightly elevated estradiol levels (see Figure 32-19). The ovarian response to high FSH level recruits increasing numbers of follicles; these follicles only partially develop, with a net effect of irregular ovulation, lower progesterone levels, and depleted follicle reserve.

The ovaries begin to decrease in size around age 30; this decrease accelerates after age 60.

Uterine changes: The increase in anovulatory cycles allows for proliferative growth of the endometrium. With this longer exposure to unopposed estrogen and greater thickness of the endometrium, 50% of perimenopausal women will experience dysfunctional uterine bleeding that is heavy and unpredictable. In the past, this has put women at high risk for hysterectomy. Newer treatment includes progesterone administration or endometrial ablation by laser or electrocautery. New methods of decreasing the function of the endometrial tissue are being developed.

Breast tissue changes: Breast tissue becomes involuted, fat deposits and connective tissue increase, and breasts are reduced in size and firmness.

Urogenital tract changes: The ovaries shrink; the uterus atrophies; and the vagina shortens, narrows, and loses some elasticity. Lubrication of the vagina diminishes and vaginal pH increases, creating higher incidence of vaginitis. The cervix atrophies; the cervical os shrinks; vaginal epithelium atrophies; labia major and minora become less prominent; some pubic hair is lost; urethral tone declines along with muscle tone throughout the pelvic area; urinary frequency or urgency, urinary tract infections, and incontinence may occur. Regular sexual activity and orgasm may diminish some of these changes. Sexually active women have less vaginal atrophy.

Skeletal changes: Bone mass is lost, leading to increased brittleness and porosity and possibly osteoporosis particularly in the lumbar spine and femoral neck (see Chapter 39).

Cardiac changes: The risk of coronary heart disease increases significantly with an increase in total and LDL-cholesterol and a decrease in HDL-cholesterol (see Chapter 24).

Systemic changes: Vasomotor flushes are characterized by a rise in skin temperature, dilation of peripheral blood vessels, increased blood flow in the hands, increased skin conductance, and transient increase in heart rate followed by a temperature drop and profuse perspiration over the area of flush distribution. This usually occurs in the face and neck and may radiate into the chest and other parts of the body. Dizziness, nausea, headaches, and palpitations may accompany the flush.[44] These flushes can vary in frequency, intensity, and duration and are experienced for 1 to 15 years (mean 1 to 5 years) by up to 85% of perimenopausal to postmenopausal women. Flushes are believed to be caused by rapid decreases in estrogen levels; estrogen replacement therapy can ameliorate these symptoms. Rapid changes in estrogen levels also can increase emotional stress with unpredictable mood swings, depression and anxiety, weight gain, migraine headaches, and insomnia. Lower estrogen levels will decrease skin thickness and diminish skin elasticity, thereby causing increased skin dryness and wrinkling.

Menopause increases the risk of ovarian, breast, and uterine cancers. The risk is greater in women who began menstruating before age 12 or experience menopause after age 55. Women who menstruate longer than normal during a lifetime are exposed to more estrogen and have more ovulations. A longer exposure to estrogen increases a woman's risk of uterine and breast cancers, and having more ovulations than normal increases a woman's risk of ovarian cancer.[45,46]

Hormone therapy can be considered to relieve severe menopausal symptoms. However, risk and benefits of such therapy must be carefully evaluated. There is increased risk for serious disorders for some women including breast cancer, heart disease, and stroke. Risks vary depending on age, timing of menopause, health history, dosage, and route of delivery (oral vs. patch). Nonhormonal therapy also may be an option for symptom relief. An individualized management plan considering risks and benefits of available alternatives can improve quality of life.[47,48]

Aging and the Male Reproductive System

Men maintain reproductive capacity longer than women. No known discrete event, comparable to menopause, characterizes aging of the male reproductive system. Changes do occur, however, in testicular structure and function and sexual behavior.[49] Emotional and physical changes associated with androgen deficiency in the aging male are known as andropause, but it occurs in only a small percentage of men.[50] Contributing factors include decreased levels of testosterone, change in responsiveness of target tissues, decreased levels of sex hormone binding globulin, and changes in the hypothalamus and pituitary gland. Obesity also contributes to decreased testosterone production in aging men.[51,52]

Male sexual behavior encompasses both sexual drive and erectile and ejaculatory capacity. Libido, or sexual drive, is a complex phenomenon that requires a baseline hormonal milieu and is significantly influenced by health status and environmental, social, and psychologic factors. However, in men older than 40 years of age, organic factors are involved in more than half of cases of male sexual dysfunction. Chronic disease and also vascular, endocrine, and neurologic disorders are common causes of organically-based dysfunction of sexual capability. Primary changes[53] are summarized as follows:

Sexual drive (libido): Influenced by changes in health status and testosterone levels.

Erectile/ejaculatory capacity: Longer stimulation needed to achieve full erection, slower and less forceful ejaculation, less pelvic muscle involvement; decreased vasocongestive response; longer refractory time, up to 24 hours.

Testicular changes: Decreased weight, atrophy, softening of testes; seminiferous tubules thicken in basement membrane area, have germ cell arrest, decrease in spermatogenic activity, and collapse; then sclerosis and fibrosis cause complete obstruction; semen volume, sperm concentration, total sperm count, sperm motility, and number of motile sperm decrease; morphologic appearance of sperm changes. Fertility decreases.[54]

Hormonal changes: Hormone synthesis decreases and target tissues decline in responsiveness; testosterone levels decline as number of Leydig cells decreases; gonadotropin levels increase.

Associated change: Functional deterioration of accessory sex organs occurs; loss of muscle mass, strength, and endurance and decrease in libido develop.

> ✔ **QUICK CHECK 32-7**
> 1. What are the physical changes associated with menopausal decreases in estrogen level?
> 2. How does andropause affect muscle mass?

■ DID YOU UNDERSTAND?

Development of the Reproductive Systems

1. Differentiation of female and male genitalia begins around 7 to 8 weeks of embryonic development when the gonads of genetically male embryos begin to secrete male sex hormones, primarily testosterone, under the influence of *SRY* gene expression and testosterone-determining factor (TDF). Female gonadal development occurs in the absence of *SRY* gene expression. Until that time, the primitive reproductive organs of males and females are homologous (the same).
2. The structure and function of both male and female reproductive systems depend on interactions among the central nervous system (hypothalamus), the endocrine system (anterior pituitary), the gonads (ovaries, testes), and the hypothalamic-pituitary-gonadal (H-P-G) axis. A set of complex neurologic and hormonal interactions accelerate at puberty and lead to sexual maturation and reproductive capability.
3. Production of primitive female gametes (ova) occurs solely during fetal life. From puberty to menopause, one female gamete matures per menstrual cycle. Production of the male gametes (sperm) begins at puberty; after that, millions are produced daily, usually for life.

4. Puberty is the onset of sexual maturation. Adolescence is a stage of human development between childhood and adulthood and includes social, psychologic, and biologic changes.
5. At puberty, extrahypothalamic factors cause the hypothalamus to secrete gonadotropin-releasing hormone (GnRH), which stimulates the anterior pituitary to secrete the gonadotropins follicle-stimulating hormone (FSH) and luteinizing hormone (LH) that stimulate the gonads (ovaries and testes) to secrete female (estrogen and progesterone) or male sex hormones (testosterone). Puberty is complete in females with the first ovulatory menstrual period and is complete in males with the first ejaculation that contains mature sperm.

The Female Reproductive System

1. The function of the female reproductive system is to produce mature ova and, when they are fertilized, to protect and nourish them through embryonic and fetal life and expel them at birth.
2. The external female genitalia are the mons pubis, labia majora, labia minora, clitoris, vestibule (urinary and vaginal openings), Bartholin glands, and Skene glands. They protect body openings and may play a role in sexual functioning.

3. The internal female genitalia are the vagina, uterus, fallopian tubes, and ovaries. Although all these organs are needed for reproduction, the ovaries are the most essential because they produce the female gametes and female sex hormones.

4. The vagina is a fibromuscular canal that receives the penis during sexual intercourse and is the exit route for menstrual fluids and products of conception. The vagina leads from the introitus (its external opening) to the cervical portion of the uterus.

5. The uterus is the hollow, muscular organ in which a fertilized ovum develops until birth. The uterine walls have three layers: the endometrium (lining), myometrium (muscular layer), and perimetrium (outer covering, which is continuous with the pelvic peritoneum). The endometrium proliferates (thickens) and is shed in response to cyclic changes in levels of female sex hormones. The cervix is the narrow, lower portion of the uterus that opens into the vagina.

6. The two fallopian tubes extend from the uterus to the ovaries. Their function is to conduct ova from the spaces around the ovaries to the uterus. Fertilization normally occurs in the distal third of the fallopian tubes.

7. From puberty to menopause, the ovaries are the site of (1) ovum maturation and release and (2) production of female sex hormones (estrogen, progesterone) and androgens. The female sex hormones are involved in sexual differentiation and development, the menstrual cycle, pregnancy, and lactation. Although they are primarily male sex hormones, androgens in women are precursors of female sex hormones and contribute to the prepubertal growth spurt, pubic and axillary hair growth, and activation of sebaceous glands.

8. Estrogen (primarily estradiol) is produced by cells in the developing ovarian follicle (structure that encloses the ovum). Progesterone is produced by cells of the corpus luteum, the structure that develops from the ruptured ovarian follicle after ovulation (ovum release). Androgens are produced within the ovarian follicle, adrenal glands, and adipose tissue.

9. The average menstrual cycle lasts 27 to 30 days and consists of three phases, which are named for ovarian and endometrial changes: the follicular/proliferative phase, the luteal/secretory phase, and menstruation.

10. Ovarian events of the menstrual cycle are controlled by gonadotropins and follicular secretion of inhibin. High follicle-stimulating hormone (FSH) levels stimulate follicle and ovum maturation (follicular phase); then a surge of luteinizing hormone (LH) causes ovulation, which is followed by development of the corpus luteum (luteal phase).

11. Uterine (endometrial) phases of the menstrual cycle are caused by ovarian hormones. During the follicular phase of the ovarian cycle, estrogen produced by the follicle causes the endometrium to proliferate (proliferative phase). During the luteal phase, estrogen maintains the thickened endometrium, and progesterone causes it to develop blood vessels and secretory glands (secretory phase). During the ischemic/menstrual phase, the corpus luteum degenerates, production of both hormones drops sharply, and the "starved" endometrium degenerates and is shed, causing menstruation.

12. Cyclic changes in hormone levels also cause thinning and thickening of the vaginal epithelium, thinning and thickening of cervical secretions, and changes in basal body temperature.

Structure and Function of the Breast

1. Until puberty, the female and male breasts are similar, consisting of a small, underdeveloped nipple, some fatty and fibrous tissue, and a few ductlike structures under the areola. At puberty, however, a variety of hormones (estrogen, progesterone, prolactin, growth hormone, insulin, cortisol) cause the female breast to develop into a system of glands and ducts that is capable of producing and ejecting milk.

2. The basic functional unit of the female breast is the lobe, a system of ducts that branches from the nipple to milk-producing units called *lobules.* Each breast contains 15 to 20 lobes, which are separated and supported by Cooper ligaments. The lobules contain *acini cells,* which are convoluted spaces lined with epithelial cells. Contraction of the subepithelial cells of each acinus moves milk into the system of ducts that leads to the nipple.

3. Milk production occurs in response to prolactin, a hormone that is secreted in larger amounts after childbirth. Milk ejection is under the control of oxytocin, another hormone of pregnancy and lactation.

4. During the reproductive years, breast tissue undergoes cyclic changes in response to hormonal changes of the menstrual cycle. At menopause, the tissue involutes, fat deposits and connective tissue increase, and the breasts reduce in size and firmness.

5. The male breast does not develop because of the absence of sufficiently high levels of estrogen and progesterone, and antagonistic effects of androgens.

The Male Reproductive System

1. The function of the male reproductive system is to produce male gametes (sperm) and deliver them to the female reproductive tract.

2. The external male genitalia are the testes, epididymides, scrotum, and penis. The internal genitalia are the vas deferens, ejaculatory duct, prostatic and membranous sections of the urethra, seminal vesicles, prostate gland, and bulbourethral glands.

3. The testes (male gonads) are paired glands suspended within the scrotum. The testes have two functions: spermatogenesis (sperm production) and production of male sex hormones (androgens, chiefly testosterone).

4. The epididymis is a long, coiled tube arranged in a comma-shaped compartment that curves over the top and rear of the testis. The epididymis receives sperm from the testis and stores them while they develop further. Sperm travel the length of the epididymis and then are ejaculated into the vas deferens, which transports sperm to the urethra.

5. The scrotum is a skin-covered, fibromuscular sac that encloses the testes and epididymides, which are suspended within the scrotum by the spermatic cord. The scrotum keeps these organs at optimal temperatures for sperm survival (about 1° to 2° C lower than body temperature) by contracting in cold environments and relaxing in warm environments.

6. The penis is a cylindric organ consisting of three longitudinal compartments (two corpora cavernosa and one corpus spongiosum) and the urethra. The urethra runs through the corpus spongiosum. The corpora cavernosa and corpus spongiosum consist of erectile tissue. Externally the penis consists of a shaft and a tip, which is called the *glans.*

7. The penis has two functions: delivery of sperm and elimination of urine.

8. Sexual intercourse is made possible by the erectile reflex, in which tactile or psychogenic stimulation of the parasympathetic nerves causes arterioles in the corpora cavernosa and corpus spongiosum to dilate and fill with blood, causing the penis to enlarge and become firm.

9. Emission, which occurs at the peak of sexual arousal, is the movement of semen from the epididymides to the penis. Ejaculation, which is a continuation of emission, is the pulsatile ejection of semen from the penis.

10. Spermatogenesis is a continuous process because spermatogonia, the primitive male gametes, undergo continuous mitosis within the seminiferous tubules of the testes. Some spermatogonia develop into primary spermatocytes, which divide meiotically into secondary spermatocytes and then spermatids. The spermatids develop into sperm with the help of nutrients and hormonal signals from Sertoli cells.

11. Production of the male sex hormones (androgens) is controlled by interactions among the hypothalamus, anterior pituitary, and gonads. The male hormones are produced steadily rather than cyclically, however.

Aging & Reproductive Function

1. Perimenopause is the transitional period between reproductive and nonreproductive years in women.

2. Menopause, the point that marks 12 consecutive months of amenorrhea, includes atrophic changes in the ovaries, vagina, and breast; loss of bone mass; and increased risk of cardiovascular disease.

3. Andropause is androgen deficiency in the aging male and occurs in about 1 in 200 men. There is a decrease in testosterone production with testicular atrophy, decreased fertility, and some loss of muscle mass and strength.

KEY TERMS

Acinus (pl., acini) of breast, 791
Activin, 790
Adrenarche, 781
Androgen, 781
Andropause, 798
Areola, 791
Breast, 791
Bulbourethral gland (Cowper gland), 796
Cervix, 785
Cornification, 791
Corpus (body of uterus), 785
Corpus cavernosum (pl., corpora cavernosa), 795
Corpus luteum, 787
Corpus spongiosum, 795
Cul-de-sac, 783
Decornification, 791
Efferent tubule, 793
Ejaculatory duct, 795
Emission, 795
Endocervical canal, 785
Endometrium, 785
Epididymis (pl., epididymides), 794
Erectile reflex, 795
Estradiol (E₂), 787

Estrogen, 787
Fallopian tube (uterine tube), 786
Fimbriae, 786
Follicle-stimulating hormone (FSH), 780
Follicular/proliferative phase, 789
Follistatin, 790
Fornix, 783
Fundus, 785
Glands of Montgomery, 791
Glans, 795
Gonad, 779
Gonadarche, 781
Gonadostat (gonadotropin-releasing hormone pulse generator), 780
Gonadotropin-releasing hormone (GnRH), 780
Granulosa cell, 787
Infundibulum, 786
Inguinal canal, 793
Inhibin, 790
Ischemic/menstrual phase, 790
Isthmus, 785
Leydig cell, 793
Libido, 797

Luteal/secretory phase, 789
Luteinizing hormone (LH), 780
Menarche, 788
Menopause, 788
Menstruation (menses), 789
Myometrium, 785
Nipple, 791
Ovarian cycle, 787
Ovarian follicle, 786
Ovary, 786
Ovulation, 789
Ovum (pl., ova), 779
Oxytocin, 792
Penis, 795
Perimetrium (parietal peritoneum), 785
Prepuce (foreskin), 795
Primary spermatocyte, 796
Progesterone, 788
Prostate gland, 796
Puberty, 780
Rete testis, 793
Ruga (pl., rugae; pertains to vagina and testes), 783
Scrotum, 794
Secondary spermatocyte, 796
Semen, 795

Seminal vesicle, 795
Seminiferous tubule, 793
Sertoli cell (nondividing support cell), 796
Sex hormone, 779
Spermatid, 796
Spermatogenesis, 796
Spermatogonium (pl., spermatogonia), 796
Spermatozoon (sperm cell), 779
Spinnbarkeit mucus, 786
Squamous-columnar junction, 786
Testis, 793
Testosterone, 780
Theca cell, 787
Thelarche, 781
Tubulus rectus, 793
Tunica albuginea, 793
Tunica dartos, 794
Tunica vaginalis, 793
Urethra, 795
Uterus, 785
Vagina, 783
Vas deferens, 794
Vasomotor flush, 797
Vulva, 782

REFERENCES

1. Alves MG et al: Hormonal control of sertoli cell metabolism regulates spermatogenesis, *Cell Mol Life Sci* 70(5):777-793, 2013.
2. Berga S, Naftolin F: Neuroendocrine control of ovulation, *Gynecol Endocrinol* 28(Suppl 1):9-13, 2012.
3. Larney C et al: Switching on sex: transcriptional regulation of the testis-determining gene *Sry*, *Development* 141(11):2195-2205, 2014.
4. Martin RJ et al: *Fanaroff and Martin's neonatal-perinatal medicine*, ed 10, Philadelphia, 2014, Saunders.
5. Tomova A et al: Influence of the body weight on the onset and progression of puberty in boys, *J Pediatr Endocrinol Metab* 2015 Mar 7. [Epub ahead of print.]
6. Biro FM et al: Puberty in girls of the 21st century, *J Pediatr Adolesc Gynecol* 25(5):289-294, 2012.

7. Burt Solorzano CM, McCartney CR: Obesity and the pubertal transition in girls and boys, *Reproduction* 140(3):399-410, 2010.
8. Lenz GM et al: *Comprehensive gynecology*, ed 6, St Louis, 2012, Mosby.
9. Labrie F: All sex steroids are made intracellularly in peripheral tissues by the mechanisms of intracrinology after menopause, *J Steroid Biochem Mol Biol* 145C:133-138, 2015.
10. Macias H, Hinck L: Mammary gland development, *Wiley Interdiscip Rev Dev Biol* 1(4):533-557, 2012.
11. Schumacher A et al: Endocrine factors modulating immune responses in pregnancy, *Front Immunol* 5:196, 2014.
12. Euling SY et al: Examination of US puberty-timing data from 1940 to 1994 for secular trends: panel findings, *Pediatrics* 121(Suppl 3):S172-S191, 2008.

13. Karapanou O, Papadimitriou A: Determinants of menarche, *Reprod Biol Endocrinol* 8:115, 2010.
14. Rogol AD: Sex steroids, growth hormone, leptin and the pubertal growth spurt, *Endocr Dev* 17:77-85, 2010.
15. Rosenfield RL: Clinical review: adolescent anovulation: maturational mechanisms and implications, *J Clin Endocrinol Metab* 98(9):3572-3583, 2013.
16. Adams Hillard PJ, Deitch HR: Menstrual disorders in the college age female, *Pediatr Clin North Am* 52(1):179-197, ix-x, 2005.
17. Pandey S, Bhattacharya S: Impact of obesity on gynecology, *Womens Health (London)* 6(1):107-117, 2010.
18. Scheid JL, De Souza MJ: Menstrual irregularities and energy deficiency in physically active women:

the role of ghrelin, PYY and adipocytokines, *Med Sport Sci* 55:82-102, 2010.

19. Yamanoto K et al: The relationship between premenstrual symptoms, menstrual pain, irregular menstrual cycles, and psychosocial stress among Japanese college students, *J Physiol Anthropol* 28(3):129-136, 2009.

20. Richards JS, Pangas SA: The ovary: basic biology and clinical implications, *J Clin Invest* 120(4): 963-972, 2010.

21. Messinis IE: Ovarian feedback, mechanism of action and possible clinical implications, *Hum Reprod Update* 12(5):557-571, 2006.

22. Makanji Y et al: Feedback regulation by inhibins A and B of the pituitary secretion of follicle-stimulating hormone, *Vitam Horm* 85:299-321, 2011.

23. Henriet P et al: The endocrine and paracrine control of menstruation, *Mol Cell Endocrinol* 358(2):197-207, 2012.

24. Curlin M, Bursac D: Cervical mucus: from biochemical structure to clinical implications, *Front Biosci (Schol Ed)* 5:507-515, 2013.

25. Pallone SR, Bergus GR: Fertility awareness-based methods: another option for family planning, *J Am Board Fam Med* 22(2):147-157, 2009.

26. Barnes C et al: From single cells to tissues: interactions between the matrix and human breast cells in real time, *PLoS One* 9(4):e93325, 2014.

27. Jesinger RA: Breast anatomy for the interventionalist, *Tech Vasc Interv Radiol* 17(1):3-9, 2014.

28. Ballard O, Morrow AL: Human milk composition: nutrients and bioactive factors, *Pediatr Clin North Am* 60(1):49-74, 2013.

29. Bachelot A, Binart N: Reproductive role of prolactin, *Reproduction* 133(2):361-369, 2007.

30. Buitrón-García-Figueroa R et al: [Contraception and breast feeding. Spacing of pregnancies. Present concepts] [Article in Spanish], *Ginecol Obstet Mex* 82(6):389-393, 2014.

31. Romero-Gutiérrez G et al: Actual use of the lactational amenorrhoea method, *Eur J Contracept Reprod Health Care* 12(4):340-344, 2007.

32. Limony Y et al: Pubertal gynecomastia coincides with peak height velocity, *J Clin Res Pediatr Endocrinol* (3):142-144, 2013.

33. Reyes JG et al: The hypoxic testicle: physiology and pathophysiology, *Oxid Med Cell Longev* 2012: 929285, 2012.

34. Dacheux JL, Dacheux F: New insights into epididymal function in relation to sperm maturation, *Reproduction* 147(2):R27-R42, 2013.

35. Giuliano F: Neurophysiology of erection and ejaculation, *J Sex Med* 8(Suppl 4):310-315, 2010.

36. Hsieh CH et al: Advances in understanding of mammalian penile evolution, human penile anatomy and human erection physiology: clinical implications for physicians and surgeons, *Med Sci Monit* 18(7):RA118-RA125, 2012.

37. Hogarth CA, Griswold MD: The key role of vitamin A in spermatogenesis, *J Clin Invest* 120(4):956-962, 2010.

38. Aitken RJ, Nixon B: Sperm capacitation: a distant landscape glimpsed but unexplored, *Mol Hum Reprod* 19(12):785-793, 2013.

39. Hiort O: The differential role of androgens in early human sex development, *BMC Med* 11:152, 2013.

40. Forman MR et al: Life-course origins of the ages at menarche and menopause, *Adolesc Health Med Ther* 4:1-21, 2013.

41. Hale GE et al: The perimenopausal woman: endocrinology and management, *J Steroid Biochem Mol Biol* 142:121-131, 2014.

42. Su HI, Freeman EW: Hormone changes associated with the menopausal transition, *Minerva Gynecol* 61(6):483-489, 2009.

43. Gold EB: The timing of the age at which natural menopause occurs, *Obstet Gynecol Clin North Am* 38(3):425-440, 2011.

44. Freedman RR: Menopausal hot flashes: mechanisms, endocrinology, treatment, *J Steroid Biochem Mol Biol* 142:115-120, 2014.

45. Collaborative Group on Hormonal Factors in Breast Cancer: Menarche, menopause, and breast cancer risk: individual participant meta-analysis, including 118,964 women with breast cancer from 117 epidemiological studies, *Lancet Oncol* 13(11): 1141-1151, 2012.

46. Cramer DW: The epidemiology of endometrial and ovarian cancer, *Hematol Oncol Clin North Am* 26(1):1-12, 2012.

47. Grant MD et al: *Comparative effectiveness review number 147. Menopausal symptoms: comparative effectiveness of therapies*, AHRQ Publication No. 15-EHC005-EF, Rockville, Md, March 2015. Available at: http://effectivehealthcare.ahrq.gov/search-for-guides-reviews-and-reports/?pageaction=displayproduct&productID=2051.

48. Neves-E-Castro M et al: EMAS position statement: the ten point guide to the integral management of menopausal health, *Maturitas* 81(1): 88-92, 2015.

49. Paul C, Robaire B: Ageing of the male germ line, *Nat Rev Urol* 10(4):227-234, 2013.

50. Pines A: Male menopause: is it a real clinical syndrome? *Climacteric* 14(1):15-17, 2011.

51. Basaria S: Reproductive aging in men, *Endocrinol Metab Clin North Am* 42(2):255-270, 2013.

52. Corona G et al: Sexual function of the ageing male, *Best Pract Res Clin Endocrinol Metab* 27(4):581-601, 2013.

53. Zirkin BR, Tenover JL: Aging and declining testosterone: past, present, and hopes for the future, *J Androl* 33(6):1111-1118, 2012.

54. Crosnoe LE, Kim ED: Impact of age on male fertility, *Curr Opin Obstet Gynecol* 25(3):181-185, 2013.

33

Alterations of the Female Reproductive System

Kathryn L. McCance and Afsoon Moktar

Alterations of the reproductive system span a wide range of concerns—from delayed sexual development and suboptimal sexual performance to structural and functional abnormalities. Many common reproductive disorders carry potentially serious physiologic or psychologic consequences. For example, sexual or reproductive dysfunction, such as impotence or infertility, can dramatically affect self-concept, relationships, and overall quality of life. Conversely, organic and psychosocial problems, such as alcoholism, depression, situational stressors, chronic illness, and medications, can affect ovulation and menstruation, sexual performance, and fertility and may be risk factors for the development of some types of reproductive tract cancers. Diagnosis and treatment of reproductive system disorders, however, are often complicated by the stigma and symbolism associated with the reproductive organs and emotion-laden beliefs and behaviors related to reproductive health.[1] Treatment or diagnosis for any problem may be delayed because of embarrassment, guilt, fear, or denial.

ABNORMALITIES OF THE FEMALE REPRODUCTIVE TRACT

Normal development of the female reproductive tract requires absence of testosterone during embryonic and fetal life (see Chapter 32). The resulting fusion of the two paramesonephric (müllerian) ducts produces the normal cervix and the uterus with an internal cavity. The distal portions of the paramesonephric ducts remain independent and form the two fallopian/uterine tubes. Alterations in the normal process include errors in cellular sensitivity to testosterone (androgen insensitivity) or failures of cell line migration resulting in changes in the structure of the reproductive organs.

Androgen insensitivity occurs in its most extreme form in about 1 in 20,000 people[2] and is discussed briefly in this chapter because of the often-resulting female phenotype despite a male genotype. **Androgen insensitivity syndrome (AIS)** is a disorder of hormone resistance characterized by a female phenotype in an individual with an XY karyotype or male genotype, and with testes producing age-appropriate normal concentrations of androgens.[3] To date, more than 1000 mutations have been reported in the androgen receptor (AR) with most of these being associated with androgen insensitivity syndrome.[4] Children with complete androgen insensitivity may have testes palpable within the labia majora, but are often not diagnosed until puberty.[5] Breast development may be normal but pubic and axillary hair is often sparse and menarche does not occur because of the absence of a cervix, uterus, and ovaries.[5] A short vagina that ends blindly also may be present. Milder forms of androgen insensitivity (also a common cause of male infertility)[2] are much more common and have less dramatic phenotypic manifestations with many having normal male genitalia.

Other abnormalities of the uterus, cervix, and fallopian/uterine tubes have multifactorial origins, often the result of an interaction between genetic predisposition and environmental factors. Such interactions result in müllerian duct abnormalities.[6] Some medications, chemicals, and toxins have been implicated as a direct cause of uterine abnormalities.

About 5% of the general female population has some sort of uterine abnormality but the rate is much higher in populations of women who have experienced infertility or miscarriage.[7] Most uterine abnormalities stem from abnormal cell migration in the müllerian ducts during key moments in fetal development (Figure 33-1). Uterine abnormalities are rarely diagnosed until the woman has trouble becoming

FIGURE 33-1 Uterine Malformations. Congenital uterine abnormalities. **A,** The normal configuration of the uterus and the ovaries. **B,** Double uterus with a double vagina and, **C,** a single vagina. **D,** Bicornuate uterus. **E,** A uterus with a midline septum. **F,** Unicornuate uterus. (From de Bruyn R: *Pediatric ultrasound,* ed 2, London, 2010, Churchill Livingstone.)

pregnant or carrying a baby to term because the uterus is capable of menstruation but may have difficulty supporting a growing fetus.[6] Uterine malformations are usually diagnosed by ultrasound during pregnancy or with magnetic resonance imaging (MRI). Their prognosis depends on the severity of the malformation and the location and size of the placenta and fetus. Some abnormalities can be surgically corrected to improve the outcome of subsequent pregnancies.[6] Abnormalities of the lower genital tract also can result in women having two vaginas or a vaginal septum (a thin membrane dividing the vaginal vault). For most women this does not create functional problems but can be surgically corrected if needed.

ALTERATIONS OF SEXUAL MATURATION

The process of sexual maturation, or *puberty,* is marked by the development of secondary sex characteristics, rapid growth, and, ultimately, the ability to reproduce. A variety of congenital and endocrine disorders can disrupt the timing of puberty. These disorders may cause puberty to occur too late *(delayed puberty)* or too early *(precocious puberty)*. Both types involve an inappropriate onset of sex hormone production by the gonads.

The age of puberty is multifactorial, involving genetic and environmental components. The study of epigenetics and the regulation of puberty is only beginning.[8,9] Girls of African descent and Hispanic/Latina girls begin puberty up to 1 year sooner than their non-African and non-Latina counterparts.[10] Obesity decreases the age at onset of puberty by about 6 months. Although many factors are associated with obesity, much research is being done on leptin-responsive pathways in the regulation of eating behaviors and the onset of puberty, follicle-stimulating hormone (FSH), and luteinizing hormone (LH).[11,12] A recent genetic study found pubertal onset in girls is strongly influenced by genetic variation affecting follicle-stimulating hormone (FSH).[13] FSH stimulates ovarian follicle maturation and estradiol synthesis, which is responsible for breast development.[13] The normal range for the onset of puberty is now 8 to 13 years of age. Although there are conflicting and inconsistent reports, the age of pubertal onset appears to be decreasing for girls.[10,14] This earlier onset appears primarily in breast development, not age of menarche. On average, breast development begins at age 10.4 for white girls and 9.5 years for black girls. The average age for menarche is 12.6 years for white girls and 12.1 for black girls. However, 5% of white girls and 15% of all girls will begin puberty before age 8.[10] Both precocious puberty and delayed

TABLE 33-1   Frequency and Common Causes of Delayed Puberty Other Than Constitutional Delay of Growth and Puberty

Delayed Puberty	Hypergonadotropic Hypogonadism	Permanent Hypogonadotropic Hypogonadism	Functional Hypogonadotropic Hypogonadism
Frequency (%)			
Boys	5-10	10	20
Girls	25	20	20
Common causes	Turner syndrome, gonadal dysgenesis, chemotherapy, or radiation therapy	Tumors or infiltrative diseases of the central nervous system, GnRH deficiency (isolated hypogonadotropic hypogonadism, Kallmann syndrome), combined pituitary-hormone deficiency, chemotherapy, or radiation therapy	Systemic illness (inflammatory bowel disease, celiac disease, anorexia nervosa, or bulimia), hypothyroidism, excessive exercise

From Palmert MR, Dunkel L: *N Engl J Med* 366(5):443-453, 2012.
GnRH, Gonadotropin-releasing hormone.

Delayed or Absent Puberty

About 3% of children living in North America experience delayed development of secondary sex characteristics. One of the first signs of puberty in girls is thelarche, or breast development; it should begin by 13 years of age. Normally, boys tend to mature later than girls, around 14 to 14.5 years of age. In boys, the first sign of maturity is enlargement of the testes and thinning of the scrotal skin. In delayed puberty, these secondary sex characteristics develop later.

In about 95% of cases, delayed puberty is a normal physiologic event. Hormonal levels are normal, the hypothalamic-pituitary-gonadal (HPG) axis is intact, and maturation is slowly occurring. Treatment is seldom needed unless the delayed puberty is causing psychosocial problems.

The other 5% of cases are caused by the disruption of the hypothalamic-pituitary-gonadal axis or by the outcomes of a systemic disease. Treatment depends on the cause (Table 33-1 and Box 33-1), and referral to a pediatric endocrinologist is recommended.

Precocious Puberty

Precocious puberty is a rare event, affecting about 1 in 10,000 girls and fewer than 1 in 50,000 boys. Precocious puberty has been defined as sexual maturation occurring before age 6 in black girls or age 7 in white girls and before age 9 in boys. Precocious puberty for boys of all ethnic/racial groups is defined as sexual maturation occurring before age 9. Precocious puberty may be caused by many conditions (Box 33-2), including obesity, an increase in protein consumption, and endocrine disruptors in common household products, pesticides, plasticizers, and pharmaceuticals[15,16] as well as lethal central nervous system tumors. All cases of precocious puberty require thorough evaluation.

All forms of precocious puberty are treated by identifying and removing the underlying cause or administering appropriate hormones (see Boxes 33-2 and 33-3). In many cases, precocious puberty can be reversed. However, complete precocious puberty is the onset and progression of all pubertal features (i.e., thelarche, pubarche, and menarche), is a challenge to treat, and causes long bones to stop growing before the child has reached normal height.

✔ **QUICK CHECK 33-1**
1. Why does puberty occur too late or too early in some individuals?
2. Define the normal age range for the onset of puberty.

BOX 33-1   Causes of Delayed Puberty

Hypergonadotropic Hypogonadism (Increased Follicle-Stimulating Hormone [FSH] and Luteinizing Hormone [LH])
1. Gonadal dysgenesis, most commonly Turner syndrome (45,X/46,XX; structural X or Y abnormalities; or mosaicism)
2. Klinefelter syndrome (47,XXY)
3. Bilateral gonadal failure
   a. Traumatic or infectious
   b. Postsurgical, postirradiation, or postchemotherapy
   c. Autoimmune
   d. Idiopathic empty-scrotum or vanishing-testes syndrome (congenital anorchia) or resistant-ovary syndrome

Hypogonadotropic Hypogonadism (Decreased LH, Depressed FSH)
1. Reversible
   a. Physiologic delay
   b. Weight loss/anorexia
   c. Strenuous exercise
   d. Severe obesity
   e. Illegal drug use, especially marijuana
   f. Primary hypothyroidism
   g. Congenital adrenal hyperplasia
   h. Cushing syndrome
   i. Prolactinomas
2. Irreversible
   a. Gonadotropin-releasing hormone (GnRH) deficiency (Kallmann syndrome) or idiopathic hypogonadotropic hypogonadism (IHH)
   b. Hypopituitarism
   c. Congenital central nervous system (CNS) defects
   d. Other pituitary adenomas
   e. Craniopharyngioma
   f. Malignant pituitary tumors

Eugonadism
These conditions are associated with amenorrhea but may have otherwise normal pubertal development:
1. Congenital anomalies
   a. Müllerian agenesis
   b. Vaginal septum or imperforate hymen
2. Androgen insensitivity syndrome
3. Inappropriate positive feedback

BOX 33-2 Primary Forms of Precocious Puberty

Complete Precocious Puberty
Premature development of appropriate characteristics for the child's gender
Hypothalamic-pituitary-ovarian axis functioning normally but prematurely
In about 10% of cases, lethal central nervous system tumor may be the cause

Partial Precocious Puberty
Partial development of appropriate secondary sex characteristics
Premature thelarche (breast budding) seen in girls between 6 months and 2 years of age
Does not progress to complete puberty (ovulation and menstruation)
Premature adrenarche (growth of axillary and pubic hair) tends to occur between 5 and 8 years of age
Can progress to complete precocious puberty; may be caused by estrogen-secreting neoplasms or may be a variant of normal pubertal development

Mixed Precocious Puberty
Causes the child to develop some secondary sex characteristics of the opposite gender
Common causes: adrenal hyperplasia or androgen-secreting tumors

Data from Burns CE et al, editors: *Pediatric primary care*, St Louis, 2009, Saunders; Osborn LM et al, editors: *Pediatrics*, Philadelphia, 2005, Mosby.

BOX 33-3 Causes of Mixed Precocious Puberty

Female (Virilization)	Male (Feminization)
Congenital adrenal hyperplasia	Estrogen-producing tumors
Androgen-secreting tumors	Adrenal
Adrenal	Teratoma
Ovarian	Hepatoma
Teratoma	Testicular
Exogenous androgens	Exogenous estrogens
	Increased peripheral conversion of androgens to estrogens

From Jospe N: Disorders of pubertal development. In Osborn LM et al, editors: *Pediatrics*, Philadelphia, 2005, Mosby.

DISORDERS OF THE FEMALE REPRODUCTIVE SYSTEM

Hormonal and Menstrual Alterations

Dysmenorrhea

Primary dysmenorrhea is painful menstruation associated with the release of prostaglandins in ovulatory cycles, but not with pelvic disease. Approximately 50% of all women experience dysmenorrhea and 10% are incapacitated for 1 to 3 days because of pain severity. Primary dysmenorrhea begins with the onset of ovulatory cycles and prevalence is highest during adolescence.[17] The incidence steadily rises, peaks in women in the late teens and early twenties, and decreases slowly thereafter. **Secondary dysmenorrhea** is related to pelvic pathologic conditions, manifests later in the reproductive years, and may occur any time in the menstrual cycle.

PATHOPHYSIOLOGY Primary dysmenorrhea results mostly from excessive prostaglandin $F_2\alpha$ ($PGF_2\alpha$), a potent myometrial stimulant and vasoconstrictor, found in secretory endometrium. Elevated levels of prostaglandins, especially $PGF_2\alpha$ and $PGE_2\alpha$, increase myometrial contractions, constrict endometrial blood vessels, and enhance nerve hypersensitivity, resulting in pain.[18] These changes can lead to ischemia and endometrial shedding. Increased synthesis of prostaglandins may result from increased cyclooxygenase (COX) enzyme activity. Inflammatory mediators produced in leukocytes (leukotrienes) also contribute to increased levels of pain.[18] The first 48 hours of menstruation correlate with higher prostaglandin levels. Women who are anovulatory because they use oral contraceptives rarely have primary dysmenorrhea. Secondary dysmenorrhea results from disorders such as endometriosis (most common cause), endometritis (infection), pelvic inflammatory disease, adhesions, obstructive uterine or vaginal anomalies, inflammation, uterine fibroids, polyps, tumors, cysts, or intrauterine devices (IUDs).[18]

CLINICAL MANIFESTATIONS The chief symptom of dysmenorrhea is pelvic pain associated with the onset of menses. The severity is directly related to length and amount of menstrual flow. The pain often radiates into the groin and may be accompanied by backache, anorexia, vomiting, diarrhea, syncope, and headache. The latter symptoms are caused by the entry of prostaglandins and their metabolites into the systemic circulation. The discomfort commonly begins shortly before the onset of menstruation and rarely persists 1 to 3 days during menstrual flow.[18]

EVALUATION AND TREATMENT Primary dysmenorrhea can be differentiated from secondary dysmenorrhea by obtaining a thorough medical history and performing a pelvic examination. Nonsteroidal anti-inflammatory drugs (NSAIDs, e.g., ibuprofen) are the treatment of choice because they reduce COX enzyme activity, and thus prostaglandin production. NSAIDs are effective in the majority of women with primary dysmenorrhea and are most effective if started at the first sign of bleeding or cramping. In women who desire contraception, dysmenorrhea may be relieved with hormonal contraceptives. Hormonal contraception stops ovulation and creates an atrophic endometrium, thereby decreasing prostaglandin synthesis and myometrial contractility. Regular exercise and stress reduction are thought to prevent or reduce symptoms. Other palliative approaches with some evidence of effectiveness in pain relief include local application of heat; acupuncture; high-frequency transcutaneous electrical nerve stimulation (TENS); supplements, such as thiamine and vitamin E; and Chinese herbal treatment.[19]

Amenorrhea

Amenorrhea means lack of menstruation; and the most common causes (aside from pregnancy) include hypothalamic dysfunction, polycystic ovarian syndrome, hyperprolactinemia, and ovarian failure. **Primary amenorrhea** is the failure of menarche and the absence of menstruation by age 13 years without the development of secondary sex characteristics or by age 15 years regardless of the presence of secondary sex characteristics[20] (see p. 804 for a discussion of delayed puberty). **Secondary amenorrhea** is the absence of menstruation for a time equivalent to three or more cycles in women who have previously menstruated.

PATHOPHYSIOLOGY One approach to understanding the pathophysiology is to compartmentalize. *Compartment I disorders* are anatomic defects, including absence of the vagina and uterus. *Compartment II disorders* involve the ovary, primarily genetic disorders (such as Turner syndrome) and androgen insensitivity syndrome (AIS). The target organs (e.g., ovaries) in AIS are completely resistant to the action

FIGURE 33-2 Causes of Secondary Amenorrhea. Of note, hypothyroidism is a relatively common condition and should be ruled out as the cause of hyperprolactinemia before more extensive evaluation (i.e., computed tomography or magnetic resonance imaging) occurs. *DHEAS,* Dehydroepiandrosterone sulfate; *PCOS,* polycystic ovary syndrome.

of androgens, resulting in a lack of estrogen. *Compartment III disorders* are of the anterior pituitary gland, including tumors, and result in failure of signaling to the ovaries through follicle-stimulating hormone (FSH) and luteinizing hormone (LH) secretion. *Compartment IV disorders* include central nervous system (CNS) disorders and primarily involve hypothalamic defects that prevent secretion of gonadotropin-releasing hormone (GnRH); thus, there is no signaling to the pituitary to release FSH and LH.

CLINICAL MANIFESTATIONS   The major clinical manifestation of primary amenorrhea is the absence of the first menstrual period. The cause of the amenorrhea determines whether secondary sex characteristics and height are affected.

EVALUATION AND TREATMENT   Diagnosis of primary amenorrhea is based on the results of a history and physical examination and determination of the presence or absence of secondary sexual characteristics. Laboratory studies may be required to document abnormal levels of gonadotropins or ovarian hormones, or the presence of genetic conditions. Diagnostic imaging, including ultrasonography and MRI, is used to document structural abnormalities.

Treatment involves correction of any underlying disorders and implementation of hormone replacement therapy to induce the development of secondary sex characteristics. Although surgical alteration of the genitalia may be undertaken to correct abnormalities, it should be postponed until the individual can make a truly informed decision.

Secondary Amenorrhea

Many disorders and physiologic conditions are associated with secondary amenorrhea. Secondary amenorrhea is common (normal) during early adolescence, pregnancy, lactation, and the perimenopausal period, primarily because of anovulation. The most common causes

(after pregnancy) are thyroid disorders (e.g., hypothyroidism); hyperprolactinemia; hypothalamic-pituitary-ovarian (HPO) interruption secondary to excessive exercise, stress, or weight loss; and polycystic ovary syndrome (PCOS).

PATHOPHYSIOLOGY   The pathophysiology is dependent on the causes of secondary amenorrhea. These causes are summarized in Figure 33-2.

CLINICAL MANIFESTATIONS   The major manifestation of secondary amenorrhea is the absence of menses after previous menstrual periods. Depending on the underlying cause of the amenorrhea, infertility, vasomotor flushes, vaginal atrophy, acne, osteopenia, and hirsutism (abnormal hairiness) may be present.

EVALUATION AND TREATMENT   Pregnancy is the most common cause of secondary amenorrhea and must be ruled out before any further evaluation. A thorough history and physical examination is important because the menstrual cycle may stop or become irregular in response to stress, extreme exercise, large dietary changes, eating disorders, or sleep abnormalities. Hypothyroidism also is a common cause and should be ruled out as well. Diagnosis of secondary amenorrhea involves identifying underlying hormonal or anatomic alterations. Evaluation of thyroid-stimulating hormone (TSH) or prolactin levels may be indicated. Depending on the cause of the amenorrhea, treatment may involve hormone replacement therapy or a corrective procedure, such as surgical removal of a pituitary tumor. The choice of treatment may be influenced by the woman's childbearing plans.

Abnormal Uterine Bleeding

Menstrual irregularity or abnormal bleeding patterns (Table 33-2) account for approximately 33% of all gynecologic visits. The most

TABLE 33-2 Abnormal Menstrual Bleeding Patterns

Term	Definition
Polymenorrhea	Cycles shorter than 3 weeks; may indicate disturbance in endocrine control of ovulation
Oligomenorrhea	Cycles longer than 6-7 weeks; may indicate disturbance in endocrine control of ovulation
Metrorrhagia	Intermenstrual bleeding or bleeding of light character occurring irregularly between cycles; may be a sign of organic disease
Hypermenorrhea	Excessive flow; may be a sign of organic disease
Menorrhea	Increased amount and duration of flow
Menorrhagia	Increased amount and duration of flow
Menometrorrhagia	Prolonged flow associated with irregular and intermittent spotting between bleeding episodes

TABLE 33-3 Common Causes of Abnormal (Vaginal/Genital) Bleeding in Descending Order of Frequency

Age Group	Cause
Prepubescence	Sexual assault
	Trauma
	Foreign bodies
	Precocious puberty
Adolescence	Anovulation (immature hypothalamic-pituitary-ovarian axis)
	Trauma and sexual abuse
Reproductive years	Pregnancy
	Pelvic inflammatory disease
	Coagulation disorder
	Hormonal contraceptives
	Endometriosis
	Anovulation
	IUDs
	Ovarian cysts
	Uterine polyps/tumors
	PCOS
	Bleeding disorders (e.g., von Willebrand)
	Trauma/rape
Perimenopause	Anovulation
	Malignancy
	Pregnancy
	Endometriosis
	Benign neoplasms (myomas, adenomyosis)
Postmenopause	Malignancy
Other: non–age-specific	Chronic conditions
	Adrenal conditions
	Thyroid disorders
	Liver disease
	Diabetes mellitus
	Obesity
	Hypertension

common cause of cycle irregularity is failure to ovulate related to age, stress, or endocrinopathy. Common causes of abnormal bleeding based on age group and frequency are presented in Table 33-3.

Dysfunctional uterine bleeding (DUB) is heavy or irregular bleeding in the absence of organic disease (i.e., uterine fibroids, polyps, infection, or systemic disease). DUB is a diagnosis of exclusion made only after other causes have been ruled out. DUB accounts for 70% of all hysterectomies, and almost all endometrial ablation procedures.[21] Perimenopausal women are by far the most affected by DUB.

PATHOPHYSIOLOGY The majority of DUB is associated with lack of ovulation.[22] Although DUB may occur at any time during the reproductive years and many conditions are associated with irregular ovulation, more than 50% of cases occur in perimenopausal women ages 40 to 50 years when they are more likely to ovulate irregularly. Women who fail to ovulate experience irregularities in their menstrual bleeding because of a lack of progesterone and, in some cases, an excess of estrogen. This results in excessive and irregular endometrial thickness and subsequent excessive and irregular bleeding. PCOS, obesity, and thyroid disease also are common contributors. Abnormal bleeding can result from defects of the corpus luteum resulting in progesterone deficiencies or from abnormalities of the uterus or cervix, such as endometrial polyps, uterine fibroids, or uterine or cervical cancers.

Abnormal menstrual bleeding in ovulatory cycles is less common, and mechanisms underlying the bleeding are unclear but can include defects of the corpus luteum and abnormalities of the uterus or cervix, such as polyps, fibroids, or cancer. Excessive fibrinolytic activity, use of anticoagulants, diseases of coagulation, infection, and changes in prostaglandin production may be implicated.

CLINICAL MANIFESTATIONS DUB is characterized by unpredictable and variable bleeding in terms of amount and duration. Especially during perimenopause, dysfunctional bleeding also may involve flooding and the passing of large clots, leading to excessive blood loss. Excessive bleeding can lead to iron deficiency anemia and associated symptoms, including fatigue or shortness of breath.

EVALUATION AND TREATMENT DUB is diagnosed after other organic conditions that could cause abnormal bleeding are eliminated. If no cause is found it is usually assumed that the bleeding is caused by lack of regular ovulation. NSAIDs are often first-line treatments for excessive menstrual bleeding because they reduce prostaglandin synthesis within the endometrial tissues, leading to vasoconstriction and decreased bleeding. For the best effect they should be taken in the few days preceding the beginning of the menstrual period and be continued through the days of heaviest bleeding. NSAIDs are not as effective in controlling menstrual blood loss as hormonal therapies but they are readily available without a prescription.

Goals of therapy are to control bleeding, prevent hyperplasia, prevent or treat anemia, and treat concurrent endocrine problems if present. Common treatments include administration of oral contraceptive pills that contain estrogen and progesterone, prescription of long-term therapy with medroxyprogesterone (Depo-Provera) (although the U.S. Food and Drug Administration [FDA] black box warning about potential bone loss has greatly curtailed the use of this therapy), and placement of a levonorgestrel intrauterine device (LNG-IUD). The LNG-IUD has a dual indication from the FDA for both birth control and suppression of abnormal menstrual bleeding. The device releases a steady amount of progesterone directly into the uterus to stabilize and suppress the uterine lining. In addition, the progesterone works to suppress the HPG axis and prevent ovulation.

Women who do not wish to have future pregnancies also can opt for treatments that permanently suppress their uterine lining. These treatments include ablation, where the lining is burned to prevent future proliferation of the endometrial cells, and complete removal of

FIGURE 33-3 Polycystic Ovary. Surgical view of polycystic ovaries. (From Symonds EM, Macpherson MBA: *Diagnosis in color: obstetrics and gynecology*, London, 1997, Mosby-Wolfe.)

FIGURE 33-4 Insulin Resistance and Hyperinsulinemia in Polycystic Ovary Syndrome (PCOS). See text for explanation. *FSH,* Follicle-stimulating hormone; *LH,* luteinizing hormone; *SHBG,* sex hormone–binding globulin.

the uterus in hysterectomy. If a woman is menopausal and has not had a menstrual period for greater than 1 year, all vaginal bleeding should be investigated to rule out uterine and other cancers.

Polycystic Ovary Syndrome

Polycystic ovary syndrome (PCOS) remains one of the most common endocrine disturbances affecting women (Figure 33-3). International criteria for the diagnosis of PCOS require at least two of the following conditions: few or anovulatory menstrual cycles, elevated levels of androgens, and polycystic ovaries. Thus polycystic ovaries do not have to be present to diagnose PCOS and their presence alone does not establish the diagnosis. Furthermore, PCOS should not be confused with benign ovarian cysts, which are common during the reproductive years and have a different etiology (see Benign Ovarian Cysts, p. 815). PCOS is a leading cause of infertility in the United States. PCOS has a large incidence of inheritability. Signs and symptoms of PCOS can vary over time, with metabolic syndrome becoming more prominent with age.[23]

PATHOPHYSIOLOGY The direct cause of PCOS is related to a genetic predisposition and an obesity-prone lifestyle related to insulin resistance and an excess of insulin and androgens. A hyperandrogenic state is a cardinal feature in the pathogenesis of PCOS. However, glucose intolerance/insulin resistance (IR) and hyperinsulinemia often occur concurrently and markedly aggravate the hyperandrogenic state, thus contributing to the severity of signs and symptoms of PCOS.[23] PCOS predisposes to obesity and preexisting obesity predisposes to more severe PCOS.

Insulin resistance and resultant compensatory hyperinsulinemia overstimulates androgen secretion by the ovarian stroma and reduces hepatic secretion of serum sex hormone–binding globulin (SHBG). The net effect is an increase in free testosterone levels. Excessive androgens affect follicular growth, and insulin affects follicular decline by suppressing apoptosis and enabling the survival of follicles that would normally disintegrate (Figure 33-4). Further, there seems to be a genetic ovarian defect in PCOS that makes the ovary either more susceptible to or more sensitive to insulin's stimulation of androgen production in the ovary.

Inappropriate gonadotropin secretion triggers the beginning of a vicious cycle that perpetuates anovulation. Typically, levels of follicle-stimulating hormone (FSH) are low or below normal, and the luteinizing hormone (LH) level is elevated. Persistent LH level elevation causes an increase in the concentration of androgens

(dehydroepiandrosterone sulfate [DHEAS] from the adrenal glands and testosterone, androstenedione, and dehydroepiandrosterone [DHEA] from the ovary). Androgens are converted to estrogen in peripheral tissues, and increased testosterone levels cause a significant reduction (approximately 50%) in SHBG level, which, in turn, causes increased levels of free estradiol. Elevated estrogen levels trigger a positive feedback response in LH and a negative feedback response in FSH. Because FSH levels are not totally depressed, new follicular growth is continuously stimulated, but not to full maturation and ovulation (see Figure 33-4).[23,24]

CLINICAL MANIFESTATIONS Clinical manifestations of PCOS usually appear within 2 years of puberty, but may appear after a period of normal menstrual function and pregnancy. Symptoms are related to anovulation and hyperandrogenism and include dysfunctional uterine bleeding or amenorrhea, hirsutism, acne, and infertility (Box 33-4). Hypertension and dyslipidemia also are frequently found in association with PCOS. PCOS is often found in association with other endocrine disorders.[24]

EVALUATION AND TREATMENT Diagnosis of PCOS is based on evidence of androgen excess (hirsutism, male pattern hair distribution, acne), chronic anovulation (as evidenced by irregular menstrual patterns, amenorrhea, and infertility), insulin resistance (obesity may be an indication, as well as abnormal glucose tolerance testing), and inappropriate gonadotropin secretion (low serum FSH concentration, and elevated levels of LH and DHEA). Treatment of PCOS often includes use of combined oral contraceptives to control irregular menstrual cycles and to oppose estrogens and androgens. Insulin sensitizers, such as metformin, may be used to decrease insulin resistance, prevent diabetes and heart disease, and restore fertility. Insulin sensitizers combined with clomiphene citrate may be effective for ovulation induction for women who are trying to become pregnant. Reductions in weight can dramatically improve insulin sensitivity and return of ovulatory cycles.

Premenstrual Disorders Syndrome

Premenstrual syndrome (PMS) and premenstrual dysphoric disorder (PMDD) are the cyclic recurrence (in the luteal phase of the

BOX 33-4   Clinical Manifestations of Polycystic Ovary Syndrome

Presenting Signs and Symptoms (% of Women Affected)

Obesity (41%)

Menstrual disturbance (70% [e.g., dysfunctional uterine bleeding])

Oligomenorrhea (47%)

Amenorrhea (19%)

Regular menstruation (48%)

Hyperandrogenism (69-74%)

Infertility (73% of anovulatory infertility)

Asymptomatic (20% of those with polycystic ovary syndrome)

Hormonal Disturbances

Increased insulin (independent of obesity)

Decreased SHBG

Increased androgens (testosterone, androstenedione)

Increased DHEA (occurs in 50% of women)

Increased LH (genetic variant LH-β subunit)

Increased prolactin

Increased leptin, especially in obesity (independent of insulin)

Suggested decreased insulin-like growth factor 1 (IGF-1) receptors on theca cells

Possible decreased estrogen receptors (intraovarian and along hypothalamic-pituitary axis)

Possible Late Sequelae

Dyslipidemia: increased low-density lipoproteins, decreased high-density lipoproteins, increased triglycerides

Diabetes mellitus (30% of women with or without obesity will develop type 2 diabetes mellitus by age 30)

Cardiovascular disease; hypertension

Endometrial hyperplasia and carcinoma (anovulatory women are hyperestrogenic)

Other

Women with PCOS are at increased risk of gestational diabetes mellitus, pregnancy-induced hypertension, preterm birth, and perinatal mortality

Adapted from Azziz R et al: *Fertil Steril* 91(2):456-488, 2009; Boomsma CM et al: *Semin Reprod Med* 26(1):72-84, 2008; Diamanti-Kandarakis E: *Expert Rev Mol Med* 10(2):e3, 2008; Spritzer PM et al: *Int J Clin Pract*, Aug. 19, 2015.
DHEA, Dehydroepiandrosterone; *LH,* luteinizing hormone; *PCOS,* polycystic ovary syndrome; *SHBG,* sex hormone–binding globulin.

menstrual cycle) of distressing physical, psychologic, or behavioral changes that impair interpersonal relationships or interfere with usual activities. The luteal phase of ovulatory cycles is linked with complex hormonal changes of the menstrual cycle. PMDD is often considered a severe, sometimes disabling extension of premenstrual syndrome (PMS). The prevalence of PMS and PMDD is difficult to determine, possibly because of the wide-ranging nature of accepted symptoms. Symptoms for PMS and PMDD begin after ovulation during the luteal phase and persist up to 4 days into the menstrual cycle.[25] It has been estimated that 91% of women experience some form of distress around their menstrual period; 30% experience enough distress to interrupt their daily routine; but a much smaller number, as low as 3.1%, meet the criteria for PMDD.

PATHOPHYSIOLOGY   There are many theories to explain PMS/PMDD and the mechanisms, including an increased vulnerability to

fluctuations in ovarian-derived hormones, and hypothalamic-pituitary-adrenal (HPA) axis changes.[26] Poorly understood are the neuroendocrine mechanisms of the hormonal environment of the menopausal transition that might trigger depression.[26] Erratic ovarian hormone fluctuation may be a mediator of risk for both vasomotor symptoms (hot flashes) and perimenopausal depression. Under investigation are the effects of changes in estradiol concentrations and the altered anti-inflammatory and neuroprotective consequences and modulation of limbic processing and memory.[26] Neurotransmitters, such as serotonin, gamma-aminobutyric acid (GABA), and norepinephrine, have demonstrated interactions with estrogen and progesterone and have established mood and behavior effects, including negative mood, irritability, aggression, and impulse control. Additionally, neurotransmitters may have mediating or moderating roles on symptom manifestation. Sex steroids also interact with the renin-angiotensin-aldosterone system (RAAS), which could explain some PMS/PMDD signs and symptoms (e.g., water retention, bloating, weight gain). Levels of inflammatory mediators may be elevated with menstrual symptom severity and PMS.[27]

A predisposition to PMS occurs in families, perhaps because of genetics or shared environment. A woman's menstrual experience is often similar to her mother's or her sister's experience. Evidence supports a relationship between severity and frequency of PMS/PMDD and reports of low well-being, major affective disorder, and personal characteristics, such as increased stress, poor nutrition, lack of exercise, low self-esteem, perfectionism, history of sexual abuse, and family conflict. In turn, when PMS/PMDD is distressing, the quality of interpersonal relationships and self-image are negatively affected.

CLINICAL MANIFESTATIONS   The pattern of symptom frequency and severity is more important than specific complaints. Nearly 300 physical, emotional, and behavioral symptoms have been attributed to PMS/PMDD. Emotional symptoms, particularly depression, anger, irritability, and fatigue, have been reported as the most prominent and the most distressing, whereas physical symptoms seem to be the least prevalent and problematic. The presence of underlying physical or psychologic disease may be aggravated premenstrually and must be diagnosed and treated independently of PMS/PMDD.

EVALUATION AND TREATMENT   Diagnosis of PMS/PMDD is based on health history and symptoms. Current treatment is symptomatic because the cause is complex and cannot be reduced to a single biologic explanation and occurrence and severity are mediated by lifestyle, social, and psychologic factors. For many women, nonpharmacologic therapies, with or without medication, can be as effective in controlling symptoms as medication alone.[28] Approaches may include stress reduction, exercise, family or individual counseling, biofeedback, diet (see *Health Alert:* Nutrition and Premenstrual Syndrome), imagery, acupuncture, and rest. Two major forms of treatment include the use of hormonal cycle regulation and use of selective serotonin reuptake inhibitor (SSRI) antidepressants.[29] If a woman does not desire immediate fertility, the oral contraceptive pill containing estrogen and progesterone has shown benefits in decreasing PMS/PMDD. In severe cases, menses can be abolished using GnRH agonists.

✔ **QUICK CHECK 33-2**

1. Why does amenorrhea occur?
2. Why do anovulatory cycles lead to dysfunctional uterine bleeding?
3. Discuss insulin resistance, hyperinsulinemia, anovulation, and androgen production in PCOS.
4. What are the current theories of pathophysiology for PMS/PMDD?

HEALTH ALERT

Nutrition and Premenstrual Syndrome

Women who are affected by premenstrual syndrome (PMS) often look for ways to decrease their symptoms. Dietary interventions that can help are multiple: eating six small meals each day; increasing intake of complex carbohydrates, fiber, and water; and decreasing caffeine, alcohol, refined sugar, and animal fat consumption. A low-fat vegetarian diet has been associated with decreased symptoms, possibly because of an increase in serum sex hormone–binding globulin concentration that lowers serum estrogen levels. It also may be helpful to limit sodium intake, and some limited evidence suggests that moderate doses (50 mg/day) of vitamin B_6 may reduce emotional symptoms of depression, irritability, and fatigue. This finding needs to be confirmed.

High food intake of thiamine and riboflavin was observed to lower risk of PMS. Thiamine, riboflavin, niacin, vitamin B_6, folate, and vitamin B_{12} are required to synthesize neurotransmitters. Limited data suggest that dietary minerals may be useful in preventing PMS. Prospective analyses suggest that higher plasma vitamin D levels may be inversely related to the development of specific menstrual symptoms. Vitamin D deficiency is associated with increased renin-angiotensin-aldosterone system (RAAS) activity, a system that regulates fluid balance and blood pressure. Vitamin D may lower the risk of unipolar depression. More research needs to confirm all of these findings.

Some researchers have suggested links between serotonin, endorphins, and high sugar intake and PMS risk. One interesting craving is chocolate. Some researchers suggest that a craving for chocolate is an unconscious desire for a compound called phenylethylamine (PEA) in chocolate that stimulates the release of the neurotransmitter dopamine, which regulates mood.

Data from Bernard ND et al: *Obstet Gynecol* 95(2):245, 2000; Bertone-Johnson E et al: *BMC Womens Health* 14:56, 2014; Chocano-Bedova PO et al: *Am J Clin Nutr* 93(5):1080-1086, 2011; Chocano-Bedova PO et al: *Am J Epidemiol* 177(10):1118-1127, 2013; Eyles DW et al: *Front Neuroendocrinol* 34:47-64, 2012; Mahan LK, Escott-Stump S: *Krause's food, nutrition, and diet therapy*, ed 10, Philadelphia, 2000, Saunders; Mura Kami K et al: *Nutrition* 24(6):554-561, 2008.

Infection and Inflammation

Infections of the genital tract may result from exogenous or endogenous microorganisms. Exogenous pathogens are most often sexually transmitted. Endogenous causes of infection include microorganisms that are normally resident in the vagina, bowel, or vulva. Infection occurs if these microorganisms migrate to a new location or overproliferate when the immune system and other defense mechanisms are impaired.

Skin disorders that can affect the vulva include reactive dermatitis, contact dermatitis, psoriasis, and impetigo. (For a discussion of skin disorders, see Chapter 41.) Most infectious disorders, however, that affect the vulva and vagina are sexually transmitted. These currently recognized sexually transmitted infections are described in Table 34-1 on p. 877.

Pelvic Inflammatory Disease

Pelvic inflammatory disease (PID) is an acute inflammatory process caused by infection (Figure 33-5). PID may involve any organ, or combination of organs, of the upper genital tract—the uterus, fallopian tubes, or ovaries—and, in its most severe form, the entire peritoneal cavity. Many infectious disorders that affect the vulva and vagina are sexually transmitted, such as chlamydia and gonorrhea that migrate from the vagina to the uterus, fallopian tubes, and ovaries.[30] However, microorganisms that comprise the vaginal flora (e.g., anaerobes, *Gardnerella vaginalis*, *Haemophilus influenzae*, enteric gram-negative rods, and *Streptococcus agalactiae*) also are implicated with PID. Additionally, cytomegalovirus (CMV), *Mycoplasma hominis*, *Ureaplasma urealyticum*, and *Mycoplasma genitalium* may be associated with PID. The risk factors for PID include infection by a *previous* sexually transmitted disease (STD) that was not treated (delaying treatment increases complications from PID); having multiple sex partners or a sex partner who has had multiple sex partners or a previous PID; being sexually active at age 25 or younger; using douches; and using an intrauterine device (IUD) for birth control.[30] Other causes of infection include spontaneous or induced abortions, normal or abnormal deliveries (called *puerperal infections*), or other surgical procedures; these infections are often polymicrobial.[31]

FIGURE 33-5 Pelvic Inflammatory Disease. A, Drawing depicting involvement of both ovaries and fallopian tubes. **B,** Total abdominal hysterectomy and bilateral salpingo-oophorectomy specimen showing unilateral pyosalpinx. (A from Ball JW et al: *Seidel's guide to physical examination*, ed 8, St Louis, 2015, Mosby; B from Morse SA et al: *Atlas of sexually transmitted diseases and AIDS*, ed 4, Edinburgh, 2010, Mosby.)

PATHOPHYSIOLOGY The development of upper genital tract infections is mediated by a number of defense mechanisms, including virulence of the microorganism, size of the inoculum, and immune defense status of the individual. PID develops when pathologic microbes ascend from an infected cervix to infect the uterus and adnexae (uterine appendages). The initial infection usually involves the endocervical mucosa, but it can start in the Bartholin gland and other glands. From these sites the infection can move upwards to involve the fallopian tubes and tubo-ovarian region (Figure 33-6). STDs from gonorrhea and chlamydia are the main infectious causes of PID; however, other infections not sexually transmitted (e.g., induced abortion, dilation and curettage of the uterus, and other surgical procedures) also can cause PID.[31] Many anaerobic bacteria have been implicated in increasing the risk of PID because they alter the pH of the vaginal environment and may decrease the integrity of the mucus blocking the cervical canal. Bacterial vaginosis (BV) is present in up to 66% of women with PID and other anaerobes, such as *Bacteroides,* and *Gardnerella vaginalis, Haemophilus influenzae,* and genital tract mycoplasmas *(Mycoplasma hominis, Mycoplasma genitalis,* and *Ureaplasma urealyticum)* are frequently isolated from women with PID. *Escherichia coli* may contribute to pelvic infections in older women. Therefore, although gonorrhea and chlamydia are the main pathogens in PID, the disease is actually polymicrobial in origin and is treated with a broad spectrum of antibiotics to ensure that all the causative agents are eliminated.[30]

Salpingitis

Salpingitis is inflammation of the fallopian tubes (see Figure 33-6). The inflammatory process develops after the infection has been established and induces changes in the columnar epithelia that line the upper reproductive tract. The inflammation causes localized edema and sometimes necrosis of the area. Gonorrhea gonococci attach to the fallopian tubes and excrete a substance toxic to the tubal mucosa, causing further inflammation and damage. Chlamydia enters the tubal cells and replicates, bursting the cell membrane as it reproduces, causing permanent scarring. Gonorrhea and chlamydia can spread to the abdominal cavity through the openings of the fallopian/uterine tubes. Other mechanisms that may contribute to PID include lymphatic drainage with parametrial spread of the infection. The acute complications of PID include peritonitis and bacteremia, which can increase the risk for endocarditis, meningitis, and infectious arthritis. The chronic consequences of PID include infertility and tubal obstruction, ectopic pregnancy, pelvic pain of varying degrees, and intestinal obstruction from adhesions between the bowel and pelvic organs.[31]

CLINICAL MANIFESTATIONS The clinical manifestations of PID vary from sudden, severe abdominal pain with fever to no symptoms at all. An asymptomatic cervicitis may be present for some time before PID develops. The first sign of the ascending infection may be the onset of low bilateral abdominal pain, often characterized as dull and steady with a gradual onset. Symptoms are more likely to develop during or immediately after menstruation. The pain of PID may worsen with walking, jumping, or intercourse. Other manifestations of PID include dysuria (difficult or painful urination) and irregular bleeding.

EVALUATION AND TREATMENT PID often has limited or vague clinical symptoms, leading to undertreatment and long-term health effects.[32] Because PID is a substantial health risk to a woman, the Centers for Disease Control and Prevention (CDC) encourage clinicians to consider PID as a likely diagnosis when a sexually active woman has abdominal or pelvic tenderness and *one* of the following: cervical motion tenderness, uterine tenderness, or adnexal tenderness.[30] Box 33-5 lists the diagnostic criteria for PID. No labs or studies are needed to begin treatment; however, additional information can improve the specificity of diagnosis. Abdominal pain in women can have many causes, and it is important to rule out other diagnoses, which can be done while treating for PID.[30]

The complications of PID can be significant; therefore, rapid treatment is recommended even before the causative pathogen can be identified. Because treatment is empiric, it needs to be effective against a broad range of pathogens, especially chlamydia, gonorrhea, and anaerobic bacteria.[30] Treatment is usually done on an outpatient basis unless the woman has symptoms of advanced infection, cannot take oral medications, is pregnant, or exhibits other pathologies that cannot be excluded. The CDC-recommended outpatient regimen is shown in Box 33-6.

Although alternative treatment regimens are available, the growing antibiotic resistance of gonorrhea limits antibiotic choices. The CDC is closely monitoring gonorrhea's antibiotic sensitivity and updates treatment guidelines periodically to reflect new information.[30] To prevent recurrence, sexual partners of women with PID should also receive treatment, even if they are asymptomatic. Women receiving treatment should be reevaluated by their care provider in 3 days to ensure antibiotic treatment is effective.[30] Because women with a history of PID are at increased risk for ectopic pregnancy, they should seek

FIGURE 33-6 Salpingitis. A, Advanced pyosalpinx. Note the swollen fallopian tubes. **B,** Bilateral, retort-shaped, swollen, sealed tubes and adhesions of ovaries are typical of salpingitis. (**A** from Ball JW et al: *Seidel's guide to physical examination,* ed 8, St Louis, 2015, Mosby. **B** from Damjanov I, Linder J, editors: *Anderson's pathology,* ed 10, St Louis, 1996, Mosby.)

BOX 33-5   Diagnostic Criteria for Pelvic Inflammatory Disease

Minimum Criteria (One or More Needed for Diagnosis)
Cervical motion tenderness, *or*
Uterine tenderness, *or*
Adnexal tenderness

Additional Criteria That Increase Specificity of Diagnosis
Body temperature >38.3° C (>101° F)
Mucopurulent cervical or vaginal discharge
Numerous white blood cells on saline wet prep
Elevated C-reactive protein
Elevated erythrocyte sedimentation rate
Documented infection with *Chlamydia trachomatis* or *Neisseria gonorrhoeae*

Definitive Criteria (*Not* Needed for Treatment)
Transvaginal ultrasound, magnetic resonance imaging, *or*
Doppler studies showing thickened and fluid-filled tubes
Laparoscopic visualization of PID-related abnormalities

Data from Centers for Disease Control and Prevention: *MMWR Morb Mortal Wkly Rep* 59(RR-12), 2010; Yudin MH, Ross JDC: Pelvic inflammatory disease. In Zenilman JM, Shahmansesh M, editors: *Sexually transmitted diseases*, pp 67-76, Sudbury, Mass, 2012, Jones & Bartlett Learning.
PID, Pelvic inflammatory disease.

BOX 33-6   CDC Outpatient Recommended Regimen for PID

Ceftriaxone 250 mg IM in a single dose
Plus
Doxycycline 100 mg orally twice a day for 14 days
With or without
Metronidazole 500 mg orally twice a day for 14 days
Or
Cefoxitin 2 g IM in a single dose and probenecid 1 g orally administered concurrently in a single dose
Plus
Doxycycline 100 mg orally twice a day for 14 days
With or without
Metronidazole 500 mg orally twice a day for 14 days
Or
Other parenteral third-generation cephalosporin (e.g., ceftizoxime or cefotaxime)
Plus
Doxcycline 100 mg orally twice a day for 14 days
With or without
Metronidazole 500 mg orally twice a day for 14 days

From Centers for Disease Control and Prevention (CDC): *Pelvic inflammatory diseases, STD sexually transmitted diseases treatment guidelines*, Atlanta, 2010, Author. Last updated August 15, 2014.

care as soon as they know they are pregnant because ectopic pregnancy is a major cause of maternal mortality.[33]

The diagnosis of PID is based on history, abdominal tenderness, the presence of uterine and cervical movement tenderness on bimanual pelvic examination, mucopurulent discharge at the cervical os, white blood cells on Gram stain or wet mount of cervical discharge, leukocytosis, and increased erythrocyte sedimentation rate. To support the diagnosis, tests for chlamydia and gonorrhea are done; sonography, laparoscopy, and culdocentesis are indicated when a woman has recurrent symptoms or symptoms unresponsive to outpatient treatment regimens, a temperature greater than 38°C (100.4°F), or an adnexal mass. Other conditions that cause pelvic pain must be excluded, including ectopic pregnancy, threatened abortion, ovarian torsion, ovarian cyst, or appendicitis. Recommendations for physical rest and avoidance of intercourse are often given as precautionary and comfort measures during initial recovery (i.e., 1 to 2 weeks).

Vaginitis

Vaginitis is irritation or inflammation of the vagina, typically caused by infection. Vaginitis is characterized by an increase in white blood cells on saline wet prep examination. Vaginal irritation without white blood cells is known as vaginosis. The major causes of vaginitis are overgrowth of normal flora, sexually transmitted diseases, and vaginal irritation related to low estrogen levels during menopause (a condition known as *atropic vaginitis*). The incidence of sexually transmitted vaginitis remains highest in women 15 to 24 years of age.

The development of vaginitis is related to alterations in the vaginal environment and includes changes with complications in local defense mechanisms, such as skin integrity, immune reaction, and particularly vaginal pH. The pH of the vagina (normally 4.0 to 4.5) depends on cervical secretions and the presence of normal flora that help maintain an acidic environment. Changes in the vaginal pH may predispose a woman to infection. Variables that affect the vaginal pH and therefore the bactericidal nature of secretions and the predisposition to infection include douching; using soaps, spermicides, feminine hygiene sprays, and deodorant menstrual pads or tampons; and having conditions associated with increased glycogen content of vaginal secretions, such as pregnancy and diabetes.

Antibiotics often destroy normal vaginal flora, facilitating overgrowth of *Candida albicans* and causing a yeast infection. Increased vaginal alkalinity also may enhance susceptibility to trichomoniasis and BV.

Diagnosis is based on history, physical examination, and examination of the discharge by wet mount. Infection is suggested with a marked change in color or if the discharge becomes copious, malodorous, or irritating.

Treatment involves developing and maintaining an acidic environment, relieving symptoms (usually pruritus and irritation), and administering antimicrobial or antifungal medications to eradicate the infectious organism. If the infection can be sexually transmitted, the woman's partner will also need to be treated. Research suggests that probiotics, especially *Lactobacillus crispatus*, can encourage proliferation of normal vaginal flora and decrease the incidence of vaginitis in women at risk for this disease.[34,35] A probiotic bacterial strain, *Lactobacillus plantarum* P17630, can attach to vaginal epithelium and reduce the adhesion of *C. albicans*, and may help reduce *Candida* recurrence.[36]

Cervicitis

Cervicitis is a nonspecific term used to describe inflammation of the cervix. The CDC defines cervicitis as having two major diagnostic signs: a purulent or mucopurulent discharge from the cervical os or endocervical bleeding induced by gently introducing a cotton swab into the cervix.[37] Either sign or both may be present. Cervicitis can have infectious or noninfectious causes. Chemicals and substances introduced into the vagina can cause cervicitis as well as disruptions in the normal vaginal flora. However, there are conflicting definitions of cervicitis used clinically and in research. Age and risk factors are important in assessing a woman with cervicitis. Younger women are at risk for sexually transmitted infections (STIs) and should be tested for chlamydia, gonorrhea, and trichomoniasis. Older women with cervicitis may have STIs but are at risk for irritation from abnormal vaginal flora related to low vaginal estrogen levels.

Mucopurulent cervicitis (MPC) is usually caused by one or more sexually transmitted pathogens, such as *Trichomonas, Neisseria, Chlamydia, Mycoplasma,* or *Ureaplasma*. Infection causes the cervix to become red and edematous. A mucopurulent (mucus- and pus-containing) exudate drains from the external cervical os, and the individual may report vague pelvic pain, bleeding, or dysuria. Bleeding can occur during sexual intercourse or with pelvic examinations, or both, and Pap smears. Because mucopurulent cervicitis is a symptom of PID, women at risk for STIs, especially those less than 26 years old, should receive treatment for PID while awaiting results of microbial testing.[38] If the woman is not at risk for STIs, a thorough evaluation often reveals another cause for the inflammation. Partners should be notified and examined if chlamydia, gonorrhea, or trichomoniasis was identified or suspected in the affected woman; these partners should then be treated for the STIs. To avoid reinfection, women and their sex partners should abstain from sexual intercourse until therapy is completed (i.e., 7 days after a single-dose regimen or after completion of a 7-day regimen).[38] The infectious microorganisms are cultured or identified by immunoassay. Definitive diagnosis is followed by oral antibiotic therapy.

Vulvodyniavestibulitis

Vulvodyniavestibulitis (VV) (also referred to as vulvitis, vestibulitis, or vulvovestibulitisdynia) is chronic vulvar pain lasting 3 months or longer without visible dermatosis; inflammation of the vulva or vaginal vestibule, or both; infection; neoplasia; or identifiable neurologic disorder.[39,40] The classification of vulvodynia is based on the location of the pain, whether it is localized or generalized, and whether the pain is provoked, unprovoked, or mixed.[39] *Localized* is characterized by pain from a cause that usually does not cause pain (allodynia) to the vulvar vestibule (entrance of vagina) area. *Generalized* is a diffuse pain pattern involving all of the pudendal nerve distribution and beyond. *Provoked* means any touch or stimulation that elicits pain, *unprovoked* is pain that occurs in the absence of touch or stimulation, and *mixed* is pain that varies with or without touch or stimulation. Individuals describe the pain as burning, stinging, irritation, or rawness. In many cases it may represent several disorders without an identifiable cause. Vulvodynia is fairly common with lifetime estimates of prevalence ranging from 10% to 28% among reproductive-aged women; in addition, it can affect girls.[41] It occurs across races and the incidence seems to decrease with increasing age.

The cause of vulvodynia is unknown. Theories suggest it is multifactorial in origin including embryonic factors, chronic inflammation, genetic immune factors, nerve pathways, increased sensitivity to environmental factors (infection, trauma, irritants), hormonal changes, human papillomavirus (HPV), and oxalates.[39] Although the inflammation of VV may be caused by contact dermatitis (i.e., exposure to soaps, detergents, lotions, sprays, shaving, menstrual pads/tampons, perfumed toilet paper, tight-fitting clothes), the condition may be more complex and represent abnormalities in three interdependent systems: vestibular mucosa, pelvic floor musculature, and central nervous system pain regulatory pathways. The condition also may represent an autoimmune reaction. The suggested pathophysiology of vulvodynia is a chronic disorder of the nerves that supply the vulva. Some evidence has documented nerve fiber proliferation or neural hyperplasia in the affected tissue.[39] An important trigger is chronic inflammation caused by contact irritants, recurrent infections, hormonal changes, and chronic skin conditions. Overall, with normal sensations there is a heightened sensitivity. Vulvodynia often occurs in the context of other pain conditions and includes irritable bowel syndrome, interstitial cystitis, recurrent yeast infections, and fibromyalgia.[40] Because the mechanisms of vulvodynia are poorly understood it is often a difficult condition to evaluate and treat.

After ruling out and treating conditions that can contribute to or cause vulvar inflammation (e.g., *Candida*, STIs, seborrhea, psoriasis), there are few treatment options. Cotton swab testing is used to identify painful areas. Studies on treatments are limited but suggest that women may benefit from topical lidocaine (Xylocaine), topical or systemic antidepressants, behavioral treatment, Botox injections into the affected nerve, or vestibulectomy. Bathing in lukewarm water in a mild baking soda solution can be soothing and ice packs may help.[39] Hot water may incite vulvar symptoms. Suggested approaches include use of hydrocortisone cream, application of a water barrier (such as thick skin cream or solid vegetable shortening) during a period of healing, behavioral treatment (35% to 83% of women benefit), or vestibulectomy (61% to 94% success rate), a procedure that is understandably unacceptable to many women. Women also are advised to avoid irritants, wear loose cotton clothing, and use appropriate antimicrobial/antifungal treatments for any recurrent vaginitis.

Bartholinitis

Bartholinitis, or Bartholin cyst, is an acute inflammation of one or both of the ducts that lead from the introitus (vaginal opening) to the Bartholin/greater vestibular glands (Figure 33-7). Most lesions of the Bartholin gland are cysts or abscesses. The usual causes are microorganisms that infect the lower female reproductive tract, such as streptococci, staphylococci, and sexually transmitted pathogens. Acute bartholinitis may be preceded by an infection, such as cervicitis, vaginitis, or urethritis.

Infection or trauma causes inflammatory changes that narrow the distal portion of the duct, leading to obstruction and stasis of glandular secretions. The obstruction, or cyst, varies from 1 to 8 cm in diameter and is located in the posterolateral portion of the vulva. The affected area is usually red and painful, and pus may be visible at the opening of the duct. This exudate should be cultured. The individual may have fever and malaise. Diagnosis is based on the clinical manifestations and the identification of infectious microorganisms.

FIGURE 33-7 Inflammation of Bartholin Gland. (Modified from Gershenson DM et al: *Operative gynecology*, ed 2, Philadelphia, 2001, W.B. Saunders. In Fuller JK: *Surgical technology*, ed 6, Philadelphia, 2013, Saunders.)

Chronic bartholinitis is characterized by the presence of a small cyst that is slightly tender but otherwise is asymptomatic. Most Bartholin cysts require no treatment. Symptoms only occur if an exacerbation of infection causes an abscess to form in the gland itself.

Diagnosis is based on the clinical manifestations and the identification of infectious microorganisms. Treatment is controversial but involves broad-spectrum antibiotics. Some clinicians attempt to drain the cyst using hot soaks, needle aspiration, insertion of a catheter, or marsupialization (cutting a slit and suturing the edges) of the infected gland. No single treatment has proved superior for both relief and prevention of recurrence. Pain is relieved with analgesics and warm sitz baths. If an abscess forms, it may be surgically drained.

Pelvic Organ Prolapse

The bladder, urethra, and rectum are supported by the endopelvic fascia and perineal muscles. This muscular and fascial tissue loses tone and strength with aging and may fail to maintain the pelvic organs in the proper position. Progressive descent of the pelvic support structures may cause pelvic floor disorders, such as urinary and fecal incontinence, and pelvic organ prolapse. Pelvic organ prolapse (POP) is the descent of one or more of the following: the vaginal wall, the uterus, or the apex of the vagina (after a hysterectomy). Although more than 50% of women have some version of POP on physical examination, most women have no symptoms. When prolapse becomes severe, the function of the surrounding organs can be altered. POP is thought be caused by direct trauma (such as childbirth); pelvic floor surgery; or damage to pelvic innervation, particularly the pudendal nerve. Risk factors in nulliparous women, however, include occupational activities that require heavy lifting or chronic medical conditions, such as chronic lung disease or refractory constipation (chronically increased intra-abdominal pressure). The most frequently cited risk factors are aging, obesity, and hysterectomy. Other risk factors include a strong familial tendency (from family and twin studies) and possibly a multifactorial genetic component.[42] Prolapse of the bladder, urethra, rectum, or uterus may occur many years after an initial injury to the supporting structure.

Uterine prolapse is descent of the cervix or entire uterus into the vaginal canal, and in severe cases the uterus falls completely through the vagina and protrudes from the introitus, creating ulceration and obvious discomfort. Figure 33-8 illustrates the different degrees (grades) of uterine prolapse, showing descent of the cervix or the entire uterus into the vaginal canal. Grade 1 prolapse is not treated unless it causes discomfort. Grades 2 and 3 prolapse usually cause feelings of fullness, heaviness, and collapse through the vagina. Symptoms of other pelvic floor disorders also may be present.

A common first-line treatment is a pessary, which is a removable mechanical device that holds the uterus in position. The pelvic fascia may be strengthened through Kegel exercises (repetitive isometric tightening and relaxing of the pubococcygeal muscles) or by estrogen therapy in menopausal women. Maintaining a healthy body mass index, preventing constipation, and treating chronic cough may help prevent prolapse. Surgical repair, with or without hysterectomy, is the treatment of last resort.

Figure 33-9 shows pelvic organ prolapse associated with cystocele and rectocele. Cystocele is descent of a portion of the posterior bladder wall and trigone into the vaginal canal and is usually caused by childbirth. In severe cases, the bladder and anterior vaginal wall bulge outside the introitus. Symptoms are usually insignificant in mild to moderate cases. Increased bulging and descent of the anterior vaginal wall and urethra can be aggravated by vigorous activity, prolonged standing, sneezing, coughing, or straining and can be relieved by rest or by assumption of a recumbent or prone position. If the prolapse is

FIGURE 33-8 Degrees of Uterine Prolapse. Grade 1 is minimal and rarely requires correction. Grade 2 prolapse has moderate symptoms, and grade 3 prolapse is severe. The uterus is so low that the cervix protrudes from the vagina. (From Phillips N: *Berry & Kohn's operating room technique,* ed 12, Philadelphia, 2013, Mosby.)

large, women may complain of vaginal pressure. Medical management can include vaginal pessary, Kegel exercises, and estrogen therapy for postmenopausal women. Surgical treatment is used for severe injury unresponsive to medical treatment (see *Health Alert:* Vaginal Mesh).

HEALTH ALERT

Vaginal Mesh

Because pelvic organ prolapse is often a result of weakened pelvic fascia and musculature, a surgical mesh was developed to improve pelvic support. This mesh was designed to be placed surgically along the area needing support. The goal was to have the woman's tissues grow through the mesh and provide consistent, long-term support. However, women who received the surgical mesh had a high rate of complications, including infection and persistent postoperative pain. In many cases the mesh eroded through the tissue, protruding into the vagina and perforating other organs. In addition, the mesh may shrink over time, causing vaginal shortening, tightening, and pain.

Some large studies have shown a benefit from mesh use for some women. However, once implanted, the mesh is difficult to remove if it is ineffective, resulting in long-term pain and the need for intensive surgeries and repairs. The U.S. Food and Drug Administration has issued several warnings about the mesh to caution women and practitioners and encourage fully informed consent about the risks and benefits of mesh placement.

Data from Maher C et al: *Cochrane Database Syst Rev* 4:CD004014, 2013; U.S. Food and Drug Administration: *FDA study communication: UPDATE on serious complications associated with transvaginal placement of surgical mesh for pelvic organ prolapse,* 2010. Available at: www.fda.gov/MedicalDevices/Safety/AlertsandNotices/ucm 2362435.htm. Accessed January 21, 2013.

A rectocele is the bulging of the rectum and posterior vaginal wall into the vaginal canal. Childbirth may increase damage, ultimately leading to a rectocele, but symptoms may not appear until after menopause. Genetic and familial predisposition and bowel habits contribute to rectocele development. Lifelong chronic constipation and straining may produce or aggravate a rectocele. A large rectocele may cause

FIGURE 33-9 Cystocele and Rectocele. A, Grade 2: anterior vaginal wall prolapse (i.e., cystocele). B, Grade 4: prolapse. C, Grade 2: posterior wall prolapse (i.e., rectocele). D, Grade 4: associated with ulceration of vaginal wall. Grades 1 and 3 not shown. (A and C from Seidel HM et al: *Mosby's guide to physical examination,* ed 4, St Louis, 1999, Mosby; B and D from Symonds EM, Macpherson MBA: *Color atlas of obstetrics and gynecology,* London, 1994, Mosby-Wolfe.)

vaginal pressure, rectal fullness, and incomplete bowel evacuation. Defecation may be difficult and can be facilitated by applying manual pressure to the posterior vaginal wall. Medical treatment focuses on the management and prevention of constipation and, if needed, the use of a pessary. Rectocele alone (without associated enterocele, uterine prolapse, and cystocele) seldom requires surgery.

An enterocele is a herniation of the rectouterine pouch into the rectovaginal septum (between the rectum and the posterior vaginal wall). It can be congenital or acquired. Although congenital enterocele rarely causes symptoms or progresses in size, those acquired can result from muscular weakness caused by previous surgery, especially those through the vagina, or from pelvic relaxation disorders, such as uterine prolapse, cystocele, and rectocele. Most large enteroceles are often found in grossly obese and older adults. Treatment is surgical. Box 33-7 summarizes the symptoms and treatment of POP.

Benign Growths and Proliferative Conditions
Benign Ovarian Cysts

Benign cysts of the ovary may occur at any time during the life span, but are most common during the reproductive years and, in particular, at the extremes of those years (Figure 33-10). An increase in benign ovarian cysts occurs when hormonal imbalances are more common, around puberty and menopause.[43] Benign ovarian cysts are quite

One or both sides, usually nontender

FIGURE 33-10 Depiction of Ovarian Cyst.

common, comprising one third of gynecologic hospital admissions. Two common causes of benign ovarian enlargement in ovulating women are follicular cysts and corpus luteum cysts. These cysts are called functional cysts because they are caused by variations of normal physiologic events. Follicular and corpus luteum cysts are unilateral. They are typically 5 to 6 cm in diameter but can grow as large as 8 to 10 cm. Most women are asymptomatic.

BOX 33-7   Pelvic Organ Prolapse: Symptoms and Treatments

Symptoms

Urinary

Sensation of incomplete emptying of bladder
Urinary incontinence
Urinary frequency/urgency
Bladder "splinting" to accomplish voiding

Bowel

Constipation or feeling of rectal fullness or blockage
Difficult defecation
Stool or flatus incontinence
Urgency
Manual "splinting" of posterior vaginal wall to accomplish defecation

Pain and Bulging

Vaginal, bladder, rectum
Pelvic pressure, bulging, pain
Lower back pain

Sexual

Dyspareunia
Decreased sensation, lubrication, arousal

Treatment

Depending on age of woman and cause and severity of condition:
Isometric exercises to strengthen pubococcygeal muscles (Kegel exercises)
Estrogen to improve tone and vascularity of fascial support (postmenopausal)
Pessary (a removable device) to hold pelvic organs in place

Surgical

Reconstructive: autologous grafts; synthetic mesh/sling
Obliterative (most extreme)
Weight loss
Avoidance of constipation
Treatment of cough/lung conditions

Benign cysts of the ovary are produced when a follicle or a number of follicles are stimulated but no dominant follicle develops and completes the maturation process. Every month about 120 follicles are stimulated, and generally, only 1 succeeds in ovulation of a mature ovum. Normally, in the early follicular phase of the menstrual cycle, follicles of the ovary respond to hormonal signals from the brain. The pituitary gland produces FSH to mature follicles in the ovary. If the dominant follicle develops properly before ovulation, the corpus luteum becomes vascularized and secretes progesterone. Progesterone arrests development of other follicles in both ovaries in that cycle. LH, proteolytic enzymes, and prostaglandins trigger follicular rupture and release of the ovum.

Follicular cysts (also called ovarian or functional cysts) are filled with fluid and can be caused by a transient condition in which the dominant follicle fails to rupture or one or more of the nondominant follicles fails to regress. This disturbance is not well understood. It may be that the hypothalamus does not receive or send a message strong enough to increase FSH levels to the degree necessary to develop or mature a dominant follicle. The hypothalamus monitors blood levels of estradiol and progesterone; when FSH level is low, estradiol concentration does not increase enough to stimulate LH surge. Research indicates that when progesterone is not being produced, the hypothalamus releases gonadotropin-releasing hormone (GnRH) to increase the FSH level. FSH continues to stimulate follicles to mature, and the granulosa cells grow and, presumably, estradiol level increases. This abnormal cycle continues to stimulate follicular size and causes follicular cysts to develop. Although individuals may experience no symptoms, some have pelvic pain, a sensation of feeling bloated, tender breasts, and heavy or irregular menses. After several subsequent cycles

in which hormone levels once again follow a regular cycle and progesterone levels are restored, cysts usually will be absorbed or will regress. Follicular cysts can be random or recurrent events.

A corpus luteum cyst may normally form by the granulosa cells left behind after ovulation. This cyst is highly vascularized but usually limited in size, and with the normal menstrual cycle it spontaneously regresses. With an imbalance in hormones, low LH and progesterone levels may cause an abnormal or hemorrhagic cyst. In some cases, large cysts can rupture and cause hemorrhage.

Corpus luteum cysts are less common than follicular cysts, but luteal cysts typically cause more symptoms, particularly if they rupture. Manifestations include dull pelvic pain and amenorrhea or delayed menstruation, followed by irregular or heavier-than-normal bleeding. Rupture occasionally occurs and can cause massive bleeding with excruciating pain; immediate surgery may be required. Corpus luteum cysts usually regress spontaneously in nonpregnant women. Oral contraceptives may be used to prevent cysts from forming in the future.

Dermoid cysts are ovarian teratomas that contain elements of all three germ layers; they are common ovarian neoplasms. These growths may contain mature tissue including skin, hair, sebaceous and sweat glands, muscle fibers, cartilage, and bone. Dermoid cysts are usually asymptomatic and are found incidentally on pelvic examination. Dermoid cysts have malignant potential and should be removed.

Torsion of the ovary is a rare complication of ovarian cysts or tumors or enlargement of the ovary; and it can occur in girls or women. If a cyst is sufficiently large, it can cause the ovary to twist on its ligaments, decreasing blood supply to the ovary and causing extreme pain. Ovarian torsion is rare but is a gynecologic emergency when present. It usually presents with acute, severe unilateral abdominal or pelvic pain and is treated surgically.

✔ QUICK CHECK 33-3

1. Why is prompt treatment of pelvic inflammatory disease (PID) critical to reproductive health?
2. Why do benign ovarian cysts develop in women who ovulate?
3. What is the difference between a follicular cyst and a corpus luteum cyst?

Endometrial Polyps

An endometrial polyp is a benign mass of endometrial tissue and contains a variable amount of glands, stroma, and blood vessels. Endometrial polyps are usually solitary and can occur anywhere within the uterus. Polyps are structurally diverse and are usually classified as hyperplastic, atrophic (or inactive), or functional. Hyperplastic polyps are often pedunculated (stalk or mushroom-like) and may be mistaken for endometrial hyperplasia or, if large, adenosarcoma (Figure 33-11). Although polyps most often develop in women between ages 40 and 50 years, they can occur at all ages. Hyperestrogenic states, obesity, tamoxifen use, and hypertension are risk factors for developing polyps.

Most polyps are asymptomatic; however, they are a common cause of intermenstrual bleeding or even excessive menstrual bleeding. Diagnosis is made by hysteroscopy or ultrasonography. The lesions can be removed with small, curved forceps but there is a high rate of spontaneous resolution. Coexistence of a separate endometrial atypical hyperplasia or adenocarcinoma is possible but malignancy is extremely rare.

Leiomyomas

Leiomyomas, commonly called myomas or uterine fibroids, are benign tumors that develop from smooth muscle cells in the myometrium. Leiomyomas are the most common benign tumors of the

FIGURE 33-11 Endometrial Polyp. Polyp is protruding through the cervical os. (From Symonds EM, Macpherson MBA: *Color atlas of obstetrics and gynecology,* London, 1994, Mosby.)

FIGURE 33-12 Leiomyomas. A, Uterine section showing whorl-like appearance and locations of leiomyomas, which are also called *uterine fibroids.* **B,** Multiple leiomyomas in sagittal section. Typical, well-circumscribed, solid, light gray nodules distort uterus. (B from Damjanov I, Linder J: *Pathology: a color atlas,* St Louis, 2000, Mosby.)

uterus, affecting 70% to 80% of all women, and most remain small and asymptomatic. Prevalence increases in women ages 30 to 50 years but decreases with menopause. The incidence of leiomyomas in black and Asian women is two to five times higher than that in white women.

The cause of uterine leiomyomas is unknown, although the size of the tumor appears to be related to hormonal fluctuations, including estrogen and progesterone, growth factors, and reduced apoptosis. Because leiomyomas are estrogen and progesterone sensitive, uterine leiomyomas are not seen before menarche, are common during the reproductive years, and generally shrink after menopause if present. Tumors in pregnant women enlarge rapidly but often decrease in size after the end of the pregnancy. Risk factors include heredity, nulliparity, obesity, PCOS, diabetes, black race, and hypertension.

PATHOPHYSIOLOGY Most leiomyomas occur in multiples in the fundus of the uterus, although often occurring singly and throughout the uterus. Leiomyomas are classified as subserous, submucous, or intramural, according to location within the various layers of the uterine wall (Figure 33-12). Most leiomyomas have normal karyotypes but some have simple chromosomal abnormalities. Recently, mutations in the Mediator Subcomplex 12 *(MED12)* gene have been identified in about 70% of uterine leiomyomas.[44] Uterine leiomyomas are usually firm and surrounded by a connective tissue layer. Degeneration and necrosis may occur when the leiomyoma outgrows its blood supply, which is more common in larger tumors and is frequently accompanied by pain.

CLINICAL MANIFESTATIONS The major clinical manifestations of leiomyomas are abnormal vaginal bleeding, pain, and symptoms related to pressure on nearby structures. Fibroids also may contribute to infertility and subfertility, as well as obstruction during birth if large enough. The leiomyoma can make the uterine cavity larger, thereby increasing the endometrial surface area. This enlargement may account for the increased menstrual bleeding associated with leiomyomas. Although pain is not an early symptom, it occurs with the devascularization of larger leiomyomas and is associated with blood vessel compression that limits blood supply to adjacent structures. Because the fibroid is relatively slow growing, enabling adjacent structures to adapt to pressure, symptoms of abdominal pressure develop slowly. Pressure

on the bladder may contribute to urinary frequency, urgency, and dysuria. Pressure on the ureter may cause it to become distended "upstream" from the pressure point; rectosigmoid pressure may lead to constipation. Larger fibroids may cause a sensation of abdominal or genital heaviness.

EVALUATION AND TREATMENT Uterine leiomyomas are suspected when bimanual examination discloses irregular, nontender nodularity of the uterus. Pelvic sonography or MRI confirms the diagnosis. Treatment depends on symptoms, tumor size, and age, reproductive status, and overall health of the individual. Most leiomyomas are asymptomatic and can be managed by observation only. Medical treatment is aimed at shrinking the myoma or reducing the symptoms. Use of hormonal contraceptives may shrink or enhance growth and should be closely monitored. Mifepristone (formerly RU-486), a progesterone receptor agonist, also may be useful as a conservative treatment, as well as GnRH agonists for temporary management. Myomectomy or removal of the fibroid from the muscle of the uterus may be less invasive than a full hysterectomy and remains the standard of cure for women wishing to preserve their fertility. Other treatments, such as uterine artery embolization (UAE), laser ablation, and levonorgestrel-intrauterine system (LNG-IUS), all hold promise. A Cochrane review found UAE appears to have an overall satisfaction rate similar to hysterectomy and myomectomy.[45] UAE is associated with a higher rate of minor complications and a much higher risk of requiring future surgical intervention within 2 to 5 years of the initial procedure.[45] Benefits and risks of all treatments should be carefully considered, as well as a woman's desire for future pregnancy.

Adenomyosis

Adenomyosis is the presence of islands of endometrial glands surrounded by benign endometrial stroma within the uterine myometrium. It commonly develops during the late reproductive years, with the highest incidence among women in their forties and in women taking tamoxifen. Parity also increases the risk for adenomyosis. Adenomyosis may be asymptomatic or may be associated with abnormal menstrual bleeding, anemia, dysmenorrhea, uterine enlargement, and uterine tenderness during menstruation. Secondary dysmenorrhea becomes increasingly severe as disease progresses. On examination, the uterus is enlarged, globular, and most tender just before or after menstruation. Diagnosis is confirmed with ultrasonography or MRI. Treatment is symptomatic, and similar to that for dysmenorrhea (i.e., nonsteroidal anti-inflammatory drugs [NSAIDs], hormonal contraceptives, or levonorgestrel-intrauterine system [LNG-IUS]). Other options include surgical resection or, if severe, hysterectomy. UAE and LNG-IUDs have shown good initial results but need further testing.

Endometriosis

Endometriosis is the presence of functioning endometrial tissue or implants outside the uterus. Like normal endometrial tissue, the ectopic (out-of-place) endometrium responds to the hormonal fluctuations of the menstrual cycle. The incidence of endometriosis is difficult to determine, especially in asymptomatic adolescent and fertile women. About 50% of women evaluated for pelvic pain, infertility, or pelvic mass are diagnosed with endometriosis. Additionally, the frequency and severity of symptoms do not correlate with the extent or site of lesions. Many theories exist on the cause of endometriosis including the implantation of endometrial cells during *retrograde menstruation*, in which menstrual fluids move through the fallopian tubes and into the pelvic cavity. It is now known, however, that retrograde menstruation occurs in almost all women, but not all women develop endometriosis. The main theories include coelomic metaplasia (peritoneal mesothelium, the müllerian ducts, and the germinal epithelium of the ovary are all derived from coelomic wall epithelium), retrograde menstruation, embryonic cell rest (primitive "at rest" embryonic cells become activated), iatrogenic mechanical transplantation, and lymphatic and vascular dissemination.[46] A genetic predisposition to endometriosis has been documented. Some genetic polymorphisms have been identified.

PATHOPHYSIOLOGY Endometriosis is a multifactorial estrogen-dependent condition that may affect 5% to 10% of women of childbearing age in developed countries (Figure 33-13).[46] Emerging evidence suggests that endometriosis can have heterogeneous characteristics and therefore the pathogenesis is modulated by many factors including genetic, epigenetic, environmental, and cellular factors.[46] The endometrium is highly dynamic tissue with regenerative tissue undergoing cyclic processes of growth, differentiation, shedding, and regeneration

FIGURE 33-13 Endometriosis. The uterus is distended, and retrograde spill of menstrual loss has led to the development of endometriosis *(dark purple patches)*. (From Symonds EM, Macpherson MBA: *Color atlas of obstetrics and gynecology,* London, 1994, Mosby-Wolfe.)

FIGURE 33-14 Pelvic Sites of Endometrial Implantation in Endometriosis. Endometrial cells may enter the pelvic cavity during retrograde menstruation.

as part of the menstrual cycle. These processes depend on steroid hormones, growth factors, and leukocytes that affect the balance between proliferation and apoptosis. Although endometriosis is considered benign, approximately 1.0% of affected women have an increased risk of malignant transformation involving multiple pathways of development.[46] The defining feature of endometriosis is the presence and proliferation of endometrial-like tissue (implants), including stromal and glandular tissue, in locations outside of the uterine cavity, primarily in the ovaries, fallopian tubes, bladder, rectosigmoid colon, and uterine myometrium (adenomyosis), often causing infertility and pain (Figure 33-14).[46]

The pathophysiology of endometriosis remains poorly understood but several characteristics are being investigated, including the following: (1) High levels of estrogen production are observed in endometriosis and a key enzyme in estrogen production is aromatase, which has been correlated with the severity of endometriosis. (2) There is evidence of switching of cell fates during development, where epithelial and mesenchymal markers highlight a contribution of the mesenchymal-epithelial transition (MET) and of the epithelial-mesenchymal transition (EMT) in endometriosis (see Chapter 10). (3) The roles of inflammation and of peritoneal leukocytes and their mediators may facilitate the progression of endometriotic lesions. (4) Some components of the innate immune system are involved in endometriosis (dendritic cells, macrophages, Toll-like receptors), and components of the adaptive immune system (T- and B-cell functions) can promote apoptosis, tissue damage, and multiorgan involvement. (5) The development of lesions is dependent on new blood vessel development (angiogenesis). (6) Genetic and epigenetic roles are present in endometriotic lesions and some ovarian cancers (clear cell carcinoma, endometrioid adenocarcinoma). (7) Stem cells play a role in the development of endometriotic lesions. Changes in stem cell populations of endometriotic lesions are associated with genetic and epigenetic alterations.

Cyclic changes depend on the blood supply of the lesions (implants) and the presence of glandular and stromal cells. Given that the blood supply is sufficient, the ectopic endometrium proliferates, breaks down, and bleeds with the normal menstrual cycle. The bleeding is one cause of inflammation, triggering a cascade of cellular inflammatory mediators, including cytokines, chemokines, growth factors, and protective factors such as secretory leukocyte protease inhibitor and superoxide dismutase.[47] The inflammation may lead to fibrosis, scarring, adhesions, and pain.

CLINICAL MANIFESTATIONS The clinical manifestations of endometriosis vary in frequency and severity and can mimic other pelvic disease (i.e., pelvic inflammatory disease, ovarian cysts, irritable bowel syndrome). Symptoms include infertility, pelvic pain, dyschezia (pain on defecation), dyspareunia, (pain on intercourse), and, less commonly, constipation and abnormal vaginal bleeding. If implants are located within the pelvis, an asymptomatic pelvic mass having irregular, movable nodules and a fixed, retroverted uterus are found on examination. Most symptoms can be explained by the proliferation, breakdown, and bleeding of the ectopic endometrial tissue with subsequent formation of adhesions. In most instances, however, the degree of endometriosis is not related to the frequency or severity of symptoms. Dysmenorrhea, for example, does not appear to be related to the degree of endometriosis. With involvement of the rectovaginal septum or the uterosacral ligaments, dyspareunia develops. Dyschezia, a hallmark symptom of endometriosis, occurs with bleeding of ectopic endometrium in the rectosigmoid musculature and subsequent fibrosis.

Up to 25% to 40% of women with infertility have endometriosis. The relationship between endometriosis and infertility is strong; however, the *degree* of disease is not as closely associated. More simply, women with untreated minimal to mild disease may have high pregnancy rates or may experience infertility. The exact reason for infertility in women with endometriosis is unknown.

EVALUATION AND TREATMENT A presumptive diagnosis is based on the previously described symptoms, but pelvic laparoscopy is required for a definitive diagnosis. A uniform classification system that includes both extent and severity has been developed including stage I, minimal; stage II, mild; and stage III, moderate. The classification, however, still does not correlate well with a woman's symptoms. Treatment is based on preventing progression of the disease, alleviating pain, and restoring fertility. Medical therapies include suppression of ovulation with various medications, such as noncyclic estrogen-progestin–combined oral contraceptive pill (COCs), depot medroxyprogesterone acetate (DMPA), danazol, GnRH agonists, mifepristone,

or gestrinone, and promotion of atrophy of the endometrium with progestins or an LNG-IUD. Conservative surgical treatment includes laparoscopic removal of endometrial implants with conventional or laser techniques and presacral neurectomy for severe dysmenorrhea. All treatments have risks or side effects and recurrent symptoms will develop in the majority of women within a few years, even with surgical treatments. Women should be fully informed of all options and understand the risk-to-benefit ratio of treatments, especially nonreversible treatments.

Cancer

Malignant tumors of the female reproductive system are common. Because the pelvis and abdomen are poorly innervated and designed to accommodate a growing fetus, cancers of the female reproductive tract can often grow large before causing pain. Reproductive cancers are likely to be diagnosed early if there are symptoms; for example, vaginal bleeding prompts women to seek treatment. Cervical cancer has minimal symptoms until late in the process, but is easy to detect early with Pap smears. Three percent of cancers in women begin in the cervix but the death rate from cervical cancer has plummeted since the advent of screening techniques.[48] Investigators are researching new biomarkers for the screening, diagnosis, and surveillance for ovarian cancer. Obtaining an early diagnosis for ovarian cancer is very challenging.

Cervical Cancer

Cervical cancer is the fourth most common cancer in women worldwide, and has the fourth highest death rate among cancers in women.[49] An estimated 12,900 new cases of invasive cervical cancer will be diagnosed in the United States for 2015, with an estimated 4100 deaths.[48] Black women have the highest rate of cervical cancer, followed by Hispanics, whites, American Indian/Alaska Natives, and Asian/American/Pacific Islanders.[48] Death rates are highest for black women. The rates of invasive cervical cancer have steadily decreased (since the 1960s) and death rates have declined significantly in the United States (and other developed countries), mainly attributed to the prevalence and frequency of screening with the Pap test.[50,51] Death rates were stable among women younger than 50 years but decreased by 1.1% per year among women aged 50 years and older[48] (*Health Alert:* Screening with the Papanicolaou [Pap] Test and with the Human Papillomavirus [HPV] DNA Test: Benefits and Harms from Cervical Cancer Screening [PDQ®]).

It is now widely known that HPV infection is a necessary condition in the development of almost all precancerous and cancerous cervical lesions. There are multiple subtypes of HPV and the "high-risk" (oncogenic) types of HPV (predominantly 16 and 18) have been most closely associated with high-grade dysplasia and cancer (also see Chapters 10 and 11). The precancerous lesion or dysplasia, also called *cervical intraepithelial neoplasia (CIN)* and *cervical carcinoma in situ (CIS)*, is a more advanced form of the cell changes and can progress to become invasive cancer. This process can be very slow. About 30% to 70% of those untreated for in situ carcinoma will develop invasive carcinoma over 10 to 12 years; but in about 10% of women, progression from in situ to invasive cancer can occur in less than 1 year.[52] Other risk factors for cervical cancer include multiple sexual partners, a male partner with multiple previous or current sexual partners, young age at first sexual intercourse, high parity, persistent infection with HPV-16 or HPV-18, immunosuppression, use of oral contraceptives, certain human leukocytic antigen (HLA) subtypes, and use of nicotine.[31,52]

PATHOGENESIS As discussed earlier, HPV-16 and HPV-18 are the most important risk factors for cervical disease progression and cancer.

HEALTH ALERT

Screening with the Papanicolaou (Pap) Test and with the Human Papillomavirus (HPV) DNA Test: Benefits and Harms from Cervical Cancer Screening (PDQ®)

Screening with the Papanicolaou (Pap) Test: Benefits

Based on solid evidence, regular screening of appropriate women for cervical cancer with the Pap test reduces mortality from cervical cancer. The benefits of screening women younger than 21 years are small because of the low prevalence of lesions that will progress to invasive cancer. Screening is not beneficial in women older than 65 years if they have had a history of recent negative tests.[1-3]

Magnitude of Effect: Regular Pap screening decreases cervix cancer incidence and mortality by at least 80%.

- Study Design: Population-based and cohort studies
- Internal Validity: Good
- Consistency: Good
- External Validity: Good

Screening with the Pap Test: Harms

Based on solid evidence, regular screening with the Pap test leads to additional diagnostic procedures (e.g., colposcopy) and treatment for low-grade squamous intraepithelial lesions (LSILs), with long-term consequences for fertility and pregnancy. These harms are greatest for younger women, who have a higher prevalence of LSILs, lesions that often regress without treatment. Harms are also increased in younger women because they have a higher rate of false-positive results.

Magnitude of Effect: Additional diagnostic procedures were performed in 50% of women undergoing regular Pap testing. Approximately 5% were treated for LSIL. The number with impaired fertility and pregnancy complications is unknown.

- Study Design: Evidence obtained from cohort or case-control studies
- Internal Validity: Good
- Consistency: Good
- External Validity: Good

Screening with the Human Papillomavirus (HPV) DNA Test: Benefits

Based on solid evidence, screening with HPV DNA or HPV RNA detects high-grade cervical dysplasia, a precursor lesion for cervical cancer. Additional clinical trials show that HPV testing is superior to other cervical cancer screening strategies. In April 2014, the U.S. Food and Drug Administration approved an HPV DNA test that can be used alone for the primary screening of cervical cancer risk in women aged 25 years and older.[4]

Magnitude of Effect: In one prospective, clustered, randomized trial, HPV testing was superior to other strategies for preventing cervical cancer mortality.[5,6]

- Study Design: Clustered randomized controlled trial (RCT)
- Internal Validity: Good
- Consistency: Good
- External Validity: Good

Screening with the HPV DNA Test: Harms

Based on solid evidence, HPV testing identifies numerous infections that will not lead to cervical dysplasia or cervical cancer. This is especially true in women younger than 30 years, in whom rates of HPV infection may be higher.

Magnitude of Effect: In one study, 86.7% of women with a positive HPV test did not develop cervical cancer or related premalignant disease after more than a decade of follow-up.[7]

- Study Design: Long-term observational trials
- Internal Validity: Good
- Consistency: Good
- External Validity: Good

Screening with the Pap Test and the HPV DNA Test (Cotesting): Benefits

Based on solid evidence, screening every 5 years with the Pap test and the HPV DNA test (cotesting) in women 30 years and older is more sensitive in detecting cervical abnormalities, compared with the Pap test alone. Screening with the Pap test and HPV DNA test reduces the incidence of cervical cancer.[3]

Magnitude of Effect: HPV-based screening provides 60% to 70% greater protection against invasive cervical carcinoma, compared with cytologic studies.[8]

- Study Design: RCTs
- Internal Validity: Good
- Consistency: Good
- External Validity: Good

Screening with the Pap Test and the HPV DNA Test (Cotesting): Harms

Based on solid evidence, HPV and Pap cotesting is associated with more false-positive results than the Pap test alone. Abnormal test results can lead to more frequent testing and invasive diagnostic procedures.[3]

Magnitude of Effect: The percentage of U.S. women undergoing cotesting who will have a normal cytologic test result and a positive HPV test result (and who will therefore require additional testing) ranges from 11% among women aged 30 to 34 years to 2.6% among women aged 60 to 65 years.[3]

- Study Design: RCTs
- Internal Validity: Good
- Consistency: Good
- External Validity: Good

Screening Women Without a Cervix

Based on solid evidence, screening is not helpful in women who do not have a cervix as a result of a hysterectomy for a benign condition.

Magnitude of Effect: Among women without cervices, fewer than 1 per 1000 had abnormal Pap test results.

- Study Design: Evidence obtained from a single cohort study
- Internal Validity: Good
- Consistency: Good
- External Validity: Good

References

1. Sasieni P et al: Effectiveness of cervical screening with age: population based case-control study of prospectively recorded data, *BMJ* 339:b2968, 2009.
2. Sawaya GF et al: Risk of cervical cancer associated with extending the interval between cervical-cancer screenings, *N Engl J Med* 349(16):1501-1509, 2003.
3. Moyer VA, U.S. Preventive Services Task Force: Screening for cervical cancer: U.S. Preventive Services Task Force recommendation statement, *Ann Intern Med* 156(12):880-891, W312, 2012.
4. *FDA approves first human papillomavirus test for primary cervical cancer screening* [News], Silver Spring, Md, 2014, FDA. Available online. Last accessed February 12, 2015.
5. Sankaranarayanan R et al: HPV screening for cervical cancer in rural India, *N Engl J Med* 360(14):1385-1394, 2009.
6. Szarewski A: Cervical screening by visual inspection with acetic acid, *Lancet* 370(9585):365-366, 2007.
7. Chen HC et al: Persistence of type-specific human papillomavirus infection and increased long-term risk of cervical cancer, *J Natl Cancer Inst* 103(18):1387-1396, 2011.
8. Ronco G et al: Efficacy of HPV-based screening for prevention of invasive cervical cancer: follow-up of four European randomised controlled trials, *Lancet* 383(9916):524-532, 2014.

FIGURE 33-15 Cervix Is Lined by Two Types of Epithelial Cells: Squamous Cells and Columnar Glandular Cells.

TABLE 33-4 Clinical Staging for Cancer of the Cervix

Stage	Characteristics
0	Cancer in situ, intraepithelial carcinoma; earliest stage of cancer; cancer confined to its original site
I	Carcinoma confined to cervix (extension to corpus disregarded)
IA	Earliest form of stage I; there is very small amount of cancer, which is visible only under a microscope
IA1	Area of invasion is <3 mm (about ⅛ inch) deep and <7 mm (about ⅓ inch) wide
IA2	Area of invasion is between 3 and 5 mm (about ⅕ inch) deep, and <7 mm (about ⅓ inch) wide
IB	Includes cancers that can be seen without a microscope; also includes cancers seen only with a microscope that have spread deeper than 5 mm (about ⅕ inch) into connective tissue of the cervix or are wider than 7 mm
IB1	IB cancer that is no larger than 4 cm (about 1⅓ inches)
IB2	IB cancer that is >4 cm
II	Cancer has spread beyond the cervix to the upper part of the vagina; cancer does not involve the lower third of the vagina
IIA	Cancer has spread beyond the cervix to the upper part of the vagina; cancer does not involve the lower third of the vagina
IIB	Cancer has spread to the tissue next to the cervix, called the *parametrial tissue*
III	Cancer has spread to the lower part of the vagina or the pelvic wall; cancer may be blocking the ureters (tubes that carry urine from the kidneys to the bladder)
IIIA	Cancer has spread to the lower third of the vagina but not to the pelvic wall
IIIB	Cancer extends to the pelvic wall, blocks urine flow to the bladder, or both
IV	Most advanced stage of cervical cancer; cancer has spread to other parts of the body
IVA	Cancer has spread to the bladder or rectum, which are organs close to the cervix
IVB	Cancer has spread to distant organs beyond the pelvic area, such as the lungs

HPV-16 accounts for about 60% of cervical cancer cases and HPV-18 for about another 10%; other types contribute less than 5% of cases. The cervix is lined by two types of epithelial cells: squamous cells at the outer aspect and columnar glandular cells along the inner canal (Figure 33-15). The site of the cellular transformation zone, called the squamocolumnar junction, is illustrated in Figure 33-16. HPVs infect immature basal cells of the squamous epithelium in the areas of epithelial breaks or injury, or immature metaplastic squamous cells present at the squamocolumnar junction. Establishing HPV infection in the mature squamous cells that cover the ectocervix, vagina, or vulva requires damage to the surface epithelium. The cervix, with its large areas of immature epithelium, is very vulnerable to HPV infection.[31] The ability of HPV to act as a carcinogen depends on the viral proteins E6 and E7 because they interfere with the activity of tumor-suppressor proteins that regulate cell growth and survival.[31]

Replication of HPV occurs in the maturing squamous cells, and studies have shown that HPV activates the cell cycle by interfering with two tumor-suppressor genes, *Rb* and *p53*.[31] Although HPV is a causative factor for cervical cancer, it is not the *only* factor. Other important cocarcinogens must play a role because in spite of the high percentage of young women infected with one or more HPV types during their reproductive years, only a few develop cancer. The other factors that appear to be associated include immune responses, hormonal responses, and other environmental factors that determine regression or persistence of the HPV infection.[31] Cervical cancer is a slowly progressive disease and moves from normal cervical epithelial cells to dysplasia to carcinoma in situ and, eventually, to invasive cancer (see Figure 33-16, *B*). Table 33-4 summarizes the staging of cervical cancer. Testing for high-risk HPV is often positive for many years (10 years or more) before dysplasia progresses to high-grade squamous

A   Normal   CIN I   CIN II   CIN III

Cervical Disease Progression[1-6]

Most HPV infections will clear, and most cervical lesions will not progress[1-3]

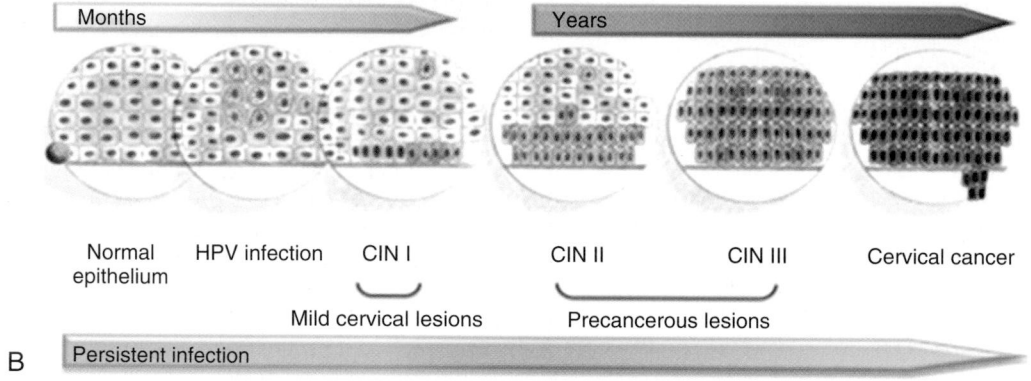

Months   Years

Normal epithelium   HPV infection   CIN I   CIN II   CIN III   Cervical cancer

Mild cervical lesions   Precancerous lesions

B   Persistent infection

- CIN 2/3 lesions are more likely to progress to cervical cancer than CIN 1 lesions[1]

1. Oster A. *Int J of Gynecol Path*, 1993, 12:186-92. 2. Moscicki A et al, *Vaccine*, 2006, 2453:42-51. 3. Einstein M. *Cancer Immunol Immunother*, 2008, 57:443-51. 4. Winer R. et al. *J Int Dis*, 2005, 191:731-38. 5. Holowaty P. et al. *J Natl Cancer Inst*, 1999, 91:252-58. 6. Solomon D. et al. *JAMA*, 2002, 287:2114-19.

FIGURE 33-16 Cervical Intraepithelial Neoplasia (CIN). A, Normal multiparous cervix including the transformation zone where precancerous and cancerous changes occur. CIN stage I note the white appearance of part of the anterior lip of the cervix associated with neoplastic changes; CIN stage II, lesions also are reflected in distant capillaries; CIN stage III, lesions are predominantly around the external os. **B,** Normal epithelium, HPV infection progressing to CIN stage I, and then with more time persistent HPV infections progressing to precancerous lesions CIN II and CIN III and eventually cervical cancer. Most cervical lesions do not progress to cervical cancer. (**A** from Kumar V et al: *Robbins & Cotran pathologic basis of disease,* ed 9, Philadelphia, 2015, Saunders; **B** from Symonds EM, Macpherson MBA: *Color atlas of obstetrics and gynecology,* London, 1994, Mosby.)

intraepithelial lesions (HSILs) that can develop into invasive cervical cancer (CIN III, Table 33-5).

CLINICAL MANIFESTATIONS Because cervical neoplasms are predominantly asymptomatic, about 90% of cervical cancers can be detected early through the use of Pap and HPV testing. If symptoms exist, they may include a change in vaginal discharge or bleeding. Bleeding varies and may occur after intercourse or between menstrual periods. At times, women will complain of abnormal menses or postmenopausal bleeding. A less common symptom may be a serosanguineous or yellowish vaginal discharge. A new or foul odor also may be present. Advanced disease may cause urinary or rectal symptoms and pelvic or back pain.

EVALUATION AND TREATMENT About 90% of cervical cancers can be detected early through the use of regular screening tests (see

TABLE 33-5   Classification System for Squamous Cervical Precursor Lesions

Dysplasia/ Carcinoma in Situ	Cervical Intraepithelial Neoplasia (CIN)	Squamous Intraepithelial Lesion (SIL), Current Classification
Mild dysplasia	CIN I	Low-grade SIL (LSIL)
Moderate dysplasia	CIN II	High-grade SIL (HSIL)
Severe dysplasia	CIN III	High-grade SIL (HSIL)
Carcinoma in situ	CIN III	High-grade SIL (HSIL)

From Kumar V et al: *Robbins & Cotran pathologic basis of disease,* ed 9, Philadelphia, 2015, Elsevier/Saunders.
CIN, Cervical intraepithelial neoplasia; *SIL,* squamous intraepithelial lesion.

Health Alert: Screening with the Papanicolaou [Pap] Test and with the Human Papillomavirus [HPV] DNA Test: Benefits and Harms from Cervical Cancer Screening [PDQ®], p. 820). When dysplasia is detected, colposcopy is usually indicated to identify lesions and obtain needed biopsies. If invasive carcinoma is found, lymphangiography, computed tomography (CT) scan, MRI, ultrasonography, or radioimmunodetection methods are used to further assess tissue involvement.

Treatment depends on the degree of neoplastic change, the size and location of the lesion, and the extent of metastatic spread. Treatment for invasive carcinoma depends on the stage of the tumor and includes surgery, radiation therapy, chemotherapy, and targeted treatment. Prognosis is excellent with early detection and treatment. The prevention of HPV infection appears to be key for substantially reducing the risk of cervical cancer and the FDA-approved vaccines for two of the high-risk types of HPV show excellent promise (see *Health Alert:* Cervical Cancer Primary Prevention).

HEALTH ALERT

Cervical Cancer Primary Prevention

Individuals not sexually active almost never develop genital HPV infections. HPV vaccination before sexual activity can reduce the risk of infection by HPV types targeted by the vaccine.

The Food and Drug Administration (FDA) has approved three vaccines to prevent HPV infection: Gardasil, Gardasil 9, and Cervarix. These vaccines provide strong protection against the HPV targeted infections but they are not effective for treating established infections or disease caused by HPV. All three vaccines prevent infections with HPV types 16 and 18, the two high-risk HPVs that cause about 70 percent of cervical cancers. Gardasil also prevents infection with HPV types 6 and 11, which causes about 90 percent of genital warts. Gardasil 9 prevents infection with the same four high-risk HPV types plus five additional high-risk types (31, 33, 45, 52, and 58). All three vaccines are given as a series of three injections into muscle tissue over a 6-month period.

Importantly, consistent and correct condom use is associated with reduced HPV transmission and less frequent use is not. The virus can infect areas not covered by the condom.

NIH National Cancer Institute Human Papillomavirus (HPV) Vaccines. Reviewed February 19, 2015. Accessed September 5, 2015.

Vaginal Cancer

Cancer of the vagina is the rarest (about 0.6 per 100,000 women yearly) of the female genital cancers. It can occur at any age but is found predominantly in women 50 years of age and older. More than 90% of women with vaginal cancer have squamous cell carcinoma. Most squamous cell carcinomas of the vagina are associated with high-risk HPVs. Risk factors include age 60 or older, diethylstilbestrol (DES) exposure in utero, HPV type 16 (cause), human immunodeficiency virus (HIV), genital warts (associated most often with the nononcogenic types HPV-6 and HPV-11, which can infect female and male genital organs and the anal area; the relationship of developing precancerous cell changes (called *vaginal intraepithelial neoplasia [VAIN])* because of also harboring oncogenic HPV types is controversial),[53,54] and previous carcinoma of the cervix or vulva. A large proportion (30% to 50%) of women with vaginal carcinomas have had a prior hysterectomy for benign, premalignant, or malignant disease.[55]

Vaginal cancer can be asymptomatic. Therefore, regular pelvic examinations, particularly for women with a history of intrauterine DES exposure, are extremely important. Clinical manifestations that occur include abnormal vaginal bleeding or discharge not related to menstrual periods, pain during intercourse, pain in the pelvic area, pain when urinating, and constipation.

Very careful biopsy techniques confirm the tumor type and determine its size, location, and extent. Treatment depends on these findings and on the age of the individual. Treatments include surgery, chemotherapy, and radiation therapy.

Vulvar Cancer

Cancer of the vulva most often affects the labia majora and less often the labia minora, clitoris, or vaginal glands.[56] An incidence for cancer of the vulva of 5100 new cases was estimated for 2015.[48] The majority (90%) are squamous cell carcinomas. Risk factors for vulvar cancer include HPV type 16 (cause), HIV, HPV-18 (probable cause), increasing age, previous cancer (untreated high-grade vulvar intraepithelial neoplasia [VIN]), cervical cancer survivor, previous cervical intraepithelial neoplasia, women with certain autoimmune conditions (increased risk of HPV-associated tumors), organ transplant recipients (perhaps because of immunosuppression to clear HPV), and tobacco use (may relate to inability to clear HPV infection).[57] The development of vulvar cancer is preceded by condyloma or squamous dysplasia.[58] Other possible risk factors include having many sexual partners, having first sexual intercourse at a young age, and having a history of abnormal Pap tests.[58] Risk factors for STIs are risk factors for vulvar cancer. Early detection is critical. Treatment includes surgery, radiation, chemotherapy, and biologic therapy.

Endometrial Cancer

Carcinoma of the endometrium is the most common type of uterine cancer and most prevalent gynecologic malignancy (Figure 33-17). Estimates in the United States include 54,870 new cases in 2015, with approximately 10,170 deaths.[48] It is the sixth most common cancer worldwide and the incidence is highest in high-income countries including North America and Northern and Western Europe.[59] Since 2002, overall *incidence* rates in the United States have not changed significantly, whereas *mortality* rates have been slowly rising since 2001.[60] The primary risk factor is unopposed estrogen exposure (without progesterone). Exposure to unopposed estrogen includes estrogen-only hormone replacement therapy, tamoxifen, early menarche, late menopause, never having children, and a failure to ovulate (i.e., PCOS and anovulatory cycles typical of the late reproductive years). Less is known about the association with other types of hormone therapy. Chronic hyperinsulinemia, hyperglycemia, body fatness and adult weight gain, chronic inflammation, and lack of physical activity confer an increased risk of endometrial cancer (Figure 33-18).[61]

FIGURE 33-17 Endometrial Cancer. Tumor fills the endometrial cavity. Obvious myometrial invasion is shown. (From Damjanov I, Linder J, editors: *Anderson's pathology,* ed 10, St Louis, 1996, Mosby.)

FIGURE 33-19 Actions of Estradiol (E$_2$) and Progesterone (P$_4$) in the Development of Endometrial Cancer. E$_2$ action through stromal ERα is critical for the development of endometrial cancer. Progesterone (P$_4$) acts through stromal PR to oppose this carcinogenic effect of E$_2$. (From Kim JJ et al: *Endocr Rev* 34[1]:130-162, 2013.)

ENDOMETRIAL CANCER		
	DECREASES RISK	INCREASES RISK
Convincing		Body fatness[1]
Probable	Physical activity[2] Coffee[3]	Glycemic load

1 The panel interpreted BMI (including BMI at age 18-25 years), measures of abdominal girth, and adult weight gain as interrelated aspects of body fatness as well as fat distribution
2 Physical activity of all types; occupational, household, transport and recreational
3 The effect is found in both caffeinated and decaffeinated coffee and cannot be attributed to caffeine

B

FIGURE 33-18 Food, Nutrition, Physical Activity, and Endometrial Cancer. **A,** Overview of the contribution of obesity to endometrial cancer progression and preventive strategies. The T-shaped bar indicates factors that decrease the risk of endometrial cancer. See text for full discussion. **B,** Convincing and probable data for decreases and increases of endometrial cancer. (**A** from Schmandt RE et al: *Am J Obstet Gynecol* 205[6]:518-525, 2011; **B** from World Cancer Research Fund/American Institute for Cancer Research: *Continuous update project report: food, nutrition, physical activity, and the prevention of endometrial cancer*, 2013. Available at: www.dietandcancerreport.org.)

Epidemiologic studies suggest an association between type 2 diabetes mellitus (T2DM) and endometrial cancer, as well as other cancers, and that T2DM increases mortality.[62-64] Diabetes mellitus and cancer share several mechanisms, including insulin and insulin-like growth factor (IGF) signaling, dysregulation of ovarian steroid hormones, and chronic inflammation.[64] Some studies have shown an elevated risk of endometrial cancer with polycystic ovary syndrome and insulin resistance.[65] Additionally, another cause may be epigenetic silencing of the tumor-suppressor gene *PTEN*.[66]

Investigators recently found the use of long-cycle estrogen and progestin hormone replacement therapy (HRT) was related to a tendency toward an elevated risk of developing endometrial cancer for exposure less than 5 years or more.[67] For exposure of more than 10 years, the risk for endometrial cancer was elevated among users of long-cycle HRT and sequential HRT. Norethisterone acetate and medroxyprogesterone acetate (MPA) (HRT) did not differ in their endometrial cancer risk.[67,68] The relationship between the use of tibolone and increased risk for endometrial cancer is controversial.[67,69] Although the numbers were small, a Cochrane review found no clear evidence of a tibolone effect on endometrial cancer compared with placebo.[70] The use of continuous HRT or estradiol plus a levonorgestrel-releasing intrauterine device system showed a decreased risk of

endometrial cancer.[67] Other risk factors not directly related to estrogen include gallbladder disease and hypertension, although being overweight may be a mediating factor for these risks. A family history of colon, endometrial, or ovarian cancer could signal hereditary nonpolyposis colorectal cancer (HNPCC, also known as Lynch syndrome); women with this family history may wish to explore genetic testing and more aggressive screening.[71]

Ninety-five percent of endometrial cancers occur in postmenopausal women, with the peak incidence occurring in the late fifties to early sixties. Although incidence rates are slightly higher in white women than in blacks, death rates in black women are nearly twice as high as those for other ethnic/racial groups. Factors related to reductions in risk of endometrial cancer include delayed menarche; history of pregnancy or breast-feeding, or both; use of combined hormonal contraception; use of progestin-containing IUDs; and engagement in physical activity. So far, the lone dietary factor that may lower risk of endometrial cancer is drinking coffee regularly.[61] A large study[72] first investigated the link between coffee and endometrial cancer risk, and then researchers looked at dietary factors in two U.S. studies—the Nurses Health Studies I and II.[73] For those in the European study, the average high coffee intake was about 3 cups a day, and in the United States it was 4.5 cups of coffee a day.

PATHOGENESIS Endometrial hyperplasia is associated with prolonged estrogenic stimulation of the endometrium. Endometrial hyperplasia and carcinoma share acquired genetic alterations in genes linked to carcinogenesis.[31] Frequent alterations in endometrial cancer include (1) altered estrogen receptor (ER) and progesterone receptor (PR) expression; (2) genetic mutation causing loss of function (inactivation) of the tumor-suppressor gene *PTEN*, which may enhance (3) the PI3K/AKT signaling pathway to become overactive, increasing the ability of the estrogen receptor to "turn on" the expression of target genes; and (4) mutations to several genes, including fibroblast growth factor receptor (FGFR) and tumor protein 53 (TP53).[74] All of these events are predicted to affect PR actions in cancer pathogenesis. Progesterone inhibits estrogen-driven growth in the uterus.[74] The antagonistic effects of progesterone on the estrogen-induced proliferation and growth occur mostly during the luteal phase and are dependent on the presence of functional PR expression.[74] Investigators are studying the importance of stromal PR and its role in progesterone inhibition of epithelial proliferation (Figure 33-19). The interactions between the epithelial and stromal cells of the endometrium may determine the eventual role in the actions of progesterone.[74] Progesterone receptor has two isoforms: PR-A and PR-B. These isoforms are both expressed in the epithelial and stromal cells of the endometrium and their expression fluctuates during the menstrual cycle as well as during pregnancy. The delicate balance of the PR isoforms can tip the scales to foster endometrial hyperplasia and atypia and enhance expression of uterine growth factors.[74] Overall, depending on isoform expression, progesterone can be either an anti- or a pro-proliferative force on the endometrium. Misregulation of isoform expression can lead to abnormal function and precancerous changes.[74]

Two broad categories of endometrial carcinoma include type I and type II. About 80% of cases are type I. Type I and type II endometrial carcinoma are summarized in Table 33-6.

CLINICAL MANIFESTATIONS, EVALUATION, AND TREATMENT

Abnormal vaginal bleeding is the most common clinical manifestation of endometrial cancer. Postmenopausal women, obese women, and women with unopposed estrogenic conditions (i.e., anovulatory cycles) should be evaluated in the event of unscheduled or persistent, irregular vaginal bleeding. Pain and weight loss are symptoms of more advanced disease. Transvaginal ultrasound (TVUS) may be used to measure endometrial thickness. If the endometrium is abnormally thick (defined as >5 mm), then further testing, such as an endometrial biopsy, is done. Treatment is based on the extent of the disease and may include curettage for carcinoma in situ, total abdominal hysterectomy, chemotherapy, radiation, and (although controversial) progestins. The data supporting the use of metformin in the prevention and treatment of cancers are increasing, including those for endometrial cancer.[75,76]

Ovarian Cancer

Among gynecologic malignancies, ovarian cancer is the leading cause of mortality in developed countries with 239,000 new cases and 152,000 estimated deaths worldwide[49] (Figure 33-20). Globally, ovarian cancer is the seventh most common cancer and the eighth cause of death from cancer in women.[49] Incidence rates are highest in more developed regions and lowest in sub-Saharan Africa.[49] In the United States, 21,290 new cases of ovarian cancer and 14,180 ovarian cancer deaths are estimated for 2015.[48] The understanding of incidence patterns both within and between populations is essential to revealing potential causes of and risk factors for ovarian cancer (Figure 33-21). Worldwide, ovarian cancer is responsible for more deaths than all other gynecologic malignancies combined.[49] Risk factors for ovarian cancer are summarized in Table 33-7.

Despite study limitations, several factors related to ovulation have been consistently associated with increased or decreased risk of developing ovarian cancer. Risk is reduced by factors that suppress ovulation (pregnancy, breast-feeding, and combined hormonal contraceptive use). Ovarian cancer has been a very difficult disease to diagnose early

TABLE 33-6 Type I and Type II Endometrial Carcinoma

Characteristics	Type I	Type II
Age	55-65 yr	65-75 yr
Clinical setting	Unopposed estrogen	Atrophy
	Obesity	Thin physique
	Hypertension	
	Diabetes	
Morphology	Endometrioid	Serous
		Clear cell
		Mixed müllerian tumor
Precursor	Hyperplasia	Serous endometrial intraepithelial carcinoma
Mutated genes/genetic abnormalities	PTEN	TP53
	ARID1A (regulator of chromatin)	Aneuploidy
	PIK3CA (PI3K)	PIK3CA (PI3K)
	KRAS	FBXW7 (regulator of MYC, cyclin F)
	FGF2 (growth factor)	CHD4 (regulator of chromatin)
	MSI	PPP2R1A (PP2A)
	CTNNB1 (Wnt signaling)	
	TP53	
Behavior	Indolent	Aggressive
	Spreads via lymphatics	Intraperitoneal and lymphatic spread

From Kumar V et al: *Robbins & Cotran pathologic basis of disease*, ed 9, Philadelphia, 2015, Elsevier/Saunders.
CTNNB1, Beta-catenin gene; *MSI*, microsatellite instability.

FIGURE 33-20 Ovarian Tumors. A serous borderline tumor displays a cyst cavity lined by papillary tumor growths (**A**). The cyst is opened (**B**) to reveal a large bulky tumor mass called cystadenocarcinoma (**C**), a tumor on the ovarian surface. Bilaterality of tumors is common, occurring in 20% of benign tumors, 30% of serous borderline tumors, and approximately 66% of serous carcinomas. A significant proportion of both borderline malignant and malignant tumors involve the surface of the ovary (**C**). (From Kumar V et al: *Robbins & Cotran pathologic basis of disease*, ed 9, Philadelphia, 2015, Saunders.)

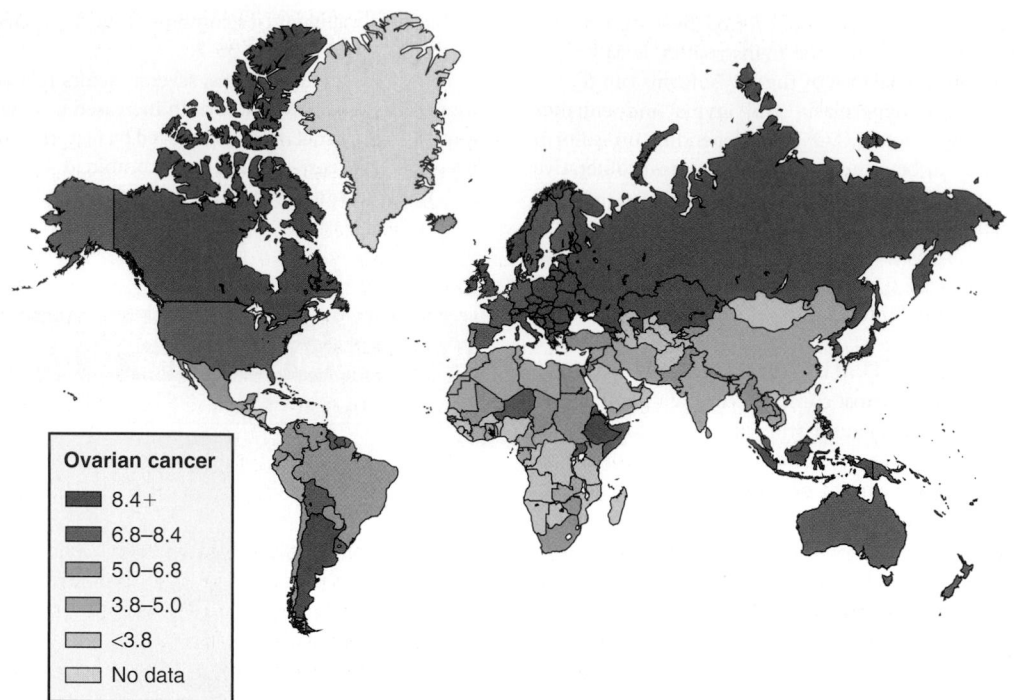

FIGURE 33-21 Map of Ovarian Cancer Worldwide. Rates are per 100,000 women and are age-standardized to the 1960 world standard population. Data were not included for white areas on the map. (From Ferlay J et al: *GLOBOCAN 2012 v1.0, Cancer incidence and mortality worldwide: IARC CancerBase No. 11,* Lyon, France, 2013, International Agency for Research on Cancer. Available at: http://globocan.iarc.fr/Default.aspx.)

and treat. The high mortality reflects a lack of early symptoms and a lack of effective screening tests (see p. 828).

PATHOGENESIS The biology of ovarian cancer is changing and it is clear that ovarian cancer is diverse in character, or *heterogeneous.* Many genetic and epigenetic changes are evident in ovarian tumors. Previously, the majority of ovarian cancers were thought to arise from just epithelial cells that cover the ovarian surface or line subserosal cysts. Newer evidence suggest that tumors arise from three ovarian components: (1) from the fimbriae of fallopian tubes and from deposits of endometriosis; (2) from germ cells, which are pluripotent and migrate to the ovary from the yolk sac; and (3) from stromal cells, including the sex cords, which precede endocrine changes of the postnatal ovary.[31,77] Some ovarian tumors remain too difficult to classify. The normal ovary contains three major cell types: (1) germ cells that are derived from the endoderm and migrate to the gonadal ridge, where they proliferate and differentiate into oocytes; (2) the endocrine and interstitial hormone producing cells that produce estrogen and progesterone; and (3) epithelial cells derived from the müllerian duct that cover the ovary and line inclusion cysts just beneath the ovarian surface. During normal ovulation, oocytes released from mature follicles enter the fallopian tube where fertilization usually occurs. The fimbriae of the fallopian tube cover the ruptured follicle and promote uptake of oocytes.[78] Both benign and malignant tumors come from each of the three ovarian cell types[78] (Figure 33-22). Epithelial ovarian cancers constitute about 90% of malignant ovarian tumors and generally develop after age 40. Sex cord–stromal tumors arise from connective tissue, often secrete hormones, can occur in women of all ages, and comprise about 7% of ovarian tumors.[78] Tumors that arise from germ cells occur in the second and third decades and account for about 3% to 5% of ovarian tumors.[78] Borderline tumors of low malignant

potential can contain structural and molecular evidence of transformed epithelial cells that do not invade the underlying stromal tissue. Approximately 10% of borderline tumors can recur after surgical resection and prove lethal.[78]

There are three major histologic types of epithelial tumors: serous, mucinous, and endometrioid. These types all have a benign, borderline, and malignant category.[31] The most common histologic subtype is high-grade serous cancers, and they may originate from a precursor lesion that arises from the fimbriae of the fallopian tubes. In women who underwent prophylactic salpingo-oophorectomies, studies showed that fallopian tubal lesions were present in almost 100% of women with early serous cancers associated with familial *BRCA* mutations. Investigators recently proposed that the fallopian tube *is* the primary site of most serous carcinomas.[79] Although historically investigators proposed that the vast majority of serous carcinomas arose from cortical inclusion cysts, a newer hypothesis is that the cysts arise from implantation of detached fallopian tube epithelium at sites where ovulation has disrupted the surface of the ovary.[31] These findings have led to changes in management of women at high risk for ovarian cancer (*BRCA* mutation carriers and women with a strong family history of breast/ovarian cancer); they are now recommended to have salpingo-oophorectomy and not just a simple oophorectomy.[31]

Additionally, histologically similar cancers diagnosed as primary peritoneal carcinomas share molecular findings (i.e., inactivation of *p53* and *BRCA1* and *BRCA2* proteins). Therefore, tumors arising from fallopian tube and other locations from the peritoneal cavity, together with most ovarian epithelial cancers, are classified as "extrauterine adenocarcinomas of Müllerian epithelial origin," and are included, staged, and treated similarly to ovarian cancer.[80]

The defining characteristics of malignant tumors are stromal invasion and increased epithelial atypia. Ovarian tumors are now classified

TABLE 33-7   Risk Factors for Ovarian Cancer

Risk Factor	Description
Advancing age	Incidence of ovarian cancer increases with advancing age. Most cases occur in postmenopausal women.
Genetic factors	About 5% to 15% of all ovarian cancers are inherited. Of these, the majority are related to mutations in *BRCA1/2* genes and others include mismatch repair genes (e.g., Lynch syndrome), TP53 in the germ line (e.g., Li-Fraumeni syndrome), and Peutz-Jeghers syndrome. Fallopian tube cancer and peritoneal carcinomas also are part of the *BRCA*-associated disease spectrum.
Family history	A family history of ovarian cancer in a first-degree relative (e.g., mother, daughter, or sister) is the most important risk factor. The highest risk appears in women who have two or more first-degree relatives with ovarian cancer. Risk may be higher if the affected relative was diagnosed at a younger age, previous breast cancer diagnosed before the age of 40, and previous breast cancer and a history of ovarian cancer. A cohort study showed ovarian cancer risk is higher in women whose sibling has/had liver, stomach, breast, prostate, connective tissue cancer, or melanoma; or whose parent has/had breast or liver cancer.
Overweight and obesity (BMI)	Meta-analysis found higher risk of ovarian cancer in premenopausal women with a BMI >30 and no effect in postmenopausal women. Another meta-analysis found a link between high BMI and ovarian cancer risk in women who had never used menopausal hormone therapy (MHT).
Height	Greater adult attained height (reflects factors that promote childhood growth) is classified by WCRF/AICR as a probable cause of ovarian cancer. A pooled analysis of Nordic data and meta-analyses showed ovarian cancer risk is 7% to 10% higher per 5-cm increment in height.
Reproductive/hormonal factors	Ovarian cancer risk is associated with factors affecting lifetime ovulations (and breaks between) or sex hormone levels (estrogens, progesterone, and androgens), or both. Structural changes to the ovary can occur with ovulation that may stimulate cancer development. These changes may be affected and enhanced by hormonal factors. Having more children, breast-feeding, or using oral contraceptives deceases the number of ovulations and therefore reduces the risk of ovarian cancer.
Menopausal hormone therapy	Current use of postmenopausal hormone replacement therapy (HRT, also known as menopausal hormone therapy [MHT]) is classified by IARC as a cause of ovarian cancer (see Table 11-1). A meta-analysis found women using MHT for just a few years were more likely to develop ovarian cancer than women who had never used MHT. For every 1000 women who take MHT for 5 years from about age 50, there will be 1 extra ovarian cancer. An estimated 1% of individuals with ovarian cancer in the United Kingdom are linked to MHT use. In long-term (5+ years) users of estrogen-only MHT, compared with never users, ovarian cancer risk is 53% higher. From a cohort study, ovarian cancer risk is 17% higher in long-term (5+ years) estrogen-progesterone MHT users when compared with never users.
Endometriosis	Recent studies have shown that women with endometriosis have an increase in ovarian cancer risk.
Diabetes	Meta-analyses have shown ovarian cancer risk is 20% to 55% higher in women with diabetes compared with those without diabetes.
Previous cancer	Ovarian cancer risk is 24% higher in breast cancer survivors compared with the general population (possibly reflects *BRCA* mutations and Lynch syndrome or shared hormonal factors). It is higher in those diagnosed with breast cancer at a younger age versus those diagnosed older; the higher risk is limited to estrogen receptor (ER) negative or ER unknown breast cancer.
Smoking	An analysis showed an increased risk for mucinous ovarian tumors in current smokers. The risk decreased to normal after cessation of smoking. Recent results from the EPIC study showed smoking increases the risk of mucinous ovarian tumors.
Asbestos (occupational exposure)	Asbestos is classified by IARC as a cause of ovarian cancer (see Table 11-1).
Talc-based powder	Talc-based powder used peritoneally is classified by the IARC as a probable cause of ovarian cancer (see Table 11-1). The risk of ovarian cancer with talc-based powders has been based on meta-analyses and pooled analyses of case-control studies. Not all body powders contain talc.
Ionizing radiation	Use of x-radiation and gamma radiation is classified by IARC as a probable cause of ovarian cancer (see Table 11-1). A small number of individuals with ovarian cancer may be associated with radiotherapy for previous cancer.
Factors that reduce risk of ovarian cancer	Taking contraceptives is classified by IARC as protective against ovarian cancer. Breast-feeding is classified by WCRF/AICR as possibly protective against ovarian cancer. Ovarian cancer risk is lower in women with the following factors supported by meta-analyses and pooled analyses: higher parity, hysterectomy, tubal ligation, use of statins, and controversial evidence of having systemic lupus erythematosus.

Cancer Research UK: *Ovarian cancer risk factors*, London, Author.

Cogliano VJ et al: *J Natl Cancer Inst* 103:1827-1839, 2011.

Ferlay J et al: *GLOBOCAN 2008 v1.2, Cancer incidence and mortality worldwide: IARC CancerBase no. 10* [Internet], Lyon, France, 2010, International Agency for Research on Cancer.

International Agency for Research on Cancer: *List of classifications by cancer sites with sufficient or limited evidence in humans*, vol 1-105; accessed December 2014.

National Cancer Institute: *PDQ®ovarian epithelial, fallopian tube, and primary peritoneal cancer treatment*, Bethesda, Md, 2015, Author. Date last modified March 27, 2015. Available at: http://cancer.gov/cancertopics/pdq/treatment/ovarianepithelial/HealthProfessional. Accessed May 2, 2015.

Parkin DM et al: *Cancer* 105(S2):S77-S81, 2011.

World Cancer Research Fund/American Institute for Cancer Research: *Food, nutrition, physical activity, and the prevention of cancer: a global perspective*, Washington, DC, 2007, AICR.

FIGURE 33-22 Heterogeneous Ovarian Tumors. A, Diverse ovarian tumors originate from different cell subtypes. **B,** Type I and type II ovarian tumors. Type I tumors progress from benign tumors through borderline tumors that give rise to low-grade carcinoma, and type II tumors arise from inclusion cysts/fallopian tube epithelium through intraepithelial precursors that often are unidentifiable. These tumors demonstrate high-grade features and are commonly of serous histology. *STIC,* Serous tubal intraepithelial carcinoma. (**B** from Kumar V et al: *Robbins & Cotran pathologic basis of disease,* ed 9, Philadelphia, 2015, Elsevier/Saunders.)

as type I (low-grade) and type II (high-grade) (see Figure 33-22, *B*). Low-grade tumors arising in serous borderline tumors have several oncogene mutations, whereas high-grade tumors have a high frequency of *TP53* mutations. Gene amplifications are noted in many tumors, as well as deletions of tumor-suppressor genes. The majority of *BRCA* mutations are high-grade serous carcinomas with *TP53* mutations. *BRCA*-associated cancer risks are determined by the mutation location and variation of the *BRCA1/2* gene function.[77] Endometrioid ovarian carcinomas may arise in the setting of endometriosis and are sometimes associated with borderline tumor.[31]

CLINICAL MANIFESTATIONS   Generally, individuals with ovarian cancer have no early symptoms. Because there are no effective screening techniques to detect it, the disease is usually advanced by the time treatment is sought. Some women may experience vague symptoms that include abdominal distention, loss of appetite, early satiety, and pelvic pain. These symptoms are important as *nonspecific* symptoms and can lead to delays in treatment. Symptoms of advanced disease include pain, abdominal swelling and distention, dyspepsia, vomiting, and alterations in bowel habits. Abnormal vaginal bleeding may occur if the postmenopausal endometrium is stimulated by a hormone-secreting tumor. The tumor also may cause ulcerations through the vaginal wall that result in bleeding. There also can be a feeling of pressure in the pelvis and leg pain. Given the location of the ovaries, assessing abnormalities on routine gynecologic examination poses difficulty, especially in obese women. Ovarian cancer is generally considered a silent disease.

Tumor obstruction of vascular channels can cause venous and, occasionally, arterial thrombosis. Alterations in coagulation also occur,

contributing to clot formation. Metastasis often causes pleural effusion (Figure 33-23).

EVALUATION AND TREATMENT   There is no sensitive and specific test for ovarian cancer for screening low-risk women, and routine screening of women without risk factors has not been shown to be beneficial and may cause harm because more women have unnecessary surgical procedures.[81] Solid evidence indicates that screening with a CA-125 blood test and transvaginal ultrasound (TVU) does not result in a decrease in ovarian cancer mortality after a research follow-up of 12.4 years.[80] Importantly, ovarian cancer deaths were higher in the screened group than in the usual care group (3.1 deaths versus 2.6 deaths/10,000 women). These effects are attributed to false-positive test results, higher rates of oophorectomy, and surgical complications. Pelvic examination may detect advanced disease.[80] Several biomarkers with potential application to screening are under investigation. A malignant tumor is confirmed by biopsy and extent of disease evaluated with imaging techniques. The International Federation of Gynecologists and Obstetricians (FIGO) staging system is described in Table 33-8.

The initial approach to treatment is surgery, which is performed to determine the stage of disease and to remove as much of the tumor as possible. Survival increases with the expertise of the surgeon. Understanding the biology of cancers and decreasing tumor implantation (seeding) have mandated highly skilled surgical and biopsy techniques.[82,83] Treatment is then customized based on the stage of the cancer, the woman's desires, the cell type, and the sensitivity of the cancer cells. Radiation and chemotherapy are common treatments. New therapies under investigation include monoclonal antibodies,

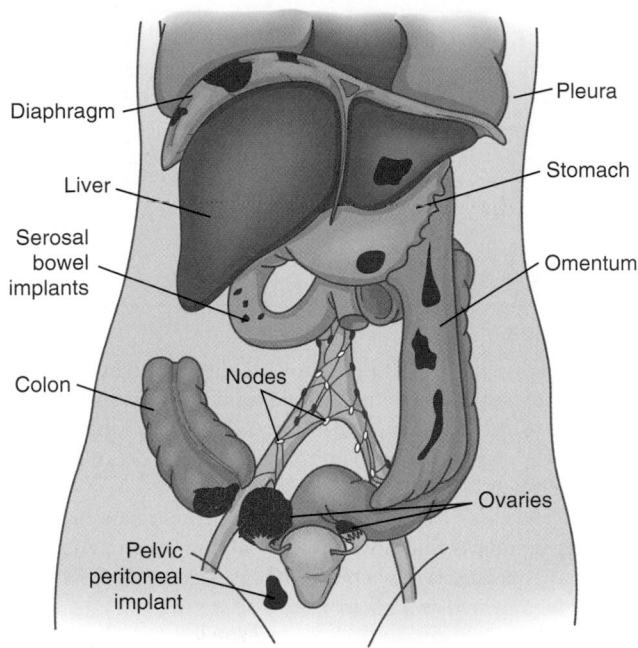

FIGURE 33-23 Metastasis of Ovarian Cancer. Pattern of spread for epithelial cancer of the ovary.

TABLE 33-8 FIGO* Staging of Carcinoma of the Ovary

Stage	Characteristics
I	Growth limited to ovaries
II	Growth involves one or both ovaries and involvement of other organs (i.e., uterus, bladder, colon)
III	Cancer involves one or both ovaries, and one or both of following are present: (1) cancer has spread beyond pelvis to lining of abdomen, (2) cancer has spread to lymph nodes
IV	Growth involves one or both ovaries with distant metastases to lungs, liver, or other organs outside peritoneal cavity
Recurrent	Cancer recurs after completion of treatment

*The International Federation of Gynecologists and Obstetricians.

epidermal growth factor receptor, gene therapy, and small-molecular-weight inhibitors. Research into prevention and treatment of ovarian cancer is ongoing and expanding.

Sexual Dysfunction

Sexual dysfunction is the lack of satisfaction with sexual function resulting from pain or a deficiency in sexual desire, arousal, or orgasm/climax.[84,85] Sexual function and dysfunction result from a complex set of personal and biologic factors that interact with culture. Both organic and psychosocial disorders can be implicated in sexual dysfunction. Additionally, studies have shown that up to 45% of adult women have some form of sexual dysfunction and adequate research is still needed.[86] Chronic medical conditions can greatly affect both sexual desire and sexual function (Table 33-9).

Disorders of desire (hypoactive sexual desire, decreased libido) are the most common sexual dysfunction in women.[86] The prevalence of hypoactive sexual desire increases with age and may be a biologic manifestation of depression, dissatisfaction with partner relationships, a history of sexual or physical abuse, alcohol or other substance abuse, prolactin-secreting pituitary tumors, or testosterone deficiency.[87] Medications, such as β-adrenergic blockers used for heart disease, may inhibit sexual desire. Treatment may include counseling, psychotherapy, and antidepressants.

Anorgasmia (orgasmic dysfunction) is the inability of a woman to reach or achieve orgasm and ranges from difficulty in arousal to lack of orgasm. Any chronic illness may affect arousal. Specific disorders that may block orgasm are diabetes, alcoholism, neurologic disturbances, hormonal deficiencies, and pelvic disorders, such as infections, trauma, and surgical scarring. Other inhibitors include drugs, such as narcotics, tranquilizers, antidepressants (especially selective serotonin reuptake inhibitors [SSRIs]), and antihypertensive medications.

Dyspareunia (painful intercourse) is common. Women may experience pain at any time from the beginning of arousal to after intercourse. The pain may have a burning, sharp, searing, or cramping quality and may be described as external, vaginal, deep abdominal, or pelvic. A variety of psychosocial and organic causes have been identified. Inadequate lubrication may make penetration or intercourse difficult or painful. Drugs with a drying effect (such as antihistamines, certain tranquilizers, and marijuana) and disorders (such as diabetes, vaginal infections, and estrogen deficiency) can decrease lubrication.

TABLE 33-9 Possible Effects of Chronic Disease on Sexual Functioning in Women

Disease	Sexual Function
Cerebral palsy	Intact genital sensations, decreased lubrication; difficulty with sexual activity/positioning because of muscle spasticity, rigidity, or weakness; pain with positioning caused by contracture of knees and hips or because of increased spasms with arousal
Cerebrovascular accident (CVA)	Difficulties in sexual positioning and sensitivity because of impaired motor strength, coordination, or paralysis; decreased libido with stroke on dominant side of brain
Diabetes	Diminished intensity of orgasm and gradual decline in ability to achieve orgasm; decreased lubrication or recurrent vaginal infections with resultant dyspareunia
Chronic renal failure	Decreased arousal; increasingly rare and less intense orgasms; decreased lubrication
Rheumatoid arthritis (RA)	Painful sexual activity/positions because of swollen, painful joints, muscular atrophy, and joint contracture; decreased libido because of pain, fatigue, or medication; genital sensations remain intact
Systemic lupus erythematosus (SLE)	Similar to RA; decreased lubrication and vaginal lesions result in painful penetration
Myocardial infarction (MI)	Most literature male-oriented; problems related to medications
Multiple sclerosis (MS)	Diminished genital sensitivity; decreased lubrication; declining orgasmic ability; difficulty with sexual activity because of muscle weakness, pain, or incontinence
Spinal cord injury	Reflex sexual response with injury above sacral area; disrupted response with lesion at or below sacrum; loss of sensation, decreased lubrication; spasticity, incontinence, or pain with arousal; continued orgasmic sensations or sensations diffused in general or to specific body parts, such as breast or lips

Other causes include skin problems around the introitus or affecting the vulva; irritation or infection of the clitoris; disorders of the vaginal opening and disorders of the urethra or anus; disorders of the vagina, such as infections, thinning of the walls caused by aging or decreased estrogen level, or irritation caused by spermicides or douches; and pelvic disorders, such as infection, tumors, and cervical or uterine abnormalities.

Vaginismus is an involuntary muscle spasm in response to attempted penetration. Common psychologic causes include prior sexual trauma and fear of sex. Organic causes are similar to those that cause dyspareunia, including vulvovestibulitis. Even after the underlying organic problem is detected and successfully treated, vaginismus may persist.

Sexual dysfunction may develop as a coping mechanism. Women with a history of sexual trauma—rape, incest, or molestation—often have problems with desire, arousal, or orgasm or experience pain with sexual activity. In extreme cases, total sexual aversion may develop. At other times, sexual dysfunction may be a symptom of marital or relationship problems. Because sexual dysfunction has many causes, assessment and treatment should be holistic and culturally sensitive.

Impaired Fertility

Infertility affects approximately 15% of all couples and is defined as the inability to conceive over 1 year of unprotected intercourse. Fertility can be impaired by factors in the man or woman, or in both partners. Female infertility results from dysfunction of the normal reproductive process: menses and ovulation, fallopian tube function (transport of the egg to the uterus and as a site of fertilization), and implantation of the fertilized egg into a receptive endometrium. Ovarian dysfunction includes defective ovulation because of hormonal effects (e.g., PCOS, depressed hypothalamic activity, secondary physical or emotional stress), diminished ovarian reserve (lack of immature eggs secondary to congenital, medical, or unexplained factors), or premature ovarian insufficiency (failure of ovarian function before the age of 40). Fallopian tube dysfunction may result from acute pelvic infections with chlamydia or gonorrhea. Adhesions from pelvic infection, abdominal surgery, or endometriosis may cause blockage of one or both fallopian tubes, preventing access of the sperm to the ovum. The fertilized ovum must implant on a receptive endometrium.[88] Receptivity may be greatly diminished by fibroids or inadequate molecular or cellular preparation of the implantation site.

A number of diagnostic procedures are required in the routine investigation of the infertile couple.[89] Initial workup includes analysis of semen, determination of ovulation, and hysterosalpingography of the fallopian tubes. Treatment of infertility is aimed towards correction of problems identified during diagnostic workup. Male infertility may be corrected surgically (varicoceles) or by artificial insemination with the husband's or donor sperm. Anovulation can be treated with hormonal medications that induce ovulation (e.g., clomiphene citrate, follicle-stimulating hormone, gonadotropin-releasing hormone). Women with fallopian tube defects, who have failed other approaches, or have no identifiable cause of their infertility are frequently treated by assisted reproductive technology (ART).[90] The basic ART procedure is in vitro fertilization (IVF), which involves collecting eggs directly from the ovary, performing fertilization and early embryonic development in the laboratory, and then transferring the eggs into the uterus. Many variations of this procedure are available. Depending on the potential cause of infertility, appropriate modifications allow for the use of donor sperm, egg, or uterus (in the case of surrogacy). An essential treatment for infertility is prevention of sexually transmitted infection, which can result in scarring and adhesion formation in the reproductive tract of either the man or the woman.

✓ QUICK CHECK 33-4
1. Why is cervical cancer considered a sexually transmitted infection?
2. What are the risk factors and pathogenesis for endometrial cancer?
3. What factors reduce the risk of ovarian cancer?
4. Discuss the new hypothesis for pathogenesis of ovarian cancer.

DISORDERS OF THE FEMALE BREAST

Galactorrhea

Galactorrhea (inappropriate lactation) is the persistent and sometimes excessive secretion of a milky fluid from the breasts of a woman who is not pregnant or nursing an infant. Galactorrhea, which also can occur in men, may involve one or both breasts, and is not associated with breast cancer.

The incidence of galactorrhea is difficult to estimate because of differences among definitions of the condition, examination techniques, and populations of women who have been studied. Prevalence has been documented as 0.1% to 32% of all women.

PATHOPHYSIOLOGY Galactorrhea is a manifestation of pathophysiologic processes elsewhere in the body, rather than a primary breast disorder. These processes are chiefly hormone imbalances caused by hypothalamic-pituitary disturbances, pituitary tumors, or neurologic damage. Exogenous causes include drugs, estrogen, and manipulation of the nipples.

The most common cause of galactorrhea is nonpuerperal hyperprolactinemia, or excessive amounts of prolactin in the blood not related to pregnancy or childbirth. Nonpuerperal hyperprolactinemia can be caused by any factor that (1) stimulates or overstimulates the prolactin-secreting units of the pituitary gland; (2) interferes with production of prolactin-inhibiting factor (PIF), a neurotransmitter (probably dopamine) that inhibits prolactin secretion; or (3) interferes with pituitary receptors for PIF.

Certain drugs can cause nonpuerperal hyperprolactinemia. They include the phenothiazines, reserpine, and methyldopa; exogenous estrogens, particularly in oral contraceptives; morphine; and the tricyclic antidepressants.

Hypothyroidism causes increased secretion of hypothalamic thyroid-stimulating hormone (TSH), which stimulates prolactin release from the pituitary. Hypothyroidism also is associated with reduced metabolic clearance of prolactin, which prolongs its effects.

Many types of pituitary tumors cause hyperprolactinemia, particularly prolactinoma. Prolactinomas cause hyperprolactinemia by secreting prolactin, decreasing production of PIF, or applying pressure to the pituitary stalk, thus preventing delivery of PIF to the anterior pituitary. Growth hormone–secreting pituitary tumors may cause galactorrhea through the intrinsic lactogenic effect that growth hormone appears to have on mammary tissue. Prolactin-secreting lung and kidney tumors also cause hyperprolactinemia.

Chronic stress may cause hyperprolactinemia by inhibiting PIF release. Head trauma, cervical spinal injuries, encephalitis, meningitis, herpes zoster, or thoracotomy scars may stimulate the suckling reflex. The suckling reflex increases prolactin secretion.

CLINICAL MANIFESTATIONS Inappropriate lactation is manifested by the appearance of a milky breast secretion from one or both breasts of nonpregnant, nonlactating women. Most women with galactorrhea experience menstrual abnormality. If a pituitary process is involved, the woman usually experiences hirsutism and infertility; if a hypothalamic lesion is present, she may report central nervous system (CNS) symptoms, such as intractable headache, visual field disturbances, sleep disturbances, and abnormal temperature, thirst, or appetite.

EVALUATION AND TREATMENT Galactorrhea in nulliparous women (women who have never been pregnant) or in parous women who have not breast-fed for 12 months must be thoroughly evaluated. Evaluation includes a variety of diagnostic tests. Serum prolactin levels are measured, and at least two positive results are needed to diagnose hyperprolactinemia. Prolactin levels higher than 25 to 30 ng/ml (measured by radioimmunoassay) are considered elevated. Those in the range of 75 to 100 ng/ml are possibly caused by a pituitary tumor until proven otherwise. Serum thyroxine (T_4) and thyroid-stimulating hormone (TSH) levels are measured to rule out hypothyroidism, and LH and FSH levels are obtained if the individual is amenorrheic. MRI may assist in locating adenomas.

Treatment for galactorrhea consists of identification and treatment of the cause. Medical therapy is typical and surgical or radiation therapy is rarely required.

Benign Breast Disease and Conditions

Benign breast disease (BBD) is a spectrum of noncancerous changes in the breast. Numerous benign alterations in ducts and lobules occur in the breast, including lumps, cysts, sensitive nipples, and itching. The most common symptoms reported by women are pain, palpable mass, or nipple discharge; the majority of these prove to have a benign cause. Major determinants of the risk of breast cancer after a diagnosis of BBD include histologic or biologic features, or both; previous biopsy; and degree of family history.[91] Benign epithelial lesions can be broadly classified as (1) nonproliferative breast lesions, (2) proliferative breast disease without atypia, and (3) atypical (atypia) hyperplasia. The majority of nonproliferative benign lesions are not precursors of cancer and generally not associated with an increased risk of breast cancer.[91,92] Some benign breast lesions, for example, atypical hyperplasia, confer an increase in risk for development of breast cancer and these women are recommended for counseling about screening recommendations and risk reduction.[91]

Nonproliferative Breast Lesions

Nonproliferative epithelial breast lesions are usually not associated with an increased risk of breast cancer. The nonproliferative lesions include (1) simple breast cysts, (2) papillary apocrine change, and (3) mild hyperplasia of the usual type. Terms such as fibrocystic changes (FCCs; or physiologic nodularity and cysts), fibrocystic disease, chronic cystic mastitis, and mammary dysplasia refer to nonproliferative lesions but are not definitive because they are a heterogeneous group of diagnoses.[91] Simple cysts (fluid-filled sacs) are the most common nonproliferative breast lesion and are a specific type of lump that commonly occurs in women in their thirties, forties, and early fifties. Cysts feel "squishy" when they occur close to the surface of the breast but when deeply embedded they can feel hard. An estimated 50% to 80% of women normally experience some of these changes. The prevalence of fibrocystic lesions is probably related to hormonal changes, which in turn are affected by genetic background, age, parity, history of lactation, and use of caffeine and exogenous hormones. Cystic changes can be induced in experimental animals by altering ratios of estrogens and progesterone. It is assumed, therefore, that breast cysts are the result of ovarian alterations, but the exact mechanism is unknown. Cysts also can be associated with unilateral nipple discharge. Cysts often rupture with release of secretory material into the adjacent tissue. The resulting chronic inflammation and scarring fibrosis contribute to the palpable firmness of the breast. Fibrous tissue increases progressively until menopause and regresses thereafter.

Papillary apocrine change is an increase in ductal epithelial cells that has apocrine changes or an eosinophilic cytoplasm. Mild hyperplasia of the usual type is an increase in the number of epithelial cells within a duct that is more than two cells, but not more than four cells, in depth.[91]

Proliferative Breast Lesions without Atypia

These disorders are characterized by proliferation of ductal epithelium or stroma, or both, without cellular signs of abnormality (atypia or deviation from normal). The following structurally diverse lesions are included and discussed next: (1) usual ductal hyperplasia, (2) intraductal papillomas, (3) sclerosing adenosis, (4) radial scar, and (5) simple fibroadenoma.[91]

1. Usual ductal hyperplasia (UDH) is additional or proliferating epithelial cells that fill and distend the ducts and lobules and are usually found as an incidental finding from mammography. The cells can vary in size and shape, but they retain features of benign cells.[91] No additional treatment is needed and chemoprevention is not recommended.[91]

2. Intraductal papillomas can occur as solitary or multiple lesions. Solitary papillomas are a monotonous (sameness) array of papillary cells that grow from the wall of the cyst into the lumen of the duct. Growth occurs within a dilated duct often near or beside the nipple, causing benign nipple discharge. These papillomas can harbor areas of atypia requiring surgical excision. Diffuse papillomatosis (multiple papillomas) may present as breast masses, nodules on ultrasound, or the cause of nipple discharge. Diffuse papillomatosis is defined as a minimum of five papillomas within a localized segment of breast tissue.[91] Although the breast cancer risk is small, these lesions require surgical excision.

3. Sclerosing adenosis is a lobular lesion with increased fibrous tissue and scattered glandular cells.[91] It is a common but poorly understood benign breast lesion.[93] A recent study found increased Ki-67 expression (a proliferation marker) carried an approximate twofold increased chance of subsequent breast cancer.[94] It is usually found as a suspicious lesion on mammography.

4. Radial scar (RS) refers to an irregular, radial proliferation of duct-like small tubules entrapped in a dense central fibrosis. The term scar refers to the structural appearance only because these lesions are not associated with prior injury, biopsy, or surgery. Radial scar also has been called radial sclerosing lesions and sclerosing papillary proliferation. RSs are usually discovered when a breast lesion or radiologic abnormality is biopsied or removed. Controversy exists about the need for surgical excision.[91]

5. Simple fibroadenomas are benign solid tumors that contain glandular and fibrous lesions.[91] In about 20% of cases, multiple fibroadenomas can occur in the same breast or bilaterally.[91] The etiology for fibroadenomas is unknown but appears to be hormonal because they can persist during the reproductive years and can increase in size during pregnancy or with estrogen therapy. They usually regress after menopause.[91] They are more common among women between 15 and 35 years of age. Fibroadenomas are now considered proliferative lesions and the histologic features influence the risk of breast cancer. There is no increased risk of breast cancer in the majority of women with a simple fibroadenoma. It is not necessary to excise all biopsy-proven fibroadenomas.[91] Disadvantages of excisional surgery include scarring at the incision site, dimpling of the breast from the removal of the tumor, damage to the breast's duct system, and mammographic changes (e.g., architectural distortion, skin thickening, increased focal density).[91] If a biopsy-proven

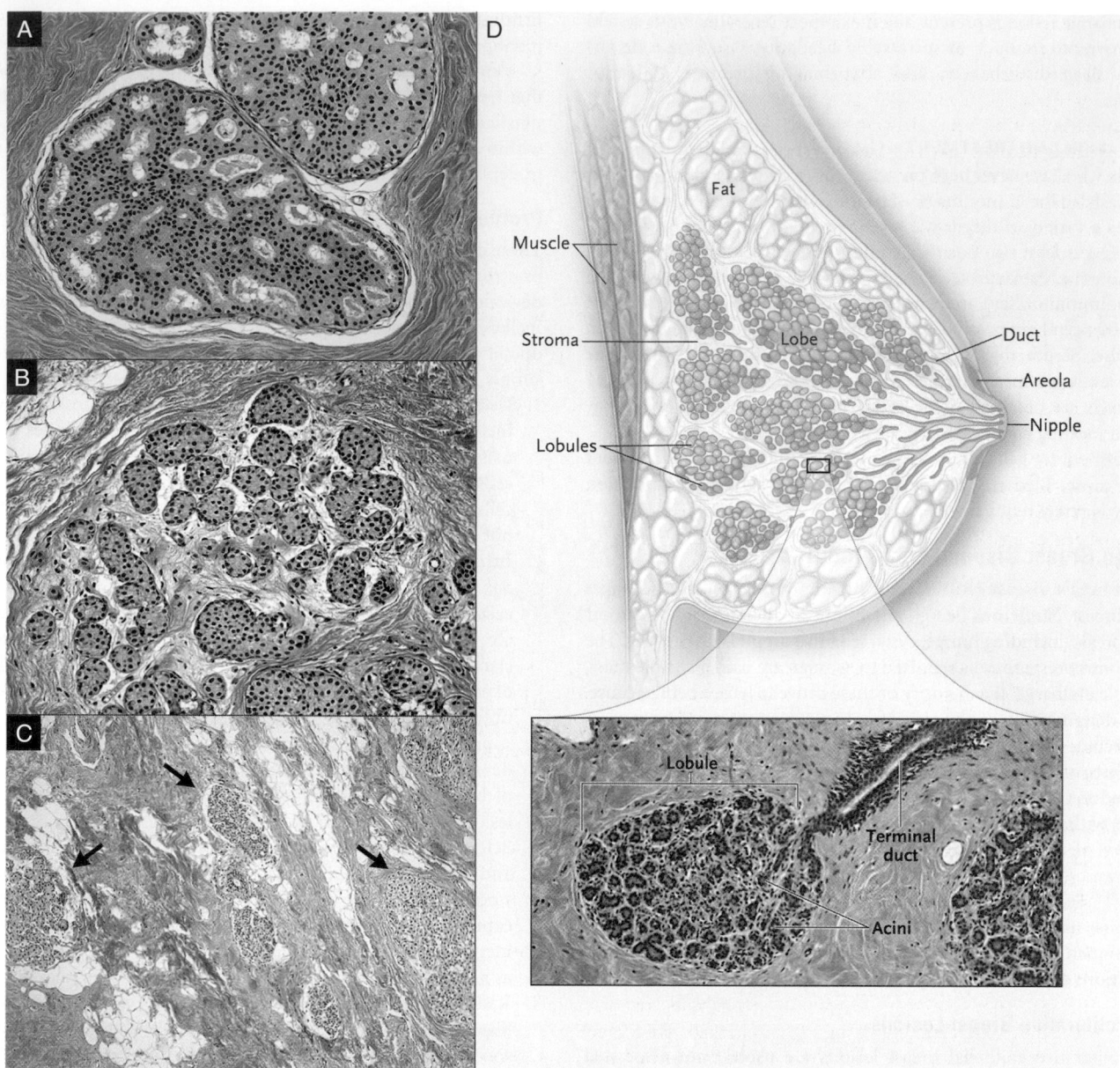

FIGURE 33-24 Anatomic and Histologic Features of Atypical Hyperplasia. Panel **A** shows atypical ductal hyperplasia with proliferation of monotonous cells in architecturally complex patterns, including secondary lumens and micropapillary formations. Panel **B** shows atypical lobular hyperplasia, with expanded acini filled with monotonous polygonal cells and a loss of acinar lumen. Panel **C** shows multifocal atypical hyperplasia (in this case atypical lobular hyperplasia). Atypical lobular hyperplasia is present in more than one terminal duct lobular unit, and units are clearly separated from one another by interlobular mammary stroma *(arrows)*. Panel **D** is an illustration of the microanatomy of the breast, including a photomicrograph of a terminal duct lobular unit. (From Hartmann LC, Degnim AC, Santen RJ, Dupont WD, Ghosh K: *N Engl J Med* 372[1]:1271-1272, 2015.)

fibroadenoma is asymptomatic, it can then be left in place, although some women wish to have the mass excised so that they will not worry further.[91]

Proliferative Breast Lesions with Atypia

Atypical hyperplasia (AH) is an increase in the number of cells (or proliferation) with the cells having some variation in structure—*atypia*. AH is a high-risk benign lesion found in about 10% of biopsies with benign findings.[92,95] These proliferative breast lesions with some atypia include atypical ductal hyperplasia and atypical lobular

hyperplasia.[92] **Atypical ductal hyperplasia (ADH)** refers to abnormal proliferating cells in breast ducts. **Atypical lobular hyperplasia (ALH)** refers to proliferation of cells in the lumen of lobular units.

Much of the next discussion will refer to just "atypical hyperplasia (AH)." Studies indicate that women with AH have an increased risk (about fourfold) of breast cancer compared with women who have nonproliferative lesions.[96-98] Ongoing studies will further determine risk estimates with such factors, for example, as breast density[92,96] (Figure 33-24). About 60% of the subsequent breast cancers in women with AH occur in the ipsilateral breast (same side) as the biopsy.[96,99,100]

From long-term studies mentioned earlier, atypical hyperplasia has been shown to confer a relative risk of 4 for future breast cancer and recently the *absolute risk* has been better defined with a cumulative incidence of breast cancer about 30% at 25 years of follow-up.[97,101] This high cumulative risk is not widely appreciated and, therefore, women with atypical hyperplasia are not included in many high-risk guidelines, for example, screening with MRI and use of chemopreventive agents.[95] Because some studies have shown a lack of concordance (agreement) among pathologists in differentiating atypical hyperplasia from carcinoma in situ,[102] it is important that pathologists follow standardized, published criteria and this may be a factor for women to seek a second opinion. It appears that menopausal status at the time of benign breast biopsy influences the magnitude of subsequent breast cancer risk. For women who were premenopausal at the time of their breast biopsy, the risk of breast cancer was greater in those with ALH than among women with ADH.[100] Overall, the younger a woman is when she receives a diagnosis of atypical hyperplasia, the higher the risk that breast cancer will develop.[97-99] Among women who were postmenopausal at the time of benign breast biopsy, the risk was similar with ALH and women with ADH.[100] Overall, ADH and ALH are viewed best as "markers" of a generalized bilateral increase in breast cancer risk.[91,100]

EVALUATION AND TREATMENT Breast problems are diagnosed from a mutimodal approach that combines physical examination, mammography, ultrasonography, thermography, possibly MRI, and biopsy. The dense breast tissue often seen in young women can make mammographic interpretation extremely difficult (see *Health Alert: Breast Cancer Screening Mammography*).

Treatment consists largely of relieving symptoms. Reduction in the consumption of caffeinated beverages (e.g., cola, root beer) and chocolate, which can cause overstimulation for some women, may reduce pain and nodularity. Given time, the cysts may disappear without treatment.

Although still controversial, isoflavone exposure was associated with a decreased risk of proliferative benign fibrocystic changes, nonproliferative changes, and breast cancer.[103] Genistein, a soy isoflavone, has been reported to down-regulate an enzyme important in cancer progression (i.e., telomerase) and contributes to inhibition in both breast benign and cancer cells.[104] Toxicologists, in perhaps the first in vitro study quantifying the proliferative effects of isoflavone metabolites, conclude soy supplement intake will not induce proliferation of normal breast tissue and may even inhibit proliferation.[105] The North American Menopause Society found that soy foods generally appear to be breast protective and recommended moderate lifelong soy consumption.[106] Although quite controversial, another preventive factor may be iodine.[107]

Breast Cancer

In 2012, 1.7 million women were diagnosed with breast cancer and there were 6.3 million women alive who had been diagnosed with breast cancer in the previous 5 years (Figure 33-25).[49] Mortality has increased by 14%. Breast cancer is the most common cause of cancer death among women (522,000 deaths in 2012) and the most frequently diagnosed cancer among women in 140 of 184 countries worldwide.[49] It now represents one in four of all cancers in women.

Breast cancer, the most common cancer in American women, is the leading cause of death in women 40 to 44 years of age and the second leading cause of cancer death in women of all ages after lung cancer. It is estimated that 234,190 women and 2350 men will be diagnosed with breast cancer, and 40,730 women and 440 men will die from breast cancer in 2015.[48] African American women have a lower

TABLE 33-10	Established Risk Factors for Breast Cancer
Relative Risk (RR)	**Risk Factor**
>4.0	Female
	Age
	Family history of breast cancer
	Personal history of breast cancer
	Inherited genetic mutations (*BRCA1/2* and others)
	High breast density
	Atypical hyperplasia
2.1-4.0	Family history (one first-degree relative)
	High-dose radiation to chest/breast
	Prior benign breast disease
1.1-2.0	No full-term pregnancies
	Late age at first full-term pregnancy (>30 years)
	Early menarche (<12 years)
	Late menopause (>55 years)
	Never breast-fed children
	High alcohol consumption
	Smoking
	Recent oral contraceptive use
	Recent or current use of combined hormone replacement therapy
	Physical inactivity
	Obesity or adult weight gain (postmenopausal)

Data from American Cancer Society: *Cancer facts & figures 2010*, Atlanta, 2010, Author.

incidence of breast cancer (118.1/100,000) than white women (123.2/100,000) but have a higher death rate (31.6/100,000) than white women (22.4/100,000). More than two thirds of breast cancer cases occur in women older than age 55. Because ductal carcinoma in situ (DCIS) is almost exclusively detected by mammography, the large increase in incidence of DCIS over the past 20 years can be attributed to screening.

Although breast cancer is a multifactorial disease involving a complex web of interacting factors, risk is related to timing, duration, and pattern of exposures. Risk factors and possible causes of breast cancer can be classified broadly as reproductive, hormonal, environmental, and familial (Table 33-10). However, two factors emerging as important are involution of the mammary gland and breast density, which are not as easily classified (see following discussion).

Reproductive Factors: Pregnancy

A clearer understanding of mammary gland structure (morphology) and function from fetal development to puberty, pregnancy, and aging will help elucidate fundamental changes to breast development and disease. A key element in that process is "branching morphogenesis," in which the mammary gland fulfills its function by producing and delivering copious amounts of milk by forming a rootlike network of branched ducts from a rudimentary epithelial bud.[108] Branching morphogenesis begins in fetal development, pauses after birth, starts again in response to estrogens at puberty, and is modified by cyclic ovarian hormonal action. This systemic hormonal action elicits local paracrine interactions between the developing epithelial ducts and their adjacent mesenchyme (embryonic) or postnatal stroma.[108] The local cellular crosstalk then directs the tissue remodeling, ultimately producing a mature ductal tree.[108]

HEALTH ALERT
Breast Cancer Screening Mammography

Joann G. Elmore, MD, MPH

The idea behind screening healthy individuals for disease is the hope that we can diagnose disease early, when more treatment options are available and when we can positively impact the life of the individual. Screening programs that cover the entire population of a country are a large undertaking and usually require extensive resources. Therefore we need to make certain that the test has a high level of accuracy with reasonable costs and disadvantages, the disease is not too rare, and the treatment is effective for individuals who are diagnosed because of the screening.

Women have been encouraged to undergo breast cancer screening for many decades. Early screening programs encouraged women to perform self-breast exams and also to have their clinician perform a breast exam in the office—subsequent data have shown that these screening techniques lead to false-positive exams and are not associated with a reduction in mortality.

Breast cancer screening with mammography continues to be recommended by many groups, although the benefits are less than we had hoped and we are learning more about the harms. Mammography is an x-ray exam that takes views of each breast (see figure). The recommended age of first mammogram and the frequency of screening vary among guidelines and countries. The U.S. Preventive Services Task Force periodically reviews the evidence and issues guidelines to help aid discussions with women about screening.

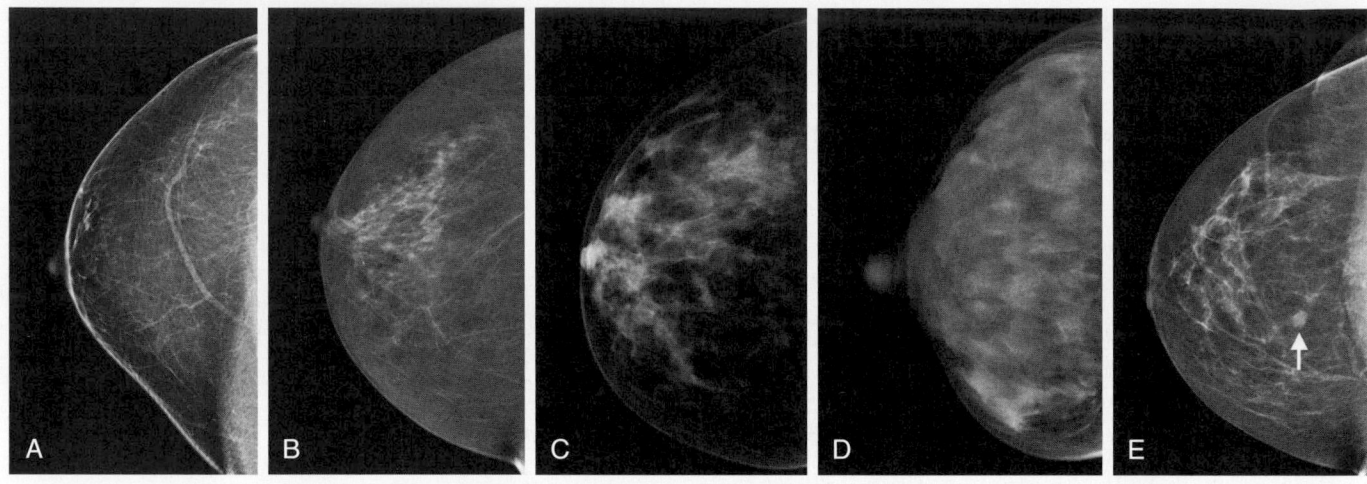

Mammograms. A-D, Mammograms depicting varying breast densities from a craniocaudal view: **A,** almost entirely fat; **B,** scattered fibroglandular densities; **C,** heterogeneously dense; and **D,** extremely dense. **E,** Mammogram showing invasive cancer. (Images provided by Christoph I. Lee, MD, MSHS. From Fuller MS et al: *Med Clin North Am* 99[3]:451-468, 2015.)

The benefits, risks, and accuracy of mammography screening depend on numerous factors, including women's age, breast density, and time interval between screening exams. Possible risks of screening are important to consider because screening at a population level involves testing healthy individuals; we are to "first, do no harm."

No medical test is perfect. About 10% of screening mammograms in the United States are interpreted as "abnormal," requiring additional testing. The great majority of women with these "abnormal" exams do not have breast cancer; this is called a false-positive result. The false-positive results lead to additional diagnostic testing, which can result in anxiety and morbidity to women. It is estimated that at least 50% of women in the United States, who are screened annually for a decade, will have experienced at least one false-positive examination.

Another harm of screening mammography is overdiagnosis—a *diagnosis* that would never have harmed the woman during her lifetime; such diagnoses can be either of a preinvasive lesion, such as ductal carcinoma in situ (DCIS), or of invasive breast cancer. With more women undergoing screening with mammography, we have seen a sharp increase in the number of women *diagnosed* with DCIS and early stage breast cancer. By definition, DCIS is not an invasive carcinoma and not an immediate life-threatening cancer—it is confined to the duct; but DCIS is almost always treated as if it is an invasive early stage breast cancer. Women with DCIS are at increased risk of a subsequent, invasive breast cancer *diagnosis;* however, the majority of women with DCIS are never

subsequently diagnosed with invasive cancer and treatment of DCIS does not alter mortality. Women with DCIS have the same death rates as women without DCIS. Some discussion has centered on changing the name of DCIS lesions to better differentiate preinvasive DCIS from invasive cancer because the term *carcinoma* is similar to the term *cancer.* However, it is not likely that the name will be changed because of its current common usage.

Unfortunately, we are not able to identify which women with a new diagnosis of DCIS or invasive breast cancer have the type of lesion that is so low risk that it will never harm them during their lifetime. Thus, most women undergo treatment with either lumpectomy and radiation therapy or mastectomy. This is overtreatment if the DCIS or invasive cancer was overdiagnosed. Estimates of the prevalence of overdiagnosis vary in the literature from <10% to 50%; more research is clearly needed.

Women with abnormalities noted on screening mammography are often offered the option of a breast biopsy versus watchful waiting with follow-up mammograms in 6 to 12 months. Some women think that a breast biopsy will provide an immediate and definitive diagnosis; however, this is not always the case. Pathologists have been noted to disagree on the diagnoses of atypia and DCIS.

Balancing the benefits and harms of breast cancer screening is not an easy task for women or their clinicians. Every woman should be encouraged to make an informed decision.

From Elmore JG et al: *J Am Med Assoc* 313(11):1122-1132, 2015; Fuller MS et al: *Med Clin North Am* 99(3):451-468, 2015; Katz DL et al: *Jekel's epidemiology, biostatistics, preventive medicine, and public health,* ed 4, Philadelphia, 2013, Elsevier Saunders; National Guideline C: *Breast cancer screening,* available at: www.guideline.gov/content.aspx?id=34275; accessed March 13, 2015; Pace LE, Keating NL: *J Am Med Assoc* 311(13):1327-1335, 2014; U.S. Preventive Services Task Force: *Ann Intern Med* 151(10):716-726, 2009.

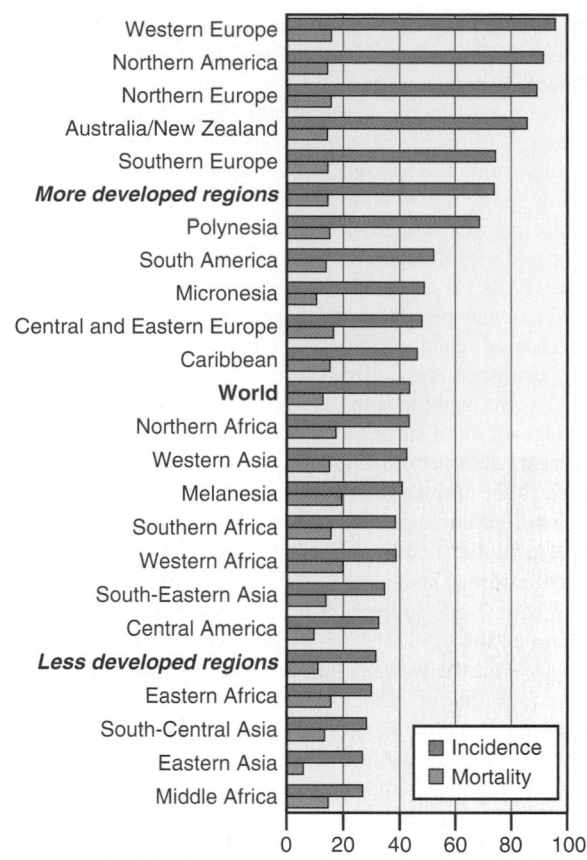

A Estimated age-standardized rates (World) per 100,000

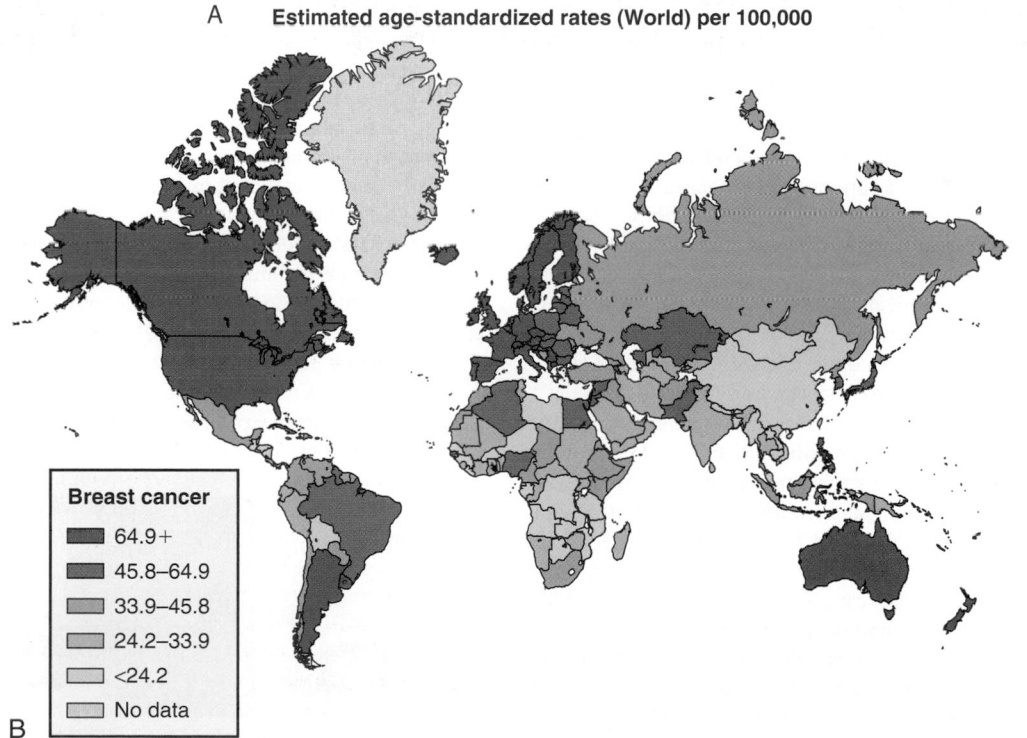

Breast cancer

- 64.9+
- 45.8–64.9
- 33.9–45.8
- 24.2–33.9
- <24.2
- No data

B

FIGURE 33-25 Breast Cancer Estimated Incidence and Mortality Worldwide in 2012. **A,** Estimated age-standardized rates (world) per 100,000 population. **B,** Incidence and mortality estimated age-standardized rates (world) per 100,000. These numbers represent a sharp rise in breast cancer incidence since the 2008 estimates by more than 20%. It is the most common cancer in women both in more and in less developed regions, with slightly more cases in less developed (883,000 cases) than in more developed (794,000) regions. Incidence rates vary nearly fourfold across the world regions. (From Ferlay J et al: *GLOBOCAN 2012 v1.0, Cancer incidence and mortality worldwide: IARC CancerBase No. 11,* Lyon, France, 2013, International Agency for Research on Cancer. Available at: http://globocan.iarc.fr/Default.aspx.)

A woman's age when her first child is born affects her risk for developing breast cancer—the younger she is, the lower the risk. Overall, lifetime risk of breast cancer is reduced in parous women compared with nulliparous women, but pregnancy must occur at a young age.[109] The influence of pregnancy on the risk of breast cancer also depends on family history, lactation postpartum, and overall parity.[110] Findings from a large prospective study found a *dual effect* from pregnancy—a transient postpartum increase in breast cancer risk followed by a long-term reduction in risk (compared with nulliparous women).[111] **Pregnancy-associated breast cancer (PABC)** is defined as breast cancers that occur during pregnancy, and risk may persist to at least 5 years postpartum and longer.[112,113] Delayed childbearing, observed in the United States and all developing countries, is expected to show a rise in diagnosed breast cancers.[110] A recent hypothesis for risk at any age is that gland *involution* after pregnancy and lactation uses some of the same tissue remodeling pathways activated during wound healing (i.e., proinflammatory pathways).[114] The proinflammatory environment, although physiologically normal, promotes tumor progression. The presence of macrophages in the involuting mammary gland may be contributing to carcinogenesis and the normal involuting gland may be in an immunosuppressed state with T-cell suppression.[114,115] Involution is discussed in the following section.

Although many mechanisms have been proposed for the *protective* effect of pregnancy, newer data on the genomic profile of parous women have shown pregnancy induces a long-lasting "genomic signature" that reveals chromatin remodeling derived from the early first pregnancy. The chromatin modifications are accompanied by higher expression of genes related to cell adhesion and differentiation, and genes only activated during the first 5 years after pregnancy may contribute to increased risk but the long-lasting genetic signature may explain pregnancy's preventive effect.[116]

Lobular Involution and Age and Postlactational Involution

Part of the uniqueness of the mammary gland is its profound physiologic changes throughout the phases of a woman's life. These phases include puberty, pregnancy, lactation, postlactational involution, and aging. The human breast is organized into 15 to 20 major lobes, each with terminal lobules containing milk-forming acini (see Figure 32-10, p. 792). **Terminal duct lobular units (TDLUs)**, structures of the breast that are responsible for lactation, are the predominant source of breast cancers.[117] With aging, breast lobules regress or involute with a decrease in the number and size of acini per lobule and with replacement of the intralobular stroma with the denser collagen of connective tissue.[118] With time, the glandular elements and collagen are replaced with fatty tissue. This process is called **lobular involution** and over many years the parenchymal elements progressively atrophy and disappear. The first study of its kind found lobular involution was associated with reduced risk of breast cancer.[118] Breast cancer risk decreased with increasing *extent* of involution in both high- and low-risk subgroups defined by family history of breast cancer, epithelial atypia, reproductive history, and age.[118] Based on pathologic and epidemiologic factors, these investigators propose that *delayed* involution (persistent glandular epithelium) is a major risk factor for breast cancer.[118] Tissue involution involves massive epithelial cell death, recruitment and activation of fibroblasts, stromal remodeling, and immune cell infiltration, including macrophages with similarities to microenvironments present during wound healing and tumor progression.[119]

Investigators suggest that the effect of lobular involution on breast cancer risk is a reduction in tissue from the involuting process, or the issue may be aging. Widely appreciated is that as women age, their risk of breast cancer increases. But, the *rate* of increase of breast cancer *slows* at about 50 years of age. This decline has been attributed to a reduction in ovarian hormone production; however, involution may contribute to this slowing rate. Importantly, investigators found an inverse association between lobular involution and parity.[118] Other investigators have reported the more children a woman has, the more likely she is to have persistent lobular tissue,[120,121] which Milanese and colleagues[118] found was associated with increased risk of breast cancer. However, multiparity also has been found to reduce the risk of breast cancer. This apparent contradiction may be explained by studies documenting that full-term pregnancies after 35 years of age are correlated with an increased risk of breast cancer.[122] In the Milanese study, the age of the mother at each child's birth was unknown.

Henson and colleagues[123] propose that late pregnancy with its concomitant increase in the proliferation of the ductal-alveolar epithelium is likely to interrupt the process of involution, which typically begins between 30 and 40 years of age. Failure to undergo TDLU involution among women with benign breast disease has been associated with progression to breast cancer, independent of other breast cancer risk factors.[117] The activated stromal environment (with the influx of immune cells similar to that which occurs during wound healing) in the process of involution is the "ideal niche" for carcinogenesis.

Major signaling pathways involved in mammary gland involution also are involved in breast cancer.[124] Certain proteases activated during involution modify the extracellular matrix and are implicated in loss of cell anchoring, providing a microenvironment for tumor growth.[124] Further, the normal involuting gland may be in an immunosuppressed state with the transient presence of immune-regulating cells that promote T-cell suppression.[115] Overall, for breast cancer, the long-term protective effects of pregnancy from hormones released (with consequent genetic and epigenetic changes) during pregnancy affect remodeling of the stromal microenvironment by causing apoptosis and involution. However, a transient increase in breast cancer risk following pregnancy may be caused by the *process* of mammary gland involution, which returns the tissue to its prepregnant state and is co-opted by the process of wound healing, resulting in a proinflammatory environment that, although physiologically normal, can promote carcinogenesis.[114] In postlactational involution, the mammary gland regresses and remodels to its prepregnant state whereby fibroblasts secrete proteases that degrade the extracellular matrix proteins. Consequently, the increased release of bioactive matrix fragments can promote tumor growth, motility, and invasion.[125] The extracellular matrix (ECM) is very different between nulliparous, lactating, and involuting glands as shown in Figure 33-26.

Oophorectomy, which is associated with a decrease in risk of breast cancer, leads to atrophy of breast parenchyma in young women, as is

FIGURE 33-26 Extracellular Matrix (ECM) Is Different in Nulliparous, Lactating, and Involuting Glands. Several ECM differences between nulliparous, lactational, and involuting mammary glands are related to collagen-fiber organization, cell motility and attachment, and cytokine regulation in a rodent model. Many protumorigenic ECM proteins are mediators of breast cancer progression specific to the involutional window, and systemic ibuprofen experimental treatment during involution decreases its tumor promotional changes. (From O'Brien JH et al: *J Proteome Res* 11:4894-4905, 2012.)

noted in older women.[123] Thus the risk reduction of oophorectomy may be caused by an accelerated involution.[123]

Investigators have shown that a benign biopsy demonstrating histologic changes consistent with incomplete or nonexistent involution or a mammogram classified as high density is independently associated with breast cancer risk, and that these factors combined are associated with an even greater risk.[126] The assessment of these "phenotypes" shows promise for improving risk prediction, particularly because they reflect the cumulative interaction of numerous genetic and environmental breast cancer risk factors over time.

Hormonal Factors

The link between breast cancer and hormones is based on six factors that affect risk: (1) the protective effect of an early (i.e., in the twenties) first pregnancy; (2) the protective effect of removal of the ovaries and pituitary gland; (3) the increased risk associated with early menarche, late menopause, and nulliparity; (4) the relationship between types of fat, free estrogen levels, and oxidative changes in estrogen metabolism; (5) the hormone-dependent development and differentiation of mammary gland structures; and (6) the efficacy of antihormone therapies for treatment and prevention of breast cancer. Throughout its existence, the mammary gland epithelium proceeds through critical "exposure periods" of rapid growth or cycles of proliferation, including neonatal growth, pubertal development, pregnancy lactation, and involution (after pregnancy and postmenopause, see p. 836).[114] Importantly, lack of TDLU involution has been associated with increased breast cancer risk, but the role of sex hormone levels and TDLU assessments has only begun to be studied (also see p. 836). Investigators suggest that hormone levels may act, in part, to delay age-appropriate TDLU involution, resulting in a higher quantity of at-risk epithelium.[117] These investigators found significant associations between higher TDLU counts, representing less involution, with higher levels of prolactin and lower levels of progesterone among premenopausal women, and higher levels of estradiol among postmenopausal women.[117] Higher testosterone levels were suggestively associated with higher TDLU counts among postmenopausal women.

The understanding of the role of systemic hormones as powerful regulators of mammary gland development is shifting. Evidence is pointing to the wide-ranging effects of systemic hormones, possibly not because of their *direct* hormone action but rather because of their *induced* actions from multiple secondary paracrine effectors—thus the term *hierarchical*. Unraveling is a complex model of hormone, paracrine, and adhesion molecule signaling pathways affecting both epithelial and stromal cell fate in both breast development and carcinogenesis (Figure 33-27). Key is *tissue remodeling* that applies not only to pubertal growth but also immediately after pregnancy and during involution (see previous section).

The female reproductive hormones (estrogens, progesterone, and prolactin) have a major role and effect on mammary gland development and breast cancer. A vast majority of breast cancers are *initially* hormone dependent (estrogen positive [ER+] and/or progesterone positive [PR+]), with estrogens playing a crucial role in their development.[127] Estrogens control processes critical for cellular functions by regulating activities and expression of key signaling molecules. These processes include regulation of receptor activity and receptor interaction with other intracellular proteins and DNA.[127] Estrogens thus play prominent roles in cellular proliferation, differentiation, and apoptosis.[127] Estrogens affect microtubules that are essential for establishing cell shape and cell polarity, processes necessary for epithelial gland organization.[127]

It is possible to consider four major hormonal hypotheses for breast cancer: (1) ovarian androgen excess (testosterone, for example);

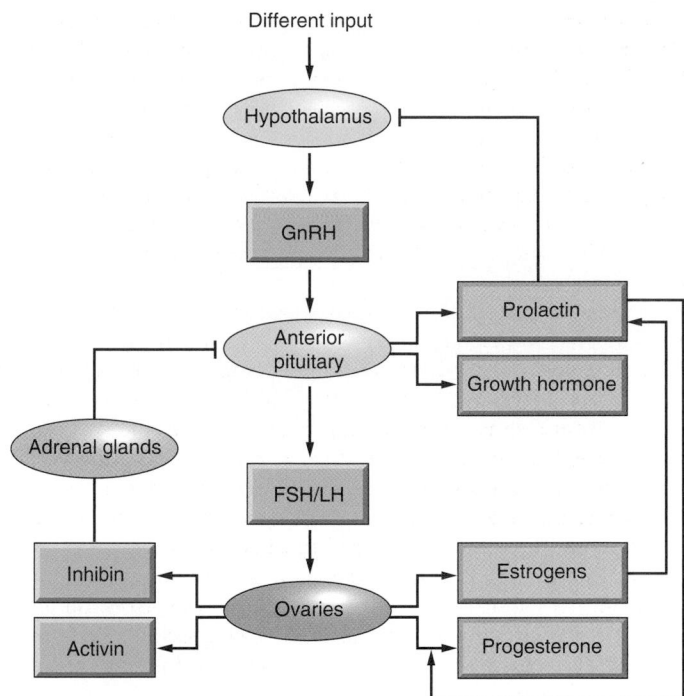

FIGURE 33-27 Female Endocrine System. The different mammary growth (mammotropic) hormone sites are shown in ovals, hormones are noted in blue boxes, and mammotropic hormones are noted in red boxes.

(2) estrogen and progesterone levels (ovarian and hormone replacement; (3) elevated estrogen levels alone (ovarian and hormone replacement); and (4) local biosynthesis of estrogens in breast tissue. These hypotheses, however, may not be mutually exclusive. Hormone replacement therapy (HRT), or the newer term menopausal hormone therapy (MHT), is discussed later in a separate section; the present discussion is concerned with endogenous levels of hormones.

The first hypothesis that breast cancer risk is increased among women who have an ovarian androgen excess also includes chronic anovulation and reduction of luteal phase (menstrual cycle) progesterone production. Therefore, it is also called the "ovarian hyperandrogenism/luteal inadequacy hypothesis." This hypothesis was based on the observation that women with breast cancer also reveal hyperplasia of the endometrium—a common symptom of ovarian androgen excess chronic anovulation and progesterone deficiency.[128] From the combination of prospective studies, case-control studies, and laboratory data the association between circulating testosterone levels in postmenopausal women and subsequent risk of breast cancer is now well established. Unclear is whether the association with testosterone level is direct or indirect (i.e., enzyme conversion by aromatase of testosterone to estradiol) (Figure 33-28).

The androgen receptor (AR) has been implicated in prostate cancer, and now in the development and progression of breast cancer.[129] Investigators used breast cancer cell lines and found that treatment of the breast cancer cells with 5α-dihydrotestosterone (DHT) promotes cell proliferation and decreases apoptosis.[129] The reduction of testosterone levels in women with oophorectomy or hysterectomy also may be a protective factor.[130]

The second hypothesis is breast cancer risk is increased among women with blood elevations of both estrogens and androgens—the "estrogen-plus-progesterone hypothesis." These observations revealed increased proliferation rates of breast epithelium during the luteal

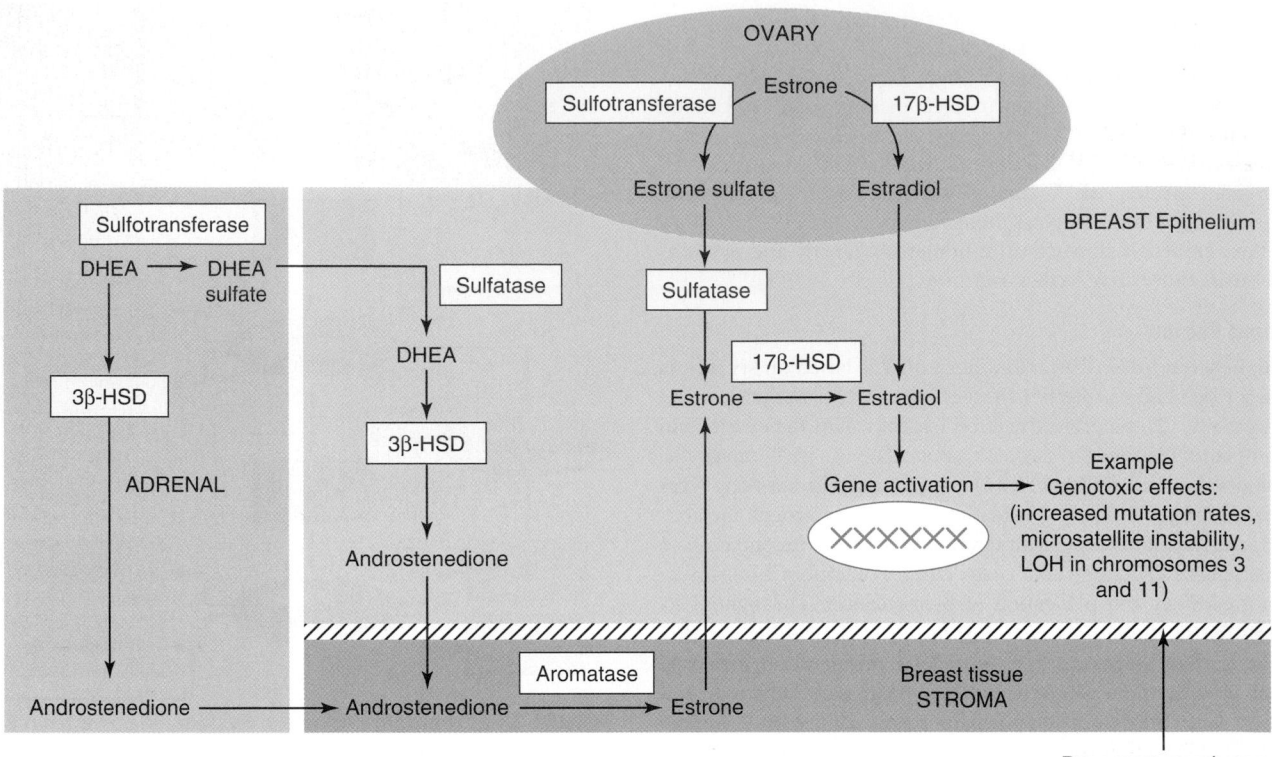

FIGURE 33-28 Local Biosynthesis of Estrogens. Three main enzyme complexes *(yellow)* involved in estrogen formation in breast tissue, including aromatase, sulfatase, and 17β-estradiol hydroxysteroid dehydrogenase *(17β-HSD)*. Thus, despite low levels of circulating estrogens in postmenopausal women with breast cancer, the tissue levels are several-fold higher than those in plasma, suggesting tumor accumulation of these estrogens. Data suggest that most abundant is sulfatase in both premenopausal and postmenopausal women with breast cancer. Numerous agents can block the aromatase action. Exploration of progesterone and various progestins to inhibit sulfatase and 17β-HSD or stimulate sulfotransferase (i.e., breast cancer cells cannot inactivate estrogens because they lack sulfotransferase) may provide new possibilities for treatment. *LOH,* Loss of heterozygosity (see Chapter 10). (Adapted from Russo J, Russo I: *Molecular basis of breast cancer: prevention and treatment,* Berlin, Heidelberg, New York, 2004, Springer-Verlag.)

phase of the menstrual cycle when the ovaries produce both estradiol and progesterone. Substantial evidence supports a positive association of circulating estrogens, androgens, and prolactin with postmenopausal breast cancer risk.[131] New data identify mammary stem cells (MaSCs) as critical targets for ovarian hormones, especially during the normal reproductive cycle when progesterone levels surge and during pregnancy when the proliferation of mammary stem cells is increased. Higher levels of progesterone among premenopausal women was associated with lower TDLU counts.[117] Among postmenopausal women, higher levels of estradiol and testosterone were associated with higher TDLU counts.[117] Select hormones may influence breast cancer risk through delaying TDLU involution (see p. 836).

The third hypothesis is often called the "estrogen-alone hypothesis." Substantial prospective data have accrued on the relationship between levels of circulating estrogens and breast cancer risk in postmenopausal women.[132,133] Overall, the positive association between levels of circulating estrogens in postmenopausal women and subsequent risk of breast cancer is now well established.

The fourth hypothesis suggests that *local* (in situ; paracrine) formation of estrogens in breast tumors may be more significant than circulating estrogens in *plasma* for the growth and survival of estrogen-dependent breast cancer in postmenopausal women.[127] Investigators measured breast sex steroids in both benign and cancerous tissue.[134] Estrogen and androgen concentrations varied greatly in both tissue and blood levels in benign and cancerous tissue.[134] The estradiol/estrone ratio was lowest in premenopausal benign tissue and much higher in premenopausal cancerous tissue and postmenopausal benign and cancerous tissue. Estradiol and estrone levels were substantially higher in tissue than in plasma in both premenopausal and postmenopausal women.[134] Hormone levels in breast adipose tissue revealed high levels of androstenedione and testosterone and significant estrone and estradiol levels in breast adipocytes from postmenopausal breast cancer patients consistent with an obesity-inflammation-aromatase axis (obesity with inflammation, cyclooxygenase [COX] elevation, and increased aromatase, which converts androgens to estrogen) occurring locally in breast tissue.[134]

Overall, two main mechanisms of carcinogenicity of estrogens involve (1) a receptor-mediated hormonal activity shown to stimulate cellular proliferation, resulting in increased opportunities for accumulation of genetic damage; and (2) oxidative catabolism of estrogens mediated by various cytochrome complexes (P450 [CYP] system) that eventually activate and generate reactive oxygen species (ROS) that can cause oxidative stress and genomic damage directly. Oxidative metabolites of estrogens can develop ultimate carcinogens that react with DNA to cause mutations leading to carcinogenesis. Thus, imbalances in estrogen metabolites in breast tissue correlate with the development of tumors and suggest possible biomarkers related to the risk of developing breast cancer.

Hormone Replacement Therapy and Breast Cancer Risk: Estrogen Plus Progesterone Therapy (MHT) and Estrogen Only Therapy (ET)

The International Agency for Research on Cancer lists estrogen-progestogen menopausal therapy and estrogen-progestrogen contraceptives as carcinogenic agents with sufficient evidence in humans for breast cancer[135] (see Table 11-1). Evidence from the Agency for Health care Research and Quality (AHRQ, United States) published a systematic review from 283 trials comparing effectiveness of treatments for menopausal symptoms.[136] From this report, they state, "Over the long term, estrogen combined with progestogen has both beneficial effects (fewer osteoporotic fractures) and harmful effects (increased risk of breast cancer, gallbladder disease, venous thromboembolic events, and stroke). Estrogens given alone do not appear to increase breast cancer risk, although endometrial cancer risk is increased." Evidence on the route of administration of MHT, oral versus transdermal (gel or patch), and the risk of breast cancer has limited research.

Insulin and Insulin-Like Growth Factors

Insulin-like growth factors (IGFs) regulate cellular functions involving cell proliferation, migration, differentiation, and apoptosis. Insulin-like growth factor 1 (IGF-1) is a protein hormone with a structure similar to that of insulin. IGF-1 is a potent mitogen, and after binding to the IGF-1R (receptor) triggers a signaling cascade leading to proliferation and anti-apoptosis.[137]

Diabetes is associated with complex physiology of insulin resistance, increased insulin level, estrogen and growth hormone levels, inflammation, and signaling pathways leading to an increased risk of breast cancer.[138] Insulin therapy and sulfonylurea were found to be mildly associated with increased breast cancer risk.[138] A United Kingdom study showed that women treated with insulin glargine were not associated with breast cancer risk in the first 5 years; however, longer use may increase the risk.[139] Metformin appears to have a protective role. Much more investigation is needed to understand the role of insulin, insulin-like growth factors, and diabetes mellitus and the risk of breast cancer and recurrence of breast cancers.

Melatonin as a regulator of circadian rhythm is the main focus of shift work and light at night and breast cancer risk. However, tumor growth (in vivo) can be accelerated by light at night in part from continuous activation of IGF-1 receptor (IGF-1R) signaling.[140] A recent case-control study of 1679 women exposed to light at night during sleep was significantly associated with breast cancer risk.[140] Although inconclusive, shift work and its disruptive effects on circadian rhythms and sleep deprivation at night have been suggested as a risk factor for breast cancer.[141,142]

Prolactin and Growth Hormone

Growth hormone (GH) induces the production of IGFs in the liver; IGF signaling is important for breast development and is implicated in breast carcinogenesis. Two studies, however, have reported a link between growth hormone level and breast cancer risk.[143,144] In the largest prospective analysis comparing circulating prolactin levels and breast cancer risk, those with the highest levels had the highest risk.[145] From an EPIC cohort, higher circulating prolactin level was associated with increased risk of in situ breast cancer.[146]

Oral Contraceptives

The International Agency for Research on Cancer (IARC) Group confirmed that combined estrogen-progestogen oral contraceptives (OCs) increase the risk for breast, cervix, and liver cancers.[135,147] However, the efficacy of OCs in protecting against ovarian cancer and endometrial

FIGURE 33-29 Breast Density Varies Among Women. The sensitivity of mammography for detecting malignancy is significantly reduced if the breast consists of a high proportion of fibroglandular (dense) breast tissue (A) compared with a breast that is fatty (B). (From O'Malley FP et al, editors: *Breast pathology*, ed 2, Philadelphia, 2011, Saunders.)

cancer is well established. Hormones are discussed further in the following Pathogenesis section (p. 842).

Mammographic Breast Density

Mammographic density (MD) is the radiologic appearance of the breast, reflecting variations in breast composition (Figure 33-29). Mammographic breast density (MBD) appears white or dense on a mammogram and is a strong and consistent risk factor for breast cancer.[126] MBD decreases with age and is associated with body mass index (BMI), family history, and postmenopausal hormone use.[148,149] Insulin-like growth factor 1 receptor (IGF-1R) may play an important role in breast cancer in individuals with mammographic breast tissue density.[150] Investigators are studying if MBD is related to reduced lobular involution of breast tissue in dense breasts (reduced involution increases cancer risk). Having a combination of dense breasts and no lobular involution was associated with higher breast cancer risk than having nondense or fatty breasts and complete involution.[126] Women with dense breasts occupying more than 60% to 75% of the breast have a fourfold to sixfold increased risk of breast cancer compared with those with little or no density.[149,151] Dense area percentage is a stronger breast cancer risk factor than absolute dense area.[152] Mammographic dense tissue has been thought to represent both epithelial and stromal components. One hypothesis is that the stromal-rich environment in MBD may have an abundance of growth factors that could stimulate the epithelium in a noninvoluted breast, thereby increasing the risk of malignant transformation.[126] Finding tumors in women with MBD is a challenge because they both appear white; as Dr. Susan Love states, "...like trying to find a polar bear in a snow storm."

Environmental Factors

The environmental causes of breast cancer possibly affect the breast the most during critical phases or "windows" of development including early differential stages—that is, undifferentiated cells to alveolar buds and then lobules, puberty, pregnancy and lactation, involution, and menopause. During these early phases, mitotic activity and cell division are greater than later in life.

Radiation. Ionizing radiation is a known mutagen and established carcinogen for breast cancer. To date, only accidentally or medically induced radiation has been demonstrated to exert a carcinogenic effect on the breast. The Institute of Medicine (IOM) reports that the two most strongly associated environmental factors are exposure to ionizing radiation and combined postmenopausal HRT.[153] There are many sources of ionizing radiation, including x-rays, CT scans, fluoroscopy, and other medical radiologic procedures (see Chapter 11). Although only about 10% of diagnostic radiologic procedures in large U.S. hospitals are CTs, they contribute an estimated 65% of the effective radiation dose to the public from all medical x-ray examinations.[154] The IOM conclusion of a causal relationship between radiation exposure in the same range as CT and cancer is consistent from a large varied literature.[155] The IOM makes it clear that *avoidance* of medical imaging is an important and concrete step that women (girls) can take to reduce their risk of breast cancer.[156] Scientists and clinicians also have expressed concern about the increasing number of CT scans performed, including on children.[156,157] Radiologic exposure of the upper spine, heart, ribs, lungs, shoulders, and esophagus also exposes breast tissue to radiation. Breast tissue may be exposed from abdominal CT scans; x-rays and fluoroscopy of infants may constitute whole-body irradiation. The duration of increased risk from radiation is unknown, but increased risk appears to have lasted at least 35 years in women treated for mastitis, those treated with fluoroscopy, and those who survived the atomic bombs during World War II. Breast cancer rates in atomic bomb survivors in Japan were highest among women younger than 20 years of age at time of exposure; importantly, those who had early full-term pregnancies were at significantly lower risk than those who had not. Thus, interacting factors can modulate the risks from radiation.

An important topic currently is the effect of low-dose ionizing radiation. The debate is that low-energy x-rays may be more hazardous per unit dose than previously reported. Conventional x-ray mammography is one of the most valuable diagnostic tools for imaging of the breast. Currently, full-field digital mammography (FFDM) is frequently used. Continuous technical development has led to several new imaging techniques, including digital breast tomosynthesis (DBT), phase contrast x-ray imaging, and computed tomography of the breast, as well as ultrasound and magnetic resonance imaging (MRI). Despite technical innovations, except for ultrasound and MRI, these modalities require exposure of breast tissue to ionizing radiation and the breast is considered a very radiosensitive organ.[158] Therefore, it is critical to compare delivered radiation doses to the breast and measure x-ray–induced DNA damage. A new technique for the detection and quantification of in vivo DNA damage has been developed. DNA double-strand breaks (DSBs) are the most relevant lesion induced by ionizing irradiation.[158] After induction of DSBs is the phosphorylation of the histone variant H2AX, named γ-H2AX. The γ-H2AX is a visible foci and a reliable and sensitive tool for the determination of DNA damage. Recently, investigators found mammography induces a slight but significant increase of γ-H2AX foci in systemic blood lymphocytes. A clear induction of DNA lesions was found both by FFDM and by DBT.[158] These data will be important to compare different breast imaging techniques. Investigators are studying mammographic radiation–induced DNA damage in mammary epithelial cells from women with low or high family risk of breast cancer, including comparisons with the number of views performed during screening.[159] Radiobiologic effects have been found in both low-risk and high-risk women, but risks are greater in high-risk women.[159,160,160A] Investigators are looking for markers that are activated by DNA damage. One new marker may be CAV1 (caveolin protein, see Chapter 1). Caveolin protein acts as a sensor and early mediator in response to DNA damage

and may be important as a biomarker for radiosensitivity.[161] New biologic understandings of low doses of radiation are presented in Chapter 11.

Women treated with chest radiation for a pediatric or young adult type of cancer have a substantially increased risk of breast cancer. Investigators from international studies have concluded that diagnostic chest irradiation or radiation therapy for benign or malignant diseases increases the risk of breast cancer for cumulative doses as low as 130 mGy. The breast cancer risk did not decrease when increasing the number of radiologic treatment fractions for delivering the same total dose, but risk decreased greatly with increasing age of exposure to ionizing radiation.[162] International agencies are assessing the utility of screening MRI and mammography in these high-risk populations. The risk of secondary lung malignancy (SLM) is an important concern for women treated with whole-breast radiation therapy after breast-conserving surgery for early-stage breast cancer.[163] Investigators studied SLM risk associated with several common methods of delivering whole-breast radiation therapy (RT). Compared with supine whole-breast irradiation (WBI), prone breast irradiation is associated with a significantly lower predicted risk of secondary lung malignancy.[163]

The United States Preventive Services Task Force (USPSTF) has updated the recommendations for mammography because of overdiagnosis and overtreatment issues related to screening mammography (*Health Alert:* Breast Cancer Screening Mammography).

Diet. Prospective epidemiologic studies on diet and breast cancer risk fail to show an association that is consistent, strong, and statistically significant except for alcohol intake, being overweight, and weight gain after menopause (see following discussion). Diet has been postulated as important for breast cancer risk because of the international correlations of consumption of specific dietary factors (e.g., fats) and breast cancer incidence and mortality and because of migrant studies showing greater incidence of breast cancer among descendants who relocated to another country compared with those in the country of origin. International variations also can occur because of differences in reproductive history, physical activity, obesity, and other factors.

Dietary fat and breast cancer risk is the subject of much study, controversy, and debate.[164] Potential biologic mechanisms between fat intake and breast cancer risk include the following: (1) fat may stimulate endogenous steroid hormone production (also affects weight gain, age of menarche), (2) fat interferes with immune or inflammatory function, and (3) fat influences gene expression. Although prospective studies and case-control studies on fat and breast cancer risk have been inconsistent, concern has been that any association with fat intake may be because of total energy intake. Moreover, there is limited evidence that modest reductions in fat intake (less than 20% of caloric intake) reduce breast cancer risk. Despite extensive investigation, there is no conclusive evidence overall that *adult* consumption of macronutrients including fat, carbohydrate, or fiber is strongly related to breast cancer incidence.

The association between individual foods and breast cancer is inconsistent, and new data on *dietary patterns* are emerging. The Mediterranean diet includes high intake of vegetables, legumes, fruits, nuts, and minimally processed cereals; moderately high intake of fish; and high intake of monounsaturated lipids coupled with low intake of saturated fat, low to moderate intake of dairy products, low intake of meat products, and moderate intake of alcohol. The Mediterranean diet may favorably influence the risk of breast cancer.[165] The Western pattern includes higher intake of red and processed meats, refined grains, sweets and desserts, and high-fat dairy products.

Most prospective studies have not supported a link between fiber intake and breast cancer. Carbohydrate quality, however, rather than absolute amount, may be important for breast cancer risk, especially for premenopausal women.

Evidence exists that alcohol consumption increases breast cancer risk. Beer, wine, and liquor all contributed to the positive association and risks did not differ by menopausal status. In large prospective studies, high intake of folic acid appeared to decrease the enhanced risk for breast cancer caused by alcohol. The mechanisms by which alcohol intake increases the risk of breast cancer are unknown; however, physiologic studies have reported an estrogen level increase in women taking hormone replacement therapy (HRT) and IGF-1 level increases with alcohol intake. Alcohol may increase breast cancer risk through increasing mammographic breast density, especially in women at high risk.[166] It is not known whether reducing or discontinuing alcohol consumption in midlife decreases the risk of breast cancer. The relationship between fruit and vegetable intake and reduction in breast cancer risk has been studied over three decades. To date, no protective effects have been firmly established.[167]

Soybeans are the main source of isoflavones. The isoflavone compounds, including daidzein and genistein, can bind estrogen receptors but are far less potent than estradiol. Soy may act like other antiestrogens (e.g., tamoxifen) by blocking the action of endogenous estrogens to reduce breast cancer risk. Thus, depending on the estradiol concentration, soy exhibits weak estrogenic or antiestrogenic activity. Many other mechanisms of action are proposed for isoflavones, including apoptosis and inhibition of angiogenesis. In 2011 the North American Menopause Society held a symposium to review the latest evidence-based science on the role of soy and found that soy foods generally appear to be breast protective and recommended moderate lifelong soy consumption.[106] A recent large study of both American and Chinese women suggested that moderate intake of soy (≥10 mg of isoflavones/day) had a significant reduction in breast cancer recurrence as well as a nonsignificant trend toward reduced all-cause mortality.[168] In addition, soy may optimize extrarenal 1,25-dihydroxycholecalciferol or vitamin D_3 (a prodifferentiating vitamin D metabolite), which could result in growth control and, conceivably, inhibition of tumor progression.

Iodine deficiency is hypothesized as contributing to the development of breast pathology and cancer.[107,169] Iodine plays a significant role in breast health.[169-172] Evidence reveals that iodine is an antioxidant and antiproliferative agent contributing to the integrity of normal mammary tissue.[173] Seaweed, which is iodine-rich, is an important dietary item in Asian communities and has been associated with the low evidence of benign and breast cancer disease in Japanese women.[173] Molecular iodine (I_2) supplementation exerts an inhibitory effect on the development and size of benign and cancerous tissue.[174] Nutrition remains an important area of study.

Obesity. Excess body fatness is known to increase cancer risk from cellular pathways that involve hormonal regulation, cellular proliferation, and immunity.[175] Obesity, measured as body mass index (BMI), has been associated with a *reduced* risk of *premenopausal* breast cancer. Recently reported (from the Nurses' Health Study I and II), however, was that weight gain or weight loss since age 18 did not significantly decrease the risk of premenopausal breast cancer.[176] Other data measuring adiposity using waist/hip ratio (WHR) have not found a reduced risk but rather no association (null) or an increased risk. Excess adiposity is positively associated with breast cancer recurrence and breast cancer specific mortality among both premenopausal and postmenopausal women.[177]

In 2002 the International Agency for Research on Cancer (IARC) concluded that excess body weight (EBW) increased the risk of developing postmenopausal breast, colorectum, endometrium, kidney, and esophageal adenocarcinoma.[178] The World Cancer Research Fund (WCRF) used a more standardized approach to evaluate studies and concluded that evidence is convincing and that a probable association exists between body fat and postmenopausal breast cancer.[179]

Despite strong links with endogenous estrogen levels, body fat has been consistently but *weakly* related to increased postmenopausal risk.[180] This observation (i.e., weakly) has been surprising because obese postmenopausal women have endogenous estrogen levels (estrone and estradiol) nearly double those of lean women.[180,181] This weak association is possibly related to two factors. First, the premenopausal reduction in breast cancer risk related to being overweight possibly persists, opposing the adverse effect of elevated levels of estrogens after menopause. Thus, *weight gain* should be more strongly related to postmenopausal breast cancer risk than attained weight. In two case-control studies and prospective studies, this was indeed true.[182-185]

Obesity is associated with poor survival among women with breast cancer and the association of obesity with mortality from breast cancer appears to be stronger than its association with incidence.[180,184] The increase in breast cancer risk with increasing BMI among postmenopausal women is most likely the result of increases in levels of estrogens by aromatase activity in adipose tissue.[175] However, studies of hormones secreted by adipose tissue, *leptin* and *adiponectin,* may underlie the association between obesity and breast cancer risk. Increasing BMI and central fat deposition are associated with increased risk for breast cancer in prospective studies, and in vitro studies have shown leptin-stimulated breast carcinogenesis.[186,187] From molecular mechanism studies, leptin enhances breast cancer cell proliferation by inhibiting cell death (pro-apoptosis) signaling pathways and by increasing in vitro sensitivity to estrogens.[188] Leptin secreted by adipocytes and fibroblasts in the microenvironment act on breast cancer cells in a paracrine fashion.[189] Adiponectin has been shown to exert antiproliferative effects in vitro on human breast cancer cells.[188] Additionally, factors that may be related to recurrence of breast cancer in women with excess adiposity at the time of diagnosis include cytokines, IGF or immune function, or both.[175]

Environmental chemicals. Evidence linking chemicals to the cause of breast cancer is difficult to obtain. It is challenging because it is a life history of exposure that is important—not just a single chemical but complex mixtures of chemicals and their interaction with endogenous hormones. With industrial development, breast cancer rates increase. An estimated 100,000 synthetic chemicals are registered for use in the United States, another 1000 or more are added each year, and toxicologic screening for these chemicals is minimal. In fact, toxicologic screening is only available for about 7% of these chemicals.[190] For chemicals other than hormonal drugs, the IARC lists only ethylene oxide as a potential risk factor with limited evidence in humans.

Chemicals persist in the environment, accumulate in adipose tissue, interact with local adipose tissue physiology in an endocrine/paracrine manner, and remain in breast tissue for decades. Estrogen receptors are some of the main targets of endocrine-disrupting chemicals (EDCs), including the plasticizer bisphenol A and the flame retardant tetrachlorobisphenol A.[191] Women who immigrate to the United States from Asian countries experience an enormous percent increase in risk within one generation. A generation later, the rate of their daughter's risk approaches that of women born in the United States. This change in risk suggests that in utero exposures affect subsequent disease risk. It is difficult to know whether these changes in risk emanate from nutritional content, pollutants, food additives, or other factors.

Xenoestrogens are synthetic chemicals that mimic the actions of estrogens and are found in many pesticides, fuels, plastics, detergents, and drugs. Because many factors correlated with breast cancer (e.g., early menarche, delayed pregnancy and breast-feeding, late menopause) are associated with lifetime exposure to estrogens, investigators reasoned that environmental chemicals affect estrogen metabolism and contribute to breast cancer. The most significant chemicals may be polychlorinated biphenyls (PCBs), such as dichlorodiphenyltrichloroethane (DDT), pesticides (dieldrin, aldrin, heptachlor, and others), bisphenol A (pervasive in polycarbonate plastics), tobacco smoke (active and passive), dioxins (vehicle exhaust, incineration, contaminated food supply), alkylphenols (detergents and cleaning products), metals, phthalates (makes plastics flexible, some cosmetics), parabens (antimicrobials), food additives (recombinant bovine somatotropin [rBST] and zeranol to enhance growth in cattle and sheep), MHT (i.e., HRT), and others.

Physical activity. Regular physical activity may reduce overall risk of breast cancer, especially in premenopausal or young postmenopausal women. Activity also may reduce the invasiveness of breast cancer.[192] A sedentary lifestyle may increase cancer risk through several mechanism including increased insulin resistance, increased inflammation, and decreased immune function.[193] Epidemiologic studies demonstrate that physical activity lowered the risk of breast cancer mortality in breast cancer survivors and improved their physiologic and immune functions.[193]

Inherited Cancer Syndromes, Genes, Epigenetic Considerations

The causes of breast cancer have been difficult to define because each woman has a different genetic profile, which is called genetic heterogeneity.[194] Genetic heterogeneity is common among individuals but also at the level of the tumor itself, involving both genetic and epigenetic processes. These genetic factors interact with environmental factors. These facts are sobering and make the understanding of the genetic driving force behind tumor initiation, progression, and metastasis very complicated. However, recently, an experiment using a mouse model of breast tumor heterogeneity allowed investigators to probe the molecular basis of stable differences in cell (clonal) populations to contribute to various aspects of the cancer process, including the ability to form circulating tumor cells (CTCs) and ultimately metastases[195] (see Pathogenesis).

A history of breast cancer in first-degree relatives (mother or sister) increases a woman's risk about two to three times. Risk increases even more if two first-degree relatives are involved, especially if the disease occurred before menopause and was bilateral. A small total proportion of breast cancers (5% to 10%, although the prevalence is significant) are the result of highly penetrant dominant genes (i.e., hereditary breast cancers). The most important of the dominant genes are the breast cancer susceptibility genes *(BRCA1, BRCA2)*. *BRCA1* (breast cancer 1 gene), located on chromosome 17, is a tumor-suppressor gene; therefore any mutation in the gene may inhibit or retard its suppressor function, leading to uncontrolled cell proliferation. *BRCA2* (breast cancer 2 gene) is located on chromosome 13. A family history of both breast cancer and ovarian cancer increases the risk that an individual with breast cancer carries a *BRCA1* mutation.[196] Carriers of the *BRCA1* gene also are at higher risk for ovarian cancer. The risks for breast or ovarian cancer, or both, however, are not equal in all mutation carriers and have been found to vary by several factors, including type of cancer, age at onset, and mutation position.[196] This observed variation in penetrance has led to the hypothesis that other genetic and/or environmental factors modify cancer risk in mutation carriers. Men who develop breast cancer are more likely to have a *BRCA2* mutation than a *BRCA1* mutation (see Chapter 34). Options for those who have a positive test for *BRCA1* or *BRCA2* mutation include surveillance to find cancers early, prophylactic surgery (i.e., bilateral salpingo-oophorectomy), risk factor avoidance, promotion of breast-feeding,

and chemoprevention. Several other genetic alterations can increase the risk of breast cancer.

PATHOGENESIS   Most breast cancers are adenocarcinomas and first arise from the ductal/lobular epithelium as carcinoma in situ. Carcinoma in situ is a proliferation of epithelial cells that is confined to the ducts and lobules by the basement membrane. Tumors of the infiltrating (invasive) ductal type do not grow to a large size, but they metastasize early. This type accounts for 70% of breast cancers. Table 33-11 summarizes some types of breast cancer. Breast cancer is a heterogeneous—not a single—disease with diverse molecular, biologic, phenotypic, and pathologic changes.[197] Heterogeneity is an important concept because the biologic attributes of a tumor as a whole are strongly influenced by its subpopulation of cells, as well as the tumor's surrounding neighborhood or microenvironment.[198] Recent research suggests that breast cancer is heterogeneous from its initial preinvasive stages[199] and within the same tumor.

The many genetic and epigenetic changes drive the sequential expansion of progressively more and more malignant cell populations.[200] Breast tissue stem cells are thought to be the cell of origin for all breast cancers. Gene expression profiling studies have identified at least four major subtypes classified as luminal A, luminal B, HER2+, and basal-like.[201] Mounting evidence shows there are "subtypes within subtypes" and emerging evidence suggests that the biology of specific subtypes reflects contributions from the microenvironment.[202] Many models of breast carcinogenesis have been suggested and three interrelated themes also have emerged and include (1) gene addiction, (2) phenotype plasticity, and (3) cancer stem cells.

Cancer gene addiction includes oncogene addiction, whereby these driver genes play key roles in breast cancer development and progression, and nononcogene addiction, whereby these genes may not initiate cancer but play roles in cancer development and progression.[203] Examples of key driver genes include *HER2* and *MYC* and examples of tumor-suppressor genes include *TP53*, *BRCA1*, and *BRCA2*. Once a founding tumor clone is established, genomic instability may assist through the establishment of other subclones and contribute to both tumor progression and therapy resistance.[92] Phenotypic plasticity is exemplified by a distinctive phenotype called epithelial-to-mesenchymal transition (EMT) (see Chapter 10). EMT is involved in the generation of tissues and organs during embryogenesis, is essential for driving tissue plasticity during development, and is an unintentional process during cancer progression. The EMT-associated reprogramming is involved in many cancer cell characteristics, including suppression of cell death or apoptosis and senescence, is reactivated during wound healing, and is resistant to chemotherapy and radiation therapy.[204] Remodeling or reprogramming of the breast during postpregnancy involution is important because it involves inflammatory and "wound healing-like" tissue reactions known as reactive stroma. These tissue reactions increase the risk for tumor invasion and may facilitate the transition of carcinoma in situ to invasive carcinoma. Activation of an EMT program during cancer development often requires signaling between cancer cells and neighboring stromal cells.[205] In advanced primary carcinomas, cancer cells recruit a variety of cell types into the surrounding stroma, including fibroblasts, myofibroblasts, granulocytes, macrophages, mesenchymal stem cells, and lymphocytes (Figure 33-30). Overall, increasing evidence suggests that interactions of cancer cells with adjacent tumor-associated stromal cells induce malignant cell phenotypes (Figure 33-31).

Research is ongoing to define cancer stem cells in breast carcinogenesis including their origin and renewability properties. Studies have begun to identify the role of mammary stem cells (MaSCs) and to

TABLE 33-11   Types of Breast Carcinomas and Major Distinguishing Features

Histologic Type	Distinguishing Features
Carcinoma of Mammary Ducts	
Papillary	Well-delineated cystic masses in multiple areas; hemorrhage often present; majority appear in 40- to 60-year age group; often involves skin
Intraductal (comedo)	Often accompanied by evidence of inflammation; well-circumscribed tumors within duct; well-differentiated tumor cells; rarely ulcerates skin
Infiltrating Carcinoma	
Ductal (no specific type [NST])	Fibrous, firm, glistening, gray-tan mass with chalky streaks, mixture of patterns; may cause discharge from nipple; represents about 70-80% of all breast cancers
Mucinous	Usually large (>3 cm in diameter), circumscribed, and encapsulated, glistening appearance, varies in color; two types: pure and mixed; pure tumor is surrounded by mucin; infrequent; found in lateral half of breast; tends to occur in women after age 70 years
Medullary	Encapsulated and grows very large (7-8 cm in diameter); commonly surrounded by lymphocytic inflammatory infiltrate; occurs after age 50 years
Tubular	Well-differentiated with orderly tubules in center (stroma) of mass; can be associated with noninfiltrating ductal carcinoma; occurs in women about 50 years of age; nodal metastasis infrequent; occurrence rare
Adenoid cystic	Very rare; well-circumscribed, painless mass arising from nipple and areola
Metaplastic	Involves cartilage or bone, mixed tumors or osteogenic sarcomas
Squamous cell	Frequent in blacks; originates in ductal epithelium
Carcinoma of Mammary Lobules	
Lobular carcinoma in situ	Found in individuals with fibrocystic disease; localized to upper breast quadrants; 15-35% risk of becoming invasive; occurs frequently in mid-40s; infiltrating variety occurs in early 50s
Infiltrating lobular	Infiltrates from duct; firm mass with chalky streaks
Paget disease	Eczema of nipple that extends to areola; cancer usually found underneath nipple; poorly circumscribed; large Paget cells arise from duct and directly invade nipple; history of scaly, red rash spreading from nipple; lesion palpable beneath nipple, often bilateral; occurs in middle age
Inflammatory carcinoma	Not a histologic type; fairly diffuse within breast tissue, diffuse edema of overlying skin; extremely undifferentiated, very rare; most metastasize to axilla
Sarcoma of the Breast	
Cystosarcoma phyllodes	Usually large (>17 cm in diameter); mostly localized but can rupture through skin; rarely metastasizes to lymph nodes; history of painless nodule present for years before it forms a large mass; ulceration and bleeding of skin often present; occurs in wide age range (13-77 years)
Fibrosarcoma	Well-circumscribed, firm, and usually does not involve skin or nipple; well-differentiated to extremely undifferentiated; arises from connective tissue; extremely rare (e.g., liposarcoma, angiosarcoma)

describe how they drive development of the gland and maintain homeostasis, the many cycles of proliferation and apoptosis needed to expand and maintain the breast during pregnancy, and return it to a quiet (quiescent) state after involution.[206] EMT generates multiple epithelial cell subsets with different states of stemness relative to more differentiated cells.[207] The extracellular matrix (ECM) and the basement membrane (BM), in particular, are no longer just considered the "bricks and mortar" of a tissue but now a place where stem cells reside; and correct tissue architecture, together with the reservoir of growth factors, cytokines, and proteinases, is critical for mammary tissue to develop and function properly.[206] Many of the biologic traits of high-grade malignancy—motility, invasiveness, and self-renewal—have been traced to subpopulations of stem cells within carcinomas.[208,209] Hormones may act as accelerators as well as initiators, delay involution, and influence the susceptibility of the breast epithelium to environmental carcinogens because hormones control the differentiation of the mammary gland epithelium and, thereby, regulate the rate of stem cell division.

Two new concepts being investigated as important to metastases are tumor dormancy and vascular mimicry. Tumor dormancy has been noted in the care of people with cancer whereby microscopic and occult cancerous lesions can enter a latent or dormant phase in various stages of tumor progression. In fact, these microscopic and occult cancerous lesions are often found in healthy people.[210] Ironically, in healthy people these are the slow-growing tumors (some called "pseudodisease") detected by present screening methods that would not advance to routine clinical presentation over the individual's lifetime.[210] The current debates are over concern that individuals often undergo unnecessary treatment for a disease they were never destined to experience.[210] Evidence exists that organ-specific molecular signaling can determine whether a metastatic lesion will expand or remain dormant. Significant to different signaling profiles that may determine this outcome are stress-activated kinases, transcription factors (such as p53), and cell cycle inhibitors. Thus, cell stress activated signaling may be increased, for example, with certain treatment modalities like surgery. Evidence has been accumulating that removal of a malignant tumor from a host is curative for many but—in some circumstances—is insufficient to prevent the cancer from reoccurring and can lead to rapid cancer recurrence.[211,212] Immune cells in the ECM or stroma and the overall immune response has been recognized for its role in regulating tumor growth and is being investigated for its role in tumor dormancy.

FIGURE 33-30 Cells of the Tumor Microenvironment. A, Distinct cell types constitute most solid tumors including breast tumors. Both the main cellular tissue, called parenchyma, and the surrounding tissue, or stroma, of tumors contain cell types that enable tumor growth and progression. For example, the immune-inflammatory cells present in tumors can include both tumor-promoting and tumor-killing subclasses of cells. **B,** The microenvironment of tumors. Multiple stromal cell types create a succession of tumor microenvironments that change as tumors invade normal tissue, eventually seeding and colonizing distant tissues. The organization, numbers, and phenotypic characteristics of the stromal cell types and the extracellular matrix *(hatched background)* evolve during progression and enable primary, invasive, and metastatic growth. (Not shown are the premalignant stages.) (Data from Hanahan D, Weinberg R: *Cell* 144:646-674, 2011.)

Cancer metastases require that primary tumor cells evolve the ability to intravasate into the lymphatic system or vasculature, and extravasate into and colonize secondary sites.[195] Investigators developed a mouse model of breast tumor heterogeneity and isolated a distinct clone of specialized cells that efficiently enter the vasculature and express two proteins, Serpine2 and Slpi, which were necessary and sufficient to program these cells for vascular mimicry. **Vascular mimicry** is a blood supply pathway in tumors that is formed by tumor cells and is independent of endothelial cell–lined blood vessels—thus it *mimics* real blood vessels (Figure 33-32). This blood supply pathway facilitates perfusion of the primary tumors and correlates with poor clinical outcome. The increase in these blood supply pathways was associated with an increase in circulating tumor cells (CTCs) and a subsequent increase in lung metastases. Additionally, treatment with the anticoagulant warfarin increased the number of CTCs and lung metastases, suggesting that the anticoagulant function of Serpine2 and Slpi both maintains blood flow through the extravascular network and promotes intravasation. These remarkable findings identify Serpine2- and Slpi-driven vascular mimicry as a critical mechanism or driver of metastatic progression in cancer.[195]

Ductal and Lobular Carcinoma in Situ

Ductal carcinoma in situ (DCIS) is a heterogeneous group of proliferations limited to breast ducts and lobules without invasion of the basement membrane. About 84% of all in situ disease is DCIS; the remainder is mostly lobular carcinoma in situ (LCIS). DCIS occurs predominantly in females but can occur in males. Since 1980 the widespread adoption of screening mammography has led to an epidemic of diagnoses of DCIS.[213] DCIS presents as microcalcifications (low grade) (Figure 33-33, *B*) or rod-shaped branching (high grade) on a mammogram (Figure 33-33, *A*).

Still controversial, DCIS does not appear to progress from sequential steps of low grade or risk types to higher grade or risk types during its route to cancer or cancer recurrence.[199,214] This property, therefore, suggests a stable population.[199] Because of these findings, some argue that the term is misleading and should be replaced by *ductal intraepithelial neoplasia*, similar to the term used in prostate cancer, and that breast cancer statistics should exclude these DCIS cases with invasive breast cancer statistics.[215] More than 60,000 women in the United States will be diagnosed with DCIS in 2015.[216] Because of the large numbers of cases diagnosed yearly in the United States, the debate is whether mammography is causing the overdiagnosis of potential pseudodisease; for example, the Canadian National Breast Screening Study-2 of women aged 50 to 59 years found a fourfold increase in DCIS cases in those screened by clinical breast examination (CBE) plus mammography compared with those screened by CBE alone, with no difference in breast cancer mortality.[213,217] The difficulty for this clinical dilemma is that the natural history of DCIS is poorly understood because nearly all cases are treated. More directed research on DCIS with genetic expression profiling, best treatment to achieve disease regression, and studies of tumor characteristics and risk profiling is needed. An important, newer mission of the DCIS Discovery Enterprise at MD Anderson Cancer Center is to prevent invasive disease while also reducing unnecessary surgery or radiation.

FIGURE 33-31 Signaling Interactions in the Tumor Microenvironment During Malignant Progression. *Upper panel:* Numerous cell types constitute the tumor microenvironment and are orchestrated and maintained by reciprocal interactions. *Lower panel:* The reciprocal interactions between the breast main tissue or parenchyma and the surrounding stroma are important for cancer progression and growth. Certain organ sites of "fertile soil" or "metastasis niches" facilitate metastatic seeding and colonization. Cancer stem cells are involved in some or all stages of tumor development and progression. (Adapted from Hanahan D, Weinberg R: *Cell* 144:646-674, 2011.)

Key to understanding the progression of breast cancer after treatment of DCIS depends on the characteristics of the lesion and on the delivered treatment. According to the National Cancer Institute (NCI), the best evidence indicates that most lesions of DCIS will not evolve to invasive cancer and those that do can be managed successfully, even after that transition.[215] The detection and treatment of nonpalpable DCIS often represents overdiagnosis and overtreatment.[215] Surprisingly, the overall death rate for women with DCIS is lower than that for women in the population as a whole.[92,215] This favorable outcome may reflect the benign nature of the condition or the benefits of

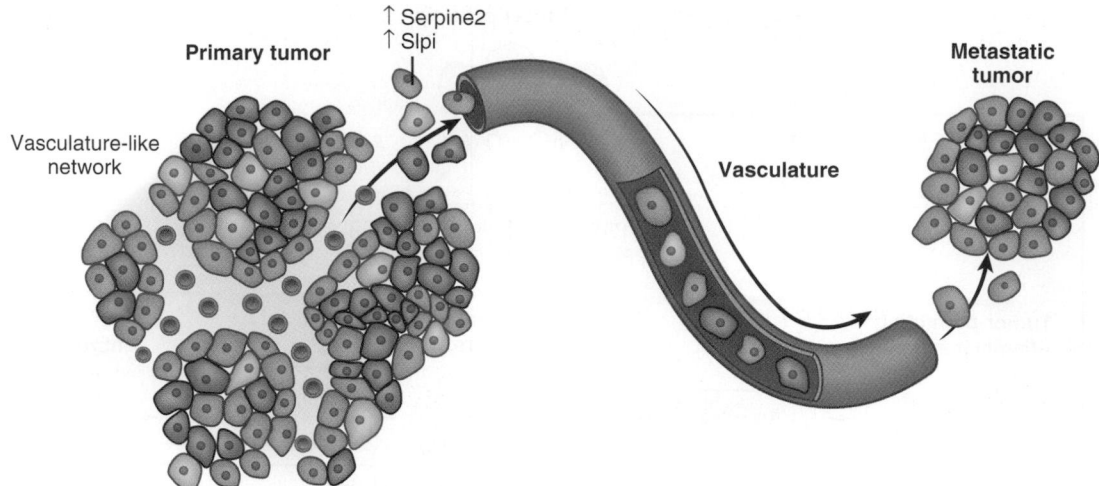

FIGURE 33-32 Vascular Mimicry Drives Metastasis. The steps to accomplish metastasis include *intravasation,* in which tumor cells escape from the primary tumor into the vasculature and move through the bloodstream; or *extravasation,* in which tumor cells escape from the vasculature to colonize in distant tissue. Metastasis is promoted by vascular mimicry, whereby tumor cells adopt characteristics similar to those of the endothelial cells that line blood vessels, and mimic vascular-like networks within tumors and between tumors and blood vessels. Wagenblast and colleagues found that two proteins, Serpine2 and Slpi, promoted metastasis by stimulating vascular mimicry. Tumor cells expressing these proteins *(green)* form the vascular-like network that allows other tumor cells *(purple, blue)* to move to secondary sites. (Adapted from Hendrix MJC: *Nature* 520:300-302, 2015; Wagenblast E et al: *Nature* 520:358-362, 2015.)

FIGURE 33-33 Ductal Carcinoma in Situ (DCIS). A, Malignant microcalcifications. Extensive area of pleomorphic microcalcifications; granular, rod-shaped, and branching microcalcifications can be identified. The appearances are typical of high-grade DCIS. **B,** Craniocaudal mammography reveals fine and coarse granular calcifications. Histopathologic analysis revealed low-grade DCIS. (**A** from O'Malley FP et al, editors: *Breast pathology,* ed 2, Philadelphia, 2011, Saunders. **B** from Donegan WL, Spratt JS: *Cancer of the breast,* ed 5, Philadelphia, 2002, Saunders.)

treatment, or is a marker for socioeconomic factors associated with longevity.[92,215] Attempts to define low-risk DCIS cases that can be managed with fewer therapies are critical.[215]

Lobular carcinoma in situ (LCIS) originates from the terminal duct lobular unit. Unlike DCIS, LCIS has a uniform appearance—the cells expand but do not distort involved spaces; thus the lobular structure is preserved. The cells grow in a noncohesive (discohesive) fashion

usually because of a loss of the tumor-suppressive adhesion protein E-cadherin.[92] LCIS is found as an incidental lesion from a biopsy and not from mammography because it is not associated with calcifications or stromal reactions that produce mammographic densities. LCIS has an incidence of about 1% to 6% of all carcinomas and did not increase with mammographic screening.[92] With biopsies in both breasts, LCIS is bilateral in 20% to 40% of cases, compared with 10% to 20% of cases

TABLE 33-12 Clinical Manifestations of Breast Cancer

Clinical Manifestation	Pathophysiology
Local pain	Local obstruction caused by tumor
Dimpling of skin	Can occur with invasion of dermal lymphatics because of retraction of Cooper ligament or involvement of pectoralis fascia
Nipple retraction	Shortening of mammary ducts
Skin retraction	Involvement of suspensory ligament
Edema	Local inflammation or lymphatic obstruction
Nipple/areolar eczema	Paget disease
Pitting of skin (similar to surface of an orange [peau d'orange])	Obstruction of subcutaneous lymphatics, resulting in accumulation of fluid
Reddened skin, local tenderness, and warmth	Inflammation
Dilated blood vessels	Obstruction of venous return by a fast-growing tumor; obstruction dilates superficial veins
Nipple discharge in a nonlactating woman	Spontaneous and intermittent discharge caused by tumor obstruction
Ulceration	Tumor necrosis
Hemorrhage	Erosion of blood vessels
Edema of arm	Obstruction of lymphatic drainage in axilla
Chest pain	Metastasis to lung

of DCIS.[92] The cells of atypical hyperplasia, LCIS, and invasive lobular carcinoma are structurally identical.[92] Loss of cellular adhesion because of dysfunction of E-cadherin results in a rounded shape without attachment to adjacent cells, increasing the risk of invasion. E-cadherin functions as a tumor-suppressor protein and may be lost in neoplastic proliferations from various mechanisms, including mutation.

LCIS is a risk factor for invasive carcinoma and develops in 25% to 35% of women over a period of 20 to 30 years. Unlike DCIS, the risk is almost as high in the contralateral breast as in the ipsilateral breast. Treatments include close clinical follow-up and mammographic screening, tamoxifen, and bilateral prophylactic mastectomy.

CLINICAL MANIFESTATIONS The majority of carcinomas of the breast occur in the upper outer quadrant, where most of the glandular tissue of the breast is located. The lymphatic spread of cancer to the opposite breast, to lymph nodes in the base of the neck, and to the abdominal cavity is caused by obstruction of the normal lymphatic pathways or destruction of lymphatic vessels by surgery or radiotherapy (see Figure 32-11). The less common inner quadrant tumors may spread to mediastinal nodes or Rotter nodes, which are located between the pectoral muscles (see Figure 32-11). Internal mammary chain nodes also are common sites of metastasis. Metastases from the vertebral veins can involve the vertebrae, pelvic bones, ribs, and skull. The lungs, kidneys, liver, adrenal glands, ovaries, and pituitary gland are also sites of metastasis.

The first sign of breast cancer is usually a painless lump. Lumps caused by breast tumors do not have any classic characteristics. Other presenting signs include palpable nodes in the axilla, retraction of tissue (dimpling) (Figure 33-34), or bone pain caused by metastasis to the vertebrae. Table 33-12 summarizes the clinical manifestations of breast cancers. Manifestations vary according to the type of tumor and stage of disease.

EVALUATION AND TREATMENT Clinical breast examination, mammography, ultrasound, thermography, MRI, biopsy, hormone receptor assays, and gene expression profiling are used in evaluating breast alterations and cancer.

Treatment is based on the extent or stage of the cancer. The extent of the tumor at the primary site, the presence and extent of lymph node metastases, and the presence of distant metastases are all

FIGURE 33-34 Retraction of Nipple Caused by Carcinoma. (From del Regato JA et al: *Ackerman and del Regato's cancer: diagnosis, treatment, and prognosis,* ed 6, St Louis, 1985, Mosby.)

evaluated to determine the stage of disease. Treatment includes surgery, radiation, chemotherapy, hormone therapy, and biologic therapy.

✔ **QUICK CHECK 33-5**
1. What types of fibrocystic breast changes increase the risk of breast cancer?
2. What is the role of hormones and growth factors in the pathophysiology of breast cancer?
3. Why are reproductive factors, such as early menarche and late menopause, important for the pathogenesis of breast cancer?
4. Why is complete breast involution important for reducing risk of breast cancer?
5. Discuss the role of the microenvironment or stromal tissue on breast cancer development.

DID YOU UNDERSTAND?

Abnormalities of the Female Reproductive Tract

1. Normal development of the female reproductive tract requires absence of testosterone during embryonic and fetal life.
2. Alterations in the normal process include errors in cellular sensitivity to testosterone (androgen insensitivity) or failures of cell line migration resulting in changes in the structure of the reproductive organs.
3. Androgen insensitivity syndrome (AIS) is a disorder of hormone resistance characterized by a female phenotype in an individual with an XY karyotype or male genotype.
4. Other abnormalities of the uterus, cervix, and fallopian/uterine tubes have multifactorial origins, often the result of an interaction between genetic predisposition and environmental factors.

Alterations of Sexual Maturation

1. Sexual maturation, or puberty, is marked by the development of secondary sex characteristics, rapid growth and ultimately, the ability to reproduce. The normal range for the onset of puberty is now 8 to 13 years of age and can vary geographically.
2. Delayed puberty is the onset of sexual maturation after these ages; precocious puberty is the onset before these ages. Treatment depends on the cause.

Disorders of the Female Reproductive System

1. The female reproductive system can be altered by hormonal imbalances, infectious microorganisms, inflammation, structural abnormalities, and benign or malignant proliferative conditions.
2. Primary dysmenorrhea is painful menstruation not associated with pelvic disease. It results from excessive synthesis of prostaglandin $F_2\alpha$. Secondary dysmenorrhea results from endometriosis, pelvic adhesions, inflammatory disease, uterine fibroids, or adenomyosis.
3. Primary amenorrhea is the continued absence of menarche and menstrual function by 13 years of age without the development of secondary sex characteristics or by 15 years of age if these changes have occurred.
4. Secondary amenorrhea is the absence of menstruation for a time equivalent to 3 or more cycles in women who have previously menstruated. Secondary amenorrhea is associated with many disorders and physiologic conditions.
5. Dysfunctional uterine bleeding (DUB) is heavy or irregular bleeding in the absence of organic disease.
6. Polycystic ovary syndrome (PCOS) is a condition in which excessive androgen production is triggered by inappropriate secretion of gonadotropins. This hormonal imbalance prevents ovulation and causes enlargement and cyst formation in the ovaries, excessive endometrial proliferation, and often hirsutism. Insulin resistance and hyperinsulinemia plays a key role in androgen excess.
7. Premenstrual syndrome (PMS) is the cyclic recurrence of physical, psychologic, or behavioral changes distressing enough to disrupt normal activities or interpersonal relationships. Emotional symptoms, particularly depression, anger, irritability, and fatigue, are reported as the most distressing symptoms; physical symptoms tend to be less problematic. Treatment is symptomatic and includes stress reduction, exercise, biofeedback, lifestyle changes, counseling, and medication.
8. Infection and inflammation of the female genitalia can result from microorganisms that are present in the environment often sexually transmitted or from overproliferation of microorganisms that normally populate the genital tract.
9. Pelvic inflammatory disease (PID) is an acute inflammatory process caused by infection. Many infections are sexually transmitted and microorganisms that comprise the vaginal flora are implicated. PID is a substantial health risk to women and untreated PID can lead to infertility.
10. Vaginitis is irritation or inflammation of the vagina, typically caused by infection. It is usually caused by sexually transmitted pathogens or *Candida albicans,* which causes candidiasis.
11. Cervicitis, which is infection of the cervix, can be acute (mucopurulent cervicitis) or chronic. Its most common cause is a sexually transmitted pathogen.
12. Vulvodyniavestibulitis (VV) is chronic vulvar pain lasting 3 months or longer. The cause of VV is unknown and theories include embryonic factors, chronic inflammation, genetic immune factors, nerve pathways, increased sensitivity to environmental factors, HPV, and hormonal changes.
13. Bartholinitis, also called Bartholin cyst, is an infection of the ducts that lead from the Bartholin glands to the surface of the vulva. Infection blocks the glands, preventing the outflow of glandular secretions.
14. The pelvic relaxation disorders—uterine displacement, uterine prolapse, cystocele, rectocele, and urethrocele—are caused by the relaxation of muscles and fascial supports, usually a result of advancing age or following childbirth or other trauma, and are more likely to occur in women with a familial or genetic predisposition.
15. Benign ovarian cysts develop from mature ovarian follicles that do not release their ova (follicular cysts) or from a corpus luteum that persists abnormally instead of degenerating (corpus luteum cyst). Cysts usually regress spontaneously.
16. Endometrial polyps consist of benign overgrowths of endometrial tissue and often cause abnormal bleeding in the premenopausal woman.
17. Leiomyomas, also called *myomas* or *uterine fibroids,* are benign tumors arising from the smooth muscle layer of the uterus, the myometrium.
18. Adenomyosis is the presence of endometrial glands and stroma within the uterine myometrium.
19. Endometriosis is the presence of functional endometrial tissue (i.e., tissue that responds to hormonal stimulation) at sites outside the uterus. Endometriosis causes an inflammatory reaction at the site of implantation and is a cause of infertility. Emerging is the relationship between endometriosis and ovarian cancer.
20. Cancers of the female genitalia involve the uterus (particularly the endometrium), the cervix, and the ovaries. Cancer of the vagina is rare.
21. Cervical cancer arises from the cervical epithelium and is triggered by human papillomavirus (HPV). The cellular transformational zone is called the squamocolumnar junction. The progressively serious neoplastic alterations are cervical intraepithelial neoplasia (cervical dysplasia), cervical carcinoma in situ, and invasive cervical carcinoma. Cocarcinogens include immune responses, hormonal responses, and other environmental factors that determine regression or persistence of the HPV infection.
22. Primary cancer of the vagina is rare. Risk factors include 60 or older, DES, HPV type 16, HIV, genital warts, and the relationship of developing precancerous cell changes called vaginal intraepithelial neoplasia (VAIN) is controversial.

23. Risk factors for vulvar cancer include HPV type 16 (cause), HIV, HPV-18 (probable cause), increasing age, previous cancer (untreated high-grade vulvar intraepithelial neoplasia [VIN]), cervical cancer survivor, previous cervical intraepithelial neoplasia, certain autoimmune conditions, organ transplant recipients (perhaps because of immunosuppression to clear HPV), and tobacco use (may relate to inability to clear HPV infection).

24. Carcinoma of the endometrium is the most common type of uterine cancer and most prevalent gynecologic malignancy. Primary risk factors for endometrial cancer include exposure to unopposed estrogen (e.g. estrogen-only hormone replacement therapy, tamoxifen, early menarche, late menopause, nulliparity, failure to ovulate), chronic hyperinsulinemia, hyperglycemia, body fatness and adult weight gain, chronic inflammation, lack of physical exercise.

25. Risk factors for ovarian cancer include advancing age, genetic factors, family history, overweight and obesity, height, reproductive/hormonal factors, HRT, endometriosis, diabetes, previous cancer, smoking, asbestos, talc-based powder, and ionizing radiation. Ovarian cancer causes more deaths than any other genital cancer in women.

26. The biology of ovarian cancer is changing and ovarian cancer is heterogeneous.

Sexual Dysfunction

1. Sexual dysfunction is the lack of satisfaction with sexual function resulting from pain or a deficiency in sexual desire, arousal, or orgasm/climax.

2. Sexual function and dysfunction result from a complex set of personal and biologic factors that interact with culture. Both organic and psychosocial disorders can be implicated in sexual dysfunction.

Impaired Fertility

1. Infertility, or the inability to conceive after 1 year of unprotected intercourse, affects approximately 15% of all couples. Fertility can be impaired by factors in the male, female, or both partners.

2. Female infertility results from dysfunction of the normal reproductive process: menses and ovulation, fallopian tube function (transport of the egg to the uterus and as a site of fertilization), ovarian dysfunction, and implantation of the fertilized egg into a receptive endometrium.

Disorders of the Female Breast

1. Most disorders of the breast are disorders of the mammary gland—that is, the female breast.

2. Galactorrhea, or inappropriate lactation, is the persistent secretion of a milky substance by the breasts of a woman who is not in the postpartum state or nursing an infant. Its most common cause is nonpuerperal hyperprolactinemia—a rise in serum prolactin levels.

3. Benign breast conditions are numerous and involve both ducts and lobules. Benign epithelial lesions can be broadly classified according to their future risk of developing breast cancer as (1) nonproliferative breast lesions, (2) proliferative breast disease, and (3) atypical (atypia) hyperplasia.

4. Nonproliferative lesions include simple breast cysts, papillary apocrine change, and mild hyperplasia of the usual type.

5. Proliferative breast lesions without atypia are diverse and include usual ductal hyperplasia, intraductal papillomas, sclerosing adenosis, radial scar, and simple fibroadenoma.

6. Proliferative breast lesions with atypia include atypical ductal hyperplasia (ADH) and atypical lobular hyperplasia (ALH).

7. Ductal carcinoma in situ (DCIS) refers to a heterogeneous group of proliferations limited to breast ducts and lobules without invasion of the basement membrane, Lobular carcinoma in situ (LCIS) originates from the duct lobular unit.

8. Breast cancer is the most common form of cancer in women and second to lung cancer as the most common cause of cancer death. However, controversial is the inclusion of DCIS with invasive breast cancer statistics. Breast cancer is a heterogeneous disease with diverse molecular, phenotypic, and pathologic changes.

9. The major risk factors for breast cancer are reproductive factors, such as nulliparity; hormonal factors and growth factors, such as excessive estradiol and IGF-1; familial factors, such as a family history of breast cancer; and environmental factors, such as ionizing radiation. Two factors emerging as important are delayed involution of the mammary gland and breast density. Physical activity and lack of postmenopausal weight gain may be risk-reducing factors.

10. A dominating movement in the field of cancer research is that epithelial function depends on the *entire* tissue including the stroma or microenvironment. Breast cancer is now known as a tissue-based disease with a possible abnormal, aberrant wound healing and inflammatory stromal (reactive stroma) component.

11. Models of breast carcinogenesis include three interrelated themes: gene addiction, phenotype plasticity, and cancer stem cells. The exact molecular events leading to breast cancer invasion are complex and not completely understood. These events involve genetic and epigenetic alterations and cancer cell and stromal interactions. New concepts for breast cancer metastases include tumor dormancy and vascular mimicry.

12. Most breast cancers arise from the ductal epithelium and then may metastasize to the lymphatics, opposite breast, abdominal cavity, lungs, bones, kidneys, liver, adrenal glands, ovaries, and pituitary glands.

13. The first clinical manifestation of breast cancer is usually a small, painless lump in the breast. Other manifestations include palpable lymph nodes in the axilla, dimpling of the skin, nipple and skin retraction, nipple discharge, ulcerations, reddened skin, and bone pain associated with bony metastases.

◼ KEY TERMS

Adenomyosis, 818
Amenorrhea, 805
Androgen insensitivity syndrome (AIS), 802
Anorgasmia (orgasmic dysfunction), 829
Atypia, 831

Atypical ductal hyperplasia (ADH), 832
Atypical hyperplasia (AH), 832
Atypical lobular hyperplasia (ALH), 832
Bartholinitis (Bartholin cyst), 813

Benign breast disease (BBD), 831
Carcinoma in situ, 842
Cervicitis, 812
Complete precocious puberty, 804
Corpus luteum cyst, 816
Cyst, 831

Cystocele, 814
Delayed puberty, 804
Dermoid cyst, 816
Diffuse papillomatosis, 831
Disorder of desire (hypoactive sexual desire, decreased libido), 829

REFERENCES

1. Greil AL et al: Variation in distress among women with infertility: evidence from a population-based sample, *Hum Reprod* 26(8):2101-2112, 2011.
2. Geffner ME: Androgen insensitivity syndrome (AIS). In Shahram Yazdano MD et al, editors: *Chronic complex diseases of childhood: a practical guide for clinicians*, Boca Raton, Fla, 2011, Universal Publishers.
3. Hughes IA et al: Androgen insensitivity syndrome, *Lancet* 380(9851):1419-1428, 2012.
4. Eisermann K et al: Androgen receptor gene mutation, rearrangement, polymorphism, *Transl Androl Urol* 2(3):137-147, 2013.
5. Galani A et al: Androgen insensitivity syndrome: clinical features and molecular defects, *Hormones (Athens)* 7(3):217-299, 2008.
6. Reichman DE, Laufer MR: Congenital uterine anomalies affecting reproduction, *Best Pract Res Clin Obstet Gynaecol* 24(2):193-208, 2010.
7. Chan YY et al: The prevalence of congenital uterine anomalies in unselected and high-risk populations: a systematic review, *Hum Reprod Update* 17(6):761-771, 2011.
8. Lomniczi A et al: Epigenetic control of female puberty, *Nat Neurosci* 16:281-289, 2013.
9. Rzeczkowska PA et al: Epigenetics: a new player in the regulation of mammalian puberty, *Neuroendocrinol* 99:139-155, 2014.
10. Bordini B, Rosenfield RL: Normal pubertal development: part II: clinical aspects of puberty, *Pediatr Rev* 32(7):281-292, 2011.
11. Farooqi IS, O'Rahilly S: 20 years of leptin: human disorders of leptin action, *J Endocrinol* 223(1):T63-T70, 2014.
12. Addo OY et al: Age at hormonal onset of puberty based on luteinizing hormone, inhibin B, and body composition in preadolescent US girls, *Pediatr Res* 76(6):564-570, 2014.
13. Hagen CP et al: Pubertal onset in girls is strongly influenced by genetic variation affecting FSH action, *Sci Rep* 4:6412, 2014.
14. Neeley EK, Crossen SS: Precocious puberty, *Curr Opin Obstet Gynecol* 26(5):332-338, 2014.
15. Baker ME, Hardiman G: Transcriptional analysis of endocrine disruption using zebrafish and massively parallel sequencing, *J Mol Endocrinol* 52(3):R241-R256, 2014.
16. Toppari J, Juul A: Trends in puberty timing in humans and environmental modifiers, *Mol Cell Endocrinol* 324(1-2):39-44, 2010.

17. Fedorowicz Z et al: Beta2-adrenoceptor agonists for dysmenorrhoea, *Cochrane Database Syst Rev* (5):CD008585, 2012.
18. Rapkin A, Nathan L: Pelvic pain and dysmenorrhea. In Berek J, editor: *Berek & Novak's gynecology*, Philadelphia, 2012, Lippincott Williams & Wilkins.
19. Khan KS et al: How effective are non-drug, non-surgical treatments for primary dysmenorrhoea? *BMJ* 344:e3011, 2012.
20. Baker VL et al: Amenorrhea. In Berek J, editor: *Berek & Novak's gynecology*, Philadelphia, 2012, Lippincott Williams & Wilkins.
21. Pitkin J: Dysfunctional uterine bleeding, *Br Med J* 334(7603):1110-1111, 2007.
22. Munro MG: FIGO classification system (PALM-COEIN) for causes of abnormal uterine bleeding in nongravid women of reproductive age, *Int J Gynaecol Obstet* 113(1):3-13, 2011.
23. Azziz R et al: The Androgen Excess and PCOS Society criteria for the polycystic ovary syndrome: the complete task force reports, *Fertil Steril* 91(2):456-488, 2009.
24. Diamanti-Kandarakis E: Polycystic ovarian syndrome: pathophysiology, molecular aspects and clinical implications, *Exp Rev Mol Med* 10(2):e3, 2008.
25. Hartlage S et al: Criteria for premenstrual dysphoric disorder: secondary analyses of relevant data sets, *Arch Gen Psychiatry* 69(3):300, 2012.
26. Gordon JL et al: Ovarian hormone fluctuation, neurosteroids, and HPA axis dysregulation in perimenopausal depression: a novel heuristic model, *Am J Psychiatry* 172(3):227-236, 2015.
27. Berone-Johnson ER et al: Association of inflammation markers with menstrual symptom severity and premenstrual syndrome in young women, *Hum Reprod* 29(9):1987-1994, 2014.
28. Jarvis CI et al: Management strategies for premenstrual syndrome/premenstrual dysphoric disorder, *Ann Pharmacother* 42(7):967-978, 2008.
29. Majorbanks J et al: Selective serotonin reuptake inhibitors for premenstrual syndrome, *Cochrane Database Syst Rev* CD001396, 2013.
30. Centers for Disease Control and Prevention (CDC): *Sexually transmitted diseases (STDs)*, Atlanta, 2015, Author.
31. Kumar V et al: *Robbins & Cotran pathologic basis of disease*, ed 9, Philadelphia, 2015, Elsevier/Saunders.

32. Wiesenfeld HC et al: Subclinical pelvic inflammatory disease and infertility, *Obstet Gynecol* 120(1):37-43, 2012.
33. Bender N et al: Chlamydia infection, pelvic inflammatory disease, ectopic pregnancy and infertility: cross-national study, *Sex Transm Infect* 87(7):601-608, 2011.
34. Nyirjesy P et al: Alternative therapies in women with chronic vaginitis, *Obstet Gynecol* 117(4):856, 2011.
35. Ray A et al: Interventions for prevention and treatment of vulvovaginal candidiasis in women with HIV infection, *Cochrane Database Syst Rev* (8):CD008739, 2011.
36. De Seta F et al: *Lactobacillus plantarum P17630* for preventing *Candida* vaginitis recurrence: a retrospective comparative study, *Eur J Obstet Gynecol Reprod Biol* 182:136-139, 2014.
37. Centers for Disease Control and Prevention (CDC): *Diseases characterized by urethritis and cervicitis, STD sexually transmitted disease treatment guidelines*, Atlanta, 2014, Author.
38. Centers for Disease Control and Prevention (CDC): *STD treatment guidelines*, Atlanta, 2014, Author.
39. Shah M, Hoffstetter S: Vulvodynia, *Obstet Gynecol Clin North Am* 41:453-464, 2014.
40. Wesselmann U et al: Vulvodynia: current state of the biological science, *Pain* 155:1696-1701, 2014.
41. Sadownik LA: Etiology, diagnosis, and clinical management of vulvodynia, *Int J Womens Health* 6:437-449, 2014.
42. Cartwright R et al: Systematic review and metaanalysis of genetic association studies of urinary symptoms and prolapse in women, *Am J Obstet Gynecol* 212(2):199, e1-e14, 2014.
43. Hoffman BL: Pelvic mass. In Schorge JO et al: *Williams gynecology*, pp 187-224, New York, 2008, McGraw-Hill.
44. Mäkinen N et al: MED12, the mediator complex subunit 12 gene, is mutated at high frequency in uterine leiomyomas, *Science* 334:252-255, 2011.
45. Gupta JK et al: Uterine artery embolization for symptomatic uterine fibroids, *Cochrane Database Syst Rev* (12):CD005073, 2014.
46. Forte A et al: Genetic, epigenetic and stem cell alterations in endometriosis: new insights and potential therapeutic perspectives, *Clin Sci* 126:123-138, 2014.
47. Giudice LC: Endometriosis, *N Engl J Med* 362(25):2389-2398, 2010.

48. American Cancer Society: *Cancer facts & figures—2015*, Atlanta, 2015, Author.
49. Ferlay J et al: *GLOBOCAN 2012 v1.0, Cancer incidence and mortality worldwide: IARC CancerBase No. 11*, Lyon, France, 2013, International Agency for Research on Cancer. Available from: http://globocan.iarc.fr.
50. Centers for Disease Control and Prevention (CDC): *Cervical cancer statistics*, Atlanta, Author, updated September 2014.
51. National Cancer Institute (NCI): *PDQ® cervical cancer screening*, Bethesda, Md, 2015, Author. Date last modified February 15, 2015. Available at: http://cancer.gov/cancertopics/pdq/screening/cervical/HealthProfessional. Accessed February 19, 2015.
52. National Cancer Institute (NCI): *PDQ® cervical cancer treatment*, Bethesda, Md, 2015, Author. Date last modified January 9, 2015. Available at: http://cancer.gov/cancertopics/pdq/treatment/cervical/HealthProfessional. Accessed February 19, 2015.
53. Blomberg M et al: Genital warts and risk of cancer: a Danish study of nearly 50,000 patients with genital warts, *J Infect Dis* 205(10):1544-1553, 2012.
54. Cancer Research UK: *Risks and causes of vaginal cancer*, London, Author. Updated October 14, 2013.
55. National Cancer Institute: *PDQ® vaginal cancer treatment*, Bethesda, Md, 2015, Author. Date last modified February 26, 2015. Available at: http://cancer.gov/cancertopics/pdq/treatment/vaginal/HealthProfessional. Accessed April 26, 2015.
56. National Cancer Institute (NCI): *PDQ® vulvar cancer treatment*, Bethesda, Md, 2015, Author. Date last modified July 23, 2014. Available at: http://cancer.gov/cancertopics/pdq/treatment/vulvar/Patient. Accessed April 22, 2015.
57. Cancer Research UK: *Vulval cancer risk factors*, London, Author. Updated July 1, 2015.
58. National Cancer Institute: *PDQ® vulvar cancer treatment*, Bethesda, Md, 2015, Author. Date last modified April 10, 2015. Available at: http://cancer.gov/cancertopics/pdq/treatment/vulvar/HealthProfessional. Accessed April 19, 2015.
59. Ferlay J et al: Cancer incidence and mortality worldwide: sources, methods and major patterns in GLOBOCAN 2012, *Int J Cancer* 136:E359-E386, 2015.
60. National Cancer Institute (NCI): *A snapshot of endometrial cancer*, Bethesda, Md, 2014, National Cancer Institute, National Institutes of Health. Updated November 5, 2014. Accessed April 26, 2015.
61. World Cancer Research Fund/American Institute for Cancer Research: *Continuous update project report. Food, nutrition, physical activity, and the prevention of endometrial cancer*, 2013. Available at: www.dietandcancerreport.org.
62. Campbell PT et al: Diabetes and cause-specific mortality in a prospective cohort of one million U.S. adults, *Diabetes Care* 35(9):1835-1844, 2012.
63. Chen H-F et al: Risks of breast and endometrial cancer in women with diabetes: a population-based cohort study, *PLoS One* 8(6):e67420, 2013.
64. Joung KH et al: The association between type 2 diabetes mellitus and women cancer: the epidemiological evidences and putative mechanisms, *Biomed Res Int* 2015:920610, 2015.
65. Gottschau M et al: Risk of cancer among women with polycystic ovary syndrome: a Danish cohort study, *Gynecol Oncol* 136(1):99-103, 2015.
66. Yoneyama K et al: miR-200a, miR-200b and miR-429 are onco-miRs that target the PTEN gene in endometrioid endometrial carcinoma, *Anticancer Res* 35(3):1401-1410, 2015.
67. Jaakkola S et al: Endometrial cancer associated with various forms of postmenopausal hormone therapy: a case control study, *Int J Cancer* 128(7):1644-1651, 2011.
68. SGO Clinical Practice Endometrial Cancer Working Group et al: Endometrial cancer: a review and current management strategies: part II, *Gynecol Oncol* 134(2):393-402, 2014.
69. Allen NE et al: Menopausal hormone therapy and risk of endometrial carcinoma among postmenopausal women in the European Prospective Investigation into cancer and nutrition, *Am J Epidemiol* 172(12):1394-1403, 2010.
70. Formoso G et al: Short- and long-term effects of tibolone in postmenopausal women, *Cochrane Database Syst Rev* CD008536, 2012.
71. Yurgelun MB et al: Impact of genetic testing on endometrial cancer risk-reducing practices in women at risk for Lynch syndrome, *Gynecol Oncol* 127(3):544-551, 2012.
72. Riboli E et al: European Prospective Investigation into Cancer and Nutrition (EPIC): study populations and data collection, *Public Health Nutr* 5(6B):1113-1124, 2002.
73. Merritt MA et al: Investigation of dietary factors and endometrial cancer risk using a nutrient-wide association study approach in the EPIC and Nurses' Health Study (NHS) and NHSII, *Cancer Epidemiol Biomarkers Prev* 24(2):466-471, 2015.
74. Diep C et al: Progesterone action in breast, uterine, and ovarian cancers, *J Mol Endocrinol* 54(2):R31-R53, 2015.
75. Banno K et al: Drug repositioning for gynecologic tumors: a new therapeutic strategy for cancer, *ScientificWorldJournal* 2015:341362, 2015.
76. Stine JE, Bae-Jump V: Metformin and gynecologic cancers, *Obstet Gynecol Surv* 69(8):477-489, 2014.
77. Desai A et al: Epithelial ovarian cancer: an overview, *World Transl Med* 3(1):1-8, 2014.
78. Romero I, Bast RC: Minireview: human ovarian cancer biology, current management, and paths to personalizing therapy, *Endocrinology* 153(4):1593-1602, 2012.
79. Nik NN et al: Origin and pathogenesis of pelvic (ovarian, tubal, and primary peritoneal) serous carcinoma, *Annu Rev Pathol* 9:27-45, 2014.
80. National Cancer Institute: *PDQ® ovarian, fallopian tube, and primary peritoneal cancer screening*, Bethesda, Md, 2015, Author. Date last modified March 3, 2015. Available at: www.cancer.gov/types/ovarian/hp/ovarian-screening-pdq. Accessed June 12, 2015.
81. U.S. Preventive Services Task Force: Screening for ovarian cancer: U.S. Preventive Services Task Force reaffirmation recommendation statement, *Ann Intern Med* 157(12):900-904, 2012.
82. Giede KC et al: Who should operate on patients with ovarian cancer? An evidence-based review, *Gynecol Oncol* 99(2):447-461, 2005.
83. Mercado C et al: Quality of care in advanced ovarian cancer: the importance of provider specialty, *Gynecol Oncol* 117(1):18-22, 2010.
84. American College of Obstetricians and Gynecologists (ACOG): *Female sexual dysfunction*, Washington, DC, 2011, Author.
85. Hatzichristou D et al: Recommendations for the clinical evaluation of men and women with sexual dysfunction, *J Sex Med* 7(1 pt 2):337-348, 2010.
86. Lewis RW et al: Definitions/epidemiology/risk factors for sexual dysfunction, *J Sex Med* 7(4 pt 2):1598-1607, 2010.
87. Kingsberg SA, Woodard T: Female sexual dysfunction: focus on low desire, *Obstet Gynecol* 125(2):477-486, 2015.
88. Timeva T et al: Recurrent implantation failure: the role of the endometrium, *J Reprod Infertil* 15(4):173-183, 2014.
89. Marshburn PB: Counseling and diagnostic evaluation for the infertile couple, *Obstet Gynecol Clin North Am* 42(1):1-14, 2015.
90. Farquhar C et al: Assisted reproductive technology: an overview of Cochrane reviews, *Cochrane Database Syst Rev* (12):CD010537, 2014.
91. Sabel MS: *Overview of benign breast disease*, 2015. Available at: UpToDate Individual Web www.uptodate.com. Accessed May 12, 2015.
92. Lester S: The breast. In Kumar V et al, editors: *Robbins & Cotran pathologic basis of disease*, ed 9, Philadelphia, 2015, Elsevier Saunders.
93. Visscher DW et al: Sclerosing adenosis and risk of breast cancer, *Breast Cancer Res Treat* 144(1):205-212, 2014.
94. Nasser A et al: Ki-67 expression in sclerosing adenosis and adjacent normal breast terminal ductal lobular units: a nested case-control study from the Mayo Benign Breast Disease Cohort, *Breast Cancer Res Treat* 151(1):89-97, 2015.
95. Hartmann LC et al: Atypical hyperplasia of the breast—risk assessment and management options, *N Engl J Med* 372(13):1271-1272, 2015.
96. Dupont WD, Page DL: Risk factors for breast cancer in women with proliferative breast disease, *N Engl J Med* 312:146-151, 1985.
97. Hartmann LC et al: Benign breast disease and the risk of breast cancer, *N Engl J Med* 353:229-237, 2005.
98. Hartmann LC et al: Understanding the premalignant potential of atypical hyperplasia through its natural history: a longitudinal cohort study, *Cancer Prev Res (Phila)* 7:211-217, 2014.
99. Page DL et al: Atypical hyperplastic lesions of the female breast. A long-term follow-up study, *Cancer* 55:2698-2708, 1985.
100. Sanders M et al: Continued observation of the natural history of low-grade ductal carcinoma in situ reaffirms proclivity for local recurrence even after more than 30 years of follow-up, *Mod Pathol* 28(5):662-669, 2015.
101. Page DL et al: Atypical lobular hyperplasia as a unilateral predictor of breast cancer risk: a retrospective cohort study, *Lancet* 361(9352):125-129, 2003 [Erratum: *Lancet* 361(9373), 1994.]
102. Elmore JG et al: Diagnostic concordance among pathologists interpreting breast biopsy specimens, *J Am Med Assoc* 313(11):1122-1132, 2015.
103. Hollowell JG et al: Iodine nutrition in the United States. Trends and public health implications: iodine excretion data from National Health and Nutrition Examination Surveys I and II (1971-1974 and 1988-1994), *J Clin Endocrinol Metab* 83(10):3401-3408, 1998.
104. Li Y et al: Genistein depletes telomerase activity through cross-talk between genetic and epigenetic mechanism, *Int J Cancer* 125(2):286-296, 2009.
105. Islam MA et al: Deconjugation of soy isoflavone glucuronides needed for estrogenic activity, *Toxicol In Vitro* 29(4):706-715, 2015.
106. North American Menopause Society (NAMS): The role of soy isoflavones in menopausal health: report of The North American Menopause Society/Wulf H. Utian Translational Science Symposium in Chicago, IL, *Menopause* 18(7):732-753, 2011.
107. Iodine monograph, *Altern Med Rev* 15(3):273-278, 2010.
108. Sternlicht MD et al: Hormonal and local control of mammary branching morphogenesis, *Differentiation* 74:365-381, 2006.
109. Lyons TR et al: Postpartum mammary gland involution drives progression of ductal carcinoma in situ through collagen and COX-2, *Nat Med* 17:1109-1115, 2011.
110. Lyons TR et al: Pregnancy and breast cancer: when they collide, *J Mammary Gland Biol Neoplasia* 14:87-98, 2009.
111. Albrektsen G et al: The short-term and long-term effect of pregnancy on breast cancer risk: a prospective study of 802,457 parous Noregian women, *Br J Cancer* 72(2):480-484, 1995.
112. Callihan EB et al: Postpartum diagnosis demonstrates a high risk for metastasis and merits an expanded definition of pregnancy-associated breast cancer, *Breast Cancer Res Treat* 138:549-559, 2013.
113. Johansson AL et al: Increased mortality in women with breast cancer detected during pregnancy and different periods postpartum, *Cancer Epidemiol Biomarkers Prev* 20(9):1865-1872, 2011.
114. Schedin P et al: Microenvironment of the involuting mammary gland mediates mammary cancer progression, *J Mammary Gland Biol Neoplasia* 12:71-82, 2007.

115. Martinson HA et al: Wound healing-like immune program facilitates postpartum mammary gland involution and tumor progression, *Int J Cancer* 136(8):1803-1813, 2015.

116. Barton M et al: Molecular pathways involved in pregnancy-induced prevention against breast cancer, *Front Endocrinol (Lausanne)* 5:213, 2014.

117. Khodr ZG et al: Circulating sex hormones and terminal duct lobular unit involution of the normal breast cancer, *Epidemiol Biomarkers Prev* 23(12):2765-2773, 2014.

118. Milanese TR et al: Age-related lobular involution and risk of breast cancer, *J Natl Cancer Inst* 98(2):1600-1607, 2006.

119. Jindal S et al: Postpartum breast involution reveals regression of secretory lobules mediated by tissue-remodeling, *Breast Cancer Res* 16(2):R31, 2014.

120. Vorrherr H, editor: *The breast: morphology, physiology, and lactation*, New York, 1974, Academic Press.

121. Geschickter CD: *Diseases of the breast*, ed 2, Philadelphia, 1945, Lippincott.

122. Trichopoulos D et al: Age at any birth and breast cancer risk, *Int J Cancer* 31:701-704, 1983.

123. Henson DE et al: Lobular involution: the physiologic prevention of breast cancer, *J Natl Cancer Inst* 98(22):1589-1590, 2006.

124. Zaragozá R et al: Involvement of different networks in mammary gland involution after the pregnancy/lactation cycle: implications in breast cancer, *IUBMB Life* 67(4):227-238, 2015.

125. Schedin P: Pregnancy-associated breast cancer and metastasis, *Nat Rev Cancer* 6:281-291, 2006.

126. Ghosh K et al: Independent association of lobular involution and mammographic breast density with breast cancer risk, *J Natl Cancer Inst* 102(22): 1716-1723, 2010.

127. Russo J, Russo I: *Molecular basis of breast cancer: prevention and treatment*, Berlin, Heidelberg, New York, 2004, Springer-Verlag.

128. Kaaks R et al: Postmenopausal serum androgens, oestrogens, and breast cancer risk: the European prospective investigation into cancer and nutrition, *Endocr Relat Cancer* 12(4):1017-1082, 2005.

129. Mehta J et al: A molecular analysis provides novel insights into androgen receptor signaling in breast cancer, *PLoS One* 10(3):e0120622, 2015.

130. Kotsopoulos J et al: The relationship between bilateral oophorectomy and plasma hormone levels in postmenopausal women, *Horm Cancer* 6(1):54-63, 2015.

131. Tworoger SS et al: Inclusion of endogenous hormone levels in risk prediction models of postmenopausal breast cancer, *J Clin Oncol* 32(28):3111-3117, 2014.

132. Hankinson SE, Eliassen H: Endogenous estrogen, testosterone, and progesterone levels in relation to breast cancer risk, *J Steroid Biochem Mol Biol* 106(1-5):24-30, 2007.

133. Key T et al: Endogenous sex hormones and breast cancer in postmenopausal women; reanalysis of nine prospective studies, *J Natl Cancer Inst* 94: 606-616, 2002.

134. Stanczyk FZ et al: Relationships of sex steroid hormone levels in benign and cancerous breast tissue and blood: a critical appraisal of current science, *Steroids* 99(Pt A):91-102, 2015.

135. World Health Organization: A review of human carcinogens. B. Biological agents IARC monographs on the evaluation of carcinogenic risks to humans, *IARC Monographs*, vol 100(B), Geneva, Switzerland, 2015, Author.

136. Grant MD et al: *Menopausal symptoms: comparative effectiveness of therapies*, Blue Cross and Blue Shield Association Technology Evaluation Center, Evidence-Based Practice Center, Rockville, Md, March 2015, Agency for Healthcare Research and Quality.

137. Christopoulos PF et al: The role of insulin-like growth factor-1 system in breast cancer, *Mol Cancer* 14(1):43, 2015.

138. Ahmadieh H, Azar ST: Type 2 diabetes oral diabetic medications, insulin therapy, and overall breast cancer risk, *ISRN Endocrinol* 2013: 181240, 2013.

139. Suissa S et al: Long-term effects of insulin glargine on the risk of breast cancer, *Diabetologia* 54(9):2254-2262, 2011.

140. Wu J et al: Light at night activates IGF-1R/PDK1 signaling and accelerates tumor growth in human breast cancer xenografts, *Cancer Res* 71(7): 2622-2631, 2011.

141. Akerstedt T et al: Night work and breast cancer in women: a Swedish cohort study, *Br Med J* 5(4):e008127, 2015.

142. Wang XS et al: Shift work and chronic disease: the epidemiological evidence, *Occup Med (Lond)* 61(2):78-89, 2011.

143. Renehen AG, Brennan BM: Acromegaly, growth hormone and cancer risk, *Best Pract Res Clin Endocrinol Metab* 22:639-657, 2008.

144. Schernhammer ES et al: Insulin-like growth factor-l, its binding protein (IGFBP-1 and IBFBP-3), and growth hormone and breast cancer risk in The Nurses Health Study II, *Endocr Relat Cancer* 13:583-592, 2006.

145. Tworoger SS et al: A prospective study of plasma prolactin concentrations and risk of premenopausal and postmenopausal breast cancer, *J Clin Oncol* 25:1482-1488, 2007.

146. Tikk K et al: Circulating prolactin and in situ breast cancer risk in the European EPIC cohort: a case-control study, *Breast Cancer Res* 17(1):49, 2015.

147. IARC Special Report: Policy: a review of human carcinogens—Part A: pharmaceuticals, *Lancet* 10:13-14, 2009.

148. Boyd NF et al: Mammographic breast density as an intermediate phenotype for breast cancer, *Lancet Oncol* 6(10):798-808, 2005.

149. Vachon CM: Mammographic density, breast cancer risk and risk prediction breast, *Cancer Res* 9(6):217, 2007.

150. Sun WY et al: Insulin-like growth factor 1 receptor expression in breast cancer tissue and mammographic density, *Mol Clin Oncol* 3(3): 572-580, 2015.

151. Boyd NF et al: Mammographic density and the risk and detection of breast cancer, *N Engl J Med* 56(3):227-236, 2007.

152. Pettersson A et al: Mammographic density phenotypes and risk of breast cancer: a meta-analysis, *J Natl Cancer Inst* 106(5), 2014.

153. Institute of Medicine of the National Academies: *Breast cancer and the environment: a life course approach*, Washington, DC, 2011, The National Academies Press.

154. National Cancer Institute: *Radiation risks and pediatric computed tomography (CT): a guide for health care providers*, 2002. Available at: www.cancer.gov. Accessed December 2012.

155. Ginsburg ON et al: Mammographic density, lobular involution, and risk of breast cancer, *Br J Cancer* 4(99):1369-1374, 2008.

156. Smith-Bindman R: Environmental causes of breast cancer and radiation from medical imaging, *Arch Intern Med* 172(13):1023-1027, 2012.

157. Brenner DJ, Hall EJ: Computed tomography—an increasing source of radiation exposure, *N Engl J Med* 357(22):2277-2284, 2007.

158. Schwab SA et al: X-ray induced formation of γ-H2AX foci after full-field digital mammography and digital breast tomosynthesis, *PLoS One* 8(7):e70660, 2013.

159. Colin C et al: DNA double-strand breaks induced by mammographic screening procedures in human mammary epithelial cells, *Int J Radiat Biol* 87(11):1103-1112, 2011.

160. Colin C, Foray N: DNA damage induced by mammography in high family risk patients: only one single view in screening, *The Breast* 21:409-410, 2012.

160A. Frankenberg-Schwager M et al: Chromosomal instability carriers, *Int J Radiat Biol* 88:846-857, 2012.

161. Pucci M et al: Caveolin-1, breast cancer and ionizing radiation, *Cancer GenomicsProteomics* 12(3):143-152, 2015.

162. Colin C et al: Update relevance of mammographic screening modalities in women previously treated with chest irradiation for Hodgkin disease, *Radiology* 265(3):669-676, 2012.

163. Ng J et al: Predicting the risk of secondary lung malignancies associated with whole-breast radiation therapy, *Int J Radiat Oncol* 83(4): 1101-1106, 2012.

164. Mourouti N et al: Diet and breast cancer, *Int J Food Sci Nutr* 66(1):1-42, 2015.

165. Demetriou CA et al: The Mediterreanean dietary pattern and breast cancer risk in Greek-Cypriot women: a case-control study, *BMC Cancer* 12:113, 2012.

166. Trinh T et al: Background risk of breast cancer influences the association between alcohol consumption and mammographic density, *Br J Can* 133(1):159-165, 2015.

167. Key TJ: Minireview: fruit and vegetables and cancer risk, *Br J Cancer* 104:6-11, 2011.

168. Nechuta SJ et al: Soy food intake after diagnosis of breast cancer and survival: an in-depth analysis of combined evidence from cohort studies of U.S. and Chinese women, *Am J Nutr* 96(1):123-132, 2012.

169. Aceves C et al: Is iodine a gatekeeper of the integrity of the mammary gland? *J Mammary Gland Biol Neoplasia* 10(2):189-196, 2005.

170. Cann SA et al: Hypothesis: iodine, selenium and the development of breast cancer, *Cancer Causes Control* 11:121-127, 2000.

171. Eskin BA et al: Different tissue responses for iodine and iodide in rat thyroid and mammary glands, *Biol Trace Elem Res* 49:9-19, 1995.

172. Ghent WR et al: Iodine replacement in fibrocystic disease of the breast, *Can J Surg* 36:453-460, 1993.

173. Funahashi H et al: Seaweed prevents breast cancer, *Jpn J Cancer Res* 92(5):483-487, 2001.

174. Smyth PP: Role of iodine in antioxidant defense in thyroid and breast disease, *Biofactors* 19(3-4): 121-130, 2003.

175. Byers T, Sedjo RL: Body fatness as a cause of cancer: epidemiologic clues to biologic mechanisms, *Endocr Relat Cancer* 22(3): R125-R134, 2015.

176. Michels KB et al: Adult weight change and incidence of premenopausal breast cancer, *Int J Cancer* 130(4):902-909, 2012.

177. Protani M et al: Effect of obesity on survival of women with breast cancer: systematic review and meta-analysis, *Breast Cancer Res Treat* 123(3): 627-635, 2010.

178. Vaino H, Bianchini F, editors: *IARC. International Agency for Research on Cancer. Weight control and physical activity*, Lyon, 2002, IARC Press.

179. World Cancer Research Fund (WCRF): *Food, nutrition, physical activity, and the prevention of cancer; a global perspective*, ed 2, Washington, DC, 2007, American Institute for Cancer Research.

180. Holmes MD, Willett WC: Does diet affect breast cancer risk? *Breast Cancer Res* 6(4):170-178, 2004.

181. Wenten M et al: Associations of weight, weight change, and body mass with breast cancer risk in Hispanic and non-Hispanic white women, *Ann Epidemiol* 12(6):435-444, 2002.

182. Trentham-Diaz A et al: Weight change and risk of postmenopausal breast cancer (United States), *Cancer Causes Control* 11(6):533-542, 2000.

183. Le Marchand L et al: Body size at different periods of life and breast cancer risk, *Am J Epidemiol* 128(1):137-152, 1998.

184. Morimoto LM et al: Obesity, body size, and risk of postmenopausal breast cancer: the Women's Health Initiative (United States), *Cancer Causes Control* 13(8):741-751, 2002.

185. Endogenous Hormones Breast Cancer Collaborative Group: Body mass index, serum sex hormones, and breast cancer risk in postmenopausal women, *J Natl Cancer Inst* 95(6):1218-1226, 2003.

186. Korner A et al: Total and high molecular weight adiponectin in breast cancer: in vitro and in vivo studies, *J Clin Endocrinol Metab* 92(3):1041-1048, 2007.

187. Surmacz E: Obesity hormone leptin: a new target in breast cancer? *Breast Cancer Res* 9(1):301, 2007.

188. Jarde T et al: Molecular mechanism of leptin and adiponectin in breast cancer, *Eur J Cancer* 47:33-43, 2011.

189. Andó S et al: The multifaceted mechanism of leptin signaling within tumor microenvironment in driving breast cancer growth and progression, *Front Oncol* 4:340, 2014.

190. Bennett LM, Davis BJ: Identification of mammary carcinogens in rodent bioassays, *Environ Mol Mutagen* 39(2-3):150-157, 2002.

191. Barrett JR: EDCs and estrogen receptor activity: a pathway to safer chemical design, *Environ Health Perspect* 122(12):A339, 2014.

192. Sprague BL et al: Lifetime recreational and occupational physical activity and risk of in situ and invasive breast cancer, *Cancer Epidemiol Biomarkers Prev* 16(2):236-243, 2007.

193. Kim J et al: The effects of physical activity on breast cancer survivors after diagnosis, *Cancer Prev* 18(3):193-200, 2013.

194. Stephens PJ et al: The landscape of cancer genes and mutational processes in breast cancer, *Nature* 486:400-404, 2012.

195. Wagenblast E et al: A model of breast cancer heterogeneity reveals vascular mimicry as a driver of metastasis, *Nature* 520:358-362, 2015.

196. National Cancer Institute: *PDQ® genetics of breast and gynecologic cancers*, Bethesda, Md, 2015, Author. Date last modified May 27, 2015. Available at: www.cancer.gov/types/breast/hp/breast-ovarian-genetics-pdq. Accessed June 3, 2015.

197. Marusyk A et al: Non-cell autonomous tumor-growth driving supports sub-clonal heterogeneity, *Nature* 514(7520):54-58, 2014.

198. Hanahan D, Weinberg R: Hallmarks of cancer: the next generation, *Cell* 144:646-674, 2011.

199. Damonte P et al: Mammary carcinoma behavior is programmed in the precancer stem cell, *Breast Cancer Res* 10(3):R50, 2008.

200. Janiszewska M, Polyak K: Clonal evolution in cancer: a tale of twisted twines, *Cell Stem Cell* 16(1):11-12, 2015.

201. Sorlie T et al: Gene expression patterns of breast carcinomas distinguish tumor subclasses with clinical implications, *Proc Natl Acad Sci U S A* 98:10869-10874, 2001.

202. Boudreau A et al: An "elite hacker:" breast tumors exploit the normal microenvironment program to instruct their progression and biological diversity, *Cell Adh Migr* 6(3):236-248, 2012.

203. Cardiff RD et al: Three interrelated themes in current breast cancer research: gene addiction, phenotypic plasticity, and cancer stem cells, *Breast Cancer Res* 13:216, 2011.

204. Craene DB, Berx G: Regulatory networks defining EMT during cancer initiation and progression, *Nat Rev Cancer* 13(2):97-110, 2013.

205. Chaffer CL, Weinberg RA: A perspective on cancer cell metastasis, *Science* 331(6024):1559-1564, 2011.

206. Inman JL et al: Mammary gland development: cell fates specification, stem cells and the microenvironment, *Development* 142(6):1028-1042, 2015.

207. Mani SA et al: The epithelial-mesenchymal transition generates cells with properties of stem cells, *Cell* 133:704-715, 2008.

208. Charafe-Jauffret E et al: Breast cancer cell lines contain functional cancer stem cells with metastatic capacity and a distinct molecular signature, *Cancer Res* 69(4):1302-1313, 2009.

209. Marcato P et al: Aldehyde dehydrogenase activity of breast cancer stem cells is primarily due to isoform ALDH1A3 and its expression is predictive of metastasis, *Stem Cell* 29(1):32-45, 2011.

210. Almog N: Genes and regulatory pathways involved in persistence of dormant micro-tumors. In Enderling H et al, editors: *System biology of tumor dormancy advances in experimental medicine and biology*, New York, 2013, Springer Science.

211. Enderling H et al, editors: *System biology of tumor dormancy advances in experimental medicine and biology*, New York, 2013, Springer Science.

212. Kim Y, Boushaba K: Regulation of tumor dormancy and role of microenvironment: a mathematical model. In Enderling H et al, editors: *System biology of tumor dormancy advances in experimental medicine and biology*, New York, 2013, Springer Science.

213. Kerlikowske K: Epidemiology of ductal carcinoma in situ, *J Natl Cancer Inst Monogr* 41:139-141, 2010.

214. Bombonati A, Sgroi DC: The molecular pathology of breast cancer progression, *J Pathol* 223:307-317, 2011.

215. National Cancer Institute (NCI): *PDQ® breast cancer screening*, Bethesda, Md, 2015, Author. Date last modified May 14, 2015. Available at: www.cancer.gov/types/breast/hp/breast-screening-pdq. Accessed June 6, 2015.

216. Siegel RL et al: Cancer statistics, 2015, *Ca Cancer J Clin* 65:5, 2015.

217. Miller AB et al: Canadian National Breast Screening Study: 2. Breast Cancer detection and death rates among women aged 50 to 59 years, *CMAJ* 147(10):1477-1488, 1992.

Alterations of the Male Reproductive System

George W. Rodway and Kathryn L. McCance

Alterations of the reproductive system span a wide range of concerns from delayed sexual development and suboptimal sexual performance to structural and functional abnormalities. Many common male reproductive disorders carry potentially serious physiologic or psychologic consequences. For example, sexual or reproductive dysfunction, such as impotence or infertility, can dramatically affect self-concept, relationships, and overall quality of life. Conversely, organic and psychosocial problems, such as alcoholism, depression, situational stressors, chronic illness, and medications, can affect sexual performance and may be risk factors for the development of some types of reproductive tract cancers. Aside from skin cancer, prostate cancer is the second leading cause of cancer deaths and is the most frequently diagnosed cancer in men. Incidence rates for prostate cancer changed substantially between the mid-1980s and mid-1990s and have since fluctuated widely from year to year, in large part reflecting changes in prostate cancer screening with the prostate-specific antigen (PSA) blood test.[1] Diagnosis and treatment of male reproductive system disorders are, like female reproductive system disorders, often complicated by the stigma and symbolism associated with the reproductive organs and emotion-laden beliefs and behaviors related to reproductive health. Treatment or diagnosis for any problem may be delayed because of embarrassment, guilt, fear, or denial.

ALTERATIONS OF SEXUAL MATURATION

The process of sexual maturation, or puberty, is marked by the development of secondary sex characteristics, rapid growth, and, ultimately, the ability to reproduce. A variety of congenital and endocrine disorders can disrupt the timing of puberty. Puberty that occurs too late (delayed puberty) or too early (precocious puberty) is caused by the inappropriate onset of sex hormone production. While the average age of pubertal onset appears to be decreasing for

girls, the age of pubertal onset has remained essentially unchanged for boys.

Delayed or Absent Puberty

About 3% of children living in North America experience delayed development of secondary sex characteristics.[2] Normally, boys tend to mature later than girls, around 14 to 14.5 years of age. In boys, the first sign of maturity is enlargement of testes and thinning of the scrotal skin. In delayed puberty, these secondary sex characteristics develop later.

In about 95% of cases, delayed puberty is a normal physiologic event. Hormonal levels are normal, the hypothalamic-pituitary-gonadal axis is intact, and maturation is slowly occurring. Treatment is seldom needed unless the delayed puberty is causing psychosocial problems.[3]

The other 5% of cases are caused by the disruption of the hypothalamic-pituitary-gonadal axis or by the outcomes of a systemic disease. Treatment depends on the cause (Box 34-1), and referral to a pediatric endocrinologist is necessary.[4]

Precocious Puberty

Precocious puberty is a rare event, affecting fewer than 1 in 50,000 boys. Precocious puberty for boys of all ethnic/racial groups is defined as sexual maturation occurring before age 9.[5] A recent study observed the mean ages of beginning male genital and pubic hair growth and early testicular volumes are leaning toward younger ages than earlier studies have suggested, although this seems to be dependent on race/ethnicity.[6] Precocious puberty may be caused by many conditions (Box 34-2), including lethal central nervous system tumors. All cases of precocious puberty require thorough evaluation.

All forms of precocious puberty are treated by identifying and removing the underlying cause or administering appropriate

BOX 34-1 Causes of Delayed Puberty

Hypergonadotropic Hypogonadism (Low Testosterone, Increased Follicle-Stimulating Hormone [FSH] and Luteinizing Hormone [LH])

1. Gonadal dysgenesis, most commonly Turner syndrome (45,X/46,XX; structural X or Y abnormalities, or mosaicism)
2. Klinefelter syndrome (47,XXY)
3. Bilateral gonadal failure
   a. Traumatic or infectious
   b. Postsurgical, postirradiation, or postchemotherapy
   c. Autoimmune
   d. Idiopathic empty-scrotum or vanishing-testes syndrome (congenital anorchia)

Hypogonadotropic Hypogonadism (Low Testosterone, Decreased LH, Depressed FSH)

1. Reversible
   a. Physiologic delay
   b. Weight loss/anorexia
   c. Strenuous exercise
   d. Severe obesity
   e. Illegal drug use, especially marijuana
   f. Primary hypothyroidism
   g. Congenital adrenal hyperplasia
   h. Cushing syndrome
   i. Prolactinomas
2. Irreversible
   a. Gonadotropin-releasing hormone (GnRH) deficiency (Kallmann syndrome) or idiopathic hypogonadotropic hypogonadism (IHH)
   b. Hypopituitarism
   c. Congenital central nervous system (CNS) defects
   d. Other pituitary adenomas
   e. Craniopharyngioma
   f. Malignant pituitary tumors

BOX 34-2 Primary Forms of Precocious Puberty

Complete Precocious Puberty

Premature development of appropriate characteristics for the child's gender
Hypothalamic-pituitary-ovarian axis functioning normally but prematurely
In about 10% of cases, lethal central nervous system tumor may be the cause

Partial Precocious Puberty

Partial development of appropriate secondary sex characteristics
Premature adrenarche (growth of axillary and pubic hair) tends to occur between 5 and 8 years of age
Can progress to complete precocious puberty; may be caused by estrogen-secreting neoplasms or may be a variant of normal pubertal development

Mixed Precocious Puberty

Causes the child to develop some secondary sex characteristics of the opposite gender
Common causes: adrenal hyperplasia or androgen-secreting tumors

Data from Burchett MLR et al: Endocrine and metabolic diseases. In Burns CE et al, editors: *Pediatric primary care,* St Louis, 2009, Saunders; Jospe N: Disorders of pubertal development. In Osborn LM et al, editors: *Pediatrics,* Philadelphia, 2005, Mosby.

hormones. In many cases, precocious puberty can be reversed. However, complete precocious puberty (development consistent with the gender of the individual) is difficult to treat and can cause long bones to stop growing before the child has reached normal height.

> **✓ QUICK CHECK 34-1**
> 1. Why does puberty occur too late or too early in some individuals?
> 2. Why do all forms of precocious puberty require evaluation?

DISORDERS OF THE MALE REPRODUCTIVE SYSTEM

Disorders of the Urethra

Urethritis and urethral strictures are common disorders of the male urethra. Urethral carcinoma, an extremely rare form of cancer, can occur in men older than 60 years.

Urethritis

Urethritis is an inflammatory process that is usually, but not always, caused by a sexually transmitted microorganism. Infectious urethritis caused by *Neisseria gonorrhoeae* is often called *gonococcal urethritis (GU);* urethritis caused by other microorganisms is called *nongonococcal urethritis (NGU).* Nonsexual origins of urethritis include inflammation or infection as a result of urologic procedures, insertion of foreign bodies into the urethra, anatomic abnormalities, or trauma.

Noninfectious urethritis is rare and is associated with the ingestion of wood or ethyl alcohol or turpentine. It is also seen with reactive arthritis.[7]

Symptoms of urethritis include urethral tingling or itching or a burning sensation, and frequency and urgency with urination. The individual may note a purulent or clear mucous-like discharge from the urethra. Nucleic acid detection amplification tests allow early detection of *N. gonorrhoeae* and *Chlamydia trachomatis* in urine studies.[8] Treatment consists of appropriate antibiotic therapy for infectious urethritis and avoidance of future exposure or mechanical irritation.

Urethral Strictures

A urethral stricture is a narrowing of the urethra caused by scarring. The scars may be congenital but can be present at any age and have a wide range of etiologic factors, including untreated urethral infection, trauma, and urologic instrumentation. Infections also can occur from long-term use of indwelling catheters. Prostatitis and infection secondary to urinary stasis are common complications. Severe and prolonged obstruction can result in hydronephrosis and renal failure.

The clinical manifestations of urethral stricture are caused by bladder outlet obstruction. Urethral stricture often manifests itself as lower urinary tract symptoms or urinary tract infections with significant impairment in the quality of life. The primary symptom is diminished force and caliber of the urinary system; other symptoms include urinary frequency and hesitancy, mild dysuria, double urinary stream or spraying, and dribbling after voiding. Urethral stricture is diagnosed on the basis of history, physical examination, flow rates, and cystoscopy. Treatment is usually surgical and may involve urethral dilation, urethrotomy, or a variety of open surgical techniques. The choice of surgical intervention depends on the age of the individual and the severity of the problem.

Disorders of the Penis
Phimosis and Paraphimosis

Phimosis and paraphimosis are both disorders in which the foreskin (prepuce) is "too tight" to move easily over the glans penis. Phimosis

FIGURE 34-1 Phimosis and Paraphimosis. A, Phimosis: the foreskin has a narrow opening that is not large enough to permit retraction over the glans. **B,** Lesions on the prepuce secondary to infection cause swelling, and retraction of foreskin may be impossible. Circumcision is usually required. **C,** Paraphimosis: the foreskin is retracted over the glans but cannot be reduced to its normal position. Here it has formed a constricting band around the penis. **D,** Ulcer on the retracted prepuce with edema. (**A** and **C** from Monahan FD et al: *Phipps' medical-surgical nursing: health and illness perspectives,* ed 8, St Louis, 2007, Mosby; **B** from Taylor PK: *Diagnostic picture tests in sexually transmitted diseases,* St Louis, 1995, Mosby; **D** from Morse SA et al: *Atlas of sexually transmitted diseases and AIDS,* ed 4, London, 2011, Saunders.)

is a condition in which the foreskin cannot be retracted back over the glans, whereas paraphimosis is the opposite: the foreskin is retracted and cannot be moved forward (reduced) to cover the glans (Figure 34-1). Both conditions can cause penile pathologic conditions.

The inability to retract the foreskin is normal in infancy and is caused by congenital adhesions. During the first 3 years of life, congenital adhesions (between the foreskin and glans) separate naturally with penile erections and are not an indication for circumcision. Phimosis can occur at any age and is most commonly caused by poor hygiene and chronic infection.[9] It rarely occurs with normal foreskin.

Reasons for seeking treatment include edema, erythema, and tenderness of the prepuce and purulent discharge; inability to retract the foreskin is a less common complaint. Circumcision, if needed, is performed after infection has been eradicated. Complications of phimosis include inflammation of the glans (balanitis) or prepuce (posthitis) and paraphimosis. There is a higher incidence of penile carcinoma in uncircumcised males, but chronic infection and poor hygiene are usually the underlying factors in such cases. Approximately 40% to 63% of invasive penile carcinomas are attributable to human papillomavirus (HPV).[10,11]

Paraphimosis, in which the foreskin is retracted, can constrict the penis, causing edema of the glans. If the foreskin cannot be reduced manually, surgery must be performed to prevent necrosis of the glans

caused by constricted blood vessels. Severe paraphimosis is a surgical emergency.

Peyronie Disease

Peyronie disease ("bent nail syndrome") is a fibrotic condition that causes lateral curvature of the penis during erection (Figure 34-2). Peyronie disease develops slowly and is characterized by tough fibrous thickening of the fascia in the erectile tissue of the corpora cavernosa. A dense, fibrous plaque is usually palpable on the dorsum of the penile shaft. The problem usually affects middle-aged men and is associated with painful erection, painful intercourse (for both partners), and poor erection distal to the involved area.[12] In some cases, impotence or unsatisfactory penetration occurs. When the penis is flaccid, there is no pain.

A local vasculitis-like inflammatory reaction occurs, and decreased tissue oxygenation results in fibrosis and calcification. The exact cause is unknown. Peyronie disease is associated with Dupuytren contracture (a flexion deformity of the fingers or toes caused by shortening or fibrosis of the palmar or plantar fascia), diabetes, tendency to develop keloids, and, in rare cases, use of beta-blocker medications.[9]

There is no definitive treatment for Peyronie disease; however, treatment can include pharmacologic agents and surgery. Spontaneous remissions occur in as many as 50% of individuals. However, men

FIGURE 34-2 Peyronie Disease. This person complained of pain and deviation of his penis to one side on erection. (From Taylor PK: *Diagnostic picture tests in sexually transmitted diseases*, London, 1995, Mosby.)

FIGURE 34-3 Priapism. (From Lloyd-Davies RW et al: *Color atlas of urology*, ed 2, London, 1994, Wolfe Medical.)

suffering with Peyronie disease and who have significant penile deformity precluding successful coitus should be appraised for surgical correction.[9]

Priapism

Priapism is an uncommon condition of prolonged penile erection. It is usually painful and is not associated with sexual arousal (Figure 34-3). Priapism is idiopathic in 60% of cases; the remaining 40% of cases can be associated with spinal cord trauma, sickle cell disease, leukemia, pelvic tumors, infections, or penile trauma.

Priapism must be considered a urologic emergency. Treatment within hours is effective and prevents impotence. Conservative approaches include iced saline enemas, ketamine administration, and spinal anesthesia. Needle aspiration of blood from the corpus through the dorsal glans is often effective and is followed by catheterization and pressure dressings to maintain decompression. More

FIGURE 34-4 Balanitis. (From Taylor PK: *Diagnostic picture tests in sexually transmitted diseases*, London, 1995, Mosby.)

aggressive surgical treatments include the creation of vascular shunts to maintain blood flow. Erectile dysfunction results in up to 50% of prolonged cases.

Balanitis

Balanitis is an inflammation of the glans penis (Figure 34-4) and usually occurs in conjunction with posthitis, an inflammation of the prepuce. (Inflammation of the glans and the prepuce is called *balanoposthitis*.) It is associated with poor hygiene and phimosis. The accumulation under the foreskin of glandular secretions (smegma), sloughed epithelial cells, and *Mycobacterium smegmatis* can irritate the glans directly or lead to infection. Skin disorders (e.g., psoriasis, lichen planus, eczema) and candidiasis must be differentiated from inflammation resulting from poor hygienic practices. Balanitis is most commonly seen in men with poorly controlled diabetes mellitus and candidiasis. The infection is treated with antimicrobials. After the inflammation has subsided, circumcision can be considered to prevent recurrences.

Tumors of the Penis

Tumors of the penis are not common. The most frequent are the benign epithelial tumor condyloma acuminatum and penile carcinomas.

Condyloma acuminatum is a benign tumor caused by human papillomavirus (HPV), a sexually transmitted infection. HPV type 6 and, less often, type 11 are the most frequent types and can cause a common wart and moist surface of the external genitalia. Giant condylomata (Buschke-Löwenstein) affect older men and may be 5 to 10 cm in size.[13] Atypia may be evident in longstanding, giant condylomata and assessment of other HPV subtypes may be indicated to distinguish from a noninvasive warty carcinoma.[13,14]

Penile Cancer

Carcinoma of the penis is rare in the United States, constituting about 1 in 100,000 men. It does account, however, for about 10% of cancers in African and South American men. It can affect men 40 to 70 years of age, with two thirds of men diagnosed at 65 years of age and older. In the United States, about four out of five cases of the disease are diagnosed in men more than 55 years of age. Although the exact cause is unknown, risk factors include HPV infection, smoking, low socioeconomic status, poor personal hygiene, and psoriasis (possibly autoimmune diseases linked to the lack of clearance of HPV). Circumcision at birth decreases the risk of penile cancer and penile cancer is more common in men with phimosis and those with acquired immunodeficiency syndrome (AIDS).[15]

Squamous cell carcinoma accounts for 95% of invasive penile cancers. Other premalignant lesions, or in situ forms of epidermal carcinoma, that occur on the penis include leukoplakia (white plaque), Paget disease (red, inflamed areas), erythroplasia of Queyrat (raised red areas), and Buschke-Löwenstein patches (large venous areas). Recently, penile intraepithelial neoplasia (PeIN, atypical cells) has been redesignated into two subcategories: differentiated PeIN and undifferentiated PeIN, including warty basaloid and mixed warty-basaloid subtypes.[13] HPV6 and HPV11 associated with genital warts (condylomata acuminata) have low cancer risks.[16] At times, the penis might be the site of metastatic spread of solid tumors from the bladder, prostate, rectum, or kidney. Early squamous cell carcinoma and pre-malignant epidermal lesions are easily treated, but delays in seeking treatment are attributed to denial, embarrassment, failure to detect lesions under a phimotic foreskin, fear, guilt, and ignorance.

Squamous cell carcinoma usually begins as a small, flat, ulcerative or papillary lesion on the glans or foreskin that grows to involve the entire penile shaft. Extensive lesions are associated with metastases and a poor prognosis.[17,18] The regional femoral and iliac lymph nodes are common metastatic sites; the urethra and bladder are rarely involved. Weight loss, fatigue, and malaise accompany chronic suppurative lesions.

The specific diagnosis is made by biopsy after examination to document the location, size, and fixation of the lesion. After a positive biopsy, the extent of cancer spread is determined by imaging studies. Distant metastases are uncommon. Stages of carcinoma of the penis are presented in Box 34-3.

Penile carcinoma is managed primarily with surgery. Newer, innovative surgical techniques can preserve as much penile tissue as possible without compromising cancer control. A multimodal approach with chemotherapy is under study.[19,20] Palliative treatment with radiation or chemotherapy may be used when the disease is inoperable and bulky inguinal metastases have occurred. Options for individuals with carcinoma in situ include local excision, radiation, laser surgery, cryosurgery, chemosurgery, or chemotherapy with topical (5%) 5-fluorouracil.[17]

✔ **QUICK CHECK 34-2**

1. Why are priapism and severe paraphimosis considered urologic emergencies?
2. What are the risk factors for cancer of the penis?

Disorders of the Scrotum, Testis, and Epididymis
Disorders of the Scrotum

Men may seek treatment for painful or painless scrotal masses. Masses may be serious (cancer or torsion) or benign (hydrocele or cyst), and may require immediate surgical intervention or allow for careful observation. Varicocele, hydrocele, and spermatocele are common intrascrotal disorders. A varicocele is an abnormal dilation of the testicular vein and the pampiniform plexus within the scrotum, and is classically described as a "bag of worms" (Figure 34-5). Varicoceles are one of the most commonly identified scrotal abnormalities and abnormal findings among infertile men. Advancements in diagnostic techniques indicate that the incidence of varicoceles is significantly greater than previously reported.[21] Most (90%) occur on the left side because of discrepancies in venous drainage and may be painful or tender. Varicocele occurs in 10% to 15% of males and is seen most often after puberty.[22] Because most develop in adolescence, physiologic changes in testosterone level may contribute to increasing blood flow to the

---

BOX 34-3 **Staging for Penile Cancer**

Stage 0: Tis or Ta, N0, M0
The cancer has not grown into tissue below the top layers of skin and has not spread to lymph nodes or distant sites.

Stage I: T1a, N0, M0
The cancer has grown into tissue just below the superficial layer of skin but has not grown into blood or lymph vessels. It is a grade 1 or 2. It has not spread to lymph nodes or distant sites.

Stage II: Any of the Following:
T1b, N0, M0
The cancer has grown into tissue just below the superficial layer of skin and is high grade or has grown into blood or lymph vessels. It has not spread to lymph nodes or distant sites.
Or

T2, N0, M0
The cancer has grown into one of the internal chambers of the penis (the corpus spongiosum or corpora cavernosa). The cancer has not spread to lymph nodes or distant sites.
Or

T3, N0, M0
The cancer has grown into the urethra. It has not spread to lymph nodes or distant sites.

Stage IIIA: T1 to T3, N1, M0
The cancer has grown into tissue below the superficial layer of skin (T1). It also may have grown into the corpus spongiosum, the corpora cavernosa, or the urethra (T2 or T3). The cancer has spread to a single groin lymph node (N1). It has not spread to distant sites.

Stage IIIB: T1 to T3, N2, M0
The cancer has grown into the tissues of the penis and may have grown into the corpus spongiosum, the corpora cavernosa, or the urethra (T1 to T3). It has spread to two or more groin lymph nodes. It has not spread to distant sites.

Stage IV: Any of the Following:
T4, any N, M0
The cancer has grown into the prostate or other nearby structures. It may or may not have spread to groin lymph nodes. It has not spread to distant sites.
Or

Any T, N3, M0
The cancer has spread to lymph nodes in the pelvis or spread in the groin lymph nodes and grown through the lymph nodes' outer covering and into surrounding tissue. The cancer has not spread to distant sites.
Or

Any T, any N, M1
The cancer has spread to distant sites.

T, Primary tumor size; N, regional lymph nodes; M, distant metastasis.

---

testicle, causing venous dilation.[23] Unilateral right-sided varicoceles are rare and result from compression or obstruction of the inferior vena cava by a tumor or thrombus. Varicoceles may be less likely to be diagnosed among obese men.[24]

The cause of varicocele is poorly understood. Blood pools in the veins rather than flowing into the venous system. Varicocele decreases blood flow through the testis, interfering with spermatogenesis and causing infertility. Varicoceles can alter testosterone and

FIGURE 34-7 Spermatocele. Retention cyst of the head of the epididymis or of an aberrant tubule or tubules of the rete testis. The spermatocele lies outside the tunica vaginalis; therefore, on palpation it can be readily distinguished and separated from the testis. (From Lloyd-Davies RW et al: *Color atlas of urology,* ed 2, London, 1994, Wolfe Medical.)

FIGURE 34-5 Depiction of a Varicocele. Dilation of veins within the spermatic cord. (From Ball JW et al: *Seidel's guide to physical examination,* ed 8, St Louis, 2015, Mosby.)

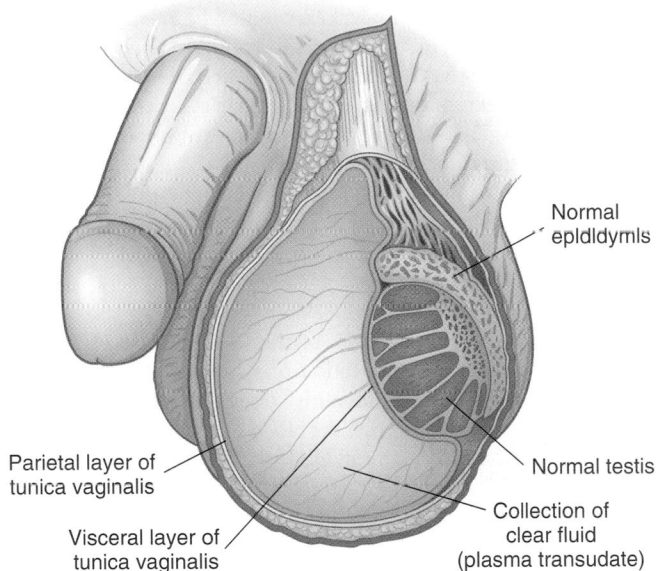

Normal epididymis

Parietal layer of tunica vaginalis

Visceral layer of tunica vaginalis

Normal testis

Collection of clear fluid (plasma transudate)

FIGURE 34-6 Depiction of a Hydrocele. Accumulation of clear fluid between the visceral (inner) and parietal (outer) layers of the tunica vaginalis.

follicle-stimulating hormone levels, cause oxidative stress, decrease sperm count, and affect sperm quality.[25] Varicocele surgical repair is generally done when the male has a grade II or III varicocele and an abnormal semen analysis and the female has no known cause of infertility. If varicocele is mild and fertility is not an issue, a scrotal support is usually sufficient to relieve symptoms of scrotal heaviness or "dragging." Color Doppler ultrasonography is used to confirm diagnosis.[25]

A **hydrocele** is a collection of fluid between the layers of the tunica vaginalis (Figure 34-6). It is the most common cause of scrotal swelling. Hydroceles occur in 6% of male newborns and are congenital malformations that often resolve spontaneously in the first year of life.[26] In North America, common infectious causes include epididymitis and viruses. Worldwide, however, filariasis is a major cause

especially with recent travel to tropical countries.[21] Other causes include trauma, torsion of the testicle or testicular appendage, and recent scrotal surgery. A man presenting with a hydrocele in his third or fourth decade needs careful evaluation for testicular cancer.[27]

Hydroceles vary in size and most are asymptomatic. The most important feature on physical examination is a tense, smooth, scrotal mass that easily transluminates. Translumination, or holding a light behind the scrotum, can help distinguish a hydrocele from a hernia or a solid mass. Treatment includes watchful waiting in infants and for those older than 1 year; 75% of hydroceles resolve within 6 months.[26,27] Symptomatic or communicating hydroceles need definitive treatment. Treatment includes surgical resection, aspiration, and sclerotherapy (injection of a sclerosing agent into the scrotal sac [cystic dilation]) to excise the tunica vaginalis.[21]

Spermatoceles (epididymal cysts) are benign cystic collections of fluid of the epididymis located between the head of the epididymis and the testis. Spermatoceles are filled with a milky fluid containing sperm and are usually painless (Figure 34-7). Spermatoceles that cause significant pain or discomfort are excised. Both spermatoceles and epididymal cysts present clinically as discrete, firm, freely mobile masses distinct from the testis that may be transilluminated. Usually, however, spermatoceles are asymptomatic or produce mild discomfort that is relieved by scrotal support. Neither hydroceles nor spermatoceles are associated with infertility.

Cryptorchidism and Ectopy

Cryptorchidism is a group of abnormalities in which the testis fails to descend completely, whereas an **ectopic testis** has strayed from the normal pathway of descent. Ectopy may be caused by an abnormal connection at the distal end of the gubernaculum testis that leads the gonad to an abnormal position, usually at the superficial inguinal site. In cryptorchidism, the descent of one or both testes is arrested with unilateral arrest occurring more often than bilateral arrest. The testes may remain in the abdomen, or testicular descent may be arrested in the inguinal canal or the puboscrotal junction. Cryptorchidism is a common congenital anomaly, with an incidence of approximately 3% in full-term infants. However, this rate increases significantly with low birth weight; for instance, the rate of cryptorchidism at 3 months has been found to be 7.7% for infants with birth weights less than 2000 g, 2.5% for birth weights of 2000 to 2500 g, and 1.41% for birth weights of 2500 g or more.[28,29] The incidence of cryptorchidism in adults is 0.7% to 0.8%.[25] Cryptorchidism is commonly associated with vasal or epididymal abnormalities. These congenital anomalies affect about 33% to 66% of newborns with cryptorchidism. Other structural anomalies include posterior urethral valves (less than 5%), upper genital tract abnormalities (less than 5%), and hypospadias. The presence of both hypospadias and cryptorchidism raises the suspicion of mixed gonadal dysgenesis (intersex infant). It has been hypothesized that cryptorchidism may result from an absence or abnormality of the gubernaculum—a cordlike structure that extends from the lower pole of the testis to the scrotum; a congenital gonadal or dysgenetic defect that makes the testis insensitive to gonadotropins (a likely explanation for unilateral cryptorchidism); or lack of maternal gonadotropins (a likely explanation for bilateral cryptorchidism of prematurity).[25]

Mechanical possibilities include a short spermatic cord, fibrous bands or adhesions in the normal path of the testes, or a narrowed inguinal canal. Chromosomal studies do not support a genetic component. Physiologic cryptorchidism, also called *retractile* or *migratory testis*, is an involuntary retraction of the testes out of the scrotum that occurs with excitement, physical activity, or exposure to cold and is caused by the small mass of prepubertal testis and the strength of the cremaster muscle. This is a common phenomenon that is self-limiting (descent occurs at puberty).

Physical examination discloses the absence of one or both testes in the scrotum and an atrophic scrotum on the affected side. If the undescended testis is in a vulnerable position, over the pubic bone for example, an individual may complain of severe pain secondary to trauma. The adult male with bilateral cryptorchidism may be infertile.

Testicular cancer also is a well-established complication of cryptorchidism. In men with a history of unilateral cryptorchidism, neoplasms also develop more commonly in the contralateral testis. This finding suggests cryptorchidism affects the testes and is a process more significant than simply the position of the testis in childhood. The risk of testicular cancer is 35 to 50 times greater for men with cryptorchidism or a history of cryptorchidism than for the general male population. Because definite histologic change occurs in the cryptorchid testis by 1 year of age, surgical correction is recommended around that age.[28,30] Treatment often begins with administration of gonadotropin-releasing hormone (GnRH) or human chorionic gonadotropin (hCG), hormones that may initiate descent and make surgery unnecessary. GnRH is available as a nasal spray in Europe and may enhance germ cell counts even when the testis does not descend.[30] If hormonal therapy is not successful (success rates range from 6% to 75%), the testis is located and moved surgically (orchiopexy) in young children or removed (orchiectomy) in adults and children more than 10 years of age.[25] The testis that is properly placed in the scrotum provides adequate hormonal function and gives the scrotum a normal appearance. A successful operation does not ensure fertility if the testis is congenitally defective. Approximately 20% of males with unilateral undescended testis remain infertile even though orchiopexy is performed by age 1 year; most individuals with treated or untreated bilateral testicular maldescent have poor fertility.

Torsion of the Testis and Testicular Appendages

In torsion of the testis, the testis rotates on its vascular pedicle, interrupting its blood supply (Figure 34-8). Torsion of the testis is one of several conditions that cause an acute scrotum, which is testicular pain and swelling. Testicular appendages include the appendix testis (a remnant of the müllerian duct) and the appendix epididymis (a remnant of the wolffian duct). Torsion of the appendages can also cause acute scrotum and be confused with testicular torsion, a urologic emergency.

Torsion of the testis can occur at any age but is most common among neonates and adolescents, particularly at puberty.[26] Onset may

FIGURE 34-8 Torsion of the Testis. The testes appear dark red and partially necrotic as a result of hemorrhagic infarction. (From Damjanov I, Linder J, editors: *Anderson's pathology*, ed 10, St Louis, 1996, Mosby.)

be spontaneous or follow physical exertion or trauma. Torsion twists the arteries and veins in the spermatic cord, reducing or stopping circulation to the testis. Vascular engorgement and ischemia develop, causing scrotal swelling and pain not relieved by rest or scrotal support. Diagnostic testing includes urinalysis (to determine infection) and color Doppler ultrasonography.[25] Torsion of the testis is a surgical emergency. If it cannot be reduced manually (scrotal elevation), surgery must be performed within 6 hours after the onset of symptoms to preserve normal testicular function.

Orchitis

Orchitis is an acute inflammation of the testes (Figure 34-9) and is uncommon except as a complication of systemic infection or as an extension of an associated epididymitis[31] (see p. 862). Infectious organisms may reach the testes through the blood or the lymphatics or, most commonly, by ascent through the urethra, vas deferens, and epididymis. Most cases of orchitis are actually cases of epididymo-orchitis (inflammation of both the epididymis and testis). Occasionally in middle-aged men, a nonspecific, apparently noninfectious, inflammatory process (called *granulomatous orchitis*) can occur, presumably a granulomatous response to spermatozoa.

Mumps is the most common infectious cause of orchitis and usually affects postpubertal males. The onset is sudden, occurring 3 to 4 days after the onset of parotitis. Signs and symptoms include high fever, reaching 40° C (104° F), marked prostration, bilateral or unilateral erythema, edema and tenderness of the scrotum, and leukocytosis. An acute hydrocele may develop. Urinary signs and symptoms, which accompany epididymitis, are absent. Atrophy with irreversible damage to spermatogenesis may result in 30% of affected testes. Bilateral orchitis does not affect hormonal function but may cause permanent sterility.

Treatment is supportive and includes bed rest, scrotal support, elevation of the scrotum, hot or cold compresses, and analgesic agents for relief of pain. If an acute hydrocele develops, it is aspirated. Testicular abscess usually requires orchiectomy (removal of the testis). Appropriate antimicrobial drugs should be used for bacterial orchitis, and

FIGURE 34-9 Depiction of Orchitis. (From Ball JW et al: *Seidel's guide to physical examination,* ed 8, St Louis, 2015, Mosby.)

FIGURE 34-10 Testicular Tumor. (From Wolfe J: *400 self-assessment picture tests in clinical medicine,* London, 1984, Wolfe Medical.)

corticosteroids are indicated in proven cases of nonspecific granulomatous orchitis.

Cancer of the Testis

Testicular cancer is a highly treatable, usually curable cancer that most often develops in young and middle-aged men. For men with seminoma (all stages combined), the cure rate exceeds 90%. For men with low stage seminoma or nonseminoma, the cure rate approaches 100%.[32] Overall, testicular cancers are uncommon, accounting for approximately 1% of all male cancers; yet they are the most common solid tumor of young adult men.[32] Cancer of the testis occurs most commonly in men between the ages of 15 and 35 years. In the United States, the lifetime probability of developing testicular cancer is 0.3% for white men, an incidence that is 4.5 times higher than that found in blacks. Testicular tumors are slightly more common on the right side than on the left, a pattern that parallels the occurrence of cryptorchidism, and they are bilateral in 1% to 3% of cases (Figure 34-10).

PATHOPHYSIOLOGY Ninety percent of testicular cancers are germ cell tumors, arising from the male gametes. Germ cell tumors include seminomas (most common), embryonal carcinomas, teratomas, and choriosarcomas. Testicular tumors also can arise from specialized cells of the gonadal stroma (Leydig, Sertoli, granulosa, theca cells).

The cause of testicular neoplasms is unknown (see *Risk Factors: Cancer of the Testis*). A genetic predisposition is suggested by the fact that the incidence is higher among brothers, identical twins, and other close male relatives. Genetic predisposition is supported statistically,

RISK FACTORS

Cancer of the Testis

- HIV and AIDS
- History of cryptorchidism
- Abnormal testicular development
- Klinefelter syndrome
- History of testicular cancer

showing that the disease is relatively rare among Africans, black Americans, Asians, and native New Zealanders. Risk factors include history of cryptorchidism, abnormal testicular development, human immunodeficiency virus (HIV) and AIDS, Klinefelter syndrome, and history of testicular cancer.[32]

CLINICAL MANIFESTATIONS Painless testicular enlargement commonly is the first sign of testicular cancer. Occurring gradually, it may be accompanied by a sensation of testicular heaviness or a dull ache in the lower abdomen. Occasionally acute pain occurs because of rapid growth resulting in hemorrhage and necrosis. Ten percent of affected men have epididymitis, 10% have hydroceles, and 5% have breast enlargement (gynecomastia). The testicular mass is usually discovered by the individual or by his sexual partner. At the time of initial diagnosis, approximately 10% of individuals already have symptoms related to metastases. Lumbar pain also may be present and usually is caused by retroperitoneal node metastasis. Signs of metastasis to the lungs include cough, dyspnea, and bloody sputum (hemoptysis). Supraclavicular node involvement may cause difficulty swallowing (dysphagia) and neck swelling. With metastasis to the central nervous system (CNS), alterations in vision or mental status, papilledema, and seizures may be experienced.

EVALUATION AND TREATMENT An incorrect diagnosis at the initial examination occurs in as many as 25% of men with testicular cancer. Epididymitis and epididymo-orchitis are the most common misdiagnoses; others include hydrocele and spermatocele. Evaluation begins with careful physical examination, including palpation of the scrotal contents with the individual in the erect and supine positions. Signs of testicular cancer include abnormal consistency, induration, nodularity, or irregularity of the testis. The abdomen and lymph nodes are palpated to seek evidence of metastasis, and tumor type is identified after orchiectomy. Although testicular self-examination has not been studied enough to be recommended by the American Cancer Society, many physicians recommend monthly examinations after puberty. Testicular biopsy is not recommended because it may cause dissemination of the

FIGURE 34-11 Epididymitis Secondary to Gonorrhea or Nongonococcal Urethritis. This infection spread to the testes, and rupture through the scrotal wall is threatened. (From Taylor PK: *Diagnostic picture tests in sexually transmitted disease,* London, 1995, Mosby.)

tumor and increase the risk of local recurrence. Primary testicular cancer can be assessed rapidly and accurately by scrotal ultrasonography. Tumor markers are higher than normal in the presence of a tumor and may help detect a tumor that is too small to be palpated during physical examination or to be visualized on imaging. Radiologic imaging and measurement of serum markers are used in clinical staging of the disease. Besides surgery, treatment involves radiation and chemotherapy singly or in combination. Factors influencing the prognosis include histologic studies of the tumor stage of the disease and selection of appropriate treatment. Most individuals treated for cancer of the testis can expect a normal life span; some have persistent paresthesias, Raynaud phenomenon, or infertility. Approximately 10% of men treated for testicular cancer will experience a relapse; if the relapse is discovered early and treated, 99% can be cured. Orchiectomy does not affect sexual function.

Epididymitis

Epididymitis, or inflammation of the epididymis, generally occurs in sexually active young males (younger than 35 years) and is rare before puberty (Figure 34-11). In young men, the usual cause is a sexually transmitted microorganism, such as *N. gonorrhoeae* or *C. trachomatis.* Coliform bacteria are the common pathogens in other age groups.[33] Men who practice unprotected anal intercourse may acquire sexually transmitted epididymitis that results from infection with *Escherichia coli, Haemophilus influenzae,* tuberculosis, or *Cryptococcus* or *Brucella* species. In men older than 35 years, Enterobacteriaceae (intestinal bacteria) and *Pseudomonas aeruginosa* associated with urinary tract infections and prostatitis also may cause epididymitis. Epididymitis also may result from a chemical inflammation caused by the reflux of sterile urine into the ejaculatory ducts, which is then called chemical epididymitis.[33] It is associated with urethral strictures, congenital posterior valves, and excessive physical straining in which increased abdominal pressure is transmitted to the bladder. Chemical epididymitis is usually self-limiting and does not require evaluation or intervention unless it persists.

PATHOPHYSIOLOGY The pathogenic microorganism usually reaches the epididymis by ascending the vasa deferentia from an already infected urethra or bladder. The resulting inflammatory response causes symptoms of bacterial epididymitis. Epididymitis caused by

heavy lifting or straining results from reflux of urine from the bladder into the vas deferens and epididymis. Urine is extremely irritating to the epididymis and initiates the inflammatory response called *chemical epididymitis.*

CLINICAL MANIFESTATIONS The main symptom of epididymitis is scrotal or inguinal pain caused by inflammation of the epididymis and surrounding tissues. The pain is usually acute and severe. Flank pain may occur if, as the urethra passes over the spermatic cord, edematous swelling of the cord obstructs the urethra. The individual may have pyuria, bacteriuria, and a history of urinary symptoms, including urethral discharge. The scrotum on the involved side is red and edematous. The tail of the epididymis near the lower pole of the testis usually swells first; then swelling ascends to the head of the epididymis. The spermatic cord also may be swollen and tender.

Complications include abscess formation, infarction of the testis, recurrent infection, and infertility. Infarction is probably caused by thrombosis (obstruction by blood clots) of the prostatic vessels secondary to severe inflammation. Recurrent epididymitis may result from inadequate initial treatment or failure to identify or treat predisposing factors. Chronic epididymitis can cause scarring of the epididymal endothelium and infertility. Once scarring has occurred, treatment with antibiotics is ineffective because adequate antibiotic levels cannot be achieved within the epididymis.

EVALUATION AND TREATMENT A history of recent urinary tract infection or urethral discharge suggests the diagnosis of epididymitis. Common physical findings include a swollen, tender epididymis or testis located in the normal anatomic position with an intact same-side cremasteric reflex.[34] The relief of pain when the inflamed testis and epididymis are elevated (Prehn sign) is also diagnostic. Definitive diagnosis is based on culture or Gram stain of a urethral swab. Epididymal aspiration may be necessary to obtain a specimen, especially if the individual has been taking antibiotics and has sterile urine.

Treatment includes antibiotic therapy for the infection itself. Analgesics, ice, and scrotal elevation can provide symptomatic relief. If the individual does not steadily improve, he should be reevaluated for possible complications, such as abscess formation, sepsis, or continued infection. Complete resolution of swelling and pain may take several weeks to months. The individual's sexual partner should be treated with antibiotics if the causative microorganism is a sexually transmitted pathogen.

> ✔ **QUICK CHECK 34-3**
> 1. Why is a genetic predisposition suggested for testicular cancer?
> 2. Why is epididymitis rare in prepubescent males?
> 3. Why is testicular torsion considered a urologic emergency?

Disorders of the Prostate Gland
Benign Prostatic Hyperplasia

Benign prostatic hyperplasia (BPH), also called benign prostatic hypertrophy, is the enlargement of the prostate gland (Figure 34-12). (Because the major prostatic changes are caused by hyperplasia, not hypertrophy, benign prostatic hyperplasia is the preferred term.) This condition becomes problematic when prostatic tissue compresses the urethra, where it passes through the prostate, resulting in frequency of lower urinary tract symptoms. Similar to prostate cancer, BPH occurs more often in Westernized countries (e.g., United States, United Kingdom, and Canada). BPH appears to be more common in black men than white men and family history may increase the risk. Being overweight or obese with central fat distribution (i.e., around the abdomen) increases the risk of developing BPH. The prevalence in the

Prostate zones

a = Central zone
b = Fibromuscular zone
c = Transitional zone
d = Peripheral zone
e = Periurethral gland region

High prevalence
Medium-high prevalence
Low prevalence
None

Ejaculatory duct

	Prostate zone		
	Peripheral	Transition	Central
Focal atrophy			
Acute inflammation			
Chronic inflammation			
Benign prostatic hyperplasia			
High-grade PIN			
Carcinoma			

FIGURE 34-12 Prostate Zones, Benign Prostatic Hyperplasia (BPH), and Prostate Cancer Locations. Benign prostatic hyperplasia (BPH) occurs in the peripheral zone of the prostate gland that can enlarge (not shown). BPH nodules and atrophy are associated with inflammation in the transition zone. Most cancer lesions occur in the peripheral zone. Carcinoma can involve the central zone but rarely occurs in isolation, suggesting that prostatic intraepithelial neoplasia (PIN) lesions do not easily progress to carcinoma in this region. (Adapted from De Marzo AM et al: *Nat Rev Cancer* 7:256-269, 2007.)

United States is about 50% in men 60 years and older and 90% among men 70 years or older.[35] BPH is common and involves a complex pathophysiology with several endocrine and local factors and remodeled microenvironment. Its relationship to aging is well documented. At birth, the prostate is pea sized, and growth of the gland is gradual until puberty. At that time, there is a period of rapid development that continues until the third decade of life when the prostate reaches adult size (see Chapter 32). Around 40 to 45 years of age, benign hyperplasia begins and continues slowly until death. Although androgens, such as dihydrotestosterone (DHT), are necessary for normal prostatic development, their role in BPH remains unclear. Among all the androgen-metabolizing enzymes within the prostate, 5α-reductase is the most powerful. This reductase corresponds to an age-dependent DHT level. Therefore, although levels of 5α-reductase and DHT in the epithelium decrease with age, they remain constant in the stroma (microenvironment) of the prostate gland.

PATHOGENESIS Current causative theories of BPH focus on aging and levels and ratios of endocrine factors such as androgens and estrogens (androgen/estrogen ratio), the role of chronic inflammation, and the effects of autocrine/paracrine growth-stimulating and growth-inhibiting factors. These factors include insulin-like growth factors (IGFs), epidermal growth factors, fibroblast factors, and transforming growth factor-beta (TGF-β) and several others. Recent data show that human prostate stromal cells can actively contribute to the

inflammatory process from the induction of inflammatory cytokines and chemokines[36] (see Cancer of the Prostate, p. 865).

With aging, circulating androgens are associated with BPH and enlargement. Other effects related to estrogens include apoptosis, aromatase expression, and paracrine regulation that may be important for stimulating inflammation.[37] BPH is a multifactorial disease and not all men respond well to currently available treatments, suggesting factors are involved other than androgens. Testosterone, the primary circulating androgen in men, also can be metabolized through CYP19/aromatase into the potent estrogen estradiol-17β. The prostate is an estrogen target tissue and estrogens directly and indirectly affect growth and differentiation of the prostate. The precise role of endogenous and exogenous estrogens in directly affecting prostate growth and differentiation in the context of BPH is an understudied area. Estrogens and selective estrogen receptor modulators have been shown to promote or inhibit prostate proliferation, signifying potential roles in BPH.[38,39] Taken together, these interactions lead to an increase in prostate volume. The remodeled stroma promotes local inflammation with altered cytokine, reactive oxygen/nitrogen species, and chemoattractants.[40] The resultant increased oxygen demands of proliferating cells cause a local hypoxia that induces angiogenesis and changes to fibroblasts.

BPH begins in the periurethral glands, which are the inner glands or layers of the prostate. The prostate enlarges as nodules form and grow (nodular hyperplasia) and glandular cells enlarge (hypertrophy).

The development of BPH occurs over a prolonged period of time, and changes within the urinary tract are slow and insidious.

CLINICAL MANIFESTATIONS As nodular hyperplasia and cellular hypertrophy progress, tissues that surround the prostatic urethra compress it, usually, but not always, causing bladder outflow obstruction. These symptoms are sometimes called the spectrum of lower urinary tract symptoms (LUTS). Symptoms include the urge to urinate often, some delay in starting urination, and decreased force of the urinary stream. As the obstruction progresses, often over several years, the bladder cannot empty all the urine, and the increasing volume leads to long-term urine retention. The volume of urine retained may be great enough to produce uncontrolled "overflow incontinence" with any increase in intra-abdominal pressure. At this stage, the force of the urinary stream is significantly reduced, and much more time is required to initiate and complete voiding.[41] Hematuria, bladder or kidney infection, bladder calculi, acute urinary retention hydroureter, hydronephrosis, and renal insufficiency are common complications.[41]

Progressive bladder distention causes diverticular outpouchings of the bladder wall. The ureters may be obstructed where they pass through the hypertrophied detrusor muscle, potentially causing hydroureter, hydronephrosis, and bladder or kidney infection.

EVALUATION AND TREATMENT Diagnosis is made from a medical history, physical examination, and laboratory tests, including urinalysis. Careful review of symptoms is necessary. Digital rectal examination (DRE) and measurement of prostate-specific antigen (PSA) level are conducted to determine hyperplasia. PSA level alone, however, cannot confirm symptoms attributable to BPH because PSA level is elevated in both BPH and prostate cancer. Annual DREs are used to screen men older than 40 years for BPH, sooner in high-risk men.[42] If marked enlargement, moderate to severe symptoms, or complications are present, transrectal ultrasound (TRUS) is used to determine bladder and prostate volume and residual urine. Urinalysis, serum creatinine and blood urea nitrogen levels, uroflowmetry, postvoid residual (PVR) urine, pressure-flow study, cystometry, and cystourethroscopy are used to determine kidney and bladder function.[41] BPH has been treated successfully with drugs. α_1-Adrenergic blockers (prazosin and tamsulosin) are used to relax the smooth muscle of the bladder and prostate. Antiandrogen agents, such as finasteride (Proscar), selectively block androgens at the prostate cellular level and cause the prostate gland to shrink.[43] By shrinking the prostate, these drugs have been shown to improve BPH-related symptoms and reduce the risk of future urinary retention and BPH-related surgery. α_1-Adrenergic blockers do not affect PSA and have no effect on prostate cancer risk; however, antiandrogen agents lower PSA by 50% after 6 months of therapy.[44] Newer, minimally invasive treatments include interstitial laser treatment, transurethral radiofrequency procedures (such as transurethral needle ablation [TUNA]), and Cooled ThermoTherapy™.

Prostatitis

Prostatitis is an inflammation of the prostate. The incidence and prevalence of prostatitis is not known. Inflammation is usually limited to a few of the gland's excretory ducts.

Prostatitis syndromes have been classified by the National Institutes of Health as (1) acute bacterial prostatitis (ABP), (2) chronic bacterial prostatitis (CBP), (3) chronic pelvic pain syndrome (CPPS), and (4) asymptomatic inflammatory prostatitis (Box 34-4). ABP and CBP are mostly caused by gram-negative Enterobacteriaceae and *Enterococci* species that originate in the gastrointestinal flora. The most common organism is *Escherichia coli,* which is identified in the majority of infections.[45] *Klebsiella* species, *Pseudomonas aeruginosa,* and *Serratia* species

---

BOX 34-4 **NIH Classification of Prostatitis Syndrome**

This system, developed for clinical research purposes, can be simplified for use in primary care practice (see text).

Category I, or acute bacterial prostatitis (ABP), is an acute infection of the prostate and is manifested by systemic signs of infection and positive urine culture.

Category II, or chronic bacterial prostatitis (CBP), is a chronic bacterial infection in which bacteria are received in significant numbers from a purulent prostatic fluid. These bacteria are thought to be the most common cause of recurrent urinary tract infection in men.

Category III, or chronic pelvic pain syndrome (CPPS), is diagnosed when no pathologic bacteria can be localized to the prostate (culture of expressed prostatic fluid or postprostatic massage urine specimen) and is further divided into IIIa and IIIb. Category IIIa refers to the inflammatory CPPS where a significant number of white blood cells (WBCs) are localized to the prostate, whereas category IIIb is noninflammatory.

Category IV refers to asymptomatic inflammatory prostatitis in which bacteria or WBCs are localized to the prostate, but individuals are asymptomatic.

---

are common gram-negative cultured microorganisms. Nonbacterial prostatitis (CP/CPPS) syndromes are caused by a cascade of inflammatory, immunologic, neuroendocrine, and neuropathic mechanisms whereby the initiating cause is unknown.

Bacterial prostatitis. Acute bacterial prostatitis (ABP, category I) is an ascending infection of the urinary tract that tends to occur in men between the ages of 30 and 50 years but is also associated with BPH in older men. Infection stimulates an inflammatory response in which the prostate becomes enlarged, tender, firm, or boggy. The onset of prostatitis may be acute and unrelated to previous illnesses, or it may follow catheterization or cystoscopy.

Clinical manifestations of acute bacterial prostatitis are those of urinary tract infection or pyelonephritis. Sudden onset of malaise, low back and perineal pain, high fever (up to 40° C [104° F]), and chills is common, as are dysuria, inability to empty the bladder, nocturia, and urinary retention. The individual also may have symptoms of lower urinary tract obstruction, such as slow, small, "narrowed" urinary stream, which may be a medical emergency. Acute inflammatory prostatic edema can compress the urethra, causing urinary obstruction. Systemic signs of infection include sudden onset of a high fever, fatigue, arthralgia, and myalgia. Prostatic pain may occur, especially when the individual is in an upright position, because the pelvic floor muscles tighten with standing and compression of the prostate gland occurs. Some individuals experience low back pain, painful ejaculation, and rectal or perineal pain. Palpation discloses an enlarged, extremely tender and swollen prostate that is firm, indurated, and warm to the touch.

Because acute bacterial prostatitis is usually associated with a bladder infection caused by the same microorganism, urine cultures disclose its identity. Prostatic massage may express enough secretions from the urethra for direct bacterial examination, but massage may be painful and increases the risk that the infection will ascend to adjacent structures or enter the bloodstream and cause septicemia.

To resolve the infection and control its spread, individuals may require antibiotics. In severe cases, the individual is hospitalized and treated with intravenous antibiotics, followed by oral antibiotics. Analgesics, antipyretics, bed rest, and adequate hydration are also therapeutic. Complications include urinary retention that resolves with antibiotic therapy; prostatic abscess that may rupture into the urethra, rectum, or perineum; epididymitis; bacteremia; and septic shock.

Urinary retention requiring drainage is best managed with a suprapubic catheter; Foley catheterization is contraindicated during acute infection.

Chronic bacterial prostatitis (CBP, category II) is characterized by recurrent urinary tract symptoms and persistence of pathogenic bacteria (usually gram negative) in urine or prostatic fluid. This form of prostatitis is the most common recurrent urinary tract infection in men. Symptoms may be similar to those of an acute bladder infection: frequency, urgency, dysuria, perineal discomfort, low back pain, myalgia, arthralgia, and sexual dysfunction. The prostate may be only slightly enlarged or boggy, but it may be fibrotic because repeated infections can cause it to be firm and irregular in shape.

When the initial urine sample is bacteria-free, prostatic massage is used to express secretions. Subsequently, the first 10 ml of voided urine is collected and examined microscopically. Prostatic secretions showing more than 10 white blood cells (WBCs) per high-power field (hpf) and macrophages containing fat are indicative of bacterial infection; diagnosis is confirmed by culture. A pelvic x-ray or transurethral ultrasound (TRUS) may show prostatic calculi.

Treatment of chronic bacterial prostatitis is difficult because it is often caused by prostatic calculi. Calculi are silent and are found in up to 50% of men with prostatitis, and infected calculi can serve as a source of bacterial persistence and relapsing urinary tract infection. Calculi harbor pathogens within the stone and, consequently, pathogens cannot be eradicated from the urinary tract. Permanent cure is achieved by surgical intervention.[46]

Chronic prostatitis/chronic pelvic pain syndrome. Chronic prostatitis/chronic pelvic pain syndrome (CP/CPPS, category III) is diagnosed when no pathogenic bacteria can be localized to the prostate, and is further subdivided into categories IIIa and IIIb (see Box 34-4). Category IIIa refers to inflammatory chronic pelvic pain syndrome in which white blood cell count is elevated and localized to the prostate. Compared with category III, symptoms tend to be milder but are persistent and annoying. Presumably, noninfectious prostatitis or pain is caused by reflux of sterile urine into the ejaculatory ducts because of high-pressure voiding.[46] Reflux may be triggered by spasms of the external or internal sphincters. Category IIIb is noninflammatory. Category IV exists when individuals are asymptomatic but have an increase in bacteria and white blood cells localized to the prostate. Microorganisms suspected of causing CP/CPPS include *Escherichia coli, Enterobacter, Pseudomonas aeruginosa,* and, a new suspect, *Helicobacter pylori.*[47]

Men with nonbacterial prostatitis may complain of pain or a dull ache that is continuous or spasmodic in the suprapubic, infrapubic, scrotal, penile, or inguinal area. Other symptoms are pain on ejaculation and urinary symptoms, such as frequency of urination. The prostate gland generally feels normal on palpation.

Nonbacterial prostatitis is a diagnosis of exclusion. Digital examination of the prostate, bacterial cultures of the urogenital tract, microscopic examination of expressed prostatic fluid, urethroscopy, and urodynamic studies are used to verify the diagnosis of nonbacterial prostatitis.

There is no generally accepted treatment for nonbacterial prostatitis. Hot sitz baths, bed rest, and pharmacologic therapies, including anti-inflammatory drugs, can relieve symptoms.

Cancer of the Prostate

Prostate cancer is the most commonly diagnosed, nonskin cancer in men in the United States with a lifetime risk for diagnosis currently estimated at 15.9%.[48] The incidence varies greatly worldwide (Figure 34-13) but it is still considered to be the second most frequently diagnosed cancer in men and the sixth leading cause of death worldwide.[49] An estimated 1.1 million cases of prostate cancer were diagnosed worldwide in 2012, accounting for 15% of the cancers diagnosed in men. Almost 70% of diagnosed cases of prostate cancer (759,000) were found to occur in more developed regions.[50] Importantly, incidence rates vary by more than 25-fold worldwide, with the highest rates recorded mostly in developed countries, such as Oceania, Europe, and North America, largely because of wide use or overuse of PSA testing. Screening with PSA can amplify the incidence of prostate cancer by allowing detection of prostate lesions that, although meeting the pathologic criteria for malignancy, may have low potential (e.g., latent, indolent, preclinical)

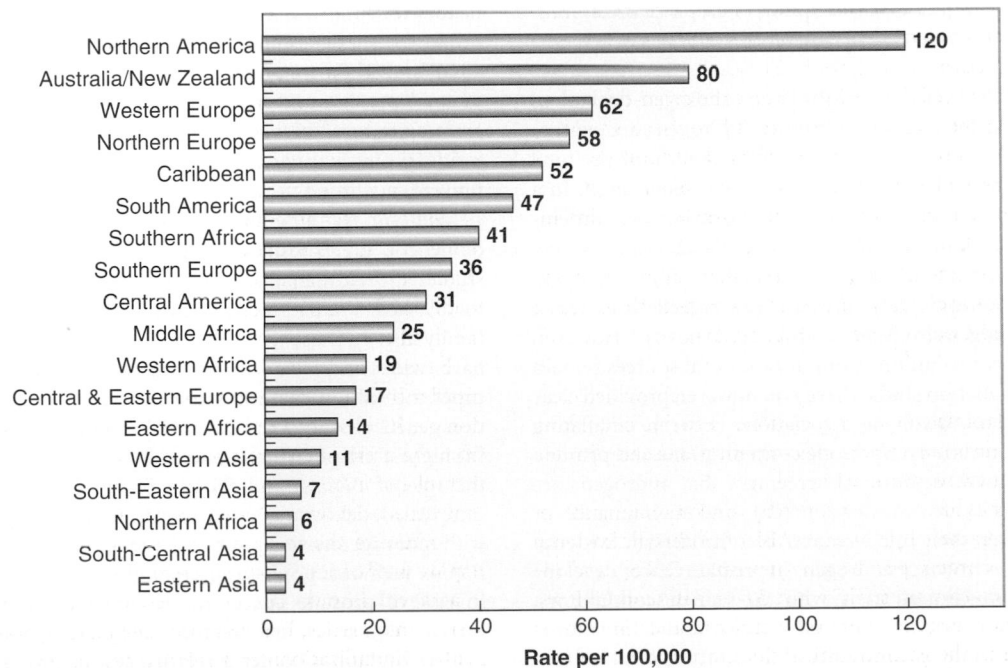

FIGURE 34-13 Selected World Population Age-Standardized (to the World Population) Incidence Rates of Prostate Cancer. (From Jemal A et al: *Biomark Prev* 19:1893, 2010.)

for growth and metastasis. In countries with higher use of PSA testing, such as United States, Canada, Australia, and the Nordic countries, trends in incidence rates follow similar patterns.[50]

Different from Western countries, incidence and death rates are rising in several Asian and Central and Eastern European countries, including Japan. Death rates have been decreasing in several countries, including Australia, Canada, the United Kingdom, the United States, Italy, and Norway, in part because of improved treatment. Males of African descent in the Caribbean region have the highest mortality from prostate cancer in the world.[50] Most cases of prostate cancer have a good prognosis even without treatment, but some cases are aggressive; the lifetime risk for dying of prostate cancer is 2.8%. Prostate cancer is rare before age 50 years and very few men die from this cancer before 60 years of age. Indeed, more than 75% of all prostate cancer is diagnosed in men older than 65.[48] With aging, most of the androgen-metabolizing enzymes undergo significant alteration and older age, race (black), and family history remain the well-established risk factors.

Dietary factors. Although evidence exists for a dietary role in prostate cancer, the epidemiologic evidence is inconsistent.[51] The problem has been confounded by the lack of biomarkers for certain nutrients, difficulties in measuring and quantifying diet, and a limitation of clinical trials to study diet over time. Important are the effects of diet on signaling pathways, hormones, oxidative stress, and reactive oxygen species (ROS). The nutrients in the epidemiology of prostate cancer that have received the most attention include carotenoids, fat, vitamin E, vitamin D/calcium, and selenium. Less studied are isoflavones, curcumin, lycopene, green tea, omega-3 polyunsaturated fats, and sulforaphane (Box 34-5). Associations between obesity and prostate cancer are not clear because there are some inconsistencies, but obesity seems to be negatively associated with more indolent prostate cancer and positively associated with more aggressive disease and a worse outcome.[52] Since adipose tissue is increasingly being regarded as hormonally active tissue, high body fat and obesity need in-depth exploration to understand the associated risk of prostate problems. Adipose tissue is now known to affect circulating levels of several bioactive messengers and therefore could affect the risk of developing prostate problems in addition to several other well-recognized health problems.[53] High-energy intake (consumption of excess calories) indicates that this may indeed increase insulin levels and levels of IGF-1, a powerful carcinogenic agent.

Hormones. Prostate cancer develops in an androgen-dependent epithelium and is usually androgen sensitive. Androgens are synthesized not only in the testis, accounting for 50% to 60% of the total testosterone in the prostate, but also in the prostate gland itself. In a process called intraprostatic conversion, the hormone dehydroepiandrosterone (DHEA) produced by the adrenal glands[54] is converted to testosterone and then into dihydrotestosterone (DHT) in the prostate (Figure 34-14). Additionally, prostate cancer cells have been reported to make androgens from cholesterol (i.e., de novo).[55] However, these overall relative contributions from intratumoral sources remain to be determined. Population studies have not, however, provided clear and convincing patterns involving associations between circulating (e.g., not tissue concentrations) hormone concentrations and prostate cancer risk.[56] Thus, there is universal agreement that androgens are important for prostatic growth, development, and maintenance of tissue balance; however, their role in cancer is controversial. Evidence in support of the involvement of androgens in prostate cancer development is derived from clinical trials with 5α-reductase inhibitors. However, the involvement of 5α-reductase, which is critical in androgen activity in the prostate, is contradictory and inconsistent[56,57] (see Figure 34-14). A prevention study has provided some of the strongest hormonal data with the drug finasteride, which inhibits 5α-reductase. The 7-year intervention study reduced prostate cancer risk in healthy

men by about 25%.[58] Important, however, was that more high-grade tumors were found in those men who developed prostate cancer while on the drug. In men younger than 50 years, circulating levels of androgens and estrogens appear to be higher in men of African descent than in European-American men.

Despite the well-documented importance of androgens, their pathophysiologic process in prostate diseases is incomplete.[59] Androgens also are metabolized to estrogens (see Figure 34-14, *B*) through the action of the enzyme aromatase, and a growing body of evidence implicates estrogens in the etiology of prostate disease (see Pathogenesis section).

Vasectomy. Vasectomy has been identified as a possible risk factor for prostate cancer in both case-controlled studies and cohort studies.[60,61] Three mechanisms by which vasectomy could increase risk are (1) elevation of circulating androgens; (2) activation of immunologic mechanisms involving antisperm antibodies; and (3) reduction of seminal fluid levels of 5α-dihydrotestosterone, the active metabolite of testosterone in the prostate, in vasectomized men. These results suggest an elevation of circulating free testosterone level following vasectomy. However, with these combined mechanisms it is unlikely that vasectomy plays a causal role.[62]

Chronic inflammation. The results of a 5-year longitudinal study of the influence of chronic inflammation and prostate cancer have been reported.[63] The study included 144 men, 33 of whom presented with chronic inflammation in their initial biopsy. Biopsies revealed prostatic hyperplasia and proliferative inflammatory atrophy in those with chronic inflammation. Upon repeat biopsy, 29 new cancers were diagnosed, representing a new cancer incidence of 20%.[63] In contrast, of the 33 men initially showing no inflammation, 2 (6%) were found to have adenocarcinoma. Certain metabolic comorbidities, including obesity, diabetes, sleep apnea, and erectile dysfunction, may be linked to both BPH and inflammation.[64] The causes of chronic inflammation are emerging (possible causes are shown in Figure 34-15). Thus, chronic inflammation may be an important risk factor for prostatic adenocarcinoma.[65] Chronic inflammation involves autocrine/paracrine growth-stimulating and growth-inhibiting factors. These factors include insulin-like growth factors (IGFs), epidermal growth factors, fibroblast factors, and transforming growth factor-beta (TGF-β) as well as several others. Recent data show that human prostate stromal cells can actively contribute to the inflammatory process from the induction of inflammatory cytokines and chemokines.[36,66] Importantly, a continuous input from TGF-β and IGF in the tumor microenvironment or stroma will result in cancer progression. Understanding of these events can help prevention, diagnosis, and therapy of prostate cancer[66] (Figure 34-16).

Genetic and epigenetic factors. Other possible causes are those of genetic predisposition (familial and hereditary forms). Genetic studies suggest that strong familial predisposition may be responsible for 5% to 10% of prostate cancers.[1] Compared with men with no family history, those with one first-degree relative with prostate cancer have twice the risk and those with two first-degree relatives have five times the risk.[67] Germline mutations in the breast cancer predisposition gene 2 *(BRCA2)* are the genetic events known to date that confer the highest risk of prostate cancer (8.6-fold in men ≤65 years). Although the role of *BRCA2* and *BRCA1* in prostate tumorigenesis remains unrevealed, deleterious mutations in both genes have been associated with more aggressive disease and poor clinical outcomes.[68,69] Men with *BRCA2* (tumor suppressor) germline mutations have a 20-fold increase in risk of prostate cancer. Using previously estimated population carrier frequencies, investigators have recently found that deleterious *BRCA1* mutations confer a relative risk of prostate cancer of ≈3.75-fold, translating to 8.6% cumulative risk by age 65.[70] A common type of somatic mutation that develops into chromosomal rearrangements is the *ETS* gene. The most common epigenetic alteration in prostate

BOX 34-5   Summary of Diet for Prostate Cancer

- Lower rates of prostate cancer are found in countries whose residents consume a low fat and high vegetable diet. When men from a low-risk country move to the United States and eat a Western diet, their rates of prostate cancer increase significantly. Inconclusive are the exact culprits that increase this risk, including fat and sugar intake.
- Obesity is linked to advanced and aggressive prostate cancer.
- High body mass index (BMI) is associated with more aggressive disease and a worse outcome.
- Calorie-dense or excessive carbohydrate intake and obesity, independent of dietary fat intake, may increase the risk of developing prostate cancer.
- Dietary fat may increase levels of androgens, increase oxidative stress, and increase reactive oxygen species (ROS).
- Monounsaturated fats may decrease the risk of prostate cancer.
- High levels of linoleic acid (found in corn oil) act as a proinflammatory eicosanoid, which is implicated in promotion of cell proliferation and angiogenesis as well as inhibition of apoptosis.
- The Western diet has increased omega-6 to omega-3 ratios and therefore is proinflammatory. Carcinogenic nitrosamines are formed after consumption of processed meat that contains nitrites and from heme iron present in large quantities of red meat.
- Even given the above knowledge, it is important to realize that studies showing an association between meat intake and prostate cancers have been largely inconclusive. Some studies reveal red meat is positively associated with increased prostate cancer risk with an association with more aggressive disease states. Despite some studies showing a 43% elevation in prostate cancer risk with high consumption of red meat, others show no association with prostate cancer risk.
- Although the role of red meat in prostate and breast cancer remains inconclusive, one explanation for the possible associations reported is the accumulation of carcinogens during the cooking process. Cooking meat at high temperatures produces heterocyclic amines and aromatic hydrocarbons that are carcinogenic.
- Vitamin E has long been considered a candidate for prostate cancer prevention from in vitro and in vivo animal studies. Vitamin E belongs to the family of tocopherols and tocotrienols that exist as α, β, γ, and δ isoforms. Among these, δ-tocopherol is the major dietary isoform, whereas supplements contain α-tocopherol. Vitamin E is a fat-soluble vitamin obtained from vegetable oils, nuts, and egg yolk. It is a potent intracellular antioxidant known to inhibit peroxidation and DNA damage. The Alpha-Tocopherol, Beta-Carotene Cancer Prevention Study (ATBC) showed that supplementation with vitamin E could reduce the incidence of prostate cancer among men who smoked. In vitro studies demonstrate that α-tocopherol succinate induces cell cycle arrest in human prostate cancer cells (i.e., induces apoptosis) and inhibits the androgen receptor. Mouse studies show vitamin E can inhibit the growth-promoting effects of a high-fat diet; however, vitamin E in combination with selenium does not reduce the incidence of prostate cancer in Lady mice models. A prospective large clinical trial, the Selenium and Vitamin E Cancer Prevention Trial (SELECT), showed no reduction in prostate cancer period prevalence but an increased risk of prostate cancer with vitamin E alone.
- Selenium is a trace mineral and exists in food as selenomethionine and selenocysteine. It is essential for the functioning of many antioxidant enzymes and proteins in the body. Humans receive selenium in their diet through plant (dependent on soil concentrations) and animal products. The SELECT trial showed that neither selenium nor vitamin E, taken alone or together, helped to prevent prostate cancer.
- Vitamin D may play an important role in prostate cancer prevention.
- Soy anticancer properties include inhibition of cell proliferation and angiogenesis and reduction in PSA and androgen receptor levels. Countries whose residents have a high intake of soy have much lower rates of prostate cancer.
- Tomatoes or tomato products ingested daily seem to reduce prostate cancer risk. In vitro studies show lycopene found in tomatoes inhibits DNA strand breaks. Unresolved is whether lycopene itself or a metabolic product is responsible for its biologic effect. In clinical studies tomato paste, which is high in lycopene, reduced plasma PSA levels in those men with benign prostatic hyperplasia. Lycopene administration is associated with cell cycle arrest (apoptosis) and growth factor signaling. In 2007 the FDA evaluated 13 available studies and found the relationship between lycopene and reduced risk of prostate cancer inadequate.
- Vegetables including broccoli, cabbage, cauliflower, brussels sprouts, Chinese cabbage, and turnips (all crucifers) may be protective (several epidemiologic studies) against prostate cancer. In particular, a diet high in broccoli reduced cancer risk. By contrast, four studies revealed no cancer preventive effects. Cruciforms have anticancer properties mediated by the phytochemicals phenethyl isothiocyanate, sulforaphane, and indole-3-carbinol. Sulforaphane is a naturally occurring isothiocyanate that was first isolated in broccoli. It protects against carcinogen-induced cancer in many rodents. Mice given 240 mg of broccoli sprouts per day showed a significant reduction in growth of prostate cancer cells. Sulforaphane treatment lowered androgen receptor protein and gene expression.
- Green tea contains polyphenols, including epigallocatechin gallate (EGCG). Green tea consumption has been associated with a reduced incidence of several cancers including prostate cancer. Green tea consumed within a balanced controlled diet in humans improved overall antioxidant potential. The anticancer effect potential of green tea from in vitro and experimental studies shows these compounds bind directly to carcinogens and induce phase II enzymes that inhibit heterocyclic amines. EGCG administration decreased NF-$\kappa\beta$ activity. Green tea was shown to inhibit IGF-1 and increase IGFBP3, leading to inhibition of prostate cancer development and progression. Yet, in two small randomized studies in individuals with high-grade prostatic neoplasia, it showed no effects. However, treatment with a mixture of bioactive compounds that share molecular anticarcinogenic targets may enhance the effect on these targets at low concentrations of individual compounds.
- Epidemiologic studies have consistently shown that regular consumption of fruits and vegetables is strongly associated with reduced risk of developing chronic diseases, such as cancer. It is now accepted that the actions of any specific phytonutrient alone do not explain the observed health benefits of diets rich in fruits and vegetables; also, clinical trials demonstrated that consumption of phytonutrients did not show consistent preventive effects. Synergistic inhibition of prostate cancer cell growth has been evident when using combinations of low concentrations of various carotenoids or carotenoids with retinoic acid and the active metabolite of vitamin D. Combinations of several carotenoids (e.g., lycopene, phytoene, and phytofluene) or carotenoids and polyphenols (e.g., carnosic acid and curcumin) and/or other compounds (e.g., vitamin E) synergistically inhibit the androgen receptor activity and activate the electrophile/antioxidant response element (EpRE/ARE) transcription system. The activation of EpRE/ARE is up to fourfold higher than the sum of activities of single ingredients.
- Examples of important potential processes that can be targeted in the regulation of tumorigenesis include cholesterol synthesis and metabolites, reactive oxygen species and hypoxia, macrophage activation and conversion, indoleamine 2,3-dioxygenase regulation of dendritic cells, vascular endothelial growth factor regulation of angiogenesis, fibrosis inhibition, and endoglin and Janus kinase signaling.
- Curcumin has anticarcinogenic potential with well-characterized antiinflammatory, antiangiogenic, and antioxidant properties. Recent studies report curcumin modulates the Wingless signaling pathway (Wnt) that supports its antiproliferative potential. Curcumin is characteristic of regulating multiple targets, a desirable feature in current drug design and drug development. Together with its potential in treating castration-resistant prostate

Continued

BOX 34-5 Summary of Diet for Prostate Cancer—cont'd

cancer and its safety profile, this feature enables curcumin to serve as an ideal compound for the design and syntheses of agents with improved potential for enhancing clinical therapies used to treat prostate cancer.

- Overall, multiple signaling pathways are involved in prostate cancer development and progression, many of which are affected by dietary and lifestyle factors.

References

Alexander DD et al: A review and meta-analysis of prospective studies of red and processed meat intake and prostate cancer, *Nutr J* 9:50, 2010.

Astorg P: Dietary N-6 and N-3 polyunsaturated fatty acids and prostate cancer risk: a review of epidemiological and experimental evidence, *Cancer Causes Control* 15:367-386, 2004.

Beier R et al: Induction of cyclin E-cdk2 kinase activity, E2F-dependent transcription and cell growth by Myc are genetically separable events, *EMBO J* 19(21):5813-5823, 2000.

Casey SC et al: Cancer prevention and therapy through the modulation of the tumor microenvironment, *Semin Cancer Biol* 2015 Apr 10. [Epub ahead of print.]

Chen QH: Curcumin-based anti-prostate cancer agents, *Anticancer Agents Med Chem* 15(2):138-156, 2015.

Dagnelie PC et al: Diet, anthropometric measures and prostate cancer risk: a review of prospective cohort and intervention studies, *BJ Int* 93(8):1139-1150, 2004.

Demark-Wahnefried W, Moyad MA: Dietary intervention in the management of prostate cancer, *Curr Opin Urol* 17:168-174, 2007; 737-743, 2001.

Freedland SJ, Aronson WJ: Obesity and prostate cancer, *Urology* 65:433-439, 2005.

Giovannucci E et al: Risk factors for prostate cancer incidence and progression in the health professionals follow-up study, *Int J Cancer* 121:1571-1578, 2007.

Greenwald P: Clinical trials in cancer prevention: current results and perspectives for the future, *J Nutr* 134(12 suppl):3507S-3512S, 2004.

Hill P et al: Diet and urinary steroids in black and white North American men and black South African men, *Cancer Res* 39:5101-5105, 1979.

Kim DJ et al: Premorbid diet in relation to survival from prostate cancer (Canada), *Cancer Causes Control* 11:65-77, 2000.

Kobayashi N et al: Effect of altering dietary omega-6/omega-3 fatty acid ratios on prostate cancer membrane composition, cyclooxygenase-2, and prostaglandin E2, *Clin Cancer Res* 12(15):4660-4670, 2006.

Kolonel LN: Fat, meat, and prostate cancer, *Epidemiol Rev* 23:72-81, 2001.

Kristal AR et al: Dietary patterns, supplement use, and the risk of symptomatic benign prostatic hyperplasia: results from the prostate cancer prevention trial, *Am J Epidemiol* 167:925-934, 2008.

Linnewiel-Hermoni K et al: The anti-cancer effects of carotenoids and other phytonutrients resides in their combined activity, *Arch Biochem Biophys* 572:28-35, 2015.

Lloyd JC et al: Effect of isocaloric low fat diet on prostate cancer xenograft progression in a hormone deprivation model, *J Urol* 183:1619-1624, 2010.

Matsumara K et al: Involvement of the estrogen receptor beta in genistein-induced expression of p21 (waf1/cip1) in PC-3 prostate cancer cells, *Anticancer Res* 28:709-714, 2008.

Ngo TH et al: Effect of diet and exercise on serum insulin, IGF-1, and IGFBP-1 levels and growth of LNCaP cells in vitro (United States), *Cancer Causes Control* 13:929-935, 2002.

Ngo TH et al: Effect of isocaloric low-fat diet on human LAPC-4 prostate cancer xenografts in severe combined immunodeficient mice and the insulin-like growth factor axis, *Clin Cancer Res* 9:2734-2743, 2003.

Ni J, Yeh S: The roles of alpha-vitamin E and its analogues in prostate cancer, *Vitam Horm* 76:493-518, 2007.

Punnen S et al: Impact of meat consumption, preparation, and mutagens on aggressive prostate cancer, *PLoS One* 6:e27711, 2011.

Rodriguez C et al: Body mass index, weight change, and risk of prostate cancer in the Cancer Prevention Study II Nutrition Cohort, *Cancer Epidemiol Biomarkers Prev* 16:63-69, 2007.

Salem S et al: Major dietary factors and prostate cancer risk: a prospective multicenter case-control study, *Nutr Cancer* 2011; 63:21-27, 2011.

Sinha R et al: Meat and meat-related compounds and risk of prostate cancer in a large prospective cohort study in the United States, *Am J Epidemiol* 170:1165-1177, 2009.

Teiten M et al: Anti-proliferative potential of curcumin in androgen dependent prostate cancer cells occurs through modulation of the Wingless signaling pathway, *Int J Oncol* 38:603-611, 2011.

Wang P et al: Increased chemopreventive effect by combining arctigenin, green tea polyphenol and curcumin in prostate and breast cancer cells, *RSC Adv* 4(66):35242-35250, 2014.

Wright JL et al: AMACR polymorphisms, dietary intake of red meat and dairy and prostate cancer risk, *Prostate* 71:498-506, 2011.

Zhou DY et al: Curcumin analogues with high activity for inhibiting human prostate cancer cell growth and androgen receptor activation, *Mol Med Rep* 10(3):1315-1322, 2014.

cancer is hypermethylation of the glutathione *S*-transferase (*GSTP1*) gene located on chromosome 11. More than 30 independent, peer-reviewed studies have reported a consistently high sensitivity and specificity of *GSTP1* hypermethylation in prostatectomy or biopsy tissue.[71] There is no clear evidence of a causal link between BPH and prostate cancer, even though they may often occur together. Variations in several other genes related to inflammatory pathways might affect the probability of developing prostate cancer.

PATHOGENESIS More than 95% of prostatic neoplasms are adenocarcinomas[72] and most occur in the periphery of the prostate (see Figures 34-12 and 34-17). Prostatic adenocarcinoma is a heterogeneous group of tumors with a diverse spectrum of molecular and pathologic characteristics and, therefore, diverse clinical behaviors and challenges.[73] The biologic aggressiveness of the neoplasm appears to be related to the degree of differentiation rather than the size of the tumor (Box 34-6). Several genetic alterations have been found for prostate carcinoma, including acquired genomic structural changes, somatic mutations, and epigenetic alterations.[74]

Hormonal factors. Just as the testicles are the male equivalent of the female ovaries, the prostate is the male equivalent of the female uterus; in both situations they originate from the same embryonic cells. This may be important in understanding the role of the associated hormones testosterone (T), dihydrotestosterone (DHT), and estrogens in prostate cancer development. Testicular testosterone synthesis and serum testosterone levels fall as men age, but the levels of estradiol do not decline, remaining unchanged or increasing with age.[75,76] The relationship between hormones and the pathophysiology of prostate

carcinogenesis is incomplete and controversial.[77] The main issues and controversies include (1) sources of androgen production outside of the testes, or extratesticular sources (e.g., from adrenal DHEA and from prostate tissue cholesterol [de novo] itself); (2) the role of prostatic androgen receptor (AR); (3) the role of estrogens, aromatase enzyme, and the estrogen receptors ERα and ERβ; and (4) the role of the surrounding microenvironment or stroma.

Prostate cancer is considered a hormone-dependent disease; cell growth and survival of early stage prostate cancer can respond to androgens and this is the background evidence for androgen-deprivation therapy (ADT). However, evidence thus far is lacking to associate *plasma* androgens with prostate cancer progression. Prostatic tissue has the ability to produce its own steroids, including androgens and estrogens.[78] Therefore, the local tissue levels of sex steroids have become a major focus of intraprostatic hormonal profiles. Prostate tissue contains many metabolizing enzymes for the local production of active androgens and estrogens. Carcinogenesis can alter these intraprostatic enzymes and alter the normal balance.

The androgenic hormone responses in the normal prostate and prostate cancer are mediated by androgen receptor (AR) signaling.[79] Exactly how AR drives the growth of prostate cancer cells is not fully known. Several mechanisms have been suggested[79] and specific pathways of signaling are important because they can provide novel therapeutic targets. A recent study using animal models found that loss of androgen receptor function prevented prostatic carcinogenesis, malignant transformation, and metastasis. Tissue-specific evaluation of androgen hormone action demonstrated that epithelial androgen receptor was not necessary for prostate cancer progression, whereas the

FIGURE 34-14 Sources of Androgens and Aromatase and Estrogen Signaling in the Prostate. A, Body sources of androgens in the prostate gland. Hypothalamic GnRH causes the release of LH from the anterior pituitary gland. LH stimulates the testes to produce testosterone, which then accumulates in the blood. Pituitary ACTH release stimulates the adrenal glands, which secrete the androgen precursor DHEA into the blood. DHEA is converted into testosterone and then into DHT in the prostate. **B,** Aromatase and estrogen signaling in the prostate. In normal and benign tissue, aromatase is expressed within the stroma and regulated by promoter PII. Estrogen then exerts its effects in an autocrine fashion through the stromal ER-α receptor and also in a paracrine fashion through both ER-α and ER-β receptors. With prostate cancer, aromatase is now expressed within the tumor cells and in stromal cells, and regulated by aromatase promoters 1.3, 1.4, and PII. Thus estrogen exerts its effects in an autocrine way through stromal and epithelial ER-α and ER-β. Consequently, the increased levels of estrogen and abnormal ER-α signaling promote inflammation, which increases aromatase expression and the development of a positive feedback cycle. Inflammation drives aromatase expression, thus increasing estrogen, which in turn promotes further inflammation. *ACTH,* Adrenocorticotropic hormone; *DHEA,* dehydroepiandrosterone; *DHT,* dihydrotestosterone; *GnRH,* gonadotropin-releasing hormone; *LH,* luteinizing hormone. (**A** adapted from Labrie F: *Nat Rev Urol* 8:73-80, 2011. **B** from Ellem SJ, Risbridger GP: *J Steroid Biochem Mol Biol* 118[4-5]:246-251, 2010.)

BOX 34-6 Determining the Grade of Prostate Cancer with the Gleason Score

Grade 1. The cancer cells closely resemble normal cells. They are small, uniform in shape, evenly spaced, and well differentiated (i.e., they remain separate from one another).

Grade 2. The cancer cells are still well differentiated, but they are arranged more loosely and are irregular in shape and size. Some of the cancer cells have invaded the neighboring prostate tissue.

Grade 3. This is the most common grade. The cells are less well differentiated (some have fused into clumps) and are more variable in shape.

Grade 4. The cells are poorly differentiated and highly irregular in shape. Invasion of the neighboring prostate tissue has progressed further.

Grade 5. The cells are undifferentiated. They have merged into large masses that no longer resemble normal prostate cells. Invasion of the surrounding tissue is extensive.

stromal androgen receptor was essential for prostate cancer progression, malignant transformation, and metastasis.[80]

Testicular testosterone provides the main source of androgens in the prostate (see Figure 34-14) and is the major *circulating* androgen, whereas DHT predominates in prostate tissue and binds to the androgen receptor (AR) with greater affinity than does T.[81] The adrenal cortex contributes the far less potent dehydroepiandrosterone (DHEA) that promotes synthesis of androgens in the prostate. In the target tissues and, to a lesser extent, in the testes themselves, testosterone is converted to dihydrotestosterone (DHT) by the enzyme 5α-reductase (Figure 34-18). Thus, DHT is the most potent intraprostatic androgen.

Normally, a small amount of estrogen is produced daily—estrone and estradiol—by the aromatization of androstenedione and testosterone, respectively. This reaction is catalyzed by the enzyme aromatase. A small quantity of estradiol is released by the testes (see Figure 34-18); the rest of the estrogens in males are produced by adipose tissue, liver, skin, brain, and other nonendocrine tissue. Thus, testosterone is a precursor of two hormones—DHT and estradiol.

A. Infectious agents

Viruses

Bacteria

B. Hormonal changes

Estradiol

E. Dietary intake of carcinogens

CH$_3$

NH$_2$

PhIP

Charred meat

Prostate

Uric acid

C. Physical trauma

Injury and blunt trauma

Bladder

Prostate

Penis

D. Urine reflux

FIGURE 34-15 Possible Causes of Prostate Inflammation. A, Infection, including viruses, bacteria, fungi, and parasites. **B,** Hormones, for example, estrogen at key times during development. **C,** Physical trauma, any type of blunt physical injury. **D,** Urine reflex. **E,** Certain dietary factors (see text).

Recent studies show aromatase is expressed in stromal tissue in the benign human prostate gland.[76] Thus it appears that both normal prostate and benign prostate have the capacity to locally metabolize androgens to estrogens through aromatase. This leads to the following question: How does aromatase gene expression contribute to the etiology and progression of prostate cancer? Investigators have demonstrated altered aromatase expression in prostate cancer[76,82,83] (see Figure 34-14, *B*, p. 869).

Accumulating evidence shows that estrogens participate in the pathogenesis and development of benign prostatic hyperplasia and prostate cancer by activating estrogen receptor α (ER-α). In contrast, estrogen receptor β (ER-β) is involved in the differentiation and maturation of prostatic epithelial cells, and thus possesses antitumor effects in prostate cancer.[84] The effect of estrogen is determined by the two receptors ER-α and ER-β. ER-α leads to abnormal proliferation, inflammation, and the development of premalignant lesions.[76] In contrast, ER-β leads to antiproliferative, anti-inflammatory, and potentially anticarcinogenic effects that act in concert or balance the actions of ER-α and androgens.[76] Increased expression of ER-α has been found to be associated with prostate cancer progression, metastasis, and the so-called castration-resistant (medical treatment that suppresses androgens) phenotype.[85] A specific oncogene is regulated by ERs, and those hormones that stimulate the ER-α receptor-like (i.e., agonists) endogenous estrogens can stimulate oncogene expression.[86]

Most of the androgen-metabolizing enzymes undergo a significant age-dependent alteration. In epithelium, both the blood levels of

5α-reductase activity and the DHT level decrease with age, whereas in stroma (prostate), not only the 5α-reductase activity but also the stromal DHT level is rather constant over the lifetime. In contrast to the relatively unaltered DHT level over time, the estrogen concentration follows an age-dependent increase. Thus the age-dependent decrease of the DHT accumulation in epithelium and the concomitant increase of the estrogen accumulation in stroma lead to a tremendous increase with age of the estrogen/androgen ratio in the human prostate. In animal studies, chronic exposure to testosterone plus estradiol is strongly carcinogenic, whereas testosterone alone is weakly carcinogenic.[57] In mice studies, elevated testosterone level in the absence of estrogen leads to the development of hypertrophy and hyperplasia but not malignancy.[76] High estrogen and low testosterone levels have been shown to lead to inflammation with aging and the emergence of precancerous lesions.[76] The mechanism is not clearly understood and may involve estrogen-generated oxidative stress and DNA toxicity, and it requires androgen-mediated and estrogen receptor–mediated processes, such as changes in sex steroid metabolism and receptor status. In addition, there are changes in the balance between autocrine/paracrine growth-stimulatory and growth-inhibitory factors, such as the insulin growth factors (IGFs).[57]

Investigators have summarized the following key findings on hormones and prostate cancer: (1) androgens are clearly involved in the progression of prostate cancer; (2) it is only with the addition of estrogen to testosterone in rats that cancer can be reliably induced; (3) in vivo and in vitro studies have identified multiple mechanisms

FIGURE 34-16 Working Model Stromal-Epithelial Interaction in Prostate Cancer Development and Progression. Normally, signaling events between TGF-β and IGF are tightly regulated, keeping the epithelial cells under homeostatic balance. TGF-β binds to receptors on the cell surface known as receptor type I (TBR-I) and type II (TBR-II). A reduction in TBRs in the stromal cells will result in an increase in IGF production. The increase of IGF has a proliferative effect on the prostate epithelial cells (which have already undergone a cancer initiation process as a result of the hormones testosterone and estradiol). TGF-β and IGF in the stromal cells adjacent to prostate epithelial cells will perpetuate a vicious cycle to promote cancer progression. (Adapted from Lee C et al: *Biomed Res* 2014:502093, 2014.)

FIGURE 34-17 Photomicrograph of Prostate Cancer Cells. Pink ruffled cells are prostate cancer cells. (From Cancer Research UK, London Research Institute, Electron Microscopy Unit.)

involving hormonal involvement with genotoxicity, epigenetic toxicity, hyperprolactinemia, chronic inflammation, and estrogen receptor–mediated changes.[77]

Prostate epithelial neoplasia. A precursor lesion, **prostatic epithelial neoplasia (PIN),** has been described. PIN may be more concentrated in prostates containing cancer and is noted in proximity to

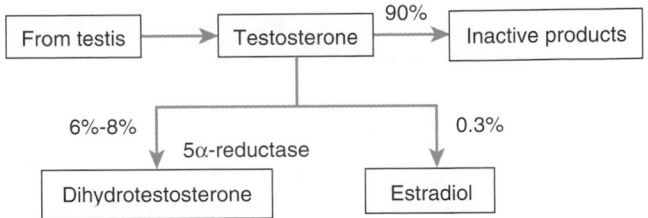

FIGURE 34-18 Testosterone and Conversion to Dihydrotestosterone (DHT).

cancer.[87] However, the final fate of PIN is unknown, including the possibilities of latency, invasion, and even regression. The current working model of prostate carcinogenesis suggests that repeated cycles of injury and cell death occur to the prostate epithelium as a result of damage (i.e., from oxidative stress) from inflammatory responses.[88] The direct injury is hypothesized as a response to infections; autoimmune disease; circulating carcinogens or toxins, or both, from the diet; or urine that has refluxed into the prostate (see Figure 34-15). The resultant manifestation of this injury is focal atrophy or prostate intraepithelial atrophy (PIA). Biologic responses cause an increase in proliferation and a massive increase in epithelial cells that possess a phenotype intermediate between basal cells and mature luminal cells (Figure 34-19).[88] In a small subset of cells, some may contain "stem cell" or tumor-initiating properties and telomere shortening (see Chapter 10). A subset of PIN cells may activate telomerase enzyme, causing the cells to become immortal.[89] Molecular genetic and epigenetic changes can increase genetic instability that might progress to high-grade PIN and early prostate cancer formation. This model of prostate carcinogenesis needs much more research.

Stromal environment. The prostate gland is composed of secretory luminal epithelium, basal epithelium, neuroendocrine cells, and various cell types comprising supportive tissue or stroma. **Stroma,** or tissue microenvironment, produces autocrine/paracrine factors as well as structural supporting molecules that help regulate normal cell behavior and organ homeostasis.[90] Stromal components in the tumor microenvironment are important contributions to tumor progression and metastasis.[91] Reciprocal interactions between tumor cells and stromal components influence the metastatic, dormancy-related, and stem cell–like potential of tumor cells.[92] The stromal compartment of the tumor is complex and includes inflammatory/immune cells, vascular endothelial cells, pericytes, fibroblasts, adipocytes, and components of the extracellular matrix.[91,93] Tumor-infiltrating inflammatory cells release a host of growth factors, chemokines, cytokines, and proinvasive matrix-degrading enzymes to promote tumor growth and progression.[91] Angiogenesis occurs in response to factors secreted from tumor cells, resulting in continued growth and progression. Adipocytes in the tumor microenvironment produce adipokines, which are important for tumor growth.[91] **Fibroblasts** in the tumor microenvironment provide the structural framework of the stroma; they remain quiet or dormant, but proliferate during wound healing, inflammation, and cancer.[91] Tumor cells release paracrine factors that activate fibroblasts to become "cancer-associated fibroblasts" (CAFs). CAFs secrete factors that modulate tumor growth and modify the stroma to enhance metastasis and dampen responses to anticancer therapies.[91] These findings suggest that alteration in the prostate microenvironment with therapeutic agents and approaches—in particular, natural products such as berberine, resveratrol, onionin A, epigallocatechin gallate, genistein, curcumin, naringenin, desoxyrhapontigenin, piperine, and zerumbone—warrants further investigation to target the tumor microenvironment for the treatment and prevention of cancer.[93]

Epithelial-mesenchymal transition (EMT) was first described in embryonic development, and is observed in a number of solid tumors[94]

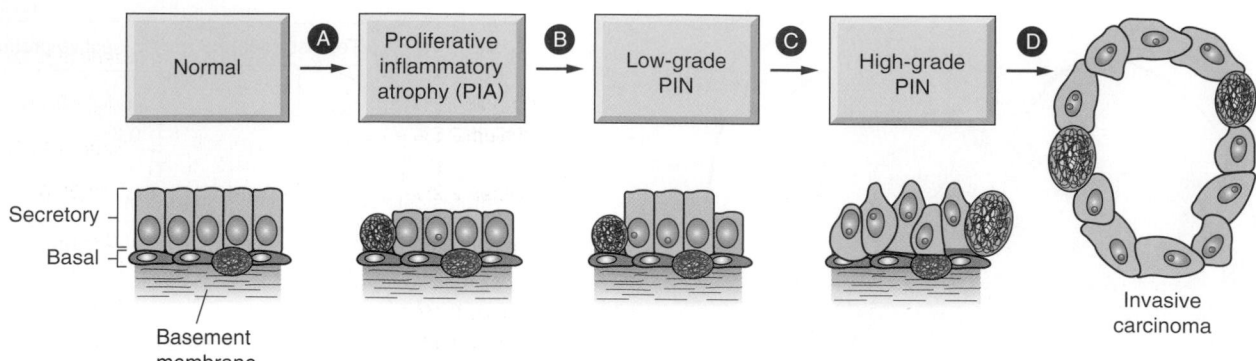

FIGURE 34-19 Cellular and Molecular Model of Early Prostate Neoplasia Progression. A, This stage includes infiltration of lymphocytes, macrophages, and neutrophils caused by repeated infections, dietary factors, urine reflux, injury, onset of autoimmunity (which triggers inflammation), and wound healing. **B,** Epigenetic alterations mediate telomere shortening. **C,** Genetic instability and accumulation of genetic alterations. **D,** Continued proliferation of genetically unstable cells leading to cancer progression. *PIN,* Prostatic intraepithelial neoplasia.

(see Chapter 10). Cells that undergo EMT become more migratory and invasive and gain access to vascular vessels.[95] Numerous studies have shown that these transition states (EMT and mesenchymal-epithelial transition [MET]) are a consequence of tumor-stromal interactions.[95,96] Investigators studying prostate cancer cells in vitro correlated EMT with increased growth, migration, and invasion.[97] These investigators demonstrated that the microenvironment is a critical site for the transition of human prostate cancer cells from epithelial to mesenchymal structure, resulting in increased metastatic potential for bone and adrenal gland.[97]

Prostate cancer is known to be diverse and composed of multiple genetically distinct cancer cell clones. Recent studies, however, indicate that most metastatic cancers arise from a single precursor cancer cell.[98]

From all of these observations, the following multifactorial general hypothesis of prostate carcinogenesis emerges: (1) androgens act as strong tumor promoters through androgen receptor–mediated mechanisms to enhance the carcinogenic activity of strong endogenous DNA toxic carcinogens, including reactive estrogen metabolites and estrogen, and prostate-generated reactive oxygen species; (2) reciprocal interactions between tumor cells and the stromal microenvironment promote prostate cancer pathogenesis; and (3) possibly unknown environmental-lifestyle carcinogens may contribute to prostate cancer. All of these factors are modulated by diet and genetic determinants, such as hereditary susceptibility genes and polymorphic genes, which encode receptors and enzymes involved in the metabolism and action of steroid hormones.[57]

The most common sites of distant metastasis are the lymph nodes, bones, lungs, liver, and adrenals. The pelvis, lumbar spine, femur, thoracic spine, and ribs are the most common sites of bone metastasis. Local extension is usually posterior, although late in the disease the tumor may invade the rectum or encroach on the prostatic urethra and cause bladder outlet obstruction (Figure 34-20). The spread of cancer through blood vessels is illustrated in Figure 34-21.

CLINICAL MANIFESTATIONS   Prostatic cancer often causes no symptoms until it is far advanced. The first manifestations of disease are those of bladder outlet obstruction: slow urinary stream, hesitancy, incomplete emptying, frequency, nocturia, and dysuria. Unlike the symptoms of obstruction caused by BPH, the symptoms of obstruction caused by prostatic cancer are progressive and do not remit. Local extension of prostatic cancer can obstruct the upper urinary tract ureters as well. Rectal obstruction also may occur, causing the

individual to experience large bowel obstruction or difficulty in defecation. Symptoms of late disease include bone pain at sites of bone metastasis, edema of the lower extremities, enlargement of lymph nodes, liver enlargement, pathologic bone fractures, and mental confusion associated with brain metastases. Prostatic cancer and its treatment can affect sexual functioning.

EVALUATION AND TREATMENT   Screening for prostatic cancer includes digital rectal examination (DRE) and prostate-specific antigen (PSA) blood tests. There is lack of evidence, however, whether screening with PSA or DRE reduces mortality from prostate cancer.[99] It is unclear if detection of prostate cancer at an early stage leads to any change in the natural history or outcome.[99] Observational studies in some countries show a trend toward lower mortality, but the relationship between the intensity and trends of screening is not clear and the associations with screening are inconsistent.[99] The observed trends may be a result of screening or improved treatment. Two randomized trials show no effect on mortality through 7 years and are inconsistent beyond 7 to 10 years.[100] Strong evidence shows implementation of PSA or DRE detects some prostate cancers that would never have caused significant clinical problems.[99] These screening tests lead to some degree of overtreatment. The screening tests can harm patients, including radical prostatectomy and radiation therapy that lead to irreversible side effects in many men.[99] The most common side effects are erectile dysfunction and urinary incontinence. The screening process can cause considerable anxiety, especially in men who have a prostate biopsy but no identified prostate cancer. Screening can lead to biopsies, which are associated with complications including fever, pain, hematuria, hematospermia, positive urine cultures for bacteria, and, rarely, sepsis. About 20% to 70% of men who had no problems before radical prostatectomy or external-beam radiation therapy will have reduced sexual function or urinary problems, or both.

Prostate cancer usually grows very slowly and is predominantly a tumor of older men with the median age at diagnosis of 72 years.[99] Until recently, many physicians and organizations encouraged yearly PSA screening for men beginning at age 50; however, with more understanding about the benefits and detriments, a number of organizations have cautioned men against routine population screening (Figure 34-22). Some organizations continue to recommend PSA screening. Some tumors found through PSA screening do not cause symptoms, grow slowly, and are unlikely to threaten a man's life. The PSA screening test often suggests that prostate cancer may be present when there

FIGURE 34-20 Carcinoma of Prostate. A, Schematic of carcinoma of the prostate. **B,** Carcinoma of the prostate extending into the rectum and urinary bladder. (**B** from Damjanov I, Linder J, editors: *Pathology: a color atlas,* St Louis, 2000, Mosby.)

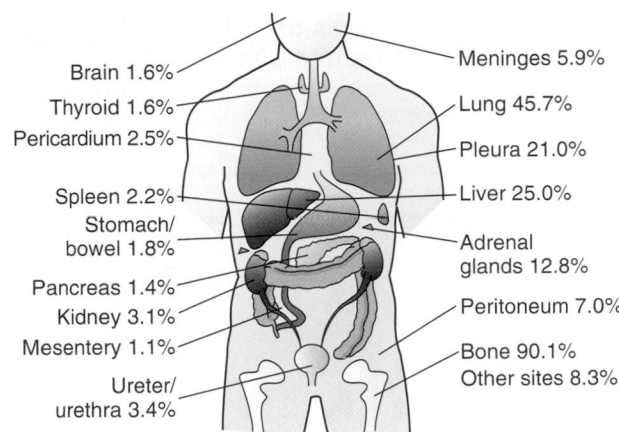

FIGURE 34-21 Distribution of Hematogenous Metastases in Prostate Cancer. Study of 556 individuals with metastatic prostate cancer. (Adapted from Budendorf L et al: *Hum Pathol* 31:578, 2000.)

is no cancer. This is called a "false positive" result. False positive results lead to unnecessary follow-up tests. Detecting these tumors is called overdiagnosis.

Across age ranges, black men and men with a family history of prostate cancer have an increased risk of developing and dying of prostate cancer. Black men are approximately twice as likely to die of prostate cancer compared with men of other races in the United States, and the reason for this disparity is unknown. Black men represent a very small minority of participants in randomized clinical trials of screening and thus no firm conclusions can be made about the balance of benefits and harms of PSA-based screening in this population. As such, it is questionable practice to selectively recommend PSA-based screening for black men in the absence of data that support a more favorable balance of risks and benefits.[48] Because of this "over-treatment" phenomenon, active surveillance with delayed intervention

is gaining traction as a viable management approach in contemporary practice.

Treatment of prostatic cancer depends on the stage of the neoplasm, the anticipated effects of treatment; and the age, general health, and life expectancy of the individual. Options include no treatment; surgical treatments, such as total prostatectomy, transurethral resection of the prostate (TURP), or cryotherapy; nonsurgical treatments, such as radiation therapy, hormone therapy, or chemotherapy; watchful waiting; and any combination of these treatment modalities.[48] In addition, new approaches are using immunotherapy. Palliative treatment is aimed at relieving urinary, bladder outlet, or colon obstruction; spinal cord compression; and pain. Box 34-7 shows staging for prostate cancer. Prognosis and survival rates have improved steadily over the past 50 years. Over the past 25 years, the 5-year relative survival rate for all stages combined has increased from 68% to almost 100%. According to the most recent data, 10- and 15-year relative survival rates are 98% and 94%, respectively.[1]

Stress incontinence can occur after surgery and mild urge incontinence can occur after radiation therapy. Prostate cancer and its treatment can affect sexual functioning. Sensation of orgasm is not usually affected, but smaller amounts of ejaculate will be produced or men may experience a "dry" ejaculate because of retrograde ejaculation.

Sexual Dysfunction

In males, the normal sexual response involves erection, emission, and ejaculation. Sexual dysfunction is the impairment of any or all of these processes and can be caused by various physiologic, psychologic, and emotional factors.

Until the late 1970s, most cases of male sexual dysfunction were considered psychogenic. Now there is evidence that 89% to 90% of cases involve organic factors and include (1) vascular, endocrine, and neurologic disorders; (2) chronic disease, including renal failure and diabetes mellitus; (3) penile diseases and penile trauma; and (4) iatrogenic factors, such as surgery and pharmacologic therapies. Most of these disorders cause erectile dysfunction (ED).[101]

PATHOPHYSIOLOGY Sexual dysfunction can have a specific physiologic cause, can be associated with many chronic diseases and their treatment, or may be related to low energy levels, stress, or depression. For example, vascular disease may cause impotence, and endocrine disorders or conditions that cause decreased testosterone levels or testicular atrophy can diminish sexual functioning or libido. In addition, neurologic disorders and spinal cord injuries can interfere with

Distribution of metastases labels:
Brain 1.6%
Thyroid 1.6%
Pericardium 2.5%
Spleen 2.2%
Stomach/bowel 1.8%
Pancreas 1.4%
Kidney 3.1%
Mesentery 1.1%
Ureter/urethra 3.4%
Meninges 5.9%
Lung 45.7%
Pleura 21.0%
Liver 25.0%
Adrenal glands 12.8%
Peritoneum 7.0%
Bone 90.1%
Other sites 8.3%

Benefits and Harms of PSA Screening for Prostate Cancer

1,000 men ages 55–69 screened every 1–4 years for 10 years with a PSA test

1,000 men screened

👤 = 10 men

Out of these:

100–120
Get false-positive results that may cause anxiety and lead to biopsy (possible side effects of biopsies include serious infections, pain, and bleeding).

110
Get a prostate cancer diagnosis.

Out of these:

At least 50
Will have treatment complications, such as infections, sexual dysfunction, or bladder or bowel control problems.

4–5
Die from prostate cancer (5 die among men who do not get screened).

0–1
Death from prostate cancer is avoided.

FIGURE 34-22 Benefits and Harms of PSA Screening for Prostate Cancer. The U.S. Preventive Services Task Force (USPSTF) recommends against PSA-based screenings for prostate cancer (grade D recommendation). (Adapted from USPSTF Recommendation Statement, Annals of Internal Medicine, 2012.)

sympathetic, parasympathetic, and CNS mechanisms required for erection, emission, and ejaculation.

Drug-induced sexual dysfunction consists of decreased desire, decreased erectile ability, or decreased ejaculatory ability. Alcohol and other CNS depressants, antihypertensives, antidepressants, antihistamines, and hormonal preparations are commonly used drugs that affect sexual functioning. Other pharmacologic agents may diminish the quality or quantity of sperm or cause priapism.

CLINICAL MANIFESTATIONS AND TREATMENT Evaluation of sexual dysfunction includes a thorough history and physical examination. Particular attention is given to drug history and examination of the genitalia, prostate, and nervous system. Basic laboratory tests are used to identify the presence of endocrinopathies or other underlying disorders that can cause dysfunction. Psychologic evaluation is indicated for younger men with a sudden onset of sexual dysfunction or for men of any age who can achieve but not maintain an erection. If no physiologic

cause is found and the condition does not improve with psychotherapy, the man is referred for further investigation of organic causes.

Treatments for organic sexual dysfunction include both medical and surgical approaches. The advent of phosphodiesterase type 5 inhibitors (PDE5i) has revolutionized the erectile dysfunction (ED) treatment landscape and provided effective, minimally invasive therapies to restore male sexual function. The original PDE5i, Viagra (sildenafil), has created much enthusiasm over its ability to help a man maintain an erection. For a small percentage of men (1%), however, this improvement in sexual function is accompanied by heart attacks and death. Whether these effects are the result of sexual performance or Viagra has been controversial. Research has shown that Viagra increases blood concentrations of the enzyme cGMP-dependent protein kinase G (PKG), which increases blood flow to the penis. PKG, however, plays a dual role: first, it increases platelet aggregation; and then, minutes later, it decreases clot size. The initial clot could cause some men with heart disease to experience cardiac arrest.

Currently available PDE5i medications in the United States include sildenafil, vardenafil, tadalafil, and avanafil, each of which has unique side effect profiles. For instance, sildenafil is associated with (in addition to the previously mentioned cardiac issues) an increased rate of visual changes, vardenafil with QT prolongation, and tadalafil with lower back pain.[102] Nonsurgical approaches include correction of underlying disorders, particularly drug-induced dysfunction and endocrinopathy-related (e.g., reduced testosterone level associated with chronic renal failure) dysfunction. Use of vasodilators and cessation of smoking can benefit individuals with vasculogenic erectile dysfunction. Surgical approaches include penile implants, penile revascularization, and correction of other anatomic defects contributing to sexual dysfunction.

Impairment of Sperm Production and Quality

Spermatogenesis requires adequate secretion of follicle-stimulating hormone (FSH) and luteinizing hormone (LH) by the pituitary and sufficient secretion of testosterone by the testes. Inadequate secretion of gonadotropins may be caused by numerous alterations (e.g., hypothyroidism, hyperadrenocortisolism, hyperprolactinemia, or hypogonadotropic hypogonadism). In the absence of adequate gonadotropin levels, the Leydig cells are not stimulated to secrete testosterone, and sperm maturation is not promoted in the Sertoli cells. Spermatogenesis also depends on an appropriate response by the testes. Defects in testicular response to the gonadotropins result in decreased secretion of testosterone and inhibin B and occur as a result of normal feedback mechanisms and high levels of circulating gonadotropins. In the absence of adequate testosterone levels, spermatogenesis is impaired. Newer studies demonstrate the importance of inhibin B as a valuable marker of the competence of Sertoli cells and spermatogenesis.[25,103] Impaired spermatogenesis also can be caused by testicular trauma, infection, atrophy of the testes, systemic illness involving high fever, ingestion of various drugs, exposure to environmental toxins, and cryptorchidism.

Fertility is adversely affected if spermatogenesis is normal but the sperm are chromosomally or morphologically abnormal or are produced in insufficient quantities. Chromosomal abnormalities are caused by genetic factors and by external variables, such as exposure to radiation or toxic substances. Because the Y chromosome plays a key role in testis determination and control of spermatogenesis, understanding how the genes interact can elucidate exact causes of infertility. The most common mutations are microdeletion of the Y chromosome (AZ [azoospermia] a, b, and c).[104] Research related to mapping the critical genes and gene pathways is the current focus of male infertility. Common mechanisms may be involved in infertility and testicular cancer. In utero environmental exposure to endocrine disruptors

BOX 34-7   Staging for Prostate Cancer

Stage I

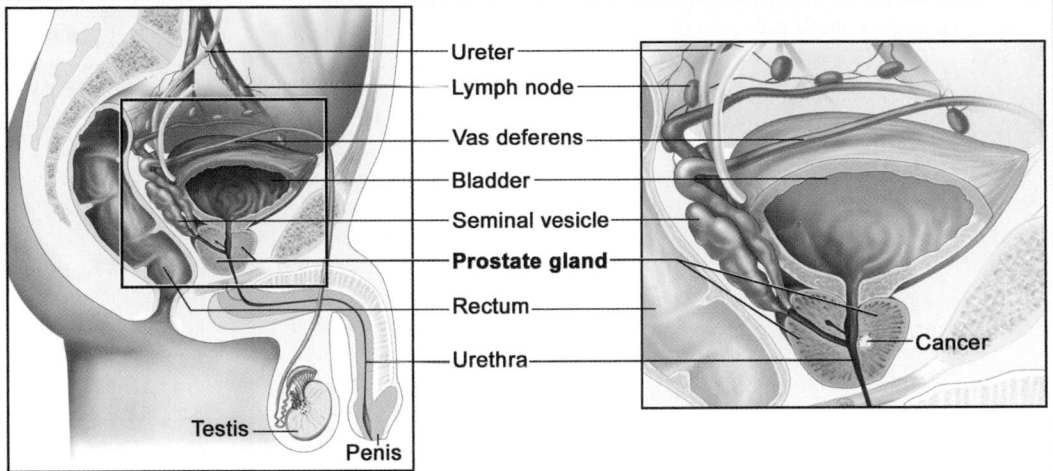

In stage I, cancer is found in the prostate only. The cancer:
- Is found by performing a needle biopsy (done for a high PSA level) or by examining a small amount of tissue during surgery for other reasons (such as benign prostatic hyperplasia). The PSA level is lower than 10 and the Gleason score is 6 or lower; *or*
- Is found on half or less of one lobe of the prostate. The PSA level is lower than 10 and the Gleason scores is 6 or lower; *or*
- Cannot be felt during a digital rectal exam and cannot be seen in imaging tests. Cancer is found in half or less of one lobe of the prostate. The PSA level and the Gleason score are not known.

Stage II
In stage II, cancer is more advanced than in stage I, but has not spread outside the prostate. Stage II is divided into stages IIA and IIB.

Stage IIA
- Is found by performing a needle biopsy (done for a high PSA level) or by examining a small amount of tissue during surgery for other reasons (such as benign prostatic hyperplasia). The PSA level is lower than 20 and the Gleason score is 7; *or*
- Is found by performing a needle biopsy (done for a high PSA level) or by examining a small amount of tissue during surgery for other reasons (such as benign prostatic hyperplasia). The PSA level is at least 10 but lower than 20 and the Gleason score is 6 or lower; *or*
- Is found in half or less of one lobe of the prostate. The PSA level is at least 10 but lower than 20 and the Gleason score is 6 or lower; *or*
- Is found in half or less of one lobe of the prostate. The PSA level is lower than 20 and the Gleason score is 7; *or*
- Is found in more than half of one lobe of the prostate.

Stage IIB
- Is found on opposite sides of the prostate. The PSA can be any level and the Gleason score can range from 2 to 10; *or*
- Cannot be felt during a digital rectal examination and cannot be seen in imaging tests. The PSA level is 20 or higher and the Gleason score can range from 2 to 10; *or*
- Cannot be felt during a digital rectal examination and cannot be seen in imaging tests. The PSA can be any level and the Gleason score is 8 or higher.

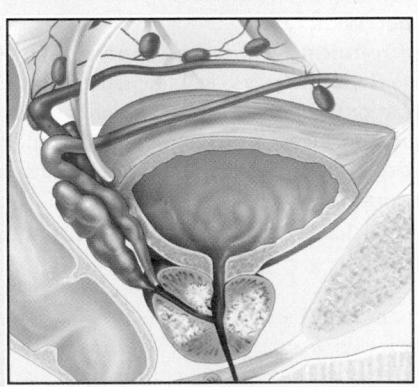

Continued

BOX 34-7 Staging for Prostate Cancer—cont'd

Stage III

- In stage III, cancer has spread beyond the outer layer of the prostate and may have spread to the seminal vesicles. The PSA can be any level and the Gleason score can range from 2 to 10.

Stage IV

In stage IV, the PSA can be any level and the Gleason score can range from 2 to 10. Also, cancer:

- Has spread beyond the seminal vesicles to nearby tissue or organs, such as the rectum, bladder, or pelvic wall; *or*
- May have spread to the seminal vesicles or to nearby tissue or organs, such as the rectum, bladder, or pelvic wall. Cancer has spread to nearby lymph nodes; *or*
- Has spread to distant parts of the body, which may include lymph nodes or bones. Prostate cancer often spreads to the bones.

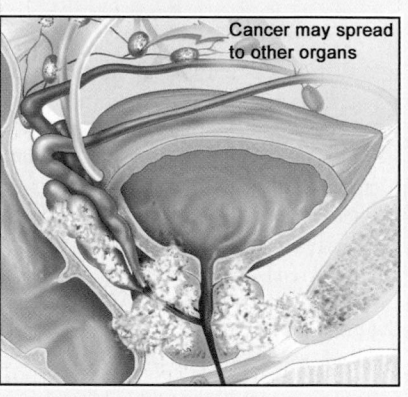

Cancer may spread to other organs

Data from National Cancer Institute: *PDQ® prostate cancer treatment,* Bethesda, Md, 2015, Author. Updated April 16, 2015. Available at: http://cancer.gov/cancertopics/pdq/treatment/prostate/Patient. Accessed May 10, 2015. Figures © Terese Winslow.

modulates the genetic makeup of the gonad and may result in both infertility and testicular cancer.[25]

Sperm motility also may affect fertility. Motility appears to be affected by the characteristics of the semen. Dysfunction of the prostate, excessive viscosity of the semen, presence of drugs or toxins in the semen, and presence of antisperm antibodies are associated with impaired sperm motility. However, new data show that motile density may not be a good indicator of infertility.[105] Approximately 17% of infertile males have antisperm antibodies in their semen. These antibodies may be (1) cytotoxic antibodies, which attack sperm and reduce their number in the semen; or (2) sperm-immobilizing antibodies, which impair sperm motility and reduce their ability to traverse the endocervical canal.

Treatment for impaired spermatogenesis involves correcting any underlying disorders, avoiding radiation and possibly electromagnetic radiation (hypothesis from cell phones) and toxins, and using hormones to enhance spermatogenesis. In addition, semen can be modified to improve sperm motility; modifications are followed by artificial insemination.

✓ QUICK CHECK 34-4

1. What is the current understanding of hormones in the pathophysiology of prostate cancer?
2. Why is the worldwide variation of prostate cancer incidence important?
3. Describe what is meant by prostate cancer cell and stromal interactions for carcinogenesis.
4. What causes impaired spermatogenesis?

DISORDERS OF THE MALE BREAST

Gynecomastia

Gynecomastia is the overdevelopment of breast tissue in a male. Gynecomastia accounts for approximately 85% of all masses that develop in the male breast and affects 32% to 40% of the male population. If only one breast is involved, it is typically the left. Incidence is greatest among adolescents and men older than 50 years.

Gynecomastia results from hormonal alterations, which may be idiopathic or caused by systemic disorders, drugs, or neoplasms. Gynecomastia usually involves an imbalance of the estrogen/testosterone ratio. The normal estrogen/testosterone ratio can be altered in one of two ways. First, estrogen levels may be excessively high, although testosterone levels are normal. This is the case in drug-induced and tumor-induced hyperestrogenism. Second, testosterone levels may be extremely low, although estrogen levels are normal, as is the case in hypergonadism. Gynecomastia also can be caused by alterations in breast tissue responsiveness to hormonal stimulation. Breast tissue may have increased responsiveness to estrogen or decreased responsiveness to androgen. Alterations of responsiveness may cause many cases of idiopathic gynecomastia.

Besides puberty and aging, estrogen/testosterone imbalances are associated with hypogonadism, Klinefelter syndrome, and testicular neoplasms. Hormone-induced gynecomastia is usually bilateral. Pubertal gynecomastia is a self-limiting phenomenon that usually disappears within 4 to 6 months. Senescent gynecomastia usually regresses spontaneously within 6 to 12 months.

Systemic disorders associated with gynecomastia include cirrhosis of the liver, infectious hepatitis, chronic renal failure, chronic

CHAPTER 34 Alterations of the Male Reproductive System   877

obstructive lung disease, hyperthyroidism, tuberculosis, and chronic malnutrition. It may be that these disorders ultimately alter the estrogen/testosterone ratio, initiating the gynecomastia.

Gynecomastia is often seen in males receiving estrogen therapy, either in preparation for a gender-change operation or in the treatment of prostatic carcinoma. Other drugs that can cause gynecomastia include digitalis, cimetidine, spironolactone, reserpine, thiazide, isoniazid, ergotamine, tricyclic antidepressants, amphetamines, vincristine, and busulfan. Gynecomastia is usually unilateral in these instances.

Malignancies of the testes, adrenals, or liver can cause gynecomastia if they alter the estrogen/testosterone ratio. Pituitary adenomas and lung cancer also are associated with gynecomastia.

PATHOPHYSIOLOGY   The enlargement of the breast consists of hyperplastic stroma and ductal tissue. Hyperplasia results in a firm, palpable mass that is at least 2 cm in diameter and located beneath the areola.

EVALUATION AND TREATMENT   The diagnosis of gynecomastia is based on physical examination. Identification and treatment of the cause are likely to be followed by resolution of the gynecomastia. The man should be taught to perform breast self-examination and is reexamined at 6- and 12-month intervals if the gynecomastia persists.

Carcinoma

Breast cancer in males accounts for 0.26% of all male cancers and 1.1% of all breast cancers. About 2350 new cases of breast cancer in men were estimated in 2015.[1] Global incidence rates were generally less than 1 per 100,000 man-years, in contrast to much higher rates in females.[106] The highest incidence rate for male breast cancer (MBC) was Israel (1.24 per 100,000), and the lowest incidence rates for males (0.16 per 100,000) and females (18.0 per 100,000) were observed in Thailand.[106] It is seen most commonly after the age of 60 years, with the peak incidence between 60 and 69 years (men tend to be diagnosed at an older age than women). It has, however, been reported in males as young as 6 years old and in adolescents. Klinefelter syndrome is the strongest risk factor for developing male breast carcinoma. Other risk factors include germline mutation in *BRCA1* or *BRCA2*, but familial cases usually have *BRCA2* rather than *BRCA1* mutations.[107-109] Obesity increases the risk of MBC. Testicular disorders, including cryptorchidism, mumps, orchitis, and orchiectomy, are related to risk.[110] The relationship between these factors and the risk of disease is not clearly defined.

Recent data on the most frequent molecular subtypes of male breast cancer appear to be different than those for female breast cancers. Luminal A and luminal B are most common; and basal-like, unclassifiable triple-negative, and *HER2*-driven male breast cancers are rare.[111,112] Male breast tumors often resemble carcinoma of the breast in women (see p. 833). The majority of MBCs express estrogen and progesterone receptors. The malignant male breast lesion is usually a unilateral solid mass located near the nipple. Because the nipple is commonly involved, crusting and nipple discharge are typical clinical manifestations. Other findings include skin retraction, ulceration of the skin over the tumor, and axillary node involvement. Patterns of metastasis are similar to those in females.

The diagnosis of cancer is confirmed by biopsy. Because of delays in seeking treatment, male breast cancer tends to be advanced at the time of diagnosis and therefore is likely to have a poor prognosis. Treatment protocols are similar to those for female breast cancer, but endocrine therapy is used more often for males because a higher percentage of male tumors are hormone-dependent. The mainstay of treatment is modified mastectomy with axillary node dissection to assess stage and prognosis. Because 90% of tumors are hormonal

receptor positive, tamoxifen is standard adjuvant therapy. Orchiectomy is performed to treat metastatic disease. For metastatic disease, hormonal therapy is the main treatment but chemotherapy also can provide palliation.[107]

SEXUALLY TRANSMITTED DISEASES

Sexually transmitted diseases (STDs) are a variety of clinical syndromes and infections caused by pathogens that can be acquired and transmitted through sexual activity.[113] Sexually contracted infections affect approximately 20 million Americans per year,[114] half among young people ages 15 to 24, and account for about one third of the reproductive mortality in the United States[114] (Table 34-1). STDs can lead to severe reproductive health problems, for example infertility and ectopic pregnancy.[114] Untreated or undertreated chlamydial infections are the primary cause of preventable infertility and ectopic pregnancy. In addition to ectopic pregnancy and infertility, other complications of STDs include pelvic inflammatory disease (PID), chronic pelvic pain, neonatal morbidity and mortality, genital cancer, and epidemiologic synergy with HIV transmission (Table 34-2). Long-term sequelae of untreated or undertreated STDs may be disastrous and can affect a

TABLE 34-1 **Currently Recognized Sexually Transmitted Infections**	
Causal Microorganism	**Infection**
Bacteria	
Campylobacter	Campylobacter enteritis
Calymmatobacterium granulomatis	Granuloma inguinale
Chlamydia trachomatis	Urogenital infections; lymphogranuloma venereum
Polymicrobial	
Gardnerella vaginalis interaction with anaerobes (*Bacteroides* and *Mobiluncus* spp.) and genital mycoplasmas	Bacterial vaginosis
Haemophilus ducreyi	Chancroid
Mycoplasma	Mycoplasmosis
Neisseria gonorrhoeae	Gonorrhea
Shigella	Shigellosis
Treponema pallidum	Syphilis
Viruses	
Cytomegalovirus	Cytomegalic inclusion disease
Hepatitis B virus (HBV)	Hepatitis
Hepatitis C virus (HCV)	Hepatitis
Herpes simplex virus (HSV)	Genital herpes
Human immunodeficiency virus (HIV)	Acquired immunodeficiency syndrome (AIDS)
Human papillomavirus (HPV)	Condylomata acuminata, cervical dysplasia, and cervical cancer
Molluscum contagiosum virus	Molluscum contagiosum
Protozoa	
Entamoeba histolytica	Amebiasis; amebic dysentery
Giardia lamblia	Giardiasis
Trichomonas vaginalis	Trichomoniasis
Ectoparasites	
Phthirus pubis	Pediculosis pubis
Sarcoptes scabiei	Scabies
Fungus	
Candida albicans	Candidiasis

TABLE 34-2   Photographs of STDs and Precursors to STDs

Bacterial Sources

Gonococcal Infections

Symptomatic Gonococcal Urethritis.[a]

Endocervical Gonorrhea.[a]

Skin Lesions of Disseminated Gonococcal Infection.[a]

Bacterial Vaginosis

Vaginal Examination Showing Mild Bacterial Vaginosis.[a]

Syphilis

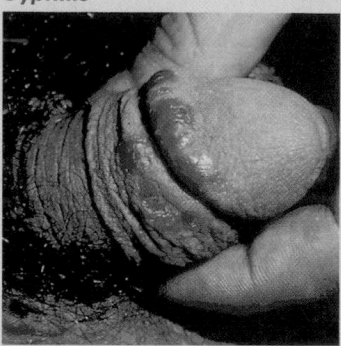

Erythematous Penile Plaques of Secondary Syphilis.[b]

Multiple Primary Syphilitic Chancres of Labia and Perineum. Courtesy Barbara Romanowski, MD.[a]

Papular Secondary Syphilis.[a]

Lymphogranuloma

"Groove Sign" in Man with Lymphogranuloma Venereum (LV).[b]

Chlamydial Infections

Beefy Red Mucosa in Chlamydial Infection.[a]

Chlamydial Epididymitis. Courtesy Richard E. Berger.[a]

Chlamydial Ophthalmia: Erythematous Conjunctiva in Infant.[a]

TABLE 34-2   **Photographs of STDs and Precursors to STDs—cont'd**

Viral Sources

Genital Herpes

Early Lesions of Primary Genital Herpes.[a]

Primary Vulvar Herpes.
Courtesy Barbara Romanowski, MD.[a]

Generalized Herpes Simplex in Patient with Atopic Dermatitis.
Courtesy of David Mandeville and Peter Lane, MD.[a]

Human Papillomavirus (HPV)

Human Papillomavirus (HPV) Infection of the Cervix.[b]

- Subclinical HPV infection
- Cervical os
- Cervical intraepithelial neoplasia
- Exophytic condyloma

Exophytic (Outward-Growing) Condyloma, Subclinical Human Papillomavirus (HPV) Infection, and High-Grade Cervical Intraepithelial Neoplasia (CIN).[b]

Condylomata Acuminata

Condylomata Acuminata: Vulva and Perineum.[a]

Condylomata Acuminata: Perianal.[a]

Condylomata Acuminata: Penile.[a]

Parasite Sources

Trichomonisasis

"Strawberry Cervix" Seen with Trichomoniasis.[a]

Scabies

Nodular Lesions of Scabies on Male Genitalia.[b]

Scabies of Palm with Secondary Pyoderma in Infant.[a]

Pediculosis Pubis (Phthirus pubis [crablouse])

Phthirus pubis Feeding on Its Host.[a]

Pubic Hair with Multiple Nits.[a]

[a]From Morse SA, Ballard RC, Holmes KK, et al: *Atlas of sexually transmitted diseases and AIDS,* ed 4, London, 2010, Elsevier.
[b]From Morse SA, Moreland AA, Holmes KK: *Atlas of sexually transmitted diseases and AIDS,* ed 2, London, 1996, Elsevier.

person's physical, emotional, and financial well-being. Treatment guidelines for STDs can be found on the CDC website (http://www.cdc.gov/std/tg2015/2015-poster-press.pdf).

Anyone can become infected with an STD, but young people and gay and bisexual men are at greatest risk.[114] Young people between the ages of 15 to 24 years continue to have the highest reported rates of chlamydia and gonorrhea compared with other groups. Both young men and women are heavily affected by STDs, but young women have the most serious long-term health consequences. Undiagnosed STDs cause 24,000 women to become infertile each year.[114] Men who have sex with men (MSM) account for about 75% of all primary and secondary syphilis cases. Primary and secondary syphilis are the most infectious stages of the disease and, if not treated adequately, can lead to visual impairment and stroke.[114] Syphilis infection raises the risk of acquiring and transmitting HIV infection. Half of MSM with syphilis also are infected with HIV.[114]

Individual risk behaviors, such as higher numbers of lifetime sex partners and environmental, social, and cultural factors, contribute to health disparities of MSM, for example, difficulty accessing health care. Homophobia and stigma also can make it difficult for gay and bisexual men to find culturally-sensitive and appropriate care and treatment.[114] STD screening is critical. It is recommended that women who are sexually active and younger than 25 years of age or have multiple sex partners annual chlamydia and gonorrhea be tested. A woman should request syphilis, HIV, chlamydia, and hepatitis B testing early in her pregnancy. These tests also should be requested if a woman has a new or multiple sex partners.[114] Recommended tests include syphilis, chlamydia, gonorrhea, and HIV once a year for gay, bisexual, or other men who have sex with men. More frequent testing is recommended for men at high risk.

> ✔ **QUICK CHECK 34-5**
> 1. What is the cause of male gynecomastia?
> 2. What are the risk factors for male breast cancer?
> 3. What factors increase the incidence of STDs?
> 4. What are the serious long-term health consequences of STDs for young women?
> 5. What are the long-term health consequences for MSM who acquire syphilis?

■ DID YOU UNDERSTAND?

Alterations of Sexual Maturation

1. Sexual maturation, or puberty, should begin in boys between the ages of 9 and 14 years.
2. Delayed puberty is the onset of sexual maturation after these ages; precocious puberty is the onset before these ages. Treatment depends on the cause.

Disorders of the Male Reproductive System

1. Disorders of the urethra include urethritis (infection of the urethra) and urethral strictures (narrowing or obstruction of the urethral lumen caused by scarring).
2. Most cases of urethritis result from sexually transmitted pathogens. Urologic instrumentation, foreign body insertion, trauma, or an anatomic abnormality can cause urethral inflammation with or without infection.
3. Urethritis causes urinary symptoms, including a burning sensation during urination (dysuria), frequency, urgency, urethral tingling or itching, and clear or purulent discharge.
4. The scarring that causes urethral stricture can be attributed to trauma or severe untreated urethritis.
5. Manifestations of urethral stricture include those of bladder outlet obstruction: urinary frequency and hesitancy, diminished force and caliber of the urinary stream, dribbling after voiding, and nocturia.
6. Phimosis and paraphimosis are penile disorders involving the foreskin (prepuce). In phimosis, the foreskin cannot be retracted over the glans. In paraphimosis, the foreskin is retracted and cannot be reduced (returned to its normal anatomic position over the glans). Phimosis is caused by poor hygiene and chronic infection and can lead to paraphimosis. Paraphimosis can constrict the penile blood vessels, preventing circulation to the glans.
7. Peyronie disease consists of fibrosis affecting the corpora cavernosa, which causes penile curvature during erection. Fibrosis prevents engorgement on the affected side, causing a lateral curvature that can prevent intercourse.
8. Priapism is a prolonged, painful erection that is not stimulated by sexual arousal. The corpora cavernosa (but not the corpus spongiosum) fill with blood that will not drain from the area, probably because of venous obstruction. Priapism is associated with spinal cord trauma, sickle cell disease, leukemia, and pelvic tumors. It can also be idiopathic.
9. Balanitis is an inflammation of the glans penis. It is associated with phimosis, inadequate cleansing under the foreskin, skin disorders, and pathogens (e.g., *Candida albicans*).
10. Cancer of the penis is rare. Penile carcinoma in situ tends to involve the glans; invasive carcinoma of the penis involves the shaft as well.
11. A varicocele is an abnormal dilation of the veins within the spermatic cord caused either by congenital absence of valves in the internal spermatic vein or by acquired valvular incompetence.
12. A hydrocele is a collection of fluid between the testicular and scrotal layers of the tunica vaginalis. Hydroceles can be idiopathic or caused by trauma or infection of the testes.
13. A spermatocele is a cyst located between the testis and epididymis that is filled with fluid and sperm.
14. Cryptorchidism is a congenital condition in which one or both testes fail to descend into the scrotum. Uncorrected cryptorchidism is associated with infertility and significantly increased risk of testicular cancer.
15. Testicular torsion is the rotation of a testis, which twists blood vessels in the spermatic cord. This interrupts the blood supply to the testis, resulting in edema and, if not corrected within 6 hours, necrosis and atrophy of testicular tissues.
16. Orchitis is an acute infection of the testes. Complications of orchitis include hydrocele and abscess formation.
17. Testicular cancer is the most common malignancy in males 15 to 35 years of age. Although its cause is unknown, high androgen levels, genetic predisposition, and history of cryptorchidism, trauma, or infection may contribute to tumorigenesis.
18. Spermatogenesis (sperm production by the testes) can be impaired by disruptions of the hypothalamic-pituitary-testicular axis that reduce testosterone secretion and by testicular trauma, infection, or atrophy from any cause. Sperm production is also impaired by neoplastic disease, cryptorchidism, or any factor that causes testicular temperature to rise (e.g., circulatory impairment, wearing tight clothing).

19. Epididymitis, an inflammation of the epididymis, is usually caused by a sexually transmitted pathogen that ascends through the vasa deferentia from an already infected urethra or bladder.

20. Benign prostatic hyperplasia (BPH), also called benign prostatic hypertrophy, is the enlargement of the prostate gland. This condition becomes symptomatic as the enlarging prostate compresses the urethra, causing symptoms of bladder outlet obstruction and urine retention.

21. Prostatitis is inflammation of the prostate. Prostatitis syndromes have been classified by the National Institutes of Health as (1) acute bacterial prostatitis (ABP), (2) chronic bacterial prostatitis (CBP), (3) chronic pelvic pain syndrome (CPPS), and (4) asymptomatic inflammatory prostatitis.

22. Prostate cancer is the most common cancer in American males, and the incidence varies greatly worldwide. Possible causes include genetic predisposition, environmental and dietary factors, inflammation, and alterations in levels of hormones (testosterone, dihydrotestosterone, and estradiol) and growth factors. Incidence is greatest among northwestern European and North American men (particularly blacks) older than 65 years.

23. Most cancers of the prostate are adenocarcinomas that develop at the periphery of the gland.

24. Sexual dysfunction in males can be caused by any physical or psychologic factor that impairs erection, emission, or ejaculation.

Disorders of the Male Breast

1. Gynecomastia is the overdevelopment (hyperplasia) of breast tissue in a male. It is first seen as a firm, palpable mass at least 2 cm in diameter and is located in the subareolar area.

2. Gynecomastia affects 32% to 40% of the male population. The incidence is greatest among adolescents and men older than 50 years of age.

3. Gynecomastia is caused by hormonal or breast tissue alterations that cause estrogen to dominate. These alterations can result from systemic disorders, drugs, neoplasms, or idiopathic causes.

4. Breast cancer is relatively uncommon in males, but it has a poor prognosis because men tend to delay seeking treatment until the disease is advanced. The incidence is greatest in men in their sixties.

5. Most breast cancers in men are estrogen receptor positive.

Sexually Transmitted Infections

1. Sexually transmitted diseases are infections contracted by intimate as well as sexual contact and include systemic infections, such as tuberculosis and hepatitis, which can spread to a sexual partner.

2. The etiology of an STI may be bacterial, viral, protozoan, parasitic, or fungal.

3. Although the majority of STIs can be treated, viral-induced STIs are considered incurable.

KEY TERMS

Acute bacterial prostatitis (ABP, category I), 864
Androgen receptor (AR) signaling, 868
Balanitis, 857
Benign prostatic hyperplasia (BPH, benign prostatic hypertrophy), 862
Bladder outflow obstruction, 864
Chemical epididymitis, 862
Chronic bacterial prostatitis (CBP, category II), 865

Chronic prostatitis/chronic pelvic pain syndrome (CP/CPPS, category III), 865
Complete precocious puberty, 855
Condyloma acuminatum, 857
Cryptorchidism, 859
Delayed puberty, 854
Ectopic testis, 859
Epididymitis, 862
Fibroblast, 871
Gynecomastia, 876

Hydrocele, 859
Intraprostatic conversion, 866
Nonbacterial prostatitis, 865
Orchitis, 860
Paraphimosis, 856
Penile intraepithelial neoplasm (PeIN), 858
Peyronie disease ("bent nail syndrome"), 856
Phimosis, 855
Precocious puberty, 854
Priapism, 857

Prostatic epithelial neoplasia (PIN), 871
Prostatitis, 864
Sexual dysfunction, 873
Spermatocele (epididymal cyst), 859
Stroma, 871
Testicular appendage, 860
Torsion of the testis, 860
Urethral stricture, 855
Urethritis, 855
Varicocele, 858

REFERENCES

1. American Cancer Society: *Cancer facts & figures 2015*, Atlanta, 2015, Author.
2. Jospe N: Disorders of pubertal development. In Osborn LM et al: *Pediatrics*, Philadelphia, 2005, Mosby.
3. Whittemore BJ et al: Endocrine and metabolic disorders. In Burns CE et al, editors: *Pediatric primary care*, St Louis, 2012, Saunders.
4. Foster DL et al: Programming of GnRH feedback controls timing puberty and adult reproductive activity, *Mol Cell Endocrinol* 254-255:109-119, 2006.
5. Euling SY et al: Examination of US puberty-timing data from 1940 to 1994 for secular trends: panel findings, *Pediatrics* 12(suppl 3):S172-S191, 2008.
6. Herman-Giddens ME et al: Secondary sexual characteristics in boys: data from the Pediatric Research in Office Settings Network, *Pediatrics* 130(5):e1058-e1068, 2012.
7. Kwiatkowska B et al: Reactive arthritis, *Pol Arch Med Wewn* 119(1-2):60-65, 2009.
8. Brill JR: Diagnosis and treatment of urethritis in men, *Am Fam Physician* 81(7):873-878, 2010.
9. McAninch JW: Disorders of the penis and male urethra. In McAninch JW, Lue TF, editors: *Smith and Tanagho's general urology*, ed 18, Norwalk, Conn, 2012, McGraw Hill Lange.
10. Anic GM, Giuliano AR: Genital HPV infection and related lesions in men, *Prev Med* 53(Suppl 1):S36-S41, 2011.
11. Centers for Disease Control and Prevention: *How many cancers are linked with HPV each year?* Atlanta, 2014, Author.
12. Gur S et al: Current status and new developments in Peyronie's disease: medical, minimally invasive and surgical treatment options, *Expert Opin Pharmacother* 12(6):931-944, 2011.
13. Downes MR: Review of in situ and invasive penile squamous cell carcinoma and associated non-neoplastic dermatological conditions, *J Clin Pathol* 68:333-340, 2015.
14. Chaux A, Cubilla AL: Advances in pathology of penile carcinoma, *Hum Pathol* 43:771-789, 2012.
15. American Cancer Society: *Penile cancer resource center*, 2015. Available at: www.cancer.org/cancer/penilecancer/index.
16. Trottler H, Burchell AN: Epidemiology of mucosal human papillomavirus infection and associated diseases, *Public Health Genomics* 12(5-6):291-307, 2009.
17. Blais N, Kassouf E: Managing advanced penile cancer in 2014, *Curr Opin Support Palliat Care* 8(3):241-249, 2014.
18. Letendre J et al: Penile cancer: what's new? *Curr Opin Support Palliat Care* 5(3):185-191, 2011.
19. Pagliaro LC et al: Neoadjuvant paclitaxel, ifosfamide, and cisplatin chemotherapy for metastatic penile cancer: a phase II study, *J Clin Oncol* 28:3851, 2010.
20. Zou B et al: Neoadjuvant therapy combined with a BMP regimen for treating penile cancer patients with lymph node metastasis: a retrospective study in China, *J Cancer Res Clin Oncol* 140(10):1733-1738, 2014.
21. Wampler SM, Llanes M: Common scrotal and testicular problems, *Prim Care* 37(3):613-626, 2010.
22. Chen SS: Differences in the clinical characteristics between young and elderly men with varicocele, *Int J Androl* 35(5):695-699, 2012.
23. Montgomery JS, Bloom DA: The diagnosis and management of scrotal masses, *Med Clin North Am* 95(1):235-244, 2011.

24. Davis JE, Silverman M: Scrotal emergencies, *Emerg Med Clin North Am* 29(3):469-484, 2011.

25. Walsh TJ, Smith JF: Male infertility. In McAninch JW, Lue TF, editors: *Smith and Tanagho's general urology*, ed 18, Norwalk, Conn, 2012, McGraw Hill Lange.

26. Günther P, Rübben I: The acute scrotum in childhood and adolescence, *Dtsch Arztebl Int* 109(25):449-457, 2012.

27. Rioja J et al: Adult hydrocele and spermatocele, *BJU Int* 107(11):1852-1864, 2011.

28. John Radcliffe Hospital Cryptorchidism Study Group: Cryptorchidism: a prospective study of 7500 consecutive male births, 1984–8, *Arch Dis Child* 67:892-899, 1992.

29. Jensen MS et al: Cryptorchidism and hypospadias in a cohort of 934,538 Danish boys: the role of birth weight, gestational age, body dimensions, and fetal growth, *Am J Epidemiol* 175(9):917-925, 2012.

30. Walsh TJ et al: Prepubertal orchiopexy for crytorchidism may be associated with lower risk of testicular cancer, *J Urol* 178(4 pt 1): 1440-1446, 2007.

31. Nguyen HT: Bacterial infections of the genitourinary tract. In McAninch JW, Lue TF, editors: *Smith and Tanagho's general urology*, ed 18, Norwalk, Conn, 2012, McGraw Hill Lange.

32. National Cancer Institute: *Testicular cancer incidence and mortality, 2014*. Available at: www.cancer.gov/cancertopics/pdq/treatment/testicular.

33. Raynor MC, Carson CC: Urinary infections in men, *Med Clin North Am* 95(1):43-54, 2011.

34. Trojian TH et al: Epididymitis and orchitis: an overview, *Am Fam Physician* 79(7):583-587, 2009.

35. Platz EA et al: Incidence and progression of lower urinary tract symptoms in a large prospective cohort of United States men, *J Urol* 188(2):496-501, 2012.

36. Timms BG, Hofkamp LE: Prostate development and growth in benign prostatic hyperplasia, *Differentiation* 82(4-5):173-183, 2011.

37. Ho CK, Habib FK: Estrogen and androgen signaling in the pathogenesis of BPH, *Nat Rev Urol* 8:29-41, 2011.

38. Nicholson TM, Ricke WA: Androgens and estrogens in benign prostatic hyperplasia: past, present and future, *Differentiation* 82(4-5):184-199, 2011.

39. Nicholson TM et al: Sex steroid receptor expression and localization in benign prostatic hyperplasia varies with tissue compartment, *Differentiation* 85:140-149. 2013.

40. Chughtai B et al: Inflammation and benign prostatic hyperplasia: clinical implications, *Curr Urol Rep* 12(4):274-277, 2011.

41. Bachmann A, de la Rosette J: *Benign prostatic hyperplasia and lower urinary tract symptoms in men*, New York, 2012, Oxford University Press.

42. Pearson R, Williams PM: Common questions about the diagnosis and management of benign prostatic hyperplasia, *Am Fam Physician* 90(11):769-774, 2014.

43. Schauer I, Madersbacher S: Medical treatment of lower urinary tract symptoms/benign prostatic hyperplasia: anything new in 2015, *Curr Opin Urol* 25(1):6-11, 2015.

44. Kapoor A: Benign prostatic hyperplasia (BPH) management in the primary care setting, *Can J Urol* 19(5 Suppl 1):10-17, 2012.

45. Touma NJ, Nickel JC: Prostatitis and chronic pelvic pain in men, *Med Clin North Am* 95:75-86, 2011.

46. Wagenlehner FM et al: Urinary tract infections and bacterial prostatitis in men, *Curr Opin Infect Dis* 27(1):97-101, 2014.

47. Karatas OF et al: Helicobacter pylori seroprevalence in patients with chronic prostatitis: a pilot study, *Scand J Urol Nephrol* 44(2):91-94, 2010.

48. Moyer VA, U.S. Preventive Services Task Force: Screening for prostate cancer: U.S. Preventive Services Task Force recommendation statement, *Ann Intern Med* 157(2):120-134, 2012.

49. Torre LA et al: Global cancer statistics, 2012, *CA Cancer J Clin* 65(2):87-108, 2015.

50. Ferlay J et al: Cancer incidence and mortality worldwide: sources, methods and major patterns in GLOBOCAN 2012, *Int J Cancer* 136(5):E359-E386, 2015.

51. Labbé DP et al: Role of diet in prostate cancer: the epigenetic link, *Oncogene* 2014 Dec 22. [Epub ahead of print.]

52. Allott EH et al: Obesity and prostate cancer: weighing the evidence, *Eur Urol* 63(5):800-809, 2013.

53. Tewari R et al: Diet, obesity, and prostate health: are we missing the link? *J Androl* 33(5):763-776, 2012.

54. Labrie F: Blockage of testicular and adrenal androgens in prostate cancer treatment, *Nat Rev Urol* 8:73-80, 2011.

55. Titus MA et al: Dominant-negative androgen receptor inhibition of intracrine androgen-dependent growth of castration-recurrent prostate cancer, *PLoS One* 7(1):e30192, 2012.

56. Bosland MC: Sex steroids and prostate carcinogenesis: integrated, multifactorial working hypothesis, *Ann N Y Acad Sci* 1089:168-176, 2006.

57. Bosland MC, Mahmoud AM: Hormones and prostate carcinogenesis: androgens and estrogens, *J Carcinog* 10:33, 2011.

58. Thompson IM et al: The influence of finasteride on the development of prostate cancer, *N Engl J Med* 349:215-224, 2003.

59. Ellem SJ, Risbridger GP: The dual, opposing roles of estrogen in the prostate, *Ann N Y Acad Sci* 1155:174-186, 2009.

60. Ganesh B et al: Risk factors for prostate cancer: a hospital-based case-control study from Mumbai, India, *Indian J Urol* 27(3):345-350, 2011.

61. van Leeuwen PJ et al: Critical assessment of prebiopsy parameters for predicting prostate cancer metastasis and mortality, *Can J Urol* 18(6): 6018-6024, 2011.

62. Köhler TS et al: Putative health risks associated with vasectomy, *Urol Clin North Am* 36(3):337-345, 2009.

63. MacLennan GT et al: The influence of chronic inflammation in prostatic carcinogenesis: a 5-year follow-up study, *J Urol* 176(3):1012-1016, 2006.

64. Jiang M et al: PPARγ: a molecular link between systemic metabolic disease and benign prostate hyperplasia, *Differentiation* 82:220-236, 2011.

65. Elkahwaji JE: The role of inflammatory mediators in the development of prostatic hyperplasia and prostate cancer, *Res Rep Urol* 5:1-10, 2012.

66. Lee C et al: Role of the adjacent stroma cells in prostate cancer development and progression: synergy between TGF-β and IGF signaling, *Biomed Res Int* 2014:502093, 2014.

67. Albright F et al: Significant evidence for a heritable contribution to cancer predisposition: a review of cancer familiality by site, *BMC Cancer* 12:138, 2012.

68. Akbari MR et al: The impact of a BRCA2 mutation on mortality from screen-detected prostate cancer, *Br J Cancer* 111(6):1238-1240, 2014.

69. Castro E, Eeles R: The role of BRCA1 and BRCA2 in prostate cancer, *Asian J Androl* 14(3):409-414, 2012.

70. Leongamornlert D et al: Germline BRCA1 mutations increase prostate cancer risk, *Br J Cancer* 106(10):1697-1701, 2012.

71. Van Neste L et al: The epigenetic promise for prostate cancer diagnosis, *Prostate* 72(11):1248-1261, 2012.

72. Lumen N et al: Screening and early diagnosis of prostate cancer: an update, *Acta Clin Belg* 67(4):270-275, 2012.

73. Mackinnon AC et al: Molecular biology underlying the clinical heterogeneity of prostate cancer: an update, *Arch Pathol Lab Med* 133(7):1033-1040, 2009.

74. Kumar V et al: *Robbins & Cotran pathologic basis of disease*, ed 9, Philadelphia, 2015, Elsevier/Saunders.

75. Bonkoff H, Berges R: The evolving role of oestrogens and their receptors in the development and progression of prostate cancer, *Eur Urol* 55:533-542, 2009.

76. Ellem SJ, Risbridger GP: Aromatase and regulating the estrogen:androgen ratio in the prostate gland, *J Steroid Biochem Mol Biol* 118(4-5):246-251, 2010.

77. Nellies JL et al: Estrogen action and prostate cancer, *Expert Rev Endocrinol Metab* 6(3):437-451, 2011.

78. Labrie A et al: Intracrinology: the basis for the rational design of endocrine therapy at all stages of prostate cancer, *Eur Urol* 24(Suppl 2):94-105, 1993.

79. Vander Griend DJ et al: Cell autonomous intracellular androgen signaling drives the growth of human prostate cancer-initiating cells, *Prostate* 70(1):90-99, 2010.

80. Ricke EA et al: Androgen hormone action in prostatic carcinogenesis: stromal androgen receptors mediate prostate cancer progression, malignant transformation and metastasis, *Carcinogenesis* 33(7):1391-1398, 2012.

81. Nakagawa H et al: Prostate cancer genomics, biology, and risk assessment through genome-wide association studies, *Cancer Sci* 103(4): 607-613, 2012.

82. Santen RJ et al: History of aromatase: saga of an important biological mediator and therapeutic target, *Endocr Rev* 30(4):343-375, 2009.

83. Risbridger GP et al: Breast and prostate cancer: more similar than different, *Nat Rev Cancer* 10(3):205-212, 2010.

84. Kawashima H, Nakatani T: Involvement of estrogen receptors in prostatic diseases, *Int J Urol* 19(6):512-522, 2012.

85. Yu Y et al: Progesterone receptor expression during prostate cancer progression suggests a role of this receptor in stromal cell differentiation, *Prostate* 75(10):1043-1050, 2015.

86. Setlur SR et al: Estrogen-dependent signaling in a molecularly distinct subclass of aggressive prostate cancer, *J Natl Cancer Inst* 100:815-825, 2008.

87. Epstein JI: The lower urinary tract and male genital system. In Kumar V et al, editors: *Robbins & Cotran pathologic basis of disease*, ed 8, Philadelphia, 2009, Saunders.

88. Taverna G et al: Inflammation and prostate cancer: friends or foe? *Inflamm Res* 64(5):275-286, 2015.

89. Marian CO, Shay JW: Prostate tumor initiating cells: a new target for telomerase inhibition therapy? *Biochim Biophys Acta* 1792:289-296, 2009.

90. Bianchi-Frias D et al: The effects of aging on the molecular and cellular composition of the prostate microenvironment, *PLoS* 5(9):e12501, 2010.

91. Feitelson MA et al: Sustained proliferation in cancer: mechanisms and novel therapeutic targets, *Semin Cancer Biol* 2015 Apr 16. [Epub ahead of print.]

92. Polyak K et al: Co-evolution of tumor cells and their microenvironment, *Trends Genet* 25(1):30-38, 2009.

93. Casey SC et al: Cancer prevention and therapy through the modulation of the tumor microenvironment, *Semin Cancer Biol* 2015 Apr 10. [Epub ahead of print.]

94. Thiery JP: Epithelial-mesenchymal transitions in tumor progression, *Nat Rev Cancer* 2(6):442-454, 2002.

95. Josson S et al: Tumor-stromal interaction influence radiation sensitivity in epithelial versus mesenchymal-like prostate cancer cell, *J Oncol* 2010: 2010.

96. Bhowmick NA, Moses HL: Tumor-stroma interactions, *Curr Opin Genet Develop* 15(1): 97-101, 2005.

97. Xu J et al: Prostate cancer metastasis: role of the host microenvironment in promoting epithelial to mesenchymal transition and increased bone adrenal gland metastasis, *Prostate* 66:1664-1673, 2006.

98. Liu W et al: Copy number analysis indicates monoclonal origin of lethal metastatic prostate cancer, *Nat Med* 15(5):559-565, 2009.

99. National Cancer Institute: *PDQ® prostate cancer treatment,* Bethesda, Md, 2015, Author. Date last modified April 2, 2015. Available at: www.cancer.gov/types/prostate/hp/prostate-treatment-pdq. Accessed May 20, 2015.

100. Ilic D et al: Screening for prostate cancer, *Cochrane Database Syst Rev* 1:CD004720, 2013.

101. Matsui H et al: Mini review: pathophysiology of erectile dysfunction, *Curr Drug Targets* 2015 Mar 9. [Epub ahead of print.]

102. Smith WB et al: PDE5 inhibitors: considerations for preference and long-term adherence, *Int J Clin Pract* 67(8):768-780, 2013.

103. Toulis KA et al: Inhibin B and anti-Mullerian hormone as markers of persistent spermatogenesis in men with non-obstructive azoospermia: a meta-analysis of diagnostic accuracy studies, *Hum Reprod Update* 16(6):713-724, 2010.

104. Zhang F et al: Clinical characteristics and treatment of azoospermia and severe oligospermia patients with Y-chromosome microdeletions, *Mol Reprod Dev* 80(11):908-915, 2013.

105. Check JH: The infertile male: diagnosis, *Clin Exp Obstet Gynecol* 33(3):133-139, 2006.

106. Ly D et al: An international comparison of male and female breast cancer incidence rates, *Int J Cancer* 132(8):1918-1926, 2012.

107. Gómez-Raposo C et al: Male breast cancer, *Cancer Treat Rev* 36(6):451-457, 2010.

108. Johansen Taber KA et al: Male breast cancer: risk factors, diagnosis, and management, *Oncol Rep* 24(5):1115-1120, 2010.

109. Ottini L et al: Male breast cancer, *Crit Rev Oncol Hematol* 73(2):141-155, 2010.

110. Zygogianni AG et al: Male breast carcinoma: epidemiology, risk factors and current therapeutic approaches, *Asian Pac J Cancer Prev* 13(1):15-19, 2012.

111. Kornegoor R et al: Molecular subtyping of male breast cancer by immunochemistry, *Mod Pathol* 25(3):398-404, 2012.

112. Sanchez-Munoz A et al: Male breast cancer: immunohistochemical subtypes and clinical outcome characterization, *Oncology* 83(4):228-233, 2012.

113. Centers for Disease Control and Prevention: Sexually transmitted diseases treatment guidelines, *MMWR Morb Mortal Wkly Rpt* 64(3) 1-140, 2015.

114. Centers for Disease Control and Prevention: *Fact sheet reported STDs in the United States 2013 national data for chlamydia, gonorrhea, and syphilis,* Atlanta, Ga, 2014, Author.

35

Structure and Function of the Digestive System

Sue E. Huether

CHAPTER OUTLINE

The digestive system includes the gastrointestinal tract and accessory organs of digestion: the salivary glands, liver, gallbladder, and exocrine pancreas (Figure 35-1). The digestive system breaks down ingested food, prepares it for uptake by the body's cells, absorbs fluid, and eliminates wastes. Food breakdown begins in the mouth with chewing and continues in the stomach, where food is churned and mixed with acid, mucus, enzymes, and other secretions. From the stomach, the fluid and partially digested food pass into the small intestine, where biochemical agents and enzymes secreted by the intestinal cells, liver, gallbladder, and exocrine pancreas break it down into absorbable components of proteins, carbohydrates, and fats. These nutrients pass through the walls of the small intestine into blood vessels and lymphatics that carry them to the liver for storage or further processing.

Ingested substances and secretions that are not absorbed in the small intestine pass into the large intestine, where fluid continues to be absorbed. Fluid wastes travel to the kidneys and are eliminated in the urine. Solid wastes pass into the rectum and are eliminated from the body through the anus Except for chewing, swallowing, and defecation of solid wastes, the movements of the digestive system (peristalsis) are all controlled by hormones and the autonomic nervous system. The autonomic innervation, both sympathetic and parasympathetic, is controlled by centers in the brain and by local stimuli that are mediated at plexuses (networks of nerve fibers) within the gastrointestinal walls. The gastrointestinal tract and gut microbiome provide important immune and protective functions. Aging can alter the structure and function of the gastrointestinal tract (see *Geriatric Considerations: Aging & the Gastrointestinal System*).

THE GASTROINTESTINAL TRACT

The gastrointestinal tract (alimentary canal) consists of the mouth, esophagus, stomach, small intestine, large intestine, rectum, and anus (see Figure 35-1). It carries out the following digestive processes:
1. Ingestion of food
2. Propulsion of food and wastes from the mouth to the anus
3. Secretion of mucus, water, and enzymes
4. Mechanical digestion of food particles
5. Chemical digestion of food particles
6. Absorption of digested food
7. Elimination of waste products by defecation
8. Immune and microbial protection against infection

Histologically, the gastrointestinal tract consists of four layers. From the inside out they are the mucosa, submucosa, muscularis, and serosa or adventitia. These concentric layers vary in thickness, and each layer has sublayers (Figure 35-2). A network of intrinsic nerves that controls mobility, secretion, sensation, and blood flow is located solely within the gastrointestinal tract and controlled by local and autonomic nervous system stimuli through the enteric (intramural) plexus located in different layers of the gastrointestinal walls (see Figure 35-2).

Mouth and Esophagus

The mouth is a reservoir for the chewing and mixing of food with saliva. There are 32 permanent teeth in the adult mouth, and they are important for speech and mastication. As food particles become smaller and move around in the mouth, the taste buds and olfactory nerves are continuously stimulated, adding to the satisfaction of eating.

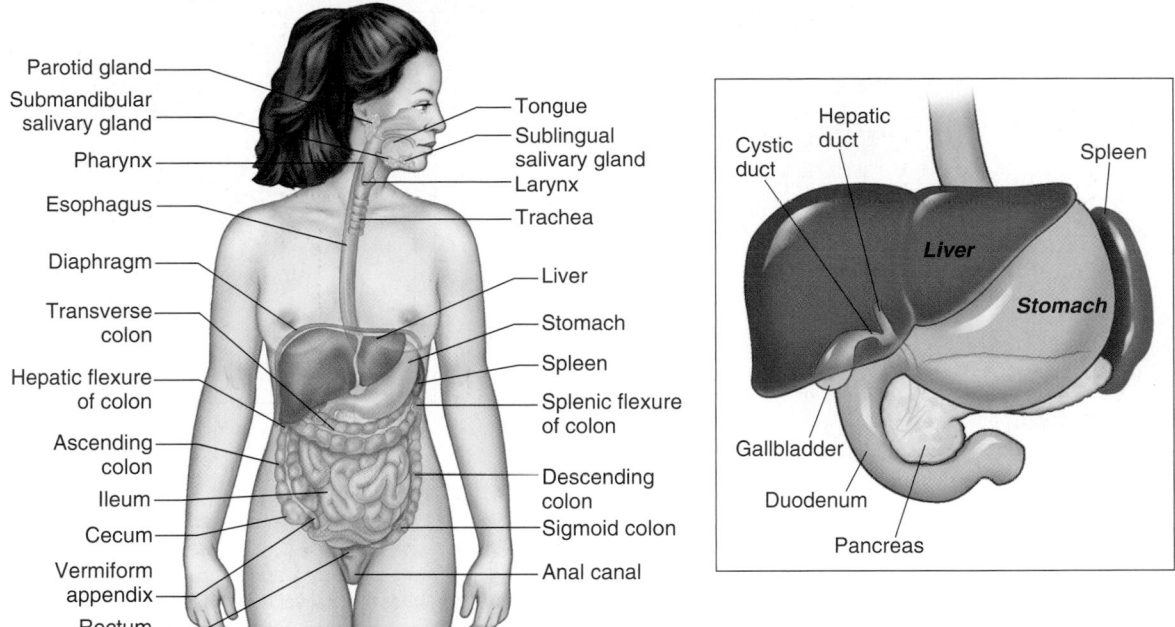

FIGURE 35-1 Structures of the Digestive System. (From Patton KT, Thibodeau GA: *The human body in health & disease,* ed 6, St Louis, 2014, Mosby.)

FIGURE 35-2 Wall of the Gastrointestinal Tract. The wall of the gastrointestinal tract is made up of four layers with a network of nerves between the layers. This generalized diagram shows a segment of the gastrointestinal tract. Note that the serosa is continuous with a fold of serous membrane called the *mesentery*. Note also that digestive glands may empty their products into the lumen of the gastrointestinal tract by way of ducts. (From Patton KT, Thibodeau GA: *Anatomy & physiology,* ed 9, St Louis, 2016, Mosby.)

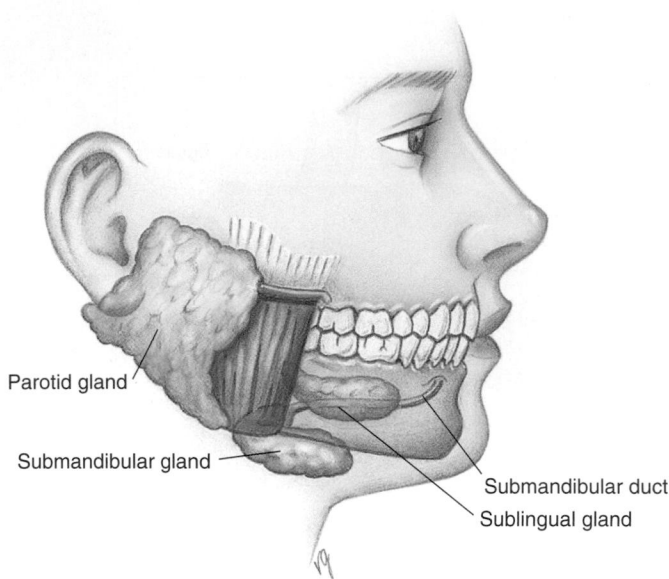

FIGURE 35-3 Salivary Glands. (From Gerdin J: *Health careers today*, ed 5, St Louis, 2012, Mosby.)

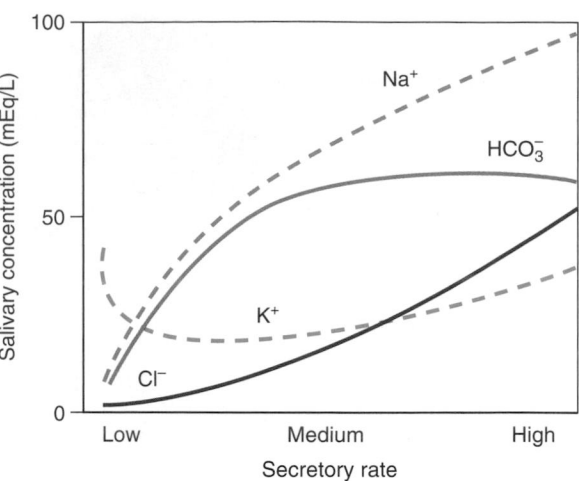

FIGURE 35-4 Salivary Electrolyte Concentrations and Flow Rate. Changes in concentrations of sodium (Na^+), potassium (K^+), chloride (Cl^-), and bicarbonate (HCO_3^-) increase flow rate of saliva. *Green line*, sodium; *orange line*, bicarbonate; *red line*, chloride; *blue line*, potassium. At low rates of salivary flow (i.e., between meals), sodium, chloride, and bicarbonate are reabsorbed in the collecting ducts of the salivary glands, and the saliva contains fewer of these electrolytes (i.e., is more hypotonic). At higher flow rates (i.e., stimulated by food), reabsorption decreases and saliva is hypertonic. By this mechanism, sodium, chloride, and bicarbonate are recycled until they are released to help with digestion and absorption.

The tongue's surface contains thousands of chemoreceptors, or taste buds, which can distinguish salty, sour, bitter, sweet, and savory (umami) tastes. Tastes and food odors help to initiate salivation and the secretion of gastric juice in the stomach.

Salivation

The three pairs of salivary glands—the submandibular, sublingual, and parotid glands (Figure 35-3)—secrete about 1 L of saliva per day. Saliva consists mostly of water with mucus, sodium, bicarbonate, chloride, potassium, and salivary α-amylase (ptyalin), an enzyme that initiates carbohydrate digestion in the mouth and stomach.

Both sympathetic and parasympathetic divisions of the autonomic nervous system control salivation. Cholinergic parasympathetic fibers stimulate the salivary glands, and atropine (an anticholinergic agent) inhibits salivation and makes the mouth dry. β-Adrenergic stimulation from sympathetic fibers also increases salivary secretion. The salivary gland secretion is not regulated by hormones.

The composition of saliva depends on the rate of secretion (Figure 35-4). Aldosterone can increase epithelial exchange of sodium for potassium, increasing sodium conservation and potassium excretion. The bicarbonate concentration of saliva sustains a pH of about 7.4, which neutralizes bacterial acids and prevents tooth decay. Saliva also contains mucin, immunoglobulin A (IgA), and other antimicrobial substances, which help prevent infection. Mucin provides lubrication. Exogenous fluoride (e.g., fluoride in drinking water) is also secreted in the saliva, providing additional protection against tooth decay.

Swallowing

The esophagus is a hollow, muscular tube approximately 25 cm long that conducts substances from the oropharynx to the stomach (see Figure 35-1). Swallowed food is moved to the stomach by peristalsis, the coordinated sequential contraction and relaxation of outer longitudinal and inner circular layers of muscles. The pharynx and upper third of the esophagus contain striated muscle (voluntary) that is directly innervated by skeletal motor neurons that control swallowing. The lower two thirds contain smooth muscle (involuntary) that is

innervated by preganglionic cholinergic fibers from the vagus nerve. The fibers are activated in a downward sequence and coordinated by the swallowing center in the medulla. Peristalsis is stimulated when afferent fibers distributed along the length of the esophagus sense changes in wall tension caused by stretching as food passes. The greater the tension, the greater the intensity of esophageal contraction. Occasionally, intense contractions cause pain similar to "heartburn" or angina.

Each end of the esophagus is opened and closed by a sphincter. The upper esophageal sphincter keeps air from entering the esophagus during respiration. The lower esophageal sphincter (cardiac sphincter) prevents regurgitation from the stomach and caustic injury to the esophagus.

Swallowing is coordinated primarily by the swallowing center in the medulla. During the oropharyngeal (voluntary) phase, the following steps occur:

1. Food is segmented into a bolus by the tongue and forced posteriorly toward the pharynx.
2. The superior constrictor muscle of the pharynx contracts so the food cannot move into the nasopharynx.
3. Respiration is inhibited, and the epiglottis slides down to prevent the food from entering the larynx and trachea.
   This entire sequence takes place in less than 1 second.
   The esophageal phase proceeds as follows:
1. The bolus of food enters the esophagus.
2. Waves of relaxation travel the esophagus, preparing for the movement of the bolus.
3. Peristalsis, the sequential waves of muscular contractions that travel down the esophagus, transports the food to the lower esophageal sphincter, which is relaxed at that point.
4. The bolus enters the stomach, and the sphincter muscles return to their resting tone.

This phase takes 5 to 10 seconds, with the bolus moving 2 to 6 cm/sec.

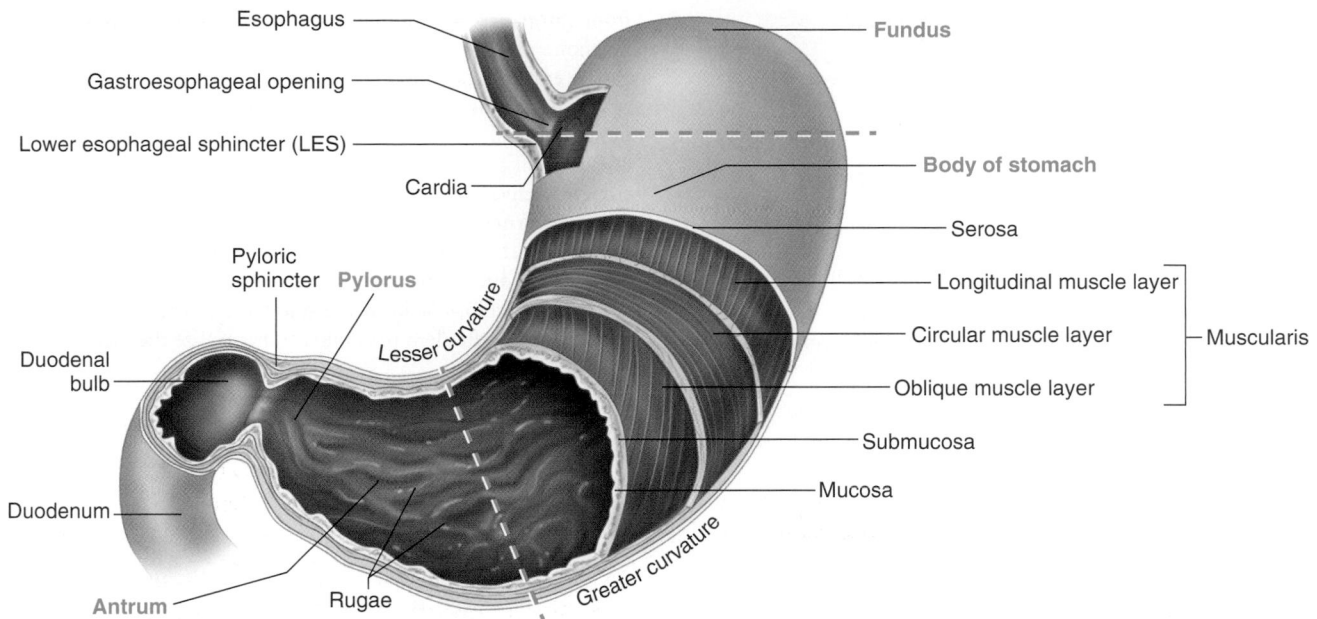

FIGURE 35-5 Stomach. A portion of the anterior wall has been excised to reveal the muscle layers of the stomach wall. Note that the mucosa lining the stomach forms folds called *rugae*. The dashed lines distinguish the fundus, body, and antrum of the stomach. (Modified from Patton KT, Thibodeau GA: *The human body in health & disease*, ed 6, St Louis, 2014, Mosby.)

Peristalsis that immediately follows the oropharyngeal phase of swallowing is called primary peristalsis. If a bolus of food becomes stuck in the esophageal lumen, secondary peristalsis—a wave of contraction and relaxation independent of voluntary swallowing—occurs. This is in response to stretch receptors stimulated by increased wall tension, which activate impulses from the swallowing center of the brain.

The lower esophageal sphincter is normally constricted and serves as a barrier between the stomach and esophagus. The muscle tone of the lower sphincter changes with neural and hormonal stimulation and relaxes with swallowing. Cholinergic vagal input and the digestive hormone gastrin increase sphincter tone. Nonadrenergic, noncholinergic vagal impulses relax the lower esophageal sphincter, as do the hormones progesterone, secretin, and glucagon.[1]

Stomach

The stomach is a hollow, muscular organ just below the diaphragm that stores food during eating, secretes digestive juices, mixes food with these juices, and propels partially digested food, called chyme, into the duodenum of the small intestine. The anatomy of the stomach is presented in Figure 35-5. Its major anatomic boundaries are the lower esophageal sphincter, where food passes through the cardiac orifice at the gastroduodenal junction into the stomach, and the pyloric sphincter, which relaxes as food is propelled through the pylorus (gastroduodenal junction) into the duodenum. Functional areas are the fundus (upper portion), body (middle portion), and antrum (lower portion).

The stomach has three layers of smooth muscle: an outer, longitudinal layer; a middle, circular layer; and an inner, oblique layer (the most prominent) (see Figure 35-5). These layers become progressively thicker in the body and antrum where food is mixed and pushed into the duodenum. The glandular epithelium is discussed under Gastric Secretion (see p. 888).

The stomach's blood supply comes from a branch of the celiac artery (Figure 35-6) and is so abundant that nearly all arterial vessels must be occluded before ischemic changes occur in the stomach wall. A series of small veins drain blood from the stomach towards the hepatic portal vein.

Sympathetic and parasympathetic divisions of the autonomic nervous system innervate the stomach. Some of the autonomic fibers are extrinsic—that is, they originate outside the stomach and are controlled by nerve centers in the brain. The vagus nerve provides parasympathetic innervation and branches of the celiac plexus innervate the stomach sympathetically. The myenteric (Auerbach) and submucosal (Meissner) plexuses are intrinsic and part of the enteric (intramural) nervous system. They originate within the stomach and respond to local stimuli.

Gastric Motility

In its resting state, the stomach is small and contains about 50 ml of fluid. There is no wall tension, and the muscle layers in the fundus contract very little. Swallowing causes the fundus to relax (receptive relaxation) to receive a bolus of food from the esophagus (see Swallowing, p. 886). Relaxation is coordinated by efferent, nonadrenergic, noncholinergic vagal fibers and is facilitated by gastrin and cholecystokinin—two polypeptide hormones secreted by the gastrointestinal mucosa. (The actions of digestive hormones are summarized in Table 35-1.) Food is stored in vertical or oblique layers as it arrives in the fundus, whereas fluids flow relatively quickly down to the antrum.

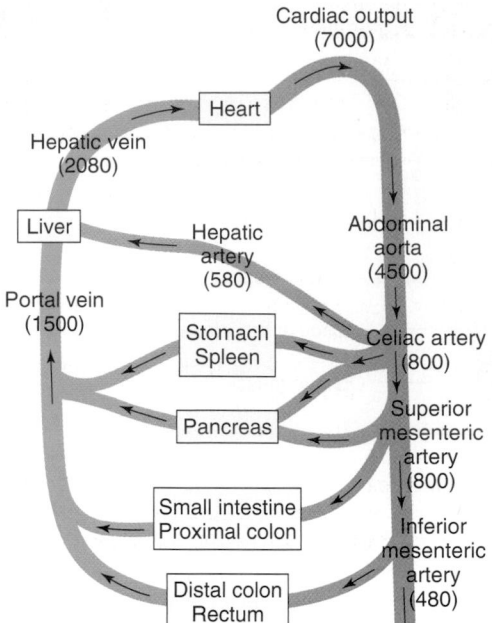

FIGURE 35-6 Major Blood Vessels and Organs Supplied with Blood in the Splanchnic Circulation. Numbers in parentheses reflect approximate blood flow values (ml/min) for each major vessel in an 80-kg normal, resting, adult human subject. Arrows indicate the direction of blood flow. (Modified from Johnson LR: *Gastrointestinal pathophysiology*, St Louis, 2001, Mosby.)

Gastric (stomach) motility increases with the initiation of peristaltic waves, which sweep over the body of the stomach toward the antrum. The rate of peristaltic contractions is approximately three per minute and is influenced by neural and hormonal activity. Gastrin, motilin (an intestinal hormone), and the vagus nerve increase the rate of contraction by lowering the threshold potential of muscle fibers. (The neural and biochemical mechanisms of muscle contraction are described in Chapter 38.) Sympathetic activity and secretin (another intestinal hormone) are inhibitory and raise the threshold potential. The rate of peristalsis is mediated by pacemaker cells that initiate a wave of depolarization (basic electrical rhythm), which moves from the upper part of the stomach to the pylorus.

Gastric mixing and emptying of gastric contents (chyme) from the stomach take several hours. Mixing occurs as food is propelled toward the antrum. As food approaches the pylorus, the velocity of the peristaltic wave increases. This forces the contents back toward the body of the stomach. This retropulsion effectively mixes food with digestive juices, and the oscillating motion breaks down large food particles. With each peristaltic wave, a small portion of the gastric contents (chyme) passes through the pylorus and into the duodenum. The pyloric sphincter is about 1.5 cm long and is always open about 2.0 mm. It opens wider during antral contraction. Normally there is no regurgitation from the duodenum into the antrum.

The rate of gastric emptying (movement of gastric contents into the duodenum) depends on the volume, osmotic pressure, and chemical composition of the gastric contents. Larger volumes of food increase gastric pressure, peristalsis, and rate of emptying. Solids, fats, and non-isotonic solutions (i.e., hypertonic or hypotonic gastric tube feedings) delay gastric emptying. (Osmotic pressure and tonicity are described in Chapters 1 and 5.) Products of fat digestion, which are formed in the duodenum by the action of bile from the liver and enzymes

from the pancreas, stimulate the secretion of cholecystokinin. This hormone inhibits food intake, reduces gastric motility, and decreases gastric emptying so that fats are not emptied into the duodenum at a rate that exceeds the rate of bile and enzyme secretion. Osmoreceptors in the wall of the duodenum are sensitive to the osmotic pressure of duodenal contents. The arrival of hypertonic or hypotonic gastric contents activates the osmoreceptors, which delay gastric emptying to facilitate formation of an isosmotic duodenal environment. The rate at which acid enters the duodenum also influences gastric emptying. Secretions from the pancreas, liver, and duodenal mucosa neutralize gastric hydrochloric acid in the duodenum. The rate of emptying is adjusted to the duodenum's ability to neutralize the incoming acidity.[2]

Gastric Secretion

The secretion of gastric juice is influenced by numerous stimuli that together facilitate the process of digestion. The phases of gastric secretion are the *cephalic phase* (stimulated by the thought, smell, and taste of food), the *gastric phase* (stimulated by distention of the stomach), and the *intestinal phase* (stimulated by histamine and digested protein). All phases promote the secretion of acid by the stomach.

Gastric secretion is stimulated by the process of eating (gastric distention), by the actions of the hormone gastrin and paracrine pathways (e.g., histamine, ghrelin, somatostatin), and by the effects of the neurotransmitter acetylcholine and other chemicals (e.g., ethanol, coffee, protein). The stomach secretes large volumes of gastric juices or gastric secretions, including mucus, acid, enzymes, hormones, intrinsic factor, and gastroferrin. Intrinsic factor is necessary for the intestinal absorption of vitamin B_{12}, and gastroferrin facilitates small intestinal absorption of iron. The hormones are secreted into the blood and travel to target tissues. The other gastric secretions are released directly into the stomach lumen.[3]

In the fundus and body of the stomach, the gastric glands of the mucosa are the primary secretory units (Figure 35-7). The composition of gastric juice depends on volume and flow rate (Figure 35-8). Potassium level remains relatively constant, but its concentration is greater in gastric juice than in plasma. The rate of secretion varies with the time of day. Generally, the rate and volume of secretion are lowest in the morning and highest in the afternoon and evening. Loss of gastric juices through vomiting, drainage, or suction may decrease body stores of sodium and potassium and result in fluid, electrolyte (e.g., hyponatremia, hypokalemia, dehydration), and acid-base imbalances (e.g., metabolic alkalosis) (see Chapters 5 and 36).[4]

Gastric secretion is inhibited by somatostatin, by unpleasant odors and tastes, and by rage, fear, or pain. A discharge of sympathetic impulses inhibits parasympathetic impulses. Increased secretions are associated with aggression or hostility and may contribute to some forms of gastric pathology.

Gastric acid. The major functions of gastric hydrochloric acid are to dissolve food fibers, act as a bactericide against swallowed microorganisms, and convert pepsinogen to pepsin. The production of acid by the **parietal cells** requires the transport of hydrogen and chloride from the parietal cells to the stomach lumen. Acid is formed in the parietal cells, primarily through the hydrolysis of water (Figure 35-9). At a high rate of gastric secretion, bicarbonate moves into the plasma, producing an "alkaline tide" in the venous blood, which also may result in a more alkaline urine.[4]

Acid secretion is stimulated by the vagus nerve, which releases acetylcholine and stimulates the secretion of gastrin; then gastrin stimulates the release of histamine from enterochromaffin cells (mast cells; see Chapter 6) in the gastric mucosa. Histamine stimulates acid secretion by activating histamine receptors (H2 receptors) on acid-secreting parietal cells. Caffeine stimulates acid secretion, as does

TABLE 35-1 **Selected Hormones* and Neurotransmitters of the Digestive System**

Source	Hormone/Neurotransmitter	Stimulus for Secretion	Action
Mucosa of stomach	Gastrin	Presence of partially digested proteins in stomach	Stimulates gastric glands to secrete hydrochloric acid, pepsinogen, and histamine; growth of gastric mucosa
	Histamine	Gastrin	Stimulates acid secretion
	Somatostatin	Acid in stomach	Inhibits acid, pepsinogen, and histamine secretion and release of gastrin
	Acetylcholine	Vagus and local nerves in stomach	Stimulates release of pepsinogen and acid secretion
	Gastrin-releasing peptide (bombesin)	Vagus and local nerves in stomach	Stimulates gastrin and release of pepsinogen and acid secretion
	Ghrelin	High during fasting	Stimulates growth hormone secretion and hypothalamus to increase appetite
Mucosa of small intestine	Motilin	Presence of acid and fat in duodenum	Increases gastrointestinal motility
	Secretin	Presence of chyme (acid, partially digested proteins, fats) in duodenum	Stimulates pancreas to secrete alkaline pancreatic juice and liver to secrete bile; decreases gastrointestinal motility; inhibits gastrin and gastric acid secretion
	Serotonin (5-hydroxytryptamine)	Intestinal distention; vagal stimulation; presence of acids, amino acids, or hypertonic fluids; released from enterochromaffin cells throughout intestine	Stimulates intestinal secretion, motility and sensation (i.e., pain and nausea), vasodilation; activates gut immune responses
	Cholecystokinin	Presence of chyme (acid, partially digested proteins, fats) in duodenum	Stimulates gallbladder to eject bile and pancreas to secrete alkaline fluid; decreases gastric motility; constricts pyloric sphincter; inhibits gastrin
	Enteroglucagon	Intraluminal fats and carbohydrates	Weakly inhibits gastric and pancreatic secretion and enhances insulin release, lipolysis, ketogenesis, and glycogenolysis
	Gastric inhibitory peptide (GIP)	Fat and glucose in small intestine	Inhibits gastric secretion and emptying; stimulates insulin release
	Peptide YY	Intraluminal fat and bile acids	Inhibits postprandial gastric acid and pancreatic secretion and delays gastric and small bowel emptying
	Pancreatic polypeptide	Protein, fat, and glucose in small intestine	Decreases pancreatic HCO_3^- and enzyme secretion
	Vasoactive intestinal peptide	Intestinal mucosa and muscle	Relaxes intestinal smooth muscle

Modified from Johnson LR. *Gastrointestinal physiology*, ed 8, St Louis, 2014, Mosby. Data from Feldman M et al: *Sleisenger and Fordtran's gastrointestinal and liver disease*, ed 10, Philadelphia, 2015, Saunders.
*NOTE: The digestive hormones are not secreted into the gastrointestinal lumen but instead into the bloodstream, where they travel to target tissues. There are more than 30 peptide hormone genes expressed in the gastrointestinal tract and more than 100 hormonally active peptides.

calcium. Acid secretion is inhibited by somatostatin, secretin, and other intestinal hormones.[3]

Pepsin. Acetylcholine, gastrin, and secretin stimulate the chief cells to release pepsinogen during eating. Pepsinogen is quickly converted to pepsin in the acidic gastric environment (optimum pH for pepsin activation = 2.0). Pepsin is a proteolytic enzyme—that is, it breaks down protein and forms polypeptides in the stomach. Once chyme has entered the duodenum, the alkaline environment of the duodenum inactivates pepsin.

Mucus. The gastric mucosa is protected from the digestive actions of acid and pepsin by intercellular tight junctions, a coating of mucus called the mucosal barrier, and gastric mucosal blood flow. Prostaglandins protect the mucosal barrier by stimulating the secretion of mucus and bicarbonate and by inhibiting the secretion of acid. A break in the protective barrier may occur from ischemia or by exposure to *Helicobacter pylori*, aspirin, nonsteroidal anti-inflammatory drugs (inhibit prostaglandin synthesis), ethanol, or regurgitated bile. Breaks cause inflammation and ulceration.

Few substances are absorbed in the stomach. The stomach mucosa is impermeable to water, but the stomach can absorb alcohol and aspirin.

✔**QUICK CHECK 35-2**

1. Why are there three layers of stomach muscle and how do they function?
2. What hormones stimulate gastric motility?
3. What are the phases of gastric secretion?

Small Intestine

The small intestine is coiled within the peritoneal cavity and is about 5 to 6 meters long. Functionally, it is divided into three segments: the duodenum, jejunum, and ileum (Figure 35-10). The duodenum

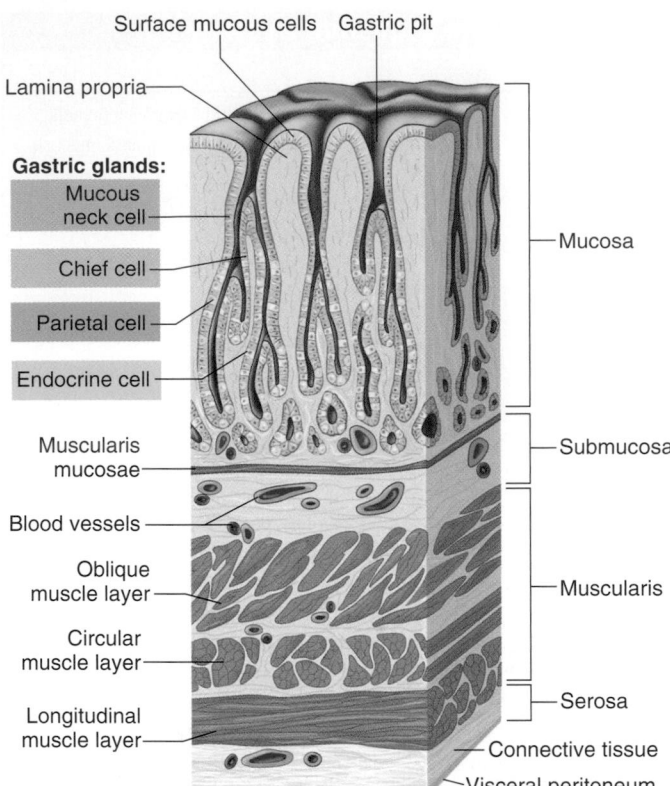

FIGURE 35-7 Gastric Pits and Gastric Glands. Gastric pits are depressions in the epithelial lining of the stomach. At the bottom of each pit are one or more tubular *gastric glands.* Chief cells produce pepsinogen, which is converted to pepsin (a proteolytic enzyme); parietal cells secrete hydrochloric acid and intrinsic factor; G cells produce gastrin; endocrine cells (enterochromaffin-like cells and D cells) secrete histamine and somatostatin. (From Patton KT, et al: *Essentials of anatomy & physiology,* St Louis, 2012, Mosby.)

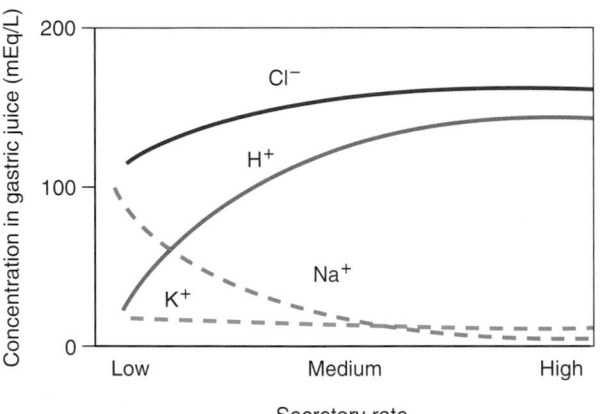

FIGURE 35-8 Gastric Electrolyte Concentrations and Flow Rate. Sodium (Na^+) concentration is lower in the gastric juice than in the plasma, whereas hydrogen (H^+), potassium (K^+), and chloride (Cl^-) concentrations are higher. *Red line,* chloride; *orange line,* hydrogen; *green line,* sodium; *blue line,* potassium.

FIGURE 35-9 Hydrochloric Acid Secretion by Parietal Cell.

the flow of digested material from the ileum into the large intestine and prevents reflux into the small intestine.

The duodenum lies behind the peritoneum, or retroperitoneally, and is attached to the posterior abdominal wall. The ileum and jejunum are suspended in loose folds from the posterior abdominal wall by a peritoneal membrane called the **mesentery.** The mesentery facilitates intestinal motility and supports blood vessels, nerves, and lymphatics.

The **peritoneum** is the serous membrane surrounding the organs of the abdomen and pelvic cavity. It is analogous to the pericardium around the heart and the pleura around the lungs. The visceral peritoneum lies on the surface of the organs, and the parietal peritoneum lines the wall of the body cavity. The space between these two layers is called the **peritoneal cavity** and normally contains just enough fluid to lubricate the two layers and prevent friction during organ movement.

The arterial supply to the duodenum arises primarily from the gastroduodenal artery, a branch of the celiac artery. The jejunum and ileum are supplied by branches of the superior mesenteric artery. The superior mesenteric vein drains blood from the entire small intestine and empties into the hepatic portal circulation. The regional lymph nodes and lymphatics drain into the thoracic duct.

Enteric nerves from both divisions of the autonomic nervous system innervate the small intestine. Secretion, motility, pain sensation, and intestinal reflexes (e.g., relaxation of the lower esophageal sphincter) are mediated parasympathetically by the vagus nerve. Sympathetic activity inhibits motility and produces vasoconstriction. Intrinsic reflexive activity is mediated by the **myenteric plexus (Auerbach plexus)** and the **submucosal plexus (Meissner plexus)** of the enteric nervous system.

The smooth muscles of the small intestine are arranged in two layers: a longitudinal outer layer and a thicker inner circular layer (see Figures 35-2 and 35-10). Circular folds of the small intestine slow the passage of food, thereby providing more time for digestion and absorption. The folds are most numerous and prominent in the jejunum and proximal ileum (see Figure 35-10).

Absorption occurs through **villi** (sing., **villus**), which cover the circular folds and are the functional units of the intestine. A villus is composed of absorptive columnar cells (**enterocytes**) and mucus-secreting goblet cells of the mucosal epithelium. Each villus (see Figure 35-10) secretes some of the enzymes necessary for digestion and absorbs nutrients. Near the surface, columnar cells closely adhere to each other at sites called *tight junctions.* Water and electrolytes are absorbed through these intercellular spaces. The surface of each columnar epithelial cell on the villus contains tiny projections called **microvilli** (sing., **microvillus**) (see Figure 35-10). Together the

begins at the pylorus and ends where it joins the jejunum at a suspensory ligament called the *Treitz ligament.* The end of the jejunum and beginning of the ileum are not distinguished by an anatomic marker. These structures are not grossly different, but the jejunum has a slightly larger lumen than the ileum. The **ileocecal valve,** or **sphincter,** controls

FIGURE 35-10 The Small Intestine.

microvilli create a mucosal surface known as the brush border. The villi and microvilli greatly increase the surface area available for absorption. Coating the brush border is an "unstirred" layer of water that is important for the absorption of water-soluble substances including emulsified micelles of fat. The lamina propria (a connective tissue layer of the mucous membrane) lies beneath the epithelial cells of the villi and contains lymphocytes and plasma cells, which produce immunoglobulins (see The Gastrointestinal Tract and Immunity).

Central arterioles ascend within each villus and branch into a capillary array that extends around the base of the columnar cells and cascades down to the venules that lead to the hepatic portal circulation (see Figure 35-10). A central lacteal, or lymphatic capillary, also is contained within each villus and is important for the absorption and transport of fat molecules. Contents of the lacteals flow to regional nodes and channels that eventually drain into the thoracic duct.[5]

Between the bases of the villi are the crypts of Lieberkühn, which extend to the submucosal layer. Undifferentiated cells arise from stem cells at the base of the crypt and move toward the tip of the villus, maturing to become columnar epithelial secretory cells (water, electrolytes, and enzymes) and goblet cells (mucus). After completing their migration to the tip of the villus, they function for a few days and then are shed into the intestinal lumen and digested. Discarded epithelial cells are an important source of endogenous protein. The entire epithelial population is replaced about every 4 to 7 days. Many factors can influence this process of cellular proliferation. Starvation, vitamin B_{12} deficiency, and cytotoxic drugs or irradiation suppress cell division and shorten the villi. Decreased absorption across the epithelial membrane can cause diarrhea and malnutrition. Nutrient intake and intestinal resection stimulate cell production.

Intestinal Digestion and Absorption

The process of digestion is initiated in the stomach by the actions of gastric hydrochloric acid and pepsin. The chyme that passes into the duodenum is a liquid with small particles of undigested food. Digestion continues in the proximal portion of the small intestine by the action of pancreatic enzymes, intestinal enzymes, and bile salts. In the proximal small intestine, carbohydrates are broken down to monosaccharides and disaccharides; proteins are degraded further to amino acids and peptides; and fats are emulsified and reduced to fatty acids (Box 35-1) and monoglycerides (Figure 35-11). These nutrients, along with water, vitamins, and electrolytes, are absorbed across the intestinal mucosa by active transport, diffusion, or facilitated diffusion. Products of carbohydrate and protein breakdown move into villus capillaries and then to the liver through the hepatic portal vein. Digested fats move into the lacteals and eventually reach the liver through the systemic circulation. Intestinal motility exposes nutrients to a large mucosal surface area by mixing chyme and moving it through the lumen. Different segments of the gastrointestinal tract absorb different nutrients. Digestion and absorption of all major nutrients and many drugs occur in the small intestine. Sites of absorption are shown in Figure 35-12. Box 35-2 outlines the major nutrients involved in this process.

BOX 35-1   Dietary Fat

Saturated Fatty Acids (e.g., Palmitic Acid [$C_{16}H_{32}O_2$])

Each carbon atom in the chain is linked by single bonds to adjacent carbon and hydrogen atoms:

1. Solid at room temperature; include animal fat and tropical oils (coconut and palm oils).
2. Increase low-density lipoprotein (LDL) cholesterol ("bad" cholesterol) blood levels.
3. Increase the risk of coronary artery disease.

Unsaturated Fatty Acids

Soft or liquid at room temperature; omega-6 fatty acids are found in plants and vegetables (olive, canola, and peanut oils); omega-3 fatty acids are found in fish and shellfish.

Monounsaturated Fatty Acids (e.g., Oleic Acid [$C_{18}H_{34}O_2$])

Contain one double bond in the carbon chain:

1. Found in both plants and animals.
2. May be beneficial in reducing blood cholesterol level, glucose level, and systolic blood pressure.

3. Do not lower high-density lipoprotein (HDL) cholesterol ("good" cholesterol) level.
4. Low HDL levels have been associated with coronary heart disease.

Polyunsaturated Fatty Acids (e.g., Linoleic Acid [$C_{18}H_{32}O_2$])

Contain two or more double bonds in the carbon chain:

1. Found in plants and fish oils.
2. Omega-6 fatty acids lower total and LDL cholesterol blood levels.
3. High levels of polyunsaturated fatty acids may lower LDL levels; omega-3 fatty acids lower blood triglyceride levels and reduce platelet aggregation and therefore blood coagulation.
4. Necessary for growth and development and may prevent coronary artery disease, hypertension, and inflammatory and immune disorders.

BOX 35-2   Major Nutrients Absorbed in the Small Intestine

Water and Electrolytes

- Approximately 85% to 90% of the water that enters the gastrointestinal tract is absorbed in the small intestine.
- Sodium passes through tight junctions and is actively transported across cell membranes; it is exchanged for bicarbonate to maintain electroneutrality in the ileum; sodium absorption is enhanced by co-transport with glucose.
- Potassium moves passively across tight junctions with changes in the electrochemical gradient.

Carbohydrates

- Only monosaccharides are absorbed by intestinal mucosa; therefore complex carbohydrates must be hydrolyzed to simplest form.
- Salivary and pancreatic amylases break down starches to oligosaccharides (sucrose, maltose, lactose) in stomach and duodenum; brush-border enzymes hydrolyze them in intestine so they can pass through the unstirred water layer by diffusion.
- Fructose diffuses into the bloodstream; glucose and galactose diffuse or are actively transported.
- Cellulose remains undigested and stimulates large intestine motility.

Proteins

- From 90% to 95% of protein is absorbed; major hydrolysis is accomplished in the small intestine by the pancreatic enzymes trypsin, chymotrypsin, and carboxypeptidase.
- Brush-border enzymes break down proteins into smaller peptides that can cross cell membranes. In the cytosol, they are metabolized into amino acids,

specifically neutral amino acids, basic amino acids, and proline and hydroxyproline.

Fats

Digestion and absorption occur in four phases:

1. Emulsification and lipolysis—agents cover small fat particles and prevent them from re-forming into fat droplets; then lipolysis divides them into diglycerides, monoglycerides, free fatty acids, and glycerol.
2. Micelle formation—products are made water soluble.
3. Fat absorption—fat products move from micelle to absorbing surface of intestinal epithelium and diffuse through resynthesis.
4. Triglycerides and phospholipids then—become chylomicrons that eventually enter the systemic circulation

Minerals

- Calcium—absorbed by passive diffusion and transported actively across cell membranes bound to a carrier protein; absorption primarily in ileum.
- Magnesium—50% absorbed by active transport or passive diffusion in jejunum and ileum.
- Phosphate—absorbed by passive diffusion and active transport in small intestine.
- Iron—absorbed by epithelial cells of duodenum and jejunum; vitamin C facilitates.

Vitamins

- Absorbed mainly by sodium-dependent active transport, with vitamin B_{12} bound to intrinsic factor and absorbed in terminal ileum.

Intestinal Motility

The movements of the small intestine facilitate digestion and absorption. Chyme leaving the stomach and entering the duodenum stimulates intestinal movements that help blend secretions from the liver, gallbladder, pancreas, and intestinal glands. A churning motion brings the luminal contents into contact with the absorbing cells of the villi. Propulsive movements then advance the chyme toward the large intestine.

Intestinal motility is affected by the following two movements:

1. Haustral segmentation. Localized rhythmic contractions of circular smooth muscles divide and mix the chyme, enabling the chyme to have contact with digestive enzymes and the absorbent mucosal surface, and then propel it toward the large intestine.
2. Peristalsis. Waves of contraction along short segments of longitudinal smooth muscle allow time for digestion and absorption. The intestinal villi move with contractions of the muscularis mucosae,

FIGURE 35-11 Digestion and Absorption of Foodstuffs.

a thin layer of muscle separating the mucosa and submucosa, with absorption promoted by the swaying of the villi in the luminal contents.

Neural reflexes along the length of the small intestine facilitate motility, digestion, and absorption. The **ileogastric reflex** inhibits gastric motility when the ileum becomes distended. This prevents the continued movement of chyme into an already distended intestine.

The **intestinointestinal reflex** inhibits intestinal motility when one part of the intestine is overdistended. Both of these reflexes require extrinsic innervation. The **gastroileal reflex**, which is activated by an increase in gastric motility and secretion, stimulates an increase in ileal motility and relaxation of the ileocecal valve (sphincter). This empties the ileum and prepares it to receive more chyme. The gastroileal reflex is probably regulated by the hormones gastrin and cholecystokinin.

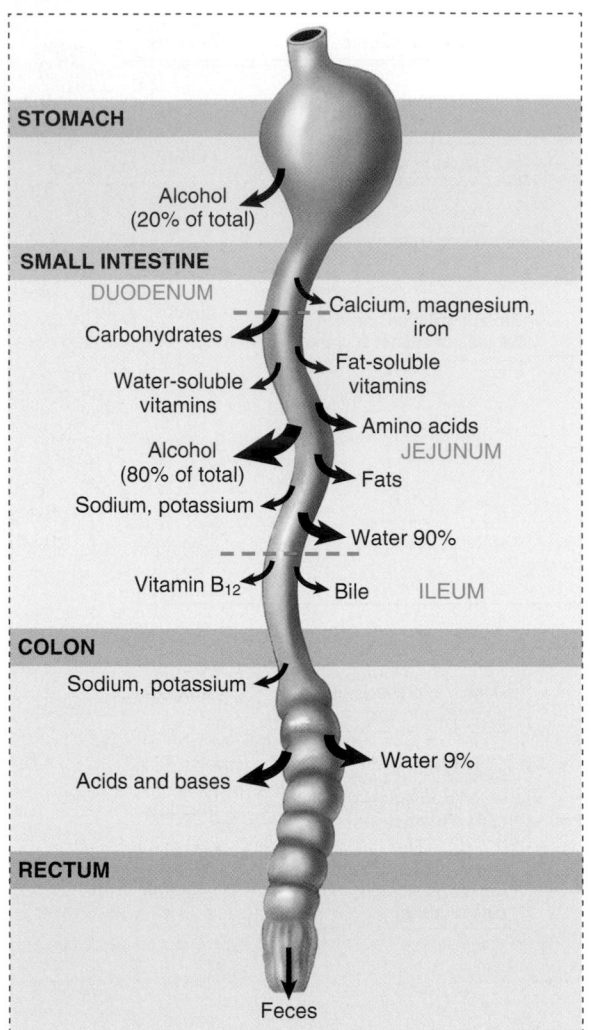

FIGURE 35-12 Sites of Absorption of Major Nutrients.

During prolonged fasting or between meals, particularly overnight, slow waves sweep along the entire length of the intestinal tract from the stomach to the terminal ileum. This interdigestive myoelectric complex appears to propel residual gastric and intestinal contents into the colon.

The **ileocecal valve (sphincter)** marks the junction between the terminal ileum and the large intestine. This valve is intrinsically regulated and is normally closed. The arrival of peristaltic waves from the last few centimeters of the ileum causes the ileocecal valve to open, allowing a small amount of chyme to pass. Distention of the upper large intestine causes the sphincter to constrict, preventing further distention or retrograde flow of intestinal contents.

✔ **QUICK CHECK 35-3**

1. What cells arise from the crypts of Lieberkühn?
2. How are fats absorbed from the small intestine?
3. Which reflexes inhibit intestinal motility? Which promote it?

Large Intestine

The **large intestine** is approximately 1.5 meters long and consists of the cecum, appendix, colon (ascending, transverse, descending, and

sigmoid), rectum, and anal canal (Figure 35-13). The **cecum** is a pouch that receives chyme from the ileum. Attached to it is the **vermiform appendix**, an appendage having little or no physiologic function. From the cecum, chyme enters the **colon**, which loops upward, traverses the abdominal cavity, and descends to the anal canal. The four parts of the colon are the **ascending colon, transverse colon, descending colon,** and **sigmoid colon**. Two sphincters control the flow of intestinal contents through the cecum and colon: the ileocecal valve, which admits chyme from the ileum to the cecum; and the **rectosigmoid (O'Beirne) sphincter**, which controls the movement of wastes from the sigmoid colon into the rectum. A thick (2.5 to 3 cm) portion of smooth muscle surrounds the anal canal, forming the **internal anal sphincter**. Overlapping it distally is the striated skeletal muscle of the **external anal sphincter** (anus).

In the cecum and colon, the longitudinal muscle layer consists of three longitudinal bands called **teniae coli** (see Figure 35-13). They are shorter than the colon and give it a gathered appearance. The circular muscles of the colon separate the gathers into outpouchings called **haustra** (sing., **haustrum**). The haustra become more or less prominent with the contractions and relaxations of the circular muscles. The mucosal surface of the colon has rugae (folds), particularly between the haustra, and Lieberkühn crypts but no villi. Columnar epithelial cells and mucus-secreting goblet cells form the mucosa throughout the large intestine. The columnar epithelium absorbs fluid and electrolytes, and the mucus-secreting cells lubricate the mucosa.

The enteric nervous system regulates motor and secretory activity independently of the extrinsic nervous system. Extrinsic parasympathetic innervation occurs through the vagus and extends from the cecum up to the first part of the transverse colon. Vagal stimulation increases rhythmic contraction of the proximal colon. Extrinsic parasympathetic fibers reach the distal colon through the sacral parasympathetic splanchnic nerves. The internal anal sphincter is usually contracted, and its reflex response is to relax when the rectum is distended. The myenteric plexus provides the major innervation of the internal anal sphincter, but responds to sympathetic stimulation to maintain contraction and parasympathetic stimulation that facilitates relaxation when the rectum is full. Sympathetic innervation of this sphincter arises from the celiac and superior mesenteric ganglia and the sphincter nerve. The external anal sphincter is innervated by the pudendal nerve arising from sacral levels of the spinal cord. Sympathetic activity in the entire large intestine modulates intestinal reflexes, conveys somatic sensations of fullness and pain, participates in the defecation reflex, and constricts blood vessels. The blood supply of the large intestine and rectum is derived primarily from branches of the superior and inferior mesenteric arteries[6] (see Figure 35-6) and venous blood drains through the inferior mesenteric vein.

The primary type of colonic movement is segmental. The circular muscles contract and relax at different sites, shuttling the intestinal contents back and forth between the haustra, most commonly during fasting. The movements massage the intestinal contents, called the **fecal mass** at that point, and facilitate the absorption of water. Propulsive movement occurs with the proximal-to-distal contraction of several haustral units. Peristaltic movements also occur and promote the emptying of the colon. The **gastrocolic reflex** initiates propulsion in the entire colon, usually during or immediately after eating, when chyme enters from the ileum. The gastrocolic reflex causes the fecal mass to pass rapidly into the sigmoid colon and rectum, stimulating defecation. Gastrin may participate in stimulating this reflex. Epinephrine inhibits contractile activity.

Approximately 500 to 700 ml of chyme flows from the ileum to the cecum per day. Most of the water is absorbed in the colon by diffusion and active transport. Aldosterone increases membrane permeability to

FIGURE 35-13 Large Intestine. A, Structure of the large intestine. **B,** Microscopic cross section illustrating cellular structures of the large intestine. The wall of the large intestine is lined with columnar epithelium in contrast to the villi characteristics of the small intestine. The longitudinal layer of muscularis is reduced to become the teniae coli. (**A,** modified from Patton KT, Thibodeau GA: *The human body in health & disease,* ed 6, St Louis, 2014, Mosby; **B,** from Gartner I P, Hiatt JL: *Color textbook of histology,* ed 3, Philadelphia, 2007, Saunders.)

sodium, thereby increasing both the diffusion of sodium into the cell and the active transport of sodium to the interstitial fluid. (See Chapters 5 and 18 for a discussion of aldosterone secretion.) The colon does not absorb monosaccharides and amino acids, but some short-chain free fatty acids, which are produced by fermentation, are absorbed.

Absorption and epithelial transport occur in the cecum, ascending colon, transverse colon, and descending colon. By the time the fecal mass enters the sigmoid colon, the mass consists entirely of wastes and is called the *feces,* composed of food residue, unabsorbed gastrointestinal secretions, shed epithelial cells, and bacteria.

The movement of feces into the sigmoid colon and rectum stimulates the defecation reflex (rectosphincteric reflex). The rectal wall stretches, and the tonically constricted internal anal sphincter (smooth muscle with autonomic nervous system control) relaxes, creating the urge to defecate. The defecation reflex can be overridden voluntarily by contraction of the external anal sphincter and muscles of the pelvic floor. The rectal wall gradually relaxes, reducing tension, and the urge to defecate passes. Retrograde contraction of the rectum may displace the feces out of the rectal vault until a more convenient time for evacuation. Pain or fear of pain associated with defecation (e.g., rectal fissures or hemorrhoids) can inhibit the defecation reflex.

Squatting and sitting facilitate defecation because these positions straighten the angle between the rectum and anal canal and increase the efficiency of straining (increasing intra-abdominal pressure). Intra-abdominal pressure is increased by initiating the Valsalva maneuver—that is, inhaling and forcing the diaphragm and chest muscles against the closed glottis to increase both intrathoracic and intra-abdominal pressure, which is transmitted to the rectum.

✔ QUICK CHECK 35-4

1. What is the major arterial blood supply to the large intestine?
2. What is the function of haustra?
3. What is the Valsalva maneuver?

The Gastrointestinal Tract and Immunity

The gastrointestinal tract plays a major role in immune defenses by killing many microorganisms.[7] The mucosa of the intestine covers a large surface area and muscosal secretions produce antibodies, particularly IgA, and enzymes that provide defenses against microorganisms. Small intestinal Paneth cells, located near the base of the crypts of Leiberkühn, produce defensins and other antimicrobial peptides and lysozymes important to mucosal immunity. Small intestinal Peyer patches (lymph nodules containing collections of lymphocytes, plasma cells, and macrophages) are most numerous in the ileum and produce antimicrobial peptides and immunoglobulin A as a component of the gut-associated lymph tissue in the small intestine (see Figures 35-2 and 7-3). Peyer patches are important for antigen processing and immune defense (see Chapter 7).

Intestinal Microbiome

The type and number of bacterial flora vary greatly throughout the normal gastrointestinal (GI) tract and among individuals. There are an increasing number of bacteria from the proximal to the distal GI tract with the highest number in the colon. Genetics, diet, environmental pollution, personal hygiene, vaccination, and antibiotics and other drugs affect the normal composition of bacterial flora. The intestinal bacteria do not have major digestive or absorptive functions but do play a role in metabolism of bile salts, estrogens, androgens, lipids, carbohydrates, various nitrogenous substances, and drugs. They produce antimicrobial peptides, hormones, neurotransmitters, anti-inflammatory metabolites, and vitamins; destroy toxins; prevent pathogen colonization; and alert the immune system to protect against infection. They are important to overall health and when altered (dysbiosis) or translocated cause disease.[8]

The intestinal tract is sterile at birth but becomes colonized within a few hours. Within 3 to 4 weeks after birth, the normal flora are established. The number and diversity of bacteria decrease with aging, increasing the risk for infection. The normal flora do not have the virulence factors associated with pathogenic microorganisms, thus permitting immune tolerances.[9]

Bacteria in the stomach are relatively sparse because of the secretion of acid that kills ingested pathogens or inhibits bacterial growth (with the exception of *Helicobacter pylori*). Bile acid secretion, intestinal motility, and antibody production suppress bacterial growth in the duodenum. In the duodenum and jejunum, there is a low concentration of aerobes (10^{-1} to 10^{-4}/ml), primarily streptococci, lactobacilli, staphylococci, and other enteric bacteria. Anaerobes are found distal to the ileocecal valve but not proximal to the ileum. They constitute about 95% of the fecal flora in the colon and contribute one third of the solid bulk of feces. *Bacteroides* and *Firmicutes* are the most common intestinal bacteria.

Splanchnic Blood Flow

The splanchnic blood flow provides blood to the esophagus, stomach, small and large intestines, liver, gallbladder, pancreas, and spleen (see Figure 35-6). Blood flow is regulated by cardiac output and blood volume, the autonomic nervous system, hormones, and local autoregulatory blood flow mechanisms. The splanchnic circulation serves as an important reservoir of blood volume to maintain circulation to the heart and lungs when needed. The superior and inferior mesenteric arteries provide the blood supply to the large intestine (see Figures 35-6 and 35-13).

ACCESSORY ORGANS OF DIGESTION

The liver, gallbladder, and exocrine pancreas all secrete substances necessary for the digestion of chyme. These secretions are delivered to the duodenum through the sphincter of Oddi at the major duodenal papilla (of Vater) (Figure 35-14). The liver produces bile, which contains salts necessary for fat digestion and absorption. Between meals, bile is stored in the gallbladder. The exocrine pancreas produces (1) enzymes needed for the complete digestion of carbohydrates, proteins, and fats; and (2) an alkaline fluid that neutralizes chyme, creating a duodenal pH that supports enzymatic action.

The liver also receives nutrients absorbed by the small intestine and metabolizes or synthesizes them into forms that can be absorbed by the body's cells. It then releases the nutrients into the bloodstream or stores them for later use.

Liver

The liver weighs 1200 to 1600 g. It is located under the right diaphragm and is divided into right and left lobes. The larger, right lobe is divided further into the caudate and quadrate lobes (Figure 35-15). The *falciform ligament* separates the right and left lobes and attaches the liver to the anterior abdominal wall. The *round ligament (ligamentum teres)* extends along the free edge of the falciform ligament, extending from the umbilicus to the inferior surface of the liver. The *coronary ligament* branches from the falciform ligament and extends

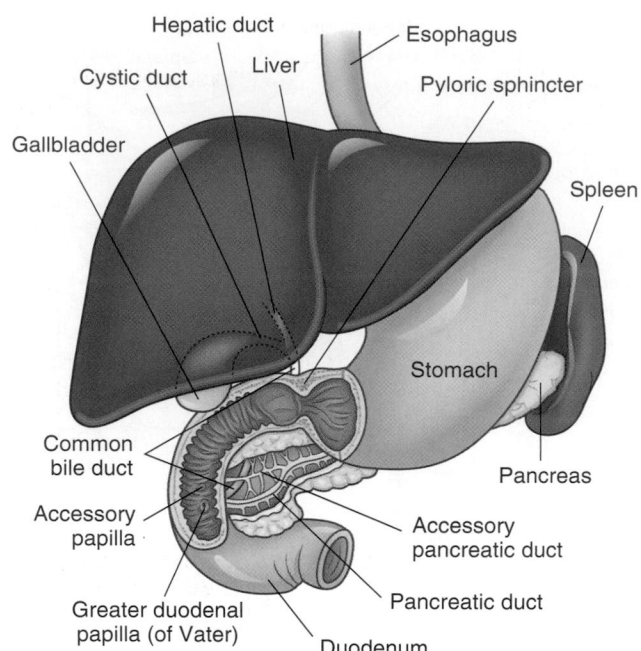

FIGURE 35-14 Location of the Liver, Gallbladder, and Exocrine Pancreas, Which Are the Accessory Organs of Digestion.

over the superior surface of the right and left lobes, binding the liver to the inferior surface of the diaphragm. The liver is covered by the Glisson capsule, which contains blood vessels, lymphatics, and nerves. When the liver is diseased or swollen, distention of the capsule causes pain because it is innervated by sensory neurons.

The metabolic functions of the liver require a large amount of blood. The liver receives blood from both arterial and venous sources. The hepatic artery branches from the celiac artery and provides oxygenated blood at the rate of 400 to 500 ml/min (about 25% of the cardiac output). The hepatic portal vein receives deoxygenated blood from the inferior and superior mesenteric veins, the splenic vein, and the gastric and esophageal veins, and delivers about 1000 to 1500 ml/min to the liver. The hepatic portal vein, which carries 70% of the blood supply to the liver, is rich in nutrients that have been absorbed from the intestinal tract (Figure 35-16).

Within the liver lobes are multiple, smaller anatomic units called liver lobules (Figure 35-17). They are formed of cords or plates of hepatocytes, which are the functional cells of the liver. These cells can regenerate; therefore damaged or resected liver tissue can regrow. Small capillaries, or sinusoids, are located between the plates of hepatocytes. They receive a mixture of venous and arterial blood from branches of the hepatic artery and portal vein. Blood from the sinusoids drains to a central vein in the middle of each liver lobule. Venous blood from all the lobules then flows into the hepatic vein, which empties into the inferior vena cava. Small channels (bile canaliculi) conduct bile, which is produced by the hepatocytes, outward to bile ducts and eventually drain into the common bile duct (see Figure 35-17). This duct empties bile into the ampulla of Vater, and then into the duodenum through an opening called the major duodenal papilla (sphincter of Oddi).

The sinusoids of the liver lobules are lined with highly permeable endothelium. This permeability enhances the transport of nutrients from the sinusoids into the hepatocytes, where they are metabolized. Immune functions of the liver are carried out by various cells. The sinusoids are lined with phagocytic Kupffer cells (tissue macrophages) and are part of the mononuclear phagocyte system. Kupffer cells are

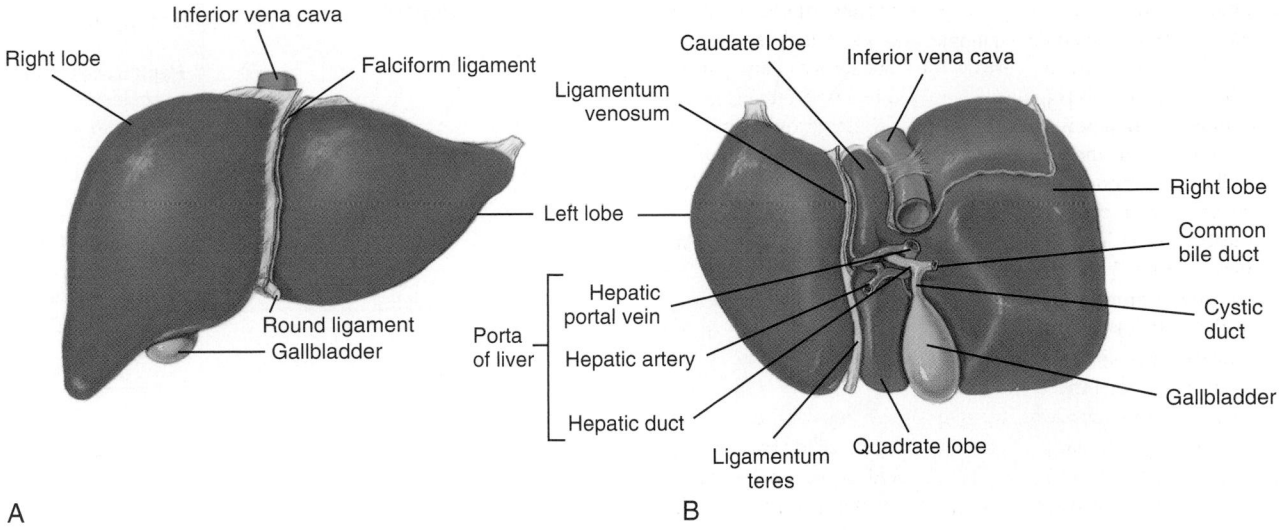

FIGURE 35-15 Gross Structure of the Liver. A, Anterior surface. B, Visceral surface. (From Applegate E: *The anatomy and physiology learning system*, ed 4, St Louis, 2011, Saunders.)

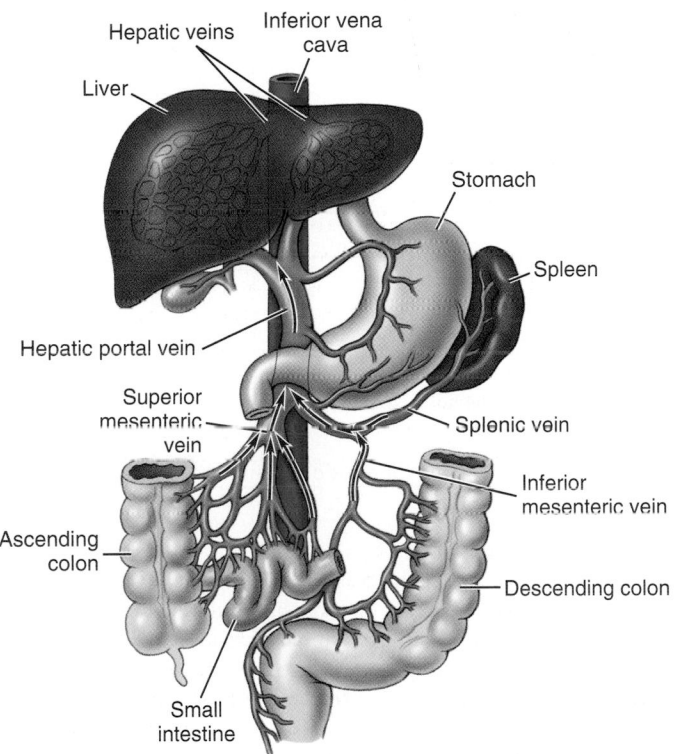

FIGURE 35-16 Hepatic Portal Circulation. In this unusual circulatory route, a vein is located between two capillary beds. The hepatic portal vein collects blood from capillaries in visceral structures located in the abdomen and empties into the liver. Hepatic veins return blood to the inferior vena cava. (From Herlihy B: *The human body in health and illness*, ed 5, St Louis, 2015, Saunders.)

important for healing of liver injury, are bactericidal, and are important for bilirubin production and lipid metabolism.[10] **Stellate cells** contain retinoids (vitamin A), are contractile in liver injury, regulate sinusoidal blood flow, may proliferate into myofibroblasts, participate in liver fibrosis, produce erythropoietin, can act as antigen-presenting cells, remove foreign substances from the blood, and trap bacteria.[11] **Natural killer cells (pit cells)** also are found in the sinusoidal lumen;

they produce interferon-γ and are important in tumor defense.[12] Between the endothelial lining of the sinusoid and the hepatocyte is the **Disse space**, which drains interstitial fluid into the hepatic lymph system.

QUICK CHECK 35-5

1. Where does blood in the portal vein originate?
2. What is the function of hepatocytes?
3. What is the function of Kupffer cells?

Secretion of Bile

The liver assists intestinal digestion by secreting 700 to 1200 ml of bile per day. **Bile** is an alkaline, bitter-tasting, yellowish green fluid that contains bile salts (conjugated bile acids), cholesterol, bilirubin (a pigment), electrolytes, and water. It is formed by hepatocytes and secreted into the canaliculi. **Bile salts**, which are conjugated bile acids, are required for the intestinal emulsification and absorption of fats. Having facilitated fat emulsification and absorption, most bile salts are actively absorbed in the terminal ileum and returned to the liver through the portal circulation for resecretion. The pathway for recycling of bile salts is termed the **enterohepatic circulation** (Figure 35-18).

Bile has two fractional components: the acid-dependent fraction and the acid-independent fraction. Hepatocytes secrete the **bile acid–dependent fraction**, which consists of bile acids, cholesterol, lecithin (a phospholipid), and bilirubin (a bile pigment). The **bile acid–independent fraction**, which is secreted by the hepatocytes and epithelial cells of the bile canaliculi, is a bicarbonate-rich aqueous fluid that gives bile its alkaline pH.

Bile salts are conjugated in the liver from primary and secondary bile acids. The **primary bile acids** are cholic acid and chenodeoxycholic (chenic) acid. These acids are synthesized from cholesterol by the hepatocytes. The **secondary bile acids** are deoxycholic and lithocholic acid. These acids are formed in the small intestine by intestinal bacteria, after which they are absorbed and flow to the liver (see Figure 35-18). Both forms of bile acids are conjugated with amino acids (glycine or taurine) in the liver to form bile salts. Conjugation makes the bile acids more water soluble, thus restricting their diffusion from

FIGURE 35-17 Schematic View of the Liver Lobule. The central vein is shown in the center of the lobule, separated by cords of hepatocytes forming sinusoids from six portal areas at the periphery. The portal areas contain a portal vein, hepatic artery, and bile duct. Blood flow is toward the center of the lobule, while bile flows toward the portal triads at the margins. Note the hepatic artery providing oxygenated blood to the hepatic sinusoids as well as the peribiliary plexus. (From Polin RA, et al: *Fetal and neonatal physiology*, ed 4, St Louis, 2011, Saunders.)

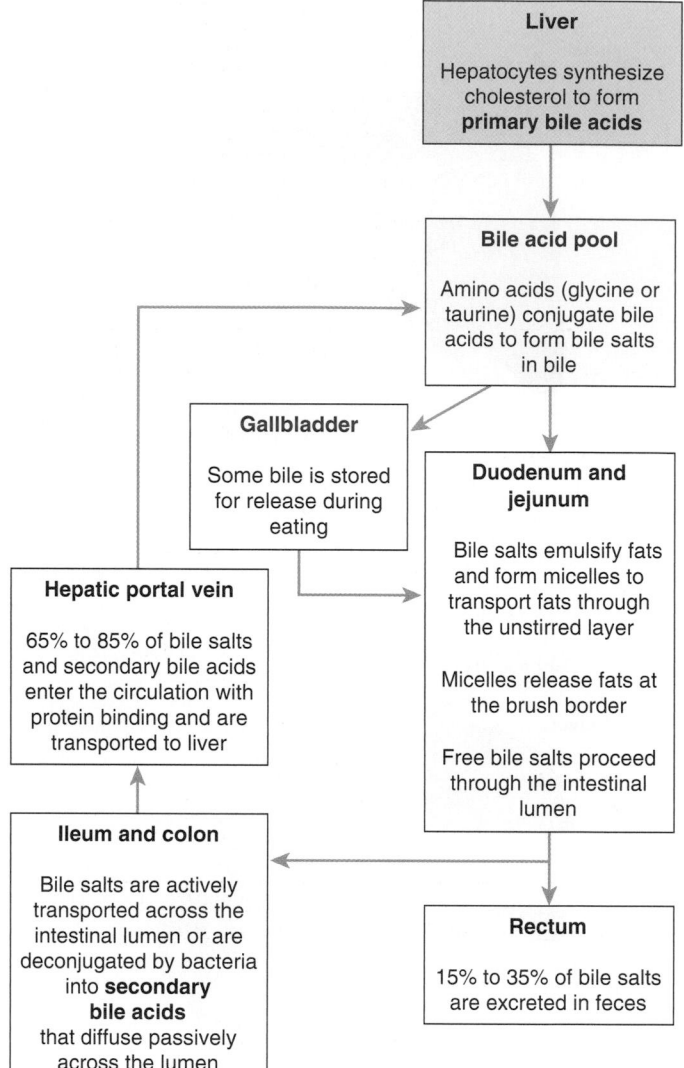

FIGURE 35-18 Enterohepatic Circulation of Bile Salts.

the duodenum and ileum. The primary and secondary bile acids together form the bile acid pool.

Some bile salts are deconjugated by intestinal bacteria to secondary bile acids. These acids diffuse passively into the portal blood from both small and large intestines. An increase in the plasma concentration of bile acids accelerates the uptake and resecretion of bile acids and salts by the hepatocytes. The cycle of hepatic secretion, intestinal absorption, and hepatic resecretion of bile acids completes the enterohepatic circulation.

Bile secretion is called choleresis. A choleretic agent stimulates the liver to secrete bile. One strong stimulus is a high concentration of bile salts. Other choleretics include cholecystokinin, vagal stimulation, and secretin, which increases the rate of bile flow by promoting the secretion of bicarbonate from canaliculi and other intrahepatic bile ducts.

Metabolism of Bilirubin

Bilirubin is a byproduct of the destruction of aged red blood cells. It gives bile a greenish black color and produces the yellow tinge of jaundice. Aged red blood cells are absorbed and destroyed by macrophages (Kupffer cells) of the mononuclear phagocyte system (also called the reticuloendothelial system), primarily in the spleen and liver. Within these cells, hemoglobin is separated into its component parts: heme and globin (Figure 35-19). The globin component is further degraded into its constituent amino acids, which are recycled to form new protein. The heme moiety is converted to biliverdin by the enzymatic (heme oxygenase) cleavage of iron. The iron

attaches to transferrin in the plasma and can be stored in the liver or used by the bone marrow to make new red blood cells. The biliverdin is enzymatically converted to bilirubin in the Kupffer cell and then is released into the plasma where it binds to albumin and is known as unconjugated bilirubin, or free bilirubin, which is lipid soluble. Bilirubin also may have a role as an antioxidant and provide cytoprotection.[13]

In the liver, unconjugated bilirubin moves from plasma in the sinusoids into the hepatocyte. Within hepatocytes, unconjugated bilirubin joins with glucuronic acid to form conjugated bilirubin, which is water soluble and is secreted in the bile. When conjugated bilirubin reaches the distal ileum and colon, it is deconjugated by bacteria and converted to urobilinogen. Urobilinogen is then reabsorbed in the intestines and excreted in the urine as urobilin. A small amount is eliminated in feces, as stercobilin, which contributes to the stool's brown pigmentation.

Vascular and Hematologic Functions

Because of its extensive vascular network, the liver can store a large volume of blood. The amount stored at any one time depends on pressure relationships in the arteries and veins. The liver also can

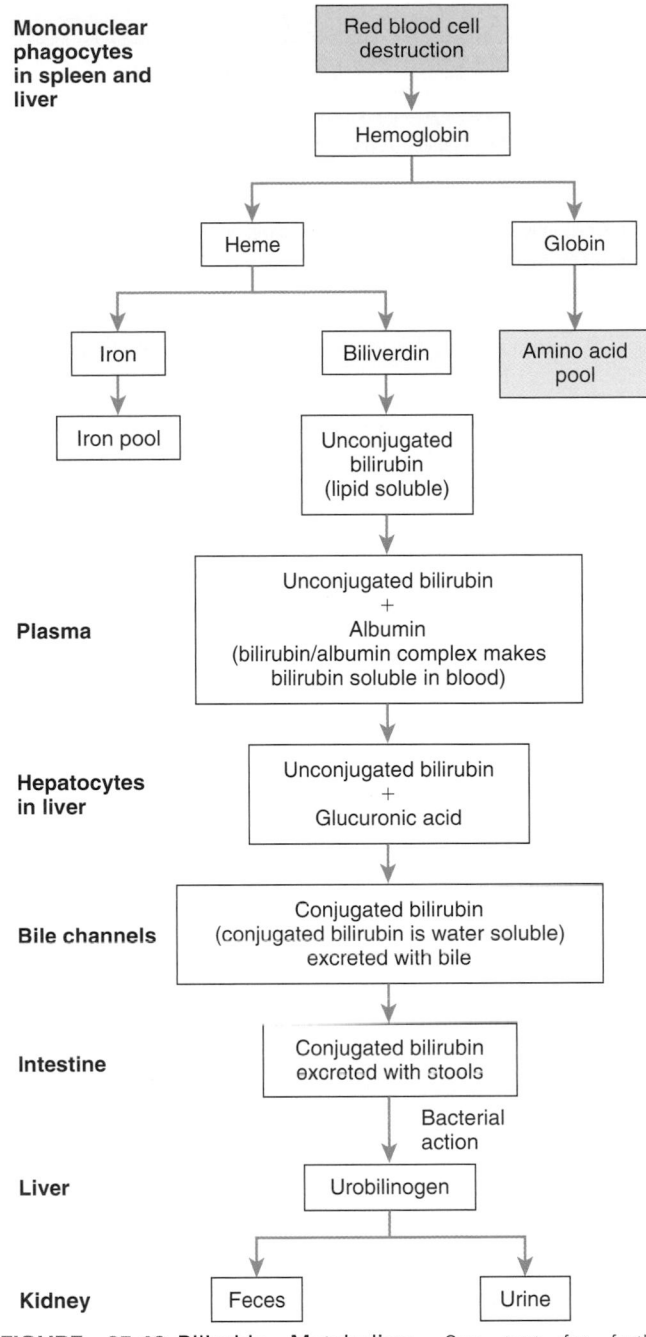

Mononuclear phagocytes in spleen and liver

Red blood cell destruction

Hemoglobin

Heme

Globin

Iron

Biliverdin

Amino acid pool

Iron pool

Unconjugated bilirubin (lipid soluble)

Plasma

Unconjugated bilirubin
+
Albumin
(bilirubin/albumin complex makes bilirubin soluble in blood)

Hepatocytes in liver

Unconjugated bilirubin
+
Glucuronic acid

Bile channels

Conjugated bilirubin
(conjugated bilirubin is water soluble)
excreted with bile

Intestine

Conjugated bilirubin excreted with stools

Bacterial action

Liver

Urobilinogen

Kidney

Feces

Urine

FIGURE 35-19 Bilirubin Metabolism. See text for further explanation.

release blood to maintain systemic circulatory volume in the event of hemorrhage.

The liver also has hemostatic functions. It synthesizes most clotting factors (see Chapter 20). Vitamin K, a fat-soluble vitamin, is essential for the synthesis of the clotting factors. Because bile salts are needed for reabsorption of fats, vitamin K absorption depends on adequate bile production in the liver.

Metabolism of Nutrients

Fats. Ingested fat absorbed by lacteals in the intestinal villi enters the liver through the lymphatics, primarily as triglycerides. In the liver the triglycerides can be hydrolyzed to glycerol and free fatty acids and

TABLE 35-2   Importance of Proteins in the Body

Function	Example
Contraction	Actin and myosin enable muscle contraction and cellular movement.
Energy	Proteins can be metabolized for energy.
Fluid balance	Albumin is a major source of plasma oncotic pressure.
Protection	Antibodies and complement protect against infection and foreign substances.
Regulation	Enzymes control chemical reactions; hormones regulate many physiologic processes.
Structure	Collagen fibers provide structural support to many parts of body; keratin strengthens skin, hair, and nails.
Transport	Hemoglobin transports oxygen and carbon dioxide in blood; plasma proteins, particularly albumin, serve as transport molecules (i.e., for hormones, cations, bilirubin, and drugs); proteins in cell membranes control movement of materials into and out of cells.
Coagulation	Hemostasis is regulated by clotting factors and proteins that balance coagulation and anticoagulation.

used to produce metabolic energy (ATP), or they can be released into the bloodstream bound to proteins (lipoproteins). The lipoproteins are carried by the blood to adipose cells for storage. The liver also synthesizes phospholipids and cholesterol, which are needed for the hepatic production of bile salts, steroid hormones, components of plasma membranes, and other special molecules.

Proteins. Protein synthesis requires the presence of all the essential amino acids (obtained only from food), as well as nonessential amino acids. Proteins perform many important functions in the body; these are summarized in Table 35-2.

Within hepatocytes, amino acids are converted to carbohydrates (keto acids) by the removal of ammonia (NH_3), a process known as deamination. The ammonia is converted to urea by the liver and passes into the blood to be excreted by the kidneys. Depending on the nutritional status of the body, the keto acids either are converted to fatty acids for fat synthesis and storage or are oxidized by the Krebs tricarboxylic acid cycle (see Chapter 1) to provide energy for the liver cells.

The plasma proteins, including albumins and globulins (with the exception of gamma globulin, which is formed in lymph nodes and lymphoid tissue), are synthesized by the liver. They play an important role in preserving blood volume and pressure by maintaining plasma oncotic pressure. The liver also synthesizes several nonessential amino acids and serum enzymes, including aspartate aminotransferase (AST; previously SGOT), alanine aminotransferase (ALT; previously SGPT), lactate dehydrogenase (LDH), and alkaline phosphatase.

Carbohydrates. The liver contributes to the stability of blood glucose levels by releasing glucose during hypoglycemia (low blood glucose level) and absorbing glucose during hyperglycemia (high blood glucose level) and storing it as glycogen (glyconeogenesis) or converting it to fat. When all glycogen stores have been used, the liver can convert amino acids and glycerol to glucose (gluconeogenesis).

Metabolic Detoxification

The liver alters exogenous and endogenous chemicals (e.g., drugs), foreign molecules, and hormones to make them less toxic or less biologically active. This process, called metabolic detoxification or biotransformation, diminishes intestinal or renal tubular reabsorption of potentially toxic substances and facilitates their intestinal and renal excretion. In this way alcohol, barbiturates, amphetamines, steroids, and hormones (including estrogens, aldosterone, antidiuretic hormone, and testosterone) are metabolized or detoxified, preventing excessive accumulation and adverse effects. Although metabolic detoxification is usually protective, the end products of metabolic detoxification sometimes become toxins (see *Health Alert:* Paracetamol [Acetaminophen] and Acute Liver Failure) or active metabolites. Toxins of alcohol metabolism, for example, are acetaldehyde and hydrogen, which can damage the liver's ability to function (see Chapter 4 and Figure 4-21).

Storage of Minerals and Vitamins

The liver stores certain vitamins and minerals, including iron and copper, in times of excessive intake and releases them in times of need. The liver can store vitamins B_{12} and D for several months and vitamin A for several years. The liver also stores vitamins E and K. Iron is stored in the liver as ferritin, an iron-protein complex, and is released as needed for red blood cell production. Common tests of liver function are listed in Table 35-3.

Gallbladder

The **gallbladder** is a saclike organ on the inferior surface of the liver (Figure 35-20). Its primary function is to store and concentrate bile

HEALTH ALERT

Paracetamol (Acetaminophen) and Acute Liver Failure

Paracetamol (acetaminophen) toxicity from chronic use or overdose is the leading cause of acute liver failure in the developed world (see Figure 4-18). Concomitant alcohol use or abuse, medications, genetics, and nutritional status can influence the susceptibility and severity of hepatotoxicity. Hepatotoxicity should be suspected when doses exceed 4 grams per day. Liver injury occurs in 17% of adults with unintentional acetaminophen overdose. The onset of toxicity is sudden and lasts for up to 24 hours. Symptoms include signs of gastrointestinal upset, nausea, vomiting, anorexia, diaphoresis, and pallor. Elevated levels of serum aminotransferase appear after 48 hours accompanied by hypoprothrombinemia, metabolic acidosis, and renal failure. Early treatment (within 8 hours) with *N*-acetylcysteine (NAC) provides a 66% chance of recovery. The acetaminophen-aminotransferase multiplication product (APAP × AT) and the Psi Parameter (acetaminophen level at 4 hours postingestion and the time-to-initiation of NAC) are predictors of acetaminophen toxicity in NAC-treated individuals. Liver transplant is lifesaving and there is about 70% survival at 1 year after liver transplantation.

Data from Blieden M et al: *Expert Rev Clin Pharmacol* 7(3):341-348, 2014; Bunchorntavakul C, Reddy KR: *Clin Liver Dis* 17(4):587-607, viii, 2013; Chomchai S, Chomchai C: *Clin Toxicol (Phila)* 52(5):506-511, 2014; Craig DG et al: *Br J Clin Pharmacol* 71(2):273-282, 2011; Hodgman MF, Garrard AR: *Crit Care Clin* 28(4):499-516, 2012.

TABLE 35-3 Common Tests of Liver Function

Test	Normal Value	Interpretation
Serum Enzymes		
Alkaline phosphatase	13-39 units/L	Increases with biliary obstruction and cholestatic hepatitis
Gamma-glutamyltranspeptidase (GGT)	Male 12-38 units/L Female 9-31 units/L	Increases with biliary obstruction and cholestatic hepatitis
Aspartate aminotransferase (AST; previously serum glutamic-oxaloacetic transaminase [SGOT])	5-40 units/L	Increases with hepatocellular injury (and injury in other tissues, such as skeletal and cardiac muscle)
Alanine aminotransferase (ALT; previously serum glutamic-pyruvic transaminase [SGPT])	5-35 units/L	Increases with hepatocellular injury and necrosis
Lactate dehydrogenase (LDH)	90-220 units/L	Isoenzyme LD_5 is elevated with hypoxic and primary liver injury
5′-Nucleotidase	2-11 units/L	Increases with increase in alkaline phosphatase and cholestatic disorders
Bilirubin Metabolism		
Serum bilirubin		
Unconjugated (indirect)	<0.8 mg/dl	Increases with hemolysis (lysis of red blood cells)
Conjugated (direct)	0.2-0.4 mg/dl	Increases with hepatocellular injury or obstruction
TOTAL	<1.0 mg/dl	Increases with biliary obstruction
Urine bilirubin	0	Increases with biliary obstruction
Urine urobilinogen	0-4 mg/24 hr	Increases with hemolysis or shunting of portal blood flow
Serum Proteins		
Albumin	3.5-5.5 g/dl	Reduced with hepatocellular injury
Globulin	2.5-3.5 g/dl	Increases with hepatitis
TOTAL	6-7 g/dl	
Albumin/globulin (A/G) ratio	1.5 : 1 to 2.5 : 1	Ratio reverses with chronic hepatitis or other chronic liver disease
Transferrin	250-300 mcg/dl	Liver damage with decreased values, iron deficiency with increased values
Alpha fetoprotein (AFP)	6-20 ng/ml	Elevated values in primary hepatocellular carcinoma
Blood-Clotting Functions		
Prothrombin time (PT)	11.5-14 sec or 90-100% of control	Increases with chronic liver disease (cirrhosis) or vitamin K deficiency
Partial thromboplastin time (PTT)	25-40 sec	Increases with severe liver disease or heparin therapy
Bromosulfophthalein (BSP) excretion	<6% retention in 45 min	Increased retention with hepatocellular injury

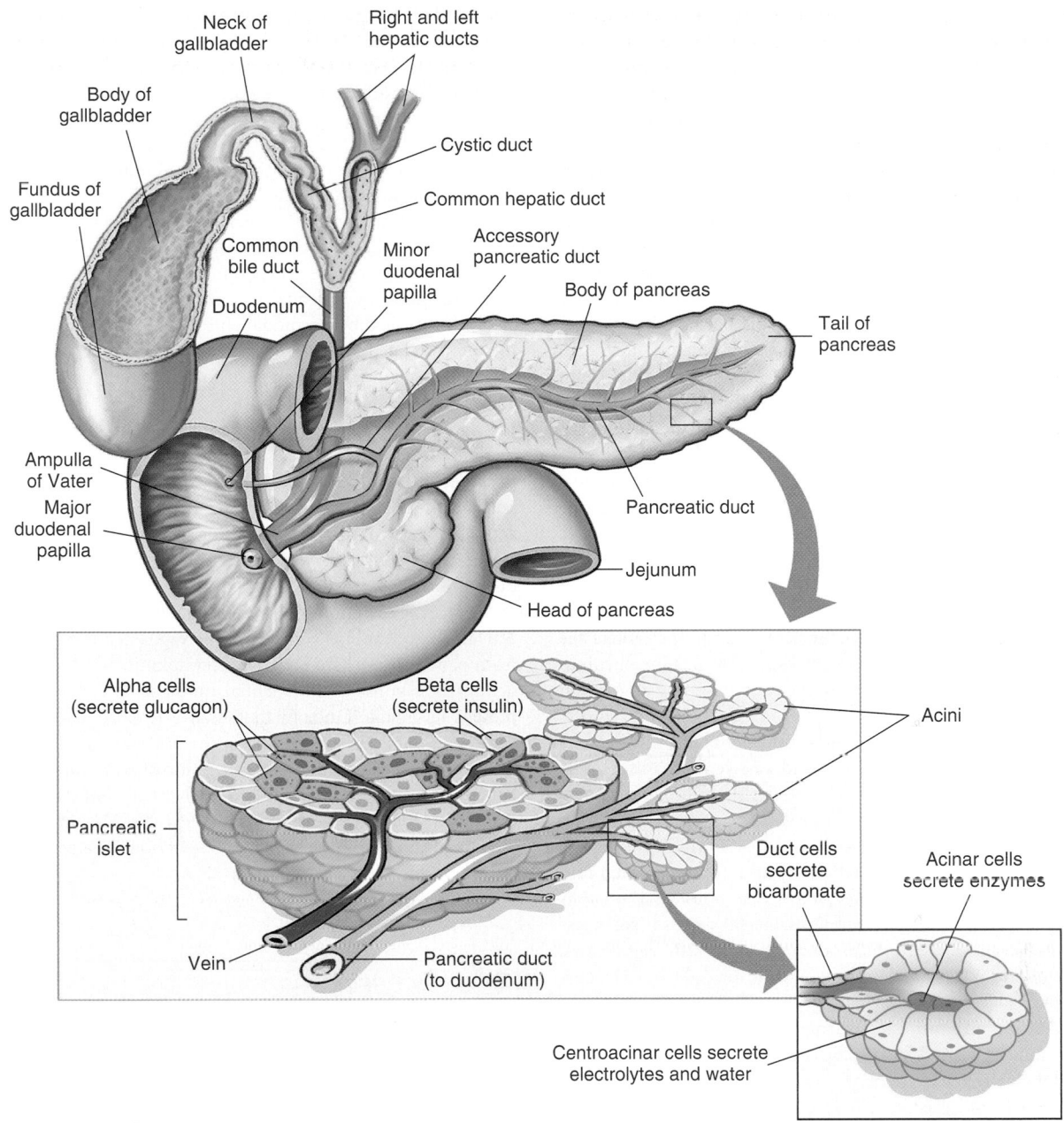

FIGURE 35-20 Associated Structures of the Gallbladder, Pancreas, and Pancreatic Acinar Cells and Duct. (Modified from Thibodeau GA, Patton KT: *Anatomy & physiology*, ed 6, St Louis, 2007, Mosby.)

between meals. During the interdigestive period, bile flows from the liver through the right or left hepatic duct into the common hepatic duct and meets resistance at the closed sphincter of Oddi (duodenal papilla), which controls flow into the duodenum and prevents backflow of duodenal contents into the pancreatobiliary system. Bile then flows through the cystic duct into the gallbladder, where it is concentrated and stored. The mucosa of the gallbladder wall readily absorbs water and electrolytes, leaving a high concentration of bile salts, bile pigments, and cholesterol. The gallbladder holds about 90 ml of bile.

Within 30 minutes after eating, the gallbladder begins to contract, forcing stored bile through the cystic duct and into the common bile duct. The sphincter of Oddi relaxes, and bile flows into the duodenum through the major duodenal papilla. During the cephalic and gastric phases of digestion, gallbladder contraction is mediated by cholinergic branches of the vagus nerve. Hormonal regulation of gallbladder contraction is derived primarily from the release of *cholecystokinin* secreted by the duodenal and jejunal mucosa in the presence of fat. Vasoactive intestinal peptide, pancreatic polypeptide, and sympathetic nerve stimulation relax the gallbladder.

Exocrine Pancreas

The pancreas is approximately 20 cm long, with its head tucked into the curve of the duodenum and its tail touching the spleen. The body of the pancreas lies deep in the abdomen, behind the stomach (see Figure 35-20). The pancreas is unique in that it has both endocrine and exocrine functions. The endocrine pancreas secretes hormones: insulin, glucagon, somatostatin, and pancreatic polypeptide (see Chapter 18).

The exocrine pancreas is composed of acinar cells that secrete enzymes and networks of ducts that secrete alkaline fluids. Both have important digestive functions. The acinar cells are organized into spherical lobules around small secretory ducts (see Figure 35-20). Secretions drain into a system of ducts that leads to the pancreatic duct (Wirsung duct), which empties into the common bile duct at the ampulla of Vater, and then into the duodenum. In some individuals, an accessory duct (the duct of Santorini) branches off the pancreatic duct and drains directly into the duodenum at the minor duodenal papilla.

Arterial blood is supplied to the pancreas by branches of the celiac and superior mesenteric arteries. Venous blood leaves the head of the pancreas through tributaries to the portal vein, with the body and tail being drained through the splenic vein. All hormonal pancreatic secretions also pass through the hepatic portal vein into the liver.

Pancreatic innervation arises from parasympathetic neurons of the vagus nerve. These fibers activate postganglionic fibers, which stimulate enzymatic and hormonal secretion. Sympathetic postganglionic fibers from the celiac and superior mesenteric plexuses innervate the blood vessels, cause vasoconstriction, and inhibit pancreatic secretion.

The aqueous secretions of the exocrine pancreas are isotonic and contain potassium, sodium, bicarbonate, and chloride. The highly alkaline pancreatic juice neutralizes the acidic chyme that enters the duodenum from the stomach and provides the alkaline medium needed for the actions of digestive enzymes and intestinal absorption of fat.

In the pancreas, transport of water and electrolytes through the ductal epithelium involves both active and passive mechanisms. The ductal cells actively transport hydrogen into the blood and bicarbonate into the duct lumen. Potassium and chloride are secreted by diffusion according to changes in electrochemical potential gradients. As the secretion flows down the duct, water is osmotically transported into the juice until it becomes isosmotic. At low flow rates bicarbonate is exchanged passively for chloride, but at higher flow rates there is less time for this exchange and bicarbonate concentration increases. Because eating stimulates the flow of pancreatic juice, the juice is most alkaline when it needs to be: during digestion.

The pancreatic enzymes can hydrolyze proteins (proteases), carbohydrates (amylases), and fats (lipases) (see Figure 35-11). The proteolytic (protein-digesting) enzymes include trypsin, chymotrypsin, carboxypeptidase, and elastase. These enzymes are secreted in their inactive forms—that is, as trypsinogen, chymotrypsinogen, procarboxypeptidase, and proelastase, respectively—to protect the pancreas from the digestive effects of its own enzymes. For further protection, the pancreas produces trypsin inhibitor, which prevents the activation of proteolytic enzymes while they are in the pancreas. Once in the duodenum, the inactive forms (proenzymes) are activated by enterokinase, an enzyme secreted by the duodenal mucosa. Trypsinogen is the first proenzyme to be activated. Its conversion to trypsin stimulates the conversion of chymotrypsinogen to chymotrypsin and procarboxypeptidase to carboxypeptidase. Each of these enzymes cleaves specific peptide bonds to reduce polypeptides to smaller peptides.

Secretion of the aqueous and enzymatic components of pancreatic juice is controlled by hormonal and vagal stimuli. Secretin stimulates the acinar and duct cells to secrete the bicarbonate-rich fluid that neutralizes chyme and prepares it for enzymatic digestion. As chyme enters the duodenum, its acidity (pH of 4.5 or less) stimulates the S cells (secretin-producing cells) of the duodenum to release secretin, which is absorbed by the intestine and delivered to the pancreas in the bloodstream. In the pancreas, secretin causes ductal and acinar cells to release alkaline fluid. Secretin also inhibits the actions of gastrin, thereby decreasing gastric hydrochloric acid secretion and motility. The overall effect is to neutralize the contents of the duodenum.

Enzymatic secretion follows, stimulated by cholecystokinin, which activates acetylcholine (Ach) from the vagus nerve and release of ACh from pancreatic stellate cells. Cholecystokinin is released in the duodenum in response to the essential amino acids and fatty acids already present in chyme. Once in the small intestine, activated pancreatic enzymes inhibit the release of more cholecystokinin and ACh. This feedback mechanism inhibits the secretion of more pancreatic enzymes. Pancreatic polypeptide is released after eating and inhibits postprandial pancreatic exocrine secretion. (See Table 35-1 for a summary of hormonal stimulation of pancreatic secretions.) Selected tests of pancreatic function are listed in Table 35-4.

✔ **QUICK CHECK 35-6**

1. Trace the route of bile salts and acids from formation to recycling.
2. What are the sources of the two types of bilirubin?
3. What is the function of the gallbladder?
4. How do pancreatic beta cells differ from acinar cells?

TABLE 35-4   Common Laboratory Tests of Exocrine Pancreatic Function

Test	Normal Value	Clinical Significance
Serum amylase	27-131 units/L	Elevated levels with pancreatic inflammation
Serum lipase	20-180 units/L	Elevated levels with pancreatic inflammation (may be elevated with other conditions; differentiates with amylase isoenzyme study)
Urine amylase	2-19 units/hr	Elevated levels with pancreatic inflammation
Secretin test	Volume 1.8 ml/kg/hr	Decreased volume with pancreatic disease because a secretin stimulates pancreatic secretion
	Bicarbonate concentration: >80 mEq/L	Decreased concentration or secretion or can occur with pancreatic injury related to pancreatitis; lack of buffering of gastric acid can lead to intestinal ulcers and decrease activation of digestive enzymes and drugs that require a higher pH
	Bicarbonate output: >10 mEq/L/30 sec	See above
Stool fat	2-5 g/24 hr	Measures fatty acids; decreased pancreatic lipase increases stool fat

GERIATRIC CONSIDERATIONS

Aging & the Gastrointestinal System

Age-related changes in gastrointestinal function vary among individuals and within organ systems. Changes can include the following:

Oral Cavity and Esophagus
1. Tooth enamel and dentin deteriorate, so cavities are more likely.
2. Teeth are lost as a result of periodontal disease and brittle roots that break easily.
3. Taste buds decline in number.
4. Sense of smell diminishes.
5. Salivary secretion decreases.
6. Dysphagia is much more common.
7. Eating is less pleasurable, appetite is reduced, and food is not sufficiently chewed or lubricated; therefore swallowing is difficult.

Stomach
1. Gastric motility, blood flow, and volume and acid content of gastric juice may be reduced, particularly with gastric atrophy, and gastric emptying may be delayed.
2. Protective mucosal barrier decreases.

Intestines
1. There is a change in the composition of the intestinal microbiota and resultant increased susceptibility to disease.
2. Size of Peyer patches and degree of mucosal immunity decline with increased risk for infection and inflammation.

3. The brain-gut axis (bidirectional neuroendocrine communication) may be disrupted and enteric neurons may degenerate with changes in gastrointestinal motility, secretion, and absorption as well as the elder person's appetite, and overall nutritional status.
4. Intestinal villi may become shorter and more convoluted, with diminished reparative capacity.
5. Intestinal absorption, motility, and blood flow may decrease, prolonging transit time and altering nutrient absorption.
6. Rectal muscle mass decreases and the anal sphincter weakens.
7. Constipation, fecal impaction, and fecal incontinence may develop and is related to immobility, low-fiber diet, and changes in enteric nervous system structure and functions.

Liver
1. There is decreased hepatic regeneration; size and weight of liver decrease.
2. Ability to detoxify drugs decreases.
3. Blood flow decreases, influencing efficiency of drug metabolism.

Pancreas and Gallbladder
1. Fibrosis, fatty acid deposits, and pancreatic atrophy occur.
2. Secretion of digestive enzymes, particularly proteolytic enzymes, decreases.
3. No changes in gallbladder and bile ducts occur, but there is an increased prevalence of gallstones and cholecystitis.

Data from Britton E, McLaughlin JT: *Proc Nutr Soc* 72(1):173-177, 2013; Lakshminarayanan B et al: *J Nutr Health Aging* 18(9):773-786, 2014; Rayner CK, Horowitz M: *Curr Opin Clin Nutr Metab Care* 16(1):33-38, 2013; Saffrey MJ: *Age (Dordr)* 36(3):9603, 2014; Saffrey MJ: *Dev Biol* 382(1):344-355, 2013.

■ DID YOU UNDERSTAND?

The Gastrointestinal Tract
1. The major functions of the gastrointestinal tract are the mechanical and chemical breakdown of food and the absorption of digested nutrients.
2. The gastrointestinal tract is a hollow tube that extends from the mouth to the anus.
3. The walls of the gastrointestinal tract have several layers: mucosa, muscularis mucosae, submucosa, tunica muscularis (circular muscle and longitudinal muscle), and serosa.
4. The peritoneum is a double layer of membranous tissue. The visceral layer covers the abdominal organs, and the parietal layer extends along the abdominal wall. The peritoneal cavity is the space between the two layers.
5. Except for swallowing and defecation, which are controlled voluntarily, the functions of the gastrointestinal tract are controlled by extrinsic and intrinsic autonomic nerves and intestinal hormones.
6. Digestion begins in the mouth, with chewing and salivation. The digestive component of saliva is α-amylase, which initiates carbohydrate digestion.
7. The esophagus is a muscular tube that transports food from the mouth to the stomach. The tunica muscularis in the upper part of the esophagus is striated muscle, and that in the lower part is smooth muscle.
8. Swallowing is controlled by the swallowing center in the reticular formation of the brain. The two phases of swallowing are the oropharyngeal phase (voluntary swallowing) and the esophageal phase (involuntary swallowing).
9. Food is propelled through the esophagus by peristalsis: waves of sequential relaxations and contractions of the tunica muscularis.
10. The lower esophageal sphincter opens to admit swallowed food into the stomach and then closes to prevent regurgitation of food back into the esophagus.
11. The stomach is a baglike structure that secretes digestive juices, mixes and stores food, and propels partially digested food (chyme) through the pylorus into the duodenum.
12. The vagus nerve stimulates gastric (stomach) secretion and motility.
13. The hormones gastrin and motilin stimulate gastric emptying; the hormones secretin and cholecystokinin delay gastric emptying.
14. Mucus is secreted throughout the stomach and protects the stomach wall from acid and digestive enzymes.
15. Gastric glands in the fundus and body of the stomach secrete intrinsic factor, which is needed for vitamin B_{12} absorption; and hydrochloric acid, which dissolves food fibers, kills microorganisms, and activates the enzyme pepsin.
16. Chief cells in the stomach secrete pepsinogen, which is converted to pepsin in the acidic environment created by hydrochloric acid.
17. Acid secretion is stimulated by the vagus nerve, gastrin, and histamine and is inhibited by sympathetic stimulation and cholecystokinin.

18. The three phases of acid secretion by the stomach are the cephalic phase (anticipation and swallowing), the gastric phase (food in the stomach), and the intestinal phase (chyme in the intestine).

19. The small intestine is 5 meters long and has three segments: the duodenum, jejunum, and ileum.

20. The duodenum receives chyme from the stomach through the pyloric valve. The presence of chyme stimulates the liver and gallbladder to deliver bile and the pancreas to deliver digestive enzymes. Bile and enzymes flow through an opening guarded by the sphincter of Oddi.

21. Enzymes secreted by the small intestine (maltase, sucrase, lactase), pancreatic enzymes, and bile salts act in the small intestine to digest proteins, carbohydrates, and fats.

22. Digested substances are absorbed across the intestinal wall and then transported to the liver, where they are metabolized further.

23. The ileocecal valve connects the small and large intestines and prevents reflux into the small intestine.

24. Villi are small fingerlike projections that extend from the small intestinal mucosa and increase its absorptive surface area.

25. Carbohydrates, amino acids, and fats are absorbed primarily by the duodenum and jejunum; bile salts and vitamin B_{12} are absorbed by the ileum. Vitamin B_{12} absorption requires the presence of intrinsic factor.

26. Bile is produced by the liver and is necessary for fat digestion and absorption. Bile's alkalinity helps to neutralize chyme, thereby creating a pH that enables the pancreatic enzymes to digest proteins, carbohydrates, and fats.

27. Bile salts emulsify and hydrolyze fats and incorporate them into water-soluble micelles, which are then transported through the unstirred water layer to the brush border of the intestinal mucosa. The fat content of the micelles readily diffuses through the epithelium into lacteals (lymphatic ducts) in the villi. From there, fats flow into lymphatics and into the systemic circulation, which delivers them to the liver.

28. Minerals and water-soluble vitamins are absorbed by both active and passive transport throughout the small intestine.

29. Peristaltic movements created by longitudinal muscles propel the chyme along the intestinal tract, and contractions of the circular muscles (haustral segmentation) mix the chyme.

30. The ileogastric reflex inhibits gastric motility when the ileum is distended.

31. The intestinointestinal reflex inhibits intestinal motility when one intestinal segment is overdistended.

32. The gastroileal reflex increases intestinal motility when gastric motility increases.

33. The large intestine consists of the cecum, appendix, colon (ascending, transverse, descending, and sigmoid), rectum, and anal canal.

34. The teniae coli are three bands of longitudinal muscle that extend the length of the colon.

35. Haustra are pouches of colon formed with alternating contraction and relaxation of the circular muscles.

36. The mucosa of the large intestine contains mucus-secreting cells and mucosal folds, but no villi.

37. The large intestine massages the fecal mass and absorbs water and electrolytes.

38. Distention of the ileum with chyme causes the gastrocolic reflex, or the mass propulsion of feces to the rectum.

39. Defecation is stimulated when the rectum is distended with feces. The tonically contracted internal anal sphincter relaxes, and if the voluntarily regulated external sphincter relaxes, defecation occurs.

40. The immune system of the GI tract consists of Paneth cells, which produce defensins and other antimicrobial peptides and lysozymes; and the lymph nodes of Peyer patches, which contain lymphocytes, plasma cells, and macrophages.

41. The largest number of intestinal bacteria (intestinal microbiome) is in the colon. The most numerous anaerobes are *Bacteroides* and *Firmicutes*. Intestinal bacteria are important for metabolism of bile salts, metabolism of selected drugs and hormones, and prevention of pathogen colonization.

42. The intestinal tract is sterile at birth and becomes totally colonized within 3 to 4 weeks.

43. The splanchnic blood flow provides blood to the esophagus, stomach, small and large intestines, gallbladder, pancreas, and spleen.

Accessory Organs of Digestion

1. The liver is the second largest organ in the body. It has digestive, metabolic, hematologic, vascular, and immunologic functions.

2. The liver is divided into the right and left lobes and smaller units called liver lobules. The liver is supported by the falciform, round, and coronary ligaments.

3. Liver lobules consist of plates of hepatocytes, which are the functional cells of the liver.

4. The hepatocytes synthesize 700 to 1200 ml of bile per day and secrete it into the bile canaliculi, which are small channels between the hepatocytes. The bile canaliculi drain bile into the common bile duct and then into the duodenum through an opening called the *major duodenal papilla (sphincter of Oddi)*.

5. Sinusoids are capillaries located between the plates of hepatocytes. Blood from the portal vein and hepatic artery flows through the sinusoids to a central vein in each lobule and then to the hepatic vein and inferior vena cava.

6. Kupffer cells, which are part of the mononuclear phagocyte system, line the sinusoids and destroy microorganisms in sinusoidal blood; they are important in bilirubin production and lipid metabolism.

7. The primary bile acids are synthesized from cholesterol by the hepatocytes. The primary acids are then conjugated to form bile salts. The secondary bile acids are the product of bile salt deconjugation by bacteria in the intestinal lumen.

8. Most bile salts and acids are recycled. The absorption of bile salts and acids from the terminal ileum and their return to the liver are known as the *enterohepatic circulation of bile*.

9. Bilirubin is a pigment liberated by the lysis of aged red blood cells in the liver and spleen. Unconjugated bilirubin is fat soluble and can cross cell membranes. Unconjugated bilirubin is converted to water-soluble, conjugated bilirubin by hepatocytes and is secreted with bile.

10. The liver produces clotting factors and can store a large volume of blood.

11. The liver plays a major role in the metabolism of fats, proteins, and carbohydrates; and stores minerals, vitamin B_{12}, and fat-soluble vitamins.

12. The liver metabolically transforms or detoxifies hormones, toxic substances, and drugs to less active substances.

13. The gallbladder is a saclike organ located on the inferior surface of the liver. The gallbladder stores bile between meals and ejects it when chyme enters the duodenum.

14. Stimulated by cholecystokinin, the gallbladder contracts and forces bile through the cystic duct and into the common bile duct. The sphincter of Oddi relaxes, enabling bile to flow through the major duodenal papilla into the duodenum.

15. The pancreas is a gland located behind the stomach. The endocrine pancreas produces hormones (glucagon, insulin) that facilitate the formation and cellular uptake of glucose. The exocrine pancreas secretes an alkaline solution and the enzymes (trypsin, chymotrypsin, carboxypeptidase, α-amylase, lipase) that digest proteins, carbohydrates, and fats.

16. Secretin stimulates pancreatic secretion of alkaline fluid, and cholecystokinin and acetylcholine stimulate secretion of enzymes. Pancreatic secretions originate in acini and ducts of the pancreas and empty into the duodenum through the common bile duct or an accessory duct that opens directly into the duodenum.

KEY TERMS

Alimentary canal (gastrointestinal tract), 884
Ampulla of Vater, 902
Antrum, 887
Ascending colon, 894
Bile, 897
Bile acid pool, 898
Bile acid–dependent fraction, 897
Bile acid–independent fraction, 897
Bile canaliculi, 896
Bile salt, 897
Bilirubin, 898
Brush border, 891
Cardiac orifice, 887
Cecum, 894
Chief cell, 889
Cholecystokinin, 887
Choleresis, 898
Choleretic agent, 898
Chyme, 887
Colon, 894
Common bile duct, 896
Conjugated bilirubin, 898
Crypts of Lieberkühn, 891
Cystic duct, 901
Deamination, 899
Defecation reflex (rectosphincteric reflex), 895
Descending colon, 894
Disse space, 897
Duodenum, 889

Enteric (intramural) plexus, 884
Enterocytes, 890
Enterohepatic circulation, 897
Enterokinase, 902
Esophageal phase of swallowing, 886
Esophagus, 886
Exocrine pancreas, 902
External anal sphincter, 894
Fecal mass, 894
Fundus, 887
Gallbladder, 900
Gastric emptying, 888
Gastric gland, 888
Gastrin, 887
Gastrocolic reflex, 894
Gastroileal reflex, 893
Glisson capsule, 896
Haustral segmentation, 892
Haustrum (pl., haustra), 894
Hepatic artery, 896
Hepatic portal vein, 896
Hepatic vein, 896
Hepatocyte, 896
Ileocecal valve (sphincter), 890
Ileogastric reflex, 893
Ileum, 889
Internal anal sphincter, 894
Intestinointestinal reflex, 893
Intrinsic factor, 888
Jejunum, 889
Kupffer cell (tissue macrophage), 896

Lacteal, 891
Lamina propria, 891
Large intestine, 894
Liver, 896
Liver lobule, 896
Lower esophageal sphincter (cardiac sphincter), 886
Major duodenal papilla, 896
Mesentery, 890
Metabolic detoxification (biotransformation), 899
Microvillus (pl., microvilli), 890
Motilin, 888
Mouth, 884
Mucosal barrier, 889
Myenteric plexus (Auerbach plexus), 890
Natural killer cells (pit cells), 897
Oropharyngeal (voluntary) phase of swallowing, 886
Pancreas, 901
Pancreatic duct (Wirsung duct), 902
Paneth cell, 895
Pepsin, 889
Peristalsis, 886
Peritoneal cavity, 890
Peritoneum, 890
Peyer patch, 895
Primary bile acid, 897
Primary peristalsis, 887
Pyloric sphincter, 887

Pylorus (gastroduodenal junction), 887
Rectosigmoid (O'Beirne) sphincter, 894
Rectum, 895
Reticuloendothelial system, 898
Retropulsion, 888
S cell, 902
Saliva, 886
Salivary α-amylase (ptyalin), 886
Salivary gland, 886
Secondary bile acid, 897
Secondary peristalsis, 887
Secretin, 888
Sigmoid colon, 894
Sinusoid, 896
Small intestine, 889
Sphincter of Oddi, 896
Splanchnic blood flow, 896
Stellate cells, 897
Stomach, 887
Submucosal plexus (Meissner plexus), 890
Swallowing, 886
Teniae coli, 894
Transverse colon, 894
Trypsin inhibitor, 902
Unconjugated bilirubin, 898
Upper esophageal sphincter, 886
Urobilinogen, 898
Valsalva maneuver, 895
Vermiform appendix, 894
Villus (pl., villi), 890

REFERENCES

1. Woodland P et al: The neurophysiology of the esophagus, *Ann N Y Acad Sci* 1300:53-70, 2013.
2. Hellström PM et al: The physiology of gastric emptying, *Best Pract Res Clin Anaesthesiol* 20(3):397-407, 2006.
3. Chu S, Schuberft ML: Gastric secretion, *Curr Opin Gastroenterol* 28(6):587-593, 2012.
4. Niv Y, Fraser GM: The alkaline tide phenomenon, *J Clin Gastroenterol* 35(1):5-8, 2002.
5. Miller MJ et al: Microanatomy of the intestinal lymphatic system, *Ann N Y Acad Sci* 1207(Suppl 1): E21-E28, 2010.
6. Bobadilla JL: Mesenteric ischemia, *Surg Clin North Am* 93(4):925-940, ix, 2013.
7. Mowat AM, Agace WW: Regional specialization within the intestinal immune system, *Nat Rev Immunol* 14(10):667-685, 2014.
8. Schippa S, Conte MP: Dysbiotic events in gut microbiota: impact on human health, *Nutrients* 6(12):5786-5805, 2014.
9. Khanna S, Tosh PK: A clinician's primer on the role of the microbiome in human health and disease, *Mayo Clin Proc* 89(1):107-114, 2014.
10. Dixon LJ et al: Kupffer cells in the liver, *Compr Physiol* 3(2):785-797, 2013.
11. Weiskirchen R, Tacke F: Cellular and molecular functions of hepatic stellate cells in inflammatory responses and liver immunology, *Hepatobiliary Surg Nutr* 3(6):344-363, 2014.
12. Tian Z et al: Natural killer cells in liver disease, *Hepatology* 57(4):1654-1662, 2013.
13. Jansen T, Daiber A: Direct antioxidant properties of bilirubin and biliverdin. Is there a role for biliverdin reductase? *Front Pharmacol* 3:30, 2012.

36

Alterations of Digestive Function

Sue E. Huether

CHAPTER OUTLINE

The gastrointestinal (GI) tract is a continuous, hollow organ that extends from the mouth to the anus. It includes the esophagus, stomach, small intestine, large intestine, and rectum. The accessory organs of digestion include the salivary glands, liver, gallbladder, and pancreas.

Disorders of the gastrointestinal tract disrupt one or more of its functions. Structural and neural abnormalities can slow, obstruct, or accelerate the movement of intestinal contents at any level of the gastrointestinal tract. Inflammatory and ulcerative conditions of the gastrointestinal wall disrupt secretion, motility, and absorption. Inflammation or obstruction of the liver, pancreas, or gallbladder can alter metabolism and result in local and systemic symptoms. Many clinical manifestations of gastrointestinal tract disorders are nonspecific and can be caused by a variety of impairments.

DISORDERS OF THE GASTROINTESTINAL TRACT

Clinical Manifestations of Gastrointestinal Dysfunction

Anorexia

Anorexia is lack of a desire to eat despite physiologic stimuli that would normally produce hunger. This nonspecific symptom is often associated with nausea, abdominal pain, diarrhea, and psychologic stress. Side effects of drugs and disorders of other organ systems, including cancer, heart disease, and renal disease, are often accompanied by anorexia.

Vomiting

Vomiting (emesis) is the forceful emptying of stomach and intestinal contents (chyme) through the mouth.[1] The vomiting center lies in the medulla oblongata. Stimuli initiating the vomiting reflex include severe pain; distention of the stomach or duodenum; the presence of ipecac or copper salts in the duodenum; stimulation of the vestibular system through the eighth cranial nerve (motion sickness); side effects of many drugs; torsion or trauma affecting the ovaries, testes, uterus, bladder, or kidney; motion; and activation of the chemoreceptor trigger zone (CTZ) (area postrema) in the medulla (e.g., morphine). Nausea and retching (dry heaves) are distinct events that usually precede vomiting. Nausea is a subjective experience associated with various conditions, including abnormal pain and labyrinthine stimulation (i.e., spinning movement). Specific neural pathways have not been identified, but hypersalivation and tachycardia are common associated symptoms. Retching is the muscular event of vomiting without the expulsion of vomitus.

Vomiting begins with deep inspiration. The glottis closes, the intrathoracic pressure falls, and the esophagus becomes distended. Simultaneously, the abdominal muscles contract, creating a pressure gradient from abdomen to thorax. The lower esophageal sphincter (LES) and body of the stomach relax, but the duodenum and antrum of the stomach spasm. The reverse peristalsis and pressure gradient force chyme from the stomach and duodenum up into the esophagus. Because the upper esophageal sphincter is closed, chyme does not enter the mouth. As the abdominal muscles relax, the contents of the esophagus drop back into the stomach. This process may be repeated several times before vomiting occurs. A diffuse sympathetic discharge causes the tachycardia, tachypnea, and diaphoresis that accompany retching and vomiting. The parasympathetic system mediates copious salivation, increased gastric motility, and relaxation of the upper and lower esophageal sphincters.

With vomiting, the duodenum and antrum of the stomach produce reverse peristalsis, while the body of the stomach and the esophagus relax. When the stomach is full of gastric contents, the diaphragm is forced high into the thoracic cavity by strong contractions of the abdominal muscles. The higher intrathoracic pressure forces the upper esophageal sphincter to open, and chyme is expelled from the mouth. Then the stomach relaxes and the upper part of the esophagus contracts, forcing the remaining chyme back into the stomach. The lower esophageal sphincter then closes. The cycle is repeated if there is a volume of chyme remaining in the stomach.

Spontaneous vomiting not preceded by nausea or retching is called *projectile vomiting*. It is caused by direct stimulation of the vomiting center by neurologic lesions (e.g., increased intracranial pressure, tumors, or aneurysms) involving the brainstem or can be a symptom of gastrointestinal obstruction (pyloric stenosis). The metabolic consequences of vomiting are fluid, electrolyte, and acid-base disturbances including hyponatremia, hypokalemia, hypochloremia, and metabolic alkalosis (see Chapter 5).

Constipation

Constipation is difficult or infrequent defecation. It is a common problem, particularly among the elderly, and usually means a decrease in the number of bowel movements per week, hard stools, and difficult evacuation. The definition must be individually determined since normal bowel habits range from one to three evacuations per day to one per week. Constipation is not significant until it causes health risks or impairs quality of life.

PATHOPHYSIOLOGY Constipation can occur as a primary or secondary condition.[2] Primary constipation is generally classified into three categories. *Normal transit (functional) constipation* involves a normal rate of stool passage but there is difficulty with stool evacuation. *Functional constipation* is associated with a sedentary lifestyle, low-residue diet (the habitual consumption of highly refined foods), or low fluid intake. *Slow-transit constipation* involves impaired colonic motor activity with infrequent bowel movements, straining to defecate, mild abdominal distention, and palpable stool in the sigmoid colon. *Pelvic floor* or *outlet dysfunction* refers to an inability or difficulty expelling stool because of dysfunction of the pelvic floor muscles or anal sphincter. Examples include pelvic floor dyssynergia, rectal fissures, strictures, or hemorrhoids.

Secondary constipation can be caused by diet, medications, or neurogenic disorders (e.g., stroke, Parkinson disease, spinal cord lesions, multiple sclerosis, Hirschsprung disease) in which neural pathways or neurotransmitters are altered and colon transit time delayed. Opiates (particularly codeine), antacids containing calcium carbonate or aluminum hydroxide, anticholinergics, iron, and bismuth tend to inhibit bowel motility. Endocrine or metabolic disorders associated with constipation include hypothyroidism, diabetes mellitus, hypokalemia, and hypercalcemia. Pelvic hiatal hernia (herniation of the bowel through the floor of the pelvis), diverticuli, irritable bowel syndrome (constipation predominant), and pregnancy are associated with constipation. Aging may result in decreased mobility, changes in neuromuscular function, use of medications, and comorbid medical conditions causing constipation.[2] Constipation as a notable change in bowel habits can be an indication of colorectal cancer.

CLINICAL MANIFESTATIONS Indicators of constipation include two of the following for at least 3 months: (1) straining with defecation at least 25% of the time; (2) lumpy or hard stools at least 25% of the time; (3) sensation of incomplete emptying at least 25% of the time; (4) manual maneuvers to facilitate stool evacuation for at least 25% of defecations; and (5) fewer than three bowel movements per week.[3] Changes in bowel evacuation patterns, such as less frequent defecation, smaller stool volume, hard stools, difficulty passing stools (straining), or a feeling of bowel fullness and discomfort, require investigation. Fecal impaction (hard, dry stool retained in the rectum) is associated with rectal bleeding, abdominal or cramping pain, nausea and vomiting, weight loss, and episodes of diarrhea. Straining to evacuate stool may cause engorgement of the hemorrhoidal veins and hemorrhoidal disease or thrombosis with rectal pain, bleeding, and itching. Passage of hard stools can cause painful anal fissures.

EVALUATION AND TREATMENT The history, current use of medications, physical examination, and stool diaries provide precise clues regarding the nature of constipation. The individual's description of frequency, stool consistency, associated pain, and presence of blood or whether evacuation was stimulated by enemas or cathartics (laxatives) is important. Palpation may disclose colonic distention, masses, and tenderness. Digital examination of the rectum and anorectal manometry are performed to assess sphincter tone and detect anal lesions. Colonic transit time and imaging techniques can assist in identifying the cause of constipation. Colonoscopy is used to visualize the lumen directly.

The treatment for constipation is to manage the underlying cause or disease for each individual. Management of constipation usually consists of bowel retraining, in which the individual establishes a satisfactory bowel evacuation routine without becoming preoccupied with bowel movements. The individual also may need to engage in moderate exercise, drink more fluids, and increase fiber intake. Fiber supplements, stool softeners, and laxative agents are useful for some individuals. Enemas can be used to establish bowel routine, but they should not be used habitually. Biofeedback may be beneficial in some instances for forming new bowel evacuation habits. When there is failure to respond to dietary or medical therapies, surgery (colectomy) is considered as a last resort.[4]

Diarrhea

Diarrhea is the presence of loose, watery stools. Acute diarrhea is more than three loose stools developing within 24 hours and lasting less than 14 days. Persistent diarrhea lasts longer than 14 to 30 days and chronic diarrhea lasts longer than 4 weeks.[5,6] Diarrhea can have high rates of morbidity and mortality in children younger than 5 years of age, particularly in developing countries (see Chapter 37) and in the elderly. Many factors determine stool volume, including water content of the colon, diet, the presence of nonabsorbed food, nonabsorbable material, and intestinal secretions. Stool volume in the normal adult averages less than 200 g/day. Stool volume in children depends on age and size. An infant may pass up to 100 g/day. The adult intestine processes approximately 9 L of luminal contents per day: 2 L are ingested and the remaining 7 L consist of intestinal secretions. Of this volume, 99% of the fluid is absorbed: 90% (7 to 8 L) in the small intestine and 9% (1 to 2 L) in the colon. Normally, approximately 150 ml of water is excreted daily in the stool.

PATHOPHYSIOLOGY Diarrhea in which the volume of feces is increased is called *large-volume diarrhea*. It generally is caused by excessive amounts of water or secretions or both in the intestines. *Small-volume diarrhea,* in which the volume of feces is not increased, usually results from excessive intestinal motility.

The three major mechanisms of diarrhea are osmotic, secretory, and motile:

1. Osmotic diarrhea. A nonabsorbable substance in the intestine draws excess water into the intestine and increases stool weight and volume, producing large-volume diarrhea. Causes include lactase and pancreatic enzyme deficiency; excessive ingestion of synthetic, nonabsorbable sugars; full-strength tube-feeding formulas; or dumping syndrome associated with gastric resection (see p. 918).
2. Secretory diarrhea. Excessive mucosal secretion of fluid and electrolytes produces large-volume diarrhea. Infectious causes include viruses (e.g., rotavirus), bacterial enterotoxins (e.g., *Escherichia coli* and *Vibrio cholerae*), exotoxins from overgrowth of *Clostridium difficile* following antibiotic therapy (see *Health Alert: Clostridium difficile* and Fecal Microbiome Transplant), or small bowel bacterial overgrowth.[7] Small-volume diarrhea is usually caused by an inflammatory disorder of the intestine, such as ulcerative colitis, Crohn disease, or microscopic colitis, but also can result from colon cancer or fecal impaction.

HEALTH ALERT

Clostridium difficile *and Fecal Microbiome Transplant*

Virulent *Clostridium difficile (C. diff)* is a gram-positive toxin producing bacteria that cause pseudomembranous colitis and *C. difficile*–associated diarrhea, particularly in hospitalized individuals treated with antibiotics. These infections are more frequent, severe, and resistant to treatment; tend to recur; and increase morbidity and mortality as well as treatment costs. Infection with *C. diff* (CDI) occurs when antibiotic therapy alters normal gut flora (dysbiosis), allowing *C. diff* to proliferate. The spore form is resistant to treatment and also can remain on dry surfaces for weeks and infect healthy individuals. New strains are more common and more virulent, and demonstrate increased resistance to treatment. Metronidazole is the first-line treatment for *C. diff*. However, it may be ineffective; then vancomycin is used, which suppresses growth of all gram-positive aerobic and anaerobic organisms, including commensal gut bacteria that are important for mucosal immunity, digestion, and control of pathogens promoting recurrence. Fidaxomicin treatment has fewer recurrences but is very costly. With resistance, spore forms remain in the gut and transition to the vegetative toxin form, causing recurrent infection and disease. Nonantibiotic treatment is being evaluated in an effort to break the cycle of recurrent infection and restore gut microbiota, protect the gut mucosa, and control *C. diff* spores. Nonantibiotic treatment includes fecal microbiota transplantation, which has been successful in about 90% of cases. The assumption is that microbiota transplant can restore the diversity and proportion of phyla that promote colonic health. The treatment is safe, efficacious, and inexpensive. Fecal microbiota transplantation is under the surveillance of the Food and Drug Administration; the FDA has approved fecal microbiota therapy in individuals not responding to standard treatment (response rates of 83% to 94% for recurrent CDI). Informed consent is required; however, fecal microbiota transplantation is not recommended for use in pregnant women. Fecal microbiome transplantation for recurrent CDI in inflammatory bowel disease has been associated with colitis exacerbation in the majority of individuals who have received this treatment. Clinical investigations are continuing, and fecal microbiome transplant is being evaluated for diseases other than recurrent CDI.

Data from Borgia G et al: *Expert Opin Biol Ther* 15(7):1001-1014, 2015; Drekonja D et al: *Fecal microbiota transplantation for clostridium difficile infection: a systematic review of the evidence* [Internet], Washington, DC, 2014, Department of Veterans Affairs (US). Available from http://www.ncbi.nlm.nih.gov/books/NBK299000/; Goldberg EJ et al: *Am J Health Syst Pharm* 72(12):1007-1012, 2015; Kelly CR et al: *Gastroenterology*. 2015 May 15. [Epub ahead of print.]

3. Motility diarrhea is caused by resection of the small intestine (short bowel syndrome), surgical bypass of an area of the intestine or fistula formation between loops of intestine, irritable bowel syndrome–diarrhea predominant, diabetic neuropathy, hyperthyroidism, and laxative abuse. Excessive motility decreases transit time and opportunity for fluid absorption, resulting in diarrhea.

CLINICAL MANIFESTATIONS   Diarrhea can be acute or chronic depending on its cause. Systemic effects of prolonged diarrhea are dehydration, electrolyte imbalance (hyponatremia, hypokalemia), and weight loss. Manifestations of acute bacterial or viral infection include fever, with or without vomiting or cramping pain. Most infectious diarrhea usually lasts less than 2 weeks. The exceptions are *Clostridium difficile, Aeromonas,* or *Yersinia enterocolitica*.[8] Fever, cramping pain, and bloody stools accompany chronic diarrhea caused by inflammatory bowel disease or dysentery. Steatorrhea (fat in the stools), bloating, and diarrhea are common signs of malabsorption syndromes. Anal and perineal skin irritation can occur.

EVALUATION AND TREATMENT   A thorough history is taken to document the onset, frequency, volume of stools, duration of diarrhea, and presence of blood in the stools. Malabsorption syndromes usually manifest steatorrhea. Exposure to contaminated food or water is indicated if the individual has traveled in foreign countries or areas where drinking water might be contaminated. Iatrogenic diarrhea is suggested if the individual has undergone abdominal radiation therapy, intestinal resection, or treatment with selected drugs (e.g., antibiotics, diuretics, antihypertensives, laxatives, anticoagulants or chemotherapy). Physical examination helps identify underlying systemic disease. Stool studies, abdominal imaging, endoscopy, and intestinal biopsies provide more specific data, particularly for persistent diarrhea.

Treatment for diarrhea includes restoration of fluid and electrolyte balance, administration of antimotility (e.g., loperamide) and/or water absorbent (e.g., attapulgite and polycarbophil) medications, and treatment of causal factors. Nutritional deficiencies need to be corrected in cases of chronic diarrhea or malabsorption.[9]

Abdominal Pain

Abdominal pain is the presenting symptom of a number of gastrointestinal diseases and can be acute or chronic.[10] The causal mechanisms of abdominal pain are *mechanical, inflammatory,* or *ischemic.* Generally, the abdominal organs are not sensitive to mechanical stimuli, such as cutting, tearing, or crushing. These organs are, however, sensitive to stretching and distention, which activate nerve endings in both hollow and solid structures. Pain accompanies rapid distention rather than gradual distention. Traction on the peritoneum caused by adhesions, distention of the common bile duct, or forceful peristalsis resulting from intestinal obstruction causes pain because of increased tension. Capsules that surround solid organs, such as the liver and gallbladder, contain pain fibers that are stimulated by stretching if these organs swell. Abdominal pain may be generalized to the abdomen or localized to a particular abdominal quadrant. The nature of the pain is often described as sharp, dull, or colicky.

Abdominal pain is usually associated with tissue injury and inflammation. Biochemical mediators of the inflammatory response, such as histamine, bradykinin, and serotonin, stimulate organic nerve endings and produce abdominal pain. The edema and vascular congestion that accompany chemical, bacterial, or viral inflammation also cause painful stretching. Hindrance of blood flow from the distention of bowel obstruction or mesenteric vessel thrombosis produces the pain of ischemia, and increased concentrations of tissue metabolites stimulate pain receptors.

Abdominal pain can be parietal (somatic), visceral, or referred. Parietal pain, from the parietal peritoneum, is more localized and intense than visceral pain, which arises from the organs themselves. Parietal pain lateralizes because, at any particular point, the parietal peritoneum is innervated from only one side of the nervous system.

Visceral pain arises from a stimulus (distention, inflammation, ischemia) acting on an abdominal organ. Inflammatory mediators associated with chronic low-grade inflammation can cause pain hypersensitivity.[11] The pain is usually poorly localized, diffuse, or vague with a radiating pattern because nerve endings in abdominal organs are sparse and multisegmented. Pain arising from the stomach, for example, is experienced as a sensation of fullness, cramping, or gnawing in the midepigastric area. Referred pain is visceral pain felt at some distance from a diseased or affected organ. It is usually well localized and is felt in the skin dermatomes or deeper tissues that share a central afferent pathway with the affected organ. For example, acute cholecystitis may have pain referred to the right shoulder or scapula.

Gastrointestinal Bleeding

Upper gastrointestinal bleeding is bleeding in the esophagus, stomach, or duodenum, and is characterized by frank, bright red bleeding or dark, grainy digested blood ("coffee grounds") that has been affected by stomach acids (Table 36-1). Upper gastrointestinal (GI) bleeding is commonly caused by bleeding varices (varicose veins) in the esophagus, peptic ulcers, arteriovenous malformations, or a Mallory-Weiss tear at the esophageal-gastric junction caused by severe retching.[12] Lower gastrointestinal bleeding, or bleeding from the jejunum, ileum, colon, or rectum, can be caused by polyps, diverticulitis, inflammatory disease, cancer, or hemorrhoids. Occult bleeding is usually caused by slow, chronic blood loss that is not obvious and results in iron deficiency anemia as iron stores in the bone marrow are slowly depleted.[13] Acute, severe GI bleeding is life-threatening depending on the volume and rate of blood loss, associated disease and age of the affected individual, and effectiveness of treatment.

Physiologic response to GI bleeding depends on the amount and rate of the loss (Figure 36-1). Changes in blood pressure and heart rate are the best indicators of massive blood loss in the GI tract. During the early stages of blood volume depletion, the peripheral arteries and arterioles constrict to shunt blood to vital organs, including the brain. Signs of large-volume blood loss are postural hypotension (a drop in blood pressure that occurs with a change from the recumbent position to a sitting or upright position), lightheadedness, and loss of vision.

Tachycardia develops as a compensatory response to maintain cardiac output and tissue perfusion. If blood loss continues, hypovolemic shock develops (see Chapter 24). Diminished blood flow to the kidneys causes decreased urine output and may lead to oliguria (low urine output), tubular necrosis, and renal failure. Ultimately, insufficient cerebral and coronary blood flow causes irreversible anoxia and death.

The presentations of GI bleeding are summarized in Table 36-1. The accumulation of blood in the gastrointestinal tract is irritating and increases peristalsis, causing vomiting or diarrhea, or both. If bleeding is from the lower GI tract, the diarrhea is frankly bloody. Bleeding from the upper GI tract also can be rapid enough to produce hematochezia (bright red stools), but generally some digestion of the blood components will have occurred, producing melena—black or tarry stools that are sticky and have a characteristic foul odor. The digestion of blood proteins originating from massive upper GI bleeding is reflected by an increase in blood urea nitrogen (BUN) levels (see Figure 36-1).

The hematocrit and hemoglobin values are not the best indicators of acute gastrointestinal bleeding because plasma volume and red cell volume are lost proportionately. As the plasma volume is replaced, the hematocrit and hemoglobin values begin to reflect the extent of blood loss. The interpretation of these values is modified to account for exogenous replacement of fluids and the hydration status of the tissues.

> ✔ **QUICK CHECK 36-1**
> 1. How is visceral pain "referred"?
> 2. How does osmotic diarrhea differ from secretory diarrhea?
> 3. What are the best clinical indicators of acute GI bleeding blood loss?

Disorders of Motility
Dysphagia

PATHOPHYSIOLOGY Dysphagia is difficulty swallowing. It can result from *mechanical obstruction* of the esophagus or a functional disorder that impairs esophageal motility. Intrinsic obstructions originate in the wall of the esophageal lumen (esophageal dysphagia) and include tumors, strictures, and diverticular herniations (outpouchings). Extrinsic mechanical obstructions originate outside the esophageal lumen and narrow the esophagus by pressing inward on the esophageal wall. The most common cause of extrinsic mechanical obstruction is tumor.

Functional dysphagia is caused by neural or muscular disorders that interfere with voluntary swallowing or peristalsis. Disorders that affect the striated muscles of the hypopharyngeal area and upper esophagus interfere with the oropharyngeal (voluntary) phase of swallowing (oropharyngeal dysphagia). Typical causes are dermatomyositis (a muscle disease) and neurologic impairments caused by cerebrovascular accidents, Parkinson disease, multiple sclerosis, muscular dystrophy, or achalasia.[14]

Achalasia is a rare form of dysphagia related to loss of inhibitory neurons in the myenteric plexus with smooth muscle atrophy in the middle and lower portions of the esophagus. The myenteric neurons are attacked by a cell-mediated and antibody-mediated immune response against an unknown antigen. This leads to altered esophageal peristalsis and failure of the lower esophageal sphincter (LES) to relax, causing functional obstruction of the lower esophagus with varying severity.[15] Food accumulates above the obstruction, distends the esophagus, and causes dysphagia (Figure 36-2). Cough and aspiration can occur. As hydrostatic pressure increases, food is slowly forced past the obstruction into the stomach. Chronic esophageal distention requires dilation or surgical myotomy of the lower esophageal sphincter (LES).

TABLE 36-1 Presentations of Gastrointestinal Bleeding

Presentations	Definition
Acute Bleeding	
Hematemesis	Bloody vomitus; either fresh, bright red blood or dark grainy digested blood with "coffee grounds" appearance
Melena	Black, sticky, tarry, foul-smelling stools caused by digestion of blood in gastrointestinal tract; should be distinguished from black stools caused by dietary iron supplements, blackberries, or bismuth (e.g., Pepto-Bismol)
Hematochezia	Fresh, bright red blood passed from rectum
Occult Bleeding	Trace amounts of blood in normal-appearing stools or gastric secretions; detectable only with positive fecal occult blood test (guaiac test)

FIGURE 36-1 Pathophysiology of Gastrointestinal (GI) Bleeding.

CLINICAL MANIFESTATIONS Distention and spasm of the esophageal muscles during eating or drinking may cause a mild or severe stabbing pain at the level of obstruction. Discomfort occurring 2 to 4 seconds after swallowing is associated with upper esophageal obstruction. Discomfort occurring 10 to 15 seconds after swallowing is more common in obstructions of the lower esophagus. If obstruction results from a growing tumor, dysphagia begins with difficulty swallowing solids and advances to difficulty swallowing semisolids and liquids. If motor function is impaired, both solids and liquids are difficult to swallow. Regurgitation of undigested food, unpleasant taste sensation, vomiting, aspiration, and weight loss are common manifestations of all types of dysphagia. Aspiration of esophageal contents can lead to cough and pneumonia.

EVALUATION AND TREATMENT Knowledge of the person's history and clinical manifestations contributes significantly to a diagnosis of dysphagia. Imaging is used to visualize the contours of the esophagus and identify structural defects. High-resolution manometry and intra-luminal impedance monitoring document the duration and amplitude of abnormal pressure changes associated with obstruction or loss of neural regulation. Esophageal endoscopy is performed to examine the esophageal mucosa and obtain biopsy specimens.

The individual is taught to manage symptoms by eating small meals slowly, taking fluid with meals, and sleeping with the head elevated to prevent regurgitation and aspiration. Food and medications may need to be formulated so they can be swallowed Anticholinergic drugs (e.g., botulinum toxin) may relieve symptoms of dysphagia. Mechanical

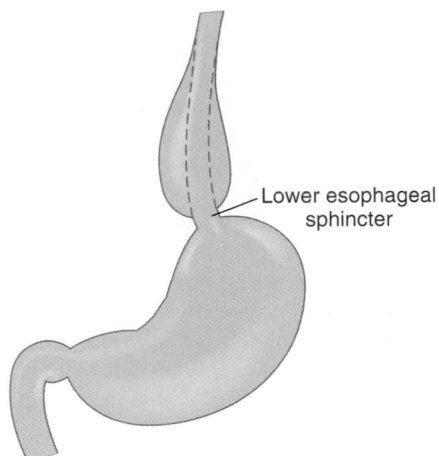

FIGURE 36-2 Achalasia. Increased lower esophageal sphincter muscle tone and loss of peristaltic function prevent food from entering the stomach, causing esophageal distention.

dilation of the esophageal sphincter and surgical separation of the lower esophageal muscles with a longitudinal incision (myotomy) are the most effective treatments for achalasia.[16]

Gastroesophageal Reflux Disease (GERD)

Gastroesophageal reflux disease (GERD) is the reflux of acid and pepsin or bile salts from the stomach into the esophagus that causes esophagitis. The prevalence of GERD is estimated at 18% to 27% in North America.[17] Risk factors for GERD include older age, obesity, hiatal hernia, and drugs or chemicals that relax the LES (anticholinergics, nitrates, calcium channel blockers, nicotine).[18] GERD may be a trigger for asthma or chronic cough. Gastroesophageal reflux that does not cause symptoms is known as *physiologic reflux*. In *nonerosive reflux disease (NERD)*, individuals have symptoms of reflux disease but no visible esophageal mucosal injury (functional heartburn).[19]

PATHOPHYSIOLOGY Abnormalities in lower esophageal sphincter function, esophageal motility, and gastric motility or emptying can cause GERD. The resting tone of the LES tends to be lower than normal from either transient relaxation or weakness of the sphincter. Vomiting, coughing, lifting, bending, obesity, or pregnancy increases abdominal pressure, contributing to the development of reflux esophagitis. Hiatal hernia can weaken the LES. Delayed gastric emptying can contribute to reflux esophagitis by (1) lengthening the period during which reflux is possible and (2) increasing gastric acid content. Disorders that delay emptying include gastroparesis, gastric or duodenal ulcers, which can cause pyloric edema and strictures that narrow the pylorus.

The severity of the esophagitis depends on the composition of the gastric contents and the esophageal mucosa exposure time. An acid pocket is an area of postprandial unbuffered gastric acid immediately distal to the gastroesophageal junction. It is enlarged in hiatal hernia and can contribute to GERD. If the gastric content is highly acidic or contains bile salts and pancreatic or intestinal enzymes, reflux esophagitis can be severe. In individuals with weak esophageal peristalsis, refluxed chyme remains in the esophagus longer than usual. This increases the amount of time the esophageal mucosa is exposed to acids, enzymes, and bile. The refluxate causes mucosal injury and inflammation with hyperemia, increased capillary permeability, edema, tissue fragility, and erosion. Fibrosis and thickening may develop. Precancerous lesions (Barrett esophagus, see p. 938) can be a long-term consequence. Precancerous lesions can progress to adenocarcinoma.[20]

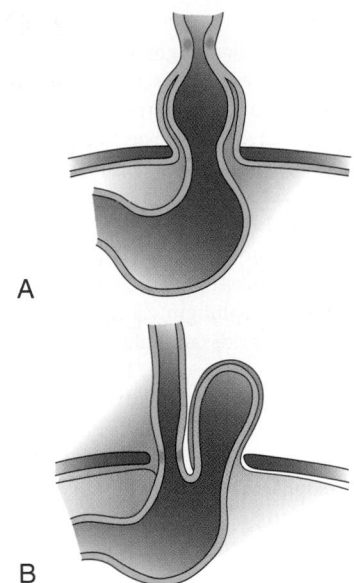

FIGURE 36-3 Types of Hiatal Hernia. A, Sliding hiatal hernia (Type 1). **B,** Paraesophageal hiatal hernia (Type 2). Not shown is mixed hiatal hernia (Type 3).

CLINICAL MANIFESTATIONS The clinical manifestations of erosive reflux esophagitis are heartburn (pyrosis), acid regurgitation, dysphagia, chronic cough, asthma attacks (see Chapter 27), laryngitis, and upper abdominal pain within 1 hour of eating. The symptoms worsen if the individual lies down or if intra-abdominal pressure increases (e.g., as a result of coughing, vomiting, or straining at stool). Edema, strictures, esophageal spasm, or decreased esophageal motility may result in dysphagia with weight loss. Alcohol or acid-containing foods, such as citrus fruits, can cause discomfort during swallowing.

EVALUATION AND TREATMENT Diagnosis of GERD is based on history and clinical manifestations. Esophageal endoscopy shows hyperemia, edema, erosion, and strictures. Dysplastic changes (Barrett esophagus) can be identified by tissue biopsy. Impedance/pH monitoring measures the movement of stomach contents upward into the esophagus and the acidity of the refluxate. Because heartburn also may be experienced as chest pain, cardiac ischemia must be ruled out.

Proton pump inhibitors are the agents of choice for controlling symptoms and healing esophagitis. Other therapies include H2-receptor antagonists or prokinetics and antacids. Weight reduction, smoking cessation, elevation of the head of the bed 6 inches, and avoiding tight clothing also help to alleviate symptoms. Laparoscopic fundoplication is the most common surgical intervention when medical treatment fails.[21]

Eosinophilic esophagitis is an idiopathic inflammatory disease of the esophagus characterized by infiltration of eosinophils associated with atopic disease, including asthma and food allergies. It occurs in adults and children. Dysphagia, food impaction, vomiting, and weight loss are common symptoms. Endoscopy with biopsy identifies the eosinophilc infiltration and differentiation from GERD. Treatment is symptomatic including elimination diets and steroids.

Hiatal Hernia

PATHOPHYSIOLOGY Hiatal hernia is a type of diaphragmatic hernia with protrusion (herniation) of the upper part of the stomach through the diaphragm and into the thorax (Figure 36-3).[22] In sliding hiatal hernia (Type 1 and the most common), the proximal portion of the stomach moves into the thoracic cavity through the esophageal hiatus, an opening in the diaphragm for the esophagus and vagus nerves. A congenitally short esophagus, fibrosis or excessive vagal nerve stimulation, or weakening of the diaphragmatic muscles at the gastroesophageal junction contributes to the hernia. GERD is associated with this type of herniation. Coughing, bending, tight clothing, ascites, obesity, and pregnancy accentuate the hernia.

Paraesophageal hiatal hernia (Type 2) is the herniation of the greater curvature of the stomach through a secondary opening in the diaphragm alongside the esophagus. The position of a portion of the stomach above the diaphragm causes congestion of mucosal blood flow, leading to gastritis and ulcer formation. Strangulation of the hernia is a major complication. It can present with vomiting and epigastric and retrosternal epigastric pain and is a surgical emergency.[23]

Mixed hiatal hernia (Type 3) is less common and is a combination of sliding and paraesophageal hiatal hernias. It tends to occur in conjunction with several other diseases, including reflux esophagitis, peptic ulcer, cholecystitis (gallbladder inflammation), cholelithiasis (gallstones), chronic pancreatitis, and diverticulosis.

CLINICAL MANIFESTATIONS   Hiatal hernias are often asymptomatic. Generally, a wide variety of symptoms develop later in life and are associated with other gastrointestinal disorders, including GERD. Symptoms include heartburn, regurgitation, dysphagia, and epigastric pain. Ischemia from hernia strangulation causes acute, severe chest or epigastric pain, nausea, vomiting, and GI bleeding.

EVALUATION AND TREATMENT   Diagnostic procedures include radiology with barium swallow, endoscopy, and high-resolution manometry. A chest x-ray film often will show the protrusion of the stomach into the thorax, indicating paraesophageal hiatal hernia.

Treatment for sliding hiatal hernia is usually conservative. The individual can diminish reflux by eating small, frequent meals and avoiding the recumbent position after eating. Abdominal supports and tight clothing should be avoided, and weight control is recommended for obese individuals. Antacids alleviate reflux esophagitis. Individuals who are uncomfortable at night benefit from sleeping with the head of the bed elevated 6 inches. Surgery (fundoplication) is performed if medical management fails to control symptoms.

Gastroparesis is delayed gastric emptying in the absence of mechanical gastric outlet obstruction. It is most commonly associated with diabetes mellitus, surgical vagotomy, or fundoplication. It can be idiopathic. The pathophysiology is not well understood but involves abnormalities of the autonomic nervous system, smooth muscle cells, enteric neurons, and gastrointestinal hormones. Diabetic gastroparesis represents a form of neuropathy involving the vagus nerve. Symptoms include nausea, vomiting, abdominal pain, and postprandial fullness or bloating. Treatment options include dietary management; prokinetic drugs; and, in some cases, gastric electrical stimulation; or surgical venting gastrostomy.[24]

Pyloric Obstruction

PATHOPHYSIOLOGY   Pyloric obstruction (gastric outlet obstruction) is the narrowing or blocking of the opening between the stomach and the duodenum. This condition can be congenital (e.g., infantile hypertrophic pyloric stenosis; see Chapter 37) or acquired. Acquired obstruction is caused by peptic ulcer disease or carcinoma near the pylorus. Duodenal ulcers are more likely than gastric ulcers to obstruct the pylorus. Ulceration causes obstruction resulting from inflammation, edema, spasm, fibrosis, or scarring. Tumors cause obstruction by growing into the pylorus.

CLINICAL MANIFESTATIONS   Early in the course of pyloric obstruction, the individual experiences vague epigastric fullness, which becomes more distressing after eating and at the end of the day. Nausea and epigastric pain may occur as the muscles of the stomach contract in attempts to force chyme past the obstruction. These symptoms disappear when the chyme finally moves into the duodenum. As obstruction progresses, anorexia develops, sometimes accompanied by weight loss. Severe obstruction causes gastric distention and atony (lack of muscle tone and gastric motility). Gastric distention stimulates gastric secretion, which increases the feeling of fullness. Rolling or jarring of the abdomen produces a sloshing sound called the *succussion splash*. At this stage, vomiting is a cardinal sign of obstruction. It is usually copious and occurs several hours after eating. The vomitus contains undigested food but no bile. Prolonged vomiting leads to dehydration, which is accompanied by a hypokalemic and hypochloremic metabolic alkalosis caused by loss of gastric potassium and acid, respectively. Because food does not enter the intestine, stools are infrequent and small. Prolonged pyloric obstruction causes severe malnutrition, dehydration, and extreme debilitation.

EVALUATION AND TREATMENT   Diagnosis is based on clinical manifestations, a history of ulcer disease, and examination of residual gastric contents. Endoscopy is performed if gastric carcinoma is the suggested cause of pyloric obstruction.

Obstructions resulting from ulceration often resolve with conservative management. A large-bore nasogastric tube is used to aspirate stomach contents and relieve distention. Then nasogastric suction is maintained for 2 to 3 days to decompress the stomach and restore normal motility. Gastric secretions that contribute to inflammation and edema can be suppressed with proton pump inhibitors or histamine$_2$ (H2) receptor antagonists. Fluids and electrolytes (saline and potassium) are given intravenously to promote rehydration and correct hypokalemia and alkalosis (see Chapter 5). Severely malnourished individuals may require parenteral hyperalimentation (intravenous nutrition). Surgery or the placement of pyloric stents may be required to treat gastric carcinoma or persistent obstruction caused by fibrosis and scarring.[25]

Intestinal Obstruction and Paralytic Ileus

Intestinal obstruction can be caused by any condition that prevents the normal flow of chyme through the intestinal lumen (Table 36-2).[26] Obstructions can occur in either the small or the large intestine (Table 36-3). The small intestine is more commonly obstructed because of its narrower lumen. Classifications of intestinal obstruction are summarized in Table 36-4. Intestinal obstruction is classified by cause as simple or functional. *Simple obstruction* is mechanical blockage of the lumen by a lesion and it is the most common type of intestinal obstruction. Paralytic ileus, or *functional obstruction*, is a failure of intestinal motility often occurring after intestinal or abdominal surgery, acute pancreatitis, or hypokalemia. Acute obstructions usually have mechanical causes, such as adhesions or hernias (Figure 36-4). Chronic or partial obstructions are more often associated with tumors or inflammatory disorders, particularly of the large intestine.

PATHOPHYSIOLOGY   The major pathophysiologic alterations are presented in Figure 36-5. Postoperative paralytic ileus results from inhibitory neural reflexes associated with inflammatory mediators, and the influence of exogenous (i.e., meperidine or morphine) and endogenous opioids (endorphins) that affect the entire GI tract. Small bowel obstruction (SBO) is caused by postoperative adhesions, tumors, Crohn disease, and hernias. SBO leads to distention caused by impaired absorption and increased secretion with accumulation of fluid and gas

TABLE 36-2 Common Causes of Intestinal Obstruction

Cause	Pathophysiology
Hernia	Protrusion of intestine through weakness in abdominal muscles or through inguinal ring
Intussusception	Telescoping of one part of intestine into another; this usually causes strangulation of blood supply; more common in infants 10-15 months of age than in adults (see Figure 36-4D)
Torsion (volvulus)	Twisting of intestine on its mesenteric pedicle, with occlusion of blood supply; often associated with fibrous adhesions; occurs most often in middle-aged and elderly men
Diverticulosis	Inflamed saccular herniations (diverticuli) of mucosa and submucosa through tunica muscularis of colon; diverticuli are interspersed between thick, circular, fibrous bands; most common in obese individuals older than 60 years (see Figure 36-9)
Tumor	Tumor growth into intestinal lumen; adenocarcinoma of colon and rectum is most common tumoral obstruction; most common in individuals older than 60 years
Paralytic (adynamic) ileus	Loss of peristaltic motor activity in intestine; associated with abdominal surgery, peritonitis, hypokalemia, ischemic bowel, spinal trauma, or pneumonia
Fibrous adhesions	Peritoneal irritation from surgery, trauma, or Crohn disease leads to formation of fibrin and adhesions that attach to intestine, omentum, or peritoneum and can cause obstruction; most common in small intestine

TABLE 36-3 Large and Small Bowel Obstruction

Type of Obstruction	Cause
Small bowel obstruction	Adhesions: secondary to previous abdominal surgeries—75%
	Hernia: inguinal, ventral, or femoral—10%
	Tumors: may be associated with intussusception—10%
	Mesenteric ischemia—3-5%
	Crohn disease—<1%
Large bowel obstruction	Colon/rectal cancer—90%
	Volvulus—4-5%
	Diverticular disease—3-5%
	Other causes (inflammatory bowel disease, adhesions, hernia)

Data from Mizell JS, Turnage RH: Chapter 123: Intestinal obstruction. In Feldman M et al, editors: *Sleisenger & Fordtran's gastrointestinal and liver disease,* ed 10, pp 2154-2170, Philadelphia, 2016, Saunders.

TABLE 36-4 Classifications of Intestinal Obstruction

Criteria for Classification	Definition
Onset	
Acute	Sudden onset; often caused by torsion, intussusception, or herniation
Chronic	Protracted onset; more commonly from tumor growth or progressive formation of strictures
Extent of Obstruction	
Partial	Incomplete obstruction of intestinal lumen
Complete	Complete obstruction of intestinal lumen
Location of Obstructing Lesion	
Intrinsic	Obstruction develops within intestinal lumen; examples: gut wall edema or hemorrhage, foreign bodies (gallstones), tumors, or gut wall fibrosis
Extrinsic	Obstruction originates outside intestine; examples: tumors, torsion, fibrosis, hernia, intussusception
Effects on Intestinal Wall	
Simple	Luminal obstruction without impairment of blood supply
Strangulated	Luminal obstruction with occlusion of blood supply
Closed loop	Obstruction at each end of a segment of intestine
Casual Factors	
Mechanical	Blockage of intestinal lumen by intrinsic or extrinsic lesions; usually treated surgically
Functional (paralytic ileus)	Paralysis of intestinal musculature caused by trauma, peritonitis, electrolyte imbalances, or spasmolytic agents; usually treated by decompression with suction or surgery if death of tissue

inside the lumen proximal to the obstruction.[27] Distention decreases the intestine's ability to absorb water and electrolytes and increases the net secretion of these substances into the lumen. Copious vomiting or sequestration of fluids in the intestinal lumen prevents their reabsorption and produces severe fluid and electrolyte disturbances. Extracellular fluid volume and plasma volume decrease, causing dehydration, increased hematocrit level, hypotension, and tachycardia. Severe dehydration leads to hypovolemic shock. Metabolic alkalosis initially develops as a result of excessive loss of hydrogen ions that would normally be reabsorbed from the gastric juice and vomiting. With prolonged obstruction or obstruction lower in the intestine, metabolic acidosis is more likely to occur because bicarbonate from pancreatic secretions and bile cannot be reabsorbed. Hypokalemia from vomiting and decreased potassium absorption can be extreme, promoting acidosis and atony of the intestinal wall. Metabolic acidosis also may be accentuated by ketosis, the result of declining carbohydrate stores caused by starvation. Lack of circulation permits the buildup of significant amounts of lactic acid, which worsen the metabolic acidosis. If pressure from the distention is severe enough, it occludes the arterial circulation and causes ischemia, necrosis, perforation, and peritonitis. Fever and leukocytosis are often associated with overgrowth of bacteria, ischemia, and bowel necrosis. Bacterial proliferation and translocation across the mucosa to the systemic circulation cause peritonitis or sepsis. The release of inflammatory mediators into the circulation causes remote organ failure.

Large bowel obstruction is less common and often related to cancer. Diverticulitis, inflammatory bowel disease, and other causes of obstruction are less common. Acute colonic pseudo-obstruction (Ogilvie syndrome) is a rare massive dilation of the large bowel that is

FIGURE 36-4 Intestinal Obstructions. A, Hernia. **B,** Constrictions from adhesions. **C,** Volvulus. **D,** Intussusception. (From Kumar V et al: *Robbins basic pathology,* ed 9, Philadelphia, 2013, Saunders.)

related to excessive sympathetic motor input or decreased parasympathetic motor input with absence of mechanical obstruction. It occurs primarily in people who are critically ill and immobilized older adults.

CLINICAL MANIFESTATIONS Signs and symptoms of *small intestine obstruction* include colicky pains caused by intestinal distention followed by nausea and vomiting. Pain intensifies for seconds or minutes as a peristaltic wave of muscle contraction meets the obstruction. Pain may be continuous with severe distention and then diminish in intensity. If ischemia occurs, the pain loses its colicky character and becomes more constant and severe. Sweating and tachycardia occur as a sympathetic nervous system response to hypotension. Fever, severe leukocytosis, abdominal distention, and rebound tenderness develop as ischemia progresses to necrosis, perforation, and peritonitis.

Obstruction at the pylorus causes early, profuse vomiting. Obstruction in the proximal small intestine causes mild distention and vomiting of bile-stained fluid. Lower obstruction in the small intestine causes more pronounced distention because a greater length of intestine is proximal to the obstruction. In this case, vomiting may not occur early but may occur later and contain fecal material. Partial obstruction can cause diarrhea or constipation, but complete obstruction usually causes constipation only. Complete obstruction increases the number of bowel sounds, which may be tinkly and accompanied by peristaltic rushes and crampy abdominal pain. Signs of hypovolemia and metabolic acidosis may be observed as early as 24 hours after the occurrence of complete obstruction. Distention may be severe enough to push against the diaphragm and decrease lung volume. This can lead to atelectasis and pneumonia, particularly in debilitated individuals.

Large intestine obstruction usually presents with hypogastric pain and abdominal distention. Pain can vary from vague to excruciating, depending on the degree of ischemia and the development of peritonitis. Vomiting occurs late in the obstructive process. Small and large

intestinal perforation presents the same with acute, persistent abdominal pain, nausea, vomiting, and fever.[28] *Acute colonic pseudo-obstruction* is characterized by abdominal distention, abdominal pain, and nausea and vomiting. Bowel sounds are usually present.

EVALUATION AND TREATMENT Evaluation is based on clinical manifestations and imaging studies. Successful management requires early identification of the site and type of obstruction. Replacement of fluid and electrolytes and decompression of the lumen with gastric or intestinal suction are essential forms of therapy. Laparoscopic procedures can release adhesions. Immediate surgical intervention is required for strangulation, complete obstruction, or perforation. Colonic stents may be placed for malignant obstruction. Neostigmine, a parasympathomimetic, is used for colonic pseudo-obstruction and colonoscopic decompression may be required.[29]

> ✔ **QUICK CHECK 36-2**
> 1. Why is heartburn associated with gastroesophageal reflux?
> 2. How does peritonitis develop with bowel obstruction?
> 3. What causes postoperative paralytic ileus?

Gastritis

Gastritis is an inflammatory disorder of the gastric mucosa; it has an incidence of less than 1% in the United States.[30] It can be acute or chronic and affect the superficial mucosa of the fundus or antrum, or both.

Acute gastritis is caused by injury of the protective mucosal barrier caused by drugs, chemicals, or *Helicobacter pylori* infection. Nonsteroidal anti-inflammatory drugs (NSAIDs; e.g., ibuprofen, naproxen, indomethacin, and aspirin) inhibit the action of cyclooxygenase-1 (COX-1) and cause gastritis because they inhibit prostaglandin synthesis, which normally stimulates the secretion of mucus. Alcohol, histamine, digitalis, and metabolic disorders, such as uremia, are contributing factors. *H. pylori*–associated acute gastritis causes inflammation, increased gastric secretion in antral gastritis, decreased gastric section in fundal gastritis, pain, nausea, and vomiting. The clinical manifestations of acute gastritis can include vague abdominal discomfort, epigastric tenderness, and bleeding. Healing usually occurs spontaneously within a few days. Discontinuing injurious drugs, using antacids, or decreasing acid secretion with H2-receptor antagonists facilitates healing.

Chronic gastritis tends to occur in older adults and causes chronic inflammation, mucosal atrophy, and epithelial metaplasia. Chronic gastritis is classified as type A, immune (fundal), or type B, nonimmune (antral), depending on the pathogenesis and location of the lesions. When both types of chronic gastritis occur, it is known as type AB, or pangastritis, and the antrum is more severely involved. Type C gastritis is associated with reflux of bile and pancreatic secretions into the stomach, causing chemical injury.

Chronic immune (fundal) gastritis is the most rare form of gastritis and is associated with loss of T-cell tolerance and development of autoantibodies to gastric H^+-K^+ ATPase. The gastric mucosa degenerates extensively in the body and fundus of the stomach, leading to gastric atrophy. Loss of parietal cells diminishes acid and intrinsic factor secretion. Pernicious anemia can develop from decreased vitamin B_{12} absorption (see Chapter 21). The feedback mechanism that normally inhibits gastrin secretion is impaired, causing elevated plasma levels of gastrin. Chronic fundal gastritis occurs in association with other autoimmune diseases (e.g., rheumatoid arthritis, autoimmune thyroid disease, or type 1 diabetes mellitus) and is a risk factor for

FIGURE 36-5 Pathophysiology of Intestinal Obstruction.

gastric carcinoma, particularly in individuals who develop pernicious anemia.

Chronic nonimmune (antral gastritis) generally involves the antrum only and is more common than fundal gastritis. It is caused by *H. pylori* bacteria and it also is associated with use of alcohol, tobacco, and nonsteroidal anti-inflammatory drugs.[31] There are high levels of hydrochloric acid secretion with an increased risk of duodenal ulcers. *H. pylori* also can progress to autoimmune atrophic gastritis and involves the fundus, thus becoming pangastritis. There is greater risk for the development of gastric cancer in these cases.[32]

Signs and symptoms of chronic gastritis often include vague symptoms: anorexia, fullness, nausea, vomiting, and epigastric pain. Gastric bleeding may be the only clinical manifestation of gastritis. Gastroscopic examination and biopsy may show a long-standing inflamma-

tory process and gastric atrophy in an individual with no history of abdominal distress. Failure to stimulate acid secretion confirms achlorhydria (diminished secretion of hydrochloric acid). The gastric secretions also can be evaluated for the presence of intrinsic factor. Symptoms can usually be managed by eating smaller meals in conjunction with a soft, bland diet and by avoiding alcohol and aspirin. *H. pylori* infection is treated with antibiotics, and vitamin B_{12} is administered to correct pernicious anemia.

Peptic Ulcer Disease

A **peptic ulcer** is a break or ulceration in the protective mucosal lining of the lower esophagus, stomach, or duodenum. Ulcers develop when mucosal protective factors are overcome by erosive factors commonly caused by NSAIDs and *H. pylori* infection. Risk factors for peptic ulcer

FIGURE 36-6 Lesions Caused by Peptic Ulcer Disease.

disease are summarized in *Risk Factors*: Peptic Ulcer. Psychologic stress may be a risk factor for peptic ulcer disease but the exact mechanism of causation is not known.[33] The prevalence of peptic ulcer in 2011 in the United States was 15.5 million people.[34]

Peptic ulcers can be single or multiple, acute or chronic, and superficial or deep. Superficial ulcerations are called *erosions* because they erode the mucosa but do not penetrate the muscularis mucosae (Figure 36-6). True ulcers extend through the muscularis mucosae and damage blood vessels, causing hemorrhage, or perforate the gastrointestinal wall.

Zollinger-Ellison syndrome is a rare syndrome that also is associated with peptic ulcers caused by a gastrin-secreting neuroendocrine tumor or multiple tumors (gastrinoma) of the pancreas or duodenum. Increased secretion of gastrin causes excess secretion of gastric acid, resulting in gastric and duodenal ulcers, gastroesophageal reflux with abdominal pain, and diarrhea.[35]

Duodenal Ulcers

Duodenal ulcers occur with greater frequency than other types of peptic ulcers and are commonly caused by *H. pylori* infection and NSAID use.[36] Idiopathic duodenal ulcers are rare and can be associated with altered mucosal defenses, rapid gastric emptying, elevated serum gastrin levels, or acid production stimulated by smoking.[37]

PATHOPHYSIOLOGY Causative factors, singly or in combination, cause acid and pepsin concentrations in the duodenum to penetrate the mucosal barrier and cause ulceration (Figure 36-7). The host response to *H. pylori* infection is activation of T and B lymphocytes with infiltration of neutrophils. Release of inflammatory cytokines damages the gastric epithelium. An *H. pylori* virulence factor (cytotoxin associated gene A *[Cag A]*) produces a vacuolating toxin *(VacA)*

causing apoptosis of gastric epithelial cells and promoting inflammation. *H. pylori* mucosal infection underlies gastric and duodenal ulcer and gastric cancer.[38]

CLINICAL MANIFESTATIONS The characteristic manifestation of a duodenal ulcer is chronic intermittent pain in the epigastric area. The pain begins 2 or 3 hours after eating, when the stomach is empty. It is not unusual for pain to occur in the middle of the night and disappear by morning. Pain is relieved rapidly by ingestion of food or antacids, creating a typical pain-food-relief pattern. Some individuals with duodenal ulcer may have no symptoms; the first manifestation may be hemorrhage or perforation, particularly with a history of NSAID or anticoagulant use.

Complications of duodenal ulcer include bleeding, perforation, and obstruction of the duodenum or outlet of the stomach. Bleeding is the most common cause of mortality, particularly among the elderly. Perforation occurs with destruction of all layers of the duodenal wall and causes sudden, severe epigastric pain.[39] Obstruction may be the result of edema from inflammation or scarring from chronic injury. It is not clear why individuals infected with *H. pylori* duodenal ulcers are negatively associated with gastric cancer.[40]

Duodenal ulcers often heal spontaneously but recur within months without treatment. Exacerbations tend to develop in the spring and fall. Relief of pain accompanies healing. Constant, unremitting pain may be caused by complications, such as intestinal obstruction or perforation. Bleeding from duodenal ulcers causes hematemesis or melena.[41]

EVALUATION AND TREATMENT Several diagnostic approaches are used to differentiate duodenal ulcers from gastric ulcers or gastric carcinoma. Endoscopic evaluation allows visualization of lesions and biopsy. Radioimmune assays of gastrin levels are evaluated to identify ulcers associated with gastric carcinomas. *H. pylori* is detected using the urea breath test, *H. pylori*–specific serum IgG and IgA antibodies, and measurement of *H. pylori* stool antigen levels. Findings from gastric biopsy detect *H. pylori* infection and confirm eradication after treatment.[42]

Management of duodenal ulcers is aimed at relieving the causes and effects of hyperacidity and preventing complications. Antacids neutralize gastric contents and relieve pain. Acid secretion can be suppressed with drugs that block H2 receptors and inhibit the secretion of acid. Proton pump inhibitors inhibit acid production. *H. pylori* is treated with a combination of antibiotics and proton pump inhibitors, but antibiotic resistance is an increasing problem.[43] Surgical resection may be required for bleeding or perforating ulcers, obstruction, or peritonitis.

FIGURE 36-7 Duodenal Ulcer. A, A deep ulceration in the duodenal wall extending as a crater through the entire mucosa and into the muscle layers. **B,** Sequence of ulcerations from normal mucosa to duodenal ulcer. **C,** Bilateral (kissing) duodenal ulcers in a person using nonsteroidal anti-inflammatory drugs (NSAIDs). (**C** courtesy David Bjorkman, MD, University of Utah School of Medicine, Department of Gastroenterology, Salt Lake City, Utah.)

Gastric Ulcers

Gastric ulcers are ulcers of the stomach and occur about equally in males and females, usually between the ages of 55 and 65 years. They are about one fourth as common as duodenal ulcers (Table 36-5).

PATHOPHYSIOLOGY Generally, gastric ulcers develop in the antral region, adjacent to the acid-secreting mucosa of the body. The primary defect is an abnormality that increases the mucosal barrier's permeability to hydrogen ions. Gastric secretion may be normal or less than normal, and there may be a decreased mass of parietal cells. Chronic gastritis is often associated with development of gastric ulcers and may precipitate ulcer formation by limiting the mucosa's ability to secrete a protective layer of mucus (Figure 36-8). Other factors include the following:

1. Decreased mucosal synthesis of prostaglandins
2. Duodenal reflux of bile and pancreatic enzymes damage the mucosal membrane
3. Use of NSAIDs (decreases prostaglandin synthesis)
4. *H. pylori* infection

A break in the mucosal barrier permits hydrogen ions to diffuse into the mucosa, where they disrupt permeability and cellular structure. A vicious cycle can be established as the damaged mucosa liberates histamine, which stimulates the increase of acid and pepsinogen production, blood flow, and capillary permeability. The disrupted mucosa becomes edematous and loses plasma proteins. Destruction of small vessels causes bleeding.

CLINICAL MANIFESTATIONS The clinical manifestations of gastric ulcers are similar to those of duodenal ulcers (see Table 36-5). The pattern of pain is common but the pain of gastric ulcers also occurs immediately after eating. Gastric ulcers also tend to be chronic rather than alternating between periods of remission and exacerbation and cause more anorexia, vomiting, and weight loss than duodenal ulcers. The evaluation and treatment of gastric ulcers are similar to the evaluation and treatment of duodenal ulcers.

TABLE 36-5　Characteristics of Gastric and Duodenal Ulcers

Characteristics	Gastric Ulcer	Duodenal Ulcer
Incidence		
Age at onset	50-70 years	20-50 years
Family history	Usually negative	Positive
Gender (prevalence)	Equal in women and men	Greater in men
Stress factors	Increased	Average
Ulcerogenic drugs	Normal use	Increased use
Cancer risk	Increased	Not increased
Pathophysiology		
Abnormal mucus	May be present	May be present
Parietal cell mass	Normal or decreased	Increased
Acid production	Normal or decreased	Increased
Serum gastrin	Increased	Normal
Serum pepsinogen	Normal	Increased
Associated gastritis	More common	Usually not present
Helicobacter pylori	May be present (60-80%) Stimulates reduced acid secretion, gastric atrophy, and risk of gastric cancer	Often present (95-100%) Stimulates acid hypersecretion
Clinical Manifestations		
Pain	Located in upper abdomen Intermittent Pain-antacid-relief pattern Food-pain pattern (when food in stomach)	Located in upper abdomen Intermittent Pain-antacid/food-relief pattern Pain when stomach empty Nocturnal pain common
Clinical course	Chronic ulcer without pattern of remission and exacerbation Heals more slowly	Pattern of remissions and exacerbation for years Heals more quickly

Stress-Related Mucosal Disease

A **stress-related mucosal disease (stress ulcer)** is an acute form of peptic ulcer that tends to accompany the physiologic stress of severe illness or major trauma. Usually multiple sites of ulceration are distributed within the stomach or duodenum. Stress ulcers may be classified as ischemic ulcers or Cushing ulcers.

Ischemic ulcers develop within hours of an event such as hemorrhage, multisystem trauma, severe burns, heart failure, or sepsis. Shock, anoxia, inflammation, and sympathetic responses cause ischemia of the stomach and duodenal mucosa, disrupting the mucosal barrier. Stress ulcers that develop as a result of burn injury are often called **Curling ulcers**. **Cushing ulcer** is a stress ulcer associated with severe brain trauma or brain surgery. Decreased mucosal blood flow and hypersecretion of acid caused by overstimulation of the vagal nuclei damage the mucosal barrier, causing erosions and ulceration.

The primary clinical manifestation of stress-related mucosal disease is bleeding, which is uncommon, but occurs more readily with the presence of coagulopathy and more than 48 hours of mechanical ventilation. Prophylactic treatment regimens are used to prevent this disease.[44] Stress ulcers seldom become chronic.

Surgical Treatment of Ulcer

Advances in the medical treatment of peptic ulcer disease with acid suppression and eradication of *H. pylori* have reduced the number of cases requiring surgery. The most common indications for ulcer surgery are recurrent or uncontrolled bleeding and perforation of the stomach or duodenum. The primary objectives of surgical treatment are to reduce stimuli for acid secretion, decrease the number of acid-secreting cells in the stomach, and correct complications of ulcer disease.

Acute complications of gastrectomy or anastomosis are relatively uncommon except in debilitated persons. Chronic complications, however, are likely to develop if a large portion of the stomach has been removed. These complications and their pathophysiologic mechanisms are described in the next section.

> ✔ **QUICK CHECK 36-3**
> 1. What is the most common cause of chronic gastritis?
> 2. Compare the three types of peptic ulcers.
> 3. What causes a stress ulcer?

Postgastrectomy Syndromes

Postgastrectomy syndromes are a group of signs and symptoms that occur after gastric resection for the treatment of peptic ulcer, gastric carcinoma, or bariatric surgery for extreme obesity. They are caused by anatomic and functional changes in the stomach and upper small intestine[45] and include the following:

1. **Dumping syndrome.** Rapid emptying of hypertonic chyme from the surgically residual stomach (the stomach component remaining after surgical resection following gastric or bariatric surgery) into the small intestine 10 to 20 minutes after eating; promoted by loss of gastric capacity, loss of emptying control when pylorus is removed, and loss of feedback control by duodenum when it is removed; responds to dietary management. Symptoms include cramping pain, nausea, vomiting, osmotic diarrhea, weakness, pallor, and hypotension.

2. **Alkaline reflux gastritis.** Stomach inflammation caused by reflux of bile and alkaline pancreatic secretions containing proteolytic enzymes that disrupt the mucosal barrier in the remnant stomach. Symptoms include nausea, bilious vomiting, and sustained epigastric pain that worsens after eating and is not relieved by antacids; responds somewhat to avoidance of aspirin and alcohol,[46] but surgical correction may be required.

3. **Afferent loop obstruction.** Intermittent severe pain and epigastric fullness after eating as a result of volvulus, hernia, adhesion, or stenosis of the duodenal stump on the proximal side of the gastrojejunostomy; vomiting relieves symptoms; management includes low-fat diet, but decompression or surgery revision is required for complete obstruction.[47]

4. **Diarrhea.** Either frequent, persistent elimination of loose stools or intermittent, precipitous, and unpredictable elimination of a large volume of stool; related to rapid gastric emptying and osmotic attraction of water into the gut, especially after large intake of high-carbohydrate liquids; small, dry meals and anticholinergic drugs are effective control measures (see p. 907).

5. **Weight loss.** Commonly caused by inadequate caloric intake because individual cannot tolerate carbohydrates or a normal-size meal; stomach is also less able to mix, churn, and break down food. In the case of bariatric surgery for extreme obesity, weight loss is the intended outcome but nutrient deficiencies, including vitamins and minerals, must be supplemented.[48]

FIGURE 36-8 Pathophysiology of Gastric Ulcer Formation. *NSAIDs,* Nonsteroidal anti-inflammatory drugs.

6. **Anemia.** Iron malabsorption may result from decreased acid secretion or lack of duodenum after Billroth II procedure (gastrojejunostomy); deficiencies of iron and vitamin B$_{12}$ or folate may result.

7. **Bone and mineral disorders.** Related to altered calcium absorption and metabolism with increased risk for fractures and deformity and malabsorption of vitamins and nutrients, such as vitamin D.

Malabsorption Syndromes

Malabsorption syndromes interfere with nutrient absorption in the small intestine. Historically they have been classified as maldigestion or malabsorption. **Maldigestion** is failure of the chemical processes of digestion that take place in the intestinal lumen or at the brush border of the intestinal mucosa. **Malabsorption** is failure of the intestinal mucosa to absorb (transport) the digested nutrients. Often these two syndromes are interrelated, or occur together, making classification difficult. Generally, however, maldigestion is caused by deficiencies of the enzymes needed for digestion or inadequate secretion of bile salts and inadequate reabsorption of bile in the ileum. Malabsorption is the result of mucosal disruption caused by gastric or intestinal resection, vascular disorders, or intestinal disease.

Pancreatic Exocrine Insufficiency

The pancreatic enzymes (lipase, amylase, trypsin, chymotrypsin) are required for the digestion of proteins, carbohydrates, and fats.

Pancreatic insufficiency is the deficient production of these enzymes, particularly lipase, by the pancreas. Causes include chronic pancreatitis, pancreatic carcinoma, pancreatic resection, and cystic fibrosis. Significant damage to or loss of pancreatic tissue must occur before enzyme levels decrease sufficiently to cause maldigestion. Although pancreatic insufficiency causes poor digestion of all nutrients, fat maldigestion is the chief problem. Absence of pancreatic bicarbonate in the duodenum and jejunum causes an acidic pH that worsens maldigestion by precipitating bile salts and preventing activation of the pancreatic enzymes that are present. A large amount of fat in the stool (steatorrhea) is the most common sign of pancreatic insufficiency. There is also a deficit of fat-soluble vitamins (A, D, E, and K) and weight loss.[49]

Lactase Deficiency (Lactose Intolerance)

Deficiency of disaccharidase at the brush border of the small intestine is caused by a genetic defect in which a single enzyme, usually lactase, is lacking. **Lactase deficiency** inhibits the breakdown of lactose (milk sugar) into monosaccharides and therefore prevents lactose digestion and absorption across the intestinal wall. Lactase deficiency is most common in blacks, Latinos, and Native Americans and usually does not develop until adulthood. Secondary (acquired) lactase deficiency can be caused by several diseases of the intestine, including gluten-sensitive enteropathy, enteritis, and bacterial overgrowth.

The undigested lactose remains in the intestine, where bacterial fermentation causes formation of gases. Undigested lactose also increases the osmotic gradient in the intestine, causing irritation and osmotic diarrhea. Clinical manifestations of lactose consumption with lactase deficiency are bloating, crampy pain, diarrhea, and flatulence. The disorder is diagnosed by a lactose-tolerance test. Avoiding milk products (more than 1 cup of milk) and adhering to a lactose-free diet relieve symptoms.[50]

Bile Salt Deficiency

Conjugated bile acids (bile salts) are necessary for the digestion and absorption of fats. Bile salts are conjugated in the bile that is secreted from the liver. When bile enters the duodenum, the bile salts aggregate with fatty acids and monoglycerides to form micelles. Micelle formation makes fat molecules more soluble and allows them to pass through the unstirred layer at the brush border of the small intestinal villi (see Chapter 35). A minimum concentration of bile salts, termed the *critical micelle concentration,* is required to allow formation of micelles. Therefore, conditions that decrease the production or secretion of bile result in decreased micelle formation and fat malabsorption. These conditions include advanced liver disease, which decreases the production of bile salts; obstruction of the common bile duct, which decreases flow of bile into the duodenum (cholestasis); intestinal stasis (lack of motility), which permits overgrowth of intestinal bacteria that deconjugate bile salts; and diseases of the ileum, which prevent the reabsorption and recycling of bile salts (enterohepatic circulation).[51]

Clinical manifestations of bile salt deficiency are related to poor intestinal absorption of fat and fat-soluble vitamins (A, D, E, and K). Increased fat in the stools (steatorrhea) leads to diarrhea and decreased levels of plasma proteins. The losses of fat-soluble vitamins and their effects include the following:

1. Vitamin A deficiency results in night blindness.
2. Vitamin D deficiency results in decreased calcium absorption with bone demineralization (osteoporosis), bone pain, and fractures.
3. Vitamin K deficiency prolongs prothrombin time, leading to spontaneous development of purpura (bruising) and petechiae.
4. Vitamin E deficiency has uncertain effects but may cause testicular atrophy and neurologic defects in children.

The most effective treatment for fat-soluble vitamin deficiency is to increase consumption of medium-chain triglycerides in the diet, for example, by using coconut oil for cooking. Vitamins A, D, and K are given parenterally. Oral bile salts are an effective therapy.

Inflammatory Bowel Disease

Ulcerative colitis (UC) and Crohn disease (CD) are chronic relapsing inflammatory bowel diseases (IBDs). The prevalence of IBD is about 1.6 million people in the United States with about 70,000 new cases per year.[52] The disease is more prevalent among white populations and Ashkenazi Jews.[53] Risk factors and theories of causation include susceptibility genes, environmental factors, alterations in epithelial cell barrier functions, and an altered immune response to intestinal microflora[54,55] (Table 36-6). Environmental factors or infections are thought to alter the barrier function of the mucosal epithelium, leading to loss of immune tolerance to normal intestinal antigens. There is possible loss of discrimination of potentially harmful pathogens from commensal microorganisms in the intestinal mucosa. The loss of tolerance activates dendritic cells, triggering their transport to mesenteric lymph nodes, where they promote differentiation of naïve T cells to Th1, Th2,

TABLE 36-6	Features of Ulcerative Colitis and Crohn Disease	
Feature	**Ulcerative Colitis**	**Crohn Disease**
Incidence		
Age at onset	Any age; 10-40 years most common	Any age; 10-30 years most common
Family history	Less common	More common
Gender	Prevalence equal in women and men	Prevalence about equal in women and men
Cancer risk	Increased	Increased
Nicotine use	Later and less severe disease; nicotine withdrawal may cause exacerbation	Increases disease risk and greater disease severity
Pathophysiology		
Location of lesions	Large intestine, continuous lesions	Mouth to anus, "skip" lesions common
	Left side more common	Right side more common
Inflammation	Mucosal layer involved	Entire intestinal wall involved
Granulomata	Rare	Transmural granulomata common; cobblestone appearance
Ulceration	Friable mucosa, superficial ulcers, crypt abscesses common	Deep fissuring ulcers and fistulae common
Anal and perianal fistulae	Rare	Common; abscesses
Narrowed lumen and possible obstruction	Rare	Common; obstruction
Clinical Manifestations		
Abdominal pain	Mild to severe	Moderate to severe
Diarrhea	Common; 4 times/day	May or may not be present
Bloody stools	Common	Less common
Weight loss	Less common	Common
Abdominal mass	Rare	Common
Small intestine malabsorption	None	Common
Clinical course	Remissions and exacerbations	Remissions and exacerbations
Comorbidities	Extraintestinal manifestations	Extraintestinal manifestations

and Th17 cells, or T-regulatory cells. Production of proinflammatory cytokines and chemokines, including tumor necrosis factor, interleukins, toxic oxygen free radicals, and interferon-gamma (IFN-γ), damages the intestinal epithelium.[56] The risk of colon cancer increases significantly after 30 to 35 years of inflammatory bowel disease, particularly in untreated disease.[57] Future research is directed at an integration of these factors to refine our understanding of disease cause and trajectory, particularly interactions between genetics, the microflora, mucosa, and immune responses.[58,59]

Ulcerative Colitis

Ulcerative colitis (UC) is a chronic inflammatory disease that causes ulceration of the colonic mucosa, most commonly in the rectum and sigmoid colon. The lesions appear in susceptible individuals between 20 and 40 years of age. UC is less common in people who smoke.[60]

PATHOPHYSIOLOGY   The primary lesion of UC begins with inflammation at the base of the crypt of Lieberkühn in the large intestine. The disease begins in the rectum (proctitis) and may extend proximally to the entire colon (pancolitis). The mucosa is hyperemic and may appear dark red and velvety, and is involved in a continuous fashion. Small erosions form and coalesce into ulcers. Abscess formation, necrosis, and ragged ulceration of the mucosa ensue. Edema and thickening of the muscularis mucosae may narrow the lumen of the involved colon. Mucosal destruction and inflammation causes bleeding, cramping pain, and an urge to defecate. Frequent diarrhea, with passage of small amounts of blood and purulent mucus, is common. Loss of the absorptive mucosal surface and rapid colonic transit time cause large volumes of watery diarrhea.

CLINICAL MANIFESTATIONS   The course of UC consists of intermittent periods of remission and exacerbation. Mild UC involves less mucosa, so that the frequency of bowel movements, bleeding, and pain is minimal. Severe forms may involve the entire colon and are characterized by abdominal pain, fever, elevated pulse rate, frequent diarrhea (10 to 20 stools/day), urgency, obviously bloody stools, and continuous, crampy pain. Dehydration, weight loss, anemia, and fever result from fluid loss, bleeding, and inflammation. Complications include anal fissures, hemorrhoids, and perirectal abscess. Severe hemorrhage is rare. Edema, strictures, or fibrosis can obstruct the colon. Perforation is an unusual but possible complication. Extraintestinal manifestations include cutaneous lesions (erythema nodosum), polyarthritis, episcleritis, uveitis, disorders of the liver, and alterations in coagulation.[61]

EVALUATION AND TREATMENT   Diagnosis of UC is based on the medical history, clinical manifestations, and laboratory, serologic, radiologic, endoscopic, and biopsy findings. Infectious causes are ruled out by stool culture. The symptoms of UC may be similar to those of Crohn disease, making differential diagnosis challenging.[62] Treatment is individualized and depends on the severity of symptoms and the extent of mucosal involvement. A goal is to promote mucosal healing and avoid surgery. Mild to moderate disease is treated with 5-aminosalicylate therapy followed by steroids. Thioprine and immunomodulatory agents (cyclosporine and tumor necrosis factor [TNF] blocking agents [i.e., tacrolimus]) or vedolizumab are used for serious disease.[63] New immunotherapies are emerging.[64] Severe, unremitting disease can require hospital admission for administration of intravenous fluids and steroids. Extreme malnutrition may require total parenteral nutrition (TPN). Surgical resection of the colon may be performed if other forms of therapy are unsuccessful or if there are acute serious complications (sepsis, hemorrhage, perforation, or obstruction). Surgical approaches for severe UC include total procto-

colectomy, with end ileostomy or ileorectal anastomosis, or ileal pouch anal anastomosis (IPAA).[65] *Pouchitis* is a complication of restorative proctocolectomy with ileal pouch–anal anastomosis performed as surgical treatment for both UC and Crohn disease. Antibiotic treatment is usually successful.[66]

Crohn Disease

Crohn disease (CD) (granulomatous colitis, ileocolitis, or regional enteritis) is an idiopathic inflammatory disorder that affects any part of the gastrointestinal tract from the mouth to the anus. In a small percentage of cases, CD is difficult to differentiate from ulcerative colitis (see Table 36-6). The distal small intestine and proximal large colon are most commonly involved.[54]

PATHOPHYSIOLOGY   Inflammation begins in the intestinal submucosa and spreads with discontinuous transmural involvement ("skip lesions"). The ascending colon and the transverse colon are the most common sites of the disease, but both the large and small intestines may be involved, particularly the ileum. One side of the intestinal wall may be affected and not the other. The ulcerations of CD can produce fissures that extend inflammation into lymphoid tissue. The typical lesion is a granuloma (granulomata are described in Chapter 6) with a cobblestone appearance from projections of inflamed tissue surrounded by ulceration. Fistulae may form in the perianal area between loops of intestine or extend into the bladder, rectum, or vagina. Strictures may develop, promoting obstruction. Smoking increases the risk of developing severe disease, and may cause a poorer response to treatment.[67]

CLINICAL MANIFESTATIONS   Individuals with CD may have no specific symptoms for several years. Symptoms vary according to the location of the disease but are similar to those for UC. Diarrhea is one of the most common symptoms and, occasionally, rectal bleeding if the colon is involved. Weight loss and abdominal pain accompany CD. If the ileum is involved, the individual may be anemic as a result of malabsorption of vitamin B_{12}. There also may be deficiencies in folic acid and vitamin D absorption. In addition, proteins may be lost, leading to hypoalbuminemia. Extraintestinal complications are similar to those occurring in ulcerative colitis.

EVALUATION AND TREATMENT   The diagnosis and treatment of CD are similar to the diagnosis and treatment of ulcerative colitis; however, imaging of the small intestine is used in the diagnosis of CD, including either a small bowel series or a capsule endoscopy (camera pill). There are no specific biomarkers or definitive treatments. Smoking cessation is a component of therapy. Immunomodulators (i.e., anti-TNF) are effective for initial therapy or for resistance to other drugs.[68] Surgery may be performed to manage complications such as fistula, abscess, or obstruction. Routine colonoscopy for cancer screening should be performed for long-standing colonic disease.

Microscopic Colitis

Microscopic colitis is a relatively common cause of diarrhea primarily in females and older adults. Although the mucosa appears normal, there are two histologic forms: lymphocytic and collagenous. Lymphocytic colitis shows an increase in the number of intraepithelial lymphocytes. Collagenous colitis is characterized by a thickened subepithelial collagen layer, alteration of the vascular mucosal pattern, and mucosal nodularity. The cause is unknown. Risk factors include age ≥50 years, female gender, weight loss, absence of abdominal pain, and use of proton pump inhibitors or nonsteroidal anti-inflammatory drugs.[69]

The symptoms of frequent, chronic daily watery diarrhea are the same for both types and can be accompanied by abdominal pain and weight loss. Antidiarrheal agents and budesonide (an anti-inflammatory steroid) are the best documented treatments. The disease is negatively associated with colorectal cancer.[70]

Irritable Bowel Syndrome

Irritable bowel syndrome (IBS) currently is a symptom-based disease characterized by recurrent abdominal pain with altered bowel habits. There is increasing evidence of organic causes of disease. In North America the prevalence is about 12% and is probably underestimated.[71] It is more common in women (1.5 to 3 times greater than men) with a higher prevalence during youth and middle age. Individuals with symptoms of IBS also are more likely to have anxiety, depression, and reduced quality of life.[72]

The pathophysiology of IBS is unknown and there are no specific biomarkers for the disease. There is increasing evidence to explain the varying symptom presentations, particularly in relation to altered gut microflora, gut immune responses, gut neuroendocrine cell function, the brain-gut axis, genetic susceptibility, and epigenetic factors.[73,74] The presentations are summarized below:

1. *Visceral hypersensitivity or hyperalgesia,* particularly with distention of the rectum but also other areas of the gut, may originate in either the peripheral or the central nervous system. The mechanism may be related to dysregulation of the bidirectional "brain-gut axis" (alterations in gut or central nervous system processing of gut nociceptive information).[75] Factors include genetic related changes in the function of serotonin-secreting cells of gut-brain pain modulation, alterations in gut microbiota metabolite production with activation of the gut immune system, increased visceral sensitivity and permeability, and altered motility.[76]

2. *Abnormal gastrointestinal permeability, motility, and secretion* are associated with IBS. Individuals with diarrhea-type IBS have more rapid colonic transit times and increased intestinal permeability. Those with bloating and constipation have delayed transit times and decreased intestinal permeability. The mechanism may be related to dysregulation of the brain-gut axis, alterations in the function of gut neuroendocrine cells or dorsal root ganglion neurons, or changes in the activity of mast cells.[77]

3. *Postinflammatory (infectious or noninfectious) IBS* is diagnosed if two or more of the following occur: fever, vomiting, diarrhea, and a positive stool culture. Intestinal infection (bacterial enteritis) and low-grade inflammation have been associated with symptoms of IBS and appear to be related to alteration of gut microbiota, immune activation in gut tissues, and changes in intestinal permeability.[78,79]

4. *Alteration in gut microbiota (dysbiosis)* influences the sensory, motor, and immune systems of the gut and interacts with higher brain centers and may contribute to symptoms of IBS.[80] Small intestine overgrowth of normal gut bacteria may be associated with IBS symptoms in some cases.[81] Nonabsorbable antibiotics and prebiotics and probiotics may be helpful in some individuals.

5. *Food allergy or food intolerance* is associated with IBS in some cases. Food antigens may activate the mucosal immune system, alter intestinal flora, or mediate hypersensitivity reactions and IBS symptoms. Food elimination approaches are helpful in some cases.[82]

6. *Psychosocial factors (epigenetic factors)*—including early life trauma or abuse or emotional stress interacting with neuroendocrine, neuroimmune, autonomic nervous system, and pain modulatory responses—contribute to the symptoms of IBS.[74,83]

BOX 36-1   Rome III—Diagnostic Criteria for Irritable Bowel Syndrome (IBS)

Recurrent abdominal pain or discomfort* at least 3 days/month in the last 3 months associated with two or more of the following:
  Improvement with defecation
  Onset associated with a change in frequency of stool
  Onset associated with a change in form (appearance) of stool[†]
  Onset of symptoms more than 6 months before diagnosis

From *Rome III diagnostic criteria for functional gastrointestinal disorders.* Available at: www.romecriteria.org/assets/pdf/19_RomeIII_apA_885-898.pdf. Accessed September 2015.
*"Discomfort" means an uncomfortable sensation not described as pain.
[†]Diagnostic criterion.

CLINICAL MANIFESTATIONS   IBS is characterized by lower abdominal pain or discomfort and bloating. Women report more abdominal pain and constipation and men report more diarrhea.[84] IBS can be grouped as diarrhea-predominant, constipation-predominant, or alternating diarrhea/constipation. Symptoms including gas, bloating, and nausea are usually relieved with defecation and do not interfere with sleep.

EVALUATION AND TREATMENT   The diagnosis of IBS is based on signs, symptoms, and personal history and includes the exclusion of structural or biochemical causes of disease. Diagnostic procedures to rule out other causes of symptoms may include endoscopic evaluations, computed tomography (CT) scans or abdominal ultrasound, blood tests, and tests for lactose intolerance, celiac disease (see Chapter 37), or other disorders. The person may be evaluated for food allergies, parasites, or bacterial growth. The Rome III criteria for diagnosing IBS guide evaluation (Box 36-1).

There is no cure for IBS and treatment is individualized. Treatment of symptoms may include laxatives and fiber, antidiarrheals, antispasmodics, prosecretory drugs, low-dose antidepressants, visceral analgesics, and serotonin agonists or antagonists. Alternative therapies include prebiotics and probiotics to manipulate the microflora, hypnosis, acupuncture, yoga, cognitive-behavioral therapy, and dietary interventions. Research continues to advance the management and understanding of the pathophysiology of this complex syndrome.[85,86]

Diverticular Disease of the Colon

Diverticula are herniations or saclike outpouchings of the mucosa and submucosa through the muscle layers, usually in the wall of the sigmoid colon (Figure 36-9). They rarely occur in the small intestine.[87] Diverticulosis is asymptomatic diverticular disease. Diverticulitis represents inflammation. The cause of diverticular disease is unknown. It is associated with increased intracolonic pressure, abnormal neuromuscular function, and alterations in intestinal motility. Approximately 300,000 hospital admissions per year are related to diverticular disease.[88] Predisposing factors include older age, genetic predisposition, obesity, smoking, diet, lack of physical activity, and medication use, such as aspirin and nonsteroidal anti-inflammatory drugs.[89] Lack of dietary fiber may or may not contribute to diverticular disease.[90]

PATHOPHYSIOLOGY   Diverticula can occur anywhere in the gastrointestinal tract, particularly at weak points in the colon wall, usually where arteries penetrate the tunica muscularis. The most common sites are the left sigmoid colon (prevalent in Western countries) and

FIGURE 36-9 Diverticular Disease. In diverticular disease, the outpouches *(arrows)* of mucosa seen in the sigmoid colon appear as slitlike openings from the mucosal surface of the opened bowel. (From Stevens A et al: *Core pathology,* ed 3, London, 2009, Mosby.)

the right colon (prevalent in Asian countries). A common associated finding is thickening of the circular muscles and shortening of the longitudinal (teniae coli) muscles surrounding the diverticula. Increased collagen and elastin deposition, not muscle hypertrophy, is associated with muscle thickening and this contributes to increased intraluminal pressure and herniation. According to the law of Laplace (see Chapter 23), wall pressure increases as the diameter of a cylindrical structure decreases. Therefore, pressure within the narrow lumen can increase enough to rupture the diverticula, causing inflammation and diverticulitis. Bacteria and local ischemia also may be contributing factors. Complicated diverticulitis includes abscess, fistula, obstruction, bleeding, or perforation.

CLINICAL MANIFESTATIONS Symptoms of uncomplicated diverticular disease may be vague or absent. Cramping pain of the lower abdomen can accompany constriction of the thickened colonic muscles. Diarrhea, constipation, distention, or flatulence may occur. If the diverticula become inflamed or abscesses form, the individual develops fever, leukocytosis (increased white blood cell count), and tenderness of the lower left quadrant.

EVALUATION AND TREATMENT Diverticula are often discovered during diagnostic procedures performed for other problems. Ultrasound, sigmoidoscopy, or colonoscopy permits direct observation of the lesions. Abdominal computed tomography is used for diagnosis of complicated cases.

An increase of dietary fiber intake often relieves symptoms and probiotics and mesalazine are being evaluated. Uncomplicated diverticulitis is usually treated with bowel rest and analgesia. Antibiotics are not required.[91] Laparoscopic resection and other minimally invasive approaches are implemented for more severe complications.[92]

Appendicitis

Appendicitis is an inflammation of the vermiform appendix, which is a projection from the apex of the cecum. It is the most common surgical emergency of the abdomen, usually occurs between 10 and 19 years of age (although it may develop at any age), and has an incidence in the United States of 7 to 10 per 10,000 persons.[93]

PATHOPHYSIOLOGY The exact mechanism of the cause of appendicitis is controversial. Obstruction of the lumen with stool, tumors, or foreign bodies with consequent bacterial infection is the most common theory. The obstructed lumen does not allow drainage of the appendix, and as mucosal secretion continues, intraluminal pressure increases. The increased pressure decreases mucosal blood flow, and the appendix becomes hypoxic. The mucosa ulcerates, promoting bacterial or other microbial invasion with further inflammation and edema. Inflammation may involve the distal or entire appendix. Gangrene develops from thrombosis of the luminal blood vessels, followed by perforation.[94]

CLINICAL MANIFESTATIONS Gastric or periumbilical pain is the typical symptom of an inflamed appendix. The pain may be vague at first and in the periumbilical area, increasing in intensity over 3 to 4 hours. It may subside and then migrate to the right lower quadrant, indicating extension of the inflammation to the surrounding tissues. Nausea, vomiting, and anorexia follow the onset of pain, and a low-grade fever is common. Diarrhea occurs in some individuals, particularly children; others have a sensation of constipation. Perforation, peritonitis, and abscess formation are the most serious complications of appendicitis.

EVALUATION AND TREATMENT In addition to clinical manifestations, there is pain with abdominal palpation and rebound tenderness, usually referred to the right lower quadrant. The white blood cell count is greater than 10,000 cells/mm^3 with increased neutrophils and C-reactive protein. Abdominal ultrasound, CT scans, and MRI (particularly for pregnant women and children) assist with diagnostic accuracy and help rule out nonappendiceal disease.[95] Antibiotics and appendectomy are the treatment for simple or perforated appendicitis. There is controversy regarding antibiotics first, then surgery.[96] Laparoscopic surgery provides quick recovery for simple appendicitis. Recovery is more complicated in cases of perforation, abscess formation, peritonitis, or older age.

Mesenteric Vascular Insufficiency

Mesenteric vascular insufficiency is rare with an incidence of about 2 to 3 cases per 100,000 persons.[97] Three branches of the abdominal aorta supply the stomach and intestines: the celiac artery and the superior and inferior mesenteric arteries (see Figure 35-6). The inferior mesenteric vein drains into the splenic vein and the splenic vein and superior mesenteric vein join the portal vein. *Mesenteric venous thrombosis* is the least common of the causes of mesenteric vascular insufficiency. Malignancies, right-sided heart failure, and deep vein thrombosis are risk factors. Mesenteric venous thrombosis presents with abdominal pain and is treated with anticoagulants.[98]

Acute mesenteric arterial insufficiency results in a significant reduction in mucosal blood flow to the large and small intestines and can be acute or chronic.[99] Preexisting morbidities include dissecting aortic aneurysms, arterial thrombi, or emboli. Embolic obstruction is associated with atrial fibrillation, mitral valve disease, heart valve prostheses, and myocardial infarction. The superior mesenteric artery has a more direct line of flow from the aorta; therefore, emboli enter it more readily than the inferior branch, causing ischemia and necrosis of the small intestine. Ischemia and necrosis (intestinal infarction) alter membrane permeability. Initially, there is increased motility, nausea and vomiting, urgent bowel evacuation, and severe abdominal pain. Ischemia leads to decreased motility and distention. The damaged intestinal mucosa cannot produce enough mucus to protect itself from digestive enzymes. Mucosal alteration causes fluid to move from the blood vessels into the bowel wall and peritoneum. Fluid loss causes hypovolemia, and further decreases intestinal blood flow. As intestinal infarction progresses, shock, fever, bloody diarrhea, and leukocytosis develop. Bacteria invade the necrotic intestinal wall, causing gangrene and peritonitis

Chronic mesenteric ischemia is rare but can develop with atherosclerotic stenosis or occlusion[100] or secondary to congestive heart failure, acute myocardial infarction, hemorrhage, thrombus formation, or any condition that decreases arterial blood flow. Chronic occlusion is often accompanied by formation of collateral circulation. The collateral vessels may be able to nourish the resting intestine, but after eating, when the intestine requires more blood, the arterial supply may be insufficient. Ischemia develops, causing cramping abdominal pain (abdominal angina), a cardinal symptom. Some individuals suffer significant weight loss because they stop eating to control the pain. Progressive vascular obstruction eventually causes continuous abdominal pain and necrosis of the intestinal tissue.

Diagnosis of acute and chronic mesenteric ischemia is based on clinical manifestations, laboratory findings, and imaging studies. A bruit can often be heard over a partially occluded artery. Treatment includes aggressive rehydration and the use of antibiotics, anticoagulants, vasodilators, and inhibitors of reperfusion injury. Surgery, including endovascular techniques, is required to remove necrotic tissue, repair sclerosed vessels, and revascularize affected tissue. Acute occlusion is a surgical emergency and mortality is high (50% to 90%). Early diagnosis and aggressive treatment result in the best survival rates.[101]

Disorders of Nutrition
Obesity

Obesity is an increase in body fat mass and a metabolic disorder that has become an epidemic worldwide with a prevalence of 35.7% in the United States in 2010, with no sex differences. The incidence is rapidly increasing among children and adolescents, and they tend to become obese adults.[102] Obesity is associated with higher all-cause mortality.[103]

Obesity is defined as a body mass index (body mass index [BMI] = kg/m^2) that exceeds 30[104] and generally develops when caloric intake exceeds caloric expenditure. Obesity is a major risk factor for morbidity, death, and high healthcare costs.[105] Three leading causes of death associated with obesity are coronary artery disease, type 2 diabetes mellitus, and cancer (colorectal, breast in postmenopausal women, endometrial, prostate, renal, and esophageal). Obesity also is a risk factor for hypertension, stroke, hyperlipidemia, gallstones, nonalcoholic steatohepatitis, gastroesophageal reflux, osteoarthritis, infectious disease, and sleep apnea.[106]

The causes and consequences of obesity are multiple and complex. Rapidly advancing research regarding risk factors, causal mechanisms, complications, and treatment is in progress. Obesity is known to occur in families and genotypes, and gene-environment interactions are important predisposing factors.[107] Environmental factors include culture, socioeconomic status, food intake habits, level of physical activity. Metabolic abnormalities associated with obesity include Cushing syndrome, Cushing disease, polycystic ovarian syndrome, hypothyroidism, and hypothalamic injury.

PATHOPHYSIOLOGY The pathophysiology of obesity involves the interaction of peripheral and central pathways and numerous cytokines, hormones, and neurotransmitters. In the periphery, white adipocytes (fat cells) store triglyceride and increase in size and number. Adipocytes also secrete hormones and cytokines, known as adipocytokines.[108] These adipocytokines and other hormones (Box 36-2) participate in regulation of food intake, lipid storage, insulin sensitivity, vascular homeostasis, blood pressure regulation, angiogenesis, coagulation, bone metabolism, inflammatory and immune responses, female

---

BOX 36-2   Examples of Adipocytokines and Other Hormones Related to Complications of Obesity

Cytokines from Adipose Cells
Adipocytokines

Leptin: Suppresses appetite at hypothalamus; promotes insulin sensitivity
Adiponectin: Insulin sensitizing for regulation of blood glucose level; promotes anti-inflammatory and anti-hypertensive vascular effects; reduces atherosclerosis and oncogenesis; increases metabolic rate
Resistin: Promotes insulin resistance and increases blood glucose levels
Visfatin: Mimics insulin and binds to insulin receptors

Proinflammatory Cytokines

Tumor necrosis factor-alpha (TNF-α): A proinflammatory hormone; suppresses appetite; induces insulin resistance
Interleukins-6, -8, and -10: Proinflammatory mediators; suppress appetite; induce insulin resistance
Monocyte chemotactic protein-1 (MCP-1): Involved in macrophage recruitment
Plasminogen activator inhibitor-1 (PAI-1): Promotes clot formation by inhibiting plasminogen and urokinase (also released by endothelial cells)
Retinol binding protein-4 (RBP-4): Promotes insulin resistance

Other Hormones

Insulin: Secreted from pancreatic beta cells; suppresses appetite at hypothalamus; promotes glucose utilization in muscle and fat
Amylin: Secreted from pancreatic beta cells; suppresses appetite and postprandial glucagon secretion
Ghrelin: Secreted from stomach; stimulates appetite and controls gastric motility and acid secretion
Peptide YY: Secreted from intestine; reduces appetite and inhibits gastric motility
Incretin: Stimulates insulin release; inhibits glucagon release; slows gastric emptying to reduce postprandial hyperglycemia
Glucagon-like peptide-1 (GLP-1): Gastric inhibitory peptide (glucose-dependent insulinotropic peptide) (GIP)

---

reproduction, and regulation of energy metabolism. Visceral white fat accumulation causes dysfunction in the regulation and interaction of these cytokines and hormones and contributes to the complications and consequences of obesity (see *Health Alert:* Types of Adipose Tissue and Obesity).

Neuroendocrine regulation of appetite, eating behavior, energy metabolism, and body fat mass are controlled by a dynamic circuit of signaling mediators from the periphery acting centrally on the hypothalamus and brainstem to regulate hunger and satiety.[109] Peripheral sources of mediators include insulin from the beta cells of the pancreas; ghrelin from the stomach; peptide YY from the intestines; glucagon-like peptide-1 from intestinal endocrine cells; and the adipokines leptin, adiponectin, and resistin. Obesity is associated with increased circulating plasma levels of leptin, insulin, resistin, and ghrelin. There are decreased levels of adiponectin and peptide YY (see Box 36-2).

Within the hypothalamus are the orexigenic neurons (increase food intake and decrease metabolism) and the anorexigenic neurons (decrease food intake and increase metabolism). They interact with peripheral mediators to control food intake and energy expenditure. The hypothalamus also communicates with higher brain centers related to reward, pleasure, and addictive behavior. These centers can override hypothalamic control of food intake and satiety, increasing

HEALTH ALERT

Types of Adipose Tissue and Obesity

Adipose tissue is often classified according to color as white (WAT), beige (bAT), or brown (BAT). WAT is located in visceral (central) and subcutaneous (peripheral) stores. Visceral adipocytes store fat as triglycerides, which are released as energy in the form of fatty acids when needed. WAT has stromal structure that contains macrophages, fibroblasts, and endothelial cells. When energy balance is positive, excess fat is stored in mature white adipocytes, which undergo hypertrophy, and adipogenesis (new fat cells) is stimulated. Chronic positive energy balance can overwhelm adipogenesis, and fat storage then depends only on hypertrophy. Visceral WAT is more likely to store fat by adipose tissue hypertrophy (visceral obesity); produce more adiponectin, less leptin, and more inflammatory cytokines; and result in central obesity. Subcutaneous fat is more likely to store fat by adipogenesis (peripheral obesity) and has higher leptin production, lower adiponectin production, and lower production of inflammatory cytokines. Visceral WAT hypertrophy is associated with greater macrophage infiltration, increased vascularity, and inflammation. Numerous adipokines are released, promoting a proinflammatory state, insulin resistance, and altered lipid metabolism, which are characteristics of the metabolic syndrome associated with obesity. Insulin resistance results in type 2 diabetes mellitus, and excess lipolysis leads to increased release of free fatty acids in the circulation. The increase in free fatty acids contributes to cardiovascular disease and nonalcoholic steatohepatitis (NASH). Adipogenesis has a lower association with inflammation and resistance. Estrogen receptors (ERs) also influence fat storage. ERa is involved in fat mass reduction and ERb is involved in fat mass expansion. ERb is more dense in subcutaneous WAT and may explain the higher incidence of peripheral obesity among premenopausal women and the increase in central obesity with menopause. The complications of obesity are related to where fat is stored, not just the accumulation of fat stores.

Chronic exposure to cold stimulates WAT transition to bAT, which is thermogenic. With warm adaptation bAT reverts to WAT. Leptin and insulin together promote bAT, increasing energy expenditure and weight loss. bAT is diminished in obesity.

BAT is located in the supraclavicular area of the neck and interscapular areas, and is rich in mitochondria containing iron (giving it a brown color). BAT produces nonshivering thermogenesis when stimulated by exposure to cold, stimulation of the sympathetic nervous system, and activation of triiodothyronine (T_3). Mitochondrial activity is uncoupled from ATP synthesis and energy production is released as heat. Leptin and adiponectin are minimally produced by BAT so there is little effect on appetite and satiety. There also is an inverse relationship between amount of BAT and body mass index and age. Interindividual differences in BAT-mediated thermogenesis may explain some of the variability in obesity susceptibility and the increased prevalence of obesity with aging. Most research related to BAT has been conducted in mouse models and research in humans is just beginning. Investigators are interested in discovering if there is a way to stimulate synthesis and activity of BAT as an approach to preventing or treating obesity and diabetes mellitus.

Data from Diaz MB et al: *Metabolism* 63(10):1238-1249, 2014; Dodd GT et al: *Cell* 160(1-2):88-104, 2015; Lanthier N, Leclercq IA: *Best Pract Res Clin Gastroenterol* 28(4):545-558, 2014; Loyd C, Obici S. *Curr Opin Clin Nutr Metab Care* 17(4):368-372, 2014; Peirce V et al: *Nature* 510(7503):76-83, 2014; Poher AL et al: *Front Physiol* 30;6:4, 2015; Roman S et al: *Transl Res* 165(4):464-479, 2015.

consumption of highly palatable foods and resulting in increased fat stores.[110,111] Interaction of altered levels of hormones and adipocytokines with hypothalamic neurons is an important determinant of excessive fat mass and the complications of obesity.

Leptin, a product of the obesity gene (*Ob* gene), acts on the hypothalamus to suppress appetite and functions to regulate body weight within a fairly narrow range. Leptin levels increase as the number of adipocytes increases; however, for unknown reasons, high leptin levels are ineffective at decreasing appetite and energy expenditure, a condition known as leptin resistance.[112] Leptin resistance fails to inhibit orexigenic hypothalamic satiety signaling and promotes overeating and excessive weight gain. Leptin resistance is also associated with insulin resistance (hyperinsulinemia/glucose intolerance) and the cardiovascular complications of obesity. Simultaneously there is an increase in ghrelin, which stimulates orexigenic neurons and increases appetite. Decreased levels of adiponectin and peptide YY decrease stimulation of anorexigenic neurons. Adiponectin also is insulin sensitizing, promotes glucose uptake, and has anti-inflammatory actions. A decrease in adiponectin is associated with insulin resistance, coronary artery disease, and hypertension, contributing to the complications of obesity.

Enlarged adipocytes increase lipolysis (with release of fatty acids) and secrete proinflammatory adipokines from T lymphocytes and activated macrophages. The result is a low-grade systemic inflammation. The inflammatory state and accelerated lipolysis contribute to the development of insulin resistance and metabolic syndrome (hypertriglyceridemia, reduced high-density lipoproteins, increased low-density lipoproteins, hypertension, and insulin resistance).[113,114] Figure 36-10 summarizes the pathophysiology and major consequences of obesity.

CLINICAL MANIFESTATIONS Obesity usually presents with two different forms of adipose tissue distribution, visceral and peripheral.[115] Visceral obesity (also known as intra-abdominal, central, or masculine obesity) occurs when the distribution of body fat is localized around the abdomen and upper body, resulting in an apple shape.[116] Visceral obesity has an increased risk for systemic inflammation, metabolic syndrome, obstructive sleep apnea syndrome, cardiovascular complications, nonalcoholic steatohepatitis cancer, osteoarthritis, and type 2 diabetes mellitus.[117,118] (Diabetes mellitus is discussed in Chapter 19.)

Peripheral obesity (also known as gluteal-femoral, feminine, or subcutaneous obesity) occurs when the distribution of body fat is extraperitoneal and distributed around the thighs and buttocks and through the muscle, resulting in a pear shape, and is more common in women. Peripheral and subcutaneous fat is less metabolically active, is less lipolytic, and releases fewer adipocytokines (particularly adiponectin) than visceral fat. Risk factors are still present for the complications of obesity but they are less severe than those for visceral obesity.

Normal weight obesity (NWO) describes individuals with normal body weight and BMI with percent of body fat greater than 30%. These individuals are at risk for metabolic dysregulation, increases in inflammatory cytokines, insulin resistance, increased risk for cardiovascular disease, and higher mortality.[119] NWO is estimated to occur in 2% to 28% of women and 3% of men.[120]

Metabolically healthy obesity (MHO) describes about 10% to 30% of individuals who are obese but have no metabolic-obesity–associated complications and decreased risk for morbidity and mortality. MHO is more prevalent among women and declines with age with adverse long-term outcomes.[121] Research is in progress to better understand the genetics, body fat distribution patterns, metabolic pathways, lifestyle practices, and therapeutic options for these individuals.

FIGURE 36-10 Pathophysiology and Common Complications of Obesity. See text for details. *CAD*, Coronary artery disease; *GERD*, gastroesophageal reflux disease; *GLP1*, glucagon-like peptide-1; *IL-6*, interleukin-6; *PYY*, intestinal peptide YY; *RBP4*, retinol-binding protein 4; *TNF-α*, tumor necrosis factor-alpha; *VLDL*, very-low-density lipoprotein.

EVALUATION AND TREATMENT There are several methods for measuring or estimating body fat mass, including computed tomography (CT) and magnetic resonance imaging (MRI) techniques; bioimpedance analysis; underwater weighing; and anthropometric measurements, such as skinfold thickness, circumferences, and various body diameters (i.e., waist-to-hip ratios and waist circumference; body mass index tables).[122] The BMI and waist-to-hip ratios are most commonly used because they are the easiest to measure and are most cost-effective. Overweight is defined as a BMI greater than 25 kg/m^2 and obesity is a BMI greater than 30 kg/m^2. BMI charts are available for children ages 2 to 20 years; these can be used for comparison during adulthood because obese children generally become obese adults.[123] No specific diagnostic criteria for obesity have been established. The complications of obesity affect nearly every body system (see Figure 36-10).

Obesity is a chronic disease for which various approaches to treatment have been used; these include correction of metabolic abnormalities, individually tailored weight reduction diets and exercise programs, psychotherapy, behavioral modification, and antiobesity drugs.[124,125]

Weight loss (bariatric) surgery is the most effective treatment for decreasing obesity-related morbidity.[126,127] Unraveling the causes of obesity will lead to more specific prevention and pharmacotherapeutic strategies.

Malnutrition and Starvation

Malnutrition is lack of nourishment from inadequate amounts of calories, protein, vitamins, or minerals and is caused by improper diet, alterations in digestion or absorption, chronic disease, or a combination of these factors. **Starvation** is a reduction in energy intake leading to weight loss. Short-term starvation and long-term starvation have different effects. Therapeutic short-term starvation is part of many weight-reduction programs because it causes an initial rapid weight loss that reinforces the individual's motivation to diet. Therapeutic long-term starvation is used in medically controlled environments to facilitate rapid weight loss in morbidly obese individuals. Pathologic long-term starvation can be caused by poverty (particularly in third-world countries); chronic diseases of the cardiovascular, pulmonary, hepatic, renal, and digestive systems; malabsorption syndromes; and cancer.

Short-term starvation, or extended fasting, consists of several days of total dietary abstinence or deprivation. Once all available energy has been absorbed from the intestine, glycogen in the liver is converted to glucose through glycogenolysis, the metabolism of glycogen into glucose. This process peaks within 4 to 8 hours, and gluconeogenesis begins. Gluconeogenesis is the formation of glucose from noncarbohydrate molecules: lactate, pyruvate, amino acids, and the glycerol portion of fats. Like glycogenolysis, gluconeogenesis takes place within the liver. Both of these processes deplete stored nutrients and thus cannot meet the body's energy needs indefinitely. Proteins continue to be catabolized to a minimal degree, providing carbon for the synthesis of glucose needed by brain and blood cells.

Long-term starvation begins after several days of dietary abstinence and eventually causes death. The major characteristics of long-term starvation are decreased energy expenditure, a decreased dependence on gluconeogenesis, and an increased use of ketone bodies (products of lipid and pyruvate metabolism) as a cellular energy source. Depressed insulin and glucagon levels promote lipolysis in adipose tissue. Lipolysis liberates fatty acids, which supply energy to cardiac and skeletal muscle cells, as well as ketone bodies, which sustain brain tissue. Fatty acid or ketone body oxidation meets most energy needs of the cells. (Some glucose is still needed as fuel for brain tissue.) Once the supply of adipose tissue is depleted, proteolysis begins. The breakdown of muscle protein is the last process to supply energy for life. Death results from severe alterations in electrolyte balance and loss of renal, pulmonary, and cardiac function.[128]

Adequate ingestion of appropriate nutrients is the obvious treatment for starvation. In medically induced starvation, the body is maintained in a ketotic state until the desired amount of adipose tissue has been lysed. Starvation imposed by chronic disease, long-term illness, or malabsorption is treated with enteral or parenteral nutrition. Care must be taken to prevent refeeding syndrome during the treatment of long-term starvation.[129] With refeeding, insulin release, hypophosphatemia, hypomagnesemia, and hypokalemia can cause life-threatening complications.

Cachexia (also known as cytokine-induced malnutrition) is physical wasting with loss of weight and muscle atrophy, fatigue, and weakness. Inflammatory cytokines induce skeletal muscle wasting and a blunted response to ghrelin. Adiponectin suppresses appetite. Cancer, acquired immunodeficiency syndrome (AIDS), tuberculosis, and other major chronic progressive diseases contribute to cachexia (see Chapter 10).[130]

> ✔ **QUICK CHECK 36-4**
> 1. Why are Crohn disease and ulcerative colitis called *inflammatory bowel diseases*?
> 2. How is leptin resistance associated with obesity?
> 3. When does proteolysis begin in long-term starvation?

DISORDERS OF THE ACCESSORY ORGANS OF DIGESTION

The accessory organs of digestion (liver, gallbladder, pancreas) secrete substances necessary for digestion and, in the case of the liver, carry out metabolic functions needed to maintain life. Disorders of these organs include inflammatory disease, obstruction of ducts, and tumors. (Cancers of the digestive system are described at the end of this chapter.)

Common Complications of Liver Disorders

Of all the accessory organ disorders, acute or chronic liver disease leads to the most significant systemic, life-threatening complications. These complications are common to all liver disorders and include portal hypertension, ascites, hepatic encephalopathy, jaundice, and hepatorenal syndrome.

Portal Hypertension

Portal hypertension is abnormally high blood pressure in the portal venous system caused by resistance to blood flow. Pressure in this system is normally 3 mm Hg; portal hypertension is an increase to at least 10 mm Hg.

PATHOPHYSIOLOGY Portal hypertension is caused by disorders that obstruct or impede blood flow through any component of the portal venous system or vena cava. *Intrahepatic causes* result from vascular remodeling with shunts, thrombosis, inflammation, or fibrosis of the sinusoids, as occurs in cirrhosis of the liver, biliary cirrhosis, viral hepatitis, or schistosomiasis (a parasitic infection). *Posthepatic causes* occur from hepatic vein thrombosis or cardiac disorders that impair the pumping ability of the right side of the heart. This causes blood to collect and increases pressure in the veins of the portal system. The most common cause of portal hypertension is fibrosis and obstruction caused by cirrhosis of the liver (see p. 931). Long-term portal hypertension causes several pathophysiologic problems that are difficult to treat and can be fatal. These problems include varices, splenomegaly, ascites, hepatic encephalopathy, and hepatopulmonary syndrome.[131]

Varices are distended, tortuous collateral veins. Prolonged elevation of pressure in the portal vein cause collateral veins to open between the portal vein and systemic veins and their transformation into varices, particularly in the lower esophagus and stomach, but also over the abdominal wall (known as the caput medusae [Medusa head]) and rectum (hemorrhoidal varices) (Figure 36-11). Rupture of varices can cause life-threatening hemorrhage.[132]

Splenomegaly is enlargement of the spleen caused by increased pressure in the splenic vein, which branches from the portal vein. Thrombocytopenia is the most common symptom of congestive splenomegaly. The enlarged spleen can be palpated. Hepatopulmonary syndrome (vasodilation, intrapulmonary shunting, and hypoxia) and portopulmonary hypertension (pulmonary vasoconstriction and vascular remodeling) are complications of liver disease and portal hypertension. The pathophysiology is complex and involves different effects of vasoactive substances. There may be no clinical manifestations, although dyspnea, cyanosis, and clubbing may occur.[133]

CLINICAL MANIFESTATIONS Vomiting of blood (hematemesis) from bleeding esophageal varices is the most common clinical manifestation of portal hypertension. Bleeding is usually from varices that have developed slowly over a period of years. Slow, chronic bleeding from varices causes anemia or melena. Rupture of esophageal varices causes hemorrhage and voluminous vomiting of dark-colored blood. The ruptured varices are usually painless. Rupture is caused by a combination of erosion by gastric acid and elevated venous pressure. Mortality from ruptured esophageal varices ranges from 30% to 60%. Recurrent bleeding of esophageal varices indicates a poor prognosis. Hemorrhoidal varices present as hematochezia and copious rectal bleeding. Most individuals die within 1 year.

EVALUATION AND TREATMENT Portal hypertension is often diagnosed at the time of variceal bleeding and confirmed by upper gastrointestinal endoscopy and evaluation of portal venous pressure. The

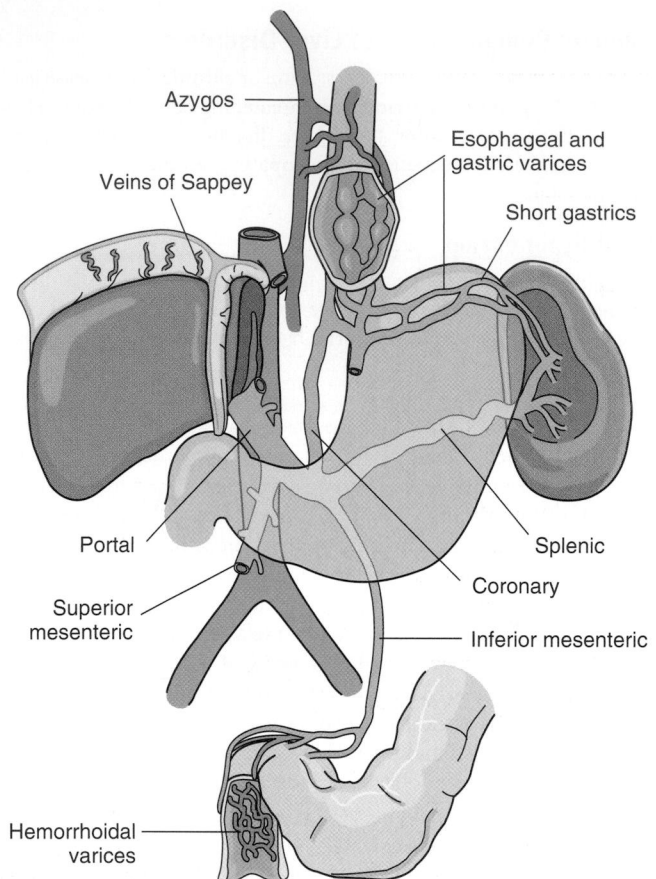

FIGURE 36-11 Varices Related to Portal Hypertension. Portal vein, its major tributaries, and the most important shunts (collateral veins) between the portal and caval systems. The shunted blood returns to the systemic venous system, bypassing the liver. (From Monahan FD et al: *Phipps' medical-surgical nursing: concepts and clinical practice*, ed 8, St Louis, 2007, Mosby.)

individual usually has a history of jaundice, hepatitis, alcoholism, or cirrhosis. Pressure in the portal venous system can be reduced with nonselective beta-blocking drugs to assist in preventing variceal bleeding.[134]

Emergency management of bleeding varices includes use of vasopressors and compression of the varices with an inflatable tube or balloon, sclerotherapy, variceal ligation, or portacaval shunt. Surgical construction of transjugular intrahepatic portosystemic shunts (TIPS procedure: anastomosis of the portal vein to the inferior vena cava) may decompress the varices. This treatment can precipitate encephalopathy. Liver transplant is the most successful option for liver failure.[135]

Ascites

Ascites is the accumulation of fluid in the peritoneal cavity. Ascites traps body fluid in the peritoneal space from which it cannot escape. The effect is to reduce the amount of fluid available for normal physiologic functions. Cirrhosis is the most common cause of ascites, but other causes include heart failure, constrictive pericarditis, abdominal malignancies, nephrotic syndrome, and malnutrition.[136] Of individuals who develop ascites caused by cirrhosis, 25% die within 1 year. Continued heavy drinking of alcohol is associated with this mortality and is related to cirrhosis.

PATHOPHYSIOLOGY Several factors contribute to the development of ascites, including portal hypertension, decreased synthesis of albumin by the liver, splanchnic arterial vasodilation, and renal sodium and water retention. Portal hypertension and reduced serum albumin levels cause capillary hydrostatic pressure to exceed capillary osmotic pressure (see Chapter 5), pushing water into the peritoneal cavity. Portal hypertension also increases the production of hepatic lymph, which "weeps" into the peritoneal cavity. Splanchnic arterial vasodilation, associated with increased nitric oxide produced by the diseased liver, can decrease effective circulating blood volume, activating aldosterone and antidiuretic hormone, which promote renal sodium and water retention. The sodium and water retention expands plasma volume, thereby accelerating portal hypertension and ascites formation. Translocation of bacteria and release of endotoxin cause peritonitis with an inflammatory response that increases mesenteric capillary permeability and fluid movement into the peritoneal cavity, promoting ascites. Figure 36-12 summarizes the mechanisms by which cirrhosis of the liver cause ascites.

CLINICAL MANIFESTATIONS The accumulation of ascitic fluid causes abdominal distention, increased abdominal girth and weight gain (Figure 36-13). Large volumes of fluid (10 to 20 L) displace the diaphragm and cause dyspnea by decreasing lung capacity. Respiratory rate increases, and the individual assumes a semi-Fowler position to relieve the dyspnea. Some peripheral edema is usually present. Approximately 10% of individuals with ascites develop bacterial peritonitis, which causes fever, chills, abdominal pain, decreased bowel sounds, and cloudy ascitic fluid.

EVALUATION AND TREATMENT Diagnosis is usually based on clinical manifestations and identification of liver disease. Dietary salt restriction and use of potassium-sparing diuretics can reduce ascites. Stronger diuretics, such as furosemide or ethacrynic acid, may be used and vasopressin receptor 2 antagonists are effective for dilutional hyponatremia. Albumin may be given. Paracentesis is used to aspirate ascitic fluid for bacterial culture, biochemical analysis, and microscopic examination. The goal of treatment is to relieve discomfort. If the restoration of liver function is possible, the ascites diminishes spontaneously. Levels of serum electrolytes are monitored carefully because the individual is at risk for hyponatremia and hypokalemia.

Palliative measures include paracentesis to remove 1 or 2 L of ascitic fluid and relieve respiratory distress. However, the removal of too much fluid relieves pressure on blood vessels and carries the risk of hypotension, shock, or death. Despite repeated paracentesis, ascitic fluid reaccumulates because of the persistent portal hypertension and reduced plasma albumin levels associated with irreversible disease. Peritonitis is treated with antibiotics. Other procedures include peritoneovenous shunt (peritoneal fluid into veins) and transjugular intrahepatic portosystemic shunt (TIPS) (bypass of blood flow from the portal venous branch to the hepatic venous branch).[137] Individuals with ascites and portal hypertension have a poor prognosis and liver transplant is the best treatment option.[137]

Hepatic Encephalopathy

Hepatic encephalopathy (portal-systemic encephalopathy) is a complex neurologic syndrome characterized by impaired behavioral, cognitive, and motor function. The syndrome may develop rapidly during acute fulminant hepatitis or slowly during the course of cirrhosis and the development of portal hypertension or after portosystemic bypass or shunting.

PATHOPHYSIOLOGY Hepatic encephalopathy results from a combination of biochemical alterations that affect neurotransmission and brain function. Liver dysfunction and the development of collateral

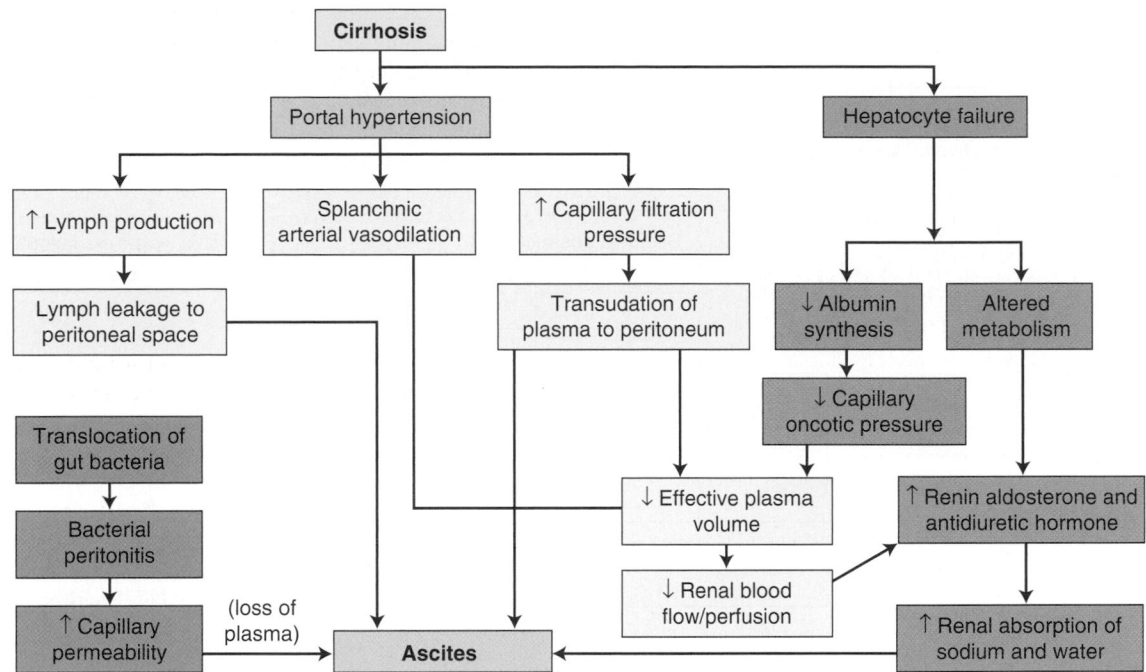

FIGURE 36-12 Mechanisms of Ascites Caused by Cirrhosis.

FIGURE 36-13 Massive Ascites in an Individual with Cirrhosis. Distended abdomen, dilated upper abdominal veins, and inverted umbilicus are classic manifestations. (From Goldman L, Schafer AI: *Goldman's Cecil medicine,* ed 24, Philadelphia, 2012, Saunders.)

vessels that shunt blood around the liver to the systemic circulation permit toxins absorbed from the gastrointestinal tract and normally removed by the liver, to accumulate and circulate freely to the brain. The accumulated toxins alter cerebral energy metabolism, interfere with neurotransmission, and cause edema. The most hazardous substances are end products of intestinal protein digestion, particularly ammonia, which cannot be converted to urea by the diseased liver. Other substances include inflammatory cytokines, short-chain fatty acids, serotonin, tryptophan, and manganese. These substances cause astrocyte swelling and alter the blood-brain barrier, promoting cerebral edema. Infection, hemorrhage, and electrolyte imbalance (including zinc deficiency), constipation and use of sedatives and analgesics can precipitate hepatic encephalopathy in the presence of liver disease.[138]

CLINICAL MANIFESTATIONS Subtle changes in personality, memory loss, irritability, disinhibition, lethargy, and sleep disturbances are common initial manifestations of hepatic encephalopathy. Symptoms then can progress to confusion, disorientation to time and space, flapping tremor of the hands (asterixis), slow speech, bradykinesia, stupor, convulsions, and coma. Coma is usually a sign of liver failure and ultimately results in death. Variceal bleeding and ascites may develop concurrently. Symptoms may be episodic, recurrent, or persistent.[139] Hepatic encephalopathy is often associated with bleeding varices and ascites.

EVALUATION AND TREATMENT Diagnosis of hepatic encephalopathy is based on a history of liver disease, clinical manifestations, psychometric tests, and exclusion of other causes of brain dysfunction. Electroencephalography and blood chemistry tests provide supportive data. Tracking levels of serum ammonia assesses treatment effectiveness and liver function.

Correction of fluid and electrolyte imbalances and withdrawal of depressant drugs metabolized by the liver are the first steps in the treatment of hepatic encephalopathy. Dietary protein is maintained to prevent malnutrition but at levels that reduce blood ammonia levels.[140] Lactulose prevents ammonia absorption in the colon. Neomycin eliminates ammonia-producing intestinal bacteria but can be nephrotoxic. Glutamase inhibitors reduce gut ammonia. Rifaximin decreases intestinal production of ammonia and is used for lactulose nonresponders. Extracorporeal liver support systems remove toxins from the blood and are an option for managing overt hepatic encephalopathy.[141]

Jaundice

Jaundice, or icterus, is a yellow or greenish pigmentation of the skin caused by hyperbilirubinemia (plasma bilirubin concentrations greater than 2.5 to 3.0 mg/dl). Hyperbilirubinemia and jaundice can result from (1) extrahepatic (posthepatic) obstruction to bile flow, (2) intrahepatic obstruction, or (3) prehepatic excessive production of unconjugated bilirubin (i.e., excessive hemolysis of red blood cells)[142]

FIGURE 36-14 Mechanisms of Jaundice.

(Figure 36-14). Jaundice in newborns is caused by impaired bilirubin uptake and conjugation (see Chapter 37).

PATHOPHYSIOLOGY Obstructive jaundice can result from extrahepatic or intrahepatic obstruction.[143] *Extrahepatic obstructive jaundice* develops if the common bile duct is occluded (e.g., by a gallstone, tumor, or inflammation). Bilirubin conjugated by the hepatocytes cannot flow through the obstructed common bile duct into the duodenum. Therefore, it accumulates in the liver and enters the bloodstream, causing hyperbilirubinemia and jaundice. *Intrahepatic obstructive jaundice* involves disturbances in hepatocyte function and obstruction of bile canaliculi. The uptake, conjugation, or excretion of bilirubin can be affected with elevated levels of both conjugated and unconjugated bilirubin. Obstruction of bile canaliculi diminishes flow of conjugated bilirubin into the common bile duct. In mild cases, some of the bile canaliculi open. Consequently, the amount of bilirubin in the intestinal tract may be only slightly decreased.

Excessive hemolysis (destruction) of red blood cells can cause hemolytic jaundice (*prehepatic* or *nonobstructive jaundice*). Increased unconjugated bilirubin is formed through metabolism of the heme component of destroyed red blood cells and exceeds the conjugation ability of the liver, causing blood levels of unconjugated bilirubin to rise. Decreased bilirubin uptake or conjugation also causes unconjugated hyperbilirubinemia, as occurs with reaction to some drugs (e.g., rifampin) and in genetic disorders such as Gilbert syndrome. Because unconjugated bilirubin is not water soluble, it is not excreted in the urine. The causes of jaundice are summarized in Table 36-7.

CLINICAL MANIFESTATIONS Conjugated bilirubin is water soluble and appears in the urine. The urine may darken several days before the onset of jaundice. The complete obstruction of bile flow from the liver to the duodenum causes light-colored stools. With partial obstruction, the stools are normal in color and bilirubin is present in the urine.

Fever, chills, and pain often accompany jaundice resulting from viral or bacterial inflammation of the liver (e.g., viral hepatitis). Yellow discoloration may first occur in the sclera of the eye and then progress to the skin as bilirubin attaches to elastic fibers. Pruritus (itching) often accompanies jaundice because bilirubin accumulates in the skin.

EVALUATION AND TREATMENT Laboratory evaluation of serum establishes whether elevated plasma bilirubin is conjugated or unconjugated, or both. The history and physical examination identify underlying disorders, such as cirrhosis, exposure to hepatitis virus, and gallbladder or pancreatic disease. The treatment for jaundice consists of correcting the cause.

Hepatorenal Syndrome

Hepatorenal syndrome is functional renal failure that develops as a complication of advanced liver disease. The renal failure is not caused by primary renal disease or other extrinsic factors but rather by portal hypertension, cardiac impairment, and other circulatory alterations associated with advanced liver disease, such as cirrhosis or fulminant hepatitis with portal hypertension. Manifestations include oliguria, sodium and water retention (usually with ascites and peripheral edema), hypotension, and peripheral vasodilation.[144] The kidney usually has a normal structure.

TABLE 36-7   Common Types of Jaundice

Type	Mechanism	Causes
Hemolytic (prehepatic) jaundice (predominantly unconjugated bilirubin)	Destruction of erythrocytes (increased bilirubin production)	Hemolytic anemias (e.g., sickle cell) Severe infection Toxic substances in circulation (e.g., snake venom) Transfusion of incompatible blood
Disorders of bilirubin metabolism (unconjugated bilirubin)	Decreased bilirubin uptake Decreased bilirubin conjugation	Drug induced (e.g., rifampin and cyclosporine) Hereditary disorder (e.g., Gilbert syndrome)
Obstructive (posthepatic) jaundice (predominantly conjugated bilirubin)	Obstruction of passage of conjugated bilirubin from liver to intestine	Obstruction of bile duct by gallstones or tumor (extrahepatic obstructive jaundice) Obstruction of bile flow through liver (intrahepatic obstructive jaundice) Drugs
Hepatocellular (intrahepatic) jaundice (both conjugated and unconjugated bilirubin)	Failure of liver cells (hepatocytes) to conjugate bilirubin and of bilirubin to pass from liver to intestine	Genetic defect of hepatocytes (decreased enzymes), such as occurs in premature infants (see Chapter 37 Severe infections (e.g., hepatitis) Alcoholic liver disease or biliary cirrhosis

PATHOPHYSIOLOGY *Type 1 hepatorenal syndrome* accompanies a sudden decrease in blood volume secondary to massive gastrointestinal or variceal bleeding and hypotension caused by bleeding and peripheral vasodilation associated with failing liver function. Hypotension also can be caused by the excessive use of diuretics to treat ascites or decreased cardiac output. The decrease in blood volume and hypotension result in decreased renal perfusion, decreased glomerular filtration, and oliguria (see Chapter 30). *Type 2 hepatorenal syndrome* develops slowly and is related to ascites. Ineffective circulating blood volume causes decreased glomerular filtration and oliguria. Intrarenal vasoconstriction may result from the selective effects of vasoactive substances that accumulate in the blood because of liver failure or a compensatory response to portal hypertension and the pooling of blood in the splanchnic circulation.[145]

CLINICAL MANIFESTATIONS The onset of hepatorenal manifestations may be acute or gradual. Oliguria and complications of advanced liver disease, including jaundice, ascites, peripheral edema, hypotension and gastrointestinal bleeding, are usually present. Systolic blood pressure is usually below 100 mm Hg. Nonspecific symptoms of hepatorenal syndrome include anorexia, weakness, and fatigue.[144]

EVALUATION AND TREATMENT Despite oliguria, serum potassium levels do not become dangerously elevated until the terminal stages of the hepatorenal syndrome. Blood urea level increases, followed by an increase in creatinine concentration. Urine osmolality increases, but urine sodium concentrations are below normal. Urine specific gravity is greater than 1.015.

The prognosis is usually poor and is related to a failing liver requiring liver transplant. Bridge treatments include albumin administration and terlipressin (a vasopressin analog).[144]

> ✔ **QUICK CHECK 36-5**
> 1. How does portal hypertension cause varices and promote formation of ascites?
> 2. What are two factors that cause hepatic encephalopathy?
> 3. Why is the concentration of unconjugated bilirubin elevated in hemolytic jaundice?
> 4. Describe how failure of liver function causes renal failure (hepatorenal syndrome).

Disorders of the Liver
Acute Liver Failure

Acute liver failure (fulminant liver failure) is a rare clinical syndrome resulting in severe impairment or necrosis of liver cells without preexisting liver disease or cirrhosis. Paracetamol (acetaminophen) overdose is a leading cause of acute liver failure in the United States[146] (see *Health Alert:* Paracetamol [Acetaminophen] and Acute Liver Failure in Chapter 35). Acute liver failure also can occur with concurrent liver disease (acute on chronic liver failure),[147] including complication of viral hepatitis, particularly hepatitis B virus (HBV) infection; compounded by infection with the delta virus; as well as metabolic liver disorders. Edematous hepatocytes and patchy areas of necrosis and inflammatory cell infiltrates disrupt the parenchyma. The death of hepatocytes may be caused by viral or toxic injury or immunologic and inflammatory damage with necrosis or apoptosis.

Acute liver failure usually develops 6 to 8 weeks after the initial symptoms of viral hepatitis or a metabolic liver disorder, or within 5 days to 8 weeks of acetaminophen overdose. Anorexia, vomiting, abdominal pain, and progressive jaundice are initial signs followed by ascites and gastrointestinal bleeding. Hepatic encephalopathy is manifested as lethargy, and altered motor functions. Coma is related to cerebral edema, ischemia, and brainstem herniation. Liver function tests show elevations in the levels of both direct and indirect serum bilirubin, serum transaminases, and blood ammonia. Prothrombin time is prolonged. Renal failure and pulmonary distress can occur.[148] Treatment of acute liver failure requires rapid evaluation and critical care. The hepatic necrosis is irreversible, and 60% to 90% of affected children die. Liver transplantation may be lifesaving.[149] Artificial liver support devices are being evaluated. Survivors usually do not develop cirrhosis or chronic liver disease.

Cirrhosis

Cirrhosis is an irreversible inflammatory, fibrotic liver disease and has a prevalence in the United States of about 633,323 with a death rate of about 26%.[150] Many disorders can cause cirrhosis and are listed in Box 36-3. The process of cellular injury depends on the cause of cirrhosis, and the pathologic mechanisms are not all clearly understood. Structural changes result from injury (e.g., viruses or toxicity from alcohol) and fibrosis, which is a consequence of infiltration of leukocytes, release of inflammatory mediators, and activation of hepatic stellate cells and myofibroblasts.[151] Chaotic fibrosis alters or obstructs biliary

---

BOX 36-3 **Causes of Cirrhosis**

Hepatitis virus—B and C (common)
Excessive alcohol intake (common)
Idiopathic (common)
Nonalcoholic fatty liver disease (NAFLD), also known as nonalcoholic steato-
   hepatitis (NASH)
Autoimmune disorders
   Autoimmune hepatitis
   Primary biliary cirrhosis
   Primary sclerosing cholangitis
Hereditary metabolic disorder
   α_1-Antitrypsin deficiency
   Hemochromatosis
   Wilson disease
   Glycogen or lipid storage diseases
Prolonged exposure to drugs or toxins (e.g., carbon tetrachloride, cleaning and
   industrial solvents, copper salts)
Hepatic venous outflow obstruction
   Budd-Chiari syndrome
   Right-sided heart failure

---

channels and blood flow, producing jaundice and portal hypertension (see pp. 927 and 929). New vascular channels form shunts, and blood from the portal vein bypasses the liver, contributing to portal hypertension, metabolic alterations, and toxin accumulation. The process of regeneration is disrupted by hypoxia, necrosis, atrophy, and (ultimately) liver failure. The formation of fibrous bands and regenerating nodules distorts the architecture of the liver parenchyma and gives the liver a cobbly appearance. The liver may be larger or smaller than normal and is usually firm or hard when palpated.

Cirrhosis develops slowly over a period of years. Its severity and rate of progression depend on the cause. If toxins, such as alcohol metabolites, are involved, the rate of cell death and the severity of inflammation depend on the amount of toxin present. Removal of the toxin slows the progression of liver damage and enhances the process of regeneration.[152]

Alcoholic liver disease. Alcoholic liver disease is related to toxic effects of alcohol (see Chapter 4) and coexisting liver disease. The incidence of alcoholic cirrhosis is greatest in middle-age men; however, women develop more severe liver injury than men.[153] Mortality resulting from cirrhosis in the United States is highest among non-whites. Although alcoholic cirrhosis is the most prevalent of the various types of cirrhosis, the occurrence of cirrhosis among persons with alcoholism is relatively low (approximately 25%). The spectrum of alcoholic liver disease includes alcoholic fatty liver, alcoholic steatohepatitis, and alcoholic cirrhosis.

PATHOPHYSIOLOGY Alcoholic fatty liver (steatosis) is the mildest form of alcoholic liver disease. It can be caused by relatively small amounts of alcohol, may be asymptomatic, and is reversible with cessation of drinking.[154] Fat deposition (deposition of triglycerides) within the liver is caused primarily by increased lipogenesis, cholesterol synthesis, and decreased fatty acid oxidation by hepatocytes. Lipids mobilized from adipose tissue or dietary fat intake may contribute to fat accumulation.

Alcoholic steatohepatitis (alcoholic hepatitis) is a precursor of cirrhosis characterized by increased hepatic fat storage, inflammation, and degeneration and necrosis of hepatocytes with infiltration of neutrophils and lymphocytes. The injured hepatocytes contain Mallory bodies (hyaline endoplasmic reticulum), indicating the onset of fibrosis. The inflammation and necrosis caused by alcoholic steatohepatitis stimulate the irreversible fibrosis characteristic of the cirrhotic stage of disease.[155]

Alcoholic cirrhosis is caused by the toxic effects of alcohol metabolism on the liver, immunologic alterations, inflammatory cytokines, oxidative stress from lipid peroxidation, and malnutrition. Alcohol is transformed to acetaldehyde, and excessive amounts significantly alter hepatocyte function and activate hepatic stellate cells, a primary cell involved in liver fibrosis. Mitochondrial function is impaired, decreasing oxidation of fatty acid. Enzyme and protein synthesis may be depressed or altered, and hormone and ammonia degradation is diminished. Acetaldehyde inhibits export of proteins from the liver, alters metabolism of vitamins and minerals, and induces malnutrition.[156,157] Kupffer cell (macrophage) activation attracts neutrophils promoting inflammation, endotoxins accumulate from translocation of gut bacteria, and cell-mediated immunity is suppressed. Cellular damage initiates an inflammatory response that, along with necrosis, results in activation of hepatic stellate cells and excessive collagen formation. Fibrosis and scarring alter the structure of the liver and obstruct biliary and vascular channels.

CLINICAL MANIFESTATIONS Fatty infiltration causes no specific symptoms or abnormal liver function test results. The liver is usually enlarged, however, and the individual has a history of continuous alcohol intake during the previous weeks or months. Anorexia, nausea, jaundice, and edema develop with advanced fatty infiltration or the onset of alcoholic steatohepatitis (Figure 36-15).

The clinical manifestations of alcoholic steatohepatitis can be mild or severe. Nonspecific symptoms include fatigue, weight loss, and anorexia. Manifestations of acute illness include nausea, anorexia, fever, abdominal pain, and jaundice. Cirrhosis is a multiple-system disease and causes hepatomegaly, splenomegaly, ascites, portal hypertension, gastrointestinal hemorrhage, hepatic encephalopathy, and esophageal varices. Anemia results from blood loss, malnutrition, and hypersplenism. Renal failure is often a late complication of hepatorenal syndrome. Toxic effects of alcohol also can cause testicular atrophy, reduced libido, azoospermia, and decreased testosterone levels in men. The presence of numerous and severe manifestations increases the risk of death. Cirrhosis increases the risk of hepatocellular carcinoma.

EVALUATION AND TREATMENT The diagnosis of alcoholic steatohepatitis or cirrhosis is based on the individual's history and clinical manifestations. The results of liver function tests are abnormal, and serologic studies show elevated levels of serum enzymes and bilirubin, decreased levels of serum albumin, and prolonged prothrombin time that is not easily corrected with vitamin K therapy. Liver biopsy can confirm the diagnosis of cirrhosis, but biopsy is not necessary if clinical manifestations of cirrhosis are evident.

There is no specific treatment for alcoholic steatohepatitis or cirrhosis. Rest, vitamin supplements, a nutritious diet, corticosteroids, antioxidants, drugs that slow fibrosis, and management of complications (such as ascites, gastrointestinal bleeding, and encephalopathy) slow disease progression. Cessation of alcohol consumption slows the progression of liver damage, improves clinical symptoms, and prolongs life. Although the liver damage is irreversible, measures that halt the inflammation and destruction of liver cells prolong life. Liver transplantation is the treatment of end-stage liver disease. Artificial liver support systems continue to be evaluated and hepatocyte transplantation is being explored.[158,159]

Nonalcoholic fatty liver disease and nonalcoholic steatohepatitis. Nonalcoholic fatty liver disease (NAFLD) is infiltration of hepatocytes with fat, primarily in the form of triglycerides, but it

FIGURE 36-15 Clinical Manifestations of Cirrhosis. *ADH,* Antidiuretic hormone; *ALT,* alanine transaminase; *AST,* aspartate transaminase.

occurs in the absence of alcohol intake. It is associated with obesity (including obese children), high levels of cholesterol and triglycerides, metabolic syndrome, and type 2 diabetes mellitus. NAFLD is the most common chronic liver disease in the United States. Some individuals with NAFLD will develop nonalcoholic steatohepatitis (NASH) with hepatocellular injury, inflammation, and fibrosis. NASH is difficult to distinguish from alcohol-induced liver fibrosis. NAFLD is usually asymptomatic and may remain undetected for years. The most severe forms of NASH progress to cirrhosis and end-stage liver disease. Treatment is individualized and includes the use of behavioral modification, dietary counseling, and regular exercise.[160,161]

Biliary cirrhosis. Biliary cirrhosis differs from alcoholic cirrhosis in that the damage and inflammation leading to cirrhosis begin in bile canaliculi and bile ducts, rather than in the hepatocytes. The two types of biliary cirrhosis are *primary* and *secondary*. Although both involve bile duct pathologic changes, they differ with respect to cause, risk factors, and mechanisms of obstruction and inflammation.

Primary biliary cirrhosis is a chronic, autoimmune, cholestatic liver disease. It is caused by autoimmune T-lymphocyte and highly specific antimitochondrial antibody destruction of the small intrahepatic bile ducts and primarily affects middle-aged women. Primary

biliary cirrhosis often accompanies other autoimmune diseases. Pathogenesis includes inflammation, destruction, fibrosis, and obstruction of the intrahepatic bile ducts. Primary biliary cirrhosis can be detected by biochemical evidence of cholestatic liver disease. Test findings include the presence of antinuclear antibodies, anticentromere antibodies, and the GP210 antinuclear antibody as well as elevated alkaline phosphatase levels for at least 6 months' duration. Ultrasound imaging of the liver, or liver biopsy, assists with diagnosis. Manifestations progress insidiously from pruritus, hyperbilirubinemia, jaundice, and light or clay-colored stools to cirrhosis, portal hypertension, and encephalopathy. Life expectancy is 5 to 10 years after onset of symptoms if not treated. Treatment with ursodeoxycholic acid slows disease progression and pruritus may be relieved by cholestyramine, which binds bile salts in the intestine. Liver transplant is highly effective.[162]

Secondary biliary cirrhosis is caused by prolonged partial or complete obstruction of the common bile duct or branches by gallstones, tumors, fibrotic strictures, or chronic pancreatitis; biliary atresia and cystic fibrosis are causative in children. Necrotic areas develop and lead to proliferation and inflammation of portal ducts, producing edema, fibrosis, and cirrhosis if not treated. Surgery or endoscopy relieves obstruction, prolongs survival, and diminishes or resolves symptoms.

Viral Hepatitis

Viral hepatitis is a relatively common systemic disease that affects primarily the liver. Different strains of viruses cause different types of hepatitis. The types and estimated incidence in the United States in 2013 were hepatitis A virus (HAV), 3473 cases; hepatitis B virus (HBV), 3050 cases; hepatitis D virus (HDV), associated with HBV unknown; hepatitis C virus (HCV), 2138 cases; and hepatitis E virus (HEV), unknown. Hepatitis A formerly was known as infectious hepatitis and hepatitis B as serum hepatitis.[163] Characteristics of the different types of viruses that cause hepatitis are presented in Table 36-8. Viral hepatitis in children is presented in Chapter 37.

PATHOPHYSIOLOGY All five types of viral hepatitis (A, B, C, D, and E) can cause acute, icteric illness. The pathologic lesions of hepatitis include hepatic cell necrosis, scarring (with chronic disease), and Kupffer cell hyperplasia, and infiltration by mononuclear phagocytes occurs with varying severity. Cellular injury is promoted by cell-mediated immune mechanisms (i.e., cytotoxic T cells, T-regulatory cells, and natural killer cells). Regeneration of hepatic cells begins within 48 hours of injury. The inflammatory process can damage and obstruct bile canaliculi, leading to cholestasis and obstructive jaundice. In milder cases, the liver parenchyma is not damaged. Damage tends to be most severe in cases of hepatitides B and C. Acute fulminating hepatitis can cause acute liver failure and severe hepatic encephalopathy, which is manifested as confusion, stupor, coma, and coagulopathy. Hepatitides B and C are the most common causes as well as hepatitis E in pregnant women.[164]

Coinfection of hepatitis B virus (HBV), hepatitis C virus (HCV), hepatitis D virus (HDV), and human immunodeficiency virus (HIV) occurs because these viruses share the same route of transmission (contact between infected body fluids and broken skin or mucous membranes, or intravenously). Progression of liver disease is more rapid in these cases.[165]

CLINICAL MANIFESTATIONS The clinical manifestations of the various types of hepatitis are very similar. The spectrum of manifestations ranges from absence of symptoms to fulminating hepatitis, with rapid onset of liver failure and coma. Acute viral hepatitis causes abnormal liver function test results. The serum aminotransferase values, aspartate transaminase (AST) and alanine transaminase (ALT), are elevated but not consistent with the extent of cellular damage.

TABLE 36-8 Characteristics of Viral Hepatitis

Characteristic	Hepatitis A	Hepatitis B	Hepatitis D	Hepatitis C	Hepatitis E
Virus	27-nm RNA virus	42-nm DNA virus	36-nm RNA virus	30- to 60-nm RNA virus	32-nm RNA virus
Antigens or antibodies	Anti-HAV	HBsAg HBcAg HbeAg	Anti-HDV	Anti-HCV	Anti-HEV
Incubation period	30 days	60-180 days	30-180 days	35-60 days	15-60 days
Route of transmission	Fecal-oral (most common), parenteral, sexual	Parenteral, sexual, across placenta	HBV coinfection Parenteral (?), fecal-oral, sexual	Parenteral, sexual, across placenta	Fecal-oral
Onset	Nonspecific Acute with fever	Insidious	Insidious	Insidious	Acute
Carrier state	Negative	Positive	Positive	Positive	Negative
Severity	Mild	Severe; may be prolonged or chronic	Severe	Unknown	Severe in pregnant women
Chronic hepatitis	No	Yes Increased risk of HCC	Yes	Yes Increased risk of HCC	No
Age group affected	Children and young adults	Any	Any	Any	Children and young adults
Prophylaxis	Hygiene, immune serum globulin, HAV vaccine	Hygiene, HBV vaccine, blood screening	Hygiene, HBV vaccine	Hygiene, blood screening, interferon-alpha	Hygiene, safe water
Pathophysiology	Hepatocyte injury caused by cellular immune responses (T cells, NK cells, and cytokines)	Viral replication, coinfection with viral mutation, inflammation, and cellular necrosis	Coinfection with HBV, severe cell injury, inflammation progressing to cirrhosis	Hepatocyte injury caused by immune response, inflammation, and fibrosis leading to cirrhosis	Viral replication, liver is cytotoxic, immune response causes inflammation and cholestasis
Treatment	Immune globulin within 2 weeks of exposure Symptomatic support	Interferon-alpha, peginterferon-alpha, antivirals (lamivudine, adefovir, entecavir, telbivudine, tenofovir)	Interferon-alpha	Interferon-alpha, peginterferon-alpha, antivirals (ribavirin, boceprevir, telaprevir, simeprevir, daclatasvir, sofosbuvir), combinations of antivirals	Symptomatic support similar to HAV

DNA, Deoxyribonucleic acid; *HAAg,* hepatitis A antigen; *HAV,* hepatitis A virus; *HBcAg,* hepatitis B core antigen; *HBeAg,* hepatitis B e antigen (a fragment derived from the same propeptide for HBcAg); *HBsAg,* hepatitis B surface antigen; *HBV,* hepatitis B virus; *HCC,* hepatocellular carcinoma; *HCV,* hepatitis C virus; *HDV,* hepatitis D virus; *HEV,* hepatitis V virus; *RNA,* ribonucleic acid.

The clinical course of hepatitis usually consists of three phases. The incubation phase and manifestations vary depending on the virus (see Table 36-8):

1. Prodromal (preicteric) phase. Begins about 2 weeks after exposure and ends with the appearance of jaundice; marked by fatigue, anorexia, malaise, nausea, vomiting, headache, hyperalgia, cough, and low-grade fever; infection is highly transmissible during this phase.

2. Icteric phase. Begins 1 to 2 weeks after the prodromal phase and lasts 2 to 6 weeks; jaundice, dark urine, and clay-colored stools are common; the liver is enlarged, smooth, and tender, and percussion or palpation of the liver causes pain; gastrointestinal and respiratory symptoms subside, but fatigue and abdominal pain may persist or become more severe. This is the actual phase of illness. Individuals who develop chronic HBV, HDV, or HCV infection do not become jaundiced and may not be diagnosed.

3. Recovery phase. Begins with resolution of jaundice, about 6 to 8 weeks after exposure; symptoms diminish, but the liver remains enlarged and tender; liver function returns to normal 2 to 12 weeks after the onset of jaundice.

Chronic active hepatitis is the persistence of clinical manifestations and liver inflammation after acute stages of HBV, HBV/HDV coinfection, and HCV infection. Liver function tests remain abnormal for longer than 6 months, and hepatitis B surface antigen (HBsAg) persists. Chronic, active HBV and HCV is a predisposition to cirrhosis and primary hepatocellular carcinoma.[166,167] Chronic active hepatitis constitutes a carrier state, and HBV and HCV can be transmitted from mothers to infants.

EVALUATION AND TREATMENT Diagnosis of HAV and HCV is based on the presence of anti-HAV and anti-HCV antibodies. The most specific diagnostic test for HBV is serologic analysis for specific hepatitis virus antigens (i.e., HBsAg, which is the marker for HBV). There are other markers for HBV including anti-HBs, HBeAg and anti-HBe, and anti-HBc IgM and IgG.[168] The assay for HDV is the measurement of total antibody to hepatitis D antigen (anti-HDV) and serum HDV RNA.[169] HCV RNA quantification is important for evaluation of viral load to evaluate antiviral therapy for chronic HCV. HEV is diagnosed from the presence of serum anti-HEV IgG and HEV RNA. HEV is usually a self-limiting disease except in undeveloped countries, where it causes chronic hepatitis with increased risk in pregnant women. Liver enzyme levels and function tests also can indicate other viral liver diseases, drug toxicity, or alcoholic hepatitis.[170]

Treatments for different types of viral hepatitis are summarized in Table 36-8. Physical activity may be restricted and a low-fat, high-carbohydrate diet is beneficial if bile flow is obstructed. For chronic hepatitis, treatment is directed at suppressing viral replication before irreversible liver cell damage or hepatic carcinoma occurs. Cyclic and combination therapy may prevent drug resistance, and new agents are being developed.[171,172]

After ingestion and gastrointestinal uptake, HAV replicates in the liver and is secreted into the bile, feces, and sera. To prevent transmission of hepatitis A, proper hand hygiene and the use of gloves for disposing of bedpans and fecal matter are imperative. HAV may be shed in the feces for up to 3 months after onset of symptoms. Molecular procedures are available for direct surveillance of HAV in food.[173] Direct contact with blood or body fluids of individuals with HBV or HBV/HDV coinfection or HCV should be avoided. The administration of immune globulin before exposure or early in the incubation period can prevent hepatitis A and hepatitis B. A combined vaccine is available to protect against HAV and HBV infection. There is no vaccine for HCV.[174] A vaccine for HEV is available in China, but no vaccine has

been approved for use in the United States.[175] Preexposure vaccination is recommended for healthcare workers, liver transplant recipients, and others who are at risk for contact with infected body fluids, particularly children.

> **QUICK CHECK 36-7**
> 1. How does hepatitis A virus (HAV) differ from hepatitis B virus (HBV)?
> 2. What vaccines are available to prevent viral hepatitis?
> 3. What are the three phases of hepatitis viral infection?
> 4. What complications are associated with chronic active viral hepatitis?

Disorders of the Gallbladder

Obstruction and inflammation are the most common disorders of the gallbladder. Obstruction is caused by gallstones, which are aggregates of substances in the bile. The gallstones may remain in the gallbladder or be ejected, with bile, into the cystic duct. Gallstones that become lodged in the cystic duct obstruct the flow of bile into and out of the gallbladder and cause inflammation. Gallstone formation is termed cholelithiasis. Inflammation of the gallbladder or cystic duct is known as cholecystitis.

Cholelithiasis (Gallstones)

Cholelithiasis (gallstones) is a prevalent disorder in developed countries, where the incidence is 10% to 15% in white adults and 60% to 70% in Native Americans. Risk factors include obesity, middle age, female gender, use of oral contraceptives, rapid weight loss, Native American ancestry, genetic predisposition, and gallbladder, pancreatic, or ileal disease.[176]

PATHOPHYSIOLOGY Gallstones are formed from impaired metabolism of cholesterol, bilirubin, and bile acids. All gallstones contain cholesterol, unconjugated bilirubin, bilirubin calcium salts, fatty acids, calcium carbonates and phosphates, and mucin glycoproteins. Gallstones are of three types depending on chemical composition: cholesterol (70% cholesterol and the most common [70% to 80%]); pigmented (black [hard] and brown [soft] with less than 30% cholesterol); and mixed.[177] Cholesterol gallstones form in bile that is supersaturated with cholesterol produced by the liver. Supersaturation sets the stage for cholesterol crystal formation, or the formation of "microstones." More crystals then aggregate on the microstones, which grow to form "macrostones." This process usually occurs in the gallbladder, which may have decreased motility. The stones may lie dormant or become lodged in the cystic or common duct, causing pain when the gallbladder contracts and cholecystitis. The stones can accumulate and fill the entire gallbladder (Figure 36-16). Pigmented brown gallstones form from calcium bilirubinate and fatty acid soaps that bind with calcium. They are associated with biliary stasis, bacterial infections, and biliary parasites. They are more common in East Asia. Black gallstones are rare. They are associated with chronic liver disease and hemolytic disease, and are composed of calcium bilirubinate with mucin glycoproteins.[178]

CLINICAL MANIFESTATIONS Cholelithiasis is often asymptomatic. Epigastric and right hypochondrium pain and intolerance to fatty foods are the cardinal manifestations of cholelithiasis. Vague symptoms include heartburn, flatulence, epigastric discomfort, and food intolerances, particularly to fats and cabbage. The pain (biliary colic) occurs 30 minutes to several hours after eating a fatty meal. It is caused by the lodging of one or more gallstones in the cystic or common duct during contraction of the gallbladder. It can be intermittent or steady and usually occurs in the right upper quadrant, radiating to the

FIGURE 36-16 Resected Gallbladder Containing Mixed Gall-stones. (From Kissane JM, editor: *Anderson's pathology*, ed 9, St Louis, 1990, Mosby.)

mid-upper area of the back. Jaundice indicates that the stone is located in the common bile duct.

EVALUATION AND TREATMENT Diagnosis is based on the medical history, physical examination, and imaging evaluation. An oral chole-cystogram usually outlines the stones. Intravenous cholangiography is used to differentiate cholelithiasis from other causes of extrahepatic biliary obstruction if the cholecystogram is negative. Endoscopic or percutaneous cholangiography and endoscopic or transabdominal ultrasonography are diagnostic options. Oral bile acids (ursodeoxy-cholic acid or chenodeoxycholic acid) may prevent or dissolve choles-terol stones, but the stones may recur when the drug is discontinued. Dietary factors may prevent the development of gallstones, including reducing the intake of polyunsaturated fat, monounsaturated fat, and caffeine and increasing the consumption of fiber.[179] Endoscopic removal of gallstones by sphincterotomy or endoscopic papillary balloon dilation is the preferred treatment for uncomplicated gall-stones causing obstruction of the bile ducts. Large stones may be managed by lithotripsy.[180]

Cholecystitis

Cholecystitis can be acute or chronic, but both forms are almost always caused by a gallstone lodged in the cystic duct.[181] Obstruction causes the gallbladder to become distended and inflamed. The pain is similar to that caused by gallstones. Pressure against the distended wall of the gallbladder decreases blood flow and may result in ischemia, necrosis, and perforation. Fever, leukocytosis, rebound tenderness, and abdomi-nal muscle guarding are common findings. Serum bilirubin and alka-line phosphatase levels may be elevated. Cholescintigraphy is the most sensitive imaging for cholecystitis. The acute abdominal pain of cho-lecystitis must be differentiated from that caused by pancreatitis, myocardial infarction, and acute pyelonephritis of the right kidney. Narcotics may be required to control pain, and antibiotics often are prescribed to manage bacterial infection in severe cases. Acute attacks usually require laparoscopic gallbladder resection (cholecystectomy). Obstruction also may lead to reflux of bile into the pancreatic duct, causing acute pancreatitis.[182]

Disorders of the Pancreas

Pancreatitis, or inflammation of the pancreas, is a relatively rare (15 cases per 100,000 people in the United States)[183] and potentially serious disorder. The incidence is about equal in men and women, is more common between 50 and 60 years of age, and is more likely to occur in blacks. Risk factors include obstructive biliary tract disease (particularly cholelithiasis), alcoholism, obesity, peptic ulcers, trauma, hyperlipidemia, hypercalcemia, smoking, certain drugs, and genetic

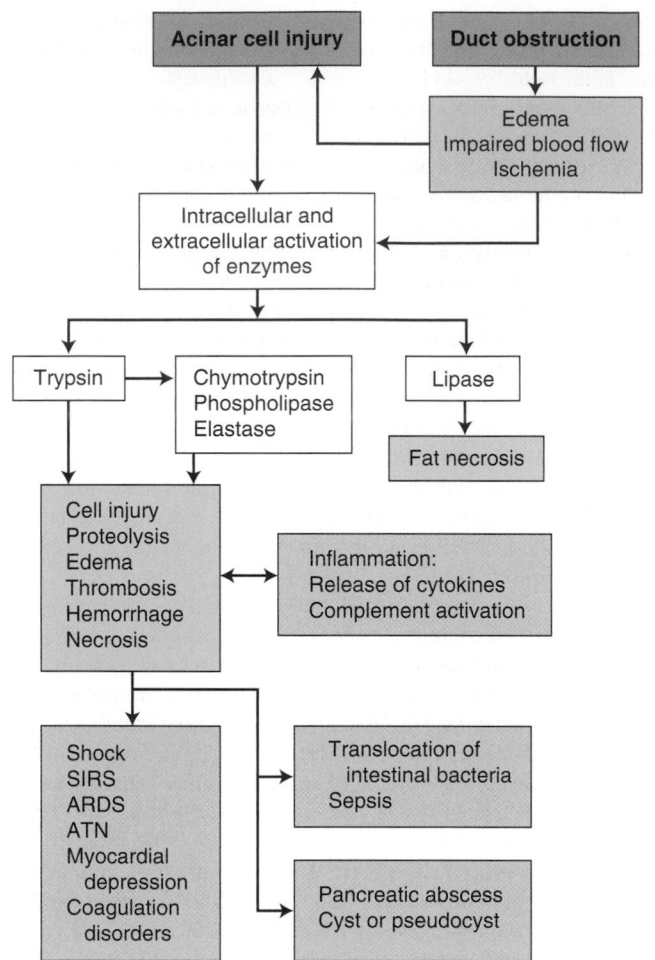

FIGURE 36-17 Pathophysiology of Acute Pancreatitis. *ARDS,* Acute respiratory distress syndrome; *ATN,* acute tubular necrosis; *SIRS,* systemic inflammatory response syndrome.

factors (hereditary pancreatitis, cystic fibrosis). The cause is unknown in 15% to 25% of cases. Pancreatitis can be acute or chronic.

Acute Pancreatitis

Acute pancreatitis is usually a mild disease and resolves spontaneously, but about 20% of those with the disease develop a severe, acute pan-creatitis requiring hospitalization. Pancreatitis develops because of obstruction to the outflow of pancreatic digestive enzymes caused by bile and pancreatic duct obstruction (e.g., gallstones). Acute pancre-atitis also results from direct cellular injury from alcohol, drugs, or viral infection.[184]

PATHOPHYSIOLOGY In obstructive disease, there is backup of pan-creatic secretions and activation and release of enzymes (activated trypsin activates chymotrypsin, lipase, and elastase) within the pancre-atic acinar cells. The activated enzymes cause autodigestion of pancre-atic cells and tissues, resulting in inflammation. The autodigestion causes vascular damage, coagulation necrosis, fat necrosis (see Chapter 4), and formation of pseudocysts (walled-off collections of pancreatic secretions). Edema within the pancreatic capsule leads to ischemia and can contribute to necrosis. There also may be independent activation of inflammation within acinar cells contributing to the local and sys-temic responses occurring in acute pancreatitis[185] (Figure 36-17). In cases of alcohol abuse, the pancreatic acinar cell metabolizes ethanol with the generation of toxic metabolites that injure pancreatic acinar cells, causing release of activated enzymes. Chronic alcohol use may also cause formation of protein plugs in pancreatic ducts and spasm of the sphincter of Oddi, resulting in obstruction. The obstruction leads to intrapancreatic release of activated enzymes, autodigestion, inflammation, and pancreatitis.

Systemic effects of acute pancreatitis are related to release of pro-inflammatory cytokines (e.g., interleukin-6, tumor necrosis factor-alpha, and platelet-activating factor) into the bloodstream. There is activation of leukocytes, injury to vessel walls, and coagulation abnormalities with development of vasodilation, hypotension, and shock. Complications can include acute respiratory distress syndrome (ARDS), heart failure, renal failure, coagulopathies, intra-abdominal hypertension, and systemic inflammatory response syndrome (SIRS) (see Chapter 24). Paralytic ileus and gastrointestinal bleeding can occur. Translocation of intestinal bacteria to the bloodstream may cause peritonitis or sepsis. Recurrent inflammation activates pancreatic stellate cells, causing pancreatic fibrosis, strictures, and duct obstruction that lead to chronic pancreatitis.[186]

CLINICAL MANIFESTATIONS   The cardinal manifestation of acute pancreatitis is epigastric or midabdominal constant pain ranging from mild abdominal discomfort to severe, incapacitating pain. The pain may radiate to the back. Pain is caused by (1) edema, which distends the pancreatic ducts and capsule; (2) chemical irritation and inflammation of the peritoneum; (3) irritation or obstruction of the biliary tract; and (4) inflammation of nerves. Fever and leukocytosis accompany the inflammatory response. Nausea and vomiting are caused by paralytic ileus secondary to the pancreatitis or peritonitis. Jaundice can occur from obstruction of the bile duct (e.g., a gallstone) or from pancreatic edema pressing on the duct. Abdominal distention accompanies bowel hypomotility and the accumulation of fluids in the peritoneal cavity. Hypovolemia, hypotension, tachycardia, myocardial insufficiency, and shock occur because plasma volume is lost as inflammatory mediators released into the circulation increase vascular permeability and dilate vessels. Tachypnea and hypoxemia develop secondary to ascites, pulmonary edema, atelectasis, or pleural effusions. Hypovolemia can decrease renal blood flow sufficiently to impair renal function and can cause renal failure. Tetany may develop as a result of hypocalcemia when calcium is deposited in areas of fat necrosis or as a decreased response to parathormone. Transient hyperglycemia also can occur if glucagon is released from damaged alpha cells in the pancreatic islets. In severe acute pancreatitis, some individuals develop flank or periumbilical ecchymosis, a sign of poor prognosis. Multiple organ failure or SIRS accounts for most deaths of those with severe acute pancreatitis.

EVALUATION AND TREATMENT   Diagnosis is based on clinical findings, identification of associated disorders, laboratory studies, and imaging results. Elevated serum amylase concentration is characteristic but is not diagnostic of severity or specificity of disease. Elevated serum lipase level is the primary diagnostic marker for acute pancreatitis.

The goal of treatment for acute pancreatitis is to stop the process of autodigestion and prevent systemic complications. Narcotic medications may be needed to relieve pain. To decrease pancreatic secretions and "rest the gland," oral food and fluids may be withheld initially and continuous gastric suction instituted. Nasogastric suction may not be necessary with mild pancreatitis, but it helps to relieve pain and prevent paralytic ileus in individuals who are nauseated and vomiting. Feeding is usually initiated within 24 to 48 hours if ileus is not present. Parenteral fluids are essential to restore blood volume and prevent hypotension and shock. In severe pancreatitis enteral nutrition with use of jejunal tube feeding usually is well tolerated, may decrease pancreatic enzyme secretion, prevents gut bacterial overgrowth, and

maintains gut barrier function. Drugs that decrease gastric acid production (e.g., H2-receptor antagonists) can decrease stimulation of the pancreas by secretin. Antibiotics are used if there is infection. The risk of mortality increases significantly with the development of infection or pulmonary, cardiac, and renal complications.[187]

Chronic Pancreatitis

Chronic pancreatitis is a process of progressive fibrotic destruction of the pancreas. Chronic alcohol abuse is the most common cause. Obstruction from gallstones, smoking, and genetic factors increase the risk of chronic pancreatitis.[188] Toxic metabolites and chronic release of inflammatory cytokines contribute to the destruction of acinar cells and islets of Langerhans. The pancreatic parenchyma is destroyed and replaced by fibrous tissues, strictures, calcification, ductal obstruction, and pancreatic cysts. The cysts are walled-off areas or pockets of pancreatic juice, necrotic debris, or blood within or adjacent to the pancreas. New imaging techniques have advanced evaluation of disease severity.[189]

Continuous or intermittent abdominal pain and weight loss are common. The pain is difficult to manage and is associated with increased intraductal pressure, ischemia, neuritis, intra-abdominal hypertension (compartment syndrome), ongoing injury, and both peripheral and central pain sensitization.[190] Manifestations of pancreatic enzyme deficiency, such as steatorrhea or a malabsorption syndrome, are present in late stages of chronic pancreatitis. To correct enzyme deficiencies and prevent malabsorption, oral enzyme replacements are taken before and during meals. Loss of islet cells can cause insulin-dependent diabetes and requires treatment. Cessation of alcohol intake is essential for the management of both acute and chronic pancreatitis. Endoscopic or surgical drainage of cysts or partial resection of the pancreas may be required to relieve pain and to prevent cystic rupture.[191] Chronic pancreatitis is a risk factor for pancreatic cancer.

CANCER OF THE DIGESTIVE SYSTEM

Cancer of the Gastrointestinal Tract

Table 36-9 contains information on the various gastrointestinal cancers by organ, percentage of death compared with all cancer deaths, risk factors, type of cell, and common manifestations. The biology of cancer is presented in Chapter 10.

Cancer of the Esophagus

Carcinoma of the esophagus is a rare type of cancer with an estimated incidence of 16,980 new cases and 15,590 deaths in the United States in 2015.[192] Risk factors are summarized in *Risk Factors:* Esophageal Cancer.

RISK FACTORS

Esophageal Cancer

- Age greater than 65 years
- Male
- Tobacco use
- Alcoholism
- Dietary factors: deficiencies of trace elements and vitamins
- Malnutrition associated with poor economic conditions or special dietary habits (e.g., very hot drinks, fish preserved in lye; diet deficient in fruits and vegetables)
- Reflux esophagitis with dysplasia
- Sliding hiatal hernia
- Obesity

TABLE 36-9   Cancer of the Gut, Liver, and Pancreas

Organ	Deaths Out of All Cancer Deaths Combined	Risks	Cell Type	Common Manifestations
Esophagus	2.5%	Malnutrition Alcohol Tobacco Chronic reflux	Squamous cell Adenocarcinoma	Chest pain Dysphagia
Stomach	1.8%	Salty food Fried red meat Nitrates-nitrosamines	Adenocarcinoma Squamous cell	Anorexia Malaise Weight loss Upper abdominal pain Vomiting Occult blood
Colorectal	8.4%	Polyps Long-term inflammatory bowel disease Diverticulitis High-refined carbohydrates; low-fiber, high-fat diets	Adenocarcinoma (left colon grows as ring; right colon grows as mass)	Pain Mass Anemia Bloody stool Obstruction Distention
Liver	4.2%	HBV, HCV, HDV Cirrhosis Intestinal parasite Aflatoxin from moldy peanuts and corn	Hepatomas Cholangiomas	Pain Anorexia Bloating Weight loss Portal hypertension Ascites Jaundice
Pancreas	6.8%	Chronic pancreatitis Cigarette smoking Alcohol (?) Diabetic women	Adenocarcinoma (exocrine part of gland, ductal epithelium)	Weight loss Weakness Nausea Vomiting Abdominal pain Depression ± jaundice May have insulin-secreting tumors with symptoms of hypoglycemia

From American Cancer Society: *Cancer facts & figures 2015*, Atlanta, 2015, Author. Available at: 5.cancer.org/research/cancerfactsstatistics/cancerfactsfigures2015/index.

PATHOPHYSIOLOGY Carcinoma of the esophagus includes squamous cell carcinoma and adenocarcinoma, which is more prevalent in the United States. Squamous cell esophageal carcinoma is more prevalent in Asia. Risk factors include chronic alcohol use combined with smoking or chewing tobacco, hot and irritant (alcohol) drinks, food containing nitrosamines, and achalasia.[193] Squamous cell carcinomas are more common in the thoracic and cervical areas of the esophagus.

Adenocarcinomas are more prevalent in males and are associated with cigarette smoking, obesity, and gastroesophageal reflux disease (GERD). Adenocarcinoma development is often secondary to infiltration by a gastric carcinoma or to the presence of Barrett dysplasia, also known as Barrett esophagus (columnar rather than squamous epithelium in the lower esophagus), and can progress to metaplasia.[194] Adenocarcinoma is more common at the gastroesophageal junction. The CagA-positive strain of *H. pylori* may be a protection against esophageal carcinoma.[195]

CLINICAL MANIFESTATIONS The two frequent symptoms of esophageal carcinoma are chest pain and dysphagia. The most common type of pain is heartburn. It is initiated by eating spicy or highly seasoned foods and by assuming the recumbent position. Odynophagia (pain on swallowing) may be initiated by the swallowing of cold liquids. Spontaneous chest pain is more difficult to diagnose positively. Some individuals with esophageal cancer complain of a constant retrosternal pain that radiates to the back. Dysphagia (difficulty swallowing) is usually pressure-like and may radiate posteriorly between the scapulae. Dysphagia usually progresses rapidly. Esophageal carcinoma is asymptomatic during the early stages and presents at an advanced stage. Esophageal cancer metastasizes rapidly and, therefore, has a poor prognosis.

EVALUATION AND TREATMENT Individuals with dysphagia undergo endoscopy so that specimens can be obtained and examined for neoplastic change. Endoscopic ultrasound and CT studies of the thorax are used for diagnosis and staging. Prevention of gastroesophageal reflux and removal of high-grade dysplasia are essential to the management of Barrett esophagus.[196] It is impossible to remove all lymph nodes with the tumor, but removal of the primary lesion and the local lymph nodes can benefit the individual with esophageal cancer. If the malignancy has not spread beyond these sites, cure is likely. If metastasis has occurred, however, an incomplete resection is of little survival benefit. Treatment is combined radiation and chemotherapy.[197,198]

Cancer of the Stomach

The incidence of gastric adenocarcinoma is estimated at 24,590 new cases and 10,720 deaths in the United States in 2015.[192] The case fatality rate is 75%.[199] The incidence is greater in males and it is more common in Asia, particularly China.[200] Loss of tumor-suppressor genes and other genetic alterations may be important in gastric cancer.[201]

PATHOPHYSIOLOGY   Gastric adenocarcinomas are associated with atrophic gastritis and *Helicobacter pylori* that carry the *CagA* gene product cytotoxin-associated vacuolating antigen A *(VacA)*. It also causes gastric B-cell mucosa-associated lymphoid tissue lymphoma. Hereditary diffuse adenocarcinoma is rare and occurs at a younger age.[202] Most adenocarcinomas are sporadic and associated with consumption of heavily salted and preserved foods (e.g., nitrates in pickled or salted foods such as bacon), low intake of fruits and vegetables, and use of tobacco and alcohol. Dietary salt enhances the conversion of nitrates to carcinogenic nitrosamines in the stomach. Salt and nitrates converted to nitrites are caustic to the stomach, delay gastric emptying, and can cause chronic atrophic gastritis. Insufficient acid secretion by the atrophic mucosa creates a relatively alkaline environment that permits bacteria to multiply and act on nitrates. The resulting increase in nitrosamines damages the deoxyribonucleic acid (DNA) of mucosal cells, further promoting metaplasia and neoplasia.

Gastric adenocarcinoma usually begins in the glands of the distal stomach mucosa. Duodenal reflux also may contribute to an intestinal-like metaplasia. The reflux contains caustic bile salts that destroy the mucosal barrier that normally protects the stomach.

CLINICAL MANIFESTATIONS   The early stages of gastric cancer are generally asymptomatic or produce vague symptoms such as loss of appetite (especially for meat), malaise, and indigestion. Later manifestations of gastric cancer include unexplained weight loss, upper abdominal pain, vomiting, change in bowel habits, and anemia caused by persistent occult bleeding. The prognosis is poor because symptoms do not occur until the tumor has spread and caused distant metastases, particularly to the liver and peritoneal structures. Generally, the first manifestations of carcinoma are caused by distant metastases, and the disease is already in an advanced stage.

EVALUATION AND TREATMENT   There are no specific biomarkers for gastric cancer. Micro RNAs are being evaluated as a specific diagnostic and prognostic marker.[203] Most symptoms suggest a problem in the upper gastrointestinal tract, and a barium x-ray film shows the lesion. Direct endoscopic visualization, lavage, and cellular examination or biopsy establish the diagnosis. Screening and treatment for *H. pylori* infection is the best preventive approach to gastric cancer. Surgery is the usual treatment for early stages of disease. Staging is determined by pathologic findings after resection. Early diagnosis and chemotherapy combined with radiation improves postsurgical outcomes.[204]

✔ **QUICK CHECK 36-8**
1. How do gallstones form?
2. Compare acute and chronic pancreatitis.
3. What factors are associated with cancer of the esophagus?
4. What dietary factors are associated with gastric cancer?

Cancer of the Colon and Rectum

Colorectal cancer (CRC) is the second most common cause of cancer and cancer death with an estimated 132,700 new cases and 49,700 deaths in the United States in 2015.[192] The incidence has been declining over the past several years because of successful screening programs. CRC tends to occur in individuals older than 50 years and is rare in children. Worldwide, the prevalence and death rate of CRC are highest in black populations, possibly because of lack of access to screening and treatment.[205] CRC occurs in women 10 years later than in men. Risk factors for CRC can be reviewed in *Risk Factors:* Cancer of the Colon and Rectum. Small intestinal carcinoma is very rare and is usually located in the duodenum.[206]

RISK FACTORS

Cancer of the Colon and Rectum

- Advanced age
- High-fat (especially egg consumption), red and processed meat, low-fiber diet
- High consumption of alcohol
- Cigarette smoking
- Obesity
- Familial polyposis or family history of colorectal cancer
- Low levels of physical activity
- Inflammatory bowel disease
- Type 2 diabetes mellitus

PATHOPHYSIOLOGY   Most CRCs are sporadic (acquired) or associated with a family history of colorectal cancer. They are caused by multiple gene alterations and environmental interactions (see Chapter 3 for epigenetics and Chapter 10 for mechanisms of oncogenesis). Familial adenomatous polyposis (FAP) is a mutation of the *APC* gene (adenomatous polyposis coli, a tumor-suppressor gene) and is the most common hereditary cause of colorectal cancer. Hereditary nonpolyposis colorectal cancer (HNPCC), or Lynch syndrome, is associated with several DNA mismatch repair (MMR). Both FAP and HNPCC have a rare, family-linked autosomal dominant inheritance trait that accounts for about 3% to 5% of colorectal cancers.[207,208] Sporadic tumors are also thought to involve the loss of function or mutation of tumor-suppressor genes (i.e., *APC, kRAS, p53* genes). CRC begins with the formation of an adenoma and is termed "tumor initiation." The progression to carcinoma is termed "tumor progression" and is a multistep process of genetic mutations that may take 8 to 10 years.

Colorectal polyps are closely associated with development of cancer. A polyp, or papilloma, is a projection arising from the mucosal epithelium. The most common types of polyps are hyperplastic (a nonneoplastic, or benign, polyp). Adenomatous polyps are neoplastic. They can be pedunculated (have a stalk) or sessile (flat with no stalk). Neoplastic polyps are premalignant lesions and are further classified as tubular (the most prevalent), villous (usually sessile), or tubulovillous adenomas (Figure 36-18). Serrated sessile polyps have a sawtooth appearance and can be difficult to detect. Serrated sessile polyps are associated with oncogene mutations and should be removed.[209] The larger the polyp, the greater the risk of colorectal cancer. Although lesions larger than 1.5 cm occur less often, they are more likely to be malignant than those smaller than 1.0 cm. Thus, screening colonoscopy with polypectomy is performed when polyps are found.

Adenocarcinomas of the colon and rectum usually arise from adenomatous polyps and undergo a multistep cascade of genetic events that leads to carcinoma and metastasis[210] (see Figure 10-6). Most colorectal cancers are moderately differentiated adenocarcinomas. These tumors have a long preinvasive phase and when they invade, they tend to grow slowly. Colorectal carcinoma begins from epithelial stem cells located in the glands at the base of the intestinal crypts. Because

FIGURE 36-18 Neoplastic Polyps. A, Tubular adenomata *(A)* are rounded lesions 0.5 to 2 cm in size that are generally red and sit on a stalk *(S)* of normal mucosa that has been dragged up by traction of the polyp in the bowel lumen. **B,** Villous adenomata are velvety lesions about 0.6 cm thick that occupy a broad area of mucosa generally 1 to 5 cm in diameter. (From Stevens A et al: *Core pathology,* ed 3, London, 2009, Mosby.)

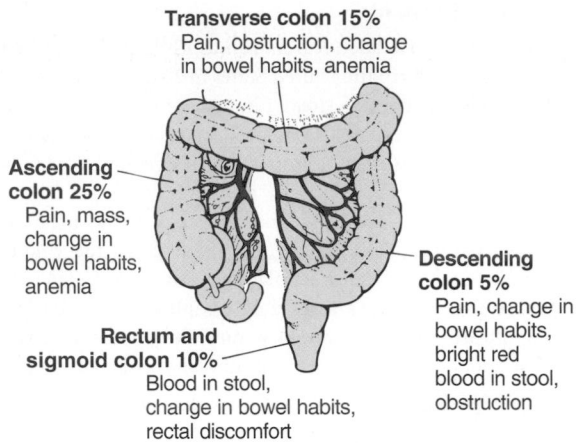

FIGURE 36-19 Signs and Symptoms of Colorectal Cancer by Location of Primary Lesion. Clinical manifestations are listed in order of frequency for each region (lymphatics of colon also shown).

the lymphatic channels are located under the muscularis mucosae, the lesions must traverse this layer before the multistep process of metastasis can occur. Once the malignant cells of an adenoma traverse the muscularis mucosae, tumor cells enter the bloodstream and lymphatics and become invasive, spreading to other organs. Adenomas can be detected early, however, because the submucosa may not be penetrated for several years.

CLINICAL MANIFESTATIONS Symptoms of colorectal cancer depend on the location, size, and shape of the lesion and are silent in the early stages (Figure 36-19). Tumors of the right (ascending) colon and left (descending) colon evolve into two distinct tumor types.[211] On the right side (proximal colon), the lesions are polypoid and extend along one wall of the cecum and ascending colon. These tumors may be silent, evolving to pain, palpable mass in the lower right quadrant, anemia, fatigue, and dark red or mahogany-colored blood mixed with the stool. These tumors can become large and bulky with necrosis and ulceration, contributing to persistent blood loss and anemia. Obstruction is unusual because the growth does not readily encircle the colon. These tumors are more common in women.

Tumors of the left, or descending, colon (distal colon) start as small, elevated, button-like masses. This type grows circumferentially, encircling the entire bowel wall, and eventually ulcerating in the middle as the tumor penetrates the blood supply. Obstruction is common but occurs slowly and stools become narrow and pencil shaped. Manifestations include progressive abdominal distention, pain, vomiting, constipation, need for laxatives, cramps, and bright red blood on the surface of the stool. These tumors are more common in men.

Systematic lymphatic distribution occurs along the aorta to the mesenteric and pancreatic lymph nodes. Liver metastasis is common and follows invasion of the mesenteric veins (left colon) or superior veins (right colon), which drain into the portal circulation.

Rectal carcinomas (about 30% of colorectal carcinomas) are defined as tumors occurring up to 15 cm from the anal opening. Tumors of the rectum can spread through the rectal wall to nearby structures: the prostate in men and the vagina in women. Penetration occurs more readily in the lower third of the rectum because it has no serosal covering. Systemic and pulmonary metastases occur through the hemorrhoidal plexus, which drains into the vena cava.

EVALUATION AND TREATMENT Individuals with hereditary polyposis should begin screening at an early age (10 to 12 years) using colonoscopy with removal of polyps when they are found. Specific, sensitive, and affordable molecular markers are being evaluated to assist with early diagnosis and evaluation of therapy. Carcinoembryonic antigen (CEA) is evaluated during and after cancer treatment. Screening procedures for detection of nonhereditary CRC are summarized in Box 36-4. Aspirin and celecoxib may reduce the incidence of CRC in the general population, but risk of GI bleeding must be considered. Vitamin D, calcium, fiber, folate, dietary modification, weight control, exercise, and other nondietary lifestyle changes can decrease the risk of colorectal cancer.[212]

The staging of colorectal cancer involves imaging and operative exploration.[213] Physical examination of the abdomen detects liver enlargement and ascites; appropriate lymph nodes are palpated. Imaging is useful for pretreatment staging.[213] Operative staging consists of careful exploration during surgery and biopsy of possible metastases. The National Cancer Institute[214] TNM classification is widely used for staging of colorectal cancer (available at: www.cancer.gov/cancertopics/pdq/treatment/colon/HealthProfessional; also see Chapter 10).

Treatment for all stages of cancer of the colon is surgical. Chemotherapy and radiation therapy may be given before surgery in the hope that they will shrink the tumor or alter the malignant cells, or both, so that these cells will not survive after surgery. Resection and anastomosis can be performed for cancer of the ascending, transverse, descending, or sigmoid colon and upper rectum. These surgeries are performed through abdominal incisions and assisted with radiofrequency ablation. Natural defecation is preserved. Growths in the lower portion of

BOX 36-4   Screening for Colorectal Cancer

Beginning at age 50, both men and women should follow one of these testing schedules:

Tests That Find Polyps and Cancer
Flexible sigmoidoscopy every 5 years,* *or*
Colonoscopy every 10 years, *or*
Double-contrast barium enema every 5 years,* *or*
CT colonography (virtual colonoscopy) every 5 years*

Tests That Primarily Find Cancer
Yearly fecal occult blood test (gFOBT),[†] *or*
Yearly fecal immunochemical test (FIT),[†] *or*
Stool DNA or RNA tests (sDNA, sRNA), interval uncertain[†]

Data from American Cancer Society: Screening guidelines for early detection of cancer in average risk asymptomatic people. In *Cancer facts & figures 2015*, p. 52, Atlanta, Ga, 2015. Available at: www.cancer.org/research/cancerfactsstatistics/cancerfactsfigures2015/index; Koga Y et al: *Expert Rev Mol Diagn* 14(1):107-120, 2014.
*All positive tests should be followed up with colonoscopy.
[†]The multiple stool take-home test should be used.

the rectum require removal of the entire rectum with the formation of a permanent colostomy. Chemotherapy, including immunotherapy, is used to treat metastatic disease and cases with a high risk of recurrence. New chemotherapeutic agents are improving personalized, first-line therapy. Immunotherapy, vaccines, and viral vectors for the treatment of colon cancer are under continuing investigation.[215,216] Resection of liver metastases or hepatic intra-arterial chemotherapy may prolong survival.[217,218]

Cancer of the Accessory Organs of Digestion
Cancer of the Liver

Cancer of the liver is a leading cause of cancer death worldwide and is highest in Eastern and Southeastern Asia.[219] The estimated number of new cases is 35,660 with 24,550 deaths in the United States in 2015.[192] In the United States, the incidence of primary liver cancer is higher in blacks than in whites and higher in males than in females. Primary liver cancer is rare before the age of 40 years and is most common after 60 years. Cancer in the liver is usually caused by metastatic spread from a primary site elsewhere in the body.[220] Risk factors for primary liver cancer are summarized in *Risk Factors: Primary Liver Cancer*. Risks associated with HBV and HCV are decreasing with antiviral therapy.[192]

RISK FACTORS
Primary Liver Cancer

- Exposure to mycotoxins (aflatoxins), particularly those produced by *Aspergillus flavus,* a mold found on spoiled corn, peanuts, and grain
- Alcohol abuse
- Obesity
- Chronic liver disease, especially cirrhosis
- Infection with hepatitis B virus (HBV), hepatitis C virus (HCV), and hepatitis D virus (HDV), particularly in conjunction with cirrhosis; these infections act either as carcinogens or as co-carcinogens in chronically infected hepatocytes

PATHOPHYSIOLOGY   Primary carcinomas of the liver are hepatocellular or cholangiocellular. **Hepatocellular carcinoma (HCC)** develops in the hepatocytes and can be nodular (consisting of multiple, discrete nodules), massive (consisting of a large tumor mass having satellite nodules), or diffuse (consisting of small nodules distributed throughout most of the liver). It is closely associated with chronic hepatitis and cirrhosis. Because carcinoma of the liver invades the hepatic and portal veins, it often spreads to the heart and lungs. Other sites of metastases are the brain, kidney, and spleen.

Cholangiocellular carcinoma (cholangiocarcinoma) is rare (less than 1% of liver cancers) and develops in the bile ducts; in the United States, it occurs less often than hepatocellular carcinoma.[221] It is associated with primary sclerosing cholangitis (a rare autoimmune disease often associated with ulcerative colitis) and is geographically associated with areas where liver fluke infestation is prevalent, such as Southeast Asia. Cholangiocellular carcinoma can occur anywhere along the bile duct and extend directly into the liver, usually as a solitary lesion. A combined form of HCC is known as combined (mixed) hepatocellular-cholangiocellular carcinoma. It is difficult to distinguish an invasion of cholangiocellular carcinoma from a metastatic adenocarcinoma except by neoplastic changes found in nearby ducts.

CLINICAL MANIFESTATIONS   HCC is usually asymptomatic. Manifestations can develop slowly or abruptly and include vague abdominal symptoms, such as nausea and vomiting, fullness, pressure, and dull ache in the right hypochondrium. In individuals with cirrhosis, deepening jaundice or abrupt lack of appetite is a sign of hepatocellular carcinoma. Obstruction by the tumor can cause sudden worsening of portal hypertension and development of ascites. As the tumor enlarges, it causes pain. Cholangiocellular carcinoma more commonly presents insidiously as pain, loss of appetite, weight loss, and gradual onset of jaundice. Some carcinomas of the liver rupture spontaneously, causing hemorrhage. Others are discovered accidentally during laboratory evaluation, imaging, or surgery for other diseases or trauma.

EVALUATION AND TREATMENT   There is no specific test for the diagnosis of liver cancer. Biopsy is not recommended because of the risk for tumor seeding. For high-risk individuals, alpha fetoprotein associated with HBV and abdominal ultrasound are common screening tools. Diagnosis is based on clinical manifestations, laboratory findings, imaging, and exploratory laparotomy. In individuals without cirrhosis, liver scans can document filling defects. CT or ultrasonography is used to detect solid tumors, but neither can distinguish benign from malignant tumors. Primary prevention may be achieved by vaccinating against HBV, preventing and treating HBV and HCV, screening all donated blood for the presence of HBV, and reducing contamination of food with aflatoxins.[222]

Surgical resection is possible only if the tumor is localized to a removable lobe of the liver. Surgery is hazardous and usually not undertaken if the individual has cirrhosis. Radiofrequency (thermal) ablation has emerged as the most effective method for local tumor destruction. Most individuals develop metastases after surgical resection, but long-term survival is possible. Chemotherapeutic agents, immunotherapy, and radiotherapy are treatment options.[223] Liver transplant offers a cure if the waiting time is short. The prognosis for those with symptomatic liver cancer is poor.[224]

Cancer of the Gallbladder

In 2015 in the United States, there were an estimated 10,910 new cases and 3700 deaths attributable to gallbladder cancer.[192] Risk factors include gallstones, advancing age, female gender (2:1), anomalous pancreaticobiliary ductal junction, and obesity. It occurs rarely before the age of 40 years and is most common between the ages of 50 and 60 years. Primary carcinoma of the gallbladder is rare and associated with larger gallstones. Most gallbladder cancer is caused by metastasis.

PATHOPHYSIOLOGY Most primary carcinomas of the gallbladder are adenocarcinomas, and more rarely squamous cell carcinomas. The pathogenesis is not clear. Chronic inflammation may trigger dysplasia and progression to metaplasia. The molecular mechanisms involve mutation of several genes, including tumor-suppressor genes and oncogenes, and alterations in the extracellular matrix.[225] Invasion of the liver and lymph nodes occurs early. Direct invasion of the stomach and the duodenum can cause pyloric obstruction. Infection often accompanies cancer of the gallbladder. Generalized peritonitis, gangrene, perforation, and liver abscesses are potential complications of infection.

CLINICAL MANIFESTATIONS Early stages of gallbladder carcinoma are asymptomatic and the disease usually presents at an advanced stage. When symptoms develop, there is usually steady, upper right quadrant pain for about 2 months. Other manifestations include diarrhea, belching, weakness, loss of appetite, weight loss, and vomiting. Obstructive jaundice can occur if an enlarging tumor presses on the extrahepatic ducts.

EVALUATION AND TREATMENT Early diagnosis of cancer of the gallbladder is rare and is often found incidentally. Therefore, older adults with gallstones, particularly women, are evaluated for disease. Inflammatory disorders, such as cholangitis (bile duct inflammation) and peritonitis, often obscure an underlying malignancy. Diagnostic procedures include ultrasonography and further imaging with suspicious findings.[226] Complete surgical resection of the gallbladder is the only effective treatment for early stages of disease, and recurrence is common. Complete removal of tumor tissue and lymph nodes with chemoradiation therapy is performed for more advanced stages. Because advanced malignancies cannot be resected, gallbladders containing stones are removed as a preventive measure. The prognosis of unresectable gallbladder cancer is extremely poor. Molecular therapies are under development.[227]

Cancer of the Pancreas

Pancreatic cancer is the fourth leading cause of cancer deaths in the United States. An estimated 48,960 new cases and 40,560 deaths occurred in the United States in 2015.[192] The incidence of pancreatic cancer rises steadily with age. Males are affected slightly more often than females, and blacks more often than whites. Mortality is nearly 100%. The cause of pancreatic cancer is not known, but there are modest risks associated with tobacco smoking, certain dietary factors (e.g., high-fat foods and processed meat), obesity, diabetes mellitus, chronic pancreatitis, family history of pancreatic cancer, hereditary nonpolyposis colon cancer (HNPCC) (Lynch syndrome), and *BRCA1* and *BRCA2* mutations.[192]

PATHOPHYSIOLOGY Pancreatic cancer can arise from exocrine or endocrine cells. Most pancreatic tumors arise from metaplastic exocrine cells in the ducts and are called *ductal adenocarcinomas*. Chronic pancreatitis and inflammatory cytokines support tumor growth.[228] There is significant expansion of the extracellular matrix (stroma) from activation of pancreatic stellate cells, a type of fibroblast in the pancreas, that contributes to therapeutic resistance.[229] Tumors arising in small ducts invade nearby glandular tissue, penetrate the covering of the pancreas, and extend into surrounding tissues.[230] Tumors of the head of the pancreas quickly spread to obstruct the common bile duct and portal vein. These tumors can then infiltrate the superior mesenteric artery, the vena cava, and the aorta and form emboli. Tumors of the body and tail of the pancreas infiltrate the posterior abdominal wall. Lymphatic invasion occurs early and rapidly. Venous invasion causes metastases to the liver. Tumor implants on the peritoneal surface can obstruct veins and promote development of ascites.

CLINICAL MANIFESTATIONS Early stages of pancreatic cancer are asymptomatic. When symptoms occur there usually has been a malignant transformation. Typically, vague upper abdominal pain that radiates to the back develops. Jaundice arises in most cases, usually caused by obstruction of the bile duct. Because obstruction impairs enzyme secretion and flow to the duodenum, pancreatic cancer causes fat and protein malabsorption, resulting in weight loss. Distant metastases are found in the cervical lymph nodes, the lungs, and the brain. Most individuals die of hepatic failure, malnutrition, or systemic diseases.

EVALUATION AND TREATMENT There is no specific biomarker for pancreatic cancer and the diagnosis is usually made after the tumor has spread. Several molecular markers are under investigation.[231] Endoscopic ultrasound and CT are used initially for diagnosis.[231] Laparotomy is often used to establish a definitive diagnosis, evaluate the extent of disease, and determine whether palliative bypass surgery (i.e., cholecystojejunostomy and gastrojejunostomy) is needed. Many surgeons recommend a total pancreatectomy because cancer of the pancreas seldom consists of a single lesion. Adjuvant chemotherapy, immunotherapy, radiochemotherapy, and combination therapy may produce favorable controls in locally advanced cancer.[232] Pain management includes opioids and celiac plexus nerve block. Supportive therapy involves an interdisciplinary team.[233] Five-year survival is about 20% with resectable disease (a small subset) and less than 6% for metastatic disease. There is a need for new approaches for earlier diagnosis and more effective treatment.

> ✔ **QUICK CHECK 36-9**
> 1. What are the primary risk factors for colorectal carcinoma?
> 2. Compare tumors of the right colon with those of the left colon.
> 3. What is the most common cause of liver cancer?

■ DID YOU UNDERSTAND?

Disorders of the Gastrointestinal Tract

1. Anorexia is lack of a desire to eat despite physiologic stimuli that would normally produce hunger.
2. Vomiting is the forceful emptying of the stomach effected by gastrointestinal contraction and reverse peristalsis of the esophagus. It is usually preceded by nausea and retching, with the exception of projectile vomiting, which is associated with direct stimulation of the vomiting center in the brain.
3. Constipation is difficult or infrequent defecation often caused by unhealthy dietary and bowel habits combined with lack of exercise. Constipation can result from a disorder that impairs intestinal motility or obstructs the intestinal lumen.

4. Diarrhea is the presence of frequent loose, watery stools and can be caused by excessive fluid drawn into the intestinal lumen by osmosis (osmotic diarrhea), excessive secretion of fluids by the intestinal mucosa (secretory or infectious diarrhea), or excessive gastrointestinal motility (motility diarrhea).

5. Abdominal pain is caused by stretching, inflammation, or ischemia (insufficient blood supply). Abdominal pain originates in the organs themselves (visceral pain) or in the peritoneum (parietal pain) and can be acute or chronic. Visceral pain is often referred to the back.

6. Obvious manifestations of gastrointestinal bleeding are hematemesis (vomiting of blood), melena (dark, tarry stools), and hematochezia (frank bleeding from the rectum). Occult bleeding can be detected only by testing stools or vomitus for the presence of blood.

7. Dysphagia is difficulty swallowing. It can be caused by a mechanical or functional obstruction of the esophagus. Functional obstruction is an impairment of esophageal motility.

8. Achalasia is a form of functional dysphagia caused by loss of esophageal innervation.

9. Gastroesophageal reflux disease is the regurgitation of chyme from the stomach into the esophagus, resulting in an inflammatory response (reflux esophagitis) when the esophageal mucosa is repeatedly exposed to acids and enzymes in the regurgitated chyme.

10. Hiatal hernia is the protrusion of the upper part of the stomach through the hiatus (esophageal opening in the diaphragm) at the gastroesophageal junction. Hiatal hernia can be sliding or paraesophageal.

11. Gastroparesis is delayed gastric emptying in the absence of mechanical gastric outlet obstruction.

12. Pyloric obstruction is the narrowing or blockage of the pylorus, which is the opening between the stomach and the duodenum. It can be caused by a congenital defect, inflammation and scarring secondary to a gastric ulcer, or tumor growth.

13. Intestinal obstruction prevents the normal movement of chyme through the intestinal tract. It can be mechanical (i.e., caused by torsion, herniation, or tumor) or functional as a result of paralytic ileus.

14. The most severe consequences of intestinal obstruction are fluid and electrolyte losses, hypovolemia, shock, intestinal necrosis, and perforation of the intestinal wall.

15. Gastritis is an acute or chronic inflammation of the gastric mucosa.

16. Regurgitation of bile, use of anti-inflammatory drugs or alcohol, *Helicobacter pylori* infection, and some systemic diseases are associated with gastritis.

17. Chronic gastritis of the fundus (immune) and antrum (nonimmune) is the most severe form of gastritis. It can result in gastric atrophy and decreased secretion of hydrochloric acid, pepsinogen, and intrinsic factor.

18. Chronic gastritis of the antrum, the most common type, is not usually associated with impaired secretion or gastric atrophy.

19. A peptic ulcer is a circumscribed area of mucosal inflammation and ulceration caused by excessive secretion of gastric acid, disruption of the protective mucosal barrier, or infection with *Helicobacter pylori*.

20. Zollinger-Ellison syndrome is a rare syndrome associated with peptic ulcers caused by a gastrin-secreting neuroendocrine tumor or multiple tumors (gastrinoma) of the pancreas or duodenum.

21. There are three types of peptic ulcers: duodenal, gastric, and stress ulcers.

22. Duodenal ulcers, the most common peptic ulcers, are associated with *H. pylori* infection, chronic use of NSAIDs, increased numbers of parietal (acid-secreting) cells in the stomach, elevated gastrin levels, and rapid gastric emptying. Pain occurs when the stomach is empty, and it is relieved with food or antacids. Duodenal ulcers tend to heal spontaneously and recur frequently.

23. Gastric ulcers develop near parietal cells, generally in the antrum, and tend to become chronic. Gastric secretions may be normal or decreased, and pain may occur after eating.

24. Stress ulcers develop suddenly after severe illness, systemic trauma, or neural injury. Ulceration follows mucosal damage caused by ischemia (decreased blood flow to the gastric mucosa).

25. Cushing ulcer is a stress ulcer caused by head trauma. Ulceration follows hypersecretion of hydrochloric acid caused by overstimulation of the vagal nuclei.

26. Curling ulcer is associated with burn trauma.

27. Postgastrectomy syndromes are long-term complications that follow gastrectomy—the resection of all or part of the stomach. The postgastrectomy syndromes include dumping syndrome, alkaline reflux gastritis, afferent loop obstruction, diarrhea, weight loss, and anemia.

28. Dumping syndrome is the rapid emptying of chyme into the small intestine. It causes an osmotic shift of fluid from the vascular compartment to the intestinal lumen, which decreases plasma volume.

29. Alkaline reflux gastritis is stomach inflammation caused by the reflux of bile and pancreatic secretions from the duodenum into the stomach. These substances disrupt the mucosal barrier and cause inflammation.

30. Afferent loop obstruction is an obstruction of the duodenal stump on the proximal side of a gastrojejunostomy. Biliary and pancreatic secretions accumulate in the stump, causing distention, intermittent pain, and vomiting.

31. Malabsorption syndromes result in impaired digestion or absorption of nutrients and usually cause diarrhea.

32. Pancreatic exocrine insufficiency causes malabsorption associated with impaired digestion. The pancreas does not produce sufficient amounts of the enzymes that digest protein, carbohydrates, and fats into components that can be absorbed by the intestine.

33. Deficient lactase production in the brush border of the small intestine inhibits the breakdown of lactose. This prevents lactose absorption and causes osmotic diarrhea.

34. Bile salt deficiency causes fat malabsorption and steatorrhea (fatty stools). Bile salt deficiency can result from inadequate secretion of bile, excessive bacterial deconjugation of bile, or impaired reabsorption of bile salts caused by ileal disease.

35. Ulcerative colitis is a chronic inflammatory bowel disease that causes ulceration, abscess formation, and necrosis of the colonic and rectal mucosa. Cramping pain, bleeding, frequent diarrhea, dehydration, and weight loss accompany severe forms of the disease. A course of frequent remissions and exacerbations is common.

36. Crohn disease is similar to ulcerative colitis but it affects the GI tract from the mouth to the anus and tends to involve all the layers of the intestinal lumen. "Skip lesion" fissures and granulomata are characteristic of Crohn disease. Abdominal tenderness, diarrhea, and weight loss are the usual symptoms.

37. Microscopic colitis is an inflammation that involves either mucosal lymphocytic infiltration or a thickened subepithelial collagen layer with symptoms of watery diarrhea.

38. Irritable bowel syndrome (IBS) is described as a functional disorder with recurring abdominal pain and bloating. IBS can be

diarrhea prevalent or constipation prevalent or may alternate between diarrhea and constipation. Alterations in the brain-gut axis, gut microflora, gut immune responses, gut neuroendocrine cell function, genetic susceptibility, and epigenetic factors contribute to intestinal hypersensitivity, intestinal inflammation, increased permeability, and symptoms caused by alterations in motility and secretion.

39. Diverticula are outpouchings of colonic mucosa through the muscle layers of the colon wall. Diverticulosis is the presence of these outpouchings; diverticulitis is inflammation of the diverticula.

40. Appendicitis is the most common surgical emergency of the abdomen. Obstruction of the lumen leads to increased pressure, ischemia, and inflammation of the appendix. Without surgical resection, inflammation may progress to gangrene, perforation, and peritonitis.

41. Vascular insufficiency in the intestine is most often associated with occlusion or obstruction of the mesenteric vessels or insufficient intestinal arterial blood flow. The resulting ischemia and necrosis produce abdominal pain, fever, bloody diarrhea, hypovolemia, and shock.

42. Obesity is a metabolic disorder with an increase in body fat mass and a BMI greater than 30.

43. The causes of obesity are complex and involve the interaction of adipokines produced by fat cells and other body weight control signals at the level of the hypothalamus. Metabolic dysregulation includes leptin resistance, insulin resistance, and a proinflammatory state that contribute to the complications of obesity.

44. Visceral obesity and normal weight obesity increase the risk of developing systemic inflammation, dyslipidemia, and insulin resistance with predisposition to atherosclerosis, hypertension, cardiovascular disease, cancer, and type 2 diabetes mellitus. Metabolically healthy obesity delays obesity-related complications until an older age.

45. Malnutrition is lack of nourishment from inadequate amounts of calories, protein, vitamins, or minerals. Starvation is an extreme state of malnutrition. Cachexia is physical wasting associated with chronic disease.

46. Short-term starvation, or lack of dietary intake for 3 or 4 days, stimulates mobilization of stored glucose by two metabolic processes: glycogenolysis (splitting of glycogen into glucose) and gluconeogenesis (formation of glucose from noncarbohydrate molecules).

47. Long-term starvation triggers the breakdown of ketone bodies and fatty acids. Eventually proteolysis (protein breakdown) begins, and death ensues if nutrition is not restored.

Disorders of the Accessory Organs of Digestion

1. Portal hypertension, ascites, hepatic encephalopathy, jaundice, and hepatorenal syndrome are complications of many liver disorders.

2. Portal hypertension is an elevation of portal venous pressure to at least 10 mm Hg. It is caused by increased resistance to venous flow in the portal vein and its tributaries, including the sinusoids and hepatic vein.

3. Portal hypertension is the most serious complication of liver disease because it can cause potentially fatal complications, such as bleeding varices, ascites, and hepatic encephalopathy.

4. Varices (esophageal, gastric, hemorrhoidal) are distended, tortuous, collateral veins resulting from prolonged elevation of pressure in the portal vein.

5. Splenomegaly is enlargement of the spleen caused by increased pressure in the splenic vein, which branches from the portal vein.

6. Hepatopulmonary syndrome and portopulmonary hypertension are complications of portal hypertension caused by release of nitric oxide and carbon monoxide in the presence of liver injury.

7. Ascites is the accumulation and sequestration of fluid in the peritoneal cavity, often as a result of portal hypertension and decreased concentrations of plasma proteins.

8. Hepatic encephalopathy (portal-systemic encephalopathy) is impaired cerebral function caused by blood-borne toxins (particularly ammonia) not metabolized by the liver. Toxin-bearing blood may bypass the liver in collateral vessels opened as a result of portal hypertension, or diseased hepatocytes may be unable to carry out their metabolic functions.

9. Manifestations of hepatic encephalopathy range from confusion and asterixis (flapping tremor of the hands) to loss of consciousness, coma, and death.

10. Jaundice (icterus) is a yellow or greenish pigmentation of the skin or sclera of the eyes caused by increases in plasma bilirubin concentration (hyperbilirubinemia).

11. Obstructive jaundice is caused by obstructed bile canaliculi (intrahepatic obstructive jaundice) or obstructed bile ducts outside the liver (extrahepatic obstructive jaundice). Bilirubin accumulates proximal to the sites of obstruction, enters the bloodstream, and is carried to the skin and deposited.

12. Hemolytic jaundice is caused by destruction of red blood cells at a rate that exceeds the liver's ability to metabolize unconjugated bilirubin.

13. Hepatorenal syndrome is functional kidney failure caused by advanced liver disease, particularly cirrhosis with portal hypertension. Renal failure is caused by a sudden decrease in blood flow to the kidneys usually caused by massive gastrointestinal hemorrhage, liver failure, or inadequate circulating blood volume associated with ascites. The chief clinical manifestation is oliguria.

14. Acute liver failure is severe impairment or necrosis of liver cells with or without preexisting liver disease or cirrhosis. It is commonly associated with acetaminophen overdose or as a complication of viral hepatitis.

15. Cirrhosis is an inflammatory disease of the liver that causes disorganization of lobular structure, fibrosis, and nodular regeneration. Cirrhosis can result from hepatitis or exposure to toxins, such as acetaldehyde (a product of alcohol metabolism). The disease causes progressive irreversible liver damage, usually over a period of years.

16. Alcoholic liver disease includes fatty liver and alcoholic steatohepatitis from accumulations of fat in the liver and is a precursor to alcoholic cirrhosis.

17. Alcoholic cirrhosis impairs the hepatocytes' ability to oxidize fatty acids, synthesize enzymes and proteins, degrade hormones, and clear portal blood of ammonia and toxins. The inflammatory response includes excessive collagen formation, fibrosis, and scarring, which obstruct bile canaliculi and sinusoids. Bile obstruction causes jaundice. Vascular obstruction causes portal hypertension, shunting, and varices.

18. Nonalcoholic fatty liver disease and nonalcoholic steatohepatitis involve accumulation of fat in the liver not associated with alcohol intake and are commonly associated with obesity.

19. Primary biliary cirrhosis is an autoimmune inflammatory destruction of intrahepatic bile ducts. Its cause is unknown.

20. Secondary biliary cirrhosis develops from prolonged obstruction of bile flow with increased pressure in the hepatic bile ducts that causes pooling of bile and necrosis of tissue. Relief of obstruction

allays symptoms of jaundice and pruritus. Continued obstruction causes cirrhosis and liver failure.

21. Viral hepatitis is an infection of the liver caused by a strain of the hepatitis virus (i.e., hepatitis A virus [HAV], hepatitis B virus [HBV], hepatitis C virus [HCV], hepatitis E virus [HEV], and HBV transmitted with HBV). Although they differ with respect to modes of transmission and severity of acute illness, all can cause hepatic cell necrosis, Kupffer cell hyperplasia, and infiltration of liver tissue by mononuclear phagocytes. These changes obstruct bile flow and impair hepatocyte function.

22. The clinical manifestations of viral hepatitis depend on the stage of infection. Fever, malaise, anorexia, and liver enlargement and tenderness characterize the prodromal phase (stage 1). Jaundice and hyperbilirubinemia mark the icteric phase (stage 2). During the recovery phase (stage 3), symptoms resolve. Recovery takes several weeks.

23. Cholelithiasis (the formation of gallstones) is a common disorder of the gallbladder. Gallstones form in the bile as a result of the aggregation of cholesterol crystals (cholesterol stones) or precipitates of unconjugated bilirubin (pigmented stones). Gallstones that fill the gallbladder or obstruct the cystic or common bile duct cause abdominal pain and jaundice.

24. Cholecystitis is an acute or chronic inflammation of the gallbladder usually associated with obstruction of the cystic duct by gallstones.

25. Acute pancreatitis (pancreatic inflammation) is a serious but relatively rare disorder. Pancreatic duct obstruction and injury permits leakage of digestive enzymes into pancreatic tissue, where they become activated and begin the process of autodigestion, inflammation, and destruction of tissues. Release of pancreatic enzymes into the bloodstream or abdominal cavity causes damage to other organs.

26. Chronic pancreatitis results from structural or functional impairment of the pancreas. It causes recurrent abdominal pain and digestive disorders.

Cancer of the Digestive System

1. Cancer of the esophagus is rare and tends to occur in people older than 60 years of age. Alcohol and tobacco use, reflux esophagitis, and nutritional deficiencies are associated with esophageal carcinoma.

2. Dysphagia and chest pain are the primary manifestations of esophageal cancer. Early treatment of tumors that have not spread into the mediastinum or lymph nodes results in a good prognosis.

3. Gastric adenocarcinoma is associated with *Helicobacter pylori* that carries the *CagA* gene product cytotoxin-associated vacuolating antigen A, a diet high in salt and food preservatives (nitrates, nitrites), and atrophic gastritis.

4. Approximately 50% of all gastric cancers are located in the prepyloric antrum. Clinical manifestations (weight loss, upper abdominal pain, vomiting, hematemesis, anemia) develop only after the tumor has penetrated the wall of the stomach.

5. Cancer of the colon and rectum (colorectal cancer) is the third most common cause of cancer death in the United States. Preexisting polyps are highly associated with adenocarcinoma of the colon. Familial adenomatous polyposis accounts for about 3% to 5% of colorectal cancer cases.

6. Tumors of the right (ascending or proximal) colon are usually large and bulky; tumors of the left (descending, sigmoid or distal) colon develop as small, button-like masses. Manifestations of colon tumors include pain, bloody stools, and a change in bowel habits.

7. Rectal carcinoma is located up to 15 cm from the opening of the anus. The tumor spreads transmurally to the vagina in women or the prostate in men.

8. Metastatic invasion of the liver is more common than primary cancer of the liver.

9. Primary liver cancers are associated with chronic liver disease (cirrhosis, hepatitis B). Hepatocellular carcinomas arise from the hepatocytes, whereas cholangiocellular carcinomas arise from the bile ducts. Primary liver cancer spreads to the heart, lungs, brain, kidney, and spleen through the circulation.

10. Cancer of the gallbladder is relatively rare and tends to occur in women older than 50 years. Adenocarcinoma is most common. Because clinical manifestations occur late in the disease, metastases to lymph channels have usually occurred by the time of diagnosis and the prognosis is poor.

11. Cancer of the pancreas is the fourth cause of cancer deaths. Most tumors are adenocarcinomas that arise in the exocrine cells of ducts in the head, body, or tail of the pancreas. Symptoms may not be evident until the tumor has spread to surrounding tissues. Treatment is palliative, and mortality is nearly 100% at 5 years.

KEY TERMS

Achalasia, 909
Acute colonic pseudo-obstruction, 913
Acute gastritis, 914
Acute liver failure (fulminant liver failure), 931
Acute pancreatitis, 936
Adiponectin, 925
Afferent loop obstruction, 918
Alcoholic cirrhosis, 932
Alcoholic fatty liver (steatosis), 932
Alcoholic steatohepatitis (alcoholic hepatitis), 932
Alkaline reflux gastritis, 918
Anemia, 919
Anorexia, 906

Appendicitis, 923
Ascites, 928
Barrett esophagus, 938
Biliary cirrhosis, 933
Bone and mineral disorder, 919
Cachexia, 927
Cholangiocellular carcinoma (cholangiocarcinoma), 941
Cholecystitis, 935
Cholelithiasis, 935
Chronic active hepatitis, 935
Chronic gastritis, 914
Chronic pancreatitis, 937
Cirrhosis, 931
Colorectal polyp, 939
Constipation, 907
Crohn disease (CD), 921

Curling ulcer, 918
Cushing ulcer, 918
Diarrhea, 907
Diverticula, 922
Diverticulitis, 922
Diverticulosis, 922
Dumping syndrome, 918
Duodenal ulcer, 916
Dysphagia, 909
Esophageal varices, 927
Familial adenomatous polyposis (FAP), 939
Gallstone, 935
Gastric ulcer, 917
Gastritis, 914
Gastroesophageal reflux disease (GERD), 911

Gastroparesis, 912
Ghrelin, 925
Gluconeogenesis, 927
Glycogenolysis, 927
Hematochezia, 909
Hemolytic jaundice, 930
Hepatic encephalopathy, 928
Hepatocellular carcinoma (HCC), 941
Hepatopulmonary syndrome, 927
Hepatorenal syndrome, 930
Hereditary nonpolyposis colorectal cancer (HNPCC: Lynch syndrome), 939
Hiatal hernia, 911

REFERENCES

1. Babic T, Browning KN: The role of vagal neurocircuits in the regulation of nausea and vomiting, *Eur J Pharmacol* 722:38-47, 2014.
2. Costilla VC, Foxx-Orenstein AE: Constipation: understanding mechanisms and management, *Clin Geriatr Med* 30(1):107-115, 2014.
3. Lacy BE et al: Chronic constipation: new diagnostic and treatment approaches, *Therap Adv Gastroenterol* 5(4):233-247, 2012.
4. Costilla VC, Foxx-Orenstein AE: Constipation in adults: diagnosis and management, *Curr Treat Options Gastroenterol* 12(3):310-321, 2014.
5. Guerrant RL et al: Practice guidelines for the management of infectious diarrhea, *Clin Infect Dis* 32(3):331-351, 2001.
6. World Gastroenterology Organisation: *Acute diarrhea in adults and children: a global perspective.* Available at: www .worldgastroenterology.org/assets/export/userfiles/ Acute%20Diarrhea_long_FINAL_120604.pdf. Accessed June, 2015
7. Dickinson B, Surawicz CM: Infectious diarrhea: an overview, *Curr Gastroenterol Rep* 16(8):399, 2014.
8. Schiller LR: Definitions, pathophysiology, and evaluation of chronic diarrhea, *Best Pract Res Clin Gastroenterol* 26(5):551-562, 2012.
9. Juckett G, Trivedi R: Evaluation of chronic diarrhea, *Am Fam Physician* 84(10):1119-1126, 2011.
10. Millham FH: Chapter 11: Acute abdominal pain. In Feldman M et al, editors: *Sleisenger and Fordtran's gastrointestinal and liver disease: pathophysiology/diagnosis/management*, ed 10, pp 161-174, Philadelphia, 2016, Elsevier.
11. Vermeulen W et al: Neuroanatomy of lower gastrointestinal pain disorders, *World J Gastroenterol* 20(4):1005-1020, 2014.
12. Feinman M, Haut ER: Upper gastrointestinal bleeding, *Surg Clin North Am* 94(1):43-53, 2014.
13. Sánchez-Capilla AD et al: New insights to occult gastrointestinal bleeding: from pathophysiology to therapeutics, *World J Gastrointest Pathophysiol* 5(3):271-283, 2014.
14. Roden DF, Altman KW: Causes of dysphagia among different age groups: a systematic review of the literature, *Otolaryngol Clin North Am* 46(6):965-987, 2013.
15. Kahrilas PJ, Boeckxstaens G: The spectrum of achalasia: lessons from studies of pathophysiology

and high-resolution manometry, *Gastroenterology* 145(5):954-965, 2013.
16. Richter JE: Esophageal motility disorder achalasia, *Curr Opin Otolaryngol Head Neck Surg* 21(6):535-542, 2013.
17. Boeckxstaens G et al: Symptomatic reflux disease: the present, the past and the future, *Gut* 63(7):1185-1193, 2014.
18. Achem SR, DeVault KR: Gastroesophageal reflux disease and the elderly, *Gastroenterol Clin North Am* 43(1):147-160, 2014.
19. Zerbib F et al: Functional heartburn: definition and management strategies, *Curr Gastroenterol Rep* 14(3):181-188, 2012.
20. Mikami DJ, Murayama KM: Physiology and pathogenesis of gastroesophageal reflux disease, *Surg Clin North Am* 95(3):515-525, 2015.
21. Hershcovici T, Fass R: Step-by-step management of refractory gastroesophageal reflux disease, *Dis Esophagus* 26(1):27-36, 2013.
22. Roman S, Kahrilas PJ: The diagnosis and management of hiatus hernia, *BMJ* 349:g6154, 2014.
23. Schweigert M et al: Gangrene of the oesophago-gastric junction caused by strangulated hiatal hernia: operative challenge or surgical dead end, *Ir J Med Sci* 183(2):323-330, 2014.
24. Camilleri M et al: Clinical guideline: management of gastroparesis, *Am J Gastroenterol* 108(1):18-37, 2013.
25. No JH et al: Long-term outcome of palliative therapy for gastric outlet obstruction caused by unresectable gastric cancer in patients with good performance status: endoscopic stenting versus surgery, *Gastrointest Endosc* 78(1):55-62, 2013.
26. Hucl T: Acute GI obstruction, *Best Pract Res Clin Gastroenterol* 27(5):691-707, 2013.
27. Taylor MR, Lalani N: Adult small bowel obstruction, *Acad Emerg Med* 20(6):528-544, 2013.
28. Brown CV: Small bowel and colon perforation, *Surg Clin North Am* 94(2):471-475, 2014.
29. Sawai RS: Management of colonic obstruction: a review, *Clin Colon Rectal Surg* 25(4):200-203, 2012.
30. Everhart JE, editor: *Digestive diseases in the United States: epidemiology and impact* (NIH Publication No. 94-1447), U.S. Department of Health and Human Services, National Institutes of Health, National Institute of Diabetes and Digestive and Kidney Diseases, Washington, DC, 1994, U.S. Government Printing Office.

31. Lahner E, Annibale B: Pernicious anemia: new insights from a gastroenterological point of view, *World J Gastroenterol* 15(41):5121-5128, 2009.
32. Smolka AJ, Backert S: How *Helicobacter pylori* infection controls gastric acid secretion, *J Gastroenterol* 47(6):609-618, 2012.
33. Levenstein S et al: Psychological stress increases risk for peptic ulcer, regardless of *Helicobacter pylori* infection or use of nonsteroidal anti-inflammatory drugs, *Clin Gastroenterol Hepatol* S1542-3565(14):01136-01137, 2014.
34. Schiller JS et al: *Summary health statistics for U.S. adults: National Health Interview Survey, 2011. Vital and Health Statistics, Series 10: Data from the National Health Interview Survey*, Centers for Disease Control and Prevention. Available at: www.niddk.nih.gov/health-information/ health-statistics/Pages/digestive-diseases-statistics-for-the-united-states.aspx#18. Accessed June 24, 2015.
35. Epelboym I, Mazeh H: Zollinger-Ellison syndrome: classical considerations and current controversies, *Oncologist* 19(1):44-50, 2014.
36. Cekin AH et al: The role of *Helicobacter pylori* and NSAIDs in the pathogenesis of uncomplicated duodenal ulcer, *Gastroenterol Res Pract* 2012:189373, 2012.
37. Gisbert JP, Cakvet X: Review article: *Helicobacter pylori*-negative duodenal ulcer disease, *Aliment Pharmacol Ther* 30(8):791-815, 2009.
38. Graham DY: History of *Helicobacter pylori*, duodenal ulcer, gastric ulcer and gastric cancer, *World J Gastroenterol* 20(18):5191-5204, 2014.
39. Nirula R: Gastroduodenal perforation, *Surg Clin North Am* 94(1):31-34, 2014.
40. Ubukata H et al: Why is the coexistence of gastric cancer and duodenal ulcer rare? Examination of factors related to both gastric cancer and duodenal ulcer, *Gastric Cancer* 14(1):4-12, 2011.
41. Najm WI: Peptic ulcer disease, *Prim Care* 38(3):383-394, vii, 2011.
42. Patel SK et al: Diagnosis of *Helicobacter pylori*: what should be the gold standard? *World J Gastroenterol* 20(36):12847-12859, 2014.
43. Federico A et al: Eradication of *Helicobacter pylori* infection: which regimen first? *World J Gastroenterol* 20(3):665-672, 2014.
44. Bardou M et al: Stress-related mucosal disease in the critically ill patient, *Nat Rev Gastroenterol Hepatol* 12(2):98-107, 2015.

45. Bolton JS, Conway WC 2nd: Postgastrectomy syndromes, *Surg Clin North Am* 91(15):1105-1122, 2011.
46. Ersan Y et al: Late results of patients undergoing remedial operations for alkaline reflux gastritis syndrome, *Acta Chir Belg* 109(3):364-370, 2009.
47. De Martino C et al: Acute afferent loop obstruction treated by endoscopic decompression. Case report and review of literature, *Ann Ital Chir* 83(6):555-558, 2012.
48. Tack J, Deloose E: Complications of bariatric surgery: dumping syndrome, reflux and vitamin deficiencies, *Best Pract Res Clin Gastroenterol* 28(4):741-749, 2014.
49. Lindkvist B: Diagnosis and treatment of pancreatic exocrine insufficiency, *World J Gastroenterol* 19(42):7258-7266, 2013.
50. Levitt M et al: Clinical implications of lactose malabsorption versus lactose intolerance, *J Clin Gastroenterol* 47(6):471-480, 2013.
51. Johnston I et al: New insights into bile acid malabsorption, *Curr Gastroenterol Rep* 13(5):418-425, 2011.
52. Crohn's and Colitis Foundation of America: *The facts about inflammatory bowel diseases*, New York, November 2014, Author. Available at: www.ccfa.org/assets/pdfs/ibdfactbook.pdf. Accessed June 24, 2015.
53. Burisch J, Munkholm P: Inflammatory bowel disease epidemiology, *Curr Opin Gastroenterol* 29(4):357-362, 2013.
54. Laass MW et al: Diagnosis and classification of Crohn's disease, *Autoimmun Rev* 13(4-5):467-471, 2014.
55. Zhang YZ, Li YY: Inflammatory bowel disease: pathogenesis, *World J Gastroenterol* 20(1):91-99, 2014.
56. Pedersen G: Development, validation and implementation of an in vitro model for the study of metabolic and immune function in normal and inflamed human colonic epithelium, *Dan Med J* 62(1):B4973, 2015.
57. Beaugerie L, Itzkowitz SH: Cancers complicating inflammatory bowel disease, *N Engl J Med* 372(15):1441-1452, 2015.
58. Kostic AD et al: The microbiome in inflammatory bowel disease: current status and the future ahead, *Gastroenterology* 146(6):1489-1499, 2014.
59. Mantzaris GJ: When can we cure Crohn's? *Best Pract Res Clin Gastroenterol* 28(3):519-529, 2014.
60. Lunney PC, Leong RW: Review article: ulcerative colitis, smoking and nicotine therapy, *Aliment Pharmacol Ther* 36(11-12):997-1008, 2012.
61. Feuerstein JD, Cheifetz AS: Ulcerative colitis: epidemiology, diagnosis, and management, *Mayo Clin Proc* 89(11):1553-1563, 2014.
62. Tontini GE et al: Differential diagnosis in inflammatory bowel disease colitis: state of the art and future perspectives, *World J Gastroenterol* 21(1):21-46, 2015.
63. Bressler B et al: Clinical practice guidelines for the medical management of nonhospitalized ulcerative colitis: the Toronto Consensus, *Gastroenterology* 2015 Mar 4. [Epub ahead of print.]
64. Papi C et al: Mucosal healing in inflammatory bowel disease: treatment efficacy and predictive factors, *Dig Liver Dis* 45(12):978-985, 2013.
65. Dayan B, Turner D: Role of surgery in severe ulcerative colitis in the era of medical rescue therapy, *World J Gastroenterol* 18(29):3833-3838, 2012.
66. Shen B: Acute and chronic Pouchitis—pathogenesis, diagnosis and treatment, *Nat Rev Gastroenterol Hepatol* 9(6):323-333, 2012.
67. Cabré E, Domènech E: Impact of environmental and dietary factors on the course of inflammatory bowel disease, *World J Gastroenterol* 18(29):3814-3822, 2012.
68. Cheifetz AS: Management of active Crohn disease, *J Am Med Assoc* 309(20):2150-2158, 2013.
69. Kane JS et al: Development and validation of a scoring system to identify patients with microscopic colitis, *Clin Gastroenterol Hepatol* 13(6):1125-1131, 2015.

70. Ohlsson B: New insights and challenges in microscopic colitis, *Therap Adv Gastroenterol* 8(1):37-47, 2015.
71. Canavan C et al: The epidemiology of irritable bowel syndrome, *Clin Epidemiol* 6:71-80, 2014.
72. Bolino CM, Bercik P: Pathogenic factors involved in the development of irritable bowel syndrome: focus on a microbial role, *Infect Dis Clin North Am* 24(4):961-975, 2010.
73. Catanzaro R et al: Irritable bowel syndrome: new findings in pathophysiological and therapeutic field, *Minerva Gastroenterol Dietol* 60(2):151-163, 2014.
74. Vaiopoulou A et al: Molecular basis of the irritable bowel syndrome, *World J Gastroenterol* 20(2):376-383, 2014.
75. Mayer EA et al: Brain-gut microbiome interactions and functional bowel disorders, *Gastroenterology* 146(6):1500-1512, 2014.
76. Coss-Adame E, Rao SS: Brain and gut interactions in irritable bowel syndrome: new paradigms and new understandings, *Curr Gastroenterol Rep* 16(4):379, 2014.
77. Nasser Y et al: Using human intestinal biopsies to study the pathogenesis of irritable bowel syndrome, *Neurogastroenterol Motil* 26(4):455-469, 2014.
78. Beatty JK et al: Post-infectious irritable bowel syndrome: mechanistic insights into chronic disturbances following enteric infection, *World J Gastroenterol* 20(14):3976-3985, 2014.
79. Piche T: Tight junctions and IBS—the link between epithelial permeability, low-grade inflammation, and symptom generation? *Neurogastroenterol Motil* 26(3):296-302, 2014.
80. Quigley EM: Small intestinal bacterial overgrowth: what it is and what it is not, *Curr Opin Gastroenterol* 30(2):141-146, 2014.
81. Ghoshal UC, Srivastava D: Irritable bowel syndrome and small intestinal bacterial overgrowth: meaningful association or unnecessary hype, *World J Gastroenterol* 20(10):2482-2491, 2014.
82. El-Salhy M et al: Interaction between ingested nutrients and gut endocrine cells in patients with irritable bowel syndrome (review), *Int J Mol Med* 34(2):363-371, 2014.
83. Fukudo S: Stress and visceral pain: focusing on irritable bowel syndrome. *Pain* 154(Suppl 1):S63-S70, 2013.
84. Lovell RM, Ford AC: Effect of gender on prevalence of irritable bowel syndrome in the community: systematic review and meta-analysis, *Am J Gastroenterol* 107(7):991-1000, 2012.
85. Chey WD et al: Irritable bowel syndrome: a clinical review, *J Am Med Assoc* 313(9):949-958, 2015.
86. Sayuk GS, Gyawali CP: Irritable bowel syndrome: modern concepts and management options, *Am J Med* 2015 Feb 27. [Epub ahead of print.]
87. Ferreira-Aparicio FE et al: Diverticular disease of the small bowel, *Case Rep Gastroenterol* 6(3):668-676, 2012.
88. Tursi A: The role of colonoscopy in managing diverticular disease of the colon, *J Gastrointestin Liver Dis* 24(1):85-93, 2015.
89. Humes DJ, Spiller RC: Review article: the pathogenesis and management of acute colonic diverticulitis, *Aliment Pharmacol Ther* 39(4):359-370, 2014.
90. Templeton AW, Strate LL: Updates in diverticular disease, *Curr Gastroenterol Rep* 15(8):339, 2013.
91. Tursi A: New physiopathological and therapeutic approaches to diverticular disease: an update, *Expert Opin Pharmacother* 15(7):1005-1017, 2014.
92. McDermott FD et al: Minimally invasive and surgical management strategies tailored to the severity of acute diverticulitis, *Br J Surg* 101(1):e90-e99, 2014.
93. Buckius MT et al: Changing epidemiology of acute appendicitis in the United States: study period 1993-2008, *J Surg Res* 175(2):185-190, 2012.
94. Vissers RJ, Lennarz WB: Pitfalls in appendicitis, *Emerg Med Clin North Am* 28(1):103-118, 2010.

95. Drake FT, Flum DR: Improvement in the diagnosis of appendicitis, *Adv Surg* 47:299-328, 2013.
96. Acute appendicitis—appendectomy or the "antibiotics first" strategy, *N Engl J Med* 372(23):2274, 2015.
97. Bobadilla JL: Mesenteric ischemia, *Surg Clin North Am* 93(4):925-940, ix, 2013.
98. Singal AK et al: Mesenteric venous thrombosis, *Mayo Clin Proc* 88(3):285-294, 2013.
99. Sise MJ: Acute mesenteric ischemia, *Surg Clin North Am* 94(1):165-181, 2014.
100. Sundermeyer A et al: Endovascular treatment of chronic mesenteric ischemia, *Interv Med Appl Sci* 6(3):118-124, 2014.
101. Acosta S, Björck M: Modern treatment of acute mesenteric ischaemia, *Br J Surg* 101(1):e100-e108, 2014.
102. Flegal KM et al: Prevalence of obesity and trends in the distribution of body mass index among US adults, 1999–2010, *J Am Med Assoc* 307(5):491-497, 2012.
103. Flegal KM et al: Association of all-cause mortality with overweight and obesity using standard body mass index categories: a systematic review and meta-analysis, *J Am Med Assoc* 309(1):71-82, 2013.
104. World Health Organization: *Obesity and overweight*. Accessed June 24, 2015. Available at: www.who.int/mediacentre/factsheets/fs311/en.
105. Wang Y et al: Will all Americans become overweight or obese? Estimating the progression and cost of the U.S. obesity epidemic, *Obesity (Silver Springs)* (10):2323-2330, 2008.
106. Dixon JB: The effect of obesity on health outcomes, *Mol Cell Endocrinol* 316(2):104-108, 2010.
107. Das UN: Obesity: genes, brain, gut, and environment, *Nutrition* 26(5):459-473, 2010.
108. Cao H: Adipocytokines in obesity and metabolic disease, *J Endocrinol* 220(2):T47-T59, 2014.
109. Ahima RS, Antwi DA: Brain regulation of appetite and satiety, *Endocrinol Metab Clin North Am* 37(4):811-823, 2008.
110. Jauch-Chara K, Oltmanns KM: Obesity—a neuropsychological disease? Systematic review and neuropsychological model, *Prog Neurobiol* 114:84-101, 2014.
111. Murray S et al: Hormonal and neural mechanisms of food reward, eating behaviour and obesity, *Nat Rev Endocrinol* 10(9):540-552, 2014.
112. Sáinz N et al: Leptin resistance and diet-induced obesity: central and peripheral actions of leptin, *Metabolism* 64(1):35-46, 2015.
113. Exley MA et al: Interplay between the immune system and adipose tissue in obesity, *J Endocrinol* 223(2):R41-R48, 2014.
114. Jung UJ, Choi MS: Obesity and its metabolic complications: the role of adipokines and the relationship between obesity, inflammation, insulin resistance, dyslipidemia and nonalcoholic fatty liver disease, *Int J Mol Sci* 15(4):6184-6223, 2014.
115. Sam S, Mazzone T: Adipose tissue changes in obesity and the impact on metabolic function, *Transl Res* 164(4):284-292, 2014.
116. Palmer BF, Clegg DJ: The sexual dimorphism of obesity, *Mol Cell Endocrinol* 2015 Jan 8. [Epub ahead of print.]
117. Goyal A et al: Is there a paradox in obesity? *Cardiol Rev* 22(4):163-170, 2014.
118. Tchernof A, Després JP: Pathophysiology of human visceral obesity: an update, *Physiol Rev* 93(1):359-404, 2013.
119. Oliveros E et al: The concept of normal weight obesity, *Prog Cardiovasc Dis* 56(4):426-433, 2014.
120. Marques-Vidal P et al: Prevalence of normal weight obesity in Switzerland: effect of various definitions, *Eur J Nutr* 47(5):251-257, 2008.
121. Kramer CK et al: Are metabolically healthy overweight and obesity benign conditions? A systematic review and meta-analysis, *Ann Intern Med* 159(11):758-769, 2013.
122. Thibault R, Pichard C: The evaluation of body composition: a useful tool for clinical practice, *Ann Nutr Metab* 60(1):6-16, 2012.

123. Biro FM, Wien M: Childhood obesity and adult morbidities, *Am J Clin Nutr* 91(5):1499S-1505S, 2010.

124. Joo JK, Lee KS: Pharmacotherapy for obesity, *J Menopausal Med* 20(3):90-96, 2014.

125. Yanovski SZ, Yanovski JA: Long-term drug treatment for obesity: a systematic and clinical review, *J Am Med Assoc* 311(1):74-86, 2014.

126. Aronne LJ: Evolving directions in obesity management, *J Fam Pract* 63(7):S27-S33, 2014.

127. Colquitt JL et al: Surgery for weight loss in adults, *Cochrane Database Syst Rev* 8:CD003641, 2014.

128. Mason JB: Nutritional principles and assessment of the gastroenterology patient. In Feldman M et al, editors: *Sleisenger and Fordtran's gastrointestinal and liver disease: pathophysiology/ diagnosis/management,* ed 10, pp 57-82, Philadelphia, 2016, Elsevier.

129. Walmsley RS: Refeeding syndrome: screening, incidence, and treatment during parenteral nutrition, *J Gastroenterol Hepatol* 28(Suppl 4): 113-117, 2013.

130. Suzuki H et al: Cancer cachexia—pathophysiology and management, *J Gastroenterol* 48(5):574-594, 2013.

131. Bloom S et al: Portal hypertension: pathophysiology, diagnosis and management, *Intern Med* 45(1):16-26, 2015.

132. Biecker E: Portal hypertension and gastrointestinal bleeding: diagnosis, prevention and management, *World J Gastroenterol* 19(31):5035-5050, 2013.

133. Møller S et al: Extrahepatic complications to cirrhosis and portal hypertension: haemodynamic and homeostatic aspects, *World J Gastroenterol* 20(42):15499-15517, 2014.

134. Tripathi D, Hayes PC: Beta-blockers in portal hypertension: new developments and controversies, *Liver Int* 34(5):655-667, 2014.

135. Liou IW: Management of end-stage liver disease, *Med Clin North Am* 98(1):119-152, 2014.

136. Hou W, Sanyal AJ: Ascites: diagnosis and management, *Med Clin North Am* 93(4):801-817, 2009.

137. Pedersen JS et al: Management of cirrhotic ascites, *Ther Adv Chronic Dis* 6(3):124-137, 2015.

138. Sturgeon JP, Shawcross DL: Recent insights into the pathogenesis of hepatic encephalopathy and treatments, *Expert Rev Gastroenterol Hepatol* 8(1):83-100, 2014.

139. Vilstrup H et al: Hepatic encephalopathy in chronic liver disease. 2014 practice guideline by the European Association for the Study of the Liver and the American Association for the Study of Liver Diseases, *J Hepatol* 61(3):642-659, 2014.

140. Amodio P et al: The nutritional management of hepatic encephalopathy in patients with cirrhosis: International Society for Hepatic Encephalopathy and Nitrogen Metabolism Consensus, *Hepatology* 58(1):325-336, 2013.

141. Bañares R et al: Molecular adsorbent recirculating system and bioartificial devices for liver failure, *Clin Liver Dis* 18(4):945-956, 2014.

142. Winger J, Michelfelder A: Diagnostic approach to the patient with jaundice, *Prim Care* 38(3):469-482, viii, 2011.

143. Roche SP, Kobos R: Jaundice in the adult patient, *Am Fam Physician* 69(2):299-304, 2004.

144. Low G et al: Hepatorenal syndrome: aetiology, diagnosis, and treatment, *Gastroenterol Res Pract* 2015:207012, 2015.

145. Barbano B et al: Pathophysiology, diagnosis and clinical management of hepatorenal syndrome: from classic to new drugs, *Curr Vasc Pharmacol* 12(1):125-135, 2014.

146. Blieden M et al: A perspective on the epidemiology of acetaminophen exposure and toxicity in the United States, *Expert Rev Clin Pharmacol* 7(3):341-348, 2014.

147. Moreau R et al: Acute-on-chronic liver failure: recent concepts, *J Clin Exp Hepatol* 5(1):81-85, 2015.

148. Shalimar, Acharya SK: Management in acute liver failure, *J Clin Exp Hepatol* 5(Suppl 1):S104-S115, 2015.

149. O'Grady J: Timing and benefit of liver transplantation in acute liver failure, *J Hepatol* 60(3):663-670, 2014.

150. Scaglione S et al: The epidemiology of cirrhosis in the United States: a population-based study, *J Clin Gastroenterol* 2014 Oct 8. [Epub ahead of print.]

151. Novo E et al: Cellular and molecular mechanisms in liver fibrogenesis, *Arch Biochem Biophys* 548:20-37, 2014.

152. Huang YW et al: Pathogenesis and management of alcoholic liver cirrhosis: a review, *Hepat Med* 3:1-11, 2011.

153. Eagon PK: Alcoholic liver injury: influence of gender and hormones, *World J Gastroenterol* 16(11):1377-1384, 2010.

154. Division of Population Health, National Center for Chronic Disease Prevention and Health Promotion: *Alcohol and public health, updated October 1, 2012,* Atlanta, Ga, 2012, Centers for Disease Control and Prevention.

155. Wiegand J, Berg T: The etiology, diagnosis and prevention of liver cirrhosis: part 1 of a series on liver cirrhosis, *Dtsch Arztebl Int* 110(6):85-91, 2013.

156. Cubero FJ et al: Alcohol and liver fibrosis, *Semin Liver Dis* 29(2):211-221, 2009.

157. Setshedi M et al: Acetaldehyde adducts in alcoholic liver disease, *Oxid Med Cell Longev* 3(3):178-185, 2010.

158. Orman ES et al: Alcoholic liver disease: pathogenesis, management, and novel targets for therapy, *J Gastroenterol Hepatol* 28(Suppl 1):77-84, 2013.

159. Struecker B et al: Liver support strategies: cutting-edge technologies, *Nat Rev Gastroenterol Hepatol* 11(3):166-176, 2014.

160. Corrado RL et al: Review of treatment options for nonalcoholic fatty liver disease, *Med Clin North Am* 98(1):55-72, 2014.

161. Rinella ME: Nonalcoholic fatty liver disease: a systematic review, *J Am Med Assoc* 313(22): 2263-2273, 2015.

162. Purohit T, Cappell MS: Primary biliary cirrhosis: pathophysiology, clinical presentation and therapy, *World J Hepatol* 7(7):926-941, 2015.

163. Centers for Disease Control and Prevention: *Surveillance for viral hepatitis—United States, 2013.* Available at: http://www.cdc.gov/hepatitis/ statistics/2013surveillance/index.htm.

164. Jayakumar S et al: Fulminant viral hepatitis, *Crit Care Clin* 29(3):677-697, 2013.

165. Price J: An update on hepatitis B, D, and E viruses, *Top Antivir Med* 21(5):157-163, 2014.

166. Aydeniz A et al: Rheumatic manifestations of hepatitis B and C and their association with viral load and fibrosis of the liver, *Rheumatol Int* 30(4):515-517, 2010.

167. Chacko EC et al: Chronic viral hepatitis and chronic kidney disease, *Postgrad Med J* 86(1018):486-492, 2010.

168. Trépo C et al: Hepatitis B virus infection, *Lancet* 384(9959):2053-2063, 2014.

169. Alvarado-Mora MV et al: An update on HDV: virology, pathogenesis and treatment, *Antivir Ther* 18(3 Pt B):541-548, 2014.

170. Pérez-Gracia MT et al: Hepatitis E: an emerging disease, *Infect Genet Evol* 22:40-59, 2014.

171. Halegoua-De Marzio D, Hann HW: Then and now: the progress in hepatitis B treatment over the past 20 years, *World J Gastroenterol* 20(2):401-413, 2014.

172. Kohli A et al: Treatment of hepatitis C: a systematic review, *J Am Med Assoc* 312(6):631-640, 2014.

173. Sánchez G et al: Hepatitis A virus detection in food: current and future prospects, *Lett Appl Microbiol* 45(1):1-5, 2007.

174. Honegger JR et al: Will there be a vaccine to prevent HCV infection? *Semin Liver Dis* 34(1):79-88, 2014.

175. Wang L et al: A dual vaccine candidate against norovirus and hepatitis E virus, *Vaccine* 32(4):445-452, 2014.

176. Stinton LM, Shaffer EA: Epidemiology of gallbladder disease: cholelithiasis and cancer, *Gut Liver* 6(2):172-187, 2012.

177. Reshetnyak VI: Concept of the pathogenesis and treatment of cholelithiasis, *World J Hepatol* 4(2):18-34, 2012.

178. O'Connell K, Brasel K: Bile metabolism and lithogenesis, *Surg Clin North Am* 94(2):361-375, 2014.

179. Gaby AR: Nutritional approaches to prevention and treatment of gallstones, *Altern Med Rev* 14(3):258-267, 2009.

180. Itoi T, Wang HP: Endoscopic management of bile duct stones, *Dig Endosc* 22(Suppl 1):S69-S75, 2010.

181. Barie PS, Eachempati SR: Acute acalculous cholecystitis, *Gastroenterol Clin North Am* 39(2):343-357, x, 2010.

182. Knab LM et al: Cholecystitis, *Surg Clin North Am* 94(2):455-470, 2014.

183. Yadav D, Lowenfels AB: The epidemiology of pancreatitis and pancreatic cancer, *Gastroenterology* 144(6):1252-1261, 2013.

184. Lankisch PG et al: Acute pancreatitis, *Lancet* 2015 Jan 20. [Epub ahead of print.]

185. Sah RP et al: New insights into the pathogenesis of pancreatitis, *Curr Opin Gastroenterol* 29(5):523-530, 2013.

186. Muniraj T et al: Chronic pancreatitis, a comprehensive review and update. Part I: epidemiology, etiology, risk factors, genetics, pathophysiology, and clinical features, *Dis Mon* 60(12):530-550, 2014.

187. Bakker OJ et al: Treatment options for acute pancreatitis, *Nat Rev Gastroenterol Hepatol* 11(8):462-469, 2014.

188. Brock C et al: Pathophysiology of chronic pancreatitis, *World J Gastroenterol* 19(42):7231-7240, 2013.

189. Sze KC et al: Current options for the diagnosis of chronic pancreatitis, *Expert Rev Mol Diagn* 14(2):199-215, 2014.

190. Poulsen JL et al: Pain and chronic pancreatitis: a complex interplay of multiple mechanisms, *World J Gastroenterol* 19(42):7282-7291, 2013.

191. Johnson MD et al: Surgical versus nonsurgical management of pancreatic pseudocysts, *J Clin Gastroenterol* 43(6):586-590, 2009.

192. American Cancer Society: *Cancer facts and figures 2015,* Atlanta, 2015, Author.

193. Shimizu M et al: Esophageal squamous cell carcinoma with special reference to its early stage, *Best Pract Res Clin Gastroenterol* 27(2):171-186, 2013.

194. Halland M et al: Recent developments in pathogenesis, diagnosis and therapy of Barrett's esophagus, *World J Gastroenterol* 21(21):6479-6490, 2015.

195. Xie FJ et al: *Helicobacter pylori* infection and esophageal cancer risk: an updated meta-analysis, *World J Gastroenterol* 19(36):6098-6107, 2013.

196. Spechler SJ: Barrett esophagus and risk of esophageal cancer: a clinical review, *J Am Med Assoc* 310(6):627-636, 2013.

197. Cowie A et al: Strategies to improve outcomes in esophageal adenocarcinoma, *Expert Rev Anticancer Ther* 14(6):677-687, 2014.

198. Nakajima M, Kato H: Treatment options for esophageal squamous cell carcinoma, *Expert Opin Pharmacother* 14(10):1345-1354, 2013.

199. Fock KM: Review article: the epidemiology and prevention of gastric cancer, *Aliment Pharmacol Ther* 40(3):250-260, 2014.

200. de Martel C et al: Gastric cancer: epidemiology and risk factors, *Gastroenterol Clin North Am* 42(2):219-240, 2013.

201. Resende C et al: Genetic and epigenetic alteration in gastric carcinogenesis, *Helicobacter* 15(Suppl 1):34-39, 2010.

202. Yakirevich E, Resnick MB: Pathology of gastric cancer and its precursor lesions, *Gastroenterol Clin North Am* 42(2):261-284, 2013.

203. Wu HH et al: Advances in molecular biomarkers for gastric cancer: miRNAs as emerging novel cancer markers, *Expert Rev Mol Med* 16:e1, 2014.

204. Blakely AM, Miner TJ: Surgical considerations in the treatment of gastric cancer, *Gastroenterol Clin North Am* 42(2):337-357, 2013.

205. Tammana VS, Laiyemo AO: Colorectal cancer disparities: issues, controversies and solutions, *World J Gastroenterol* 20(4):869-876, 2014.

206. Aparicio T et al: Small bowel adenocarcinoma: epidemiology, risk factors, diagnosis and treatment, *Dig Liver Dis* 46(2):97-104, 2014.

207. Cunningham D et al: Colorectal cancer, *Lancet* 375(9719):1030-1047, 2010.

208. Jasperson K et al: Hereditary and familial colon cancer, *Gastroenterology* 138(6):2044-2058, 2010.

209. Kalady MF: Sessile serrated polyps: an important route to colorectal cancer, *J Natl Compr Canc Netw* 11(12):1585-1594, 2013.

210. Zoratto F et al: Focus on genetic and epigenetic events of colorectal cancer pathogenesis: implications for molecular diagnosis, *Tumour Biol* 35(7):6195-6206, 2014.

211. Lee GH et al: Is right-sided colon cancer different to left-sided colorectal cancer? A systematic review, *Eur J Surg Oncol* 41(3):300-308, 2014.

212. Song M et al: Nutrients, foods, and colorectal cancer prevention, *Gastroenterol* 148(6):1244-1260.e16, 2015.

213. Tan YN et al: The accuracy of computed tomography in the pretreatment staging of colorectal cancer, *Hepatogastroenterology* 61(133):1207-1212, 2014.

214. National Cancer Institute: *Stages of colon cancer.* Updated December 11, 2014. Available at: http://www.cancer.gov/types/colorectal/patient/colon-treatment-pdq#section/_112. Accessed June 24, 2015.

215. Grady WM, Pritchard CC: Molecular alterations and biomarkers in colorectal cancer, *Toxicol Pathol* 42(1):124-139, 2014.

216. Linnekamp JF et al: Colorectal cancer heterogeneity and targeted therapy: a case for molecular disease subtypes, *Cancer Res* 75(2):245-249, 2015.

217. Allard MA, Malka D: Place of hepatic intra-arterial chemotherapy in the treatment of colorectal liver metastases, *J Vasc Surg* 151(Suppl 1):S21-S24, 2014.

218. Sorbye H: Recurrence patterns after resection of liver metastases from colorectal cancer, *Recent Results Cancer Res* 203:243-252, 2014.

219. Bosetti C et al: Hepatocellular carcinoma epidemiology, *Best Pract Res Clin Gastroenterol* 28(5):753-770, 2014.

220. Nault JC: Pathogenesis of hepatocellular carcinoma according to aetiology, *Best Pract Res Clin Gastroenterol* 28(5):937-947, 2014.

221. Razumilava N, Gores GJ: Cholangiocarcinoma, *Lancet* 2014 383(9935):2168-2179, 2014.

222. Colombo M, Iavarone M: Role of antiviral treatment for HCC prevention, *Best Pract Res Clin Gastroenterol* 28(5):771-781, 2014.

223. Rasool M et al: New possibilities in hepatocellular carcinoma treatment, *Anticancer Res* 34(4):1563-1571, 2014.

224. Weledji EP et al: How grim is hepatocellular carcinoma? *Ann Med Surg (Lond)* 3(3):71-76, 2014.

225. Maurya SK et al: Genetic aberrations in gallbladder cancer, *Surg Oncol* 21(1):37-43, 2012.

226. Wernberg JA, Lucarelli DD: Gallbladder cancer, *Surg Clin North Am* 94(2):343-360, 2014.

227. Marino D et al: Biliary tract carcinomas: from chemotherapy to targeted therapy, *Crit Rev Oncol Hematol* 85(2):136-148, 2013.

228. Roshani R et al: Inflammatory cytokines in human pancreatic cancer, *Cancer Lett* 345(2):157-163, 2014.

229. Lunardi S et al: The stromal compartments in pancreatic cancer: are there any therapeutic targets? *Cancer Lett* 343(2):147-155, 2014.

230. Pinho AV et al: Chronic pancreatitis: a path to pancreatic cancer, *Cancer Lett* 345(2):203-209, 2014.

231. Poruk KE et al: Screening for pancreatic cancer, *Adv Surg* 48:115-136, 2014.

232. Mian OY et al: Management options in locally advanced pancreatic cancer, *Curr Oncol Rep* 16(6):388, 2014.

233. Erdek MA et al: Pain management and palliative care in pancreatic cancer, *Curr Probl Cancer* 37(5):266-272, 2013.

Alterations of Digestive Function in Children

Sharon Sables-Baus and Sara J. Fidanza

EVOLVE WEBSITE

http://evolve.elsevier.com/Huether/

Student Review Questions
Audio Key Points

Case Studies
Animations
Quick Check Answers

Disorders of the gastrointestinal tract, liver, and pancreas in children include congenital anomalies with structural and functional alterations, enzyme deficiencies, and infections. These disorders lead to impairment of motility, digestion, absorption, nutrition, and normal growth and development.

DISORDERS OF THE GASTROINTESTINAL TRACT

Congenital Impairment of Motility

Cleft Lip and Cleft Palate

There are numerous types of congenital orofacial anomalies, the most common of which is cleft lip (CL) or cleft palate (CP), or both (CL/P). The incidence of cleft lip, with or without cleft palate, is about 1 in 1000 live births. In the United States, the incidence varies significantly by racial group,[1,2] with Asian and Native American populations have the highest prevalence and African-derived populations have the lowest.[3] CL and CP can occur in isolation or as part of a broad range of chromosomal, mendelian, or teratogenic syndromes. When this occurs, the defect may be referred to as syndromic CLP. If CP occurs alone, the defect may be referred to as nonsyndromic or isolated CP and is more common in females. CL with or without CP is more common in males. Both anomalies can be unilateral or bilateral, or partial or complete.[4] Periconceptional intake of B vitamins, folate, and folic acid and reduced tobacco and alcohol use may prevent orofacial clefts.[5]

PATHOPHYSIOLOGY Cleft lip (CL) and cleft palate (CP) are embryonic developmental anomalies and vary in severity (Figure 37-1). There may be genetic and environmental triggers for syndromic and nonsyndromic CLP. Epigenetic influences include maternal smoking, alcohol steroid or statin use; folate deficiency, or disordered metabolism. Cleft lip and cleft palate also may be associated with other malformations (i.e., cardiac, skeletal, or central nervous system). This phenomenon, called *multifactorial inheritance,* is discussed in Chapter 2. Together, the genetic and epigenetic factors reduce the amount of neural crest mesenchyme that migrates into the area that will develop into the face of the embryo.[6]

Cleft lip is caused by the incomplete fusion of the nasomedial or intermaxillary process beginning the fourth week of embryonic development, a period of rapid development. The cleft causes structures of the face and mouth to develop without the normal restraints of encircling lip muscles. The facial cleft may affect not only the lip but also the external nose, nasal cartilages, nasal septum, and alveolar processes. The cleft is usually just beneath the center of one nostril. The defect may occur bilaterally and may be symmetric or asymmetric. The more complete the cleft lip, the greater the chance that teeth in the line of the cleft will be missing or malformed.

Cleft palate is often associated with cleft lip but may occur without it. The fissure may affect only the uvula and soft palate or may extend forward to the nostril and involve the hard palate and the maxillary alveolar ridge. It may be unilateral or bilateral, with the cleft occupying the midline posteriorly and as far forward as the alveolar process, where it deviates to the involved side. Clefts involving the palate only are usually but not necessarily in the midline. In some cases, the vomer and nasal septum are partly or completely undeveloped. When these facial bones are involved, the nasal cavity may freely communicate with the oral cavity. Teeth in the cleft palate area may be missing or deformed. There is increased risk for middle ear infections.

CLINICAL MANIFESTATIONS Clefts of the lip or palate, or both, are immediately recognizable disruptions of normal facial structure. Feeding difficulty is the most significant clinical manifestation because of the oronasal communication and inability to generate negative pressure needed for normal sucking.[7] There also may be swallowing difficulty.

FIGURE 37-1 Variations in Clefts of the Lip and Palate. **A,** Notch in vermilion border. **B,** Unilateral cleft lip and palate. **C,** Bilateral cleft lip and cleft palate. **D,** Cleft palate.

EVALUATION AND TREATMENT Prenatal diagnosis is made by ultrasound, and postnatal imaging confirms the extent of bone deformity. Soft tissue alterations are evaluated by history and physical examination. The nature and extent of the cleft, the infant's condition, and the method of surgical correction proposed determine the course of treatment. Surgical correction is planned at about the third to sixth month and may be performed in stages.[8,9] There are limited long-term outcome studies.[10]

Feeding the infant with cleft lip usually presents no difficulty if the cleft lip is simple and the palate intact. A baby with a complete cleft palate requires consultation with a feeding and swallowing specialist to ensure adequate and safe nutritional intake. Bottles with nipples specialized for feeding an infant with a cleft palate are required. Breastfeeding may be possible for some infants.[7] An orthodontic prosthesis for the roof of the mouth may facilitate sucking for some infants. Parental education and support is required for the long-term care of children with cleft palate. Longitudinal monitoring requires a cleft/

orofacial multidisciplinary team including a plastic surgeon, speech therapist, orthodontist, and nurse.[11]

Esophageal Atresia

Congenital malformations of the esophagus occur in 1 of 3000 to 4500 live births. **Esophageal atresia (EA)** is the most common congenital atresia of the esophagus. The esophagus ends in a blind pouch. EA is usually accompanied by a fistula between the esophagus and the trachea (**tracheoesophageal fistula [EA/TEF]**).[12] Either defect can occur alone (Figure 37-2). There is a high frequency of anomalies and syndromes associated with esophageal atresias.[13] Environmental risk factors include maternal exposure to methimazole, exogenous sex hormones, infectious diseases, alcohol, or smoking; maternal diabetes; advanced maternal age; and maternal employment in agriculture.[14] Many genes and chromosomal abnormalities have been implicated; 10% to 30% of infants with EA/TEF have associated *v*ertebral, *a*nal, *c*ardiovascular, *t*racheo*e*sophageal, *r*enal, and *l*imb anomalies (VACTERL).[15]

PATHOPHYSIOLOGY The pathogenesis of esophageal abnormalities is unknown. Defective growth of endodermal cells and impaired embryonic foregut development of the trachea and esophagus lead to atresia.[12]

CLINICAL MANIFESTATIONS Antenatal diagnosis of EA/TEF increases with the findings of polyhydramnios (excessive amniotic fluid).[13,14] Swallowed amniotic fluid is usually absorbed into the placental circulation; therefore if the fetus cannot swallow, amniotic fluid accumulates in the uterus. EA will be diagnosed at birth on the basis of drooling, inability to swallow secretions or choking with feeding, and respiratory distress. Confirmation is established by inability to pass a gastric tube into the stomach. If a fistula connects the trachea with the distal esophagus, the abdomen fills with air and becomes distended, possibly interfering with breathing (see Figure 37-2, *C* to *E*). Intermittent cyanosis may result.

Pulmonary complications are compounded by reflux of air and gastric secretions into the tracheobronchial tree through the fistula, causing severe chemical irritation. Infants with esophageal atresia but no fistulae have scaphoid (boat-shaped), gasless abdomens. In infants with fistulae but without atresia (see Figure 37-2, *E*), the usual symptoms are recurrent aspiration, pneumonia, and atelectasis that remains unexpressed for days or even months.

EVALUATION AND TREATMENT Infants presenting with esophageal atresia are evaluated with ultrasound, echocardiogram, and vertebral and limb radiographs. Following diagnosis, a tube should be placed into the upper pouch and continuous suction applied to decrease risk of aspiration. The head of the bed should be elevated slightly to assist drainage of the upper pouch. The infant should not be fed orally. Surgical repair is completed in the majority of cases.[16] The overall survival rate for infants with esophageal defects is 95%.[17]

Infantile Hypertrophic Pyloric Stenosis

Infantile hypertrophic pyloric stenosis (IHPS) is an acquired narrowing and distal obstruction of the pylorus and a common cause of postprandial vomiting. The incidence of pyloric stenosis is approximately 2 to 5 in 1000 live births for males and 1 in 1000 live births for females.[18] The etiology is unclear but probably multifactorial, involving genetic and environmental factors.

PATHOPHYSIOLOGY Individual muscle fibers thicken, so the entire pyloric sphincter becomes enlarged and inflexible. The mucosal lining

FIGURE 37-2 Five Types of Esophageal Atresia and Tracheoesophageal Fistulae. A, Simple esophageal atresia. Proximal esophagus and distal esophagus end in blind pouches, and there is no tracheal communication. Nothing enters the stomach; regurgitated food and fluid may enter the lungs. **B,** Proximal and distal esophageal segments end in blind pouches, and a fistula connects the proximal esophagus to the trachea. Nothing enters the stomach; food and fluid enter the lungs from the mouth. **C,** Proximal esophagus ends in a blind pouch, and a fistula connects the trachea to the distal esophagus. Air enters the stomach; regurgitated gastric secretions enter the lungs through the fistula. **D,** Fistula connects both proximal and distal esophageal segments to the trachea. Air, food, and fluid enter the stomach and the lungs from the mouth; regurgitated gastric secretions enter the lungs through the fistula. **E,** Simple tracheoesophageal fistula between otherwise normal esophagus and trachea. Air, food, and fluid enter the stomach and the lungs from the mouth through the fistula; and regurgitated gastric secretions enter the lungs through the fistula. Between 85% and 90% of esophageal anomalies are type **C**; 6% to 8% are type **A**; 3% to 5% are type **E**; and fewer than 1% are type **B** or **D.**

of the pyloric opening is folded and narrowed by the encroaching muscle. Because of the extra peristaltic effort necessary to force the gastric contents through the narrow pylorus, the muscle layers of the stomach may become hypertrophied as well.

CLINICAL MANIFESTATIONS Between 2 and 8 weeks after birth, an infant who has fed well and gained weight begins forceful, nonbilious vomiting immediately after feeding.[19,20] The infant then demands to be refed. Constipation occurs because little food reaches the intestine.

In severe, untreated cases, increased gastric peristalsis and vomiting lead to severe fluid and electrolyte imbalances, malnutrition, and weight loss that can be fatal within 4 to 6 weeks. Infants with pyloric stenosis are irritable because of hunger, and they may have esophageal discomfort caused by repeated vomiting and esophagitis. The vomitus may be blood-streaked because of rupture of gastric and esophageal vessels.

EVALUATION AND TREATMENT Diagnosis is based on the history, clinical manifestations, and findings on abdominal ultrasound. The force and timing of the vomiting can help distinguish IHPS from gastroesophageal reflux, for which episodes of vomiting are not forceful and occur 10 minutes or more after a feeding. The hypertrophied pylorus is palpable as a firm, small, movable mass, approximately the size of an olive, and is felt in the right upper quadrant in 70% to 90% of infants with pyloric stenosis. The hypertrophied pyloric muscles and narrowed pyloric channel are identified with ultrasound and radiographs.

The standard treatment for hypertrophic pyloric stenosis is a laparoscopic pyloromyotomy, in which the muscles of the pylorus are split and separated. Preoperative and postoperative medical management to correct fluid and electrolyte imbalance has been the key to the high success rate and low complication rates associated with this surgery.[21]

Obstructions of the Duodenum, Jejunum, and Ileum

High intestinal obstruction should be considered whenever persistent vomiting occurs. With duodenal obstruction there will be upper abdominal distention, visible peristaltic waves, a decrease in the size and frequency of meconium stools, progressive weight loss, persistent vomiting, and dehydration. Congenital obstruction of the duodenum can be caused by intrinsic malformations, such as atresia (complete blockage), stenosis (partial obstruction or narrowing), or external pressure, and occurs in 2.5 to 10 per 100,000 live births.[22] The obstruction may be partial or complete and is usually located at or near the major duodenal papilla. The classic "double bubble" sign is seen on imaging of the abdomen and represents duodenal obstruction. The larger, proximal "bubble" is air in a dilated stomach. The more distal, smaller "bubble" is air in a dilated proximal duodenum. There is usually little or no air in the bowel distal to the obstruction. Double bubble also may be seen on prenatal ultrasounds. An annular pancreas—a defect in which the head of the pancreas surrounds part of the duodenum—can obstruct the duodenum. Congenital obstructions of the jejunum and ileum can be attributable to atresia, stenosis, meconium ileus, megacolon (Hirschsprung disease), intussusception, Meckel diverticulum, intestinal duplication, or strangulated hernia. In ileal or jejunal atresia, the intestine ends blindly, proximal and distal to an interruption in its continuity, with or without a gap in the mesentery. Stenosis (narrowing of the lumen) causes dilation proximal to the obstruction and luminal collapse distal to it.

Malrotation

Malrotation is the term used to describe the spectrum of abnormalities of embryonic development of the midgut associated with abnormal intestinal rotation or fixation, or both. The incidence is between 1 in 500 and 1 in 600 live births.[22]

PATHOPHYSIOLOGY In malrotation, the small intestine lacks a normal posterior attachment. The mobile loops of intestine can twist upon themselves (volvulus), leading to symptoms of bowel obstruction (see Figure 36-4). The twisting can partly or completely occlude the superior mesenteric artery, causing infarction and necrosis of the entire midgut. Peritoneal (Ladd) bands may press against and obstruct the duodenum.

CLINICAL MANIFESTATIONS Most cases of malrotation-associated volvulus and infarction develop during the neonatal period (90% are younger than 1 year). Some develop during childhood or adulthood. Classic symptoms in infants are intermittent or persistent bile-stained vomiting after feedings and epigastric distention. Dehydration and electrolyte imbalance may occur rapidly. Fever usually ensues with pain and scanty stools. Diarrhea and bloody stools are associated with progressive volvulus, vascular compression, and infarction of the intestine. Intermittent or partial volvulus is more common in older children and adults. It may be asymptomatic or cause minor abdominal discomfort and be discovered during unrelated abdominal surgery.

EVALUATION AND TREATMENT Diagnosis of malrotation with volvulus and infarction is based on clinical manifestations. Radiographic films of the abdomen and barium studies show intestinal gas bubbles and distention proximal to the site of obstruction.

Treatment includes laparoscopic or open surgery to reduce the volvulus.[23] Necrotic bowel may be resected and a primary anastomosis performed. An enterostomy may be created. Most children have a good outcome; however, there is risk for adhesion-related bowel obstruction in about 15% of cases. Resection of large segments of the small intestine results in short bowel syndrome and its long-term sequelae.[24,25]

Meckel Diverticulum

Diverticula are small outpouches, or sacs, that have formed and pushed outward through weak spots of the intestinal wall. Meckel diverticulum is a remnant of the embryonic yolk sac and the most prevalent congenital abnormality of the small bowel (usually in the ileum). It is a true diverticulum in that it contains all layers of the intestinal wall. Ectopic gastric mucosal cells are contained in the diverticuli and may cause peptic ulcer and painless bleeding or mimic colonic diverticulitis. Often referred to as "the rule of 2s," a Meckel diverticulum occurs in approximately 2% of the general population, is typically located within 2 feet of the ileocecal valve (on the antimesenteric border of the ileum), is 2 inches in length on average, and its clinical symptomatology often occurs before 2 years of age.[26] Although most Meckel diverticuli are asymptomatic, the most common symptom is painless rectal bleeding. Intestinal obstruction, intussusception, and volvulus can occur, more commonly in adults. Diagnosis is made by symptom presentation and radionucleotide scintigraphy. The scan shows the gastric mucosal cells in the diverticuli. Treatment in those with symptoms is surgical resection.[27-30]

> **✓ QUICK CHECK 37-1**
> 1. What structures are affected in cleft palate and cleft lip?
> 2. What is esophageal atresia?
> 3. What produces pyloric stenosis?

Meconium Syndromes

Meconium is a substance that fills the entire intestine before birth. It is a dark greenish mass of desquamated cells, mucus, and bile that accumulates in the bowel of a fetus and is typically discharged during the first 12 to 48 hours after birth.

Meconium ileus (MI) is an intestinal obstruction in the neonatal period caused by meconium formed in utero that is abnormally thick and sticky, which leads to a partial or complete obstruction at the level of the terminal ileum. There are two forms of MI: simple and complex. Complex MI is a surgical emergency and there is usually an associated gastrointestinal pathology, such as bowel atresia, necrosis, or perforation. MI occurs in up to 20% of infants with cystic fibrosis, and is thought to result from abnormal mucus production in the intestine or impaired pancreatic enzymes, or both[31,32] (see Chapter 28 and p. 956).

Meconium plug syndrome (MPS), also termed functional immaturity of the colon, is a transient disorder of the newborn colon characterized by delayed passage (>24 to 48 hours) of meconium and intestinal dilatation. Meconium disease (MD) is often associated with severe prematurity and low birth weight. It results from a combination of extremely sticky meconium in the colon or terminal ileum and poor intestinal motility, resulting in mechanical bowel obstruction. In both MPS and MD, plugs of meconium are found in the distal ileum and proximal colon, resulting in obstruction of passage of meconium from the rectum.

Distal intestinal obstruction syndrome (DIOS), formerly called meconium ileus equivalent, is seen in about 7.4% of children and adults with cystic fibrosis.[33] It is characterized by complete or incomplete intestinal obstruction of viscid fecal accumulation in the terminal ileum and proximal colon.[34]

PATHOPHYSIOLOGY The terminal ileum is plugged with thick, viscous meconium resulting from the formation of an insoluble, calcium-glycoprotein compound in abnormal mucus. The segment of the ileum proximal to the obstruction is distended with liquid contents, and its walls may be hypertrophied. The segment distal to the obstruction is collapsed and filled with small pellets of pale-colored stool. Meconium in the obstructed segment has the consistency of thick syrup or glue. Peristalsis fails to propel this viscous material through the ileum, and it becomes impacted. Volvulus, atresia, or perforation of the bowel sometimes accompanies meconium ileus.

CLINICAL MANIFESTATIONS Abdominal distention usually develops during the first few hours after birth. As air is swallowed, the distention increases and the infant begins to vomit bile-stained material. Infants with cystic fibrosis may have signs of pulmonary involvement, such as tachypnea, intercostal retractions, and grunting respirations. The distended abdomen shows patterns of dilated intestinal loops that feel doughlike when palpated. Some of the loops contain scattered, firm, movable masses. Despite hyperactive peristalsis, the rectal ampulla is empty.

EVALUATION AND TREATMENT Radiologic examination confirms the presence of meconium in the ileum or ileocecum. The sweat test measures the amount of chloride in the sweat, is performed to detect or rule out cystic fibrosis, and is accurate in 90% of infants. Defective chloride channels in cystic fibrosis cause increased chloride concentration in sweat. About 50% of cases are complicated with volvulus or perforation. In most cases, the obstruction is relieved by intestinal lavage and administration of oral laxatives.[34,35] If this is not possible, the meconium is removed surgically.[36] Survival of infants with simple meconium ileus is improving, with rates approaching 100%. Mortality of infants with complex meconium ileus with perforation and subsequent peritonitis or septicemia is about 70%.[31,35] DIOS is treated with hydration and stool softeners.

Idiopathic Intestinal Pseudo-obstruction

Idiopathic intestinal pseudo-obstruction is a disorder of impaired intestinal motility. The pseudo-obstruction is caused by nerve or peristaltic muscle dysfunction that affects the movement of food, fluid, or air through the intestine. Children present with abdominal swelling or bloating, crampy abdominal pain, nausea, vomiting, constipation, or diarrhea. Idiopathic intestinal pseudo-obstruction is difficult to diagnose and treatment includes intestinal decompression, nutritional support, and symptom management.[37-39]

Hirschsprung Disease

Hirschsprung disease, or aganglionic megacolon, is a functional obstruction of the colon. It is the most common cause of colon obstruction, accounting for about one third of all gastrointestinal obstructions in infants. The incidence is approximately 1 in 5000 live births, and varies among ethnic groups. There is a predominance in males. Hirschsprung disease is a multifactorial malformation.[40-42]

PATHOPHYSIOLOGY   Hirschsprung disease is characterized by the absence of parasympathetic intrinsic ganglion cells in the submucosal and myenteric plexuses along with the absence of peristaltic movement in the bowels (see Figure 35-13 for normal colon structure). In 80% of cases, the aganglionic segment is limited to the rectal end of the sigmoid colon. In rare cases, the entire colon lacks ganglion cells. The abnormally innervated colon impairs fecal movements, causing the proximal colon to become distended—hence the term megacolon (Figure 37-3).

CLINICAL MANIFESTATIONS   The infant typically becomes symptomatic during the first 24 to 72 hours after birth with delayed passage of meconium. Mild to severe constipation is the usual manifestation of Hirschsprung disease, with poor feeding, poor weight gain, and progressive abdominal distention. However, diarrhea may be the first sign because only water can travel around the impacted feces.

The most serious complication in the neonatal period is enterocolitis related to fecal impaction. Bowel dilation stretches and partly occludes the encircling blood and lymphatic vessels, causing edema, ischemia, infarction of the mucosa, and significant outflow of fluid into the bowel lumen. Copious liquid stools result. Infarction and destruction of the mucosa enable enteric microorganisms to penetrate the bowel wall. Frequently, gram-negative sepsis occurs, accompanied by fever and vomiting. Severe and rapid fluid and electrolyte changes may take place, causing hypovolemic or septic shock or death.

EVALUATION AND TREATMENT   Radiocontrast enema and anorectal manometry are screening tools for the diagnosis of Hirschsprung disease. The definitive diagnosis is made by rectal biopsy showing an absence of ganglion cells in the submucosa of the colon.[43] Surgery is the definitive treatment in all cases of Hirschsprung disease. In general, the prognosis of congenital megacolon is satisfactory for children who undergo surgical treatment. Bowel training may be prolonged; most children achieve bowel continence before puberty but some have long-term constipation or fecal incontinence.[44-48]

Anorectal Malformations

Anorectal malformations (ARMs) represent a spectrum of anomalies of the anus and rectum (Figure 37-4). ARMs include anorectal stenosis, imperforate anus, anorectal atresia, and rectal atresia. Persistent cloaca is the most severe type of anorectal malformation and occurs exclusively in girls. The rectum, urethra, and vagina fail to develop separately; instead, they drain through a single, common channel onto the perineum.[49-51] Approximately 40% of infants with anorectal malformations have other developmental anomalies (i.e., Down syndrome, Hirschsprung disease, and duodenal atresia).[52]

Most ARMs are identified in routine physical examination during the neonatal period. Types of imperforate anus include an anal opening that is narrow or misplaced, a membrane (covering) may be present over the anal opening, the rectum may not connect to the anus, the rectum may connect to part of the urinary tract or to the reproductive system through an opening called a fistula, or the anal opening is not present. Treatment recommendations depend on the type of imperforate anus, the presence and type of associated abnormalities, and the child's overall health status. Anal stenosis can be treated by dilations. Infants with an imperforate anus and other anorectal malformations require surgical correction. Overall mortality is approximately 10%. Lower lesions have better functional outcomes than higher lesions.[51,53]

Acquired Impairment of Motility
Gastroesophageal Reflux

Gastroesophageal reflux (GER) is the passage of gastric contents into the esophagus independent of swallowing. GER is normal and nonpathologic in healthy infants and may be asymptomatic or exhibited by regurgitation and vomiting.[54] The frequency of GER is highest in premature infants and occurs in about 70% of healthy infants; however, GER resolves without treatment in 95% of infants by 12 to 14 months of age.[55] **Gastroesophageal reflux disease (GERD)** is different from GER and occurs when it is the cause of troublesome symptoms or complications, or both, described as esophageal or extraesophageal in nature.[56] Children at greatest risk for complicated GERD are those with prematurity, neurologic impairment, esophageal atresia, obesity, hiatal hernia, achalasia, chronic lung diseases, and certain genetic disorders, including cystic fibrosis.

PATHOPHYSIOLOGY   GERD is influenced by genetic, environmental, anatomic, hormonal, and neurogenic factors. Although transient lower esophageal sphincter relaxations (TLESRs) are the most common pathophysiologic cause of GER, inadequate adaptation of sphincter tone to changes in abdominal pressure also may be implicated. Factors that maintain lower esophageal sphincter integrity in children include the location of the gastroesophageal junction in a high-pressure zone

Distended
sigmoid
colon

Aganglionic portion

Rectum

FIGURE 37-3 Hirschsprung Disease.

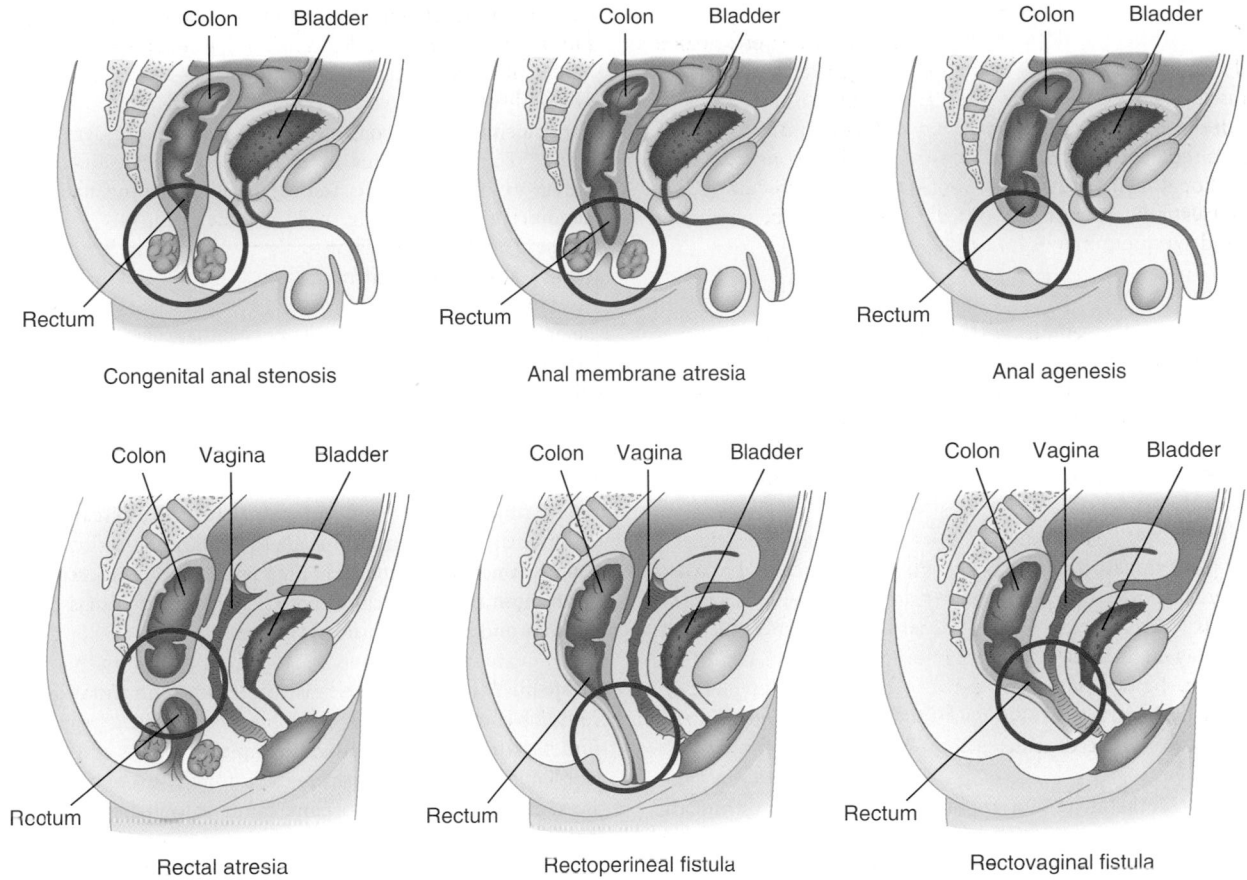

FIGURE 37-4 Anorectal Stenosis and Imperforate Anus. NOTE: With the exception of the rectovaginal fistula, all of the malformations shown occur in both males and females.

within the abdomen, mucosal gathering within the sphincter, and the angle at which the esophagus is inserted into the stomach. Reflux persists if any one of these pressure-maintaining factors is altered. Other mediators of GER are esophageal peristalsis or clearance, mucosal resistance that mediates the noxiousness of the refluxate, and delayed gastric emptying. Reflux of acidic gastric contents results in inflammation of the esophageal epithelium (esophagitis) and stimulation of the vomiting reflex.

Esophageal inflammation resulting from GERD is differentiated from eosinophilic esophagitis (EoE), which can occur in children. EoE is thought to be an allergic esophageal disease involving both immediate and delayed hypersensitivity reactions to food ingestion. An eosinophilic infiltrate is associated with inflammation of the entire esophagus that is nonresponsive to acid-suppression therapy. The hallmark symptoms of EoE are dysphagia, food refusal or impaction, and throat and chest pain. Treatment involves food elimination and oral steroids.[57]

CLINICAL MANIFESTATIONS The clinical manifestations of GERD include excessive regurgitation or vomiting; food refusal/anorexia; unexplained crying, choking, or gagging; sleep disturbance; dysphagia; and abdominal or epigastric pain, or both.[56] Esophageal complications of GER can be significant, such as esophagitis, hemorrhage, stricture, Barrett esophagus (metaplasia) (see Chapter 36) and, rarely, adenocarcinoma. Extraesophageal symptoms include cough and wheezing, laryngitis, pharyngitis, dental erosions, sinusitis, recurrent otitis media, and Sandifer syndrome (a neurologic disorder).[58] This constellation of symptoms is often indistinguishable from those of cow's milk protein allergy, which may coexist with or overlap GERD.

EVALUATION AND TREATMENT The clinical manifestations are often adequate to confirm a diagnosis of GERD. Esophageal pH monitoring with a probe for 24 hours and endoscopy are routinely used for diagnosis.

Normal physiologic GER resolves without treatment. In breast-fed babies, maternal elimination of cow's milk protein is recommended whereas formula-fed infants may require feeding volume and frequency adjustments using extensively hydrolyzed protein or amino acid–based formulas. Using thickened feedings has shown to improve symptoms of GER. Prone positioning is only recommended for infants older than 1 year of age because of the risk of sudden infant death syndrome. Lifestyle changes for children and adolescents include weight loss, smoking cessation, and avoidance of caffeine, chocolate, alcohol, and spicy foods.

Medications are used to buffer or decrease gastric acid secretion, increase motility, or increase lower esophageal sphincter pressure to treat GER.[59] If no improvement is seen with medical management or the child has life-threatening events with reflux, an antireflux surgical procedure, including gastropexy and fundoplication, is performed. More evidence is needed to evaluate long-term surgical outcomes.[60]

Intussusception

Intussusception is the telescoping of a proximal segment of intestine into a distal segment, causing an obstruction. It is the most common cause of small bowel obstruction in children and occurs in about 56 of 100,000 children yearly in the United States.[61] Most cases occur between 5 and 7 months of age. Intussusception is more common in males and can occur in children with polyps or tumors (lead points),

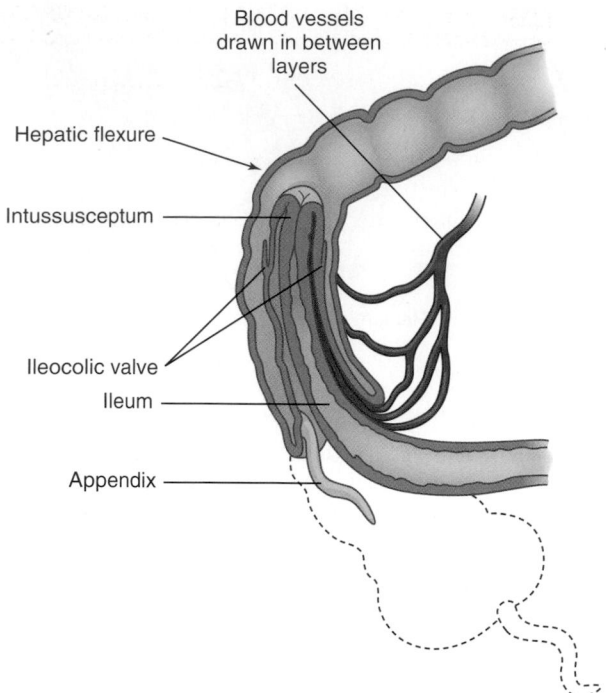

Blood vessels drawn in between layers

Hepatic flexure

Intussusceptum

Ileocolic valve

Ileum

Appendix

FIGURE 37-5 Ileocolic Intussusception.

cystic fibrosis, Meckel diverticulum, intestinal adhesions, or immediately after abdominal surgery.[62] There is a small risk of intussusception associated with rotovirus vaccination but the vaccine is generally safe.[63]

PATHOPHYSIOLOGY   In intussusception, the ileum commonly telescopes into the cecum and part of the ascending colon by collapsing through the ileocecal valve, although intussusception can occur anywhere from the duodenum to the rectum. The proximal portion of the intestine (the intussusceptum) collapses into the distal portion (the intussuscipiens) in the direction of peristaltic flow (Figure 37-5). The intussusceptum then drags its mesentery into the enveloping lumen, causing an intussusception. Initially, the mesentery is constricted, obstructing venous return. Compression of the mesenteric vessels between the two layers of intestinal wall and at the U-shaped angle at either end of the intussusceptum leads within hours to venous stasis, engorgement, edema, exudation, and further vascular compression. The tension of the mesentery on the intussusceptum tends to arch the bowel in a curve having its center at the mesenteric root. Edema and compression obstruct the flow of chyme through the intestine. Unless the intussusception is treated, ischemia and necrosis ensue.

CLINICAL MANIFESTATIONS   The classic symptoms of intussusception include colicky abdominal pain, irritability, knees drawn to the chest, abdominal mass, vomiting, and bloody (currant-jelly) stools. All of these symptoms may not occur, and intussusception has been discovered incidentally by computed tomography (CT) or magnetic resonance imaging (MRI) scan for other indications. Abdominal tenderness and distention develop as intestinal obstruction becomes more acute.

EVALUATION AND TREATMENT   Diagnosis is based on clinical manifestations, onset of symptoms, and ultrasonographic or radiologic imaging studies. An enema reduction is usually effective for large bowel intussusception and avoids the progression to ischemia and perforation. Laparotomy remains the treatment of choice for small bowel intussusception.[64] Untreated intussusception in infants is nearly always

fatal. Most infants recover if the intussusception is reduced within 24 hours.[65]

Appendicitis

Appendicitis is common in children between the ages of 10 and 11 years.[66] The mechanisms of disease, symptoms, and treatment are similar to those for adults and can be reviewed in Chapter 36.

> ✔ **QUICK CHECK 37-2**
> 1. Describe the pathologic defect in meconium ileus.
> 2. Why is there poor bowel motility with Hirschsprung disease?
> 3. Describe the defect in intussusception.

Impairment of Digestion, Absorption, and Nutrition
Cystic Fibrosis

Cystic fibrosis (CF) is an autosomal recessive disease that involves multiple organ systems and leads to death at an earlier age, although new treatments are extending life expectancy. This section focuses on gastrointestinal complications of CF; Chapter 28 discusses CF's epidemiology and pulmonary involvement.

PATHOPHYSIOLOGY   The gastrointestinal presentation of CF is caused by a dysfunction of the CF transmembrane regulator (CFTR) protein, which is located on epithelial membranes and regulates chloride and sodium ion channels. It is found throughout the airways, sweat glands, digestive tract, pancreas, hepatobiliary system, and reproductive system (also called *mucoviscidosis* or *fibrocystic disease of the pancreas*). The hallmark pathophysiologic triad of CF includes obstruction, infection, and inflammation that are evident throughout the gastrointestinal tract and within the airways. The full spectrum of involvement is summarized in Table 37-1.

Dysfunction of the CFTR protein results in altered sodium, chloride, and potassium resorption, all of which remain external to the surface of the epithelial membrane with reduced clearance from tubular structures lined by affected epithelia.[67] Maldigestion of proteins, carbohydrates, fats, and fat-soluble vitamins occurs because mucus obstruction of the pancreatic ducts blocks the flow of pancreatic enzymes, causing intestinal malabsorption and degenerative and fibrotic changes in the pancreas and gastrointestinal tract. Diabetes mellitus commonly develops from damage to insulin-producing beta cells and insulin resistance.[68]

CLINICAL MANIFESTATIONS   Clinical manifestations are summarized in Table 37-1. Gastrointestinal symptoms often precede pulmonary manifestations. Approximately 85% of those with CF present early in life with pancreatic insufficiency (PI). PI is the cause of nutrient malabsorption and failure to thrive in children with CF. Steatorrhea and abdominal distention are common symptoms with potential sequelae that include distal intestinal obstruction syndrome (DIOS) (see p. 953), fibrotic colonopathy, or focal biliary cirrhosis. Children who are pancreatic sufficient (PS) are at greater risk of developing pancreatitis.[69] Those with CF are at greater risk for many gastrointestinal complications, including gastrointestinal cancers and hepatobiliary abnormalities, which may lead to pancreatic transplant or death.

EVALUATION AND TREATMENT   All states in the United States screen newborns for cystic fibrosis using a blood test to detect immunoreactive trypsinogen. Genetic screening and the sweat test are required for diagnosis. Evaluation of pancreatic sufficiency also is essential. The extent of pancreatic function is determined by 72-hour fecal fat

TABLE 37-1 Pathophysiology, Clinical Manifestations, and Complications of Cystic Fibrosis

Organ Involved	Secretory Dysfunction	Clinical Manifestations	Complications
Sweat glands	Elevated concentration of sodium and chloride in sweat	Hyponatremia; hypochloremia	Heat prostration; shock
Intestine			
Newborn	Viscid meconium	Meconium ileus with intestinal obstruction	Meconium peritonitis; growth failure
Older child and adult	Inspissated (dried out) mucofecal masses (intestinal sludging)	Partial intestinal obstruction with severe cramping pains	Volvulus (obstruction), intussusception (prolapse) Distal intestinal obstruction syndrome Growth failure
Pancreas (enzyme deficiency)	Inspissation and precipitation of pancreatic secretions, causing obstruction of pancreatic ducts Insulin deficiency	Absence of pancreatic enzymes, causing malabsorption of food and fatty, bulky stools Decreased vitamin A, D, E, and K absorption Glucose intolerance	Hypoproteinemia; iron deficiency anemia; malnutrition Vitamins A, D, E, and K deficiency and rectal prolapse Diabetes mellitus (see Chapter 19)
Liver	Inspissation and precipitation of bile and biliary system	Focal biliary cirrhosis; shrunken, "hobnail" liver; fatty liver	Portal hypertension with esophageal varices and hematemesis
Salivary glands	Inspissation and precipitation of secretions in small ducts of submaxillary and sublingual salivary glands	Mild patchy fibrosis of salivary glands	None
Respiratory Tract			
Paranasal structures	Viscid mucus	Retention of mucus; clouding seen on sinus roentgenograms	Mucopyoceles (pus accumulations) with nasal deformity or orbital cavity extension
Nose	Nasal polyps	Obstruction of nasal air flow	Sinusitis
Lungs	Viscid mucus in bronchioles and bronchi	Obstruction of bronchioles causing bronchiolectasis, bronchiectasis, and chronic lung infection	Atelectasis, hemoptysis; pneumothorax; cor pulmonale; respiratory failure
Reproductive Tract			
Male	Viscid genital tract secretions during embryologic development, causing failure of formation of normal vas deferens; aspermia	Sterility	None
Female	Distention of endocervical epithelial cells with cytoplasmic mucin	Decreased fertility	Polypoid cervicitis (cervical inflammation) while taking oral contraceptives

Data from Marcdante KJ, Kliegman RM: *Nelson essentials of pediatrics*, ed 7, Philadelphia, 2015, Saunders.

measurements, which are not easily obtained. Therefore, the most common measurement of fat malabsorption is fecal elastase. A serum test for trypsinogen also can be used to detect pancreatic insufficiency in children older than 8 years of age.

The goal of treatment for PI is to reduce malabsorption of nutrients and improve growth. Most children with CF take pancreatic enzyme replacement therapy (PERT) for the rest of their lives. PERT is administered before or with every meal, snack, or enteral feeding supplementation. High doses of PERT are associated with DIOS; therefore, minimal effective doses are indicated. High-caloric, high-protein diets with frequent snacks and vitamin supplements are used to treat malnutrition. Nutritional status and growth should be carefully monitored, and growth hormone may be included with nutritional supplements.[70]

Celiac Disease

Celiac disease (CD), formerly called celiac sprue, is an autoimmune disease that damages small intestinal villous epithelium when there is ingestion of gluten (gliadin), the protein component of cereal grains. CD is a common multiorgan disease with a strong genetic predisposition associated with human leukocyte antigen DQ2 (HLA-DQ2) and HLA-DQ8.[71] The disease has a prevalence of about 1% worldwide, although evidence suggests only 10% to 15% of the population have been diagnosed and treated.[72] Nonceliac gluten sensitivity (GS), or wheat allergy, should not be confused with CD; although it presents similarly after the ingestion of gluten, the individual does not have positive autoantibodies or classic intestinal villous atrophy but instead has variable HLA status with similar symptoms as CD.[73]

The pathogenesis of CD is complex and involves genetic and immunologic factors. Environmental factors include early infections, gut microbiota in infants, feeding patterns, and timing and amount of gluten. CD presents with greater frequency in children with type 1 diabetes mellitus, autoimmune thyroid or liver disease, Down syndrome, Turner syndrome, Williams syndrome, selective IgA deficiency, Addison disease, and first-degree relatives with CD.[72]

PATHOPHYSIOLOGY The major pathophysiologic characteristic of celiac disease is T-cell–mediated autoimmune injury to the small intestinal epithelial cells of genetically susceptible individuals. There is atrophy and flattening of villi, crypt hyperplasia in the upper small

FIGURE 37-6 Pathophysiology of Celiac Disease.

intestine, and malabsorption of most nutrients in the presence of cereal gluten, particularly wheat, rye, and barley (Figure 37-6).[74]

Damage to the mucosa of the duodenum and jejunum exacerbates malabsorption. The secretion of intestinal hormones, such as secretin and cholecystokinin-pancreozymin, may be diminished; consequently, secretion of pancreatic enzymes and expulsion of bile from the gallbladder decrease, contributing to malabsorption.

Destruction of mucosal cells causes inflammation, and water and electrolytes are secreted, leading to watery diarrhea. Potassium loss leads to muscle weakness. Magnesium and calcium malabsorption can cause seizures or tetany. Unabsorbed fatty acids combine with calcium, and secondary hyperparathyroidism increases phosphorus excretion, resulting in bone reabsorption. Calcium is no longer able to bind oxalate in the intestine and is absorbed, which causes hyperoxaluria. Gallbladder function may be abnormal, and bile salt conjugation may decrease.

Fat malabsorption in the jejunum is the major cause of steatorrhea (fatty stools). Deficiencies of fat-soluble vitamins are common in children with CD. Vitamin K malabsorption leads to hypoprothrombinemia. In one third of cases, iron and folic acid malabsorption is manifested as cheilosis, anemia, and a smooth red tongue. Vitamin B_{12} absorption is impaired in those with extensive ileal disease, and folate and iron deficiencies are common.

CLINICAL MANIFESTATIONS The onset of clinical manifestations of celiac disease depends on the age of the infant when gluten-containing substances are added to the diet. Although in 50% of affected children onset occurs by 18 months of age, it is not uncommon to be diagnosed later in life. Severity of symptoms can vary tremendously and many children older than 3 years of age present with nongastrointestinal symptoms.[72] Gastrointestinal and extraintestinal symptoms of CD are listed in Box 37-1.

An unusual complication of celiac disease in infancy is celiac crisis. Celiac crisis is characterized by severe diarrhea, dehydration, and hypoproteinemia as a result of malabsorption and protein loss.

BOX 37-1	Symptoms of Celiac Disease
Gastrointestinal Symptoms	**Extraintestinal Symptoms**
Diarrhea	Fatigue
Abdominal pain and distention	Weight loss, growth failure
Vomiting	Delayed puberty
	Dermatitis herpetiformis
Anorexia	Dental enamel hypoplasia, aphthous stomatitis
Constipation	Arthritis
	Osteoporosis
	Fractures
	Neurologic manifestations: ataxia, neuropathy, seizures

Data from Ferraz EG et al: *Pediatr Dent* 34(7):485-488, 2012; Guandalini S, Assiri A: *JAMA Pediatr* 168(3):274, 2014; Hadjivassiliou M et al: *Handb Clin Neurol* 120:607-619, 2014.

EVALUATION AND TREATMENT Diagnosis includes confirmation with serologic autoantibody measurement against tissue transglutaminase IgA (tTG IgA) (most sensitive and specific), anti-endomysium (EMA) IgA, or deaminated gliadin peptides (DGPs), which are more sensitive in children younger than 2 years of age. A negative genetic screening for HLA haplotypes would rule out CD.[75] Currently, there is controversy regarding treatment for those children who are HLA-positive but asymptomatic. If an autoantibody or genetic screen is positive, a small intestinal biopsy is obtained to detect the classic mucosal changes caused by gluten-induced enteropathy. A wide variety of screening tests for malabsorption also may be useful. Even though there are very useful screening tools to diagnose CD, many children remain undiagnosed.

Treatment consists of lifelong adherence to a gluten-free diet (GFD), which includes elimination of wheat, rye, barley, and malt.

Lactose intolerance also may be present from damage to villi; therefore, lactose (milk sugar) also may be excluded from the diet but should be resumed after treatment. Infants are routinely given vitamin D, iron, and folic acid supplements to treat deficiencies. Bone mineral density (BMD) screening is required. For most children the long-term prognosis is excellent. There is an increased incidence of malignant disease, particularly lymphoma, in individuals who fail to respond or are nonadherent to a GFD.[76]

Malnutrition

Pediatric malnutrition is an imbalance between nutrient requirements and intake that results in energy, protein, and micronutrient deficits that negatively impact growth and development. Malnutrition also involves impaired absorption and altered nutrient utilization. Kwashiorkor (deficiency of dietary protein) and marasmus (all forms of inadequate nutrient intake) are the two most common types of malnutrition in children. Collectively they are known as protein-energy malnutrition (PEM). PEM describes the effects of malnutrition but not the etiology or interactions that contribute to nutrient depletion.

Both kwashiorkor and marasmus are states of long-term starvation and are the result of widespread nutritional deficiencies among children in developing countries and economically destitute populations, particularly when associated with human immunodeficiency virus (HIV) infection.[77] Kwashiorkor usually occurs in infants or children from 1 to 4 years of age who have been weaned from breast milk to a high-starch, protein-deficient diet. The death rate of kwashiorkor is higher than that for marasmus.

Marasmus can occur at any age but it is common in children younger than 1 year. In marasmus, starvation is attributable to lack of protein and carbohydrates, and in neglected children it can have a psychogenic basis. In developing countries and impoverished populations, early weaning of breast-fed infants to overdiluted commercial formulas is a risk factor for marasmus.

Although PEM is common in developing countries, it is underestimated in hospitalized children. A new paradigm used to define pediatric malnutrition and includes etiology (illness or environmental), identification of pathogenesis and chronicity, associations with inflammation, and resulting impact on functional outcomes.[78] PEM is a known complication of chronic diseases, such as chronic fever; infectious diseases like tuberculosis; malignancy; digestive and malabsorptive disorders; cardiac, pulmonary, renal, and neurologic diseases; burns or hypermetabolic states; anorexia and bulimia; and psychogenic illness. Treatments such as radiation therapy and chemotherapy also can contribute to malnutrition. PEM contributes to hospital-acquired conditions (HACs), longer time on mechanical ventilation, increased hospital length of stay, and increased morbidity and mortality rates.[79]

PATHOPHYSIOLOGY The pathogenesis of kwashiorkor is uncertain but includes inadequate dietary protein, leaky gut syndrome (compromised gut barrier), and intestinal inflammation. Recent studies are now implicating alterations in gut microbiota as the central cause of kwashiorkor.[78] There is evidence that children with kwashiorkor show stunting of gut microbiota maturation, which may generate products, such as inhibitors of enzymes in the tricarboxylic acid cycles, that compromise energy metabolism.[80] Support for this theory of causation includes an antibiotic treatment study that demonstrated significant improvement in recovery and mortality rates of malnourished Malawian children.[81]

The lack of sufficient plasma proteins results in generalized edema with a substantial loss of potassium. The liver swells with stored fat because no hepatic proteins are synthesized to form and release lipoproteins. Pancreatic atrophy and fibrosis may be present. Kwashiorkor also causes malabsorption, reduced bone density, and impaired renal function. If the condition is not reversed, the prognosis is very poor.

The metabolic response in marasmus is different, allowing sustained protein and lipid supply during periods of decreased dietary intake. Metabolic processes, including liver function, are preserved, but growth is severely retarded. Caloric intake is too low to support protein synthesis for growth or the storage of fat. Muscle and fat wasting occur and anemia is common and can be severe.[82]

CLINICAL MANIFESTATIONS Children with kwashiorkor have appropriate stores of protein and fat that are mobilized inadequately. They have marked generalized edema, dermatoses, hypopigmented hair, distended abdomen, hepatomegaly, and almost normal weight for age (because of edema). Children with marasmus demonstrate greater wasting of protein and fat stores yet have improved survival. Marasmus is characterized by muscle wasting, fatty liver and hepatomegaly, diarrhea, dermatosis, low hemoglobin level, and infection. There is loss of subcutaneous fat and an absence of edema. Both conditions lead to delays in physical, behavioral, and cognitive development and academic performance. Lastly, micronutrient deficiencies, especially with zinc, selenium, iron, and antioxidant vitamins, can lead to immune deficiency and infections. Severe vitamin A deficiency commonly results in blindness.[83]

EVALUATION AND TREATMENT Evaluation of PEM is based on nutritional history and clinical manifestations, including anthropometric measurements. Laboratory monitoring is used to assess for macro- and micronutrient deficiencies, aminotransaminase alterations, and response to refeeding. The provision of deficient nutrients will resolve clinical symptoms in 4 to 6 weeks. Use of antibiotics has been shown to improve recovery of PEM and decrease mortality.[84] Developmental sequelae of PEM may be irreversible; therefore early intervention is recommended. Nutritional rehabilitation with appropriate environmental stimulation for infants and young children has been shown to resolve or improve cerebral shrinkage, physical growth, and psychomotor development.

Failure to Thrive or Growth Faltering

Failure to thrive (FTT) or growth faltering (GF) is a physical sign demonstrating that a child is receiving inadequate nutrition for optimal growth and development. It is manifested as a deceleration in weight gain, a low weight/height or BMI ratio, or a low weight/height/head circumference ratio. FTT is a common problem and can present at any time in childhood.[85] Approximately 80% of children with FTT present before 18 months of age.[85]

PATHOPHYSIOLOGY Currently, there is a move away from describing FTT as organic versus nonorganic; instead, it is considered a multifactorial condition that includes biologic, psychosocial, and environmental contributions that are illness related or nonillness related (Box 37-2). An underlying medical condition is never found in more than 80% of cases of FTT. Categories of FTT include inadequate caloric intake, inadequate caloric absorption, or excessive caloric expenditure. Infants and children are at risk for FTT if their parents or primary caregivers are unable to provide nurturance.

CLINICAL MANIFESTATIONS Clinical manifestations of FTT are delayed growth accompanied by manifestations of malnutrition or an underlying disease, or both. Infants who present with FTT frequently have feeding problems. Symptoms include delayed growth; pallid or dry, cracked skin; sparse hair; poorly developed musculature; decreased subcutaneous fat; and swollen abdomen with malabsorption, diarrhea, anorexia, and signs of vitamin deficiencies such as rickets. Social or emotional manifestations include reduced energy level, reduced responsiveness and interaction with the environment, social isolation, spasticity and rigidity when held or touched, inability to make eye contact or smile, refusal to eat, and rejection of foods. There may be long-term adverse effects on cognitive, behavioral, and academic performance.[86]

EVALUATION AND TREATMENT FTT is suggested if a child falls below the 3rd percentile for weight, or shows stagnation in length or weight.[87] Underlying medical conditions are evaluated. If illness is ruled out, a thorough review of psychosocial, emotional, and environmental components of care is necessary. Screening tools are available to assist with evaluation of nutrition status and to guide therapy, particularly in hospitalized children.[88]

Treatment of FTT includes treating an underlying illness if found, increasing volume or caloric density of formula, increasing frequency of breast-feeding (if found to be insufficient), structuring meals and snacks, and adding high-calorie foods and additives. Eliminating fruit juice, soda, or excessive milk also will improve appetite and absorption of nutrients. Medications are used to stimulate appetite. Nutrient deficiencies are supplemented. If unable to gain weight, an oral enteral supplement may be added to the diet or a nasogastric or gastrostomy tube can be used to supplement oral intake.

If the cause is not medical, management then involves the immediate total care of the child and measures to address (1) the psychosocial and emotional problems of the caregivers and (2) parent-child interactions. Counseling, parental modeling, and long-term family support are sometimes required.[89]

Hospital admission and evaluation is recommended if the diagnosis is unclear or the child is in nutritional or emotional jeopardy. Eating patterns, food preferences, caloric intake, and family interactions can be assessed and treatment plans implemented during the hospital stay.

Necrotizing Enterocolitis

Necrotizing enterocolitis (NEC) is an ischemic, inflammatory condition that causes bowel necrosis and perforation. NEC is not a specific diagnosis but a constellation of signs and symptoms with several proposed etiologies. It is the most common severe neonatal gastrointestinal emergency that predominantly affects the smallest and most premature infants.[90,91] Approximately 12% of infants born weighing less than 1500 g will develop NEC; of those, about 30% will not survive.[92] Isolated or focal intestinal perforation is sometimes confused with NEC and generally is not accompanied by an inflammatory component or by diffuse necrosis.[93]

PATHOPHYSIOLOGY The exact etiology of NEC is unclear. Factors contributing to the development of NEC include infections, abnormal bacterial colonization, intestinal ischemia, immature immune responses, exaggerated inflammatory responses, immature intestinal motility and barrier function, perinatal stress, effects of medications and feeding practices, and genetic predisposition. The immature mucosal barrier delays digestion and motility is slower, allowing for the accumulation of noxious substances that damage the intestine, increase permeability, and increase the risk for infection. Translocation of intestinal bacteria and other substances contributes to injury, inflammation, and development of systemic inflammatory disease. Immature intestinal innate immunity and an unfavorable balance between normal and pathogenic bacteria promote intestinal inflammation and release of proinflammatory cytokines. Accumulation of gas in the intestine can cause pressure that decreases blood flow, and an imbalance between vasodilator and vasoconstrictor inputs in the immature gut may lead to vasoconstriction promoting ischemia, injury, and necrosis.[94]

CLINICAL MANIFESTATIONS Manifestations of NEC usually appear suddenly and within weeks of premature birth, and sooner for term neonates. Signs and symptoms of "classic" NEC include feeding intolerance, abdominal distention and bloody stools after 8 to 10 days of age, septicemia with elevated white blood cell count, and falling platelet levels. Unstable temperature, bradycardia, and apnea are nonspecific signs. In late preterm or term infants, NEC is more likely to be associated with other predisposing factors, such as low Apgar scores, chorioamnionitis, exchange transfusions, prolonged rupture of membranes, congenital heart disease, or neural tube defects.

EVALUATION AND TREATMENT Abdominal radiographs show pneumatosis intestinalis or portal venous gas, or both. Symptoms usually progress rapidly, often within hours, from subtle signs to abdominal discoloration, intestinal perforation, and peritonitis or even death. Systemic hypotension requires intensive medical support or bowel resection, or both. A study is in progress to identify predictive biologic markers for early diagnosis.[94] Preventive strategies include encouragement of breast milk feeding, judicious fluid management to prevent vascular fluid overload, confirmation of patent ductus arteriosus (see Chapter 25), administration of arginine and glutamine supplements to support intestinal epithelial cell growth, and utilization of enteral probiotics to support normal gut bacteria.[90,95] The rapid onset of symptoms makes primary prevention difficult.

Treatments include cessation of feeding, implementation of gastric suction to decompress the intestines, maintenance of fluid and electrolyte balance, and administration of antibiotics to control sepsis. Surgical resection is the treatment of choice for perforation, and peritoneal drainage may be used as an adjunct to laparotomy.[96] Overall mortality is high, particularly for infants who have surgery.[91]

✔ QUICK CHECK 37-3

1. Why do individuals with cystic fibrosis have pancreatic insufficiency?
2. Why does loss of villi occur with gluten-sensitive enteropathy?
3. Compare kwashiorkor and marasmus.

Diarrhea

Diarrhea is an increase in the water content, volume, or frequency of stools and can be acute or chronic. Diarrhea is usually defined as three or more watery or loose stools in 24 hours.[97] Children with acute gastroenteritis often remain mildly symptomatic for up to 4 weeks; therefore, diarrhea that persists longer than 4 weeks is considered chronic. Diarrhea is a common gastrointestinal problem during infancy and early childhood and is the leading cause of death in young children, particularly among preterm infants and children in developing countries, with 760,000 deaths per year.[98,99] Severe, acute infectious diarrhea occurs one to three times during the first 3 years of life. Most episodes are self-limiting and resolve within 72 hours.

The pathophysiologic mechanisms of diarrhea in children are similar to those described for adults—osmotic, secretory, intestinal dysmotility, or inflammatory (see Chapter 36). Prolonged diarrhea is more dangerous in infants and children, however, because they have much smaller fluid reserves and more rapid peristalsis and metabolism than adults. Therefore dehydration can develop rapidly if any disturbance increases fluid secretion into the gastrointestinal lumen (secretory diarrhea), draws fluid into the lumen by osmosis (osmotic diarrhea), reduces intestinal transit time with luminal fluid retention (intestinal dysmotility), or causes inflammation that results in malabsorption and increased luminal osmotic load from nutrients, fluid, and blood, which may increase gut motility (inflammatory diarrhea).[100]

Diarrhea in Infants and Children

There are numerous causes of diarrhea in infants and young children, including bacterial and systemic infections, malabsorption syndromes, autoimmune disorders, congenital malformations, and genetic disorders.[100] Acute infection is a common cause of childhood diarrhea worldwide.

Acute infectious diarrhea in infants and young children is usually associated with viral or bacterial gastroenteritis. Viruses include rotaviruses, noroviruses, and adenoviruses. **Rotavirus** is the most common cause in young children and is associated with a higher death rate in low-income countries. Rotavirus vaccine is an effective preventive strategy.[101] Numerous bacteria or parasites can contaminate food or water and cause diarrhea. Specific bacteria can be identified using molecular analysis or stool culture. *Clostridium difficile* is often associated with previous antibiotic therapy.

Infectious diarrhea has a rapid onset, with watery stools sometimes mixed with blood, abdominal cramping, fever, vomiting, and weight loss. Severe dehydration, acidosis, and shock can occur quickly from diarrhea and vomiting.[102] Hemolytic uremic syndrome and renal failure can develop when diarrhea is associated with *Shigella* toxin and *Escherichia coli* infection (see Chapter 31). Other causes of acute diarrhea in the older child include antibiotic therapy, appendicitis, chemotherapy, inflammatory bowel disease, parasitic infestation, parenteral infections, and ingestion of toxic substances.

Treatment of diarrhea requires evaluation of cause through history, stool testing for common pathogens, and laboratory analysis. Treatment of underlying illness is warranted when identified. Other treatments include fluid and electrolyte replacement, and antibiotics if a pathogen is found. Antispasmodics may relieve abdominal cramping, and probiotics can reduce duration and improve morbidity and mortality.[103] Intravenous solutions are used only when oral solutions are not tolerated.[104] Prevention includes clean water, environmental sanitation, and good hygiene.

Primary lactose intolerance. **Lactose malabsorption** and **intolerance**, the inability to digest milk sugar, is caused by inadequate production or impaired activity of the enzyme lactase. It is a common cause of diarrhea, particularly in nonwhite children under the age of 7 years. The malabsorption of lactose results in osmotic diarrhea accompanied by abdominal pain, bloating, and flatulence. Systemic manifestations include skin disease, rheumatologic complaints, chronic

fatigue, and failure to thrive.[105] Diagnosis includes elimination of dietary lactose or implementation of hydrogen lactose breath testing. Treatment consists of reducing milk consumption or supplementing the diet with oral lactase. Some children can tolerate lactose in fermented forms, such as cheese and yogurt, or by adding soy food. Utilization of a diet low in fermentable oligosaccharides, disaccharides, and monosaccharides and polyols (FODMAPs) or administration of probiotics to alter intestinal flora has been found to be effective in lactose-intolerant irritable bowel syndrome children with persistent symptoms.[105]

DISORDERS OF THE LIVER

Disorders of Biliary Metabolism and Transport

Neonatal Jaundice

Jaundice (icterus) is a yellow pigmentation of the skin caused by an increased level of bilirubin in the bloodstream (total serum bilirubin [TSB]) that exceeds the 95th percentile for the infant's age in hours or greater than 20 mg/dl, except in the low birth weight population. Jaundice usually becomes clinically apparent when the serum bilirubin concentration is greater than 2 mg/dl (34 μmol/L). **Physiologic jaundice (hyperbilirubinemia) of the newborn**, or neonatal bilirubinemia, is a frequently encountered problem in otherwise healthy newborns caused by lack of maturity of bilirubin uptake and conjugation. Poor caloric intake or dehydration, or both, associated with inadequate breast-feeding also may contribute to the high levels of bilirubin. Although up to 60% of term newborns have clinical jaundice in the first week of life, with a higher percentage in the preterm population, few have significant underlying disease. High bilirubin levels in the newborn period can be associated with hemolytic disease, metabolic and endocrine disorders, anatomic abnormalities of the liver, and infections. For older infants and children, the most common causes of unconjugated hyperbilirubinemia are hemolytic processes resulting in bilirubin overproduction. *Pathologic jaundice* is a bilirubin concentration greater than 20 mg/dl in the newborn period associated with a severe illness, or a total serum bilirubin level that rises by more than 5 mg/dl during the newborn period.

Risk factors for development of pathologic jaundice include fetal-maternal blood type incompatibility (ABO and Rh incompatibility, hemolytic disease in the newborn), premature birth, exclusive breast-feeding in some infants, maternal age greater than or equal to 25 years, male gender, delayed meconium passage, glucose-6-phosphate dehydrogenase deficiency, and excessive birth trauma such as bruising or cephalohematomas.[106,107]

PATHOPHYSIOLOGY Pathologic jaundice results from the complex interaction of factors that cause (1) increased bilirubin production (e.g., hemolysis), (2) impaired hepatic uptake or excretion of unconjugated bilirubin, or (3) delayed maturation of liver bilirubin conjugating mechanisms.[108] The most common cause is hemolytic disease of the newborn (ABO blood incompatibility) (see Chapters 8 and 22), and all pregnant women should be tested for ABO and Rh incompatibility. Unconjugated bilirubin (indirect bilirubin) is lipid soluble and bound to albumin in the blood, and in the free form it readily crosses the blood-brain barrier in infants. Chronic bilirubin encephalopathy **(kernicterus)** is caused by the deposition of toxic, unconjugated bilirubin in brain cells and usually does not occur in healthy, full-term infants. The mechanism of injury is not clearly known. Elevated conjugated bilirubin level is a sign of underlying disease.

CLINICAL MANIFESTATIONS Physiologic jaundice develops during the second or third day after birth and usually subsides in 1 to 2 weeks in full-term infants and in 2 to 4 weeks in premature infants. After this, increasing bilirubin values and persistent jaundice indicate pathologic hyperbilirubinemia. Manifestations include yellowing of skin, dark urine, light-colored stools, and weight loss. Premature infants with respiratory distress, acidosis, or sepsis are at greater risk for kernicterus (brain damage related to unconjugated hyperbilirubinemia) and the development of athetoid cerebral palsy and speech and hearing impairment.[109]

EVALUATION AND TREATMENT Jaundice is detected by clinical assessment. Both total and direct (conjugated) bilirubin levels are monitored as described previously. Other causes of jaundice must be eliminated to confirm physiologic jaundice. Treatment depends on the degree of hyperbilirubinemia. Physiologic jaundice is commonly treated by phototherapy and several techniques are available.[110] Pathologic jaundice requires an exchange transfusion and treatment of the underlying disorder.

Biliary Atresia

Biliary atresia (BA) is a rare congenital malformation (from 1 in 8000 to 1 in 18,000 live births) characterized by the absence or obstruction of intrahepatic or extrahepatic bile ducts; the most common cause of BA is neonatal cholestasis.[111] The etiology of duct injury is not clear but is thought to be related to an embryonic, congenital, or genetic abnormality or an acquired, perinatal viral-induced progressive inflammation with innate autoimmune destruction. The disease expression is a continuum in which the principal process is one of bile duct destruction.[112] The atresia or obstruction of the bile ducts leads to plugging, inflammation, fibrosis of the bile canaliculi, and cholestasis. Progressive obstruction leads to secondary biliary cirrhosis (see Chapter 36), portal hypertension, or liver failure.

Jaundice is the primary clinical manifestation of biliary atresia, along with hepatomegaly and acholic (clay-colored) stools. Fat absorption is impaired because of the lack of bile salts. Abdominal distention caused by hepatomegaly and ascites may cause anorexia and failure to thrive. Fat-soluble vitamin (A, D, E, K) deficiencies require supplementation. Manifestations of cirrhosis and liver failure include ascites, hypoalbuminemia, hypercoagulation, pruritus, esophageal varices, and gastrointestinal bleeding that may lead to death.

Early diagnosis of biliary atresia is essential with the best outcome occurring when diagnosed and treated in the first 30 to 45 days of life. Late diagnosis of BA does not respond well to current surgical treatment. Diagnosis of BA is based on clinical manifestations, abnormal liver function tests, liver biopsy results, and intraoperative cholangiogram. Serum aminotransaminase and alkaline phosphatase levels are elevated and conjugated (direct) serum bilirubin levels rise progressively. BA can be relieved by hepatoportoenterostomy (HPE or Kasai procedure). Even with initial restoration of bile flow, however, obliteration of intrahepatic bile ducts can continue and cirrhosis results. Liver transplantation is a successful long-term therapy for biliary atresia.[113] Eighty percent of children with biliary atresia die before the age of 3 years if not treated.

Inflammatory Disorders
Hepatitis

Details related to viral hepatitis are presented in Chapter 36, including differentiation of types of viruses (see Table 36-8).

Hepatitis A virus (HAV). Approximately 30% to 50% of the reported cases of hepatitis A virus (HAV) occur in children,[114] particularly children of nursery school age. Outbreaks tend to occur in daycare centers with large numbers of children who are not toilet trained and staff members who practice poor handwashing techniques.[115]

Vertical transmission from mother to newborn or from a transfusion is rare. HAV in children is usually mild and asymptomatic, but it may involve nausea, vomiting, and diarrhea. Jaundice appears in more than 70% of older children. Almost all children recover from hepatitis A without residual liver damage. Relapse HAV occurs in 3% to 20% of individuals.[116] Vaccination programs have successfully reduced the incidence of HAV in the United States by 92% since their introduction.[117]

Hepatitis B virus (HBV). Risk factors for hepatitis B virus (HBV) include infants of mothers who are chronic hepatitis B virus (HBV) surface antigen (HBsAg) carriers, children from families that immigrated to the United States or are adopted from endemic areas, infection from HBsAg-positive household contacts, and children who abuse parenteral drugs or engage in unprotected sex. Ninety percent of newborns are infected by their mothers (vertical transmission); 25% to 50% of children between the ages of 1 and 5 years of age who are acutely infected will develop chronic infection.[118] Chronic hepatitis may develop because the infant's immune system is immature. Infected infants are at risk for cirrhosis and hepatocellular carcinoma.[119] The most serious consequence of HBV infection is fulminant hepatitis, which occurs in 1% of cases. Hepatitis D virus (HDV) infection depends on active infection with HBV. Exacerbation of HBV is more common in children with superinfected HDV. There is evidence that the risk of fulminant hepatitis is higher in individuals with combined infection of HBV and HDV than in those with HBV infection alone.[120] There also is a higher risk of hepatocellular carcinoma and increased mortality in this group. Aggressive HBV vaccination programs have reduced the incidence of HBV; HDV reduction has mirrored this response.[121] To prevent perinatal transmission of HBV, immunoprophylaxis and HBV vaccination within the first 12 hours of birth are recommended with close follow-up visits.[122] Treatment is conservative and antivirals are used for chronic disease. Children ages 2 to 17 years who are hepatitis B surface antigen (HBsAg) seropositive for more than 6 months with elevated serum alanine transaminase (ALT) and HBV DNA levels for more than 3 months may be eligible for treatment with antivirals. Maternal antiviral therapy may be given during the third trimester when there is impending liver decompensation.[123]

Hepatitis C virus (HCV). Hepatitis C virus (HCV) in children is most commonly transmitted vertically and is enhanced with maternal coinfection with human immunodeficiency virus (HIV). Risk factors for vertical transmission include internal fetal monitoring, prolonged rupture of membranes, and fetal anoxia.[124] HCV transmission also can occur through exposure to infected blood or contaminated materials (as in injection drug use or tattooing and body piercing) and, less commonly, following sexual encounters with HCV-infected partners. Transmission from blood transfusions has become a negligible risk with universal HCV screening of blood. With vertical transmission, spontaneous resolution of HCV is high, up to 40%; otherwise, the disease is usually mild in children and cirrhosis is rare.[124] Because of adverse drug events, only children with persistently elevated serum aminotransferases or those with progressive liver disease are treated with antiviral drugs.

Chronic hepatitis. Hepatitis B virus (HBV) and hepatitis C virus (HCV) are the main causes of chronic hepatitis in children. Manifestations of chronic hepatitis include malaise, anorexia, fever, gastrointestinal bleeding, hepatomegaly, edema, and transient joint pain. Often there are no symptoms. Serum alanine aminotransferase and bilirubin levels are elevated. There may be evidence of impairment of synthetic functions of the liver: prolonged prothrombin time, thrombocytopenia, and hypoalbuminemia. Diagnosis is based on the clinical manifestations and liver biopsy results. There is no curative therapy for chronic

HBV or chronic HCV. Children are treated with antiviral drugs and should continue to be monitored.[125] Liver transplant may ultimately be required for chronic hepatitis.

There also is an autoimmune form of chronic hepatitis, known as autoimmune hepatitis (AIH) or autoimmune primary sclerosing cholangitis (PSC), with unknown etiology. The pathogenic mechanism is thought to be immunologic, environmental, or genetic in nature. These diseases present with elevations in the levels of aminotransferases, autoantibodies, and immunoglobulin G (IgG). AIH is more common in female children, and both are treated with immunosuppressive therapy; about 50% to 80% will achieve remission and long-term survival.[126]

Cirrhosis

Cirrhosis is fibrotic scarring of the liver in response to inflammation and tissue damage resulting in obstruction to the flow of blood and bile. Most forms of chronic liver diseases in children can progress to cirrhosis, but they seldom do so. The complications of cirrhosis in children are the same as those in adults: portal hypertension, the opening of collateral vessels between the portal and systemic veins, and varices. In addition, children with cirrhosis experience growth failure caused by nutritional deficits, as well as developmental delay, particularly in gross motor function because of ascites and weakness. The cause of cirrhosis may influence its severity and course. Some types of cirrhosis can be stabilized if the cause is identified and treated early.[127] The risk of cirrhosis is increasing in obese children with nonalcoholic fatty liver disease (see *Health Alert:* Childhood Obesity and Nonalcoholic Fatty Liver Disease).

HEALTH ALERT

Childhood Obesity and Nonalcoholic Fatty Liver Disease

Nonalcoholic fatty liver disease (NAFLD) is the most common cause of chronic liver disease in children and is associated with obesity, insulin resistance, genetic predisposition, the gut microbiome, and environmental factors. The rise in childhood obesity worldwide is contributing to the increasing prevalence of NAFLD. The disease usually presents in prepubertal children and is predominant in males and in children of Hispanic origin. Diagnosis is made by exclusion of other disease causes. Liver biopsy is required for definitive diagnosis of steatosis (hepatic fat accumulation greater than 5%), and there are differences in the extent of fat, inflammation, and fibrosis in children compared with adults. There is no consensus regarding treatment. Exercise and slow, consistent weight loss with a low glycemic index diet have been shown to be more effective than a low-fat diet in lowering body weight. Pharmacologic agents are being evaluated to control insulin resistance and prevent progression of liver disease, and cirrhosis and vitamin E may be a specific therapy. Research is in progress to define the pathophysiology, noninvasive diagnostic procedures, and prevention of this disease.

Data from Berardis S, Sokal E: *Eur J Pediatr* 173(2):131-139, 2014; Bozic MA et al: *Nutr Clin Pract* 28(4):448-458, 2013; Giorgio V et al: *BMC Pediatr* 13:40, 2013; Nobili V et al: *JAMA Pediatr* 169(2):170-176, 2015.

Portal Hypertension

Portal hypertension is increased pressure in the portal venous system (see Chapter 36) and a major cause of morbidity and mortality in children with liver disease. There are two basic causes of portal hypertension in children: (1) increased resistance to blood flow within the portal system and (2) increased volume of portal blood flow. The second cause is rare in children and is not discussed here. Increased resistance to flow can occur anywhere in the portal circulatory system. Portal hypertension can accompany cirrhosis, intra-abdominal infections, portal vein thrombosis, congenital anomalies of the portal vein, and congenital hepatic fibrosis.

Types of Portal Hypertension

Extrahepatic portal hypertension. Extrahepatic (prehepatic) portal venous obstruction causes 50% to 70% of the cases of extrahepatic portal hypertension in children. In approximately two thirds of these children, no specific cause can be found.[128] Obstruction is almost always in the portal vein and is usually caused by thrombosis as a complication of abdominal trauma, pancreatitis, abdominal infections, and some systemic disorders; however, these causes are rare. Life-threatening bleeding and coagulation disorders can occur. Mesoportal bypass (anastomosis of portal vein to mesenteric vein) restores normal physiologic portal flow to the liver and corrects portal hypertension.[129]

Intrahepatic portal hypertension. Liver fibrosis is the primary cause of intrahepatic portal hypertension. The fibrosis can lead to cirrhosis with increased resistance to portal blood flow by constricting and reducing the compliance of hepatic sinusoids. Chronic hepatitis, biliary atresia, nonalcoholic fatty liver disease, and congenital hepatic fibrosis are causes of liver fibrosis in children.[130-132]

The clinical manifestations of portal hypertension are (1) splenomegaly, (2) upper gastrointestinal tract bleeding, (3) ascites, (4) hepatopulmonary syndrome, (5) hepatorenal syndrome, and (6) hepatic encephalopathy (see Chapter 36).

The objectives of the clinical investigation are to (1) locate the site of the venous block and (2) identify the disease responsible for the portal hypertension. Thorough physical examination; laboratory evaluation of liver function, white blood count, and platelet count; ultrasonographic imaging; endoscopic evaluation; and biopsy may be included in the diagnostic evaluation. Treatment in children is the same as that in adults (see Chapter 36).

The outcome of portal hypertension depends almost entirely on its cause. Children with extrahepatic disease are expected to recover with little morbidity. For children with intrahepatic disease, the prognosis varies.

Metabolic Disorders

More than 5000 genetically determined metabolic pathways have been identified in liver tissue. The earliest possible identification of metabolic disorders is essential because (1) early treatment may prevent permanent damage to vital organs, such as the liver or brain; (2) precise genetic counseling may be possible with prenatal diagnosis; and (3) complications can be minimized, even if cure is not possible. Galactosemia, fructosemia, glycogen storage disease (GSD), and Wilson disease are treatable metabolic disorders that have hepatic clinical manifestations. The mechanisms of disease, clinical manifestations, and evaluation and treatment of these disorders are presented in Table 37-2.

✔ QUICK CHECK 37-4

1. Why is diarrhea such a serious disorder in infants and children?
2. What is biliary atresia?
3. What are the three most common metabolic disorders that cause liver damage in children?

TABLE 37-2 Galactosemia, Fructosemia, and Wilson Disease

	Galactosemia	Fructosemia	Wilson Disease
Mechanism of disease	Deficiency of galactose-1-phosphate uridylyltransferase Autosomal recessive trait Cannot convert galactose to glucose Toxic accumulation of galactose in body tissues, liver, and brain	Deficiency of fructose-1-phosphate aldolase Autosomal recessive trait Cannot metabolize fructose, sucrose, or honey; occurs when breast milk is replaced with cow's milk Toxic accumulation of fructose in body tissues	Autosomal recessive: defect on chromosome 13 (ATP 7B) Defect in copper excretion by liver Impaired transport of copper into bile/blood caused by diminished transport protein (ceruloplasmin) Toxic accumulations of copper in liver, brain, kidney, corneas
Clinical manifestation	High levels of blood galactose Vomiting Hypoglycemia May have failure to thrive Symptoms of cirrhosis at 2-6 months—jaundice Intellectual disabilities if not treated Cataracts if not treated	High levels of blood fructose Vomiting Hypoglycemia May have failure to thrive Hepatomegaly Jaundice Seizures	Intention tremors Indistinct speech Dystonia Greenish yellow rings in cornea Hepatomegaly Jaundice Anorexia Renal tubular defects
Evaluation	Newborn screening Presence of reducing substances in urine when infant is receiving lactose	Detailed dietary history Liver or intestinal mucosa biopsy	Low plasma ceruloplasmin level
Treatment	Galactose-free diet	Fructose, sucrose, honey-free diet Vitamin C supplementation	Chelation therapy to remove copper from body Decreased dietary intake of copper Liver transplant

▌DID YOU UNDERSTAND?

Disorders of the Gastrointestinal Tract

1. Alterations of digestive function in children include congenital obstructions of the intestinal tract; disorders of digestion, absorption, or nutrition; or liver disease.
2. Cleft lip and cleft palate (failure of the bony palate to fuse in the midline) may occur separately or together. The fissure may affect the uvula, soft palate, hard palate, nostril, and maxillary alveolar ridge, with difficulty sucking and swallowing.
3. Esophageal atresia, a condition in which the esophagus ends in a blind pouch, may occur with or without tracheoesophageal fistula. As the infant swallows oral secretions or ingests milk, the pouch fills, causing either drooling or aspiration into the lungs.
4. Infantile hypertrophic pyloric stenosis is an obstruction of the pyloric outlet caused by hypertrophy of circular muscles in the pyloric sphincter.
5. In intestinal malrotation, the small intestine lacks a normal posterior attachment during fetal development, causing volvulus (twisting of the bowel on itself) that may partly or completely occlude the gastrointestinal tract and its blood vessels.
6. Meckel diverticulum is a congenital malformation of the gastrointestinal tract involving all layers of the small intestinal wall; it usually occurs in the ileum.
7. Meconium ileus is a newborn condition in which intestinal secretions and amniotic waste products produce a thick, tarry plug that obstructs the intestine; it occurs in 10% to 15% of newborns with cystic fibrosis.
8. Idiopathic intestinal pseudo-obstruction is a disorder of impaired intestinal motility.
9. Congenital aganglionic megacolon (Hirschsprung disease) is caused by a malformation of the parasympathetic nervous system in a segment of the colon needed for peristalsis, resulting in colon obstruction.
10. Malformations of the anus and rectum range from mild congenital stenosis of the anus to complex deformities, all of which are classified as imperforate anus.
11. Intussusception is a condition in which one portion of the bowel telescopes, or invaginates, into another, most commonly in the area of the ileocecal junction, and causes obstruction.
12. Gastroesophageal reflux disease is the presence of symptoms related to the return of stomach contents into the esophagus caused by relaxation or incompetence of the lower esophageal sphincter that results from immaturity of the gastroesophageal sphincter.
13. Intussusception is the telescoping of a proximal segment of intestine into a distal segment, causing an obstruction.
14. Cystic fibrosis is an inherited fibrocystic disease that involves mucosal chloride and sodium ion channels in many organs, including the GI tract and pancreas; CF causes pancreatic enzyme deficiency with maldigestion.
15. Celiac disease is caused by hypersensitivity to gluten protein, with autoimmune injury and loss of the villous epithelium. It results in malabsorption and growth failure.
16. Pediatric malnutrition is an imbalance between nutrient requirements and intake that results in energy, protein, and micronutrient deficits, which negatively impact growth and development.
17. Kwashiorkor is a severe protein deficiency. Marasmus is a deficiency of all dietary nutrients, including carbohydrates.
18. Failure to thrive or growth faltering is a multifactorial condition that includes biologic, psychosocial, and environmental contributions; may or may not be illness related; and results in inadequate physical growth and development of a child.
19. Necrotizing enterocolitis is an ischemic, inflammatory disorder in neonates, particularly premature infants, thought to result from immaturity, infection, stress, and anoxia of the bowel wall.

20. Acute diarrhea in infants and children is three or more watery or loose stools in 24 hours; it is commonly caused by viral or bacterial enterocolitis.

21. Chronic diarrhea (diarrhea persisting longer than 4 weeks) can be caused by a wide variety of underlying conditions and often leads to growth failure and slow development.

22. Primary lactose intolerance is the inability to digest milk sugar because of a lack of the enzyme lactase, resulting in osmotic diarrhea.

Disorders of the Liver

1. Physiologic jaundice of the newborn is caused by mild hyperbilirubinemia that subsides in 1 or 2 weeks. Pathologic jaundice is caused by severe hyperbilirubinemia and can cause brain damage (kernicterus).

2. Biliary atresia is a congenital malformation of the bile ducts that obstructs bile flow and causes jaundice, cirrhosis, and liver failure.

3. Acute hepatitis is usually caused by a virus, and hepatitis A is the most common form of childhood hepatitis. Chronic hepatitis B or C usually occurs by maternal transmission.

4. Cirrhosis results from fibrotic scarring of the liver and is rare in children, but it can develop from most forms of chronic liver disease.

5. Portal hypertension in children usually is caused by extrahepatic obstruction and the cause is often unknown. Intrahepatic obstruction is related to diseases that cause liver fibrosis.

6. The four most common metabolic disorders that cause liver damage in children are galactosemia, fructosemia, glycogen storage disease, and Wilson disease. All three are inherited as genetic traits and allow toxins to accumulate in the liver.

KEY TERMS

Anorectal malformation (ARM), 954
Biliary atresia (BA), 962
Celiac crisis, 958
Celiac disease (CD; celiac sprue), 957
Cirrhosis, 963
Cleft lip (CL), 950
Cleft palate (CP), 950
Cystic fibrosis (CF), 956
Diarrhea, 960
Distal intestinal obstruction syndrome (DIOS), 953
Eosinophilic esophagitis (EoE), 955
Esophageal atresia (EA), 951

Extrahepatic portal hypertension, 963
Failure to thrive (FTT), 959
Fructosemia, 963
Galactosemia, 963
Gastroesophageal reflux (GER), 954
Gastroesophageal reflux disease (GERD), 954
Glycogen storage disease (GSD), 963
Growth faltering (GF), 959
Hepatitis A virus (HAV), 962
Hepatitis B virus (HBV), 962
Hepatitis C virus (HCV), 962
Hepatitis D virus (HDV), 962
Hirschsprung disease, 954

Idiopathic intestinal pseudo-obstruction, 954
Infantile hypertrophic pyloric stenosis (IHPS), 951
Intrahepatic portal hypertension, 963
Intussusception, 955
Jaundice (icterus), 961
Kernicterus, 961
Kwashiorkor, 959
Lactose intolerance, 961
Lactose malabsorption, 961
Malrotation, 952
Marasmus, 959
Meckel diverticulum, 953
Meconium, 953
Meconium disease, 953

Meconium ileus (MI), 953
Meconium plug syndrome (MPS), 953
Necrotizing enterocolitis (NEC), 960
Nonceliac gluten sensitivity, 957
Nonsyndromic (isolated) CP, 950
Physiologic jaundice (hyperbilirubinemia) of the newborn, 961
Protein-energy malnutrition (PEM), 959
Rotavirus, 961
Syndromic CLP, 950
Tracheoesophageal fistula (EA/TEF), 951
Wilson disease, 963

REFERENCES

1. Arosarena OA: Cleft lip and palate, Otolaryngol Clin North Am 40(1):27-60, 2007.
2. National Institute of Dental and Craniofacial Research: Prevalence (number of cases) of cleft lip and palate, updated October 13, 2011. Available at: www.nidcr.nih.gov/DataStatistics/FindDataByTopic/CraniofacialBirthDefects/PrevalenceCleft+LipCleftPalate.htm.
3. Dixon MJ et al: Cleft lip and palate: understanding genetic and environmental influences, Nat Rev Genet 12(3):167-178, 2011.
4. Leslie EJ, Marazita ML: Genetics of cleft lip and cleft palate, Am J Med Genet C Semin Med Genet 163C(4):246-258, 2013.
5. Molina-Solana R et al: Current concepts on the effect of environmental factors on cleft lip and palate, Int J Oral Maxillofac Surg 42(2):177-184, 2013.
6. Mossey PA et al: Cleft lip and palate, Lancet 374(9703):1773-1785, 2009.
7. Reilly S et al: ABM Clinical Protocol #17: guidelines for breastfeeding infants with cleft lip, cleft palate, or cleft lip and palate, Breastfeed Med 2(4):243-250, 2007.
8. Farronato G et al: How various surgical protocols of the unilateral cleft lip and palate influence the facial growth and possible orthodontic problems? Which is the best timing of lip, palate and alveolus repair? Literature review, Stomatologija 16(2):53-60, 2014.

9. Jayaram R, Huppa C: Surgical correction of cleft lip and palate, Front Oral Biol 16:101-110, 2012.
10. Shaye D: Update on outcomes research for cleft lip and palate, Curr Opin Otolaryngol Head Neck Surg 22(4):255-259, 2014.
11. Sitzman TJ et al: Measuring outcomes in cleft lip and palate treatment, Clin Plast Surg 41(2):311-319, 2014.
12. El-Gohary Y et al: Congenital anomalies of the esophagus, Semin Pediatr Surg 19(3):186-193, 2010.
13. Holland AJ, Fitzgerald DA: Oesophageal atresia and tracheo-oesophageal fistula: current management strategies and complications, Paediatr Respir Rev 11(2):100-106, 2010; quiz 106-107.
14. de Jong EM et al: Etiology of esophageal atresia and tracheoesophageal fistula: "mind the gap," Curr Gastroenterol Rep 12(3):215-222, 2010.
15. Solomon BD et al: An approach to the identification of anomalies and etiologies in neonates with identified or suspected VACTERL (vertebral defects, anal atresia, tracheo-esophageal fistula with esophageal atresia, cardiac anomalies, renal anomalies, and limb anomalies), J Pediatr 164(3):451-457, 2014.
16. Pinheiro PF et al: Current knowledge on esophageal atresia, World J Gastroenterol 18(28):3662-3672, 2012.

17. Alberti D et al: Esophageal atresia: pre and post-operative management, J Matern Fetal Neonatal Med 24(Suppl 1):4-6, 2011.
18. Krogh C et al: Pre- and perinatal risk factors for pyloric stenosis and their influence on the male predominance, Am J Epidemiol 176(1):24-31, 2012.
19. Askew N: An overview of infantile hypertrophic pyloric stenosis, Paediatr Nurs 22(8):27-30, 2010.
20. Peters B et al: Advances in infantile hypertrophic pyloric stenosis, Expert Rev Gastroenterol Hepatol 8(5):533-541, 2014.
21. Ranells JD et al: Infantile hypertrophic pyloric stenosis: epidemiology, genetics, and clinical update, Adv Pediatr 58(1):195-206, 2011.
22. Kliegman RM et al: Nelson textbook of pediatrics, ed 19, Philadelphia, 2011, Saunders.
23. Ooms N et al: Laparoscopic treatment of intestinal malrotation in children, Eur J Pediatr Surg 2015 Jun 18, [Epub ahead of print.]
24. Daneman A: Malrotation: the balance of evidence, Pediatr Radiol 39(Suppl 2):S164-S166, 2009.
25. El-Gohary Y et al: Long-term complications following operative intervention for intestinal malrotation: a 10-year review, Pediatr Surg Int 26(2):203-206, 2010.
26. Kotecha M et al: Multimodality imaging manifestations of the Meckel diverticulum in children, Pediatr Radiol 42(1):95-103, 2012.

27. St-Vil D et al: Meckel's diverticulum in children: a 20-year review, *J Pediatr Surg* 26(11):1289-1292, 1991.
28. Thurley PD et al: Radiological features of Meckel's diverticulum and its complications, *Clin Radiol* 64(2):109-118, 2009.
29. Uppal K et al: Meckel's diverticulum: a review, *Clin Anat* 24(4):416-422, 2011.
30. Yahchouchy EK et al: Meckel's diverticulum, *J Am Coll Surg* 192(5):658-662, 2001.
31. Carlyle BE et al: A review of pathophysiology and management of fetuses and neonates with meconium ileus for the pediatric surgeon, *J Pediatr Surg* 47(4):772-781, 2012.
32. Karimi A et al: Issues in the management of simple and complex meconium ileus, *Pediatr Surg Int* 27(9):963-968, 2011.
33. Lavie M et al: Long-term follow-up of distal intestinal obstruction syndrome in cystic fibrosis, *World J. Gastroenterol* 21(1):318-325, 2015.
34. van der Doef HP et al: Intestinal obstruction syndromes in cystic fibrosis: meconium ileus, distal intestinal obstruction syndrome, and constipation, *Curr Gastroenterol Rep* 13(3):265-270, 2011.
35. Colombo C et al: Guidelines for the diagnosis and management of distal intestinal obstruction syndrome in cystic fibrosis patients, *J Cyst Fibros* 10(Suppl 2):S24-S28, 2011.
36. Copeland DR et al: Diminishing role of contrast enema in simple meconium ileus, *J Pediatr Surg* 44(11):2130-2132, 2009.
37. Ambartsumyan L, Rodriguez L: Gastrointestinal motility disorders in children, *Gastroenterol Hepatol (N Y)* 10(1):16-26, 2014.
38. Gariepy CE, Mousa H: Clinical management of motility disorders in children, *Semin Pediatr Surg* 18(4):224-238, 2009.
39. Mallick S et al: Chronic intestinal pseudo-obstruction: systematic histopathological approach can clinch vital clues, *Virchows Arch* 464(5):529-537, 2014.
40. Amiel J, Lyonnet S: Hirschsprung disease, associated syndromes, and genetics: a review, *J Med Genet* 38(11):729-739, 2001.
41. McKeown SJ et al: Hirschsprung disease: a developmental disorder of the enteric nervous system, *Wiley Interdisc Rev Dev Biol* 2(1):113-129, 2013.
42. Moore SW: Chromosomal and related Mendelian syndromes associated with Hirschsprung's disease, *Pediatr Surg Int* 28(11):1045-1058, 2012.
43. Butler Tjaden NE, Trainor PA: The developmental etiology and pathogenesis of Hirschsprung disease, *Transl Res* 162(1):1-15, 2013.
44. Amiel J et al: Hirschsprung disease, associated syndromes and genetics: a review, *J Med Genet* 45(1):1-14, 2008.
45. Chumpitazi BP, Nurko S: Defecation disorders in children after surgery for Hirschsprung disease, *J Pediatr Gastroenterol Nutr* 53(1):75-79, 2011.
46. Dillon PW: *Congenital pediatric colorectal disorders*, American Society of Colon & Rectal Surgeons. Available at: www.fascrs.org/physicians/education/core_subjects/2002/congenital_pediatric_colorectal_disorders/. Published 2002. Accessed July 10, 2014.
47. Feichter S et al: The histopathology of gastrointestinal motility disorders in children, *Semin Pediatr Surg* 18(4):206-211, 2009.
48. Gourlay DM: Colorectal considerations in pediatric patients, *Surg Clin North Am* 93(1):251-272, 2013.
49. Bischoff A et al: Laparoscopy and its use in the repair of anorectal malformations, *J Pediatr Surg* 46(8):1609-1617, 2011.
50. Bischoff A et al: Update on the management of anorectal malformations, *Pediatr Surg Int* 29(9):899-904, 2013.
51. Herman RS, Teitelbaum DH: Anorectal malformations, *Clin Perinatol* 39(2):403-422, 2012.

52. Levitt MA, Pena A: Anorectal malformations, *Orphanet J Rare Dis* 2:33, 2007.
53. England RJ et al: Laparoscopic repair of anorectal malformations at the Red Cross War Memorial Children's Hospital: taking stock, *J Pediatr Surg* 47(3):565-570, 2012.
54. Lightdale JR, Gremse DA, Section on Gastroenterology, Hepatology, and Nutrition: Gastroesophageal reflux: management guidance for the pediatrician, *Pediatrics* 131(5):e1684-e1695, 2013.
55. Wyllie R et al: *Pediatric gastrointestinal and liver disease*, ed 4, p 233, Philadelphia, 2011, Elsevier Saunders.
56. Vandenplas Y et al: Pediatric gastroesophageal reflux clinical practice guidelines: joint recommendations of the North American Society for Pediatric Gastroenterology, Hepatology, and Nutrition (NASPGHAN) and the European Society for Pediatric Gastroenterology, Hepatology, and Nutrition (ESPGHAN), *J Pediatr Gastroenterol Nutr* 49(4):498-547, 2009.
57. Gupta SK: Diagnostic and therapeutic challenges in pediatric eosinophilic esophagitis: past, present and future, *Dig Dis* 32(1-2):107-109, 2014.
58. Sherman PM et al: A global, evidence-based consensus on the definition of gastroesophageal reflux disease in the pediatric population, *Am J Gastroenterol* 104(5):1278-1295, 2009.
59. Tighe M et al: Pharmacological treatment of children with gastro-oesophageal reflux, *Cochrane Database Syst Rev* 11:CD008550, 2014.
60. Martin K et al: Outcomes of pediatric laparoscopic fundoplication: a critical review of the literature, *Can J Gastroenterol Hepatol* 28(2):97-102, 2014.
61. Applegate KE: Intussusception in children: evidence-based diagnosis and treatment, *Pediatr Radiol* 39(Suppl 2):S140-S143, 2009.
62. Parikh M et al: Does all small bowel intussusception need exploration? *Afr J Paediatr Surg* 7(1):30-32, 2010.
63. Yih WK et al: Intussusception risk after rotavirus vaccination in U.S. infants, *N Engl J Med* 370(6):503-512, 2014.
64. Apelt N et al: Laparoscopic treatment of intussusception in children: a systematic review, *J Pediatr Surg* 48(8):1789-1793, 2013.
65. Gray MP et al: Recurrence rates after intussusception enema reduction: a meta-analysis, *Pediatrics* 134(1):110-119, 2014.
66. Pepper VK et al: Diagnosis and management of pediatric appendicitis, intussusception, and Meckel diverticulum, *Surg Clin North Am* 92(3):505-26, vii, 2012.
67. Gelfond D, Borowitz D: Gastrointestinal complications of cystic fibrosis, *Clin Gastroenterol Hepatol* 11(4):333-342, 2013.
68. Ode KL, Moran A: New insights into cystic fibrosis-related diabetes in children, *Lancet Diabetes Endocrinol* 1(1):52-58, 2013.
69. Borowitz D, Gelfond D: Intestinal complications of cystic fibrosis, *Curr Opin Pulm Med* 19(6):676-680, 2013.
70. Phung OJ et al: Recombinant human growth hormone in the treatment of patients with cystic fibrosis, *Pediatrics* 126(5):e1211-e1226, 2010.
71. Husby S et al: European Society for Pediatric Gastroenterology, Hepatology, and Nutrition guidelines for the diagnosis of coeliac disease, *J Pediatr Gastroenterol Nutr* 54(1):136-160, 2012.
72. Guandalini S, Assiri A: Celiac disease: a review, *JAMA Pediatr* 168(3):272-278, 2014.
73. Kabbani TA et al: Celiac disease or non-celiac gluten sensitivity? An approach to clinical differential diagnosis, *Am J Gastroenterol* 109(5):741-746, 2014.
74. Kaukinen K et al: Coeliac disease—a diagnostic and therapeutic challenge, *Clin Chem Lab Med* 48(9):1205-1216, 2010.
75. Liu E et al: Risk of pediatric celiac disease according to HLA haplotype and country, *N Engl J Med* 371(1):42-49, 2014.
76. Elli L et al: Does gluten intake influence the development of celiac disease-associated

complications? *J Clin Gastroenterol* 48(1):13-20, 2014.
77. Fergusson P, Tomkins A: HIV prevalence and mortality among children undergoing treatment for severe acute malnutrition in sub-Saharan Africa: a systematic review and meta-analysis, *Trans R Soc Trop Med Hyg* 103(6):541-548, 2009.
78. Garrett WS: Kwashiorkor and the gut microbiota, *N Engl J Med* 368(18):1746-1747, 2013.
79. Prieto MB, Cid JL: Malnutrition in the critically ill child: the importance of enteral nutrition, *Int J Environ Res Public Health* 8(11):4353-4366, 2011.
80. Smith MI et al: Gut microbiomes of Malawian twin pairs discordant for kwashiorkor, *Science* 339(6119):548-554, 2013.
81. Trehan I et al: Antibiotics as part of the management of severe acute malnutrition, *N Engl J Med* 368(5):425-435, 2013.
82. Grover Z, Ee LC: Protein energy malnutrition, *Pediatr Clin North Am* 56(5):1055-1068, 2009.
83. Maida JM et al: Pediatric ophthalmology in the developing world, *Curr Opin Ophthalmol* 19(5):403-408, 2008.
84. Kismul H et al: Diet and kwashiorkor: a prospective study from rural DR Congo, *Peer J* 2:e350, 2014.
85. Cole SZ, Lanham JS: Failure to thrive: an update, *Am Fam Physician* 83(7):829-834, 2011.
86. Jaffe AC: Failure to thrive: current clinical concepts, *Pediatr Rev* 32(3):100-107, 2011.
87. Nützenadel W: Failure to thrive in childhood, *Dtsch Arztebl Int* 108(38):642-649, 2011.
88. Joosten KF, Hulst JM: Nutritional screening tools for hospitalized children: methodological considerations, *Clin Nutr* 33(1):1-5, 2014.
89. Black MM et al: Early intervention and recovery among children with failure to thrive: follow-up at age 8, *Pediatrics* 120(1):59-69, 2007.
90. Neu J, Mihatsch W: Recent developments in necrotizing enterocolitis, *JPEN J Parenter Enteral Nutr* 36(1 Suppl):30S-35S, 2012.
91. Srinivasan PS et al: Necrotizing enterocolitis, *Clin Perinatol* 35(1):251-272, 2008.
92. Caplan MS: Neonatal necrotizing enterocolitis [introduction], *Semin Perinatol* 32(2):69, 2008.
93. Gordon PV, Swanson JR: Necrotizing enterocolitis is one disease with many origins and potential means of prevention, *Pathophysiology* 21(1):13-19, 2014.
94. Kim JH: Necrotizing enterocolitis: the road to zero, *Semin Fetal Neonatal Med* 19(1):39-44, 2014.
95. Alfaleh K et al: Probiotics for prevention of necrotizing enterocolitis in preterm infants, *Cochrane Database Syst Rev* 3, 2011:CD005496.
96. Sola JE et al: Peritoneal drainage versus laparotomy for necrotizing enterocolitis and intestinal perforation: a meta-analysis, *J Surg Res* 161(1):95-100, 2010.
97. Churgay CA, Aftab Z: Gastroenteritis in children: part 1. Diagnosis, *Am Fam Physician* 85(11):1059-1062, 2012.
98. Mehal JM et al: Risk factors for diarrhea-associated infant mortality in the United States, 2005-2007, *Pediatr Infect Dis J* 31(7):717-721, 2012.
99. World Health Organization: *Diarrhoeal disease*, Fact sheet No. 330, April 2013. Available at: www.who.int/mediacentre/factsheets/fs330/en/.
100. Zella GC, Israel EJ: Chronic diarrhea in children, *Pediatr Rev* 33(5):207-217, 2012.
101. Kollaritsch H et al: Rotavirus vaccines: a story of success, *Clin Microbiol Infect* 2015 Feb 11. [Epub ahead of print.]
102. Pawlowski SW et al: Diagnosis and treatment of acute or persistent diarrhea, *Gastroenterology* 136(6):1874-1886, 2009.
103. Bernaola Aponte G et al: Probiotics for treating persistent diarrhoea in children, *Cochrane Database Syst Rev* 8:CD007401, 2013.
104. Grimwood K, Forbes DA: Acute and persistent diarrhea, *Pediatr Clin North Am* 56(6):1343-1361, 2009.

105. Misselwitz B et al: Lactose malabsorption and intolerance: pathogenesis, diagnosis and treatment, *United European Gastroenterol J* 1(3):151-159, 2013.

106. Maisels MJ: What's in a name? Physiologic and pathologic jaundice: the conundrum of defining normal bilirubin levels in the newborn, *Pediatrics* 118(2):805-807, 2006.

107. Porter ML, Dennis BL: Hyperbilirubinemia in the term newborn, *Am Fam Physician* 65(4):599-606, 2002.

108. Colletti JE et al: An emergency medicine approach to neonatal hyperbilirubinemia, *Emerg Med Clin North Am* 25(4):1117-1135, 2007.

109. Shapiro SM: Chronic bilirubin encephalopathy: diagnosis and outcome, *Semin Fetal Neonatal Med* 15(3):157-163, 2010.

110. Watson RL: Hyperbilirubinemia, *Crit Care Nurs Clin North Am* 21(1):97-120, 2009.

111. Bassett MD, Murray KF: Biliary atresia: recent progress, *J Clin Gastroenterol* 42(6):720-729, 2008.

112. Petersen C, Davenport M: Aetiology of biliary atresia: what is actually known? *Orphanet J Rare Dis* 8:128, 2013.

113. Tessier ME et al: Beyond the pediatric end-stage liver disease system: solutions for infants with biliary atresia requiring liver transplant, *World J Gastroenterol* 20(32):11062-11068, 2014.

114. Degertekin B, Lok AS: Update on viral hepatitis: 2008, *Curr Opin Gastroenterol* 25(3):180-185, 2009.

115. Klevens RM et al: The evolving epidemiology of hepatitis A in the United States: incidence and molecular epidemiology from population-based surveillance, 2005-2007, *Arch Intern Med* 170(20):1811-1818, 2010.

116. Suchy FJ et al: *Liver disease in children,* ed 4, Cambridge, United Kingdom, 2014, Cambridge University Press.

117. Matheny SC, Kingery JE: Hepatitis A, *Am Fam Physician* 86(11):1027-1034, 2012.

118. Haber BA et al: Recommendations for screening, monitoring, and referral of pediatric chronic hepatitis B, *Pediatrics* 124(5):e1007-e1013, 2009.

119. Slowik MK, Jhaveri R: Hepatitis B and C viruses in infants and young children, *Semin Pediatr Infect Dis* 16(4):296-305, 2005.

120. Grabowski J, Wedemeyer H: Hepatitis delta: immunopathogenesis and clinical challenges, *Dig Dis* 28(1):133-138, 2010.

121. Jonas MM et al: Hepatitis B Foundation. Treatment of children with chronic hepatitis B virus infection in the United States: patient selection and therapeutic options, *Hepatology* 52(6):2192-2205, 2010.

122. Sorrell MF et al: National Institutes of Health consensus development conference statement: management of hepatitis B, *Hepatology* 49(5 Suppl):S4-S12, 2009.

123. Pan CQ, Lee HM: Antiviral therapy for chronic hepatitis B in pregnancy, *Semin Liver Dis* 33(2):138-146, 2013.

124. Mack CL et al: NASPGHAN practice guidelines: diagnosis and management of hepatitis C infection in infants, children, and adolescents, *J Pediatr Gastroenterol Nutr* 54(6):838-855, 2012.

125. El-Shabrawi M, Hassanin F: Treatment of hepatitis B and C in children, *Minerva Pediatr* 66(5):473-489, 2014.

126. Floreani A et al: Autoimmune hepatitis: contrasts and comparisons in children and adults—a comprehensive review, *J Autoimmun* 46:7-16, 2013.

127. Badizadegan K et al: Histopathology of the liver in children with chronic hepatitis C viral infection, *Hepatology* 28(5):1416-1423, 1998.

128. Mack CL et al: Surgically restoring portal blood flow to the liver in children with primary extrahepatic portal vein thrombosis improves fluid neurocognitive ability, *Pediatrics* 117(3):e405-e412, 2006.

129. Sharif K et al: Mesoportal bypass for extrahepatic portal vein obstruction in children: close to a cure for most! *J Pediatr Surg* 45(1):272-276, 2010.

130. Brunt EM: Histopathology of non-alcoholic fatty liver disease, *Clin Liver Dis* 13(4):533-544, 2009.

131. Haafiz AB: Liver fibrosis in biliary atresia, *Exp Rev Gastroenterol Hepatol* 4(3):335-343, 2010.

132. Peters L, Rockstroh JK: Biomarkers of fibrosis and impaired liver function in chronic hepatitis C: how well do they predict clinical outcomes? *Curr Opin HIV AIDS* 5(6):517-523, 2010.

38

Structure and Function of the Musculoskeletal System

Christy L. Crowther-Radulewicz and Kathryn L. McCance

ⓔ EVOLVE WEBSITE

http://evolve.elsevier.com/Huether/
Student Review Questions
Audio Key Points

Case Studies
Animations
Quick Check Answers

CHAPTER OUTLINE

The way an individual functions in daily life, moves about, or manipulates objects physically depends on the integrity of the musculoskeletal system. The musculoskeletal system is actually two systems: (1) the skeleton composed of bones and joints and (2) soft tissues (skeletal muscles, tendons, and ligaments). Each system contributes to mobility. The skeleton supports the body and provides leverage to the skeletal muscles so that movement of various parts of the body is possible. Contraction of the skeletal muscles and bending or rotation at the joints facilitate movements of the various body parts.

STRUCTURE AND FUNCTION OF BONES

Bones give form to the body, support tissues, and permit movement by providing points of attachment for muscles. Many bones meet in movable joints that determine the type and extent of movement possible. Bones also protect many of the body's vital organs. For example, the bones of the skull, thorax, and pelvis are hard exterior shields that protect the brain, heart and lungs, and reproductive and urinary organs, respectively.

The marrow cavities within certain bones serve as sites of blood cell formation. In adults, blood cells originate exclusively in the marrow cavities of the skull, vertebrae, ribs, sternum, shoulders, and pelvis. The development of blood cells is discussed in Chapter 20. Bones also have a crucial role in mineral homeostasis (storing minerals [i.e., calcium, phosphate, carbonate, magnesium] that are essential for the proper performance of many delicate cellular mechanisms), play a role in hormone homeostasis, and assist in maintaining normal immunologic function.

Elements of Bone Tissue

Mature bone is a rigid connective tissue consisting of cells, fibers, a gelatinous material termed ground substance, and large amounts of crystallized minerals, mainly calcium, that give bone its rigidity. Ground substance consists of proteoglycans and hyaluronic acid secreted by chondroblasts. The structural elements of bone are summarized in Table 38-1.

Bone cells enable bone to grow, repair itself, change shape, and continuously synthesize new bone tissue and resorb (dissolve or digest) old tissue. The fibers in bone are made of collagen, which gives bone its tensile strength (the ability to hold itself together). Ground substance acts as a medium for the diffusion of nutrients, oxygen, metabolic wastes, biochemicals, and minerals between bone tissue and blood vessels.

Bone formation begins during fetal life with the growth of cartilage—the precursor of bone tissue. In mature bone, the formation of new tissue begins with the production of an organic matrix by the bone cells. This bone matrix consists of ground substance, collagen, and other proteins (see Table 38-1) that take part in bone formation and maintenance.

The next step in bone formation is calcification, in which minerals are deposited and then crystallize. Minerals bind tightly to collagen fibers, producing tensile and compressional strength in bone and allowing it to withstand pressure and weightbearing.

Bone Cells

Bone contains three types of cells: osteoblasts, osteocytes, and osteoclasts (Figure 38-1). Both osteoblasts and osteocytes originate from

TABLE 38-1 Structural Elements of Bone

Structural Elements	Function
Bone Cells	
Osteoblasts	Synthesize collagen and proteoglycans, mineralize osteoid matrix; produce RANKL, which in turn stimulates osteoclast resorption of bone; also produce osteoprotegerin (OPG), which inhibits osteoclast formation by binding to RANKL
Osteoclasts	Resorb bone; major role in bone homeostasis
Osteocytes	Transform osteoblasts trapped in osteoid; signal both osteoblasts and osteoclasts; maintain bone matrix; mechanosensory receptors to reduce or augment bone mass; produce sclerostin (SOST), which inhibits bone growth
Bone Matrix	
Bone morphogenic proteins (BMPs)	Subfamily of TGF-β cytokine growth factors; induce and regulate bone and cartilage formation; affect all other organ systems
BMP-1	Unrelated to other BMPs (is a metalloprotease); key role in extracellular matrix (ECM) formation
BMP-2	Promotes chondrogenesis, bone formation; clinically used to enhance bone formation in spine surgery
BMP-3 (osteogenin)	Inhibits bone formation
BMP-4	Osteoblast differentiation; involved in cartilage repair, endochondral bone formation; enhances chondrogenesis
BMP-6	Found in human plasma; promotes osteoblast differentiation from mesenchymal stem cells (MSCs)
BMP-7	Osteogenic cell formation from MSCs; enhances bone formation in spine surgery; induces formation of brown fat
BMP-9	Promotes osteoblast formation from MSCs
BMP-13	Inhibits bone formation by reducing calcium mineralization
Collagen fibers	Lend support and tensile strength
Proteoglycans	Control transport of ionized materials through matrix
Glycoproteins	
Albumin	Transports essential elements to matrix; maintains osmotic pressure of bone fluid
α-Glycoproteins	Promote calcification
Laminin	Stabilizes basement membranes in bones
Osteocalcin	Vitamin K–dependent protein present in bone; inhibits calcium phosphate precipitation (attracts calcium ions to incorporate into hydroxyapatite crystals); serum osteocalcin is a sensitive marker of bone formation
Osteonectin	Binds calcium in bone; necessary for normal bone formation
Sialoprotein	Promotes calcification, osteoblast formation
Minerals	
Calcium	Crystallizes, providing bone rigidity and compressive strength
Phosphate	Balance of organic and inorganic phosphate required for proper bone mineralization; regulates vitamin D, promoting mineralization
Alkaline phosphatase	Promotes mineralization
Vitamins	
Vitamin D	Assists with differentiation, mineralization of osteoblasts
Vitamin K	Increases bone calcification; reduces serum osteocalcin

FIGURE 38-1 Bone Cells. A, Osteoblasts are responsible for the production of collagenous and noncollagenous proteins that compose osteoid. Active osteoblasts are aligned on the osteoid. Note the eccentrically located nuclei. **B,** Electron photomicrograph of an osteocyte. Osteocytes reside within the lacunae of compact bone. **C,** Osteoclasts actively resorb mineralized tissue. The scalloped surface in which the multinucleated osteoclasts rest is termed *Howship lacuna*. (**A** and **C** from Damjanov I, Linder J, editors: *Anderson's pathology,* ed 10, St Louis, 1996, Mosby; **B** from Wikimedia Commons, courtesy Robert M. Hunt.)

osteoprogenitor cells found in the mesenchymal stem cell lineage. Unlike osteoblasts and osteocytes, osteoclasts originate from hematopoietic stem cells. Osteoblasts are the bone-forming cells. Once this function is complete, osteoblasts become osteocytes. Osteocytes, the most numerous cells within bone, are osteoblasts that have become imprisoned within the mineralized bone matrix. They have multiple important duties in maintaining bone homeostasis, including synthesizing new bone matrix molecules and initiating osteoclast function. Osteoclasts primarily resorb (remove) bone during processes of growth and repair.

Osteoblasts. Originating from mesenchymal stem cells (MSCs), osteoblasts are the primary bone-producing cells, and are involved in many functions related to the skeletal system (see Table 38-1). Osteoblasts are responsive to parathyroid hormone (PTH) and produce osteocalcin when stimulated by 1,25-dihydroxy-vitamin D$_3$.[1] Osteoblasts are active on the outer surfaces of bones, where they form a single layer of cells. Osteoblasts initiate new bone formation by their synthesis of osteoid (nonmineralized bone matrix). Osteoblasts also mineralize newly formed bone matrix. Stimulation of new bone formation and orderly mineralization of bone matrix occur by concentrating some of the plasma proteins (growth factors) found in the bone matrix and by facilitating the deposit and exchange of calcium and other ions at the site. Enzymes, signaling proteins, and growth factors, including bone morphogenic proteins (BMPs) and other members of the transforming growth factor-beta (TGF-β) superfamily, are critical components of bone formation, maintenance, and remodeling (Table 38-2).

Osteoblasts use intercellular calcium signaling to include osteoclastic activity. One of the most important discoveries linking osteoblast and osteoclast function is that of the cytokine receptor activator nuclear factor kappa-B ligand, or RANKL (see below). RANKL is expressed by osteoblasts and osteocytes and is necessary for forming osteoclasts[2-4] (see Osteoclasts). Thus, the cells of the osteoblastic lineage (osteoblasts, osteocytes) form a network of cells in bone that sense the shape and structure of bone and determine where it is appropriate that bone be formed or resorbed, according to Wolff law (bone is shaped according to its function).

Osteoblasts synthesize and secrete osteoid when active, and in the resting state they are termed *satellite cells*. If appropriately stimulated, however, the resting osteoblasts are capable of resuming activity.

Osteocytes. Osteocytes, the most abundant cells in bone, are transformed osteoblasts trapped or surrounded in osteoid as it hardens because of minerals that enter during calcification (see Figure 38-1, *B*). The osteocyte is within a space in the hardened bone matrix called a lacuna. Each osteocyte contains long, thin cytoplasmic extensions, called processes, which run through the canaliculi, providing communication with osteoblasts lying on the bone surface. Another form of extracellular communication used by osteocytes is through transmembrane channels called gap junctions, which connect the cytoplasm of adjacent cells.

Osteocytes are the most abundant cells found in bone and have numerous functions, including acting as mechanoreceptors and synthesizing certain matrix molecules, playing a major role in controlling osteoblast differentiation and production of growth factors, and maintaining bone homeostasis.[5] As the major source of sclerostin, RANKL, and osteoprotegerin (OPG), osteocytes are thought to be key regulators of both bone formation and bone resorption.[6-8] They also help concentrate nutrients in the matrix. Osteocytes obtain nutrients from capillaries in the canaliculi, which contain nutrient-rich fluids. Through exchanges among these cells, hormone catalysts, and minerals, optimal levels of calcium, phosphorus, and other minerals are maintained in blood plasma.

One of the osteocyte's primary functions is to act as a mechanoreceptor, responding to changes in weightbearing or other stressors ("loading") on bone. Lying within the lacunae are the osteocyte's primary cilia, which are likely the primary mechanoreceptors in bone.[9,10] Once changes in bone, such as mechanical stress, hormonal imbalance, loading, or unloading, are detected by the osteocyte's mechanoreceptors, multiple molecular signals are produced and the process of bone remodeling begins.[4,11] Remodeling is described on p. 974.

Osteoclasts. Osteoclasts are large (typically 20 to 100 μm in diameter), multinucleated cells that develop from the hematopoietic monocyte-macrophage lineage. Osteoclasts are the major resorptive cells of bone. They migrate over bone surfaces to resorption areas that have been prepared and stripped of osteoid by enzymes, such as collagenases produced by osteoblasts in the presence of PTH, which is necessary for the resorptive process. Osteoclasts travel over the prepared bone surfaces, creating irregular, scalloped cavities known as *Howship lacunae* or *resorption bays,* as they resorb bone areas and then acidify hydroxyapatite in order to dissolve it.

A specific area of the cell membrane forms adjacent to the bone surface and develops multiple infoldings to permit intimate contact with the resorption bay. These infoldings, known as the ruffled border, greatly increase the surface areas of cells under their scalloped or ruffled borders. Osteoclasts resorb bone by secretion of hydrochloric acid, acid proteases (such as cathepsin K), and matrix metalloproteinases (MMPs) that help digest collagen, along with the action of cytokines (see Table 38-2). Osteoclasts also resorb bone through the action of lysosomes (digestive vacuoles) filled with hydrolytic enzymes in their mitochondria.

Osteoclasts bind to the bone surfaces through attachments called podosomes, which are foot-like structures that cluster together along a sealing membrane that forms a "belt" containing multiple proteins, enzymes, and integrin receptors.[12,13] Once resorption is complete, the osteoclasts retract and loosen from the bone surface under the ruffled border through the action of calcitonin. Calcitonin binds to receptor areas of the osteoclasts' cell membranes to effectively loosen the osteoclasts from the bone surfaces. Once resorption is completed, osteoclasts disappear by the process of degeneration, either by reverting to the form of their parent cells or by undergoing cell movements away from the site, in which the osteoclast becomes an inactive or resting osteoclast.

In addition to resorption of bone, osteoclasts assist the endocrine and renal systems in maintaining appropriate serum calcium and phosphorus levels. Osteoclasts also appear to have a role in the body's immune response.[12]

OPG/RANKL/RANK System

Osteoprotegerin (OPG) is a glycoprotein belonging to the tumor necrosis factor superfamily and inhibits bone remodeling/resorption, inhibiting osteoclast formation. Numerous cells, including osteoblasts and osteocytes, produce it. OPG is key in the interaction between osteoblasts and osteoclasts.[14] Osteoblasts and osteoclasts cooperate (a process called *coupling*) to maintain normal bone homeostasis. RANKL is an essential cytokine needed for the formation and activation of osteoclasts. RANKL, like an automobile's accelerator, increases bone loss. OPG, similar to an automobile's brakes, decreases bone loss because when it is activated it promotes bone formation. When RANKL binds to its receptor RANK on osteoclast precursor cells, it triggers their proliferation and increases bone resorption. OPG is secreted by osteoblasts and B lymphocytes[15] and serves as a decoy by binding to RANK, preventing RANKL binding to RANK, and thus preventing bone resorption. Therefore, the overall balance between RANKL

TABLE 38-2 Selected Factors Affecting Bone Formation, Maintenance, and Remodeling

Factor	Function
Transforming growth factor-beta (TGF-β)	Superfamily of polypeptides; regulates bone formation, many other cellular processes through signaling
Platelet-derived growth factor (PDGF)	Increases number of osteoblasts
Fibroblast growth factor (FGF)	FGF-2 increases osteoblast population, but not function; inhibits alkaline phosphatase activity, osteocalcin, type I collagen, and osteopontin
Insulin-like growth factor (IGF)	
IGF-1	Increases peak bone mass during adolescence; decreases osteoblast apoptosis; maintains bone matrix
IGF-2	Increases BMP-9–induced endochondral ossification
Smad proteins	Mediate signaling cascade of TGF-β, especially in embryonic bone development; play role in crosstalk between BMP/TGF-β and Wnt signaling pathways
Bone morphogenic proteins (BMPs)	Members of TGF-β superfamily of polypeptides; have many functions outside skeletal system; stimulate endochondral bone and cartilage formation and function, promote osteoblast maturation; augment bone remodeling by affecting both osteoblasts and osteoclasts
Tumor necrosis factors (TNFs)	Superfamily of cytokines; play major role in regulating bone metabolism, especially osteoclast function
Osteoprotegerin (OPG)	Inhibits bone remodeling/resorption; produced by several cells, including osteoblasts; is a decoy receptor for RANKL (binds to RANKL, inhibiting RANK/RANKL interactions, suppressing osteoclast formation and bone resorption); also may directly interfere with ability of osteoclasts' podosomes to attach to bone matrix
Receptor activator of nuclear factor-κB (RANK)	Stimulates differentiation of osteoclast precursors; activates mature osteoclasts
Receptor activator of nuclear factor-κB ligand (RANKL)	Promotes osteoclast differentiation/activation; inhibits osteoclast apoptosis
Bone morphogenic protein antagonists	Prevent BMP signaling
Noggin	Binds BMP-2 and -4, reducing osteoblast function
Gremlin	Multiple effects in and out of skeletal system, but also binds BMP-2, -4, and -7, thus reducing BMP signaling; may play role in development of osteoporosis
Twisted gastrulation	Acts as either a BMP agonist or a BMP antagonist
Activin (a BMP-related protein)	Affects both osteoblasts and osteoclasts; may promote bone formation and fracture healing; expressed by both osteoblasts and chondrocytes; helps regulate bone mass
Annexins	Class of calcium-binding proteins; help mineralize matrix vesicles; may influence bone formation
Inhibin	Dominant over activin and BMPs; helps regulate bone mass and strength by affecting formation of osteoblasts and osteoclasts
Leptin	Plays role in bone formation and resorption
Wnt antagonists	
Dickkopf family (Dkk)	Disrupt Wnt signaling, leading to reduced bone mass
Sclerostin	A protein secreted by osteocytes, osteoblasts, and osteoclasts; binds to BMP-6 and BMP-7; interferes with Wnt signaling pathway, inhibiting bone formation by osteoblasts
Transcription factors	
β-Catenin pathway	Protein with multiple functions, one of most important is activation of genetic transcription factors; balance between Wnt/β-catenin signaling promotes normal bone formation/resorption
Wnts (complex signaling pathway)	Important in differentiating osteoblasts, bone formation; has overlapping effects with BMPs, helps regulate bone formation and remodeling; crosstalks with other signaling pathways
Nuclear factor of activated B cells (NF-κB)	Affects embryonic osteoclastogenesis; plays role in certain osteoclast, osteoblast, and chondroblast functions
Matrix metalloproteinases (MMPs)	
Family of endopeptidases (enzymes) that includes collagenases, gelatinases, stromelysins, matrilysins	Help maintain equilibrium of extracellular matrix (ECM); breakdown almost all components of ECM
A disintegrin and metalloproteinase (ADAM)	Proteolytic enzymes; also have cell-signaling functions, usually linked to cell membrane
A disintegrin and metalloproteinase with thrombospondin motifs (ADAMTs)	Similar to ADAMs but are secreted into circulation, are found around cells; various subgroups affect multiple tissues
Cysteine protease	Cathepsin K expressed by osteoclasts; assists in bone remodeling by cleaving proteins, such as collagen type I, collagen type II, and osteonectin
MMP inhibitors	
Tetracyclines (especially doxycycline), bisphosphonates	Block enzymatic function of MMPs
Tissue inhibitors of metalloproteinases (TIMPs)	Balance effect of MMPs in maintaining ECM equilibrium

From Boyce BF et al: *Ann N Y Acad Sci* 1192:367-375, 2010; Genetos DC et al: *PLoS One* 9(9):e107482, 2015; Kim Y-S et al: *J Korean Med Sci* 25:985-991, 2010; Norrie JL et al: *Dev Biol* 393 (2):270-281, 2014; Stewart A et al: *J Cell Physiol* 223(3):658-666, 2010; Wang RN et al: *Genes Dis* 1(1):87-105, 2014; Zhao H et al: *Cytokine* 71(2):199-206, 2014.

and OPG determines the amount of bone loss. The balance between RANKL and OPG is regulated by cytokines and hormones.[16] Alterations of the RANKL/RANK/OPG system can lead to dysregulation and pathologic conditions, including primary osteoporosis, immune-mediated bone diseases, malignant bone disorders, and inherited skeletal diseases (see Figure 38-5).

Bone Matrix

Bone matrix is made of the *extracellular elements* of bone tissue, specifically collagen fibers, structural proteins (such as proteoglycans and certain glycoproteins), carbohydrate-protein complexes, ground substance, and minerals.

Collagen fibers. Collagen fibers make up the bulk of bone matrix. They are formed as follows:

1. Osteoblasts synthesize and secrete type I collagen and osteocalcin.
2. Collagen molecules assemble into three thin chains (alpha chains) to form fibrils.
3. Fibrils organize into the staggered pattern, with each fibril overlapping its nearest neighbor by about one fourth its length. This creates gaps into which mineral crystals are deposited.
4. After mineral deposition, fibrils interlink and twist to form ropelike fibers.
5. The fibers join to form the framework that gives bone its tensile and supportive strength.

Proteoglycans. Proteoglycans are large complexes of numerous polysaccharides attached to a common protein core. They strengthen bone by forming compression-resistant networks between the collagen fibers. Proteoglycans also control the transport and distribution of electrically charged particles (ions), particularly calcium, through the bone matrix, thereby playing a role in bone calcium deposition and calcification. Proteoglycans are important constituents of ground substance.

Glycoproteins. Glycoproteins are carbohydrate-protein complexes that control the collagen interactions that lead to fibril formation. They also may function in calcification. Four glycoproteins are present in bone: sialoprotein, which binds easily with calcium; osteocalcin, which binds preferentially to crystallized calcium; bone albumin, which is identical to serum albumin and possibly transports essential nutrients to and from bone cells and maintains the osmotic pressure of bone fluid; and alpha-glycoprotein (α-glycoprotein), which probably plays a significant role in calcification and also may facilitate bone resorption by activating osteoclasts (see Table 38-1).

Bone Minerals

After collagen synthesis and fiber formation, mineralization, the final step, occurs in areas known as matrix vesicles that "bud" from the surfaces of osteoblasts, chondrocytes (cartilage cells), and odontoblasts (cells that form dentin in teeth).[17] Mineralization has two distinct phases: (1) formation of the initial mineral deposit (initiation) and (2) proliferation or accretion of additional mineral crystals on the initial mineral deposits (growth). The majority of the minerals in the body are an analog of the naturally occurring mineral hydroxyapatite (HAP). The HAP crystals then penetrate the matrix vesicle membrane and enter into the extracellular space.[17]

Table 38-3 lists the sequence in which calcium and phosphate form amorphous (fluid) calcium phosphate compounds that are converted, in stages, to solid hexagonal crystals of HAP. As the calcium and phosphorus concentrations increase in the bone matrix, the first precipitate to form is dicalcium phosphate dihydrate (DCPD). Once DCPD precipitation begins, the remaining phases of bone crystal formation proceed until insoluble HAP is produced, with approximately 80% to 90% of the HAP incorporated into the collagen fibers. Amorphous calcium phosphate is distributed throughout the bone matrix.

TABLE 38-3 Sequence of Calcium and Phosphate Compound Formation and Crystallization*

Formula	Name	Abbreviation
$Ca(HPO_4) \cdot 2H_2O$	Dicalcium phosphate dihydrate	DCPD
$Ca_4H(PO_4)_3$	Octacalcium phosphate	OCP
$Ca_9(PO_4)_6$ (var.)	Amorphous calcium phosphate	ACP
$Ca_3(PO_4)_2$	Tricalcium phosphate	TCP
$Ca_5(PO_4)_3OH$	Hydroxyapatite	HAP

*Compounds are listed in the order in which precipitation and crystal formation occur.

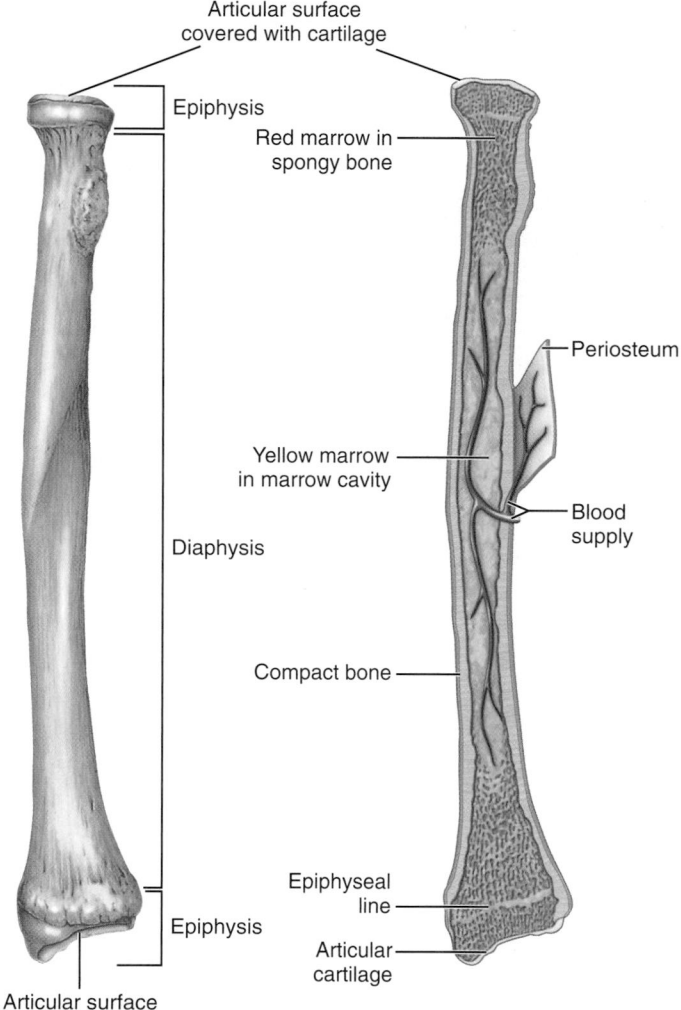

FIGURE 38-2 Anatomy of the Bone. **A,** External anatomy of a long bone. **B,** Internal structure of a long bone showing spongy (cancellous) and compact bone. (From Solomon E: *Introduction to human anatomy and physiology,* ed 4, St Louis, 2016, Saunders.)

Types of Bone Tissue

Bone is composed of two types of bony (osseous) tissue: compact bone (cortical bone) and spongy bone (cancellous bone) (Figure 38-2). Cortical bone is about 85% of the skeleton; cancellous bone makes up the remaining 15%. Both types of bone tissue contain the same structural elements, with a few exceptions. In addition, both compact tissue and spongy tissue are present in every bone. The major

FIGURE 38-3 Structure of Compact and Cancellous Bone. A, Magnified view of compact bone. **B,** Longitudinal section of a long bone showing both cancellous and compact bone. **C,** Section of a flat bone. Outer layers of compact bone surround cancellous bone. Fine structure of compact and cancellous bone is shown in the electron photomicrograph. (From Patton KT, Thibodeau GA: *Anatomy & physiology*, ed 9, St Louis, 2016, Mosby. Photo courtesy Dennis Strete.)

difference between the two types of tissue is the organization of the elements.

Compact bone is highly organized, solid, and extremely strong. The basic structural unit in compact bone is the haversian system (Figure 38-3). Each haversian system consists of the following:

1. A central canal called the haversian canal
2. Concentric layers of bone matrix called lamellae (sing., lamella)
3. Tiny spaces (lacunae) between the lamellae
4. Bone cells (osteocytes) within the lacunae
5. Small channels or canals called canaliculi (sing., canaliculus)

Spongy bone is less complex and lacks haversian systems. In spongy bone, the lamellae are not arranged in concentric layers but in plates or bars termed trabeculae (sing., trabecula) that branch and unite with one another to form an irregular meshwork. The pattern of the meshwork is determined by the direction of stress on the particular bone. The spaces between the trabeculae are filled with red bone marrow. The osteocyte-containing lacunae are distributed between the trabeculae and interconnected by canaliculi. Capillaries pass through the marrow to nourish the osteocytes.

All bones are covered with a double-layered connective tissue called the periosteum. The outer layer of the periosteum contains blood vessels and nerves, some of which penetrate to the inner structures of the bone through channels called *Volkmann canals* (see Figure 38-3). The inner layer of the periosteum is anchored to the bone by collagenous fibers (Sharpey fibers) that penetrate the bone. Sharpey fibers also help hold or attach tendons and ligaments to the periosteum of bones.

Characteristics of Bone

The 206 bones of the human skeleton are distributed between the axial skeleton and the appendicular skeleton. The axial skeleton—the skull, vertebral column, and thorax—consists of 80 bones. The other 126 bones of the appendicular skeleton comprise the upper and lower extremities, the shoulder girdle (pectoral girdle), and the pelvic girdle

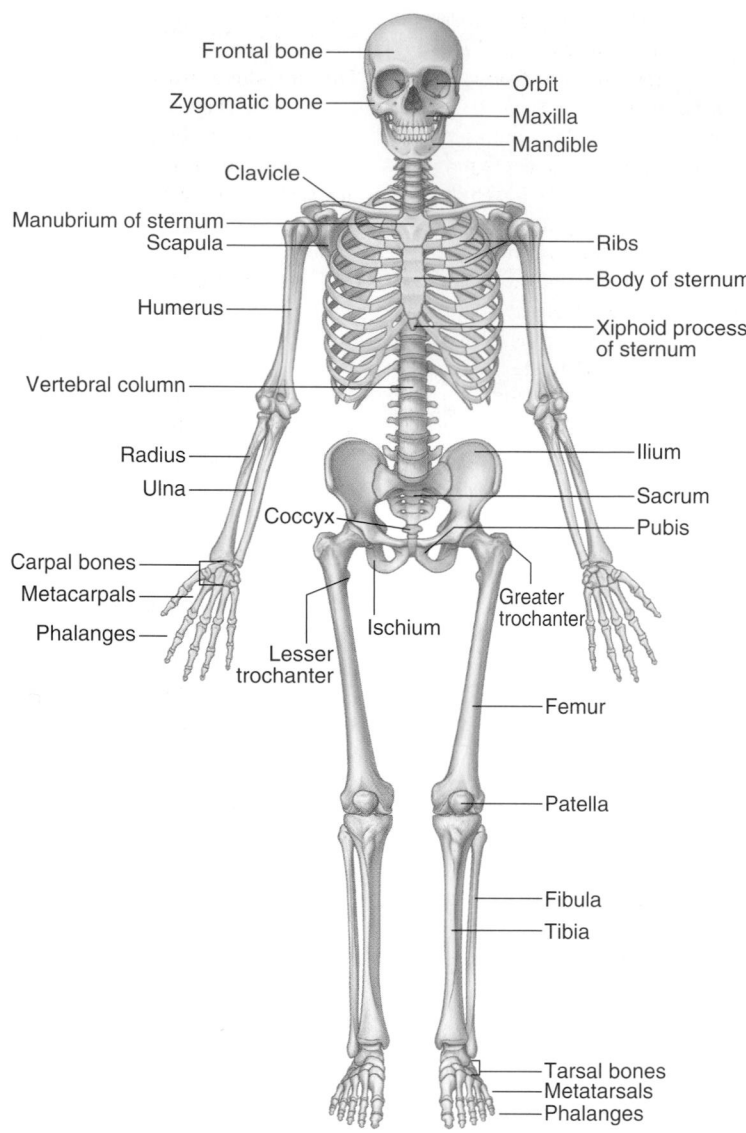

FIGURE 38-4 Anterior View of the Skeleton. (From Drake R, et al: *Gray's atlas of anatomy,* ed 2, Philadelphia, 2015, Churchill Livingstone.)

(os coxae) (Figure 38-4). The skeleton contributes approximately 14% of an adult's body weight.

Bones can be classified by shape as long, flat, short (cuboidal), or irregular. Long bones are longer than they are wide and consist of a narrow tubular midportion (diaphysis) that merges into a broader neck (metaphysis) and a broad end (epiphysis) (see Figure 38-2).

The diaphysis consists of a shaft of thick, rigid compact bone that is able to tolerate bending forces. Contained within the diaphysis is the elongated marrow (medullary) cavity. The marrow cavity of the diaphysis contains primarily fatty tissue, which is referred to as *yellow marrow.* The yellow marrow assists red bone marrow in hematopoiesis only during times of stress. The yellow marrow cavity of the diaphysis is continuous with marrow cavities in the spongy bone of the metaphysis and diaphysis. The marrow contained within the epiphysis is red because it contains primarily blood-forming tissue (see Chapter 20). A layer of connective tissue, the endosteum, lines the outer surfaces of both types of marrow cavity.

The broadness of the epiphysis allows weightbearing to be distributed over a wide area. The epiphysis is made up of spongy bone covered by a thin layer of compact bone. In a child, the epiphysis is separated from the metaphysis by a cartilaginous growth plate (epiphyseal plate). After puberty, the epiphyseal plate calcifies and the epiphysis and metaphysis merge. By adulthood, the line of demarcation between the epiphysis and metaphysis is undetectable.

In flat bones, such as the ribs and scapulae, two plates of compact bone are nearly parallel to each other. Between the compact bone plates is a layer of spongy bone. Short bones, such as the bones of the wrist or ankle, are often cuboidal. They consist of spongy bone covered by a thin layer of compact bone.

Irregular bones, such as the vertebrae, mandibles, or other facial bones, have various shapes that include thin and thick segments. The thin part of an irregular bone consists of two plates of compact bone surrounding spongy bone. The thick part consists of spongy bone surrounded by a layer of compact bone.

Maintenance of Bone Integrity
Remodeling

The internal structure of bone is maintained by remodeling, a three-phase process in which existing bone is resorbed and new bone is laid down to replace it. Clusters of bone cells, termed basic multicellular units, carry out remodeling. The basic multicellular units are made up of bone precursor cells that differentiate into osteoclasts and osteoblasts. Precursor cells are located on the free surfaces of bones and along the vascular channels (especially the marrow cavities).

In phase 1 (activation) of the remodeling cycle, a stimulus (e.g., hormone, drug, vitamin, physical stressor) activates the cytokine system, particularly the tumor necrosis factor (TNF) superfamily, to form osteoclasts.[14] Osteoclasts attach to the bone matrix by actin microfilaments and multiple other proteins that form foot-like structures called podosomes. Once attached, the osteoclasts' integrin receptors anchor its microfilaments to the extracellular matrix, thus providing receptor pathways between the osteocyte and bone matrix. Lysosomal enzymes produced by osteoclasts "digest" bone; the osteoclasts then release the degraded bone products into the vascular system.[12] After bone is resorbed, the osteoclast leaves behind an elongated cavity termed a *resorption cavity*. The resorption cavity in compact bone follows the longitudinal axis of the haversian system, whereas the resorption cavity in spongy bone parallels the surface of the trabeculae.

New bone formation begins as osteoblasts lining the walls of the resorption cavity express osteoid and alkaline phosphatase, forming sites for calcium and phosphorus deposition. As the osteoid mineralizes, new bone is formed. Successive layers (lamellae) in compact bone are laid down, until the resorption cavity is reduced to a narrow haversian canal around a blood vessel. In this way, old haversian systems are destroyed and new haversian systems are formed. New trabeculae are formed in spongy bone. The entire process of remodeling takes about 3 to 6 months.

Repair

The remodeling process can repair microscopic bone injuries, but gross injuries, such as fractures and surgical wounds (osteotomies), heal by the same stages as soft tissue injuries, except that new bone, instead of scar tissue, is the final result (see Chapter 6). The stages of bone healing are listed here and shown in Figure 38-5:

1. Inflammation/hematoma formation
2. Procallus formation
3. Callus formation
4. Replacement, by basic multicellular units, of the callus with lamellar or trabecular bone
5. Remodeling of the periosteal and endosteal surfaces of the bone to the size and shape of the bone before injury

The speed with which bone heals depends on the severity of the bone disruption; the type and amount of bone tissue that need to be replaced (spongy bone heals faster); the blood and oxygen supply available at the site; the presence of growth and thyroid hormones, insulin, vitamins, and other nutrients; the existence of systemic disease; the effects of aging (see Osteoporosis in Chapter 39 on p. 1000); and the availability of effective treatment, including immobilization and the prevention of complications such as infection. In general, however, hematoma formation occurs within hours of fracture or surgery, formation of procallus by osteoblasts within days, callus formation within weeks, and replacement and contour modeling within years—up to 4 years in some cases.

✔ QUICK CHECK 38-1
1. Name the different types of bone cells.
2. What are the major cells involved in bone resorption?
3. What are the stages of bone wound healing?
4. Briefly describe the process of remodeling.

STRUCTURE AND FUNCTION OF JOINTS

The site where two or more bones are attached is called a joint, or articulation (Figure 38-6). The primary function of joints is to provide stability and mobility to the skeleton. A joint's function depends on both its location and its structure. Generally, joints that stabilize the skeleton have a simpler structure than those that enable the skeleton to move. Most joints provide both stability and mobility to some degree.

Joints are classified based on the degree of movement they permit or on the connecting tissues that hold them together. Based on movement, a joint is classified as a synarthrosis (immovable joint), an amphiarthrosis (slightly movable joint), or a diarthrosis (freely movable joint). On the basis of connective structures, joints are classified broadly as fibrous, cartilaginous, or synovial. Each of these three structural classifications can be subdivided according to the shape and contour of the articulating surfaces (ends) of the bones and the type of motion the joint permits.

Fibrous Joints

A joint in which bone is united directly to bone by fibrous connective tissue is called a fibrous joint. These joints have no joint cavity and allow little, if any, movement.

Fibrous joints are further subdivided into three types: sutures, syndesmoses, and gomphoses. A suture has a thin layer of dense fibrous tissue that binds together interlocking flat bones in the skulls of young children. Sutures form an extremely tight union that permits no motion. By adulthood, the fibrous tissue has been replaced by bone. A syndesmosis is a joint in which the two bony surfaces are united by a ligament or membrane. The fibers of ligaments are flexible and stretch, permitting a limited amount of movement. The paired bones of the lower arm (radius and ulna) and the lower leg (tibia and fibula) and their ligaments are syndesmotic joints. A gomphosis is a special type of fibrous joint in which a conical projection fits into a complementary socket and is held in place by a ligament. The teeth held in the maxilla or mandible are gomphosis joints.

Cartilaginous Joints

There are two types of cartilaginous joints: symphyses and synchondroses. A symphysis is a cartilaginous joint in which bones are united by a pad or disk of fibrocartilage. A thin layer of hyaline cartilage usually covers the articulating surfaces of these two bones, and the thick pad of fibrocartilage acts as a shock absorber and stabilizer. Examples of symphyses are the symphysis pubis, which joins the two pubic bones, and the intervertebral disks, which join the bodies of the vertebrae. A synchondrosis is a joint in which hyaline cartilage, rather than fibrocartilage, connects the two bones. The joints between the ribs and the sternum are synchondroses. The hyaline cartilage of these joints is called *costal cartilage*. Slight movement at the synchondroses between the ribs and the sternum allows the chest to move outward and upward during breathing.

Joint (Articular) Capsule

The joint (articular) capsule is fibrous connective tissue that covers the ends of bones where they meet in a joint; Sharpey fibers firmly attach the proximal and distal capsule to the periosteum, and ligaments and tendons also may reinforce the capsule. It is composed of parallel, interlacing bundles of dense, white fibrous tissue richly supplied with nerves, blood vessels, and lymphatic vessels. Nerves in and around the joint capsule are sensitive to rate and direction of motion, compression, tension, vibration, and pain.

FIGURE 38-5 Bone Remodeling. All bone cells participate in bone remodeling. In the remodeling sequence bone sections are removed by bone-resorbing cells (osteoclasts) and replaced with a new section laid down by bone-forming cells (osteoblasts). Bone remodeling is necessary because it allows the skeleton to respond to mechanical loading, maintains quality control (repair and prevent microdamage), and allows the skeleton to release growth factors and minerals (calcium and phosphate) stored in bone matrix to the circulation. The cells work in response to signals generated in the environment (see **F**). Only the osteoclastic cells mediate the first phase of remodeling. They are activated, scoop out bone (**A**), and resorb it; then the work of the osteoblasts begins (**B**). They form new bone that replaces bone removed by the resorption process (**C**). The sequence takes 4 to 6 months. **D,** Micrograph of active bone remodeling seen in the settings of primary or secondary hyperparathyroidism. Note the active osteoblasts surmounted on red-stained osteoid. Marrow fibrosis is present. **E,** Bone remodeling cycle in normal bone with (**F**). Numerous signaling factors are necessary for remodeling. Factors most important for resorption include granulocyte macrophage-colony stimulating factor (GM-CSF), interleukin-1 (IL-1) and IL-6, receptor activator for nuclear factor-κB ligand (RANKL), prostaglandin E_2 (PGE_2), and tumor necrosis factor-alpha (TNF-α). Important factors for bone formation include osteoprotegerin (OPG), transforming growth factor-beta (TGF-β), and estrogen. (Adapted from Nucleus Medical Art. D from Damjananov I, Linder J, editors: *Anderson's pathology,* ed 10, St Louis, 1996, Mosby.)

Synovial Membrane

The synovial membrane is a smooth, delicate inner lining of joint capsule found in the nonarticular portion of the synovial joint and any ligaments or tendons that traverse this cavity. It is composed of two layers: the vascular subintima and the thin cellular intima. The vascular subintima merges with the fibrous joint capsule and is composed of loose fibrous connective tissue, elastin fibers, fat cells, fibroblasts, macrophages, and mast cells; the cellular intima consists of rows of synovial cells embedded in fiber-free intercellular matrix and contains two types of cells—**A** and **B**. **A** cells (macrophages) ingest and remove (phagocytose) bacteria and particles of debris in the joint cavity; **B** cells

FIGURE 38-6 **Various Kinds of Joints.** *Fibrous:* **A,** syndesmosis (tibiofibular); **B,** suture (skull). *Cartilaginous:* **C,** symphysis (vertebral bodies); **D,** synchondrosis (first rib and sternum). *Synovial:* **E,** condyloid (wrist); **F,** gliding (radioulnar); **G,** hinge or ginglymus (elbow); **H,** ball and socket (hip); **I,** saddle (carpometacarpal of thumb); **J,** pivot (atlantoaxial). (From Dorland: *Dorland's medical illustrated dictionary,* ed 32, St Louis, 2012, Saunders.)

(fibroblasts) are the most numerous and secrete hyaluronate, which gives synovial fluid its viscous quality. The synovial membrane is richly supplied with blood and lymphatic vessels and is capable of rapid repair and regeneration.

Joint (Synovial) Cavity

The joint (synovial) cavity is an enclosed, fluid-filled space between articulating surfaces of two bones, also called *joint space*. It enables two bones to move "against" one another and is surrounded by synovial membrane and filled with synovial fluid.

Synovial Fluid

Synovial fluid is superfiltrated plasma from blood vessels that lubricates the joint surfaces, nourishes the pad of the articular cartilage, and covers the ends of the bones. Hyaluronic acid in the synovial fluid gives it important biomechanical properties. It also contains free-floating synovial cells and various leukocytes that phagocytose joint debris and microorganisms.

Articular Cartilage

Articular cartilage is a layer of hyaline cartilage that covers the end of each bone; it may be thick or thin, depending on the size of the joint, the fit of the two bone ends, and the amount of weight and shearing force the joint normally withstands. The function of articular cartilage is to reduce friction in the joint and to distribute the forces of weight-bearing. Articular cartilage is composed of chondrocytes (cartilage cells) (about 2% of the tissue) and an intercellular matrix consisting of type II collagen (about 10% to 30% of weight), proteoglycans (about 5% to 10% of weight), and water. The water content ranges from 60% to almost 80% of the net weight of the cartilage, and individual molecules rapidly enter or exit the articular cartilage to contribute to the resiliency of the tissue.

At the surface of articular cartilage, the collagen fibers run parallel to the joint surface and are closely compacted into a dense, protective mat. (Loss of this dense, compacted configuration at the surface subjects the underlying fibers to splitting and thinning, in which case the cartilage is unable to tolerate weightbearing.) In the middle layer (the proliferative zone) of the cartilage, the fibers are arranged tangential to the surface, which allows them to deform and absorb some of the weightbearing (Figure 38-7). In the bottom layer (the hypertrophic zone) of the cartilage, the fibers are perpendicular to the joint surface, allowing them to resist shear forces, and are embedded in a calcified layer of cartilage called the *tidemark*.[18] The tidemark anchors the collagen fibers to the underlying (subchondral) bone. Collagen fibers are important components of the cartilage matrix because they account for approximately 60% of the dry weight and because they (1) anchor the cartilage securely to underlying bone, (2) provide a taut framework for the cartilage, (3) control the loss of fluid from the cartilage, and (4) prevent the escape of protein polysaccharides (proteoglycans) from the cartilage. The proteoglycans give articular cartilage its stiff quality and regulate the movement of synovial fluid through the cartilage. The proteoglycans are macromolecules consisting of proteins, carbohydrates (glycosaminoglycans), and hyaluronic acid.

Synovial Joints
Structure of Synovial Joints

Synovial joints (diarthroses) are the most movable and the most complex joints in the body (Figure 38-8).

Movement of Synovial Joints

Synovial joints are described as uniaxial, biaxial, or multiaxial according to the shapes of the bone ends and the type of movement occurring at the joint (Figure 38-9). Usually, one of the bones is stable and serves as an axis for the motion of the other bone. The body

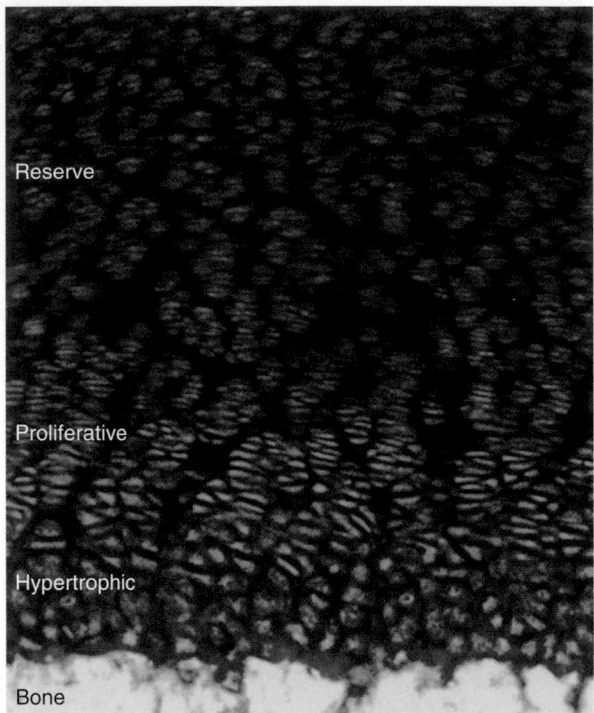

FIGURE 38-7 Collagen Zones. The three collagen zones (reserve, proliferative, and hypertrophic) are distinctly shown in a growth plate. (From Hjorten R et al: *Bone* 41[4]:535, 2007.)

movements made possible by various synovial joints are either circular or angular (Figure 38-10).

STRUCTURE AND FUNCTION OF SKELETAL MUSCLES

Skeletal muscles arise from mesodermal precursor cells that then form myoblasts. The millions of individual fibers of skeletal muscle contract and relax to perform the work necessary to move the body (Figure 38-11). Muscle constitutes 40% of an adult's body weight and 50% of a child's weight. Muscle is 75% water, 20% protein, and 5% organic and inorganic compounds. Thirty-two percent of all protein stores for energy and metabolism are contained in muscle. Between the ages of 30 and 60, muscle mass decreases by about 0.5 pound of muscle each year. For each 0.5 pound of muscle lost, almost 1 pound of fat is typically gained.

Whole Muscle

There are more than 600 skeletal muscles in the body. The body's muscles vary dramatically in size and shape. They range from 2 to 60 cm in length and are shaped according to function. Fusiform muscles are elongated muscles shaped like straps and can run from one joint to another. The biceps brachii and psoas major are examples

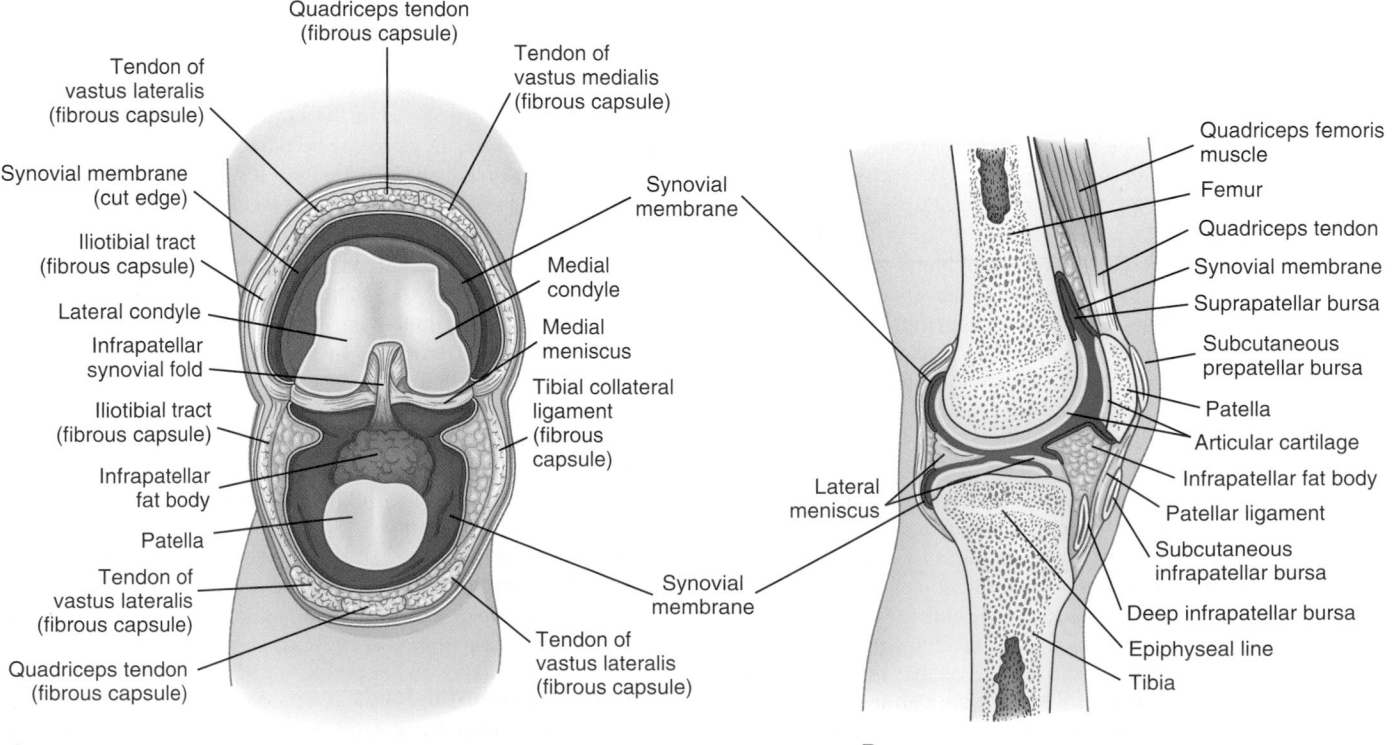

FIGURE 38-8 Knee Joint (Synovial Joint). A, Frontal view. **B,** Lateral view.

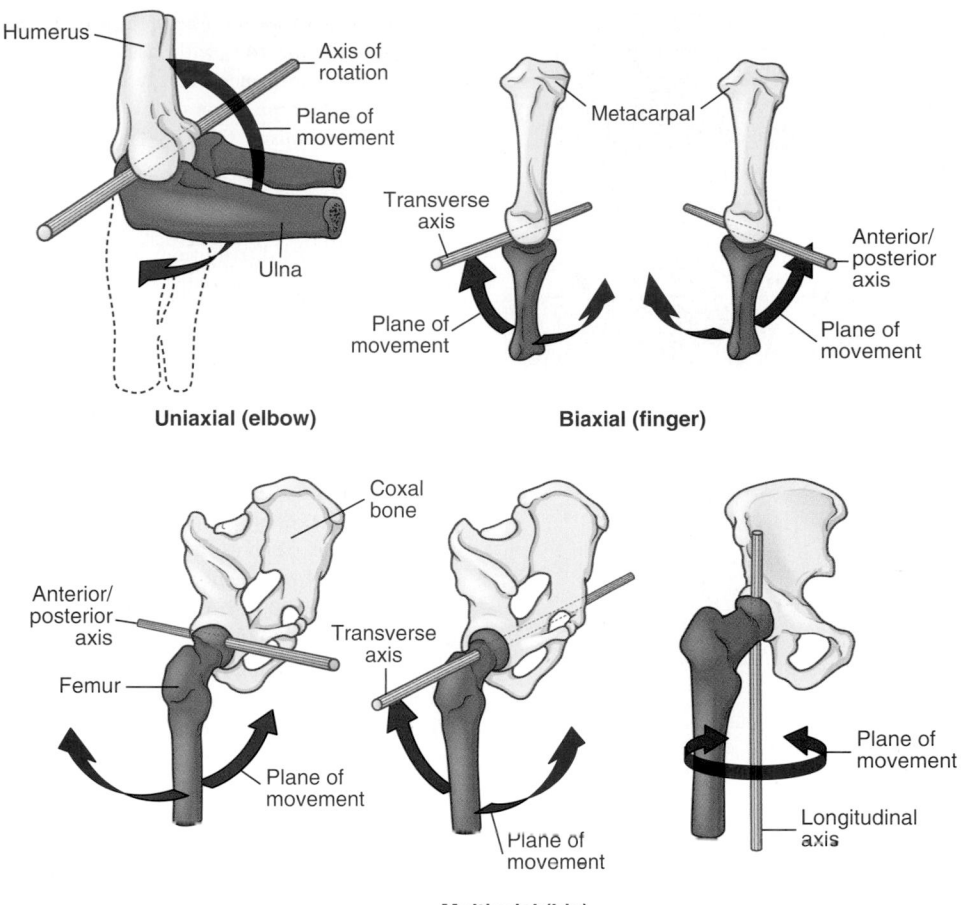

FIGURE 38-9 Movements of Synovial (Diarthrodial) Joints.

of fusiform muscles. **Pennate muscles** are broad, flat, and slightly fan shaped, with fibers running obliquely to the muscle's long axis. The multipennate deltoid muscle, which flexes and extends the arm, is a good example of a muscle shaped according to its function.

Each skeletal muscle is a separate organ, encased in a three-part connective tissue framework called **fascia**. The layers of connective tissue protect the muscle fibers, attach the muscle to bony prominences, and provide a structure for a network of nerve fibers, blood vessels, and lymphatic channels. The layers are as follows:

1. The outermost layer, the **epimysium**, is located on the surface of the muscle and tapers at each end to form the **tendon** (Figure 38-12, also see p. 986 for a discussion of tendons). Tendons allow short muscles to exert power on a distant joint, whereas a thick muscle would interfere with the joint's mobility.
2. The **perimysium** further subdivides the muscle fibers into bundles of connective tissue, or **fascicles**.
3. The smallest unit of muscle visible without a microscope is the **endomysium**, which surrounds the muscle.

The ligaments, tendons, and fascia are made up of connective tissue that also buffers the limbs from the effects of sudden strains or changes in speed. The rapid recovery necessary for strenuous exercise is supported by the elastic property of muscle and its connective tissue.

Skeletal muscle has been designated as **voluntary** (controlled directly by the nervous system), **striated** (has a striped pattern when viewed under a light microscope), or **extrafusal** (to distinguish from other contractile fibers in the sensory organ of the muscle). Components that are visible on gross inspection of the whole muscle include the motor and sensory nerve fibers. These function together with the muscle, innervating portions of it and providing the electrical impulses needed for motor function.

Motor Unit

From the anterior horn cell of the spinal cord, the axons of motor nerves branch to innervate a specific group of muscle fibers. Each anterior horn cell, its axon (part of the lower motor neuron; see Chapter 13), and the muscle fibers innervated by it are called a **motor unit** (Figure 38-13). The motor units are composed of lower motor neurons, which extend to skeletal muscles. Often termed the *functional unit* of the neuromuscular system, the motor unit behaves as a single entity and contracts as a whole when it receives an electrical impulse.

The whole muscle may be controlled by several motor nerve axons. These branch to innervate many motor units within the muscle. The whole muscle then may be made up of many motor units. The number of motor units per individual muscle varies greatly. In the calf, for example, 1 motor axon innervates approximately 2000 muscle fibers, out of a total of 1,200,000 muscle fibers. This is a high innervation ratio of muscle fibers to axons, and it contrasts markedly with the low innervation ratio found in laryngeal muscles, where two to three muscle fibers constitute each motor unit and the innervation ratio can be of great functional significance. The greater the innervation ratio of a particular organ, the greater its endurance. Higher innervation ratios prevent fatigue, whereas lower innervation ratios allow for precision of movement.

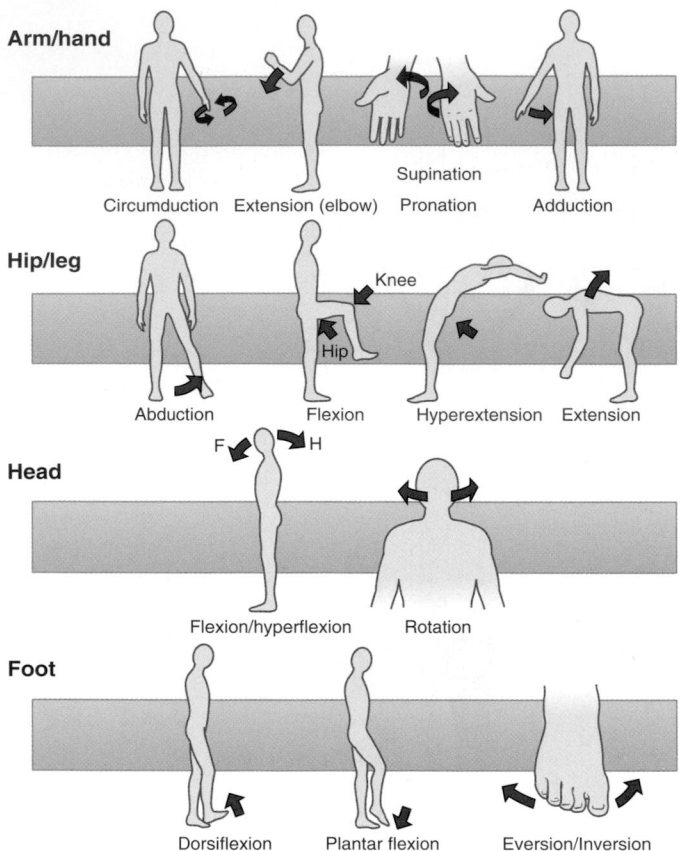

Arm/hand

Circumduction   Extension (elbow)   Supination Pronation   Adduction

Hip/leg

Knee
Hip

Abduction   Flexion   Hyperextension   Extension

Head

F   H

Flexion/hyperflexion   Rotation

Foot

Dorsiflexion   Plantar flexion   Eversion/Inversion

FIGURE 38-10 Body Movements Made Possible by Synovial (Diarthrodial) Joints.

Sensory receptors. Although muscles function as effector organs, they also contain sensory receptors and are involved in sending different signals to the central nervous system. Among these are the muscle spindles and Golgi tendon organs. Spindles are mechanoreceptors that lie parallel to muscle fibers and respond to muscle stretching. Golgi tendon organs are dendrites that terminate and branch to tendons near the neuromuscular junction. The muscle spindles, Golgi tendon organs, and free nerve endings provide a means of reporting changes in length, tension, velocity, and tone in the muscle. This system of afferent signals is responsible for the muscle stretch response and maintenance of normal muscle tone.

Muscle fibers. Each muscle fiber is a single muscle cell that is cylindrical in structure and surrounded by a membrane capable of excitation and impulse propagation. The muscle fiber contains bundles of myofibrils, the fiber's functional subunits, in a parallel arrangement along the longitudinal axis of the muscle (Figure 38-14). At birth, the muscle fibers have completed development from precursor cells called myoblasts. All voluntary muscles are derived from the mesodermal layer of the embryo. Genetic transcription factors, most notably MyoD, induce skeletal muscle differentiation. Myoblasts are the main cells responsible for muscle growth and regeneration. Myoblasts are termed *satellite cells* when in a dormant state. Satellite cells are crucial in muscle growth, maintenance, repair, and regeneration. Once muscle is injured, satellite cells become activated and increase the number of transcriptional factors necessary to form myoblasts and assist in repair.[19]

The type of peripheral nerve influences the muscle fiber and motor unit considerably. Whether motor nerves are fast or slow determines the type of muscle fibers in the motor unit. White muscle (type II

fibers [white fast-twitch fibers]) is innervated by relatively large type II alpha motor neurons with fast conduction velocities. These fibers rely on a short-term anaerobic glycolytic system for rapid energy transfer. Red muscle (type I fibers [slow-twitch fibers]) depends on aerobic oxidative metabolism. Table 38-4 describes the specific characteristics of type I and type II fibers.

The overlap of muscle fibers that appears with staining gives a checkerboard appearance to muscle biopsy specimens. This overlap provides an equal distribution of fiber types throughout the muscle and also helps to compensate for muscle fiber loss and fatigue of individual motor units during activity. In spite of this, some muscles contain proportionally more of one fiber type than another. Postural muscles have more type I fibers, allowing them the high resistance to fatigue that is necessary to maintain the same position for extended periods. The ocular muscles have more type II muscle fibers, allowing them to respond rapidly to visual changes.

The number of muscle fibers varies according to location. Large muscles, such as the gastrocnemius, have more fibers (1,200,000) than smaller muscles, such as the lumbrical muscles in the hand (10,000). The diameter of muscle fibers also varies. The closely packed polygons are small (10 to 20 μm) until puberty, when they attain the normal adult diameter of 40 to 80 μm. Women usually have smaller-diameter fibers than men. Small muscles, such as the ocular muscles, are 15 μm in diameter; larger, more proximal muscles are 40 μm in diameter. Fiber size can have functional significance. Studies have shown that larger fiber diameter is associated with generation of greater forces. Fiber diameter can be increased by exercise or occupational overuse, activities that cause hypertrophied muscle.

The major components of the muscle fiber include the muscle membrane, myofibrils, sarcotubular system, sarcoplasm, and mitochondria (see Figure 38-14). The muscle membrane is a two-part membrane. It includes the sarcolemma, which contains the plasma membrane of the muscle cell, and the cell's basement membrane. The sarcolemma is 7.5 μm thick and is capable of propagating electrical impulses to initiate contraction. At the motor nerve end plate, where the nerve impulse is transmitted, the sarcolemma forms the highly convoluted synaptic cleft. The sarcolemma is made up of lipid molecules and protein systems. The protein systems perform special functions, such as transport of nutrients and protein synthesis. They also provide the sodium-potassium pump and include the cell's cholinergic receptor. The basement membrane is 50 μm thick and is composed primarily of proteins and polysaccharides. It also serves as the cell's microskeleton and maintains the shape of the muscle cell. The basement membrane also may function in some way to restrict further diffusion of electrolytes once they have crossed the sarcolemma.

The sarcoplasm is the cytoplasm of the muscle cell and contains myoglobin plus the intracellular components that are common to all cells (see Chapter 1). Myoglobin is a protein found primarily in skeletal and heart muscle. Related to hemoglobin in the blood, myoglobin stores oxygen and iron in the muscle. The sarcoplasm is an aqueous substance that provides a matrix that surrounds the myofibrils. It contains numerous enzymes and proteins that are responsible for the cell's energy production, protein synthesis, and oxygen storage. The mitochondria house enzyme systems for energy production, particularly those that regulate processes such as the citric acid cycle and adenosine triphosphate (ATP) formation. Many other structures are present in the sarcoplasm. The ribosomes are composed of primarily ribonucleic acid (RNA) and participate in the process of protein synthesis. The cell nucleus, satellite cells, glycogen granules, and lipid droplets are suspended in the sarcoplasmic matrix. Blood vessels, nerve endings, muscle spindles, and Golgi tendon organs are also directly located within this structure.

FIGURE 38-11 Skeletal Muscles of Body. A, Anterior view. B, Posterior view.

TABLE 38-4 Characteristics of Human Skeletal Muscle Fibers

Characteristics	Type I (Red) (Oxidative Fibers [OFs])	Type II (White) Type II-1A (Fast Oxidative Glycolic Fibers [FOGs])
Anatomic location	Deep axial portion of muscle	Surface portion of muscle
Fiber diameter	Small	Large
Motor neuron size	Small	Large
Contraction speed	Slow	Fast
Motor neuron type	Type I, α	Type II-A, II-B, II-X, and II-D
		II-A: fatigue resistant; II-B: fast fatigable; II-X and II-D: intermediate fatigability
Glycogen content (at rest)	Low	High
Oxidative capacity	High	High (for short periods)
Myosin-ATPase activity	Low	High
Metabolism	Oxidative (also most effective in removing glucose from bloodstream)	Some oxidative pathways, mostly glycolysis
Used for	Maintaining body posture, skeletal support, aerobic activity	Short, intense activity (e.g., sprinting)
Aerobic metabolic capacity	High	Low
Fatigue resistance	High	Intermediate to low
Myoglobin content	High	Low
Capillary supply	Profuse	Intermediate to low
Mitochondria	Many	Few
Intensity of contraction	Low	High
Example (most muscles are mixed)	Soleus muscle	Laryngeal
Satellite cell content	High	Low

From Schiaffino S, Reggiani C: *Physiol Rev* 91:1447-1531, 2011; Verdijk LB et al: *Age* 36(2):545-547, 2014.

FIGURE 38-12 Levels of Organization within a Skeletal Muscle Showing Muscle Fibers and Their Coverings. (From Standring S: *Gray's anatomy*, ed 40, Edinburgh, 2008, Churchill Livingstone.)

Unique to the muscle is the sarcotubular system, a network that includes the transverse tubules and the sarcoplasmic reticulum, which crosses the interior of the cell. The sarcoplasmic reticulum is constructed like the endoplasmic reticulum in other cells. The sarcoplasmic reticulum is composed of tubules that run parallel to the myofibrils. The longitudinal tubules are termed sarcotubules. In muscle cells, the sarcoplasmic reticulum contains a network of intracellular receptors known as ryanodine receptors (RyRs). In response to a nerve impulse, RyR1 (found in skeletal muscle cells) releases intracellular calcium and initiates muscle contraction at the sarcomere, a portion of the myofibril. The transverse tubules, which also contain calcium release channels and are closely associated with the sarcotubules, run across the sarcoplasm and communicate with the extracellular space. Together, the tubules of this membrane system allow for uptake and regulation of intracellular calcium, release of calcium during muscle contraction, and storage of calcium during muscle relaxation.[20-22]

Myofibrils. The myofibrils are the functional units of muscle contraction. Each myofibril contains sarcomeres, which appear at intervals (see Figure 38-14). The speed with which sarcomeres lengthen and shorten during movement directly influences the strength and function of skeletal muscles. Sprinters tend to have more fast-twitch (FT) fibers than slow-twitch (ST) fibers in their leg muscles, and endurance runners have more ST fibers in their leg muscles. Sarcomeres are composed of several proteins. The two most abundant are actin and myosin, but three other giant, muscle-specific proteins (titin, nebulin, and obscurin) play important roles in myofibril formation and function (see Table 38-5).

The myofibrils are the most abundant subcellular muscle component, equaling 85% to 90% of the total volume. On cross section, they are seen to be irregular polygons with a mean diameter of less than 1 μm. Each myofibril is composed of serially repeating sarcomeres, separated by Z bands, which give the muscle its striped, cross-striated appearance. Each sarcomere has a dark A band and is flanked by two light I bands (Figure 38-15). The A band is 1.5 to 1.6 μm long and contains the thick myosin filaments. Included in the A band is a lighter zone called the *H band,* and in the center of the H band is the dark *M band,* or *M line.* The *I band,* which contains actin, is divided at the midpoint of each sarcomere by the *Z band.* Its length varies with the start of muscle contraction. The *Z disk* (made up of different layers of Z bands, depending on muscle type) marks the boundaries of the sarcomere.[23]

Myofibrils are composed of myofilaments. Each myofilament is structured in a closely packed hexagonal arrangement, with two thin filaments for every thick filament. The thick filament, along with C protein and M line protein, is made up of myosin. Myosin has two subunits—heavy and light meromyosin, which resemble twisted golf club shafts. The thin filaments are twisted double strands consisting of actin, troponin, and tropomyosin (see Chapter 23 and Figure 23-13).

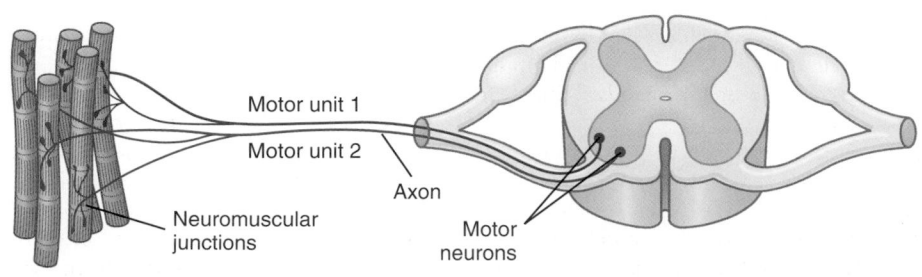

Muscle fibers   **Spinal cord**

FIGURE 38-13 Motor Units of a Muscle. Each motor unit consists of a motor neuron and all the muscle fibers (cells) supplied by the neuron and its axon branches.

TABLE 38-5 Contractile Proteins of Skeletal Muscle Sarcomere

Protein	Location	Function
Actinin	Z disk	Attaches actin to Z disks; helps coordinate sarcomere contraction; cross-links thin filaments in adjacent sarcomeres
Actin	I band (thin filaments)	Contraction; activates myosin-ATPase; interacts with myosin
α-Actin	Z disk	Main ligand of titin; links and controls filament length
β-Actin	Z disk	Regulatory and structural function; links filaments, controls filament length
Myosin	A band (thick filament)	Contraction force; two distinct types: myosin heavy chain (MyHC) and myosin light chain (MyLC); hydrolyzes ATP and develops tension
Titin* (largest and third most abundant muscle protein)	Half of sarcomere (from Z disk to M band)	Coordinates assembly of proteins that comprise sarcomere; regulates resting length of sarcomere; important for myofibril assembly, stabilization, and maintenance
Nebulin*	I band (with α-actin)	Interacts with myosin to produce contraction; binding site for actin, desmin, titin, other proteins; stabilizes and regulates length of actin filaments; plays role in assembly, structure, and maintenance of Z disks
Obscurin*	Surrounds sarcomere (mainly at Z disk and M band)	May mediate interaction of sarcoplasmic reticulum and myofibrils; plays role in muscle response to injury; has role in formation and stabilization of M bands and A band

Data from Herzog JA et al: *Mol Cell Biomech* 11(1):1-17, 2014; Luther PK: *J Muscle Res Cell Motil* 30:171-185, 2009; Pappas CT et al: *J Cell Biol* 189(5):858-870, 2010; Schiaffino S, Reggiani C: *Physiol Rev* 91:1447-1531, 2011.
ATP, Adenosine triphosphate; *ATPase,* adenosinetriphosphatase.
*Also may function as molecular scaffolds for myofibril formation.

FIGURE 38-14 **Muscle Structure.** A skeletal muscle consists of fascicles (bundles) of muscle fibers. Each fiber is a cell containing myofibrils that consist of actin and myosin filaments. The filaments are organized into repeating units called sarcomeres. (From Solomon E: *Introduction to human anatomy and physiology,* ed 4, St Louis, 2016, Saunders.)

Muscle proteins. A multitude of muscle proteins have been identified and their functions are still being discovered. Table 38-5 summarizes the location and function of some of the important muscle proteins.

Nonprotein constituents of muscle. Substances such as nitrogen, creatine, creatinine, phosphocreatine, purines, uric acid, and amino acids all serve in the complex process of muscle metabolism. Energy is provided by glycogen and its derivatives.

Creatine metabolism and creatinine metabolism have been used to measure muscle mass. Plasma creatine is taken up by muscle and converted into the high-energy phosphate compound phosphocreatine by the enzyme creatine kinase. Creatinine is formed in muscle from creatine at a constant rate of 2% per day. (Tests for measurement of plasma creatine level are discussed in Chapter 30.) Creatine excretion is increased in muscle wasting. This change reflects the reduction in total body creatine stores and the loss of muscle mass.

Inorganic compounds, anions (phosphate, chloride), and cations (calcium, magnesium, sodium, potassium) are important in the regulation of protein synthesis, muscle contraction, and enzyme systems as well as in the stabilization of cell membranes. Total body potassium (TBK) level, measured by the K40 method, has been used to measure muscle mass, also called *lean body mass.* Total body potassium levels reflect changes in muscle mass seen during growth, malnutrition, and muscle wasting.

Components of Muscle Function

The ultimate function of muscle is to accomplish work. Although variously expressed in such measures as foot-pounds or kilogram-meters, work usually refers to the amount of energy liberated or force exerted over a distance (work = force × distance). Muscles usually contract or tense while doing work. Muscle contraction occurs on the molecular level and leads to the observable phenomenon of muscle movement.

Muscle Contraction at the Molecular Level

The four steps of muscle contraction are (1) excitation, (2) coupling, (3) contraction, and (4) relaxation. The process involves the electrical properties of all cells and the movement of ions across the plasma membrane (see Chapter 1). The muscle fiber is an excitable tissue. At rest, an electrical charge of −90 mV is continually maintained across the sarcolemma. This resting potential, generated by the separation of positive and negative charges on either side of the membrane, creates an electrochemical equilibrium caused by the selective permeability of the sarcolemma to electrolytes in the intracellular and extracellular fluids, particularly potassium and sodium.

Excitation, the first step of muscle contraction, begins with the spread of an action potential from the nerve terminal to the neuromuscular junction. The rapid depolarization of the membrane initiates an electrical impulse in the muscle fiber membrane called the **muscle fiber action potential.** As the action potential advances along the sarcolemmal membrane, it spreads to the transverse tubules. (The velocity of conduction is much slower in muscle fibers than in myelinated nerve fibers—only 3 to 5 m/sec compared with 54 to 90 m/sec in nerve fibers.) A receptor on the transverse tubule opens, allowing calcium to enter the cell.[24]

FIGURE 38-15 Muscle Fibers. A, The Z disks define the end of an individual sarcomere. The M line (which lies within the H band) is made of cross-connecting elements of the cytoskeleton. **B,** Actin is the primary protein of the I band (thin filament). Nebulin also extends along the I band and contains binding sites for actin and myosin. Myosin (thick filament) extends through the A band. Titin extends from the Z disk to the M band, binding with myosin; strong titin anchoring within the I band is necessary for proper muscle function. During contraction, the I bands and H bands shorten, moving the Z disks closer together. **C,** Electron photomicrograph of human muscle tissue corresponding to schematics in **A** and **B.** (A modified from Thompson JM et al: *Mosby's clinical nursing,* ed 5, St Louis, 2002, Mosby; **C** courtesy Louisa Howard.)

The second stage, coupling, follows the depolarization of the transverse tubules. This triggers the release of calcium ions from the sarcoplasmic reticulum through RyR1 channels into the sarcoplasm. The calcium then binds to a protein on the actin filament. (Calcium affects troponin and tropomyosin, muscle proteins that bind with actin when the muscle is at rest.) In the presence of calcium, however, both these proteins are attracted to calcium ions, leaving the actin free to bind with myosin. The release of intracellular calcium ions is the critical link between a nerve impulse (electrical excitation) and muscle contraction.[25]

Contraction begins as the calcium ions combine with troponin, a reaction that overcomes the inhibitory function of the troponin-tropomyosin system. Myosin binds to actin, forming cross-bridges. The myosin heads attach to the exposed actin-binding sites, pulling actin (the thin filament) inward. The thin filament, actin, then slides toward the thick filament, myosin. The two ends of the myofibril shorten after contraction when the myosin heads attach to the actin molecules, forming a cross-bridge that constitutes an actin-myosin complex. ATP, located on the actin-myosin complex, is released when the cross-bridges attach. The process of contraction was first described by A.F. Huxley in the 1950s. It is commonly known as the cross-bridge theory because the actin and myosin proteins form cross-bridges as they contract. The useful distance of contraction of a skeletal muscle is approximately 25% to 35% of the muscle's length.

The last step, relaxation, begins as calcium ions are actively transported back into the sarcoplasmic reticulum, removing ions from interaction with troponin. The cross-bridges detach, and the sarcomere lengthens. (The cross-bridge theory of muscle contraction is discussed in Chapter 23.)

Muscle Metabolism

Skeletal muscle requires a constant supply of ATP and phosphocreatine. These substances are necessary to fuel the complex processes of muscle contraction, driving the cross-bridges of actin and myosin together and transporting calcium from the sarcoplasmic reticulum to the myofibril. Other internal processes of the muscular system that require ATP include protein synthesis, which replenishes muscle constituents and accommodates growth and repair. The rate of protein synthesis is related to hormone levels (particularly insulin), the presence of amino acid substrates, and overall nutritional status. At rest, the rate of ATP formation by oxidation of glucose or acetoacetate is sufficient to maintain internal processes, given normal nutritional status. During activity, the need for ATP increases 100-fold. The metabolic pathways for muscle activity in Table 38-6 show reactions to the immediate need for increased ATP caused by contraction. Activity

lasting longer than 5 seconds expends the available stored ATP and phosphocreatine.

Stored glycogen and blood glucose are converted anaerobically to sustain brief activity without increasing the demand for oxygen. Anaerobic glycolysis is much less efficient than aerobic glycolysis, using six to eight times more glycogen to produce the same amount of ATP. With increased activity, such as intense exercise, or with ischemia, an increase in the amount of lactic acid occurs because of the breakdown of glycogen, thus causing a shift in muscle pH (see Table 38-6). This short-term mechanism buys time by allowing ATP formation in spite of inadequate energy stores or oxygen supply. When the anaerobic threshold is reached and more oxygen is required, physiologic changes occur, including an increase in lactic acid level and increases in oxygen consumption, heart rate, respiratory rate, and muscle blood flow.

Strenuous exercise requires oxygen, which activates the aerobic glycogen pathway for ATP formation. During maximal exercise, free fatty acid mobilization and the aerobic glycogen pathways provide ATP over an extended time. These pathways require oxygen both to maintain maximal activity and to return the muscle to the resting state. Maximal exercise increases oxygen uptake by 15 to 20 times over the resting state. When this system becomes exhausted or inadequate to respond to the need for ATP, fatigue and weakness finally force the muscle to reduce activity with a resultant buildup of lactic acid in muscle fibers. Creatine supplementation may provide some protective effects on muscle in older adult athletes as well as after strenuous physical activity.[26]

Sustaining maximal muscular activity accumulates an oxygen debt, which is the amount of oxygen needed to oxidize the residual lactic acid, convert it back to glycogen, and replenish ATP and phosphocreatine stores. For example, after running at maximal speed for 10 seconds, the average person has consumed 1 L of oxygen. At rest, oxygen consumption for the same period is approximately 40 ml. As the person recovers, the measured oxygen debt is 4 L greater than the amount used during activity.

Oxygen consumption is measured to calculate the metabolic cost of activity in normal and diseased muscle. It is an indirect measure of energy expenditure, along with timed tests of activity, heart rate, and respiratory quotient (ratio of carbon dioxide to expired oxygen consumed). Energy expenditure is measured directly by heat production because heat is released whenever work is accomplished.

Another factor that changes energy requirements is muscle fiber type. Type II fibers rely on anaerobic glycolytic metabolism and fatigue readily. Type I fibers can resist fatigue for longer periods because of their capacity for oxidative metabolism.

Muscle Mechanics

Muscle contraction cannot be viewed in isolation. Several factors determine how force is transmitted from the cross-bridges on individual muscle fibers to accomplish whole-muscle contraction. First, when a motor unit responds to a single nerve stimulus, it develops a phasic contraction, also called a *twitch*. Because the motor unit contracts in an all-or-nothing manner, the contraction that is generated will be a maximal contraction. The central nervous system smoothly grades the force generated by recruiting additional motor units and varying the discharge frequency of each active motor unit. This adding of motor units within the muscle is called repetitive discharge.

Recruitment and repetitive discharge of motor units allow the muscle to activate the number of motor units needed to generate the desired force. The total force developed is the sum of the force generated by each motor unit. If the motor units are stimulated again and the muscle unit has not been able to relax between stimulation and the next contraction, the second contraction will fuse with the

TABLE 38-6	Energy Sources for Muscular Activity
Sources	**Reactions**
Short-term (anaerobic) sources	Adenosine triphosphate (ATP) → Adenosine diphosphate (ADP) + Inorganic phosphate (P_i) + Energy
	Phosphocreatine + ADP $\rightleftharpoons$ Creatine + ATP
	Glycogen/glucose + P_i + ADP → Lactate + ATP
Long-term (aerobic) sources	Glycogen/glucose + ADP + P_i + O_2 → H_2O + CO_2 + ATP
	Free fatty acids + ADP + P_i + O_2 → H_2O + CO_2 + ATP
	Creatine kinase catalyzes reversible reaction of ATP to ADP:
	Creatine phosphate + ATP $\xrightarrow{\text{Creatine Kinase}}$ Creatine + ATP

From Spence AP, Mason EE: *Human anatomy and physiology*, ed 4, St Paul, Minn, 1992, West Publishing.

first, causing **physiologic tetanus** (not to be confused with the disease tetanus).

Other variables, such as fiber type, innervation ratio, muscle temperature, and muscle shape, influence the efficiency of muscular contraction. The two muscle fiber types differ in their responses to electrical activity. Tetanus and duration of phasic contractions, which take microseconds to accomplish, are achieved more rapidly in type II (white fast-twitch) than in type I (red slow-twitch) muscle fibers. Low innervation ratios promote control and coordination, whereas high ratios promote strength and endurance. Muscles work best at normal body temperature, 98.6° F (37° C). Finally, muscles with a large cross-sectional area, such as the fan-shaped pennate muscles, develop greater contractile forces than smaller-diameter muscles. The initial length of a muscle and the range of shortening that occur when the muscle contracts also determine the force it can generate. The long fusiform muscles have a greater range of shortening and can contract up to 57% of their resting length. A certain amount of elongation is necessary to generate sufficient tension and muscular force. The elongation that occurs during the swing of a golf club or tennis racket is an example of how stretch improves contractile force.

Types of Muscle Contraction

During **isometric** (or **static**) **contraction**, the muscle maintains constant length as tension is increased (Figure 38-16). Isometric contraction occurs, for example, when the arm or leg is pushed against an immovable object. The muscle contracts, but the limb does not move. Isometric contraction is also called **static (holding) contraction**.

During **dynamic** (formerly known as **isotonic**) **contraction**, the muscle maintains a constant tension as it moves. Isotonic contractions can be **eccentric (lengthening)** or **concentric (shortening)**. Positive

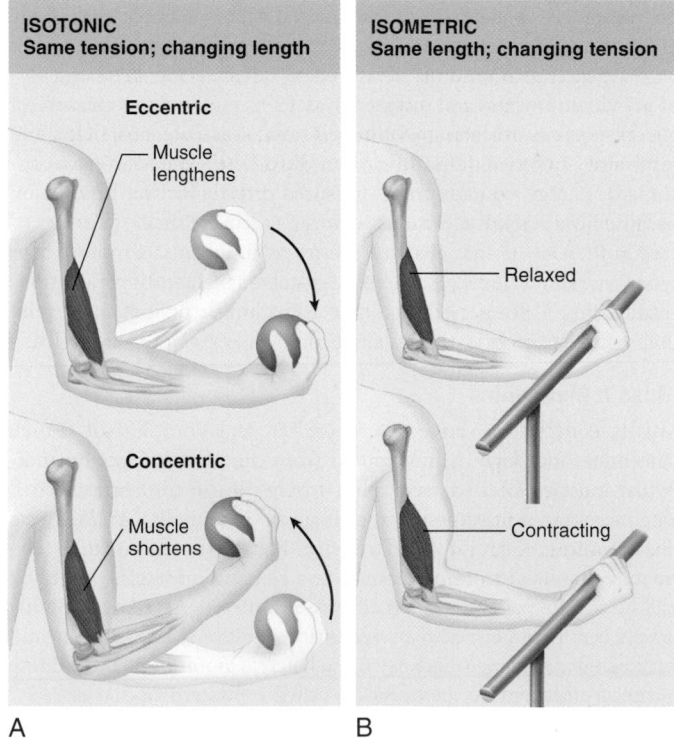

A   B

FIGURE 38-16 Isotonic and Isometric Contraction. A, In isotonic contraction, the muscle shortens, producing movement. **B,** In isometric contraction, the muscle pulls forcefully against a load but does not shorten. (From Patton KT, Thibodeau GA: *Structure & function of the body,* ed 15, St Louis, 2016, Mosby.)

work is accomplished during concentric contraction, and energy is released to exert force or lift a weight. In contrast, during an eccentric contraction the muscle lengthens and absorbs energy (such as extending the elbow while lowering a weight). Eccentric contraction requires less energy to accomplish and has been said to result in the development of pain and stiffness after unaccustomed exercise.

Movement of Muscle Groups

Muscles do not act alone but in groups, often under automatic control. When a muscle contracts and acts as a prime mover, or **agonist**, its reciprocal muscle, or **antagonist**, relaxes. To illustrate this, hold the right arm in the horizontal position in front of the body and bend the elbow; use the other hand to feel the biceps on the top and the triceps on the bottom of the arm. When the elbow is bent, the biceps are firm, and the triceps are soft. As the arm is extended, the muscles change. When the elbow is completely extended, the biceps is soft and the triceps firm. Completing this movement causes the agonist and antagonist to change automatically; only the movement is commanded, not the alternate contraction and relaxation of the specific muscle groups.

Other associated actions may be seen during walking; as the foot leaves the ground, the paravertebral and gluteal muscles on the opposite sides of the body contract to maintain balance. One notices the loss of the associated muscle's action when paralysis offsets this process and decreases balance. If a person is paralyzed, difficulty in maintaining balance is noticeable.

Tendons and Ligaments

Tendons are important musculoskeletal structures that attach muscle to bone at a site called an **enthesis**. **Ligaments** attach bone to bone, helping to form joints as well as stabilizing them against excessive movement. Both tendons and ligaments are primarily composed of types III, IV, V, and VI collagen and fibroblasts (termed tenocytes in tendons).[27] The fibroblasts in tendon are arranged in parallel rows; fibroblasts appear less organized in ligaments. Collagen fibers and fibroblasts form fascicles, with multiple fascicles then forming whole tendon or ligament. In the proteoglycan matrix of tendons, collagen oligomeric matrix protein (COMP) assists in providing gliding and viscoelastic properties. Compared with tendons, ligament fibers typically contain a greater proportion of elastin.

Two main functions of tendons are (1) transferring forces from muscle to bone and (2) acting as a type of biologic spring for muscles to allow additional stability during movement. Ligaments stabilize joints by restricting movement. Although both tendons and ligaments can withstand significant distraction (stretching) force, they tend to buckle when compressive force is applied.

Both tendons and ligaments have complex structures at the attachment site of two dissimilar tissues. Figure 38-17 illustrates the transition of tissue between tendon/ligament and bone. These complex structures and differences in mechanical and structural characteristics (either tendon and bone or ligament and bone) make healing and repair of damaged tissue complicated (see *Health Alert:* Tendon and Ligament Repair).

AGING & THE MUSCULOSKELETAL SYSTEM

Aging of Bones

Aging is accompanied by the loss of bone tissue. Bones become less dense, less strong, and more brittle with aging. The bone remodeling cycle takes longer to complete, and the rate of mineralization also slows. With aging, women experience loss of bone density, accelerated with the rapid bone loss that occurs during early menopause from

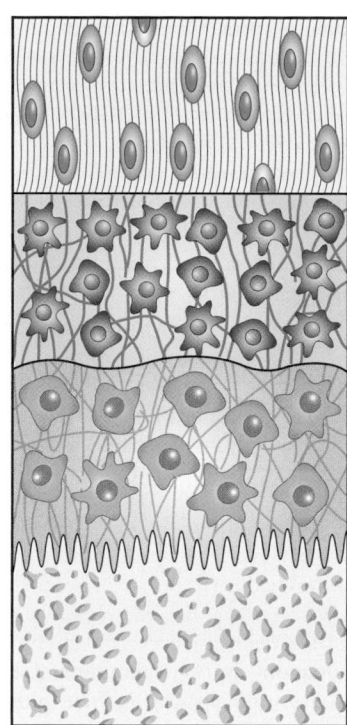

Tendon/ligament
Aligned collagen fibrils (lines)
Fibroblasts embedded throughout (blue oval cells)
Collagen fibrils extend into uncalcified fibrocartilage

Uncalcified fibrocartilage
Larger, less parallel collagen bundles (vertical blue lines)
Collagen types I and II, aggrecan (irregular-shaped cells)
Avascular (yellow background)
Ovoid-shaped, aligned cells (smooth-edged cells)

Wavy tidemark (marks beginning of calcification)

Calcified fibrocartilage
Mineralized tissue
Hypertrophic, more circular chondrocytes
Consists of collagen types I, II, and X

Bone
Interdigitation at surface (zig-zag line)
Calcified tissue

FIGURE 38-17 Cartilage-Bone, Tendon/Ligament-Bone, Meniscus-Bone, and Muscle-Tendon Interfaces. This diagram depicts the cartilage-bone, tendon/ligament-bone, meniscus-bone, and muscle-tendon interfaces and their compositions. Gradients of matrix composition, interdigitation of tissue zones, and interconnecting collagen fibers all enable load transfer between disparate tissues. (From Yang PJ, Temenoff JS: *Tissue Eng Part B Rev* 15(2):128, 2009.)

HEALTH ALERT

Tendon and Ligament Repair

Injury of tendons and ligaments constitutes one of the greatest challenges in musculoskeletal rehabilitation. When these types of structures are damaged, attempts to engineer suitable tissue replacements have proved disappointing. The structures and intricate protein composition of tendons and ligaments are the basis for their complex biomechanical properties. One reason for poor clinical outcome in synthetic tendon structures has been the inability to replicate any material that can bear the high mechanical stresses that occur at the interface between two dissimilar materials (i.e., either tendon and bone or ligament and bone). One promising area of investigation is finding or engineering a biodegradable material, or "scaffold," implanted with specific cells that would regenerate into normal tendon or ligament. The scaffold must be strong enough to withstand the forces at the tissue/bone interface and then gradually break down as it is completely replaced by new cells. Currently, investigators are using synthetic polymers, silk, and collagen as scaffolds, with tendon or ligament fibroblasts and mesenchymal stem cells as the implanted cells. Once these biochemical hurdles are overcome, the repair of damaged tendons and ligaments will be revolutionized.

Data from Jahr H et al: *Curr Rheumatol Rep* 17(3):22, 2015.

increased osteoclastic bone resorption, fewer osteocytes, and decreased numbers of osteoblasts.[28] By age 70 years, susceptible women have, on average, lost 50% of their peripheral cortical bone mass (see Chapter 39). Bone mass losses to such an extent can lead to deformity, pain, stiffness, and high risk for fractures. Men experience bone loss also but at later ages and much slower rates than seen in women. Also, initial bone mass in men is approximately 30% higher than in women;

therefore bone loss in men causes less risk of disability than that found in women. Men's peak bone mass is related to their race, heredity, hormonal factors, physical activity, and calcium intake during childhood. Bone loss in both genders is related to smoking, calcium deficiency, alcohol intake, and physical inactivity. Bone mass can be gained in healthy young women up to the third decade through participation in physical activity, intake of dietary calcium and other minerals, and use of oral contraceptives. Height is also lost with aging because of intervertebral disk degeneration and, sometimes, osteoporotic spinal fractures.

Stem cells in the bone marrow perform less efficiently with aging, predisposing older persons to acute and chronic illnesses. Such illnesses cause weakness and confusion in older persons and may increase the risk of injury or falling.

Aging of Joints

With aging, cartilage becomes more rigid, fragile, and susceptible to fraying because of increased cross-linking of collagen and elastin, decreased water content in the cartilage ground substance, and reduced concentrations of glycosaminoglycans. Decreased range of motion of the joint is related to the changes in ligaments and muscles. Bones in joints develop evidence of osteoporosis with fewer trabeculae and thinner, less dense bones, making them prone to fractures. Intervertebral disk spaces decrease in height. The rate of loss of height accelerates at age 70 years and beyond. Tendons shrink and harden.

Aging of Muscles

The function of skeletal muscle depends on many influences that are affected by cellular factors, such as reduced mitochondrial volume associated with aging.[29] Other influences include the nervous, vascular, and endocrine systems. In the young child, the development of muscle tissue depends greatly on continuing neurodevelopmental maturation. Muscle loss begins at about age 50; however, muscle function remains trainable even into advanced age. Maintaining musculoskeletal fitness at any age can improve overall health.[30,31]

Age-related loss in skeletal muscle is referred to as sarcopenia and is a direct cause of the age-related decrease in muscle strength. As the body ages, muscle mass and strength decline slowly; thus, strength is maintained through the fifth decade, with a slow decline in dynamic and isometric strength evident after age 70. The amount of type II fibers also decreases. There is reduced synthesis of RNA, loss of mitochondrial function,[29,32] and reduction in the size of motor units. The regenerative function of muscle tissue remains normal in aging persons. As much as 30% to 40% of skeletal muscle mass and strength may be lost from the third to ninth decades. Muscle fatigue also may contribute to loss of function with aging.[32] Sarcopenia is thought to be secondary to progressive neuromuscular changes and diminishing levels of anabolic hormones. There is an age-related decline in the synthesis of mixed proteins, myosin heavy chains, and mitochondrial protein.[33] Changes in these muscle proteins are related to reduced levels of insulin-like growth factor-1 (IGF-1), testosterone, and dehydroepiandrosterone (DHEA) sulfate.

Maximal oxygen intake declines with age. Basal metabolic rate is reduced and lean body mass decreases in the aged population.

✔ QUICK CHECK 38-3

1. Name three differences between slow-twitch and fast-twitch muscle fibers.
2. Why is adenosine triphosphate (ATP) used for muscle contraction?
3. Define the differences between tendons and ligaments.
4. Describe significant changes in the musculoskeletal system with aging.

DID YOU UNDERSTAND?

Structure and Function of Bones

1. Bones provide support and protection for the body's tissues and organs and are important sources of minerals and blood cells.
2. Bone formation begins with the production of an inorganic matrix by bone cells. Bone minerals crystallize in and around collagen fibers in the matrix, giving bone its characteristic hardness and strength.
3. Bone tissue is continuously being resorbed and synthesized by basic multicellular units of osteoclasts and osteoblasts, respectively.
4. Bones in the body are made up of compact bone tissue and spongy bone tissue. Compact bone is highly organized into haversian systems that consist of concentric layers of crystallized matrix surrounding a central canal that contains blood vessels and nerves. Dispersed throughout the concentric layers of crystallized matrix are small spaces containing osteocytes. Smaller canals, called *canaliculi,* interconnect the osteocyte-containing spaces. The crystallized matrix in spongy bone is arranged in bars or plates. Spaces containing *osteocytes* are dispersed between the bars or plates and interconnected by canaliculi.
5. Osteoblasts are multifunctional mononuclear cells derived from osteogenic mesenchymal stromal cells; they are the primary bone-producing cells and are involved in many functions related to the skeletal system.
6. Osteocytes are the most numerous cells in bone and represent the final stage of an osteoblast's life. Though imbedded in the bone matrix, osteocytes have important functions in directing bone remodeling.
7. Osteoclasts are large (typically 20 to 100 μm in diameter), multinucleated cells that develop from the hematopoietic monocyte-macrophage lineage. Osteoclasts are the major resorptive cells of bone.
8. There are 206 bones in the body divided into the axial skeleton and the appendicular skeleton. Bones are classified by shape as long, short, flat, or irregular. Long bones have a broad end (epiphysis), broad neck (metaphysis), and narrow midportion (diaphysis) that contains the medullary cavity.
9. Bone injuries are repaired in stages. Hematoma formation provides the fibrin framework for formation strand organization of granulation tissue. The granulation tissue provides a cartilage model for the formation and crystallization of bone matrix. Remodeling restores the original shape and size to the injured bone.

Structure and Function of Joints

1. A joint is the site where two or more bones attach. Joints provide stability and mobility to the skeleton.
2. Joints are classified as synarthroses, amphiarthroses, or diarthroses, depending on the degree of movement they allow. Joints are also classified by the type of connecting tissue holding them together. Fibrous joints are connected by dense fibrous tissue, ligaments, or membranes. Cartilaginous joints are connected by fibrocartilage or hyaline cartilage. Synovial joints are connected by a fibrous joint capsule. Within the capsule is a small fluid-filled space. The fluid in the space nourishes the articular cartilage that covers the ends of the bones meeting in the synovial joint.
3. Articular cartilage is a highly organized system of collagen fibers and proteoglycans. The fibers firmly anchor the cartilage to the bone, and the proteoglycans control the loss of fluid from the cartilage.
4. Joints help move bones and muscle.

Structure and Function of Skeletal Muscles

1. Skeletal muscle is made up of millions of individual fibers.
2. Whole muscles vary in size (2 to 60 cm) and shape (fusiform, pennate). They are encased in a three-part connective tissue framework. The fundamental concept of muscle function is the motor unit, defined as those muscle fibers innervated by a single motor nerve, its axon, and anterior horn cell.
3. Satellite cells are dormant myoblasts; however, when activated, they can regenerate muscle.
4. Muscle fibers contain bundles of myofibrils arranged in parallel along the longitudinal axis and include the muscle membrane, myofibrils, sarcotubular system, sarcoplasm, and mitochondria. There are two types of muscle fibers, type I and type II, determined by motor nerve innervation.
5. Myofibrils and myofilaments contain the major muscle proteins actin and myosin, which interact to form cross-bridges during muscle contraction. The nonprotein muscle constituents provide an energy source for contraction and regulate protein synthesis and enzyme systems as well as stabilize cell membranes.

6. Muscle contraction includes excitation, coupling, contraction, and relaxation.

7. Muscle strength is graded by the all-or-nothing phenomenon and recruitment. Speed of contraction is affected by several factors: muscle fiber type, temperature, stretch, and weight of the load.

8. There are two types of muscle contraction: static (isometric) and dynamic (isotonic). Muscle shortening occurs during contraction but can be seen also during pathologic and physiologic contracture.

9. Skeletal muscle requires a constant supply of adenosine triphosphate (ATP) and phosphocreatine to fuel muscle contraction and for growth and repair. ATP and phosphocreatine can be generated aerobically or anaerobically.

10. Tendon attachment sites of muscle to bone are called entheses.

11. Ligaments attach bone to bone, helping to form joints as well as stabilizing them against excessive movement. Both tendons and ligaments are mostly composed of types III, IV, V, and VI collagen and fibroblasts (termed tenocytes in tendons).

Aging & the Musculoskeletal System

1. Sarcopenia, or age-related loss in skeletal muscle, is a direct cause of decrease in muscle strength. A slow decline in dynamic and isometric strength is evident after age 70 years.

2. The regenerative function of muscle tissue remains normal in elderly persons.

3. On average, people lose about one third of a pound of muscle every year after age 40 years and gain at least as much body fat.

4. Reduced basal metabolic rate and decreased lean body mass are also noted in the elderly population.

KEY TERMS

Agonist, 986
Alpha-glycoprotein (α-glycoprotein), 972
Amphiarthrosis (slightly movable joint), 975
Antagonist, 986
Appendicular skeleton, 973
Articular cartilage, 977
Axial skeleton, 973
Basement membrane, 980
Basic multicellular unit, 974
Bone albumin, 972
Bone fluid, 972
Bone matrix, 968
Calcification, 968
Canaliculus (pl., canaliculi), 973
Chondrocyte, 977
Collagen fiber, 972
Compact bone (cortical bone), 972
Concentric (shortening) contraction, 986
Contraction, 985
Coupling, 985
Cross-bridge theory, 985
Diaphysis, 974
Diarthrosis (freely movable joint), 975
Dynamic (isotonic) contraction, 986
Eccentric (lengthening) contraction, 986
Endomysium, 979

Endosteum, 974
Enthesis, 986
Epimysium, 979
Epiphysis, 974
Excitation, 983
Fascia, 979
Fascicle, 979
Fibril, 972
Fibrous joint, 975
Flat bone, 974
Fusiform muscle, 978
Glycoprotein, 972
Golgi tendon organ, 980
Gomphosis, 975
Ground substance, 968
Growth plate (epiphyseal plate), 974
Haversian canal, 973
Haversian system, 973
Hydroxyapatite (HAP), 972
Integrin, 970
Irregular bone, 974
Isometric (static) contraction, 986
Joint (articular) capsule, 975
Joint (articulation), 975
Joint (synovial) cavity, 977
Lacuna, 970
Lamella (pl., lamellae), 973
Ligament, 986
Long bone, 974
Metaphysis, 974
Mineralization, 972

Motor unit, 979
Muscle fiber (muscle cell), 980
Muscle fiber action potential, 983
Muscle membrane, 980
Myoblast, 980
Myofibril, 980
Myoglobin, 980
Osteoblast, 970
Osteocalcin, 972
Osteoclast, 970
Osteocyte, 970
Osteoid, 970
Osteoprotegerin (OPG), 970
Oxygen debt, 985
Pennate muscle, 979
Perimysium, 979
Periosteum, 973
Physiologic tetanus, 986
Podosome, 970
Proteoglycan, 972
Receptor activator nuclear factor kappa-B ligand (RANKL), 970
Relaxation, 985
Remodeling, 974
Repetitive discharge, 985
Resorb, 968
Ruffled border, 970
Sarcolemma, 980
Sarcomere, 982
Sarcopenia, 988
Sarcoplasm, 980
Sarcoplasmic reticulum, 982

Sarcotubular system, 982
Sarcotubule, 982
Satellite cell, 980
Short bone, 974
Sialoprotein, 972
Skeletal muscle (voluntary, striated, or extrafusal muscle), 979
Spindle, 980
Spongy bone (cancellous bone), 972
Static (holding) contraction, 986
Suture, 975
Symphysis, 975
Synarthrosis (immovable joint), 975
Synchondrosis, 975
Syndesmosis, 975
Synovial fluid, 977
Synovial joint, 977
Synovial membrane, 976
Tendon, 979
Tidemark, 977
Trabecula (pl., trabeculae), 973
Transverse tubule, 982
Type I fiber (slow-twitch fiber), 980
Type II fiber (white fast-twitch fiber), 980
Voluntary muscle, 980

REFERENCES

1. van der Meijden K et al: Primary human osteoblasts in response to 25-hydroxyvitamin D3, 1,25-dihydroxyvitamin D3, and 24R,25-dihydroxyvitamin D3, *PLoS One* 9(10):e110283, 2014.

2. Boyce BF et al: Functions of NF κB in bone, *Ann N Y Acad Sci* 1192:367-375, 2010.

3. Nakashima T et al: Evidence for osteocyte regulation of bone homeostasis through RANKL expression, *Nat Med* 17:1231-1234, 2011.

4. Xiong J, O'Brien CA: Osteocyte RANKL: New insights into control of bone remodeling, *J Bone Miner Res* 27:499-505, 2012.

5. Hughes JM, Petit MA: Biological underpinnings of Frost's mechanostat thresholds: the important role

of osteocytes, *J Musculosklet Neuronal Interact* 10(2):128-135, 2010.

6. Bellido T: Osteocyte-driven bone remodeling, *Calcif Tissue Int* 94:25-34, 2014.

7. Komori T: Functions of the osteocyte network in the regulation of bone mass, *Cell Tissue Res* 352:191-198, 2013.

8. Sapir-Koren R, Livshits G: Osteocyte control of bone remodeling: is sclerostin a key molecular coordinator of the balanced bone resorption-formation cycles? *Osteoprors Int* 25:2685-2700, 2014.

9. Nguyen AM, Jacobs CR: Emerging role of primary cilia as a mechanoreceptor in osteocytes, *Bone* 54(2):196-204, 2013.

10. Schaffler MB, Kennedy OD: Osteocyte signaling in bone, *Curr Osteoporos Rep* 19(2):118-125, 2012.

11. Hambli R: Connecting mechanics and bone cell activities in the bone remodeling process: an integrated finite element modeling, *Front Bioeng Biotechnol* 2:6, 2014.

12. Cappariello A et al: The great beauty of the osteoclast, *Arch Biochem Biophys* 561:13-21, 2014.

13. Luenburg C et al: Involvement of actin polymerization in podosomes dynamics, *J Cell Sci* 125:1666-1672, 2012.

14. Martin TJ: Historically significant events in the discovery of RANK/RANKL/OPG, *World J Orthop* 4(4):186-197, 2013.

15. Manilay JO, Zouali M: Tight relationships between B lymphocytes and the skeletal system, *Trends Mol Med* 20:405-412, 2014.

16. Weitzman MN: The role of inflammatory cytokines, the RANKL/OPG axis and the immunoloskeletal interface in physiological bone turnover and osteoporosis, *Scientifica (Cairo)* 2013:125705, 2013.

17. Orimo H: The mechanism of mineralization and the role of alkaline phosphatase in health and disease, *J Nippon Med Sch* 77(1):4-12, 2010.

18. Li X, Majumdar S: Quantitative MRI of articular cartilage and its clinical applications, *J Magn Reson Imaging* 38:991-1008, 2013.

19. Tsivites S: Notch and Wnt signaling, physiological stimuli and postnatal myogenesis, *Int J Biol Sci* 6(3):268-281, 2010.

20. Catterall WA: Voltage-gated calcium channels, *Cold Spring Harb Perspect Biol* 3(8):a003947, 2011.

21. Lanner JT: Ryanodine receptor physiology and its role in disease, *Adv Exp Med Biol* 1(74):217-234, 2012.

22. Ramachandran S et al: Structural determinants of skeletal muscle ryanodine receptor gating, *J Biol Chem* 288(9):6154-6165, 2013.

23. Luther PK: The vertebrate muscle Z-disc: sarcomere anchor for structure and signaling, *J Muscle Res Cell Motil* 30:171-185, 2009.

24. Rebbeck RT et al: Skeletal muscle excitation-contraction coupling: who are the dancing partners? *Int J Biochem Cell Biol* 48:28-38, 2014.

25. Prosser BL et al: S100A1 and calmodulin regulation of ryanodine receptor in striated muscle, *Cell Calcium* 50(4):323-331, 2011.

26. Bassit RA et al: Effect of short-term creatine supplementation on markers of skeletal muscle damage after strenuous contractile activity, *Eur J Appl Physiol* 108(5):945-955, 2010.

27. Kuo CK et al: Novel strategies in tendon and ligament tissue engineering: advanced biomaterials and regeneration motifs, *Sports Med Arthrosc Rehabil Ther Technol* 2:20, 2010.

28. Almeida M, O'Brien CA: Basic biology of skeletal aging: role of stress response pathways, *J Gerontol A Biol Sci Med Sci* 68(10):1197-1208, 2013.

29. Konopka AR, Streekumaran NK: Mitochondrial and skeletal muscle health with advancing age, *Mol Cell Endocrinol* 397(1-2):19-29, 2013.

30. Pratesi A et al: Skeletal muscle: an endocrine organ, *Clin Cases Miner Bone Metab* 10(1):11-14, 2013.

31. Waters DL et al: Advances of dietary, exercise-related, and therapeutic interventions to prevent and treat sarcopenia in adult patients: an update, *Clin Interv Aging* 5:259-270, 2010.

32. Burton LA, Sumukadas D: Optimal management of sarcopenia, *Clin Interv Aging* 5:217-228, 2010.

33. Lang T et al: Sarcopenia: etiology, clinical consequences, intervention, and assessment, *Osteoporos Int* 21(4):543-559, 2010.

39

Alterations of Musculoskeletal Function

Christy L. Crowther-Radulewicz and Kathryn L. McCance

ⓔ EVOLVE WEBSITE

http://evolve.elsevier.com/Huether/

Student Review Questions
Audio Key Points

Case Studies
Animations
Quick Check Answers

Musculoskeletal injuries include fractures, dislocations, sprains, and strains. Metabolic disorders, infections, inflammatory or noninflammatory diseases, or tumors may cause alterations in bones, joints, and muscles. The most common disease affecting bone is osteoporosis; much attention and debate has been focused on its risk factors and pathophysiology. Soft tissue disorders—including muscle, tendon, and ligament injuries; tumors; and metabolic derangements—also affect the musculoskeletal system.

MUSCULOSKELETAL INJURIES

Trauma is referred to as the "neglected disease." It is the leading cause of death in people ages 1 to 44 years of all races and socioeconomic levels. Each year, more than 120,000 persons in the United States die from unintentional injuries.[1]

Musculoskeletal injuries have a major impact on the affected individuals, families, and society in general because of the physical and psychologic effects of limitation on mobility and daily activities, pain, and decreased quality of life. In addition, there are direct costs of diagnosis and treatments, and indirect economic costs related to loss of employment and decreased productivity.

Skeletal Trauma
Fractures
A fracture is a break in the continuity of a bone. A break occurs when force is applied that exceeds the tensile or compressive strength of the bone. The incidence of fractures varies for individual bones according to age and gender, with the highest incidence of fractures in young males (between the ages of 15 and 24 years) and older persons (65 years of age and older). Fractures of healthy bones, particularly the tibia, clavicle, and lower humerus, tend to occur in young persons as the result of trauma. Fractures of the hands and feet are often caused by accidents in the workplace. The incidence of fractures of the upper femur, upper humerus, vertebrae, and pelvis is highest in older adults and is often associated with osteoporosis (see p. 1000). Hip fractures, the most serious outcome of osteoporosis, have a wide variation in geographic occurrence.[2]

Classification of fractures. There are numerous classification systems for various types of fractures, but the simplest systems describe the basic features of the broken bone. Fractures can be classified as complete or incomplete and as open or closed (Figure 39-1). In a **complete fracture** the bone is broken entirely, whereas in an **incomplete fracture** the bone is damaged but is still in one piece. Complete and incomplete fractures also can be called **open** (formerly referred to as **compound**) if the skin is open and **closed** (formerly called simple or **incomplete**) if it is not. A fracture in which a bone breaks into more than two fragments is termed a **comminuted fracture**. Fractures are also classified according to the direction of the fracture line. A **linear fracture** runs parallel to the long axis of the bone. An **oblique fracture** occurs at a slanted angle to the shaft of the bone. A **spiral fracture** encircles the bone, and a **transverse fracture** occurs straight across the bone.

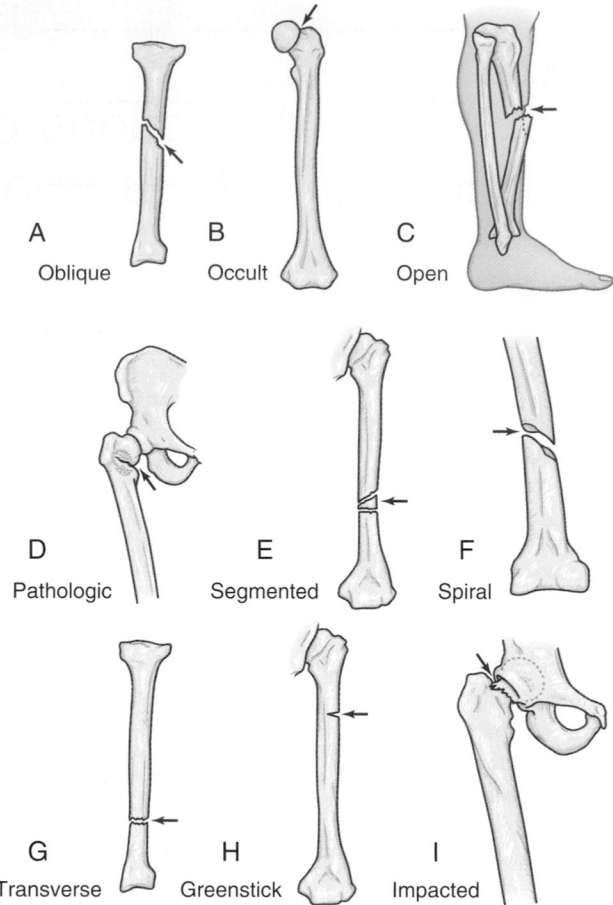

FIGURE 39-1 Examples of Types of Bone Fractures. **A,** Oblique: fracture at oblique angle across both cortices. *Cause:* Direct or indirect energy, with angulation and some compression. **B,** Occult: fracture that is hidden or not readily discernible. *Cause:* Minor force or energy. **C,** Open: skin broken over fracture; possible soft tissue trauma. *Cause:* Moderate to severe energy that is continuous and exceeds tissue tolerance. **D,** Pathologic: transverse, oblique, or spiral fracture of bone weakened by tumor pressure or presence. *Cause:* Minor energy or force, which may be direct or indirect. **E,** Segmented: fracture with two or more pieces or segments. *Cause:* Direct or indirect moderate to severe force. **F,** Spiral: fracture that curves around cortices and may become displaced by twist. *Cause:* Direct or indirect twisting energy or force with distal part held or unable to move. **G,** Transverse: horizontal break through bone. *Cause:* Direct or indirect energy toward bone. **H,** Greenstick: break in only one cortex of bone. *Cause:* Minor direct or indirect energy. **I,** Impacted: fracture with one end wedged into opposite end of inside fractured fragment. *Cause:* Compressive axial energy or force directly to distal fragment. (Redrawn from Mourad L: Musculoskeletal system. In Thompson JM et al, editors: *Mosby's clinical nursing,* ed 7, St Louis, 2002, Mosby.)

Incomplete fractures tend to occur in the more flexible, growing bones of children. The three main types of incomplete fractures are greenstick, torus, and bowing fractures. A **greenstick fracture** perforates one cortex and splinters the spongy bone. The name is derived from the damage sustained by a young tree branch (a green stick) when it is bent sharply. The outer surface is disrupted, but the inner surface remains intact. Greenstick fractures typically occur in the metaphysis or diaphysis of the tibia, radius, and ulna. In a **torus fracture,** the cortex buckles but does not break. **Bowing fractures** usually occur when longitudinal force is applied to bone. This type of fracture is common in children and usually involves the paired radius-ulna or the

TABLE 39-1	Types of Fractures
Type of Fracture	**Definition**
Typical Complete Fractures	
Closed	Noncommunicating wound between bone and skin
Open	Communicating wound between bone and skin
Comminuted	Multiple bone fragments
Linear	Fracture line parallel to long axis of bone
Oblique	Fracture line at an angle to long axis of bone
Spiral	Fracture line encircling bone (as a spiral staircase)
Transverse	Fracture line perpendicular to long axis of bone
Impacted	Fracture fragments pushed into each other
Pathologic	Fracture at a point where bone has been weakened by disease, for example, by tumors or osteoporosis
Avulsion	Fragment of bone connected to a ligament or tendon detaches from main bone
Compression	Fracture wedged or squeezed together on one side of bone
Displaced	Fracture with one, both, or all fragments out of normal alignment
Extracapsular	Fragment close to joint but remains outside joint capsule
Intracapsular	Fragment within joint capsule
Typical Incomplete Fractures	
Greenstick	Break in one cortex of bone with splintering of inner bone surface; commonly occurs in children and elderly persons
Torus	Buckling of cortex
Bowing	Bending of bone
Stress	Microfracture
Transchondral	Separation of cartilaginous joint surface (articular cartilage) from main shaft of bone

fibula-tibia. A complete diaphyseal fracture occurs in one of the bones of the pair, which disperses the stress sufficiently to prevent a complete fracture of the second bone, which bows rather than breaks. A bowing fracture resists correction **(reduction)** because the force necessary to reduce it must be equal to the force that bowed it. Treatment of bowing fractures is also difficult because the bowed bone interferes with reduction of the fractured bone. Types of fractures are summarized in Table 39-1.

Fractures may be further classified by cause as pathologic, stress, or transchondral fractures. A **pathologic** (also known as **insufficiency** or **fragility) fracture** is a break at the site of a preexisting abnormality, resulting from force that would not fracture a normal bone. In any bone that lacks normal ability to deform and recover, these fractures can occur with normal weightbearing or activity. Rheumatoid arthritis, osteoporosis, Paget disease, osteomalacia, rickets, hyperparathyroidism, and radiation therapy all cause bone to lose its normal ability to deform and recover. Pathologic fractures are generally a result of bone weakness caused by another disease such as cancer, metabolic bone disorders, or infection. Although usually considered insufficiency fractures, breaks in the bone attributable to osteoporosis can also be referred to as pathologic fractures. Any disease process that weakens a bone (especially the cortex) predisposes the bone to pathologic fracture.

During activities that subject a bone to repeated strain, such as certain athletics, a **stress fracture** can occur in normal or abnormal bone. The forces placed on the bone are cumulative, eventually causing a fracture. A fatigue fracture is caused by repetitive, sometimes abnormal stress or torque applied to a bone with normal ability to deform and recover. Fatigue fractures usually occur in individuals who engage in a new or different activity that is both strenuous and repetitive (e.g., joggers, skaters, dancers, military recruits). Because gains in muscle strength occur more rapidly than gains in bone strength, the newly developed muscles place exaggerated stress on the bones that are not yet ready for the additional stress. The imbalance between muscle and bone development causes microfractures to develop in the cortex. If the activity is controlled and increased gradually, new bone formation catches up to the increased demands and microfractures do not occur.

A transchondral fracture consists of fragmentation and separation of a portion of the articular cartilage. (Joint structures are defined in Chapter 38.) Single or multiple sites may be fractured, and the fragments may consist of cartilage alone or cartilage and bone. Typical sites of transchondral fracture are the distal femur, the ankle, the patella, the elbow, and the wrist. Transchondral fractures are most prevalent in adolescents.

PATHOPHYSIOLOGY Fracture healing is a complex process that occurs primarily in one of two ways: direct or indirect healing.[3] Both types of healing require integration of cells, signaling pathways, and various molecules. In direct (or primary) healing, intramembranous bone formation occurs when adjacent bone cortices are in contact with one another. This most often occurs when surgical fixation is used to repair a broken bone. No callus formation occurs with direct bone healing. Indirect (or secondary) healing involves both intramembranous and endochondral bone formation, development of callus, and eventual remodeling of solid bone.[4] Bone formation that begins with an underlying cartilage scaffold is termed endochondral bone formation.

A hallmark of indirect fracture healing is the formation of callus. Indirect fracture healing is most often observed when a fracture is treated with a cast or other nonsurgical method. When a bone is broken, the periosteum and blood vessels in the cortex, marrow, and surrounding soft tissues are disrupted. Bleeding occurs from the damaged ends of the bone and from the neighboring soft tissue. A clot (hematoma) forms within the medullary canal, between the fractured ends of the bone, and beneath the periosteum (Figure 39-2). Bone tissue immediately adjacent to the fracture dies. This dead tissue (along with any debris in the fracture area) stimulates an intense inflammatory response characterized by vasodilation, exudation of plasma and leukocytes, and infiltration by inflammatory leukocytes, growth factors, and mast cells that simultaneously decalcify the fractured bone ends. Within 48 hours after injury, vascular tissue from surrounding soft tissue and the marrow cavity invades the fracture area, and blood flow to the entire bone increases. Bone-forming cells in the periosteum, endosteum, and marrow are activated to produce subperiosteal procallus along the outer surface of the shaft and over the broken ends of the bone (see Figure 39-2). Osteoblasts within the procallus synthesize collagen and matrix, which becomes mineralized to form callus. As the repair process continues, remodeling occurs, during which unnecessary callus is resorbed and trabeculae are formed along lines of stress as the repair tissues align with the tissue cells of the host (Figure 39-3). Except for the liver, bone is unique among all body tissues in that it will form new bone, not scar tissue, when it heals after a fracture.

CLINICAL MANIFESTATIONS The signs and symptoms of a fracture include unnatural alignment (deformity), swelling, muscle spasm, tenderness, pain and impaired sensation, and decreased mobility. The position of the broken bone segments is determined by the pull of

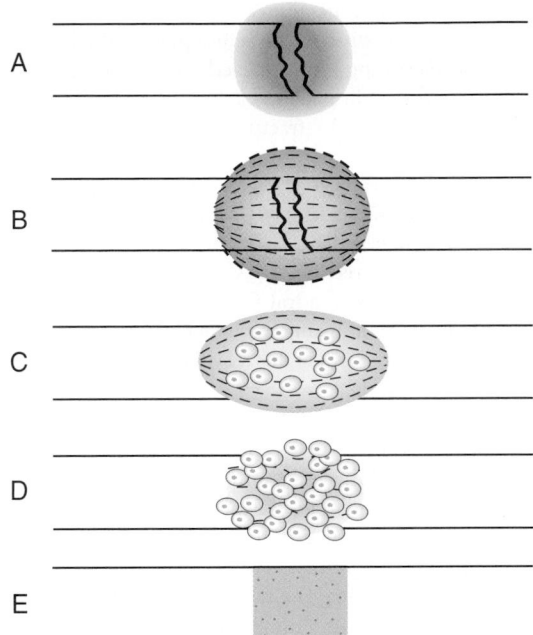

FIGURE 39-2 Bone Healing (Schematic Representation). **A,** Bleeding at broken ends of the bone with subsequent hematoma formation. **B,** Organization of hematoma into fibrous network. **C,** Invasion of osteoblasts, lengthening of collagen strands, and deposition of calcium. **D,** Callus formation; new bone is built while osteoclasts destroy dead bone. **E,** Remodeling is accomplished while excess callus is reabsorbed and trabecular bone is deposited. (From Monahan FD et al: *Phipps' medical-surgical nursing: health and illness perspectives,* ed 8, St Louis, 2007, Mosby.)

FIGURE 39-3 Exuberant Callus Formation Following Fracture. (From Rosai J: *Ackerman's surgical pathology,* ed 8, St Louis, 1996, Mosby.)

attached muscles, gravity, and the direction and magnitude of the force that caused the fracture.

Immediately after a bone is fractured, there often is numbness at the fracture site because of trauma to the nerve or nerves at the injury site. The numbness may last several minutes, during which time the injured person can continue to use the fractured bone. However, once the numbness dissipates, the subsequent pain is quite severe and may be incapacitating until relieved with medication and treatment of the fracture. Pain can be caused by muscle spasms at the fracture site, overriding of the fracture segments, or damage to adjacent soft tissues.

Pathologic fractures can cause angular deformity, painless swelling, or generalized bone pain. Stress fractures are painful because of accelerated remodeling; initially, pain occurs during activity and is usually relieved by rest. Stress fractures also cause local tenderness and soft tissue swelling. Transchondral fractures may be entirely asymptomatic or may be painful during movement. Range of motion in the joint is limited, and movement may evoke audible clicking sounds (crepitus).

EVALUATION AND TREATMENT Adequate immobilization with a splint or cast is often all that is required for healing of fractures that are *not* misaligned. Treatment of a displaced fracture involves realigning the bone fragments (reduction) close to their normal or anatomic position and holding the fragments in place (immobilization) so that bone union can occur. Several methods are available to reduce a fracture: closed manipulation, traction, and open reduction. Many displaced fractures can be reduced by closed manipulation and reduction. The bone is moved or manipulated into place without opening the skin. Closed reduction is used when the contour of the bone is in fair anatomic alignment and can be manually placed into normal alignment, and then maintained with immobilization. Splints and casts are used to immobilize and hold a closed reduction in place.

Traction may be used to accomplish or maintain reduction. When bone fragments are displaced (not in their anatomic position), weights may be used to apply firm, steady traction (pull) and countertraction to the long axis of the bone. Traction stretches and fatigues muscles that have pulled the bone fragments out of place, more readily allowing the distal fragment to align with the proximal fragment. Traction can be applied to the skin (skin traction) or directly to the involved bone (skeletal traction). Skin traction is used when only a few pounds of pulling force are needed to realign the fragments or when the traction will be used only for a brief time, such as before surgery or, for children with femoral fractures, for 3 to 7 days before applying a cast. In skeletal traction, a pin or wire is drilled through the bone distal to the fracture site, and a traction bow, rope, and weights are attached to the pin or wire to apply tension and to provide the pulling force required to overcome the muscle spasm and help realign the fracture fragments. More often, surgical repair (open reduction and internal fixation) or external fixation devices are used to realign displaced fractures.

Open reduction is a surgical procedure that exposes the fracture site; the fragments are then manipulated into alignment under direct visualization. Some form of hardware, such as a screw, plate, nail, or wire, is used to maintain the reduction (internal fixation). External fixation, a procedure in which pins or rods are surgically placed into uninjured bone near the fracture site and then stabilized with an external frame of bars, is another method used to treat fractures that would not be adequately stabilized with a cast. Bone grafts—using donor bone from the individual (autograft), a cadaver (allograft), or bone substitutes (ceramic composites, bioactive cement)—can fill voids in the bone.

Improper reduction or immobilization of a fractured bone may result in nonunion, delayed union, or malunion. Nonunion is failure of the bone ends to grow together. The gap between the broken ends of the bone fills with dense fibrous and fibrocartilaginous tissue instead of new bone. Occasionally, the fibrous tissue contains a fluid-filled space that resembles a joint and is termed a *false joint,* or *pseudoarthrosis.* Delayed union is union that does not occur until approximately 8 to 9 months after a fracture. Malunion is the healing of a bone in an incorrect anatomic position.

Dislocation and Subluxation

Dislocation and subluxation are usually caused by trauma. Dislocation is the displacement of one or more bones in a joint in which the opposing joint surfaces entirely lose contact with one another. If contact between the opposing joint surfaces is only partially lost, the injury is called a subluxation.

Dislocation and subluxation are most common in persons younger than 20 years of age and are generally associated with fractures. However, they may be the result of congenital or acquired disorders that cause (1) muscular imbalance, as occurs with congenital dislocation of the hip or neurologic disorders; (2) incongruities in the articulating surfaces of the bones, as occur with rheumatoid arthritis (see p. 1012); or (3) joint instability.

The joints most often dislocated or subluxated are the joints of the shoulder, elbow, wrist, finger, hip, and knee. The shoulder joint most often injured is the glenohumeral joint. Finger dislocations are common injuries in contact sports such as basketball, football, and rugby.

Traumatic dislocation of the elbow joint is common in the immature skeleton. In adults, an elbow dislocation is usually associated with a fracture of the ulna or head of the radius. Traumatic dislocation of the wrist usually involves the distal ulna and carpal bones. Any one of the eight carpal bones can be dislocated after an injury. Dislocation in the hand usually involves the metacarpophalangeal and interphalangeal joints.

Considerable trauma is needed to dislocate the hip. Anterior hip dislocation is rare in healthy persons; it is caused by forced abduction—for example, when an individual lands on his or her feet after falling from an elevated height. Posterior dislocation of the hip can occur as a result of an automobile accident in which the flexed knee strikes the dashboard, causing the head of the femur to be pushed posteriorly from the hip joint.

The knee is an unstable weightbearing joint that depends heavily on the soft tissue structures around it for support. It is exposed to many different types of motion (flexion, extension, rotation) and is one of the most commonly injured joints. A knee dislocation can be anterior, posterior, lateral, medial, or rotary. It is often the result of an injury that occurs during contact sports activities, such as soccer, lacrosse, or football.

PATHOPHYSIOLOGY Dislocations and subluxations are often accompanied by fracture because stress is placed on areas of bone not usually subjected to stress. In addition, as the joint loses its normal congruity, there may be bruising or tearing of adjacent nerves, blood vessels, ligaments, supporting structures, and soft tissue. Dislocations of the shoulder may damage the shoulder capsule and the axillary nerve. Damage to axillary nerves can cause anesthesia or dysesthesia in the sensory distribution of the nerve and paralysis of the deltoid muscle. Dislocations also may disrupt circulation, leading to ischemia and possibly even permanent disability of the affected extremity tissues.

CLINICAL MANIFESTATIONS Signs and symptoms of dislocations or subluxations include pain, swelling, limitation of motion, and joint deformity. Pain may be caused by effusion of inflammatory exudate into the joint or by associated tendon and ligament injury. Joint deformity is typically caused by muscle contractions that exert pull on the dislocated or subluxated joint. Limitation of motion results from effusion into the joint or the displacement of bones.

EVALUATION AND TREATMENT Evaluation of dislocations and sub-luxations is based on clinical manifestations and radiographic evaluation. Treatment consists of reduction and immobilization for 2 to 6 weeks to allow healing of damaged structures, followed by exercises to restore normal range of motion in the joint. Depending on the joint and severity of injury, complete healing can take months to sometimes years.

Support Structures
Sprains and Strains of Tendons and Ligaments

Tendon and ligament injuries often accompany fractures and dislocations. A tendon is fibrous connective tissue (composed primarily of type I collagen) that attaches skeletal muscle to a bone or other structure; the area of attachment on a bone is called an enthesis. The enthesis serves to evenly distribute tension differences between the bone and tendon. The zone where muscle transitions into tendon is known as the myotendinous junction. Functionally, muscles and tendons work together as a single, integrated unit allowing motion.[5,6] A ligament is a band of fibrous connective tissue that connects bones where they meet in a joint. Ligaments are structurally quite similar to tendons, although ligaments have a higher proportion of small-diameter collagen fibrils. The primary difference between tendons and ligaments is their anatomic location.[7] Tendons and ligaments support the bones and joints and either facilitate or limit motion, respectively. Either structure can be completely separated from bone at their points of attachment, torn, lacerated, or ruptured.

Tearing or stretching of a muscle or tendon is commonly known as a strain. Major trauma can tear or rupture a tendon at any site in the body. Most commonly injured are the tendons of the hands and feet, the knee (patellar), the upper arm (biceps and triceps), the thigh (hamstring), the ankle, and the heel (Achilles).

Ligament tears are commonly known as sprains. Ligament tears and ruptures can occur at any joint but are most common in the wrist, ankle, elbow, and knee joints. A complete separation of a tendon or ligament from its bony attachment site is known as an avulsion and is commonly seen in young athletes, especially sprinters, hurdlers, and distance runners.

Strains and sprains are classified as first degree (mild), second degree (moderate), and third degree (severe). In first-degree injuries, the fibers are stretched but the muscle (strain) or joint (sprain) remains stable. In second-degree strains or sprains, there is more tearing of the tendon or ligament fibers, with muscle weakness (strain) or some joint instability (sprain) but incomplete tearing of fibers. Third-degree strains and sprains result in an inability to contract the muscle normally (strain) and cause significant joint instability (sprain).

PATHOPHYSIOLOGY When a tendon or ligament is torn, an inflammatory exudate develops between the torn ends. Multiple growth factors that direct the repair process are released. Later, granulation tissue containing macrophages, fibroblasts, and capillary buds grows inward from the surrounding soft tissue and cartilage to begin the repair process. Within 4 to 5 days after the injury, collagen formation begins. At first, collagen formation is random and disorganized. As the collagen fibers interweave and connect with preexisting tendon fibers, they become organized parallel to the lines of the musculotendinous unit. Eventually vascular fibrous tissue fuses the new and surrounding tissues into a single mass. Collagen fibers reconnect the tendon and bone, forming a type of enthesis.[7] Usually a healing tendon or ligament lacks sufficient strength to withstand some stress for 4 to 5 weeks after the injury; it may take more than 3 months to achieve mechanical stability of a joint.[8] If powerful muscle pull does occur during healing, the tendon or ligament ends may separate again, which causes the tendon or ligament to heal in a lengthened shape or with an excessive amount of scar tissue, resulting in poor tendon or ligament function.

CLINICAL MANIFESTATIONS Tendon and ligament injuries are painful and are usually accompanied by soft tissue swelling, changes in tendon or ligament contour, and dislocation or subluxation of bones. Pain is generally sharp and localized, and tenderness persists over the distribution of the tendon or ligament. Movement or weight-bearing increases pain. Even with prompt treatment, depending on the tendon or ligament involved, significant injuries may result in decreased mobility, instability, and weakness of the affected joints.

EVALUATION AND TREATMENT Evaluation is based on mechanism of injury, clinical manifestations, stress radiography, arthroscopy, or arthrography. Initial treatment consists of PRICE (Protection, Rest, Ice, Compression, and Elevation) for the first 48 to 72 hours. Once swelling and acute pain subside, in most cases, support of the affected tendon or ligament with a compression dressing or brace will provide appropriate reinforcement while the tissues heal. Rehabilitation is crucial to regaining good functional outcome.[9] In severe (third-degree) injuries, treatment may include suturing the tendon or ligament ends in close approximation. If this is not feasible because of the extent of damage, tendon or ligament grafting may be necessary. Prolonged, functional rehabilitation programs help ensure return of near-normal functions, but recovery may be complicated by posttraumatic arthritis.

Tendinopathy, Epicondylopathy, and Bursitis

Trauma also can cause painful inflammation of tendons (tendinopathy [tendonitis]) and bursae (bursitis). Other causes of damage to tendons include reduced tissue perfusion, mechanical irritation, crystal deposits, postural misalignment, and hypermobility of a joint. Thus, tendinopathy is a more accurate term than tendonitis in most cases. Studies have shown that vascular ingrowth in tendinopathy (neovascularization) is accompanied with nerve ingrowth, facilitating pain transmission in Achilles and patellar tendinopathy.[10]

The histopathology of common conditions, such as lateral epicondylopathy ("tennis elbow") or medial epicondylopathy ("golfer's elbow"), is a degenerative process[11,12] (Figure 39-4). A bony prominence at the end of a bone where tendons or ligaments attach is termed an epicondyle. When force is sufficient to cause microscopic tears (microtears) in tissue, the result is known as tendinopathy or epicondylopathy. Microtears in the tendon, the presence of disorganized collagen fibers, and neovascularization are indicative of incomplete tissue repair. Initial inflammatory changes cause thickening of the tendon sheath, limiting movements and causing pain.[13] Microtears cause bleeding, edema, and pain (because of the presence of substance P) in the involved tendon or tendons. At times, after repeated microtears, calcium may be deposited in the tendon origin area.

Lateral epicondylopathy (tennis elbow) is caused by irritation and overstretching of the extensor carpi radialis brevis (ECRB) tendon and forearm extensor muscles, resulting in tissue degradation, loss of grip strength, and pain.[14] Medial epicondylopathy (golfer's elbow) is the result of similar forces affecting the forearm muscles responsible for forearm flexion and pronation (see Figure 39-4). Repetitive load-bearing activities or acute injuries that involve flexion, extension, pronation, or supination of the elbow and forearm can lead to either lateral or medial elbow symptoms.

Clinical manifestations of epicondylopathy are usually localized to one side of the joint. In general, there is local tenderness and more pain with active motion than with passive motion. With tendinopathy or tendonitis, the pain is localized over the involved tendon. Stressing the

FIGURE 39-4 Epicondylopathy and Tendinopathy. **A,** Lateral and medial epicondyles of the distal humerus, sites of tennis elbow (lateral) and golfer's elbow (medial). **B,** Achilles tendon, common site of tendinopathy.

FIGURE 39-5 Olecranon Bursitis. Note swelling at the point of the elbow (olecranon). A smaller, rheumatoid nodule also is present. (From Hochberg MC et al: *Rheumatology,* ed 6, Philadelphia, 2015, Elsevier.)

tendon with simple activities, such as lifting even a few pounds of weight, can increase pain. Pain and sometimes weakness limit joint movement.

Bursae are small sacs lined with synovial membrane and filled with synovial fluid that are located between bony prominences and soft tissues such as tendons, muscles, and ligaments (Figure 39-5). Bursae can be either "constant" (those formed during embryologic development) or "adventitious" (bursae that develop as a result of chronic friction and degeneration of fibrous tissue between adjacent structures). The primary function of a bursa is to separate, lubricate, and cushion these structures. When irritated or injured, these sacs become inflamed and swell. Because most bursae lie outside joints, joint movement is rarely compromised with bursitis. Acute bursitis occurs primarily in middle age and is caused by trauma. Chronic bursitis can result from repeated trauma. Septic bursitis is caused by wound infection or bacterial infection of the skin overlying the bursae. Bursitis commonly occurs in the shoulder, hip, knee, and elbow but also can affect the spine, wrist, foot, and ankle.

PATHOPHYSIOLOGY   Bursitis usually is an inflammation that is reactive to overuse or excessive pressure but also can be caused by infection, autoimmune diseases, crystal deposition, or acute trauma. The inflamed bursal sac becomes engorged, and the inflammation can spread to adjacent tissues. The inflammation may decrease with rest, ice, and aspiration of the fluid. (Inflammation is discussed in Chapter 6.)

CLINICAL MANIFESTATIONS   Joint motion is rarely limited in bursitis, except by pain. Shoulder pain may impair arm abduction. Bursitis in the knee produces pain when climbing stairs, and crossing the legs is painful in bursitis of the hip. Lying on the side of the inflamed trochanteric bursa is also very painful. Signs of infectious bursitis may include the presence of pain, a puncture site, warmth and erythema, prior corticosteroid injection, severe inflammation, or an adjacent source of infection, such as from total joint replacement surgery.

EVALUATION AND TREATMENT   The diagnosis of tendinopathy, epicondylopathy, and bursitis is primarily based on clinical history and physical examination. Other imaging techniques, such as ultrasound or magnetic resonance imaging (MRI), may be used to evaluate the severity of the problem. Treatment may include temporary immobilization of the joint with a sling, splint, or cast; administration of systemic analgesics; application of ice or heat; or local injection of an anesthetic, a corticosteroid, platelet-rich plasma (PRP), or a combination local anesthetic/corticosteroid. Physical therapy to prevent loss of function begins after acute inflammation subsides (see *Health Alert:* Managing Tendinopathy).

Muscle Strains

Muscle strain is a general term for local muscle damage. Mild injury such as **muscle strain** is usually seen after traumatic or sports injuries. It is often the result of sudden, forced motion causing the muscle to become stretched beyond normal capacity. Strains often involve the tendon as well. Penetrating injuries, such as knife and gunshot wounds, can cause traumatic rupture (see Chapter 4). Muscles are ruptured more often than tendons in young people; the opposite is true in the older population. Muscle strain may be chronic when the muscle is repeatedly stretched beyond its usual capacity. There is evidence of tissue disruption with subsequent signs of muscle regeneration and connective tissue repair when a biopsy is performed. Hemorrhage into the surrounding tissue and signs of inflammation also may be present.

Muscle healing occurs in three phases:

1. Destruction, in which the myofibers of the damaged muscle contract and necrose, beginning an inflammatory reaction. The gap between torn fibers is filled by a hematoma.

HEALTH ALERT

Managing Tendinopathy

Tennis and golfer's elbow, Achilles tendinopathy, and other tendon problems account for a large percentage of sports-related overuse injuries. Successful treatment of these conditions is challenging because of the mechanisms of tendon healing as well as inconsistent results, with many interventions still not completely understood. Chronic pain is common and may be the result of ingrowth of nerves that accompanies ingrowth of new blood vessels during the healing process. Recent studies suggest that the traditional approach of corticosteroid injections is helpful only for the short term. Other therapies that show promise include the following:

Prolotherapy: An irritant such as glucose or lidocaine is injected into the affected tendon, inducing an inflammatory response, thereby stimulating growth of new tendon fibers.

Eccentric exercises: The tendon is "prestretched," increasing its resting length and resulting in less strain during movement. The load on the tendon is gradually increased, causing the tendon, itself, to strengthen.

Extracorporeal shockwave therapy (SWT): External acoustic or sonic waves are focused on the affected area. The shockwaves stimulate soft tissue healing and inhibit pain receptors.

Needling: This treatment involves multiple insertions of a sterile needle into affected tissue. It is thought the pain sensation is reduced by stimulating A-nerve fibers. This technique is often referred to as "dry needling" since no fluid is introduced.

Platelet-rich plasma (PRP): This autologous source of concentrated platelets is obtained by centrifugation of plasma. The resulting solution contains high concentrations of cytokines and growth factors, such as platelet-derived growth factor (PDGF) and transforming growth factor-beta (TGF-β), which are thought to promote the growth of new, healthy tissue.

Autologous tenocyte injections: Autologous injection of tenocytes at the site of tendinopathy is thought to provide necessary mediators of tissue healing.

From Andarawis-Puri N et al: *J Orthop Res* 33(6):780-784, 2015; Krey D et al: *Phys Sportsmed* 43(1):80-86, 2015; Langer PR: *Clin Podiatr Med Surg* 32(2):183-193, 2015; Mautner K, Kneer L: *Phys Med Rehabil Clin North Am* 25(4):865-880, 2014; Wang A et al: *Am J Sports Med* 43(7):1775-1783, 2015.

TABLE 39-2 Muscle Strain

Type	Manifestations	Treatment
First degree (example: bench press in untrained athlete)	Muscle overstretched, pain but no muscle deformity	Ice should be applied 5 or 6 times in first 24-48 hr; gradual resumption of full weightbearing after initial rest for up to 2 weeks Exercises individualized to specific injury
Second degree (example: any muscle strain with bruising and pain)	Muscle intact with some tearing of fibers, swelling, pain	Treatment similar to that for first-degree strains
Third degree (example: traumatic injury)	Caused by tearing of fascia, marked weakness, deformity	Surgery to approximate ruptured edges; immobilization and non-weightbearing status for 6 weeks

2. Repair, which begins with monocytes phagocytizing the dead tissue and activating satellite cells, which become myoblasts. The myoblasts infiltrate the scar tissue and new capillary formation begins at the site of injury. The first two phases occur within a week of injury.

3. Remodeling occurs as the myofibers mature, form contractile tissue, and attach to the ends of scar tissue.[15] Regeneration may take up to 6 weeks, and the affected muscle should be protected during that time.

Degrees of acute muscle strain, together with their manifestations and treatment, are summarized in Table 39-2.

A late complication of some muscle injuries is myositis ossificans, also known as heterotopic ossification (HO). Its exact pathophysiology remains unknown, but the basic problem seems to be the inability of mesenchymal cells to differentiate into osteoblastic stem cells and inappropriate differentiation of fibroblasts into bone-forming cells. Though uncommon, HO is associated with burns, joint surgery, and trauma to the musculoskeletal system or central nervous system. HO may involve the muscle or tendons, ligaments, or bones near the muscle, causing stiffness or deformity of an extremity. Soft tissue calcifications may be seen on plain radiographs.

Rhabdomyolysis

Once used interchangeably with the term *myoglobinuria*, rhabdomyolysis is the rapid breakdown of muscle that causes the release of intracellular contents, including the protein pigment myoglobin, into the extracellular space and bloodstream. Physical interruptions in the sarcolemma membrane, called delta lesions, are the route by which muscle constituents are released. (The sarcolemma membrane, the plasma membrane of the muscle cell, is described in Chapter 38.) Myoglobinuria, first described in victims of crush injuries in London during World War II, refers to the presence of the muscle protein myoglobin in the urine.

PATHOPHYSIOLOGY Rhabdomyolysis is sometimes incorrectly used interchangeably with *crush injury* (a description of injuries resulting from crushing of a body part), *compartment syndrome* (the consequences of increased intracompartmental pressures of a muscle), or *crush syndrome* (the systemic pathophysiologic events caused by rhabdomyolysis, primarily involving the kidneys and coagulation syndrome).[16,17] Although relatively rare, rhabdomyolysis has many causes (Box 39-1) and can result in serious complications, including hyperkalemia (because of the release of intracellular potassium into the circulation) and cardiac dysrhythmias. The most clinically significant complication is acute renal failure (myoglobin precipitates in the tubules, obstructing flow through the nephron and producing injury).[18] Other complications include metabolic acidosis (from liberation of intracellular phosphorus and sulfate) and even disseminated intravascular coagulation (DIC) (likely caused by activation of the clotting cascade by sarcolemma damage and release of intracellular components from the damaged muscles).

CLINICAL MANIFESTATIONS A *classic triad* of muscle pain, weakness, and dark urine is considered typical of rhabdomyolysis, but those

BOX 39-1   Selected Causes of Rhabdomyolysis

Direct Trauma

Blunt trauma or crush injury (motor vehicle crashes, collapsed buildings)

Burns (thermal)

Electrical injury

Excessive compression (from immobility attributable to stroke, alcohol or drug intoxication)

Drugs

Alcohol

Amphetamines

Anesthetic and paralytic agents (halothane, propofol, succinylcholine—malignant hyperthermia syndrome)

Antihistamines (diphenhydramine, doxylamine)

Anti-hyperlipidemic agents (statins, clofibrate, bezafibrate)

Antipsychotics and antidepressants (amitriptyline, doxepin, fluoxetine, haloperidol, lithium, protriptyline, perphenazine, promethazine, chlorpromazine, trifluoperazine, venlafaxine)

Caffeine

Cocaine

Corticosteroids

Fibrinates (antilipid agents: bezafibrate, ciprofibrate, clozfibrate, clofibrate, ezetimibe, gemfibrozil)

Heroin

HIV integrase inhibitor (raltegravir)

Hypnotics and sedatives (benzodiazepines, barbiturates)

LSD (lysergic acid diethylamide)

Methadone

Methamphetamine

Methylenedioxymethamphetamine (MDMA; "ecstasy")

Miscellaneous medications (amphotericin B, azathioprine, ε-aminocaproic acid, quinidine, penicillamine, salicylates, theophylline, terbutaline, thiazides, vasopressin)

Phencyclidine

Protease inhibitors

Statins (atorvastatin, fluvastatin, lovastatin, pravastatin, rosuvastatin, simvastatin)

Miscellaneous drugs (amphotericin B, arsenic, azathioprine, halothane, naltrexone, quinidine, penicillamine, propofol, salicylates, succinylcholine, theophylline, terbutaline, thiazides, vasopressin)

Excessive Muscular Contraction

Status epilepticus

Delirium tremens

Acute psychosis

Severe dystonia

Sporadic strenuous exercise (e.g., marathons, squats)

Tetanus

Infectious Agents

Bacteria (group B streptococci, *Streptococcus pneumoniae, Staphylococcus epidermidis, Borrelia burgdorferi, Escherichia coli, Clostridium perfringens, Clostridium tetani, Streptococcus viridans; Bacillus, Brucella, Legionella, Listeria, Leptospira, Mycoplasma, Plasmodium, Rickettsia, Salmonella,* and *Vibrio* species)

Fungal organisms (*Aspergillus, Candida* species)

Viruses (influenza types A and B, coxsackievirus, dengue, Epstein-Barr, HIV, cytomegalovirus, parainfluenza, varicella-zoster, West Nile)

Toxins

Carbon monoxide

Envenomation (black widow spider, Africanized honey bees, vipers)

Hemlock

Methanol

Toluene

Hereditary Enzyme Disorders (Rare)

McArdle disease (myophosphorylase deficiency)

Tarui disease (type VII glycogen storage disease)

Phosphoglycerate mutase deficiency (glycogen storage disease type X)

Carnitine palmitoyltransferase deficiency (CPT1 deficiency)

Miscellaneous Causes

Diabetic ketoacidosis

Endocrinopathy

Heatstroke

Hypothermia

Nonketotic hyperosmolar coma

Polymyositis

Severe electrolyte disorders (near-drowning or water intoxication, severe vomiting or diarrhea)

Data from Cervellin G et al: *Clin Chem Lab Med* 48(6):749-756, 2010; Croche F et al: *Int J STD AIDS* 21(11):783-785, 2010; Halpern P et al: *Hum Exp Toxicol* 30(4):259-266, 2011; Keltz E et al: *Muscles Ligaments Tendons J* 3(4):303-312, 2014; Torres PA et al: *Ochsner J* 15(1):58-69, 2015; Zutt R et al: *Neuromuscul Disord* 24(8):651-659, 2014.

affected may have no complaint of pain or muscle weakness.[16] Abnormally dark urine caused by myoglobinuria may be the first and only symptom; however, the presence of myoglobin in urine is not a reliable test for rhabdomyolysis.[19] The renal threshold for myoglobin is low (approximately 0.5 mg/dl of urine); therefore only 200 g of muscle need to be damaged to cause visible changes in the urine. Myoglobin is rapidly cleared and levels may return to normal within 24 hours of injury. Along with the release of myoglobin, creatine kinase (CK) and other serum enzymes are released in massive quantities (normal CK levels are 5 to 25 international units/L for women and 5 to 35 international units/L for men). The efflux of intracellular proteins and enzymes includes loss of potassium, phosphate, nucleotides, creatinine, and creatine. Serum hypocalcemia is seen early in the course of myoglobinuria and is followed by late hypercalcemia. The risk of renal failure increases proportionately to the increase in the levels of serum CK, potassium, and phosphorus.

EVALUATION AND TREATMENT   The most important and clinically useful measurement in rhabdomyolysis is serum creatine kinase (CK) level. A level 5 to 10 times the upper limit of normal (about 1000 units/L) is used to identify rhabdomyolysis.[18] Once CK levels exceed 15,000 units/L, acute renal failure is likely. Other laboratory tests may include electrolytes (elevated serum potassium level [hyperkalemia] can cause life-threatening cardiac abnormalities) and BUN/creatinine ratio (decreased ratio because of creatine released from damaged muscle being converted to creatinine). Additional laboratory tests—such as measurement of hemoglobin, hematocrit, and platelet levels and determination of activated partial thromboplastin time—may be indicated in the presence of other trauma or suspected bleeding. A recent study evaluated the ultrasonographic appearance of rhabdomyolysis in damaged muscle from earthquake victims and found abnormalities in muscle texture and subcutaneous tissue, as well as liquid areas in the damaged tissue.[20]

Maintaining adequate urinary flow and prevention of kidney failure are goals of treatment. Rapid intravenous hydration maintains adequate kidney flow. Other issues, such as hyperkalemia, may require temporary hemodialysis. Treatments such as using mannitol to cause an osmotic diuresis or bicarbonate to alkalinize the urine have not been shown to consistently improve outcomes, though in most instances these types of therapy are unlikely to cause additional complications.[16,17]

Compartment Syndrome

Compartment syndrome is the result of increased pressure within a muscle compartment. Several layers of fibrous fascia (that do not expand) surround skeletal muscles. Increased pressure on the muscle tissue causes diminished capillary blood flow, resulting in local tissue hypoxia and necrosis. Causes of compartment syndrome include conditions that increase the contents of the compartment (such as bleeding after a fracture), decrease the compartment volume (such as a tight bandage or cast), or a combination of both conditions that result in disturbing the muscle's microvasculature (Box 39-2).[21-23] Any condition that disrupts the vascular supply to an extremity (such as severe burns, bleeding disorders, crush injury, snake or insect bites, extremely tight bandages, or casts) can cause increased pressure within the muscle compartments.

BOX 39-2 Factors Affecting Development of Compartment Syndrome

Increased Intracompartmental Pressure

Fracture (open or closed)
Traction
Crush syndrome
Vigorous exercise or nonroutine activity/overuse in nonathletes
High-energy soft tissue injury (blast injuries, blunt force trauma)
Fluid infusion
Arterial puncture
Ruptured abdominal aortic aneurysm
Ruptured ganglion/other cyst
Envenomation (venomous snakes, black widow spiders)
Nephrotic syndrome
Viral myositis
Acute hematogenous osteomyelitis
Orthopedic procedures (e.g., osteotomy, joint replacement)
Seizures
Tetany

Reduced Compartment Volume

Burns
Repair of muscle herniation
Circumferential dressings
Casts that are too tight

Conditions That Disturb Microcirculation

Diabetes
Hypothyroidism
Bleeding disorders (hemophilia, von Willebrand disease, leukemia, vitamin K deficiency, viral hemorrhagic fevers [dengue])
Excessive anticoagulation
Malignancies

Data from Raza H, Mahapatra A: *Adv Orthop* 2015:543412, 2015; Shadgan B et al: *Can J Surg* 53(5):329-334, 2010.

PATHOPHYSIOLOGY The weight of a limb extremity can generate enough pressure to produce muscle ischemia (Figures 39-6 and 39-7). This causes edema, rising compartment pressure, and tamponade that lead to muscle infarction and neural injury and eventually result in cell loss.

CLINICAL MANIFESTATIONS Compartments often affected are the anterior and deep posterior tibial compartments in the leg, the forearm, the gluteal compartments in the buttocks, and the abdominal wall. Diagnosis is initiated by clinical examination. The "6 Ps" of compartment syndrome are *Pain* (out of proportion to the injury), *Pressure* (swelling, tenseness of the affected area), *Pallor*, *Paresthesia*, *Paresis* (of the involved extremity), and *Pulselessness*. None of these signs is truly dependable, although pain with passive extension of the fingers or toes in the affected extremity and paresthesia tend to be most suggestive of compartment syndrome.[21,24]

A condition known as Volkmann ischemic contracture can develop when compartment syndrome is unrecognized or is not adequately treated. Irreversible neurovascular damage can occur. Contracture deformities of the fingers, hand, and wrist can lead to partial or complete disability of the affected limb.

EVALUATION AND TREATMENT Direct measurement of intracompartmental pressure, using a manometer or an electronic transducer, is essential to confirm the diagnosis.[25,26] Laboratory tests, ultrasonography, and imaging studies may help exclude other conditions but generally are not helpful in diagnosing compartment syndrome. Once intracompartmental pressures reach 30 mm Hg, surgical intervention is warranted to relieve pressure within the compartment.

Surgical intervention consists of performing a fasciotomy of the affected area to decompress the compartment and allow return of normal blood supply. Skin grafts are often required to close the resultant opening, but vacuum-assisted wound closure devices also have been used successfully in accelerating wound closure.

Malignant Hyperthermia

Malignant hyperthermia (MH) is an autosomal dominant inherited muscle disorder characterized by a hypermetabolic reaction to certain volatile anesthetics or certain depolarizing muscle relaxants (such as succinylcholine) that activate a prolonged release of intracellular calcium from the sarcoplasmic reticulum. Recently, advances in molecular genetics have shown that a mutation in the ryanodine receptor of skeletal muscle (RyR1) is responsible for the majority of cases, though other genetic mutations also may be involved.[27,28] The normal excitation-coupling process of muscle contraction is altered in MH. Mutations of RyR1 receptors release uncontrolled amounts of calcium from the sarcoplasmic reticulum into the cytoplasm, causing continuous muscle contraction.[29] This process also causes hypermetabolism with extremely high body temperature, muscle rigidity, rhabdomyolysis, and death if not quickly treated with dantrolene infusion.[30]

Though reported in all countries, ages, and both genders, young males tend to be more susceptible to MH. Common signs and symptoms are respiratory acidosis (with elevated end tidal CO_2), tachycardia, masseter and skeletal muscle spasm, and elevated body temperature.[29,31]

EVALUATION AND TREATMENT Careful and thorough preoperative assessment should alert the anesthesiologist to the possibility of an individual being susceptible to malignant hyperthermia. A family history of anesthetic problems and previous untoward anesthetic experiences (muscle cramping, unexplained fevers, dark urine) are criteria that require further clarification before administration of a volatile

FIGURE 39-6 Pathogenesis of Compartment Syndrome and Crush Syndrome Caused by Prolonged Muscle Compression. *ECF,* Extracellular fluid.

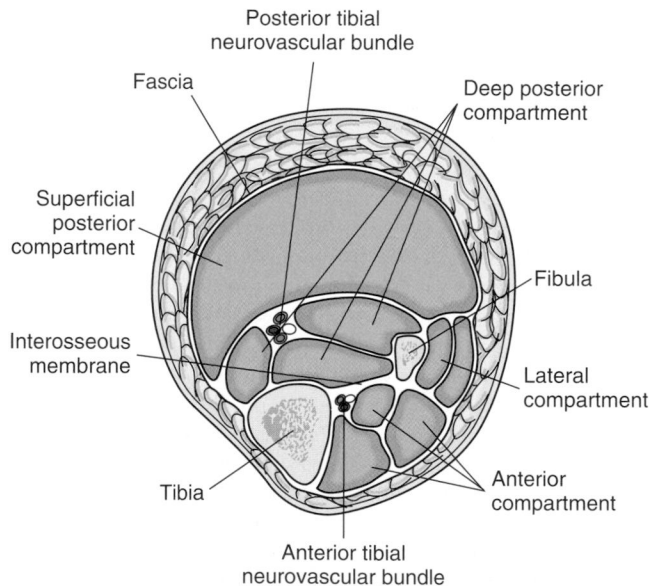

FIGURE 39-7 Muscle Compartments of the Lower Leg. (From Mohahan FD et al: *Phipps' medical-surgical nursing: health and illness perspectives,* ed 8, St Louis, 2007, Mosby.)

anesthetic, such as halothane, or of the muscle relaxant succinylcholine. Currently, the muscle contracture test is considered the best predictor of developing MH. A muscle biopsy is obtained from the individual and then separately exposed to standardized amounts halothane and caffeine. If the muscle bundles exhibit a contracture at

specified limits, the individual is considered susceptible to MH.[31] Molecular and DNA testing are promising future means of identifying at-risk individuals.

Priorities in treatment of MH include identifying and treating the underlying disorder and preventing life-threatening renal failure. Malignant hyperthermia and myoglobinuria can be treated by infusing dantrolene sodium (Dantrium). Secondary problems include electrolyte imbalance, volume depletion, acidosis, hyperuricemia, hyperkalemia, and calcium imbalance; these need specific treatment. Short-term dialysis also may be necessary.

✔ **QUICK CHECK 39-1**
1. How are fractures classified?
2. What is the primary pathology of epicondylopathy?
3. What are some causes of compartment syndrome?
4. Why is myoglobinuria a dangerous complication of rhabdomyolysis?

DISORDERS OF BONES

Metabolic Bone Diseases

Metabolic bone disease is characterized by abnormal bone structure that is caused by altered or inadequate biochemical reactions, which may be attributable to genetics, diet, or hormones.

Osteoporosis

Osteoporosis, or porous bone, is generally described as decreased bone mineral density (BMD) and an increased risk of fractures because of alterations in bone microarchitecture. It is a complex, multifactorial,

FIGURE 39-8 Vertebral Body. Osteoporotic vertebral body *(right)* shortened by compression fractures compared with a normal vertebral body. Note that the osteoporotic vertebra has a characteristic loss of horizontal trabeculae and thickened vertical trabeculae. (From Kumar V et al: *Robbins & Cotran pathologic basis of disease,* ed 9, Philadelphia, 2015, Saunders.)

FIGURE 39-9 Electron Microscopic Comparison of Normal and Osteoporotic Bone. A, Normal trabecular structure. **B,** Osteoporotic bone; note the loss of supporting trabeculae. (From Golob AL, Laya MB: *Med Clin North Am* 99[3]:587-606, 2015.)

TABLE 39-3	T-Score and World Health Organization Diagnosis of Bone Density
T-Score	**Diagnosis**
0 to −0.99 SD	Normal BMD
−1.0 to −2.49 SD	Low bone density (osteopenia)
≤2.5 SD	Osteoporosis
≤2.5 SD with any fracture	Severe osteoporosis

BMD, Bone mineral density; *SD,* standard deviation.

chronic disease that often progresses silently for decades until fractures occur. It is the most common disease that affects bone but is not necessarily a consequence of the aging process because some elderly people retain strong, relatively dense bones. In osteoporosis, old bone is being resorbed faster than new bone is being made, causing the bones to lose density, becoming thinner and more porous. A progressive loss of bone mass may continue until the skeleton is no longer strong enough to support itself. Eventually, bones can fracture spontaneously. As bone becomes more fragile, falls or bumps that would not have caused a fracture previously now cause bone to break (a fragility fracture). The most common sites for osteoporosis-related fractures are the spine, femoral neck, and wrist.[32]

Bone tissue can be normally mineralized in osteoporosis but the mass (density) of bone is decreased and the structural integrity of trabecular bone is impaired. Cortical bone becomes more porous and thinner, making bone weaker and prone to fractures (Figures 39-8 and 39-9). The World Health Organization (WHO) has defined osteoporosis as "a systematic skeletal disease characterized by low bone density and microarchitectural deterioration of bone tissue with a consequent increase in bone fragility."[33]

Bone density is based on the number of standard deviations that differ from the mean bone mineral density of a young-adult reference population (a T-score). Table 39-3 lists these categories. Bone density between 1.5 and 2.5 standard deviations below normal is considered osteopenia. A T-score of 2.5 or more standard deviations below normal bone density is considered osteoporotic. Severe or established osteoporosis is identified when there has been a fragility fracture associated

with low bone density. The disease can be (1) generalized, involving major portions of the axial skeleton, or (2) regional, involving one segment of the appendicular skeleton.

Skeletal homeostasis depends on a narrow range of plasma calcium and phosphate concentrations, which are maintained by the endocrine system. Therefore, endocrine dysfunction ultimately can cause metabolic bone disease. In addition to declining levels of sex steroids, the hormones most commonly associated with osteoporosis are parathyroid hormone, cortisol, thyroid hormone, and growth hormone. (Endocrine function is discussed in Chapters 18 and 19.)

Other factors that can adversely affect normal bone homeostasis include multiple medications (such as glucocorticoids, proton pump inhibitors, thiazolidinediones, antiseizure medications, aromatase inhibitors, selective serotonin reuptake inhibitors [SSRIs], and anticoagulants), vitamin D deficiency, underlying diseases (rheumatoid disease, Paget disease, cancer, diabetes), low physical activity, and abnormal body mass index.[34-38]

Throughout a lifetime, old bone is removed (resorption) and new bone is added (formation) to the skeleton. During childhood and teenage years, new bone is added faster than old bone is removed. Consequently, bones become larger, heavier, and denser. Bone formation continues at a pace faster than resorption until peak bone mass or maximum bone density and strength is reached, around age 30. Up to 90% of peak bone mass is obtained by age 20. After age 30, bone resorption slowly exceeds bone formation. In women, bone loss is most rapid in the first years after menopause but persists throughout the postmenopausal years. In 2011, the U.S. Preventive Services Task Force (USPSTF) issued a new recommendation that women age 65 and older be routinely screened for osteoporosis.[39] Fractures are the major complication of osteoporosis and it has been estimated that nearly one in two white American women older than age 50 will sustain at least one fragility fracture in her lifetime.[40] Hospitalization admissions and costs for osteoporosis-related fractures in the United States are more than those from myocardial infarction, stroke, or breast cancer.[41] Osteoporosis is a worldwide problem with significant economic and health implications.[42-44] Hip fractures, in particular, can have devastating effects on an individual's life. In addition to direct medical costs, studies have shown decreased quality of life as well as excess loss of life-years for those experiencing hip or osteoporotic fractures.[45-47] The major complications for persons with osteoporosis are fractures (see *Health Alert:* Osteoporosis Facts and Figures at a Glance). Bone structure in men allows for improved torque strength and although men lose bone density with aging, it is at a slower, steadier rate than that of women.[48] Nevertheless, men are more likely to die after a hip fracture than are women.[49,50]

Vertebral fractures tend to occur in the later years of life; however, they are more difficult to ascertain because people may be unaware of the fracture. The degree of compression necessary to define a vertebral fracture is not standardized, although attempts have been made to standardize the definition and diagnosis of vertebral fractures. Thus,

HEALTH ALERT

Osteoporosis Facts and Figures at a Glance

- Osteoporosis is the most common bone disease of adults and the foremost cause of fractures in the elderly.
- Nearly 10 million Americans have osteoporosis (T-score ≥ 2.5 SD below normal peak bone mass) and nearly 43.1 million have low bone density (T-score 1.5 to 2.5 SD below normal peak bone mass).
- The National Osteoporosis Foundation (NOF) estimates that only about 40% of individuals with a hip fracture return to their prefracture level of functioning.
- Hip fractures account for only 14% of fractures in osteoporosis, but are responsible for 72% of fracture costs.
- Osteoporosis-related fractures result in approximately 180,000 nursing home admissions, more than 432,000 hospital admissions, and nearly 2.5 million medical office visits annually.
- By 2025, fractures are estimated to increase to 3 million annually, with medical costs escalated to $25.3 billion.
- It is estimated that one in two white women and one in five white men will experience a hip, spine, or wrist fracture sometime in their lives.
- By 2025, Hispanics are predicted to account for 20% of fractures in Arizona and California, with Asians and other non-white ethnic groups sustaining 27% of fractures in New York.

Data from National Osteoporosis Foundation: *Clinician's guide to prevention and treatment of osteoporosis*, Washington, DC, 2014, Author.

TABLE 39-4 Comparison of Fracture Risk Assessment Tools Not Utilizing Bone Mineral Density

Risk Factor	FRAX	SCORE	OSIRIS	ORAI	OST
Age	X	X	X	X	X
Weight	X	X	X	X	X
Previous low-energy fracture	X	X	X		
Estrogen therapy		X	X	X	
Rheumatoid arthritis	X	X			
Height	X				
Parental hip fracture	X				
Smoking	X				
Alcohol	X				
Glucocorticoid therapy	X				
Secondary osteoporosis	X				
Sex	X				
Ethnicity		X			

Chart from Rubin KH et al: *Bone* 56:18, 2013.
FRAX, World Health Organization's "Fracture Risk Assessment Tool"; *ORAI*, osteoporosis risk assessment instrument; *OSIRIS*, osteoporosis index of risk; *OST*, osteoporosis self-assessment tool; *SCORE*, simple calculated osteoporosis risk estimation.

the true prevalence is unknown but fractures do increase in frequency by the sixth and seventh decades. Approximately 1 in 6 women and 1 in 12 men will sustain a vertebral fracture.[51]

Age-related loss of bone density and osteoporosis is most common in white women but affects all races. Asian and black women have only about half the fracture rate of whites, but that percentage is expected to increase with improved life expectancy.[52] In spite of lower incidence, mortality in black women after a hip fracture is higher than among white women. Other factors may include lower calcium intake, a high percentage of lactose intolerance, and increased prevalence of diseases such as sickle cell disease and lupus that increase the risk of developing osteoporosis.[53] Both black women and black men have generally been undertreated for osteoporosis.

Fracture prevention is a primary goal of osteoporosis treatment. Measuring bone mineral density (BMD) by using dual x-ray absorptiometry (DXA) to calculate an individual's T-score continues to be the most common method of evaluating bone health and predicting fracture risk. Unfortunately, the technology to perform DXA scans is not available in all areas of the world. As a result, several tools that do not require BMD testing have been developed and validated to predict future fracture risk. These tools are summarized in Table 39-4. Interestingly, when BMD measurement is not available, there is little difference in fracture prediction between the Internet-based FRAX® and the other tools, including the simplest screening tool—the Osteoporosis Self-assessment Tool, or OST.[54]

Bone quality is not defined by bone mass alone (as measured by BMD) but also by the microarchitecture of the bone. Thus, other variables include crystal size and shape, brittleness, vitality of bone cells, structure of the bone proteins, integrity of the trabecular network, and the ability to repair tiny cracks. Because bone density relates to *quantity* of bone, *quality* of bone is not accurately identified by bone density testing alone. As a result, bone density testing may not accurately identify those who will eventually be susceptible to fractures.

Postmenopausal osteoporosis is bone loss that occurs in middle-aged and older women. It can occur because of estrogen deficiency as well as from estrogen-independent age-related mechanisms (e.g., secondary causes such as hyperparathyroidism and decreased mechanical stimulation). Estrogen deficiency can also increase with stress, excessive exercise, and low body weight. Postmenopausal changes include alterations in the RANKL/OPG/RANK system resulting in a substantial increase in bone turnover—that is, a remodeling imbalance between the activity of osteoclasts (bone destroyers) and osteoblasts (bone formers). Increased formation and activity of osteoclasts causes removal or resorption of bone and results in a cascade of proinflammatory cytokines. Increased cytokine activation, especially tumor necrosis factor (TNF), can occur with declining estrogen levels.[55] In addition, estrogen helps osteoclast apoptosis (programmed cell death) so a decrease in estrogen levels is associated with *survival* of the bone-removing osteoclasts. Biologically, these processes involve the receptor activator nuclear factor κB ligand (RANKL), osteoprotegerin (OPG) signaling pathways, and insulin-like growth factor (IGF) (see Chapter 38, p. 975, and Figures 38-5 and 39-10). Other causes may include a combination of inadequate dietary calcium intake and lack of vitamin D (and possibly decreased magnesium), lack of exercise, low body mass, and family history. IGF is known to help in fracture healing and collagen synthesis and improves conditions for bone mineralization. IGF levels significantly decline by age 60. Excessive phosphorus intake, chiefly through the intake of highly processed foods, hampers the calcium/phosphorus balance by interfering with parathyroid hormone and fibroblast growth factor 23 (FGF-23).[56,57]

Sex hormones, particularly estradiol (estrogen), are major determinants of bone density in both females and males.[58,59] Androgens (i.e., testosterone and dihydrotestosterone) have long been recognized as stimulants of bone formation. Increasing age in both men and women is associated with declining levels of estradiol and androgen, leading to losses in BMD. Other factors, such as inadequate dietary calcium intake, decreases in weightbearing exercise, and sarcopenia, also are associated with osteoporosis. Other risk factors are identified in *Risk Factors: Osteoporosis*.

RISK FACTORS
Osteoporosis

Genetic
Family history of osteoporosis
White race
Increased age
Female gender

Anthropometric
Small stature
Fair or pale skinned
Thin build
Low bone mineral density

Hormonal and Metabolic
Early menopause (natural or
  surgical)
Late menarche
Nulliparity
Obesity
Hypogonadism
Gaucher disease
Cushing syndrome
Weight below healthy range
Acidosis

Dietary
Low dietary calcium and vitamin D
Low endogenous magnesium
Excessive protein*
Excessive sodium intake
Anorexia
Malabsorption

Lifestyle
Sedentary
Smoker
Alcohol consumption (excessive)
Low-impact fractures as an adult
Inability to rise from a chair without
  using one's arms

Concurrent
Hyperparathyroidism

Illness and Trauma
Renal insufficiency, hypocalciuria
Rheumatoid arthritis
Spinal cord injury
Systemic lupus erythematosus

Liver Disease
Marrow disease (myeloma, masto-
  cytosis, thalassemia)

Drugs
Corticosteroids
Dilantin
Gonadotropin-releasing hormone
  agonists
Loop diuretics
Methotrexate
Thyroid medications
Heparin
Cyclosporin
Medroxyprogesterone acetate
  (Depo-Provera)
Retinoids

*Low levels of protein intake also have been reported.

Insufficient intake or malabsorption of dietary minerals is a factor in the development of osteoporosis. Calcium absorption from the intestine decreases with age, and studies of individuals with osteoporosis show that their calcium intake is lower than that of age-matched controls. Other mineral deficiencies, including magnesium, also may be important. Vitamin deficiencies, particularly vitamin D, as well as either deficiencies or excesses of protein also contribute to bone loss. Decreased serum levels of trace elements (zinc, copper, iron, magnesium, and manganese) have been associated not only with lower peak bone mass in developing bone but also with later development of osteoporosis.[60-62] Excessive intake of caffeine, phosphorus, alcohol, and nicotine along with low body fat (weight less than 125 pounds) has been shown to lower bone mineral density.[63-65] **Secondary osteoporosis** is osteoporosis caused by other conditions, including hormonal imbalances (endocrine disease, diabetes, hyperparathyroidism, hyperthyroidism), medications (e.g., heparin, corticosteroids, phenytoin, barbiturates, lithium), and other substances (e.g., tobacco, ethanol). Other conditions, including rheumatoid disease, human immunodeficiency virus (HIV), malignancies, malabsorption syndrome, and liver or kidney disease, also increase the risk for developing osteoporosis (see *Risk Factors:* Osteoporosis).

Secondary osteoporosis sometimes develops temporarily in individuals receiving large doses of heparin by decreasing osteoblast formation and increasing bone resorption by reducing OPG and, thus, increasing osteoclast formation.[66] Osteoporosis caused by heparin therapy usually resolves when therapy ceases. Other medications increasing risk of osteoporosis include glucocorticoids, proton pump inhibitors, aromatase inhibitors, lithium, methotrexate, anticonvulsants, cyclophosphamide, thiazolidinediones, and cyclosporine.

Regional osteoporosis—osteoporosis confined to a segment of the appendicular skeleton—often has no known cause. Classic regional osteoporosis is associated with disuse or immobilization of a limb because of fractures or bone or joint inflammation. A negative calcium balance develops early and continues throughout the period of immobilization. After 8 weeks of immobilization, significant osteoporosis is present. One result of weightlessness has been a uniform distribution of osteoporosis observed in astronauts and in individuals treated with air suspension therapy.

Transient regional osteoporosis has no known etiology and is characterized by bone marrow edema and, sometimes, severe pain. Transient regional osteoporosis is usually self-limiting, and tends to occur in middle-aged men and in women during their late second or third trimester of pregnancy.[67,68] Bone marrow edema can be seen on magnetic resonance imaging (MRI) and areas of localized bone demineralization are seen in plain radiographs.[69] The lower extremity is most often affected but other areas also can be involved. Treatment is primarily symptomatic and the condition usually resolves spontaneously over 3 to 6 months, with no long-term adverse effects.

PATHOPHYSIOLOGY   Osteoporosis develops when the remodeling cycle (coupling)—bone resorption and bone formation—is disrupted, leading to an imbalance in the coupling process. Osteoclasts are differentiated cells that function to resorb bone. The explosion of new information in the field of bone biology has led to new understandings of osteoclast biology and bone pathophysiology. Of primary importance is the osteoclast differentiation pathway that is dependent on various processes including proliferation, maturation, fusion, and activation. These processes, in turn, are dependent on the availability of stem cells to allow differentiation to occur and are controlled by hormones, cytokines, and paracrine stromal cell interactions. Thus, proper intracellular communication within bone among its molecular regulators is necessary for normal bone homeostasis. Numerous interleukins, tumor necrosis factor (TNF), transforming growth factor-beta (TGF-β), prostaglandin E_2, and hormones interact to control osteoclasts (Figure 39-10). Staggering in its importance to understanding osteoclast biology is the cytokine **receptor activator of nuclear factor κB ligand (RANKL)**; its **receptor activator nuclear factor κB (RANK)**; and its decoy receptor **osteoprotegerin (OPG)**, a glycoprotein (see Chapter 36 and Figure 36-5).

Glucocorticoid-induced osteoporosis (e.g., prednisone, cortisone) is the most common type of secondary osteoporosis. Glucocorticoids have a direct impact on bone quality by improving osteoclast survival, inhibiting osteoblast formation and function, and increasing osteocyte apoptosis.[70-72] Glucocorticoids increase RANKL expression and inhibit OPG production by osteoblasts. Overall, these alterations result in decreased thickness of the bone cortex and fewer, thinner, and more widely spaced trabeculae in the marrow.[73]

Age-related bone loss begins in the third to fourth decade.[74] The cause remains unclear, but it is known that decreased serum growth hormone (GH) and insulin-like growth factor 1 (IGF-1) levels, along with increased binding of RANKL and decreased OPG production, affect osteoblast and osteoclast function.[75] Loss of trabecular bone in men proceeds in a linear fashion with thinning of trabecular bone

FIGURE 39-10 OPG/RANKL/RANK System. Expression of RANKL, a cytokine and part of the TNF family, and OPG, a glycoprotein receptor antagonist, is modulated by various cytokines, hormones, drugs, and mechanical strains (see inserts). In bone RANKL is expressed by both stromal cells and osteoblasts. RANKL stimulates the receptor RANK on osteoclast precursor cells and mature osteoclasts and activates intracellular signaling pathways to promote osteoclast differentiation and activation as well as cytoskeletal reorganization and survival (PKB/Akt pathway), which increase resorption and bone loss. OPG, secreted by stromal cells and osteoblasts, acts as a "decoy" receptor and blocks RANKL binding to and activation of RANK. *BMP,* Bone morphogenic protein; *IL,* interleukin; *OPG,* osteoprotegerin; *PTH,* parathyroid hormone; *RANK,* receptor activator nuclear factor κB; *RANKL,* receptor activator nuclear factor κB ligand; *TGF-β,* transforming growth factor-beta; *TNF-α,* tumor necrosis factor-alpha. (Adapted from Hofbauer LC, Schoppet M: *JAMA* 292[4]:490-495, 2004.)

FIGURE 39-11 Mechanism of Loss of Trabecular Bone in Women and Trabecular Thinning in Men. Bone thinning predominates in men because of reduced bone formation. Loss of connectivity and complete trabeculae predominates in women.

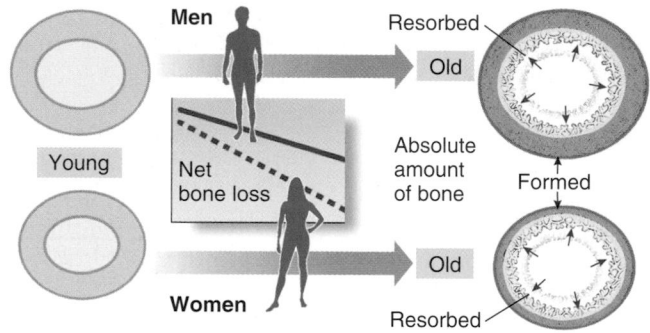

FIGURE 39-12 Bone Loss in Men and Women. Absolute amount of bone resorbed on the inner bone surface and formed on the outer bone surface is more in men than women during aging.

rather than complete loss, as is noted in women (Figure 39-11).[76] Men have approximately 30% greater bone mass than women, which may be a factor in their later involvement with osteoporosis (Figure 39-12). In addition, men have a more gradual decrease in the levels of testosterone and estradiol (and possibly progesterone), thereby maintaining their bone mass longer than women. Reduced physical activity in older persons is also a likely factor.

CLINICAL MANIFESTATIONS The specific clinical manifestations of osteoporosis depend on the bones involved. The most common manifestations, however, are pain and bone deformity because of fracture. Unfortunately, these manifestations occur only in an advanced disease state. Fractures are likely to occur because the trabeculae of spongy bone become thin and sparse, and compact bone becomes porous. As

the bones lose volume, they become brittle and weak and may collapse or become misshapen. Vertebral collapse causes **kyphosis** (hunchback) and diminishes height (Figure 39-13). Fractures of the long bones (particularly the femur),[77] distal radius, ribs, and vertebrae are most common. Fracture of the neck of the femur—the so-called broken hip—tends to occur in older or elderly women with osteoporosis. Fatal complications of fractures include fat or pulmonary embolism, pneumonia, hemorrhage, and shock. Approximately 20% of persons may die as a result of surgical complications. Osteoporosis in men, as in women, also may be related to hypogonadism, with estradiol levels being more clinically important than testosterone levels in both genders. Adequate dietary intake of calcium, vitamin D, magnesium, and other trace minerals (see *Health Alert:* Calcium, Vitamin D, and Bone Health); adherence to a regular regimen of weightbearing exercise; and avoidance of alcoholism, tobacco, and glucocorticoids seem to help prevent primary osteoporosis.

FIGURE 39-13 Kyphosis. This elderly woman's condition was caused by a combination of spinal osteoporotic vertebral collapse and chronic degenerative changes in the vertebral column. (From Kamal A, Brocklehurst JC: *Color atlas of geriatric medicine,* ed 2, St Louis, 1992, Mosby.)

EVALUATION AND TREATMENT In general, osteoporosis is detected radiographically as increased radiolucency of bone. By the time abnormalities are detected by radiologic examination, up to 25% to 30% of bone tissue may have been lost.

Dual x-ray absorptiometry (DXA) is the current gold standard for detecting and monitoring osteoporosis; however, bone density is not necessarily indicative of bone quality. The utility of DXA in predicting fracture risk has recently been enhanced by development of a trabecular bone score (TBS). TBS evaluates pixel variations in the gray-level areas of lumbar spine images from DXA scans and has been shown to correlate with high-resolution peripheral quantitative computed tomography (HRpQCT) and be a reliable predictor of fractures.[78-81] High-resolution imaging techniques, such as quantitative computed tomography (QCT) scans and HRpQCT imaging, show changes of trabecular and cortical microarchitecture in osteopenic women.[82] Newer magnetic resonance imaging techniques also show promise for providing more detailed information about cortical and trabecular bone and have the added safety of no radiation exposure.[40,82] Other evaluation procedures include measurement of serum and urinary biochemical markers to monitor bone turnover (Box 39-3).

The goals of osteoporosis treatment are risk reduction and the prevention of fractures. Bisphosphonates are first-line medications for treating osteoporosis; they primarily work by inhibiting hydroxyapatite breakdown, reducing bone resorption. New medications formulated to prevent or treat osteoporosis are currently being prescribed and evaluated. There are new treatments that help rebuild the skeleton (see *Health Alert:* New Treatments for Osteoporosis). Selective steroid agents—for example, raloxifene—also may be prescribed (see Chapter 33). Regular, moderate weightbearing exercise can slow the rate of bone loss and, in some cases, reverse demineralization because the mechanical stress of exercise stimulates bone formation. An exercise program to enhance strength and balance has the added benefits of reducing the risk of falls and promoting bone quality.

BOX 39-3 Biochemical Markers of Bone Turnover

Biochemical markers of bone turnover are useful in monitoring osteoporosis treatment. Markers of resorption include urinary N-telopeptide (NTx), C-telopeptide (CTx), and deoxypyridinoline. Markers of bone formation include bone-specific alkaline phosphatase (BSAP) and osteocalcin. However, these tests have diurnal variability within the same individual, so there must be significant changes in levels to indicate a difference in bone turnover.

HEALTH ALERT

New Treatments for Osteoporosis

Although bisphosphonates remain the first line of osteoporosis therapy, not all individuals are able to tolerate them and side effects can include bisphosphonate-related osteonecrosis of the jaw (BRONJ), atrial fibrillation, and fractures. Zoledronic acid, a third-generation bisphosphonate, is given as an annual intravenous infusion and has demonstrated efficacy in treating glucocorticoid-associated osteoporosis, in addition to reducing vertebral and nonvertebral fractures in women and men. However, it can cause an acute phase response in recipients and still carries some risk of BRONJ. Several new treatment options promise progress in treating osteoporosis and may be better tolerated than bisphosphonates.

Denosumab is the first commercially available human monoclonal antibody for treatment of osteoporosis. It binds to the receptor activator nuclear factor κB ligand (RANKL) (see Chapter 38), preventing activation of osteoclasts. By reducing osteoclast activity, bone density is increased and bone resorption is reduced, thus lessening the incidence of fractures. Because denosumab is not cleared by the kidneys (as are bisphosphonates), it has the potential to be useful in those with chronic kidney disease. It is given every 6 months as a 60-mg subcutaneous injection.

Raloxifene, a selective estrogen receptor modulator (SERM), has been in use for several years to treat postmenopausal osteoporosis. It has been effective in reducing vertebral fractures but not hip or other nonspinal fractures. Newer SERMs, including lasofoxifene (which is approved for use in Europe, but not the United States), have been shown to reduce both vertebral and nonvertebral fractures. Bazedoxifene, in combination with estrogen, has been designated as a tissue-selective estrogen complex (TSEC), and is approved for use in Japan and Europe. It has been shown to reduce both vertebral and nonvertebral fractures in postmenopausal women. Neither of these agents, given as daily oral doses, stimulates endometrial or breast tissue.

Other biologic agents for treating osteoporosis include odanacatib, a cathepsin K inhibitor. By affecting this enzyme (produced by osteoclasts), bone density is increased. It is given as a once weekly oral agent. Agents directed at signaling pathways of bone formation and homeostasis are another target of osteoporosis intervention. One of the main signaling targets is the Wnt pathway (see Chapter 38). Wnt stimulates osteoblast function and bone formation but is blocked by sclerostin (which is produced by the osteocyte gene *SOST*). Parathyroid hormone (PTH) inhibits sclerostin expression, which may result in increased numbers of osteoblasts. The development of monoclonal antibodies to sclerostin may provide another means to increase bone formation and density.

Data from Bone HG et al: *Osteoporosis Int* 26(2):699-712, 2015; Choi HJ: *J Menopausal Med* 21(1):1-11, 2015; Reid IR: *Nat Rev Endocrinol* 11(7):418-428, 2015; Reyes C et al: *J Cell Biochem* 20 Jun2015 [Epub ahead of print]; Suresh E, Abrahamsen B: *Cleve Clin J Med* 82(2):105-114, 2015.

The anabolic or bone-building drug parathyroid hormone (PTH) has been widely studied and is a major regulator of calcium homeostasis. PTH acts directly on osteocytes, stimulates bone formation, and promotes migration of progenitor bone cells from the marrow into the bloodstream, increasing the production of osteoblasts when intermittently administered[83,84] (see *Health Alert:* New Treatments for Osteoporosis).

Osteomalacia

Osteomalacia is a metabolic disease characterized by inadequate and delayed mineralization of osteoid in mature compact and spongy bone.

In osteomalacia, the remodeling cycle proceeds normally through osteoid formation, but mineral calcification and deposition do not occur. Bone volume remains unchanged, but the replaced bone consists of soft osteoid instead of rigid bone. Rickets is similar to osteomalacia in pathogenesis, but it occurs in the growing bones of children, whereas osteomalacia occurs in adult bone. (Rickets is described in Chapter 40.)

Both osteomalacia and rickets are relatively rare in the United States and Western Europe but are significant health problems in Great Britain, Ethiopia, Pakistan, Iran, and India. Concomitant diseases, such as HIV, chronic kidney or liver disease, certain cancers, and impaired nutrient absorption from bariatric surgery, can result in vitamin D deficiency and secondary osteomalacia. In the United States, other causes include prematurity with very low birth weight and adhering to a rigid macrobiotic vegetarian diet. Breast-fed black infants who do not receive vitamin D supplementation have been shown to be at risk for developing nutritional rickets.[85,86]

Many factors contribute to the development of osteomalacia, but the most important is a deficiency of vitamin D. The major risk factors in vitamin D deficiency are diets deficient in vitamin D, decreased endogenous production of vitamin D, intestinal malabsorption of vitamin D, renal tubular diseases, certain types of tumors (particularly of mesenchymal origin), and anticonvulsant therapy. Classic vitamin D deficiency is rare in the United States because of the addition of synthetic vitamin D to dairy products and bread.

Disorders of the small bowel, hepatobiliary system, and pancreas are causes of vitamin D deficiency in the United States. In malabsorptive disease of the small bowel, both vitamin D and calcium absorption are decreased, so vitamin D is lost in feces. Liver disease interferes with the metabolism of vitamin D to its more active form, and diseases of the pancreas and biliary system cause a deficiency of bile salts, which are necessary for normal intestinal absorption of vitamin D.

The mechanism by which anticonvulsant drug therapy results in vitamin D deficiency is not completely understood, but researchers think that the anticonvulsants phenobarbital and phenytoin interfere with calcium absorption and increase degradation of vitamin D metabolism in the liver. Renal osteodystrophy is another cause of osteomalacia.

PATHOPHYSIOLOGY Crystallization of minerals in osteoid requires adequate concentrations of calcium and phosphate. When the concentrations are too low, crystallization (and hence ossification) does not proceed normally.

Vitamin D deficiency disrupts mineralization because vitamin D normally regulates and enhances the absorption of calcium ions from the intestine. A lack of vitamin D causes the plasma calcium concentrations to fall. Low plasma calcium levels stimulate increased synthesis and secretion of PTH. Although the increase in circulating PTH level raises the plasma calcium concentration, it also stimulates increased renal clearance of phosphate. When the concentration of phosphate in the bone decreases below a critical level, mineralization cannot proceed normally. Newer research has identified a complex interplay of matrix proteins, hormones, metallopeptidases, and certain proteins as also being involved in the development of osteomalacia.

Abnormalities occur in both spongy and compact bone. Trabeculae in spongy bone become thinner and fewer, whereas haversian systems in compact bone develop large channels and become irregular. Because osteoid continues to be produced but not mineralized, abnormal quantities of osteoid accumulate, coating the trabeculae and the linings of the haversian canals. Excessive osteoid also can accumulate in areas beneath the periosteum. The excess of osteoid leads to gross deformities of the long bones, spine, pelvis, and skull.

CLINICAL MANIFESTATIONS Osteomalacia causes varying degrees of diffuse muscular and skeletal pain and tenderness. Pain is noted particularly in the hips, and the individual may be hesitant to walk.[87] Muscular weakness is common and may contribute to a waddling gait. Facial deformities and bowed legs or "knock-knees" may be present. Bone fractures and vertebral collapse occur with minimal trauma. Low back pain may be an early complaint, but pain may also involve ribs, feet, other areas of the vertebral column, and other sites. Fragility fractures may occur. Uremia may be present in renal osteodystrophy.

EVALUATION AND TREATMENT Laboratory data may include elevated blood urea nitrogen (BUN) and creatinine levels, normal or low serum calcium levels, and a serum inorganic phosphate level that is usually more than 5.5 mg. Alkaline phosphatase and PTH levels are usually elevated. Radiographic findings may show symmetric bowing deformities and fractures with callus formation, particularly in the lower extremities. These types of fractures, known as pseudofractures, along with radiolucent bands perpendicular to the surface of involved bones can help differentiate osteomalacia from fragility fractures that are seen in osteoporosis. A bone biopsy is used to obtain information on bone structure and remodeling and evaluate the presence of subclinical renal osteodystrophy to determine bone architecture, turnover, and even aluminum deposits.[88,89]

Treatment of osteomalacia may vary, depending on its etiology, but the following general principles are included:
1. Adjustment of serum calcium and phosphorus levels to normal
2. Suppression of secondary hyperthyroidism
3. Chelation of bone aluminum if needed
4. Administration of calcium carbonate to decrease hyperphosphatemia
5. Administration of vitamin D supplements (oral or infusion)
6. Administration of bisphosphonate
7. Implementation of renal dialysis, if indicated

Paget Disease

Paget disease of bone (PDB, or osteitis deformans), the second most common bone disease after osteoporosis, is a state of increased metabolic activity in bone characterized by localized abnormal and excessive bone remodeling. Chronic accelerated remodeling eventually enlarges and softens the affected bones, causing bowing deformity, fracture, or neurologic problems.

Paget disease can occur in any bone but most often affects the vertebrae, skull, sacrum, sternum, pelvis, and femur. The disease process may occur in one or more bones without causing significant clinical manifestations.

Paget disease occurs with equal frequency in men more than 55 years of age and women older than 40 years of age. It is often symptomless and diagnosis is often suspected when an elevated serum alkaline phosphatase level or abnormal x-ray is noted.[90] Radioisotope bone scan, x-rays, and CT are used to confirm the diagnosis.[91] Serum plasma procollagen-1 N-peptide (PINP) is another serum marker that may provide a more accurate diagnosis.[92] Autopsy data from England and Germany indicate that approximately 3% to 4% of the population older than 40 years of age has Paget disease. It is most prevalent in Australia, Great Britain, New Zealand, and the United States. Paget disease affects several members of the same family in 5% to 25% of individuals.

The cause of PDB is not yet fully known, but studies have implicated both genetic and environmental factors. Environmental factors that seem to be implicated are primarily viruses, particularly the paramyxovirus family (that includes mumps, parainfluenza, and measles viruses), but no definitive microorganism has yet been identified.[93,94]

Of individuals diagnosed with PDB, 10% to 30% have mutations of a specific gene, *sequestosome-1 (SQSTM1)*.[95,96] Interaction between genetic and environmental factors appears to increase osteoclast activity in PDB.

PATHOPHYSIOLOGY Certain chromosomes on *SQSTM1* are known to affect osteoclast differentiation and function, although the exact locus of the genetic abnormality has yet to be identified.[94,97] Paget disease begins with excessive resorption of spongy bone and deposition of disorganized bone. The trabeculae diminish, and bone marrow is replaced by extremely vascular fibrous tissue.

The resorption phase of Paget disease is followed by the formation of abnormal new bone at an accelerated rate. The collagen fibers are disorganized, and glycoprotein levels in the matrix decrease. Mineralization may extend into the bone marrow. Bone formation is excessive around partially resorbed trabeculae, causing them to thicken and enlarge. The net result of this accelerated remodeling process is increased bone fragility and an increased risk for bone tumors.[98]

CLINICAL MANIFESTATIONS In the skull, abnormal remodeling is first evident in the frontal or occipital regions; then it encroaches on the outer and inner surfaces of the entire skull. The skull thickens and assumes an asymmetric shape. Thickened segments of the skull may compress areas of the brain, producing altered mentality and dementia. Impingement of new bone on cranial nerves causes sensory abnormalities, impaired motor function, deafness (because of involvement of the middle ear ossicles or compression of the auditory nerve), atrophy of the optic nerve, and obstruction of the lacrimal duct. Headache is commonly noted.

Extensive alterations of the facial bones are rare except in the jaw, where sclerosis and thickening of the maxilla and mandible displace teeth and produce malocclusion. In long bones, resorption begins in the subchondral regions of the epiphysis and extends into the metaphysis and diaphysis. Occasionally, Paget disease affects both ends of a tubular bone. In the femur, Paget disease produces an exaggerated lateral curvature. In the tibia, anterior curvature is also exaggerated. Stress fractures are common in the lower extremities.

Clinical manifestations of Paget disease in the vertebral column depend on the level of involvement and are caused by compression of adjacent structures. In the cervical spine, cord compression can lead to spastic quadriplegia. Approximately 1% of persons with Paget disease develop osteogenic sarcoma.

EVALUATION AND TREATMENT Evaluation of Paget disease is made on the basis of radiographic findings of irregular bone trabeculae with a thickened and disorganized pattern. Early disease is detected by bone scanning that shows increased uptake of bone radionuclides. Plasma alkaline phosphatase and urinary hydroxyproline levels are elevated.

Many individuals require no treatment if the disease is localized and does not cause symptoms. Treatment during active disease is for relief of pain and prevention of deformity or fracture. Bisphosphonates are the treatment of choice; a one-time infusion of zoledronic acid can provide long-term reduction of biochemical markers and even remission.[99-102] Newer agents, including monoclonal antibodies (denosumab), interleukin-6 receptor inhibitors (tocilizumab), cathepsin K inhibitors (odanacatib), and Dickkopf-1 inhibitors, are under study for treatment of PDB.[91,98]

Infectious Bone Disease: Osteomyelitis

Osteomyelitis is a bone infection most often caused by bacteria; however, fungi, parasites, and viruses also can cause bone infection (Figure 39-14). Multiple classification systems have been used to

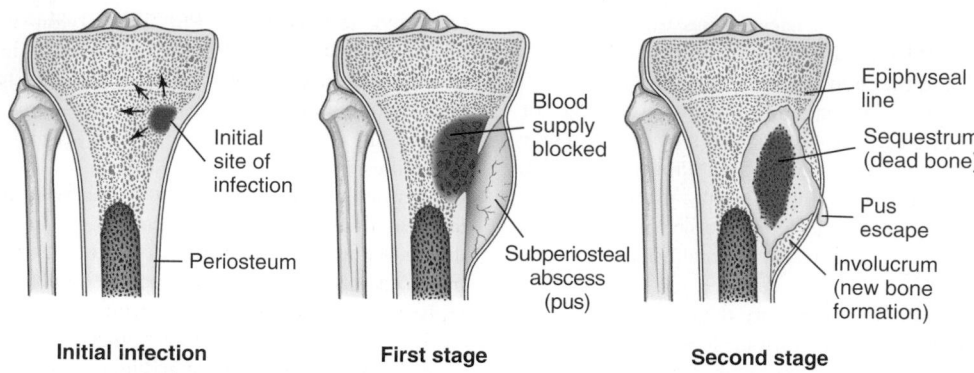

Initial infection   First stage   Second stage

FIGURE 39-14 Osteomyelitis Showing Sequestration and Involucrum.

describe osteomyelitis; the simplest refers to the mode of infection. A bone infection caused by pathogens carried through the bloodstream is termed hematogenous osteomyelitis. Acute hematogenous osteomyelitis is more often seen in children and is characterized by fever, pain, and voluntary immobility of the affected limb. (Osteomyelitis in children is discussed in Chapter 40.) Contiguous osteomyelitis occurs when infection spreads to an adjacent bone and is often caused by open fractures, penetrating wounds, or surgical procedures. Other causes of osteomyelitis include metabolic and vascular diseases (diabetes, peripheral vascular disease), lifestyle risks (smoking, alcohol or drug abuse), and advanced age.[103] In infants, incidence rates among males and females are approximately equal. In children and older adults, however, males are most commonly affected. A new category of autoimmune, noninfectious osteomyelitis, known as chronic nonbacterial osteomyelitis (CNO), has recently been identified as a cause of chronic bone pain in children.[104]

Staphylococcus aureus remains the primary microorganism responsible for osteomyelitis.[105-107] Other microorganisms include group B streptococcus, Haemophilus influenzae, Salmonella, and gram-negative bacteria. Group B streptococcus and H. influenzae tend to infect young children; Salmonella infection is associated with sickle cell anemia; and gram-negative infections are most common in older adults and immunocompromised individuals with impaired immunity. Mycobacterial, viral, and fungal infections occur in immunocompromised individuals.

Cutaneous, sinus, ear, and dental infections are the primary sources of bacteria in hematogenous bone infections. Soft tissue infections, disorders of the gastrointestinal tract, infections of the genitourinary system, and respiratory tract infections are also sources of bacterial contamination. In addition, infections that occur after total joint replacement procedures are sometimes the cause. The vulnerability of specific bone depends on the anatomy of its vascular supply.

In adults, hematogenous osteomyelitis is more common in the spine, pelvis, and small bones. Microorganisms reach the vertebrae through arteries, veins, or lymphatic vessels. The spread of infection from pelvic organs to the vertebrae is well documented. Vaginal, uterine, ovarian, bladder, and intestinal infections can lead to iliac or sacral osteomyelitis.

Superficial animal or human bites inoculate local soft tissue with bacteria that later spread to underlying bone. Deep bites can introduce microorganisms directly onto bone. The most common infecting organism in human bites is Staphylococcus aureus. In animal bites, the most common infecting organism is Pasteurella multocida, which is part of the normal mouth flora of cats and dogs.

Direct contamination of bones with bacteria can also occur in open fractures or dislocations with an overlying skin wound. Intervertebral

disk surgery and operative procedures involving implantation of large foreign objects, such as metallic plates or artificial joints, are associated with contiguous osteomyelitis. Osteomyelitis of the arm and hand bones tends to occur in persons who abuse drugs. In general, persons who are chronically ill, have diabetes or alcoholism, or are receiving large doses of steroids or immunosuppressive drugs are particularly susceptible to chronic osteomyelitis or recurring episodes of this disease.

PATHOPHYSIOLOGY Regardless of the source of the pathogen, the pathologic features of bone infection are similar to those in any other body tissue (see Chapter 6). First, the invading pathogen provokes an intense inflammatory response. S. aureus, in addition to producing toxins that destroy neutrophils, also forms colonies of microorganisms, called biofilms, that adhere to surfaces (such as implants) and increase antibiotic resistance. Biofilms also can reduce the duration of osteoblast activity while enhancing osteoclast activity and promoting inflammation[108-110] (also see Chapter 8). Primarily through activation of the cytokine pathway, the biofilm and inflammation alter the normal balance between osteoblast and osteoclast activity.[107,111] Inflammation in bone is characterized by vascular engorgement, edema, leukocyte activity, and abscess formation. Once inflammation is initiated, the small terminal vessels thrombose and exudate seals the bone's canaliculi. Inflammatory exudate extends into the metaphysis and the marrow cavity and through small metaphyseal openings into the cortex. In children, exudate that reaches the outer surface of the cortex forms abscesses that lift the periosteum of underlying bone. Lifting of the periosteum disrupts blood vessels that enter bone through the periosteum, which deprives underlying bone of its blood supply. This leads to necrosis and death of the area of bone infected, producing sequestrum, an area of devitalized bone. Lifting of the periosteum also stimulates an intense osteoblastic response. Osteoblasts lay down new bone that can partially or completely surround the infected bone. This layer of new bone surrounding the infected bone is called an involucrum (Figure 39-15). Openings in the involucrum allow the exudate to escape into surrounding soft tissue and ultimately through the skin by way of sinus tracts.

In adults, this complication is rare because the periosteum is firmly attached to the cortex and resists displacement. Instead, infection disrupts and weakens the cortex, which predisposes the bone to pathologic fracture.

CLINICAL MANIFESTATIONS Clinical manifestations of osteomyelitis vary with the age of the individual, the site of involvement, the initiating event, the infecting organism, and the type of infection—acute, subacute, or chronic. Osteomyelitis is generally considered acute

FIGURE 39-15 Resected Femur in a Person with Draining Osteomyelitis. The drainage tract in the subperiosteal shell of viable new bone (involucrum) reveals the inner native necrotic cortex (sequestrum). (From Kumar V et al: *Robbins & Cotran pathologic basis of disease*, ed 9, Philadelphia, 2015, Saunders.)

if diagnosed within 2 weeks after symptom onset and is associated with abrupt onset of inflammation (see Figure 39-15). Subacute osteomyelitis is disease that has been present for 1 to several months, and chronic disease is that which has been present for many months to even years.[103,112]

If an acute infection is not completely eliminated, the disease may become subacute or chronic. In subacute osteomyelitis, signs and symptoms are usually vague. In the chronic stage, infection is indolent or silent between exacerbations. The microorganisms persist in small abscesses or fragments of necrotic bone and produce occasional exacerbations of acute osteomyelitis. The progression from acute to subacute osteomyelitis may be the result of inadequate or inappropriate therapy, or the development of drug-resistant microorganisms.

In the adult, hematogenous osteomyelitis has an insidious onset. The symptoms are usually vague and include fever, malaise, anorexia, weight loss, and pain in and around the infected areas. Edema may or may not be evident. Recent infection (urinary, respiratory, cutaneous) or instrumentation (catheterization, cystoscopy, myelography, diskography) usually precedes onset of symptoms.

Single or multiple abscesses (Brodie abscesses) characterize subacute or chronic osteomyelitis. Brodie abscesses are circumscribed lesions 1 to 4 cm in diameter that are found usually in the ends of long bones and surrounded by dense ossified bone matrix. The abscesses are thought to develop when the infectious microorganism has become less virulent or the individual's immune system is resisting the infection somewhat successfully.

In contiguous osteomyelitis, signs and symptoms of soft tissue infection predominate. Inflammatory exudate in the soft tissues disrupts muscles and supporting structures and forms abscesses. Low-grade fever, lymphadenopathy, local pain, and swelling usually occur within days of contamination by a puncture wound.

EVALUATION AND TREATMENT Laboratory data show an elevated white cell count and an elevated level of noncardiac C-reactive protein (CRP). Radiographic studies include radionuclide bone scanning, CT, functional imaging using a combination of radionuclide scanning (using fluorodeoxyglucose [FDG]) and single photon emission

computed tomography (SPECT), positron emission tomography (PET), and MRI. MRI scanning with gadolinium contrast shows both bone and soft tissue, providing more accurate assessment of infection. MRI also shows early changes of bone marrow edema. FDG-SPECT imaging is highly sensitive for evaluating osteomyelitis of the extremities.[113]

Treatment of osteomyelitis includes bone biopsy to identify the causative organism, use of antimicrobial agents, and débridement of infected bone.[106,114] Biodegradable antibiotic-impregnated bioabsorbable beads have also benefited many individuals; newer therapies include the promise of injectable scaffolds impregnated with antibiotics and other antimicrobial substances.[115] Chronic conditions may require surgical removal of the inflammatory exudate followed by continuous wound irrigation with antibiotic solutions in addition to systemic treatment with antibiotics. The ideal antibiotic regimen for treating osteomyelitis has not yet been developed. Hyperbaric oxygen therapy of 100% oxygen may stimulate healing by suppressing proinflammatory cytokines and prostaglandins. Implants for total joint replacements may be removed to treat the infected joint more thoroughly.

> ✔ **QUICK CHECK 39-2**
> 1. What are the causes associated with osteoporosis in women and men?
> 2. How does osteoporosis differ from osteomalacia? Name three differences.
> 3. What are the risk factors for osteomyelitis?

DISORDERS OF JOINTS

The American College of Rheumatology (ACR) recognizes several groups of joint disease (arthropathies). Most of these disorders can be placed into two major categories: noninflammatory joint disease and inflammatory joint disease. With the improvement in detection methods, however, inflammatory pathways are now being identified in conditions previously classified as noninflammatory, such as osteoarthritis.

Osteoarthritis

Osteoarthritis (OA) is the most common, age-related disorder of synovial joints. Affecting the entire joint, OA is characterized by local areas of loss and damage of articular cartilage, inflammation, new bone formation of joint margins (osteophytosis), subchondral bone changes, variable degrees of mild synovitis, and thickening of the joint capsule (Figure 39-16). Pathology centers on load-bearing areas. Advancing disease shows narrowing of the joint space attributable to cartilage loss, bone spurs (osteophytes), and sometimes changes in the subchondral bone. OA can arise in any synovial joint but is commonly found in the knees, hips, hands, and spine. It is less common in people younger than 40 years of age and its prevalence increases with age. Although the exact causes of OA are unclear, obesity and trauma are well-known risk factors.[116] Recent research has identified specific microRNAs that affect gene expression in chondrocytes, and that may play a role in developing OA.[117,118] OA involves a complex interaction of transcription factors, cytokines, growth factors, matrix molecules, the immune system, mechanical stresses on joints, and enzymes[119-121] (see the following Pathophysiology section). Emerging understanding of synovitis and inflammation in OA has led to the recognition of the role played by the body's immune system in OA.[122]

Although incidence rates are quite similar in men and women, after age 50, women typically are more severely affected. OA usually occurs

FIGURE 39-16 Osteoarthritis (OA). **A,** Cartilage and degeneration of the hip joint from osteoarthritis. **B,** Heberden nodes and Bouchard nodes. **C,** Severe osteoarthritis with small islands of residual articular cartilage next to exposed subchondral bone. (**C** from Kumar V et al: *Robbins & Cotran pathologic basis of disease,* ed 9, Philadelphia, 2015, Saunders.)

in those persons who put exceptional stress (or joint loading) on joints (e.g., obese persons, gymnasts, long-distance runners or marathoners); persons participating in such sports as basketball, soccer, or football have been shown to develop osteoarthritis at earlier ages than usual. Obesity itself seems to be an independent risk factor for developing OA of the knee.[123-126] Chondrocyte death because of mitochondrial release of reactive oxygen species (ROS) is thought to be caused by increased stress on joints.[120] A previously torn anterior cruciate ligament or meniscectomy increases the risk for accelerated osteoarthritis of the knee.[127,128]

Types of Osteoarthritis

PATHOPHYSIOLOGY   The primary defect in OA is loss of articular cartilage.[129] Early in the disease, the articular cartilage loses its glistening appearance, becoming yellow-gray or brownish gray. As the disease progresses, surface areas of the articular cartilage flake off and deeper layers develop longitudinal fissures (fibrillation). The cartilage becomes thin and may be absent over some areas, leaving the underlying bone

(subchondral bone) unprotected. Consequently, the unprotected subchondral bone becomes sclerotic (dense and hard). Cysts sometimes develop within the subchondral bone and communicate with the longitudinal fissures in the cartilage. Pressure builds in the cysts until the cystic contents are forced into the synovial cavity, breaking through the articular cartilage on the way. As the articular cartilage erodes, cartilage-coated osteophytes may grow outward from the underlying bone and alter the bone contours and joint anatomy. These spurlike bony projections enlarge until small pieces, called *joint mice,* break off into the synovial cavity. If osteophyte fragments irritate the synovial membrane, synovitis and joint effusion result. Interestingly, joint pain may be more related to inflammation of the synovium than subsequent cartilage damage or the radiographic extent of arthritis.[130,131] The joint capsule also becomes thickened and at times adheres to the deformed underlying bone, which may contribute to the limited range of motion of the joint (see Figure 39-16).

Articular cartilage is lost through a cascade of signaling, cytokine, and anabolic growth factor pathways.[132,133] Enzymatic processes (including matrix metalloproteinases) assist in breaking the macro-molecules of proteoglycans, glycosaminoglycans, and collagen into large, diffusible fragments. Then the fragments are taken up by the cartilage cells (chondrocytes) and digested by the cell's own lysosomal enzymes. (Processes of cellular uptake and lysosomal digestion are described in Chapter 1.) The loss of proteoglycans from articular cartilage is a hallmark of the osteoarthritic process.

Enzymatic destruction of articular cartilage begins in the matrix, with destruction of proteoglycans and collagen fibers. Enzymes, particularly stromelysin and acid metalloproteinases, affect proteoglycans by interfering with assembly of the proteoglycan subunit or the proteoglycan aggregate (see Chapter 38); levels of these enzymes are markedly elevated in OA. Changes in the conformation of proteoglycans disrupt the pumping action that regulates movement of water and synovial fluid into and out of the cartilage. Without the regulatory action of the proteoglycan pump, cartilage imbibes too much fluid and becomes less able to withstand the stresses of weightbearing. With aging, the proteoglycan content is decreased, and water content in cartilage can be increased by as much as 8%, affecting the strength of the cartilage. Persons with OA, even those with fairly extensive cartilage destruction, have elevated levels of proteoglycans/fragments in their synovial fluid, perhaps indicative of the degree of disease activity. MicroRNAs, small nucleic acids that do not code for proteins (but appear to regulate the RNAs that do), may have a direct effect on developing OA by targeting specific genes involved in cartilage development and homeostasis.[118,134,135] Disruptions in cellular signaling pathways, particularly the transforming growth factor-beta (TGF-β) superfamily, play a significant role in developing OA.[136] Other studies indicate that cytokines, such as interleukin-1 and tumor necrosis factor (TNF) (see Chapter 7 for discussion of cytokines), play a major role in cartilage degradation[132] as a result of release and activation of proteolytic and collagenolytic enzymes associated with an imbalance of cell responses to growth factor activity.[137,138]

Cell-signaling proteins, particularly adipokines such as adiponectin and collagenases (enzymes that degrade collagen), contribute to collagen breakdown in cartilage.[139] Collagen breakdown destroys the fibrils that give articular cartilage its tensile strength and exposes the chondrocytes to mechanical stress and enzyme attack. The osteochondral junction formed by cartilage and its underlying subchondral bone allows alterations in one tissue to affect the adjacent one (biomechanical coupling). When articular cartilage is damaged, abnormal subchondral bone remodeling occurs.[140,141] Thus, a cycle of destruction begins that involves all the components of a joint: cartilage, bone, and the synovium.

CLINICAL MANIFESTATIONS   Clinical manifestations of OA typically appear during the fifth or sixth decade of life; although often asymptomatic, articular surface changes are common after the age of 40 years. Pain in one or more joints—usually with weightbearing, use of the joint, or load bearing—is the first and most predominant symptom of the disease. Resting the joint often relieves pain. If present, nocturnal pain is usually not relieved by rest and may be accompanied by paresthesias (numbness, tingling, or prickling sensations). Sometimes pain is referred to another part of the body. For example, osteoarthritis of the lumbosacral spine may mimic sciatica, causing severe pain in the back of the thigh along the course of the sciatic nerve. OA in the lower cervical spine may cause brachial neuralgia (pain in the arm) and is aggravated by movement of the neck. Osteoarthritic conditions in the hip cause pain that may be referred to the lower thigh and knee area. Sleep deprivation adds to the stress of the chronic pain of OA. Physical examination of the person with OA usually shows general involvement of both peripheral and central joints. Peripheral joints most often involved are in the hands, wrists, knees, and feet. Central joints most often afflicted are in the lower cervical spine, lumbosacral spine, shoulders, and hips.

Joint structures are capable of generating a limited number of signs and symptoms. The primary signs and symptoms of osteoarthritic joint disease are pain, stiffness, enlargement or swelling, tenderness, limited range of motion, muscle wasting, partial dislocation, and deformity (see *Risk Factors:* Osteoarthritis).

RISK FACTORS
Osteoarthritis

- Trauma, sprains, strains, joint dislocations, and fractures
- Long-term mechanical stress—athletics, ballet dancing, repetitive physical tasks, and obesity
- Inflammation in joint structures
- Joint instability from damage to supporting structures
- Neurologic disorders (e.g., diabetic neuropathy, Charcot neuropathic joint) in which pain and proprioceptive reflexes are diminished or lost
- Congenital or acquired skeletal deformities
- Hematologic or endocrine disorders, such as hemophilia, which causes chronic bleeding into the joints, or hyperparathyroidism, which causes bone to lose calcium
- Drugs (e.g., colchicine, indomethacin, steroids) that stimulate the collagen-digesting enzymes in the synovial membrane

The origin of joint stiffness is unknown. Joint stiffness is generally defined as difficulty initiating joint movement, immobility, or a loss of range of motion. The stiffness usually occurs as joint movement begins, and it dissipates rapidly after a few minutes. Stiffness lasting longer than 30 minutes is uncommon in OA. Enlargement and bulging of bone contour, commonly described as swelling, may be caused by bone enlargement or the proliferation of osteophytes around the margins of the joint. In the hands, these areas are called Heberden and Bouchard nodes, where they are typical features of OA (see Figure 39-16). Inflammation of the joint lining, known as synovitis, is thought to be initiated by the release of cartilage extracellular matrix into the joint, which then activates the body's complement system.[142] Swelling also occurs if inflammatory exudate or blood enters the joint cavity, thereby increasing the volume of synovial fluid. This condition, termed joint effusion, is caused by (1) the presence of osteophyte fragments in the synovial cavity, (2) drainage of cysts from diseased subchondral bone, or (3) acute trauma to joint structures, resulting in hemorrhage and inflammatory exudation into the synovial cavity (see Figure 39-16, *C*).

Range of motion is limited to some degree, depending on the extent of cartilage degeneration. Frequently, joint motion is accompanied by sounds of crepitus, creaking, or grating. Hypermobility and subluxation of joints occur in OA secondary to a neurologic disorder. Abnormal knee alignment (either varus or valgus) has been shown to be a risk factor for and can increase progression of the disease.[143,144]

As OA of the lower extremity progresses, the person may begin to noticeably limp (Figure 39-17). Having a limp is distressing because it affects the person's independence and ability to perform usual activities of daily living. The affected joint is also more symptomatic after use, such as at the end of a period of strenuous activity.

EVALUATION AND TREATMENT   Evaluation consists primarily of clinical assessment and radiologic studies. More expensive studies,

FIGURE 39-17 Typical Varus Deformity of Knee Osteoarthritis. (From Doherty M: *Color atlas and text of osteoarthritis,* London, 1994, Wolfe.)

including CT scan, arthroscopy, and MRI, are rarely needed. Newer imaging technologies, such as compositional MRI, are showing promise in identifying structural changes in cartilage; improvements in technology may also allow better monitoring of OA treatment.

Treatment is either conservative or surgical. Conservative treatment includes both pharmacologic and nonpharmacologic therapies; surgery is a last resort. Both exercise and weight loss have been shown to be two of the most important nonpharmacologic treatments in improving knee OA symptoms. Exercise can reduce pain and improve physical function in people with knee OA.[145-149] Exercises to improve muscle tone, range of motion, and balance; stretch the joint capsule; and decrease fear of falling also have shown promise in reducing OA symptoms.[150,151] Braces and foot orthoses may help correct biomechanical abnormalities, thereby reducing pain and improving mobility.[152] Dietary and nutritional supplements can sometimes also improve symptoms. Nutraceuticals, such as chondroitin and glucosamine, have shown success in relieving OA pain in some individuals.[153] Other nonsurgical therapies include analgesic and anti-inflammatory drug therapy to reduce swelling and pain. Acetaminophen was once considered first-line treatment, but it has been shown to be less effective than nonsteroidal anti-inflammatory drugs (NSAIDs), such as ibuprofen. However, prolonged use significantly increases the risk of serious associated side effects that are common.[154] Intra-articular injection of corticosteroids and high-molecular-weight viscose supplements, such as hyaluronic acid, also decreases knee pain with OA.[155,156] Recently, because of its high concentration of growth factors, platelet-rich plasma (PRP) also has been injected into osteoarthritic knee joints with some success in reducing pain and markers of inflammation.[157] Current evidence does not support low-level laser therapy for knee osteoarthritis.[158] Newer agents, including inhibitors of cytokines, matrix metalloproteinases (MMPs), and leptin, are under investigation and may prove more effective in treating OA. Surgery is used to improve joint movement, correct deformity or malalignment, or create a new joint with artificial implants. It has been estimated by some researchers that one in four individuals has a lifetime risk of developing symptomatic OA of the hip.[159] More than 280,000 total hip and more than 600,000 total knee replacement surgeries are performed yearly in the United States, most of which are related to OA.[160]

Classic Inflammatory Joint Disease

Inflammatory joint disease is commonly called arthritis. Inflammatory joint disease is characterized by inflammatory damage or destruction in the synovial membrane or articular cartilage and by systemic signs of inflammation (fever, leukocytosis, malaise, anorexia, hyperfibrinogenemia).

Inflammatory joint disease can be infectious or noninfectious. Infectious inflammatory joint disease is caused by invasion of the joint by bacteria, mycoplasmas, viruses, fungi, or protozoa. These agents can invade the joint through a traumatic wound, surgical incision, or contaminated needle, or they can be delivered by the bloodstream from sites of infection elsewhere in the body—typically bones, heart valves, or blood vessels. Noninfectious inflammatory joint disease, the most common form, is caused by immune reactions or the deposition of crystals of monosodium urate in and around the joint. Rheumatoid arthritis, psoriatic arthritis, and ankylosing spondylitis are noninfectious inflammatory diseases caused by immune reactions and possibly hypersensitivity reactions; gouty arthritis is a noninfectious inflammatory disease caused by crystal deposition.

Rheumatoid Arthritis

Rheumatoid arthritis (RA) is a chronic, systemic, inflammatory autoimmune disease distinguished by joint swelling and tenderness and destruction of synovial joints leading to disability and premature death.[161] (Autoimmune disease is described in Chapter 8.) The first joint tissue to be affected is the synovial membrane, which lines the joint cavity (see Chapter 36, Figure 36-9). The two primary types of synovial cells are fibroblast-like synovial cells and macrophage-like synovial cells. Though the initiating mechanism of RA is still unknown, its pathology is fairly well understood. Some factor activates the synovial fibroblasts (SFs) that line the joint cavity.[162-164] The SFs undergo significant changes and develop an exaggerated immune response. Once activated, both types of SF abnormally proliferate and produce proinflammatory cytokines, enzymes, and prostaglandins that perpetuate the inflammatory process,[165] including increasing their lining depth from the normal 1 to 2 cells deep up to 10 to 20 cells thick. This thickened synovial tissue, called "pannus," invades the bone and acts like a localized tumor, where other factors (including increased osteoclast activity) cause bone destruction.[166] Some of the most significant synovial changes involve altered signaling pathways for immune reactions, where SFs attach to articular cartilage and attack it, causing more inflammation; the release of enzymes, such as metal metalloproteinases, inflammatory chemokines, and cytokines (interleukins and tumor necrosis factor); and ingrowth of blood vessels. Increased blood vessel formation improves the opportunity for activated SFs to enter the bloodstream and affect other joints.[1,167,168] Eventually, inflammation spreads to the fibrous joint capsule and surrounding ligaments and tendons, causing pain, joint deformity, and loss of function (Figure 39-18). The joints most commonly affected are in the fingers, feet, wrists, elbows, ankles, and knees, but the shoulders, hips, and cervical spine also may be involved, as well as the tissues of the lungs, heart, kidneys, and skin.

The incidence and prevalence of RA have decreased over the past five decades; RA now affects about 1% of the adult population in developed countries.[169] The frequency of RA increases with age. Besides inflammation and destruction of the joints, RA can cause fever, malaise,

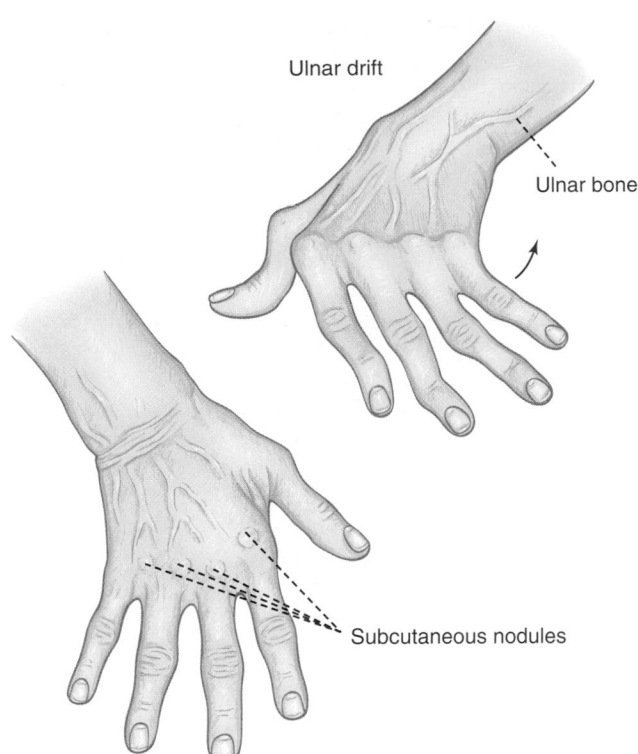

FIGURE 39-18 Rheumatoid Arthritis of the Hand. Note swelling from chronic synovitis of metacarpophalangeal joints, marked ulnar drift, subcutaneous nodules, and subluxation of metacarpophalangeal joints with extension of proximal interphalangeal joints and flexion of distal joints. Note also deformed position of thumb. Hand has wasted appearance. (From Mourad LA: *Orthopedic disorders,* St Louis, 1991, Mosby.)

FIGURE 39-19 Synovitis. Inflamed synovium showing typical arrangements of macrophages and fibroblastic cells.

rash, lymph node or spleen enlargement, and Raynaud phenomenon (transient lack of circulation to the fingertips and toes).

Despite intensive research, the exact cause of RA remains obscure. It is likely a combination of genetic factors interacting with inflammatory mediators. There is a strong genetic predisposition to developing RA. The chronic inflammation characteristics of RA result from an intricate interplay of chemokines that are powerful mediators of inflammation. Ligand/receptor chemokines attract T cells and produce inflammatory changes.[1] A key genetic element has been localized to the human leukocyte antigen (HLA) areas of the major histocompatibility complex in all ethnic groups. Recent research reveals the possibility of specific amino acid malpositions in the (HLA) molecule as a major factor in developing rheumatic diseases.[170] A surprising new discovery is the presence of T-cell abnormalities in individuals with RA, indicating a defect in telomere repair that may result in faster aging of telomeres and consequent less efficient immune function. With long-term or intensive exposure to the antigen, normal antibodies (immunoglobulins [Igs]) become autoantibodies—antibodies that attack host tissues (self-antigens). Because they are usually present in individuals with RA, the altered antibodies are termed **rheumatoid factors (RFs)**. The RFs usually consist of two classes of immunoglobulin antibodies (antibodies for IgM and IgG) but occasionally involve antibodies for IgA. Their main antigenic targets are portions of the immunoglobulin molecules. RFs bind with their target self-antigens in blood and synovial membrane, forming immune complexes (antigen-antibody complexes). (See Chapter 7 for a discussion about antigen-antibody binding in the immune response.)

Environmental factors, including geographic area of birth, diet, socioeconomic status, and especially smoking, have been identified as risk factors for developing and having higher disease activity of RA.[171,172] RA and other autoimmune diseases have a higher prevalence among women. Additionally, because disease symptoms lessen during pregnancy and are increased again in the postpartal period, researchers are including hormonal involvement in their studies.

PATHOPHYSIOLOGY Although no specific events (such as trauma, illness, or environmental conditions) have been identified that would cause immune abnormalities to develop into localized tissue and joint inflammation, the pathology of RA is fairly well understood. During inflammation, arginine (an α-amino acid) can be enzymatically modified into another α-amino acid, citrulline. This process (citrullination) changes the structure and function of the protein. Other proteins, like fibrin and vimentin, become citrullinated during cell death and tissue inflammation.[173] In turn, the citrullinated proteins can be seen as antigens by the body's immune system.[174] Thus both T and B cells play a role in the autoimmune response. T cells express receptor activator of nuclear factor κB ligand (RANKL), which promotes osteoclast formation and causes bony erosion.

Basically, cartilage damage in RA is the result of at least three processes: (1) neutrophils and other cells in the synovial fluid become activated, degrading the surface layer of articular cartilage; (2) inflammatory cytokines, particularly tumor necrosis factor-alpha (TNF-α), interleukin-1beta (IL-1β), interleukin-6 (IL-6), interleukin-7 (IL-7), and interleukin-21 (IL-21), induce enzymatic (metalloproteinase) breakdown of cartilage and bone; and (3) T cells also interact with synovial fibroblasts through TNF-α, converting synovium into a thick, abnormal layer of granulation tissue known as **pannus** (see Chapter 7). Macrophages, components of pannus (Figure 39-19), stimulate the release of IL-1, platelet-derived growth factor (PDGF), and fibronectin. The B lymphocytes are stimulated to produce more RFs. The newly

FIGURE 39-20 Emerging Model of Pathogenesis of Rheumatoid Arthritis. Rheumatoid arthritis is an autoimmune disease of a genetically susceptible host triggered by an unknown antigenic agent. Chronic autoimmune reaction with activation of CD4+ helper T cells and possibly other lymphocytes and the local release of inflammatory cytokines and mediators eventually destroy the joint. T cells stimulate cells in the joint to produce cytokines that are key mediators of synovial damage. Apparently, immune complex deposition also plays a role. Tumor necrosis factor (TNF) and interleukin-1 (IL-1), as well as some other cytokines, stimulate synovial cells to proliferate and produce other mediators of inflammation, such as prostaglandin E_2 *(PGE₂)*, matrix metalloproteinases, and enzymes that all contribute to destruction of cartilage. Activated T cells and synovial fibroblasts also produce receptor activator of nuclear factor κB ligand *(RANKL)*, which activates the osteoclasts and promotes bone destruction. Pannus is a mass of synovium and synovial stroma with inflammatory cells, granulation tissue, and fibroblasts that grows over the articular surface and causes its destruction.

targeted self-antigens (immunoglobulins) are in relatively constant supply and can thus perpetuate inflammation and the formation of immune complexes indefinitely (Figure 39-20).

Inflammatory and immune processes have several damaging effects on the synovial membrane. Along with the swelling caused by leukocyte infiltration, the synovial membrane undergoes hyperplastic thickening as its cells proliferate and abnormally enlarge. As synovial inflammation progresses to involve its blood vessels, small venules become occluded by hypertrophied endothelial cells, fibrin, platelets, and inflammatory cells, which decrease vascular flow to the synovial tissue. Compromised circulation, coupled with increased metabolic needs as a result of hypertrophy and hyperplasia, causes hypoxia and metabolic acidosis. Acidosis stimulates the release of hydrolytic enzymes from synovial cells into the surrounding tissue, initiating erosion of the articular cartilage and inflammation in the supporting

ligaments and tendons. Pannus formation does not lead to synovial or articular regeneration but rather to formation of scar tissue that immobilizes the joint.

CLINICAL MANIFESTATIONS The onset of RA is usually insidious, although as many as 15% of cases have an acute onset. RA begins with general systemic manifestations of inflammation, including fever, fatigue, weakness, anorexia, weight loss, and generalized aching and stiffness. Local manifestations also appear gradually over a period of weeks or months. Typically, the joints become painful, tender, and stiff. Pain early in the disease is caused by pressure from swelling. Later in the disease, pain is caused by sclerosis of subchondral bone and new bone formation. Pain and inability to perform normal functions are the main reasons people seek medical help.[175] Stiffness usually lasts for about 1 hour after rising in the morning and is thought to be related to synovitis. Initially the joints most commonly involved are the metacarpophalangeal (MCP) joints, proximal interphalangeal (PIP) joints, and wrists, with later involvement of larger weightbearing joints.

Widespread, symmetric joint swelling is caused by increasing amounts of inflammatory exudate (leukocytes, plasma, plasma proteins) in the synovial membrane, hyperplasia of inflamed tissues, and formation of new bone. On palpation, the swollen joint feels warm and the synovial membrane feels boggy. The skin over the joint may have a ruddy, cyanotic hue and may look thin and shiny.

An inflamed joint may lose some of its mobility. Even mild synovitis can lead to reduced range of motion, which becomes evident after inflammation subsides. Extension becomes limited and is eventually lost if flexion contractures develop. Limited range of motion can progress to permanent deformities of the fingers, toes, and limbs, including ulnar deviation of the hands, boutonnière and swan neck deformities of the finger joints, plantar subluxation of the metatarsal heads of the foot, and hallux valgus (angulation of the great toe toward the other toes). Flexion contractures of the knees and hips are also common.

Joint deformities cause the physical limitations experienced by persons with RA (see Figure 39-18). Loss of joint motion is quickly followed by secondary atrophy of the surrounding muscles. With secondary muscle atrophy, the joint becomes unstable, which further aggravates joint pathology.

Two complications of chronic RA are caused by excessive amounts of inflammatory exudate in the synovial cavity. One complication is the formation of cysts in the articular cartilage or subchondral bone. Occasionally, these cysts communicate with the skin surface (such as in the sole of the foot) and can drain through passages called *fistulae*. The second complication is rupture of a cyst or of the synovial joint itself, usually caused by strenuous physical activity that places excessive pressure on the joint. Rupture releases inflammatory exudate into adjacent tissues, thereby spreading inflammation.

Extrasynovial rheumatoid nodules, seen in up to 30% of individuals with RA, are the most common extra-articular manifestations. Each nodule is a collection of inflammatory cells surrounding a central core of fibrinoid and cellular debris. T lymphocytes are the predominant leukocytes in the nodule. B lymphocytes, plasma cells, and phagocytes are found around the periphery. Nodules are most often found in subcutaneous tissue over the extensor surfaces of elbows and fingers. Less common sites are the scalp, back, feet, hands, buttocks, and knees.

Rheumatoid nodules also may invade the skin, cardiac valves, pericardium, pleura, lung parenchyma, and spleen. These nodules are identical to those encountered in some individuals with rheumatic fever and are characterized by central tissue necrosis surrounded by proliferating connective tissue. Also noted are large numbers of lymphocytes and occasional plasma cells. Acute glaucoma may result with nodules forming on the sclera. Pulmonary involvement may result in diffuse pleuritis or multiple intraparenchymal nodules. Together, the occurrence of pulmonary nodules and pneumoconiosis (chronic inflammation of the lungs from inhalation of dust) creates the syndrome called Caplan syndrome. Diffuse pulmonary fibrosis may occur because of immunologically mediated immune complex deposition.

Rheumatoid nodules within the heart may cause valvular deformities, particularly of the aortic valve leaflets, and pericarditis. Lymphadenopathy of the nodes close to the affected joints may develop. Rheumatoid nodules within the spleen result in splenomegaly. Involvement of blood vessels results in an acute necrotizing vasculitis, characteristic of that noted in other immunologic/inflammatory states. Thromboses of such involved vessels may lead to myocardial infarctions, cerebrovascular occlusions, mesenteric infarction, kidney damage, and vascular insufficiency in the hands and fingers (Raynaud

phenomenon). Fortunately, the development of vascular changes (particularly systemic vasculitis) is decreasing in frequency as more effective RA treatments are becoming available.[176] Changes in skeletal muscle are often noted in the form of nonspecific atrophy secondary to joint dysfunction.

EVALUATION AND TREATMENT   The diagnosis of RA relies on clinical evaluation of joint swelling; however, limitation of movement and control of pain often prevent identification of individuals who would benefit from treatment in early stages of the disease. Early treatment can be effective in preventing the systemic and joint abnormalities of chronic disease. Research has shown that the autoantibodies rheumatoid factor (RF) and anti-citrullinated protein antibody (ACPA) can be present for years to decades before synovial or radiographic involvement becomes apparent.[177,178] Compared with RF, ACPA is a much more specific serum marker for RA. The American College of Rheumatology (ACR) and the European League Against Rheumatism (EULAR) revised their RA classification criteria in 2010 in order to better identify the early stage of RA.[161] These new criteria are shown in Table 39-5. Clinical examination and history are the mainstays of RA diagnosis, but new imaging techniques show promise for earlier diagnosis, leading to earlier treatment with a better chance for avoiding disability and joint destruction (see *Health Alert:* Musculoskeletal Molecular Imaging).

HEALTH ALERT
Musculoskeletal Molecular Imaging

With improved understanding of the molecular and cellular mechanisms responsible for the effects of rheumatoid arthritis (RA), new imaging techniques promise benefits in earlier and more accurate diagnosis and monitoring of cartilage and bone involvement. Imaging on that same molecular level can provide a "biological read-out" of disease progression and response to treatment. Nuclear medicine imaging, positron emission tomography (PET), and magnetic resonance imaging (MRI) all incorporate some element of molecular imaging.

New modalities of molecular imaging use various probes and contrast agents that have an affinity for specific targets, such as cells, hormones, antigens, and enzymes. Certain monoclonal antibodies have already been successfully labeled with various nuclides and could be used to identify disease progression. Bioluminescent and fluorescent imaging techniques have the advantage of being radiation-free tests and are being used to view in vivo activity, osteoblast activity, osteocalcin expression in bone damage, and osteoclast activity and gene expression during inflammation. A significant area of promise for molecular imaging in RA is recognition of the initial molecular events that occur before cartilage and joint damage becomes apparent. Better monitoring of response to medications also may allow more accurate dosing with the potential for fewer side effects. Because certain bioluminescent and fluorescent agents have specific affinities for particular cells, more efficient bone regeneration may be possible by targeted delivery of appropriate growth factors or stem cells to damaged bone and cartilage.

Data from Malviya G et al: *Eur J Med Mol Imaging* 37(2):386-398, 2010; Reumann MK et al: *Trends Biotechnol* 28(2):93-1001, 2010.

Early treatment of RA begins with disease-modifying antirheumatic drugs (DMARDs), such as methotrexate (MTX), azathioprine, sulfasalazine, hydroxychloroquine, leflunomide, and cyclosporine. These agents have been shown to slow the progression of RA and may prevent complications such as joint deformities and extra-articular complications. MTX remains the first line of treatment. More recently, targeted treatment for RA has involved use of agents aimed at

TABLE 39-5   The 2010 American College of Rheumatology/European League Against Rheumatism Classification Criteria for Rheumatoid Arthritis

Target population to be tested:
1. Persons who have at least one joint with definite clinical synovitis (swelling)[a]
2. Persons who have synovitis not better explained by another disease[b]

Classification criteria for RA (score-based algorithm: add scores of categories A to D; a score of ≥6/10 is needed for positive RA diagnosis)[c]

Clinical Finding	Score
A. Joint involvement[d]	
1 large joint[e]	0
2-10 large joints	1
1-3 small joints (with or without involvement of large joints)[f]	2
4-10 small joints (with or without involvement of large joints)	3
>10 joints (at least 1 small joint)[g]	5
B. Serology (at least 1 test result is needed for classification)[h]	
Negative RF *and* negative ACPA	0
Low-positive RF *or* low-positive ACPA	2
High-positive RF *or* high-positive ACPA	3
C. Acute-phase reactants (at least 1 test result is needed for classification)[i]	
Normal CRP *and* normal ESR	0
Abnormal CRP *or* abnormal ESR	1
D. Duration of symptoms[j]	
<6 weeks	0
≥6 weeks	1

Data from Aletaha D et al: *Arthritis Rheum* 62(9):2574, 2010.

[a]The criteria are aimed at classification of newly presenting persons. In addition, persons with erosive disease typical of rheumatoid arthritis (RA) with a history compatible of prior fulfillment of the 2010 criteria should be classified as having RA. Persons with longstanding disease—including those whose disease is inactive (with or without treatment) and who, based on retrospectively available data, have previously fulfilled the 2010 criteria—should be classified as having RA.

[b]Differential diagnoses vary among persons with different presentations, but may include conditions such as systemic lupus erythematosus, psoriatic arthritis, and gout. If it is unclear about the relevant differential diagnoses to consider, an expert rheumatologist should be consulted.

[c]Although persons with a score <6/10 are not classifiable as having RA, their status can be reassessed and the criteria might be fulfilled cumulatively over time.

[d]Joint involvement refers to any *swollen* or *tender* joint on examination, which may be confirmed by imaging evidence of synovitis. Distal interphalangeal joints, first metacarpophalangeal joints, and first metatarsophalangeal joints are *excluded from assessment*. Categories of joint distribution are classified according to the location and number of involved joints, with placement into the highest category possible based on the pattern of joint involvement.

[e]"Large joints" refer to shoulders, elbows, hips, knees, and ankles.

[f]"Small joints" refer to the metacarpophalangeal joints, proximal interphalangeal joints, second through fifth metatarsophalangeal joints, thumb interphalangeal joints, and wrists.

[g]In this category, at least one of the involved joints must be a small joint; the others can include any combination of large and additional small joints, as well as other joints not specifically listed elsewhere (e.g., temporomandibular, acromioclavicular, sternoclavicular).

[h]Negative refers to international unit (IU) values that are less than or equal to the upper limit of normal (ULN) for the laboratory and assay; low-positive refers to values that are higher than the ULN but ≤3 times the ULN for the laboratory and assay; high-positive refers to IU values that are >3 times the ULN for the laboratory and assay. Where rheumatoid factor (RF) information is only available as positive or negative, a positive result should be scored as low-positive for RF. *ACPA,* Anti-citrullinated protein antibody.

[i]Normal/abnormal is determined by local laboratory standards. *CRP,* C-reactive protein; *ESR,* erythrocyte sedimentation rate.

[j]Duration of symptoms refers to individual's self-report of the duration of signs and symptoms of synovitis (e.g., pain, swelling, tenderness) of joints that are clinically involved at the time of assessment, regardless of treatment status.

interrupting the pathogenesis of the disease. Known as biologic DMARDs (bDMARDs), these medications affect specific processes in the development of RA and include tumor necrosis factor inhibitors, such as etanercept, adalimumab, and infliximab. They have recently been augmented by the monoclonal antibodies golimumab and certolizumab. Other agents interfere with cytokine function (anakinra inhibits IL-1 function and tocilizumab targets IL-6), inhibit T-cell activation (abatacept), or deplete B cells (rituximab).

Education for individuals with RA is fundamental to treatment. Other treatments and therapies include nonsteroidal anti-inflammatory drugs (NSAIDs), glucocorticoids, intra-articular steroid injections, physical and occupational therapy with therapeutic exercise, and use of assistive devices. Surgery is used to treat deformities or mechanical deficiencies of joints and can include synovectomy or joint replacement surgery.

Ankylosing Spondylitis

Ankylosing spondylitis (AS) is the most common of a group of inflammatory arthropathies known as *spondyloarthropathies* (SpAs). The Assessment of SpondyloArthritis International Society (ASAS) has recommended classifying spondyloarthropathies to include individuals who do not have visible radiographic changes of the skeleton, as well as those who do. There would then be two subgroups: (1) mainly axial disease, including AS; and (2) peripheral SpA.[179] AS is a chronic, inflammatory joint disease characterized by stiffening and fusion (ankylosis) of the spine and sacroiliac joints. Like RA, ankylosing spondylitis is a systemic, autoimmune inflammatory disease. Although inflammation is the primary pathologic process in both RA and ankylosing spondylitis, the two diseases differ in the primary site of inflammation and the end result. In RA, the primary site of inflammation is the synovial membrane, resulting in the destruction and instability of synovial joints. In ankylosing spondylitis, excessive bone formation occurs. The primary pathologic site is the enthesis (the point at which ligaments, tendons, and the joint capsule are inserted into bone), and the end result is fibrosis, ossification, and fusion of the joint, primarily the sacroiliac joints and the vertebral column (axial skeleton).

AS occurs worldwide, with the lowest prevalence in South Asian countries and highest in North America and Europe; it affects men more often than women.[180] In women, AS may affect the peripheral joints of the appendicular skeleton rather than the axial skeleton, progress less rapidly, and cause less dramatic spinal changes. Primary AS usually develops in late adolescence and young adulthood, with peak incidence at about 20 years of age. Secondary AS affects older age groups and is often associated with other inflammatory diseases (e.g., psoriatic arthropathy, inflammatory bowel disease, Reiter syndrome).

The exact cause of AS is unknown, but its high association with histocompatibility antigen human leukocyte antigen (HLA-B27) has been known for decades. Misfolding of HLA-B27 in the endoplasmic reticulum (ER) may play a key role in developing AS. As misfolded proteins accumulate, they may cause an unfolded protein response (UPR) that disrupts normal cellular functions and causes a stress response of the ER (also see Chapter 4). That stress response increases production of interleukins-17 and -23 (IL-17, IL-23), potent cytokines that also may act on T-helper 17 (Th17) cells, promoting their survival.[181,182] Th17 cells are important mediators in human immune diseases. Additional studies have revealed that HLA-B27, itself, has many forms; to date more than 100 subtypes have been identified.[183] Certain variations in the endoplasmic reticulum aminopeptidase 1 (ERAP1) protein appear to increase the likelihood of developing AS in people who are HLA-B27 positive.

PATHOPHYSIOLOGY Ankylosing spondylitis begins with inflammation of fibrocartilage in cartilaginous joints. In men, the sacroiliac joint is often affected first, usually before any damage can be radiographically detected.[181] Knee pain may be the initial symptom in women.[184] Inflammatory cells infiltrate the fibrous tissue of the joint capsule, the cartilage that surrounds intervertebral disks, the entheses, and the periosteum. As inflammatory cells (chiefly macrophages) and lymphocytes infiltrate and erode bone and fibrocartilage in joint structures, repair begins. Repair of cartilaginous structures begins with the proliferation of fibroblasts. Fibroblasts synthesize and secrete collagen. The collagen becomes organized into fibrous scar tissue that eventually undergoes calcification and ossification. With time, all the cartilaginous structures of the joint are replaced by ossified scar tissue, causing the joint to fuse, or lose flexibility.

Repair of eroded bone begins with osteoblast activation and proliferation. Osteoblasts lay down new bone (callus), which is remodeled and replaced by compact, lamellar bone. Bone repair changes the contour of the bone's surface because the new bone grows outward (outside the normal border of unaffected bone) to form a new enthesis with the end of the eroded ligament. The new enthesis, which forms on top of the old one, is called a syndesmophyte. As calcification of the spinal ligaments progresses, the vertebral bodies lose their concave

Ossification of disks, joints, and ligaments of spinal column

FIGURE 39-21 Ankylosing Spondylitis. Characteristic posture and primary pathologic sites of inflammation and resulting damage. (Redrawn from Mourad LA: *Orthopedic disorders,* St Louis, 1991, Mosby.)

anterior contour and appear square. The spine assumes the classic bamboo spine appearance of ankylosing spondylitis.

CLINICAL MANIFESTATIONS The most common signs and symptoms of early AS are low back pain and stiffness. Typically, the individual with primary disease develops low back pain during the early twenties. The pain is at first insidious but progressively becomes persistent. It is often worse after prolonged rest and is alleviated by physical activity. Early morning stiffness usually accompanies the low back pain, and the individual typically has difficulty sitting up or twisting the spine. Forward flexion, rotation, and lateral flexion of the spine are restricted and painful. Early pain and resultant loss of motion are caused by the underlying inflammation and reflex muscle spasm rather than by soft tissue or bony fusion.

As the disease progresses, the normal convex curve of the lower spine (lumbar lordosis) diminishes and concavity of the upper spine (kyphosis) increases. The individual becomes increasingly stooped. The thoracic spine becomes rounded, the head and neck are held forward on the shoulders, and the hips are flexed (Figure 39-21).

Inflammation in the tendon insertions of the many costosternal and costovertebral muscles can cause pleuritic chest pain and restricted chest movement. The pain is usually worse on inspiration. Movement of the diaphragm is normal and full. Pressure on the anterior chest wall over the sternum, ribs, and costal cartilages may cause tenderness. Tenderness over the pelvic brim may cause discomfort at night and interfere with sleep because turning onto the iliac crests causes pain. Tenderness over the ischial tuberosities may make sitting on hard seats unbearable. Tenderness in the heels may contribute to a limp or cautious placement of the feet during walking.

Along with low back pain and sacroiliac pain, inflammation of the bowels, anterior uveitis, aortic regurgitation, fibrosis of the upper lobes of the lung, Achilles tendonitis, and immune-related (IgA) kidney disease frequently accompany AS.[185] Elevated sedimentation rate (ESR) and elevated level of C-reactive protein (CRP) also are common.

EVALUATION AND TREATMENT Diagnosis of AS is based on specific criteria. One of the previous problems with diagnosing AS has been a requirement for radiographic (x-ray) evidence of sacroiliitis; MRI can discover sacroiliitis an average of 7.7 years before there is evidence on x-rays.[186] Both MRI and plain radiographic findings are important in detecting early disease and for evaluating individuals younger than 45 years of age with back pain of at least 3 months' duration.[187]

In addition to sacroiliitis being present on imaging, one or more of the following features allow a diagnosis of spondyloarthritis (SpA): inflammatory back pain, arthritis, anterior uveitis, heel pain, dactylitis, psoriasis, Crohn disease or ulcerative colitis, good response to NSAIDs, family history of SpA, positive HLA-B27, or elevated CRP. If the individual has a positive HLA-B27, at least two of the previously mentioned items must be present along with sacroiliitis on MRI or radiographic imaging in order to make a diagnosis.[188]

Treatment of individuals with AS consists of education about the disease, as well as physical therapy to maintain skeletal mobility and prevent the natural progression of contractures. Prevention of deformity and maintenance of mobility require a continuous program of physical therapy. Supervised group exercises have been shown to reduce pain and to maintain and improve chest expansion and respiratory function, spine mobility, and complete range of motion in the proximal joints.[189]

Nonsteroidal anti-inflammatory drugs (NSAIDs) will often provide temporary symptom relief within 48 hours. Analgesic medications are prescribed to suppress some of the pain and stiffness and to facilitate exercise. The medications do not prevent disease progression, but they do provide relief from symptoms. Biologic response modifying agents, such as tumor necrosis factor inhibitors (certolizumab, golimumab) or B-cell depleting agents (rituximab), are increasingly being used to treat AS. Newer agents that target cytokines of Th17 and small nano particles that alter certain inflammatory pathways are showing promise in treating AS.[190,191] Surgical procedures, such as osteotomy, total hip replacement, and cervical spinal fusion, and radiation therapy are sometimes used to provide relief for individuals with end-stage disease or intolerable deformity. Individuals should stop smoking to lessen pulmonary problems.

Gout

The prevalence of gout has steadily increased over the past several decades and is now considered the most common inflammatory arthritis worldwide.[192,193] **Gout** is a syndrome caused by either overproduction or underexcretion of uric acid and is characterized by inflammation and pain of the joints. Incomplete purine metabolism results in excess serum uric acid levels (hyperuricemia). Either excessive uric acid production or underexcretion of uric acid by the kidneys will cause hyperuricemia. Underexcretion of uric acid is responsible for about 90% of the cases of elevated uric acid level and appears to have a strong genetic basis.[194,195]

When uric acid reaches a certain concentration in fluids, it crystallizes, forming insoluble precipitates that are deposited in connective tissues throughout the body. Crystallization in synovial fluid triggers the TNF-α inflammatory pathway, causing the release of various chemokines and interleukins, resulting in painful inflammation of the joint, a condition known as **gouty arthritis**. Urate crystal deposits cause oxidative stress reactions in other tissues as well. With time, crystal deposition in subcutaneous tissues causes the formation of small, white nodules, or **tophi**, that are visible through the skin. Tophi are associated with joint damage and an increased death rate, primarily because of cardiovascular events.[196] Hyperuricemia is associated with hypertension, heart disease, type 2 diabetes, kidney disease, and metabolic syndrome.[197]

TABLE 39-6 **Mean Urate Concentrations by Age and Gender**	
Characteristic	Mean Urate Levels (mg/dl)
Prepuberty	3.5
Males (at puberty)	Steep rise to 5.2
Females (puberty to after premenopause)	Slow rise to ≈4.0
Females (after menopause)	4.7
Hyperuricemia	
Males	7.0
Females	6.0

In classic gouty arthritis, monosodium urate crystals form and are deposited in joints and their surrounding tissues, initiating a powerful inflammatory response.[198] Pseudogout is caused by the formation of calcium pyrophosphate-dihydrate crystals. The effect of either crystal is the same—the onset of an acute inflammatory response (see Chapter 6).

Gout is rare in children and premenopausal women and is uncommon in males younger than 30 years. Male gender, increasing age, and high intake of alcohol, red meat, and fructose are all risk factors for gout.[193] The peak age of onset in males is between 40 and 50 years. The risk of developing gouty arthritis is similar in males and females for a particular urate concentration. Females tend to have onset at a later age and have greater use of diuretics, more coexisting diseases (hypertension, renal insufficiency), more frequent involvement of other joints, and fewer recurrent episodes.[199] Plasma urate concentration is the single most important determinant of the risk of developing gout (Table 39-6).

Uric acid is a weak acid that is ionized at normal body pH and thus occurs in the blood or tissues in the form of urate ion. When ionized, uric acid can form salts with various cations, but 98% of extracellular uric acid is in the form of monosodium urate (uric acid salt). At any time the proportion of uric acid or urate is pH dependent, so the ratio of these two forms varies considerably in urine.

The solubility of urate and uric acid is critical to the development of crystals. Urate is more soluble in plasma, synovial fluid, and urine than in aqueous solutions. The solubility of uric acid in urine rises dramatically as the pH increases. There is little change, however, in the solubility of urate within the normal pH range that exists in the plasma, synovial fluid, and other tissues. The pH can be 5.0 in the collecting tubules of the kidney, thus favoring formation of uric acid. Decreasing temperatures cause both urate and uric acid solubility to fall. The pathways of production of uric acid are shown in Figure 39-22.

PATHOPHYSIOLOGY The pathophysiology of gout is closely linked to purine metabolism (or cellular metabolism of purines) and kidney function. Most mammals, except humans, have the enzyme uricase, which catalyzes the conversion of uric acid to allantoin, thus preventing overproduction of uric acid. Environmental and genetic factors also play a role in an individual's urate concentration. At the cellular level, purines are synthesized to purine nucleotides, which are used in the synthesis of nucleic acids, adenosine triphosphate (ATP), cyclic adenosine monophosphate (cAMP), and cyclic guanosine monophosphate (cGMP). Uric acid is a breakdown product of purine nucleotides (urate synthesis and elimination are illustrated in Figure 39-23).

Most uric acid is eliminated from the body through the kidneys. Urate is filtered at the glomerulus and undergoes both reabsorption and excretion within the renal tubules. In primary gout, urate excretion

Synthesis **Metabolism** **Elimination**

FIGURE 39-22 Uric Acid Synthesis and Elimination. Uric acid is derived from purines ingested or synthesized from ingested foods, as well as being recycled after cell breakdown. Uric acid is then eliminated through the kidneys and gastrointestinal tract. (Redrawn from Klippel JH, Dieppe PA, editors: *Rheumatology,* ed 2, St Louis, 1998, Mosby.)

by the kidneys is sluggish. The sluggish excretion may be the result of a decrease in glomerular filtration of urate or acceleration in urate reabsorption. In addition, monosodium urate (MSU) crystals are deposited in renal interstitial tissues, causing impaired urine flow. (Kidney function is described in Chapter 29.)

The exact process by which crystals of monosodium urate are deposited in joints and induce gouty arthritis is unknown, but several mechanisms may be involved, including the following:

1. Monosodium urate precipitates at the periphery of the body, where lower body temperatures may reduce the solubility of monosodium urate.
2. Albumin or glycosaminoglycan levels decrease, which causes decreased urate solubility.
3. Changes in ion concentration and decreases of pH enhance urate deposition.
4. Trauma promotes urate crystal precipitation.

The monosodium urate crystals may form in the synovial fluid or in the synovial membrane, cartilage, or other connective tissues in joints and elsewhere, such as in the heart, earlobes, and kidneys. Evidence suggests that an acute attack of gout is the result of the *formation* of crystals rather than the release of crystals from connective tissues into the synovial fluid.

Monosodium urate crystals can stimulate and perpetuate the inflammatory response (see Figure 39-23, *A, B*). The presence of the crystals triggers the acute inflammatory response, releasing proinflammatory cytokines and tumor necrosis factors, during which neutrophils are attracted out of the circulation and begin to phagocytose (ingest) the crystals.

Importantly, deposits of MSU in joints and other tissues can be present years before an acute gout attack occurs. Early identification and intervention in treating gout can reduce morbidity and mortality associated with the disease. Traditionally, plain radiographs (x-rays) have been used to assess joints affected by gout, but only damaged joints can be seen. Newer technologies, including high-resolution ultrasound, dual-energy computed tomography (DECT), and MRI, can assess the presence of MSU crystals before joint, tendon, or ligament damage occurs.[200] Imaging modalities also can be used when

joints cannot be aspirated to look for MSU crystals microscopically. Earlier identification allows timely as well as ongoing evaluation of treatment.[201]

CLINICAL MANIFESTATIONS Gout is manifested by (1) an increase in serum urate concentration (hyperuricemia); (2) recurrent attacks of monoarticular arthritis (inflammation of a single joint); (3) deposits of monosodium urate monohydrate (tophi) in and around the joints; (4) renal disease involving glomerular, tubular, and interstitial tissues and blood vessels; and (5) the formation of renal stones. These manifestations appear in three clinical stages:

1. **Asymptomatic hyperuricemia.** The serum urate level is elevated but arthritic symptoms, tophi, and renal stones are not present; this stage may persist throughout life.
2. **Acute gouty arthritis.** Attacks develop with increased serum urate concentrations; tends to occur with sudden or sustained increases of hyperuricemia but also can be triggered by trauma, drugs, and alcohol.
3. **Tophaceous gout.** The third and chronic stage of the disease; can begin as early as 3 years or as late as 40 years after the initial attack of gouty arthritis. Progressive inability to excrete uric acid expands the urate pool until monosodium urate crystal deposits (tophi) appear in cartilage, synovial membranes, tendons, and soft tissue.

Trauma is the most common aggravating factor of an acute gouty exacerbation. Attacks of gouty arthritis occur abruptly, usually in a peripheral joint (see Figure 39-23, *C*). The primary symptom is severe pain. Approximately 50% of the initial attacks occur in the metatarsophalangeal joint of the great toe (a condition known as podagra). The other 50% can occur in almost any joint, but most often involve the heel, ankle, instep of the foot, knee, wrist, or elbow. The pain is usually noted at night. Within a few hours the affected joint becomes hot, red, and extremely tender and may be slightly swollen. Lymphangitis and systemic signs of inflammation (leukocytosis, fever, elevated sedimentation rate) are occasionally present. Untreated, mild attacks usually subside in several hours but may persist for 1 or 2 days. Severe attacks may persist for several days or weeks. When the individual recovers, the symptoms resolve completely.

Tophaceous deposits produce irregular swellings of the fingers, hands, knees, and feet. The helix of the ear is the most common site of tophi, which are the characteristic diagnostic lesions of chronic gout. Tophi also may develop along the ulnar surface of the forearm, the tibial surface of the leg, the Achilles tendon, olecranon bursa, or other areas. Tophi may produce marked limitation of joint movement and can eventually cause grotesque deformities of the hands and feet (see Figure 39-23, *C*). Although the tophi themselves are painless, they often cause progressive stiffness and persistent aching of the affected joint. Tophi in the extremities can cause nerve compression—carpal tunnel syndrome in the wrists, tarsal tunnel syndrome in the ankles. Tophi also may erode and drain through the skin.

Renal stones are 1000 times more prevalent in individuals with primary gout than in the general population. The stones can be the size of a grain of sand or a piece of gravel, or they can accumulate in massive deposits called *staghorn calculi.* They range in color from pale yellow to brown to reddish black, depending on their composition. Some stones consist of pure monosodium urate; others consist of calcium oxalate or calcium phosphate. Renal stones can form in the collecting tubules, pelvis, or ureters, causing obstruction, dilation, and atrophy of the more proximal tubules and leading eventually to acute renal failure. Stones deposited directly in renal interstitial tissue initiate an inflammatory reaction that leads to chronic renal disease and progressive renal failure.

FIGURE 39-23 Pathogenesis of Acute Gouty Arthritis. A, Depending on the urate crystal coating, a variety of cells may be stimulated to produce a wide range of inflammatory mediators. *Apo-E,* Apolipoprotein E; *IgG,* immunoglobulin G; *IL,* interleukin; LTB_4, leukotriene B_4; PGE_2, prostaglandin E_2. **B,** Sequence of events in the production of the inflammatory response to urate crystals. **C,** Gouty tophus on right foot. **D,** Bone destruction of first metatarsal because of gout. (**C** from Dieppe PA et al: *Arthritis and rheumatism in practice,* London, 1991, Gower; **D** from Chhana A, Dalbeth N: *Rheum Dis Clin North Am* 40[2]:291-309, 2014.)

EVALUATION AND TREATMENT   Evaluation of gout may include history and physical examination, blood tests, joint fluid test, ultrasound, and other imaging. The goals of treatment are to terminate the acute gouty attack as promptly as possible, decrease serum uric acid levels (to dissolve monosodium urate crystals), prevent acute attacks of gout by removing tophi, and, finally, cure gout.[202] Acute gouty arthritis should be treated with anti-inflammatory drugs within 24 hours after the attack. The drugs of choice are nonsteroidal anti-inflammatory drugs (NSAIDs), corticosteroids, and colchicine.[203] Newer medications include interleukin inhibitors.[204] In persons unable to tolerate NSAIDs, colchicine is useful but can be poorly tolerated because of a number of side effects. Once infection has been ruled out, steroids may be injected into the joint to relieve pain. Local application of ice reduces pain during an acute attack.[205] Weightbearing on the involved joint is avoided until the acute attack subsides. A diet that includes mostly vegetables and fruit with little meat, avoidance of alcohol, and weight loss can help lower serum uric acid concentration.[206] Current recommendations are to decrease serum urate levels to less than 6 mg/dl (or less than 5 mg/dl if the individual has marked monosodium urate crystal deposits on clinical examination or imaging studies).[200] High fluid intake, particularly water, can increase urinary output. Long-term use of anti-hyperuricemic drugs, including newer agents such as pegloticase, helps reduce serum urate concentrations. Allopurinol and febuxostat are both used to lower serum urate levels by inhibiting the activity of xanthine oxidase.

> ✔ QUICK CHECK 39-3
> 1. How does noninflammatory joint disease differ from inflammatory joint disease? Describe two principal features of each.
> 2. How does rheumatoid arthritis affect the skin, heart, lungs, and kidneys?
> 3. How do monosodium urate crystals cause gout to develop?

DISORDERS OF SKELETAL MUSCLE

Muscle diseases (myopathies) encompass many entities. Muscle weakness and muscle fatigue are common symptoms. In many cases, neural, traumatic, and psychogenic causes provide an adequate explanation for the failure to generate force (weakness) or sustain force (fatigue) seen in myopathies. The pathophysiologic mechanisms in some of the metabolic and inflammatory muscle diseases have been explored, but the cause of many of the myopathies remains obscure. The complex interaction between muscles and nerves affects muscular function as well. Only inherited and acquired disorders of skeletal muscles are discussed here.

Secondary Muscular Dysfunction

Muscular symptoms arise from a variety of causes unrelated to the muscle itself. Secondary muscular phenomena (contracture, stress-related muscle tension, immobility) are common disorders that influence muscular function.

Contractures

Contractures are described as the loss of full passive range of motion secondary to joint, muscle, or other soft tissue limitations[207] and can be pathologic or physiologic. A physiologic muscle contracture occurs in the absence of a muscle action potential in the sarcolemma. Muscle shortening is explained on the basis of failure of the calcium pump in the presence of plentiful adenosine triphosphate (ATP). A physiologic contracture is seen in McArdle disease (muscle myophosphorylase deficiency) and malignant hyperthermia. The contracture is usually temporary if the underlying pathology is reversed.

A pathologic contracture is a permanent muscle shortening caused by muscle spasm or weakness. Heel cord (Achilles tendon) contractures are examples of pathologic contractures. They are associated with plentiful ATP and occur in spite of a normal action potential. The most common contractures are seen in stroke, neuromuscular diseases (such as muscular dystrophy), Charcot-Marie-Tooth disease, amyotrophic lateral sclerosis, and central nervous system (CNS) injury. Lower extremity contractures are more common than those in the upper extremity. Prolonged splinting in a single position or an imbalance

between agonist-antagonist muscles also can cause joint stiffness and contractures. Contractures also may develop secondary to scar tissue contraction in the flexor tissues of a joint, as in scarring of burned tissues in the antecubital area of the forearm, leading to a flexion contracture.

Stress-Induced Muscle Tension

Abnormally increased muscle tension has been associated with chronic anxiety as well as a variety of stress-related muscular symptoms including neck stiffness, back pain, and headache.[208] Abnormalities in the CNS, reticular activating system, and autonomic nervous system (ANS) have been implicated. For example, as an individual progressively relaxes, the amplitude of the knee jerk reflex diminishes. Conversely, individuals with absent reflexes increase tension by such maneuvers as clenching the teeth or strengthening the handgrip. The underlying pathophysiology may be related to the fact that as a muscle contracts, the muscle spindle is activated. This gamma-feedback system produces a series of impulses that are transmitted to the brain by the sensitive 1A afferent fibers. Unconscious tension is thought to increase the activity of the reticular activating system as well, which stimulates firing of the efferent loop of the gamma fibers, produces further muscle contraction, and increases muscle tension. ANS function that regulates increased blood flow to the muscle during sympathetic activity may be related to increased muscle contraction tension.

Various forms of treatment have been used to reduce the muscle tension associated with stress. Progressive relaxation training, yoga, meditation, and biofeedback are examples of stress reduction therapies. Biofeedback uses integrated electromyography (EMG) to make recordings from the skin surface. The goal is to teach the individual to control maladaptive tension. It is particularly useful in individuals who have a connection between skeletal muscle tension and pain. Progressive relaxation training emphasizes the individual's ability to perceive the difference between tension and relaxation. This technique involves sequential tensing and a relaxing environment. The individual is taught to practice this routine daily, often with the use of audiotaped instructions. By teaching the individual to recognize excessive contraction of skeletal muscle, one hopes to enhance the person's ability to relax specific muscle groups to relieve tension and thus reduce CNS arousal as well as ANS arousal.

Disuse Atrophy

The term disuse atrophy describes the pathologic reduction in normal size of muscle fibers after prolonged inactivity from bed rest, trauma (casting), or local nerve damage as can be seen with spinal cord trauma or poliomyelitis. Decreased muscle activity reduces muscle mass through both decreased muscle protein synthesis and increased muscle protein breakdown.[209] Reduced protein synthesis is primarily responsible for muscle atrophy. The effects of muscular deconditioning associated with lack of physical activity may be apparent in a matter of days. A normal individual prescribed bed rest loses muscle strength from baseline levels at a rate of 3% per day. Bed rest also is associated with cardiovascular, skeletal, and other organ system changes. Likewise, as people age, their muscles atrophy and become weaker (sarcopenia).

Measures to prevent atrophy include frequent forceful isometric muscle contractions and passive lengthening exercises. Artificial gravity (through the use of a "human centrifuge") has shown benefit in maintaining muscle strength. One of the simplest ways to improve disuse atrophy is to restore a load to the muscle, such as returning to walking, starting active motion to a limb, and adding resistance to movements.[210] If reuse is not restored within 1 year, regeneration of muscle fibers becomes impaired.

Fibromyalgia

Fibromyalgia (FM) is a chronic musculoskeletal syndrome character-ized by diffuse pain, fatigue, increased sensitivity to touch (i.e., tender points), the absence of systemic or localized inflammation, and the presence of fatigue and nonrestorative sleep; anxiety and depression also are frequently present. FM has often been misdiagnosed or com-pletely dismissed by clinicians because there are few objective clinical findings on examination. A common misdiagnosis has been chronic fatigue syndrome. Of affected individuals, 80% to 90% are women, and the peak age is 30 to 50 years. New research supports the possible role of inflammation in FM.[211-213] FM and its symptoms are viewed as the result of central nervous system dysfunction, where pain transmission and interpretation are amplified, a condition called central sensitiza-tion. Although the incidence is unknown, the prevalence is reported to be 2% to 8% and increases with age.[214] Certain autoimmune dis-eases, especially systemic lupus erythematosus (SLE) and irritable bowel syndrome (IBS), are often seen in association with FM and may coexist if not initially present with fibromyalgia.

PATHOPHYSIOLOGY Genetic factors are increasingly being suggested as important in developing FM. Relatives of individuals with FM have an increased risk of developing FM. Studies of genetic factors have implicated alterations in genes affecting serotonin, catecholamines, and dopamine—all of these substances are involved in the stress response and sensory processing.[215-217] In spite of these studies, the role of genetic factors has not yet been fully identified in FM. External stressors, such as infection, psychosocial stress, and physical or emo-tional trauma, have been proposed as mechanisms precipitating FM; however, as yet, there is no definitive scientific evidence supporting these theories.[218]

Functional magnetic resonance imaging (fMRI) and positron emis-sion tomography (PET) scans of the brains of individuals with FM have shown activity in different areas of the brain than normally seen in healthy individuals exposed to painful stimuli.[219] These functional abnormalities within the central nervous system (CNS) are shown in Figure 39-24. Other pathophysiologic evidence includes hypothalamic-pituitary axis alterations that show abnormal response to stress.[220]

CLINICAL MANIFESTATIONS The prominent symptom of fibromy-algia is diffuse, chronic pain. Chronic pain is defined as being present more than 3 months. Traditionally, to be classified as FM, tenderness in 11 of 18 specific points was required along with widespread pain. In 2010 the classification of FM was simplified and expanded to include other important non–pain symptoms.[221] The pain often begins in one location, especially the neck and shoulders, but then becomes more generalized. People describe the pain as *burning* or *gnawing*. Fatigue is profound. The effect on everyday life is considerable. Fatigue is most notable when arising from sleep and in midafternoon. Headaches and memory loss are common complaints. There is a strong association between fibromyalgia, Raynaud phenomenon, and irritable bowel syndrome. Individuals with fibromyalgia are light sleepers and awake frequently, which may explain why individuals feel nonrefreshed upon waking.

Almost 25% of individuals seek psychologic support for depression. Anxiety, particularly with regard to their diagnosis and future, is almost universal.

EVALUATION AND TREATMENT Because the manifestations of chronic, generalized pain and fatigue are present in many musculo-skeletal (e.g., rheumatic) disorders, these disorders should be consid-ered in the differential diagnosis of FM. In an effort to simplify and more accurately diagnose FM, the American College of Rheumatology (ACR) recently expanded the diagnostic criteria to include a wide-spread pain index (WPI) definition as "axial pain, left- and right-sided pain, and upper and lower segment pain"[221] and a symptom severity (SS) score. The SS score includes symptoms such as fatigue, waking unrefreshed, and cognitive difficulty. The WPI and SS scores are then tabulated to identify or exclude the diagnosis of FM in individuals who also meet the following criteria:

1. Symptoms have been present at a similar level for at least 3 months.
2. The individual does not have a disorder that would otherwise explain the pain.[221]

The 2010 FM classification criteria were further updated in 2011 so that FM can be classified solely by patient-report using a questionnaire and scale.[222] Treatment should be highly individualized and can include mind-body interventions (such as biofeedback), movement therapies,

FIGURE 39-24 Theoretic Pathophysiologic Model of Fibromyalgia.

BOX 39-4 Educating and Providing Reassurance for Individuals with Fibromyalgia

Stress that the illness is real, not imagined.

Explain that fibromyalgia is presumably not caused by infection.

Explain that fibromyalgia is not a deforming or deteriorating condition.

Explain that fibromyalgia is neither life-threatening nor markedly debilitating, although it is an irritating presence.

Discuss the role of sleep disturbances and the relationship of neurohormones to pain, fatigue, abnormal sleep, and mood.

Reassure that although the cause is unknown, some information is known about the physiologic changes responsible for the symptoms.

Use muscle "spasms" and, perhaps, "low muscle blood flow" to lay the groundwork for exercise recommendations.

Assist the individual to use aerobic exercise to reduce stress and increase rapid eye movement (REM) sleep.

and relaxation techniques as well as medication.[223] No one regimen of medication has proved successful for FM. Exercise regimens are beneficial in reducing symptoms. Recommended exercises for individuals with FM include aerobic activities (including kickboxing and weight-lifting), stretching, and gentle strengthening programs. Medications also are helpful. The FDA has currently approved three medications specifically to treat FM: pregabalin, duloxetine, and milnacipran. Pregabalin reduces the release of several neurochemicals, decreasing pain. Duloxetine and milnacipran are norepinephrine and serotonin reuptake inhibitor antidepressants that also improve pain and depression. Milnacipran also improves fatigue, cognition, and other FM symptoms. Two of the most important aspects of treatment are physical activity and patient education (Box 39-4).[224-226]

Chronic Fatigue Syndrome

Chronic fatigue syndrome (CFS) is a chronic debilitating disease that is likely best described as neuroimmunoendocrine disease that is characterized by cognitive impairment, severe postexertional fatigue (including physical, emotional, or cognitive activity), unrefreshing sleep, and decreased physical activity that affects daily functioning.[227,228] Other frequent symptoms include sore throat, tender lymph nodes, pain, and psychiatric complaints. CFS has often been a diagnosis of exclusion because it cannot be objectively identified by any laboratory or specific clinical tests.[229] Because of the difficulty finding objective data to diagnose CFS, the disease also has been termed myalgic encephalomyelitis (ME) and has been considered a psychiatric disorder. CFS/ME has remained a controversial diagnosis until recently.

Though there seems to be some psychologic involvement in CFS/ME, there is emerging evidence for a physiologic basis. New research has revealed a number of physiologic abnormalities associated with CFS/ME. Some of these processes include skeletal muscle abnormalities, mitochondrial dysfunction, diminished activity of several types of immune cells, abnormal cytokine regulation, and dysfunction of the hypothalamic-pituitary-adrenal (HPA) axis.[230-233] Because of the continued controversy surrounding CFS/ME and the difficulties diagnosing and treating it, the U.S. Institute of Medicine recommended a new term for the condition in 2015, systemic exertional intolerance disease (SEID).[234] Treatment for SEID remains challenging and must be individualized, because there both physical and psychologic components to the disease. Learning how to adapt to stressors and improving physical activity may assist in improving symptoms.[235,236]

Muscle Membrane Abnormalities

Two defects of the muscle membrane (plasma membrane of the muscle fiber) have been linked to clinical syndromes: the hyperexcitable membrane seen in myotonic disorders and the intermittently unresponsive membrane seen in periodic paralyses. Although these are rare disorders, research into their pathologic processes has led to an improved understanding of cell membrane channelopathies (ion channels are described in Chapter 13).

Myotonia

Myotonias are genetically inherited diseases caused by alterations in skeletal muscle sodium and calcium ion channels that result in delayed relaxation after voluntary muscle contraction, such as handgrip, eye closure, or muscle percussion.[237,238] Definitive diagnosis is made by genetic testing. Needle electromyography (EMG) is useful in determining likelihood of disease; the distinctive "dive bomber" noise, audible on needle EMG, is caused by the prolonged depolarization of the muscle membrane.

Myotonia comprises various disorders: myotonia congenita, paramyotonia congenita, myotonic muscular dystrophy, and some forms of periodic paralysis. With the exception of myotonic muscular dystrophy, most are mild in symptomatology. Treatment includes sodium channel blocking agents, such as mexiletine, but no pharmacologic agents have yet received FDA approval for treating myotonia.[239,240] Other treatment modalities include genetic counseling as well as lifestyle and dietary modifications.[241]

Periodic Paralysis

Periodic paralysis encompasses a rare group of muscle diseases characterized by episodes of flaccid weakness. Most are hereditary (autosomal dominant) and caused by calcium or sodium channel abnormalities (pore gating anomalies) because of specific genetic mutations. In normal skeletal muscle, the cellular inflow and outflow of potassium are balanced to maintain the cell's resting potential. Sodium channels, in response to nerve stimulation, create the action potentials that initiate muscle contraction. Calcium channels interact with ryanodine receptors to initiate fast muscle contraction.[242] In susceptible individuals, some instigating factor (such as hyperthyroidism, strenuous exercise, or intake of a high carbohydrate meal) allows increased muscle uptake of potassium from the plasma. This results in slightly decreased plasma potassium levels but it triggers depolarization of the sarcolemma and allows more potassium to enter the cell, causing hypokalemia.[243] Hypokalemic periodic paralysis also can be triggered by exposure to cold or by rest after strenuous exercise. During an attack of hypokalemic periodic paralysis, the resting muscle membrane potential both is unresponsive to neural stimuli and is reduced from −90 to −45 mV. This condition can last hours to days.

Thyrotoxic hypokalemic periodic paralysis (TPP) is caused by a potassium channelopathy that causes increased flow of potassium into the cell; it does not indicate a potassium deficiency.[244,245] Most common in Asian males, TPP is increasingly being seen in all ethnic groups.[245] The main consequence of increased concentration of intracellular potassium is depolarization of the muscle and resulting weakness. Prevention is aimed at correcting the hyperthyroidism. β-Adrenergic blockers, such as propranolol, are sometimes given until thyroid function is normal. Oral and intravenous administration of potassium can relieve acute hypokalemic attacks.

Hyperkalemic periodic paralysis is another genetic disorder and is characterized by episodes of flaccid paralysis. It can be activated by several factors, including pregnancy, alcohol, illness, certain medications, eating potassium-rich foods, exposure to cold, and rest after exercising.[246] Although the most striking feature of the condition is flaccid paralysis, many individuals have myotonia present on examination.[246] The sodium channel fails to completely inactivate, causing more sodium to enter the cell and forcing potassium into the extracellular space, thus blocking sodium channels from depolarizing. Though hyperkalemic PP episodes are typically of shorter duration than those in hypokalemic PP, there is often a lifelong trend to have increasing frequency of attacks. In addition, hyperkalemic PP can cause permanent muscle weakness. Respiratory insufficiency can be a life-threatening situation.

Preventive measures include avoiding alcohol and diet soda, potassium-rich foods, or activities that provoke symptoms. Maintaining adequate water intake, eating carbohydrate-rich foods, and keeping warm seem to help some individuals.[247] In acute hyperkalemic periodic paralysis, inhaled albuterol or glucose/insulin therapy can reduce symptoms. Preventive medications include potassium-lowering agents, such as hydrochlorothiazide or mexiletine.

Metabolic Muscle Diseases

Disorders in muscle metabolism can be caused by endocrine abnormalities or diseases of energy metabolism, such as glycogen storage disease, enzyme deficiencies, and abnormalities in lipid metabolism and mitochondrial function. The term *metabolic myopathies* refers to a group of hereditary muscle disorders caused by defective genes.

Endocrine Disorders

Often the systemic effects of hormonal imbalance overshadow the individual's muscular symptoms. For example, individuals with thyrotoxicosis may have signs of proximal weakness, paresis of the extraocular muscles (exophthalmic ophthalmoplegia), and, rarely, hypokalemic periodic paralysis. Hypothyroidism is often associated with a decrease in muscle mass and strength, with weak, flabby skeletal muscles and sluggish movements.

Thyroid hormone is believed to regulate muscle protein synthesis and electrolyte balance. Alterations in muscle protein synthesis and electrolyte balance may therefore explain the changes in muscle mass and contractility seen in endocrine disorders. The muscular symptoms subside with appropriate treatment of the primary hormonal disorder.

Diseases of Energy Metabolism

Muscles rely on carbohydrates (such as glycogen) and lipids (free fatty acids) for energy. When stored glycogen or lipids cannot be metabolized because of lack of enzymes necessary to generate ATP for muscle contraction, the individual experiences cramps, fatigue, and exercise intolerance. Disorders of muscle metabolism can be self-limiting, such as McArdle disease and some lipid disorders, or they can cause widespread irreparable muscle destruction, as in acid maltase deficiency.

McArdle disease. McArdle disease (MD), or myophosphorylase deficiency, is also known as glycogen storage disease type V. It was the first myopathy in which a single enzyme defect was identified. It is now one of nine diseases identified to date that have in common an underlying defect in glycogen synthesis, glycogenolysis, or glycolysis. These diseases are often referred to as glycogen storage diseases (GSDs) because each defect results in the abnormal deposition and accumulation of glycogen in skeletal muscle. Individuals with McArdle disease lack muscle phosphorylase, an enzyme responsible for the breakdown of glycogen in muscle. Normally, after the body uses the short-term ATP and phosphocreatine stores, intramuscular lactic acid accumulated as glycogen is used (see Chapter 18). The individual with McArdle disease is not able to metabolize glycogen or produce lactic acid.

The altered energy production manifests itself in exercise intolerance, fatigue, and painful muscle cramps. When exercise is carried to an extreme, painful muscle contracture and myoglobinuria can develop. Some individuals describe a "second wind" phenomenon, in which exercise tolerance increases if they slow their pace once the initial sensation of fatigue commences.[248] The muscles of persons with McArdle disease are able to readily utilize glucose and lactate from the bloodstream. After it is converted to pyruvate, lactate has been shown to be an energy substrate that is oxidized more quickly than either fructose or glucose.[249,250] Higher levels of lactate found in skeletal muscles of those with MD may account for this "second wind." As the disease progresses, some individuals have pronounced muscle weakness and wasting. Other organs are not involved, because the absence of phosphorylase is limited to muscle. In general, individuals with McArdle disease learn to adapt their daily routine to avoid muscle symptoms.

Acid maltase deficiency. Acid maltase deficiency (glycogen storage disease type II or Pompe disease) is an autosomal recessive neuromuscular disease because of mutations of the acidic α-glucosidase (GAA) gene. This results in an accumulation of glycogen in the lysosomes of muscle cells and other tissues because of the lack of the enzyme acid maltase (also known as acid α-glucosidase).[251,252] The exact mechanism of disease progression is still unknown, but mitochondrial dysfunction and abnormal autophagy of cells appear to play a major role in the disease's clinical manifestations.

The infantile form, which is more severe, is called Pompe disease (PD) and is recognized shortly after birth by hypotonia, dysreflexia, and an enlarged heart, tongue, and liver. Hypertrophy of these tissues is thought to be the result of glycogen deposition. Muscle biopsy is an important diagnostic tool in identifying PD.[253] In the past, children died of cardiac or respiratory failure within 1 year of diagnosis, but new treatments have improved survival. Late-onset Pompe disease (LOPD) occurs from childhood into adulthood. Muscular symptoms of LOPD are highly variable and can range from muscle cramping and weakness to varying degrees of respiratory insufficiency.[254] The mainstay of treatment is enzyme replacement therapy with recombinant GAA but dietary modifications also may improve the course of the disease.[255]

Myoadenylate deaminase deficiency. An enzyme deficiency that produces changes in skeletal muscle and is associated with exercise intolerance is myoadenylate deaminase deficiency (MDD). More often referred to as adenosine monophosphate deaminase deficiency (AMDD), this autosomal recessive condition has a wide variation in symptoms.[256] Because these individuals lack myoadenylate deaminase, they have a poor capacity for sustained energy production, yet some with the condition have been able to perform as high-level athletes. The most common symptoms appear to be postexercise muscle cramping or pain, or both, and easy fatigability. Myoadenylate deaminase is the catalytic enzyme that forms phosphocreatine and ATP during exercise through a metabolic pathway that binds the purine and phosphate molecules that constitute ATP. Persons with MDD differ from those with McArdle disease in that, during the ischemic exercise test, lactate production is normal in MDD when ATP and phosphocreatine are synthesized. The enzyme defect has been reported to be quite common, but in practice it may be rarely recognized as a cause of exercise intolerance.

Lipid deficiencies. Disorders of lipid metabolism are uncommon but account for severe changes in muscle metabolism. These disorders are caused by abnormalities in the transport and processing of fatty acids for energy. The lipid content of muscle cells consists of free fatty acids, which are oxidized in the mitochondria. These acids require carnitine and the enzyme carnitine palmitoyltransferase (CPT) to transport long-chain fatty acids to the mitochondria. There are two types of CPT: CPT1 is found in liver, muscle, and brain tissue; only deficiencies of the liver type have been found in humans. Children younger than 18 months are most often affected. CPT2 deficiency, most often seen in adolescents or young adults, is an autosomal recessive disorder that invariably causes attacks of severe myalgia and may cause myoglobinuria.[257] Carnitine deficiency causes abnormal lipid deposition in skeletal muscles.

Measuring the CPT and carnitine content in muscle is essential to diagnosis. Cells in the muscle biopsy show vacuoles and lipid deposits. Treatments with riboflavin, medium-chain triglycerides, oral carnitine, prednisone, and propranolol have been beneficial to some individuals. Bezafibrate, a drug to lower lipid levels, also has shown promise in treating CPT2 deficiency.[257]

Inflammatory Muscle Diseases: Myositis
Viral, Bacterial, and Parasitic Myositis

Viral, bacterial, and parasitic infections of varying severity are known to produce inflammatory changes in skeletal muscle, a group of conditions collectively described by the term myositis. In tuberculosis and sarcoidosis, chronic inflammatory changes and granulomata are found in muscle as well as in other affected tissues. In the parasitic infection trichinellosis, *Trichinella* larvae reside in infected meat (primarily pork, but wildlife and even horses can carry the microorganism), migrate to the intestinal mucosa after ingestion, and then travel through the circulatory system to various tissues. The larvae that penetrate into skeletal muscle are able to survive and grow, causing symptoms such as severe pain, rash, and muscle stiffness. Treatment includes the administration of corticosteroids, immunotherapeutic agents, and the antiparasitic agent thiabendazole. Toxoplasmosis, a common parasitic infection, is also associated with a generalized polymyositis that responds rapidly to therapy.

In the tropics, more prevalent disorders include bacterial infections with *Staphylococcus aureus* and parasites such as cysticercus, the larva of the tapeworm *Taenia solium*. Viral infections can be associated with an acute myositis. Muscle pain, tenderness, signs of inflammation, and creatine kinase (CK) elevation are common manifestations of viral myositis. The self-limiting symptoms of muscle aches and pains during a bout of influenza may actually be a subacute form of viral myopathy.

Polymyositis, Dermatomyositis, and Inclusion Body Myositis

Idiopathic inflammatory myopathies (IIMs) are a group of autoimmune diseases that target skeletal muscle in both children and adults. There are generally four diseases included in this group: dermatomyositis (DM), polymyositis (PM), necrotizing myopathy (NM), and sporadic inclusion body myositis (IBM). The most common form, DM, has been further subclassified into additional subgroups, including the juvenile form—juvenile dermatomyositis (JDM). The exact cause of IIM is unknown, but recent investigations have uncovered strong links between genetic, environmental, and immunologic factors.[258,259] Though still relatively rare, IIMs seem to have a geographic distribution, with greater incidence in Northern latitudes, further supporting the hypotheses of genetic and environmental influences in their development.[260,261] The pathophysiology of IIMs remains fully unknown, but it involves interplay between specific autoantibodies, cytokine-mediated inflammation of muscle, and genetic factors.[262,263]

Several characteristics differentiate IBM from the other IIMs in that IBM affects men more often than women and can cause asymmetric weakness. Compared with DM and PM, IBM does not respond as well to anti-inflammatory and immunosuppressive medications.

CLINICAL MANIFESTATIONS IIMs are characterized by progressive, symmetric proximal (shoulder girdle and quadriceps) muscle weakness and myalgia that develops over weeks to months. Because of their progressive nature, these illnesses can be initially confused with other myopathies. A thorough evaluation is required to exclude other disorders. Clinical features common in both PM and DM are joint pain, dysphagia, reduced esophageal motility, vasculitis, Raynaud phenomenon, cardiomyopathy, and interstitial pulmonary fibrosis. Reduced mobility with frequent falls is a common symptom in IBM because both proximal and distal muscles are affected. Some individuals have other coexisting collagen vascular disorders, such as rheumatoid arthritis, systemic lupus erythematosus, and progressive systemic sclerosis (formerly called scleroderma).

Although PM and DM have similar histories of onset, DM includes cutaneous manifestations. The presence of skin involvement is significant in that it can precede muscle involvement by months or even years.[264] The two most classic signs of skin involvement are (1) rashes— a typical heliotrope (reddish purple) rash that generally covers the eyelids and periorbital tissue (Figure 39-25); and (2) erythematous,

FIGURE 39-25 Clinical Manifestations of Dermatomyositis. A and **B,** Heliotrope (violaceous) discoloration around the eyes and periorbital edema. **C,** Gottron lesions. **D,** Increased erythema around nail beds. (**A, C, D** from Dimachkie MM et al: *Neurol Clin* 32[3]:595-628, 2014. **B** from Habif TP: *Clinical dermatology,* ed 3, St Louis, 1996, Mosby.)

scaly lesions that cover joints such as the knees and elbows, known as Gottron lesions. Other differences between PM and DM include their suspected pathology. PM may be caused by T-cell invasion of the muscle fibers.[265] DM, PM, and NM are associated with an increased risk of malignancy.[266] Both PM and DM seem to respond to prednisone, with or without the addition of immunosuppressives as well as intravenous immunoglobulin administration.[267]

Inclusion body myositis (IBM) is the most common acquired muscle disease affecting individuals older than age 50. IBM differs from both PM and DM in several important ways. Muscle biopsy and histopathologic studies of IBM show degenerative changes of muscle, accumulation of multiple proteins within muscle fibers, and evidence of endoplasmic reticular stress with misfolding of proteins.[268,269] Clinical presentation may show earlier onset of asymmetric atrophy and weakness of the quadriceps as well as the wrists and finger flexors. Additionally, IBM generally does not improve with standard immunosuppressants or immune-modifying drugs.[270]

EVALUATION AND TREATMENT   Muscle biopsy results are striking in DM, with most individuals showing inflammatory cells grouped around blood vessels and atrophy of cells in muscle fascicles. This change, perifascicular atrophy, is absent in PM. Creatinine kinase (CK) level is often extremely elevated in both disorders and is a helpful indicator of disease activity. Levels of other muscle enzymes, including aldolase, aspartate aminotransferase (AST), alanine aminotransferase (AST), and lactate dehydrogenase (LDH), are also found to be elevated in most individuals. The presence of serum antinuclear antibodies (ANAs) also may be helpful in diagnosis. Muscle biopsy is indispensable for a diagnosis of PM or DM as opposed to other myotonic disease.[266] MRI reveals inflammation and edema of the muscles, as well as changes in muscles that may not show clinical evidence of disease.

Contrast-enhanced ultrasound can differentiate between IBM and myositis.[271,272] Electromyography (EMG) is useful in guiding the site for muscle biopsy.

Treatment primarily includes immunosuppressive drugs, although they are not always successful, particularly in the case of IBM. Most clinicians choose corticosteroids initially, usually prednisone on a daily or alternating day schedule, tapering the dosage as the symptoms subside. Successful treatment with azathioprine, methotrexate, creatine, and cyclosporine also has been reported.[266,273] High-dose intravenous immunoglobulin administration is sometimes used during active disease. Individuals with muscle weakness require careful physiotherapy to design a regular exercise program that prevents contractures and maximizes functional ability.

Toxic Myopathies

Muscle damage caused by drugs or toxins is also called toxic myopathy. Alcohol, lipid-lowering agents (fibrates and statins), antimalarial drugs, steroids, thiol derivatives, and narcotics (particularly heroin) can all cause symptoms. Many drugs, diseases, and infectious and environmental agents can cause myopathy. The combination of certain medications can also cause muscle injury.[274] Box 39-5 lists some of the causes of toxic myopathy.

Alcohol remains the most common cause of toxic myopathy. Two clinical syndromes are prevalent: (1) an acute attack of muscle weakness, pain, and swelling after a drinking binge; or (2) a more chronic, progressive proximal weakness in a long-term drinker.[275] The incidence of acute alcoholic myopathy has been estimated as being up to 20% of individuals admitted with acute alcoholic withdrawal.

The pathologic abnormalities include necrosis of individual muscle fibers; whole segments can be found in the same stage of degeneration. The mechanism by which alcohol affects the muscle fiber is uncertain,

---

BOX 39-5   Agents That Can Cause Toxic Myopathy

Drug-Induced

Alcohol
Amiodarone (and others that inhibit CYP3A4 when combined with a statin)
Amphotericin B
Azathioprine
Chloroquine
Clofibrate
Cocaine
Colchicine
Diuretics
Ethanol
Finasteride
Illicit drugs and drugs of abuse (heroin, cocaine, amphetamine, meperidine, pentazocine)
Ipecac (withdrawn from U.S. markets)
Isotretinoin
Labetalol
3,4-Methylenedioxymethamphetamine (MDMA, "ecstasy")
Omeprazole
Pentachlorophenol (PCP)
Propofol
Retrovirals (AZT [zidovudine])
Statins
Steroids (especially with prolonged high doses; doses >25 mg/day; fluorinated steroids)
Vincristine

Endocrine Disorders

Adrenal disorders (Addison disease, Cushing disease)
Hyperparathyroidism
Hyperthyroidism (CK may be normal)
Hypothyroidism (CK may be mildly elevated)

Infectious Agents

Coxsackie A and B viruses
Human immunodeficiency virus (HIV)
Influenza
Lyme disease
Staphylococcus aureus muscle infection (frequent cause of pyomyositis)
Toxoplasmosis
Trichinosis

Miscellaneous

Licorice
Certain edible wild mushrooms
Lead poisoning
Malignant hyperthermia
Organophosphates
Red yeast rice
Snake venom
European migratory quail (quail eat toxic hemlock, hellebore seeds)
Any medication that alters serum concentrations of sodium, potassium, calcium, phosphorus, or magnesium

Data from Pasnoor M et al: *Neurol Clin* 32:647-670, 2014; Valiyil VR, Christopher-Stine O: *Curr Rheumatol Rep* 12(3):213-220, 2010.

but a direct toxic effect and nutritional deficiency have both received experimental support.

Acute alcoholic myopathy can range from benign cramps and pain resolving in a matter of hours to severe weakness and markedly increased CK level associated with myoglobinuria and renal failure. Individuals are prone to repeated attacks following recovery. The only treatment is abstinence from alcohol and improved nutrition. The individual with chronic alcoholic myopathy often has coexisting peripheral neuropathy that complicates the diagnosis.

The most severe complication of toxic myopathy is rhabdomyolysis (acute muscle fiber necrosis with leakage of muscle protein into the bloodstream) that leads to myoglobinuria and acute renal failure. Most individuals with toxic myopathy present with acute muscle weakness. Pain is an unreliable indicator because many toxic myopathies are painless, but necrotizing toxic myopathies can cause severe pain. Dark-colored urine may indicate rhabdomyolysis, a serious complication that can lead to death (see p. 997). Other serious complications can include involvement of respiratory and cardiac muscles.

Measurement of serum creatine levels is helpful in determining muscle damage. Other tests such as electromyography (EMG) may show characteristic changes in function. Magnetic resonance imaging (MRI) can demonstrate muscle edema. Features of myopathy can be seen on muscle biopsy.

Repeated intramuscular injections have also been associated with changes in muscle fibers. Local necrosis of muscle fibers and elevated CK level have been reported after intramuscular injections of cephalothin, lidocaine, diazepam, and digoxin; these effects were not produced with injections of saline. When drugs are injected over long periods, a chronic focal myopathy develops. Proliferation of connective tissue in both the muscle fiber and the overlying skin and subcutaneous tissue has been reported. Over time, segments of the muscles, particularly the deltoid and quadriceps, are converted into fibrotic bands. Pathophysiologic mechanisms for these changes include repeated needle trauma and infection, along with the nonphysiologic acidity or alkalinity of the injected material.

Treatment primarily consists of removing or stopping the offending agent and providing supportive care. Supportive care may include hemodialysis and respiratory or cardiovascular support, depending on severity of symptoms.

MUSCULOSKELETAL TUMORS

Bone Tumors

Many different types of tumors involve the skeleton. Although the skeleton is the major site for metastatic spread of multiple myeloma and breast, lung, and prostate cancers, primary bone tumors are relatively rare. Bone tumors may originate from bone cells, cartilage, fibrous tissue, marrow, or vascular tissue. Based on the tissue of origin, bone tumors are classified as osteogenic, chondrogenic, collagenic, or myelogenic. Box 39-6 contains the classification of primary bone tumors. Each of the types arises from one of the four stem cells that are ultimately derived from the primitive mesoderm (Figure 39-26). In addition, bone tumors may be classified as being of histiocytic, notochordal, lipogenic, or neurogenic origin.

The mesoderm contributes the primitive fibroblast and reticulum cells. The fibroblast is the progenitor of the osteoblast and chondroblast cells. Each cell synthesizes a specific type of intercellular ground substance, and the type of ground substance produced by the cell generally characterizes the tumor derived from that cell. For example, osteogenic tumors usually contain cells that have the appearance of osteoblasts and produce an intercellular substance that can be recognized as osteoid. Chondrogenic tumors contain chondroblasts and produce an intercellular substance similar to chondroid (cartilage). Collagenic tumors contain fibrous tissue cells and produce an intercellular substance similar to the type of collagen found in fibrous connective tissue.

Tumors are also classified as benign or malignant, based on characteristics of the tumor cells (see Chapter 10). The criteria used to identify tumor cells as malignant are (1) an increased nuclear/cytoplasmic ratio, (2) an irregular nuclear border, (3) an excess of chromatin, (4) a prominent nucleolus, and (5) an increase in the number of cells undergoing mitosis. However, many young, rapidly

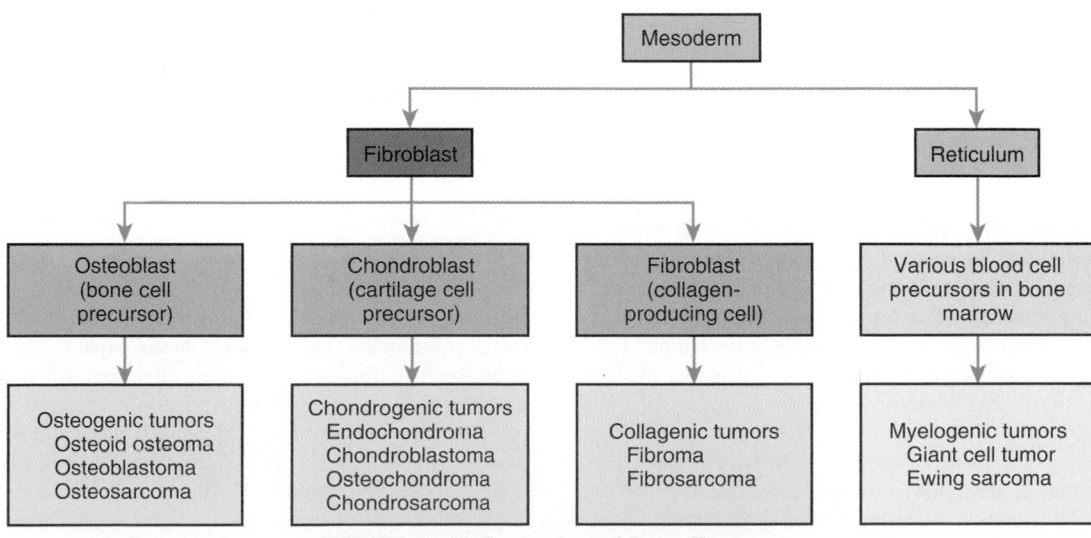

FIGURE 39-26 Derivation of Bone Tumors.

BOX 39-6 Classification of Major Primary Tumors Involving Bone

Category and Fraction (%)	Behavior	Tumor Type	Common Locations	Age (yr)	Morphology
Hematopoietic (20)	Malignant	Myeloma Lymphoma	Vertebrae, pelvis	50-60	Malignant plasma cells or lymphocytes replacing marrow space
Cartilage forming (30)	Benign	Osteochondroma	Metaphysis of long bones	10-30	Bony excrescence with cartilage cap
		Chondroma	Small bones of hands and feet	30-50	Circumscribed hyaline cartilage nodule in medulla
		Chondroblastoma	Epiphysis of long bones	10-20	Circumscribed, pericellular calcification
		Chondromyxoid fibroma	Tibia, pelvis	20-30	Collagenous to myxoid matrix, stellate cells
	Malignant	Chondrosarcoma (conventional)	Pelvis, shoulder	40-60	Extends from medulla through cortex into soft tissue, chondrocytes with increased cellularity and atypia
Bone forming (26)	Benign	Osteoid osteoma	Metaphysis of long bones	10-20	Cortical, interlacing microtrabeculae of woven bone
		Osteoblastoma	Vertebral column	10-20	Posterior elements of vertebrae, histology similar to osteoid osteoma
	Malignant	Osteosarcoma	Metaphysis of distal femur, proximal tibia	10-20	Extends from medulla to lift periosteum, malignant cells producing woven bone
Unknown origin (15)	Benign	Giant cell tumor	Epiphysis of long bones	20-40	Destroys medulla and cortex, sheets of osteoclasts
		Aneurysmal bone cyst	Proximal tibia, distal femur, vertebrae	10-20	Vertebral body, hemorrhagic spaces separated by cellular, fibrous septae
	Malignant	Ewing sarcoma	Diaphysis of long bones	10-20	Sheets of primitive small round cells
		Adamantinoma	Tibia	30-40	Cortical, fibrous, bone matrix with epithelial islands
Notochordal (4)	Malignant	Chordoma	Clivus, sacrum	30-60	Destroys medulla and cortex, foamy cells in myxoid matrix

From Kumar V et al: *Robbins & Cotran pathologic basis of disease,* ed 9, Philadelphia, 2015, Saunders. Adapted from Unni KK, Inwards CY: *Dahlin's bone tumors,* ed 6, Philadelphia, 2010, Lippincott Williams & Wilkins; by permission of Mayo Foundation.

growing normal cells and cells subjected to inflammation and change in their blood supply also exhibit many of these same characteristics. (Tumor characteristics in general are described in Chapter 10.)

Epidemiology

The incidence rate of bone tumors varies with age. In children younger than 15 years, the rate of bone tumors is relatively low, constituting approximately 5% of all malignancies. Adolescents have the highest incidence of bone tumors, and adults between the ages of 30 and 35 have the lowest incidence. After age 35 years, the incidence rate slowly increases until at age 60 years it nearly equals the incidence rate in adolescents, primarily related to secondary metastatic tumors.

Patterns of Bone Destruction

The general pathologic features of bone tumors include bone destruction, erosion or expansion of the cortex, and periosteal response to changes in underlying bone. The least amount of pathologic damage occurs with benign bone tumors, which push against neighboring tissue. Because they usually have a symmetric, controlled growth pattern, benign bone tumors tend to compress and displace neighboring normal bone tissue, which weakens the bone's structure until it is incapable of withstanding the stress of ordinary use, leading to pathologic fracture. Other tumors invade and destroy adjacent normal bone tissue by producing substances that promote resorption by increasing osteoclast activity or by interfering with a bone's blood supply. Three patterns of bone destruction by bone tumors have been identified: (1) the geographic pattern, (2) the moth-eaten pattern, and (3) the permeative pattern (Table 39-7).

Tumors that erode the cortex of the bone usually stimulate a periosteal response—that is, new bone formation at the interface between the surface of the bone and the periosteum. Slow erosion of the cortex usually stimulates a uniform periosteal response. Additional layers of

TABLE 39-7 Patterns of Bone Destruction Caused by Bone Tumors

Type	Features
Geographic pattern	Least aggressive type
	Generally indicative of slow-growing or benign tumor
	Well-defined margins on tumor, easily separated from surrounding normal bone
	Uniform and well-defined lytic area in bone
	Margin smooth or irregular, demarcated by short zone of transition between normal and abnormal bone tissue
Moth-eaten pattern	Characteristic of rapidly growing, malignant bone tumors
	More aggressive pattern
	Tumor margin less defined or demarcated; cannot easily be separated from normal bone
	Areas of partially destroyed bone adjacent to completely lytic areas
Permeative pattern	Caused by aggressive malignant tumor with rapid growth potential
	Margins of tumor poorly demarcated
	Abnormal bone merges imperceptibly with normal bone

bone are added to the exterior surface of the bone to buttress the cortex. Eventually, the additional layers expand the bone's contour. Aggressive penetration of the cortex, often seen with malignant tumors, usually elevates the periosteum and stimulates erratic patterns of new bone formation. Examples of erratic patterns include concentric layers of new bone; a sunburst pattern, in which delicate rays of new bone radiate toward the periosteum from a single focus on the underlying surface; and rays of new bone that grow perpendicularly, creating a brush or bristle pattern.

EVALUATION   A malignant bone tumor must be identified early to allow survival of the individual and preservation of the affected limb. However, individuals often have only vague symptoms that may be attributed to minor trauma, degenerative changes, or inflammatory conditions. In addition, other conditions may obscure the diagnosis.

Thorough diagnostic studies are needed to determine the exact type and extent of bone tumor present, which also helps determine the optimal treatment regimen. Serum alkaline phosphatase levels are elevated in bone lytic tumors and significantly elevated in osteosarcoma. Radiologic studies, including plain radiographic films, radionucleotide bone scans, CT scan, MRI, and positron emission tomography combined with CT (PET/CT), are used to evaluate bone lesions. MRI and PET/CT have become the examination of choice for the local staging of bone tumors, especially the staging of peripheral osteosarcomas (Table 39-8). MRI and PET/CT are used to monitor the response of osteosarcomas to radiation or chemotherapy and to detect recurrent disease. A PET/CT, particularly when augmented by injection of the radioisotope fluorodeoxyglucose (FDG), provides earlier, more detailed information on tumor location, differentiation, metastases, and response to therapy than other imaging modalities.[276] (Tumor staging is discussed in Chapter 10.)

Additional diagnostic studies done for specific bone tumors include a complete blood count and erythrocyte sedimentation rate (to rule out infection or myeloma) and measurement of serum levels of calcium and phosphorus to detect hypercalcemia. Serum glucose levels may be elevated in chondrosarcoma. Bone-specific alkaline phosphatase is elevated when there is bone metastasis.[277] Acid phosphatase level may be moderately elevated in bone metastases, multiple myeloma, and advanced Paget disease. Serum protein electrophoresis and immunoelectrophoresis are performed to exclude other diseases. To determine the exact tumor type, core needle biopsy is usually done at the time of surgery.[278]

Types

A large number of lesions are classified as bone tumors. Bone tumors are typically classified according to their origin—osteogenic, chondrogenic, collagenic, and myelogenic tumors. They are described in the following sections (Figure 39-27).

Osteogenic tumors: osteosarcoma. Osteogenic (bone-forming) tumors are characterized by the formation of bone or osteoid tissue with a sarcomatous tissue. The tissue can have the appearance of callus or compact or spongy bone. The most common malignant bone-forming tumor is the osteosarcoma.

The incidence of osteosarcomas, the most commonly diagnosed primary bone tumor, peaks around the second decade, with a slight preference for males.[279,280] Sixty percent of osteosarcomas occur in persons younger than 20 years. A secondary peak incidence for osteosarcoma occurs in the 50- to 60-year age group, primarily in individuals with a history of radiation therapy several years previously for pelvic or other malignancies or for Paget disease of bone.[281,282] Though considered a bone-forming tumor because of formation of immature osteoid that shows a "lace-like" pattern of bone growth, the radiologic appearance of sarcoma is quite variable and often shows a moth-eaten (lytic) pattern of destruction with the tumor extending into the adjacent soft tissue.[283] Occasionally, the tumor may spread to nonadjacent bone or across a joint with normal-appearing areas of bone between tumors (i.e., "skip lesions"). Radionuclide bone scans are used to find skip lesions. MRI and PET/CT are useful in determining bony changes associated with the tumor.

The borders of the tumor are indistinct and merge into adjacent normal bone. Osteosarcomas contain osteoid produced by anaplastic stromal cells, which are atypical, abnormal cells not seen in normal developing bone; they are neither normal nor embryonal. Many

TABLE 39-8   Surgical Staging System for Bone Tumors of Mesenchymal Origin

Stage	Grade	Site (T)	Metastasis (M)
IA	Low (G_1)	Intracompartmental (T_1)	None (M_0)
IB	Low (G_1)	Extracompartmental (T_2)	None (M_0)
IIA	High (G_2)	Intracompartmental (T_1)	None (M_0)
IIB	High (G_2)	Extracompartmental (T_2)	None (M_0)
IIIA	Low (G_1)	Intracompartmental or extracompartmental (T_1 or T_2)	Regional or distant (M_1)
IIIB	High (G_2)	Intracompartmental or extracompartmental (T_1 or T_2)	Regional or distant (M_1)

Data from Jawad MU, Scully SP: *Clin Orthop Relat Res* 468(7):2000-2002, 2010; Simon SR, editor: *Orthopaedic basic science*, Chicago, 1994, American Academy of Orthopaedic Surgeons.

FIGURE 39-27 Osteosarcoma. **A,** Common locations of Ewing sarcoma and osteosarcoma. *Blue,* osteosarcoma; *red,* Ewing sarcoma. **B,** Comparison of plain radiograph, MRI, and nuclear bone scan appearances of osteosarcoma of the distal femur. Note destruction of the bone cortex and soft tissue component. (**A** adapted from Bontrager KL, Lampignanno JP, editors: *Textbook of radiographic positioning and related anatomy,* St Louis, 2013, Elsevier. **B** from HaDuong JH et al: *Pediatr Clin N Am* 62:179-200, 2015.)

tumors are heterogeneous; for example, the osteosarcoma also may contain chondroid (cartilage) and fibrinoid tissue that may form the bulk of the tumor. The osteoid is deposited as thick masses or "streamers," which infiltrate the normal compact bone, destroy it, and replace it with masses of osteoid. Bone tissue produced by osteosarcomas never matures to compact bone.

Ninety percent of osteosarcomas are located in the metaphyses of long bones, especially the distal femoral metaphysis, with 50% around the knee area. The tumor typically impregnates the cortex, lifts the periosteum, and forms a soft tissue mass that is not covered by a smooth shell of new bone. Lifting of the periosteum stimulates bizarre patterns of new bone formation called a *periosteal reaction*. Distinct osteosarcomas occur on the surface of long bones, called parosteal, periosteal, and high-grade surface osteosarcomas; dedifferentiated parosteal and central osteosarcomas also occur.

The most common initial symptoms are pain and an enlarging mass.[284] Initially, the pain is slight and intermittent, but within a short time the pain increases in severity and duration. Pain is usually worse at night and gradually requires medication. Systemic symptoms are uncommon. Often, a coincidental history of trauma is noted. Occasionally, the individual may present with a pathologic fracture.

Bone biopsy is critical to diagnosis. Because the most frequent site of metastasis is the lung, a chest CT or MRI of the thorax also should be performed. There are no specific laboratory tests that aid in diagnosing sarcoma but laboratory studies are helpful in assessing overall health before beginning treatment. Once osteosarcoma has been diagnosed, measuring serum alkaline phosphatase and LDH levels can be useful in following response to treatment. The best clinical outcomes occur in those who receive both preoperative and postoperative chemotherapy in addition to surgery.[285,286] Surgery is directed at salvaging the affected limb.[280,284]

Surgery is the major treatment of choice, with the tumor's location and size, the extent of malignancy, and evidence of metastasis dictating the type and extent of surgery (see Table 39-8). Preoperative chemotherapy has greatly increased the number of individuals qualifying for limb salvage surgery. Limb-salvaging procedures have been made possible by advances in reconstructive techniques and endoprosthetics. If an amputation is done, individuals are monitored closely with chest radiographs and CT. Pulmonary metastases are surgically resected, and chemotherapy is now a common therapy given both before and after surgery, using combinations of chemotherapeutic agents. Despite advances in chemotherapy and surgical techniques, overall long-term survival in osteosarcoma with metastases has not significantly improved in the past 30 to 40 years. Osteosarcomas are very difficult to treat with current chemotherapeutic agents.[287,288]

Other sarcomas include Ewing sarcoma and synovial sarcoma, each of which demonstrates specific genetic alterations.[289,290] Others include rhabdomyosarcoma (a soft tissue sarcoma that likely originates in the skeleton but with features more like skeletal muscle) and sarcomas that have no definite morphologic pattern, such as leiomyosarcoma and pleomorphic liposarcoma.

Chondrogenic tumors: chondrosarcoma. **Chondrogenic (cartilage-forming) tumors** produce cartilage or chondroid, a primitive cartilage or cartilage-like substance. The most common chondrogenic tumor is chondrosarcoma.

Chondrosarcoma is the second most common primary malignant bone tumor[291] and is a tumor of middle-aged and older adults. Chondrosarcomas that develop from a preexisting benign bone lesion (such as an enchondroma) are known as secondary chondrosarcomas. Individuals with certain conditions, such as multiple osteochondromas, may be at greater risk for developing secondary chondrosarcoma. Secondary chondrosarcomas are rare, occurring most often in young

adults between 20 and 30 years of age. The tumor is more common in men than in women.

A chondrosarcoma is a large, cartilage-producing, ill-defined malignant tumor that infiltrates trabeculae in spongy bone. It occurs most often in the metaphysis or diaphysis of long bones, especially the femur or proximal humerus, and in the bones of the pelvis.[292] If located near the end of the bone, the tumor will infiltrate into the joint space. The tumor expands and enlarges the contour of the bone, causes extensive erosion of the cortex, and grows into the soft tissues.

Symptoms associated with a chondrosarcoma have an insidious onset. Local swelling and pain are the usual presenting symptoms. At first the pain is dull and intermittent, then gradually intensifies and becomes constant; it may awaken the person at night.

Diagnostic studies include radiographs, which must be reviewed carefully for an accurate diagnosis. MRI is useful in determining the extent of soft tissue involvement.[293,294] Biopsy is done at the time of surgery. (If biopsy is conducted before scheduled surgical incision, seeding of tumor cells could occur.) Sufficient tumor material must be obtained to facilitate an accurate diagnosis.

Surgical excision is generally regarded as the treatment of choice because chemotherapy is generally ineffective.[291] Tumors more centrally located (in the appendicular skeleton) are more likely to metastasize. Consequently, individuals with tumors located in the limbs may have a better prognosis than those with pelvic lesions. Recent advances in understanding the pathophysiology of bone sarcomas has led to development of targeted therapies that show promise for improving outcomes.[295,296]

Collagenic tumors: fibrosarcoma. **Collagenic (collagen-forming) tumors** originate from mesenchymal cells and produce fibrous connective tissue. Fibrosarcoma is the most common collagenic tumor and can affect bone or soft tissue.

Fibrosarcomas represent 4% of the primary malignant bone tumors, with a broad age distribution. They may occur at any age but are most common in adults between 30 and 50 years of age. The incidence is slightly greater in females. Fibrosarcoma also may be a secondary complication of radiation therapy, Paget disease, and long-standing osteomyelitis.

Fibrosarcoma is a rare, malignant, solitary tumor that most often affects the metaphyseal region of the femur or tibia. The tumor is composed of a firm, fibrous mass of tissue that contains collagen, malignant fibroblasts, and occasional osteoclast-like giant cells. Secondary fibrosarcoma, which tends to have a worse prognosis, can occur after prior radiation to an area.

The tumor begins in the marrow cavity of the bone and infiltrates the trabeculae. It demonstrates a permeative growth pattern, destroys the cortex, and extends into the soft tissue. Metastasis to the lung is common.

Symptoms associated with the tumor have an insidious onset, which delays diagnosis. Pain and swelling are the usual presenting symptoms and usually indicate that the tumor has infiltrated the cortex. Local tenderness, a palpable mass, and limitation of motion also may be present. A pathologic fracture in the affected bone is often the reason for seeking medical help. Diagnostic studies include radiographs and MRI.

Radical surgery and amputation are the treatments of choice for fibrosarcoma. There is a high probability of metastases. Radiation therapy is generally considered ineffective treatment for this tumor. Promising investigations of matrix metalloproteinase inhibitors and even injectable compounds may alter future treatment of fibrosarcoma.[297,298]

Giant cell tumor. Giant cell tumor, along with myeloma (see Chapter 21), are **myelogenic tumors**, ones that originate from various bone marrow cells. Giant cell tumor (GCT) is the sixth most common of the primary bone tumors, accounting for 4% to 5% of bone tumors. It is generally benign but can become malignant after radiation treatment. Giant cell tumors have a wide age distribution; however, they are rare in persons younger than 10 years or older than 70 years. Most giant cell tumors are found in persons between 20 and 40 years of age. Unlike most other bone tumors, giant cell tumors affect females more often than males.

The giant cell tumor is a solitary, circumscribed tumor that causes extensive bone resorption because of its osteoclastic origin and RANKL overexpression.[299] GCTs are typically located in the epiphyseal regions of the femur, tibia, radius, or humerus.[300] The tumor has a slow, relentless growth rate and is usually contained within the original contour of the affected bone. It may, however, extend into the articular cartilage. When the tumor extends, it is usually covered by periosteum or periosteal bone growth; it may extend into surrounding soft tissue. GCTs have a low rate of metastasis to other organs or tissues, although they have a high rate of recurrence.

The most common symptoms associated with GCT are pain, local swelling, and limitation of movement. Diagnostic studies include radiographs, CT, and MRI. Cryosurgery and resection of the tumor with the use of adjuvant polymethylmethacrylate (PMMA) for bone grafts decrease recurrence and are more successful treatments than curettage and radiation.[299] The monoclonal antibody denosumab has been approved for treating GCTs in cases of recurrence or where surgery is not feasible.[301,302] Depending on the extent of the tumor and its recurrence, amputation may be necessary.

Muscle Tumors
Rhabdomyoma

Rhabdomyoma is an extremely rare benign tumor of muscle that generally occurs in the tongue, neck muscles, larynx, uvula, nasal cavity, axilla, vulva, and heart. These tumors are usually treated by surgical excision and typically do not recur.

Rhabdomyosarcoma

About 3% to 5% of childhood cancers are malignant tumors of striated muscle called rhabdomyosarcoma. Infants, children, and teenagers account for more than 85% of cases; there is a slight preference in males. This tumor is highly malignant with rapid metastasis. Rhabdomyosarcomas are located in the muscle tissue of the head, neck, and genitourinary tract in 75% of cases, with the remainder found in the trunk and extremities. Recent animal studies have established a link between chemical, biologic, and physical triggers of rhabdomyosarcoma.[303] Recent advances in treatment have improved the 5-year survival for children to greater than 80% in cases of localized tumors.[304] Unfortunately, survival in adults remains poor.

Three types of rhabdomyosarcoma are differentiated on pathologic section: anaplastic (formerly known as pleomorphic), embryonal, and alveolar. Each type differs from the other molecularly; they are all aggressive tumors and are typically more resistant to therapy. Although rare, the anaplastic, or spindle cell, type is considered to be one of the most highly malignant tumors of the extremities seen in adulthood. Microscopically, embryonal tumors resemble a tadpole or tennis racquet and are most often seen in infancy and childhood. Alveolar-type tumors appear lattice-like, similar to lung tissue alveoli, and are more often found in adolescents and adults.

The diagnosis of rhabdomyosarcoma is made by careful incisional biopsy or core needle aspiration and examination of the specimen by a pathologist. CT scan also helps define the tissue borders. PET/CT is useful in identifying involvement of bones, lymph nodes, and bone marrow. Staging is based on the tumor's size, location, presence of metastases, and lymph node involvement. Pathologic grading of the tumor is helpful in determining prognosis and treatment.

Treatment consists of a combination of surgical excision, systemic chemotherapy, and radiation therapy. Cure is unlikely when distant metastases are present.

Other Tumors

Metastatic tumors in muscles are rare in spite of the extensive vascular supply of skeletal muscles. It is suggested that local pH or metabolic changes within muscles prevent metastatic involvement from other tumors. When adjacent carcinomas do cause muscle damage, it is usually related to the compression of tissue and resultant muscle atrophy.

✔ **QUICK CHECK 39-5**
1. From what cells do bone tumors originate?
2. Compare five major characteristics of benign bone tumors with those of malignant bone tumors.
3. How does the presence of metastatic tumors affect treatment options and prognosis of persons with osteosarcoma?

■ DID YOU UNDERSTAND?

Musculoskeletal Injuries

1. The most serious musculoskeletal injury is a fracture. A bone can be completely or incompletely fractured. A closed fracture leaves the skin intact. An open fracture has an overlying skin wound. The direction of the fracture line can be linear, oblique, spiral, or transverse. Greenstick, torus, and bowing fractures are examples of incomplete fractures that occur in children. Stress fractures occur in normal or abnormal bone that is subjected to repeated stress. Fatigue fractures occur in normal bone subjected to abnormal stress. Normal weightbearing can cause an insufficiency (or fragility) fracture in abnormal bone.
2. Dislocation is complete loss of contact between the articular surfaces of two bones. Subluxation is partial loss of joint contact between two bones. As a bone separates from a joint, it may damage adjacent nerves, blood vessels, ligaments, tendons, and muscle.

3. Tendon tears are called strains, and ligament tears are called sprains. A complete separation of a tendon or ligament from its attachment is called an avulsion.
4. Rhabdomyolysis, often manifested by the presence of myoglobinuria, can be a life-threatening complication of severe muscle trauma, genetic predisposition, or toxic effects of certain medications.

Disorders of Bones

1. Metabolic bone diseases are characterized by abnormal bone structure. In osteoporosis, the density or mass of bone is reduced because the bone remodeling cycle is disrupted. Osteomalacia is a metabolic bone disease characterized by inadequate bone mineralization. Excessive and abnormal bone remodeling occurs in Paget disease.
2. Osteomyelitis is a bone infection caused *most often* by bacteria. Bacteria can enter bone from outside the body (exogenous

osteomyelitis) or from infection sites within the body (hematogenous osteomyelitis).

Disorders of Joints

1. Because of improved imaging technology, inflammation has been identified as an important feature of osteoarthritis.
2. Osteoarthritis (OA) is a common, age-related disorder of synovial joints. The primary defect in OA is loss of articular cartilage.
3. Rheumatoid arthritis is an inflammatory joint disease characterized by inflammatory destruction of the synovial membrane, articular cartilage, joint capsule, and surrounding ligaments and tendons. Rheumatoid nodules also may invade the skin, lung, and spleen and involve small and large arteries. Rheumatoid arthritis is a systemic disease that affects the heart, lungs, kidneys, and skin, as well as the joints.
4. Ankylosing spondylitis is a chronic, systemic autoimmune disease characterized by stiffening and fusion of the sacroiliac and spine joints.
5. Gout is a syndrome caused by defects in uric acid metabolism with high levels of uric acid in the blood and body fluids. Uric acid crystallizes in the connective tissue of a joint where it initiates inflammatory destruction of the joint.

Disorders of Skeletal Muscle

1. A pathologic contracture is permanent muscle shortening caused by muscle spasticity, as seen in central nervous system (CNS) injury or severe muscle weakness.
2. Stress-induced muscle tension is presumably caused by increased activity in the reticular activating system and gamma loop in the muscle fiber. The use of progressive relaxation training and biofeedback has been advocated to reduce muscle tension.
3. Fibromyalgia is a chronic musculoskeletal syndrome characterized by diffuse pain and tender points. Theories have proposed that the muscle is the end organ responsible for the pain and fatigue, although this has not been confirmed. Most cases of FM involve women, and the peak age is 30 to 50 years. Genetic factors are being increasingly recognized as agents in developing fibromyalgia.
4. Atrophy of muscle fibers and overall diminished size of the muscle are seen after prolonged inactivity. Isometric contractions and passive lengthening exercises decrease atrophy to some degree in immobilized persons.
5. Because of ion channel disorders, hyperexcitable membranes cause the physical and electrical phenomenon of myotonia. The disorder is treated with drugs that reduce muscle fiber excitability. The biochemical defect is related to changes in the muscle membrane and sarcoplasmic reticulum.

6. Metabolic muscle diseases are caused by endocrine disorders, glycogen storage diseases, enzyme deficiencies, and abnormal lipid function. The muscle depends on a complex system of carbohydrates and fats converted by enzymes to produce energy for the muscle cell. Abnormalities in these pathways can inhibit function or cause damage to the muscle fiber. These illnesses are rare, yet they account for significant functional abnormalities.
7. Viral, bacterial, and parasitic infections of muscles produce the characteristic clinical and pathologic changes associated with inflammation. These are usually treatable and self-limiting disorders.
8. Polymyositis (generalized muscle inflammation) and dermatomyositis (polymyositis accompanied by skin rash) are characterized by inflammation of connective tissue and muscle fibers and muscle fiber necrosis. Cell-mediated and humoral immune factors have been implicated. Treatment with immunosuppressive agents is effective in many cases.
9. The most common cause of toxic myopathy is alcohol abuse. It has been suggested that alcohol use affects muscle fibers both directly (by causing necrosis) and indirectly (by the concomitant nutritional deficiencies typically associated with excessive use of alcohol). Drug administration can also lead to toxic myopathy; a needle used during an injection, secondary infection, and alterations in the acidity and alkalinity of muscle fibers can mechanically damage muscle fibers.

Musculoskeletal Tumors

1. Sarcomas of muscle tissue are rare. Rhabdomyosarcoma has a uniformly poor prognosis, particularly in adults, because of an aggressive invasion and early, widespread dissemination. The usual treatment includes surgical excision, radiation therapy, and systemic chemotherapy.
2. Bone tumors originate from bone cells, cartilage cells, fibrous tissue cells, or vascular marrow cells. Each cell produces a specific type of ground substance that is used to classify the tumor as osteogenic (bone cell), chondrogenic (cartilage cell), collagenic (fibrous tissue cell), or myelogenic (vascular marrow cell). Malignant bone tumors are usually large, aggressively destroy surrounding bone, invade surrounding tissue, and initiate independent growth outside the site of origin. Benign bone tumors are generally less destructive, limit their growth to the anatomic confines of the bone, and have a well-demarcated border. Certain benign tumors can become malignant.

KEY TERMS

Acid maltase deficiency, 1024
Acute gouty arthritis, 1019
Age-related bone loss, 1003
Ankylosing spondylitis (AS), 1016
Asymptomatic hyperuricemia, 1019
Avulsion, 995
Biofeedback, 1021
Bone tumor, 1027
Bowing fracture, 992
Bursa (pl., bursae), 996
Caplan syndrome, 1015

Central sensitization, 1022
Chondrogenic (cartilage-forming) tumor, 1030
Chondrosarcoma, 1030
Chronic fatigue syndrome (CFS), 1023
Closed (incomplete) fracture, 991
Collagenic (collagen-forming) tumor, 1030
Comminuted fracture, 991
Compartment syndrome, 999

Complete fracture, 991
Contiguous osteomyelitis, 1008
Contracture, 1021
Delayed union, 994
Direct (primary) healing, 993
Dislocation, 994
Disuse atrophy, 1021
Dual x-ray absorptiometry (DXA), 1005
Endochondral bone formation, 993
Enthesis, 995

Epicondyle, 995
Epicondylopathy, 995
External fixation, 994
Fatigue fracture, 993
Fibromyalgia (FM), 1022
Fibrosarcoma, 1030
Fracture, 991
Giant cell tumor (GCT), 1031
Glucocorticoid-induced osteoporosis, 1003
Glycogen storage disease (GSD), 1024

REFERENCES

1. Roeleveld DM, Koenders MI: The role of the Th17 cytokines IL-17 and IL-22 in rheumatoid arthritis pathogenesis and developments in cytokine immunotherapy, Cytokine 74(1):101-107, 2014.
2. Kanis JA et al: Systematic review of hip fracture incidence and probability of fracture worldwide, Osteoporos Int 23:2239-2256, 2012.
3. Marsell R, Einhorn TA: The biology of fracture healing, Injury 42(6):551-555, 2011.
4. Secreto FJ et al: Wnt signaling during fracture repair, Curr Osteoporos Rep 7(2):64-69, 2009.
5. Bunker DLJ et al: Tendon to bone healing and its implications for surgery, Muscles Ligaments Tendons J 4(3):343-350, 2014.
6. Charvet B et al: The development of the myotendinous junction. A review, Muscles Ligaments Tendons J 2(2):53-63, 2012.
7. Birch HL et al: Specialisation of extracellular matrix for function in tendons and ligaments, Muscles Ligaments Tendons J 3(1):12-22, 2013.
8. Hubbard TJ, Hicks-Little CA: Ankle ligament healing after an acute ankle sprain: an evidence-based approach, J Athl Train 43(5):523-529, 2008.
9. Kaminski TW et al: National Athletic Trainers' Association position statement: conservative management and prevention of ankle sprains in athletes, J Athl Train 48(4):528-545, 2013.
10. Knobloch K: The role of tendon microcirculation in Achilles and patellar tendinopathy, J Orthop Surg Res 3:18, 2008.
11. Luk JK et al: Lateral epicondylalgia: midlife crisis of a tendon, Hong Kong Med J 20(2):145-151, 2014.
12. Orchard J, Kountouris A: The management of tennis elbow, Br Med J 342:d2687, 2011.
13. Waseem M et al: Lateral epicondylitis: a review of the literature, J Back Musculoskelet Rehabil 25(2):131-142, 2012.
14. Chourasia AO et al: Relationships between biomechanics, tendon pathology, and function in individuals with lateral epicondylosis, J Orthop Sports Phys Ther 43(6):368-378, 2013.

15. Järvinen TAH et al: Regeneration of injured skeletal muscle after the injury, Muscles Ligaments Tendons J 3(4):337-345, 2013.
16. Cervellin G et al: Rhabdomyolysis: historical background, clinical, diagnostic, and therapeutic features, Clin Chem Lab Med 48(6):749-756, 2010.
17. Genthon A, Wilcox SR: Crush syndrome: a case report and review of the literature, J Emerg Med 46(2):313-319, 2014.
18. Zutt R et al: Rhabdomyolysis: review of the literature, Neuromuscul Disord 24:651-659, 2014.
19. Young SE et al: Urine dipstick testing to rule out rhabdomyolysis in patients with suspected heat injury, Am J Emerg Med 27(7):875-877, 2009.
20. Su B-H et al: Ultrasonic appearance of rhabdomyolysis in patients with crush injury in the Wenchuan earthquake, Chin Med J 122(16):1872-1876, 2009.
21. Ali P et al: Assessment and diagnosis of acute limb compartment syndrome: a literature review, Int J Orthop Trauma Nurs 18(4):180-190, 2014.
22. McDonald S, Bearcroft P: Compartment syndromes, Semin Musculoskelet Radiol 14(2):236-244, 2010.
23. Shadgan B et al: Current thinking about acute compartment syndrome of the lower extremity, Can J Surg 53(5):329-334, 2010.
24. Raza H, Mahapatra A: Acute compartment syndrome in orthopedics: causes, diagnosis, and management, Adv Orthop 2015:543412, 2015.
25. Collinge C, Kuper M: Comparison of three methods for measuring intracompartmental pressure in injured limbs of trauma patients, J Orthop Trauma 24(6):364-368, 2010.
26. Hammerberg EM et al: The reliability of measurement of tissue pressure in compartment syndrome, J Orthop Trauma 26(1):24-31, 2012.
27. Bandschapp O, Girard T: Malignant hyperthermia, Swiss Med Wkly 142:13652, 2012.
28. Stowell KM: DNA testing for malignant hyperthermia: the reality and the dream, Anesth Analg 118(2):397-406, 2014.

29. Schneiderbanger D et al: Management of malignant hyperthermia: diagnosis and treatment, Ther Clin Risk Manag 10:355-362, 2014.
30. Correia ACC et al: Malignant hyperthermia: clinical and molecular aspects, Rev Bras Anestesiol 62(6):820-837, 2012.
31. Kim DC: Malignant hyperthermia, Korean J Anesthesiol 65(5):391-401, 2012.
32. Chen H, Kubo KY: Bone three-dimensional microstructural features of the common osteoporotic fracture sites, World J Orthop 5(4):486-495, 2014.
33. World Health Organization (WHO) Scientific Group on the Prevention and Management of Osteoporosis: WHO technical report series, no. 921, Geneva, Switzerland, 2000, Author.
34. Dede AD et al: Bone disease in anorexia nervosa, Hormones (Athens) 13(1):38-56, 2014.
35. Gonnelli S et al: Obesity and fracture risk, Clin Cases Miner Bone Metab 11(1):9-14, 2014.
36. Jackuliak P, Payer J: Osteoporosis, fractures, and diabetes, Int J Endocrinol 2014:820615, 2014.
37. Misra M, Klibanski A: Anorexia nervosa and bone, J Endocrinol 221(3):R163-R176, 2014.
38. Panday K et al: Medication-induced osteoporosis: screening and treatment strategies, Ther Adv Musculoskel Dis 6(5):185-202, 2014.
39. U.S. Preventive Services Task Force: Screening for osteoporosis: U.S. Preventive Services Task Force recommendation statement, Ann Intern Med 154(5):356-364, 2011.
40. Honig S: Osteoporosis—new treatments and updates, Bull NYU Hosp Jt Dis 68(3):166-170, 2010.
41. Singer A et al: Burden of illness for osteoporotic fractures compared with other serious diseases among postmenopausal women in the United States, Mayo Clin Proc 90(1):53-62, 2015.
42. Lange A et al: One-year disease-related health care costs of incident vertebral fractures in osteoporotic patients, Osteoporos Int 25(10):2435-2443, 2014.

43. Svedbom A et al: Osteoporosis in the European Union: a compendium of country-specific reports, *Arch Osteoporos* 8(1-2):137, 2013.

44. Viswanathan HN et al: Direct healthcare costs of osteoporosis-related fractures in managed care patients receiving pharmacological osteoporosis therapy, *Appl Health Econ Health Policy* 10(3):163-173, 2012.

45. Adachi JD et al: Impact of prevalent fractures on quality of life: baseline results from the global longitudinal study of osteoporosis in women, *Mayo Clin Proc* 5(9):806-813, 2010.

46. Leslie WD, Morin SN: Osteoporosis epidemiology 2013: implications for diagnosis, risk assessment, and treatment, *Curr Opin Rheumatol* 26(4):440-446, 2014.

47. Rao SS et al: Osteoporosis in men, *Am Fam Physician* 82(5):503-508, 2010.

48. Dy CJ et al: Sex and gender considerations in male patients with osteoporosis, *Clin Orthop Relat Res* 469(7):1906-1912, 2011.

49. Cawthorn PM: Gender differences in osteoporosis and fractures, *Clin Orthop Relat Res* 469(7):1900-1905, 2011.

50. Haentjens P et al: Meta-analysis: excess mortality after hip fracture among older women and men, *Ann Intern Med* 152:380-390, 2010.

51. Gerdhem P: Osteoporosis and fragility fractures: vertebral fractures, *Best Pract Res Clin Rheumatol* 27(6):743-755, 2013.

52. Cauley JA: Defining ethnic and racial differences in osteoporosis and fragility fractures, *Clin Orthop Relat Res* 469(7):1891-1899, 2011.

53. NIH Osteoporosis and Related Bone Diseases National Resource Center: *Osteoporosis and African American women*, June 2010. Available at: www.niams.nih.gov/Health_Info/Bone/Osteoporosis/Background/default.asp. Accessed January 20, 2011.

54. Rubin KH et al: Comparison of different screening tools (FRAX®, OST, ORAI, OSIRIS, SCORE and age alone) to identify women with increased risk of fracture. A population-based prospective study, *Bone* 56:16-22, 2013.

55. Khosla S: Pathogenesis of age-related bone loss in humans, *J Gerontol A Biol Sci Med Sci* 68(10):1226-1235, 2013.

56. Calvo MS, Tucker KL: Is phosphorus intake that exceed dietary requirements a risk factor in bone health? *Ann N Y Acad Sci* 1301:29-35, 2013.

57. Calvo MS, Uribarri J: Public health impact of dietary phosphorus excess on bone and cardiovascular health in the general population, *Am J Clin Nutr* 98(1):6-13, 2013.

58. Cauley JA: Estrogen and bone health in men and women, *Steroids* 99(Pt A):11-15, 2015.

59. Vandenput L et al: Serum estradiol levels are inversely associated with cortical porosity in older men, *J Clin Endocrinol Metab* 99(7):E1322-E1326, 2014.

60. Aaseth J et al: Osteoporosis and trace elements—an overview, *J Trace Elem Med Biol* 26(2-3):149-152, 2012.

61. Okyay E et al: Comparative evaluation of serum levels of main minerals and postmenopausal osteoporosis, *Maturitas* 76(4):320-325, 2013.

62. Zofkova I et al: Trace elements and bone health, *Clin Chem Lab Med* 51(8):1555-1561, 2013.

63. Body JJ et al: Non-pharmacological management of osteoporosis: a consensus of the Belgian Bone Club, *Osteoporos Int* 22(11):2769-2788, 2011.

64. Celec P, Behuliak M: Behavioural and endocrine effects of chronic cola intake, *J Psychopharmacol* 24(10):1569-1572, 2010.

65. Hallström H et al: Long-term coffee consumption in relation to fracture risk and bone mineral density in women, *Am J Epidemiol* 178(8):898-909, 2013.

66. Panday K et al: Medication-induced osteoporosis: screening and treatment strategies, *Ther Adv Musculoskel Dis* 6(5):185-202, 2014.

67. Cano-Marquina A et al: Transient regional osteoporosis, *Maturitas* 77(4):324-329, 2014.

68. Rocchietti March M et al: Transient osteoporosis of the hip, *Hip Int* 20(3):297-300, 2010.

69. Klontzas ME et al: MR imaging of transient regional osteoporosis of the hip: an update on 155 hip joints, *Eur J Radiol* 84(3):431-436, 2015.

70. Dore RK: How to prevent glucocorticoid-induced osteoporosis, *Clev Clin Med J* 77(8):529-536, 2010.

71. Henneicke H et al: Glucocorticoids and bone: local effects and systemic implications, *Trends Endocrinol Metab* 25:97-211, 2014.

72. Seibel MJ et al: Glucocorticoid-induced osteoporosis: mechanisms, management, and future perspectives, *Lancet Diabetes Endocrinol* 1(1):59-70, 2013.

73. Sutter S et al: Abnormalities in cortical bone, trabecular plates, and stiffness in postmenopausal women treated with glucocorticoids, *J Clin Endocrinol Metab* 99(11):4231-4241, 2014.

74. Khosla S: Pathogenesis of age-related bone loss in humans, *J Gerontol A Biol Sci Med Sci* 68(10):1226-1235, 2012.

75. Perrini S et al: The GH/IGF1 axis and signaling pathways in the muscle and bone: mechanism underlying age-related skeletal muscle wasting and osteoporosis, *J Endocrinol* 205(3):201-210, 2010.

76. Giusti A, Bianchi G: Treatment of primary osteoporosis in men, *Clin Interv Aging* 10:105-115, 2015.

77. Warriner AH et al: Which fractures are most attributable to osteoporosis? *J Clin Epidemiol* 64(1):46-53, 2011.

78. Hans D et al: Bone microarchitecture assessed by TBS predicts osteoporotic fractures independent of bone density: the Manitoba study, *J Bone Miner Res* 26(11):2762-2769, 2011.

79. Popp AW et al: Microstructural parameters of bone evaluated using HR-pQCT correlate with the DXA-derived cortical index and the trabecular bone score in a cohort of randomly selected premenopausal women, *PLoS One* 9(2):e88946, 2014.

80. Silva BC et al: Trabecular bone score: a noninvasive analytical method based upon the DXA image, *J Bone Miner Res* 29(3):518-530, 2014.

81. Ulivieri FM et al: Utility of the trabecular bone score (TBS) in secondary osteoporosis, *Endocrine* 47(2):435-438, 2014.

82. Link YM: The founder's lecture 2009: advances in imaging of osteoporosis and osteoarthritis, *Skelet Radiol* 39:943-955, 2010.

83. Bellido T et al: Effects of PTH on osteocyte function, *Bone* 54(2):250-257, 2013.

84. Huber BC et al: Impact of parathyroid hormone on bone marrow-derived stem cell mobilization and migration, *World J Stem Cells* 6(5):637-643, 2014.

85. Thacher TD, Clarke BL: Vitamin D deficiency, *Mayo Clin Proc* 86(1):50-60, 2011.

86. Unuvar T, Buyukgebiz A: Nutritional rickets and vitamin D deficiency in infants, children and adolescents, *Pediatr Endocrinol Rev* 7(3):283-291, 2011.

87. Bhan A et al: Osteomalacia as a result of vitamin D deficiency, *Endocrinol Metab Clin North Am* 39(2):321-331, 2010.

88. Babayev R, Nickolas TL: Can one evaluate bone disease in chronic kidney disease without a biopsy? *Curr Opin Nephrol Hypertens* 23(4):431-437, 2014.

89. Kulak CA, Dempster DW: Bone histomorphometry: a concise review for endocrinologists and clinicians, *Arq Bras Endocrinol Metabol* 54(2):87-98, 2010.

90. Ferraz-de-Souza B, Correa PH: Diagnosis and treatment of Paget's disease of bone: a mini-review, *Arq Bras Endocrinol Metabol* 57(8):577-582, 2013.

91. Michou L, Brown JP: Emerging strategies and therapies for treatment of Paget's disease of bone, *Drug Dis Devel Ther* 5:225-239, 2011.

92. Cundy T, Reid IR: Paget's disease of bone, *Clin Biochem* 45(1-2):43-48, 2012.

93. Galson DL, Roodman GD: Pathobiology of Paget's disease of bone, *J Bone Metab* 21(2):85-98, 2014.

94. Ralston SH, Layfield R: Pathogenesis of Paget disease of bone, *Calcif Tissue Int* 91(2):97-113, 2012.

95. Roodman GD: Insights into the pathogenesis of Paget's disease, *Ann N Y Acad Sci* 1192:176-180, 2010.

96. Visconti MR et al: Mutations of SQSTM1 are associated with severity and clinical outcome in Paget disease of bone, *J Bone Miner Res* 25(11):2368-2373, 2010.

97. Chung PY, Van Hul W: Paget's disease of bone: evidence for complex pathogenic interactions, *Semin Arthritis Rheum* 41(5):619-641, 2012.

98. Brandi ML: Current treatment approaches for Paget's disease of bone, *Discov Med* 10(52):209-212, 2010.

99. Baykan EK et al: Efficacy of zoledronic acid treatment in Paget disease of bone, *Osteoporos Int* 25(9):2221-2223, 2014.

100. Bolland MJ, Cundy T: Republished: Paget's disease of bone: clinical review and update, *Postgrad Med J* 90(1064):328-331, 2014.

101. Seton M: Paget disease of bone: diagnosis and drug therapy, *Cleve Clin J Med* 80(7):452-462, 2013.

102. Wat WZ: Current perspectives on bisphosphonate treatment in Paget's disease of bone, *Ther Clin Risk Manag* 10:977-983, 2014.

103. Romanò CL et al: Bone and joint infections in adults: a comprehensive classification proposal, *Eur Orthop Traumatol* 1(6):207-217, 2011.

104. Stern SM, Ferguson PJ: Autoinflammatory bone diseases, *Rheum Dis Clin North Am* 39(4):735-749, 2013.

105. Jorge LS et al: Osteomyelitis: a current challenge, *Braz J Infect Dis* 14:310-315, 2010.

106. Kim BN et al: Oral antibiotic treatment of staphylococcal bone and joint infections in adults, *J Antimicrob Chemother* 69(2):309-322, 2014.

107. Wright JA, Nair SP: Interaction of staphylococci with bone, *Int J Med Microbiol* 300(2-3):193-204, 2010.

108. Aman AJ, Adhikari RP: Staphylococcal biocomponent pore-forming toxins: targets for prophylaxis, *Toxins (Basel)* 6(3):950-972, 2014.

109. Chung PY, Toh YS: Anti-biofilm: recent breakthrough against multi-drug resistant *Staphylococcus aureus*, *Pathog Dis* 79(3):231-239, 2014.

110. Dapunt U et al: The macrophage inflammatory proteins MIP1α (CCL3) and MIP2α (CXCL2) in implant-associated osteomyelitis: linking inflammation to bone degradation, *Mediators Inflamm* 2014:728619, 2014.

111. Sanchez CJ Jr et al: *Staphylococcus aureus* biofilms decrease osteoblast viability, inhibits osteogenic differentiation, and increases bone resorption in vitro, *BMC Musculoskelet Disord* 14:187, 2013.

112. Prieto-Pérez L et al: Osteomyelitis: a descriptive study, *Clin Orthop Surg* 6(1):20-25, 2014.

113. Gotthardt M et al: Imaging of inflammation by PET, conventional scintigraphy, and other imaging techniques, *J Nucl Med Technol* 41(3):157-169, 2013.

114. Conterno LO, Turchi MD: Antibiotics for treating chronic osteomyelitis in adults, *Cochrane Database Syst Rev* 9:CD004439, 2013.

115. McLaren JS et al: A biodegradable antibiotic-impregnated scaffold to prevent osteomyelitis in a contaminated in vivo bone defect model, *Eur Cell Mater* 27:332-349, 2014.

116. Losina E et al: Lifetime risk and age at diagnosis of symptomatic knee osteoarthritis in the US, *Arthritis Care Res (Hoboken)* 65(5):703-711, 2013.

117. Evangelou E et al: Meta-analysis of genome-wide association studies confirms a susceptibility locus for knee osteoarthritis on chromosome 7q22, *Ann Rheum Dis* 70(2):349-355, 2011.

118. Tsezou A: Osteoarthritis year in review 2014: genetics and genomics, *Osteoarthritis Cartilage* 22(12):2017-2024, 2014.

119. Andriacchi TP et al: A systems view of risk factors for knee osteoarthritis reveals insights into the pathogenesis of the disease, *Ann Biomed Eng* 43(2):376-387, 2015.

120. Buckwalter JA et al: The roles of mechanical stresses in the pathogenesis of osteoarthritis: implications for treatment of joint injuries, *Cartilage* 4(4):286-294, 2013.

121. Orlowsky EW, Kraus VB: The role of innate immunity in osteoarthritis: when our first line of defense goes on the offensive, *J Rheumatol* 42(3): 363-371, 2015.

122. Sokolove J, Lepus CM: Role of inflammation in the pathogenesis of osteoarthritis: latest findings and interpretations, *Ther Adv Musculoskelet Dis* 5(2):77-94, 2013.

123. Karlsson MK et al: Patients with knee osteoarthritis have a phenotype with higher bone mass, higher fat mass, and lower lean body mass, *Clin Orthop Relat Res* 473(1):258-264, 2015.

124. Losina E et al: Impact of obesity and knee osteoarthritis on morbidity and mortality in older Americans, *Ann Intern Med* 154(4):217-226, 2011.

125. Silverwood V et al: Current evidence on factors for knee osteoarthritis in older adults: a systematic review and meta-analysis, *Osteoarthritis Cartilage* 23(4):507-515, 2015.

126. Wang X et al: Metabolic triggered inflammation in osteoarthritis, *Osteoarthritis Cartilage* 23(1): 22-30, 2015.

127. Dare D, Rodeo S: Mechanisms of post-traumatic osteoarthritis after ACL injury, *Curr Rheumatol Rep* 16(10):448, 2014.

128. Stein V et al: Pattern of joint damage in persons with knee osteoarthritis and concomitant ACL tears, *Rheumatol Int* 32(5):1197-1208, 2013.

129. Amoako AO, Pujalte GA: Osteoarthritis in young, active, and athletic individuals, *Clin Med Insights Arthritis Musculoskel Disord* 7:27-32, 2014.

130. Hall M et al: Synovial pathology on ultrasound correlates with the severity of radiographic knee osteoarthritis more than with symptoms, *Osteoarthritis Cartilage* 22(10):1627-1633, 2014.

131. Haugen IK et al: Increasing synovitis and bone marrow lesions are associated with incident joint tenderness in hand osteoarthritis, *Ann Rheum Dis* 2015 Mar 9. [Epub ahead of print]

132. Kapoor M et al: Role of proinflammatory cytokines in the pathophysiology of osteoarthritis, *Nat Rev Rheumatol* 7:33-42, 2011.

133. van der Kraan PM: Age-related alterations in TGF beta signaling as a causal factor of cartilage degeneration in osteoarthritis, *Biomed Mater Eng* 24(1 Suppl):75-80, 2014.

134. Clement T et al: Identification of new microRNAs targeting genes regulating the Pi/PPi balance in chondrocytes, *Biomed Mater Eng* 24(1 Suppl): 3-16, 2014.

135. Trzeciak T, Czarny-Ratajczak M: MicroRNAs: Important epigenetic regulators in osteoarthritis, *Curr Genomics* 15(6):481-484, 2014.

136. van der Kraan PM: Age-related alterations in TGF beta signaling as a causal factor of cartilage degeneration in osteoarthritis, *Biomed Mater Eng* 24(1 Suppl):75-80, 2014.

137. Mrosewski I et al: Regulation of osteoarthritis-associated key mediators by TNFα and IL-10; effects of IL-10 overexpression in human synovial fibroblasts and a synovial cell line, *Cell Tissue Res* 357(1):207-223, 2014.

138. Sauerschnig M et al: Diverse expression of selected cytokines and proteinases in synovial fluid obtained from osteoarthritic and healthy human knee joints, *Eur J Med Res* 19(1):65-71, 2014.

139. Francin P-J et al: Association between adiponectin and cartilage degradation in human osteoarthritis, *Osteoarthritis Cartilage* 22(3):519-526, 2014.

140. Findlay DM, Atkins GJ: Osteoblast-chondrocyte interactions in osteoarthritis, *Curr Osteoporos Rep* 12(1):127-134, 2014.

141. Li G et al: Subchondral bone in osteoarthritis: insight into risk factors and microstructural changes, *Arthritis Res Ther* 15:223, 2013.

142. Liu-Bryan R: Synovium and the innate inflammatory network in osteoarthritis progression, *Curr Rheumatol Rep* 15(5):323, 2013.

143. Felson DT et al: Valgus malalignment is a risk factor for lateral knee osteoarthritis incidence and progression: findings from the Multicenter Osteoarthritis Study and the Osteoarthritis Initiative, *Arthritis Rheum* 65(2):355-362, 2013.

144. Stief F et al: Effect of lower limb malalignment in the frontal plane on transverse plane mechanics during gait in young individuals with varus knee alignment, *Knee* 21(3):688-693, 2014.

145. Felson DT et al: Physical activity, alignment and knee osteoarthritis: data from MOST and the OAI, *Osteoarthritis Cartilage* 21(6):789-795, 2013.

146. Fransen M et al: Exercise for osteoarthritis of the knee, *Cochrane Database Syst Rev* 1:CD004376, 2015.

147. Juhl C et al: Impact of exercise type and dose on pain and disability in knee osteoarthritis: a systematic review and meta-regression analysis of randomized controlled trials, *Arthritis Rheumatol* 66(3):622-636, 2014.

148. Koonce RC, Bravman JT: Obesity and osteoarthritis: more than just wear and tear, *J Am Acad Orthop Surg* 21(3):161-169, 2013.

149. Messier SP et al: Effects of intensive diet and exercise on knee joint loads, inflammation, and clinical outcomes among overweight and obese adults with knee osteoarthritis, *J Am Med Assoc* 310(12):1263-1273, 2013.

150. Chyu MC et al: Complementary and alternative exercises for management of osteoarthritis, *Arthritis* 2011:364319, 2011.

151. Yan JH et al: Efficacy of Tai Chi on pain, stiffness and function in patients with osteoarthritis: a meta-analysis, *PLoS One* 8(4):e61671, 2013.

152. Raja K, Dewan N: Efficacy of knee braces and foot orthoses in conservative management of knee osteoarthritis: a systematic review, *Am J Phys Med Rehabil* 90(3):247-262, 2011.

153. Fransen M et al: Glucosamine and chondroitin for knee osteoarthritis: a double-blind randomized placebo-controlled clinical trial evaluating single and combination regimens, *Ann Rheum Dis* 74(5):851-858, 2015.

154. Fibel KH et al: State-of-the-art management of knee osteoarthritis, *World J Clin Cases* 3(2): 89-101, 2015.

155. Ayhan E et al: Intraarticular injections (corticosteroid, hyaluronic acid, platelet rich plasma) for the knee osteoarthritis, *World J Orthop* 5(3):351-361, 2014.

156. Bannuru RR et al: Comparative effectiveness of pharmacologic interventions for knee osteoarthritis: a systematic review and network meta-analysis, *Arch Int Med* 162(1):203, 2015.

157. Sundman EA et al: The anti-inflammatory and matrix restorative mechanisms of platelet-rich plasma in osteoarthritis, *Am J Sports Med* 42(1): 35-41, 2014.

158. Huang Z et al: Effectiveness of low-level laser therapy in patients with knee osteoarthritis: a systemic review and meta-analysis, *Osteoarthritis Cartilage* 2015 Apr 23. [Epub ahead of print.]

159. Murphy LB et al: One in four people may develop symptomatic hip osteoarthritis in his or her lifetime, *Osteoarthritis Cartilage* 18(11):1372-1379, 2010.

160. Kurtz SM et al: Impact of the economic downturn on total joint replacement demand in the United States: updated projections to 2021, *J Bone Joint Surg Am* 96(8):624-630, 2014.

161. Aletaha D et al: The 2010 American College of Rheumatology/European League Against Rheumatism classification criteria for rheumatoid arthritis: an American College of Rheumatology/ European League Against Rheumatism collaborative initiative, *Arthritis Rheum* 62(9): 2569-2581, 2010.

162. Klein K et al: Epigenetic contributions in the development of rheumatoid arthritis, *Arthritis Res Ther* 14(6):227, 2012.

163. Korczowska I: Rheumatoid arthritis susceptibility genes: an overview, *World J Orthop* 5(4):544-549, 2014.

164. Mohan VK et al: Association of susceptible genetic markers and autoantibodies in rheumatoid arthritis, *J Genet* 93(2):597-605, 2014.

165. You S et al: Identification of key regulators for the migration and invasion of rheumatoid synoviocytes through a systems approach, *Proc Natl Acad Sci U S A* 111(1):550-555, 2015.

166. Choy E: Understanding the dynamics: pathways involved in the pathogenesis of rheumatoid arthritis, *Rheumatology (Oxford)* 51(Suppl 5):v3-v11. 2012.

167. Bartok B, Firestein GS: Fibroblast-like synoviocytes: key effector cells in rheumatoid arthritis, *Immunol Rev* 233(1):233-255, 2010.

168. Lefevre S et al: Role of synovial fibroblasts in rheumatoid arthritis, *Curr Pharm Des* 21(2): 130-141, 2015.

169. Gibofsky A: Overview of epidemiology, pathophysiology, and diagnosis of rheumatoid arthritis, *Am J Manag Care* 18(13 Suppl):S295-302, 2012.

170. van Heemst J et al: Fine-mapping the human leukocyte antigen locus in rheumatoid arthritis and other rheumatic diseases: identifying causal amino acid variants? *Curr Opin Rheumatol* 27(3):256-261, 2015.

171. Klein K, Gay S: Epigenetics and rheumatoid arthritis, *Curr Opin Rheumatol* 27(1):76-82, 2015.

172. Putrik P et al: Lower education and living in countries with lower wealth are associated with higher disease activity in rheumatoid arthritis: results from the multinational COMORA study, *Ann Rheum Dis* 2015 Jan 28. [Epub ahead of print.]

173. Song YW, Kang EH: Autoantibodies in rheumatoid arthritis: rheumatoid factors and anticitrullinated protein antibodies, *Q J Med* 103(3):139-146, 2010.

174. Valesini G et al: Citrullination and autoimmunity, *Autoimmun Rev* 14(6):490-497, 2015.

175. Gong G et al: Pain experiences and self-management strategies among middle-aged and older adults with arthritis, *J Clin Nurs* 22(13-14):1857-1869, 2013.

176. Ntatsaki E et al: Systemic rheumatoid vasculitis in the era of modern immunosuppressive therapy, *Rheumatology (Oxford)* 53(1):145-152, 2015.

177. Goronzy JJ, Weyand CM: Developments in the scientific understanding of rheumatoid arthritis, *Arthritis Res Ther* 11(5):249, 2009.

178. Pruijn GJ et al: The use of citrullinated peptides and proteins for the diagnosis of rheumatoid arthritis, *Arthritis Res Ther* 12(1):203, 2010.

179. Raychaudhuri SP, Deodhar A: The classification and diagnostic criteria of ankylosing spondylitis, *J Autoimmun* Feb-Mar(48-19):128-133, 2014.

180. Dean L et al: Global prevalence of ankylosing spondylitis, *Rheumatology (Oxford)* 53(4):650-657, 2014.

181. Colbert RA et al: From HLA-B27 to spondyloarthritis: a journey through the ER, *Immunol Rev* 233(1):181-202, 2010.

182. Colbert RA et al: HLA-B27 misfolding and ankylosing spondylitis, *Mol Immunol* 57(1):44-51, 2015.

183. Khan MA: Polymorphism of HLA-B27: 105 subtypes currently known, *Curr Rheumatol Rep* 15(10):362, 2013.

184. Rossou E, Sultana S: Early spondyloarthropathies in multiracial society: differences between gender, race, and disease subgroups with regard to symptoms at presentation, main problem that the disease is causing to patients, and employment status, *Rheumatol Int* 32(6):1597-1604, 2012.

185. Rozin AP et al: Seronegative polyarthritis as severe systemic disease, *Neth J Med* 68(6):236-241, 2010.

186. Haroon N, Inman RD: Ankylosing spondylitis: new criteria, new treatments, *Bull NYU Hosp Jt Dis* 68(3):171-174, 2010.

187. Rudwaleit M et al: The development of assessment of SpondyloArthritis International Society classification criteria for axial spondyloarthritis (part II): validation and final selection, *Ann Rheum Dis* 68(6):777-783, 2009.

188. Golder V, Schachna L: Ankylosing spondylitis: an update, *Austral Fam Phys* 42(11):780-784, 2013.

189. O'Dwyer T et al: Exercise therapy for spondyloarthropathies: a systematic review, *Rheumatol Int* 34(7):887-902, 2014.

190. Braun J et al: Emerging drugs for the treatment of axial and peripheral spondyloarthritis, *Expert Opin Emerg Drugs* 20(1):1-14, 2015.

191. Van den Bosch F, Dodhar A: Treatment of spondyloarthritis beyond TNF-alpha blockade, *Best Pract Res Clin Rheumatol* 28(5):819-827, 2014.

192. Rees F et al: Optimizing current treatment of gout, *Nat Rev Rheumatol* 10(5):271-283, 2014.

193. Roddy E, Choi HK: Epidemiology of gout, *Rheum Dis Clin North Am* 40(2):155-175, 2014.

194. Merriman TR et al: The genetic basis of gout, *Rheum Dis Clin North Am* 40(2):279-290, 2014.

195. Richette P, Bardin T: Gout, *Lancet* 375(9711):318-328, 2010.

196. Sriranganathan MK et al: Interventions for tophi in gout, *Cochrane Database Syst Rev* 10:CD010069, 2014.

197. Perez-Ruiz F et al: Tophaceous gout and high level of hyperuricaemia are both associated with increased risk of mortality in patients with gout, *Ann Rheum Dis* 73:177-182, 2014.

198. VanItallie TB: Gout: epitome of painful arthritis, *Metabolism* 59(Suppl 1):S32-S36, 2010.

199. Dirken-Heukensfeldt KJ et al: Clinical features of women with gout arthritis: a systemic review, *Clin Rheumatol* 29(6):575-582, 2010.

200. Perez-Ruiz F et al: A review of uric acid, crystal deposition disease, and gout, *Adv Ther* 32:31-41, 2015.

201. Chowalloor PV et al: Imaging in gout: a review of recent developments, *Ther Adv Musculoskelet Med* 6(4):131-143, 2014.

202. Sivera F et al: Multinational evidence-based recommendations for the diagnosis and management of gout: integrating systematic literature review and expert opinion of a broad panel of rheumatologists in the 3e initiative, *Ann Rheum Dis* 73(2):328-335, 2014.

203. Crittendon DB, Pillinger MH: The year in gout: a walk through the 2012 ACR treatment guidelines, *Bull Hosp Joint Dis* 71(3):189-193, 2013.

204. Edwards NL, So A: Emerging therapies for gout, *Rheum Dis Clin North Am* 40(2):375-387, 2014.

205. Moi JH et al: Lifestyle interventions for gout, *Cochrane Database Syst Rev* 11:CD010519, 2013.

206. Kanbara A et al: Urine alkalization facilitates uric acid excretion, *Nutr J* 9:45, 2010.

207. Skalsky AJ, McDonald CM: Prevention and management of limb contractures in neuromuscular diseases, *Phys Med Rehabil Clin North Am* 23(3):675-687, 2012.

208. Larsman P et al: Psychosocial work conditions, perceived stress, perceived muscular tension, and neck/shoulder symptoms among medical secretaries, *Int Arch Occup Environ Health* 86(1):57-63, 2013.

209. Powers SK: Can antioxidants protect against disuse muscle atrophy? *Sports Med* 44(Suppl 2):S155-165, 2014.

210. Brooks NE, Myburgh KH: Skeletal muscle wasting with disuse atrophy is multi-dimensional: the response and interaction of myonuclei, satellite cells and signaling pathways, *Front Physiol* 5:99, 2014.

211. Pernambuco AP et al: Increased levels of IL-17A in patients with fibromyalgia, *Clin Exp Rheumatol* 31(6 Suppl 79):S60-63, 2013.

212. Rodriguez-Pintò I et al: Fibromyalgia and cytokines, *Immunol Lett* 161(2):200-203, 2014.

213. Sturgill J et al: Unique cytokine signature in the plasma of patients with fibromyalgia, *J Immunol Res* 2014:938576, 2014.

214. Clauw DJ: Fibromyalgia: a clinical review, *J Am Med Assoc* 311(15):1547-1555, 2014.

215. Arnold LM et al: The fibromyalgia family study: a genome-wide linkage scan study, *Arthritis Rheum* 65(4):1122-1128, 2013.

216. Diatchenko L et al: The phenotypic and genetic signatures of common musculoskeletal pain conditions, *Nat Rev Rheumatol* 9(6):340-350, 2013.

217. Docamp E et al: Genome-wide analysis of single nucleotide polymorphisms and copy number variants in fibromyalgia suggest a role for the central nervous system, *Pain* 15(6):1102-1109, 2014.

218. Wolfe F et al: Fibromyalgia and physical trauma: the concepts we invent, *J Rheumatol* 41(9):1737-1745, 2014.

219. Cagnie B et al: Central sensitization in fibromyalgia? A systematic review on structural and functional brain MRI, *Semin Arthritis Rheum* 44(1):68-75, 2014.

220. Harbeck B et al: High prevalence of fibromyalgia-associated symptoms in patients with hypothalamic-pituitary disorders, *Clin Exp Rheumatol* 31(6 Suppl 79):S16-21, 2013.

221. Wolfe F et al: The American College of Rheumatology preliminary diagnostic criteria for fibromyalgia and measurement of symptom severity, *Arthritis Care Res (Hoboken)* 62(5):600-610, 2010.

222. Wolfe F et al: Fibromyalgia criteria and severity scales for clinical and epidemiological studies: a modification of the ACR preliminary diagnostic criteria for fibromyalgia, *J Rheumatol* 38(6):1113-1122, 2011.

223. Theadom A et al: Mind and body for fibromyalgia, *Cochrane Database Syst Rev* 4:CD001980, 2015.

224. Bidone JM et al: Aquatic exercise training for fibromyalgia, *Cochrane Database Syst Rev* 10:CD011336, 2014.

225. Bidone J et al: Exercise for adults with fibromyalgia: an umbrella systematic review with synthesis of best evidence, *Curr Rheumatol Rev* 10(1):45-79, 2014.

226. O'Connor SR et al: Walking exercise for chronic musculoskeletal pain: systemic review and meta-analysis, *Arch Phys Med Rehabil* 96(4):724-734, 2014.

227. Aerenhouts D et al: Sleep characteristics, exercise capacity and physical activity in patients with chronic fatigue syndrome, *Disabil Rehabil* 16:1-7, 2014.

228. Kallestad H et al: The role of insomnia in the treatment of chronic fatigue, *J Psychosom Res* 78(5):427-432, 2015.

229. Rosenblum H et al: The common immunogenic etiology of chronic fatigue syndrome: from infections to vaccines via adjuvants to the ASIA syndrome, *Infect Dis Clin North Am* 25:851-863, 2011.

230. Brown AE et al: Abnormalities of AMPK activation and glucose uptake in cultured skeletal muscle cells from individuals with chronic fatigue syndrome, *PLoS One* 10(4):e0122982, 2015.

231. Gambuzza ME et al: The role of Toll-like receptors in chronic fatigue syndrome/myalgic encephalomyelitis: a new promising therapeutic approach? *CNS Neurol Disord Drug Targets* 2015 Mar 25. [Epub ahead of print.] Accessed April 10, 2015.

232. Kempke S et al: Effects of early childhood trauma on hypothalamic-pituitary-adrenal axis function in patients with chronic fatigue syndrome, *Psychoneuroendocrinology* 52:14-21, 2015.

233. Romano GE et al: Fibromyalgia and chronic fatigue: the underlying biology and related theoretical issues, *Adv Psychosom Med* 34:61-77, 2015.

234. Committee on the Diagnostic Criteria for Myalgic Encephalomyelitis/Chronic Fatigue Syndrome, Board on the Health of Select Populations, Institute of Medicine: *Beyond myalgic encephalomyelitis/chronic fatigue syndrome: redefining and illness*, Washington, DC, 2015, National Academies Press.

235. Bourke J: Fibromyalgia and chronic fatigue syndrome: management issues, *Adv Psychosom Med* 34:78-91, 2015.

236. Olson K et al: The nature of fatigue in chronic fatigue syndrome, *Qual Health Res* 2015 Feb 26. [Epub ahead of print.]

237. Drost G et al: Myotonic discharges discriminate chloride from sodium muscle channelopathies, *Neuromuscul Disord* 25(1):73-80, 2015.

238. Statland JM, Barohn RJ: Muscle channelopathies: the nondystrophic myotonias and periodic paralyses, *Continuum (Minneap Minn)* 19(6 Muscle Disease):1598-1614, 2013.

239. Novak KR et al: Sodium channel slow inactivation as a therapeutic target for myotonia congenita, *Ann Neurol* 77(2):320-322, 2015.

240. Sharp L, Trivedi JR: Treatment and management of neuromuscular channelopathies, *Curr Treat Options Neurol* 16(10):313, 2014.

241. Statland J et al: Muscle channelopathies, *Neurol Clin* 32(3):601-615, 2014.

242. Catterall WA: Voltage-gated calcium channels, *Cold Spring Harb Perspect Biol* 3(8):a003947, 2011.

243. Cheng C-J et al: Extracellular potassium homeostasis: insights from hypokalemic periodic paralysis, *Semin Nephrol* 33(3):237-247, 2013.

244. Lin SH, Huang C-L: Mechanism of thyrotoxic periodic paralysis, *J Am Soc Nephrol* 23(6):985-988, 2012.

245. Rolim AL et al: Ion channelopathies in endocrinology: recent genetic findings and pathophysiological insights, *Arq Bras Endocrinol Metabol* 54(8):673-681, 2010.

246. Jurkat-Rott K et al: Sodium channelopathies of skeletal muscle result from gain or loss of function, *Pflugers Arch Eur J Physiol* 460:239-248, 2010.

247. Charles G et al: Characterization of hyperkalemic periodic paralysis: a survey of genetically diagnosed individuals, *J Neurol* 260(10):2606-2613, 2013.

248. Das AM et al: Inborn errors of energy metabolism associated with myopathies, *J Biomed Biotechnol* 2010:340849, 2010.

249. Kitaoka Y: McArdle disease and exercise physiology, *Biology* 3:157-166, 2014.

250. Kitaoka Y et al: Monocarboxylate transporter and lactate metabolism, *J Phys Fitness Sports Med* 1:247-252, 2012.

251. Bhengu L et al: Diagnosis and management of Pompe disease, *S Afr Med J* 104(4):273-274, 2014.

252. Kishnani PS et al: The new era of Pompe disease: advances in the detection, understanding of the phenotypic spectrum, pathophysiology and management, *Am J Genet C Semin Med Genet* 160C(1):1-7, 2012.

253. Werneck LC et al: Muscle biopsy in Pompe disease, *Arq Nueropsiquiatr* 71(5):284-289, 2013.

254. Lachmann R, Schoser B: The clinical relevance of outcomes used in late-onset Pompe disease: can we do better? *Orphanet J Rare Dis* 8:160, 2013.

255. Pascual JM, Roe CR: Systemic metabolic abnormalities in adult-onset acid maltase deficiency: beyond muscle glycogen accumulation, *J Am Med Assoc Neuro* 70(6):756-763, 2013.

256. Hayes LD et al: Genetic predictors of adenosine monophosphate deaminase deficiency, *J Sports Medicine Doping Stud* 3:124, 2014.

257. Bonnefont JP et al: Long-term follow-up of bezafibrate treatment in patients with the myopathic form of carnitine palmitoyltransferase 2 deficiency, *Clin Pharmacol Ther* 88(1):101-108, 2010.

258. Lu X et al: Discovery of new biomarkers of idiopathic inflammatory myopathy, *Clin Chim Acta* 444:117-125, 2015.

259. van der Kooi AJ, de Visser M: Idiopathic inflammatory myopathies, *Handb Clin Neurol* 119:495-512, 2014.

260. Dobloug GC et al: High prevalence of inclusion body myositis in Norway: a population-based clinical epidemiology study, *Eur J Neurol* 22(4):672-e41, 2015.

261. Meyer A et al: Incidence and prevalence of inflammatory myopathies: a systematic review, *Rheumatology (Oxford)* 54(1):50-63, 2015.

262. Rothwell S et al: Entering a new phase of immunogenetics in the idiopathic inflammatory myopathies, *Curr Opin Rheumatol* 25(6):735-741, 2013.

263. Tansley S, Gunawardena H: The evolving spectrum of polymyositis and dermatomyositis—moving towards clinicoserological syndromes: a critical review, *Clin Rev Allergy Immunol* 47(3):264-273, 2014.

264. Auriemma M et al: Cutaneous signs of classical dermatomyositis, *G Ital Dermatol Venereol* 149(5):505-517, 2014.

265. Dalakas MC: Inflammatory muscle diseases: a critical review on pathogenesis and therapies, *Curr Opin Pharmacol* 10(3):346-352, 2010.

266. Carstens PO, Schmidt J: Diagnosis, pathogenesis and treatment of myositis: recent advances, *Clin Exp Immunol* 175(3):349-358, 2014.

267. Dalakas MC: Immunotherapy of myositis: issues, concerns and future prospects, *Nat Rev Rheumatol* 6(3):129-137, 2010.

268. Dimachkie MM, Barohn RJ: Inclusion body myositis, *Curr Neurol Neurosci Rep* 13(1):321, 2013.

269. Schmidt J, Dalakas MC: Inclusion body myositis: from immunopathology and degenerative mechanisms to treatment perspectives, *Expert Rev Clin Immunol* 9(11):1125-1133, 2013.

270. Mastaglia FL, Needham M: Inclusion body myositis: a review of clinical and genetic aspects, diagnostic criteria and therapeutic approaches, *J Clin Neurosci* 22(1):6-13, 2015.

271. Iaccarino L et al: The clinical features, diagnosis and classification of dermatomyositis, *J Autoimmun* 48-49:122-127, 2014.

272. Schiffenbauer A: Imaging: seeing muscle in new ways, *Curr Opin Rheumatol* 25(6):712-716, 2014.

273. Kley RA et al: Creatine for treating muscle disorders, *Cochrane Database Syst Rev* 6:CD0044760, 2013.

274. Kuncl RW: Agents and mechanisms of toxic myopathy, *Curr Opin Neurol* 22(5):506-515, 2009.

275. Pasnoor M et al: Toxic myopathies, *Neurol Clin* 32:647-670, 2014.

276. Peller PJ: Role of positron emission tomography/computed tomography in bone malignancies, *Radiol Clin North Am* 51:845-864, 2013.

277. Du WX et al: Serum bone-specific alkaline phosphatase as a biomarker for osseous metastases in patients with malignant carcinomas: a systematic review and meta-analysis, *J Cancer Res Ther* 10(Suppl C):140-143, 2014.

278. Traina F et al: Current concepts in the biopsy of musculoskeletal tumors, *J Bone Joint Surg Am* 97(1):e7, 2015.

279. Berner K et al: Time-trends on incidence and survival in a nationwide and unselected cohort of patients with skeletal osteosarcoma, *Acta Oncol* 54(1):25-33, 2015.

280. HaDuong JH et al: Sarcomas, *Pediatr Clin North Am* 62:179-200, 2015.

281. Burningham Z et al: The epidemiology of sarcoma, *Clin Sarcoma Res* 2(1):14, 2012.

282. Moore DD, Luu HH: Osteosarcoma, *Cancer Treat Res* 162:65-92, 2014.

283. Green JT, Mills AM: Osteogenic tumors of bone, *Semin Diagn Pathol* 31(1):21-29, 2014.

284. Lietman SA, Joyce MJ: Bone sarcomas: overview of management, with a focus on surgical treatment considerations, *Clev Clin J Med* 77(Suppl 1):S8-S12, 2010.

285. Knops RR et al: The volume effect in paediatric oncology: a systematic review, *Ann Oncol* 24(7):1749-1753, 2013.

286. Luetke A et al: Osteosarcoma treatment—where do we stand? A state of the art review, *Cancer Treat Rev* 40(4):523-532, 2014.

287. Forscher C et al: Targeted therapy for osteosarcomas, *Biologics* 8:91-105, 2014.

288. Kansara M et al: Translational biology of osteosarcoma, *Nat Rev Cancer* 14(11):722-735, 2014.

289. Choi EY et al: Ewing sarcoma, *Semin Diagn Pathol* 31(1):39-47, 2014.

290. Moore DD, Haydin RC: Ewing's sarcoma of bone, *Cancer Treat Res* 162:93-115, 2014.

291. Leddy LR, Holmes RE: Chondrosarcoma of bone, *Cancer Treat Res* 162:117-130, 2014.

292. Bindiganaville S et al: Long-term outcome of chondrosarcoma: a single institutional experience, *Cancer Res Treat* 2015 Feb 12. [Epub ahead of print.]

293. Choi BB et al: MR differentiation of low-grade chondrosarcoma from enchondroma, *Clin Imaging* 37(3):542-547, 2013.

294. Logie CI et al: Chondrosarcoma: a diagnostic imager's guide to decision making and patient management, *Semin Musculoskelet Radiol* 17(2):101-115, 2013.

295. Heymann D, Rédini F: Targeted therapies for bone sarcomas, *Bonekey Rep* 2:378, 2013.

296. Radaelli S et al: Emerging therapies for adult soft tissue sarcoma, *Expert Rev Anticancer Ther* 14(6):689-704, 2014.

297. Bao Q et al: Recombinant TIMP-1-GPI inhibits growth of fibrosarcoma and enhances tumor sensitivity to doxorubicin, *Target Oncol* 9(3):251-261, 2014.

298. Li L et al: Injectable and biodegradable pH-responsive hydrogels for localized and sustained treatment of human fibrosarcoma, *ACS Appl Mater Interfaces* 7(15):8033-8040, 2015.

299. van der Heijden L et al: The clinical approach toward giant cell tumor of bone, *Oncologist* 19(5):550-561, 2014.

300. Raskin KA et al: Giant cell tumor of bone, *J Am Acad Orthop Surg* 21(2):118-126, 2013.

301. Lewin J, Thomas D: Denosumab: a new treatment option for giant cell tumor of bone, *Drugs Today (Barc)* 49(11):693-700, 2013.

302. Xu SF et al: Denosumab and giant cell tumor of bone—a review and future management considerations, *Curr Oncol* 20(5):e442-3447, 2013.

303. Zanola A et al: Rhabdomyosarcomas: an overview on the experimental animal models, *J Cell Mol Med* 16(7):1377-1391, 2012.

304. Sultan I et al: Comparing adult and pediatric rhabdomyosarcomas in the surveillance, epidemiology and end results program, 1973 to 2005: an analysis of 2600 patients, *J Clin Oncol* 27(20):3391-3397, 2009.

40

Alterations of Musculoskeletal Function in Children

Kristen Lee Carroll, Lynne M. Kerr, and Kathryn L. McCance

EVOLVE WEBSITE

CHAPTER OUTLINE

Musculoskeletal problems in children can be either congenital or acquired. Both pathology and treatment can cause long-term sequelae because of the growing nature of the immature skeleton. In addition, the emotional trauma of an injured or malformed child is substantial and requires that careful attention be paid to the emotional health of both the child and his or her family.

CONGENITAL DEFECTS

Clubfoot

Clubfoot describes a range of foot deformities in which the foot turns inward and downward. It can affect one or both feet. Technically called congenital equinovarus (Table 40-1), the heel is positioned varus (inwardly deviated) and equinus (plantar flexed) (Figures 40-1 and 40-2). The clubfoot deformity can be positional (correctable passively), idiopathic, or teratologic (as a result of another syndrome, such as spina bifida). The idiopathic clubfoot occurs in 1 per 1000 live births, with males twice as likely as females to be affected.

The clubfoot deformity can be corrected by an above-knee casting regimen popularized by Ponseti.[1] In almost 90% of idiopathic and up to 70% of teratologic clubfeet, the Ponseti method of serial casting infants' feet is effective (see Figure 40-1, *B*). The hindfoot equinus portion of the deformity often requires lengthening of the Achilles tendon, which can be performed in a clinic with the use of a local anesthetic. Achilles tenotomy (complete transection of the tendon) can be safely performed with local anesthetic until 8 or 9 months after birth. After this age, a formal lengthening and repair procedure using a general anesthetic is required. Bracing is required until age 3.

Idiopathic feet resistant to these procedures require repeat casting or, in very rare cases, a surgical posteromedial release (PMR). The posteromedial release includes lengthening of the Achilles, posterior tibialis, and flexor tendons, and surgical release of the capsules of the ankle, subtalar, and midfoot joints. Teratologic clubfeet require surgical intervention more often than idiopathic clubfeet (see Figure 40-1, *B*) and more prolonged bracing, often through childhood. The Ponseti technique has revolutionized clubfoot treatment around the world. The ability to correct such a crippling deformity without the need for surgery has helped countless children.[2]

Developmental Dysplasia of the Hip

Developmental dysplasia of the hip (DDH) describes imperfect development of the hip joint and can affect the femur, the acetabulum, or both (Figure 40-3). Although most often present congenitally, dysplasia may develop later in the newborn or infant period. Like clubfoot, DDH can be idiopathic or teratologic. Teratologic hips (i.e., those attributable to another disorder such as cerebral palsy, spina bifida, or arthrogryposis) are more difficult to treat and often need operative intervention. In idiopathic DDH, 70% of cases involve the left side only and 10% to 15% are bilateral. Girls are four times as likely as boys to be affected. Positive family history, breech presentation, and oligohydramnios (low levels of intrauterine fluid) all predispose children to DDH. Children in these groups are considered high risk and must be carefully evaluated with physical examination and, possibly, ultrasound.[3,3A] Variants of idiopathic DDH are dislocated hip (no contact between the femoral head and acetabulum), subluxated hip (partial contact only), and acetabular dysplasia (the femoral head is

TABLE 40-1 Terms Used to Describe Foot Abnormalities

Term	Definition
Position*	
Abduction	Lateral deviation away from the midline of the body
Adduction	Lateral deviation toward the midline of the body
Eversion	Twisting of the foot outward along its long axis
Inversion	Twisting of the foot inward on its long axis
Dorsiflexion	Bending of the foot upward and backward
Plantar flexion	Bending of the foot downward and forward
Abnormality	
Talipes	Congenital abnormality of the foot (clubfoot)
Pes	Acquired deformity of the foot
Varus	Inversion and adduction of the heel and forefoot
Valgus	Eversion and abduction of the heel and forefoot
Equinus	Plantar flexion of the foot in which the heel is lower than the toes
Calcaneus	Dorsiflexion of the foot in which the heel is lower than the toes
Planus	Flattening of the medial longitudinal arch of the foot (flatfoot)
Cavus	Elevation of the medial longitudinal arch of the foot (high arch)
Equinovarus	Coexistent equinus and varus deformities
Calcaneovarus	Coexistent calcaneus and varus deformities
Equinovalgus	Coexistent equinus and valgus deformities
Calcaneovalgus	Coexistent calcaneus and valgus deformities

*NOTE: The positions listed can all be achieved by voluntary movement of the normal foot; an abnormality exists if the foot is fixed in one or more of the positions while at rest.

FIGURE 40-1 A, Infant with Bilateral Congenital Talipes Equinovarus. B, Ponseti Casting. (A courtesy Dr. A.E. Chudley, Section of Genetics and Metabolism, Department of Pediatrics and Child Health, Children's Hospital and University of Manitoba, Winnipeg, Manitoba, Canada. In Moore KL et al, editors: *The developing human,* ed 10, Philadelphia, 2016, Saunders.)

located properly but the acetabulum is shallow). Idiopathic instability of the hip ranges from 3 to 7 per 1000 live births, but a true dislocation is present in only 1 of 1000 live births.

Clinical examination is the mainstay of diagnosis. The examination must be performed on a relaxed infant for accuracy. Absolute indications for treatment include a positive Barlow sign (hip reduced, but dislocatable) (Figure 40-4, A) or positive Ortolani sign (hip dislocated, but reducible) (Figure 40-4, B). Other indicators for further evaluation are limitation of abduction[4] or apparent shortening of the femur (Galeazzi sign). Asymmetric skin folds at the groin also can be a clinical sign of hip pathology.

In children younger than 4 months old, bracing with a Pavlik harness is successful in 90% of DDH cases. A Barlow positive hip (hip reduced, but dislocatable) is easier to treat with a Pavlik harness, and success rates approach 95% to 98% (Figure 40-5). An Ortolani positive hip (hip dislocated, but reducible) must be followed closely with ultrasound and exam; the success rate with Pavlik harness is 70% in this situation. If a stable reduction is not attained within 2 to 3 weeks of treatment, the Pavlik harness should be abandoned and casting or surgery pursued instead. A partially reduced hip applies pressure on the rim of the acetabulum by the femoral head and can worsen dysplasia and make treatment more difficult. In older children (6 to 12 months), or those who failed bracing with a Pavlik harness, closed reduction of the hip and spica (body) casting performed using a general anesthetic are required. The spica cast is worn for 3 months. Children older than 12 months require surgery on the joint, the femur, or the acetabulum, or all three (see Figure 40-3). The incidence of good

or excellent outcome falls to only 20% by age 4, underscoring the need for early diagnosis and treatment.[5]

Osteogenesis Imperfecta

Osteogenesis imperfecta (OI; brittle bone disease) is a spectrum of disease caused by genetic mutation in the gene that encodes for type I collagen, the main component of bone and blood vessels. The Sillence classification defines six types. Types I and IV are milder forms and are inherited in an autosomal dominant pattern. Types II and III are more severe and are inherited in a recessive pattern. Types V and VI are very rare and are autosomal recessive. Children with type II often die during infancy because of extreme bone fragility.

The classic clinical manifestations of osteogenesis imperfecta (OI) are osteopenia (decreased bone mass) and an increased rate of fractures. Children can also have fatigue, pain, hearing loss, and abnormal dentition. With recurrent fractures, bone deformity (bowing) often occurs. In type III OI, the most severe form compatible with life, children have short stature and triangular faces, possibly blue sclerae, and poor dentition. Because type I collagen also is the main component of blood vessels, vascular deformity, such as aortic aneurysm, can occur. Type IV OI can be subtle with the child presenting with more normal stature and with fractures often not occurring until the child is older;

FIGURE 40-2 Idiopathic Clubfoot. Idiopathic clubfoot displaying forefoot adduction (toward midline of body) and supination (upturning) and hindfoot equinus (pointed downward). Note skin creases along arch and back of heel.

FIGURE 40-3 Hip Dysplasia in Children. Development dysplasia of the hip (DDH) with residual acetabular dysplasia. Radiographs at birth, 3, 10, and 19 years (top to bottom) show persisting dysplasia.

FIGURE 40-4 Congenital Dislocation of the Hip. A, Barlow maneuver *(left side).* With one hand pressing the symphysis in front and the sacral spine in back, lateral pressure is applied to the thigh with the thumb of the other hand while pressure is applied with the palm to the knee on the side being examined. The hip that has been flexed to 90 degrees is then adducted. A positive sign is a sensation of abnormal movement, indicating dislocation of the femoral head from the acetabulum. The hands are reversed for examining the other hip. This sign and Ortolani sign may be found only in the first weeks of life. **B,** Ortolani maneuver *(right side).* Sign of jerking into correct position. After Barlow maneuver **(A),** the hip should be abducted to about 80 degrees while the femur is lifted anteriorly with the fingers along the thigh. A positive sign is a sensation of a jerk or snap with reduction into the joint socket. (Adapted from Specht EE: *Am Fam Physician* 9:88-96, 1974.)

FIGURE 40-5 Pavlik Harness for Bilateral Hip Dislocation. (From Wheaton Brace Co., Carol Stream, Ill.)

FIGURE 40-6 Osteogenesis Imperfecta Treated with Osteotomies and Telescoping Medullary Rods. **A,** Severe deformity of both femurs. **B,** Same individual after multiple osteotomies with telescoping medullary rod fixation. **C,** Same individual 4 years later demonstrating growth of femurs, no recurrence of deformity, and elongation of rods. (Plaster casts are in place for immobilization of tibial osteotomies.) (From Crenshaw AH, editor: *Campbell's operative orthopaedics,* ed 8, vol 3, St Louis, 1992, Mosby.)

it can be misdiagnosed as child abuse. Analysis of skin fibroblasts is diagnostic in 85% of children with OI.

Treatment is a combination of medical and surgical approaches (Figure 40-6). For fractures and deformity, intramedullary rodding of the long bones improves position and also splints new fractures. Telescoping rods, which grow with the child, are improving in efficacy. Unfortunately, these children may have to undergo multiple surgeries and re-roddings with growth. The medical treatment, classically involving calcium and vitamin D supplementation, is under intense study. Pamidronate and other bisphosphates, such as alendronate (Fosamax), which decrease bone resorption by inhibiting osteoclasts, are now frequently used. In a multicenter trial,[6] pamidronate was given at 2- to 4-month intervals to children with severe (type III) and mild (type IV) OI. In the 30 children in the study, bone mineral density increased by 41.9%, fractures decreased by 1.7% per year, and mobility increased in 51% of the children. All children claimed their fatigue and chronic bone pain improved.[7] A Cochrane review, however, states it is unclear whether oral or intravenous bisphosphonate treatment consistently decreases fractures and no studies report an increased fracture rate with treatment.[7A] Further long term studies are needed. Fracture healing remained unchanged. A large multicenter study is now trying to refine these treatments for all children with OI.

BONE INFECTION

Osteomyelitis

Osteomyelitis, or bone infection, is caused by either bacterial or granulomatous (e.g., tuberculosis) infective processes (Box 40-1, Figures 40-7 and 40-8). Antibiotic drugs and often surgical interventions are used to treat these infections. Morbidity and mortality resulting from osteomyelitis declined drastically until the 1980s. Unfortunately, with the escalation of methicillin-resistant *Staphylococcus aureus* (MRSA) infections, serious increases in morbidity and mortality have developed.

Acute hematogenous osteomyelitis is the most common form in children. The infection usually begins as an abscess in the metaphysis of a long bone where blood flow is sluggish and bacteria can collect.

BOX 40-1   Causative Microorganisms of Osteomyelitis According to Age

Newborns

Staphylococcus aureus (both methicillin-sensitive [MSSA] and methicillin-resistant [MRSA])
Group B streptococcus
Gram-negative enteric rods

Infants

Staphylococcus aureus (MSSA and MRSA)
Haemophilus influenzae (decreasingly less common secondary to immunization)

Older Children

Staphylococcus aureus (MSSA and MRSA)
Pseudomonas
Salmonella
Neisseria gonorrhoeae

Adolescents and Adults

Pseudomonas
Mycobacterium tuberculosis

A

B

FIGURE 40-7 Pathogenesis of Acute Osteomyelitis Differs with Age. **A,** In infants younger than 1 year the epiphysis is nourished by arteries penetrating through the physis, allowing development of the condition within the epiphysis. **B,** In children up to 15 years of age, the infection is restricted to below the physis because of interruption of the vessels.

With increasing pressure, the infection will rupture out of the periosteum and spread along the diaphysis of the bone. A new shell of bone can develop under the elevated periosteum and can become an **involucrum**. The portion of bone that is separated from adequate blood supply by the infection can die, thereby leading to an involucrum. All three of these changes are apparent on radiograph and signify the need for surgical débridement as well as antibiotic treatment.

These radiographic bone changes take 2 to 3 weeks to develop. Initially, osteomyelitis presents as pain, swelling, and warmth. Children often will have fever, decreased appetite, fatigue, elevated white blood cell (WBC) count (50% to 70%), elevated C-reactive protein (CRP) (98%) level, and elevated erythrocyte sedimentation rate (ESR) (90%). Blood culture is positive in only 40% to 60% of cases. Without changes on plain radiograph, magnetic resonance imaging (MRI) can help define the location and extent of the infectious process. In infants, where osteomyelitis can be multifocal in up to 40% of cases, bone scan identifies other locations of infection that may need surgical intervention.

Treatment of osteomyelitis consists of appropriate antibiotic management for 6 weeks. If blood cultures are negative, bone aspirate must be analyzed to determine the bacterial source of the infection. With MRSA or bone changes on MRI, surgical débridement is required. MRSA often leads to more systemic illness, such as endocarditis (infection of the heart valves), organ failure, and infected thrombotic events.[8]

Septic Arthritis

Septic arthritis is a bacterial or granulomatous infection of the joint space. This is always a surgical emergency. The bacteria, and the lysosomes created by white blood cells fighting the bacteria, can quickly destroy the articular cartilage of the joint and affect the blood supply to the epiphyseal bone nearby. Both of these complications have poor outcomes and can lead to a lifetime of disability.

Septic arthritis can occur primarily or secondary to osteomyelitis that spreads from the metaphysis of the bone into the joint space. The metaphyses of the pediatric hip, shoulder, proximal radius, and distal lateral tibia are all located within the joint capsule, and therefore osteomyelitis in these regions must be carefully monitored for secondary septic arthritis. The most common sites for septic arthritis are knees, hips, ankles, and elbows.

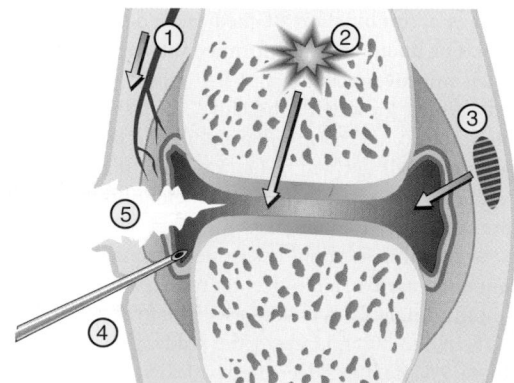

FIGURE 40-8 Routes of Infection to the Joint. **1,** Hematogenous route. **2,** Dissemination from osteomyelitis. **3,** Spread from an adjacent soft tissue infection. **4,** Diagnostic or therapeutic measures. **5,** Penetrating damage by puncture or cutting.

Children with septic arthritis present with severe joint pain, "pseudoparalysis" or marked guarding to motion of the joint, inability to bear weight, and malaise, often with anorexia. Children appear quite ill with this diagnosis. Nonpyogenic arthritis, such as juvenile idiopathic arthritis, can be difficult to distinguish clinically from septic arthritis because both can lead to malaise and elevated ESR. The Kocher criteria are often used to distinguish septic joints from joint pain of another cause. There is a greater than 90% chance of a septic joint if three of the five following criteria are met[9,10]:

1. WBC >12,000 cells/μL
2. Inability to bear weight on the joint
3. Fever >101.3° F (38.5° C)
4. ESR >40 mm/hr
5. CRP >2 mg/dl

Fever and CRP level >2 mg/dl appear to have the most influence in the differential diagnosis.

Blood cultures are positive in 30% to 40% of cases. Joint aspirate positive for a white blood cell (WBC) count of greater than 7000 per high-power field (HPF) defines the diagnosis, and culture of this fluid often determines bacterial etiology. As in osteomyelitis, *Staphylococcus aureus* is the most common bacteria; however, MRSA is now present in up to 30% of affected children.[8,8A] Emerging is the understanding that Kingella kingae is an important pathogen, occurs in children between 6 months and 4 years of age, and can involve many joints and bone, less frequently the endocardium and other locations.[8A]

After surgical débridement of the joint, antibiotics are required for 2 to 3 weeks. Long-term follow-up to assess articular or physeal damage is required.

JUVENILE IDIOPATHIC ARTHRITIS

Juvenile idiopathic arthritis (JIA) is the childhood form of rheumatoid arthritis (see Chapter 39) and accounts for 5% of all cases of rheumatoid arthritis. Juvenile idiopathic arthritis has three distinct modes of onset: oligoarthritis (fewer than three joints), polyarthritis (more than three joints), and Still disease (severe systemic onset) (Table 40-2). JIA differs from rheumatoid arthritis in several ways:

1. Large joints are most commonly affected.
2. Chronic uveitis (inflammation of the anterior chamber of the eye) is common if the blood test for antinuclear antibody (ANA) is positive; slit lamp examination by a trained ophthalmologist is required every 6 months to avoid vision loss.
3. Serum tests may be negative for rheumatoid factor (RF); RF-positive children have a worse prognosis.
4. Subluxation and ankylosis may occur in the cervical spine if disease progresses.
5. Rheumatoid arthritis that continues through adolescence can have severe effects on growth and adult morbidity.

Many children with oligoarthritis who are "seronegative" (blood tests negative for RF or ANA) will resolve their symptoms over time. Systemic onset, or "seropositivity," of the disease is more likely consistent with lifelong arthritis. Therefore, treatment is supportive, not curative. Nonsteroidal anti-inflammatory drugs are a mainstay of treatment, and methotrexate is also being used with success. The goals are to minimize inflammation and deformity.

> **✔ QUICK CHECK 40-1**
> 1. Why is an early diagnosis of developmental dysplasia of the hip imperative?
> 2. How does osteomyelitis develop?
> 3. How does juvenile idiopathic arthritis differ from the adult form?
> 4. How has MRSA changed musculoskeletal infections in children?

TABLE 40-2	**Characteristics of Juvenile Idiopathic Arthritis Related to Mode of Onset**		
	Systemic Onset	**Pauciarticular (Two or Three Subtypes)**	**Polyarticular (Two Subtypes)**
Percentage of patients	30	45	25
Age at onset	Bimodal distribution 1-3 yr of age 8-10 yr of age	Type I: younger than 10 yr Type II: older than 10 yr	Throughout childhood and adolescence
Gender ratio (female/male)	1.5:1	Type I: almost all female Type II: 1:9	Mostly female
Joints involved	Any Only 20% have joint involvement at time of diagnosis	Usually confined to lower extremities—knee, ankle, and eventually sacroiliac; sometimes elbow	Any joint; usually symmetric involvement of small joints Hip involvement in 50% Spine involvement in 50%
Extra-articular manifestations	Fever, malaise, myalgia, rash, pleuritis or pericarditis, adenomegaly, splenomegaly, hepatomegaly Systemic signs minimal	Type I: chronic iridocyclitis; mucocutaneous lesions Type II: acute iridocyclitis; sacroiliitis common; eventual ankylosing spondylitis in many	Possible low-grade fever, malaise, weight loss, rheumatoid nodules, or vasculitis
Laboratory test results	Elevated ESR, CRP levels; RF negative; ANA rarely positive; anemia; leukocytosis	Elevated ESR, CRP levels; ANA positive Type I: HLA-DRW5 positive Type II: HLA-B27 positive Type III: HLA-TMo positive	Elevated ESR, CRP levels Type I: RF positive Type II: RF negative
Long-term prognosis	Mortality: 1-2% of all JIA patients Joint destruction in 40%	Continuous disease; eventual remission in 60% Type I: ocular damage; functional blindness in 10% Type II: ankylosing spondylitis Type III: best outlook for recovery	Longer duration; more crippling; remission in 25% Type I: high incidence of crippling arthritis Type II: outlook good

From Hockenberry MJ, Wilson D: *Wong's nursing care of infants and children*, ed 8, St Louis, 2007, Mosby.
ANA, Antinuclear antibody; *CRP*, C-reactive protein; *ESR*, erythrocyte sedimentation rate; *HLA*, human leukocyte antigen; *JIA*, juvenile idiopathic arthritis; *RF*, rheumatoid factor.

OSTEOCHONDROSES

The osteochondroses are a series of childhood diseases involving areas of significant tensile or compressive stress (e.g., tibial tubercle, Achilles insertion, hip epiphysis). The pathophysiology is partial loss of blood supply, death of bone (osseous necrosis), progressive bony weakness, and then microfracture. The cause of the decreased blood supply is controversial; trauma, a change in clotting sensitivity, vascular injury, genetic predisposition, or a combination of these factors is presently considered most likely. Additionally, during the years of rapid bone growth, blood supply to the growing ends of bones (epiphyses) may become insufficient, resulting in necrotic bone, usually near joints. Because bone is normally undergoing a continuous rebuilding process, the necrotic areas can self-repair over a period of weeks or months.

Use of anti-inflammatory medications, modification of activities, immobilization, and rest are recommended during active stages of the disease. Reparative correction by revascularization is the rule, although years may be required for full healing, and deformity from compression during the period of osseous necrosis can persist.

Legg-Calvé-Perthes Disease

Legg-Calvé-Perthes (LCP) disease is a common osteochondrosis usually occurring in children between the ages of 3 and 10 years, with a peak incidence at 6 years. The disorder is bilateral in 10% to 20% of children, and boys are affected five times more often than girls. Boys have a more poorly developed blood supply to the femoral head than do girls of the same age, and this is thought to be the reason for male predilection. The role of genetics is unclear, but LCP is more common in northern European and Japanese children and rare in black children; family history is positive in 20% of cases. This self-limited disease of the hip, which runs its natural course in 2 to 5 years, is presumably created by recurrent interruption of the blood supply to the femoral head. The ossification center first becomes necrotic (osteonecrosis) and then is gradually replaced by live bone.

PATHOPHYSIOLOGY   Several causative theories have been proposed, including a generalized disorder of epiphyseal cartilage growth, thyroid hormone deficiency, trauma, infection, and blood clotting disorders. However, a Harvard study did not show increases in thrombotic disorders in consecutive children with LCP.[11] Boys with a hypercoagulable state are three times more likely to acquire LCP than girls with the same disorder.[12] Another study has shown the risk of LCP is five times greater in children exposed to passive smoke as opposed to children living in a smoke-free environment.[13] Increased risk has been associated with smoke from indoor use of a wood stove.[13A]

In the first stage of LCP, the soft tissues of the hip (synovial membrane and joint capsule) are swollen, edematous, and hyperemic, often with fluid present in the joint (Figure 40-9). In the second necrotic stage, the anterior 50% or more of the epiphysis of the femoral head dies because of a lack of blood supply, and the metaphyseal bone at the junction of the femoral neck and capital epiphyseal plate is softened because of increased blood supply and decalcification. Granulation tissue (procallus) and blood vessels then invade the dead bone. The third, or regenerative healing, stage ordinarily lasts 2 to 4 years. The dead bone in the femoral head is replaced by procallus, and new bone is established (see Figure 40-9). In the fourth, or residual, stage, remodeling takes place and the newly formed bone is organized into a live spongy bone.

CLINICAL MANIFESTATIONS   Injury or trauma precedes the onset of LCP in approximately 30% to 50% of children with Legg-Calvé-Perthes disease. For several months the child complains of a limp and pain that can be referred to the knee, inner thigh, and the groin, following the path of the obturator nerve. The pain is usually aggravated by activity and relieved by rest and administration of anti-inflammatory medications.

The typical physical findings include spasm on rotation of the hip, limitation of internal rotation and abduction, and hip flexion–adduction deformity. If the child is walking, an early abnormal gait termed an antalgic (painful) abductor lurch, or a "Trendelenburg gait" (gluteus medius gait pattern), is apparent. If the hip pain or limp has been present for a prolonged period, muscles of the hip and thigh atrophy.

EVALUATION AND TREATMENT   The goals of treatment are to preserve normal congruity of the femoral head and acetabulum and maintain spasm-free and pain-free range of motion in the hip joint. Currently, most children can be managed with anti-inflammatory medications and activity modification during periods of synovitis. Serial radiographs are obtained to monitor the progress of the disease and to ensure that the femoral head remains congruent in the acetabulum. Surgery may be necessary if the femoral head becomes subluxated or incongruent with the acetabulum (Figure 40-10).[14-16] Children older than age 6 (by bone age) have a worse prognosis attributable to poorer remodeling potential. Older children require surgery more often to avoid poor congruence of the hip. Poor congruence predisposes to early osteoarthritis, with nearly 50% requiring hip replacement surgery by age 40.

Osgood-Schlatter Disease

Osgood-Schlatter disease consists of osteochondrosis of the tibia tubercle and associated patellar tendonitis. Osgood-Schlatter disease occurs most often in preadolescents and adolescents who participate in sports and is more prevalent in boys than in girls. Osgood-Schlatter disease is one of the most common ailments reported in the 30 million children who are involved in sports.[17]

The severity of the lesion varies from mild tendonitis to a complete separation of the anterior tibial apophysis, a part of the tibial tubercle.

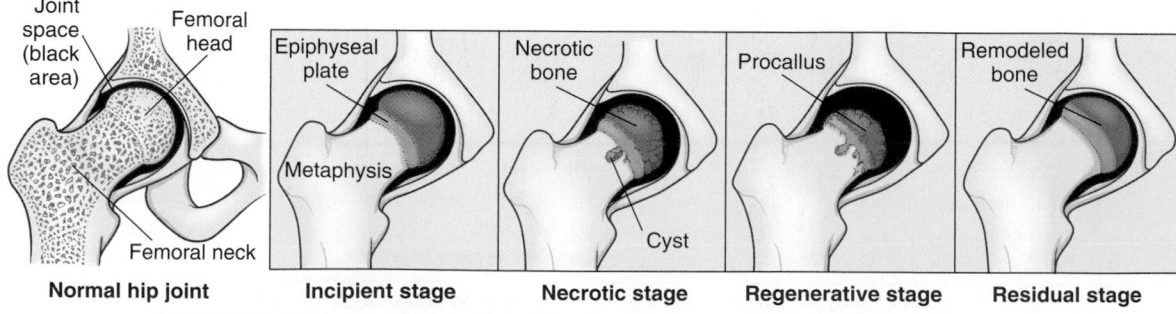

FIGURE 40-9 Stages of Legg-Calvé-Perthes Disease, a Form of Osteochondrosis.

FIGURE 40-10 Pelvis of a 7-Year-Old Boy with Legg-Calvé-Perthes Disease. A, The femoral head is flat and extruded from the edge of the joint. This hip is at risk for early arthritis if left to revascularize and heal in this position. **B,** Surgical replacement of the femoral head. As the Perthes heals, the ball has assumed a round shape that matches the socket well.

The mildest form of Osgood-Schlatter disease causes ischemic (avascular) necrosis in the region of the bony tibial tubercle, with hypertrophic cartilage formation during the stages of repair. In more severe cases, the abnormality involves a true apophyseal separation of the tibial tubercle with avascular necrosis.

The child complains of pain and swelling in the region around the patellar tendon and tibial tubercle, which becomes prominent and is tender to direct pressure. The pain is most severe after physical activity that involves vigorous quadriceps contraction (jumping or running) or direct local trauma to the tibial tubercle area.

The goal of treatment for Osgood-Schlatter disease is to decrease the stress at the tubercle. Often a period of 4 to 8 weeks of restriction from strenuous physical activity, administration of anti-inflammatory medications, and stretching of the quadriceps muscle are sufficient. Bracing with a tubercle band can be very helpful. If the pain is not relieved, a cast or knee immobilizer is required, a situation that is particularly difficult if the condition is bilateral.

Gradual resumption of activity is permitted after 8 weeks, but return to unrestricted athletic participation requires an additional 8 weeks to allow for revascularization, healing, and ossification of the tibial tubercle.[14,18] With skeletal maturity and closure of the apophysis, Osgood-Schlatter disease resolves.

Sever Disease

Sever disease is the "Osgood-Schlatter" of the calcaneus (heel bone). The insertion of the Achilles pulls on the cartilaginous apophysis of the calcaneus, causing pain. It is more common in athletic children and children who have underlying Achilles tendon tightness, for example, soccer players between the ages of 8 and 12. It is relieved by a heel lift in the shoe, rest, stretching, and anti-inflammatory medications.

SCOLIOSIS

Scoliosis is a rotational curvature of the spine most obvious in the anteroposterior plane (Figure 40-11). It can be classified as nonstructural or structural. Nonstructural scoliosis results from a cause other than the spine itself, such as posture, leg length discrepancy, or splinting from pain. Structural scoliosis is a curvature of the spine associated with vertebral rotation. Nonstructural scoliosis can become structural if the underlying cause is not found and treated.

FIGURE 40-11 Scoliosis in Children. Normal spine alignment and abnormal spinal curvatures associated with scoliosis. **A,** Normal. **B,** Mild. **C,** Severe. **D,** Rotation and curvature of scoliosis.

There are three main types of structural scoliosis: idiopathic; congenital (attributable to bony deformity such as hemivertebrae); and teratologic (caused by another systemic syndrome such as cerebral palsy). Eighty percent of all scoliosis is idiopathic, which may have a genetic component. Although girls and boys are equally affected, once the curve becomes more than 20 degrees, girls are five times more likely to be affected. Ninety-eight percent of curves are apex right thoracic. If a left thoracic curve appears in the adolescent with idiopathic scoliosis, MRI is performed to rule out a neurologic cause. MRI should be performed in scoliotic children with loss of abdominal reflexes and those who have exertional headaches or a congenital curve.[18,19]

Idiopathic curves progress while a child is growing, and progression can be very rapid during growth spurts. When idiopathic curves progress to 25 degrees or greater, and the child is skeletally immature, bracing is required. The total number of hours a brace is worn correlates to efficacy of treatment; 82% of children who wore the brace as prescribed had minimal progression.[20] In braced curves, 72% required no surgery compared with only 48% of those who wore no brace.[21]

Curves of more than 50 degrees will progress after skeletal maturity, so spinal fusion is required to stop progression. Bracing is the only nonoperative measure known to slow scoliotic progression. Chiropractic manipulation, physical therapy, exercise, and diet regimens have not been shown to alter natural history. Bracing is less successful in teratologic or congenital curves; therefore, these conditions may require surgical intervention more often.

MUSCULAR DYSTROPHY

The muscular dystrophies are a group of inherited disorders that cause progressive muscle fiber loss leading to weakness, mostly of the voluntary muscles. Some dystrophies cause disease in infancy, others in childhood, and others not until adulthood. Muscular dystrophies have different inheritance patterns and different biochemical alterations that cause each specific type. Three are discussed in detail in this chapter. Individuals with Duchenne muscular dystrophy (DMD) have a mutation in a specific gene that leads to alterations in the muscle protein dystrophin. Individuals with myotonic muscular dystrophy (MMD) have a genetic alteration that leads to systemic disease. Although there is no cure for any of the muscular dystrophies, aggressive preventive management has increased the life expectancy and quality of life of children with these disorders. Common forms of muscular dystrophy are described in Table 40-3.

Duchenne Muscular Dystrophy

PATHOPHYSIOLOGY   Duchenne muscular dystrophy (DMD) is X-linked, generally occurring in boys, and is present in about 1 in 3500 male births. It is the most common childhood dystrophy. DMD is caused by mutations in the dystrophin gene, which lead to alterations or deletions of the muscle protein dystrophin.

The protein dystrophin mediates anchorage of the actin cytoskeleton of skeletal muscle fibers to the basement membrane through a membrane-glycoprotein complex. With lack of dystrophin, the poorly anchored fibers tear themselves apart under the repeated stress of contraction. Free calcium then enters the muscle cells, causing cell death and fiber necrosis (Figure 40-12).

CLINICAL MANIFESTATIONS   Boys with DMD will present in the preschool years with muscle weakness, difficulty walking, and large calves (pseudohypertrophy) caused by normal muscle fiber replacement with fat and connective tissue (see Figure 40-12, *B* and *C*). Although the calves are large the muscle is actually weak. Clinical weakness starts in the pelvic girdle, initially causing difficulty rising from the floor (Gower sign) and climbing stairs, and a waddling gait because of weakness in the lumbar and gluteal muscles. Boys with DMD often toe-walk because of weakness of the anterior tibial and peroneal muscles, causing the feet to assume a talipes equinovarus position. The weakness worsens over the subsequent few years, resulting in the loss of ability to ambulate by 8 to 13 years of age. Muscle weakness also leads to contractures of the knees, hips, and other joints, and scoliosis develops in most boys with DMD. Once scoliosis begins, it is relentlessly progressive. Curves of more than 20 degrees are treated surgically to maintain pulmonary function. Muscle weakness and inactivity, particularly once a person is in a wheelchair full time, lead to osteoporosis and pathologic fractures. If fracture occurs, bisphosphonates may be used to strengthen bone, although long-term studies on safety have not been performed in this population.

As children age, muscle weakness progresses and respiratory weakness leads to breathing difficulty, particularly when sleeping. Susceptibility to respiratory tract infections and progressive deterioration of pulmonary function generally lead to premature death, usually in the twenties. Cardiomyopathy also may occur and, despite treatment, is generally progressive. Bowel and bladder functions are often mildly affected, with constipation and urinary urgency as frequent symptoms. Mild to moderate cognitive problems are common but not universal.

EVALUATION AND TREATMENT   Diagnosis is suggested (a high creatine kinase [CK] level does not confirm the diagnosis because many other alterations can also increase CK) by measuring the blood creatine kinase level, which can be 100 times the normal level, with confirmation by genetic testing for mutations in the dystrophin gene.

Management involves maintaining function for as long as possible. Treatment with steroids can prolong the ability to walk by several years and improves life expectancy.[22] Prednisone is used in the United States, although many families prefer to use deflazacort (however, it is not currently approved in the United States but is available from the internet), which is a steroid that may have fewer side effects than prednisone. Treatment also involves range-of-motion exercises, bracing, and surgical release of contracture deformities and scoliosis when necessary. Children with DMD require a multidisciplinary approach to care, including attention to heart and breathing problems, weight loss/gain, constipation, rehabilitative/developmental problems, psychosocial needs, and neurologic and orthopedic problems (Figure 40-13). New guidelines for the evaluation and treatment of Duchenne muscular dystrophy were developed after reviewing thousands of clinical

TABLE 40-3   Major Muscular Dystrophy Syndromes

Disease	Mode of Inheritance	Age at Clinical Onset	Distribution of Weakness
Duchenne muscular dystrophy/Becker muscular dystrophy (DMD/BMD)	X-linked, sporadic	2-3 years/5-7 years	Proximal with pseudohypertrophy
Facioscapulohumeral (FSH) muscular dystrophy	Autosomal dominant	Early adolescence	Face, arms, legs
Myotonic muscular dystrophy (MMD)	Autosomal dominant	Variable—birth to adulthood	Distal muscles, face

From Moxley RT III et al: *Neurology* 64(1):13-20, 2005.

FIGURE 40-12 Duchenne Muscular Dystrophy. A, Young boy with DMD but on horseback. **B,** Transverse section of gastrocnemius muscle from a healthy boy. **C,** Transverse section of gastrocnemius muscle from a boy with Duchenne muscular dystrophy. Normal muscle fiber is replaced with fat and connective tissue. (From Jorde LB et al: *Medical genetics*, ed 4, Philadelphia, 2010, Mosby.)

scenarios and are presented as a multisystem, two-part approach. One part is for diagnosis and the other part for management.

If appropriate, families should receive genetic counseling for recurrence risk and prenatal screening. Family support is necessary throughout the life span of the child because needs vary depending on the stage of the disease.

Becker Muscular Dystrophy

Although Becker muscular dystrophy (BMD) has been designated historically as a separate muscular dystrophy, it is actually caused by alterations of the same dystrophin gene (i.e., dystrophinopathies) and protein as seen in DMD. Children with BMD present later and have a longer life expectancy than those with DMD; however, they are part of the same clinical spectrum.

Facioscapulohumeral Muscular Dystrophy

Facioscapulohumeral (FSH) muscular dystrophy, one of the most common muscular dystrophies, is inherited in an autosomal dominant fashion. It is more variable in presentation than Duchenne muscular dystrophy. FSH muscular dystrophy is usually observed in *late* childhood. Progression is usually slow and life span is normal or near normal. FSH muscular dystrophy occurs because of a deletion on chromosome 4 that is not associated with any particular gene and causes disease by still unknown mechanisms.

Muscle weakness, which is often asymmetric, usually begins in the face and is then observed in the shoulders and legs. Individuals with FSH muscular dystrophy often have weak eye closure, are not able to whistle or inflate a balloon, and have scapular winging.

Diagnosis is by genetic testing, although sometimes biopsies or electrodiagnostic testing may also be performed as part of the diagnostic evaluation. FSH muscular dystrophy also may be associated with mild hearing loss, retinal abnormalities, and mild cardiac problems. Unlike DMD or BMD, children with FSH muscular dystrophy often have muscle pain, particularly in their arms and shoulders.

Treatment involves administration of nonsteroidal anti-inflammatory drugs to decrease pain and inflammation. Massage and heat treatments also may be helpful. Bracing may be performed for function; for example, dorsiflexion of the feet with ankle-foot orthotics to prevent tripping or to provide support and comfort.

Myotonic Muscular Dystrophy

PATHOPHYSIOLOGY   Myotonic muscular dystrophy (MMD) is a multisystem disease that can occur because of mutations in either of two genes resulting in type 1 (*DMPK* gene) and type 2 (*CNBP* gene) MMD. MMD1 may demonstrate a genetic mechanism called *anticipation*, in which children born to a mother with MMD usually have a more severe form of the disease.

CLINICAL MANIFESTATIONS   MMD affects the brain, skeletal and smooth muscles, the eyes, the heart, and the endocrine system, manifesting as distal muscle weakness, learning problems or intellectual disability, or both. Additionally, children can have dysphagia, constipation, cardiac dysrhythmias that if untreated may be life-threatening, diabetes, and cataracts. Boys with MMD also may manifest testicular atrophy and early male pattern baldness. A hallmark of the disease is myotonia—individuals have difficulty relaxing muscles; for example,

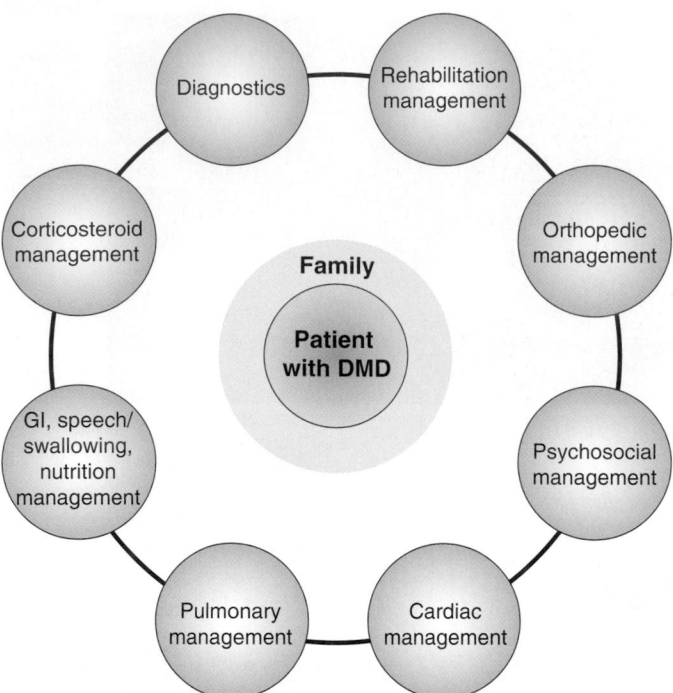

FIGURE 40-13 Multisystem Approach for Evaluation and Treatment of Duchenne Muscular Dystrophy. (Adapted from Bushby K: *Diagnosis and management of Duchenne muscular dystrophy part 1: diagnosis and pharmacological and psychosocial management,* 2009; Bushby K: *Diagnosis and management of Duchenne muscular dystrophy part 2: implementation of multidisciplinary care,* 2009. Available at: www.thelancet.com/neurology. Published online November 30, 2009 [doi:10.1016/S1474-4422(09)70271].)

they may have difficulty relaxing their hand grip after a handshake or opening their eyes after closing them tightly.

Children with mild disease do not develop symptoms until adolescence or older and may display mild muscle weakness (usually more pronounced in the distal muscles), cataracts, and myotonia, but have normal life spans. Children with a more classic form of the disease also have onset of symptoms in the teenage years but have progressive muscle weakness, cataracts, and cardiac conduction abnormalities; they may have a shortened life span and require a wheelchair for mobility. The congenital form, the most severe, may be present at birth or become obvious over the first few years of life.

EVALUATION AND TREATMENT   Diagnosis is made by genetic testing for the two genes known to cause MMD. In each case, an abnormal segment of DNA, caused by an abnormally large trinucleotide, repeat expansion (CTG) in an untranslated region of a gene, causes abnormal functioning of muscle and other cells. Type 1 is more common and can present in infancy (the congenital form). Infants with MMD may have life-threatening breathing and swallowing problems and developmental delay or intellectual disability, although MMD is not observed until childhood or even adolescence.

Steroids are not useful for the treatment of MMD; however, maintaining muscle function is important, including range-of-motion exercises, bracing, and surgical release of contractures when necessary. Children need to be followed closely by neurologists and primary care providers with treatment for the various aspects of the disease, such as dysphagia, heart dysrhythmias, and constipation, as well as other problems.

MUSCULOSKELETAL TUMORS

Benign Bone Tumors

The two most common forms of benign bone tumors are osteochondroma and nonossifying fibroma.

Osteochondroma

Osteochondroma (or exostosis) can occur as a solitary lesion or as an inherited syndrome of hereditary multiple exostoses (HME). HME is an autosomal dominant condition with exostoses occurring throughout the skeleton. Osteochondromas appear as bony protuberances because of *EXT1* and *EXT2* genetic anomalies near active growth plates of the proximal humerus, distal femur, or proximal tibia. The most common presentation is a palpable mass that is painful when traumatized. Rarely, the lesion can cause neurologic or vascular problems, or tendon rupture from local compression. The lesions can lead to growth disturbance and mildly short stature. Knee valgus (knock-knee), ankle valgus, and hip problems are common. Upper extremity lesions can lead to a pronounced deformity in the forearm with a very short ulna bone. These lesions grow until skeletal maturity; growth or pain after skeletal maturity is a sign of possible malignant transformation, especially in the pelvis or scapular region. Transformation to chondrosarcoma is very rare, occurring in less than 1% of children.

Treatment involves minimizing growth disturbance, local tissue compression, and pain by resection of symptomatic lesions. The regrowth rate is 30% when lesions are removed in early childhood; therefore only symptomatic lesions should be surgically addressed in the growing child.[23]

Nonossifying Fibroma

Of all benign bone tumors, 50% are nonossifying fibromas or fibrous cortical defects. Nonossifying fibromas are sharply demarcated, cortically based lesions of fibrocytes that have replaced normal bone. The lesion can occur in any bone, at any age. Nearly 30% of all children have at least one.

Microscopically, these benign nonmetastasizing lesions appear as whorled bundles of fibroblasts and osteoclast-like giant cells. As the tumor grows, lipids make the fibroblasts foamy in appearance, and they are known as *foam cells*.

Treatment is observational only. If these lesions grow too large, however, they will compromise the biomechanical strength of the bone and lead to pathologic fractures. Curettage and bone grafting is suggested after pathologic fracture or if impending fracture (nonossifying fibroma greater than 50% of the diameter of the bone or greater than 3 or 4 cm) is noted radiographically.

Malignant Bone Tumors

Malignant bone tumors are uncommon tumors in childhood, accounting for fewer than 5% of childhood malignancies and occurring mostly during adolescence. The two main tumors are osteosarcoma and Ewing sarcoma.

Osteosarcoma

Osteosarcoma is the most common malignant bone tumor found during childhood and originates in bone-producing mesenchymal cells. Tumors can be broadly classified as those arising within the bone and those arising on the surface of bone. Approximately 75% of these tumors occur in persons between the ages of 10 and 25 years, with most being diagnosed between 15 and 19 years of age during the adolescent growth spurt. Incidence is the same for males and females.

Osteosarcoma may develop as a result of rapid local growth, which increases the likelihood of mutation. It can be induced by ionizing radiation, even with relatively low doses, and can be a tragic consequence of therapeutic radiation for other forms of cancer. The latent period after radiation exposure is 5 to 40 years. There also has been a link to individuals with retinoblastoma (a hereditary eye tumor).

Osteosarcoma has not been linked to chemical carcinogens or viruses. No deoxyribonucleic acid (DNA) or ribonucleic acid (RNA) virus has been isolated.

Molecular analysis has demonstrated deletion of genetic material on the long arm of chromosome 13, which led to the identification of a tumor-suppressor gene as being part of the mechanism for tumor development. The oncogene *src* also has been associated with osteosarcoma.

PATHOPHYSIOLOGY Osteosarcoma occurs mainly in the metaphyses of long bones near sites of active physeal growth. The tumor most commonly occurs at the distal femur, proximal tibia, or proximal humerus. As a tumor of mesenchymal cells, osteosarcoma demonstrates production of osteoid cells.

Osteosarcoma is a bulky tumor that extends beyond the bone into a soft tissue mass. It may encircle the bone and destroy the trabeculae of the diseased area. Osteosarcoma disseminates through the bloodstream, usually to the lung. As many as 25% of children diagnosed with osteosarcoma exhibit lung metastases at diagnosis. Other sites of metastatic spread include other bones and visceral organs.

CLINICAL MANIFESTATIONS The most common presenting complaint is pain. Night pain, awakening a child from sleep, is a particularly foreboding sign. There may be swelling, warmth, and redness caused by the vascularity of the tumor. Symptoms also may include cough, dyspnea, and chest pain if lung metastasis is present. If a lower extremity is involved, a child may limp or suffer a pathologic fracture. Although osteosarcoma is not the result of trauma, trauma may call attention to a preexisting tumor.

EVALUATION AND TREATMENT The five histologic types of osteosarcoma are determined by the predominant cell type. The tumor is graded according to degree of malignancy; the higher the grade, the worse the prognosis.

Surgery and chemotherapy are the primary treatments for osteosarcoma. The tumor is resistant to radiation. Traditionally, surgery includes amputation at the joint above the involved bone; however, more recent limb salvage procedures have gained acceptance, and amputation may be avoided in many children.

Chemotherapy is an important component of treatment. Children routinely receive chemotherapy preoperatively; then the disease is restaged with MRI and surgical biopsy to determine rate of "tumor kill." If more than 90% of tumor cells are killed by chemotherapy, the prognosis is markedly improved. Chemotherapy is then used after surgery for any additional cell spill during surgery. The use of chemotherapy with surgery has increased the 5-year survival rate to 60% or more.[24]

FIGURE 40-14 Ewing Sarcoma. **A**, Most common anatomic sites. **B**, Close-up view of Ewing sarcoma of the distal end of the tibia. Tumor extends into the soft tissue. (From Damjanov I, Linder J, editors: *Anderson's pathology*, ed 10, St Louis, 1996, Mosby.)

A number of approaches have been used to treat pulmonary metastases. Because pulmonary metastases are generally solitary, thoracotomy with wedge resection has proven to be the most effective treatment.

Ewing Sarcoma

Ewing sarcoma is the second most common and most lethal malignant bone tumor that occurs during childhood. This tumor is named after James Ewing, who first identified it as a separate clinical diagnosis in 1921. The most common period of diagnosis is between 5 and 15 years of age; it is rare after age 30 years. Ewing sarcoma is slightly more common in males than females. Cytogenic studies have shown a translocation of chromosomes 11 and 22 resulting in a fusion protein (EWS-FLI 1) forming at the chromosomal junction.

PATHOPHYSIOLOGY Ewing sarcoma is most commonly located in the midshaft of long bones or in flat bones. The most common sites include the femur, pelvis, and humerus (Figure 40-14).

Arising from bone marrow, Ewing sarcoma can penetrate the cortex of the bone to form a soft tissue mass. Unlike osteosarcoma, Ewing sarcoma does not make bone and radiographically appears as a permeative, destructive lesion (Figure 40-15). Ewing sarcoma metastasizes to nearly every organ. Metastasis occurs early and is usually apparent at diagnosis or within 1 year. The most common sites are the lung, other bones, lymph nodes, bone marrow, liver, spleen, and central nervous system.

CLINICAL MANIFESTATIONS As with osteosarcoma, the most common complaint is pain that increases in severity. A soft tissue mass is often present. Additional symptoms may include fever, malaise, and anorexia. The radiographic appearance is similar to that of osteomyelitis, and diagnosis is only confirmed with biopsy.

EVALUATION AND TREATMENT Evaluation is determined from genetic testing, elevated sedimentation rate, and lactic acid

FIGURE 40-15 Ewing Sarcoma of the Distal Radius. Radiograph of an 8-year-old boy showing a permeative lesion of the distal radius. Note the loss of bone cortex on the ulnar border, suggesting an aggressive process. Bone biopsy revealed Ewing sarcoma.

FIGURE 40-16 Corner Fracture. Bilateral knee radiograph showing healing corner fractures of bilateral proximal tibias and distal femurs. Note the varying amount of callus formation signifying fractures at different stages of healing.

dehydrogenase (LDH) levels. Biopsy is used to conclusively establish the diagnosis of a small round cell tumor.

Treatment includes radiation, chemotherapy, and, if possible, surgical débridement. Chemotherapy is continued for 12 to 18 months after resection. Present 5-year survival with this tritherapeutic approach is 60%; however, tumors of the pelvis have a markedly worse prognosis. Metastasis at diagnosis is another poor prognostic indicator, with 5-year survival rate dropping to less than 40%.

> ✔ **QUICK CHECK 40-3**
> 1. What are the most common benign bone tumors of children?
> 2. What are the two malignant bone tumors found in children?
> 3. What is the most lethal bone tumor in children?

NONACCIDENTAL TRAUMA

It is estimated that more than 2.0 million children are abused per year in the United States. Maltreatment may be psychologic, sexual, or physical.[25] Thirty percent of children who have been physically abused are seen by an orthopedist. Accurate and appropriate referrals to child protection agencies not only are legally mandated but also are essential for the well-being of the child. An abused child who is returned to the same situation without intervention has a 10% to 15% chance of subsequent mortality.

Fractures in Nonaccidental Trauma

Children who are not yet ambulatory and present with a long bone fracture have more than a 75% chance of that fracture being caused by nonaccidental trauma (NAT).[26] "Corner" metaphyseal fractures are nearly always from abuse but occur only 25% of the time (Figure 40-16). Fractures at multiple stages of healing also suggest abuse;

however, osteogenesis imperfecta or other causes of systemic osteomalacia must be ruled out. The most common presentation is a transverse tibia fracture. After walking age, only 2% of long bone fractures are the result of nonaccidental trauma.[27]

EVALUATION Nonaccidental trauma necessitates early consultation with child protective services. The child should undergo skeletal survey (especially if less than 2 years of age) and have a complete physical examination to evaluate for pattern bruising, burns, or multiple soft tissue injuries. A thorough history must be obtained for all identified injuries. It is important to remember that social isolation can lead to an increased likelihood of abuse, but no social status is immune. One study reported that racial differences may exist in the evaluation and reporting of nonaccidental trauma. Skeletal trauma is present in a significant number of abused children.[28-30]

When the cause of injury is unclear, bone scan can be helpful in diagnosing subtle injuries, especially rib fractures. Posterior rib fractures are especially likely to be the result of abuse. MRI/CT of the brain to check for subdural hematoma and retinal examination to look for hemorrhages are essential.

TREATMENT The treating healthcare provider must have a nonjudgmental attitude. The child and family involved in nonaccidental trauma are emotionally delicate and require not only physical but also emotional care. Social workers need to be involved early to ensure that the child receives appropriate medical care. Fortunately, fractures tend to heal quickly for those in this age group. Neurologic injury and social disease, however, are much more difficult to cure.

> ✔ **QUICK CHECK 40-4**
> 1. Describe the incidence and types of child maltreatment or abuse.
> 2. What is the most common orthopedic injury in NAT?

DID YOU UNDERSTAND?

Congenital Defects

1. Clubfoot is a common deformity in which the foot is twisted out of its normal shape or position. Clubfoot can be positional, idiopathic, or teratologic.
2. Developmental dysplasia of the hip (DDH) is an abnormality in the development of the femoral head, acetabulum, or both. Like clubfoot, DDH can be idiopathic or teratologic. It is a serious and disabling condition in children if not diagnosed and treated early, with best outcomes when treated before walking age.
3. Osteogenesis imperfecta (brittle bone disease) is an inherited disorder of collagen that affects primarily bones and results in serious fractures of many bones.

Bone Infection

1. Osteomyelitis is a local or generalized bacterial or granulomatous (e.g., tuberculosis) infection of bone and bone marrow. Bacteria are usually introduced by direct extension from a nearby infection, through the bloodstream, or by trauma.
2. Septic arthritis can occur de novo or secondary to osteomyelitis in very young children in which the metaphysis is still located within the joint capsule of certain joints.

Juvenile Idiopathic Arthritis

1. Juvenile idiopathic arthritis is an inflammatory joint disorder characterized by pain and swelling. Large joints are most commonly affected.

Osteochondroses

1. Avascular diseases of the bone are collectively referred to as osteochondroses and are caused by an insufficient blood supply to growing bones.
2. Legg-Calvé-Perthes disease is one of the most common osteochondroses. This disorder is characterized by epiphyseal necrosis or degeneration of the head of the femur followed by regeneration or recalcification. Children older than age 7 years at onset have a worse prognosis.
3. Osgood-Schlatter disease is characterized by tendonitis of the anterior patellar tendon and inflammation or partial separation of the tibial tubercle caused by chronic irritation, usually as a result of overuse of the quadriceps muscles. The condition is seen primarily in muscular, athletic adolescent males.

Scoliosis

1. Scoliosis is a rotational curvature of the spine most obvious in the anteroposterior plane, and can be classified as nonstructural or structural. Nonstructural scoliosis results from a cause other than the spine itself, such as posture, leg length discrepancy, or splinting from pain. Structural scoliosis is a curvature of the spine associated with vertebral rotation.

Muscular Dystrophy

1. The muscular dystrophies are a group of genetically transmitted diseases characterized by progressive atrophy of skeletal muscles. There is an insidious loss of strength in all forms of the disorder with increasing disability and deformity. The most common type in childhood is Duchenne muscular dystrophy.

Musculoskeletal Tumors

1. The two most common forms of benign bone tumors are osteochondroma and nonossifying fibroma.
2. The two main types of malignant childhood bone tumors are osteosarcoma and Ewing sarcoma.
3. Osteosarcoma, the most common malignant childhood bone tumor, originates in bone-producing mesenchymal cells and is most often located near active growth plates, such as the distal femur, proximal tibia, or proximal humerus.
4. Most children with osteosarcoma are diagnosed between 15 and 19 years of age, and osteosarcoma occurs equally in males and females.
5. Ewing sarcoma originates from cells within the bone marrow space and is most often located in the midshaft of long bones or in flat bones. The most common sites include the femur, pelvis, and humerus.
6. Ewing sarcoma is more common in males and is diagnosed most often between the ages of 5 and 15 years.
7. Pain is the usual presenting symptom for either osteosarcoma or Ewing sarcoma.
8. The primary treatments for osteosarcoma are surgery and chemotherapy. The primary treatment for Ewing sarcoma is a combination of chemotherapy, radiation, and surgery.

Nonaccidental Trauma

1. Nonaccidental trauma must be considered with any long bone injury in the preambulatory child.
2. The presence of soft tissue injury, corner fractures, and multiple fractures at different stages of healing is extremely helpful for making a diagnosis of nonaccidental trauma.
3. When nonaccidental trauma is suspected, a child must be evaluated radiographically for other fractures, heat trauma, and retinal hemorrhage.
4. All social strata are at risk.
5. The healthcare provider is legally responsible to report suspected nonaccidental trauma.

KEY TERMS

Acetabular dysplasia, 1038
Acute hematogenous osteomyelitis, 1041
Antalgic abductor lurch, 1044
Becker muscular dystrophy (BMD), 1047
Clubfoot, 1038

Congenital equinovarus, 1038
Developmental dysplasia of the hip (DDH), 1038
Dislocated hip, 1038
Duchenne muscular dystrophy (DMD), 1046
Dystrophin, 1046

Ewing sarcoma, 1049
Facioscapulohumeral (FSH) muscular dystrophy, 1047
Hereditary multiple exostoses (HME), 1048
Involucrum, 1042

Juvenile idiopathic arthritis (JIA), 1043
Legg-Calvé-Perthes (LCP) disease, 1044
Malignant bone tumor, 1048
Muscular dystrophy, 1046

REFERENCES

1. Morcuende JA et al: Plaster cast treatment of clubfoot: the Ponseti method of manipulation and casting, *J Pediatr Orthop* 3(2):161-167, 1994.
2. Janicki JA et al: Treatment of neuromuscular and syndrome-associated (nonidiopathic) clubfeet using the Ponseti method, *J Pediatr Orthop* 29(4): 393-397, 2009.
3. Woolacott NF et al: Ultrasonography in screening for developmental dysplasia of the hip in newborns: systematic review, *Br Med J* 330(7505): 1413, 2005.
3A. Le Ba TB et al: Ultrasound for infants at risk for developmental dysplasia of the hip. *Orthopedics* 38(8):e722-e726, 2015.
4. Jari S et al: Unilateral limitation of abduction of the hip: a valuable clinical sign for DDH? *J Bone Joint Surg Br* 84(1):104-107, 2002.
5. Holman J et al: Long term follow-up of open reduction surgery for developmental dysplasia of the hip, *J Pediatr Orthop* 32(2):121-124, 2012.
6. Glorieux FH et al: Cyclic administration of pamidronate in children with severe osteogenesis imperfecta, *N Engl J Med* 339(14):947-952, 1998.
7. Poyrazoglu S et al: Successful results of pamidronate treatment in children with osteogenesis imperfecta with emphasis on interpretation of bone mineral density for local standards, *J Pediatr Orthop* 28(4):483-487, 2008.
7A. Dwan K et al: Bisphosphonate therapy for osteogensis imperfecta. *Cochrane Database Syst Rev:* CD005008, pub 3, 2014.
8. Vaderhave KL et al: Community-associated methicillin-resistant *Staphylococcus aureus* in acute musculoskeletal infection in children: a game changer, *J Pediatr Orthop* 29(8):927-931, 2009.
8A. Principi N et al: Kingella kingae infections in children. *BMC Infect Dis* 15:260, 2015.

9. Caird MS et al: Factors distinguishing septic arthritis from transient synovitis of the hip in children. A prospective study, *J Bone Joint Surg Am* 88(6):1251-1257, 2006.
10. Kocher MS et al: Differentiating between septic arthritis and transient synovitis of the hip in children: an evidence-based clinical prediction algorithm, *J Bone Joint Surg Am* 81(12):1662-1670, 1999.
11. Hresko MT et al: Prospective reevaluation of the association between thrombotic diathesis and Legg-Perthes disease, *J Bone Joint Surg Am* 84(9): 1613-1618, 2002.
12. Vosmaer A et al: Coagulation abnormalities in Legg-Calvé-Perthes disease, *J Bone Joint Surg Am* 92(1):121-128, 2010.
13. Mata SG et al: Legg-Calvé-Perthes disease and passive smoking, *J Pediatr Orthop* 20(3):326-330, 2000.
13A. Daniel AB et al: Environmental tobacco and wood smoke increase the risk of Legg-Calvé-Perthes disease. *Clin Orthop Rel Res* 470(9):2369-2375, 2012.
14. McCullough L, Lyman KS: Musculoskeletal considerations across the life span. In Gates SJ, Mooar PA, editors: *Musculoskeletal primary care*, Philadelphia, 1998, Lippincott.
15. Morrissy R, Weinstein S, editors: *Lovell and Winter's pediatric orthopaedics*, ed 4, Philadelphia, 1996, Lippincott-Raven.
16. Jorde LB et al: *Medical genetics*, ed 3, St Louis, 2006, Mosby.
17. Cassas KJ, Cassettari-Wayhs A: Childhood and adolescent sports-related overuse injuries, *Am Fam Physician* 73(6):1014-1022, 2006.
18. Kaeding CC, Whitehead R: Musculoskeletal injuries in adolescents, *Prim Care* 25(1):211-223, 1998.

19. Davis JR et al: Indications for magnetic resonance imaging in presumed adolescent idiopathic scoliosis, *J Bone Joint Surg Am* 86:2187-2195, 2004.
20. Katz DE et al: Brace wear control of curve progression in adolescent idiopathic scoliosis, *J Bone Joint Surg Am* 92:1343-1352, 2010.
21. Stuart L et al: Effects of bracing in adolescents with idiopathic scoliosis, *N Engl J Med* 369:1512-1521, 2013.
22. Moxley RT III et al: Practice parameter: corticosteroid treatment of Duchenne dystrophy: report of the Quality Standards Subcommittee of the American Academy of Neurology and the Practice Committee of the Child Neurology Society, *Neurology* 64(1):13-20, 2005.
23. Cummings JR et al: Congenital clubfoot, *Instr Course Lect* 51:385-400, 2002.
24. Heyden JB, Hoang BH: Osteosarcoma: basic science and clinical implications, *Orthop Clin North Am* 37(1):1-7, 2006.
25. Administration for Children and Families Children's Bureau: *Child maltreatment 2009*, Washington, DC, 2010, U.S. Department of Health and Human Services. Available at: www.acf.hhs.gov/programs/cb/stats_research/index.htm#can.
26. Rex C, Kay PR: Features of femoral fractures in nonaccidental injury, *J Pediatr Orthop* 20(3): 411-413, 2000.
27. Thomas SA et al: Long-bone fractures in young children: distinguishing accident injuries from child abuse, *Pediatrics* 88(3):471-476, 1991.
28. Lane WG et al: Racial differences in the evaluation of pediatric fractures for physical abuse, *JAMA* 288(13):1603-1609, 2002.
29. Swoboda SL et al: Skeletal trauma in child abuse. *Pediatr Ann* 42(11):e245-e252, 2013.
30. Wood JN et al: Evaluation for occult fractures in injured children. *Pediatrics* 136(2):232-240, 2015.

41

Structure, Function, and Disorders of the Integument

Sue Ann McCann, Noreen Heer Nicol, and Sue E. Huether

CHAPTER OUTLINE

The skin covers the entire body and is the largest organ of the body, accounting for about 20% of body weight. Combined with the accessory structures of hair, nails, and glands, it forms the integumentary system. The skin's primary function is protection from the environment by serving as a barrier against microorganisms, ultraviolet radiation, loss of body fluids, and the stress of mechanical forces. The skin regulates body temperature and is involved in immune surveillance and the activation of vitamin D. Touch and pressure receptors provide important protective functions and pleasurable sensations. The commensal (normal) microorganisms of the skin protect against pathologic bacteria.

STRUCTURE AND FUNCTION OF THE SKIN

Layers of the Skin

The skin is formed of two major layers: (1) a superficial or outer layer of epidermis and (2) a deeper layer of dermis (the true skin) (Figure 41-1). The subcutaneous layer (hypodermis) is the lowest lying layer of connective tissue that contains macrophages, fibroblasts, fat cells, nerves, fine muscles, blood vessels, lymphatics, and hair follicle roots. Each skin layer contains cells that represent progressive stages of skin cell differentiation and function as the skin grows. These are summarized in Table 41-1.

Dermal Appendages

The dermal appendages include the nails, hair, sebaceous glands, and the eccrine and apocrine sweat glands. The nails are protective keratinized plates that appear at the ends of fingers and toes. They have the

following structures: (1) the proximal nail fold, (2) the eponychium (cuticle), (3) the matrix from which the nail grows and its nail root, (4) the hyponychium (nail bed), (5) the nail plate, and (6) the paronychium (lateral nail fold) (Figure 41-2). Nail growth continues throughout life at 1 mm or less per day.

Hair color, density, grain, and pattern of distribution vary considerably among people and depend on age, sex, and race. Hair follicles arise from the matrix (or bulb) located deep in the dermis. They extend from the dermis at an angle and have an erector pili muscle attached near the mid-dermis that straightens the follicle when contracted, causing the hair to stand up. Hair growth begins in the bulb, with cellular differentiation occurring as the hair progresses up the follicle. Hair is fully hardened, or cornified, by the time it emerges at the skin surface. Hair color is determined by melanin-secreting follicular melanocytes. Hair growth is cyclic, with periods of growth and rest that vary over different body surfaces.

The sebaceous glands open onto the surface of the skin through a canal. They are found in greatest numbers on the face, chest, and back, with modified glands on the eyelids, lips, nipples, glans penis, and prepuce. Sebaceous glands secrete sebum, composed primarily of lipids, which oils the skin and hair and prevents drying. Androgens stimulate the growth of sebaceous glands, and their enlargement is an early sign of puberty.

The eccrine sweat glands are distributed over the body, with the greatest numbers in the palms of the hands, soles of the feet, and forehead. They open onto the surface of the skin and are important in thermoregulation and cooling of the body through evaporation. The apocrine sweat glands are fewer in number but produce significantly

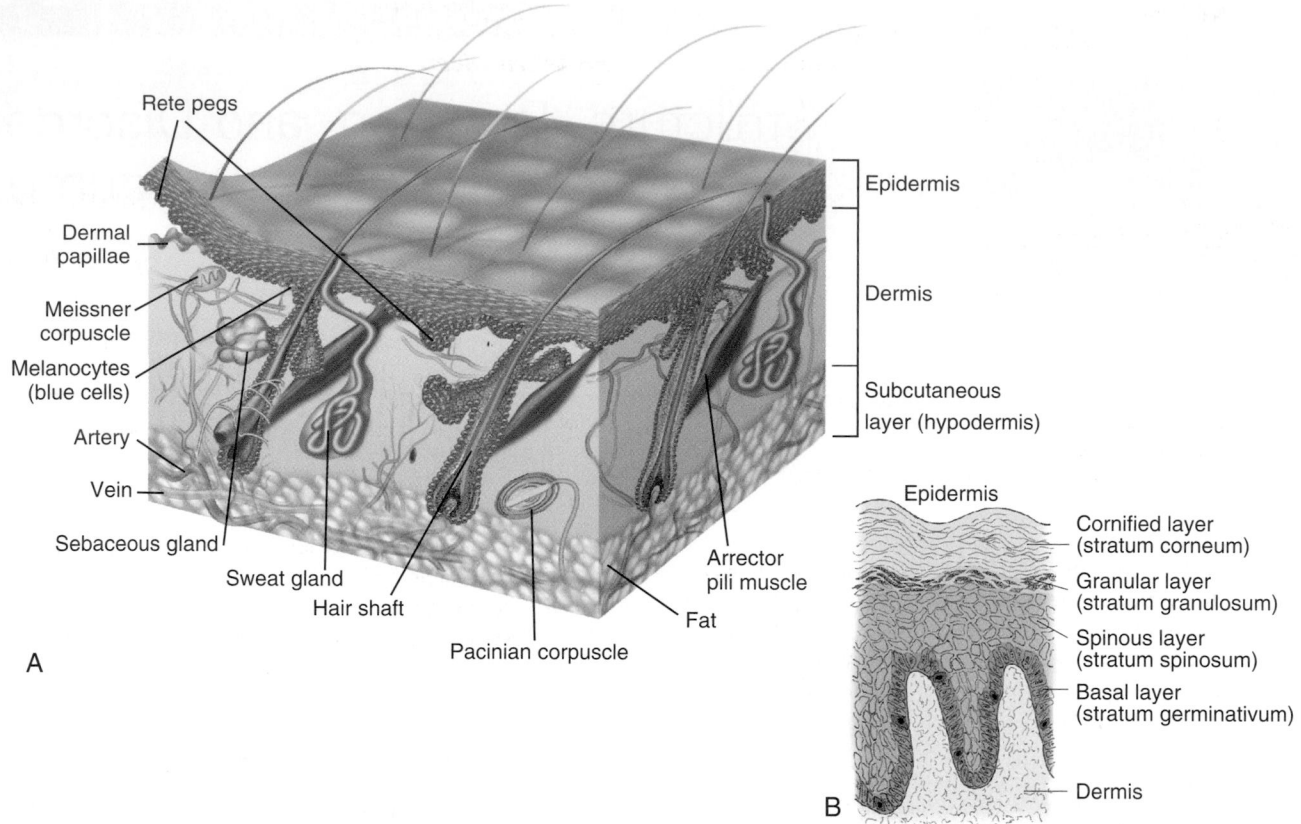

FIGURE 41-1 Structure of the Skin. A, Cross section showing major skin structures. **B,** Layers of the epidermis. (**A** from Kumar V et al: *Robbins & Cotran pathologic basis of disease,* ed 9, Philadelphia, 2015, Saunders; **B** from Baker SR: *Local flaps in facial reconstruction,* ed 3, Philadelphia, 2007, Saunders.)

TABLE 41-1   Layers of the Skin

Structure	Cell Types	Characteristics
Epidermis	Keratinocytes	Most important layer of skin; normally very thin (0.12 mm) but can thicken and form corns or calluses with constant pressure or friction; includes rete pegs that extend into papillary layer of dermis
	Langerhans cells	Cells with dendrite process and immune functions
Stratum corneum	Keratinocytes	Tough superficial layer covering body
Stratum lucidum	Keratinocytes	Clear layers of cells containing eleidin, which becomes keratin as cells move up to corneum layer
Stratum granulosum	Keratinocytes	Keratohyalin gives granular appearance to this layer
	Melanocytes	
Stratum spinosum	New keratinocytes	Polygonal shaped with spinous processes projecting between adjacent keratinocytes
Stratum basale	Keratinocytes	Basal layer where keratinocytes divide and move upward to replace cells shed from surface
(germinativum)	Melanocytes	Melanocytes synthesize pigment melanin
	Merkel cells	Function of Merkel cells is not clearly known; they are associated with sensory nerve endings
Dermis	Macrophages	Irregular connective tissue layer with rich blood, lymphatic, and nerve supply; contains sensory receptors and
Papillary layer (thin)	Mast cells	sweat glands (apocrine, eccrine, sebaceous), macrophages (phagocytic and important for wound healing), and mast cells (release histamine and have immune functions) (see Chapter 6)
Reticular layer (thick)	Histiocytes	Histiocytes are wandering macrophages that collect pigments and inflammatory debris
Subcutaneous layer (hypodermis)		Subcutaneous tissue or superficial fascia of varying thickness that connects overlying dermis to underlying muscle; contains macrophages, fibroblasts, fat cells, nerves, blood vessels, lymphatics, and hair follicle roots

more sweat than the eccrine glands. They are located near the bulb of hair follicles in the axillae, scalp, face, abdomen, and genital area. Their ducts open into the hair follicle. The interaction of sweat with commensal (normal) flora bacteria contributes to the odor of perspiration.

Blood Supply and Innervation

The blood supply to the skin is limited to the papillary capillaries, or plexus, of the dermis. These capillary loops are supplied by a deeper arterial plexus. Branches from the deep plexus also supply hair follicles and sweat glands. A subpapillary network of veins drains the capillary

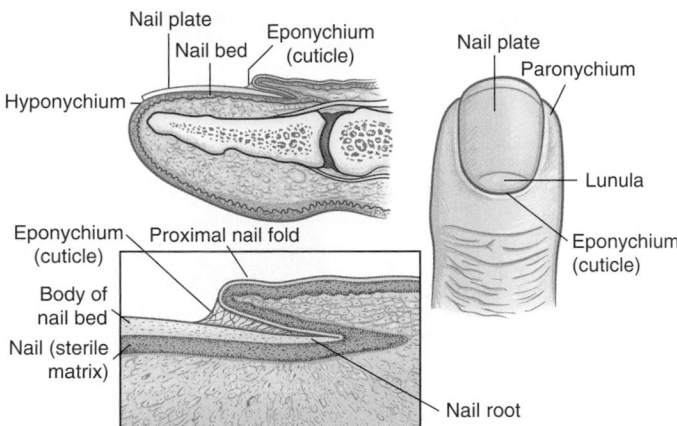

FIGURE 41-2 Structures of the Nail. (Redrawn from Thompson JM et al: *Mosby's clinical nursing,* ed 5, St Louis, 2002, Mosby.)

loops. Arteriovenous anastomoses in the dermis facilitate the regulation of body temperature. Heat loss is regulated by (1) variations in skin blood flow through the opening and closing of arteriovenous anastomoses and (2) the evaporative heat loss of sweat. The sympathetic nervous system regulates both vasoconstriction and vasodilation through α-adrenergic receptors in the skin. The lymphatic vessels of the skin arise in the papillary dermis and drain into larger subcutaneous trunks, removing cells, proteins, and immunologic mediators.

The structure and function of the skin change with advancing age. A summary of aging changes is included in the box titled *Geriatric Considerations:* Aging and Changes in Skin Integrity (p. 1079).

✔ **QUICK CHECK 41-1**
1. Describe the two layers of the skin.
2. How do the skin blood vessels and sweat glands regulate body temperature?
3. What are some changes that occur in skin with aging?

Clinical Manifestations of Skin Dysfunction
Lesions

Identification of the morphologic structure of the skin, including differentiation between primary and secondary lesions, and assessment of the appearance of the skin in combination with obtaining a health history are essential to identify underlying pathophysiology. Tables 41-2 and 41-3 describe and illustrate the basic lesions of the skin. Clinical manifestations of select skin lesions are described in Table 41-4.

Pressure ulcers. Pressure ulcers are ischemic ulcers resulting from unrelieved pressure, shearing forces, friction, and moisture. The term *decubitus ulcer* refers to ulcers or pressure sores that develop when unrelieved pressure interrupts normal blood flow to the skin and its underlying tissues. The risks for pressure ulcers are summarized in *Risk Factors:* Pressure Ulcer.[1]

Pressure sores usually develop over bony prominences, such as the sacrum, heels, ischia, and greater trochanters. Continuous pressure on tissue between the bony prominence and a resistant outside surface distorts capillaries and occludes the blood supply. Pressure ulcers also can occur in soft tissues from unrelieved pressure, for example, from nasal cannulas or endotracheal tubes. If the pressure is relieved within a few hours, a brief period of reactive hyperemia (redness) occurs and there may be no lasting tissue damage. If the pressure continues

---

External Factors
- Prolonged pressure
- Immobilization
- Lying in bed or sitting in chair or wheelchair without changing position or relieving pressure over an extended period
- Lying for hours on hard x-ray, emergency department, and operating room tables
- Prolonged moisture exposure
- Neurologic disorders (coma, spinal cord injuries, cognitive impairment, or cerebrovascular disease)
- Fractures or contractures
- Debilitation: elderly persons in hospitals and nursing homes
- Pain
- Sedation
- Friction and shearing forces
- Coarse bed sheets used for turning by dragging, which produces friction and a shearing force
- Inadequate caretaking staff
- Lack of communication/education regarding pressure ulcer care

Disease/Tissue Factors
- Impaired perfusion; ischemia
- Fecal or urinary incontinence; prolonged exposure to moisture
- Malnutrition, dehydration
- Chronic diseases accompanied by anemia, edema, renal failure, malnutrition, peripheral vascular disease, or sepsis
- Previous history of pressure ulcers
- Thin skin associated with aging or prolonged use of steroids

Data from Bogie K et al: *Handb Clin Neurol* 109:235-246, 2012; Coleman S et al: *Int J Nurs Stud* 50(7):974-1003, 2013; García-Fernández FP et al: *Nurs Scholarsh* 46(1):28-38, 2014; Michel JM et al: *Ann Phys Rehabil Med* 55(7):454-465, 2012.

---

unrelieved, the endothelial cells lining the capillaries become disrupted with platelet aggregation, forming microthrombi that block blood flow and cause anoxic necrosis of surrounding tissues (Figure 41-3). Shearing and friction are mechanical forces moving parallel to the skin (dragging) and can extend to the bony skeleton, causing detachment and injury of tissues. Pressure ulcers are staged or graded and one classification scheme is as follows[2]:

Stage 1—Nonblanchable erythema of intact skin, usually over a bony prominence; darkly pigmented skin may not have visible blanching

Stage 2—Partial-thickness skin loss (erosion or blistering) involving epidermis or dermis

Stage 3—Full-thickness skin loss involving damage or necrosis of subcutaneous tissue that may extend to, but not through, underlying fascia

Stage 4—Full-thickness tissue loss with exposure of muscle, bone, or supporting structures (tendons or joint capsules); can include undermining and tunneling

Suspected deep tissue injury—Localized in an area of purple or maroon discolored intact skin or blood-filled blister caused by underlying soft tissue damage from pressure and/or shear

Unstageable—Full-thickness tissue loss with base of ulcer covered by slough or eschar, or both, in the wound bed

Superficial damage results in a layer of dead tissue that forms as an abrasion, blister, erosion, or nonblanchable red/darkened skin or as a

Text continued on p. 1060

TABLE 41-2 Primary Skin Lesions

Macule
A flat, circumscribed area that is a change in color of skin; less than 1 cm in diameter
Examples: Freckles, flat moles (nevi), petechiae, measles, scarlet fever

Macules[a]

Papule
An elevated, firm, circumscribed area less than 1 cm in diameter
Examples: Wart (verruca), elevated moles, lichen planus, fibroma, insect bite

Lichen planus[b]

Patch
A flat, nonpalpable, irregular-shaped macule more than 1 cm in diameter
Examples: Vitiligo, port-wine stains, mongolian spots, café au lait spots

Vitiligo[c]

Plaque
Elevated, firm, and rough lesion with flat top surface greater than 1 cm in diameter
Examples: Psoriasis, seborrheic and actinic keratoses

Plaque[d]

Wheal
Elevated, irregular-shaped area of cutaneous edema; solid, transient; variable diameter
Examples: Insect bites, urticaria, allergic reaction

 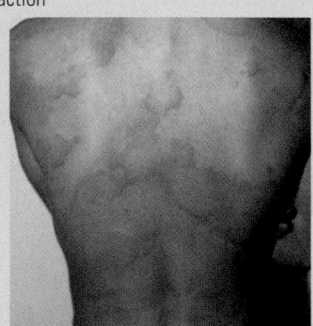

Wheal[e]

Nodule
Elevated, firm, circumscribed lesion; deeper in dermis than a papule; 1-2 cm in diameter
Examples: Erythema nodosum, lipomas

Lipoma[f]

TABLE 41-2 Primary Skin Lesions—cont'd

Tumor
Elevated, solid lesion; may be clearly demarcated; deeper in dermis; more than 2 cm in diameter

Examples: Neoplasms, benign tumor, lipoma, neurofibroma, hemangioma

Neurofibroma[f]

Vesicle
Elevated, circumscribed, superficial; does not extend into dermis; filled with serous fluid; less than 1 cm in diameter

Examples: Varicella (chickenpox), herpes zoster (shingles), herpes simplex

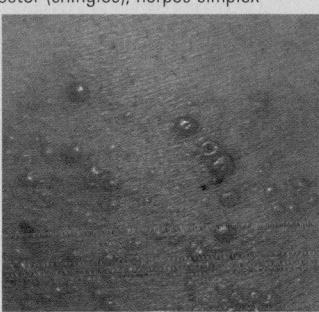

Vesicles[g]

Bulla
Vesicle more than 1 cm in diameter

Examples: Blister, pemphigus vulgaris

Bulla[h]

Pustule
Elevated, superficial lesion; similar to a vesicle but filled with purulent fluid

Examples: Impetigo, acne

Acne[c]

Cyst
Elevated, circumscribed, encapsulated lesion; in dermis or subcutaneous layer; filled with liquid or semisolid material

Examples: Sebaceous cyst, cystic acne

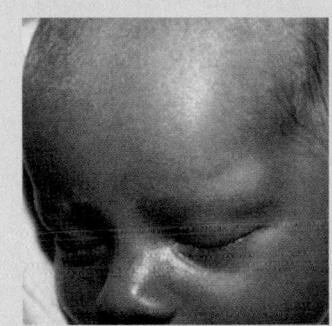

Sebaceous cyst[c]

Telangiectasia
Fine (0.5-1.0 mm), irregular red lines produced by capillary dilation; can be associated with acne rosacea (face), venous hypertension (spider veins in legs), systemic sclerosis, or developmental abnormalities (port-wine birthmarks)

Example: Telangiectasia in rosacea

Telangiectasia[e]

[a]Farrar WE et al: *Infectious diseases,* ed 2, London, 1992, Gower.

[b]James WD et al: *Andrews' diseases of the skin,* ed 11, Philadelphia, 2011, Saunders.

[c]Weston WL, Lane AT: *Color textbook of pediatric dermatology,* ed 3, Philadelphia, 2002, Mosby.

[d]Habif TP: *Clinical dermatology: a color guide to diagnosis and therapy,* ed 5, Philadelphia, 2010, Mosby.

[e]Bolognia JL et al: *Dermatology,* ed 3, Philadelphia, 2012, Saunders.

[f]Weston WL et al: *Color textbook of pediatric dermatology,* ed 4, Philadelphia, 2007, Mosby.

[g]Black MM et al: *Obstetric and gynecologic dermatology,* ed 3, Philadelphia, 2008, Mosby.

[h]Marks JG, Miller JJ: *Lookingbill & Marks' principles of dermatology,* ed 4, London, 2006, Saunders.

TABLE 41-3 Secondary Skin Lesions

Scale
Heaped-up, keratinized cells; flaky skin; irregular-shape; thick or thin; dry or oily; variation in size

Examples: Flaking of skin with seborrheic dermatitis following scarlet fever, or flaking of skin following a drug reaction; dry skin

Fine scaling[a]

Lichenification
Rough, thickened epidermis secondary to persistent rubbing, itching, or skin irritation; often involves flexor surface of extremity

Example: Chronic dermatitis

 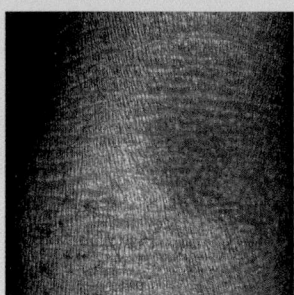

Atopic dermatitis of arm[b]

Keloid
Irregular-shaped, elevated, progressively enlarging scar; grows beyond boundaries of wound; caused by excessive collagen formation during healing

Examples: Keloid formation following surgery

Keloid[c]

Scar
Thin to thick fibrous tissue that replaces normal skin following injury or laceration to the dermis

Examples: Healed wound or surgical incision

Hypertrophic scar[d]

Excoriation
Loss of epidermis; linear, hollowed-out, crusted area

Examples: Abrasion or scratch, scabies

 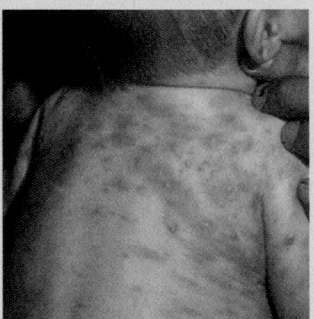

Scabies[c]

Fissure
Linear crack or break from the epidermis to the dermis; may be moist or dry

Examples: Athlete's foot, cracks at the corner of mouth, anal fissure, dermatitis

Fissures from infected dermatitis[c]

TABLE 41-3 Secondary Skin Lesions—cont'd

Erosion

Loss of part of the epidermis; depressed, moist, glistening; follows rupture of a vesicle or bulla or chemical injury

Example: Chemical injury

Erosion on leg[e]

Ulcer

Loss of epidermis and dermis; concave; varies in size

Examples: Pressure ulcer, stasis ulcers

Pressure ulcer on heel[f]

Atrophy

Thinning of skin surface and loss of skin markings; skin appears translucent and paper-like

Examples: Aged skin, striae

Aged skin[g]

[a]Baran R et al: *Color atlas of the hair, scalp, and nails,* St Louis, 1991, Mosby.
[b]James WD et al: *Andrews' diseases of the skin,* ed 11, Philadelphia, 2011, Saunders.
[c]Weston WL et al: *Color textbook of pediatric dermatology,* ed 4, St Louis, 2007, Mosby.
[d]Nouri K, Leal-Khouri S: *Techniques in dermatologic surgery,* Philadelphia, 2003, Mosby.
[e]Bolognia JL et al: *Dermatology,* ed 3, Philadelphia, 2012, Saunders.
[f]Robinson JK et al: *Surgery of the skin,* ed 3, Philadelphia, 2015, Saunders.
[g]Seidel HM et al: *Seidel's guide to physical examination,* ed 8, St Louis, 2015, Mosby.

TABLE 41-4 Clinical Manifestations of Select Skin Lesions

Type	Clinical Manifestation
Comedone	Plug of sebaceous and keratin material lodged in opening of hair follicle; open comedone has dilated orifice (blackhead) and closed comedone has narrow opening (whitehead)
Burrow	Narrow, raised, irregular channel caused by parasite
Petechiae	Circumscribed area of blood less than 0.5 cm in diameter
Purpura	Circumscribed area of blood greater than 0.5 cm in diameter
Telangiectasia	Dilated, superficial blood vessels

FIGURE 41-3 **Progression of Pressure Ulcer.** Sustained pressure over a bony prominence compresses the tissue and reduces blood flow, resulting in progressive ischemia and necrosis of tissue.

reddish blue discoloration when there is deeper tissue damage. Superficial sores are more common on the sacrum as a result of shearing or friction forces (forces parallel to the skin). Deep sores develop closer to the bone as a result of tissue distortion and vascular occlusion from pressure perpendicular to the tissue (over the heels, trochanter, and ischia). Bacteria colonize the dead tissue, and infection is usually localized and self-limiting. Proteolytic enzymes from bacteria and macrophages dissolve necrotic tissues and cause a foul-smelling discharge that resembles, but is not, pus. The necrotic tissue initiates an inflammatory response with potential pain, fever, and leukocytosis. If the ulceration is large, toxicity and pain lead to a host of possible complications, including loss of appetite, debility, local/systemic infections, and renal insufficiency.

The primary goal for those at risk for pressure ulcers is prevention and early detection. Preventive techniques include frequent assessment of the skin with repositioning and turning of the individual; promotion of movement; implementation of pressure reduction (type of positioning and use of specialty beds), pressure removal (positioning interval), and pressure distribution (positioning aids) devices; and elimination of excessive moisture and drainage. Adequate nutrition, oxygenation, and fluid balance must be maintained.[3,4]

Superficial ulcers should be covered with flat, moisture-retaining dressings (e.g., hydrogel dressings) that cannot wrinkle and cause increased pressure or friction. Successful healing requires continued adequate relief of pressure, débridement of necrotic tissue, opening of deep pockets for drainage, and repair of damaged tissue by construction of skin flaps for large, deep ulcers. Infection requires treatment with antibiotics, and pain should be controlled.[5,6]

Keloids and Hypertrophic Scars

Keloids are rounded, firm elevated scars with irregular clawlike margins that extend beyond the original site of injury. They are most common in darkly-pigmented skin types and generally appear weeks to months after a stable scar has formed. Hypertrophic scars are elevated erythematous fibrous lesions that do not extend beyond the border of injury. Hypertrophic scars appear within 3 to 4 months and usually regress within 1 year. Both lesions are caused by abnormal wound healing with excessive fibroblast activity and collagen formation, and loss of control of normal tissue repair and regeneration.[7] Genetic susceptibility is likely.[8]

Excessive or poorly aligned tension on a wound, introduction of foreign material into the skin, infection, and certain types of trauma (e.g., burns) are all provocative factors. Those parts of the body at risk include shoulders, back, chin, ears, and lower legs. Individuals 10 to 30 years of age develop lesions much more commonly than do prepubescent children or older adults.

Keloids start as pink or red, firm, well-defined, rubbery plaques that persist for several months after trauma. Later, uncontrolled overgrowth causes extension beyond the site of the original wound, and the overgrowth becomes smoother, irregularly shaped, hyperpigmented, harder, and more symptomatic. The fibrous tissue that accumulates in keloids is associated with increased cellularity and metabolic activity of fibroblasts. The tendency to form clawlike prolongations is typical (Figure 41-4).

Various treatments are available for the management of keloids and hypertrophic scars. There also is a need for research to improve treatment outcome.[7]

Pruritus

Pruritus, or itching, is a symptom associated with many primary skin disorders, such as eczema, psoriasis, or insect infestations, or it can be a manifestation of systemic disease (e.g., chronic renal failure,

FIGURE 41-4 Keloid. (Courtesy Department of Dermatology, School of Medicine, University of Utah, Salt Lake City, Utah.)

cholestatic liver disease, thyroid disorders, iron deficiency, neuropathies, or malignancy) or the use of opiate drugs. It may be acute or chronic (neuropathic itch), localized or generalized, and migratory (moves from one location to another).[9] Multiple stimuli can produce itching, and there is interaction between itch and pain sensations. There are many itch mediators, including histamine, serotonin, prostaglandins, bradykinins, neuropeptides, acetylcholine, and interleukins-2 and -31. Small unmyelinated type C nerve fibers transmit itch sensations and specific spinal pathways may carry itch sensations to the brain.[10]

Management of pruritus is challenging and depends on the cause, and the primary condition must be treated. Both topical and systemic therapies are used.[11]

> ### ✔ QUICK CHECK 41-2
> 1. What areas are at greatest risk of pressure ulcers?
> 2. How does a keloid differ from a normal scar?
> 3. What stimulates pruritus?

DISORDERS OF THE SKIN

Disorders of the skin may be precipitated by trauma, abnormal cellular function, infection, immune responses and inflammation, and systemic diseases.

Inflammatory Disorders

The most common inflammatory disorders of the skin are eczema and dermatitis. Eczema and dermatitis are general terms that describe a particular type of inflammatory response in the skin and can be used interchangeably. Eczematous disorders are generally characterized by pruritus, lesions with indistinct borders, and epidermal changes. These lesions can appear as erythema, papules, or scales; they can present in an acute, subacute, or chronic phase. Edema, serous discharge, and crusting occur with continued irritation and scratching. In chronic eczema, the skin becomes thickened, leathery, and hyperpigmented from recurrent irritation and scratching. The location of eczema is related to the underlying cause. Eczematous inflammations need to be differentiated from other rashes and dermatoses, particularly psoriasis.

Allergic Contact Dermatitis

Allergic contact dermatitis is a common form of T-cell–mediated or delayed hypersensitivity. (See Chapter 8 for different types of allergic responses.) The response is an interaction of skin barrier function,

FIGURE 41-5 Poison Ivy. A, Poison ivy on knee. **B,** Poison ivy dermatitis. (Courtesy Department of Dermatology, School of Medicine, University of Utah, Salt Lake City, Utah.)

FIGURE 41-6 Stasis Ulcer. (Courtesy Department of Dermatology, School of Medicine, University of Utah, Salt Lake City, Utah.)

reaction to irritants, and neuronal responses, such as pruritus. Genetic susceptibility involves several genes including loss-of-function mutations in the gene encoding the epidermal protein filaggrin. Various allergens (e.g., microorganisms, chemicals, foreign proteins, latex, drugs, metals) can form the sensitizing antigen. Contact with poison ivy is a common example (Figure 41-5). As the allergen contacts the skin, the allergen is bound to a carrier protein, forming a sensitizing antigen. The Langerhans cells (antigen presenting dendritic cells) process the antigen and present it to T cells. T cells then become sensitized to the antigen, inducing the release of inflammatory cytokines and the symptoms of dermatitis.[12] In latex allergy, there is either a type IV hypersensitivity reaction to chemicals used in latex rubber processing or a type I immediate hypersensitivity reaction with immunoglobulin E (IgE) antibodies formed in response to latex rubber protein.[13]

In delayed hypersensitivity (type IV), several hours pass before an immunologic response is apparent. The T cells play an important role because they differentiate and secrete lymphokines that affect macrophage (Langerhans cells) movement and aggregation, coagulation, and other inflammatory responses (see Chapter 8). Sensitization usually develops with first exposure to the antigen, and symptoms of dermatitis occur with reexposure.

The manifestations of allergic contact dermatitis include erythema and swelling with pruritic (itching) vesicular lesions in the areas of allergen contact. The pattern of distribution provides clues to the source of the antigen (e.g., hands exposed to chemical solutions or boundaries from rings and bracelets). The antigen must be removed for the inflammatory response to resolve and tissue repair to begin. Treatment may require topical or systemic steroids.

Irritant Contact Dermatitis

Irritant contact dermatitis is a nonspecific inflammatory dermatitis caused by activation of the innate immune system by proinflammatory properties of chemicals. The severity of the inflammation is related to the concentration of the irritant, length of exposure, and disruption of the skin barrier.[14] Chemical irritation from acids and prolonged exposure to soaps, detergents, and various agents used in industry can cause inflammatory lesions. The skin lesions resemble allergic contact dermatitis. Removing the source of irritation and using topical agents provide effective treatment.

Atopic Dermatitis

Atopic dermatitis (allergic dermatitis) is common in individuals with a history of hay fever or asthma and is associated with IgE antibodies. It is more common in infancy and childhood; however, some individuals are affected throughout life. Specific details of this disorder are presented in Chapter 42.

Stasis Dermatitis

Stasis dermatitis usually occurs on the lower legs as a result of chronic venous stasis and edema and is associated with varicosities, phlebitis, and vascular trauma (see Chapter 24). Pooling of venous blood traps neutrophils that may release oxidants and proteolytic enzymes. Increased venous pressure widens interendothelial pores with deposition of red blood cells, fibrin, and other macromolecules, making them unavailable for repair while promoting inflammation.[15] First, erythema and pruritus develop followed by scaling, petechiae, and hyperpigmentation. Progressive lesions become ulcerated, particularly around the ankles and pretibial surface (Figure 41-6).

Treatment includes elevating the legs as often as possible, not wearing tight clothes around the legs, and not standing for long periods. Defined infections are treated with antibiotics. Chronic lesions with ulceration are treated with moist dressings, external compression/dressings, and vein ablation surgery.[16]

Seborrheic Dermatitis

Seborrheic dermatitis is a common chronic inflammation of the skin involving the scalp, eyebrows, eyelids, ear canals, nasolabial folds, axillae, chest, and back (Figure 41-7). In infants it is known as *cradle cap*. The cause is unknown. Proposed theories include genetic predisposition, phospholipases from *Malassezia* yeasts, immunosuppression, and epidermal hyperproliferation.[17]

The lesions develop from infancy to old age with periods of remission and exacerbation. The lesions appear as scaly, white or yellowish inflammatory plaques with mild pruritus. Topical therapy includes antifungal shampoos, calcineurin inhibitors, and low-dose steroids for acute flares. Corticosteroids should not be used for maintenance therapy.

FIGURE 41-7 Seborrheic Dermatitis. (Courtesy Department of Dermatology, School of Medicine, University of Utah, Salt Lake City, Utah.)

FIGURE 41-8 Psoriasis. Typical oval plaque with well-defined borders and silvery scale. (Courtesy Department of Dermatology, School of Medicine, University of Utah, Salt Lake City, Utah.)

Papulosquamous Disorders

Psoriasis, pityriasis rosea, lichen planus, acne vulgaris, acne rosacea, and lupus erythematosus are characterized by papules, scales, plaques, and erythema. Collectively they are described as papulosquamous disorders.

Psoriasis

Psoriasis is a chronic, relapsing, proliferative, inflammatory disorder that involves the skin, scalp, and nails and can occur at any age. Psoriasis affects about 1% to 4% of the population in countries north of the equator. The onset is generally established by 40 years of age. A family history of psoriasis is common and the genetic mechanisms are complex. The onset of psoriasis later in life is less familial and more secondary to comorbidities, such as obesity, smoking, hypertension, and diabetes.[18,19]

The inflammatory cascade of psoriasis involves the complex interactions between macrophages, fibroblasts, dendritic cells, natural killer cells, T helper cells, and regulatory T cells. These immune cells lead to the secretion of numerous inflammatory mediators, such as interferon (IFN), tumor necrosis factor-alpha (TNF-α), and various other cytokines including interleukin-12 (IL-12), IL-23, and IL-17. These inflammatory markers are the target for several therapeutic drugs known as the biologics (biotherapy).[20]

Both the dermis and the epidermis are thickened because of cellular hyperproliferation, altered kerotinocyte differentiation, and expanded dermal vasculature. The turnover time for shedding the epidermis is decreased to 3 to 4 days from the normal of 14 to 20 days, with many more germinative cells and increased transit time through the dermis. Cell maturation and keratinization are bypassed, and the epidermis thickens and plaques form. The loosely cohesive keratin gives the lesion a silvery appearance. Capillary dilation and increased vascularization accommodate the increased cell metabolism but also cause erythema. The disease can be mild, moderate, or severe, depending on the size, distribution, and inflammation of the lesions. Psoriasis is marked by remissions and exacerbations.

The types of psoriasis include plaque (psoriasis vulgaris), inverse, guttate, pustular, and erythrodermic. Plaque psoriasis is the most common and affects 80% to 90% of individuals with psoriasis. The typical plaque psoriatic lesion is a well-demarcated, thick, silvery, scaly, erythematous plaque surrounded by normal skin (Figure 41-8). Small erythematous papules enlarge and coalesce into larger inflammatory lesions on the face, scalp, elbows, and knees and at sites of trauma (Koebner phenomenon).

Inverse psoriasis is rare and involves lesions that develop in skin folds (i.e., axilla or groin). In guttate psoriasis, small papules appear

FIGURE 41-9 Guttate Psoriasis Following Streptococcal Infection. Numerous uniformly small lesions may abruptly occur following streptococcal pharyngitis. (Courtesy Department of Dermatology, School of Medicine, University of Utah, Salt Lake City, Utah.)

suddenly on the trunk and extremities (Figure 41-9) a few weeks after a streptococcal respiratory tract infection. Guttate psoriasis may resolve spontaneously in weeks or months. Pustular psoriasis appears as blisters of noninfectious pus (collections of neutrophils), and erythrodermic (exfoliative) psoriasis is often accompanied by pruritus or pain with widespread red, scaling lesions that cover a large area of the body.

Psoriatic arthritis of hands, feet, knees, and ankle joints develops in 5% to 30% of cases. Psoriatic nail disease can occur in all psoriasis subtypes with pitting, onycholysis, subungal hyperkeratosis, and nail plate dystrophy. A number of comorbidities are associated with the inflammatory mechanisms of psoriasis (see *Health Alert:* Psoriasis and Comorbidities).

Treatment is individualized and related to maintaining skin moisture, reducing epidermal cell turnover and pruritus, and promoting immunomodulation. Mild psoriasis is treated with skin-directed therapy, such as medium- to high-strength topical corticosteroids, vitamin D analogs, emollients, and keratolytic agents (such as salicylic acid), and narrow-band ultraviolet light therapy. Systemic therapy is indicated for moderate to severe disease or in the presence of psoriatic arthritis. Current FDA-approved medications include methotrexate,

FIGURE 41-10 Pityriasis Rosea Herald Patch. A collarette pattern has formed around the margins *(arrows).* (Courtesy Department of Dermatology, School of Medicine, University of Utah, Salt Lake City, Utah.)

FIGURE 41-11 Hypertrophic Lichen Planus on Arms. (Courtesy Department of Dermatology, School of Medicine, University of Utah, Salt Lake City, Utah.)

acitretin, and cyclosporine (short term). Newer FDA-approved biologics are being used with more frequency as our understanding of the pathophysiology of psoriasis continues to grow. These biologics include the anti-TNF medications infliximab, adalimumab, and etanercept. Ustekinumab is the most recent FDA-approved injectable biologic targeting IL-12 and IL-23. The IL-17 inhibitors are currently under investigation for their safety and efficacy.[21,22] A potential complication of biotherapy is the development of anti–drug antibodies.[23]

Pityriasis Rosea

Pityriasis rosea is a self-limiting inflammatory disorder that occurs more often in young adults. The cause is thought to be a herpes-like virus (e.g., human herpesvirus 6 [HHV6] and HHV7).[24] Pityriasis rosea begins as a single lesion (herald patch) that is circular, demarcated, and salmon-pink, approximately 3 to 10 cm in diameter, and usually located on the trunk. Early lesions are macular and papular. Secondary lesions develop within 14 to 21 days and extend over the trunk and upper part of the extremities (Figure 41-10), although rarely on the face. The small erythematous rose-colored papules expand into characteristic oval lesions that are bilateral and symmetrically distributed. The pattern of distribution on the back follows the skin lines around the trunk and resembles a drooping pine tree. The scales are sloughed from the margin of the lesions, forming a collarette pattern. Itching is the most common symptom. Occasionally headache, fatigue, or sore throat precedes the development of the lesions.

The diagnosis of pityriasis rosea follows the clinical appearance of the lesion. Secondary syphilis, psoriasis, drug eruption, nummular eczema, and seborrheic dermatitis are among the differential diagnosis considerations. The disorder is usually self-limiting and resolves in a few months with symptomatic treatment for pruritus or cosmetic concerns. Ultraviolet light (with some risk for hyperpigmentation) or systemic corticosteroids may be used to control pruritus. Acyclovir and erythromycin also may be used for treatment.[25]

Lichen Planus

Lichen planus (LP) is a benign autoimmune inflammatory disorder of the skin and mucous membranes.[26] The age of onset is usually between 30 and 70 years. The cause is unknown but T cells, adhesion molecules,

inflammatory cytokines, perforin, and antigen-presenting cells are involved. LP also is linked to numerous drugs and hepatitis C virus.[27] The disorder begins with nonscaling, purple-colored, flat-topped, polygonal pruritic papules 2 to 4 mm in size, usually located symmetrically on the wrists, ankles, lower legs, and genitalia (Figure 41-11). New lesions are pale pink and evolve into a dark violet color. Persistent lesions may be thickened and red, forming hypertrophic lichen planus. Oral lesions (oral lichen planus) appear as lacy white rings that must be differentiated from leukoplakia or oral candidiasis.[28] Usually, oral lesions do not ulcerate, but localized or extensive painful ulcerations can occur, and there may be increased risk for oral cancer.[28] Chronic ulcerated lesions become malignant in 1% of individuals with the disease. Thinning and splitting of nails are common, and part or the entire nail may be shed.

Pruritus is the most distressing symptom. The lesions are self-limiting and may last for months or years, with an average duration of 6 to 18 months. Postinflammatory hyperpigmentation is a common consequence of the lesion. Approximately 20% of individuals have a recurrence. Diagnosis is made by the clinical appearance and histopathology of the lesion. Treatment is individualized and includes topical, intralesional, or systemic corticosteroids (second line for resistant LP), and systemic acitretin with or without adjuvant light therapy. Antihistamines are given for itching, and short-term use of topical or systemic corticosteroids may be used to control inflammation. Mucous membrane lesions are treated with topical steroids, topical retinoids or immunomodulators (or both), and systemic glucocorticoids.[29]

Acne Vulgaris

Acne vulgaris is an inflammatory disorder of the pilosebaceous follicle (the sebaceous gland contiguous with a hair follicle) that usually occurs during adolescence. It is discussed in Chapter 42.

Acne Rosacea

Acne rosacea is a chronic inflammation of the skin that develops in middle-aged adults. There are four subtypes of lesions: erythematotel-angiectatic, papulopustular, phymatous, and ocular (eyelids and ocular surface). The exact cause is unknown but factors that trigger an altered innate immune response are involved (i.e., sun exposure and damage, drinking alcohol or hot beverages, hormonal fluctuations, and *Demodex folliculorum* [mites]).[30] The most common lesions are erythema, papules, pustules, and telangiectasia. They occur in the middle third of the face, including the forehead, nose, cheeks, and chin (Figure 41-12). The lesions are associated with chronic, inappropriate vasodilation resulting in flushing and sun sensitivity. Sebaceous hypertrophy, fibrosis, and telangiectasia may be severe enough to produce an irreversible bulbous appearance of the nose (rhinophyma). Disorders of the eye often accompany rosacea, particularly conjunctivitis and keratitis, which can result in visual impairment. Facial application of fluorinated topical steroids may increase the severity of telangiectasias.

Photoprotection, using sunscreens, is essential along with avoidance of other triggers. Both topical (metronidazole, azelaic acid) and oral drugs (tetracyclines and doxycline) may be effective. Surgical excision of excessive tissue may be required for rhinophyma.[31]

Lupus Erythematosus

Lupus erythematosus is a systemic inflammatory, autoimmune disease with cutaneous manifestations (see Chapter 8). Discoid (or cutaneous) lupus erythematosus (DLE) is limited to the skin and can progress to systemic lupus erythematosus.[32]

Discoid (cutaneous) lupus erythematosus. Discoid (cutaneous) lupus erythematosus (DLE) usually occurs in genetically susceptible adults, particularly women in their late thirties or early forties, but people of any age can be affected. The disease can be acute, subacute, intermittent, or chronic. Differentiation of subtypes is by physical examination, laboratory studies, histologic analysis, and antibody serology direct immunofluorescence.[33] The lesions may be single or multiple and vary in size. Often the lesions are located on light-exposed areas of the skin, and photosensitivity is common. The face is the most common site of lesion involvement with a butterfly pattern of distribution found over the nose and cheeks.

The cause is unknown but is related to genetic and environmental factors and an altered immune response to an unknown antigen or to ultraviolet B wavelengths. There is development of self-reactive T and B cells, decreased number of regulatory T cells, and increased levels of proinflammatory cytokines. Autoantibodies and immune complexes cause tissue damage and inflammation[34] (Figure 41-13). On skin biopsy with immunofluorescent observation, there are lumpy deposits of immunoglobulins, especially IgM (lupus band test).[35]

The early lesion is asymmetric, with a 1- to 2-cm raised red plaque with a brownish scale. The scale penetrates the hair follicle and leaves a visible follicle opening (carpet-tack appearance) when removed. The lesions persist for months and then resolve spontaneously or atrophy. Healing progresses outward from the center of the lesion, with residual telangiectasia and hypopigmented scarring. Atrophy of the dermis and epidermis can cause a depressed scar. Treatment options include protection from the sun and use of topical steroids, calcineurin inhibitors, antimalarial drugs (e.g., hydroxychloroquine sulfate), and

FIGURE 41-12 Granulomatous Rosacea. Pustules and erythema occur on the forehead, cheeks, and nose. (From Habif TP: *Clinical dermatology*, ed 6, Philadelphia, 2016, Saunders.)

FIGURE 41-13 Subacute Cutaneous Lupus (Discoid Lupus Erythematosus). (Courtesy Department of Dermatology, School of Medicine, University of Utah, Salt Lake City, Utah.)

immunosuppressors. These medications must be used with caution to prevent serious side effects.[35]

Vesiculobullous Diseases

Vesiculobullous skin diseases share a common characteristic of vesicle, or blister, formation. Two such diseases are pemphigus and erythema multiforme.

Pemphigus

Pemphigus (meaning to blister or bubble) is a group of rare autoimmune blistering diseases of the skin and oral mucous membranes caused by circulating autoantibodies directed against the cell surface adhesion molecule desmoglein at the desmosomal cell junction in the suprabasal layer of the epidermis. Immunoglobulin G (IgG) autoantibodies and C3 complement bind to the desmoglein adhesion molecules, resulting in the destruction of cell-to-cell adhesion (acantholysis) in the basal layer of the epidermis (see Table 41-1) with fluid accumulation and the resulting symptom of blister formation (Figure 41-14). Pemphigus can occur in all age groups but is more prevalent in persons between 40 and 50 years of age. There is a genetic predisposition as well as environmental (viral infections, drug-induced, dietary intake, or physical effects such as radiation or surgery) and endogenous (emotional or hormonal stressors) influences. Pemphigus presents in varying forms often with painful, superficial erosions prone to infection[36,37]:

- **Pemphigus vulgaris** is the most common form. Oral lesions precede the onset of skin blistering, which is more prominent on the face, scalp, and axilla. The blisters rupture easily because of the thin, fragile overlying portion of the epidermis.
- **Pemphigus vegetans** is a variant of pemphigus vulgaris in which large blisters develop in tissue folds of the axilla and groin.
- **Pemphigus foliaceus** is a milder form of the disease and involves acantholysis at the more superficial, subcorneal level of the epidermis (see Table 41-1) with blistering, erosions, scaling, crusting, and erythema usually of the face and chest. Oral mucous membranes are rarely involved.
- **Pemphigus erythematosus** is a subset of pemphigus foliaceus often associated with system lupus erythematosus with positive antinuclear antibodies. The lesions are generally less widely distributed.
- **Paraneoplastic pemphigus** is the most severe form of pemphigus and is associated with lymphoproliferative neoplasms.
- **IgA pemphigus** is the most benign form of pemphigus characterized by tissue-bound and circulating IgA antibodies targeting

desmosomal or nondesmosomal cell surface components in the basement membrane of the epidermis.

- **Pemphigus herpetiformis** is a very rare form of pemphigus that resembles dermatitis herpetiformis (blistering lesions that have the appearance of herpes lesions) but with immunologic and histologic findings consistent with pemphigus.

The diagnosis of pemphigus is made from the clinical and histologic findings of the skin. Immunofluorescence demonstrates the presence of antibodies at the site of blister formation. The clinical course of the disease may range from rapidly fatal to relatively benign. The primary treatment for pemphigus is systemic corticosteroids in combination with adjuvant immunosuppressants. Newer methods of treatment and a clearer understanding of the pathogenesis have improved the prognosis and decreased mortality.[38]

Erythema Multiforme

Erythema multiforme is a syndrome characterized by inflammation of the skin and mucous membranes, often associated with a T-cell–mediated immunologic reaction to a drug or microorganisms (e.g., herpes simplex virus) that targets small blood vessels in the skin or mucosa.[39] Bullous erythema multiforme involves the mucous membranes. It is relatively rare and occurs more often during the second to fourth decade of life; however, it can occur at any age. Immune complex formation and deposition of C3, IgM, and fibrinogen around the superficial dermal blood vessels, basement membrane, and keratinocytes are common histologic findings. Edema develops in the superficial dermis, so vesicles and bullae form. The lesions vary in clinical presentation and may involve the skin or mucous membranes, or both. The characteristic "bull's-eye," or "target," lesions occur on the skin surface with a central erythematous region surrounded by concentric rings of alternating edema and inflammation. The lesions usually occur suddenly in groups over a period of 2 to 3 weeks. Urticarial plaques, 1 to 2 cm in diameter, can develop without the target lesion. A vesiculobullous form is characterized by mucous membrane lesions and erythematous plaques on the extensor surfaces of the extremities. Single or multiple vesicles or bullae may arise on a part of the plaque accompanied by pruritus and burning. The lesions heal within 3 to 4 weeks.

The most common forms of erythema multiforme are usually associated with severe drug reactions and include Stevens-Johnson syndrome (severe mucocutaneous bullous form involving 10% of body surface area) and toxic epidermal necrolysis (TEN) (severe mucocutaneous bullous form involving 30% of body surface area). Cytotoxic T lymphocytes (CTLs) in an HLA-restricted fashion mediate the immune mechanism related to drug reactions[40,41] (see Chapter 42 for pediatric considerations).

Prodromal symptoms of erythema multiforme, including fever, headache, malaise, sore throat, and cough, develop in approximately one third of the cases. The bullous lesions form erosions and crusts when they rupture. There is necrosis of the epidermis in TEN. The mouth, air passages, esophagus, urethra, and conjunctiva may be involved when mucous membranes are affected. Blindness can result from corneal ulcerations. Difficulty eating, breathing, and urinating may develop with severe consequences. The disease can involve the kidneys and extend from the upper respiratory passages into the lungs. Severe forms of the disease can be fatal.

Recognizing the person's medication history that preceded the target lesion and performing a skin biopsy are required to establish the diagnosis. Mild acute forms of the disease last 10 to 14 days and require no treatment. Any ongoing drug therapy should be withdrawn and reevaluated and underlying infections treated. Fluid and electrolyte balance should be monitored in severe forms of the disease, and

FIGURE 41-14 Bullous Pemphigoid. Generalized eruption with blisters arising from an edematous, erythematous annular base. (Courtesy Department of Dermatology, School of Medicine, University of Utah, Salt Lake City, Utah.)

mucous membranes should be carefully managed with a bland diet, warm saline eyewashes, topical anesthetics, or corticosteroids to maintain comfort and prevent infection. Cutaneous blisters can be treated with wet compresses of Burow solution. Ophthalmic, kidney, and lung involvement require special care. Resolution occurs in 8 to 10 days, usually without scarring. Mucosal lesions may take 6 weeks to heal.

✔ QUICK CHECK 41-4
1. Describe the inflammatory lesion associated with lupus erythematosus.
2. Compare the three forms of pemphigus.
3. What is the characteristic lesion of erythema multiforme?

Infections

Cutaneous infections are common forms of skin disease. They generally remain localized, although serious complications can develop with systemic involvement that can be life-threatening. The types of skin infection include bacterial, viral, and fungal. The commensal (normal) flora of the skin consists of aerobes, yeast, and anaerobes and often provides protection against pathogens that cause skin infections, including *Staphylococcus* and *Streptococcus*.

Bacterial Infections

Most bacterial infections of the skin are caused by local invasion of pathogens. Coagulase-positive *Staphylococcus aureus* and, less often, beta-hemolytic streptococci are the common causative microorganisms. Community-acquired methicillin-resistant *Staphylococcus aureus* (CA-MRSA [see Chapter 8]) also is a cause of serious skin infection, particularly skin abscesses.[42]

Folliculitis. Folliculitis is an infection of the hair follicle and can be caused by bacteria, viruses, or fungi, although *S. aureus* is the common culprit. The infection develops from proliferation of the microorganism around the opening and inside the follicle. Inflammation is caused by the release of chemotactic factors and enzymes from the bacteria. The lesions appear as pustules with a surrounding area of erythema. They are most prominent on the scalp and extremities and rarely cause systemic symptoms. Prolonged skin moisture, skin trauma (e.g., shaving facial hair), occlusive clothing, topical agents, and poor hygiene are associated contributing factors. Cleaning with soap and water and topical application of antibiotics are effective treatments.

Furuncles and carbuncles. Furuncles, or "boils," are inflammations of hair follicles (Figure 41-15). They may develop after folliculitis

FIGURE 41-15 Furuncle of the Forearm. (Courtesy Department of Dermatology, School of Medicine, University of Utah, Salt Lake City, Utah.)

that spreads through the follicular wall into the surrounding dermis. The invading microorganism is usually *S. aureus*, including community-acquired methicillin-resistant *S. aureus* (CA-MSRA [see Chapter 8]). The infecting strain may spread to the skin from the anterior nares. Any skin area with hair can be infected, and one or several lesions may be present. The initial lesion is a deep, firm, red, painful nodule 1 to 5 cm in diameter. Within a few days, the erythematous nodules change to a large, fluctuant, and tender cystic nodule accompanied by cellulitis. No systemic symptoms are present, and the lesion may drain large amounts of pus and necrotic tissue.

Carbuncles are a collection of infected hair follicles and usually occur on the back of the neck, the upper back, and the lateral thighs. The lesion begins in the subcutaneous tissue and lower dermis as a firm mass that evolves into an erythematous, painful, swollen mass that drains through many openings. Abscesses may develop. Chills, fever, and malaise can occur during the early stages of lesion development.

Furuncles and carbuncles are treated with warm compresses to provide comfort and promote localization and spontaneous drainage. Abscess formation, recurrent infections, extensive lesions, or lesions associated with cellulitis or systemic symptoms require incision and drainage and are treated with systemic antibiotics.

Cellulitis. Cellulitis is an infection of the dermis and subcutaneous tissue usually caused by *Staphylococcus aureus*, CA-MRSA, or group B streptococci.[43] Cellulitis can occur as an extension of a skin wound, as an ulcer, or from furuncles or carbuncles. The infected area is warm, erythematous, swollen, and painful. The infection is usually in the lower extremities and responds to systemic antibiotics, as well as therapy to relieve pain. Cellulitis also can be associated with other diseases including chronic venous insufficiency and stasis dermatitis.

Cellulitis must be differentiated from necrotizing fasciitis. Necrotizing fasciitis is a rare, rapidly spreading infection. It is commonly caused by *Streptococcus pyogenes* starting in the fascia, muscles, and subcutaneous fat with subsequent necrosis of the overlying skin. Treatment requires antibiotics and often surgical débridement.[44]

Erysipelas. Erysipelas is an acute superficial infection of the upper dermis most often caused by *Streptococcus pyogenes, beta-hemolytic streptococci,* and *Staphylococcus aureus.* The face, ears, and lower legs are involved. Chills, fever, and malaise precede the onset of lesions by 4 hours to 20 days. The initial lesions appear as firm, red spots that enlarge and coalesce to form a clearly circumscribed, advancing, bright red, hot lesion with a raised border. Vesicles may appear over the lesion and at the border. Pruritus, burning, and tenderness are present. Cold compresses provide symptomatic relief, and systemic antibiotics are required to arrest the infection.[45]

Impetigo. Impetigo is a superficial lesion of the skin that is caused by coagulase-positive *Staphylococcus* or beta-hemolytic streptococci. The disease occurs in adults but is more common in children (see Chapter 42).

Lyme disease. Lyme disease is a multisystem inflammatory disease caused by the spirochete *Borrelia burgdorferi* transmitted by *Ixodes* tick bites and is the most frequently reported vector-borne illness. The highest incidence of Lyme disease is among children. The microorganism is difficult to culture, escapes immunodefenses, and hides in tissue. It spreads to other tissues by entering capillary beds.[46]

Symptoms of the disease occur in three stages, although 50% of infected individuals are symptom free.[47] *Localized infection* occurs soon after the bite (within 3 to 32 days) with erythema migrans (bull's-eye rash), a T-cell–mediated response usually with fever. Within days to weeks after the onset of the illness, there is *disseminated infection* with secondary erythema migrans, usually with myalgias, arthralgias, and more rarely meningitis, neuritis, or carditis. *Late persistent infection* (more common in Europe) can continue for years with arthritis, encephalopathy, polyneuropathy, or heart failure. The diagnosis of Lyme disease is based on the clinical presentation and history of the tick bite, if known. Serologic tests are used to confirm the diagnosis, although there is a delayed antibody response and the test may be negative during the first 3 weeks after infection.[48] Antibiotics (e.g., doxycycline [not used in children younger than 8 years or in pregnant or breast-feeding women] or amoxicillin) are used for treatment.[49] Reinfection can occur. There is currently no vaccine for Lyme disease.[50]

Viral Infections

Herpes simplex virus. Skin infections with **herpes simplex virus (HSV)** are commonly caused by two types of HSV: HSV-1 and HSV-2. Either type can occur in different parts of the body, including oral and genital locations. Their differences are distinguished by laboratory tests. HSV-1, transmitted by contact with infected saliva, is generally associated with oral infections (cold sore or fever blister) or infection of the cornea (herpes keratitis), mouth (gingivostomatitis), and orolabia (lips/labialis), but it can also cause genital herpes. With initial (primary) infection, the virus is imbedded in sensory nerve endings and it moves by retrograde axonal transport to the dorsal root ganglion, where the virus develops lifelong latency. During the secondary phase, the lesions occur at the same site from reactivation of the virus. The virus travels down the peripheral nerve to the site of the original infection, where it is shed. Exposure to ultraviolet light, skin irritation, fever, fatigue, or stress may cause reactivation.[51]

The lesions for HSV-1 appear as a rash or clusters of inflamed and painful vesicles (e.g., within the mouth, over the tongue, on the lips, around the nose) (Figure 41-16). Increased sensitivity, paresthesias, pruritus, and mild burning may occur before onset of the lesions. The vesicles rupture, forming a crust. Lesions may last from 2 to 6 weeks but usually resolve within 2 weeks. Treatment is symptomatic and includes topical or oral antiviral agents.[52]

Genital infections are more commonly caused by HSV-2. The virus is spread by skin-to-skin mucous membrane contact during viral shedding. Risk of infection is high in immunosuppressed persons or in persons who have sexual contact with infected individuals. Vertical transmission from mother to neonate is associated with significant neonatal neurologic morbidity and mortality.[53] The initial infection is asymptomatic. With recurrent exposure, the lesions begin as small vesicles that progress to ulceration within 3 to 4 days with pain, itching, and weeping. Treatment is symptomatic and includes topical or oral antiviral agents. A vaccine has been effective in controlling recurrent infection, and progress is being made with prophylactic vaccines.[54]

Herpes zoster and varicella. **Herpes zoster (shingles)** and **varicella (chickenpox,** see Chapter 42) are caused by the same herpesvirus—varicella-zoster virus (VZV). VZV occurs as a primary infection followed years later by activation of the virus to cause herpes zoster (shingles). During this time, the virus remains latent in trigeminal and dorsal root ganglia.

Herpes zoster has initial symptoms of pain and paresthesia localized to the affected dermatome (the cutaneous area innervated by a single spinal nerve; see Chapter 13), followed by vesicular eruptions that follow a facial, cervical, or thoracic lumbar dermatome (Figure 41-17). Local symptoms are alleviated with compresses, calamine lotion, or baking soda. Approximately 15% to 20% of individuals experience postherpetic neuralgia (pain) with reactivation of the virus.[55] Antiviral drugs, tricyclic antidepressants, and analgesics are helpful treatments. The varicella vaccine is safe and effective in both children and adults, particularly those older than age 60. In children, the vaccine is given to prevent chickenpox; and in adults, particularly the elderly, the vaccine is given to prevent herpes zoster (shingles).[56]

Warts. **Warts (verrucae)** are benign lesions of the skin caused by the many different types of **human papillomavirus (HPV)** that infect the stratified epithelium of skin and mucous membranes. The lesions can occur anywhere and are flat, round, or fusiform and elevated with a rough, grayish surface. Warts are transmitted by touch. Common warts (verruca vulgaris) occur most often in children and are usually on the fingers (Figure 41-18). Plantar warts are usually located at pressure points on the bottom of the feet. Warts are commonly treated with cryotherapy or topical salicylic acid; new agents are being investigated.[57,58]

Condylomata acuminata (venereal warts) are highly contagious and sexually transmitted. The cauliflower-like lesions occur in moist areas, along the glans of the penis, vulva, and anus. Oncogenic types of HPV are a primary cause of cervical and other types of cancer[59] (see Chapter 33).

FIGURE 41-16 Herpes Simplex of the Lips (Labialis). Typical presentation with tense vesicles appearing on the lips and extending onto the skin. (From Habif TP: *Clinical dermatology: a color guide to diagnosis and therapy,* ed 4, St Louis, 2004, Mosby.)

FIGURE 41-17 Herpes Zoster. Diffuse involvement of a dermatome. (Courtesy Department of Dermatology, School of Medicine, University of Utah, Salt Lake City, Utah.)

FIGURE 41-18 Verruca Vulgaris (Near Toes). (Courtesy Department of Dermatology, School of Medicine, University of Utah, Salt Lake City, Utah.)

FIGURE 41-19 Tinea Pedis. Inflammation has extended from the web area onto the dorsum of the foot. (Courtesy Department of Dermatology, School of Medicine, University of Utah, Salt Lake City, Utah.)

TABLE 41-5 Common Sites of Tinea Infections

Site	Clinical Manifestations
Tinea capitis (scalp)	Scaly, pruritic scalp with bald areas; hair breaks easily
Tinea corporis (skin areas, excluding scalp, face, hands, feet, groin)	Circular, clearly circumscribed, mildly erythematous scaly patches with slightly elevated ringlike border; some forms are dry and macular, and other forms are moist and vesicular
Tinea cruris (groin, also known as "jock itch")	Small, erythematous, and scaling vesicular patches with well-defined borders that spread over inner and upper surfaces of thighs; occurs with heat and high humidity
Tinea pedis (foot; also known as "athlete's foot")	Occurs between toes and may spread to soles of feet, nails, and skin or toes; slight scaling; macerated, painful skin, occasionally with fissures and vesiculation
Tinea manus (hand)	Dry, scaly, erythematous lesions, or moist, vesicular lesions that begin with clusters of intensely pruritic, clear vesicles; often associated with fungal infection of feet
Tinea unguium or onychomycosis (nails)	Superficial or deep inflammation of nail that develops yellow-brown accumulations of brittle keratin over all or portions of nail

Fungal Infections

The fungi causing superficial skin infections are called *dermatophytes,* and they thrive on keratin (stratum corneum, hair, nails). Fungal disorders are known as *mycoses;* when caused by dermatophytes, the mycoses are termed *tinea* (dermatophytosis or ringworm).

Tinea infections. Tinea infections are classified according to their location on the body. The most common sites are summarized in Table 41-5 (Figure 41-19).

Tinea is diagnosed by culture, microscopic examination of skin scrapings prepared with potassium hydroxide wet mount, or observation of the skin with an ultraviolet light (Wood's lamp). Cultures establish the particular type of fungus; identification is necessary for diagnosis of hair and nail infections. Fungi have characteristic spores and filaments known as *hyphae* that are more prominent when prepared in potassium hydroxide. The spores fluoresce blue-green when exposed to ultraviolet light. Treatment is related to the type of fungi and includes both topical and systemic antifungal medication.[60]

Candidiasis. Candidiasis is caused by the yeastlike fungus *Candida albicans* and normally can be found on mucous membranes, on the skin, in the gastrointestinal tract, and in the vagina. *C. albicans* can, under certain circumstances, change from a commensal (normal) microorganism to a pathogen, particularly in the critically ill and those who are immunosuppressed.[61]

Factors that predispose to infection include (1) local environment of moisture, warmth, maceration, or occlusion; (2) systemic administration of antibiotics; (3) pregnancy; (4) diabetes mellitus; (5) Cushing disease; (6) debilitated states; (7) infants younger than 6 months of age, as a result of decreased immune reactivity; (8) immunosuppressed persons; and (9) certain neoplastic diseases of the blood and monocyte/macrophage system. The commensal (normal) bacteria on the skin, mainly cocci, inhibit proliferation of *C. albicans. C. albicans* can activate the complement system by the alternative pathway and produce small abscesses. Candidiasis affects only the outer layers of mucous membranes and skin and occurs in the mouth, vagina, uncircumcised penis, nail folds, interdigital areas, and large skin folds. Table 41-6 lists the points of differentiation of various sites of candidiasis habitation.

The initial lesion is a thin-walled pustule that extends under the stratum corneum with an inflammatory base that may burn or itch. The accumulation of inflammatory cells and scale produces a whitish yellow curdlike substance over the infected area. The lesion ceases to spread when it reaches dry skin.[62] Topical antifungal agents are commonly used for treatment.

Vascular Disorders

Vascular abnormalities are commonly associated with skin diseases; they may be congenital or may involve vascular responses to local or systemic vasoactive substances. Blood vessels may increase in number, dilate, constrict, or become obliterated by disease processes.

Cutaneous Vasculitis

Vasculitis (angiitis) is an inflammation of the blood vessel wall that can result in bleeding aneurysm formation, or occlusion with ischemia or infection of surrounding tissue. The extensive vascular bed in the

TABLE 41-6 Sites of Candidiasis Infection

Site	Risk Factors	Clinical Manifestations	Treatment

Vagina (vulvovaginitis)	Heat, moisture, occlusive clothing
	Pregnancy
	Systemic antibiotic therapy
	Diabetes mellitus
	Sexual intercourse with infected male
		Vaginal itching; white, watery, or creamy
		  discharge
		Red, swollen vaginal and labial membranes
		  with erosions
		Lesions may spread to anus and groin
			Miconazole cream
			Clotrimazole tablets or cream
			Nystatin tablets
			Ketoconazole cream
			Loose cotton clothing

Penis (balanitis)	Uncircumcised Sexual intercourse with infected female	Pinpoint, red, tender papules and pustules on glans and shaft of penis	Any of creams listed above Topical steroids for severe inflammation

Mouth	Diabetes mellitus
	Immunosuppressive therapy
	Inhaled steroid therapy
		Red, swollen, painful tongue and oral mucous
		  membranes
		Localized erosions and plaques appear with
		  chronic infection
			Nystatin oral suspension
			Clotrimazole troches
			Ketoconazole

skin results in vasculitic syndromes that may be localized and self-limiting or generalized with multiorgan involvement. The initiating site may be the blood, the vessel wall, or the adjacent tissue. Small vessels are usually affected.

Cutaneous vasculitis develops from the deposit of immune complexes in small blood vessels as a toxic response to drugs (phenothiazines, barbiturates, sulfonamides), allergens, or streptococcal or viral infection, or as a component of systemic vasculitic syndromes. The deposits activate complement, which is chemotactic for polymorphonuclear leukocytes, and proinflammatory cytokines.

The disorder is also known as *cutaneous leukocytoclastic angiitis* (from the presence of leukocytes [i.e., neutrophils] in and around vessel walls). A systemic form (cutaneous systemic vasculitis) can involve other organs, including the kidneys, lungs, and gastrointestinal tract. The pattern of skin involvement includes palpable purpura in the lower legs and feet (from the leakage of blood from damaged vessels) that may progress to hemorrhagic bullae with necrosis and ulceration from occlusion of the vessel. Lesions appear in clusters and persist for 1 to 4 weeks. The disease may be self-limiting and occur as a single episode. Biopsy confirms the diagnosis.

Identifying and removing the antigen (chemical, drug, or source of infection) is the first step of treatment. Corticosteroids and immunosuppressants may be used when symptoms are severe.[63]

Urticaria

Urticaria (hives) is a circumscribed area of raised erythema and edema of the superficial dermis. Urticarial lesions are most commonly associated with type I hypersensitivity reactions to drugs (penicillin, aspirin), certain foods (strawberries, shellfish, food dyes), environmental exposure (pollen, animal dander, insect bites), systemic diseases (intestinal parasites, lupus erythematosus), or physical agents (heat or cold) (see Chapter 8). The lesions are mediated by histamine release from sensitized mast cells or basophils, or both, which causes the endothelial cells of skin blood vessels to contract. The leakage of fluid from the vessel appears as wheals, welts, or hives, and there may be few or many that may be distributed over the entire body. Most lesions resolve spontaneously within 24 hours, but new lesions may appear. All possible causes of the reaction should be removed. Antihistamines usually reduce hives and provide relief of itching. Corticosteroids and β-adrenergic agonists may be required for severe attacks. Chronic urticaria (recurrent wheals for more than 6 weeks) is either idiopathic or autoimmune in origin and involves inappropriate activation of mast cells.[64] Angioedema (welts or swelling deeper within the skin or mucous membranes) is associated with both groups and more commonly affects the eyes and mouth.

Scleroderma

Localized scleroderma (morphea) means sclerosis of the skin and underlying tissue. The disease is rare, more common in females, and the cause is unknown. Genetic predisposition, autoimmunity, and an immune reaction to a toxic substance are possible initiating mechanisms of the disease. Autoantibodies are often recovered from the skin and serum of individuals with scleroderma. Impaired regulation of collagen gene expression by fibroblasts probably underlies the persistent fibrosis. There are subtypes of localized scleroderma but all involve thickening of the skin. Localized scleroderma is differentiated from the systemic form of the disease by the absence of the following: sclerodactyly, Raynaud phenomenon, abnormalities of the nail bed capillaries, or internal organ involvement.[65]

Systemic scleroderma involves the connective tissues of the skin and many organs, including the kidneys, gastrointestinal tract, and lungs. There are massive deposits of type I collagen with progressive fibrosis accompanied by inflammatory reactions as well as vascular changes in the capillary network with a decrease in the number of capillary loops, dilation of the remaining capillaries, formation of perivascular infiltrates, and development of occlusion and ischemia.[66]

The clinical features of systemic scleroderma can be summarized using the CREST acronym as a guide:

Calcinosis—calcium deposits in the subcutaneous tissue that cause pain

Raynaud phenomenon—episodes of arteriolar vasoconstriction or spasm in response to cold or stress

Esophageal changes—swallowing difficulty related to acid reflux and increased esophageal fibrosis

Sclerodactyly—tightening of skin over the fingers and toes leading to tapering of the digits with scarring and tissue atrophy

Telangiectasias—dilation of capillaries causing small (0.5-cm), weblike red marks on skin surface

The cutaneous lesions are most often on the face and hands, the neck, and the upper chest, although the entire skin can be involved. The skin is hard, hypopigmented, taut, shiny, and tightly connected to the underlying tissue. The tightness of the facial skin projects an immobile masklike appearance, and the mouth may not open completely. The nose may assume a beaklike appearance. The hands are shiny and sometimes red and edematous (Figure 41-20). Progression to body organs may occur, and death is caused by subsequent respiratory failure, renal failure, cardiac dysrhythmias, or esophageal or intestinal obstruction or perforation.[67]

Suitable clothing and a warm environment are essential for protecting the hands. Trauma and smoking should be avoided. Treatment is individualized and based on severity and progression of the disease.

FIGURE 41-20 Scleroderma. Note inflammation and shiny skin resulting from a combination of Raynaud phenomena and scleroderma affecting the fingers (acrosclerosis). (Courtesy Department of Dermatology, School of Medicine, University of Utah, Salt Lake City, Utah.)

FIGURE 41-21 Seborrheic Keratosis. Typical lesion that is broad, flat, and comparatively smooth surfaced. (Courtesy Department of Dermatology, School of Medicine, University of Utah, Salt Lake City, Utah.)

Immunosuppression, ultraviolet treatment, and other therapies are prescribed.[68]

> **QUICK CHECK 41-5**
> 1. Name two bacterial skin infections, and describe the typical lesions.
> 2. Compare herpes zoster and varicella.
> 3. What features distinguish urticarial lesions?

Benign Tumors

Most benign tumors of the skin are associated with aging. Benign tumors include seborrheic keratosis, keratoacanthoma, actinic keratosis, and moles.

Seborrheic Keratosis

Seborrheic keratosis is a benign proliferation of cutaneous basal cells that produces flat or slightly elevated lesions that may be smooth or warty in appearance. The pathogenesis is unknown. These benign tumors are usually seen in older people and occur as multiple lesions on the chest, back, and face. The color varies from tan to waxy yellow, flesh colored, or dark brown-black. Lesion size varies from a few millimeters to several centimeters, and they are often oval and greasy appearing with a hyperkeratotic scale (Figure 41-21). Cryotherapy with liquid nitrogen and laser therapy are effective treatments.

Keratoacanthoma

A keratoacanthoma is a benign, self-limiting tumor of squamous cell differentiation arising from hair follicles. It usually occurs on sun-damaged skin of elderly individuals. Incidence is highest among smokers and males. The most commonly affected sites are the face, back of the hands, forearms, neck, and legs. The lesion develops in stages (proliferative, mature, and involution) over a period of 1 to 2 months with a histologic pattern resembling squamous cell carcinoma.

Although the lesions will resolve spontaneously, they can be removed by curettage or excision to improve cosmetic appearance and reduce the risk of evolution to squamous cell carcinoma (SCC). A biopsy is performed to rule out SCC.

Actinic Keratosis

Actinic keratosis is a premalignant lesion composed of aberrant proliferations of epidermal keratinocytes caused by prolonged exposure to ultraviolet radiation. The prevalence is highest in individuals with unprotected, light-colored skin and is rare in those with black skin. The lesions appear as rough, poorly defined papules, which may be felt more than seen. Surrounding areas may have telangiectasias. Treatment options include cryoablation, photodynamic therapy, laser surgery, and topical therapies, such as 5-fluorouracil, diclofenac, imiquimod cream, and ingenol mebutate.[69]

Excisions also may be performed, providing tissue for cellular analysis. The lesions should continue to be evaluated for progression to squamous cell carcinoma. Protection from the sun with clothing or a sun-blocking agent to prevent lesions from developing elsewhere is advised.

Nevi (Moles)

Nevi (sing., nevus) (also known as moles or birthmarks) are benign pigmented or nonpigmented lesions. Melanocytic nevi, formed from melanocytes, may be congenital or acquired and small (less than 1 cm) or large (greater than 20 cm). Congenital melanocytic nevi may be removed to reduce risk of cutaneous malignant melanoma.[70] During the early stages of development, the cells accumulate at the junction of the dermis and epidermis and are macular lesions. Over time, the cells move deeper into the dermis and the nevi become nodular and symmetric without irregular borders. Nevi may appear on any part of the skin, vary in size, occur singly or in groups, and may undergo transition to malignant melanoma (see p. 1072). Classification of nevi is summarized in Table 41-7. Nevi irritated by clothing or trauma or large lesions may be excised. Multiple and changing moles require regular evaluation.[71]

> **QUICK CHECK 41-6**
> 1. List two diseases caused by insect bites.
> 2. Compare keratoacanthoma and actinic keratosis.

Skin Cancer

Basal cell carcinoma and squamous cell carcinoma (collectively known as nonmelanoma skin cancers) are the most prevalent forms of cancer. Malignant melanoma is the most serious and most common cause of death from skin cancer. Important trends related to skin cancer are described in Box 41-1.

Chronic exposure to ultraviolet (UV) radiation causes most skin cancers. Lesions are most common on the face, neck, hands, and other areas with intense sunlight exposure. Protection from the sun and

BOX 41-1   Important Trends for Skin Cancer

Incidence
- Skin cancer is the most commonly diagnosed cancer in the United States. An estimated 3.5 million cases of squamous and basal cell carcinoma were diagnosed in 2006
- Malignant melanoma is the most serious form of skin cancer; it is not as common as the other forms of skin cancer; an estimated 73,870 new cases were predicted in 2015

Mortality
- Total estimated deaths from skin cancer in 2015 were 13,340—9940 from malignant melanoma and 3400 from other nonepithelial skin cancers

Survival
- Basal and squamous cell carcinoma can be cured when detected early
- 5-year survival for melanoma: localized 98%, regional metastasis 63%, distant metastasis 16%

Risk Factors
- Excessive exposure to ultraviolet radiation from the sun or tanning salons
- Fair complexion
- Occupational exposure to coal tar, pitch, creosote, arsenic compounds, and radium
- In people of color, skin cancer is less common, is diagnosed at a more advanced stage, and has higher morbidity and mortality than in people with light-colored skin; it is often found on the palms of hands and soles of feet
- Immunosuppression

Warning Signs
- Any unusual skin condition, especially a change in the size, borders, or color of a mole or other darkly pigmented growth or spot

Prevention and Early Detection
- Avoid the sun when ultraviolet light is strongest (e.g., 10 AM to 3 PM), avoid sun tanning beds, seek shade, use sunscreen preparations, especially those containing ingredients such as PABA (*para*-aminobenzoic acid), and wear protective clothing
- Basal and squamous cell skin cancers often form a pale, waxlike pearly nodule or a red, scaly, sharply outlined patch
- Melanomas usually have dark brown or black pigmentation; they start as small molelike growths that increase in size, change color, become ulcerated, and bleed easily from slight injury

Treatment
- Options for treatment include surgery, electrodesiccation (tissue destruction by heat), radiation therapy, cryosurgery (tissue destruction by freezing)
- Malignant melanomas require wide and often deep excisions and removal of nearby lymph nodes; selective lymphadenectomy or immunotherapy can be used; vaccines and gene therapy are in development

Survival
- For basal cell and squamous cell cancers, cure is virtually ensured with early detection and treatment; malignant melanoma, however, metastasizes quickly and accounts for a lower 5-year survival rate

Data from American Cancer Society: *Cancer facts & figures 2015,* Atlanta, 2015, Author.

TABLE 41-7   Classification of Nevi

Type	Common Characteristics
Junctional nevus	Flat, well-circumscribed; vary in size up to 2 cm; dark color hairs may be present; originate in basal layer of epidermis and can eventually reach cutaneous surface; most likely to develop into melanoma
Compound nevus	Most common in adolescents; majority of pigmented lesions in children; rarely does this lesion develop into melanoma; usually 1 cm in size; hairs may be present; surface is elevated and smooth
Intradermal nevus	Small, less than 1 cm, with regular edges and bristle-like hairs; color ranges from fair skin tone to light brown; has slight likelihood of developing into melanoma

avoidance of tanning beds, particularly during childhood, significantly reduce the risk of skin cancer in later years. Genetic mutations in oncogenes and tumor-suppressor genes (see Chapter 10) are associated with skin cancers. This leads to loss of keratinocyte repair functions and apoptosis resistance of DNA-damaged cells.[72] Dark-skinned persons and those avoiding sunlight are significantly less likely to develop these malignant tumors. In dark-skinned persons, basal cells contain more of the pigment melanin, a protective factor against sun exposure. Vitamin D may be an important tumor-suppressor for the skin but more research is needed.[73]

Basal Cell Carcinoma

Basal cell carcinoma (BCC) of the skin is the most common cancer in the world, making it the most common skin cancer by default. BCC is thought to be caused by UV radiation exposure and also is associated with arsenic in food or water.

BCCs have numerous subtypes, including superficial, nodular, pigmented, morpheaform, and combinations of each; thus, they can have very different clinical presentations—from superficial erythematous papules; to thick, pigmented nodules resembling melanomas; to erosive, necrotic, and ulcerating lesions (Figure 41-22). As the tumor grows it usually has a depressed center, a rolled border, and small blood vessels on the surface (telangiectasias) (see Figure 41-22). Early tumors are so small they are not clinically apparent. The lesion grows slowly, often ulcerates, develops crusts, and is firm to the touch. If left untreated, basal cell lesions invade surrounding tissues and, over months or years, can destroy a nose, eyelid, or ear (for treatment, see Box 41-1). Metastasis is rare because these tumors do not invade blood or lymph vessels.

Squamous Cell Carcinoma

Squamous cell carcinoma (SCC) of the skin is a tumor of the epidermis and is the second most common human cancer. Two types are characterized: in situ (including Bowen disease) and invasive. Ultraviolet radiation exposure causes SCC and actinic keratosis is a precursor lesion. Other risk factors include arsenic at a higher level in drinking water, exposure to x-rays and gamma rays, immunosuppression, and light-colored skin. *P53* gene mutations are common in SCC and produce tumor cells resistant to apoptosis.[72]

Premalignant lesions include actinic keratosis, leukoplakia (whitish discolored areas), scars, radiation-induced keratosis, tar and oil keratosis, and chronic ulcers,. In situ SCC is usually confined to the epidermis (intraepidermal) but may extend into the dermis. Bowen disease is a dysplastic epidermal lesion often found on unexposed areas of the body such as the penis and demonstrated by flat, reddish, scaly

FIGURE 41-22 Types of Basal Cell Carcinoma. A, Superficial. **B,** Nodular. **C,** Pigmented. **D,** Morpheaform—recurrent tumor. (**A** and **D** from Bolognia JL et al: *Dermatology,* ed 3, Philadelphia, 2012, Saunders. **B** and **C** from James WD et al: *Andrews' diseases of the skin: clinical dermatology,* ed 11, Philadelphia, 2009, Saunders.)

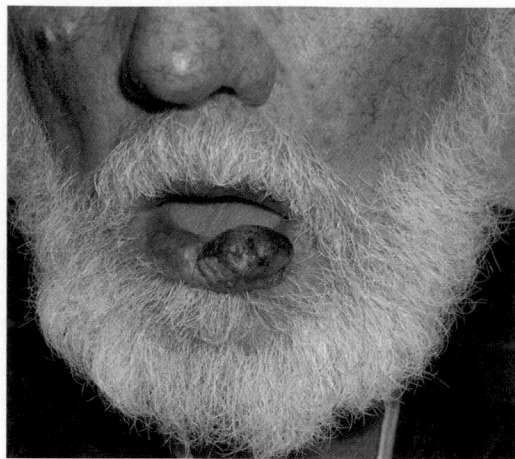

FIGURE 41-23 Lip Cancer. Biopsy confirmed squamous cell carcinoma. Lip vermilion shows diffuse actinic keratosis. (From Bagheri SC et al: *Current therapy in oral and maxillofacial surgery,* Philadelphia, 2012, Saunders.)

FIGURE 41-24 Squamous Cell Carcinoma. The sun-exposed ear is a common site for squamous cell carcinoma. (Courtesy Department of Dermatology, School of Medicine, University of Utah, Salt Lake City, Utah.)

patches. These lesions rarely invade surrounding tissue and, although they rarely metastasize, they do so more often than BCCs. Other components of the skin (e.g., sweat glands, hair follicles) can develop into skin cancer, but this is relatively uncommon.

SCC is the most common cause of lip cancer, prevalent in older white men, with about 3000 new cases per year.[74] The lower lip is the most common site. Long-term environmental exposure results in dryness, chapping, hyperkeratosis, and predisposition to malignancy. Immunosuppression, pipe smoking, and chronic alcoholism increase the risk for lip cancer. The most common lesion is termed *exophytic* and usually develops in the outer part of the lip along the vermilion border. The lip becomes thickened and evolves to an ulcerated center with a raised border (Figure 41-23). These lesions have an irregular surface, follow cracks in the lip, and tend to extend toward the inner surface.

Invasive SCC can arise from premalignant lesions of the skin; it rarely develops from normal-appearing skin and is usually confined to the epidermis (intraepidermal), but may extend into the reticular layer of the dermis (see Table 41-1). Invasive SCCs grow more rapidly than basal cell carcinomas and can spread to regional lymph nodes. These tumors are firm and increase in both elevation and diameter. The surface may be granular and bleed easily (Figure 41-24). Treatment includes surgical excision and radiotherapy with consideration of adjuvant chemotherapy or epithelial growth factor receptor inhibitors for advanced disease.[75]

Cutaneous Melanoma

Cutaneous melanoma is a malignant tumor of the skin originating from melanocytes, cells that synthesize the pigment melanin, and arise from the neural crest. Malignant melanoma is the most serious skin cancer with an estimated 73,870 new cases and 9940 deaths in the United States in 2015.[74] Melanoma also can arise in the uvea of the eye and on mucous membranes.[76] The incidence is increasing worldwide.

Risk factors include a personal or family history, or both, ultraviolet radiation (UVR) exposure (including sunbed use before age 30 years), immunosuppression, fair hair, light skin with repeated sunburns, freckles, younger females and older males, geographic location, past pesticide exposure, and three or more clinically atypical (dysplastic) nevi[77] (see *Health Alert:* Melanoma in Non-White People). Melanoma is the most common cancer in white women 25 to 29 years old.[78]

Cutaneous melanomas arise as a result of malignant degeneration of melanocytes located either along the basal layer of the epidermis (see Figure 41-1) or in a benign melanocytic nevus. The clinical varieties of cutaneous melanoma include *superficial spreading melanoma* (SSM), the most common; *lentigo malignant melanoma* (LMM) (Figure 41-25), frequently found in the elderly and confused with age spots; *primary nodular melanoma* (PNM), an aggressive tumor; and *acral lentiginous melanoma* (ALM). It is rare and aggressive and occurs on non–hair-bearing surfaces (i.e., palms of the hands and soles of the feet) and mucous membranes in black people.

The pathogenesis of malignant melanoma is complex. Most familial melanomas are associated with cyclin-dependent kinase 4 gene (*CDK4*) and cyclin-dependent kinase inhibitor 2A gene (*p16/CDKN2A*), located on chromosome 9p21. The *CDKN2A* gene encodes two potent tumor-suppressor proteins (p16 and p14[ARF]) that are cell-cycle inhibitors. Both *CDNKN2A* and *CDK4* are highly penetrant susceptibility

FIGURE 41-25 Lentigo Malignant Melanoma. A, Superficial spreading melanoma. **B,** Nodular melanoma. **C,** Lentigo malignant melanoma. **D,** Acral lentiginous melanoma on plantar surface of foot. (From Bolognia JL et al: *Dermatology essentials,* Philadelphia, 2014, Saunders.)

FIGURE 41-26 Kaposi Sarcoma. The purple lesion commonly seen on the skin. (Courtesy Department of Dermatology, School of Medicine, University of Utah, Salt Lake City, Utah.)

HEALTH ALERT

Melanoma in Non-White People

The risk of melanoma is lower in non-white people. However, they have more advanced disease when diagnosed and a higher death rate. Associated factors include location of the lesion on palms, soles, and subungual sites (e.g., acral lentiginous melanoma) and lower socioeconomic status and education level. These melanomas may represent molecular distinct cancers that are inherently more aggressive. The location of the lesions may contribute to delayed detection or misdiagnosis. The role of ultraviolet radiation in the risk for melanoma in non-white people is not clear and research is needed. Genetic mutations may be a contributing factor. Educational programs to increase awareness of risk for melanoma among non-white people, screening, and self-examination can improve outcomes.

Data from Alexandrescu DT et al: *Dermatol Surg* 39(9):1291-1303, 2013; Rouhani P et al: *Cancer Control* 15(3):248-253, 2008; Stubblefield J, Kelly B: *Surg Clin North Am* 94(5):1115-1126, 2014.

genes and result in melanomas. A number of proto-oncogenes have been identified, including BRAF point mutations and genes involved in the regulation of mitogen-activated protein kinase (MAPK), and other signaling pathways. Melanomas have a high mutation rate stimulated by UVR, making gene sequencing difficult.[79]

The relationship between nevi and melanoma makes it important for the clinician to understand the various forms of nevi (see Table 41-7). Most nevi never become suspicious; however, suspicious pigmented nevi need to be evaluated and removed.[71] Indications for biopsy, including sentinel lymph node biopsy, are color change, size change, irregular notched margin, itching, bleeding or oozing, nodularity, scab formation, and ulceration or an unusual pattern of presentation. The ABCDE rule is used as a guide: **A**symmetry, **B**order irregularity, **C**olor variation, **D**iameter larger than 6 mm, and Elevation or **E**volving, which includes raised appearance or rapid enlargement. Staging is determined by lesion thickness (presence of **t**umor), lymph **n**ode involvement, and presence of **m**etastasis (TNM staging).[80]

Treatment of melanoma with no evidence of metastatic disease involves a wide surgical excision of the primary lesion site. A lymph node biopsy of the peripherally draining lymph node (sentinel node) is warranted for lesions greater than 1 mm deep. Lesions on the extremities have the best surgical prognosis. Radiation therapy, chemotherapy, and immunotherapy inhibiting the MAPK pathway and BRAF mutations are used to treat metastatic disease and have demonstrated long-term improvement in disease outcome.[81] Promising new immunotherapies are used for advanced disease, including checkpoint inhibitors (anti-PD1 antibodies [pembrolizumab, nivolumab], anti-CTLA4 antibody [ipilimumab]), and targeted therapy (BRAF and/or MEK inhibition).[82] Vaccines, cell therapy, and biomarkers are under continuing investigation.[83] Early detection is critical to decreasing mortality from metastatic disease.

Kaposi Sarcoma

Kaposi sarcoma (KS) is a vascular malignancy associated with immunodeficiency states and occurs among transplant recipients taking immunosuppressive drugs. Genetic and environmental cofactors determine disease progression. Human herpesvirus type 8 (HHV8) is found in the lesions of KS. Four forms of the disease have been described: classic (more benign), epidemic (rapidly progressive and associated with AIDS), African endemic, and iatrogenic (associated with immunosuppressant treatment including organ transplant).[84]

The endothelial cell is thought to be the progenitor of KS. The lesions emerge as purplish brown macules and develop into plaques and nodules with angioproliferation. They tend to be multifocal rather than spreading by metastasis. The lesions initially appear over the lower extremities in the classic form (Figure 41-26). The rapidly progressive form associated with AIDS tends to spread symmetrically over the upper body, particularly the face and oral mucosa. The lesions are often pruritic and painful. About 75% of individuals with epidemic KS have involvement of lymph nodes, particularly in the gastrointestinal tract and lungs. Organ involvement is much less common in the classic form. The rapidly progressive form has a poor prognosis and shorter survival rates than the classic form. (See Chapter 8 for a further discussion of AIDS.)

Diagnosis is by medical history, physical examination, and skin biopsy, with a high index of suspicion for those with immunodeficiency. Chest x-ray reveals lesions in the lungs. Local lesions can be excised. Multiple disseminated lesions may be treated with a combination of α-interferon, radiotherapy, and cytotoxic drugs. Antiangiogenic agents are being tested. Individuals receiving highly active antiretroviral therapy (HAART) have a markedly reduced incidence of KS.[85]

Primary Cutaneous Lymphomas

Primary cutaneous lymphomas are cutaneous T-cell and B-cell lymphomas present in the skin without evidence of extracutaneous disease at the time of diagnosis (see Chapter 21 for classification and general pathophysiology of lymphomas). Cutaneous lymphomas are rare but are the second most common site of extranodal non-Hodgkin lymphoma. The incidence rate is about 1 per 100,000 and the cause of these lesions is unknown.[86] Cutaneous lymphomas are more common in men and generally present after age 50 years.

Cutaneous lymphomas develop from clonal expansion of B cells, T-helper cells, and rarely T-suppressor cells. The most common is cutaneous T-cell lymphoma (66%), and mycosis fungoides is the most prominent subtype. Mycosis fungoides can present as focal or widespread erythematous patches or plaques, follicular papules, comedone-like lesions, and tumors. There may be patches of alopecia. The lesions progress over a period of months or years.

The differential diagnosis of the different types of cutaneous lymphomas is based on clinical manifestations, histologic appearance, immunologic and cytogenetic features, and response to appropriate treatment. Treatment is based on staging of the disease and includes topical and systemic drugs and phototherapy.[87,88]

✔ **QUICK CHECK 41-7**
1. What is the most common skin cancer?
2. What malignancy can arise from melanocytes?
3. How is Kaposi sarcoma related to AIDS?

Burns

The incidence of burn injuries has declined in the past several years. About 1 million people are burned in the United States each year, with 486,000 visits to hospital emergency departments, 40,000 hospitalizations, and 3240 smoke inhalation or burn-related deaths with a 96.7% survival rate. Most burns occur in the home, and the highest percentage (69%) occurs in men.[89] Burns may be caused by thermal or nonthermal sources including chemical, electrical, or radioactive sources. Thermal injuries result from thermal contact, scalds, or radiation. Direct contact, inhalation, and ingestion of acids, alkalis, or blistering agents cause chemical burns. Electrical burns occur with the passage of electrical current through the body to the ground or electrical flames or flashes. In addition to cutaneous injury, burns can be associated with smoke inhalation and other traumatic injuries that exacerbate local and systemic responses. Ventilatory support is often needed with inhalation injury.[90]

Burn Wound Depth

The depth of injury identifies the level of tissue destruction; the extent of injury determines clinical management, healing, and mortality. The depth of the burn is divided into four categories and is summarized in Table 41-8.

First-degree burns require no treatment unless the person is elderly or an infant, in which case severe nausea and vomiting may lead to inadequate fluid intake and dehydration. Fluid therapy may be required in these cases. First-degree burns heal in 3 to 5 days without scarring.

TABLE 41-8 Depth of Burn Injury

Characteristic	First Degree	SECOND DEGREE Superficial Partial Thickness	SECOND DEGREE Deep Partial Thickness	THIRD DEGREE Full Thickness	FOURTH DEGREE Full Thickness and Deeper Tissue
Morphology	Destruction of epidermis only; local pain and erythema	Destruction of epidermis and some dermis	Destruction of epidermis and dermis, leaving only skin appendages	Destruction of epidermis, dermis, and underlying subcutaneous tissue	Destruction of epidermis, dermis, and underlying subcutaneous tissue, tendons, muscle, and bone
Skin function	Intact	Absent	Absent	Absent	Absent
Tactile and pain sensors	Intact	Intact	Intact but diminished	Absent	Absent
Blisters	Usually none or present after first 24 hr	Present within minutes; thin walled and fluid filled	May or may not appear as fluid-filled blisters; often is layer of flat, dehydrated tissue paper–like skin that lifts off in sheets	Blisters rare; usually is layer of flat, dehydrated tissue paper–like skin that lifts off easily	None
Appearance of wound after initial débridement	Skin peels at 24-48 hr; normal or slightly red underneath	Red to pale ivory, moist surface	Mottled with areas of waxy, white, dry surface	White, cherry red, or black; may contain visible thrombosed veins; dry, hard, leathery surface	Black and charred appearing wound
Healing time	3-5 days	21-28 days	30 days to many months	Will not heal; may close from edges as secondary healing if wound is small	Will not heal; requires skin grafting; may require amputation and/or reconstructive surgery
Scarring	None	May be present; low incidence influenced by genetic predisposition	Highest incidence because of slow healing rate promoting scar tissue development; also influenced by genetic predisposition	Skin graft; scarring minimized by early excision and grafting; influenced by genetic predisposition	Degree of scarring associated with reconstruction and grafting success

FIGURE 41-27 Superficial Partial-Thickness Burn. Scald injury following débridement of overlying blister and nonadherent epithelium. (Courtesy Intermountain Burn Center, University of Utah, Salt Lake City, Utah.)

FIGURE 41-29 Axillary Burn Scar Contracture. Note the blanching of the anterior axillary fold and small ulceration from a deep partial-thickness burn, both indicating the diminished range of motion. (Courtesy Intermountain Burn Center, University of Utah, Salt Lake City, Utah.)

FIGURE 41-28 Deep Partial-Thickness Burn. Note pale appearance and minimal exudates. (Courtesy Intermountain Burn Center, University of Utah, Salt Lake City, Utah.)

FIGURE 41-30 Full-Thickness Burn. The wound is dry and insensate. (Courtesy Intermountain Burn Center, University of Utah, Salt Lake City, Utah.)

Second-degree burns involve thin-walled, fluid-filled blisters that develop within just a few minutes after injury (Figure 41-27). Tactile and pain sensors remain intact throughout the healing process, and wound care can cause extreme pain. Wounds heal in 3 to 4 weeks with adequate nutrition and no wound complications. Scar formation is unusual and is genetically determined.

Deep partial-thickness burns (Figure 41-28) look waxy white and take weeks to heal. Necrotic tissue is surgically removed followed by an application of the person's own unburned skin from another body area (autograft). Healing commonly results in hypertrophic scarring with poor functional and cosmetic results (Figure 41-29).

Third-degree burns, or **full-thickness burns**, have a dry, leathery appearance from loss of dermal elasticity (Figure 41-30). In areas of circumferential burns, distal circulation may be compromised from pressure caused by edema. **Escharotomies** (tissue decompression by cutting through burned skin) are performed to release pressure and prevent compartment syndrome (the compression of blood vessels, veins, muscles, or abdominal organs resulting in ischemia, necrosis, and irreversible injury).[91] Full-thickness burns are painless because all

nerve endings have been destroyed by the injury. **Fourth-degree burns** require skin grafting or reconstructive surgery.

The extent of **total body surface area (TBSA)** burned is estimated using either the "rule of nines" (Figure 41-31) or the modified Lund and Browder chart.[92] The severity of burn injury also considers many factors, including age, medical history, extent and depth of injury, and body area involved. The American Burn Association has defined criteria to assist healthcare professionals in identifying who should be referred to a specialized multidisciplinary burn center (available at: http://ameriburn.org/BurnCenterReferralCriteria.pdf).

PATHOPHYSIOLOGY AND CLINICAL MANIFESTATIONS Burn injury results in dramatic changes in many physiologic functions of the body within the first few minutes after the event. Burns exceeding 20% of TBSA in most adults are considered to be major burn injuries and are associated with massive evaporative water losses and fluctuations of large amounts of fluids, electrolytes, and plasma proteins into the body tissues, manifested as generalized edema, circulatory hypovolemia, and hypotension.

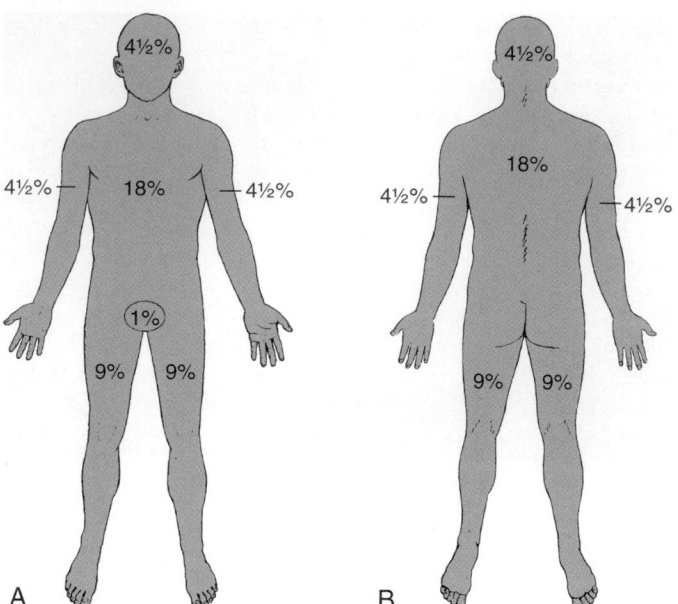

FIGURE 41-31 Estimation of Burn Injury: Rule of Nines. A commonly used assessment tool with estimates of the percentages (in multiples of 9) of the total body surface area burned. **A,** Adults *(anterior view).* **B,** Adults *(posterior view).*

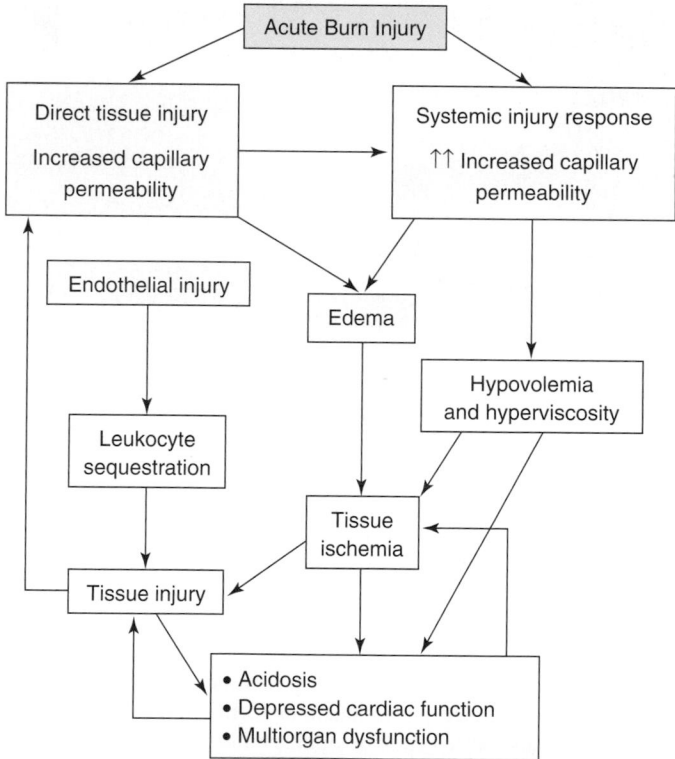

FIGURE 41-32 Immediate Cellular and Immunologic Alterations of Burn Shock.

The immediate (acute) systemic physiologic consequences of major burn injury focus on the profound, life-threatening hypovolemic shock that occurs in conjunction with cellular and immunologic disruption within a few minutes of injury (Figure 41-32). **Burn shock** is a condition consisting of a hypovolemic cardiovascular component and a cellular component.

Hypovolemia associated with burn shock results from massive fluid losses and shifts to the interstitial space from the circulating blood volume. The losses are caused by an increase in capillary permeability that persists for approximately 24 hours after burn injury. There is decreased cardiac contractility and decreased blood volume. Blood is shunted away from the liver, kidney, and gut—known as the "ebb phase" of the burn response. This phase lasts during the first 24 hours after burn injury and most organ systems are affected. Decreased perfusion of the viscera can decrease gut barrier function and result in translocation of bacteria and endotoxemia with sepsis. Intravenous **fluid resuscitation** is critical to restore the circulating blood volume during this phase, often using lactated Ringer solution. The rate of fluid replacement must be carefully monitored to prevent complications associated with fluid overload. Formulas are available (i.e., Parkland formula or the modified Brooke formula) to guide calculation of fluid volume replacement.[93,94]

Cellular metabolism is disrupted with onset of the burn wound, resulting in altered cell membrane permeability and loss of normal electrolyte homeostasis. Many cytokines and inflammatory mediators in burn serum play a role in these cellular processes. The cardiovascular and systemic responses to burn injury are integrated with the cellular response but are described separately for clarification.

Cardiovascular and Systemic Response to Burn Injury

The clinical manifestations of burn shock are the result of multiple physiologic alterations related to burn injury and release of inflammatory cytokines, in addition to the loss of fluid. The hallmark of burn shock is decreased cardiac contractility and decreased cardiac output with inadequate capillary perfusion in most tissues. Decreased cardiac output is related to myocardial depressant factor, as well as decreased intravascular volume.

Fluid and protein movement out of the vascular compartment results in an elevated hematocrit level and white blood cell count, and hypoproteinemia. If not treated immediately, profound hypovolemic shock and inadequate perfusion lead to irreversible shock and death within a few hours. Restoration of capillary integrity and renewal of a functional lymphatic system are required for resolution of the edema. Usually this occurs within 24 hours, but in extensive burns, it may take days or weeks. After the individual has reached the endpoint of burn shock, the term used to describe the person's condition is **capillary seal.**

The liver, with its metabolic, inflammatory, immune, and acute phase functions, plays a pivotal role in burn injury survival and recovery by modulating multiple metabolic pathways. Hepatic changes are common following a major burn, including fatty changes and hepatomegaly, which can influence burn wound recovery.[95] The hepatic response also alters clotting factors, leads to a hypercoagulable state, and can increase the risk for disseminated intravascular coagulation (systemic formation of microthrombi and abnormal bleeding).[96]

Cellular Response to Burn Injury

In addition to capillary endothelial permeability changes resulting in vascular fluid, electrolyte, and protein losses, there are transmembrane potential changes in cells not directly damaged by heat.[97] Cellular dysfunction resulting from burn injury impairs the sodium-potassium pump and results in increased amounts of intracellular sodium and water and decreased potassium level with disruption of the transmembrane potential. Intracellular calcium concentration also may be elevated, thereby influencing myocardial function.[98] Loss of intracellular magnesium and phosphate, hypocalcemia,[99] and elevated serum lactic dehydrogenase (LDH) level occur.[100]

Metabolic Response to Burn Injury

Major burn injury (greater than 40% of total body surface area) initiates a systemic hypermetabolic response with an increase in metabolic rate and a hyperdynamic circulation that begins 24 hours after burn injury—known as the "flow phase."[101] This phase can persist for up to 2 years following a burn.[102] Metabolic responses involve the sympathetic nervous system and other homeostatic regulators. Levels of catecholamines, cortisol, glucagon, and insulin (insulin resistance) are elevated with a corresponding increase in energy expenditure and increased gluconeogenesis, glycogenolysis, lipolysis, proteolysis, and lactic acidosis. Myocardial oxygen consumption is elevated and there is catabolic loss of muscle mass.[103] Hyperglycemia and insulin resistance can be prolonged in severe burns and require management with intensive insulin therapy to improve postburn morbidity and mortality.[104,105]

Burn injury initiates an inflammatory response with local activation and recruitment of inflammatory cells, such as leukocytes and monocytes, at the site of injury. These cells release inflammatory cytokines that contribute to the hypermetabolic state.[106] The metabolic rate increases in proportion to burn size and compensates for the profound water and heat loss associated with the burn. The inflammatory response and the release of cytokines at the wound level are magnified into a generalized systemic inflammatory response syndrome that can lead to multiple organ dysfunction.[107] Acute kidney injury is associated with hypovolemia, hypervolemia, and the inflammatory response.[108]

Hypermetabolism also increases the thermal regulatory set point and core and skin temperatures. There is persistent tachycardia, hypercapnia, and body wasting. Wound healing may be impaired, contributing to increased risk for infection and sepsis. Increasing the ambient temperature and early excision and grafting can decrease resting energy expenditure and improve mortality after major burns.[109] Inflammatory mediators circulating to the lung result in pulmonary edema that can be life-threatening.[110]

Immunologic Response to Burn Injury

The immunologic/inflammatory response to burn injury is immediate, prolonged, and severe. The result in individuals surviving burn shock is *immunosuppression* with increased susceptibility to potentially fatal systemic burn wound sepsis. White blood cells are altered at a time when their need to inhibit sepsis is vital.[111] Phagocytosis is impaired, and cellular and humoral immunity is abnormal. Individuals with altered immunocompetence or chronic disease before burn injury are at additional risk for complications, including wound sepsis.[112]

Macrophages, neutrophils, lymphocytes, and platelets release large amounts of inflammatory cytokines and antibodies, with their levels remaining elevated for weeks after burn injury. When combined with bacterial products, they produce peripheral vasodilation, pulmonary vasoconstriction, increased capillary permeability, and local tissue ischemia in the burn wound. There is distant organ dysfunction and multiple organ failure.[113]

Evaporative Water Loss

With major burn injury, there is loss of the skin's barrier function and ability to regulate evaporative water loss. Normally, the skin is the major source of insensible water loss (75%), and the lungs are minor sources (25%), with a total loss of only approximately 600 to 800 ml/day. This changes dramatically with burns because both the skin and the lungs have increased loss of water as a result of hypermetabolism and hyperventilation, especially in an intubated individual. Total evaporative losses exceed many liters per day in an adult with large burn wounds. Replacement of the loss is mandatory to prevent volume deficit and shock.

EVALUATION AND TREATMENT   Burn recovery is complex and prolonged with complications being the rule rather than the exception. Severity of inhalation injury is also a significant morbidity and mortality factor. The goal of burn management is wound débridement and closure in a manner that promotes survival. Scar formation with contractures is often a consequence of healing in deep partial-thickness and third-degree burns (Figure 41-33).

The essential elements of survival of major burn injury are (1) provision of adequate fluids and nutrition, (2) meticulous management of wounds with early surgical excision and grafting (Figure 41-34), (3) aggressive treatment of infection or sepsis, and (4) promotion of thermoregulation.[113] Several drugs are used for the management of severe burns, including β-adrenergic antagonists, β-adrenergic agonists, recombinant human growth hormone, insulin, androgenic steroids, and antibiotics.[101] Burn pain is almost always acute and severe, and treatment strategies are aggressive.[114] The risk of developing stress ulcers (Curling ulcers) is reduced with antacids or histamine H2-receptor antagonists.

Nutritional therapy focuses on early enteral therapy to reduce gut-mediated sepsis and to reduce the catabolic state.[115,116] Advancements in skin replacement procedures promote wound closure and healing.[117,118] Reconstructive surgery reduces complications associated with scarring and contractures.[119]

FIGURE 41-33 Hypertrophic Scarring. Deep partial-thickness thermal injury can result in extensive hypertrophic scarring. (Courtesy Intermountain Burn Center, University of Utah, Salt Lake City, Utah.)

FIGURE 41-34 Application of Cultured Epithelial Autografts. Thin sheets of keratinocytes are attached to gauze backing to allow application onto the clean, excised thigh. (Courtesy Intermountain Burn Center, University of Utah, Salt Lake City, Utah.)

Cold Injury

Exposure to extreme cold includes a spectrum of injuries[120]:

1. *Frostnip*—mild and completely reversible injury characterized by skin pallor and numbness
2. *Chilblains*—more serious than frostnip; violaceous skin color with plaques or nodules, pain, and pruritus, but no ice crystal formation; chronic vasculitis can develop and is usually located on the face, anterior lower leg, hands, and feet
3. *Frostbite*—tissues freeze and form ice crystals at temperatures less than 28° F (−2° C); progresses from distal to proximal and potentially reversible
4. *Flash freeze*—rapid cooling with intracellular ice crystals associated with contact with cold metals or volatile liquids

The most common areas affected are fingers, toes, ears, nose, and cheeks. Mild frostbite (frostnip) is cold exposure without tissue freezing. It causes pallor and pain followed by redness and discomfort during rewarming, with no tissue damage. Frostbite occurs when tissues freeze slowly with ice crystal formation. Frozen skin becomes white or yellowish and has a waxy texture. There is numbness and no sensation of pain. Frostbite injury is related to direct cold injury to cells, indirect injury from ice crystal formation, and endothelial cell damage. During rewarming, there is progressive microvascular thrombosis followed by reperfusion injury with release of inflammatory mediators (including thromboxanes, prostaglandins, bradykinins, and histamines) and with impaired circulation and anoxia to the exposed area. Cyanosis and mottling develop followed by redness, edema, and burning pain on rewarming in more severe cases. Edema can cause capillary compression and vascular stasis. Within 24 to 48 hours, vesicles and bullae appear that resolve into crusts that eventually slough, leaving thin, newly formed skin. Frostbite may be classified by depth of injury: superficial includes partial skin freezing (first degree) and full-thickness skin freezing (second degree); deep includes full-thickness and subcutaneous freezing (third degree) and deep tissue freezing (fourth degree). Third-degree and fourth-degree frostbite result in gangrene with loss of tissue.[121]

Immediate treatment of frostbite is to cover affected areas with other body surfaces and warm clothing. The area should not be rubbed or massaged. Rewarming for severe frostbite should occur after emergency transport. Immersion in a warm water bath (40° to 42° C, or 104° to 107.6° F) until frozen tissue is thawed is the best treatment. Pain is severe and should be treated with potent analgesics. Antibiotics may be given. Vasodilators, thrombolytics, hyperbaric oxygen, and sympathectomy may improve healing responses. Débridement or amputation of necrotic tissue occurs when there is a clear line of demarcation.[122]

DISORDERS OF THE HAIR

Alopecia

Alopecia means loss of hair from the head or body. Hair loss occurs when there is disruption in the growth phase of the hair follicle. Hair loss can be associated with systemic disorders such as hypothyroidism and iron deficiency, chemotherapy for cancer, malnutrition, compulsive hair pulling (trichotillomania), traction on hair from braiding and ponytails, use of hair treatment chemicals, hormonal alterations, and immune reactions.[123]

Androgenic Alopecia

Androgenic alopecia is localized hair loss and occurs in about 80% of men. It is not a disease but a genetically predisposed response to androgens that clusters in families. Within the distribution of hair over the scalp, androgen-sensitive hair follicles are on top and androgen-insensitive follicles are on the sides and back. In genetically predisposed men, the androgen-sensitive follicles are transformed into vellus follicles. Male-pattern baldness begins with frontotemporal recession and progresses to loss of hair over the top of the scalp. Minoxidil may be used to stimulate hair growth and finasteride (a 5α-reductase inhibitor) may decrease the effect of androgens on hair follicles.[124]

Female-Pattern Alopecia

Some genetically susceptible women in their twenties and thirties experience progressive thinning and loss of hair over the central part of the scalp, and prevalence increases with advancing age. Contrary to male-pattern baldness, there is usually no loss of hair along the frontal hairline but the hairs are shorter and thinner (follicular miniaturization). The mechanism of hair loss is unknown but related to genetic and hormonal changes.[125]

Alopecia Areata

Alopecia areata is an autoimmune T-cell–mediated chronic inflammatory disease directed against hair follicles and results in hair loss. There is rapid onset of hair loss in multiple areas of the scalp, usually in round patches. The eyebrows, eyelashes, beard, and other areas of body hair are rarely involved. Stressful events, cell-mediated immune cytokines, genetic susceptibility, and metabolic disorders, such as Addison disease, thyroid disease, and lupus erythematosus, are associated with alopecia areata.[126]

The affected areas of skin are smooth or may have short shafts of poorly developed hair that breaks at the surface ("exclamation mark" hair). Regrowth occurs within 1 to 3 months, but hair loss may recur at the same site. Permanent regrowth of hair usually occurs. Diagnosis is made by observation of the pattern of hair loss. Biopsy may show a lymphocytic infiltrate around the follicle. There are several treatments for alopecia areata, including corticosteroids and topical immunotherapy, and new treatments are being tested.[127,128]

Hirsutism

Hirsutism occurs in women and is the abnormal growth and distribution of hair on the face, body, and pubic area in a male pattern. There is also frontotemporal hair recession. These areas of hair growth are androgen sensitive. Variations of hair growth in women are great, and a male pattern may be normal. Women who develop hirsutism may be secreting hormones associated with polycystic ovarian syndrome, adrenal hyperplasia, or adrenal tumors; and these disorders require treatment. If no hormonal pathologic conditions exist, treatment may include cosmetic removal of hair, suppression of excessive androgen production, or blockage of peripheral androgen receptors.[129]

DISORDERS OF THE NAIL

Paronychia

Paronychia is an acute or chronic infection of the cuticle. One or more fingers or toes may be involved. Individuals whose hands are frequently exposed to moisture are at greatest risk. The most common causative microorganisms are staphylococci and streptococci. Occasionally *Candida* will be present. Acute paronychia is manifested by the rapid onset of painful inflammation of the cuticle, usually after minor trauma. An abscess may develop requiring incision and drainage for relief of pain. The skin around the nail becomes more edematous and painful with progressive infection. Pus may be expressed from the proximal nail fold and an abscess may develop. The nail plate is usually not affected, although it can become discolored with ridges. Chronic paronychia develops slowly, with tenderness and swelling around the proximal or lateral nail folds.[130]

Treatment includes prevention by keeping the hands dry. Oral antifungals are not effective because they do not penetrate the affected tissues. Topical application of thymol is usually effective.[131]

Onychomycosis

Onychomycosis (tinea unguium) is a fungal or dermatophyte infection of the nail unit. The most common pattern is a nail plate that turns yellow or white and becomes elevated with the accumulation of hyperkeratotic debris within the plate. Fungal infections of the nail are differentiated from psoriasis, lichen planus, and trauma by culture and microscopy and the absence of pitting on the nail surface, which is characteristic of psoriasis. Treatment is difficult because topical or systemic antifungal agents do not penetrate the nail plate readily. Systemic antifungal drugs are more effective. Surgical excision of the nail may be required. Education is essential to preventing recurrence.[132]

> ✔ **QUICK CHECK 41-8**
> 1. Describe the three degrees of burn injury.
> 2. What dangers accompany frostbite?
> 3. What is alopecia? Compare the different types.
> 4. What disorders of the nail are seen?

GERIATRIC CONSIDERATIONS

Aging & Changes in Skin Integrity

- Skin becomes thinner, dryer, and more wrinkled.
- DNA repair of damaged skin decreases.
- Epidermal cells contain less moisture and change shape.
- The dermis thins, producing translucent, paper-thin quality that is more susceptible to tearing.
- Dermis becomes more permeable and less able to clear substances, so they accumulate and cause irritation.
- There is a loss of epidermal rete pegs, which weakens the connection to the dermis and gives skin a smooth, shiny, and wrinkled appearance with an increased likelihood to tear from shearing forces.
- There is a loss of elastin, contributing to wrinkling.
- There is a loss of flexibility of collagen fibers, so skin cannot stretch and regain shape as readily.
- The barrier function of the stratum corneum is reduced, increasing risk for injury and infection.
- Significantly decreased number of Langerhans cells reduces the skin's immune response.

- The dermoepidermal border flattens, shortening and decreasing the number of capillary loops.

Other Skin Changes with Aging

- Wound healing decreases as a result of decreased estrogen in both men and women, decreased blood flow, and slower rate of basal cell and fibroblast turnover.
- There are fewer melanocytes; pigmentation becomes irregular, giving decreased protection from ultraviolet radiation and leading to graying of hair.
- Atrophy of eccrine, apocrine, and sebaceous glands causes dry skin.
- Pressure and touch receptors and free nerve endings decrease in number, causing reduced sensory perception.
- With compromised temperature regulation, loss of cutaneous vasomotion, and decreased eccrine sweat production, there is an increased risk of heat stroke and hypothermia.
- The nail plate thins and nails are more brittle.

Data from Amaro-Ortiz A et al: *Molecules* 19(5):6202-6219, 2014; Chang AL et al: *J Am Med Dir Assoc* 14(10):724-730, 2013; Emmerson E, Hardman MJ: *Biogerontol* 13(1):3-20, 2012; Kottner J et al: *Br J Dermatol* 169(3):528-542, 2013; Ramos-e-Silva M et al: *Clin Dermatol* 30(3): 274-276, 2012.

▌DID YOU UNDERSTAND?

Structure and Function of the Skin

1. Skin is the largest organ of the body and equals 20% of body weight. The major functions are to provide a protective barrier and to regulate body temperature.
2. The skin has two layers—the dermis and epidermis. The underlying hypodermis contains connective tissue, fat cells, fibroblasts, and macrophages.
3. The epidermis contains basal and spinous layers with melanocytes, Langerhans cells, and Merkel cells.
4. The dermis is composed of connective tissue elements, hair follicles, sweat glands, sebaceous glands, blood vessels, nerves, and lymphatic vessels.
5. The dermal appendages include nails, hair, and eccrine and apocrine sweat glands.
6. The papillary capillaries provide the major blood supply to the skin, arising from deeper arterial plexuses.
7. Heat loss and heat conservation are regulated by arteriovenous anastomoses that lead to the papillary capillaries in the dermis.

8. Pressure ulcers develop from pressure and shearing forces that occlude capillary blood flow with resulting ischemia and necrosis. Areas at greatest risk are pressure points over bony prominences, such as the greater trochanters, sacrum, ischia, and heels.
9. Keloids are sharply elevated scars that extend beyond the border of traumatized skin. Hypertrophic scars do not extend beyond the border of injury.
10. Pruritus is itching and is associated with many skin disorders. Small unmyelinated type C nerve fibers transmit itch sensation.

Disorders of the Skin

1. Allergic contact dermatitis is a form of delayed hypersensitivity that develops with sensitization to allergens, such as metal, chemicals, or poison ivy.
2. Irritant contact dermatitis develops from prolonged exposure to chemicals, such as acids or soaps, with disruption of the skin barrier.
3. Atopic or allergic dermatitis is associated with a family history of allergies, hay fever, elevated IgE levels, and increased histamine

sensitivity. Pruritus and scratching predispose the skin to infection, scaling, and thickening.

4. Stasis dermatitis occurs on the legs and results from chronic venous stasis and edema.

5. Seborrheic dermatitis involves scaly, yellowish, inflammatory plaques of the scalp, eyebrows, eyelids, ear canals, chest, axillae, and back. The cause is unknown but *Malassezia* yeasts have been implicated.

6. Papulosquamous disorders are characterized by papules, scales, plaques, and erythema.

7. Psoriasis is a chronic inflammatory skin disease associated with a complex inflammatory cascade involving multiple immune cells resulting in cellular proliferation of both the epidermis and the dermis; it is characterized by scaly, erythematous, pruritic plaques.

8. Pityriasis rosea is a self-limiting inflammatory disease characterized by oval lesions with scales around the edges; it is located along skin lines of the trunk and may be caused by a herpes-like virus.

9. Lichen planus is an autoimmune papular, violet-colored inflammatory lesion of unknown origin manifested by severe pruritus.

10. Acne vulgaris is an inflammation of the pilosebaceous follicle.

11. Acne rosacea develops on the middle third of the face with hypertrophy and inflammation of the sebaceous glands and is associated with altered innate immune responses.

12. Discoid (cutaneous) lupus erythematosus is an autoimmune disease that can affect only the skin. The systemic form also presents cutaneous lesions. The cutaneous inflammatory lesions usually occur in sun-exposed areas with a butterfly distribution over the nose and cheeks.

13. Pemphigus is a chronic, autoimmune, blistering disease that begins in the mouth or on the scalp and spreads to other parts of the body, often with a fatal outcome.

14. Erythema multiforme is an acute inflammation of the skin and mucous membranes (bullous form) with lesions that appear target-like with alternating rings of edema and inflammation; it is often associated with T-cell–mediated allergic reactions to drugs.

15. Folliculitis is a bacterial infection of the hair follicle.

16. A furuncle is an infection of the hair follicle that extends to the surrounding tissue.

17. A carbuncle is a collection of infected hair follicles that forms a draining abscess.

18. Cellulitis is a diffuse infection of the dermis and subcutaneous tissue.

19. Erysipelas is a superficial streptococcal infection of the skin commonly affecting the face, ears, and lower legs.

20. Impetigo may have a bullous or an ulcerative form and is caused by *Staphylococcus* or *Streptococcus*.

21. Herpes simplex virus type 1 (HSV-1) causes cold sores but can infect the cornea, mouth, and labia. HSV-2 causes genital lesions and is usually spread by sexual contact.

22. Herpes zoster (shingles) and varicella (chickenpox) are both caused by the varicella-zoster virus.

23. Warts are benign, rough, elevated lesions caused by human papillomavirus. Condylomata acuminata, or venereal warts, are spread by sexual contact.

24. Tinea infections (fungal infections) can occur anywhere on the body and are classified by location (i.e., tinea pedis, tinea corporis, tinea capitis).

25. Candidiasis is a yeastlike fungal infection (*Candida albicans*) occurring on skin and mucous membranes and in the gastrointestinal tract.

26. Cutaneous vasculitis is an inflammation of skin blood vessels related to immune complex deposition with purpura, ischemia, and necrosis resulting from vessel necrosis.

27. Urticarial lesions are commonly associated with type I hypersensitivity responses and appear as wheals, welts, or hives.

28. Scleroderma is an autoimmune-mediated sclerosis of the skin that may also affect systemic organs and cause renal failure, bowel obstruction, or cardiac dysrhythmias.

29. Ticks transmit numerous diseases including Lyme disease caused by an immune response to the spirochete *Borrelia burgdorferi*.

30. Seborrheic keratosis is a proliferation of basal cells that produce elevated, smooth, or warty lesions of varying size. They are most common among the elderly population.

31. Keratoacanthoma arises from hair follicles on sun-exposed areas. Three stages of development characterize the lesion, which results in a dome-shaped, crusty lesion filled with keratin that resolves in 3 to 4 months.

32. Actinic keratosis is a pigmented scaly lesion that develops in sun-exposed individuals with fair skin. The lesion may become malignant in the form of a squamous cell carcinoma.

33. Nevi arise from melanocytes and may be pigmented or fleshy pink. They occur singly or in groups and may undergo transition to malignant melanoma.

34. Basal cell carcinoma is the most common skin cancer and occurs most often on ultraviolet-exposed areas of the skin.

35. Squamous cell carcinoma is a tumor of the epidermis and can be localized (in situ) or invasive.

36. Cutaneous malignant melanoma arises from melanocytes, and if not excised early, metastasis occurs through the lymph nodes.

37. Kaposi sarcoma is a vascular malignancy associated with herpesvirus-8 and immunodeficiency.

38. Burns are classified according to depth and extent of injury as first-, second-, third-, or fourth-degree burns.

39. Severe burns cause profound edema and burn shock related to an inflammatory response throughout the cardiovascular system with loss of capillary seal. Fluid resuscitation is critical to prevent shock and death.

40. Burns cause a hypermetabolic response with increased cortisol, glucagon, and insulin levels and with gluconeogenesis.

41. Immune suppression associated with inflammatory cytokine release from burned tissue increases risk for infection and can delay wound healing.

42. Cold injury usually occurs on the face and digits, with direct injury to cells and impaired circulation.

Disorders of the Hair

1. Alopecia is loss of hair from the head or body.

2. Male-pattern alopecia is an inherited form of irreversible baldness with hair loss in the central scalp and recession of the frontotemporal hairline.

3. Female-pattern alopecia is a thinning of the central hair of the scalp beginning in women at 20 to 30 years of age.

4. Alopecia areata is an autoimmune-mediated loss of hair and may be associated with stress or metabolic diseases; it is usually reversible.

5. Hirsutism is a male pattern of hair growth in women that may be normal or the result of excessive secretion of androgenic hormones.

Disorders of the Nail

1. Paronychia is an inflammation of the cuticle that can be acute or chronic and is usually caused by staphylococci, streptococci, or fungi.

2. Onychomycosis is a fungal infection of the nail plate.

KEY TERMS

Acne rosacea, 1064
Acne vulgaris, 1064
Actinic keratosis, 1070
Allergic contact dermatitis, 1060
Alopecia, 1078
Alopecia areata, 1078
Androgenic alopecia, 1078
Apocrine sweat gland, 1053
Atopic dermatitis (allergic dermatitis), 1061
Basal cell carcinoma (BCC), 1071
Bullous erythema multiforme, 1065
Burn shock, 1076
Candidiasis, 1068
Capillary seal, 1076
Carbuncle, 1066
Cellulitis, 1066
Chronic uticaria, 1069
Clawlike prolongation, 1060
Condylomata acuminata (venereal warts), 1067
Cutaneous melanoma, 1072
Cutaneous vasculitis, 1069
Deep partial-thickness burn, 1075
Dermal appendage, 1053
Dermatitis, 1060

Dermis, 1053
Discoid (cutaneous) lupus erythematosus (DLE), 1064
Eccrine sweat gland, 1053
Eczema, 1060
Epidermis, 1053
Erysipelas, 1066
Erythema multiforme, 1065
Erythrodermic (exfoliative) psoriasis, 1062
Escharotomy, 1075
First-degree burn, 1074
Fluid resuscitation, 1076
Folliculitis, 1066
Fourth-degree burn, 1075
Furuncle, 1066
Guttate psoriasis, 1062
Herald patch, 1063
Herpes simplex virus (HSV), 1067
Herpes zoster (shingles), 1067
Hirsutism, 1078
Human papillomavirus (HPV), 1067
Hypertrophic scar, 1060
IgA pemphigus, 1065
Impetigo, 1066
Inverse psoriasis, 1062
Irritant contact dermatitis, 1061

Kaposi sarcoma (KS), 1073
Keloid, 1060
Keratoacanthoma, 1070
Lichen planus (LP), 1063
Lip cancer, 1072
Localized scleroderma (morphea), 1069
Lupus erythematosus, 1064
Lyme disease, 1066
Mycosis fungoides, 1074
Nails, 1053
Necrotizing fasciitis, 1066
Nevus (pl., nevi), 1070
Onychomycosis (tinea unguium), 1079
Papillary capillary, 1054
Papulosquamous disorder, 1062
Paraneoplastic pemphigus, 1065
Paronychia, 1078
Pemphigus, 1065
Pemphigus erythematosus, 1065
Pemphigus foliaceus, 1065
Pemphigus hepatiformis, 1065
Pemphigus vegetans, 1065
Pemphigus vulgaris, 1065
Pityriasis rosea, 1063
Plaque psoriasis, 1062
Pressure ulcer, 1055

Primary cutaneous lymphoma, 1074
Psoriasis, 1062
Psoriatic arthritis, 1062
Psoriatic nail disease, 1062
Pustular psoriasis, 1062
Sebaceous gland, 1053
Seborrheic dermatitis, 1061
Seborrheic keratosis, 1070
Second-degree burn, 1075
Squamous cell carcinoma (SCC), 1071
Stasis dermatitis, 1061
Stevens-Johnson syndrome, 1065
Subcutaneous layer (hypodermis), 1053
Systemic scleroderma, 1069
Third-degree burn (full-thickness burn), 1075
Tinea infection, 1068
Total body surface area (TBSA), 1075
Toxic epidermal necrolysis (TEN), 1065
Urticaria (hives), 1069
Urticarial lesion, 1069
Varicella (chickenpox), 1067
Wart, 1067

REFERENCES

1. de Laat EH et al: Epidemiology, risk and prevention of pressure ulcers in critically ill patients: a literature review, *J Wound Care* 15(6):269-275, 2006.
2. National Pressure Ulcer Advisory Panel: *Pressure ulcer stages revised by NPUAP, Feb 2007.* Accessed February 10, 2015. Available at: www.npuap.org/resources/educational-and-clinical-resources/npuap-pressure-ulcer-stagescategories/.
3. Thomas DR: Role of nutrition in the treatment and prevention of pressure ulcers, *Nutr Clin Pract* 29(4):466-472, 2014.
4. Black J et al: Dressings as an adjunct to pressure ulcer prevention: consensus panel recommendations, *Int Wound J* 2014 Mar 3. [Epub ahead of print.]
5. Cushing CA, Phillips LG: Evidence-based medicine: pressure sores, *Plast Reconstr Surg* 132(6):1720-1732, 2013.
6. Smith ME et al: Pressure ulcer treatment strategies: a systematic comparative effectiveness review, *Ann Intern Med* 159(1):39-50, 2013.
7. Arno AI et al: Up-to-date approach to manage keloids and hypertrophic scars: a useful guide, *Burns* 40(7):1255-1266, 2014.
8. Shih B, Bayat A: Genetics of keloid scarring, *Arch Dermatol Res* 302(5):319-339, 2010.
9. Ikoma A: Updated neurophysiology of itch, *Biol Pharm Bull* 36(8):1235-1240, 2013.
10. Hassan I, Haji MI: Understanding itch: an update on mediators and mechanisms of pruritus, *Indian J Dermatol Venereol Leprol* 80:106-114, 2014.
11. Tominaga M, Takamori K: An update on peripheral mechanisms and treatments of itch, *Biol Pharm Bull* :36(8):1241-1247, 2013.

12. Peiser M: Role of Th17 cells in skin inflammation of allergic contact dermatitis, *Clin Dev Immunol* 2013:261037, 2013.
13. Cabañes N et al: Latex allergy: position paper, *J Investig Allergol Clin Immunol* 22(5):313-330, 2012.
14. Lee HY et al: Cytokines and chemokines in irritant contact dermatitis, *Mediators Inflamm* 2013:916497, 2013.
15. McDaniel JC et al: Neutrophil activity in chronic venous leg ulcers—a target for therapy? *Wound Repair Regen* 21(3):339-351, 2013.
16. White-Chu EF, Conner-Kerr TA: Overview of guidelines for the prevention and treatment of venous leg ulcers: a US perspective, *J Multidiscip Healthc* 7:111-117, 2014.
17. Dessinioti C, Katsambas A: Seborrheic dermatitis: etiology, risk factors, and treatments: facts and controversies, *Clin Dermatol* 31(4):343-351, 2013.
18. Boehncke WH, Schön MP: Psoriasis, *Lancet* 386(9997):983-994, 2015.
19. Lynde CW et al: Interleukin 17A: toward a new understanding of psoriasis pathogenesis, *J Am Acad Dermatol* 71(1):141-150, 2014.
20. Baliwag J et al: Cytokines in psoriasis, *Cytokine* 73(2):342-350, 2015.
21. Brezinski EA, Armstrong AW: Strategies to maximize treatment success in moderate to severe psoriasis: establishing treatment goals and tailoring of biologic therapies, *Semin Cutan Med Surg* 33(2):91-97, 2014.
22. Olivieri I et al: Advances in the management of psoriatic arthritis, *Nat Rev Rheumatol* 10(9): 531-542, 2014.

23. Jullien D et al: Immunogenicity of biotherapy used in psoriasis: the science behind the scenes, *J Invest Dermatol* 135(1):31-38, 2015.
24. Rebora A et al: Pityriasis rosea and herpesviruses: facts and controversies, *Clin Dermatol* 28(5): 497-501, 2010.
25. Amatya A et al: Comparative study of effectiveness of oral acyclovir with oral erythromycin in the treatment of Pityriasis rosea, *Kathmandu Univ Med J (KUMJ)* 10(37):57-61, 2012.
26. Sharma A et al: Lichen planus: an update and review, *Cutis* 90(1):17-23, 2012.
27. Carrozzo M, Scally K: Oral manifestations of hepatitis C virus infection, *World J Gastroenterol* 20(24):7534-7543, 2014.
28. Di Stasio D et al: Oral lichen planus: a narrative review, *Front Biosci (Elite Ed)* 6:370-376, 2014.
29. Le Cleach L, Chosidow O: Clinical practice. Lichen planus, *N Engl J Med* 366(8):723-732, 2012.
30. Tüzün Y et al: Rosacea and rhinophyma, *Clin Dermatol* 32(1):35-46, 2014.
31. Layton A, Thiboutot D: Emerging therapies in rosacea, *J Am Acad Dermatol* 69(6 Suppl 1): S57-S65, 2013.
32. Chong BF et al: Determining risk factors for developing systemic lupus erythematosus in patients with discoid lupus erythematosus, *Br J Dermatol* 166(1):29-35, 2012.
33. Kuhn A, Landmann A: The classification and diagnosis of cutaneous lupus erythematosus, *J Autoimmun* 48-49:14-19, 2014.
34. Yu C et al: Immunologic and genetic considerations of cutaneous lupus erythematosus: a comprehensive review, *J Autoimmun* 41:34-45, 2013.

35. Okon LG, Werth VP: Cutaneous lupus erythematosus: diagnosis and treatment, *Best Pract Res Clin Rheumatol* 27(3):391-404, 2013.

36. Porro AM et al: Non-classical forms of pemphigus: pemphigus herpetiformis, IgA pemphigus, paraneoplastic pemphigus and IgG/IgA pemphigus, *Ann Bras Dermatol* 89(1):96-106, 2014.

37. Ruocco V et al: Pemphigus: etiology, pathogenesis, and inducing or triggering factors: facts and controversies, *Clin Dermatol* 31(4):374-381, 2013.

38. Ruocco E et al: Pemphigus: associations and management guidelines: facts and controversies, *Clin Dermatol* 31(4):382-390, 2013.

39. Samim F et al: Erythema multiforme: a review of epidemiology, pathogenesis, clinical features, and treatment, *Dent Clin North Am* 57(4):583-596, 2013.

40. Cheng CY et al: HLA associations and clinical implications in T-cell mediated drug hypersensitivity reactions: an updated review, *J Immunol Res* 2014:565320, 2014.

41. Tomasini C et al: From erythema multiforme to toxic epidermal necrolysis. Same spectrum or different diseases? *G Ital Dermatol Venereol* 149(2):243-261, 2014.

42. Mistry RD: Skin and soft tissue infections, *Pediatr Clin North Am* 60(5):1063-1082, 2013.

43. Chira S, Miller LG: *Staphylococcus aureus* is the most common identified cause of cellulitis: a systematic review, *Epidemiol Infect* 138(3):313-317, 2010.

44. Al Shukry S, Ommen J: Necrotizing fasciitis—report of ten cases and review of recent literature, *J Med Life* 6(2):189-194, 2013.

45. Gunderson CG, Martinello RA: A systematic review of bacteremias in cellulitis and erysipelas, *J Infect* 64(2):148-155, 2012.

46. Radolf JD et al: Of ticks, mice and men: understanding the dual-host lifestyle of Lyme disease spirochaettes, *Nat Rev Microbiol* 10(2):98-99, 2012.

47. Bratton RL et al: Diagnosis and treatment of Lyme disease, *Mayo Clin Proc* 83(5):566-571, 2008.

48. Eshoo MW et al: Achieving molecular diagnostics for Lyme disease, *Expert Rev Mol Diagn* 13(8):875-883, 2013.

49. Stanek G et al: Lyme borreliosis, *Lancet* 379(9814):461-473, 2012.

50. Embers ME, Narasimhan S: Vaccination against Lyme disease: past, present, and future, *Front Cell Infect Microbiol* 3:6, 2013.

51. Bloom DC et al: Epigenetic regulation of latent HSV-1 gene expression, *Biochim Biophys Acta* 1799(3-4):246-256, 2010.

52. Vere Hodge RA, Field HJ: Antiviral agents for herpes simplex virus, *Adv Pharmacol* 67:1-38, 2013.

53. Pinninti SG, Kimberlin DW: Neonatal herpes simplex virus infections, *Pediatr Clin North Am* 60(2):351-365, 2013.

54. Zhu XP et al: HSV-2 vaccine: current status and insight into factors for developing an efficient vaccine, *Viruses* 6(2):371-390, 2014.

55. Ruocco V et al: Beyond zoster: sensory and immune changes in zoster-affected dermatomes: a review, *Acta Derm Venereol* 92(4):378-382, 2012.

56. Kim SR et al: Varicella zoster: an update on current treatment options and future perspectives, *Expert Opin Pharmacother* 15(1):61-71, 2014.

57. Bruggink SC et al: Monochloroacetic acid application is an effective alternative to cryotherapy for common and plantar warts in primary care: a randomized controlled trial, *J Invest Dermatol* 135(5):1262-2367, 2015.

58. On SC et al: A single-blinded randomized controlled study to assess the efficacy of twice daily application of sinecatechins 15% ointment when used sequentially with cryotherapy in the treatment of external genital warts, *J Drugs Dermatol* 13(11):1400-1405, 2014.

59. Grce M, Mravak-Stipetić M: Human papillomavirus-associated diseases, *Clin Dermatol* 32(2):253-258, 2014.

60. Del Rosso JQ, Kircik LH: Optimizing topical antifungal therapy for superficial cutaneous fungal infections: focus on topical naftifine for cutaneous dermatophytosis, *J Drugs Dermatol* 12(11 Suppl):s165-s171, 2013.

61. Yapar N: Epidemiology and risk factors for invasive candidiasis, *Ther Clin Risk Manag* 10:95-105, 2014.

62. Habif TP: *Clinical dermatology*, ed 5, p 523, St Louis, 2009, Mosby.

63. Marzano AV et al: Skin involvement in cutaneous and systemic vasculitis, *Autoimmun Rev* 12(4):467-476, 2013.

64. Jain S: Pathogenesis of chronic urticaria: an overview, *Dermatol Res Pract* 2014:674709, 2014.

65. Bielsa Marsol I: Update on the classification and treatment of localized scleroderma, *Actas Dermosifiliogr* 104(8):654-666, 2013.

66. Wigley FM: Vascular disease in scleroderma, *Clin Rev Allergy Immunol* 36(2-3):150-175, 2009.

67. Hudson M, Fritzler MJ: Diagnostic criteria of systemic sclerosis, *J Autoimmun* 48-49:38-41, 2014.

68. Kreuter A: Localized scleroderma, *Dermatol Ther* 25(2):135-147, 2012.

69. Chetty P et al: Primary care review of actinic keratosis and its therapeutic options: a global perspective, *Dermatol Ther (Heidelb)* 5(1):19-35, 2015.

70. Ibrahimi OA et al: Congenital melanocytic nevi: where are we now? Part II. Treatment options and approach to treatment, *J Am Acad Dermatol* 67(4):515, 2012.

71. Puig S, Malvehy J: Monitoring patients with multiple nevi, *Dermatol Clin* 31(4):565-577, 2013.

72. Emmert S et al: Molecular biology of basal and squamous cell carcinomas, *Adv Exp Med Biol* 810:234-252, 2014.

73. Reichrath J, Rass K: Ultraviolet damage, DNA repair and vitamin D in nonmelanoma skin cancer and in malignant melanoma: an update, *Adv Exp Med Biol* 810:208-233, 2014.

74. American Cancer Society: *Cancer facts & figures 2015*, Atlanta, 2015, Author.

75. Bejar C, Maubec E: Therapy of advanced squamous cell carcinoma of the skin, *Curr Treat Options Oncol* 15(2):302-320, 2014.

76. Sondak VK, Messina JL: Unusual presentations of melanoma: melanoma of unknown primary site, melanoma arising in childhood, and melanoma arising in the eye and on mucosal surfaces, *Surg Clin North Am* 94(5):1059-1073, 2014.

77. Azoury SC, Lange JR: Epidemiology, risk factors, prevention, and early detection of melanoma, *Surg Clin North Am* 94(5):945-962, 2014.

78. Little EG, Eide MJ: Update on the current state of melanoma incidence, *Dermatol Clin* 30(3):355-361, 2012.

79. Lo JA, Fisher DE: The melanoma revolution: from UV carcinogenesis to a new era in therapeutics, *Science* 346(6212):945-949, 2014.

80. Kauffmann RM, Chen SL: Workup and staging of malignant melanoma, *Surg Clin North Am* 94(5):963-972, 2014.

81. Robert C et al: Improved overall survival in melanoma with combined dabrafenib and trametinib, *N Engl J Med* 372(1):30-39, 2015.

82. Hao M et al: Advances in targeted therapy for unresectable melanoma: new drugs and combinations, *Cancer Lett* 359(1):1-8, 2015.

83. Ozao-Choy J et al: Melanoma vaccines: mixed past, promising future, *Surg Clin North Am* 94(5):1017-1030, 2014.

84. Ruocco E et al: Kaposi's sarcoma: etiology and pathogenesis, inducing factors, causal associations, and treatments: facts and controversies, *Clin Dermatol* 31(4):413-422, 2013.

85. Luu HN et al: Age patterns of Kaposi's sarcoma incidence in a cohort of HIV-infected men, *Cancer Med* 3(6):1635-1643, 2014.

86. Klemke CD: Cutaneous lymphomas, *J Dtsch Dermatol Ges* 12(1):7-28, 2014.

87. Jawed SI et al: Primary cutaneous T-cell lymphoma (mycosis fungoides and Sézary syndrome). Part II: prognosis, management, and future directions, *J Am Acad Dermatol* 70(2):223, 2014.

88. Kempf W et al: Cutaneous lymphomas: an update. Part 1: T-cell and natural killer/T-cell lymphomas and related conditions, *Am J Dermatopathol* 36(2):105-123, 2014.

89. American Burn Association: *Burn incidence and treatment in the United States: 2015 fact sheet.* Available at: http://ameriburn.org/resources_factsheet.php.

90. Dries DJ, Endorf FW: Inhalation injury: epidemiology, pathology, treatment strategies, *Scand J Trauma Resusc Emerg Med* 21:31, 2013.

91. Sheridan RL, Chang P: Acute burn procedures, *Surg Clin North Am* 94(4):755-764, 2014.

92. Yu CY et al: Human body surface area database and estimation formula, *Burns* 36(5):616-629, 2010.

93. Cancio LC: Initial assessment and fluid resuscitation of burn patients, *Surg Clin North Am* 94(4):741-754, 2014.

94. Pruitt BA Jr: Reflection: evolution of the field over seven decades, *Surg Clin North Am* 94(4):721-740, 2014.

95. Jeschke MG: The hepatic response to thermal injury: is the liver important for postburn outcomes? *Mol Med* 15(9-10):337-351, 2009.

96. Lippi G et al: Disseminated intravascular coagulation in burn injury, *Semin Thromb Hemost* 36(4):429-436, 2010.

97. Kramer GC: Pathophysiology of burn shock and burn edema. In Herndon DN, editor: *Total burn care*, ed 4, Philadelphia, 2012, Saunders.

98. White DJ et al: Cardiomyocyte intracellular calcium and cardiac dysfunction after burn trauma, *Crit Care Med* 30(1):14-22, 2002.

99. Klein GL et al: Effects of burn injury on bone and mineral metabolism. In Herndon DN, editor: *Total burn care*, ed 4, Philadelphia, 2012, Saunders.

100. Liu ZJ et al: Comparison of serum and plasma lactate dehydrogenase in postburn patients, *Burns* 26(1):46-48, 2000.

101. Pruitt BA Jr, Wolf SE: An historical perspective on advances in burn care over the past 100 years, *Clin Plast Surg* 36(4):527-545, 2009.

102. Jeschke MG et al: Long-term persistence of the pathophysiologic response to severe burn injury, *PLoS One* 6(7):e21245, 2011.

103. Mecott GA et al: The role of hyperglycemia in burned patients: evidence-based studies, *Shock* 33(1):5-13, 2010.

104. Ballian N et al: Glucose metabolism in burn patients: the role of insulin and other endocrine hormones, *Burns* 36(5):599-605, 2010.

105. Williams FN et al: What, how, and how much should patients with burns be fed? *Surg Clin North Am* 1(3), 2011:609–629, 2011.

106. Gerd GG et al: Modulation of the hypermetabolic response after burn injury. In Herndon DN, editor: *Total burn care*, ed 4, Philadelphia, 2012, Saunders.

107. Kallinen O et al: Multiple organ failure as a cause of death in patients with severe burns, *J Burn Care Res* 33(2):206-211, 2012.

108. Fagan SP et al: Burn intensive care, *Surg Clin North Am* 94(4):765-779, 2014.

109. Saaiq M et al: Early excision and grafting versus delayed excision and grafting of deep thermal burns up to 40% total body surface area: a comparison of outcome, *Ann Burns Fire Disasters* 25(3):143-147, 2012.

110. Turnage RH et al: Mechanisms of pulmonary microvascular dysfunction during severe burn injury, *World J Surg* 26(7):848-853, 2002.

111. Xiu F, Jeschke MG: Perturbed mononuclear phagocyte system in severely burned and septic patients, *Shock* 40(2):81-88, 2013.

112. Mann-Salinas EA et al: Novel predictors of sepsis outperform the American Burn Association sepsis criteria in the burn intensive care unit patient, *J Burn Care Res* 34(1):31-43, 2013.

113. Rex S: Burn injuries, *Curr Opin Crit Care* 18(6):671-676, 2012.

114. Gamst-Jensen H et al: Acute pain management in burn patients: appraisal and thematic analysis of four clinical guidelines, *Burns* 40(8):1463-1469, 2014.

115. Nordlund MJ et al: Micronutrients after burn injury: a review, *J Burn Care Res* 35(2):121-133, 2014.

116. Rousseau AF et al: ESPEN endorsed recommendations: nutritional therapy in major burns, *Clin Nutr* 32(4):497-502, 2013.

117. Mogoșanu GD, Grumezescu AM: Natural and synthetic polymers for wounds and burns dressing, *Int J Pharm* 463(2):127-136, 2014.

118. Wasiak J et al: Dressings for superficial and partial thickness burns, *Cochrane Database Syst Rev* 3:CD002106, 2013.

119. Orgill DP, Ogawa R: Current methods of burn reconstruction, *Plast Reconstr Surg* 131(5):827e-836e, 2013.

120. Mohr WJ et al: Cold injury, *Hand Clin* 25(4): 481-496, 2009.

121. Petrone P et al: Management of accidental hypothermia and cold injury, *Curr Probl Surg* 51(10):417-431, 2014.

122. Handford C et al: Frostbite: a practical approach to hospital management, *Extrem Physiol Med* 3:7, 2014.

123. Qi J, Garza LA: An overview of alopecias, *Cold Spring Harb Perspect Med* 4(3):a013615, 2014.

124. Piraccini BM, Alessandrini A: Androgenetic alopecia, *G Ital Dermatol Venereol* 149(1):15-24, 2014.

125. Vujovic A, Del Marmol V: The female pattern hair loss: review of etiopathogenesis and diagnosis, *Biomed Res Int* 2014:767628, 2014.

126. Alkhalifah A et al: Alopecia areata update: part I. Clinical picture, histopathology, and pathogenesis, *J Am Acad Dermatol* 62(2):177-188, 2010.

127. Alkhalifah A et al: Alopecia areata update: part II. Treatment, *J Am Acad Dermatol* 62(2):191-202, 2010.

128. Hordinsky MK: Overview of alopecia areata, *J Investig Dermatol Symp Proc* 16(1):S13-S15, 2013.

129. Blume-Peytavi U: How to diagnose and treat medically women with excessive hair, *Dermatol Clin* 31(1):57-65, 2013.

130. Relhan V et al: Management of chronic paronychia, *Indian J Dermatol* 59(1):15-20, 2014.

131. Rigopoulos D et al: Acute and chronic paronychia, *Am Fam Physician* 77(3):339-346, 2008.

132. Westerberg DP, Voyack MJ: Onychomycosis: current trends in diagnosis and treatment, *Am Fam Physician* 88(11):762-770, 2013.

42

Alterations of the Integument in Children

Noreen Heer Nicol and Sue E. Huether

Children frequently develop alterations of the skin, which may be minor or severe and localized or generalized. Skin diseases in children may have different causative mechanisms and different patterns of distribution than those found in adults, although there may be similarities. Some skin diseases resolve spontaneously and require no treatment. Diagnosis is commonly made from the history, appearance, and distribution of the lesion or lesions. Common skin diseases of childhood are presented here.

ACNE VULGARIS

Acne vulgaris is the most common skin disease and occurs primarily between the ages of 12 and 25 years. Acne tends to occur in families, and genetic susceptibility may determine the severity of the disease. The incidence of acne is the same in both genders, although severe disease affects males more often.[1] Diets high in simple carbohydrates and dairy products are associated with acne.[2-4]

Acne develops at distinctive pilosebaceous units known as *sebaceous follicles*. Located primarily on the face and upper parts of the chest and back, these follicles have many large sebaceous glands, a small vellus hair (very short, nonpigmented, and very thin hair), and a dilated follicular canal that is visible as a pore on the skin surface. Acne lesions may be noninflammatory or inflammatory (cystic) (Figure 42-1). In **noninflammatory acne**, the comedones are open (blackheads) and closed (whiteheads), with the accumulated material causing distention of the follicle and thinning of follicular canal walls. **Inflammatory (cystic) acne** develops in closed comedones when the follicular wall ruptures, expelling sebum into the surrounding dermis and initiating inflammation. Pustules form when the inflammation is close to the surface; papules and cystic nodules can develop when the inflammation is deeper, causing mild to severe scarring. Both types of lesions may exist in the same individual.

The principal causative factors are (1) hyperkeratinization of the follicular epithelium, (2) excessive sebum production, (3) follicular proliferation of anaerobic *Propionibacterium acnes,* and (4) inflammation and rupture of a follicle from accumulated debris and bacteria (see Figure 42-1). *P. acnes* shifts from being symbiotic to pathogenic and from being noninflammatory to inflammatory. The causal mechanism is unknown.[5] Androgens (dehydroepiandrosterone sulfate and testosterone), synthesized in increasing amounts during puberty, increase the size and productivity of the sebaceous glands, which promotes *P. acnes*. *P. acnes* produces extracellular porphyrins and proinflammatory molecules, including chemotactic factors and lipolytic and proteolytic enzymes. The hydrolytic action of the enzymes converts triglycerides into free fatty acids (FFAs). FFAs activate Toll-like receptors, T-cell–associated and Th17-associated inflammation, and edema that results in pus formation and breakdown of the follicle wall.[6]

The treatment of acne should be individualized according to severity. Combinations of a topical retinoid, benzoyl peroxide, and antimicrobial agents are preferred. Retinoids are anticomedogenic and comedolytic and have some anti-inflammatory effects. Benzoyl peroxide is antimicrobial with some keratolytic effects. Antibiotics have anti-inflammatory and antimicrobial effects. Use of systemic therapies, including oral antibiotics, sex hormones, corticosteroids,

FIGURE 42-1 Acne. **A,** Inflammatory papules and pustules. **B,** Severe nodular cystic acne. (From Kliegman RM et al, editors: *Nelson textbook of pediatrics,* ed 19, Philadelphia, 2011, Saunders.)

and isotretinoin (requires pregnancy prevention), may be limited by side effects.[7] Acne surgery, including comedo extraction, intralesional steroids, and cryosurgery, is useful in selected individuals. Severe scarring may be treated with dermabrasion, lasers, and resurfacing techniques. Diets should avoid high glycemic index foods. Psychologic support is important because acne negatively affects quality of life, self-esteem, and mood in adolescents and is associated with an increased risk of anxiety, depression, and suicidal ideation.[8] Special consideration must be given to treatment for those with darker skin because they have greater risk for hyperpigmentation and keloidal scarring.[9] Research is continuing on the development of vaccines to prevent acne.[10]

Acne conglobata is a highly inflammatory form of acne with communicating cysts and abscesses beneath the skin that can cause scarring. Remissions tend to occur during the summer, perhaps from more exposure to sunlight. This type of acne requires the use of systemic and combination therapies to prevent drug resistance.

Hydradinitis suppurativa (inverse acne) is a chronic, inflammatory disease characterized by recurrent abscesses, sinus tract formation, and scarring. There is hyperkeratosis and occlusion of the pilosebaceous follicular ducts involving areas of skin where there are folds, hair follicles, and apocrine (sweat) glands (i.e., axillary, inguinal, inframammary, genital, buttocks, and perineal areas of the body). The cause is unknown but the incidence is estimated at 1% to 4% of the population and is more common in females. Aggravating factors include obesity, stress, and smoking. The lesions present as deep, firm, painful subcutaneous nodules that track and rupture horizontally under the skin. Treatment can include incision and drainage of nodules, culture of exudate, and administration of antibiotics (with concern about the presence of methicillin-resistant *Staphylococcus aureus* [MRSA]), topical or intralesional corticosteroids, and retinoids. The disease can recur for years with negative effects on quality of life.[11]

DERMATITIS

Atopic Dermatitis

Atopic dermatitis (AD), also known as atopic eczema, is the most common cause of eczema in children. The prevalence is up to 20% in children and approximately 3% of adults in the United States and other industrialized countries.[12] More than half of these individuals develop asthma and allergies later in life.[13] Onset is usually from 2 to 6 months of age, and 85% of cases develop within the first 5 years of life.

The cause of this chronic relapsing form of pruritic eczema involves an interplay of genetic predisposition; altered skin barrier function associated with filaggrin gene mutations and filaggrin deficiency (proteins that bind keratin in the epidermis); reduced ceramide (a stratum corneum lipid) levels; decreased antimicrobial peptides; altered innate immunity; and altered immune responses to allergens, irritants, and microbes.[14] Filaggrin gene mutations also are associated with increased

FIGURE 42-2 Atopic Dermatitis. Characteristic lesions with crusting from irritation and scratching over knees and around ankles. (Courtesy Department of Dermatology, School of Medicine, University of Utah, Salt Lake City, Utah.)

risk for asthma in AD and ichthyosis vulgaris (dry, scaly skin)[15] (Figure 42-2). There is an altered skin microbiome with formation of biofilm by *S aureus* that may act as super-antigens causing exacerbations of eczema.[16]

AD has a constellation of clinical features that include severe pruritus and a characteristic eczematoid appearance with redness, edema, and scaling. The skin becomes increasingly dry, itchy, sensitive, and easily irritated because the barrier function of the skin is impaired. Itching is the hallmark of atopic dermatitis and rubbing and scratching to relieve the itch are responsible for many of the clinical skin changes of AD. In young children, a rash appears primarily on the face, scalp, trunk, and extensor surfaces of the arms and legs (Figure 42-2). In older children and adults, the rash tends to be found on the neck, antecubital and popliteal fossae, and hands and feet. Individuals with AD also tend to develop viral, bacterial, and fungal skin infections in the eczematous areas. There are no specific laboratory features of AD that can be used for diagnostic and treatment purposes.[17] Most affected individuals show increased serum levels of immunoglobulin E (IgE) level, interleukin-4, eosinophils (eosinophilia), and positive skin tests to a variety of common food and inhalant allergens.

Management of individuals with AD includes accurate diagnosis and comprehensive evaluation of triggers and response to treatment; management of confounding factors, including sleep disruption; and education of individuals and caregivers. Avoidance of triggers and promotion of skin hydration, including soaking baths and emollients, are key to good therapy.[18] Anti-inflammatory agents, such as topical corticosteroids and calcineurin inhibitors, are necessary during active flare-ups of eczema. Immunomodulator therapy and wet wrap therapy[19] are used for severe eczema. Systemic therapy includes the use of sedating antihistamines and antibiotics. Research is in progress to develop molecule-specific targets to produce long-term disease remission.[20]

Diaper Dermatitis

Diaper dermatitis (diaper rash) is a form of irritant contact dermatitis initiated by a combination of factors including prolonged exposure to and irritation by urine and feces as well as maceration by wet diapers or airtight plastic diaper covers. Disposable diaper designs have decreased the incidence of diaper dermatitis in infants. Often, diaper dermatitis is secondarily infected with *Candida albicans*. The resulting inflammation affects the lower aspect of the abdomen, genitalia, buttock, and upper portion of the thigh.

The lesions vary from mild erythema to erythematous papular lesions. Candidal (monilial) diaper dermatitis is usually very erythematous, with sharp margination and pustulovesicular satellite lesions (Figure 42-3).

Treatment involves frequent diaper changes to keep the affected area clean and dry or regular exposure of the perineal area to air, use of superabsorbent diapers, and topical protection with a product containing petrolatum or zinc oxide, or both. Topical antifungal medication is used to treat *C. albicans* when present.[21]

> ✔ **QUICK CHECK 42-1**
> 1. What causes the inflammation of acne vulgaris?
> 2. What lesions are typical of atopic dermatitis in children?
> 3. What causes diaper dermatitis?

FIGURE 42-3 Diaper Dermatitis. A, Diaper dermatitis with erosions. **B,** Diaper dermatitis with *Candida albicans* secondary infection. (Courtesy Department of Dermatology, School of Medicine, University of Utah, Salt Lake City, Utah.)

INFECTIONS OF THE SKIN

Infectious diseases caused by bacteria, viruses, and fungi constitute the major forms of skin disease. Breaks in the skin integrity, particularly those that inoculate pathogens into the dermis and epidermis, may cause or exacerbate infections. Most infections tend to occur superficially; however, systemic signs and symptoms develop occasionally and can be life-threatening in immunosuppressed children.

Bacterial Infections
Impetigo Contagiosum

Impetigo is the most common bacterial skin infection in children 2 to 5 years of age. *Staphylococcus aureus (S. aureus)* and, less commonly, *Streptococcus pyogenes* cause impetigo. The mode of transmission is by both direct and indirect contact. The disease is more common in midsummer to late summer, with a higher incidence in hot, humid climates. Impetigo is particularly infectious among people living in crowded conditions with poor sanitary facilities or in settings such as day-care facilities. It affects children in good health, but conditions such as anemia and malnutrition are predisposing factors.

Bacterial invasion occurs through minor breaks in the cutaneous surface or as a secondary infection of a preexisting dermatosis or infestation. The staphylococci produce bacterial toxins called *exfoliative toxins (ETs)* that cause a disruption in desmosomal adhesion molecules with blister formation. There are two types of impetigo: nonbullous and, more rarely, bullous (caused only by *S. aureus*), where blisters enlarge or coalesce to form bullae (Box 42-1). Both forms of impetigo begin as vesicles with a thin vesicular roof composed of stratum corneum that ruptures to form a honey-colored crust (Figure 42-4). The lesions are often located on the face, around the nose and mouth, but the hands and other exposed areas also are involved.

BOX 42-1 Impetigo

Vesicular Impetigo
- Contagious, acute, superficial, vesiculopustular, and most common form
- Caused by group A *Streptococcus pyogenes* (alone or with *S. aureus*)
- Spread by direct physical contact with other infected individuals or through insect bites
- Presents as small vesicles with a honey-colored serum; yellow to white-brown crusts form as vesicles rupture and extend radially
- Untreated lesions last for weeks and cover large area
- Regional lymphadenitis common
- Most significant complication is acute glomerulonephritis
- Treatment is aggressive in light of this complication

Bullous Impetigo
- Caused by *Staphylococcus aureus*
- Bacterial toxin produced (exfoliative toxin [ET]) causes disruption in cellular adhesion with blister formation
- Occurs in neonates
- Highly contagious
- Source is family member with pustule or asymptomatic carrier with pathogen in anterior nares, perineal region, or fingernails
- Transmitted by contact with individual or contaminated equipment
- Presents with vesicles that enlarge or coalesce to form superficial bullae, few localized lesions, or many lesions scattered over the skin surface; as bullae rupture, thin, flat, honey-colored crust appears (hallmark of impetigo)
- Lesions found on face around the nose and mouth; hands and other exposed areas also susceptible

FIGURE 42-4 Impetigo. Multiple crusted and oozing lesions of impetigo. (From Kliegman RM et al, editors: *Nelson textbook of pediatrics,* ed 19, Philadelphia, 2011, Saunders.)

FIGURE 42-5 Staphylococcal Scalded-Skin Syndrome (SSSS). The skin lesions, showing desquamation and wrinkling of the skin margins, appeared 1 day after drainage of a staphylococcal abscess. (From Kliegman RM et al: *Nelson textbook of pediatrics,* ed 19, St Louis, 2011, Saunders.)

Impetigo is clinically characterized by crusted erosions or ulcers that may arise as a primary infection or as a secondary infection of a preexisting dermatosis or infestation.

The treatment of choice for both types of impetigo is topical mupirocin or fusidic acid for uncomplicated lesions. For extensive or complicated impetigo, systemic antibiotics may be warranted but β-lactam antibiotics should be avoided if methicillin-resistant *S. aureus* (MRSA) is suspected.[22] Prompt treatment avoids complications, such as glomerulonephritis, necrotizing fasciitis, and septic shock syndrome. Lesions usually resolve in 2 to 3 weeks without scarring. Using good handwashing techniques and isolating the infected child's washcloth, towels, drinking glass, and linen are important for prevention.[23]

Staphylococcal Scalded-Skin Syndrome

Staphylococcal scalded-skin syndrome (SSSS) is the most serious staphylococcal infection that affects the skin and is usually seen in infants and children younger than 5 years of age. SSSS is caused by virulent group II strains of staphylococci that produce an exfoliative toxin. The toxin attacks desmoglein and adhesion molecules and causes a separation of the skin just below the granular layer of the epidermis (see Figure 41-1).[24] The toxin is usually produced at body sites other than the skin and arrives at the epidermis through the circulatory system. Staphylococci typically are not found in the skin lesions themselves. Adults have circulating antistaphylococcal antibodies and are better able to metabolize and excrete the toxin. Neonates are at the highest risk because of their lack of immunity with no prior exposure to the toxin.[25] A source of the infection in neonates may be from healthcare workers who are nasal carriers of the microorganism. This reinforces the need for good infection control practices with all neonates.[26]

The clinical symptoms begin with fever, malaise, rhinorrhea, and irritability followed by generalized erythema with exquisite tenderness of the skin. There may be an associated impetigo, but the infection often begins in the throat or chest. The erythema spreads from the face and trunk to cover the entire body except for the palms, soles, and mucous membranes. Within 48 hours, blisters and bullae may form, giving the child the appearance of being scalded. The pain is severe (Figure 42-5). Fluid loss from ruptured blisters and water evaporation from denuded areas may cause dehydration. Perioral and nasolabial crusting and fissures develop. In severe cases, the skin of the entire body may slough. When secondary infection can be prevented, healing of the involved skin occurs in 10 to 14 days, usually without scarring.

Before medical intervention is initiated, culture and histologic or exfoliative cytologic studies must be performed to differentiate SSSS from *erythema multiforme* and *toxic epidermal necrolysis* (TEN), both of which are usually caused by an immune reaction to drugs.[27] When SSSS infection is confirmed, treatment with oral or intravenous antibiotics begins. The skin should be treated in the same manner as a severe burn, with meticulous aseptic technique. Skin substitutes may be used for adjuvant therapy.[28] Special care is required when there is involvement of the lips and eyelids.

Fungal Infections
Tinea Capitis

Tinea capitis, a fungal infection of the scalp (scalp ringworm), is the most common fungal infection of childhood. It rarely affects infants and is seen in children between 2 and 10 years of age. The primary microorganism responsible for this disease is *Trichophyton tonsurans*.[29] *Microsporum canis* also continues to be a pathogenic microorganism in this disease and is found on cats, dogs, and certain rodents. Humans appear to be a terminal host for *M. canis*. Children who handle such animals are possible hosts. Direct transmission between humans does not occur. However, there is direct human transmission of *T. tonsurans* in crowded areas, the most prevalent environment of the fungus.[30]

The lesions are often circular and manifested by broken hairs 1 to 3 mm above the scalp, leaving a partial area of alopecia from 1 to 5 cm in diameter (Figure 42-6). A slight erythema and scaling with raised borders can be observed.

Diagnosis is best confirmed by potassium hydroxide (KOH) examination, and fungal culture. Tinea capitis always requires systemic treatment because topical antifungal agents do not penetrate the hair follicle. Several oral antifungal agents, particularly griseofulvin, are available for treatment.[31] Use of Wood's light examination has become less popular because there are a number of dermatophytes that fluoresce under an ultraviolet light.

Tinea Corporis

Tinea corporis (ringworm) is a common superficial dermatophyte infection in children. The organisms most commonly responsible for this disease are *M. canis* and *Trichophyton mentagrophytes*. As in tinea capitis, contact with young kittens and puppies is a common source of

FIGURE 42-6 Tinea Capitis. (Courtesy Department of Dermatology, School of Medicine, University of Utah, Salt Lake City, Utah.)

FIGURE 42-7 Molluscum Contagiosum. Waxy pink globules with umbilicated centers. (From Habif TP: *Clinical dermatology: a color guide to diagnosis and therapy,* ed 4, St Louis, 2004, Mosby.)

the disorder. Tinea corporis preferentially affects the nonhairy parts of the face, trunk, and limbs. Lesions are often erythematous, round or oval scaling patches that spread peripherally with clearing in the center, creating the ring appearance, which is why this disease is commonly referred to as *ringworm*. The lesions are distributed asymmetrically, and multiple lesions, when present, overlap. Transmission occurs by direct contact with an infected lesion and through indirect contact with personal items used by the infected person. Potassium hydroxide examination of the scale from the border of the lesions confirms the diagnosis. Most lesions respond well to applications of appropriate topical antifungal medications.[32]

Thrush

Thrush is the term used to describe the presence of *Candida albicans* in the mucous membranes of the mouths of infants. It occurs less commonly in adults, and infected adults are usually immunocompromised. *C. albicans* penetrates the epidermal barrier more easily than other microorganisms because of its keratolytic proteases and other enzymes. Thrush is characterized by the formation of white plaques or spots in the mouth that lead to shallow ulcers caused by keratolytic proteases from the microorganism. The tongue may have a dense, white covering. The underlying mucous membrane is red and tender and may bleed when the plaques are removed. The disease is often accompanied by fever and gastrointestinal irritation. The infection commonly spreads to the groin, buttocks, and other parts of the body. Treatment may be difficult and includes oral antifungal washes, such as nystatin oral suspension. Simultaneous treatment of a *Candida* nipple infection or vaginitis in the mother is helpful in reducing the *C. albicans* surface colonization of the infant. Feeding bottles and nipples should be sterilized to prevent reinfection. The diaper area should be kept clean and dry.

Viral Infections

Viral infections of the skin in children are caused by poxvirus, papovavirus, and herpesvirus.

Molluscum Contagiosum

Molluscum contagiosum is a common, highly contagious viral infection of the skin and, occasionally, conjunctiva that affects school-aged children, sexually active young adults, and immunocompromised individuals. The incidence is higher among children who swim or have eczema; however, the mechanism of disease is not clear.[33] The disease is transmitted by skin-to-skin contact or from autoinoculation.[34]

The poxvirus proliferates within the follicular epithelium and induces epidermal cell proliferation. The epidermis grows down into the dermis to form saccules containing clusters of virus. The characteristic molluscum body is composed of mature, immature, and incomplete viruses and cellular debris.[35]

The lesions of molluscum are discrete, slightly umbilicated, dome-shaped papules 1 to 5 mm in diameter that appear anywhere on the skin or conjunctiva. The lesions are mainly on the trunk, face, and extremities in children (Figure 42-7). There is usually no inflammation surrounding molluscum lesions unless they are traumatized or secondary infection occurs. Scarring may occur with healing.

The three best diagnostic procedures are (1) staining smears of the expressed molluscum body, (2) examining a biopsy specimen, or (3) inoculating a molluscum suspension into cell cultures to demonstrate the cytotoxic reactions. Most lesions are self-limiting and clear in 6 to 9 months if not manipulated.

Treatment options include immunomodulatory and antiviral therapy and destructive procedures (cryotherapy, curettage, or laser ablation); however, no treatment is universally effective. Potassium hydroxide solution applications can be safe, effective, and inexpensive.[36] Treatment is recommended for genital molluscum to prevent sexual transmission and autoinoculation.[37] Measures to prevent spread of infection must be taken. Recurrences are common.

Rubella (German or 3-Day Measles)

Rubella is a common communicable disease of children and young adults caused by a ribonucleic acid (RNA) virus that enters the bloodstream through the respiratory route. This disease is mild in most children. The incubation period ranges from 14 to 21 days. Prodromal symptoms include enlarged cervical and postauricular lymph nodes, low-grade fever, headache, sore throat, rhinorrhea, and cough. A faint-pink to red coalescing maculopapular rash develops on the face with spread to the trunk and extremities 1 to 4 days after the onset of initial symptoms (Figure 42-8). The rash is thought to be the result of virus dissemination to the skin. The rash subsides after 2 to 3 days, usually without complication. Children are usually not contagious after development of the rash (Table 42-1).

Vaccination for rubella is usually combined with vaccines for mumps and measles (rubeola) (MMR). Measles is known to occur in previously immunized children. The Centers for Disease Control and Prevention vaccine recommendations are available at www.cdc.gov/

TABLE 42-1 Differential Presentation of Viral Diseases Producing Rashes

Viral Disease	Incubation Period	Prodromal Symptoms	Duration/Characteristics	Clinical Symptoms
Rubella (German measles)	14-21 days	1-2 days Mild fever Malaise Respiratory symptoms	1-3 days Pink-red maculopapular Face and trunk	Enlarged and tender occipital and periauricular lymph nodes
Rubeola (red measles)	7-12 days	2-5 days Fever Cough Respiratory symptoms	3-5 days Purple-red to brown maculopapular Face, trunk, extremities	Koplik spots 1-3 days before rash
Roseola (exanthema subitum)	5-15 days	2-5 days High fever	1-3 days Red macular Neck and trunk	Rash develops when fever subsides
Varicella (chickenpox)	11-20 days	1-2 days Low-grade fever Cough May be asymptomatic	7-14 days Red papules, vesicles, pustules in clusters	Eruption of new lesions for 4-5 days Occasional ulcerative lesion in mouth
Fifth disease (human parvovirus B19, erythrovirus)	4-28 days	May be asymptomatic Low-grade fever, malaise before rash	7-10 days "Slapped-cheek" rash on face; lacy red rash on trunk and limbs; may itch	Rash develops when fever subsides

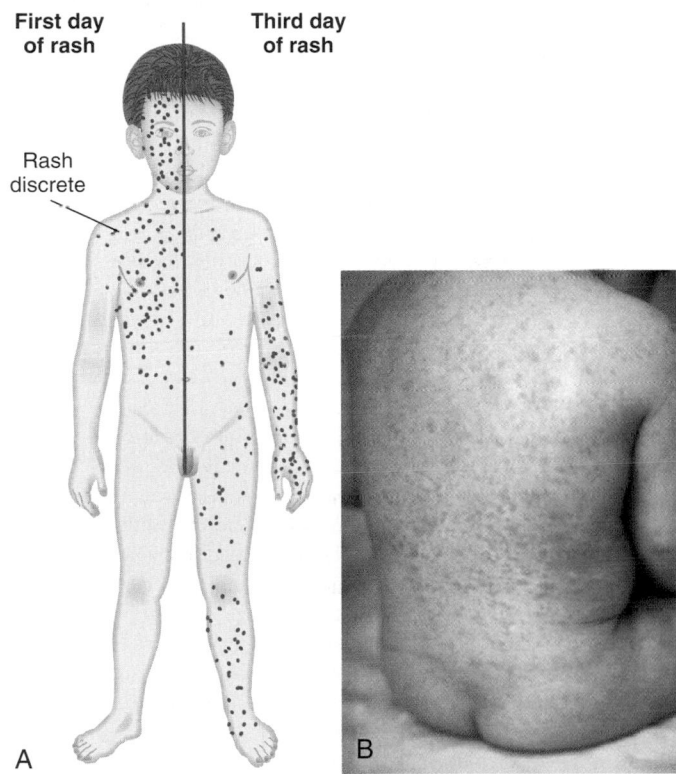

First day of rash

Third day of rash

Rash discrete

A

B

FIGURE 42-8 Rubella (3-Day Measles). A, Typical distribution of full-blown maculopapular rash with tendency to coalesce. **B,** Rash of rubella. (From Centers for Disease Control and Prevention Image Bank, Figure #712. Available at: http://phil.cdc.gov/phil/. Accessed June 8, 2015.)

vaccines/recs/schedules/default.htm. Rubella has almost been eliminated in the United States because of vaccination campaigns. However, challenges to maintain elimination include large outbreaks of measles in highly traveled developed countries, frequent international travel, and clusters of U.S. residents who remain unvaccinated because of

personal belief exemptions.[38] Although MMR vaccine may rarely be associated with adverse neurologic events, studies conclude that MMR immunization does not cause autism.[39] Lack of vaccination, however, leads to significant morbidity and mortality with pneumonia, croup, and encephalitis being causes of death worldwide.

Women of childbearing age are immunized if their rubella hemagglutination-inhibition titer is low. Pregnancy should be avoided for 3 months after vaccination because the attenuated virus in the vaccine may remain viable for this period. Pregnant women who have rubella early in the first trimester may have a fetus who develops congenital defects.

There is no specific treatment for rubella. Recovery is spontaneous, although lymph nodes may remain enlarged for weeks. Supportive therapy includes rest, fluids, and use of a vaporizer. In rare cases, a mild encephalitis or peripheral neuritis may follow rubella.

Rubeola (Red Measles)

Rubeola is a highly contagious, acute viral disease of childhood. Transmitted by direct contact with droplets from infected persons, rubeola is caused by an RNA-containing paramyxovirus with an incubation period of 7 to 12 days, during which there are no symptoms. The virus enters the respiratory tract and attaches to dendritic cells and alveolar macrophages, amplifies in local lymphatic tissue, and progresses to systemic disease.[40] Prodromal symptoms include high fever (up to 40.5° C [104.9° F]), malaise, enlarged lymph nodes, rhinorrhea, conjunctivitis, and barking cough. Within 3 to 4 days, an erythematous maculopapular rash develops over the head and spreads distally over the trunk, extremities, hands, and feet. Early lesions blanch with pressure, followed by a brownish hue that does not blanch as the rash fades. Characteristic pinpoint white spots surrounded by an erythematous ring develop over the buccal mucosa and are known as *Koplik spots.* These spots precede the rash by 1 to 2 days. The rash then subsides within 3 to 5 days.

Complications associated with measles may be caused by the primary infection or by a secondary bacterial infection. Measles encephalitis occurs in about 1 of 800 cases, and most children recover completely. Only a small minority of children develop permanent brain damage or die. Bacterial complications include otitis media and pneumonia, usually caused by group A hemolytic streptococcus, *Haemophilus influenzae,* or *S. aureus* infection.

Measles is prevented by vaccination. As discussed in the Rubella section (p. 1088), immunization is key to prevention. There is no specific treatment for measles, and supportive therapy is the same as that recommended for rubella. Antibiotic therapy is initiated if secondary bacterial infections develop.

Roseola (Exanthema Subitum)

Roseola is a presumed viral infection of children between 6 months and 2 years of age and can be seen in children up to 4 years of age. The incubation period is 5 to 15 days, followed by the sudden onset of fever (38.9° to 40.5°C [102° to 104.9°F]) that lasts 3 to 5 days. Following the fever, an erythematous macular rash that lasts about 24 hours develops primarily over the trunk and neck. Children usually feel well, eat normally, and have few other symptoms. There is usually no treatment.

Small Pox

Smallpox (variola) was a highly contagious and deadly, but also preventable, disease caused by poxvirus variolae. Smallpox was eradicated worldwide in 1977. Routine vaccination in the United States was discontinued in 1972, and a new vaccine, ACAM2000, has been produced for the U.S. Strategic National Stockpile. Information is available from the Food and Drug Administration at www.fda.gov/BiologicsBlood Vaccines/Vaccines/QuestionsaboutVaccines/ucm078041.htm.

Chickenpox and Herpes Zoster

Chickenpox (varicella) and herpes zoster (shingles) are both produced by the varicella-zoster virus (VZV). VZV is a complex deoxyribonucleic acid (DNA) virus of the herpes group. The incubation period is 10 to 27 days, averaging 14 days. Vesicular lesions occur in the epidermis as infection occurs within keratinocytes. An inflammatory infiltrate is often present. Vesicles eventually rupture, followed by crust formation or the development of transient ulcers on mucous membranes. Varicella occurs in people not previously exposed to VZV, whereas herpes zoster (shingles) occurs in individuals who had varicella in the past. The virus enters the dorsal root ganglia and remains latent. Since the introduction of live attenuated varicella-zoster virus (VZV) vaccine in 1995, there has been a significant reduction in varicella incidence and its associated complications.[41]

Chickenpox. Chickenpox (varicella) is a disease of early childhood, with 90% of children contracting the disease during the first decade of life. Being a highly contagious virus, chickenpox is spread by close person-to-person contact and by airborne droplets. Introduction of an infected person into a household results in a 90% possibility of susceptible persons developing the disease within the incubation period, usually 14 days. Children are contagious for at least 1 day before development of the rash. Transmission of the virus may occur until approximately 5 to 6 days after the onset of the first skin lesions in healthy children. In immunocompromised children, the virus is recoverable for a longer period, but infected children must be considered contagious for at least 7 to 10 days. Transmission occurs more readily in temperate climates than in tropical climates.

Normally, children who develop chickenpox have no prodromal symptoms. The first sign of illness may be pruritus or the appearance of vesicles, usually on the trunk, scalp, or face. The rash later spreads to the extremities. Characteristically, lesions can be seen in various stages of maturation with macules, papules, and vesicles present in a particular area at the same time (Figure 42-9). The vesicular lesions are superficial and rupture easily. New lesions will erupt for 4 to 5 days, until there are approximately 100 to 300 in different stages of

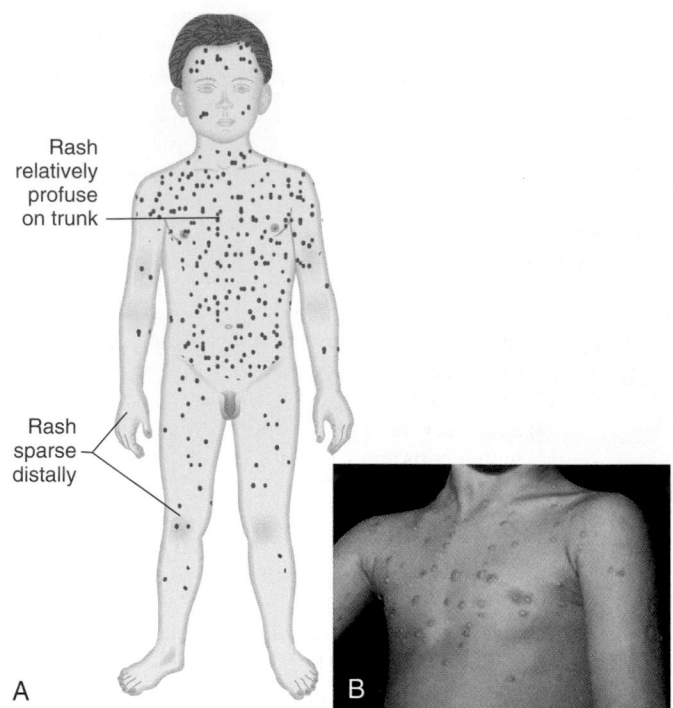

FIGURE 42-9 Chickenpox. **A,** Pattern of generalized, polymorphous eruption. **B,** Chickenpox lesions on fifth day of illness. (From Centers for Disease Control and Prevention Image Bank, Figure #2882. Available at: http://phil.cdc.gov/phil/. Accessed June 8, 2015.)

development. The vesicles become crusted, and over time only the crust remains, although there may be an occasional vesicle on the palm later in the disease. Although uncommon, ulcerative lesions are sometimes seen in the mouth and, less commonly, on the conjunctiva and pharynx. Fever usually lasts 2 to 3 days, with body temperature ranging from 38.5° to 40°C (101.3° to 104°F).

Complications are rare in children but more common in adults. They can include transient hematuria (from rupture of vesicles in the bladder), epistaxis, laryngeal edema, and varicella pneumonia. One case of chickenpox produces almost complete immunity against a second attack. Rarely, the fetus may be malformed (congenital varicella syndrome) if chickenpox develops in the first half of pregnancy. Infants whose mothers have chickenpox at any stage of pregnancy have a higher risk of developing herpes zoster during the first few years of life.[42] Varicella-zoster immunoglobulin should be administered to neonates whenever the onset of maternal disease is between 5 days before and 2 days after delivery.[43]

Uncomplicated chickenpox requires no specific therapy. Baths, wet dressings, and oral antihistamines occasionally help to relieve pruritus and to prevent secondary infection from developing as a result of scratching. Oral antistaphylococcal drugs should be given if secondary bacterial infection is present. Zoster immune globulin may be administered to immunodeficient individuals if given within 72 hours after exposure to chickenpox. Oral acyclovir may be valuable in immunosuppressed or other select groups of children. The varicella vaccine protects against both varicella and herpes zoster. However, wild-type (vaccine-resistant) viruses are a continuing threat.[44]

Herpes zoster. Although herpes zoster (shingles) occurs mainly in adults, approximately 5% of cases are in children younger than 15 years. The pathophysiology and treatment are reviewed in Chapter 41.

INSECT BITES AND PARASITES

Insect bites and infestations are common causes of skin disorders in children and adults. Skin damage occurs by various mechanisms, including trauma of bites and stings, allergic reactions, transmission of disease, injection of substances that cause local or systemic reactions, and inflammatory reactions resulting from embedded and retained insect mouth parts and scratching of the skin.

Scabies

Scabies is a contagious disease caused by the itch mite *Sarcoptes scabiei* (Figure 42-10, *A*), which can colonize the human epidermis. Scabies is a common skin infection in tropical settings, affecting large numbers of people, particularly children. It is transmitted by close personal contact and by infected clothing and bedding. Scabies is often epidemic in areas of overcrowded housing and poor sanitation. Immunocompromised individuals are at greater risk. Scabies can facilitate *Streptococcus pyogenes* and *Staphylococcus aureus* skin coinfections with systemic complications. The scabies mite has adapted mechanisms to overcome host defenses including complement inhibitors.[45] Infestation is initiated by a female mite that tunnels into the stratum corneum, depositing eggs and creating a burrow several millimeters to 1 cm long.

FIGURE 42-10 Scabies. A, Scabies mite, as seen clinically when removed from its burrow. **B,** Characteristic scabies bites. (Courtesy Department of Dermatology, School of Medicine, University of Utah, Salt Lake City, Utah.)

Over a 3-week period, the eggs mature into adult mites, which sometimes are recognized as tiny dots at the ends of intact burrows.

Symptoms appear 3 to 5 weeks after infestation. The primary lesions are burrows, papules, and vesicular lesions, with severe pruritus that worsens at night. Pruritus is thought to be related to sensitization to the larval stages of the parasite. In older children and adults, the lesions occur in the webs of fingers; in the axillae; in the creases of the arms and wrists; along the belt line; and around the nipples, genitalia, and lower buttocks. Infants and young children have a different pattern of distribution, with involvement of the palms, soles, head, neck, and face (Figure 42-10, *B*). Secondary infections and crusting develop as a result of scratching and eczematous changes.

Diagnosis of scabies is made by observation of the tunnels and burrows and by microscopic examination of scrapings of the skin to identify the mite or its eggs or feces. Treatment involves the application of a scabicide, which is curative. All clothing and linens should be washed and dried in hot cycles or dry-cleaned.[46]

Pediculosis (Lice Infestation)

The three known types of human lice are (1) the head louse *(Pediculus capitis),* (2) the body louse *(Pediculus corporis),* and (3) the crab or pubic louse *(Phthirus pubis).* They are parasites and survive by sucking blood. The female louse reproduces every 2 weeks, producing hundreds of nits as newly hatched lice mate with older lice. The mouthparts are shaped for piercing and sucking and are attached to the skin of the host while the louse is feeding. When piercing the skin, the louse secretes toxic saliva, and the mechanical trauma and toxin produce a pruritic dermatitis. Head and body lice are acquired directly by personal contact or indirectly by sharing of combs, brushes, or towels or contact with infested clothes, toys, furniture, carpets, or bedding. Crab lice are spread by close body contact, usually with an infected adult. Other common sources of transmission include sharing clothing or headphones.

Pruritus is the major symptom of lice infestation. With head lice, the ova attach to hairs above the ears and in the occipital region. The primary lesion caused by the body louse is a pinpoint red macule, papule, or wheal with a hemorrhagic puncture site. The primary lesion often is not seen, because it is masked by excoriations, wheals, and crusts. The crab louse is found on pubic hairs but also may be found in other body hair, such as eyelashes, mustache, beard, and underarm hair. Young children in particular may become infected with crab lice on their eyebrows or eyelashes.

The live louse, 2 to 3 mm long, is rarely observed. The ova, or nits, can be observed as oval, yellowish, pinpoint specks fastened to a hair shaft. The ova fluoresce under an ultraviolet light (Wood's lamp) and are observed best with a microscope. Nits are removed with a nit comb, and pediculicides, such as lindane shampoo or lotion, are the most effective treatment. Success or failure of therapy for ectoparasitic infestation depends much more on proper use of the topical preparation than on the type of scabicide or pediculicide used.[47]

All clothes, towels, bedding, combs, and brushes should be washed and dried in hot air or instead washed in boiling water, or clothes can be ironed to rid them of lice. Individuals who have close personal contact with the infected person also should be treated.

Fleas

Young children are very susceptible to fleabites. Bites occur in clusters along the arms and legs or where clothing is tight fitting, such as near elastic bands that circle the thigh or waist. The bite produces a urticarial wheal with a central hemorrhagic puncture (Figure 42-11). Itching can be controlled with antihistamines.[48] Treatment includes spraying carpets, crevices, and furniture with malathion or lindane

FIGURE 42-11 Fleabites. Fleabite producing a urticarial wheal with central puncture.

powder. Infected animals should be treated, and clothes and bedding should be washed in hot water.

Bedbugs

Bedbugs *(Cimex lectularius)* are blood-sucking parasites that live in the crevices and cracks of floors, walls, and furniture and in bedding or furniture stuffing. They are 3 to 5 mm long and reddish brown. Bedbugs are nocturnal, emerging to feed in darkness by attaching to the skin to suck blood, and are attracted by warmth and carbon dioxide. Feeding occurs for 5 to 15 minutes, and the bedbug then leaves. It will move long distances to search for food and can travel from house to house.

Immunologic reactions to bedbug saliva vary, but bites typically yield erythematous and pruritic papules. The face and distal extremities, areas uncovered by sleeping clothes or blankets, are preferentially involved. If the host has not been previously sensitized, the only symptom is a red macule that develops into a nodule, lasting up to 14 days. In sensitized children and adults, pruritic wheals, papules, and vesicles may form. Most lesions respond to oral antihistamines or topical corticosteroids, or both. Secondary infections require antibiotic treatment. Bedbugs are eliminated by inspecting and cleaning or disposing of bedding, mattresses, furniture, and other contaminated items and by using applications of approved insecticides, usually by a professional.[49]

CUTANEOUS HEMANGIOMAS AND VASCULAR MALFORMATIONS

Cutaneous vascular anomalies are frequent tumors of early infancy and are categorized as either hemangiomas or vascular malformations.

FIGURE 42-12 Superficial (Capillary) Hemangioma. (Courtesy Department of Dermatology, School of Medicine, University of Utah, Salt Lake City, Utah.)

Cutaneous Hemangiomas

Cutaneous hemangiomas are benign tumors that form from the rapid growth of vascular endothelial cells, which results in formation of extra blood vessels. Hemangiomas can be superficial or deep.[50] *Superficial hemangiomas* are known as infantile (capillary) or strawberry hemangiomas. Deep lesions are known as cavernous or congenital hemangiomas. The etiology may be related to embolization of fetal placental endothelial cells with placental trauma or loss of placental angiogenic inhibitor of placental and maternal origin. Superficial hemangiomas are associated with endothelial glucose transporter 1 (GLUT1). There is proliferation of mast cells, which are thought to promote the angiogenesis. Infiltration of fat cells, fibrosis, and the rich vascular network give the lesions a firm, rubbery feel. Females are affected more often than males.

About 30% of infantile hemangiomas are apparent at birth, but usually emerge 3 to 5 weeks after birth. They grow rapidly during the first few years of life and become bright red and elevated with minute capillary projections that give them a strawberry appearance. Only one lesion is usually present and is located on the head and neck area or trunk (Figure 42-12). After the initial growth, the lesion grows at the same rate as the child and then starts to involute at 12 to 16 months of age. Approximately 90% of strawberry hemangiomas involute by 5 to 9 years of age, usually without scarring. Most superficial hemangiomas require no treatment. Hemangiomas located over the eye, ear, nose, mouth, urethra, or anus may require treatment because they interfere with function and have a higher risk for infection or injury.

Cavernous hemangiomas are a rare variant of superficial hemangiomas and are GLUT1-negative (Figure 42-13). They are present and fully grown at birth and are usually solitary lesions on the head or limbs that appear as a spongy purplish mass of tissue. They have larger and more mature vessels within the lesion. There are two groups of cavernous hemangiomas: rapidly involuting and noninvoluting. Rapidly involuting cavernous hemangiomas disappear by 12 months to 14 months of age, leaving an area of thin skin. Noninvoluting cavernous hemangiomas do not undergo involution.

Rapidly progressing hemangiomas are treated with a beta-blocker (e.g., propranolol) with regression occurring within 2 weeks and should be considered a first-line agent.[51] Other therapies include systemic or intralesional steroids. Cryosurgery, laser surgery, sclerotherapy, and embolization are alterative treatment options.

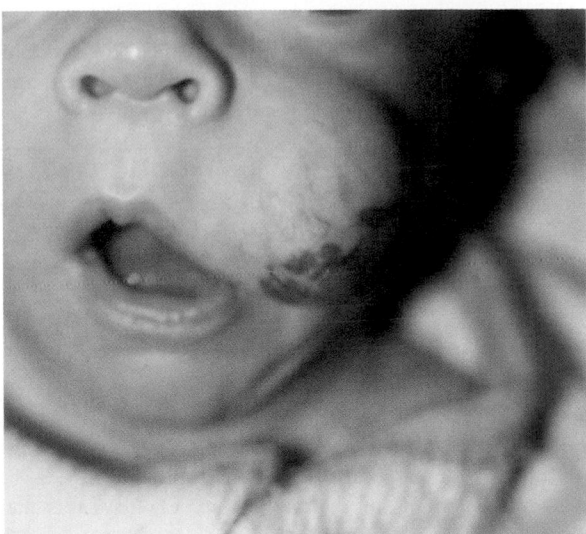

FIGURE 42-13 Cavernous Hemangioma. (Courtesy Department of Dermatology, School of Medicine, University of Utah, Salt Lake City, Utah.)

FIGURE 42-14 Port-Wine Hemangioma. Port-wine hemangioma in a child. (Courtesy Department of Dermatology, School of Medicine, University of Utah, Salt Lake City, Utah.)

Interferons, vincristine, cyclophosphamide, and radiotherapy can suppress angiogenesis.[52]

Cutaneous Vascular Malformations

Cutaneous vascular malformations are rare congenital anomalies of blood vessels present at birth but may not be apparent for several years.[53] They grow proportionately with the child and never regress. The malformations occur equally among males and females. Occasionally they expand rapidly, particularly during the hormonal changes of puberty or pregnancy and in association with trauma. Vascular malformations are classified as low flow or high flow. *Low-flow malformations* involve capillaries, veins, and lymphatics. *High-flow malformations* involve arteries. In addition to locations within the skin, they may involve the gastrointestinal tract, bone (Maffucci syndrome or Sturge-Weber syndrome),[54] facial capillary malformation, skin, eye, or brain (leptomeningeal hemangioma). *Overgrowth syndromes* can occur with either high-flow or low-flow malformations, with overgrowth of the underlying structures (i.e., legs, arms, facial bones). The most common vascular malformations are nevus flammeus (port-wine stains) and salmon patches (stork bite, angel kiss).

Port-wine (nevus flammeus) stains are congenital malformations of the dermal capillaries. The lesions are flat, and their color ranges from pink to dark reddish purple. They are present at birth or within a few days after birth and do not fade with age. Involvement of the face and other body surfaces is common, and the lesions may be large (Figure 42-14). Treatments using cryosurgery or tattooing are not satisfactory. The pulsed dye laser is the treatment of choice to successfully lighten the color and flatten the more nodular and cavernous lesions. Waterproof cosmetics may be used to cover the lesions.

Salmon patches are macular pink lesions present at birth and located on the nape of the neck, forehead, upper eyelids, or nasolabial fold region. They are a variant of nevus flammeus, more superficial, and one of the most common congenital malformations in the skin. The pink color results from distended dermal capillaries, and 95% of patches fade by 1 year of age. Those located at the nape of the neck may persist for a lifetime. They generally do not present a cosmetic problem.

FIGURE 42-15 Miliaria Rubra. Note discrete erythematous papules or papulovesicles. (Courtesy Department of Dermatology, School of Medicine, University of Utah, Salt Lake City, Utah.)

OTHER SKIN DISORDERS

Miliaria

Miliaria is a dermatosis commonly seen in infants that is characterized by a vesicular eruption after prolonged exposure to perspiration with subsequent obstruction of the eccrine ducts. There are two forms of miliaria: miliaria crystallina and miliaria rubra. In miliaria crystallina, ductal rupture occurs within the stratum corneum and appears as 1- to 2-mm clear vesicles without erythema. They rupture within 24 to 48 hours and leave a white scale. In miliaria rubra, the ductal rupture occurs in the lower epidermis with inflammatory cells attracted to the site of the rupture. Miliaria rubra (prickly heat) is characterized by 2- to 4-mm discrete erythematous papules or papulovesicles (Figure 42-15). Both forms may become secondarily infected, requiring systemic antibiotics. The key to management is avoidance of excessive heat and humidity, which cause sweating. Light clothing, cool baths, and air conditioning assist in keeping the skin surface dry and cool.

Erythema Toxicum Neonatorum

Erythema toxicum neonatorum (toxic erythema of the newborn) is a benign, erythematous accumulation of macules, papules, or pustules that appears at birth or 3 to 4 days after birth. The lesions first appear as a blotchy, macular erythematous rash. The macules vary from 1 mm to 1 cm in diameter. When papules or pustules develop, they are light yellow or white and 1 to 3 mm in diameter. There may be a few or several hundred lesions, and any body surface can be affected, with the exception of the palms and soles, where there are no pilosebaceous follicles. The cause of the lesion is unknown but may be related to an innate immune response to the first commensal microflora with release of mast cell mediators. It is self-limiting and resolves spontaneously within a few weeks after birth. No treatment is required.

✔ QUICK CHECK 42-3

1. Give two examples of insect bites or parasites that affect children. What features are observed in each?
2. Compare a strawberry hemangioma with a cavernous hemangioma.

DID YOU UNDERSTAND?

Acne Vulgaris

1. Acne vulgaris is a common disorder related to obstruction of pilosebaceous follicles and proliferation of *Propionibacterium acnes,* primarily of the face, neck, and upper trunk. It is characterized by both noninflammatory and inflammatory lesions.
2. Hydradinitis suppurativa is a chronic, inflammatory disease with occlusion of the pilosebaceous follicles, primarily where there are folds of skin. The lesions include inflammatory nodules, sinus tracts, fistulae, and scarring.

Dermatitis

1. Atopic dermatitis is an alteration in the skin barrier; occurs as red, scaly lesions on the face, cheeks, and flexor surfaces of the extremities in infants and young children; and is associated with inflammatory cytokines, elevated IgE levels, and a family history of asthma and hay fever.
2. Diaper dermatitis is a type of irritant contact dermatitis that develops from prolonged exposure to urine and feces and often becomes secondarily infected with *Candida albicans.*

Infections of the Skin

1. Impetigo is a contagious bacterial disease occurring in two forms: bullous and vesicular. The toxins from the bacteria produce a weeping lesion with a honey-colored crust.
2. Staphylococcal scalded-skin syndrome (SSSS) is a staphylococcal skin infection that produces an exfoliative toxin with painful blisters and bullae formation over large areas of the skin, requiring systemic antibiotic treatment.
3. Tinea capitis and tinea corporis are fungal infections of the scalp and body caused by dermatophytes.
4. Thrush is a fungal infection of the mouth caused by *Candida albicans.*
5. Molluscum contagiosum is a poxvirus of the skin that produces pale papular lesions filled with viral and cellular debris.
6. Rubella (German or 3-day measles) is a communicable viral disease characterized by fever, sore throat, enlarged cervical and postauricular lymph nodes, and a generalized maculopapular rash that lasts 1 to 4 days.
7. Rubeola is a viral contagious disease with symptoms of high fever, enlarged lymph nodes, conjunctivitis, and a red rash that begins on the head, spreads to the trunk and extremities, and lasts 3 to 5 days. Both bacterial and viral complications may accompany rubeola.
8. Roseola is a benign disease of infants with a sudden onset of fever that lasts 3 to 5 days, followed by a rash that lasts 24 hours.
9. Smallpox (variola) was a highly contagious, deadly viral disease that has been eradicated worldwide by vaccination but may be a bioterrorist threat.
10. Chickenpox (varicella) is a highly contagious disease caused by the varicella-zoster virus. Vesicular lesions occur on the skin and mucous membranes. Individuals are contagious from 1 day before the development of the rash until about 5 to 6 days after the rash develops.
11. Herpes zoster (shingles) is a viral eruption of vesicles on the skin along the distribution of a sensory nerve caused by chickenpox virus that persists in sensory nerve ganglia.

Insect Bites and Parasites

1. Scabies is a pruritic lesion caused by the itch mite, which burrows into the skin and forms papules and vesicles. The mite is very contagious and is transmitted by direct contact.
2. Pediculosis (lice infestation) is caused by blood-sucking parasites that secrete toxic saliva and damage the skin to produce pruritic dermatitis. Lice are spread by direct contact and are recognized by the ova or nits that attach to the shafts of body hairs.
3. Fleabites produce a pruritic wheal with a central puncture site and occur as clusters in areas of tight-fitting clothing.
4. Bedbugs are blood-sucking parasites that live in cracks of floors, furniture, or bedding and feed at night. They produce pruritic wheals and nodules.

Cutaneous Hemangiomas and Vascular Malformations

1. Cutaneous hemangiomas are benign tumors that form from the rapid growth of vascular endothelial cells and result in formation of extra blood vessels.
2. Cutaneous vascular malformations are rare congenital anomalies of blood vessels present at birth.
3. A strawberry hemangioma is a vascular lesion present at birth that proliferates in size and then grows at the same rate as the child. Most lesions resolve spontaneously by 5 years of age.
4. A cavernous hemangioma is present at birth, with larger vessels than a strawberry hemangioma, and is bluish red. Cavernous hemangiomas usually involute by 9 years of age and may require surgical removal if located near the eyes, nares, or genitalia.
5. Salmon patches are macular pink lesions with dilated capillaries that usually resolve by 1 year of age.
6. Port-wine stains are congenital malformations of dermal capillaries that do not fade with age.

Other Skin Disorders

1. Miliaria are small pruritic papules or vesicles that result from obstruction of the sweat duct opening in infants.
2. Erythema toxicum neonatorum is a benign accumulation of macules, papules, and pustules that spontaneously resolves within a few weeks after birth.

KEY TERMS

REFERENCES

1. Bate K, Williams HC: Epidemiology of acne vulgaris, *Br J Dermatol* 168(3):474-485, 2013.
2. Grossi E et al: The constellation of dietary factors in adolescent acne: a semantic connectivity map approach, *J Eur Acad Dermatol Venereol* 2014 Dec 2. [Epub ahead of print.]
3. Mahmood SN, Bowe WP: Diet and acne update: carbohydrates emerge as the main culprit, *J Drugs Dermatol* 13(4):428-435, 2010.
4. Melnik BC et al: Acne: risk indicator for increased body mass index and insulin resistance, *Acta Derm Venereol* 93(6):644-649, 2013.
5. Harvey A, Huynh TT: Inflammation and acne: putting the pieces together, *J Drugs Dermatol* 13(4):459-463, 2014.
6. Lwin SM et al: Acne, quorum sensing and danger, *Clin Exp Dermatol* 39(2):162-167, 2014.
7. Eichenfield LF et al: Evidence-based recommendations for the diagnosis and treatment of pediatric acne, *Pediatrics* 131(Suppl 3): S163-S186, 2013.
8. Bhate K, Williams HC: What's new in acne? An analysis of systematic reviews published in 2011-2012, *Clin Exp Dermatol* 39(3):273-277, 2014.
9. Yin NC, McMichael AJ: Acne in patients with skin of color: practical management, *Am J Clin Dermatol* 15(1):7-16, 2014.
10. Simonart T: Immunotherapy for acne vulgaris: current status and future directions, *Am J Clin Dermatol* 14(6):429-435, 2013.
11. Gill L et al: Update on hidradenitis suppurativa: connecting the tracts, *F1000Prime Rep* 6:112, 2014.
12. Odhiambo JA et al: Global variations in prevalence of eczema symptoms in children from ISAAC phase three, *J Allergy Clin Immunol* 124:1251-1258, 2009.
13. Darlenski R et al: Atopic dermatitis as a systemic disease, *Clin Dermatol* 32(3):409-413, 2014.
14. Lyons JJ et al: Atopic dermatitis in children: clinical features, pathophysiology, and treatment, *Immunol Allergy Clin North Am* 35(1):161-183, 2015.
15. McAleer MA, Irvine AD: The multifunctional role of filaggrin in allergic skin disease, *J Allergy Clin Immunol* 131(2):280-291, 2013.
16. Oranje AP, de Waard-van der Spek FB: Recent developments in the management of common childhood skin infections, *J Infect* 71(Suppl 1): S76-S79, 2015.
17. Eichenfield LF et al: Guidelines of care for the management of atopic dermatitis: section 1. Diagnosis and assessment of atopic dermatitis, *J Am Acad Dermatol* 70(2):338-351, 2014.
18. Kanchongkittiphon W et al: Child with atopic dermatitis, *Ann Allergy Asthma Immunol* 114(1): 6-11, 2015.

19. Nicol NH et al: M.D. (2014) wet wrap therapy in children with moderate to severe atopic dermatitis in a multidisciplinary treatment program, *J Allergy Clin Immunol Pract* 2(4):400-407, 2014.
20. Schäkel K et al: Future treatment options for atopic dermatitis—small molecules and beyond, *J Dermatol Sci* 73(2):91-100, 2014.
21. Shin HT: Diagnosis and management of diaper dermatitis, *Pediatr Clin North Am* 61(2):367-382, 2014.
22. Hartman-Adams H et al: Impetigo: diagnosis and treatment, *Am Fam Physician* 90(4):229-235, 2014.
23. Pereira LB: Impetigo—review, *An Bras Dermatol* 89(2):293-299, 2014.
24. Aalfs AS et al: Staphylococcal scalded skin syndrome: loss of desmoglein 1 in patient skin, *Eur J Dermatol* 20(4):451-456, 2010.
25. Neylon O et al: Neonatal staphylococcal scalded skin syndrome: clinical and outbreak containment review, *Eur J Pediatr* 169(12):1503-1509, 2010.
26. Paranthaman K et al: Nosocomial outbreak of staphylococcal scalded skin syndrome in neonates in England, December 2012 to March 2013, *Euro Surveill* 19(33), 2014.
27. Williams PM, Conklin RJ: Erythema multiforme: a review and contrast from Stevens-Johnson syndrome/toxic epidermal necrolysis, *Dent Clin North Am* 49(1):67-76, 2005: viii.
28. Baartmans MG et al: Use of skin substitute dressings in the treatment of staphylococcal scalded skin syndrome in neonates and young infants, *Neonatology* 100(1):9-13, 2011.
29. Mirmirani P, Tucker LY: Epidemiologic trends in pediatric tinea capitis: a population-based study from Kaiser Permanente Northern California, *J Am Acad Dermatol* 69(6):916-921, 2013.
30. Abdel-Rahman SM et al: The prevalence of infections with *Trichophyton tonsurans* in schoolchildren: the CAPITIS study, *Pediatrics* 125(5):966-973, 2010.
31. Kakourou T, Uksal U: European Society for Pediatric Dermatology. Guidelines for the management of tinea capitis in children, *Pediatr Dermatol* 27(3):226-228, 2010.
32. Andrews MD, Burns M: Common tinea infections in children, *Am Fam Physician* 77(10):1415-1420, 2008.
33. Olsen JR et al: Epidemiology of molluscum contagiosum in children: a systematic review, *Fam Pract* 31(2):130-136, 2014.
34. Butala N et al: Molluscum BOTE sign: a predictor of imminent resolution, *Pediatrics* 131(5):e1650-e1653, 2013.
35. Smith KJ, Skelton H: Molluscum contagiosum: recent advances in pathogenic mechanisms, and

new therapies, *Am J Clin Dermatol* 3(8):535-545, 2002.
36. Can B et al: Treatment of pediatric molluscum contagiosum with 10% potassium hydroxide solution, *J Dermatolog Treat* 25(3):246-248, 2014.
37. Zichichi L, Maniscalco M: The challenges of a neglected STI: *Molluscum contagiosum*, *G Ital Dermatol Venereol* 147(5):447-453, 2012.
38. Parker Fiebelkorn A et al: Measles in the United States during the postelimination era, *J Infect Dis* 202(10):1520-1528, 2010.
39. Maglione MA et al: Safety of vaccines used for routine immunization of U.S. children: a systematic review, *Pediatrics* 134(2):325-337, 2014.
40. de Vries RD et al: The pathogenesis of measles, *Curr Opin Virol* 2(3):248-255, 2012.
41. Gershon AA, Gershon MD: Pathogenesis and current approaches to control of varicella-zoster virus infections, *Clin Microbiol Rev* 26(4):728-743, 2013.
42. Smith CK, Arvin AM: Varicella in the fetus and newborn, *Semin Fetal Neonatal Med* 14(4):209-217, 2009.
43. Shrim A et al: Management of varicella infection (chickenpox) in pregnancy, *J Obstet Gynaecol Can* 34(3):287-292, 2012.
44. Quinlivan M, Breuer J: Clinical and molecular aspects of the live attenuated Oka varicella vaccine, *Rev Med Virol* 24(4):254-273, 2014.
45. Swe PM et al: Parasitic scabies mites and associated bacteria joining forces against host complement defense, *Parasite Immunol* 36(11): 585-593, 2014.
46. Mounsey KE, McCarthy JS: Treatment and control of scabies, *Curr Opin Infect Dis* 26(2):133-139, 2013.
47. Wolf R, Davidovici B: Treatment of scabies and pediculosis: facts and controversies, *Clin Dermatol* 28(5):511-518, 2010.
48. Juckett G: Arthropod bites, *Am Fam Physician* 88(12):841-847, 2013.
49. Studdiford JS et al: Bedbug infestation, *Am Fam Physician* 86(7):653-658, 2012.
50. Elluru RG: Cutaneous vascular lesions, *Facial Plast Surg Clin North Am* 21(1):111-126, 2013.
51. Gunturi N et al: Propranolol therapy for infantile hemangioma, *Indian Pediatr* 50(3):307-313, 2013.
52. Greene AK: Management of hemangiomas and other vascular tumors, *Clin Plast Surg* 38(1):45-63, 2011.
53. Huang JT, Liang MG: Vascular malformations, *Pediatr Clin North Am* 57(5):1091-1110, 2010.
54. Chen JK et al: An overview of clinical and experimental treatment modalities for port wine stains, *J Am Acad Dermatol* 67(2):289-304, 2012.

Page numbers followed by "*f*" indicate figures, "*t*" indicate tables, and "*b*" indicate boxes. Syndromes and disorders appear in boldface.

1096

PREFIXES AND SUFFIXES USED IN MEDICAL TERMINOLOGY

Prefix	Meaning	Suffix	Meaning
a-	Without, not	-al, -ac	Pertaining to
acantho-	Spiny, thorny	-algia	Pain
af-	Toward	-aps, -apt	Fit; fasten
an-	Without, not	-arche	Beginning; origin
ante-	Before	-ase	Signifies an enzyme
anti-	Against; resisting	-blast	Sprout; make
auto-	Self	-centesis	A piercing
bi-	Two; double	-cide	To kill
blast-	Immature cell, embryonic	-clast	Break; destroy
circum-	Around	-crine	Release; secrete
co-, con-	With; together	-cytosis	Increase in number
contra-	Against	-ectomy	A cutting out
crine-	Secrete, separate	-emesis	Vomiting
de-	Down from, undoing	-emia	Refers to blood condition
dia-	Across; through	-flux	Flow
dipl-	Twofold, double	-gen	Creates; forms
dys-	Bad; disordered; difficult	-genesis	Creation, production
ecto-	Displaced, outside	-gram	Something written
ef-	Away from	-graph(y)	To write, draw
em-, en-	In, into	-hydrate	Containing H_2O (water)
endo-	Within	-ia, -sia	Condition; process
epi-	Upon, above	-iasis	Abnormal condition
eu-	Good	-ic, -ac	Pertaining to
ex-, exo-	Out of, out from	-in	Signifies a protein
extra-	Outside of	-ism	Signifies "condition of"
hapl-	Single	-itis	Signifies "inflammation of"
hem-, hemat-	Blood	-lemma	Sheath, covering
hemi-	Half	-lepsy	Seizure
hom(e)o-	Same; equal	-lith	Stone; rock
hyper-	Over; above	-logy	Study of
hypo-	Under; below	-lunar	Moon; moonlike
infra-	Below, beneath	-malacia	Softening
inter-	Between	-megaly	Enlargement
intra-	Within	-metric, -metry	Measurement, length
iso-	Same, equal	-oid	Like; in the shape of
juxta-	Near	-oma	Tumor
macro-	Large	-opia	Vision, vision condition
mega-	Large; million(th)	-oscopy	Viewing
mes-	Middle	-ose	Pertaining to, sugar
meta-	Beyond, change, after	-osis	Condition, process
micro-	Small; millionth	-ostomy	Formation of an opening
milli-	Thousandth	-otomy	Cut
mono-	One (single)	-penia	Lack
necro-	Death	-philic	Loving
neo-	New	-phobic	Fearing
non-	Not	-phragm	Partition
oligo-	Few, scanty	-plasia	Growth, formation
ortho-	Straight; correct, normal	-plasm	Substance, matter
para-	By the side of; near	-plasty	Shape; make
per-	Through	-plegia	Paralysis
peri-	Around; surrounding	-pnea	Breath, breathing
poly-	Many	-(r)rhage, -(r)rhagia	Breaking out, discharge
post-	After	-(r)rhaphy	Sew, suture
pre-	Before	-(r)rhea	Flow
pro-	First; promoting	-some	Body
quadri-	Four	-tensin, -tension	Pressure
re-	Back again	-tonic	Pressure, tension
retro-	Behind	-tripsy	Crushing
semi-	Half	-ule	Small, little
sub-	Under	-uria	Refers to urine condition
super-, supra-	Over, above, excessive		
trans-	Across; through		
tri-	Three; triple		